THE NUTRIBASE
NUTRITION FACTS
DESK REFERENCE

The NutriBase
NUTRITION FACTS
DESK REFERENCE

DR. ART ULENE

Avery Publishing Group
Garden City Park, New York

The information in this book is based upon the latest data made available by government agencies, food manufacturers, and trade associations. It is important to note that all nutrient breakdowns for processed foods are subject to change by manufacturers without notice and may therefore vary from printing to printing.

Cataloging-in-Publication Data

Ulene, Art.
    The Nutribase nutrition facts desk reference : the single encyclopedic source for the most complete, up-to-date and comprehensive collection of food values / Art Ulene.
        p. cm.
        ISBN 0-89529-623-3

        1. Nutrition—Tables. 2. Food—Composition—Tables.
    3. Nutribase (Computer file)   I. Title.

TX551.U44 1995   641.1'04
                                        QBI94-2205

Printed in the United States of America

10   9   8   7   6   5   4   3   2   1

CONTENTS

ACKNOWLEDGMENTS

The creation of this book was no easy feat. The fact that it was completed at all is due to the dedication and perseverance of many people.

First, let me acknowledge the good people at CyberSoft Corporation for their tireless dedication in collecting and updating the enormous amount of material needed to produce such a complete volume. Thanks are especially due to group leader Ed Prestwood and his team of data specialists: Jan Gamble, Maggy Russo, Jacqueline Hadley, Jodie Smith, Theresa Porty, Carla Rigoni, Lisa Hernandez, Kim Dodds, Anne Jackson, and Carol Havell, who gathered and organized data from a wide range of sources, and to CyberSoft's nutritional consultant, Sally Mills. Special thanks go to Robyn Freeman, whose software wizardry helped bring this ambitious project to fruition.

Second, I would like to thank the editors at Avery Publishing Group for taking the raw data and turning it into an accessible, easy-to-use reference. Their innovative ideas regarding the book's structure have helped to create one of the best volumes of nutritional data now available. Thanks go to team leader Marie Caratozzolo, and to editors Elaine Will Sparber, Amy Tecklenburg, Karen Hay, Joanne Abrams, Shoshana Shur, and David Porello. No less thanks go to William Gonzalez, Bonnie Freid, Nuno Faisca, Kerri Jenal, and Janet Pospisil for their typesetting skills, and to Susan McDonnell and Ken Rajman for their data-processing expertise. Finally, I would like to thank Avery's managing editor, Rudy Shur, for his patience, his numerous phone calls, and his persistence in seeing the project through to completion.

I would like to thank the hundreds of corporations and individuals who responded to our requests for nutritional information. Included among this list are the unsung heroes of the United States Department of Agriculture, who work inexhaustibly to establish accurate nutritional data. Three people at the USDA who deserve special thanks are Dr. Jacob Exler, Karen W. Andrews, and David Haydowitz, who gave generously of their time and knowledge.

During my work on this project, I have been fortunate enough to come into contact with many people who have provided me with important bits and pieces of information at crucial times. While I may not have named these individuals, I would nevertheless like to express my thanks to each and every one of them.

INTRODUCTION

For thousands of years, people have recognized the life-sustaining nature of food. But only during the last four or five decades have we begun to understand the many ways in which our choices of foods can affect the quality of our health and the length of our life. And only during the last four or five years have we really begun to appreciate how profound the effects of those choices can be.

Now we know that some of the so-called "inevitable" diseases like atherosclerosis, osteoporosis, and even cancer are often the consequence of poor nutritional choices. Research has clearly shown the relationship between poor nutritional intake and many of these diseases. The studies prove that high-fat diets can—and often do—contribute to the development of coronary heart disease; that low-fiber intake promotes the development of colon cancer; that folic acid deficiency increases the risk of birth defects; and that inadequate calcium intake fosters the onset of osteoporosis and bone fractures. The list of nutrition-related disorders goes on and on.

But there is also a hopeful side to this story. New studies have clearly demonstrated the positive effects that good nutritional choices can have on our health. Coronary heart disease can be prevented—even reversed—through dietary changes. The incidence of cancer can be reduced with diets that are low in fat and high in cruciferous vegetables (broccoli and cauliflower, for instance), and through the use of the antioxidant nutrients, such as vitamins C and E. Bone strength can be increased and fracture rates decreased with a diet rich in calcium and vitamin D. Blood cholesterol levels can be reduced with dietary fiber, niacin, and garlic. Blood pressure can be lowered with sodium restriction and calcium supplementation. The list of

health-promoting nutritional interventions is lengthy, and constantly growing.

THE NEW NUTRITION

Modern research studies are giving rise to a "new" nutrition, one that is both scientifically sound and practical. The new nutrition differs from the old in at least two important ways. First, the old nutrition dealt in generalities, such as the four food groups, and created minimum recommendations designed to prevent deficiency-related disorders. The new nutrition seeks to achieve *optimal* levels of health, and creates specific recommendations based on individual differences, such as age, sex, lifestyle, and medical factors. Second, the old nutrition left many nutritional decisions up to the health professionals and food marketers, while the new nutrition puts *you* in control. It empowers you with the information necessary to evaluate confusing and conflicting claims, and enables you to reject foods that do not meet your nutritional needs and goals.

This book is designed to provide you with that empowering information. It will help you make wiser choices when you buy food and when you dine out. It will help you interpret nutritional stories in the media so you can distinguish useful information from nonsense. It will give you the control you need over your personal nutrition.

Many people refer to books of this sort as "counter" books, because of the nutritional numbers that fill the pages. But this is not a book about counting. This is a book about *control* and *choices*. Use this book to learn more about the foods you should consume—or avoid—so you can meet your particular nutritional needs. Don't be intimidated by the huge number of choices listed or by the impossible-tomemorize nutritional value numbers that accompany the lists. It is not necessary to memorize these numbers. Instead, just try to familiarize yourself with the foods and food categories that are best suited to your needs. Begin by looking up the foods that you eat most often or in the largest quantities. If these foods are not providing you with the nutrients you need, use the book to find better alternatives that are just as tasty. Once you are familiar with the nutritional content of your most common food choices, gradually look up the remainder of the foods in your diet. You'll be surprised by how easy it is to learn about these foods and to make any necessary changes.

As you take more control over the foods you are eating and put more thought into your choices, keep in mind that good nutrition is just one element of a healthy lifestyle. To achieve maximum benefits from the new nutrition, your life should be filled with physical activity and free of cigarette smoke and other toxic substances. In addition, the stress in your life should be under control. Even the best diet can't overcome the problems caused by smoking, an immoderate use of alcohol, poorly managed stress, and other health-compromising habits.

Finally, keep in mind that research is constantly adding to our knowledge of nutrition, and, in the process, changing some of our beliefs. As best you can, try to keep up with the new information and, when appropriate, make whatever dietary changes are necessary. But also be skeptical about nutritional news that seems too good to be true. (More often than not, it isn't true.) Be wary of nutritional claims made by people who are trying to sell you something. And be cautious—don't make any drastic changes in your nutritional program without first talking to a health professional who is knowledgeable about nutrition and about your particular medical circumstances. Don't forget: If the *right* nutritional choices are powerful enough to keep you well, it is only logical that the *wrong* ones could make you sick.

The following section will explain some of the basics of nutrition. After that, you will learn how to use this book to locate the information you need to improve your diet.

A QUICK LOOK AT THE BASIC NUTRIENTS AND MICRONUTRIENTS

Everyone's diet must contain the four basic *nutrients*—water, complex carbohydrates, proteins, and fats—as well as the *micronutrients,* which are the vitamins and minerals. These nutrients and micronutrients fuel the body and enable all bodily functions to occur. A proper balance of these essentials is necessary for optimum health.

This book presents the nutrient values of a wide range of foods, both whole and processed. In order to wisely use this information, it is important to have a basic understanding of the function of the nutrients and micronutrients needed by the body.

The Nutrients

Water, complex carbohydrates, proteins, and fats are the basic building blocks of a healthy diet. Each works in different ways to fuel the body, build and repair the cells that make up the body, and provide the environment in which the cells live.

Water

The human body is two-thirds water by weight. Indeed, water is an essential nutrient that is involved in every function of the body. It helps transport nutrients and waste products in and out of cells. It is necessary for all digestive, absorption, circulatory, and excretory functions, and for the utilization of the water-soluble vitamins. And it is needed to maintain proper body temperature.

Most of us are aware of some of the early signs of dehydration: scant or dark urine, thirst, and a dry mouth. If the body continues to be denied adequate water, serious health problems occur, requiring hospitalization.

Complex Carbohydrates

Complex carbohydrates provide the body with the energy it needs to function. Signs of an inadequate supply of complex carbohydrates include lack of energy and the breakdown of proteins in tissues.

One type of carbohydrate you may have heard a good deal about is *fiber*. Referred to in the past as roughage, fiber is actually the part of plant materials that our body cannot digest. Yet, fiber is known to perform a number of important functions. It promotes feelings of fullness; prevents constipation, hemorrhoids, and other intestinal problems; and is associated with a reduced incidence of colon cancer. In addition, fiber may help lower blood cholesterol levels, reducing the risk of heart disease. (To learn about the difference betwen *crude fiber* and *dietary fiber,* see page xx.)

Proteins

Protein is essential for growth and development. It provides the body with energy, and is needed for the manufacture of hormones, antibodies, enzymes, and muscle tissues. It also helps maintain the proper acid-alkali balance. Inadequate protein intake can result in stunted growth, diarrhea, vomiting, lack of appetite, and edema, a buildup of fluids in the tissues.

Fats

Recently, much attention has been focused on the need to reduce dietary fat. Nevertheless, the body does need fats—but only the right fats, and only in appropriate quantities. Specifically, it needs fatty acids, which perform a variety of vital bodily functions. Fatty acids carry the fat-soluble vitamins. They are essential for growth and development, and for the maintenance of healthy skin, hair, and nails. And they provide the body with energy. A variety of problems occur when the body fails to receive adequate fatty acids. Signs of the deficiency may include retarded growth; skin, hair, and nail disorders; and an impaired metabolism of fats and fat-soluble vitamins.

Although fat is necessary, most of us are now aware that there are several kinds of dietary fat—saturated, polyunsaturated, and monounsaturated—and that some are better than others. To understand the difference between these three fats, it is helpful to first learn a little about cholesterol.

Cholesterol is a white, waxy, fatty substance found in all foods that come from animal sources.

Cholesterol is essential to our well-being, as it helps to build cell membranes, to produce hormones, and to manufacture bile acids. The liver is capable of manufacturing all of the cholesterol needed for good health.

The cholesterol manufactured by our liver is carried through our bloodstream by LDLs (low-density lipoproteins). High levels of LDLs in the bloodstream can result in clogged arteries, causing high blood pressure, stroke, or heart disease. This is why LDL is referred to as the "bad" cholesterol. Fortunately, in many people, LDL levels can be reduced to healthy levels through proper diet.

HDLs (high-density lipoproteins) carry excess cholesterol from different body tissues to the liver, where it is converted to bile acids and then eliminated through the intestines. High levels of HDLs are linked with a decreased risk of coronary heart disease. This is why HDL is often called the "good" cholesterol. To a limited extent, HDL levels can be raised through regular exercise.

How are the three types of fat related to cholesterol? *Saturated fats*—which come from animal foods like meat, fish, poultry, milk, butter, and cheese, as well as from palm, coconut, and palm kernel oil—have been shown to increase total blood cholesterol levels, especially the undesirable LDL portion. *Polyunsaturated fats*—found mainly in vegetable oils like corn, sunflower, safflower, and soybean—tend to lower levels of both HDL and LDL. *Monounsaturated fats*—found mainly in vegetable and nut oils such as olive, peanut, and canola—have been shown to reduce total blood cholesterol without lowering levels of the good cholesterol, HDL. Indeed, some monounsaturated fats have been shown to raise HDL levels.

Most experts agree that it is best to limit fat consumption, and to choose mostly monounsaturated fats, which increase the levels of HDL while lowering total blood cholesterol. There is, in fact, no biological need for saturated fat!

A Word About Calories

When we talk about foods, we often mention the number of calories a certain food has. As you have soon, calories are not among the four basic nutrients, nor are they considered micronutrients. What, then, are calories?

A calorie is an energy unit. As already discussed, carbohydrates, protein, and fat provide the body with the energy it needs to function. This energy is measured in calories. There are, for instance, 4 calories in every gram of protein, 4 calories in every gram of carbohydrate, and 9 calories in every gram of fat. It is no wonder, then, that when people try to lose weight, they are often advised to cut down on fatty foods. On a gram-for-gram basis, fat is more than twice as fattening as carbohydrates or protein.

In addition to fat's having more calories than protein or carbohydrates, it is important to understand that the way in which our body metabolizes dietary fat is different from the way it metabolizes the other two nutrients. Because dietary fat is similar in chemical composition to body fat, it takes less energy to convert it to body fat. In fact, it takes only *3 percent* of the calories in the fat we eat to turn that food into body fat, while it takes at least *25 percent* of the carbohydrates and protein calories we eat to convert them into body fat. Remember, though, that if you eat more calories than your body needs, regardless of the nutrient providing these calories, the excess will be stored as body fat.

The Micronutrients

Like water, carbohydrates, protein, and fats, vitamins and minerals are essential to life. As such, they are considered nutrients, and are often referred to as "micronutrients" simply because they are needed in relatively small amounts compared with the four basic nutrients.

Vitamins

Vitamins are organic compounds, meaning that they occur naturally in plants and animals. Generally, vitamins function as coenzymes. Enzymes are the catalysts or activators in all of the chemical reactions that are continually taking place in the human body. As coenzymes, vitamins work with the enzymes and allow all activities that occur within the body to happen quickly and accurately. In addition to this role, some vitamins have other functions. For instance, vitamin D functions as a hormone.

Each vitamin is classified as either water-soluble or fat-soluble, depending on whether fat- or water-based molecules transport that vitamin in the bloodstream. Water-soluble vitamins include all of the B-complex vitamins and vitamin C. These vitamins are either used by the body in a short period of time—two to four days—or excreted. As a result, they must be replenished daily through diet or supplements. Fat-soluble vitamins stay in the body longer, and are stored in the body's fat tissues and in some organs, especially the liver. Vitamins A, D, E, and K are all fat-soluble vitamins.

Each vitamin has specific functions. Even a brief look at the major functions performed by each of these nutrients shows just how important they are to our health.

Vitamin A plays an important role in strengthening the mucous membranes, the immune system, the adrenal glands, and the eyes. Moreover, beta-carotene—a compound that the body converts to vitamin A—is an antioxidant, and thus works to "neutralize" harmful substances known as free radicals. As such, beta-carotene appears to help protect the body against a variety of disorders, including cancer and heart disease. A deficiency of this vitamin can lead to visual problems, including night blindness; an increased susceptibility to infection; impaired growth; and impaired function of the reproductive organs.

Thiamine (Vitamin B₁) supports the healthy functioning of the heart, muscles, and nerves, and plays a role in the breakdown of carbohydrates. Too little thiamine can result in fatigue, constipation, loss of appetite, memory loss, irritability, and depression. In the most severe cases of thiamine deprivation, a now-rare disease known as beriberi may result.

Riboflavin (Vitamin B₂) plays a role in the breakdown and use of carbohydrates, fats, and proteins; is involved in cell energy production; supports the production of adrenal hormones; and helps the body utilize other vitamins. Riboflavin deficiency may be signaled by light-sensitivity and other eye problems, loss of appetite, impaired growth, anemia, dry skin, and depression.

Niacin (Vitamin B₃) is necessary for the breakdown of carbohydrates and fats, the healthy functioning of the nervous and digestive systems, the production of sex hormones, and the maintenance of healthy skin. Signs of niacin deficiency include fatigue, irritability, depression, confusion, insomnia, blood sugar fluctuations, and arthritis. In the case of severe deficiencies, the now-rare disease known as pellagra may result.

Pantothenic Acid (Vitamin B₅) is involved in the breakdown and use of carbohydrates and fats, in normal growth and development, in the production of adrenal and sex hormones, and in the body's use of other vitamins. Headaches, nausea, abdominal cramps, fatigue, depression, an increased susceptibility to colds, insomnia, and numbness and tingling in the hands and feet are all possible signs of pantothenic acid deficiency.

Pyridoxine (Vitamin B₆) is used in the breakdown of proteins, carbohydrates, and fats; in the healthy functioning of the nervous and digestive systems; in the production of red blood cells and antibodies; and in the maintenance of healthy skin. Some of the most common symptoms of pyridoxine deficiency are an impaired immune system, anemia, inflammation of the tongue, weakness, dizziness, nausea and vomiting, and depression.

Cobalamin (Vitamin B₁₂) is needed for growth and development, the production of red blood cells, the body's use of folic acid, and healthy nervous system function. Too little of this nutrient can lead to pernicious anemia, a disorder signaled by weakness, weight loss, and pale skin; loss of coordination; tingling in the hands and feet; moodiness; and depression.

Biotin, also a B-complex vitamin, is involved in the metabolism of fatty acids, carbohydrates, and protein; and in the maintenance of healthy skin, hair, sweat glands, nerves, and bone marrow. Biotin deficiency may result in dry and scaly skin, loss of appetite, muscle pain, nausea and vomiting, hair loss, insomnia, and depression.

Folic acid, another B-complex vitamin, is needed for growth, development, and reproduction; in the production of red blood cells; and in the functioning of the nervous system. It also supports the hair and skin. Signs of folic acid deficiency include anemia, digestive problems, and fatigue. In addition, maternal folic acid deficiency has been implicated as a cause of fetal nervous system abnormalities.

Vitamin C, also known as ascorbic acid, has many functions. It helps maintain normal enzyme function; is important for the healthy growth of teeth, bones, gums, ligaments, and blood vessels; plays an important role in the immune system's response to infection and in healing; and helps in the absorption of iron from the digestive tract. In its role as an antioxidant, this nutrient also protects the body against a variety of disorders, including cancer. Vitamin C deficiency may result in slow wound healing, bleeding gums, recurrent infections, and allergies. Severe deficits of vitamin C can result in scurvy, a now-rare disease.

Vitamin D supports bone and tooth formation, muscle function, and thyroid gland function; and is necessary for the proper absorption of calcium, phosphorus, magnesium, and zinc. In severe cases, vitamin D deficiency can cause rickets, a disease whose symptoms include loss of appetite, slowed growth, and a softening of the bones.

Vitamin E aids in tissue healing, is essential for normal cell structure, helps maintain normal enzyme function, and is involved in the formation of red blood cells. In its role as an antioxidant, vitamin E protects the lungs against injury from air pollution and helps preserve tissues throughout the body. In addition, several major studies have shown that this nutrient may offer protection from heart disease. Recognized signs of vitamin E deficiency include loss of appetite, difficulty in walking, anemia, nausea, eye problems, and impairment of reproductive function.

Vitamin K is essential for blood clotting and bone formation. A lack of this vitamin is signaled by blood clotting difficulty.

Minerals

Minerals are inorganic elements, meaning that they are not produced by plants and animals. Like vitamins, many minerals are needed for proper body function. For instance, minerals are essential in nerve responses and muscle contractions, and are needed to maintain proper fluid balance and for the internal processing of nutrients. Some minerals have other functions, as well. Calcium and phosphorus, for instance, serve as building blocks for bones and teeth.

Depending on the amount in which they are needed in the body, each mineral is categorized as either a "macro" or "micro" mineral. The macro minerals, which include calcium, magnesium, phosphorus, potassium, and sodium, are needed in larger amounts than are the micro minerals, which include chromium, cobalt, copper, iron, selenium, silicon, and zinc. Each mineral, like each vitamin, performs specific functions in the body.

Calcium plays a role in bone and tooth formation, blood clotting, heart rhythm, nerve transmission, muscle growth and contraction, and the proper functioning of cell membranes. In addition, calcium contributes to lower blood pressure and may protect against colon cancer. Calcium deficiency can result in muscle cramps, irritability, and insomnia. The most common problem related to long-term calcium deficiency is osteoporosis, a condition in which bones lose their normal density and strength.

Chromium helps to maintain proper blood sugar levels and healthy functioning of the circulatory system. Too little of this mineral can result in blood sugar fluctuations and high cholesterol levels.

Cobalt is involved in the healthy functioning of red blood cells. An inadequate intake of cobalt can result in anemia, weakness, nausea, loss of appetite, and bleeding gums.

Copper plays a role in bone formation, hair and skin color, the healing processes, red blood cell production, and mental and emotional processes. Copper deficiency can show itself as anemia, inflammation, and arthritis.

Iron supports growth and development in children, is needed to produce hemoglobin, and supports a healthy immune system. The most common condition related to inadequate amounts of iron is iron deficiency anemia, a disorder whose symptoms include

fatigue, irritability, headache, shortness of breath, intolerance to cold, and an increased vulnerability to infection.

Magnesium is involved in blood sugar metabolism and energy maintenance, plays a role in the metabolism of calcium and vitamin C, and is used in the structuring of basic genetic material. Too little magnesium can cause depression, fatigue, irritability, muscle weakness or tremors, constipation, nausea, and rapid heartbeat.

Phosphorus is involved in bone and tooth formation, cell growth and repair, energy maintenance, heart contraction, kidney function, the healthy activity of nerves and muscles, and the body's use of vitamins. Phosphorus deficiency may be indicated by stunted growth, bone malformation and pain, weakness, and loss of appetite.

Potassium is needed for the healthy, steady functioning of the nervous system, and supports the normal function of the heart, muscles, kidneys, and blood. Too little potassium can cause muscle weakness, irregular heartbeat, loss of appetite, nausea and vomiting, and irritability.

Selenium is involved in the healthy functioning of cell membranes, may be involved in increasing resistance to cancer, and supports pancreatic function. Also, as an antioxidant, selenium appears to work with vitamin E to prevent injuries to cells, and thus may help protect the body from several serious disorders. Poor growth, dry flaky scalp, muscular weakness and discomfort, and skin problems are all possible signs of selenium deficiency.

Silicon is used in bone formation, and supports the skin, the major blood vessels, the connective tissue, and the thymus gland. A deficiency of this mineral may cause bone deformities, connective tissue disorders, muscle cramps, irritability, and insomnia.

Sodium helps maintain normal fluid levels in the body, is involved in healthy muscle functioning, and supports the blood and lymph systems. Fainting, intolerance to heat, headaches, muscle cramps, and swelling in the extremities may all result from an inadequate intake of sodium. It is important to note, though, that most people get too much sodium in their diet. Nutritionists recommend a maximum intake of about 3,000 milligrams of sodium per day.

Zinc promotes burn and wound healing, supports the immune system, is involved in carbohydrate and protein digestion, and plays a role in reproductive organ growth and development. Possible signs of zinc deficiency include white spots on the fingernails, stretch marks on the skin, hair loss, loss of the sense of smell or taste, joint pain, poor sexual development, menstrual irregularities, slow wound healing, and recurrent infections.

THE FOOD GUIDE PYRAMID

Because the four basic nutrients and the many micronutrients are essential to life, and because most of them cannot be made by the body, we must get these nutrients from food or from nutritional supplements. Over the years, the United States Department of Agriculture (USDA) has tried to insure adequate nutrition by encouraging Americans to eat a "well-balanced diet"—a concept that has changed dramatically over the years. Most of us still remember the four food groups that the USDA once promoted. These food groups—fruits and vegetables; breads and cereals; meat, poultry, fish, and eggs; and dairy products—were developed to encourage a balanced diet that was rich in meat, poultry, and dairy products. Clearly, we now have a greater understanding of how such a diet affects our health, and the government now recommends a diet high in complex carbohydrates and low in fat. With this in mind, in May 1992, the government abandoned the four food groups in favor of the Food Guide Pyramid, which has dramatically changed the recommended amounts of foods in each group.

At the base of the Food Guide Pyramid is the bread, cereal, rice and pasta group. Six to eleven servings from this group are recommended daily—more servings than from any other food group. The next level of the pyramid is occupied by the vegetable group, with three to five daily servings recommended daily, and the fruit group, with two to four servings recommended daily. Moving upward, the next pyramid level is shared by the milk, yogurt, and cheese

group—two to three servings—and the meat, poultry, fish, dry beans, eggs, and nuts group—two to three servings. Finally, at the peak of the pyramid are fats, oils, and sweets, a group of foods that is to be eaten only sparingly.

How Americans Measure Up

How many Americans are now following the government's lead and using the Food Guide Pyramid as their model? Unfortunately, most Americans—97 percent, by some estimates—are not eating a balanced diet by any definition. One survey showed that the vast majority of Americans have significant shortages of vitamin A, the B vitamins, vitamin C, calcium, iron, niacin, and magnesium. Still other reports have documented dietary deficiencies of fiber, folic acid, and zinc.

What *are* Americans eating? The Standard American Diet—appropriately nicknamed SAD—consists of 40 to 45 percent fat, mostly animal fat from meat and dairy products. Because of this emphasis on meat products, many Americans also get twice as much protein as they need. Even worse, some have days when they do not get even one serving of fruits or vegetables!

Scaling the Pyramid

To insure that you have adequate servings of healthful foods, it is best to follow the Food Guide Pyramid and, within each group, to choose foods that are high in the nutrients needed for good health. The remainder of this book shows how each food rates in terms of its nutrient values. To make sure that these foods are still high in nutrients when they reach your table, and to help keep your diet low in fat and high in fiber, certain additional guidelines should be followed when selecting foods from each group.

■ When eating foods from the important bread, cereal, rice, and pasta group, always choose whole-grain, high-fiber, low-fat breads and cereals—preferably without added sugar, coloring, or unnecessary preservatives. Choose brown rice over white rice, and whole-wheat or other whole-grain pastas over pastas made from white flour.

■ When eating fruits and vegetables, eat fresh raw produce as often as possible. Water-soluble vitamins, such as vitamin C, may leach out of foods during cooking, be damaged by overprocessing, or be destroyed when foods are overcooked. Even fat-soluble vitamins, which are fairly stable during low-temperature cooking, can be affected by frying. For this reason, it is best to steam or microwave vegetables rather than boiling or frying them. And, unless the produce was grown organically, be sure to peel or thoroughly wash it to eliminate pesticide residues and waxes.

■ When choosing foods from the milk, yogurt, and cheese group, select low-fat and nonfat brands, which provide the most nutrients and the least amount of fat. When eating meat, poultry, and fish, choose the leanest cuts available, trim off any excess fat, and bake or broil the foods instead of frying them.

■ Select as few foods as possible from the fats, oils, and sweets group. When you do use fats and oils, though, choose monounsaturated and polyunsaturated fats instead of saturated fats. Limit your intake of sweets, choosing fresh fruits instead of cakes, cookies, and other high-fat desserts.

THE NEW FOOD LABELING

For many years, consumers and consumer groups alike complained about the confusing nature of food labels. For instance, the word "light" might mean light in calories when used by one manufacturer, and light in taste or color when used by another. Serving sizes, too, varied greatly, making it nearly impossible to compare the nutrient values of one product with those of another.

Because of this confusion, as of 1994, new food labels were required on all processed foods regulated by the Food and Drug Administration (FDA) and on all processed meat products regulated by the USDA. Let's take a look at the most significant features of the new food label.

Nutrition Facts

One of the new label's features is a revamped nutrition panel, identified by its "Nutrition Facts" heading. The new nutrition panel features more consistent serving sizes, in both household and metric measures, and states how many servings are found in each container. In addition, the panel lists the following dietary components:

- Total calories
- Calories from fat
- Total fat
- Saturated fat
- Cholesterol
- Sodium
- Total carbohydates
- Dietary fiber
- Sugars
- Protein
- Vitamin A
- Vitamin C
- Calcium
- Iron

For the last four nutrients listed above—vitamin A, vitamin C, calcium, and iron—the amount is expressed only as a percentage of its Daily Value—a recommended daily amount based on a 2,000-calorie diet. For most of the other nutrients listed, the amount is expressed both in grams or milligrams and as a percentage of its Daily Value. To educate the consumer, reference values are provided at the bottom of the label to show how much total fat, saturated fat, cholesterol, sodium, total carbohydrates, and dietary fiber should be included in both a 2,000-calorie and a 2,500-calorie diet.

Nutrient Content Descriptions

On the new food label, terms once used inconsistently, and often misleadingly, now must be applied uniformly to insure that such terms mean the same on each product on which they apppear. Following are definitions of some of the most frequently used terms.

■ **Free.** The product contains no amount of, or only "physiologically inconsequential" amounts of one or more of these components: fat, saturated fat, cholesterol, sodium, sugars, and calories. For instance, "calorie free" means that there are fewer than 5 calories per serving, and "sugar free" and "fat free" indicate that there are less than 0.5 grams per serving.

   Low. This food could be eaten frequently without exceeding dietary guidelines for one or more of the following components: fat, saturated fat, cholesterol, sodium, and calories. Thus, the following terms are used:

   Low fat. 3 grams or less per serving.

   Low saturated fat. 1 gram or less per serving.

   Low sodium. Less than 140 mgs per serving.

   Very low sodium. Less than 35 mgs per serving.

   Low cholesterol. Less than 20 mgs per serving.

   Low calorie. 40 calories or less per serving.

   Lean and extra lean. The following terms can be used to describe the fat content of meat, poultry, seafood, and game meats:

   Lean. Less than 10 grams of fat, less than 4 grams of saturated fat, and less than 95 mgs of cholesterol per serving and per 100 grams.

   Extra lean. Less than 5 grams of fat, less than 2 grams of saturated fat, and less than 95 mgs of cholesterol per serving and per 100 grams.

   High. One serving of the food contains 20% or more of the Daily Value for a particular nutrient.

■ **Good source.** One serving of the food contains 10% to 19% of the Daily Value for a particular nutrient.

   Reduced. A nutritionally altered product contains 25% less of a nutrient or of calories than the regular, or reference, product.

   Less. A food, whether altered or not, contains 25% less of a nutrient or of calories than the reference food.

   Light. A nutritionally altered product contains one-third fewer calories or half of the fat of the reference food, or the sodium content of a low-calorie, low-fat food has been reduced by 50%.

   More. One serving of the food, altered or not, contains a nutrient in a quantity that is at least 10% of the Daily Value more than the reference food.

How Helpful Is the New Food Label?

Certainly, the new label is helpful in that it provides more consistent serving sizes. In addition, it makes it a great deal easier for consumers to budget their dietary fat, a major concern for many people. However, problems still remain. For instance, the Daily Values are based on a diet of 2,000 calories. However, many people—including older people and smaller people—need only 1,200 to 1,800 calories per day, making the Daily Values of questionable worth. In addition, amounts of many nutrients known to be insufficient in the SAD diet—the B vitamins and magnesium, for instance—are not listed on the new label. Also the Daily Values for vitamins and minerals are based on the old RDAs (Recommended Dietary Allowances), which are the *minimum* amounts needed by an average healthy person. For some vitamins—vitamins C and E, for example—much higher levels may be necessary to realize the *optimum* benefits these nutrients have to offer. Clearly, for those who are trying to choose foods that are high in the nutrients needed for optimum health, a more comprehensive listing of nutrient values is needed not only for those foods covered by the new labeling laws, but for all foods.

   The following section should provide you with the details you need to better access and understand the data contained in this volume. I hope that this book will inspire you to learn more about your unique nutritional needs and the foods you are using to meet those needs. You will enjoy the sense of control this knowledge gives you. More important, you will make better food choices and take a major step toward better health.

   Should you have any comments about this book, feel free to write to the following address: Nutribase Comments, c/o Avery Publishing Group, 120 Old Broadway, Garden City Park, NY 11040.

Best wishes for good health always.

Arthur Ulene, MD

How to Use This Book

This book was designed to provide comprehensive nutritional information on a wide range of foods, both generic and brand name, raw and prepared. The information provided here was gleaned from a number of government agencies, from hundreds of manufacturers, and from food trade associations. This information was compiled and later supplemented through countless hours of follow-up that involved hundreds of additional sources. Because scientific techniques are constantly being improved, this book will be continuously updated to reflect the most current nutritional data available.

FINDING THE LISTING YOU WANT

This easy-to-use guide is divided into three parts. Part One is an A-to-Z reference to the general nutrients provided by foods. In this section, you will find the amount of calories, protein, carbohydrates, sodium, fiber, fat, saturated fat, and cholesterol, as well as the percentage of calories that come from fat.

Part Two is an A-to-Z reference to the vitamins and minerals provided by foods. This section states the amount of vitamin A, thiamine, riboflavin, niacin, vitamin B_6, folic acid, vitamin B_{12}, vitamin C, calcium, iron, magnesium, potassium, and zinc.

Part Three is an A-to-Z reference to the nutrient values of restaurant-chain foods. In this section, foods are listed alphabetically under the name of the appropriate restaurant, and each food item is accompanied by the amounts of the general nutrients found in that item.

All of the foods in this reference have been listed alphabetically. For instance, if you were looking for the nutrient values of ground beef, you would turn to the B's and look under *Beef*. For convenience, similar foods have been grouped together in categories such as *Baby Foods, Breads, Candies, Cereals, Cheese, Cookies, Pasta,* and *Sauces*. Therefore, if the food you are looking for is not listed individually by its own name, you should try looking it up under a logical category.

Always be sure to look in the appropriate part of the book. For instance, if you want to know the amount of a general nutrient—fat, for instance—look the product up in Part One. If you want to know whether a particular food is high in vitamin A, look in Part Two.

Some foods are known by two or more names. In most cases, the food is listed under just one name, and cross-references have been provided to guide you to the proper listing. For instance, garbanzo beans are also called chick peas and ceci beans. In this book, you will find the nutrient information under *Garbanzo beans*, with cross-references under *Ceci beans* and *Chick peas*.

If you are unable to find a particular food, look for the listing of a similar food. The nutritional data should be close, if not exact, for any product not listed.

After you locate the listing of the food you are interested in, you may find that abbreviations have been used to provide you with the information you need. Refer to page xxii for a complete key to the abbreviations used throughout this book.

UNDERSTANDING FISH, MEAT, AND VEGETABLE LISTINGS

When examining the nutrient values of *cooked* fish, meat, poultry, and vegetables, keep in mind that unless otherwise noted, no additional ingredients have been added. Also be aware that unless otherwise noted, the food values for fish, meats, and poultry are for meat only, and do not include skin or bones.

UNDERSTANDING FIBER VALUES

When looking at the fiber values of foods, it is important to understand that as a result of two different methods of analysis, two different types of fiber have been listed in this book. For many years, the acid-based process used to measure the fiber content of foods actually destroyed some of the fiber it was designed to measure. Referred to as "crude fiber," the results of this type of analysis are inaccurate, and almost always show an amount that is lower than the actual amount of fiber present in the food. Later, a more precise enzyme-related process for measuring this nutrient was devised. The fiber analyzed with this system is referred to as "dietary fiber."

In the interest of accuracy, whenever possible, we have provided the most up-to-date, accurate measure of total dietary fiber. You will know that the value reflects *total fiber* when the number is not accompanied by a qualifying symbol. For instance, the amount of fiber found in 1/2 cup of boiled sliced carrots is listed as *2.6*. This means that according to the most accurate techniques of analysis now available, 2.6 grams of fiber are present in this amount of carrots. Unfortunately, in the case of some foods, only the *crude fiber* value is available at this time. You will know that the value reflects crude fiber when it is preceded by the symbol > — meaning "greater than"— and followed by the letter *c* — meaning "crude." For instance, the amount of fiber found in 1/2 cup of boiled garbanzo beans is listed as *>2.0c*. This means that according to crude analysis, *at least* 2 grams of fiber can be found in this amount of beans. Of course, as techniques of analysis are improved and as additional foods are tested, the listings in this book will be updated.

UNDERSTANDING FAT PERCENTAGES

One feature that sets this book apart from many other nutrition books is the inclusion of the column called *% Fat Calories*. Although scientists and nutritionists can use any of several methods to determine the per-

centage of calories derived from fat, the simplest and most popular one is the "4-4-9 method." This technique assumes that 1 gram of protein contains 4 calories, that 1 gram of carbohydrate contains 4 calories, and that 1 gram of fat contains 9 calories. In beverages or other foods containing alcohol, it is assumed that each gram of alcohol contains 7 calories. Once you know the total calories and the calories from fat, the calculations used to determine the percentage of calories from fat is, in theory, fairly straightforward and accurate.

When applied to actual published nutrition data, however, several factors make the 4-4-9 method less than ideal. For one thing, many manufacturers consider any nutrient containing fewer than 5 calories to be "nutritionally insignificant." For this reason, the manufacturers "round off" their published values for protein, carbohydrates, and fats. Sometimes they publish a value of "<1.0 gram" of fat, which means that the fat content might be anywhere from 0.0 grams to 0.99 grams. When a food item contains only a few calories, the "insignificant" rounding of fat values can have significant and misleading consequences.

One consequence of this practice of rounding off values is that when the calorie values for protein, carbohydrates, and fat are added up, they very rarely match the calorie values published by the manufacturer or restaurant. This means that to simply multiply fat grams by 9 will often result in a misleading value for percentage of calories from fat.

To more accurately represent the percentage of calories from fat, we developed a simple method called the "compensated 4-4-9 method." Here is how this method was used to calculate the percentage-of-calories-from-fat values that appear in this book.

1. We calculated the total calories from each of the calorie sources by multiplying protein grams by 4, carbohydrate grams by 4, and fat grams by 9. We added these values together to get a "total derived calories" value.

2. We made the assumption that the manufacturer's total calorie value was correct. We then compared our total derived calorie value to the manufacturer's published total calorie value. If our derived value was lower or higher, we adjusted all of the nonzero nutrient values—maintaining the 4-4-9 ratio—to match the manufacturer's total.

3. Using the adjusted nutrient values, we calculated the percentage of calories from fat.

The compensated 4-4-9 method results in percentage-of-calories values for protein, carbohydrates, and fat that both match the manufacturer's total calorie figure and add up to 100 percent of the total calories. Using the nutritional information provided by manufacturers at this time, we feel that this method is the best means of determining accurate values.

SPECIAL FEATURES

You will find that in an effort to make all information as accessible and understandable as possible, this book has been designed with several special features.

First, boxed insets scattered throughout the listings have been used to provide additional information about or insight into a number of foods. For instance, if you are interested in finding the nutrient value of ground beef for the purpose of making hamburgers, you will find that the *Beef, Ground* listing contains a handy Quick-Reference inset. This inset gives you an at-a-glance look at other ingredients that you may use to make your hamburger—ingredients such as hamburger buns, ketchup, and mayonnaise. This feature will make it easy for you to realistically evaluate the calories, fat grams, and other nutrients found in the hamburger that you plan to serve to your family. Or perhaps you want to know the nutrient values of different types of pork with the goal of choosing the lowest-fat pork available. A Quick-Reference inset found within the pork listings explains which cuts and grades of pork are leanest, allowing you to easily identify and purchase the most healthful food available. These and other insets will either save you time by integrating data from various sections of the book, or provide information that cannot be presented in the listings themselves.

A second feature of this book makes it easy to find and compare alternative food products. In some cases, alternative or substitute products have been created by food manufacturers to provide vegetarian versions of meat products. For instance, vegetarian bacon bits have been made out of soy or other nonmeat bases. In other cases, alternative or substitute products have been created to provide lower-fat versions of a relatively high-fat food. Turkey bacon, for example, is a lower-fat—but not vegetarian—version of regular bacon. In still other instances, alternative products have been created to provide lower-priced versions of comparatively expensive items. For instance, substitutes are now available for crab meat, shrimp, and a variety of other seafoods. In each such case, an *Alternatives* heading—found within the listing of the product you wish to replace—will alert you to alternative products and provide the nutrient information you are looking for.

The third feature is a separate, clearly marked *Serving Size* column, which appears directly to the right of the food name. This column—which may, for instance, specify that the portion of rice being evaluated is 1/2 cup—makes it possible to quickly and easily compare different *products,* while reducing the likelihood of your inadvertently comparing different *portion sizes.*

Finally, this book includes an easy-to-use table that will help you to understand the measurements used within the listings, and to apply all nutrient value information to the amount of food you are actually using. The Table of Measurement Conversions on page xxiii will enable you to easily translate teaspoons into tablespoons, tablespoons into cups, and grams into ounces, as well as perform many other simple calculations. Thus, if the listings provide the nutrient values for 1 tablespoon of a food, but you are using 1/2 cup, you will have the information you need to determine the nutrient values for the amount you have. This table should take some of the mystery out of metric measures and the confusion out of a variety of calculations.

Codes and Abbreviations

To provide the most comprehensive nutritional information possible, a number of codes and abbreviations have been used throughout this book. A complete translation is given below.

>	greater than[1]	(mq)	may contain a measurable quantity[3]
<	less than	na	not available
%	percentage	nia	niacin
approx	approximately	pkg	package
c	crude fiber[1]	pot	potassium
cal	calories	prep	prepared according to directions
calc	calcium	prot	protein
carbs	carbohydrates	rib	riboflavin
chol	cholesterol	sat fat	saturated fat
diam	diameter	sod	sodium
fl	fluid	tbsp	tablespoon
fol	folic acid	thi	thiamine
gm	gram	tr	trace
I.U.	international units[2]	(tr)	may contain a trace amount
lb	pound	tsp	teaspoon
mag	magnesium	w/	with
mcg	microgram(s)	w/o	without
med	medium-sized	wt	weight
mgs	milligrams	zn	zinc

[1] The symbols > and *c*, which are used only in fiber value listings, indicate that the amount shown is the result of crude analysis, and that the actual amount of fiber present most probably is greater than the amount shown. For further explanation, see page xx.

[2] International units, which are used throughout this book to express vitamin A content, are a measure of fat-soluble vitamin activity. The amounts of all other nutrients are expressed in grams or milligrams, which are units of mass and weight.

[3] The food item may contain a quantity ranging from a trace amount to a substantial amount. This quantity depends upon any one of a number of variables—such as soil condition and mineral content of fertilizer used—that may have affected the food item during growing, processing, and/or preparation.

TABLE OF MEASUREMENT CONVERSIONS

VOLUME MEASUREMENT EQUIVALENTS

Pinch or dash	= less than $\frac{1}{8}$ teaspoon		
1 teaspoon	= $\frac{1}{3}$ tablespoon		= $\frac{1}{6}$ fluid ounce
1 tablespoon	= 3 teaspoons		= $\frac{1}{2}$ fluid ounce
2 tablespoons	= $\frac{1}{8}$ cup	= $\frac{1}{16}$ pint	= 1 fluid ounce
4 tablespoons	= $\frac{1}{4}$ cup		= 2 fluid ounces
8 tablespoons	= $\frac{1}{2}$ cup		= 4 fluid ounces
12 tablespoons	= $\frac{3}{4}$ cup		= 6 fluid ounces
16 tablespoons	= 1 cup	= $\frac{1}{2}$ pint	= 8 fluid ounces
$\frac{1}{8}$ cup	= 2 tablespoons		= 1 fluid ounce
$\frac{1}{4}$ cup	= 4 tablespoons		= 2 fluid ounces
$\frac{1}{2}$ cup	= 8 tablespoons		= 4 fluid ounces
$\frac{3}{4}$ cup	= 12 tablespoons		= 6 fluid ounces
1 cup	= 16 tablespoons	= $\frac{1}{2}$ pint	= 8 fluid ounces
2 cups	= 1 pint	= $\frac{1}{2}$ quart	= 16 fluid ounces
4 cups	= 2 pints	= 1 quart	= 32 fluid ounces
8 cups	= 4 pints	= 2 quarts	= 64 fluid ounces
16 cups	= 8 pints	= 4 quarts = 1 gallon	= 128 fluid ounces
$\frac{1}{2}$ pint	= 1 cup		= 8 fluid ounces
1 pint	= 2 cups		= 16 fluid ounces
2 pints	= 4 cups	= 1 quart	= 32 fluid ounces
4 pints	= 8 cups	= 2 quarts	= 64 fluid ounces
8 pints	= 16 cups	= 4 quarts = 1 gallon	= 128 fluid ounces
$\frac{1}{2}$ quart	= 2 cups	= 1 pint	= 16 fluid ounces
1 quart	= 4 cups	= 2 pints	= 32 fluid ounces

WEIGHT MEASUREMENT EQUIVALENTS

1 gram	= 0.035 ounce	
100 grams	= 3.57 ounces	
1 ounce		= 28.35 grams
$\frac{1}{2}$ pound	= 8 ounces	= 226.8 grams
1 pound	= 16 ounces	= 453.6 grams

PART ONE

GENERAL NUTRIENT VALUES

Calories • Protein • Carbohydrates • Sodium •
Fiber • Fat •Saturated Fat • Cholesterol •
Percentage of Calories From Fat

A

Food Name	Serving Size	Calories	Prot. gms	Carbs gms	Sod. mgs	Fiber gms	Fat gms	Sat. Fat gms	Chol. mgs	% Fat Cal.
ABALONE, MIXED SPECIES, raw	3 oz	89	14.5	5.1	256	0	0.7	0.1	72	7%
ABALONE MUSHROOM. See MUSHROOM, OYSTER.										
ACEROLA CHERRY/Barbados cherry										
trimmed	1 cup	31	0.4	7.5	7	1.1	0.3	na	0	8%
trimmed	1 oz	9	0.1	2.2	2	>.1 c	0.1	(tr)	0	9%
trimmed	1 fruit	2	0.0	0.4	0	0.1	0.0	na	0	0%
untrimmed	1 lb	114	1.5	27.9	26	>1.5 c	1.1	na	0	8%
ACEROLA CHERRY JUICE/Barbados cherry juice										
	1 cup	51	1.0	11.6	7	.7	0.7	na	0	11%
	1 oz	6	0.1	1.5	1	.1	0.1	na	0	12%
ACORN										
dried	1 oz	145	2.3	15.2	0	>1.0 c	8.9	1.2	0	53%
dried, in shell	1 lb	1432	22.8	150.9	1995	>9.5 c	88.3	11.5	0	53%
raw, in shell	1 lb	1037	17.3	114.6	1515	>7.2 c	67.1	8.7	0	53%
raw, shelled	1 oz	105	1.8	11.6	0	>.7 c	6.8	0.9	0	53%
ACORN FLOUR, full fat	1 oz	142	2.1	15.5	0	>.8 c	8.6	1.1	0	52%
ACORN SQUASH. See SQUASH, ACORN.										
ADZUKI BEAN										
boiled, mature seeds	1/2 cup	147	8.6	28.5	9	>2.3 c	0.1	0.0	0	1%
raw	1 oz	93	5.6	17.8	1	>1.5 c	0.2	tr	0	2%
raw (Arrowhead Mills)	2 oz	190	13.0	35.0	3	14.3	1.0	tr	0	5%
raw, mature seeds	1/2 cup	322	19.5	61.6	5	12.5	0.5	0.2	0	1%
yokan, mature seeds, 1/4-inch slice	1 slice	36	0.5	8.5	12	>.2	0.0	0.0	0	0%
ADZUKI BEAN, CANNED										
mature seeds, sweetened	1/2 cup	351	5.6	81.4	323	>2.3 c	0.0	0.0	0	0%
organic, no salt added (Eden Foods)	1/2 cup	80	7.0	18.0	10	5.0	<1.0	na	0	<8%
organic, w/liquid (Eden Foods)	1/2 cup	100	6.0	17.0	20	4.3	<1.0	na	0	<9%
AGAR										
dried	100 gm	306	6.2	80.9	102	7.7	0.3	0.1	0	1%
raw	1 lb	116	2.5	30.6	40	>2.0 c	0.1	<.1	0	1%
raw	100 gm	26	0.5	6.8	9	.5	0.0	0.0	0	0%
raw	1 oz	7	0.2	1.9	3	>.1 c	tr	tr	0	0%
AHI. See TUNA, YELLOWFIN.										
AKU. See TUNA, SKIPJACK.										
ALBACORE. See TUNA, CANNED; TUNA, FROZEN.										
ALCOHOL-FREE BEVERAGES										
BEER										
(Cutter)	12 oz	76	0.5	19.6	<1	0	0.0	0.0	0	0%
(Kaliber)	12 oz	71	1.2	10.6	3	na	0.0	0.0	na	0%
(Sharp's)	12 oz	86	1.0	9.5	5	0	0.0	0.0	0	0%
MIXED-DRINK MIXERS										
Banana Daiquiri, frozen, diluted w/water (Bacardi)	7 oz	150	0.0	35.0	0	na	1.0	na	na	6%
Bloody Mary										
bottled (Mr. & Mrs. T)	4.5 oz	20	1.0	4.0	670	0	0.0	na	0	0%
bottled, rich & spicy (Mr. & Mrs. T)	4.5 oz	30	1.0	6.0	500	0	0.0	na	0	0%
bottled 'Smooth N' Spicy' (Holland House)	1 oz	3	0.0	<1.0	329	(tr)	0.0	0.0	0	0%
Daiquiri										
bottled (Holland House)	1 oz	36	0.0	9.0	111	(tr)	0.0	0.0	0	0%
instant, dry (Holland House)	.56 oz	65	0.0	16.0	21	(tr)	0.0	0.0	0	0%
Grenadine										
syrup (Roses)	1 oz	65	0.0	16.0	27	(tr)	0.0	0.0	0	0%

Food Name	Serving Size	Calories	Prot. gms	Carbs gms	Sod. mgs	Fiber gms	Fat gms	Sat. Fat gms	Chol. mgs	% Fat Cal.
syrup *(Roses)*	.5 oz	32	1.0	8.0	14	na	<1.0	na	na	<20%
Lime Daiquiri, shelf stable, w/water *(Bacardi)*	7 oz	130	0.0	33.0	10	na	0.0	na	na	0%
Mai Tai										
bottled *(Holland House)*	1 oz	32	0.0	8.0	60	(tr)	0.0	0.0	0	0%
instant, dry *(Holland House)*	.56 oz	64	0.0	16.0	4	(tr)	0.0	0.0	0	0%
Manhattan, bottled *(Holland House)*	1 oz	28	0.0	7.0	5	0	0.0	0.0	0	0%
Margarita										
bottled *(Holland House)*	1 oz	27	0.0	6.0	92	(tr)	0.0	0.0	0	0%
bottled *(Mr. & Mrs. T)*	3 oz	80	<1.0	20.0	35	na	<1.0	na	na	<10%
frozen, diluted w/water *(Bacardi)*	7 oz	90	0.0	24.0	0	na	0.0	na	na	0%
instant, dry *(Holland House)*	.5 oz	57	0.0	14.0	4	(tr)	0.0	0.0	0	0%
shelf stable, w/water *(Bacardi)*	7 oz	130	0.0	33.0	10	na	0.0	na	na	0%
Old Fashioned, bottled *(Holland House)*	1 oz	33	0.0	8.0	6	0	0.0	0.0	0	0%
Peach Daiquiri, frozen, diluted w/water *(Bacardi)*	7 oz	130	0.0	33.0	5	na	0.0	na	na	0%
Piña Colada										
bottled *(Holland House)*	1 oz	33	0.0	8.0	4	na	0.0	0.0	0	0%
bottled *(Mr. & Mrs. T)*	4 oz	150	<1.0	39.0	120	na	<1.0	na	na	<5%
frozen, diluted w/water *(Bacardi)*	7 oz	200	1.0	37.0	25	na	6.0	na	na	26%
instant, dry *(Holland House)*	.56 oz	82	0.0	12.0	<1	na	3.0	na	0	36%
shelf stable, w/water *(Bacardi)*	7 oz	170	0.0	36.0	20	na	2.0	na	na	11%
Raspberry Daiquiri, bottled *(Holland House)*	1 oz	30	0.0	7.0	4	(tr)	0.0	0.0	0	0%
Rum Runner, shelf stable, w/water *(Bacardi)*	7 oz	140	0.0	33.0	15	na	0.0	na	na	0%
Strawberry Colada, shelf stable, w/water *(Bacardi)*	7 oz	150	0.0	34.0	15	na	1.0	na	na	6%
Strawberry Daiquiri										
bottled *(Holland House)*	1 oz	31	0.0	7.0	3	(tr)	0.0	0.0	0	0%
frozen, diluted w/water *(Bacardi)*	7 oz	140	0.0	34.0	0	na	0.0	na	na	0%
shelf stable, w/water *(Bacardi)*	7 oz	130	0.0	31.0	15	na	0.0	na	na	0%
Strawberry Margarita										
bottled *(Holland House)*	1 oz	31	0.0	7.0	3	na	0.0	0.0	0	0%
bottled *(Mr. & Mrs. T)*	3.5 oz	100	<1.0	24.0	10	na	<1.0	na	na	<8%
instant, dry *(Holland House)*	.56 oz	66	0.0	16.0	<1	(tr)	0.0	0.0	0	0%
Sweet and Sour										
bottled *(Mr. & Mrs. T)*	3 oz	70	<1.0	17.0	45	na	<1.0	na	na	<11%
liquid *(Holland House)*	1 oz	34	0.0	8.0	107	na	0.0	0.0	0	0%
Tom Collins										
bottled *(Holland House)*	1 oz	47	0.0	11.0	96	na	0.0	0.0	0	0%
instant, dry *(Holland House)*	.56 oz	65	0.0	16.0	14	na	0.0	0.0	0	0%
Whiskey Sour										
bottled *(Holland House)*	1 oz	37	0.0	9.0	105	na	0.0	0.0	0	0%
instant, dry *(Holland House)*	.56 oz	64	0.0	16.0	16	na	0.0	0.0	0	0%
ALCOHOLIC BEVERAGES. See also ALCOHOL-FREE BEVERAGES.										
BEER, ALE, and MALT LIQUOR										
(Anheuser Marzen)	12 oz	168	2.3	15.2	12	0	0.0	0.0	0	0%
(Beck's)	12 oz	148	1.7	10.0	14	0	0.0	0.0	0	0%
(Budweiser)	12 oz	144	1.2	11.3	12	0	0.0	0.0	0	0%
(Budweiser) 'Bud Light'	12 oz	110	1.1	6.9	12	0	0.0	0.0	0	0%
(Busch)	12 oz	144	1.2	11.9	12	0	0.0	0.0	0	0%
(Carlsberg)	12 oz	149	1.2	11.9	12	0	0.0	0.0	0	0%
(Carlsberg) 'Light'	12 oz	110	1.1	6.5	12	0	0.0	0.0	0	0%
(Coors)	12 oz	137	0.6	11.6	<1	0	0.0	0.0	0	0%
(Coors) 'Dry'	12 oz	119	0.4	6.0	<1	0	0.0	0.0	0	0%
(Coors) 'Dry' 3.2%	12 oz	101	0.6	5.3	<1	0	0.0	0.0	0	0%
(Coors) 'Extra Gold'	12 oz	151	1.3	12.5	<1	0	0.0	0.0	0	0%
(Coors) 'Extra Gold' 3.2%	12 oz	121	0.6	10.2	<1	0	0.0	0.0	0	0%

Food Name	Serving Size	Calories	Prot. gms	Carbs gms	Sod. mgs	Fiber gms	Fat gms	Sat. Fat gms	Chol. mgs	% Fat Cal.
(Coors) 'Light'	12 oz	103	0.7	4.7	<1	0	0.0	0.0	0	0%
(Coors) 'Light' 3.2%	12 oz	98	0.7	4.7	<1	0	0.0	0.0	0	0%
(Coors) 3.2%	12 oz	119	0.7	9.7	<1	0	0.0	0.0	0	0%
(Coqui)	12 oz	208	1.7	9.8	13	0	0.0	0.0	0	0%
(Dribeck's)	12 oz	94	1.0	7.0	14	0	0.0	0.0	0	0%
(Elephant)	12 oz	208	1.6	16.9	12	0	0.0	0.0	0	0%
(Keystone)	12 oz	121	0.6	6.8	<1	0	0.0	0.0	0	0%
(Keystone) 'Dry'	12 oz	121	0.6	6.4	<1	0	0.0	0.0	0	0%
(Keystone) 'Light'	12 oz	100	0.6	4.4	<1	0	0.0	0.0	0	0%
(Keystone) 'Light' 3.2%	12 oz	99	0.4	5.0	<1	0	0.0	0.0	0	0%
(Keystone) 3.2%	12 oz	104	0.5	6.1	<1	0	0.0	0.0	0	0%
(Killian's)	12 oz	161	1.0	15.0	<1	0	0.0	0.0	0	0%
(Killian's) 3.2%	12 oz	128	1.2	11.4	<1	0	0.0	0.0	0	0%
(King Cobra)	12 oz	182	1.4	15.2	12	0	0.0	0.0	0	0%
(Knickerbocker)	12 oz	140	0.9	12.3	9	0	0.0	0.0	0	0%
(LA) light alcohol	12 oz	114	0.8	16.4	12	0	0.0	0.0	0	0%
(Lite) 'Genuine Draft'	12 oz	98	0.8	3.5	6	0	0.0	0.0	0	0%
(Lite) 'Lite'	12 oz	96	0.8	2.8	6	0	0.0	0.0	0	0%
(Lowenbräu) 'Dark Special'	12 oz	158	1.4	14.3	7	0	0.0	0.0	0	0%
(Lowenbräu) 'Special'	12 oz	158	1.4	14.3	7	0	0.0	0.0	0	0%
(McSorley's)	12 oz	166	1.7	14.7	6	0	0.0	0.0	0	0%
(Meister Brau)	12 oz	141	1.0	12.8	6	0	0.0	0.0	0	0%
(Meister Brau) 'Light'	12 oz	98	0.8	3.5	6	0	0.0	0.0	0	0%
(Michelob)	12 oz	156	1.5	13.6	12	0	0.0	0.0	0	0%
(Michelob) 'Classic Dark'	12 oz	158	1.5	14.4	12	0	0.0	0.0	0	0%
(Michelob) 'Dry'	12 oz	133	1.3	7.8	12	0	0.0	0.0	0	0%
(Michelob) 'Light'	12 oz	134	1.2	11.9	12	0	0.0	0.0	0	0%
(Miller) 'Genuine Draft'	12 oz	147	1.0	13.1	7	0	0.0	0.0	0	0%
(Miller) 'High Life'	12 oz	147	1.0	13.1	7	0	0.0	0.0	0	0%
(Miller) 'Magnum'	12 oz	162	1.3	10.2	8	0	0.0	0.0	0	0%
(Milwaukee) 'Milwaukee's Best'	12 oz	133	0.9	11.4	6	0	0.0	0.0	0	0%
(Milwaukee) 'Milwaukee's Best Light'	12 oz	98	0.8	3.5	6	0	0.0	0.0	0	0%
(Natural Light)	12 oz	110	1.1	6.6	12	0	0.0	0.0	0	0%
(Ortlieb's)	12 oz	140	0.9	12.3	9	0	0.0	0.0	0	0%
(Prior) 'Double Dark'	12 oz	171	1.4	15.4	10	0	0.0	0.0	0	0%
(Rheingold)	12 oz	148	1.0	12.9	9	0	0.0	0.0	0	0%
(Rheingold) 'Light'	12 oz	96	0.7	2.8	7	0	0.0	0.0	0	0%
(Rolling Rock) 'Light'	12 oz	104	0.4	8.0	<1	0	0.0	0.0	0	0%
(Rolling Rock) 'Premium'	12 oz	145	0.4	10.0	<1	0	0.0	0.0	0	0%
(Schmidt's)	12 oz	148	1.0	12.9	9	0	0.0	0.0	0	0%
(Schmidt's) 'Classic'	12 oz	144	1.0	12.8	10	0	0.0	0.0	0	0%
(Schmidt's) 'Light'	12 oz	96	0.7	2.8	7	0	0.0	0.0	0	0%
(Tiger Head)	12 oz	166	1.7	14.7	6	0	0.0	0.0	0	0%
(Zima)	12 oz	148	0.2	14.0	2	na	na	na	na	0%
CHAMPAGNE										
brut (Jacques Bonet)	4 oz	92	0.0	2.1	4	0	0.0	0.0	0	0%
brut (Lejon)	4 oz	92	0.0	3.4	4	0	0.0	0.0	0	0%
extra dry (Jacques Bonet)	4 oz	97	0.0	3.4	4	0	0.0	0.0	0	0%
extra dry (Lejon)	4 oz	97	0.0	2.1	4	0	0.0	0.0	0	0%
pink (Jacques Bonet)	4 oz	98	0.0	3.7	4	0	0.0	0.0	0	0%
pink (Lejon)	4 oz	98	0.0	3.7	4	0	0.0	0.0	0	0%
LIQUOR AND LIQUEUR										
Bourbon										
80 proof, distilled	1 oz	65	0.0	tr	tr	0	0.0	0.0	0	0%

Food Name	Serving Size	Calories	Prot. gms	Carbs gms	Sod. mgs	Fiber gms	Fat gms	Sat. Fat gms	Chol. mgs	% Fat Cal.
86 proof, distilled	1 oz	70	0.0	tr	tr	0	0.0	0.0	0	0%
90 proof, distilled	1 oz	74	0.0	tr	tr	0	0.0	0.0	0	0%
94 proof, distilled	1 oz	77	0.0	tr	tr	0	0.0	0.0	0	0%
100 proof, distilled	1 oz	83	0.0	tr	tr	0	0.0	0.0	0	0%
Brandy										
80 proof, distilled	1 oz	65	0.0	tr	tr	0	0.0	0.0	0	0%
86 proof, distilled	1 oz	70	0.0	tr	tr	0	0.0	0.0	0	0%
90 proof, distilled	1 oz	74	0.0	tr	tr	0	0.0	0.0	0	0%
94 proof, distilled	1 oz	77	0.0	tr	tr	0	0.0	0.0	0	0%
100 proof, distilled	1 oz	83	0.0	tr	tr	0	0.0	0.0	0	0%
Coffee Liqueur										
53 proof	1 oz	117	0.0	16.3	3	0	0.1	0.0	0	1%
63 proof	1 oz	107	0.0	11.2	3	0	0.1	0.0	0	1%
Creme de Menthe, 72 proof	1 oz	125	0.0	14.0	2	0	0.1	0.0	0	1%
Gin										
80 proof, distilled	1 oz	64	0.0	0.0	0	0	0.0	0.0	0	0%
86 proof, distilled	1 oz	69	0.0	0.0	0	0	0.0	0.0	0	0%
90 proof, distilled	1 oz	73	0.0	0.0	0	0	0.0	0.0	0	0%
94 proof, distilled	1 oz	76	0.0	0.0	0	0	0.0	0.0	0	0%
100 proof, distilled	1 oz	82	0.0	0.0	0	0	0.0	0.0	0	0%
Rum										
80 proof, distilled	1 oz	64	0.0	0.0	0	0	0.0	0.0	0	0%
86 proof, distilled	1 oz	69	0.0	0.0	0	0	0.0	0.0	0	0%
90 proof, distilled	1 oz	73	0.0	0.0	0	0	0.0	0.0	0	0%
94 proof, distilled	1 oz	76	0.0	0.0	0	0	0.0	0.0	0	0%
100 proof, distilled	1 oz	82	0.0	0.0	0	0	0.0	0.0	0	0%
Rye Whiskey										
80 proof, distilled	1 oz	65	0.0	tr	tr	0	0.0	0.0	0	0%
86 proof, distilled	1 oz	70	0.0	tr	tr	0	0.0	0.0	0	0%
90 proof, distilled	1 oz	74	0.0	tr	tr	0	0.0	0.0	0	0%
94 proof, distilled	1 oz	77	0.0	tr	tr	0	0.0	0.0	0	0%
100 proof, distilled	1 oz	83	0.0	tr	tr	0	0.0	0.0	0	0%
Scotch										
80 proof, distilled	1 oz	65	0.0	tr	tr	0	0.0	0.0	0	0%
86 proof, distilled	1 oz	70	0.0	tr	tr	0	0.0	0.0	0	0%
90 proof, distilled	1 oz	74	0.0	tr	tr	0	0.0	0.0	0	0%
94 proof, distilled	1 oz	77	0.0	tr	tr	0	0.0	0.0	0	0%
100 proof, distilled	1 oz	83	0.0	tr	tr	0	0.0	0.0	0	0%
Tequila										
80 proof, distilled	1 oz	65	0.0	tr	tr	0	0.0	0.0	0	0%
86 proof, distilled	1 oz	70	0.0	tr	tr	0	0.0	0.0	0	0%
90 proof, distilled	1 oz	74	0.0	tr	tr	0	0.0	0.0	0	0%
94 proof, distilled	1 oz	77	0.0	tr	tr	0	0.0	0.0	0	0%
100 proof, distilled	1 oz	83	0.0	tr	tr	0	0.0	0.0	0	0%
Vodka										
80 proof, distilled	1 oz	64	0.0	0.0	0	0	0.0	0.0	0	0%
86 proof, distilled	1 oz	69	0.0	0.0	0	0	0.0	0.0	0	0%
90 proof, distilled	1 oz	73	0.0	0.0	0	0	0.0	0.0	0	0%
94 proof, distilled	1 oz	76	0.0	0.0	0	0	0.0	0.0	0	0%
100 proof, distilled	1 oz	82	0.0	0.0	0	0	0.0	0.0	0	0%
Whiskey										
80 proof, distilled	1 oz	64	0.0	0.0	0	0	0.0	0.0	0	0%
86 proof, distilled	1 oz	69	0.0	0.0	0	0	0.0	0.0	0	0%
90 proof, distilled	1 oz	73	0.0	0.0	0	0	0.0	0.0	0	0%

Food Name	Serving Size	Calories	Prot. gms	Carbs gms	Sod. mgs	Fiber gms	Fat gms	Sat. Fat gms	Chol. mgs	% Fat Cal.
94 proof, distilled	1 oz	76	0.0	0.0	0	0	0.0	0.0	0	0%
100 proof, distilled	1 oz	82	0.0	0.0	0	0	0.0	0.0	0	0%
MIXED DRINKS. See also ALCOHOL-FREE BEVERAGES, MIXED-DRINK MIXERS.										
Banana Daiquiri										
frozen, prepared w/1/2 can rum, diluted as directed										
(Bacardi)	7 oz	210	0.0	35.0	0	na	1.0	na	na	4%
Bloody Mary, prepared from recipe	5 oz	115	0.7	4.9	332	>.3 c	0.2	0.0	0	2%
Bourbon and Soda, prepared from recipe	4 oz	104	0.0	0.0	16	0	0.0	0.0	0	0%
Daiquiri										
instant, prepared as directed (Bar-Tender's)	3.5 oz	177	0.0	18.0	50	0	0.0	0.0	0	0%
prepared from recipe	1 oz	56	0.0	2.0	2	0	0.0	0.0	0	0%
Gin and Tonic, prepared from recipe	1 oz	23	0.0	2.1	1	0	0.0	0.0	0	0%
Lime Daiquiri, mix, shelf stable, prepared w/1/2 can rum										
(Bacardi)	7 oz	210	0.0	33.0	10	na	0.0	na	na	0%
Manhattan, prepared from recipe	1 oz	64	0.0	0.9	1	0	0.0	0.0	0	0%
Margarita										
frozen, prepared w/1/2 can rum, diluted as directed										
(Bacardi)	7 oz	160	0.0	24.0	5	na	0.0	na	na	0%
shelf stable, prepared w/1/2 can rum (Bacardi)	7 oz	210	0.0	33.0	10	na	0.0	na	na	0%
Martini, prepared from recipe	1 oz	63	0.0	0.1	1	0	0.0	0.0	0	0%
Peach Daiquiri										
frozen, prepared w/1/2 can rum, diluted as directed										
(Bacardi)	7 oz	200	0.0	33.0	5	na	0.0	na	na	0%
Piña Colada										
frozen, prepared w/1/2 can rum, diluted as directed										
(Bacardi)	7 oz	260	1.0	37.0	25	na	6.0	na	na	21%
mix, shelf stable, prepared w/1/2 can rum (Bacardi)	7 oz	240	0.0	36.0	20	na	2.0	na	na	8%
prepared from recipe	1 oz	58	0.1	8.9	2	>.1 c	0.6	0.3	0	9%
Rum Runner, shelf stable, prepared w/1/2 can rum										
(Bacardi)	7 oz	210	0.0	33.0	15	na	0.0	na	na	0%
Screwdriver, prepared from recipe	1 oz	25	0.2	2.6	0	0	0.0	0.0	0	0%
Strawberry Colada										
mix, shelf stable, prepared w/1/2 can rum (Bacardi)	7 oz	230	0.0	34.0	15	na	1.0	na	na	4%
Strawberry Daiquiri										
frozen, prepared w/1/2 can rum, diluted as directed										
(Bacardi)	7 oz	200	0.0	34.0	0	na	0.0	na	na	0%
mix, shelf stable, prepared w/1/2 can rum (Bacardi)	7 oz	200	0.0	31.0	15	na	0.0	na	na	0%
Tequila Sunrise, prepared from recipe	1 oz	34	0.1	2.7	1	0	0.0	0.0	0	0%
Tom Collins, prepared from recipe	1 oz	16	0.0	0.4	5	0	0.0	0.0	0	0%
Whiskey Sour										
mix, powder, instant, prepared w/whiskey (Bar-Tender's)	3.5 oz	177	0.0	18.0	50	0	0.0	0.0	0	0%
prepared from recipe	1 oz	41	0.1	1.7	3	0	0.0	0.0	0	0%
WINE. See also WINE, COOKING.										
'Arriba' (Mission Bell)	2 oz	95	0.0	6.8	4	0	0.0	0.0	0	0%
'Diamond Red' (Mission Bell)	2 oz	95	0.0	6.8	4	0	0.0	0.0	0	0%
'Silver Satin' (Mission Bell)	2 oz	83	0.0	5.4	4	0	0.0	0.0	0	0%
'Silver Satin Bitter Lemon' (Mission Bell)	2 oz	83	0.0	5.5	4	0	0.0	0.0	0	0%
'Swiss Up' (Mission Bell)	2 oz	84	0.0	5.6	4	0	0.0	0.0	0	0%
Barbera, white (Colony)	4 oz	91	0.0	3.5	4	0	0.0	0.0	0	0%
Burgundy										
(Bravo)	4 oz	91	0.0	1.7	4	0	0.0	0.0	0	0%
(Carlo Rossi)	4 oz	92	0.0	1.6	na	0	0.0	0.0	0	0%
(Colony) 'Classic'	4 oz	90	0.0	1.2	4	0	0.0	0.0	0	0%
(Gallo)	4 oz	88	0.0	0.8	na	0	0.0	0.0	0	0%

Food Name	Serving Size	Calories	Prot. gms	Carbs gms	Sod. mgs	Fiber gms	Fat gms	Sat. Fat gms	Chol. mgs	% Fat Cal.
(Gallo) 'Hearty'	4 oz	92	0.0	1.6	na	0	0.0	0.0	0	0%
(Gambarelli & Davitto) 'Parma'	4 oz	91	0.0	1.7	4	0	0.0	0.0	0	0%
(Petri)	4 oz	91	0.0	1.7	4	0	0.0	0.0	0	0%
Cabernet Sauvignon										
(Colony)	4 oz	88	0.0	0.7	4	0	0.0	0.0	0	0%
(Gallo)	4 oz	88	0.0	0.0	na	0	0.0	0.0	0	0%
Carbonated										
(Carlo Rossi) 'Paisano'	4 oz	92	0.0	1.6	na	0	0.0	0.0	0	0%
(Jacques Bonet) almond	4 oz	104	0.0	7.7	4	0	0.0	0.0	0	0%
(Jacques Bonet) apricot	4 oz	111	0.0	9.5	4	0	0.0	0.0	0	0%
(Jacques Bonet) cherry	4 oz	106	0.0	8.3	4	0	0.0	0.0	0	0%
(Jacques Bonet) peach	4 oz	111	0.0	9.5	4	0	0.0	0.0	0	0%
(Jacques Bonet) raspberry	4 oz	106	0.0	8.3	4	0	0.0	0.0	0	0%
Chablis										
(Bravo)	4 oz	86	0.0	1.7	4	0	0.0	0.0	0	0%
(Carlo Rossi)	4 oz	84	0.0	2.0	na	0	0.0	0.0	0	0%
(Carlo Rossi) pink	4 oz	92	0.0	3.6	na	0	0.0	0.0	0	0%
(Colony)	4 oz	98	0.0	4.5	4	0	0.0	0.0	0	0%
(Colony) 'Classic'	4 oz	84	0.0	1.8	4	0	0.0	0.0	0	0%
(Colony) emerald	4 oz	102	0.0	5.3	4	0	0.0	0.0	0	0%
(Colony) gold	4 oz	97	0.0	4.3	4	0	0.0	0.0	0	0%
(Colony) ruby	4 oz	104	0.0	5.9	4	0	0.0	0.0	0	0%
(Gallo)	4 oz	80	0.0	4.0	na	0	0.0	0.0	0	0%
(Gallo) 'Blanc'	4 oz	80	0.0	0.6	na	0	0.0	0.0	0	0%
(Gambarelli & Davitto) 'Parma'	4 oz	86	0.0	1.7	4	0	0.0	0.0	0	0%
(Petri)	4 oz	98	0.0	4.5	4	0	0.0	0.0	0	0%
(Petri) 'Blanc'	4 oz	86	0.0	1.7	4	0	0.0	0.0	0	0%
Chardonnay (Gallo)	4 oz	88	0.0	na	na	0	0.0	0.0	0	0%
Chenin Blanc										
(Colony)	4 oz	86	0.0	2.4	4	0	0.0	0.0	0	0%
(Gallo)	4 oz	88	0.0	1.6	na	0	0.0	0.0	0	0%
Chianti										
(Carlo Rossi) 'Light'	4 oz	92	0.0	2.4	na	0	0.0	0.0	0	0%
(Petri)	4 oz	91	0.0	1.7	4	0	0.0	0.0	0	0%
Cold duck										
(Jacques Bonet)	4 oz	108	0.0	5.9	4	0	0.0	0.0	0	0%
(Lejon)	4 oz	108	0.0	5.9	4	0	0.0	0.0	0	0%
French colombard										
(Colony)	4 oz	84	0.0	1.8	4	0	0.0	0.0	0	0%
(Gallo)	4 oz	88	0.0	2.0	na	0	0.0	0.0	0	0%
Gewurztraminer (Gallo)	4 oz	88	0.0	1.6	na	0	0.0	0.0	0	0%
Marsala (Gambarelli & Davitto)	4 oz	77	0.0	4.0	4	0	0.0	0.0	0	0%
Moselle (Colony) 'Rhineskeller'	4 oz	97	0.0	4.3	4	0	0.0	0.0	0	0%
Muscatel (Italian Swiss Colony)	2 oz	122	0.0	5.9	4	0	0.0	0.0	0	0%
Pastoso (Petri)	4 oz	92	0.0	1.8	4	0	0.0	0.0	0	0%
Port										
(Gallo)	2 oz	64	0.0	2.0	na	0	0.0	0.0	0	0%
(Gallo) white	2 oz	86	0.0	5.6	na	0	0.0	0.0	0	0%
(Italian Swiss Colony)	2 oz	85	0.0	5.7	4	0	0.0	0.0	0	0%
(Italian Swiss Colony) white	2 oz	86	0.0	6.3	4	0	0.0	0.0	0	0%
(Livingston Cellars) tawny	2 oz	86	0.0	6.4	na	0	0.0	0.0	0	0%
Rhine										
(Bravo)	4 oz	97	0.0	4.3	4	0	0.0	0.0	0	0%
(Carlo Rossi)	4 oz	84	0.0	4.4	na	0	0.0	0.0	0	0%

Food Name	Serving Size	Calories	Prot. gms	Carbs gms	Sod. mgs	Fiber gms	Fat gms	Sat. Fat gms	Chol. mgs	% Fat Cal.
(Colony) 'Classic'	4 oz	89	0.0	3.8	4	0	0.0	0.0	0	0%
(Gallo)	4 oz	80	0.0	4.0	na	0	0.0	0.0	0	0%
(Gambarelli & Davitto) 'Parma'	4 oz	92	0.0	1.2	4	0	0.0	0.0	0	0%
(Petri)	4 oz	97	0.0	4.3	4	0	0.0	0.0	0	0%
Reisling (Gallo) 'Johannisberg'	4 oz	84	0.0	1.6	na	0	0.0	0.0	0	0%
Rosé										
(Bravo)	4 oz	92	0.0	3.1	4	0	0.0	0.0	0	0%
(Carlo Rossi) 'Vin Rosé'	4 oz	88	0.0	2.8	na	0	0.0	0.0	0	0%
(Colony) 'Classic'	4 oz	89	0.0	3.0	4	0	0.0	0.0	0	0%
(Gallo) 'Grenache'	4 oz	88	0.0	2.4	na	0	0.0	0.0	0	0%
(Gallo) 'Red Rosé'	4 oz	112	0.0	6.4	na	0	0.0	0.0	0	0%
(Gallo) 'Vin Rosé'	4 oz	88	0.0	2.8	na	0	0.0	0.0	0	0%
(Gambarelli & Davitto) 'Parma'	4 oz	92	0.0	3.1	4	0	0.0	0.0	0	0%
(Petri)	4 oz	92	0.0	3.1	4	0	0.0	0.0	0	0%
Sauvignon Blanc, (Gallo)	4 oz	80	0.0	0.8	na	0	0.0	0.0	0	0%
Sherry										
(Gallo)	2 oz	64	0.0	2.0	na	0	0.0	0.0	0	0%
(Italian Swiss Colony) cream	2 oz	85	0.0	6.8	4	0	0.0	0.0	0	0%
(Italian Swiss Colony) dry	2 oz	63	0.0	1.2	4	0	0.0	0.0	0	0%
(Livingston Cellars) cream	2 oz	78	0.0	5.6	na	0	0.0	0.0	0	0%
(Livingston Cellars) 'Very Dry'	2 oz	60	0.0	1.0	na	0	0.0	0.0	0	0%
Tokay (Italian Swiss Colony)	2 oz	82	0.0	5.1	4	0	0.0	0.0	0	0%
Vermouth										
(Gallo) dry	2 oz	56	0.0	0.8	na	0	0.0	0.0	0	0%
(Gallo) sweet	2 oz	90	0.0	9.4	na	0	0.0	0.0	0	0%
(Gambarelli & Davitto) dry	2 oz	64	0.0	1.5	4	0	0.0	0.0	0	0%
(Gambarelli & Davitto) sweet	2 oz	77	0.0	8.4	4	0	0.0	0.0	0	0%
(Lejon) dry	2 oz	64	0.0	1.5	4	0	0.0	0.0	0	0%
(Lejon) sweet	2 oz	77	0.0	8.4	4	0	0.0	0.0	0	0%
Zinfandel										
(Colony)	4 oz	91	0.0	0.7	4	0	0.0	0.0	0	0%
(Colony) white	4 oz	82	0.0	2.7	4	0	0.0	0.0	0	0%
(Gallo)	4 oz	92	0.0	0.0	na	0	0.0	0.0	0	0%
WINE COOLERS										
(Bartles & Jaymes) Berry Cooler 'Light'	12 oz	150	0.0	32.0	na	na	0.0	0.0	na	0%
(Bartles & Jaymes) Black Cherry Cooler 'Light'	12 oz	139	0.0	30.0	na	na	0.0	0.0	na	0%
(Bartles & Jaymes) Citrus Cooler 'Light'	6 oz	67	<1.0	12.0	na	na	<1.0	na	na	<13%
(Bartles & Jaymes) Tropical Cooler 'Light'	12 oz	151	0.0	32.0	na	na	0.0	0.0	na	0%
ALE. See ALCOHOLIC BEVERAGES.										
ALFALFA SEEDS										
(Arrowhead Mills)	1 cup	40	5.0	4.0	na	(mq)	1.0	na	0	20%
sprouted, raw	1 lb	132	18.1	17.1	29	10.0	3.1	0.3	0	17%
sprouted, raw	1/2 cup	5	0.7	0.6	1	.4	0.1	<.1	0	15%
sprouted, raw	1 tbsp	1	0.1	0.1	0	.1	0.0	0.0	0	0%
sprouted, raw	1 oz	8	1.1	1.1	2	.6	0.2	<.1	0	17%
ALLIGATOR	1 oz	41	8.3	na	na	na	0.8	0.2	18	18%
ALLSPICE										
ground	1 oz	75	1.7	20.4	22	>6.1 c	2.5	0.7	0	20%
ground	1 tbsp	16	0.4	4.3	5	1.3	0.5	0.2	0	tr
ground	1 tsp	5	0.1	1.4	1	.4	0.2	0.1	0	tr
ground (Durkee)	1 tsp	7	0.0	0.0	0	0.0	tr	na	na	tr
ground (Laurel Leaf)	1 tsp	7	0.0	0.0	0	0.0	tr	na	na	tr
ground (Spice Islands)	1 tsp	6	0.1	1.3	1	>.4 c	0.1	tr	0	tr

Food Name	Serving Size	Calories	Prot. gms	Carbs gms	Sod. mgs	Fiber gms	Fat gms	Sat. Fat gms	Chol. mgs	% Fat Cal.
ALMOND										
(Beer Nuts)	1 oz	180	5.0	7.0	51	(mq)	14.4	(mq)	0	73%
(Dole)	1 oz	170	6.0	12.0	4	(mq)	14.0	(mq)	0	64%
(Fisher)	1 oz	170	3.0	3.0	0	na	15.0	1.0	0	85%
chopped	1 cup	766	25.9	26.5	14	6.1	67.9	6.4	0	75%
in shell	1 lb	1069	36.2	37.0	19	>4.9 c	94.7	9.0	0	74%
sliced	1 cup	554	18.8	19.2	10	4.4	49.1	4.7	0	74%
slivered, tightly packed	1 cup	795	26.9	27.5	15	6.4	70.5	6.7	0	75%
whole kernels	1 cup	836	28.3	29.0	16	15.5	74.1	7.0	0	74%
whole kernels, approx 24	1 oz	167	5.7	5.8	3	>.8 c	14.8	1.4	0	74%
Blanched										
sliced	1 cup	615	21.4	19.5	11	>2.4 c	55.2	5.2	0	75%
whole kernels	1 cup	850	29.6	26.9	15	9.7	76.2	7.2	0	75%
whole kernels	1 oz	166	5.8	5.3	3	>.7 c	14.9	1.4	0	75%
Dry roasted										
(Planters)	1 oz	170	6.0	6.0	200	(mq)	15.0	2.0	0	74%
whole kernels	1 cup	810	22.5	33.4	15	>6.8 c	71.2	6.8	0	74%
whole kernels	1 oz	167	4.6	6.9	3	>1.4 c	14.7	1.4	0	74%
Honey roasted										
(Planters)	1 oz	170	5.0	9.0	180	na	13.0	1.0	0	68%
whole kernels	1 cup	855	26.2	40.2	187	na	71.9	6.8	0	71%
whole kernels	1 oz	168	5.2	7.9	37	na	14.1	1.3	0	71%
Oil roasted										
whole kernels	1 cup	970	32.0	24.9	16	17.6	90.5	8.6	0	78%
whole kernels, approx 22	1 oz	176	5.8	4.5	3	3.2	16.4	1.6	0	78%
Oil roasted and blanched										
approx 24 whole kernels	1 oz	174	5.4	5.1	3	3.2	16.1	1.5	0	78%
toasted	1 cup	870	27.0	25.6	17	15.9	80.3	7.6	0	78%
toasted	1 oz	167	5.8	6.5	3	>1.4 c	14.4	1.4	0	73%
Raw										
blanched (Planters)	1 oz	170	6.0	6.0	0	na	15.0	2.0	0	74%
sliced (Planters)	1 oz	170	6.0	6.0	0	(mq)	15.0	2.0	0	74%
slivered (Planters)	1 oz	170	6.0	6.0	0	(mq)	15.0	2.0	0	74%
whole (Planters)	1 oz	170	6.0	6.0	0	na	15.0	2.0	0	74%
Toasted										
(Dole)	1 oz	170	6.0	5.0	4	na	14.0	na	na	74%
unblanched	1 oz	167	5.8	6.5	3	>1.4 c	14.4	1.4	0	73%
ALMOND BUTTER										
Plain										
	1/2 cup	791	18.9	26.5	14	4.65	73.9	7.0	0	79%
	1 oz	179	4.3	6.0	3	>.4 c	16.8	1.6	0	79%
blanched, toasted (Hain)	2 tbsp	220	8.0	3.0	10	(mq)	19.0	2.0	0	80%
gourmet (Roaster Fresh)	1 oz	184	5.0	6.0	4	na	16.0	1.6	na	77%
no salt, crunchy 'Natural' (Westbrae)	2 tbsp	190	7.0	7.0	0	na	17.0	na	na	73%
no salt, smooth 'Natural' (Westbrae)	2 tbsp	190	7.0	7.0	0	na	17.0	na	0	73%
raw 'Natural' (Hain)	2 tbsp	190	8.0	3.0	5	(mq)	18.0	2.0	0	79%
raw, organic (Maranatha Natural)	2 tbsp	190	7.0	8.0	5	na	15.0	na	0	69%
roasted (Maranatha Natural)	2 tbsp	190	7.0	8.0	5	na	15.0	na	na	69%
salted	1 cup	791	18.9	26.5	563	4.65	73.9	7.0	0	79%
salted	1 oz	179	4.3	6.0	128	>.4 c	16.8	1.6	0	79%
salted	1 tbsp	101	2.4	3.4	72	>.2 c	9.5	0.9	0	79%
Honey and cinnamon										
	1/2 cup	753	19.8	33.7	14	4.65	65.3	6.2	0	73%
	1 oz	171	4.5	7.6	3	>.4 c	14.8	1.4	0	73%

Food Name	Serving Size	Calories	Prot. gms	Carbs gms	Sod. mgs	Fiber gms	Fat gms	Sat. Fat gms	Chol. mgs	% Fat Cal.
salted	1/2 cup	753	19.8	33.7	213	4.65	65.3	6.2	0	73%
salted	1 oz	171	4.5	7.6	48	>.4 c	14.8	1.4	0	73%
ALMOND MEAL										
partially defatted	4 oz	463	44.8	32.8	8	>2.6 c	20.8	2.0	0	38%
partially defatted, salted	4 oz	463	44.8	32.8	846	>2.6 c	20.8	2.0	0	38%
ALMOND OIL										
	1/2 cup	964	0.0	0.0	0	0	109.0	9.0	0	100%
	1 oz	251	0.0	0.0	0	0	28.4	2.3	0	100%
	1 tbsp	120	0.0	0.0	0	0	13.6	1.1	0	100%
(Hain)	1 tbsp	120	0.0	0.0	0	0	14.0	1.0	0	100%
(Spectrum Naturals)	1 tbsp	120	0.0	0.0	0	(tr)	14.0	1.0	(tr)	100%
ALMOND PASTE										
	4 oz	506	13.4	49.4	10	16.8	30.8	2.9	0	53%
	1 oz	127	3.4	12.4	3	4.2	7.7	0.7	0	52%
firmly packed	1 cup	1012	26.9	98.9	20	33.8	61.7	5.8	0	53%
ALMOND POWDER										
full-fat	1 oz	168	5.6	6.3	2	>.5 c	14.7	1.4	0	74%
full-fat, not packed	1 cup	385	12.9	14.5	4	>1.2 c	33.6	3.2	0	73%
partially defatted	1 oz	112	10.6	9.0	3	>.8 c	4.5	0.4	0	34%
partially defatted, not packed	1 cup	255	24.4	20.7	7	>1.8 c	10.4	1.0	0	34%
ALOE VERA JUICE										
sodium free, certified 100% juice (Sunburst)	2 oz	5	0.0	1.0	<3	na	0.0	na	na	0%
ALPINE SPICED CIDER (Krusteaz)	8 oz	80	0.0	21.0	20	na	0.0	0.0	0	0%
AMARANTH										
boiled, drained	1/2 cup	14	1.4	2.7	14	>.9 c	0.1	0.0	0	5%
raw	1 cup	7	0.7	1.1	6	>.3 c	0.1	0.0	0	11%
AMARANTH DINNER, CANNED										
w/garden vegetables 'Fast Menu' fat-free (Health Valley)	7.5 oz	120	8.0	16.0	138	8.3	3.0	(mq)	0	22%
w/garden vegetables 'Fast Menu' fat-free (Health Valley)	5 oz	70	6.0	11.0	90	5.5	0.0	na	0	0%
AMARANTH FLOUR (Arrowhead Mills)	2 oz	200	8.0	35.0	<1	3.9	3.0	(mq)	0	14%
AMARANTH SEED (Arrowhead Mills)	2 oz	200	8.0	35.0	1	3.9	3.0	(mq)	0	14%
AMBERJACK										
raw	1 lb	386	82.1	0.0	(mq)	0	4.1	(mq)	(mq)	10%
raw	1 oz	24	5.1	0.0	(mq)	0	0.3	tr	(mq)	12%
AMBROSIA SALAD (Sunfresh) in light syrup	2/3 cup	70	0.0	18.0	30	1.0	0.0	0.0	0	0%
AMBROSIA JUICE (Knudsen & Sons)	8 oz	110	<1.0	27.0	na	na	0.0	na	na	0%
ANASAZI BEAN raw (Arrowhead Mills)	2 oz	200	13.0	35.0	3	12.1	1.0	na	0	5%
ANCHOVY, European, meat only, raw	1 oz	37	5.8	0.0	29	0	1.4	0.4	(mq)	35%
ANCHOVY, CANNED										
in olive oil, drained	1 oz	60	8.2	0.0	1040	0	2.8	0.6	(mq)	43%
in olive oil, drained, 5 medium	.7 oz	42	5.8	0.0	734	0	1.9	0.4	(mq)	42%
in olive oil, drained, yield from 2-oz can	1.6 oz	94	13.0	0.0	1651	0	4.4	1.0	38	43%
ANGLER FISH. See MONKFISH.										
ANISE SEED										
whole	1 oz	95	5.0	14.2	5	>4.1 c	4.5	na	0	35%
whole	1 tbsp	23	1.2	3.3	1	>1.0 c	1.1	na	0	36%
whole	1 tsp	7	0.4	1.0	0	>.3 c	0.3	na	0	33%
ANTELOPE										
raw	1 oz	32	6.3	0.0	14	na	0.6	0.2	27	18%
roasted	3 oz	127	25.0	0.0	46	na	2.3	0.8	107	17%
roasted, diced	1 cup	210	41.2	0.0	76	0	3.7	1.4	176	17%
APPLE										
boiled, peeled slices	1/2 cup	60	0.3	15.5	1	2.2	0.4	0.1	0	5%
boiled, unpeeled slices	1/2 cup	46	0.2	11.7	1	>.5 c	0.3	0.1	0	5%

Food Name	Serving Size	Calories	Prot. gms	Carbs gms	Sod. mgs	Fiber gms	Fat gms	Sat. Fat gms	Chol. mgs	% Fat Cal.
microwaved, peeled slices	1/2 cup	64	0.3	16.3	1	2.7	0.5	0.1	0	6%
microwaved, unpeeled slices	1/2 cup	48	0.2	12.3	1	>.5 c	0.4	0.1	0	7%
raw, peeled	1 oz	16	<.1	4.2	tr	.5	0.1	<.1	0	5%
raw, peeled slices	1 cup	63	0.2	16.3	0	2.1	0.3	0.1	0	4%
raw, peeled whole fruit, approx 3 per lb	1 med	73	0.2	19.0	0	2.4	0.4	0.1	0	5%
raw, unpeeled	1 oz	17	0.1	4.3	tr	.6	0.1	<.1	0	5%
raw, unpeeled slices	1 cup	65	0.2	16.8	0	3.0	0.4	0.1	0	5%
raw, unpeeled whole fruit, approx 3 per lb	1 med	81	0.3	21.0	0	3.7	0.5	0.1	0	5%
raw, unpeeled whole fruit	1 lb	244	0.8	63.7	2	11.1	1.5	0.2	0	5%
APPLE, CANNED										
Chipped										
(Lucky Leaf)	4 oz	50	0.0	12.0	10	(mq)	0.0	0.0	0	0%
(Musselman's)	4 oz	50	0.0	12.0	10	(mq)	0.0	0.0	0	0%
(White House) in water	4 oz	50	0.0	12.0	5	(mq)	0.0	0.0	0	0%
Diced										
(Lucky Leaf)	4 oz	50	0.0	12.0	10	(mq)	0.0	0.0	0	0%
(Musselman's)	4 oz	50	0.0	12.0	10	(mq)	0.0	0.0	0	0%
Rings, spiced										
(Lucky Leaf) green	4 oz	100	0.0	24.0	20	(mq)	0.0	0.0	0	0%
(Lucky Leaf) red	4 oz	100	0.0	24.0	20	(mq)	0.0	0.0	0	0%
(Musselman's) green	4 oz	100	0.0	24.0	20	(mq)	0.0	0.0	0	0%
(Musselman's) red	4 oz	100	0.0	24.0	20	(mq)	0.0	0.0	0	0%
(White House)	3.5 oz	180	0.0	44.0	25	(mq)	0.0	0.0	0	0%
Sliced										
(Lucky Leaf) dessert	4 oz	70	0.0	16.0	25	(mq)	0.0	0.0	0	0%
(Lucky Leaf) sweetened, in syrup	4 oz	50	0.0	13.0	35	(mq)	0.0	0.0	0	0%
(Lucky Leaf) sweetened, in water	4 oz	50	0.0	12.0	10	(mq)	0.0	0.0	0	0%
(Lucky Leaf) sweetened, unpeeled	4 oz	90	0.0	22.0	15	(mq)	0.0	0.0	0	0%
(Musselman's) dessert	4 oz	70	0.0	16.0	25	(mq)	0.0	0.0	0	0%
(Musselman's) sweetened, in syrup	4 oz	50	0.0	13.0	35	(mq)	0.0	0.0	0	0%
(Musselman's) sweetened, in water	4 oz	50	0.0	12.0	10	(mq)	0.0	0.0	0	0%
(Musselman's) sweetened, unpeeled	4 oz	90	0.0	22.0	15	(mq)	0.0	0.0	0	0%
(White House) sweetened	4 oz	54	0.0	14.0	10	(mq)	0.0	0.0	0	0%
(White House) sweetened, in water	4 oz	40	0.0	12.0	5	(mq)	0.0	0.0	0	0%
Whole										
(Lucky Leaf) baked	1 apple	110	0.0	28.0	35	(mq)	0.0	0.0	0	0%
(Lucky Leaf) sweetened, peeled, cored	1 apple	90	0.0	21.0	10	(mq)	0.0	0.0	0	0%
(Musselman's) baked	1 apple	110	0.0	28.0	35	(mq)	0.0	0.0	0	0%
(Musselman's) sweetened, peeled, cored	1 apple	90	0.0	21.0	10	(mq)	0.0	0.0	0	0%
(White House) baked	3.5 oz	118	0.0	29.0	11	(mq)	0.0	0.0	0	0%
APPLE, DEHYDRATED/SULFURED										
chips (Weight Watchers)	.75-oz pkg	70	0.0	19.0	200	4.0	0.0	0.0	0	0%
cooked	4 oz	84	0.3	22.6	29	>1.0 c	0.1	<.1	0	1%
stewed, low moisture	1/2 cup	72	0.3	19.3	25	>.8 c	0.1	0.0	0	1%
uncooked	4 oz	392	1.5	111.7	141	>4.6 c	0.7	0.1	0	1%
uncooked, low moisture	1/2 cup	104	0.4	28.1	37	3.7	0.2	0.0	0	2%
APPLE, DRIED										
chunks (Sun•Maid)	2 oz	150	1.0	42.0	40	(mq)	0.0	0.0	0	0%
chunks (SunSweet)	2 oz	150	1.0	42.0	40	(mq)	0.0	0.0	0	0%
sliced, uncooked (Del Monte)	2 oz	140	0.0	37.0	50	(mq)	0.0	0.0	0	0%
sulfured, stewed	1/2 cup	73	0.3	19.6	26	2.6	0.1	0.0	0	1%
sulfured, uncooked	4 oz	276	1.1	74.7	99	>3.3 c	0.4	0.1	0	1%
sulfured, uncooked	1 cup	209	0.8	56.7	75	7.5	0.3	0.0	0	1%
sulfured, uncooked, approx 2.3 oz	10 rings	155	0.6	42.2	56	5.6	0.2	<.1	0	1%

Food Name	Serving Size	Calories	Prot. gms	Carbs gms	Sod. mgs	Fiber gms	Fat gms	Sat. Fat gms	Chol. mgs	% Fat Cal.
APPLE, FROZEN										
escalloped (Stouffer's)	4 oz	130	0.0	27.0	15	na	2.0	(mq)	na	14%
glazed, in raspberry sauce 'Side Dish' (Budget Gourmet)	5 oz	110	0.0	22.0	210	(mq)	3.0	(mq)	10	24%
unsweetened	4 oz	54	0.3	14.0	3	2.3	0.4	0.1	0	6%
unsweetened, heated	4 oz	53	0.3	13.6	3	2.2	0.4	0.1	0	6%
unsweetened, heated, sliced	1/2 cup	48	0.3	12.4	3	>.6 c	0.3	0.1	0	5%
unsweetened, sliced	1/2 cup	41	0.2	10.6	3	1.8	0.3	<.1	0	6%
APPLE APRICOT JUICE (Knudsen & Sons)	8 oz	120	<1.0	29.0	na	na	0.0	na	na	0%
APPLE BANANA JUICE (Knudsen & Sons)	8 oz	85	<1.0	21.0	na	na	0.0	na	na	0%
APPLE BLACKBERRY JUICE										
(Knudsen & Sons)	8 oz	100	<1.0	24.0	na	na	0.0	na	na	0%
(Santa Cruz Natural) organic	8 oz	120	<1.0	29.0	na	na	1.0	na	na	7%
APPLE BOYSENBERRY JUICE										
(Knudsen & Sons)	8 oz	110	<1.0	28.0	na	na	0.0	na	na	0%
(Santa Cruz Natural) organic	8 oz	120	<1.0	29.0	na	na	1.0	na	na	7%
APPLE BUTTER										
	1 cup	519	0.3	134.5	0	3.7	0.9	na	0	2%
	1 tbsp	33	0.0	8.6	0	.2	0.1	na	0	3%
APPLE CHERRY BERRY DRINK (Veryfine)	8 oz	130	0.1	33.0	25	(mq)	0.0	0.0	0	0%
APPLE CHERRY CIDER										
(Indian Summer)	6 oz	100	<1.0	25.0	10	(mq)	<1.0	(tr)	0	<8%
(McCain) 100% juice 'Junior'	4.2 oz	50	0.0	13.0	5	na	0.0	na	na	0%
(Musselman's) 'Breakfast Cocktail'	6 oz	100	1.0	26.0	5	(mq)	0.0	0.0	0	0%
(Red Cheek) 'Naturally 100%'	6 oz	113	0.2	28.0	11	(mq)	0.0	0.0	0	0%
APPLE CIDER										
(Indian Summer) can or bottle	6 oz	80	<1.0	20.0	10	(mq)	<1.0	(tr)	0	<10%
(Indian Summer) can or bottle, cinnamon	6 oz	90	<1.0	21.0	10	(mq)	<1.0	(tr)	0	<9%
(Lucky Leaf) can or bottle	6 oz	90	0.0	21.0	0	(mq)	0.0	0.0	0	0%
(Lucky Leaf) can or bottle, sparkling	6 oz	80	0.0	18.0	45	(mq)	0.0	0.0	0	0%
(Musselman's) can or bottle	6 oz	90	0.0	21.0	0	(mq)	0.0	0.0	0	0%
(S. Martinelli) 'Sparkling'	6 oz	100	0.0	25.0	5	na	0.0	na	0	0%
(Tree Top) canned or frozen, diluted as directed	6 oz	90	0.0	22.0	10	na	0.0	0.0	0	0%
APPLE CIDER MIX (Swiss Miss)	.776 oz	84	0.0	20.3	58	.9	0.3	0.0	0	3%
APPLE CITRUS JUICE (Tree Top) canned or frozen	6 oz	90	1.0	22.0	10	(mq)	0.0	0.0	0	0%
APPLE CRANBERRY CIDER (Indian Summer)	6 oz	100	<1.0	24.0	10	(mq)	<1.0	(tr)	0	<8%
APPLE CRANBERRY DRINK										
(Mott's)	10 oz	176	0.0	44.0	3	(tr)	0.0	0.0	0	0%
(Mott's)	9.5 oz	167	0.0	42.0	3	(tr)	0.0	0.0	0	0%
(Tropicana)	6 oz	110	<1.0	27.0	15	na	<1.0	na	na	<7%
(Tropicana) 'Single Serve'	10 oz	175	(tr)	43.0	3	(tr)	0.0	0.0	0	0%
APPLE CRANBERRY JUICE										
(Apple & Eve)	6 oz	80	0.0	19.0	5	(mq)	0.0	0.0	0	0%
(Knudsen & Sons)	8 oz	110	<1.0	28.0	na	na	0.0	na	na	0%
(Lucky Leaf)	6 oz	130	0.0	32.0	10	(mq)	0.0	0.0	0	0%
(Mott's)	9.5 oz	147	0.0	38.0	27	(mq)	0.0	0.0	0	0%
(Mott's)	6 oz	83	0.0	24.0	17	(mq)	0.0	0.0	0	0%
(Mott's) aseptic box	8.45 oz	136	0.0	34.0	24	(mq)	0.0	0.0	0	0%
(Santa Cruz Natural) organic	8 oz	115	<1.0	28.0	na	na	<1.0	na	na	<7%
(Smucker's) 'Naturally 100%'	8 oz	120	0.0	32.0	10	(tr)	0.0	0.0	0	0%
(Tree Top) canned	6 oz	100	0.0	25.0	10	(mq)	0.0	0.0	0	0%
(Tree Top) frozen	6 oz	100	0.0	25.0	10	(mq)	0.0	0.0	0	0%
(Veryfine) cocktail	8 oz	130	0.1	33.0	10	(tr)	0.0	0.0	0	0%
APPLE DRINK										
(Hi-C) 'Candy Apple Cooler'	8.45 oz	132	<.1	32.6	25	(tr)	<.1	0.0	0	<1%

Food Name	Serving Size	Calories	Prot. gms	Carbs gms	Sod. mgs	Fiber gms	Fat gms	Sat. Fat gms	Chol. mgs	% Fat Cal.
(Hi-C) 'Candy Apple Cooler'	6 oz	94	<.1	23.1	17	(tr)	<.1	0.0	0	<1%
(Hi-C) 'Jamin' Apple Drink,' aseptic box	6 oz	90	0.0	23.0	20	na	0.0	na	na	0%
(10-K)	8 oz	60	0.0	15.0	55	na	0.0	na	na	0%
APPLE DUMPLING, frozen (Pepperidge Farm)	3 oz	260	2.0	33.0	230	(mq)	13.0	(mq)	na	46%
APPLE GRAPE CHERRY JUICE										
(Welch's) 'Orchard Cocktail'	6 oz	110	0.0	27.0	20	(tr)	0.0	0.0	0	0%
(Welch's) 'Orchard Cocktail-in-a-Box'	8.45 oz	150	0.0	38.0	20	(tr)	0.0	0.0	0	0%
(Welch's) 'Orchard Cocktail' frozen	6 oz	90	0.0	22.0	10	(tr)	0.0	0.0	0	0%
APPLE GRAPE JUICE										
(Juicy Juice)	6 oz	90	0.0	22.0	10	(mq)	0.0	0.0	0	0%
(Juicy Juice) box	8.45 oz	120	1.0	29.0	10	na	0.0	na	na	0%
(Mott's)	9.5 oz	139	0.0	37.0	27	(mq)	0.0	0.0	0	0%
(Mott's)	6 oz	86	0.0	23.0	17	(mq)	0.0	0.0	0	0%
(Mott's) aseptic box	8.45 oz	128	0.0	32.0	24	(mq)	0.0	0.0	0	0%
(Musselman's) 'Breakfast Cocktail'	6 oz	110	0.0	28.0	5	(tr)	0.0	0.0	0	0%
(Red Cheek)	6 oz	109	0.3	27.0	9	(mq)	0.0	0.0	0	0%
(Tree Top) canned	6 oz	100	0.0	25.0	10	(mq)	0.0	0.0	0	0%
(Tree Top) frozen	6 oz	100	0.0	25.0	10	(mq)	0.0	0.0	0	0%
(Welch's) 'Orchard Cocktail'	6 oz	110	0.0	27.0	20	(tr)	0.0	0.0	0	0%
(Welch's) 'Orchard Cocktail,' frozen	6 oz	110	0.0	27.0	10	(tr)	0.0	0.0	0	0%
(Welch's) 'Orchard Cocktail,' frozen, w/raspberry	6 oz	90	0.0	22.0	10	(tr)	0.0	0.0	0	0%
(Welch's) 'Orchard Cocktail-in-a Box' w/raspberry	8.45 oz	140	0.0	35.0	20	(tr)	0.0	0.0	0	0%
APPLE JUICE										
Can, bottle, or box										
(Heinz) strained, 'Saver Size'	4.2 oz	70	0.0	17.0	15	na	0.0	0.0	na	0%
(IGA) 'Unsweetened'	6 oz	74	0.0	18.0	10	(mq)	0.0	0.0	0	0%
(Indian Summer)	6 oz	90	<1.0	21.0	10	(mq)	<1.0	(tr)	0	<9%
(J. Hungerford)	9.03 oz	128	0.1	32.2	6	0	0.0	0.0	0	0%
(J. Hungerford) 50% juice	9.03 oz	119	0.2	29.9	8	0	0.0	0.0	0	0%
(J. Hungerford) 100% juice	9.03 oz	112	0.3	28.0	17	0	0.0	0.0	0	0%
(Juicy Juice)	6 oz	90	0.0	21.0	5	(mq)	0.0	0.0	0	0%
(Knudsen & Sons) Gravenstein	8 oz	110	<1.0	28.0	na	na	0.0	na	na	0%
(Knudsen & Sons) 'Natural'	8 oz	85	<1.0	21.0	na	na	0.0	na	na	0%
(Kraft) 'Pure 100%'	6 oz	80	0.0	20.0	5	(mq)	0.0	0.0	0	0%
(Lucky Leaf) 'Individual Portion Control'	3.8 oz	60	0.0	14.0	0	(mq)	0.0	0.0	0	0%
(Lucky Leaf) 100% vitamin C enriched	6 oz	90	0.0	21.0	0	(mq)	0.0	0.0	0	0%
(Lucky Leaf) regular	6 oz	90	0.0	21.0	0	(mq)	0.0	0.0	0	0%
(McCain) 100% juice 'Junior'	4.2 oz	50	0.0	13.0	5	na	0.0	na	na	0%
(Minute Maid) aseptic box	6 oz	80	0.0	21.0	30	na	0.0	na	na	0%
(Minute Maid) 'Juices to Go'	6 oz	80	0.0	21.0	30	na	0.0	na	na	0%
(Mott's)	10 oz	148	0.0	37.0	22	(mq)	0.0	0.0	0	0%
(Mott's)	9.5 oz	141	0.0	35.0	20	(mq)	0.0	0.0	0	0%
(Mott's)	8.45 oz	124	0.0	31.0	18	(mq)	0.0	0.0	0	0%
(Mott's)	6 oz	88	0.0	22.0	13	(mq)	0.0	0.0	0	0%
(Mott's) natural style	6 oz	76	0.0	19.0	28	(mq)	0.0	0.0	0	0%
(Musselman's) 'Individual Portion Control'	3.8 oz	60	0.0	14.0	0	(mq)	0.0	0.0	0	0%
(Musselman's) 100% vitamin C enriched	6 oz	90	0.0	21.0	0	(mq)	0.0	0.0	0	0%
(Musselman's) regular	6 oz	90	0.0	21.0	0	(mq)	0.0	0.0	0	0%
(Ocean Spray)	6 oz	90	0.0	23.0	15	(mq)	0.0	0.0	0	0%
(Red Cheek) 'Natural'	6 oz	97	0.2	24.0	16	(mq)	0.0	0.0	0	0%
(Red Cheek) '100% Pure'	6 oz	97	0.2	24.0	7	(mq)	0.0	0.0	0	0%
(S&W) '100% Pure Unsweetened'	6 oz	85	0.0	20.0	5	(mq)	0.0	0.0	0	0%
(S. Martinelli)	6 oz	100	0.0	25.0	5	na	0.0	na	0	0%
(S. Martinelli) 'Sparkling'	6 oz	100	0.0	25.0	5	na	0.0	na	0	0%

Food Name	Serving Size	Calories	Prot. gms	Carbs gms	Sod. mgs	Fiber gms	Fat gms	Sat. Fat gms	Chol. mgs	% Fat Cal.
(Sippin' Pak) 100% pure, from concentrate	8.45 oz	110	0.0	28.0	25	na	0.0	na	na	0%
(Snapple) 'Apple Crisp'	8 oz	140	0.0	36.0	30	na	0.0	0.0	0	0%
(Tree Top)	6 oz	90	0.0	22.0	10	>.2 c	0.0	0.0	0	0%
(TreeSweet)	6 oz	90	0.0	22.0	15	(mq)	0.0	0.0	0	0%
(Tropicana) '100% Pure'	8 oz	116	(tr)	28.5	17	(mq)	0.0	0.0	0	0%
(Tropicana) 100% pure	6 oz	80	<1.0	20.0	15	na	<1.0	na	na	<10%
(Veryfine) '100%'	8 oz	107	0.2	27.0	10	(mq)	0.0	0.0	0	0%
(Welch's) sparkling	6 oz	100	0.0	24.0	5	0	0.0	0.0	0	0%
(White House)	6 oz	87	0.0	22.0	5	(mq)	0.0	0.0	0	0%
Chilled or frozen										
(A&P) diluted as directed	6 oz	90	<1.0	22.0	0	(mq)	<1.0	(tr)	0	<9%
(Knudsen & Sons) clear	8 oz	90	<1.0	22.0	na	na	0.0	na	na	0%
(Minute Maid) diluted as directed	6 oz	80	0.0	21.0	15	na	0.0	na	na	0%
(Sunkist) diluted as directed	8 oz	79	0.2	19.4	12	(mq)	0.2	0.0	0	2%
(Tree Top) diluted as directed	6 oz	90	0.0	22.0	10	(mq)	0.0	0.0	0	0%
(Welch's) 'Orchard Cocktail'	10 oz	170	0.0	42.0	95	0	0.0	0.0	0	0%
APPLE KIT										
Candy (Concord) microwaveable	1 apple	50	0.0	14.0	0	na	0.0	na	na	0%
Caramel (Concord) microwaveable	1 apple	150	2.0	27.0	105	0.0	3.0	1.5	<5	19%
APPLE ORANGE PINEAPPLE COCKTAIL										
(Welch's) 'Orchard Tropical Cocktails'	8.45 oz	140	0.0	35.0	20	(tr)	0.0	0.0	0	0%
(Welch's) 'Orchard Tropical Cocktails'	6 oz	100	0.0	25.0	20	(tr)	0.0	0.0	0	0%
APPLE PASTRY										
Fresh										
(Entenmann's) 'Apple Puffs'	1 puff	280	4.0	39.0	320	na	13.0	na	na	41%
(Tastykake) pocket	3 oz	323	4.3	38.3	222	1.5	17.6	4.0	11	48%
Frozen										
(Hormel) 'Apple Dulcita'	4 oz	290	5.0	44.0	350	(mq)	10.0	(mq)	na	32%
(Mrs. Paul's) 'Apple Fritter'	2 pieces	240	4.0	35.0	500	na	9.0	(mq)	5	34%
(Pepperidge Farm) 'Apple Dumpling'	3 oz	260	2.0	33.0	230	(mq)	13.0	(mq)	na	46%
(Pepperidge Farm) apple fruit square	1 piece	220	2.0	27.0	170	(mq)	12.0	(mq)	na	48%
(Pepperidge Farm) 'Berkshire' apple crisps	1 ramekin	250	2.0	43.0	130	1.0	8.0	4.0	4	29%
(Weight Watchers) 'Sweet Celebrations' apple crisps	3.5 oz	190	1.0	40.0	190	(mq)	5.0	<1.0	na	22%
APPLE PEACH JUICE (Knudsen & Sons)	8 oz	140	<1.0	34.0	na	na	0.0	na	na	0%
APPLE PEAR JUICE (Tree Top) frozen	6 oz	90	0.0	22.0	10	(mq)	0.0	0.0	0	0%
APPLE PIE. See PIE.										
APPLE PIE FILLING. See PIE FILLING.										
APPLE PIE SPICE (Tone's)	1 tsp	9	0.2	2.4	1	.7	0.2	0.1	0	15%
APPLE PUNCH										
(Minute Maid) chilled	6 oz	90	0.0	23.0	20	na	0.0	na	na	0%
(Minute Maid) frozen concentrate	6 oz	90	0.0	23.0	0	na	0.0	na	na	0%
APPLE PUNCH DRINK (Red Cheek)	6 oz	113	0.3	28.0	7	(tr)	0.0	0.0	0	0%
APPLE RASPBERRY DRINK										
(Mott's)	10 oz	158	0.0	40.0	17	(tr)	0.0	0.0	0	0%
(Mott's)	9.5 oz	150	0.0	38.0	16	(tr)	0.0	0.0	0	0%
APPLE RASPBERRY JUICE										
(Knudsen & Sons)	8 oz	110	<1.0	28.0	na	na	0.0	na	na	0%
(Mott's)	9.5 oz	134	0.0	35.0	76	(mq)	0.0	0.0	0	0%
(Mott's)	6 oz	83	0.0	22.0	48	(mq)	0.0	0.0	0	0%
(Mott's) aseptic box	8.45 oz	124	0.0	31.0	67	(mq)	0.0	0.0	0	0%
(Red Cheek)	6 oz	113	0.3	28.0	8	(mq)	0.0	0.0	0	0%
(Santa Cruz Natural) organic	8 oz	120	<1.0	29.0	na	na	1.0	na	na	7%
(Tree Top) canned or frozen	6 oz	80	0.0	21.0	10	(mq)	0.0	0.0	0	0%
(Veryfine) cocktail	8 oz	110	0.0	27.0	15	(tr)	0.0	0.0	0	0%

Food Name	Serving Size	Calories	Prot. gms	Carbs gms	Sod. mgs	Fiber gms	Fat gms	Sat. Fat gms	Chol. mgs	% Fat Cal.
APPLE STICKS, frozen, breaded, fried *(Farm Rich)* .... 4 oz		260	2.0	44.0	565	(mq)	8.0	(mq)	0	28%
APPLE STRAWBERRY JUICE										
(Knudsen & Sons) .... 8 oz		110	<1.0	28.0	na	na	0.0	na	na	0%
(Santa Cruz Natural) organic .... 8 oz		120	<1.0	29.0	na	na	<1.0	na	na	<7%
APPLE STRAWBERRY NECTAR *(Kern's)* can or bottle ..... 6 oz		110	0.0	26.0	0	na	0.0	na	na	0%
APPLE STRUDEL										
(Aunt Fanny's) individual .... 3 oz		330	4.0	38.0	210	na	18.0	7.0	na	49%
(Entenmann's) old fashioned .... 1.5 oz		120	1.0	17.0	110	na	5.0	na	na	39%
APPLE SYRUP *(Knudsen & Sons)* .... 1 oz		75	<1.0	15.0	na	na	<1.0	na	na	<12%
APPLE-WHITE GRAPE JUICE										
(Welch's) 'No Sugar Added' frozen cocktail .... 6 oz		40	0.0	10.0	5	(tr)	0.0	0.0	0	0%
APPLESAUCE										
(A&P)										
regular .... 1/2 cup		110	<1.0	25.0	15	(mq)	<1.0	(tr)	0	<8%
unsweetened .... 1/2 cup		50	<1.0	10.0	0	(mq)	<1.0	(tr)	0	<17%
(Del Monte)										
'Lite' .... 1/2 cup		50	0.0	13.0	10	(mq)	0.0	0.0	0	0%
regular .... 1/2 cup		90	0.0	24.0	5	(mq)	0.0	0.0	0	0%
(Featherweight) .... 1/2 cup		50	0.0	12.0	3	(mq)	0.0	0.0	0	0%
(Finast)										
regular .... 1/2 cup		105	0.0	25.0	10	(mq)	0.0	0.0	0	0%
unsweetened .... 1/2 cup		56	0.4	15.0	na	(mq)	0.2	(tr)	0	3%
(Lucky Leaf)										
chunky .... 4 oz		80	0.0	20.0	20	(mq)	0.0	0.0	0	0%
'Juice Pack' .... 4 oz		50	0.0	12.0	0	(mq)	0.0	0.0	0	0%
'Natural' individual portion control .... 4 oz		50	0.0	13.0	0	(mq)	0.0	0.0	0	0%
regular .... 4 oz		80	0.0	20.0	20	(mq)	0.0	0.0	0	0%
'Regular' individual portion control .... 4 oz		80	0.0	20.0	0	(mq)	0.0	0.0	0	0%
unsweetened .... 4 oz		50	0.0	12.0	0	(mq)	0.0	0.0	0	0%
(Mott's)										
chunky .... 6 oz		86	0.0	21.0	11	(mq)	0.0	0.0	0	0%
cinnamon .... 6 oz		152	0.0	36.0	<1	(mq)	0.0	0.0	0	0%
'Natural' .... 6 oz		80	0.0	20.0	3	(mq)	0.0	0.0	0	0%
'Natural Single Serve' .... 4 oz		53	0.0	13.0	2	(mq)	0.0	0.0	0	0%
regular .... 6 oz		150	0.0	36.0	<1	(mq)	0.0	0.0	0	0%
'Single Serve' .... 4 oz		100	0.0	24.0	<1	(mq)	0.0	0.0	0	0%
'Single Serve' cinnamon .... 4 oz		101	0.0	24.0	<1	(mq)	0.0	0.0	0	0%
(Musselman's)										
chunky .... 4 oz		80	0.0	20.0	20	(mq)	0.0	0.0	0	0%
'Juice Pack' .... 4 oz		50	0.0	12.0	0	(mq)	0.0	0.0	0	0%
'Natural' individual portion control .... 4 oz		50	0.0	13.0	0	(mq)	0.0	0.0	0	0%
regular .... 4 oz		80	0.0	20.0	20	(mq)	0.0	0.0	0	0%
'Regular' individual portion control .... 4 oz		80	0.0	20.0	0	(mq)	0.0	0.0	0	0%
unsweetened .... 4 oz		50	0.0	12.0	0	(mq)	0.0	0.0	0	0%
(S&W)										
regular .... 1/2 cup		90	0.0	24.0	10	(mq)	0.0	0.0	0	0%
unsweetened .... 1/2 cup		55	0.0	14.0	5	(mq)	0.0	0.0	0	0%
(S&W Nutradiet) .... 1/2 cup		55	0.0	14.0	10	(mq)	0.0	0.0	0	0%
(Stokely)										
regular .... 1/2 cup		90	0.0	23.0	30	(mq)	0.0	0.0	0	0%
unsweetened .... 1/2 cup		45	0.0	12.0	5	(mq)	0.0	0.0	0	0%
(Tree Top) 'Original' .... 1/2 cup		80	0.0	21.0	0	(mq)	0.0	0.0	0	0%
(White House)										
chunky .... 4 oz		80	0.0	22.0	5	(mq)	0.0	0.0	0	0%

Food Name	Serving Size	Calories	Prot. gms	Carbs gms	Sod. mgs	Fiber gms	Fat gms	Sat. Fat gms	Chol. mgs	% Fat Cal.
in apple juice	4 oz	50	0.0	13.0	5	(mq)	0.0	0.0	0	0%
'Regular'	4 oz	80	0.0	22.0	5	(mq)	0.0	0.0	0	0%
unsweetened	4 oz	50	0.0	12.0	5	(mq)	0.0	0.0	0	0%
APRICOT										
candied	100 gm	338	0.6	86.5	1	>.6 c	0.2	0.0	0	1%
pitted	1 oz	14	0.4	3.2	<1	.4	0.1	tr	0	6%
raw, halves	1 cup	74	2.2	17.2	2	3.7	0.6	0.0	0	7%
untrimmed	1 lb	202	5.9	46.9	2	5.6	1.7	0.1	0	7%
APRICOT, CANNED										
In extra heavy syrup										
peeled	4 oz	109	0.6	28.2	15	>.4 c	<.1	tr	0	<1%
peeled, whole	1/2 cup	118	0.7	30.6	16	>.4 c	0.1	tr	0	1%
In extra light syrup										
unpeeled	4 oz	56	0.7	14.2	2	>.5 c	0.1	tr	0	2%
unpeeled, halves	1/2 cup	61	0.7	15.4	3	>.5 c	0.1	tr	0	1%
In heavy syrup										
peeled	4 oz	94	0.6	24.3	12	>.4 c	0.1	tr	0	1%
peeled, halves	1 cup	214	1.4	55.4	10	>1.0 c	0.2	0.0	0	1%
peeled, whole	1/2 cup	107	0.7	27.7	14	>.5 c	0.1	tr	0	1%
peeled, whole (S&W)	1/2 cup	100	0.0	26.0	15	(mq)	0.0	0.0	0	0%
unpeeled	4 oz	94	0.6	24.3	5	>.5 c	0.1	tr	0	1%
unpeeled (A&P)	1/2 cup	110	<1.0	28.0	15	(mq)	1.0	na	0	7%
unpeeled, halves	1/2 cup	107	0.7	27.7	5	1.65	0.1	tr	0	1%
unpeeled, halves (IGA)	1 cup	220	1.0	56.0	15	(mq)	0.0	0.0	0	0%
unpeeled, halves (S&W)	1/2 cup	110	0.0	28.0	15	(mq)	0.0	0.0	0	0%
In juice										
peeled (Featherweight)	1/2 cup	50	1.0	12.0	10	(mq)	0.0	0.0	0	0%
unpeeled	4 oz	54	0.7	14.0	5	.5	<.1	tr	0	<2%
unpeeled, halves	1/2 cup	60	0.8	15.3	5	.6	<.1	tr	0	<1%
unpeeled, 'Lite' (Libby's)	1/2 cup	60	0.0	17.0	5	(mq)	0.0	0.0	0	0%
In light syrup										
unpeeled	4 oz	71	0.6	18.7	5	1.65	0.1	tr	0	1%
unpeeled, halves	1/2 cup	80	0.7	20.9	5	>.5 c	0.1	tr	0	1%
unpeeled, halves 'No Frills' (Pathmark)	1/2 cup	80	0.0	20.0	5	(mq)	0.0	0.0	0	0%
In water										
peeled	1/2 cup	25	0.8	6.2	12	>.4 c	<.1	tr	0	<3%
peeled, whole (S&W Nutradiet)	1/2 cup	28	0.0	7.0	5	(mq)	0.0	0.0	0	0%
unpeeled	4 oz	31	0.8	7.2	3	>.5 c	0.2	<.1	0	5%
unpeeled, halves	1/2 cup	33	0.9	7.8	4	1.6	0.2	<.1	0	5%
unpeeled, halves (S&W)	1/2 cup	35	0.0	9.0	5	(mq)	0.0	0.0	0	0%
unpeeled, halves (S&W Nutradiet)	1/2 cup	35	0.0	9.0	5	(mq)	0.0	0.0	0	0%
APRICOT, DEHYDRATED/SULFURED										
cooked	4 oz	143	2.2	37.0	6	>1.8 c	0.3	<.1	0	2%
stewed, low-moisture	1/2 cup	156	2.4	40.4	6	>1.9 c	0.3	0.0	0	2%
uncooked	4 oz	363	5.6	94.0	15	>4.5 c	0.7	<.1	0	2%
uncooked, low-moisture	1/2 cup	192	2.9	49.7	8	>2.4 c	0.4	0.0	0	2%
APRICOT, DRIED										
sulfured, cooked	4 oz	96	1.5	24.8	3	>1.2 c	0.2	<.1	0	2%
sulfured, stewed, halves	1/2 cup	106	1.6	27.4	4	>1.3 c	0.2	0.0	0	2%
sulfured, uncooked	4 oz	270	4.1	70.0	11	8.8	0.5	<.1	0	2%
sulfured, uncooked, approx 1.2 oz	10 halves	83	1.3	21.6	3	3.2	0.2	<.1	0	2%
sulfured, uncooked, halves	1 cup	309	4.7	80.3	13	11.7	0.6	0.0	0	2%
(Del Monte)	2 oz	140	2.0	35.0	10	(mq)	0.0	0.0	0	0%
(Mariani) California, sun dried, premium	1/4 cup	140	2.0	35.0	10	4.0	0.0	na	0	0%

Food Name	Serving Size	Calories	Prot. gms	Carbs gms	Sod. mgs	Fiber gms	Fat gms	Sat. Fat gms	Chol. mgs	% Fat Cal.
(Mariani) Mediterranean, sun dried, premium	1/4 cup	140	2.0	35.0	10	4.0	0.0	na	0	0%
(Sun•Maid)	2 oz	140	2.0	35.0	10	(mq)	0.0	0.0	0	0%
(SunSweet)	2 oz	140	2.0	35.0	10	(mq)	0.0	0.0	0	0%
APRICOT, FROZEN										
sweetened	4 oz	111	0.8	28.5	5	>.7 c	0.1	tr	0	1%
sweetened, unthawed	1 cup	237	1.7	60.7	10	4.1	0.2	0.0	0	1%
APRICOT KERNEL OIL										
. . . .	1/2 cup	964	0.0	0.0	0	0	109.0	6.9	0	100%
. . . .	1 oz	251	0.0	0.0	0	0	28.4	1.8	0	100%
. . . .	1 tbsp	120	0.0	0.0	0	0	13.6	0.9	0	100%
(Hain)	1 tbsp	120	0.0	0.0	0	0	14.0	1.0	0	100%
(Spectrum Naturals)	1 tbsp	120	0.0	0.0	0	(tr)	14.0	1.0	(tr)	100%
APRICOT NECTAR										
(Del Monte)	6 oz	100	1.0	26.0	10	(mq)	0.0	0.0	0	0%
(Kern's)	6 oz	110	1.0	27.0	0	na	0.0	na	na	0%
(Knudsen & Sons)	8 oz	105	<1.0	24.0	na	na	0.0	na	na	0%
(Libby's)	6 oz	110	0.0	26.0	0	(mq)	0.0	0.0	0	0%
(S&W)	6 oz	100	0.0	26.0	10	(mq)	0.0	0.0	0	0%
APRICOT PIE FILLING. See PIE FILLING.										
APRICOT PINEAPPLE NECTAR										
(Kern's)	6 oz	110	0.0	27.0	5	na	0.0	na	na	0%
(S&W Nutradiet)	4 oz	35	0.0	12.0	20	(mq)	0.0	0.0	0	0%
ARCTIC BONITO. See TUNA, SKIPJACK.										
ARROWHEAD										
boiled, drained	4 oz	88	5.1	18.3	20	>1.7 c	0.1	(tr)	0	1%
boiled, drained	1 med	9	0.5	1.9	2	>.2 c	0.0	na	0	0%
raw	1 large	25	1.3	5.1	6	>.2 c	0.1	na	0	3%
raw	1 med	12	0.6	2.4	3	>.1 c	0.0	na	0	0%
raw, trimmed	1 oz	28	1.5	5.7	6	>.2 c	0.1	(tr)	0	3%
raw, untrimmed	1 lb	337	18.2	68.8	75	>2.8 c	1.0	na	0	3%
ARROWROOT, powdered *(Tone's)*	1 tsp	10	0.0	2.3	1	0	0.0	0.0	0	0%
ARROWROOT FLOUR										
. . . .	1/3 cup	154	0.1	37.9	1	(mq)	(mq)	(mq)	0	0%
. . . .	1 oz	101	0.1	25.0	1	(mq)	(mq)	(mq)	0	0%
ARTICHOKE HEARTS										
boiled, drained	4 oz	57	3.9	12.7	108	>1.4 c	0.2	<.1	0	3%
boiled, drained	1/2 cup	42	2.9	9.4	80	>1.1 c	0.1	<.1	0	2%
canned, marinated *(S&W)*	3.5 oz	225	2.0	6.0	15	(mq)	26.0	(mq)	0	88%
frozen, boiled, drained	4 oz	51	3.5	10.4	60	>1.0 c	0.6	0.1	0	9%
frozen, 'Deluxe' *(Birds Eye)*	3 oz	30	2.0	7.0	140	(mq)	0.0	0.0	0	0%
frozen *(Seabrook)*	3 oz	25	3.0	4.0	6	>1.0 c	0.0	0.0	0	0%
ARTICHOKES, FRENCH										
boiled, drained	1 med	60	4.2	13.4	114	>1.5 c	0.2	0.0	0	3%
boiled, drained, hearts	1/2 cup	42	2.9	9.4	80	4.5	0.1	0.0	0	2%
frozen, boiled, drained	3 oz	36	2.5	7.3	42	>.7 c	0.4	0.1	0	8%
raw	1 large	76	5.3	17.0	152	8.8	0.2	0.1	0	2%
raw	1 med	60	4.2	13.4	120	6.7	0.2	0.0	0	3%
ARTICHOKES, GLOBE										
boiled, drained	1 med	60	4.2	13.4	114	>1.5 c	0.2	0.0	0	3%
boiled, drained, hearts	1/2 cup	42	2.9	9.4	80	4.54	0.1	0.0	0	2%
boiled, drained, trimmed	4 oz	57	3.9	12.7	108	>1.4 c	0.2	<.1	0	3%
boiled, drained, untrimmed	4 oz	23	1.6	5.1	43	>.6 c	0.1	<.1	0	3%
fresh *(Dole)*	1 large	23	2.0	5.0	65	3.0	0.1	na	na	3%
frozen, boiled, drained	3 oz	36	2.5	7.3	42	>.7 c	0.4	0.1	0	8%

Food Name	Serving Size	Calories	Prot. gms	Carbs gms	Sod. mgs	Fiber gms	Fat gms	Sat. Fat gms	Chol. mgs	% Fat Cal.
frozen, unprepared	9 oz	97	6.7	19.8	120	9.94	1.1	0.3	0	9%
raw	1 large	76	5.3	17.0	152	8.8	0.2	0.1	0	2%
raw	1 med	60	4.2	13.4	120	6.9	0.2	0.0	0	3%
raw, untrimmed	1 lb	85	5.9	19.1	171	9.4	0.3	0.1	0	3%
ARTICHOKES, JERUSALEM										
raw, slices	1/2 cup	57	1.5	13.1	3	1.2	0.0	0.0	0	0%
trimmed	1 oz	22	0.6	4.9	na	>.2 c	tr	tr	0	0%
untrimmed	1 lb	238	6.3	54.6	na	>2.5 c	<.1	tr	0	0%
ARUGULA/rocket/roquette/ruculo/rugula										
raw	1 leaf	1	0.1	0.1	1	na	0.0	na	0	0%
raw	1/2 cup	3	0.3	0.4	3	na	0.1	na	0	24%
(Frieda's)	1 lb	104	10.0	17.7	68	4.1	1.4	na	0	10%
(Frieda's)	1 oz	7	0.6	1.1	4	.3	<.1	(tr)	0	<12%
ASPARAGUS										
boiled, drained	1/2 cup	22	2.3	3.8	10	1.9	0.3	0.1	0	10%
boiled, drained, cuts and spears	4 oz	28	2.9	5.0	5	>.9 c	0.4	0.1	0	10%
fresh (Dole)	5 spears	18	2.0	2.0	0	2.0	0.0	na	na	0%
raw, cuts and spears	1/2 cup	15	2.1	2.5	1	1.41	0.2	<.1	0	9%
raw, trimmed	1 oz	6	0.9	1.0	1	.3	0.1	<.1	0	11%
raw, untrimmed	1 lb	54	7.3	8.9	5	2.4	0.5	0.1	0	7%
ASPARAGUS, CANNED										
Cuts and tips (Finast)	1 cup	35	4.0	6.0	720	(mq)	0.0	0.0	0	0%
Points, all green (S&W Nutradiet)	1/2 cup	17	4.0	3.0	10	(mq)	0.0	0.0	0	0%
Spears										
and tips, all green (Del Monte)	1/2 cup	20	2.0	3.0	355	(mq)	0.0	0.0	0	0%
colossal, all green 'Fancy' (S&W)	1/2 cup	20	2.0	4.0	320	(mq)	0.0	0.0	0	0%
cut (Green Giant)	1/2 cup	18	2.0	3.0	420	1.0	0.0	0.0	0	0%
cut, 50% less salt (Green Giant)	1/2 cup	18	2.0	3.0	210	1.0	0.0	0.0	0	0%
cut, green (Pathmark)	1/2 cup	20	3.0	2.0	450	(mq)	0.0	0.0	0	0%
cut, green 'No Salt Added' (Pathmark)	1/2 cup	20	3.0	2.0	5	(mq)	0.0	0.0	0	0%
green (Stokely)	1/2 cup	20	2.0	3.0	380	(mq)	0.0	0.0	0	0%
green 'Fancy' (S&W)	1/2 cup	18	2.0	3.0	320	(mq)	0.0	0.0	0	0%
green, w/liquid (Green Giant)	1/2 cup	20	2.0	3.0	420	1.0	0.0	0.0	0	0%
'No Salt or Sugar Added' (Stokely)	1/2 cup	20	2.0	3.0	5	(mq)	0.0	0.0	0	0%
white (Green Giant)	1/2 cup	16	2.0	3.0	410	1.0	0.0	0.0	0	0%
white, w/liquid (Green Giant)	1/2 cup	16	2.0	3.0	410	1.0	0.0	0.0	0	0%
w/liquid, 50% less salt (Green Giant)	1/2 cup	20	2.0	3.0	210	1.0	0.0	0.0	0	0%
w/liquid, green, tipped (Del Monte)	1/2 cup	20	2.0	3.0	355	(mq)	0.0	0.0	0	0%
ASPARAGUS, FROZEN										
boiled, drained	10-oz pkg	82	8.6	14.3	12	>2.5 c	1.2	0.3	0	11%
boiled, drained, cuts and spears	4 oz	32	3.3	5.5	5	>1.0 c	0.5	0.1	0	11%
cuts (Birds Eye)	3.3 oz	25	3.0	4.0	5	(mq)	0.0	0.0	0	0%
cuts (Seabrook)	3.3 oz	25	3.0	4.0	6	(mq)	0.0	0.0	0	0%
cuts 'Harvest Fresh' (Green Giant)	1/2 cup	25	3.0	4.0	95	2.0	0.0	0.0	0	0%
cuts and spears (Frosty Acres)	3.3 oz	25	3.0	4.0	6	(mq)	0.0	0.0	0	0%
spears (Birds Eye)	3.3 oz	25	3.0	4.0	0	(mq)	0.0	0.0	0	0%
spears (Finast)	3.3 oz	25	3.0	4.0	5	(mq)	0.0	0.0	0	0%
spears (Frosty Acres)	3.3 oz	25	3.0	4.0	4	>1.0 c	0.0	0.0	0	0%
spears (Seabrook)	3.3 oz	25	3.0	4.0	4	>1.0 c	0.0	0.0	0	0%
spears (Southern)	3.5 oz	27	3.3	4.1	20	(mq)	0.2	0.0	0	6%
unprepared	10-oz pkg	68	9.2	11.6	23	6.0	0.7	0.2	0	7%

ASPARAGUS BEAN. See YARDLONG BEAN.

AUBERGINE. See EGGPLANT.

AU JUS. See GRAVY.

Food Name	Serving Size	Calories	Prot. gms	Carbs gms	Sod. mgs	Fiber gms	Fat gms	Sat. Fat gms	Chol. mgs	% Fat Cal.
AVOCADO										
All commercial varieties										
puréed	1/2 cup	185	2.3	8.5	12	>2.4 c	17.6	2.8	0	79%
trimmed	1 oz	46	0.6	2.1	3	>.6 c	4.3	0.7	0	78%
untrimmed	1 lb	540	6.7	24.8	35	>7.1 c	51.4	8.2	0	79%
California										
puréed	1/2 cup	204	2.4	8.0	14	3.1	19.9	3.0	0	81%
trimmed	1 oz	50	0.6	2.0	3	.8	4.9	0.7	0	81%
untrimmed	1 lb	610	7.3	23.8	42	9.3	59.8	8.9	0	81%
Florida										
puréed	1/2 cup	129	1.8	10.3	6	>2.4 c	10.2	2.0	0	66%
trimmed	1 oz	32	0.5	2.5	1	>.6 c	2.5	0.5	0	65%
untrimmed	1 lb	339	4.8	27.1	14	>6.4 c	26.9	5.3	0	66%
AVOCADO OIL										
	1/2 cup	964	0.0	0.0	0	0	109.0	12.6	0	100%
	1 oz	251	0.0	0.0	0	0	28.4	3.3	0	100%
	1 tbsp	124	0.0	0.0	0	0	14.0	1.6		100%
(Hain)	1 tbsp	120	0.0	0.0	0	0	14.0	1.0	0	100%
(Spectrum Naturals)	1 tbsp	120	0.0	0.0	0	(tr)	14.0	2.0	(tr)	100%
AWA / milkfish										
dry-heat cooked	3 oz	161	22.4	0.0	78	0	7.3	na	57	42%
raw	1 lb	673	93.1	0.0	(mq)	0	30.5	(mq)	235	42%
raw	1 oz	42	5.8	0.0	(mq)	0	1.9	(mq)	15	42%

B

Food Name	Serving Size	Calories	Prot. gms	Carbs gms	Sod. mgs	Fiber gms	Fat gms	Sat. Fat gms	Chol. mgs	% Fat Cal.
BABASSU OIL. See PALM KERNEL OIL.										
BABY FOOD										
CEREAL										
Barley										
dry	1 tbsp	9	2.4	9.0	42	0.2	2.3	0.8	81	31%
dry	.5 oz	52	1.6	10.7	7	1.2	0.5	na	na	8%
instant, dry, '1st Foods' (Gerber)	.5 oz	60	1.0	11.0	na	na	1.0	na	na	16%
instant, dry, 'Stage 1' (Beech-Nut)	.5 oz	60	1.0	12.0	10	na	0.0	na	na	0%
instant, .5 oz cereal prepared w/2.4 oz formula, 'Stage 1' (Beech-Nut)	1 serving	120	2.0	18.0	25	na	4.0	na	na	31%
instant, .5 oz cereal prepared w/2.4 oz whole milk (Gerber)	1 serving	100	3.0	14.0	na	(mq)	4.0	(mq)	(mq)	35%
instant, .5 oz cereal prepared w/2.4 oz formula	1 serving	110	2.0	16.0	na	na	4.0	na	na	33%
instant (Heinz)	3.5 oz	370	8.9	78.5	15	na	3.7	na	na	9%
prepared w/whole milk	3.5 oz	111	4.6	16.3	49	>.2 c	3.3	na	na	26%
Cereal w/applesauce and bananas, '3rd Foods' (Gerber)	7 tbsp	82	1.3	17.9	3	na	0.6	na	na	7%
Cereal w/egg yolks										
junior	7.5 oz	111	4.1	15.1	70	1.9	3.8	1.3	na	31%
junior	1 oz	15	0.5	2.0	9	0.3	0.5	0.2	na	31%
strained	1 oz	14	0.5	2.0	9	0.3	0.5	0.2	18	31%
w/bacon, junior	4.5 oz	101	3.2	7.9	61	1.1	6.4	na	na	57%
w/bacon, junior	1 oz	22	0.7	1.8	14	0.3	1.4	na	na	56%
w/bacon, strained	7.5 oz	179	5.3	15.1	98	1.9	11.1	na	na	55%
w/bacon, strained	1 oz	24	0.7	2.0	13	0.3	1.5	na	na	56%

Food Name	Serving Size	Calories	Prot. gms	Carbs gms	Sod. mgs	Fiber gms	Fat gms	Sat. Fat gms	Chol. mgs	% Fat Cal.
Cereal w/eggs										
strained	4.5 oz	74	2.8	10.2	49	>.1 c	1.9	0.6	66	25%
strained	1 oz	16	0.6	2.3	11	tr	0.4	0.1	15	24%
Corn										
instant, dry, 'Tropical Foods' *(Gerber)*	.5 oz	60	1.0	12.0	na	na	1.0	na	na	15%
instant, dry, 'Tropical Foods' *(Gerber)*	3.5 oz	390	6.3	80.8	55	na	4.6	na	na	11%
instant, prepared w/milk, 'Tropical Foods' *(Gerber)*	2.4 oz	110	3.0	15.0	na	na	4.0	na	na	33%
Grits and egg yolks										
strained	4.5 oz	73	2.3	9.5	45	>.1 c	2.9	na	na	36%
strained	1 oz	16	0.5	2.1	10	tr	0.7	na	na	38%
High-protein										
instant, dry	1 tbsp	9	0.9	1.1	1	.2	0.1	na	na	10%
instant, dry	.5 oz	51	5.1	6.6	7	1.0	0.8	na	na	13%
instant, 1 oz cereal prepared w/whole milk	1 serving	31	2.5	3.3	14	>.1 c	1.1	na	na	30%
instant, w/apple and orange, dry	1 tbsp	9	0.6	1.4	3	.2	0.2	na	na	18%
instant, w/apple and orange, dry	.5 oz	53	3.6	8.2	15	1.0	0.9	na	na	15%
instant, w/apple and orange, 1 oz cereal prepared w/whole milk	1 serving	32	2.0	3.8	16	>.1 c	1.1	na	na	30%
Mixed										
dry	1 tbsp	9	0.3	1.8	1	.2	0.1	na	na	10%
dry	.5 oz	54	1.7	10.4	6	1.1	0.6	na	na	10%
instant, dry *(Earth's Best)*	.5 oz	60	2.0	11.0	0	(mq)	0.0	0.0	0	0%
instant, dry, '2nd Foods' *(Gerber)*	.5 oz	60	1.0	11.0	na	na	1.0	na	na	16%
instant, dry, 'Stages 2' *(Beech-Nut)*	.5 oz	60	1.0	12.0	10	na	0.0	na	na	0%
instant, .5 oz cereal prepared w/2.4 oz formula, 'Stages 2' *(Beech-Nut)*	1 serving	120	2.0	17.0	25	na	4.0	na	na	32%
instant, .5 oz cereal prepared w/2.5 oz formula *(Earth's Best)*	1 serving	110	3.0	16.0	15	(mq)	3.0	(mq)	na	26%
instant, .5 oz cereal prepared w/2.4 oz whole milk, 'Stages 2' *(Beech-Nut)*	1 serving	100	4.0	14.0	50	(mq)	3.0	(mq)	(mq)	27%
instant *(Heinz)*	3.5 oz	373	12.8	71.9	12	na	4.9	na	na	12%
instant, prepared w/apple juice, '2nd Foods' *(Gerber)*	2.4 oz	90	1.0	20.0	na	na	1.0	na	na	10%
1 oz cereal prepared w/whole milk	1 serving	32	1.4	4.5	13	>.1 c	1.0	na	na	28%
w/apples and bananas, 'Stages 2' *(Beech-Nut)*	4.5 oz	90	2.0	19.0	0	(mq)	1.0	(tr)	0	10%
w/apples and bananas, strained *(Heinz)*	3.5 oz	70	1.1	15.7	3	na	0.3	na	na	4%
w/applesauce and bananas, junior	7.75 oz	183	2.6	40.5	79	2.6	0.9	na	na	5%
w/applesauce and bananas, junior	1 oz	24	0.3	5.2	10	.3	0.1	na	na	4%
w/applesauce and bananas, '2nd Foods' *(Gerber)*	4 oz	90	1.0	20.0	na	na	1.0	na	na	10%
w/applesauce and bananas, '2nd Foods' *(Gerber)*	7 tbsp	81	1.2	17.8	2	na	0.6	na	na	7%
w/applesauce and bananas, strained	4.75 oz	111	1.6	24.2	3	1.6	0.7	na	na	6%
w/applesauce and bananas, strained	1 oz	23	0.3	5.1	1	.3	0.1	na	na	4%
w/applesauce and bananas, '3rd Foods' *(Gerber)*	7 tbsp	82	1.3	18.9	3	na	0.6	na	na	6%
w/bananas, dry	1 tbsp	9	0.3	1.9	3	.2	0.1	na	na	9%
w/bananas, dry	.5 oz	56	1.5	10.9	17	1.1	0.7	na	na	11%
w/bananas, instant, dry, '2nd Foods' *(Gerber)*	.5 oz	60	1.0	11.0	na	na	1.0	na	na	16%
w/bananas, 1 oz cereal prepared w/whole milk	1 serving	33	1.3	4.7	17	(mq)	1.0	na	na	27%
w/fruit and nuts, no sugar added, 1-4 yr., dry *(Familia)*	1.5 oz	170	4.0	31.0	4	na	3.0	na	na	16%
w/fruit and nuts, no sugar added, 1-4 yr., 1.5 oz cereal prepared w/whole milk *(Familia)*	1 serving	270	9.0	38.0	77	na	8.0	na	na	28%
w/fruit and nuts, 1-4 yr., 1.5 oz cereal prepared w/2/3 cup milk *(Familia)*	1 serving	270	9.0	39.0	74	na	8.0	na	na	27%
w/fruit and nuts, 100% natural, 1-4 yr., dry *(Familia)*	1.5 oz	170	4.0	32.0	1	na	3.0	na	na	16%
w/honey, dry	1 tbsp	9	0.3	1.8	1	(mq)	0.1	na	na	10%
w/honey, dry	.5 oz	56	2.0	10.4	6	(mq)	0.7	na	na	11%

Food Name	Serving Size	Calories	Prot. gms	Carbs gms	Sod. mgs	Fiber gms	Fat gms	Sat. Fat gms	Chol. mgs	% Fat Cal.
w/honey, 1 oz cereal prepared w/whole milk	1 serving	33	1.4	4.5	14	(mq)	1.0	na	na	28%
Oatmeal										
instant, dry	1 tbsp	10	0.3	1.7	1	.2	0.2	na	na	18%
instant, dry	.5 oz	57	1.9	9.8	5	.9	1.1	na	na	18%
prepared w/whole milk	1 oz	33	1.4	4.3	13	>.1 c	1.2	na	na	32%
w/apples and bananas, 'Stages 2' (Beech-Nut)	4.5 oz	90	2.0	17.0	5	(mq)	1.0	(tr)	0	11%
w/apples and bananas, strained (Heinz)	3.5 oz	76	1.5	16.1	3	.5	0.6	na	na	7%
w/apples and cinnamon, instant, '3rd Foods' (Gerber)	1 pkt	90	2.0	16.0	50	na	2.0	na	na	20%
w/applesauce and bananas, '2nd Foods' (Gerber)	4 oz	90	1.0	20.0	na	(mq)	1.0	(tr)	0	10%
w/applesauce and bananas, '2nd Foods' (Gerber)	7 tbsp	83	1.4	17.6	2	na	0.8	na	na	9%
w/applesauce and bananas, '3rd Foods' (Gerber)	7 tbsp	80	1.4	17.0	3	na	0.8	na	na	9%
w/applesauce and bananas, junior	7.75 oz	165	2.9	34.5	68	1.8	1.5	na	na	8%
w/applesauce and bananas, junior	1 oz	21	0.4	4.4	9	.2	0.2	na	na	9%
w/applesauce and bananas, strained	4.75 oz	99	1.8	20.8	3	1.1	0.9	na	na	8%
w/applesauce and bananas, strained	1 oz	21	0.4	4.4	1	.2	0.2	na	na	9%
w/bananas, dry	1 tbsp	9	0.3	1.8	3	.1	0.1	na	na	10%
w/bananas, dry	.5 oz	56	1.7	10.4	17	.7	0.9	na	na	14%
w/bananas, instant, '3rd Foods' (Gerber)	1 pkt	90	2.0	16.0	50	na	2.0	na	na	20%
w/bananas, prepared w/whole milk	1 oz	33	1.3	4.5	17	>.1 c	1.1	na	na	30%
w/bananas, prepared w/whole milk	3.5 oz	116	4.7	16.0	61	>.2 c	3.8	na	na	29%
w/bananas, 100% natural, organic, dry (Healthy Times) ..	.5 oz	60	2.0	12.0	0	na	0.0	0.0	na	0%
w/bananas, organic, .5 oz cereal prepared w/2.4 oz formula (Healthy Times)	.5 oz	100	3.0	17.0	15	na	3.0	na	na	25%
w/honey, dry	1 tbsp	9	0.3	1.7	1	(mq)	0.2	na	na	18%
w/honey, dry	.5 oz	56	1.9	9.8	7	>.1 c	1.0	na	na	16%
w/honey, prepared w/whole milk	1 oz	33	1.4	4.3	14	(mq)	1.1	na	na	30%
Rice										
dry	1 tbsp	9	0.2	1.9	1	(mq)	0.1	na	na	10%
dry	.5 oz	56	1.0	11.0	5	.1	0.7	na	na	12%
dry (Earth's Best)	.5 oz	60	1.0	12.0	0	(mq)	0.0	0.0	0	0%
dry (Health Valley)	1 tbsp	60	1.0	10.0	5	.7	1.0	(tr)	0	17%
dry, .5 oz cereal prepared w/2.5 oz formula (Earth's Best)	3 oz	110	2.0	17.0	15	(mq)	3.0	(mq)	na	26%
dry, prepared w/whole milk	1 oz	33	1.1	4.7	13	(mq)	1.0	na	na	28%
instant, dry, '1st Foods' (Gerber)	.5 oz	60	1.0	11.0	na	na	1.0	na	na	16%
instant, dry, '1st Foods' (Gerber)	3.5 oz	380	8.3	79.3	7	na	3.3	na	na	8%
instant, dry, 'Stages 1' (Beech-Nut)	.5 oz	60	1.0	12.0	15	(mq)	0.0	0.0	0	0%
instant, .5 oz cereal prepared w/2.4 oz formula (Beech-Nut)	.5 oz	120	2.0	18.0	20	na	4.0	na	na	31%
instant, .5 oz cereal prepared w/2.4 oz whole milk (Beech-Nut)	2.9 oz	110	2.0	17.0	30	(mq)	3.0	(mq)	na	26%
instant (Heinz)	3.5 oz	376	7.9	78.0	12	na	4.1	na	na	10%
sprouted (Health Valley)	1 tbsp	60	1.0	10.0	5	2.1	1.0	(tr)	0	17%
w/apples, instant, dry, 'Stages 2' (Beech-Nut)	.5 oz	60	0.0	13.0	15	(mq)	0.0	0.0	0	0%
w/apples, instant, .5 oz cereal prepared w/2.4 oz formula (Beech-Nut)	.5 oz	120	1.0	19.0	20	na	4.0	na	na	31%
w/apples, instant, .5 oz cereal prepared w/2.4 oz whole milk (Beech-Nut)	2.9 oz	110	3.0	17.0	50	(mq)	3.0	(mq)	na	25%
w/apples and bananas, 'Stages 2' (Beech-Nut)	4.5 oz	100	2.0	24.0	25	(mq)	0.0	0.0	0	0%
w/apples and bananas, strained (Heinz)	3.5 oz	70	0.6	16.2	5	na	0.2	na	na	3%
w/applesauce and bananas, '2nd Foods' (Gerber)	4 oz	90	1.0	21.0	na	(mq)	0.0	(tr)	0	0%
w/applesauce and bananas, '2nd Foods' (Gerber)	7 tbsp	79	0.9	18.2	9	na	0.2	na	na	2%
w/applesauce and bananas, strained	4.75 oz	107	1.6	23.1	38	1.4	0.5	na	na	4%
w/applesauce and bananas, strained	1 oz	22	0.3	4.8	8	.3	0.1	na	na	4%
w/bananas, dry	1 tbsp	10	0.2	1.9	2	(mq)	0.1	na	na	10%

Food Name	Serving Size	Calories	Prot. gms	Carbs gms	Sod. mgs	Fiber gms	Fat gms	Sat. Fat gms	Chol. mgs	% Fat Cal.
w/bananas, dry	.5 oz	57	1.2	11.4	14	.1	0.6	na	na	10%
w/bananas, instant, dry, '2nd Foods' (Gerber)	.5 oz	60	1.0	11.0	na	na	1.0	na	na	16%
w/bananas, instant, dry, 'Stages 2' (Beech-Nut)	.5 oz	60	1.0	13.0	15	(mq)	0.0	0.0	0	0%
w/bananas, instant, .5 oz cereal prepared w/2.4 oz formula (Beech-Nut)	.5 oz	120	1.0	19.0	20	na	4.0	na	na	31%
w/bananas, instant, .5 oz cereal prepared w/2.4 oz whole milk (Beech-Nut)	2.9 oz	100	3.0	17.0	50	(mq)	3.0	(mq)	(mq)	25%
w/bananas, prepared w/whole milk	1 oz	33	1.2	4.8	16	(mq)	1.0	na	na	27%
w/formula, instant, '1st Foods' (Gerber)	2.4 oz	110	2.0	16.0	na	na	4.0	na	na	33%
w/honey, dry	1 tbsp	9	0.2	1.9	1	(mq)	0.1	na	na	10%
w/honey, dry	.5 oz	56	1.0	11.5	7	(mq)	0.4	na	na	7%
w/honey, prepared w/whole milk	1 oz	33	1.1	4.8	14	(mq)	0.9	na	na	26%
w/mango, instant, dry, 'Tropical Foods' (Gerber)	3.5 oz	386	6.4	84.3	20	na	2.6	na	na	6%
w/mango, instant, prepared w/milk, 'Tropical Foods' (Gerber)	2.4 oz	100	3.0	15.0	na	na	3.0	na	na	27%
w/mixed fruit, junior	7.75 oz	185	2.2	41.1	24	2.2	0.4	na	na	2%
w/mixed fruit, junior	1 oz	24	0.3	5.3	3	.3	0.1	na	na	4%
w/mixed fruit, junior (Gerber)	6 oz	140	1.0	31.0	17	(mq)	1.0	(tr)	0	7%
w/mixed fruit, '3rd Foods' (Gerber)	7 tbsp	79	0.9	18.3	10	na	0.2	na	na	2%
DESSERTS AND SNACKS										
Apple betty										
junior	7.75 oz	154	0.9	41.8	20	2.2	0.0	na	na	0%
junior	1 oz	20	0.1	5.4	3	.3	0.0	na	na	0%
strained	4.75 oz	97	0.5	26.5	14	1.4	0.0	na	na	0%
strained	1 oz	20	0.1	5.6	3	.3	0.0	na	na	0%
Apple Juice Dessert, w/yogurt, '2nd Foods' (Gerber)	4 oz	100	2.0	18.0	na	na	2.0	na	na	18%
Apple yogurt										
apple yogurt dessert, 'Stages 2' (Beech-Nut)	4.5 oz	120	1.0	25.0	25	na	2.0	na	na	15%
'Breakfast' (Earth's Best)	4.5 oz	100	3.0	17.0	20	na	2.0	na	na	18%
Banana yogurt										
'2nd Foods' (Gerber)	7 tbsp	74	1.1	16.4	22	na	0.4	na	na	5%
'Stages 2' (Beech-Nut)	4.5 oz	120	1.0	26.0	30	na	2.0	na	na	14%
strained (Heinz)	3.5 oz	83	1.0	18.7	20	na	0.5	na	na	5%
Banana-apple dessert, '2nd Foods' (Gerber)	7 tbsp	68	0.2	16.4	7	na	0.1	na	na	1%
Banana-pineapple dessert, 'Stages 2' (Beech-Nut)	4.5 oz	110	0.0	27.0	15	na	0.0	na	na	0%
Banana-vanilla dessert, 'Tropical Foods' (Gerber)	7 tbsp	85	0.5	18.7	11	na	0.9	na	na	10%
Blueberry yogurt, 'Breakfast' (Earth's Best)	4.5 oz	100	3.0	16.0	20	na	2.0	na	na	19%
Cereal snack										
apple-banana finger snacks, 'Graduates' (Gerber)	3.2 oz	405	8.2	82.6	86	na	4.8	na	na	11%
apple-cinnamon finger snacks, 'Graduates' (Gerber)	3.2 oz	407	7.9	82.6	84	na	5.0	na	na	11%
Cherry vanilla dessert										
junior	7.75 oz	152	0.4	40.5	33	.7	0.4	na	na	2%
junior	1 oz	20	0.1	5.2	4	.1	0.1	na	na	4%
strained	4.75 oz	92	0.3	24.0	22	.4	0.4	na	na	4%
strained	1 oz	19	0.1	5.1	5	.1	0.1	na	na	4%
Cookies and crackers										
animal-shaped, baked, chunky (Gerber)	3.5 oz	443	6.5	74.8	187	na	13.1	na	na	27%
apple, organic, 'Hugga Bears' (Healthy Times)	1 oz	120	2.0	17.0	38	na	3.0	na	0	26%
arrowroot	1 oz	125	2.2	20.2	105	1.1	4.1	0.9	0	29%
arrowroot, baked finger snacks, 'Graduates' (Gerber)	3.5 oz	452	8.4	70.3	324	na	15.3	na	na	30%
arrowroot, w/maple, wheat-free (Healthy Times)	1 cookie	120	2.0	17.0	38	na	3.0	na	0	26%
baked, chunky, 'Biter Biscuit' (Gerber)	1 biscuit	50	1.0	9.0	na	na	1.0	na	na	18%
cinnamon animal crackers, baked, 'Graduates' (Gerber)	3.5 oz	449	5.9	78.7	369	na	12.3	na	na	25%
pretzel	1 oz	113	3.1	23.3	76	.7	0.6	na	na	5%

Food Name	Serving Size	Calories	Prot. gms	Carbs gms	Sod. mgs	Fiber gms	Fat gms	Sat. Fat gms	Chol. mgs	% Fat Cal.
pretzel, baked, finger snacks, 'Graduates' *(Gerber)*	3.5 oz	403	10.5	83.0	597	na	3.3	na	na	7%
strawberry, organic, 'Hugga Bears' *(Healthy Times)*	1 oz	120	2.0	17.0	38	na	3.0	na	0	26%
teething biscuit	1 biscuit	43	1.2	8.4	40	.2	0.5	na	na	11%
teething biscuit	1 oz	111	3.0	21.7	103	.4	1.2	na	na	10%
zwieback, baked, chunky *(Gerber)*	3.5 oz	432	12.9	69.4	210	na	11.5	na	na	24%
Cottage cheese w/pineapple										
junior	7.75 oz	172	6.6	35.0	112	>2.2 c	1.5	na	na	8%
junior	1 oz	22	0.9	4.5	14	>.3 c	0.2	na	na	8%
strained	4.75 oz	93	3.9	17.8	70	>1.8 c	1.1	na	na	10%
strained	1 oz	20	0.8	3.7	15	>.4 c	0.2	na	na	9%
'Stages 2' *(Beech-Nut)*	4.5 oz	130	2.0	26.0	15	(mq)	1.0	(mq)	(mq)	7%
'Stages 3' *(Beech-Nut)*	6 oz	170	3.0	36.0	20	na	2.0	na	na	10%
Custard / pudding										
banana pudding, 'Stages 2' *(Beech-Nut)*	4.5 oz	100	0.0	25.0	10	na	0.0	na	na	0%
banana pudding, strained *(Heinz)*	3.5 oz	74	0.7	16.8	9	na	0.5	na	na	6%
caramel pudding, junior	7.75 oz	168	3.0	36.2	60	>.2 c	1.9	na	na	10%
caramel pudding, junior	1 oz	22	0.4	4.8	8	(mq)	0.3	na	na	12%
caramel pudding, strained	4.75 oz	104	1.8	23.2	36	>.1 c	0.9	na	na	8%
caramel pudding, strained	1 oz	22	0.4	4.9	8	(mq)	0.2	na	na	8%
cherry vanilla pudding, '2nd Foods' *(Gerber)*	7 tbsp	69	0.3	16.6	9	na	0.2	na	na	3%
cherry vanilla pudding, strained *(Gerber)*	4.5 oz	90	0.0	21.0	12	(mq)	1.0	na	3	10%
chocolate custard, junior	7.75 oz	196	4.2	38.3	55	1.5	3.5	na	na	16%
chocolate custard, junior	1 oz	25	0.5	4.9	7	.2	0.5	na	na	17%
chocolate custard, junior *(Heinz)*	3.5 oz	75	2.0	14.0	27	na	1.2	na	na	14%
chocolate custard, strained	4.75 oz	108	2.4	20.6	29	.9	2.2	na	na	18%
chocolate custard, strained	1 oz	24	0.5	4.6	7	.2	0.5	na	na	18%
orange pudding, strained	4.75 oz	108	1.5	23.9	27	.8	1.2	na	na	10%
orange pudding, strained	1 oz	23	0.3	5.0	6	.2	0.3	na	na	11%
pineapple pudding, junior	7.75 oz	191	3.1	47.5	48	1.8	0.9	na	na	4%
pineapple pudding, junior	1 oz	25	0.4	6.1	6	.2	0.1	na	na	3%
pineapple pudding, strained	4.75 oz	104	1.7	26.0	24	.9	0.4	na	na	3%
pineapple pudding, strained	1 oz	23	0.4	5.8	5	.2	0.1	na	na	4%
vanilla custard, junior	7.75 oz	196	3.5	35.6	64	>.4 c	5.1	2.6	na	23%
vanilla custard, junior	1 oz	25	0.5	4.6	8	>.1 c	0.7	0.3	na	24%
vanilla custard, junior *(Gerber)*	6 oz	150	3.0	31.0	41	na	2.0	(mq)	23	12%
vanilla custard, '2nd Foods' *(Gerber)*	7 tbsp	88	1.8	18.2	25	na	0.9	na	na	9%
vanilla custard, 'Stages 2' *(Beech-Nut)*	4.5 oz	140	2.0	24.0	60	na	4.0	(mq)	na	26%
vanilla custard, 'Stages 3' *(Beech-Nut)*	6 oz	180	3.0	30.0	80	na	5.0	(mq)	na	25%
vanilla custard, strained	4.75 oz	109	2.0	20.6	36	>.3 c	2.6	1.3	na	21%
vanilla custard, strained	1 oz	24	0.5	4.6	8	>.1 c	0.6	0.3	na	21%
vanilla custard, strained *(Gerber)*	4.5 oz	100	2.0	22.0	32	na	1.0	(mq)	14	9%
vanilla custard, '3rd Foods' *(Gerber)*	7 tbsp	89	1.7	18.4	24	na	0.9	na	na	9%
vanilla custard, strained *(Heinz)*	3.5 oz	75	2.0	14.0	27	na	1.2	na	na	14%
Dutch apple dessert										
junior	7.75 oz	152	0.0	37.0	35	2.0	2.2	1.4	na	12%
junior	1 oz	20	0.0	4.8	5	.3	0.3	0.2	na	12%
junior *(Heinz)*	3.5 oz	69	0.1	16.3	5	na	0.4	na	na	5%
'2nd Foods' *(Gerber)*	7 tbsp	79	0.1	17.4	14	na	1.0	na	na	11%
'Stages 2' *(Beech-Nut)*	4.5 oz	100	0.0	24.0	15	(mq)	0.0	0.0	0	0%
strained	4.75 oz	92	0.0	22.5	22	1.2	1.2	0.8	na	11%
strained	1 oz	19	0.0	4.7	5	.3	0.3	0.2	na	13%
strained *(Heinz)*	3.5 oz	69	0.1	16.3	5	na	0.4	na	na	5%
'3rd Foods' *(Gerber)*	7 tbsp	77	0.1	16.9	14	na	0.9	na	na	11%

Food Name	Serving Size	Calories	Prot. gms	Carbs gms	Sod. mgs	Fiber gms	Fat gms	Sat. Fat gms	Chol. mgs	% Fat Cal.
Fruit dessert										
junior *(Gerber)*	6 oz	130	0.0	30.0	12	(mq)	1.0	(tr)	0	7%
junior *(Heinz)*	3.5 oz	65	0.2	15.7	14	na	0.2	na	na	3%
'2nd Foods' *(Gerber)*	7 tbsp	82	0.4	19.7	9	na	0.2	na	na	2%
'Stages 2' *(Beech-Nut)*	4.5 oz	80	0.0	20.0	0	(mq)	0.0	0.0	0	0%
'Stages 3' *(Beech-Nut)*	6 oz	120	0.0	28.0	5	(mq)	0.0	0.0	0	0%
strained *(Gerber)*	4.5 oz	100	0.0	24.0	13	(mq)	1.0	(tr)	0	9%
strained *(Heinz)*	3.5 oz	66	0.3	15.8	11	na	0.2	na	na	3%
'3rd Foods' *(Gerber)*	7 tbsp	73	0.3	17.6	7	na	0.2	na	na	3%
w/o ascorbic acid, junior	7.75 oz	139	0.7	37.8	29	1.3	0.0	na	na	0%
w/o ascorbic acid, junior	1 oz	18	0.1	4.9	4	.2	0.0	na	na	0%
w/o ascorbic acid, strained	4.75 oz	80	0.4	21.6	19	.8	0.0	na	na	0%
w/o ascorbic acid, strained	1 oz	17	0.1	4.5	4	.2	0.0	na	na	0%
Guava dessert, w/tapioca, 'Tropical Foods' *(Gerber)*	7 tbsp	69	0.1	16.8	3	na	0.1	na	na	1%
Hawaiian dessert										
junior *(Gerber)*	6 oz	150	2.0	33.0	32	(mq)	1.0	na	3	6%
'2nd Foods' *(Gerber)*	7 tbsp	86	1.3	19.7	17	na	0.2	na	na	2%
'3rd Foods' *(Gerber)*	7 tbsp	87	1.3	20.2	15	na	0.1	na	na	1%
strained *(Gerber)*	4.5 oz	120	2.0	25.0	23	(mq)	1.0	na	2	8%
Mango dessert, w/tapioca 'Tropical Foods' *(Gerber)*	7 tbsp	75	0.2	18.2	2	na	0.2	na	na	2%
Mango-banana dessert, w/passion fruit, 'Tropical Foods' *(Gerber)*	7 tbsp	73	0.2	17.7	9	na	0.1	na	na	1%
Mixed fruit yogurt, '2nd Foods' *(Gerber)*	7 tbsp	79	1.0	18.0	15	na	0.3	na	na	3%
Papaya dessert, w/tapioca, 'Tropical Foods' *(Gerber)*	7 tbsp	62	0.2	15.1	7	na	0.2	na	na	3%
Papaya-pineapple dessert, 'Tropical Foods' *(Gerber)*	7 tbsp	76	0.2	18.6	8	na	0.0	na	na	0%
Peach cobbler										
junior	7.75 oz	147	0.7	40.3	20	1.5	0.0	na	na	0%
junior	1 oz	19	0.1	5.2	3	.2	0.0	na	na	0%
'2nd Foods' *(Gerber)*	7 tbsp	77	0.5	18.2	8	na	0.2	na	na	2%
strained	4.75 oz	88	0.4	24.0	9	.9	0.0	na	na	0%
strained	1 oz	18	0.1	5.1	2	.2	0.0	na	na	0%
strained *(Heinz)*	3.5 oz	72	0.5	16.9	6	.3	0.3	na	na	4%
'3rd Foods' *(Gerber)*	7 tbsp	77	0.6	18.4	9	na	0.1	na	na	1%
Peach melba										
junior	7.75 oz	132	0.7	36.1	20	>.2 c	0.0	na	na	0%
junior	1 oz	17	0.1	4.7	3	(mq)	0.0	na	na	0%
strained	4.75 oz	81	0.3	22.3	12	>.3 c	0.0	na	na	0%
strained	1 oz	17	0.1	4.7	3	>.1 c	0.0	na	na	0%
Peach yogurt										
'2nd Foods' *(Gerber)*	7 tbsp	76	1.0	17.2	14	na	0.4	na	na	5%
'Stages 2' *(Beech-Nut)*	4.5 oz	120	1.0	25.0	30	na	2.0	na	na	15%
Peach-mango dessert, 'Tropical Foods' *(Gerber)*	7 tbsp	60	0.3	16.8	7	na	0.2	na	na	3%
Pear yogurt										
'Stages 2' *(Beech-Nut)*	4.5 oz	130	1.0	29.0	35	na	2.0	na	na	13%
strained *(Heinz)*	3.5 oz	80	0.8	18.1	19	na	0.4	na	na	5%
pineapple-banana dessert, 'Tropical Foods' *(Gerber)*	7 tbsp	79	0.3	19.3	9	na	0.1	na	na	1%
Pineapple-orange dessert										
strained	4.75 oz	90	0.3	24.4	13	.5	0.0	na	na	0%
strained	1 oz	20	0.1	5.4	3	.1	0.0	na	na	0%
Tropical fruit dessert										
junior	7.75 oz	132	0.4	36.1	15	>.2 c	0.0	na	na	0%
junior	1 oz	17	0.1	4.7	2	(mq)	0.0	na	na	0%
medley, 'Tropical Foods' *(Gerber)*	7 tbsp	64	0.2	15.4	6	na	0.1	na	na	1%
w/tapioca, strained	4.5 oz	80	0.0	20.0	6	(mq)	0.0	0.0	0	0%

Food Name	Serving Size	Calories	Prot. gms	Carbs gms	Sod. mgs	Fiber gms	Fat gms	Sat. Fat gms	Chol. mgs	% Fat Cal.
Tropical yogurt, 'Breakfast' (Earth's Best)	4.5 oz	110	3.0	19.0	20	na	2.0	na	na	17%
Tutti frutti dessert, junior (Heinz)	3.5 oz	67	0.3	15.7	12	.3	0.4	na	na	5%
DINNERS AND MAIN DISHES										
Apples and chicken dinner, 'Simple Recipe'										
'2nd Foods' (Gerber)	7 tbsp	66	2.4	11.0	13	na	1.4	na	na	19%
Apples and ham dinner, 'Simple Recipe'										
'2nd Foods' (Gerber)	7 tbsp	67	2.7	12.2	9	na	0.8	na	na	11%
Apples and turkey dinner										
'Simple Recipe,' '2nd Foods' (Gerber)	4 oz	80	3.0	13.0	20	na	2.0	na	na	22%
'Simple Recipe,' '2nd Foods' (Gerber)	7 tbsp	67	2.9	11.3	13	na	1.2	na	na	16%
Beans and rice dinner										
'Tropical Foods' (Gerber)	7 tbsp	52	2.1	7.4	8	na	1.5	na	na	26%
w/green beans (Earth's Best)	4.5 oz	70	2.0	14.0	0	(mq)	0.0	0.0	0	0%
Beef and egg noodle dinner										
'2nd Foods' (Gerber)	7 tbsp	62	2.7	8.3	10	na	2.0	na	na	29%
'3rd Foods' (Gerber)	7 tbsp	64	2.7	8.9	14	na	1.9	na	na	27%
strained (Heinz)	3.5 oz	49	2.0	6.3	15	.3	1.8	na	na	33%
Beef and rice dinner										
toddler	6.25 oz	145	8.9	15.6	632	>.5 c	5.1	na	na	32%
toddler	1 oz	23	1.4	2.5	101	>.1 c	0.8	na	na	32%
Beef dinner										
junior (Gerber)	2.5 oz	80	11.0	1.0	38	0	4.0	(mq)	20	43%
'Stages 1' (Beech-Nut)	2.8 oz	90	10.0	0.0	40	0	5.0	(mq)	(mq)	53%
'Stages 3' (Beech-Nut)	6 oz	150	6.0	14.0	45	(mq)	8.0	(mq)	(mq)	47%
supreme, 'Stages 2' (Beech-Nut)	4.5 oz	120	3.0	13.0	40	na	6.0	(mq)	(mq)	46%
'3rd Foods' (Gerber)	7 tbsp	103	15.1	0.2	52	na	4.6	na	na	40%
w/vegetables, lean meat, junior (Gerber)	4.5 oz	100	8.0	10.0	29	(mq)	3.0	(mq)	12	27%
w/vegetables, lean meat, strained (Gerber)	4.5 oz	90	7.0	9.0	32	(mq)	3.0	(mq)	11	30%
Beef lasagna dinner										
toddler	6.25 oz	136	7.4	17.7	804	>.4 c	3.7	na	na	25%
toddler	1 oz	22	1.2	2.8	129	>.1 c	0.6	na	na	25%
Beef noodle dinner										
junior	7.5 oz	121	5.3	15.8	36	2.3	4.1	na	na	30%
junior	1 oz	16	0.7	2.1	5	.3	0.5	na	na	29%
strained	4.5 oz	68	2.9	9.0	37	1.4	2.2	na	na	29%
strained	1 oz	15	0.7	2.0	8	.3	0.5	na	na	29%
Beef stew										
'Stages Table Time' (Beech-Nut)	6 oz	150	10.0	16.0	380	(mq)	6.0	(mq)	(mq)	34%
toddler	6.25 oz	90	9.0	9.7	611	2.0	2.1	1.0	22	20%
toddler	1 oz	14	1.5	1.6	98	.3	0.3	0.2	4	18%
Beef vegetable dinner										
high-meat, junior	4.5 oz	109	8.1	6.8	42	1.1	5.9	na	na	47%
high-meat, junior	1 oz	24	1.8	1.5	9	.3	1.3	na	na	47%
high-meat, strained	4.5 oz	96	7.3	5.4	46	1.1	5.4	na	na	49%
high-meat, strained	1 oz	21	1.6	1.2	10	.3	1.2	na	na	49%
Beef vegetable entrée										
'Stages 2' (Beech-Nut)	4.5 oz	90	2.0	10.0	35	(mq)	4.0	(mq)	(mq)	43%
'Stages 3' (Beech-Nut)	6 oz	160	6.0	16.0	70	(mq)	7.0	(mq)	(mq)	42%
Broccoli-chicken dinner, 'Simple Recipe'										
'2nd Foods' (Gerber)	7 tbsp	42	3.7	3.4	20	na	1.5	na	na	32%
Carrots and beef dinner, 'Simple Recipe'										
'2nd Foods' (Gerber)	7 tbsp	59	3.4	5.7	40	na	2.5	na	na	38%
Chicken dinner										
junior (Gerber)	2.5 oz	110	11.0	1.0	28	0	7.0	(mq)	42	57%

Food Name	Serving Size	Calories	Prot. gms	Carbs gms	Sod. mgs	Fiber gms	Fat gms	Sat. Fat gms	Chol. mgs	% Fat Cal.
'3rd Foods' (Gerber)	7 tbsp	132	15.0	0.2	39	na	7.9	na	na	54%
vegetable entrée, 'Stages 2' (Beech-Nut)	4.5 oz	90	3.0	14.0	65	(mq)	3.0	(mq)	(mq)	28%
vegetable entrée, 'Stages 3' (Beech-Nut)	6 oz	90	7.0	13.0	70	(mq)	2.0	(mq)	(mq)	18%
w/vegetables, lean meat, junior (Gerber)	4.5 oz	90	7.0	10.0	32	(mq)	3.0	(mq)	19	28%
w/vegetables, lean meat, strained (Gerber)	4.5 oz	90	7.0	8.0	31	(mq)	3.0	(mq)	18	31%
Chicken noodle dinner										
junior	7.5 oz	109	4.1	16.0	36	2.3	3.0	na	na	25%
junior	1 oz	14	0.5	2.1	5	.3	0.4	na	na	26%
'2nd Foods' (Gerber)	7 tbsp	55	2.5	8.6	14	na	1.2	na	na	20%
strained	4.5 oz	67	2.7	9.6	20	1.4	1.9	na	na	26%
strained	1 oz	15	0.6	2.1	5	.3	0.4	na	na	25%
'3rd Foods' (Gerber)	7 tbsp	56	2.5	8.6	14	na	1.3	na	na	21%
Chicken rice dinner										
'Stages 2' (Beech-Nut)	4.5 oz	80	2.0	11.0	40	(mq)	3.0	(mq)	(mq)	34%
'Tropical Foods' (Gerber)	7 tbsp	48	2.3	6.9	14	na	1.3	na	na	24%
Chicken stew dinner										
toddler	6 oz	133	8.8	10.9	683	1.0	6.3	1.9	49	42%
toddler	1 oz	22	1.5	1.8	114	.2	1.0	0.3	8	41%
w/noodles, 'Graduates'	3.2 oz	69	4.4	8.5	308	na	2.0	na	na	26%
Chicken vegetable dinner										
high-meat, junior	4.5 oz	118	9.0	5.4	33	1.1	7.0	na	na	52%
high-meat, junior	1 oz	26	2.0	1.2	7	.3	1.6	na	na	53%
high-meat, strained	4.5 oz	100	7.9	7.6	35	1.1	4.6	na	na	40%
high-meat, strained	1 oz	22	1.8	1.7	8	.3	1.0	na	na	39%
Green bean dinner, w/turkey, 'Simple Recipe,' '2nd Foods' (Gerber)	7 tbsp	55	4.1	6.5	11	na	1.5	na	na	24%
Ham dinner										
ham and vegetable entrée, 'Stages 2' (Beech-Nut)	4.5 oz	80	3.0	12.0	30	(mq)	3.0	(mq)	(mq)	31%
w/vegetables, lean meat, junior (Gerber)	4.5 oz	110	8.0	11.0	27	(mq)	4.0	(mq)	11	32%
w/vegetables, lean meat, strained (Gerber)	4.5 oz	100	7.0	10.0	26	(mq)	4.0	(mq)	12	35%
Ham vegetable dinner										
high-meat, junior	4.5 oz	99	8.2	7.8	28	1.1	4.2	1.4	23	37%
high-meat, junior	1 oz	22	1.8	1.7	6	.3	0.9	0.3	5	37%
high-meat, strained	4.5 oz	97	8.1	7.0	28	1.1	4.5	1.5	na	40%
high-meat, strained	1 oz	22	1.8	1.6	6	.3	1.0	0.3	na	40%
Lamb and vegetable entrée, 'Stages 2' (Beech-Nut)	4.5 oz	90	2.0	13.0	40	(mq)	4.0	(mq)	(mq)	38%
Lamb noodle dinner										
junior	7.5 oz	138	4.9	18.5	38	>.4 c	4.7	na	na	31%
junior	1 oz	18	0.7	2.5	5	>.1 c	0.6	na	na	30%
Macaroni dinner										
tomato beef, '2nd Foods' (Gerber)	7 tbsp	57	2.6	9.1	32	na	1.1	na	na	18%
tomato beef, '3rd Foods' (Gerber)	7 tbsp	60	2.5	10.2	12	na	0.9	na	na	14%
tomatoes and beef, junior (Heinz)	3.5 oz	52	2.0	8.2	14	.3	1.2	na	na	21%
w/bacon, junior	7.5 oz	160	5.3	18.3	166	>.2 c	7.0	na	na	40%
w/bacon, junior	1 oz	21	0.7	2.4	22	(mq)	0.9	na	na	40%
w/beef, 'Stages 2' (Beech-Nut)	4.5 oz	90	2.0	13.0	40	(mq)	4.0	(mq)	(mq)	38%
w/beef, 'Stages 3' (Beech-Nut)	6 oz	160	6.0	17.0	85	(mq)	8.0	(mq)	(mq)	44%
w/cheese (Earth's Best)	4.5 oz	100	4.0	12.0	10	na	4.0	na	na	36%
w/cheese, junior	7.5 oz	130	5.5	17.5	162	.6	4.3	na	na	30%
w/cheese, junior	1 oz	17	0.7	2.3	22	.1	0.6	na	na	31%
w/cheese, strained	4.5 oz	76	3.3	9.6	93	.4	2.7	na	na	32%
w/cheese, strained	1 oz	17	0.7	2.1	21	.1	0.6	na	na	33%
w/cheese, '2nd Foods' (Gerber)	7 tbsp	63	2.8	8.6	88	na	2.0	na	na	28%

Food Name	Serving Size	Calories	Prot. gms	Carbs gms	Sod. mgs	Fiber gms	Fat gms	Sat. Fat gms	Chol. mgs	% Fat Cal.
Macaroni main dish										
alphabets w/beef and tomato sauce, chunky *(Gerber)* ...	7 tbsp	80	4.2	11.4	199	na	2.0	na	na	22%
w/beef, in sauce, 'Graduates' *(Gerber)*	3.2 oz	78	4.7	11.1	302	na	1.7	na	na	20%
w/ham, junior	7.5 oz	128	6.8	18.1	100	>.4 c	3.0	na	na	21%
w/ham, junior	1 oz	17	0.9	2.4	13	>.1 c	0.4	na	na	21%
w/tomato and beef, junior	7.5 oz	126	5.3	20.0	36	2.3	2.3	na	na	17%
w/tomato and beef, junior	1 oz	17	0.7	2.7	5	.3	0.3	na	na	17%
w/tomato and beef, strained	4.5 oz	70	2.8	11.3	22	1.4	1.4	na	na	18%
w/tomato and beef, strained	1 oz	16	0.6	2.5	5	.3	0.3	na	na	18%
Mixed vegetable dinner										
junior	7.5 oz	70	2.1	16.8	19	>.4 c	0.0	na	na	0%
junior	1 oz	9	0.3	2.2	3	>.1 c	0.0	na	na	0%
strained	4.5 oz	52	1.5	12.2	10	>.4 c	0.1	na	na	2%
strained	1 oz	12	0.3	2.7	2	>.1 c	0.0	na	na	0%
Noodle main dish										
w/beef, chunky, 'Homestyle' *(Gerber)*	7 tbsp	88	4.4	9.8	216	na	3.5	na	na	36%
w/chicken, carrots, and peas, chunky *(Gerber)*	7 tbsp	65	4.1	8.8	207	na	1.5	na	na	21%
Pasta dinner *(Earth's Best)*	4.5 oz	90	3.0	13.0	20	na	3.0	na	na	30%
Potato dinner, w/green beans *(Earth's Best)*	4.5 oz	100	4.0	13.0	25	na	3.0	na	na	28%
Ravioli										
beef, w/tomato sauce, 'Graduates' *(Gerber)*	3.2 oz	97	3.4	16.3	322	na	2.0	na	na	19%
beef, w/tomato sauce, 'Graduates' micro cup *(Gerber)* ...	6 oz	170	6.0	28.0	590	na	4.0	na	na	21%
cheese, w/tomato sauce, 'Graduates' *(Gerber)*	3.2 oz	99	3.6	16.3	297	na	2.2	na	na	20%
cheese, w/tomato sauce, 'Graduates' micro cup *(Gerber)*	6 oz	170	6.0	28.0	510	na	4.0	na	na	21%
rice and lentil dinner, *(Earth's Best)*	4.5 oz	80	3.0	13.0	25	na	2.0	na	na	22%
Rice main dish										
saucy, w/chicken, chunky *(Gerber)*	7 tbsp	67	3.3	10.1	222	na	1.5	na	na	20%
w/beef and tomato sauce, chunky *(Gerber)*	7 tbsp	79	3.8	11.7	202	na	1.9	na	na	22%
Spaghetti										
rings, in meat sauce, 'Stages Table Time' *(Beech-Nut)* ...	6 oz	160	7.0	22.0	390	(mq)	4.0	(mq)	(mq)	24%
w/beef, 'Stages 3' *(Beech-Nut)*	6 oz	170	6.0	17.0	75	(mq)	8.0	(mq)	(mq)	44%
w/mini meatballs and sauce,'Graduates' *(Gerber)*	6 oz	160	7.0	21.0	590	na	5.0	na	na	29%
w/mini meatballs and sauce, 'Graduates' *(Gerber)*	3.2 oz	91	4.4	12.0	300	na	2.8	na	na	28%
w/tomato and meat, junior	7.5 oz	134	5.3	21.5	43	2.3	2.8	na	na	19%
w/tomato and meat, junior	1 oz	18	0.7	2.9	6	.3	0.4	na	na	20%
w/tomato and meat, toddler	6.25 oz	133	9.4	19.1	634	>.7 c	1.8	na	na	12%
w/tomato and meat, toddler	1 oz	21	1.5	3.1	101	>.1 c	0.3	na	na	13%
w/tomato sauce and beef, chunky *(Gerber)*	7 tbsp	85	4.4	12.5	223	na	1.9	na	na	20%
w/tomato sauce and beef, junior *(Gerber)*	6 oz	120	5.0	19.0	41	(mq)	3.0	(mq)	7	22%
w/tomato sauce and beef, '3rd Foods' *(Gerber)*	7 tbsp	64	2.8	10.6	20	na	1.2	na	na	17%
w/tomato sauce and meat, junior *(Heinz)*	3.5 oz	58	2.2	9.6	19	.4	1.3	na	na	20%
Split pea and ham dinner										
junior	7.5 oz	151	7.0	24.1	30	2.3	2.8	na	na	17%
junior	1 oz	20	0.9	3.2	4	.3	0.4	na	na	18%
sweet potato dinner, w/chicken *(Earth's Best)*	4.5 oz	90	3.0	13.0	30	na	2.0	na	na	22%
Turkey dinner										
junior *(Gerber)*	2.5 oz	100	10.0	1.0	37	0	6.0	(mq)	38	55%
supreme, 'Stages 2' *(Beech-Nut)*	4.5 oz	120	4.0	11.0	35	(mq)	0.0	(mq)	(mq)	17%
Turkey rice dinner										
junior	7.5 oz	104	3.8	15.3	32	2.3	3.0	0.9	na	26%
junior	1 oz	14	0.5	2.0	4	.3	0.4	0.1	na	27%
junior *(Gerber)*	6 oz	110	4.0	14.0	34	(mq)	4.0	(mq)	19	33%
'2nd Foods' *(Gerber)*	7 tbsp	55	2.7	7.5	15	na	1.5	na	na	25%
'Stages 2' *(Beech-Nut)*	4.5 oz	70	2.0	12.0	35	(mq)	2.0	(mq)	(mq)	24%

Food Name	Serving Size	Calories	Prot. gms	Carbs gms	Sod. mgs	Fiber gms	Fat gms	Sat. Fat gms	Chol. mgs	% Fat Cal.
'Stages 3' (Beech-Nut)	6 oz	110	6.0	14.0	65	(mq)	4.0	(mq)	(mq)	31%
strained	4.5 oz	63	2.4	9.3	22	1.4	1.7	0.5	13	25%
strained	1 oz	14	0.5	2.1	5	.3	0.4	0.1	3	26%
strained (Gerber)	4.5 oz	80	3.0	10.0	20	(mq)	3.0	(mq)	15	34%
'3rd Foods' (Gerber)	7 tbsp	55	2.7	7.8	17	na	1.4	na	na	23%
w/vegetables, junior (Heinz)	3.5 oz	42	1.5	7.9	20	.2	0.6	na	na	13%
w/vegetables, strained (Heinz)	3.5 oz	47	1.2	8.2	21	.6	1.1	na	na	21%
Turkey stew main dish, w/rice, 'Graduates' (Gerber)	3.2 oz	59	4.9	7.6	298	na	1.0	na	na	15%
Turkey vegetable dinner										
high-meat, junior	4.5 oz	115	7.6	7.6	55	1.1	6.4	na	na	49%
high-meat, junior	1 oz	26	1.7	1.7	12	.3	1.4	na	na	48%
high-meat, strained	4.5 oz	111	7.2	7.7	38	1.1	6.1	na	na	48%
high-meat, strained	1 oz	25	1.6	1.7	9	.3	1.4	na	na	49%
lean meat, junior (Gerber)	4.5 oz	100	7.0	10.0	31	(mq)	4.0	(mq)	16	35%
lean meat, strained (Gerber)	4.5 oz	100	7.0	9.0	31	(mq)	4.0	(mq)	17	36%
Veal vegetable dinner										
high-meat, junior	4.5 oz	93	7.8	7.4	32	1.1	4.0	na	na	37%
high-meat, junior	1 oz	21	1.7	1.6	7	.3	0.9	na	na	38%
high-meat, strained	4.5 oz	88	7.6	7.8	31	1.1	3.5	na	na	34%
high-meat, strained	1 oz	20	1.7	1.7	7	.3	0.8	na	na	35%
Vegetable bacon dinner										
junior	7.5 oz	151	3.8	16.2	96	2.3	8.3	3.0	na	48%
junior	1 oz	20	0.5	2.2	13	.3	1.1	0.4	na	48%
'2nd Foods' (Gerber)	7 tbsp	73	2.0	8.8	49	na	3.3	na	na	41%
strained	4.5 oz	88	2.0	11.0	55	1.4	4.2	1.5	4	42%
'3rd Foods' (Gerber)	7 tbsp	77	2.3	9.3	52	na	3.4	na	na	40%
Vegetable beef dinner										
(Earth's Best)	4.5 oz	90	3.0	11.0	15	na	3.0	na	na	33%
junior	7.5 oz	113	5.1	15.8	51	2.3	3.6	na	na	28%
junior	1 oz	15	0.7	2.1	7	.3	0.5	na	na	29%
'2nd Foods' (Gerber)	7 tbsp	65	2.3	8.5	11	na	2.4	na	na	33%
strained	4.5 oz	68	2.6	9.0	27	1.4	2.6	na	na	34%
strained	1 oz	15	0.6	2.0	6	.3	0.6	na	na	34%
'3rd Foods' (Gerber)	7 tbsp	62	2.6	9.2	16	na	1.6	na	na	23%
Vegetable chicken dinner										
junior	7.5 oz	107	4.1	18.1	19	2.3	2.3	na	na	19%
junior	1 oz	14	0.5	2.4	3	.3	0.3	na	na	19%
'2nd Foods' (Gerber)	7 tbsp	58	2.3	9.4	10	na	1.3	na	na	20%
strained	4.5 oz	55	2.4	8.4	14	1.4	1.4	na	na	23%
strained	1 oz	12	0.5	1.9	3	.3	0.3	na	na	22%
'3rd Foods' (Gerber)	7 tbsp	51	2.1	8.1	17	na	1.1	na	na	20%
vegetable dinner, 'Summer' (Earth's Best)	4.5 oz	90	3.0	12.0	15	na	3.0	na	na	31%
Vegetable dumpling dinner										
w/beef, junior	7.5 oz	102	4.5	17.0	111	>.6 c	1.7	na	na	15%
w/beef, junior	1 oz	14	0.6	2.3	15	>.1 c	0.2	na	na	13%
w/beef, junior (Heinz)	3.5 oz	47	1.9	7.2	16	.4	1.2	na	na	23%
w/beef, strained	4.5 oz	61	2.6	9.9	63	>.4 c	1.1	na	na	17%
w/beef, strained	1 oz	14	0.6	2.2	14	>.1 c	0.3	na	na	19%
w/beef, strained (Heinz)	3.5 oz	49	1.9	8.6	15	.4	1.3	na	na	22%
Vegetable ham dinner										
junior	7.5 oz	111	5.1	14.9	38	2.3	3.6	na	na	29%
junior	1 oz	15	0.7	2.0	5	.3	0.5	na	na	29%
'2nd Foods' (Gerber)	7 tbsp	59	1.9	8.6	9	na	1.9	na	na	29%
strained	4.5 oz	61	2.3	8.8	15	1.4	2.2	na	na	31%

Food Name	Serving Size	Calories	Prot. gms	Carbs gms	Sod. mgs	Fiber gms	Fat gms	Sat. Fat gms	Chol. mgs	% Fat Cal.
strained	1 oz	14	0.5	2.0	3	.3	0.5	na	na	31%
'3rd Foods' *(Gerber)*	7 tbsp	61	2.1	9.2	12	na	1.8	na	na	26%
toddler	6.25 oz	127	7.4	14.0	531	2.0	5.3	1.9	14	36%
toddler	1 oz	20	1.2	2.2	85	.3	0.9	0.3	2	37%
Vegetable lamb dinner										
junior	7.5 oz	109	4.5	15.1	28	2.3	3.6	na	na	29%
junior	1 oz	14	0.6	2.0	4	.3	0.5	na	na	30%
strained	4.5 oz	67	2.6	8.8	26	1.4	2.6	na	na	34%
strained	1 oz	15	0.6	2.0	6	.3	0.6	na	na	34%
Vegetable liver dinner										
junior	7.5 oz	94	3.8	17.5	28	2.3	1.3	na	na	12%
junior	1 oz	12	0.5	2.3	4	.3	0.2	na	na	14%
strained	4.5 oz	50	2.8	8.8	23	1.4	0.5	na	na	9%
strained	1 oz	11	0.6	2.0	5	.3	0.1	na	na	8%
Vegetable main dish										
w/beef, chunky *(Gerber)*	7 tbsp	70	3.8	9.2	201	na	2.0	na	na	26%
w/chicken, chunky *(Gerber)*	7 tbsp	66	3.8	9.5	202	na	1.4	na	na	19%
w/ham, chunky *(Gerber)*	7 tbsp	70	3.7	8.7	200	na	2.3	na	na	29%
w/turkey, chunky *(Gerber)*	7 tbsp	61	3.6	8.4	190	na	4.4	na	na	45%
Vegetable noodle dinner										
w/chicken, junior	7.5 oz	136	3.6	19.4	55	2.3	4.7	na	na	32%
w/chicken, junior	1 oz	18	0.5	2.6	7	.3	0.6	na	na	30%
w/chicken, junior *(Heinz)*	3.5 oz	57	1.6	8.7	21	.3	1.8	na	na	28%
w/chicken, strained	4.5 oz	81	2.6	10.1	26	1.4	3.2	na	na	36%
w/chicken, strained	1 oz	18	0.6	2.2	6	.3	0.7	na	na	36%
w/chicken, strained *(Heinz)*	3.5 oz	54	2.2	7.5	24	.2	1.7	na	na	28%
w/turkey, junior	7.5 oz	111	3.8	16.2	36	2.3	3.2	na	na	27%
w/turkey, junior	1 oz	15	0.5	2.2	5	.3	0.4	na	na	25%
w/turkey, junior *(Heinz)*	3.5 oz	48	1.2	6.4	21	na	2.0	na	na	37%
w/turkey, strained	4.5 oz	56	1.5	8.7	27	1.4	1.5	na	na	25%
w/turkey, strained	1 oz	12	0.3	1.9	6	.3	0.3	na	na	24%
w/turkey, strained *(Heinz)*	3.5 oz	47	1.3	6.7	22	.3	1.6	na	na	31%
Vegetable stew										
w/beef, 'Graduates' *(Gerber)*	3.2 oz	71	5.8	8.8	290	na	1.4	na	na	18%
w/beef, 'Graduates' micro cup *(Gerber)*	6 oz	130	10.0	15.0	500	na	3.0	na	na	21%
w/chicken, 'Stages Table Time' *(Beech-Nut)*	6 oz	190	5.0	23.0	340	(mq)	8.0	(mq)	(mq)	39%
Vegetable turkey dinner										
(Earth's Best)	4.5 oz	60	3.0	11.0	15	na	1.0	na	na	14%
junior	7.5 oz	100	3.6	16.4	36	2.3	2.6	na	na	23%
junior	1 oz	13	0.5	2.2	5	.3	0.3	na	na	20%
'2nd Foods' *(Gerber)*	7 tbsp	49	2.2	7.5	12	na	1.2	na	na	22%
'3rd Foods' *(Gerber)*	7 tbsp	53	2.2	8.7	13	na	1.0	na	na	17%
strained	4.5 oz	54	2.2	8.4	17	1.4	1.5	na	na	24%
strained	1 oz	12	0.5	1.9	4	.3	0.3	na	na	22%
toddler	6.25 oz	142	8.5	14.2	591	>.9 c	6.0	na	na	37%
toddler	1 oz	23	1.4	2.3	95	>.1 c	1.0	na	na	38%
EGG YOLK										
'2nd Foods' *(Gerber)*	7 tbsp	193	9.5	1.0	42	na	10.0	na	na	78%
strained	3.3 oz	191	9.4	0.9	37	0	16.3	4.9	691	78%
strained	1 oz	58	2.8	0.3	11	0	4.9	1.5	208	78%
FRUIT										
Apple *(Earth's Best)*	4.5 oz	60	0.0	14.0	5	(mq)	1.0	(tr)	0	14%
Apple, peach, and strawberry, 'Stages 2' *(Beech-Nut)*	4.5 oz	100	0.0	24.0	0	(mq)	0.0	0.0	0	0%
Apple, pear, and banana, 'Stages 2' *(Beech-Nut)*	4.5 oz	100	0.0	24.0	0	(mq)	0.0	0.0	0	0%

Food Name	Serving Size	Calories	Prot. gms	Carbs gms	Sod. mgs	Fiber gms	Fat gms	Sat. Fat gms	Chol. mgs	% Fat Cal.
Apple and apricot										
(Earth's Best)	4.5 oz	70	0.0	15.0	5	(mq)	1.0	(tr)	0	13%
strained (Heinz)	3.5 oz	55	0.3	12.9	3	na	0.3	na	na	5%
Apple and banana										
(Earth's Best)	4.5 oz	80	0.0	18.0	15	(mq)	1.0	(tr)	0	11%
'2nd Foods' (Gerber)	4 oz	60	0.0	15.0	na	na	0.0	na	na	0%
Apple and blueberry										
(Earth's Best)	4.5 oz	60	0.0	14.0	na	(mq)	1.0	(tr)	0	14%
junior	7.75 oz	136	0.4	36.5	29	4.0	0.4	na	na	2%
junior	1 oz	18	0.1	4.7	4	.5	0.1	na	na	5%
junior (Gerber)	6 oz	80	0.0	19.0	2	(mq)	1.0	(tr)	0	11%
'2nd Foods' (Gerber)	7 tbsp	51	0.2	12.1	0	na	0.2	na	na	4%
strained	4.75 oz	82	0.3	22.0	3	2.4	0.3	na	na	3%
strained	1 oz	17	0.1	4.6	1	.5	0.1	na	na	5%
strained (Gerber)	4.5 oz	60	0.0	14.0	1	(mq)	1.0	(tr)	0	14%
'3rd Foods' (Gerber)	7 tbsp	50	0.2	11.8	1	na	0.2	na	na	4%
Apple and cranberry, w/tapioca, strained (Heinz)	3.5 oz	66	0.1	15.9	6	na	0.3	na	na	4%
Apple and pear										
(Heinz)	3.5 oz	56	0.2	13.4	2	na	0.2	na	na	3%
junior	3.5 oz	57	0.2	12.9	1	.6	0.2	na	na	3%
Apple and plum (Earth's Best)	4.5 oz	70	0.0	16.0	10	(mq)	1.0	(tr)	0	12%
Apple and raspberry										
w/sugar, junior	7.75 oz	128	0.4	34.1	4	4.6	0.4	na	na	3%
w/sugar, junior	1 oz	16	0.1	4.4	1	.6	0.1	na	na	5%
w/sugar, strained	4.75 oz	78	0.3	21.2	3	2.8	0.3	na	na	3%
w/sugar, strained	1 oz	16	0.1	4.4	1	.6	0.1	na	na	5%
Applesauce										
'Beginner Foods' (Heinz)	3.5 oz	73	0.1	18.0	1	na	0.1	na	na	1%
'1st Foods' (Gerber)	2.5 oz	35	0.0	9.0	0	(mq)	0.0	0.0	0	0%
'1st Foods' (Gerber)	7 tbsp	56	0.2	13.2	0	na	0.2	na	na	3%
golden delicious, 'Baby's First' (Beech-Nut)	2.5 oz	50	0.0	11.0	0	na	0.0	na	na	0%
golden delicious, 'Stages 1' (Beech-Nut)	4.5 oz	70	0.0	17.0	0	(mq)	0.0	0.0	0	0%
golden delicious, 'Stages 1' (Beech-Nut)	2.8 oz	50	0.0	13.0	0	(mq)	0.0	0.0	0	0%
junior	7.5 oz	79	0.0	21.9	4	3.6	0.0	na	na	0%
junior	1 oz	10	0.0	2.9	1	.5	0.0	na	na	0%
junior (Gerber)	6 oz	90	0.0	20.0	3	(mq)	1.0	(tr)	0	10%
junior (Heinz)	3.5 oz	53	0.2	12.4	2	na	0.2	na	na	3%
'2nd Foods' (Gerber)	7 tbsp	52	0.2	12.3	22	na	0.2	na	na	4%
'Stages 3' (Beech-Nut)	6 oz	90	0.0	22.0	0	(mq)	0.0	0.0	0	0%
strained	4.5 oz	52	0.3	14.0	3	2.2	0.3	na	na	5%
strained	1 oz	12	0.1	3.1	1	.5	0.1	na	na	7%
strained (Gerber)	4.5 oz	60	0.0	14.0	3	(mq)	1.0	(tr)	0	14%
strained (Heinz)	3.5 oz	53	0.2	12.4	2	na	0.2	na	na	3%
'3rd Foods' (Gerber)	7 tbsp	51	0.2	12.1	1	na	0.2	na	na	4%
w/apricot, junior	7.75 oz	103	0.4	27.3	7	4.0	0.4	na	na	3%
w/apricot, junior	1 oz	13	0.1	3.5	1	.5	0.1	na	na	6%
w/apricot, '2nd Foods' (Gerber)	7 tbsp	53	0.3	12.5	1	na	0.2	na	na	3%
w/apricot, 'Stages 2' (Beech-Nut)	4.5 oz	80	0.0	19.0	0	(mq)	0.0	0.0	0	0%
w/apricot, strained	4.75 oz	61	0.3	15.7	4	2.4	0.3	na	na	4%
w/apricot, strained	1 oz	13	0.1	3.3	1	.5	0.1	na	na	6%
w/apricot, strained (Gerber)	4.5 oz	70	0.0	15.0	3	(mq)	1.0	(tr)	0	13%
w/banana, 'Stages 2' (Beech-Nut)	4.5 oz	80	0.0	18.0	0	(mq)	0.0	0.0	0	0%
w/banana, 'Stages 3' (Beech-Nut)	6 oz	100	0.0	25.0	0	(mq)	0.0	0.0	0	0%
w/cherry, junior	7.75 oz	106	0.7	29.0	7	3.3	0.0	na	na	0%

Food Name	Serving Size	Calories	Prot. gms	Carbs gms	Sod. mgs	Fiber gms	Fat gms	Sat. Fat gms	Chol. mgs	% Fat Cal.
w/cherry, junior	1 oz	14	0.1	3.7	1	.4	0.0	na	na	0%
w/cherry, 'Stages 2' (Beech-Nut)	4.5 oz	70	0.0	18.0	5	(mq)	0.0	0.0	0	0%
w/cherry, 'Stages 3' (Beech-Nut)	6 oz	100	0.0	24.0	0	(mq)	0.0	0.0	0	0%
w/cherry, strained	4.75 oz	65	0.4	17.7	3	2.0	0.0	na	na	0%
w/cherry, strained	1 oz	14	0.1	3.7	1	.4	0.0	na	na	0%
w/pineapple, junior	7.5 oz	83	0.2	22.4	4	3.2	0.2	na	na	2%
w/pineapple, junior	1 oz	11	0.0	3.0	1	.4	0.0	na	na	0%
w/pineapple, strained	4.5 oz	47	0.1	12.9	3	1.9	0.1	na	na	2%
w/pineapple, strained	1 oz	10	0.0	2.9	1	.4	0.0	na	na	0%
Apricot										
w/pear, 'Stages 3' (Beech-Nut)	6 oz	120	1.0	27.0	0	(mq)	0.0	0.0	0	0%
w/pear and applesauce, 'Stages 2' (Beech-Nut)	4.5 oz	90	0.0	21.0	0	(mq)	0.0	0.0	0	0%
w/tapioca, junior	7.75 oz	139	0.7	38.1	13	3.3	0.0	na	na	0%
w/tapioca, junior	1 oz	18	0.1	4.9	2	.4	0.0	na	na	0%
w/tapioca, junior (Gerber)	6 oz	130	1.0	29.0	9	(mq)	1.0	(tr)	0	7%
w/tapioca, junior (Heinz)	3.5 oz	66	0.2	15.9	10	na	0.2	na	na	3%
w/tapioca, '2nd Foods' (Gerber)	7 tbsp	67	0.3	16.2	6	na	0.2	na	na	3%
w/tapioca, strained	4.75 oz	81	0.4	22.0	11	2.0	0.0	na	na	0%
w/tapioca, strained	1 oz	17	0.1	4.6	2	.4	0.0	na	na	0%
w/tapioca, strained (Gerber)	4.5 oz	90	0.0	20.0	8	(mq)	1.0	(tr)	0	10%
w/tapioca, strained (Heinz)	3.5 oz	64	0.2	15.3	7	.2	0.2	na	na	3%
w/tapioca, '3rd Foods' (Gerber)	7 tbsp	71	0.3	17.1	5	na	0.2	na	na	3%
Banana										
'Beginner Foods' (Heinz)	3.5 oz	107	1.2	25.0	3	na	0.2	na	na	2%
Chiquita, 'Baby's First' (Beech-Nut)	2.5 oz	70	0.0	16.0	0	na	0.0	na	na	0%
Chiquita, 'Stages 1' (Beech-Nut	4.5 oz	110	1.0	26.0	0	(mq)	0.0	0.0	0	0%
Chiquita, 'Stages 1' (Beech-Nut)	2.8 oz	70	0.0	16.0	0	(mq)	0.0	0.0	0	0%
(Earth's Best)	4.5 oz	100	2.0	22.0	60	(mq)	0.0	0.0	0	0%
'1st Foods' (Gerber)	2.5 oz	70	1.0	17.0	na	(mq)	0.0	0.0	0	0%
'1st Foods' (Gerber)	7 tbsp	100	1.2	23.3	3	na	0.3	na	na	3%
w/pineapple and tapioca, '2nd Foods' (Gerber)	7 tbsp	52	0.4	12.3	na	na	0.1	6.0	na	2%
w/pineapple and tapioca,'3rd Foods' (Gerber)	7 tbsp	52	0.4	12.3	4	na	0.1	na	na	2%
w/tapioca, junior	7.75 oz	147	0.9	39.2	20	3.5	0.4	na	na	2%
w/tapioca, junior	1 oz	19	0.1	5.1	3	.5	0.1	na	na	4%
w/tapioca, junior (Gerber)	6 oz	140	1.0	31.0	15	(mq)	1.0	(tr)	0	7%
w/tapioca, junior (Heinz)	3.5 oz	73	0.2	17.6	8	na	0.2	na	na	3%
w/tapioca, '2nd Foods' (Gerber)	7 tbsp	78	0.5	18.5	5	na	0.2	na	na	2%
w/tapioca, '3rd Foods' (Gerber)	7 tbsp	77	0.5	18.4	5	na	0.2	na	na	2%
w/tapioca, strained	4.75 oz	77	0.5	20.7	12	2.2	0.1	na	na	1%
w/tapioca, strained	1 oz	16	0.1	4.3	3	.5	0.0	na	na	0%
w/tapioca, strained (Gerber)	4.5 oz	110	1.0	24.0	12	(mq)	1.0	(tr)	0	8%
w/tapioca, strained (Heinz)	3.5 oz	73	0.2	17.6	8	na	0.2	na	na	3%
Banana and apple, strained (Gerber)	4.5 oz	90	0.0	20.0	9	(mq)	1.0	(tr)	0	10%
Banana and pear, w/applesauce, 'Stages 2' (Beech-Nut)	4.5 oz	100	0.0	24.0	0	(mq)	0.0	0.0	0	0%
Banana and pineapple										
'Stages 2' (Beech-Nut)	4.5 oz	110	0.0	27.0	15	(mq)	0.0	0.0	0	0%
w/tapioca, junior	4.75 oz	92	0.3	24.8	11	2.2	0.1	na	na	1%
w/tapioca, junior	1 oz	19	0.1	5.2	2	.5	0.0	na	na	0%
w/tapioca, junior (Gerber)	6 oz	90	1.0	20.0	7	(mq)	1.0	(tr)	0	10%
w/tapioca, strained	7.75 oz	143	0.4	39.2	13	3.5	0.0	na	na	0%
w/tapioca, strained	1 oz	18	0.1	5.1	2	.5	0.0	na	na	0%
w/tapioca, strained (Gerber)	4.5 oz	60	1.0	15.0	5	(mq)	0.0	0.0	0	0%
w/tapioca, strained (Heinz)	3.5 oz	64	0.2	15.3	8	.1	0.2	na	na	3%

Food Name	Serving Size	Calories	Prot. gms	Carbs gms	Sod. mgs	Fiber gms	Fat gms	Sat. Fat gms	Chol. mgs	% Fat Cal.
Guava										
w/tapioca, strained	4.5 oz	86	0.4	23.4	3	2.3	0.0	na	na	0%
w/tapioca, strained	1 oz	19	0.1	5.2	1	.5	0.0	na	na	0%
w/tapioca, strained (Gerber)	4.5 oz	90	0.0	20.0	3	(mq)	1.0	na	0	10%
w/tapioca, strained, 'Stages 2' (Beech-Nut)	4.5 oz	100	0.0	24.0	10	(mq)	0.0	0.0	0	0%
Guava and papaya										
w/tapioca, strained	4.5 oz	81	0.3	21.8	5	>.6 c	0.1	na	na	1%
w/tapioca, strained	1 oz	18	0.1	4.8	1	>.1 c	0.0	na	na	0%
Mango										
tropical fruit dessert, 'Stages 2' (Beech-Nut)	4.5 oz	100	0.0	25.0	15	(mq)	0.0	0.0	0	0%
w/tapioca, strained	4.75 oz	108	0.4	29.2	5	1.4	0.3	na	na	2%
w/tapioca, strained	1 oz	23	0.1	6.1	1	.3	0.1	na	na	4%
w/tapioca, strained (Gerber)	4.5 oz	90	0.0	21.0	4	(mq)	1.0	(tr)	0	10%
Mango and banana, w/passion fruit and tapioca,										
strained (Gerber)	4.5 oz	100	0.0	25.0	12	(mq)	0.0	0.0	0	0%
Papaya										
'Stages 2' (Beech-Nut)	4.5 oz	100	0.0	24.0	15	(mq)	0.0	0.0	0	0%
w/tapioca, strained (Gerber)	4.5 oz	80	0.0	19.0	9	(mq)	1.0	(tr)	0	11%
Papaya and applesauce										
w/tapioca, strained	4.5 oz	90	0.3	24.2	6	1.8	0.1	na	na	1%
w/tapioca, strained	1 oz	20	0.1	5.4	1	.4	0.0	na	na	0%
Peach										
'Beginner Foods' (Heinz)	3.5 oz	80	1.2	18.3	2	na	0.2	na	na	2%
'1st Foods' (Gerber)	2.5 oz	30	0.0	7.0	na	(mq)	0.0	0.0	0	0%
'1st Foods' (Gerber)	7 tbsp	43	0.7	9.6	1	na	0.2	na	na	4%
junior (Gerber)	6 oz	110	1.0	25.0	5	(mq)	1.0	(tr)	0	8%
junior (Heinz)	3.5 oz	68	0.9	15.4	7	.7	0.3	na	na	4%
'2nd Foods' (Gerber)	7 tbsp	66	0.7	15.3	3	na	0.2	na	na	3%
'Stages 3' (Beech-Nut)	6 oz	90	1.0	22.0	0	(mq)	0.0	0.0	0	0%
strained (Gerber)	4.5 oz	90	1.0	19.0	4	(mq)	1.0	(tr)	0	10%
strained (Heinz)	3.5 oz	68	0.9	15.4	7	.7	0.3	na	na	4%
'3rd Foods' (Gerber)	7 tbsp	65	0.7	15.1	2	na	0.2	na	na	3%
w/mango and tapioca, strained (Gerber)	4.5 oz	100	0.0	24.0	9	(mq)	1.0	(tr)	0	9%
w/oatmeal and banana (Earth's Best)	4.5 oz	70	2.0	15.0	5	(mq)	1.0	na	0	12%
w/sugar, junior	7.75 oz	156	1.1	41.6	11	3.3	0.4	na	na	2%
w/sugar, junior	1 oz	20	0.1	5.4	1	.4	0.1	na	na	4%
w/sugar, strained	4.75 oz	96	0.7	25.5	8	2.0	0.3	na	na	3%
w/sugar, strained	1 oz	20	0.1	5.4	2	.4	0.1	na	na	4%
w/yogurt, 'Stages 2' (Beech-Nut)	4.5 oz	120	1.0	25.0	30	(mq)	2.0	(mq)	(mq)	15%
yellow cling, 'Baby's First' (Beech-Nut)	2.5 oz	45	0.0	10.0	0	na	0.0	na	na	0%
yellow cling, 'Stages 1' (Beech-Nut)	4.5 oz	70	0.0	15.0	0	(mq)	0.0	0.0	0	0%
yellow cling, 'Stages 1' (Beech-Nut)	2.8 oz	50	0.0	12.0	0	(mq)	0.0	0.0	0	0%
Pear										
Bartlett, 'Baby's First' (Beech-Nut)	2.5 oz	50	0.0	12.0	0	na	0.0	na	na	0%
Bartlett, 'Stages 1' (Beech-Nut)	4.5 oz	70	0.0	18.0	0	(mq)	0.0	0.0	0	0%
Bartlett, 'Stages 1' (Beech-Nut)	2.8 oz	50	0.0	13.0	0	(mq)	0.0	0.0	0	0%
Bartlett, 'Stages 3' (Beech-Nut)	6 oz	100	0.0	24.0	5	(mq)	0.0	0.0	0	0%
Bartlett, w/applesauce, 'Stages 2' (Beech-Nut)	4.5 oz	80	0.0	20.0	0	(mq)	0.0	0.0	0	0%
Bartlett, w/pineapple, 'Stages 2' (Beech-Nut)	4.5 oz	90	0.0	21.0	0	(mq)	0.0	0.0	0	0%
'Beginner Foods' (Heinz)	3.5 oz	76	0.5	18.0	3	na	0.2	na	na	2%
(Earth's Best)	4.5 oz	60	0.0	14.0	11	(mq)	0.0	0.0	0	0%
'1st Foods' (Gerber)	2.5 oz	40	0.0	11.0	2	(mq)	0.0	0.0	0	0%
'1st Foods' (Gerber)	7 tbsp	57	0.4	13.2	1	na	0.3	na	na	5%
junior	7.5 oz	92	0.6	24.7	4	7.7	0.2	na	na	2%

Food Name	Serving Size	Calories	Prot. gms	Carbs gms	Sod. mgs	Fiber gms	Fat gms	Sat. Fat gms	Chol. mgs	% Fat Cal.
junior	1 oz	12	0.1	3.3	1	1.0	0.0	na	na	0%
junior *(Gerber)*	6 oz	100	1.0	21.0	2	(mq)	1.0	(tr)	0	9%
junior *(Heinz)*	3.5 oz	60	0.4	14.1	3	na	0.2	na	na	3%
'2nd Foods' *(Gerber)*	7 tbsp	55	0.4	12.9	0	na	0.2	na	na	3%
strained	4.5 oz	52	0.4	13.8	3	4.6	0.3	na	na	5%
strained	1 oz	12	0.1	3.1	1	1.0	0.1	na	na	7%
strained *(Gerber)*	4.5 oz	80	1.0	16.0	3	(mq)	1.0	(tr)	0	12%
strained *(Heinz)*	3.5 oz	60	0.4	14.1	3	na	0.2	na	na	3%
'3rd Foods' *(Gerber)*	7 tbsp	55	0.4	12.9	2	na	0.2	na	na	3%
Pear and pineapple										
junior	7.5 oz	94	0.6	24.3	2	5.5	0.4	na	na	4%
junior	1 oz	12	0.1	3.2	0	.7	0.1	na	na	6%
junior *(Gerber)*	6 oz	100	1.0	21.0	3	(mq)	1.0	(tr)	0	9%
'2nd Foods' *(Gerber)*	7 tbsp	55	0.4	12.8	1	na	0.2	na	na	3%
strained	4.5 oz	52	0.4	14.0	5	3.3	0.1	na	na	2%
strained	1 oz	12	0.1	3.1	1	.7	0.0	na	na	0%
strained *(Gerber)*	4.5 oz	80	1.0	16.0	3	(mq)	1.0	(tr)	0	12%
'3rd Foods' *(Gerber)*	7 tbsp	54	0.4	12.7	2	na	0.2	na	na	3%
Pears and raspberries, *(Earth's Best)*	4.5 oz	60	0.0	15.0	0	na	0.0	na	na	0%
Plum										
w/banana and rice *(Earth's Best)*	4.5 oz	90	2.0	19.0	15	(mq)	0.0	0.0	0	0%
w/rice, 'Stages 2' *(Beech-Nut)*	4.5 oz	150	1.0	34.0	0	(mq)	0.0	0.0	0	0%
w/tapioca, junior *(Gerber)*	6 oz	130	1.0	30.0	3	(mq)	1.0	(tr)	0	7%
w/tapioca, '2nd Foods' *(Gerber)*	7 tbsp	74	0.3	17.7	3	na	0.2	na	na	2%
w/tapioca, strained *(Gerber)*	4.5 oz	90	0.0	22.0	5	(mq)	0.0	0.0	0	0%
w/tapioca, strained *(Heinz)*	3.5 oz	67	0.2	16.2	9	na	0.2	na	na	3%
w/tapioca, '3rd Foods' *(Gerber)*	7 tbsp	75	0.3	18.1	2	na	0.2	na	na	2%
w/tapioca, w/o ascorbic acid, junior	7.75 oz	163	0.2	44.9	18	2.6	0.0	na	na	0%
w/tapioca, w/o ascorbic acid, junior	1 oz	21	0.0	5.8	2	.3	0.0	na	na	0%
w/tapioca, w/o ascorbic acid, strained	4.75 oz	96	0.1	26.6	8	1.6	0.0	na	na	0%
w/tapioca, w/o ascorbic acid, strained	1 oz	20	0.0	5.6	2	.3	0.0	na	na	0%
Prune										
'1st Foods' *(Gerber)*	2.5 oz	70	1.0	17.0	na	(mq)	0.0	0.0	0	0%
'1st Foods' *(Gerber)*	7 tbsp	101	1.0	23.8	6	na	0.2	na	na	2%
w/oatmeal *(Earth's Best)*	4.5 oz	100	1.0	24.0	20	(mq)	0.0	0.0	0	0%
w/pear, 'Stages 2' *(Beech-Nut)*	4.5 oz	90	0.0	22.0	0	(mq)	0.0	0.0	0	0%
w/tapioca, '2nd Foods' *(Gerber)*	7 tbsp	77	0.7	18.1	4	na	0.2	na	na	2%
w/tapioca, strained *(Gerber)*	4.5 oz	100	1.0	22.0	5	(mq)	1.0	(tr)	0	9%
w/tapioca, strained *(Heinz)*	3.5 oz	90	0.5	21.5	8	na	0.2	na	na	2%
w/tapioca, w/o ascorbic acid, junior	7.75 oz	154	1.3	41.1	4	5.9	0.2	na	na	1%
w/tapioca, w/o ascorbic acid, junior	1 oz	20	0.2	5.3	1	.8	0.0	na	na	0%
w/tapioca, w/o ascorbic acid, strained	4.75 oz	94	0.8	25.0	7	3.7	0.1	na	na	1%
w/tapioca, w/o ascorbic acid, strained	1 oz	20	0.2	5.2	1	.8	0.0	na	na	0%
INFANT FORMULA										
Mix										
liquid, iron-fortified, prepared, 'Follow-Up' *(Carnation)*	5 oz	100	2.6	13.2	39	na	4.1	na	na	37%
liquid, iron-fortified, prepared, 'Good Start' *(Carnation)*	5 oz	100	2.4	11.0	24	na	5.1	na	na	46%
liquid, low-iron, prepared *(Enfamil)*	5 oz	100	2.2	10.3	27	na	5.6	na	na	50%
liquid, low-iron, prepared *(Gerber)*	5 oz	100	3.0	10.0	47	na	5.3	na	na	48%
liquid, low-iron, prepared *(Similac)*	5 oz	100	2.1	10.7	27	na	5.4	na	na	49%
liquid, soy, iron-fortified, milk-free *(Nursoy)*	5 oz	100	2.7	10.2	30	na	5.3	na	na	48%
liquid, soy, iron-fortified, milk-free, prepared *(Gerber)*	5 oz	100	3.0	10.0	47	na	5.3	na	na	48%
liquid, soy, iron-fortified, milk-free, prepared *(ProSobee)*	5 oz	100	3.0	10.0	36	na	5.3	na	na	48%
liquid, soy, w/iron, milk-free, prepared *(Isomil)*	5 oz	100	2.5	10.3	44	na	5.4	na	na	49%

Food Name	Serving Size	Calories	Prot. gms	Carbs gms	Sod. mgs	Fiber gms	Fat gms	Sat. Fat gms	Chol. mgs	% Fat Cal.
liquid, w/iron, prepared (Enfamil)	5 oz	100	2.2	10.3	27	na	5.6	na	na	50%
liquid, w/iron, prepared (Gerber)	5 oz	100	2.2	10.7	33	na	5.4	na	na	49%
liquid, w/iron, prepared (Similac)	5 oz	100	2.1	10.7	27	na	5.4	na	na	49%
powder, iron-fortified, prepared, 'Follow-Up' (Carnation)	5 oz	100	2.6	13.2	39	na	4.1	na	na	37%
powder, iron-fortified, prepared, 'Good Start' (Carnation)	5 oz	100	2.4	11.0	24	na	5.1	na	na	46%
powder, low-iron, prepared (Enfamil)	5 oz	100	2.2	10.3	27	na	5.6	na	na	50%
powder, low-iron, prepared (Gerber)	5 oz	100	3.0	10.0	47	na	5.3	na	na	48%
powder, low-iron, prepared (Similac)	5 oz	100	2.1	10.7	27	na	5.4	na	na	49%
powder, soy, iron-fortified, milk-free, prepared (Gerber)	5 oz	100	3.0	10.0	47	na	5.3	na	na	48%
powder, soy, iron-fortified, milk-free, prepared (ProSobee)	5 oz	100	3.0	10.0	36	na	5.3	na	na	48%
powder, soy, w/iron, milk-free, prepared (Isomil)	5 oz	100	2.5	10.3	44	na	5.5	na	na	49%
powder, w/iron, prepared (Enfamil)	5 oz	100	2.2	10.3	27	na	5.6	na	na	50%
powder, w/iron, prepared (Gerber)	5 oz	100	2.2	10.7	33	na	5.4	na	na	49%
powder, w/iron, prepared (Similac)	5 oz	100	2.1	10.7	27	na	5.4	na	na	49%
Ready to use										
iron-fortified, 'Follow-Up' (Carnation)	5 oz	100	2.6	13.2	39	na	4.1	na	na	37%
iron-fortified, 'Good Start' (Carnation)	5 oz	100	2.4	11.0	24	na	5.1	na	na	46%
low-iron (Enfamil)	5 oz	100	2.2	10.3	27	na	5.6	na	na	50%
low-iron (Gerber)	5 oz	100	3.0	10.0	47	na	5.3	na	na	48%
low-iron (Similac)	5 oz	100	2.1	10.7	27	na	5.4	na	na	49%
soy, iron-fortified, milk-free (Gerber)	5 oz	100	3.0	10.0	47	na	5.3	na	na	48%
soy, iron-fortified, milk-free (ProSobee)	5 oz	100	3.0	10.0	36	na	5.3	na	na	48%
soy, w/iron, milk-free (Isomil)	5 oz	100	2.5	10.3	44	na	5.4	na	na	49%
w/iron (Enfamil)	5 oz	100	2.2	10.3	27	na	5.6	na	na	50%
w/iron (Gerber)	5 oz	100	2.2	10.7	33	na	5.4	na	na	49%
w/iron (Similac)	5 oz	100	2.1	10.7	27	na	5.4	na	na	49%
JUICE										
Apple										
	4.2 oz	61	0.0	15.2	4	.1	0.1	na	na	2%
	1 oz	15	0.0	3.6	1	tr	0.0	na	na	0%
(Earth's Best)	4.2 oz	60	0.0	14.0	20	(mq)	0.0	0.0	0	0%
'Graduates' (Gerber)	6 oz	80	0.0	21.0	0	na	0.0	na	na	0%
'Graduates' (Gerber)	3.2 oz	48	0.1	11.7	2	na	0.1	na	na	2%
100% juice, 'Junior' (McCain)	4.2 oz	50	0.0	13.0	5	na	0.0	na	na	0%
'Stages 1' (Beech-Nut)	4.2 oz	60	0.0	14.0	5	(mq)	0.0	0.0	0	0%
strained, '1st Foods' (Gerber)	4 oz	60	0.0	14.0	2	(mq)	0.0	0.0	0	0%
strained, '1st Foods' (Gerber)	3.2 oz	46	0.1	11.0	1	na	0.1	na	na	2%
strained (Heinz)	3.5 oz	48	0.1	11.7	5	.1	0.2	na	na	4%
strained, 'Saver Size' (Heinz	4.2 oz	70	0.0	17.0	15	na	0.0	0.0	na	0%
w/yogurt, 2nd Foods' (Gerber)	3.2 oz	73	2.0	14.2	32	na	0.9	na	na	11%
Apple-apricot, strained (Heinz)	3.5 oz	47	0.2	11.2	8	.2	0.2	na	na	4%
Apple-banana										
(Earth's Best)	4.2 oz	60	0.0	14.0	2	(mq)	0.0	0.0	0	0%
'Graduates' (Gerber)	6 oz	90	0.0	23.0	10	na	0.0	na	na	0%
'Graduates' (Gerber)	3.2 oz	51	0.1	12.5	2	na	0.1	na	na	2%
'2nd Foods' (Gerber)	3.2 oz	51	0.2	12.3	2	na	0.1	na	na	2%
strained (Heinz)	3.5 oz	52	0.1	12.5	6	na	0.2	na	na	3%
Apple-carrot										
'3rd Foods' (Gerber)	4 oz	50	0.0	12.0	15	na	0.0	na	na	0%
'3rd Foods' (Gerber)	3.2 oz	42	0.1	10.0	10	na	0.1	na	na	2%
Apple-cherry										
	4.2 oz	53	0.1	12.9	4	.1	0.3	na	na	5%
	1 oz	13	0.0	3.1	1	tr	0.1	na	na	7%
'Graduates' (Gerber)	6 oz	80	0.0	21.0	25	na	0.0	na	na	0%

Food Name	Serving Size	Calories	Prot. gms	Carbs gms	Sod. mgs	Fiber gms	Fat gms	Sat. Fat gms	Chol. mgs	% Fat Cal.
'Graduates' *(Gerber)*	3.2 oz	51	0.1	12.4	3	na	0.1	na	na	2%
100% juice, 'Junior' *(McCain)*	4.2 oz	50	0.0	13.0	5	na	0.0	na	na	0%
'2nd Foods' *(Gerber)*	4 oz	60	0.0	14.0	na	na	0.0	na	na	0%
'2nd Foods' *(Gerber)*	3.2 oz	48	0.2	11.5	5	na	0.1	na	na	2%
'Stages 2' *(Beech-Nut)*	4 oz	60	0.0	14.0	5	(mq)	0.0	0.0	0	0%
strained *(Heinz)*	3.5 oz	45	0.1	10.7	7	.1	0.2	na	na	4%
Apple-cranberry										
'Stages 2' *(Beech-Nut)*	4 oz	60	0.0	14.0	5	(mq)	0.0	0.0	0	0%
strained *(Heinz)*	3.5 oz	48	0.1	11.5	7	na	0.2	na	na	4%
Apple-grape										
	4.2 oz	60	0.1	14.8	4	.1	0.3	na	na	4%
	1 oz	14	0.0	3.5	1	tr	0.1	na	na	6%
(Earth's Best)	4.2 oz	60	0.0	14.0	15	(mq)	0.0	0.0	0	0%
'Graduates' *(Gerber)*	6 oz	90	0.0	22.0	40	na	0.0	na	na	0%
'Graduates' *(Gerber)*	3.2 oz	51	0.0	12.4	3	na	0.1	na	na	2%
'2nd Foods' *(Gerber)*	4 oz	60	0.0	15.0	na	na	0.0	na	na	0%
'2nd Foods' *(Gerber)*	3.2 oz	48	0.1	11.7	7	na	0.1	na	na	2%
'Stages 2' *(Beech-Nut)*	4 oz	70	0.0	16.0	15	(mq)	0.0	0.0	0	0%
strained *(Heinz)*	3.5 oz	47	0.1	11.3	7	na	0.2	na	na	4%
Apple-peach										
	4.2 oz	55	0.3	13.6	1	.1	0.1	na	na	2%
	1 oz	13	0.1	3.3	0	tr	0.0	na	na	0%
'2nd Foods' *(Gerber)*	3.2 oz	47	0.2	11.3	5	na	0.1	na	na	2%
'2nd Foods' *(Gerber)*	4 oz	60	0.0	14.0	na	na	0.0	na	na	0%
strained *(Heinz)*	3.5 oz	44	0.2	10.4	7	.2	0.2	na	na	4%
Apple-pineapple, strained *(Heinz)*	3.5 oz	47	0.2	11.1	6	na	0.2	na	na	4%
Apple-plum										
	4.2 oz	64	0.1	16.0	1	.1	0.0	na	na	0%
	1 oz	15	0.0	3.8	0	tr	0.0	na	na	0%
'2nd Foods' *(Gerber)*	4 oz	60	0.0	15.0	na	na	0.0	na	na	0%
'2nd Foods' *(Gerber)*	3.2 oz	48	0.2	11.7	8	na	0.1	na	na	2%
Apple-prune										
	4.2 oz	95	0.3	23.4	7	.1	0.1	na	na	1%
	1 oz	23	0.1	5.6	2	tr	0.0	na	na	0%
'2nd Foods' *(Gerber)*	4 oz	60	0.0	16.0	na	na	0.0	na	na	0%
'2nd Foods' *(Gerber)*	3.2 oz	53	0.2	12.8	4	na	0.1	na	na	2%
strained *(Heinz)*	3.5 oz	50	0.2	11.9	7	na	0.2	na	na	4%
Apple-sweet potato, '3rd Foods' *(Gerber)*	3.2 oz	48	0.3	11.4	5	na	0.1	na	na	2%
Banana										
w/yogurt, '2nd Foods' *(Gerber)*	4 oz	110	3.0	21.0	na	na	2.0	na	na	16%
w/yogurt, '2nd Foods' *(Gerber)*	3.2 oz	84	2.2	16.5	37	na	1.0	na	na	11%
Grape										
'Juice Plus,' 'Stages 2' *(Beech-Nut)*	4 oz	90	0.0	22.0	10	(mq)	0.0	0.0	0	0%
red, '1st Foods' *(Gerber)*	4 oz	80	0.0	20.0	na	na	0.0	na	na	0%
red, '1st Foods' *(Gerber)*	3.2 oz	65	0.4	15.4	5	na	0.1	na	na	1%
white, '1st Foods' *(Gerber)*	4 oz	80	0.0	19.0	na	na	0.0	na	na	0%
white, '1st Foods' *(Gerber)*	3.2 oz	65	0.4	15.6	6	na	0.1	na	na	1%
white, 'Stages 1' *(Beech-Nut)*	4.2 oz	80	0.0	20.0	10	(mq)	0.0	0.0	0	0%
white, strained *(Heinz)*	3.5 oz	58	0.4	13.8	6	.2	0.2	na	na	3%
Guava, w/mixed fruit, 'Tropical Foods' *(Gerber)*	3.2 oz	58	0.3	13.8	6	na	0.1	na	na	2%
Mango, w/mixed fruit 'Tropical Foods' *(Gerber)*	3.2 oz	59	0.2	14.2	5	na	0.1	na	na	2%
Mango nectar, w/grape and pear juice										
'Stages 2' *(Beech-Nut)*	4 oz	80	0.0	19.0	5	na	0.0	na	na	0%

Food Name	Serving Size	Calories	Prot. gms	Carbs gms	Sod. mgs	Fiber gms	Fat gms	Sat. Fat gms	Chol. mgs	% Fat Cal.
Mixed fruit										
. . . .	4.2 oz	61	0.1	15.1	5	.1	0.1	na	na	2%
. . . .	1 oz	15	0.0	3.6	1	tr	0.0	na	na	0%
100% juice, 'Junior' (McCain)	4.2 oz	60	0.0	15.0	5	na	0.0	na	na	0%
'2nd Foods' (Gerber)	4 oz	60	0.0	14.0	na	na	0.0	na	na	0%
'2nd Foods' (Gerber)	3.2 oz	49	0.3	11.8	4	na	0.1	na	na	2%
'Stages 2' (Beech-Nut)	4 oz	70	0.0	16.0	10	(mq)	0.0	0.0	0	0%
strained (Heinz)	3.5 oz	50	0.3	11.7	6	na	0.2	na	na	4%
w/yogurt, '2nd Foods' (Gerber)	4 oz	100	3.0	18.0	na	na	2.0	na	na	18%
w/yogurt, '2nd Foods' (Gerber)	3.2 oz	75	2.2	14.4	36	na	0.9	na	na	11%
Orange										
. . . .	4.2 oz	57	0.8	13.3	1	.1	0.4	na	na	6%
. . . .	1 oz	14	0.2	3.2	0	tr	0.1	na	na	6%
'2nd Foods' (Gerber)	4 oz	60	1.0	13.0	na	na	0.0	na	na	0%
'2nd Foods' (Gerber)	3.2 oz	46	0.7	10.3	2	na	0.3	na	na	6%
'Stages 3' (Beech-Nut)	4 oz	60	0.0	14.0	0	(mq)	0.0	0.0	0	0%
strained (Heinz)	3.5 oz	48	0.7	10.7	5	na	0.3	na	na	6%
Orange-apple										
. . . .	4.2 oz	56	0.5	13.1	4	.1	0.3	na	na	5%
. . . .	1 oz	13	0.1	3.1	1	tr	0.1	na	na	7%
strained (Heinz)	3.5 oz	50	0.4	11.4	8	na	0.3	na	na	5%
w/banana	4.2 oz	61	0.5	14.9	5	.1	0.1	na	na	1%
w/banana	1 oz	15	0.1	3.6	1	tr	0.0	na	na	0%
Orange-apricot										
. . . .	4.2 oz	60	1.0	14.2	8	.1	0.1	na	na	2%
. . . .	1 oz	14	0.3	3.4	2	tr	0.0	na	na	0%
Orange-banana										
. . . .	4.2 oz	65	0.9	15.5	4	.1	0.1	na	na	1%
. . . .	1 oz	15	0.2	3.7	1	tr	0.0	na	na	0%
Orange-carrot, '3rd Foods' (Gerber)	3.2 oz	43	0.5	9.9	10	na	0.1	na	na	2%
Orange-pineapple										
. . . .	4.2 oz	62	0.7	15.2	3	.1	0.1	na	na	1%
. . . .	1 oz	15	0.2	3.6	1	tr	0.0	na	na	0%
Papaya, w/mixed fruit, 'Tropical Foods' (Gerber)	3.2 oz	57	0.3	13.5	5	na	0.2	na	na	3%
Papaya nectar, w/pear and grape juice,										
'Stages 2' (Beech-Nut)	4 oz	70	0.0	17.0	10	na	0.0	na	na	0%
Peach nectar, w/pear and grape juice,										
'Stages 2' (Beech-Nut)	4 oz	70	0.0	17.0	10	na	0.0	na	na	0%
Pear										
(Earth's Best)	4.2 oz	60	0.0	15.0	0	(mq)	0.0	0.0	0	0%
'Stages 1' (Beech-Nut)	4 oz	60	0.0	15.0	5	(mq)	0.0	0.0	0	0%
strained (Heinz)	3.5 oz	49	0.2	11.7	9	na	0.2	na	na	4%
strained, '1st Foods' (Gerber)	4 oz	60	0.0	14.0	6	(mq)	0.0	0.0	0	0%
strained, '1st Foods' (Gerber)	3.2 oz	46	0.1	11.1	1	na	0.1	na	na	2%
strained, 'Saver Size' (Heinz)	4.2 oz	70	0.0	15.0	25	na	1.0	na	na	13%
Pear-grape, strained (Heinz)	3.5 oz	43	0.1	10.5	4	na	0.1	na	na	2%
Pear-peach										
w/yogurt, '2nd Foods' (Gerber)	4 oz	90	3.0	18.0	na	na	1.0	na	na	10%
w/yogurt, '2nd Foods' (Gerber)	3.2 oz	72	2.2	14.0	34	na	0.9	na	na	11%
Pineapple-carrot										
'3rd Foods' (Gerber)	4 oz	60	1.0	13.0	15	na	0.0	na	na	0%
'3rd Foods' (Gerber)	3.2 oz	47	0.4	11.0	10	na	0.1	na	na	2%
Prune-orange										
. . . .	4.2 oz	91	0.8	21.8	3	.1	0.4	na	na	4%

Food Name	Serving Size	Calories	Prot. gms	Carbs gms	Sod. mgs	Fiber gms	Fat gms	Sat. Fat gms	Chol. mgs	% Fat Cal.
....	1 oz	22	0.2	5.2	1	tr	0.1	na	na	4%
Tropical blend, 'Stages 2' (Beech-Nut)	4 oz	70	0.0	17.0	5	(mq)	0.0	0.0	0	0%
Tropical blend nectar, 'Stages 2' (Beech-Nut)	4 oz	90	0.0	21.0	10	na	0.0	na	na	0%
MEAT										
Beef										
junior	3.5 oz	105	14.4	0.0	65	0	4.8	2.6	na	43%
junior	1 oz	30	4.1	0.0	19	0	1.4	0.7	na	43%
'2nd Foods' (Gerber)	7 tbsp	100	14.4	0.1	52	na	4.7	na	na	42%
strained	3.5 oz	106	13.5	0.0	80	0	5.3	2.5	na	47%
strained	1 oz	30	3.9	0.0	23	0	1.5	0.7	na	46%
'3rd Foods' (Gerber)	7 tbsp	103	15.1	0.2	52	na	4.6	na	na	40%
w/beef heart, strained	3.5 oz	93	12.6	0.0	62	0	4.4	2.1	na	44%
w/beef heart, strained	1 oz	27	3.6	0.0	18	0	1.3	0.6	na	45%
w/broth, junior (Heinz)	3.5 oz	123	14.6	0.3	53	.4	7.2	na	na	52%
w/broth, 'Stages 1' (Beech-Nut)	2.5 oz	80	9.0	0.0	40	na	5.0	na	na	56%
w/broth, strained (Heinz)	3.5 oz	123	14.6	0.3	53	.4	7.2	na	na	52%
w/egg yolks, strained (Gerber)	2.5 oz	80	10.0	0.0	38	0	4.0	(mq)	21	47%
Chicken										
junior	3.5 oz	148	14.5	0.0	50	0	9.5	2.5	na	60%
junior	1 oz	42	4.2	0.0	14	0	2.7	0.7	na	59%
'2nd Foods' (Gerber)	7 tbsp	128	14.1	0.0	40	na	7.9	na	na	56%
'Stages 1' (Beech-Nut)	2.8 oz	80	10.0	0.0	55	0	4.0	(mq)	(mq)	47%
strained	3.5 oz	129	13.6	0.1	47	0	7.8	2.0	na	56%
strained	1 oz	37	3.9	0.0	13	0	2.2	0.6	na	56%
'3rd Foods' (Gerber)	7 tbsp	132	15.0	0.2	39	na	7.9	na	na	54%
w/broth, junior (Heinz)	3.5 oz	143	13.5	0.7	59	.1	9.7	na	na	61%
w/broth, 'Stages 1' (Beech-Nut)	2.5 oz	70	9.0	0.0	55	na	4.0	na	na	50%
w/broth, strained (Heinz)	3.5 oz	143	13.5	0.7	59	.1	9.7	na	na	61%
Chicken sticks										
finger snacks, 'Graduates' (Gerber)	10 sticks	143	15.4	1.6	445	na	8.3	na	na	52%
junior	1 stick	19	1.5	0.1	48	0	1.4	na	na	66%
Ham										
junior	3.5 oz	124	14.9	0.0	66	0	6.6	2.2	na	50%
junior	1 oz	35	4.3	0.0	19	0	1.9	0.6	na	50%
junior (Gerber)	2.5 oz	90	11.0	0.0	30	0	5.0	(mq)	21	51%
'2nd Foods' (Gerber)	7 tbsp	120	13.7	0.2	42	na	7.1	na	na	54%
strained	3.5 oz	110	13.8	0.0	41	0	5.7	1.9	na	48%
strained	1 oz	31	3.9	0.0	12	0	1.6	0.6	na	48%
'3rd Foods' (Gerber)	7 tbsp	123	14.5	0.1	42	na	7.2	na	na	53%
w/egg yolks, strained (Gerber)	2.5 oz	90	10.0	1.0	30	0	5.0	(mq)	17	51%
Lamb										
junior	3.5 oz	111	15.1	0.0	72	0	5.2	2.5	na	44%
junior	1 oz	32	4.3	0.0	21	0	1.5	0.7	na	44%
'2nd Foods' (Gerber)	7 tbsp	104	15.1	0.0	51	na	4.8	na	na	42%
'Stages 1' (Beech-Nut)	2.8 oz	70	9.0	0.0	50	0	3.0	(mq)	(mq)	43%
strained	3.5 oz	102	14.0	0.1	61	0	4.7	2.3	na	43%
strained	1 oz	29	4.0	0.0	18	0	1.3	0.7	na	42%
w/broth, 'Stages 1' (Beech-Nut)	2.5 oz	60	9.0	0.0	50	na	3.0	na	na	43%
w/broth, strained (Heinz)	3.5 oz	129	15.3	0.2	59	.2	7.6	na	na	53%
w/egg yolks, strained (Gerber)	2.5 oz	70	10.0	1.0	36	0	3.0	(mq)	27	38%
Liver										
strained	3.5 oz	100	14.2	1.4	73	0	3.8	1.4	182	35%
strained	1 oz	29	4.1	0.4	21	0	1.1	0.4	52	36%
w/liver broth, strained (Heinz)	3.5 oz	100	14.3	3.6	49	.1	3.2	na	na	29%

Food Name	Serving Size	Calories	Prot. gms	Carbs gms	Sod. mgs	Fiber gms	Fat gms	Sat. Fat gms	Chol. mgs	% Fat Cal.
Meat sticks										
finger snacks, 'Graduates' (Gerber)	10 sticks	150	14.5	1.5	451	na	9.6	na	na	57%
junior	1 stick	18	1.3	0.1	55	0	1.5	0.6	na	71%
Pork										
strained	3.5 oz	123	13.9	0.0	42	0	7.0	2.4	na	53%
strained	1 oz	35	4.0	0.0	12	0	2.0	0.7	na	53%
Turkey										
junior	3.5 oz	128	15.2	0.0	71	0	7.0	2.3	na	51%
junior	1 oz	37	4.4	0.0	20	0	2.0	0.7	na	51%
'2nd Foods' (Gerber)	7 tbsp	109	13.7	0.2	54	na	5.9	na	na	49%
'Stages 1' (Beech-Nut)	2.8 oz	100	9.0	0.0	50	0	6.0	(mq)	(mq)	60%
strained	3.5 oz	113	14.2	0.1	54	0	5.7	1.9	na	47%
strained	1 oz	32	4.1	0.0	16	0	1.6	0.5	na	47%
'3rd Foods' (Gerber)	7 tbsp	115	14.8	0.1	52	na	6.1	na	na	48%
w/broth, 'Stages 1' (Beech-Nut)	2.5 oz	90	8.0	0.0	40	na	6.0	na	na	63%
w/broth, strained (Heinz)	3.5 oz	137	14.9	0.4	49	.8	8.6	na	na	56%
w/egg yolks, strained (Gerber)	2.5 oz	100	10.0	1.0	38	0	6.0	(mq)	42	55%
Turkey sticks										
finger snacks, 'Graduates' (Gerber)	10 sticks	141	14.5	1.5	425	na	8.5	na	na	54%
junior	1 stick	18	1.4	0.1	48	.1	1.4	na	na	68%
Veal										
junior	3.5 oz	109	15.1	0.0	68	0	4.9	2.4	na	42%
junior	1 oz	31	4.3	0.0	20	0	1.4	0.7	na	42%
junior (Gerber)	2.5 oz	80	11.0	0.0	39	0	4.0	(mq)	19	45%
'2nd Foods' (Gerber)	7 tbsp	102	14.1	0.1	55	na	5.1	na	na	45%
'Stages 1' (Beech-Nut)	2.8 oz	60	10.0	0.0	50	0	2.0	(mq)	(mq)	31%
strained	3.5 oz	100	13.4	0.0	63	0	4.8	2.3	na	45%
strained	1 oz	29	3.8	0.0	18	0	1.4	0.7	na	45%
'3rd Foods' (Gerber)	7 tbsp	108	15.5	0.0	56	na	5.0	na	na	42%
w/broth, 'Stages 1' (Beech-Nut)	2.5 oz	70	10.0	0.0	50	na	3.0	na	na	40%
w/broth, strained (Heinz)	3.5 oz	130	15.1	0.2	57	.5	7.9	na	na	54%
w/egg yolks, strained (Gerber)	2.5 oz	80	10.0	1.0	38	0	4.0	(mq)	18	45%
Veal and beef										
junior (Gerber)	6 oz	110	4.0	16.0	31	(mq)	3.0	(mq)	7	25%
strained (Gerber)	4.5 oz	90	3.0	11.0	17	(mq)	4.0	(mq)	5	39%
Veal and ham										
junior (Gerber)	6 oz	120	3.0	17.0	24	(mq)	4.0	(mq)	7	31%
strained (Gerber)	4.5 oz	80	2.0	11.0	14	(mq)	3.0	(mq)	4	34%
Veal and turkey										
junior (Gerber)	6 oz	100	3.0	15.0	24	(mq)	3.0	(mq)	19	27%
strained (Gerber)	4.5 oz	70	2.0	10.0	17	(mq)	2.0	(mq)	12	27%
SOUP										
Chicken										
hearty, w/stars, 'Stages Table Time' (Beech-Nut)	6 oz	180	4.0	20.0	350	(mq)	9.0	(mq)	(mq)	46%
strained	4.5 oz	64	2.0	9.2	20	1.4	2.2	na	na	31%
strained	1 oz	14	0.5	2.0	5	.3	0.5	na	na	31%
strained (Heinz)	3.5 oz	49	1.5	7.2	20	.3	1.7	na	na	31%
Cream of broccoli, '3rd Foods' (Gerber)	3.2 oz	26	1.4	2.7	83	na	1.1	na	na	38%
Cream of chicken										
strained	4.5 oz	74	3.2	10.8	24	0	2.0	na	na	24%
strained	1 oz	16	0.7	2.4	5	0	0.5	na	na	27%
Cream of potato, '3rd Foods' (Gerber)	3.2 oz	33	1.2	5.2	69	na	0.8	na	na	22%
Cream of tomato, '3rd Foods' (Gerber)	3.2 oz	41	1.4	7.3	73	na	0.7	na	na	15%
Cream of vegetable, '3rd Foods' (Gerber)	3.2 oz	29	1.2	4.4	48	na	0.8	na	na	24%

Food Name	Serving Size	Calories	Prot. gms	Carbs gms	Sod. mgs	Fiber gms	Fat gms	Sat. Fat gms	Chol. mgs	% Fat Cal.
VEGETABLES										
Beet										
'2nd Foods' (Gerber)	7 tbsp	39	1.2	8.1	91	na	0.2	na	na	5%
strained	4.5 oz	44	1.7	9.9	106	2.4	0.1	na	na	2%
strained	1 oz	10	0.4	2.2	24	.5	0.0	na	na	0%
strained (Gerber)	4.5 oz	60	1.0	11.0	115	(mq)	1.0	na	0	16%
strained (Heinz)	3.5 oz	40	1.1	8.3	34	na	0.2	na	na	5%
Broccoli, carrot, and cheese, '3rd Foods' (Gerber)	7 tbsp	44	1.6	7.2	46	na	1.0	na	na	20%
Carrot										
(Earth's Best)	4.5 oz	40	1.0	7.0	70	(mq)	1.0	0.0	0	22%
'Beginner Foods' (Heinz)	3.5 oz	30	0.8	6.1	32	na	0.3	na	na	9%
buttered, junior	7.5 oz	70	1.7	14.3	34	>.9 c	1.3	na	na	16%
buttered, junior	1 oz	9	0.2	1.9	5	>.1 c	0.2	na	na	18%
buttered, strained	4.5 oz	46	1.0	9.5	23	>.4 c	0.8	na	na	15%
buttered, strained	1 oz	10	0.2	2.1	5	>.1 c	0.2	na	na	16%
diced, 'Graduates' (Gerber)	3.2 oz	22	0.5	4.7	26	na	0.1	na	na	4%
'1st Foods' (Gerber)	2.5 oz	25	1.0	5.0	na	(mq)	0.0	0.0	0	0%
'1st Foods' (Gerber)	7 tbsp	34	0.9	6.9	78	na	0.3	na	na	8%
junior	7.5 oz	68	1.7	15.3	104	3.6	0.4	na	na	5%
junior	1 oz	9	0.2	2.0	14	.5	0.1	na	na	9%
junior (Gerber)	6 oz	80	3.0	16.0	83	(mq)	1.0	na	0	11%
junior (Heinz)	3.5 oz	23	0.5	4.9	44	na	0.2	na	na	8%
'Regal Imperial,' 'Baby's First' (Beech-Nut)	2.5 oz	25	0.0	6.0	80	na	0.0	na	na	0%
'Regal Imperial,' 'Stages 1' (Beech-Nut)	4.5 oz	40	1.0	9.0	130	(mq)	0.0	0.0	0	0%
'Regal Imperial,' 'Stages 1' (Beech-Nut)	2.8 oz	30	0.0	7.0	80	(mq)	0.0	0.0	0	0%
'2nd Foods' (Gerber)	7 tbsp	30	0.8	6.1	40	na	0.2	na	na	6%
'Stages 3' (Beech-Nut)	6 oz	60	1.0	13.0	170	(mq)	0.0	0.0	0	0%
strained	4.5 oz	35	1.0	7.7	47	2.2	0.1	na	na	3%
strained	1 oz	8	0.2	1.7	10	.5	0.0	na	na	0%
strained (Gerber)	4.5 oz	35	1.0	8.0	46	(mq)	0.0	0.0	0	0%
strained (Heinz)	3.5 oz	23	0.5	4.9	44	na	0.2	na	na	8%
'3rd Foods' (Gerber)	7 tbsp	29	0.8	6.0	49	na	0.2	na	na	6%
Carrot and parsnip (Earth's Best)	4.5 oz	60	0.0	14.0	30	na	0.0	na	na	0%
Corn, creamed										
junior	7.5 oz	138	3.0	34.7	111	4.5	0.9	na	na	5%
junior	1 oz	18	0.4	4.6	15	.6	0.1	na	na	4%
junior (Heinz)	3.5 oz	65	0.9	14.1	14	.4	0.5	na	na	7%
'2nd Foods' (Gerber)	7 tbsp	62	1.8	12.7	8	na	0.5	na	na	7%
'Stages 2' (Beech-Nut)	4.5 oz	100	2.0	20.0	25	(mq)	1.0	na	na	9%
strained	4.5 oz	73	1.8	18.0	55	2.7	0.5	na	na	5%
strained	1 oz	16	0.4	4.0	12	.6	0.1	na	na	5%
strained (Gerber)	4.5 oz	80	2.0	16.0	12	(mq)	1.0	na	na	11%
strained (Heinz)	3.5 oz	63	0.8	14.0	16	.3	0.4	na	na	6%
Garden vegetable										
(Earth's Best)	4.5 oz	70	1.0	15.0	15	na	0.0	na	na	0%
'2nd Foods' (Gerber)	7 tbsp	39	2.3	6.4	20	na	0.4	na	na	9%
'Stages 2' (Beech-Nut)	4.5 oz	60	2.0	11.0	35	(mq)	0.0	0.0	0	0%
strained	4.5 oz	47	2.9	8.7	45	1.9	0.3	na	na	6%
strained	1 oz	10	0.7	1.9	10	.4	0.1	na	na	8%
strained (Gerber)	4.5 oz	50	3.0	8.0	26	(mq)	1.0	(tr)	0	17%
Green bean										
'Beginner Foods' (Heinz)	3.5 oz	30	1.2	5.9	3	na	0.3	na	na	9%
buttered, junior	7.25 oz	66	2.7	12.6	4	>.8 c	1.9	na	na	22%
buttered, junior	1 oz	9	0.4	1.7	1	>.1 c	0.3	na	na	24%

Food Name	Serving Size	Calories	Prot. gms	Carbs gms	Sod. mgs	Fiber gms	Fat gms	Sat. Fat gms	Chol. mgs	% Fat Cal.
buttered, strained	4.5 oz	42	1.5	8.4	4	>.5 c	1.0	na	na	19%
buttered, strained	1 oz	9	0.3	1.9	1	>.1 c	0.2	na	na	17%
creamed, junior	7.5 oz	68	2.1	15.3	26	3.4	0.9	na	na	10%
creamed, junior	1 oz	9	0.3	2.0	3	.5	0.1	na	na	9%
creamed, junior (Gerber)	6 oz	80	3.0	16.0	14	(mq)	1.0	na	na	11%
creamed, junior (Heinz)	3.5 oz	41	1.4	6.6	13	na	1.0	na	na	22%
creamed, '3rd Foods' (Gerber)	7 tbsp	45	1.6	9.1	8	na	0.2	na	na	4%
diced, 'Graduates' (Gerber)	3.2 oz	21	0.8	4.2	23	na	0.1	na	na	4%
'1st Foods' (Gerber)	2.5 oz	25	1.0	5.0	na	(mq)	0.0	0.0	0	0%
'1st Foods' (Gerber)	7 tbsp	32	1.3	6.2	1	na	0.2	na	na	6%
junior	7.25 oz	52	2.5	11.7	4	3.9	0.2	na	na	3%
junior	1 oz	7	0.3	1.6	1	.5	0.0	na	na	0%
'2nd Foods' (Gerber)	7 tbsp	30	1.3	5.8	1	na	0.2	na	na	6%
'Stages 3' (Beech-Nut)	6 oz	45	2.0	10.0	80	(mq)	0.0	0.0	0	0%
'Stages 1' (Beech-Nut)	4.5 oz	35	1.0	8.0	0	(mq)	0.0	0.0	0	0%
strained	4.5 oz	32	1.7	7.6	3	2.4	0.1	na	na	2%
strained	1 oz	7	0.4	1.7	1	.5	0.0	na	na	0%
strained (Heinz)	3.5 oz	25	1.0	4.9	2	.7	0.2	na	na	7%
Mixed										
junior	7.5 oz	87	3.0	17.5	77	3.2	0.9	na	na	9%
junior	1 oz	12	0.4	2.3	10	.4	0.1	na	na	8%
junior (Gerber)	6 oz	70	2.0	14.0	32	(mq)	1.0	(tr)	0	12%
'2nd Foods' (Gerber)	7 tbsp	42	1.2	8.4	17	na	0.4	na	na	9%
'Stages 2' (Beech-Nut)	4.5 oz	50	1.0	12.0	30	(mq)	0.0	0.0	0	0%
strained	4.5 oz	52	1.5	10.2	17	1.9	0.6	na	na	10%
strained	1 oz	12	0.3	2.3	4	.4	0.1	na	na	8%
strained (Gerber)	4.5 oz	60	1.0	11.0	15	(mq)	1.0	(tr)	0	16%
strained (Heinz)	3.5 oz	44	1.4	8.8	21	na	0.4	na	na	8%
'3rd Foods' (Gerber)	7 tbsp	39	1.3	8.0	14	na	0.2	na	na	5%
Peas										
'Beginner Foods' (Heinz)	3.5 oz	55	3.6	9.5	13	1.4	0.5	na	na	8%
buttered, junior	7.25 oz	124	7.2	23.3	10	>2.3 c	2.7	na	na	17%
buttered, junior	1 oz	17	1.0	3.2	1	>.3 c	0.4	na	na	18%
buttered, strained	4.5 oz	72	4.7	13.6	10	>.9 c	1.4	na	na	15%
buttered, strained	1 oz	16	1.0	3.0	2	>.2 c	0.3	na	na	14%
buttered, tender, sweet, 'Stages 1' (Beech-Nut)	4.5 oz	60	4.0	10.0	0	(mq)	0.0	0.0	0	0%
buttered, tender, sweet, 'Stages 1' (Beech-Nut)	2.8 oz	40	2.0	6.0	0	(mq)	0.0	0.0	0	0%
creamed, strained	4.5 oz	68	2.8	11.4	18	2.4	2.4	na	na	28%
creamed, strained	1 oz	15	0.6	2.5	4	.5	0.5	na	na	27%
creamed, strained (Heinz)	3.5 oz	52	2.0	7.6	11	na	1.5	na	na	26%
diced, 'Graduates' (Gerber)	3.2 oz	44	2.7	8.4	9	na	0.1	na	na	2%
'1st Foods' (Gerber)	2.5 oz	30	2.0	6.0	na	(mq)	0.0	(tr)	0	0%
'1st Foods' (Gerber)	7 tbsp	47	3.0	7.7	6	na	0.4	na	na	8%
junior (Gerber)	6 oz	90	5.0	16.0	5	(mq)	1.0	(tr)	0	10%
'2nd Foods' (Gerber)	7 tbsp	47	3.0	7.7	5	na	0.5	na	na	10%
strained	4.5 oz	51	4.5	10.4	5	2.7	0.4	na	na	6%
strained	1 oz	11	1.0	2.3	1	.6	0.1	na	na	6%
strained (Gerber)	4.5 oz	60	4.0	10.0	6	(mq)	1.0	(tr)	0	14%
tender, sweet, 'Baby's First' (Beech-Nut)	2.5 oz	40	2.0	7.0	0	na	0.0	na	na	0%
'3rd Foods' (Gerber)	7 tbsp	47	3.0	7.8	6	na	0.4	na	na	8%
Peas and brown rice (Earth's Best)	4.5 oz	80	5.0	16.0	10	na	0.0	na	na	0%
Peas and carrots, 'Stages 2' (Beech-Nut)	4.5 oz	60	2.0	11.0	35	(mq)	0.0	0.0	0	0%
Potato, diced, 'Graduates' (Gerber)	3.2 oz	38	1.0	8.5	6	na	0.1	na	na	2%

Food Name	Serving Size	Calories	Prot. gms	Carbs gms	Sod. mgs	Fiber gms	Fat gms	Sat. Fat gms	Chol. mgs	% Fat Cal.
Spinach, creamed										
junior	7.5 oz	89	6.4	13.6	117	3.8	3.0	na	na	25%
junior	1 oz	12	0.9	1.8	16	.5	0.4	na	na	25%
'2nd Foods' (Gerber)	7 tbsp	47	3.1	7.3	57	na	0.6	na	na	12%
strained	4.5 oz	47	3.2	7.3	63	2.3	1.7	na	na	27%
strained	1 oz	10	0.7	1.6	14	.5	0.4	na	na	28%
strained (Gerber)	4.5 oz	60	4.0	9.0	73	(mq)	1.0	na	na	15%
Spinach and potato (Earth's Best)	4.5 oz	60	2.0	8.0	25	na	2.0	na	na	31%
Squash										
'Beginner Foods' (Heinz)	3.5 oz	36	1.2	7.3	5	na	0.2	na	na	5%
buttered, junior	7.5 oz	64	1.5	13.6	4	>.4 c	1.3	na	na	16%
buttered, junior	1 oz	9	0.2	1.8	1	>.1 c	0.2	na	na	18%
buttered, strained	4.5 oz	37	0.8	8.8	3	>.3 c	0.4	na	na	9%
buttered, strained	1 oz	8	0.2	2.0	1	>.1 c	0.1	na	na	9%
butternut, 'Baby's First' (Beech-Nut)	2.5 oz	30	0.0	7.0	0	na	0.0	na	na	0%
butternut, 'Stages 1' (Beech-Nut)	4.5 oz	50	1.0	11.0	0	(mq)	0.0	0.0	0	0%
butternut, 'Stages 1' (Beech-Nut)	2.8 oz	30	0.0	7.0	0	(mq)	0.0	0.0	0	0%
'1st Foods' (Gerber)	2.5 oz	25	1.0	5.0	na	(mq)	0.0	0.0	0	0%
'1st Foods' (Gerber)	7 tbsp	33	0.8	7.0	1	na	0.3	na	na	8%
junior	7.5 oz	51	1.7	11.9	2	4.5	0.4	na	na	6%
junior	1 oz	7	0.2	1.6	0	.6	0.1	na	na	11%
junior (Gerber)	6 oz	60	1.0	11.0	3	(mq)	1.0	(tr)	0	16%
'2nd Foods' (Gerber)	7 tbsp	32	0.8	6.8	1	na	0.2	na	na	6%
strained	4.5 oz	31	1.0	7.2	3	2.7	0.3	na	na	8%
strained	1 oz	7	0.2	1.6	1	.6	0.1	na	na	11%
strained (Gerber)	4.5 oz	35	1.0	8.0	3	(mq)	0.0	0.0	0	0%
strained (Heinz)	3.5 oz	32	0.9	6.6	2	.8	0.3	na	na	8%
'3rd Foods' (Gerber)	7 tbsp	33	0.9	6.8	1	na	0.2	na	na	6%
winter (Earth's Best)	4.5 oz	50	1.0	12.0	10	(mq)	0.0	0.0	0	0%
Sweet potato										
(Earth's Best)	4.5 oz	60	1.0	12.0	15	(mq)	1.0	(tr)	0	15%
'Baby's First' (Beech-Nut)	2.5 oz	50	0.0	11.0	10	na	0.0	na	na	0%
'Beginner Foods' (Heinz)	3.5 oz	69	1.0	15.7	14	na	0.2	na	na	3%
buttered, junior	7.75 oz	125	1.8	26.8	18	>.4 c	1.5	na	na	11%
buttered, junior	1 oz	16	0.2	3.5	2	>.1 c	0.2	na	na	11%
buttered, strained	4.75 oz	76	1.2	15.9	11	>.1 c	0.9	na	na	11%
buttered, strained	1 oz	16	0.3	3.3	2	(mq)	0.2	na	na	11%
'1st Foods' (Gerber)	2.5 oz	45	1.0	10.0	na	(mq)	0.0	0.0	0	0%
'1st Foods' (Gerber)	7 tbsp	67	1.2	15.0	15	na	0.2	na	na	3%
junior	7.75 oz	132	2.4	30.6	48	3.3	0.2	na	na	1%
junior	1 oz	17	0.3	3.9	6	.4	0.0	na	na	0%
junior (Gerber)	6 oz	110	1.0	24.0	39	(mq)	1.0	(tr)	0	8%
junior (Heinz)	3.5 oz	69	1.0	15.6	11	na	0.3	na	na	4%
'2nd Foods' (Gerber)	7 tbsp	62	1.0	14.1	17	na	0.2	na	na	3%
'Stages 1' (Beech-Nut)	2.8 oz	60	0.0	14.0	10	(mq)	0.0	0.0	0	0%
'Stages 1' (Beech-Nut)	4.5 oz	90	1.0	20.0	80	(mq)	0.0	0.0	0	0%
'Stages 3' (Beech-Nut)	0 oz	110	1.0	26.0	80	(mq)	0.0	0.0	0	0%
strained	4.75 oz	77	1.5	17.8	27	2.0	0.1	na	na	1%
strained	1 oz	16	0.3	3.7	6	.4	0.0	na	na	0%
strained (Gerber)	4.5 oz	80	1.0	18.0	22	(mq)	1.0	(tr)	0	11%
strained (Heinz)	3.5 oz	69	1.0	15.6	11	na	0.3	na	na	4%
'3rd Foods' (Gerber)	7 tbsp	63	1.1	14.2	23	na	0.2	na	na	3%
WATER, w/fluoride, sodium-free (Beech-Nut)	4 oz	0	0.0	0.0	0	na	0.0	na	na	0%

Food Name	Serving Size	Calories	Prot. gms	Carbs gms	Sod. mgs	Fiber gms	Fat gms	Sat. Fat gms	Chol. mgs	% Fat Cal.
BACON										
cooked, yield from 1 lb raw	4.5 oz	732	38.7	0.8	2026	0	62.5	22.1	107	78%
cured, approx 20 slices per lb, cooked	3 slices	109	5.8	0.1	303	0	9.4	3.3	16	78%
cured, breakfast strips, cooked	3 slices	156	9.8	0.4	714	0	12.5	4.3	36	73%
cured, broiled	4.5 oz	732	38.7	0.8	2027	0	62.5	22.1	108	78%
cured, broiled	3 med slices	109	5.8	0.1	303	0	9.4	3.3	16	78%
cured, canned	100 gm	685	8.5	1.0	680	0	71.5	22.9	89	94%
cured, pan-fried	4.5 oz	732	38.7	0.8	2027	0	62.5	22.1	108	78%
cured, pan-fried	3 med slices	109	5.8	0.1	303	0	9.4	3.3	16	78%
cured, roasted	4.5 oz	732	38.7	0.8	2027	0	62.5	22.1	108	78%
cured, roasted	3 med slices	109	5.8	0.1	303	0	9.4	3.3	16	78%
cured, strips, cooked	6 oz	780	49.2	1.8	3568	0	62.4	21.7	178	73%
cured, 12 slices per lb, raw	1 slice	211	3.3	0.0	277	0	21.9	8.1	25	94%
cured, strips, 15 slices per 12 oz, raw	3 slices	264	8.0	0.5	671	0	25.3	8.8	47	87%
raw	1 oz	158	2.5	<.1	194	0	16.3	6.0	19	93%
(Hormel)										
'Black Label' cooked	1 oz	142	3.0	2.0	192	na	14.0	6.0	18	86%
'Black Label' low salt, cooked	1.76 oz	250	5.0	2.0	260	na	25.0	10.0	32	89%
'Black Label' sliced, cooked	2 slices	60	4.0	0.0	298	0	5.0	(mq)	(mq)	74%
'Range' thick sliced, cooked	1 oz	152	2.0	2.0	199	na	16.0	6.0	17	90%
(JM)										
cooked	2 slices	100	4.0	1.0	370	0	9.0	(mq)	12	80%
'Lower Sodium' cooked	2 slices	100	4.0	1.0	260	0	9.0	(mq)	(mq)	80%
'Lower Sodium' raw	2 slices	290	5.0	1.0	250	0	30.0	(mq)	(mq)	92%
raw	2 slices	280	4.0	1.0	530	0	29.0	(mq)	38	93%
(Jones Dairy Farm), raw	1 slice	165	2.3	tr	187	0	17.0	(mq)	25	94%
(Kahn's), 'American Beauty,' cooked	2 slices	100	5.0	na	(mq)	0	9.0	(mq)	(mq)	80%
(Oscar Mayer)										
'Center Cut' cooked, approx .2-oz slices	1 slice	25	2.0	0.1	113	0	1.8	0.8	6	66%
'Center Cut' cooked, yield from 1 lb raw	6 oz	852	68.8	3.5	3813	0	62.5	27.5	189	66%
cooked, approx .2-oz slices	1 slice	33	2.0	0.1	138	0	2.8	1.2	5	75%
cooked, yield from 16-oz pkg raw	5 oz	784	47.1	3.0	3236	0	64.9	25.8	127	75%
'Lower Salt' cooked, approx .2-oz slices	1 slice	33	2.2	0.1	104	0	2.6	0.9	6	72%
'Lower Salt,' cooked, yield from 1 lb raw	5.6 oz	870	57.2	2.3	2768	0	70.3	25.1	170	73%
thick sliced, cooked, approx .4-oz slices	1 slice	58	3.6	0.1	259	0	4.8	1.9	9	75%
thick sliced, cooked, yield from 1 lb raw	5 oz	811	50.6	1.1	3656	0	67.1	25.8	123	75%
(Range Brand) 'Sliced,' cooked	2 slices	110	6.0	0.0	392	0	9.0	(mq)	(mq)	77%
(Red Label) cooked	3 slices	110	6.0	0.0	(mq)	0	10.0	(mq)	(mq)	79%
BACON, ALTERNATIVE										
BEEF										
heated *(JM)*	2 slices	100	7.0	1.0	320	0	7.0	(mq)	20	66%
heated *(Sizzlean)*	2 strips	70	6.0	0.0	480	0	5.0	(mq)	(mq)	65%
heated, yield from 12-oz pkg	6 oz	764	53.2	2.4	700	0	58.5	24.4	202	70%
raw	1 oz	115	2.8	0.2	271	0	11.0	4.5	23	89%
raw *(JM)*	2 slices	200	9.0	1.0	430	0	18.0	(mq)	53	80%
unheated	1 oz	115	2.8	0.2	271	0	11.0	4.5	23	89%
PORK										
80% fat-free *(Louis Rich)*	1 slice	35	2.0	<1.0	185	na	2.0	na	10	60%
heated *(Sizzlean)*	2 strips	90	6.0	0.0	530	0	8.0	(mq)	(mq)	75%
heated, brown sugar cured *(Sizzlean)*	2 strips	110	6.0	2.0	490	0	9.0	(mq)	(mq)	72%
heated, yield from 12-oz pkg	6 oz	780	49.2	1.8	3568	0	62.4	21.7	179	73%
raw	1 oz	110	3.3	0.2	280	0	10.5	3.7	20	87%
TURKEY, heated *(Louis Rich)*	1 slice	32	2.4	0.3	186	0	2.4	0.7	10	67%

Food Name	Serving Size	Calories	Prot. gms	Carbs gms	Sod. mgs	Fiber gms	Fat gms	Sat. Fat gms	Chol. mgs	% Fat Cal.
VEGETARIAN										
....	1 cup	446	15.4	9.1	2110	3.7	42.5	6.7	0	80%
....	1 oz	88	3.0	1.8	415	.2	8.4	1.3	0	80%
(Morningstar Farms) 'Breakfast Strips' frozen	3 strips	80	3.0	4.0	350	na	6.0	1.0	0	66%
(White Wave SoyFood) 'Healthy'	1 oz	27	4.0	4.0	310	3.3	1.0	na	0	22%
(Worthington) 'Stripples' frozen	4 strips	120	4.0	6.0	460	na	9.0	1.0	0	67%
Canadian style										
(Heartline)	2 oz	176	19.0	9.0	260	na	7.0	na	0	36%
(Heartline) 'Canadian Bacon Style' lite	.5 oz	22	5.0	1.0	135	3.0	0.0	0.0	0	0%
BACON, CANADIAN-STYLE										
cured, grilled	2 slices	86	11.3	0.6	719	0	3.9	1.3	27	42%
cured, grilled, yield from 6 oz raw	4.9 oz	257	33.7	1.9	2149	0	11.7	4.0	81	43%
cured, packed 6 slices per 6 oz, unheated	2 slices	89	11.7	1.0	799	0	4.0	1.3	28	42%
cured, unheated	6 oz	267	35.1	2.9	2395	0	11.9	3.8	85	41%
unheated	1 oz	45	5.9	0.5	399	0	2.0	0.6	14	41%
(Hormel) 'Sliced'	1 oz	45	6.0	0.0	315	0	2.0	(mq)	(mq)	43%
(Jones Dairy Farm) unheated	1 slice	25	3.2	tr	144	0	1.0	(mq)	7	41%
(Light & Lean)	2 slices	35	6.0	0.0	(mq)	0	1.0	(mq)	(mq)	27%
(Oscar Mayer)	.8 oz	28	4.7	0.1	305	0	1.0	0.3	11	32%
BACON BITS										
(Hormel)	1 oz	117	12.0	1.0	1008	na	7.0	3.0	16	55%
(Hormel)	1 tbsp	30	3.0	0.0	313	0	2.0	na	na	60%
(Libby's) 'Bacon Crumbles'	1 tbsp	25	2.0	2.0	(mq)	0	1.0	na	na	36%
(Oscar Mayer)	3 oz	248	31.6	2.5	2224	0	12.4	4.3	67	45%
(Oscar Mayer)	1 tbsp	20	2.6	0.2	183	0	1.0	0.3	6	45%
BACON BITS, ALTERNATIVE										
(Bac•Os)	2 tsp	25	2.0	2.0	90	na	1.0	na	na	36%
(McCormick) 'Bac'N Pieces' no cholesterol	1 1/2 tbsp	30	3.0	2.0	240	na	1.0	na	0	30%
(Schilling) 'Bac'N Pieces'	1 tsp	26	2.0	2.0	51	na	0.4	na	na	18%
BACON PIECES (Hormel)	1 oz	94	12.0	2.0	654	na	5.0	2.0	26	45%
BAGEL										
BLUEBERRY										
(Earth Grains) 3 oz	1 bagel	245	9.0	48.0	210	na	0.0	0.0	0	0%
(Western Bagel)	1 bagel	240	8.0	43.0	410	2.0	4.0	1.0	0	15%
CINNAMON-RAISIN										
(Dunkin' Donuts)	1 bagel	250	8.0	49.0	370	na	2.0	na	0	7%
(Earth Grains) 3 oz	1 bagel	245	9.0	48.0	210	na	0.0	0.0	0	0%
(Thomas') Deli Style'	1 bagel	170	6.0	33.0	230	2.0	2.0	na	0	10%
(Western Bagel)	1 bagel	230	8.0	40.0	410	4.0	4.0	1.0	0	16%
EGG										
....	1 oz	79	3.0	15.0	143	na	0.6	0.1	7	7%
(Dunkin' Donuts)	1 bagel	250	9.0	47.0	380	na	2.0	na	15	7%
(Lender's) 'Bagel Shop'	1 bagel	230	9.0	41.0	460	2.0	2.5	0.5	15	10%
(Lender's) 'Bakery Style'	1 bagel	210	9.0	41.0	450	2.0	2.0	na	5	8%
HONEY WHEAT (Earth Grains) 3 oz	1 bagel	240	9.0	45.0	210	na	0.0	0.0	0	0%
ONION										
enriched, 3.5 inch diam	1 bagel	195	7.5	37.9	379	1.5	1.1	0.2	0	5%
enriched, w/calcium proprianate, 3.5 inch diam	1 bagel	195	7.5	37.9	379	1.5	1.1	0.2	0	5%
enriched, w/calcium proprianate, toasted	1 oz	84	3.2	16.3	163	na	0.5	0.1	0	6%
unenriched, 3.5 inch diam	1 bagel	195	7.5	37.9	379	1.5	1.1	0.2	0	5%
unenriched, w/calcium proprianate, 3.5 inch diam	1 bagel	195	7.5	37.9	379	1.5	1.1	0.2	0	5%
(Dunkin' Donuts)	1 bagel	230	9.0	46.0	480	na	1.0	na	0	4%
(Earth Grains) 3 oz	1 bagel	240	9.0	45.0	210	na	0.0	0.0	0	0%

Food Name	Serving Size	Calories	Prot. gms	Carbs gms	Sod. mgs	Fiber gms	Fat gms	Sat. Fat gms	Chol. mgs	% Fat Cal.
(Lender's) 'Bagel Shop'	1 bagel	220	9.0	40.0	460	2.0	2.0	0.0	0	8%
(Western Bagel)	1 bagel	220	8.0	39.0	430	4.0	4.0	1.0	0	16%
PLAIN										
enriched, 3.5 inch diam	1 bagel	195	7.5	37.9	379	1.5	1.1	0.2	0	5%
enriched, w/calcium proprianate, 3.5 inch diam	1 bagel	195	7.5	37.9	379	1.5	1.1	0.2	0	5%
unenriched, 3.5 inch diam	1 bagel	195	7.5	37.9	379	1.5	1.1	0.2	0	5%
unenriched, w/calcium proprianate, 3.5 inch diam	1 bagel	195	7.5	37.9	379	1.5	1.1	0.2	0	5%
(Dunkin' Donuts)	1 bagel	240	9.0	47.0	450	na	1.0	na	0	4%
(Earth Grains) 3 oz	1 bagel	240	9.0	45.0	210	na	0.0	0.0	0	0%
(Lender's) 'Bagel Shop'	1 bagel	210	10.0	40.0	350	1.0	1.5	0.0	0	6%
(Lender's) 'Bakery Style'	1 bagel	210	8.0	42.0	450	2.0	2.0	na	0	8%
POPPY SEED										
enriched, 3.5 inch diam	1 bagel	195	7.5	37.9	379	1.5	1.1	0.2	0	5%
enriched, w/calcium proprianate, 3.5 inch diam	1 bagel	195	7.5	37.9	379	1.5	1.1	0.2	0	5%
enriched, w/calcium proprianate, toasted	1 oz	84	3.2	16.3	163	na	0.5	0.1	0	6%
unenriched, 3.5 inch diam	1 bagel	195	7.5	37.9	379	1.5	1.1	0.2	0	5%
unenriched, w/calcium proprianate, 3.5 inch diam	1 bagel	195	7.5	37.9	379	1.5	1.1	0.2	0	5%
RAISIN										
(Lender's) 'Bagel Shop'	1 bagel	240	8.0	44.0	350	2.0	3.0	0.0	0	11%
(Lender's) 'Bakery Style'	1 bagel	220	8.0	44.0	380	2.0	2.0	0.0	na	8%
RAISIN-HONEY CINNAMON (Finast) 2.5 oz	1 bagel	200	8.0	40.0	305	(mq)	1.0	na	0	5%
SESAME										
enriched, 3.5 inch diam	1 bagel	195	7.5	37.9	379	1.5	1.1	0.2	0	5%
enriched, w/calcium proprianate, 3.5 inch diam	1 bagel	195	7.5	37.9	379	1.5	1.1	0.2	0	5%
enriched, w/calcium proprianate, toasted	1 oz	84	3.2	16.3	163	na	0.5	0.1	0	6%
unenriched, 3.5 inch diam	1 bagel	195	7.5	37.9	379	1.5	1.1	0.2	0	5%
unenriched, w/calcium proprianate, 3.5 inch diam	1 bagel	195	7.5	37.9	379	1.5	1.1	0.2	0	5%
WATER (Western Bagel)	1 bagel	230	8.0	41.0	420	2.0	4.0	1.0	0	16%
BAGEL, FROZEN										
BLUEBERRY (Lender's) 2.5 oz	1 bagel	190	7.0	38.0	250	(mq)	1.0	na	0	5%
CINNAMON-RAISIN										
(Lender's) 'Big'n Crusty' 3 1/8 oz	1 bagel	250	8.0	49.0	370	(mq)	2.0	(mq)	0	7%
(Sara Lee) 3.1 oz	1 bagel	240	8.0	48.0	280	(mq)	2.0	(mq)	0	7%
(Sara Lee) 2.5 oz	1 bagel	200	7.0	39.0	230	(mq)	2.0	(mq)	0	9%
EGG										
(Lender's) 2 oz	1 bagel	150	7.0	29.0	360	(mq)	1.0	na	5	6%
(Lender's) 'Big'n Crusty' 3 1/8 oz	1 bagel	250	9.0	47.0	380	(mq)	2.0	(mq)	15	7%
(Sara Lee) 3.1 oz	1 bagel	250	9.0	48.0	450	(mq)	2.0	(mq)	20	7%
(Sara Lee) 2.5 oz	1 bagel	200	8.0	38.0	360	(mq)	2.0	(mq)	15	9%
GARLIC										
(Lender's) 2 oz	1 bagel	160	6.0	32.0	340	(mq)	1.0	na	0	6%
(Lender's) 'Big'n Crusty' 3 1/8 oz	1 bagel	250	9.0	50.0	530	(mq)	1.0	na	0	4%
OAT BRAN										
(Lender's) 2.5 oz	1 bagel	170	7.0	36.0	290	3.0	2.0	(mq)	0	10%
(Sara Lee) 3 oz	1 bagel	220	9.0	47.0	450	(mq)	1.0	na	0	4%
(Sara Lee) 2.5 oz	1 bagel	180	8.0	38.0	360	(mq)	1.0	na	0	5%
ONION										
(Lender's) 2 oz	1 bagel	160	7.0	31.0	290	(mq)	1.0	na	0	6%
(Lender's) 'Bagelettes' .9 oz	1 bagel	70	3.0	14.0	135	<.1 c	<1.0	na	0	<12%
(Lender's) 'Big'n Crusty' 3 1/8 oz	1 bagel	230	9.0	46.0	480	(mq)	1.0	na	0	4%
(Sara Lee) 3.1 oz	1 bagel	230	9.0	45.0	560	(mq)	1.0	na	0	4%
(Sara Lee) 2.5 oz	1 bagel	190	7.0	37.0	450	(mq)	1.0	na	0	5%
PLAIN										
(Lender's) 2 oz	1 bagel	150	6.0	30.0	320	(mq)	1.0	na	0	6%

Food Name	Serving Size	Calories	Prot. gms	Carbs gms	Sod. mgs	Fiber gms	Fat gms	Sat. Fat gms	Chol. mgs	% Fat Cal.
(Lender's) 'Bagelettes' .9 oz	1 bagel	70	3.0	13.0	170	(mq)	<1.0	na	0	<12%
(Lender's) 'Big'n Crusty'	1 bagel	240	9.0	47.0	450	(mq)	1.0	na	0	4%
(Lender's) soft, 2.5 oz	1 bagel	210	7.0	36.0	350	(mq)	3.0	(mq)	12	14%
(Sara Lee) 3.1 oz	1 bagel	230	9.0	46.0	580	(mq)	1.0	na	0	4%
(Sara Lee) 2.5 oz	1 bagel	190	8.0	38.0	460	(mq)	1.0	na	0	5%
POPPY SEED										
(Lender's) 2 oz	1 bagel	160	7.0	29.0	370	(mq)	1.0	na	0	6%
(Sara Lee) 3.1 oz	1 bagel	230	9.0	46.0	560	(mq)	1.0	na	na	4%
(Sara Lee) 2.5 oz	1 bagel	190	8.0	37.0	450	(mq)	1.0	na	0	5%
PUMPERNICKEL (Lender's) 2 oz	1 bagel	160	6.0	31.0	330	(mq)	1.0	na	0	6%
RAISIN, 'Bagelettes' (Lender's) .9 oz	1 bagel	70	2.0	14.0	110	(mq)	<1.0	na	0	<12%
RAISIN-HONEY (Lender's) 2.5 oz	1 bagel	200	8.0	40.0	310	(mq)	1.0	na	0	5%
RYE (Lender's) 2 oz	1 bagel	150	6.0	30.0	310	(mq)	1.0	na	0	6%
SESAME										
(Lender's) 2 oz	1 bagel	160	7.0	31.0	320	(mq)	1.0	na	0	6%
(Sara Lee) 3.1 oz	1 bagel	240	9.0	46.0	550	(mq)	2.0	(mq)	0	8%
(Sara Lee) 2.5 oz	1 bagel	190	8.0	37.0	440	(mq)	1.0	na	0	5%
WHEAT-RAISIN (Lender's) 2.5 oz	1 bagel	190	6.0	39.0	310	(mq)	1.0	na	0	5%
BAGEL CHIP										
(Burns & Ricker) cinnamon raisin 'Original Bagel Crisps'	1 oz	130	4.0	20.0	170	1.0	4.0	1.0	0	27%
(Burns & Ricker) garlic 'Original Bagel Crisps'	1 oz	130	4	20.0	190	1.0	4.0	1.0	0	27%
BAKED BEANS, CANNED. See also BEANS, CANNED.										
(Allens)	1/2 cup	170	6.0	21.0	330	(mq)	6.0	(mq)	na	33%
(Grandma Brown's)	1 cup	301	14.6	53.9	655	15.5	3.0	(mq)	<1	9%
(Green Giant)	1/2 cup	150	5.0	28.0	670	na	2.0	na	na	12%
(Open Range)	4.656 oz	152	6.6	30.5	425	6.7	2.3	0.7	1	12%
(Van Camp's)	1 cup	260	11.0	52.0	1020	(mq)	2.0	(mq)	na	7%
bacon and brown sugar, 'Premium' (Van Camp's)	6 oz	170	8.0	36.0	790	8.3	2.0	na	na	9%
barbecue (B&M)	8 oz	260	15.0	48.0	1000	11.0	6.0	(mq)	5	18%
barbecue (Campbell's)	7 7/8 oz	210	10.0	43.0	900	(mq)	4.0	(mq)	na	15%
Boston (Health Valley)	4 oz	213	11.0	43.0	74	22.3	1.0	na	0	4%
Boston, 'No Salt Added' (Health Valley)	4 oz	213	11.0	43.0	25	22.3	1.0	na	0	4%
Boston, w/ham 'Homestyle' (Hunt's)	9.03 oz	248	15.9	41.8	740	9.8	1.9	0.5	9	7%
'Brick Oven' (S&W)	1/2 cup	160	7.0	28.0	560	(mq)	2.0	(mq)	na	11%
brown sugar (Van Camp's)	1 cup	290	11.6	51.0	640	>3.2 c	5.1	(mq)	na	16%
'Deluxe' (Van Camp's)	1 cup	320	13.0	57.0	970	(mq)	4.0	(mq)	na	11%
'Dry Beans in Sauce' (Green Giant)	1/2 cup	130	6.0	30.0	570	6.0	1.0	0.0	2	6%
'Dry Beans in Sauce' (Joan of Arc)	1/2 cup	130	6.0	30.0	570	6.0	1.0	0.0	2	6%
'Home Style' (Campbell's)	8 oz	220	11.0	48.0	820	(mq)	4.0	(mq)	na	13%
honey (B&M)	8 oz	240	15.0	50.0	940	11.0	2.0	(mq)	0	7%
hot 'n spicy (B&M)	8 oz	240	14.0	50.0	990	12.0	3.0	1.0	3	10%
in homestyle sauce (Bush's Best)	4 oz	110	5.0	25.0	350	6.0	1.0	na	na	7%
in molasses, brown sugar, 'Old Fashioned' (Campbell's)	8 oz	230	11.0	49.0	730	(mq)	3.0	(mq)	na	10%
in tomato sauce (B&M)	8 oz	230	12.0	48.0	1010	10.0	3.0	1.0	1	10%
in tomato sauce (Campbell's)	8 oz	200	10.0	43.0	770	(mq)	3.0	(mq)	na	11%
in tomato sauce (Pathmark)	1/2 cup	150	7.0	23.0	440	(mq)	2.0	(mq)	na	13%
in tomato sauce, 40-oz can (Finast)	1/2 cup	120	7.0	21.0	930	(mq)	1.0	na	na	7%
in tomato sauce, 'No Frills' (Pathmark)	1/2 cup	160	7.0	28.0	390	(mq)	2.0	(mq)	na	11%
in tomato sauce, 16-oz can (Finast)	1 cup	270	13.0	50.0	1180	(mq)	3.0	(mq)	na	10%
maple (B&M)	8 oz	240	14.0	52.0	890	11.0	2.0	1.0	5	6%
maple (Friends)	8 oz	240	14.0	52.0	890	11.0	2.0	1.0	5	6%
no salt added, fat-free (Health Valley)	7.5 oz	190	8.0	41.0	20	5.0	0.0	na	0	0%
pea beans (B&M)	8 oz	270	14.0	50.0	750	11.0	6.0	(mq)	5	17%
pea, small (Friends)	8 oz	360	17.0	62.0	1040	15.0	4.0	3.0	6	10%

Food Name	Serving Size	Calories	Prot. gms	Carbs gms	Sod. mgs	Fiber gms	Fat gms	Sat. Fat gms	Chol. mgs	% Fat Cal.
pea, small, w/pork (Friends)	8 oz	260	14.0	53.0	890	11.0	5.0	na	5	14%
pork & beans, 'Deluxe' (Bush's Best)	4 oz	110	5.0	25.0	350	6.0	1.0	na	na	7%
pork and beans, 'Showboat' (Bush's Best)	4 oz	80	6.0	19.0	470	na	<1.0	na	na	<8%
regular, fat-free (Health Valley)	7.5 oz	190	8.0	41.0	290	5.0	0.0	na	0	0%
'Saucepan' (Grandma Brown's)	1 cup	307	13.7	52.3	592	14.8	4.8	(mq)	<1	14%
vegetarian	1/2 cup	118	6.1	26.0	504	9.8	0.6	0.2	0	4%
vegetarian (A&P)	1/2 cup	130	7.0	25.0	420	(mq)	<1.0	na	0	<7%
vegetarian (Allens)	1/2 cup	110	6.0	19.0	380	(mq)	1.0	na	0	8%
vegetarian (B&M)	8 oz	230	14.0	50.0	370	11.0	3.0	(mq)	0	10%
vegetarian (Campbell's)	7.75 oz	170	11.0	40.0	780	(mq)	1.0	na	0	4%
vegetarian 'Vegetarian Style' (Van Camp's)	1 cup	206	10.0	42.0	950	(mq)	0.6	na	0	3%
vegetarian, w/miso 'Vegetarian' (Health Valley)	4 oz	90	6.0	19.0	134	6.5	1.0	na	0	8%
w/beef	1/2 cup	161	8.5	22.5	632	>1.4 c	4.6	2.2	29	25%
w/franks	1/2 cup	182	8.6	19.7	550	8.8	8.4	3.0	8	40%
w/franks, 'Beanee Weenee' (Van Camp's)	1 cup	326	15.2	31.7	990	7.0	15.4	5.0	15	43%
w/onions, approx 1/2 cup (Bush's Best)	4 oz	110	6.0	27.0	550	7.0	1.0	na	na	6%
w/pork	1/2 cup	134	6.5	25.2	522	6.9	2.0	0.8	9	12%
w/pork (A&P)	1/2 cup	150	7.0	25.0	440	(mq)	2.0	(mq)	(mq)	12%
w/pork (Hunt's)	4 oz	140	6.0	26.0	400	(mq)	1.0	(mq)	(mq)	7%
w/pork (S&W)	1/2 cup	130	5.0	22.0	135	(mq)	2.0	(mq)	(mq)	14%
w/pork (Van Camp's)	1 cup	216	10.9	41.0	1000	9.9	1.9	1.0	(mq)	8%
w/pork 'Extra Fancy' (Allens)	1/2 cup	125	5.0	24.0	540	(mq)	1.0	(mq)	(mq)	7%
w/pork, 'Extra Standard' (Allens)	1/2 cup	90	5.0	15.0	350	(mq)	1.0	(mq)	(mq)	10%
w/pork,'Fancy' (Allens)	1/2 cup	110	6.0	18.0	430	(mq)	1.0	(mq)	(mq)	9%
w/pork, 'Micro-Cup' (Hormel)	7.5 oz	254	11.0	41.0	650	(mq)	5.0	(mq)	30	18%
w/pork and sweet sauce	1/2 cup	140	6.7	26.5	423	6.9	1.8	0.7	9	11%
w/pork and tomato sauce	1/2 cup	123	6.5	24.4	554	6.9	1.3	0.5	9	9%
w/pork and tomato sauce (Green Giant)	1/2 cup	90	5.0	21.0	420	5.0	1.0	0.0	0	8%
w/pork and tomato sauce (Joan of Arc)	1/2 cup	90	5.0	21.0	420	5.0	1.0	0.0	0	8%

BAKING POWDER

Food Name	Serving Size	Calories	Prot. gms	Carbs gms	Sod. mgs	Fiber gms	Fat gms	Sat. Fat gms	Chol. mgs	% Fat Cal.
	1 tbsp	11	0.0	2.6	1050	0	0.0	0.0	0	0%
	1 tsp	3	0.0	0.7	290	0	0.0	0.0	0	0%
commercial	3 1/2 oz	109	0.1	26.5	16804	0	0.0	0.0	0	0%
commercial (Calumet)	1/4 tsp	0	0.0	0.0	100	0	0.0	0.0	0	0%
cream of tartar, w/tartaric acid	1 tbsp	7	0.0	1.8	694	0	0.0	0.0	0	0%
double-acting, sodium aluminum sulfate	1 tsp	2	0.0	1.3	488	na	0.0	na	0	0%
double-acting, straight phosphate	1 tsp	2	0.0	1.1	363	na	0.0	na	0	0%
'Low Salt' (Featherweight)	1 tsp	8	0.0	2.0	2	0	0.0	0.0	0	0%
low-sodium	1 tsp	5	0.0	2.3	5	na	0.0	na	0	0%
low-sodium, commercial	1 tbsp	23	0.0	5.6	1	0	0.0	0.0	0	0%
low-sodium, commercial	1 tsp	7	0.0	1.8	0	0	0.0	0.0	0	0%
low-sodium, non-commercial	1 tsp	2	0.0	0.6	0	0	0.0	0.0	0	0%
w/monohydrate	1 tbsp	14	0.0	3.4	1205	0	0.0	0.0	0	0%
w/monohydrate	1 tsp	4	0.0	0.9	329	0	0.0	0.0	0	0%
w/straight phosphate	1 tbsp	15	0.0	3.7	1028	0	0.0	0.0	0	0%
w/straight phosphate	1 tsp	5	0.0	1.1	312	0	0.0	0.0	0	0%

BAKING SODA

Food Name	Serving Size	Calories	Prot. gms	Carbs gms	Sod. mgs	Fiber gms	Fat gms	Sat. Fat gms	Chol. mgs	% Fat Cal.
	1 tsp	0	0.0	0.0	1259	na	0.0	na	0	0%
(Arm & Hammer)	1/2 tsp	0	0.0	0.0	476	0	0.0	0.0	0	0%

BALSAM PEAR / bitter melon
Leafy tips

Food Name	Serving Size	Calories	Prot. gms	Carbs gms	Sod. mgs	Fiber gms	Fat gms	Sat. Fat gms	Chol. mgs	% Fat Cal.
boiled, drained	4 oz	40	4.1	7.7	15	2.1	0.2	(tr)	0	4%
boiled, drained	1/2 cup	10	1.0	2.0	4	.6	0.1	na	0	7%
raw	1/2 cup	7	1.3	0.8	3	>.6 c	0.2	na	0	18%

Food Name	Serving Size	Calories	Prot. gms	Carbs gms	Sod. mgs	Fiber gms	Fat gms	Sat. Fat gms	Chol. mgs	% Fat Cal.
raw, trimmed	1 oz	9	1.5	0.9	3	>.6 c	0.2	(tr)	0	16%
raw, untrimmed	1 lb	52	9.1	5.7	18	>3.9 c	1.2	na	0	15%
Pods										
boiled, drained	4 oz	22	1.0	4.9	7	2.5	0.2	(tr)	0	7%
boiled, drained, 1/2-inch pieces	1/2 cup	12	0.5	2.7	4	1.2	0.1	na	0	7%
raw	1 pear	21	1.2	4.6	6	3.5	0.2	na	0	7%
raw, approx 9 3/8 inch x 1 1/2 inch, 5.3 oz each	1 pod	21	1.2	4.6	6	3.5	0.2	(tr)	0	7%
raw, 1/2-inch pieces	1 cup	16	0.9	3.4	5	2.6	0.2	na	0	10%
raw, trimmed	1 oz	5	0.3	1.1	1	>.4 c	0.1	(tr)	0	14%
raw, untrimmed	1 lb	64	3.8	13.9	20	>5.3 c	0.6	na	0	7%
BAMBOO SHOOTS										
boiled, drained	4 oz	14	1.7	2.2	5	>.7 c	0.2	0.1	0	10%
boiled, drained, 1/2-inch slices	1 cup	14	1.8	2.3	5	>.8 c	0.3	0.1	0	14%
canned (LaChoy)	1.5 oz	8	0.7	1.4	3	(mq)	0.2	na	0	18%
canned (LaChoy)	2 tbsp	3	0.2	0.7	0	>.4 c	0.1	0.0	0	20%
canned, drained solids, 1/8-inch slices	1 cup	25	2.3	4.2	9	3.9	0.5	0.1	0	15%
raw, 1/2-inch slices	1 cup	41	3.9	7.8	6	3.3	0.5	0.1	0	9%
raw, trimmed	1 oz	8	0.7	1.5	1	.7	0.1	0.1	0	9%
raw, w/sheath	1 lb	36	3.4	6.8	6	3.4	0.4	0.1	0	8%
BANANA										
fresh (Dole)	1 fruit	120	1.0	28.0	na	3.0	1.0	na	0	7%
mashed	1/2 cup	104	1.2	26.4	1	1.8	0.5	<.1	0	4%
peeled	1 oz	26	0.3	6.6	<1	.5	0.1	0.1	0	3%
powdered	1 oz	98	1.1	25.0	1	>.5 c	0.5	0.2	0	4%
powdered	1/4 cup	87	1.0	22.1	1	>.5 c	0.5	0.2	0	5%
powdered	1 tbsp	21	0.2	5.5	tr	>.1 c	0.1	<.1	0	4%
raw, w/o skin and seeds	1 fruit	105	1.2	26.7	1	1.8	0.6	0.2	0	5%
unpeeled	1 lb	271	3.1	69.1	3	4.7	1.4	0.5	0	4%
BANANA, COOKING. See PLANTAIN.										
BANANA, DEHYDRATED										
	1 oz	98	1.1	25.0	1	1.8	0.5	0.2	0	4%
	1/4 cup	87	1.0	22.1	1	1.8	0.5	0.2	0	5%
BANANA, RED										
raw	100 gm	90	1.2	23.4	1	>.4 c	0.2	0.0	0	2%
raw, approx 7.25 inch x 1.5 inch	1 med	118	1.6	30.7	1	(mq)	0.3	na	0	2%
raw, sliced	1/2 cup	68	0.9	17.6	1	(mq)	0.2	na	0	2%
BANANA BERRY DRINK										
'Stompin' Banana Berry Drink' (Hi-C)	6 oz	90	0.0	22.0	25	na	0.0	na	na	0%
BANANA BREAD. See BREAD, QUICK.										
BANANA CHIPS										
	1 oz	147	0.7	16.6	2	>.7 c	9.5	8.2	0	55%
freeze-dried (Mountain House)	1/2 cup	248	2.0	15.0	na	(mq)	8.0	(mq)	0	51%
premium (Mariani)	1 oz	150	1.0	17.0	<10	na	9.0	na	0	54%
BANANA NECTAR (Libby's)	6 oz	110	0.0	26.0	15	na	0.0	na	na	0%
BANANA PEPPER. See PEPPER, BANANA.										
BANANA PINEAPPLE NECTAR (Kern's)	6 oz	110	1.0	27.0	0	na	0.0	na	na	0%
BANANA SQUASH. See SQUASH, BANANA.										
BANNER BEAN SEED, whole, dried	1 oz	95	6.3	17.4	na	>2.2 c	0.3	na	0	3%
BARBADOS CHERRY. See ACEROLA CHERRY.										
BARBADOS CHERRY JUICE. See ACEROLA CHERRY JUICE.										
BARBECUE SAUCE										
(Bull's Eye)	.5 oz	22	0.0	5.0	47	na	0.0	0.0	0	0%
(Cattleman's) mild	1 tbsp	25	0.0	5.0	260	na	0.0	0.0	0	0%
(Enrico's) 'Original'	1 tbsp	18	1.0	3.0	4	na	1.0	na	0	36%

Food Name	Serving Size	Calories	Prot. gms	Carbs gms	Sod. mgs	Fiber gms	Fat gms	Sat. Fat gms	Chol. mgs	% Fat Cal.
(Healthy Choice) original	1.1 oz	25	0.3	5.7	229	.5	0.2	0.0	0	7%
(Heinz) 'Old Fashioned'	1 tbsp	18	0.2	4.1	180	tr	0.1	(tr)	0	5%
(Heinz) 'Select'	1 oz	40	0.0	9.0	275	na	0.0	0.0	0	0%
(Heinz) 'Thick and Rich' old fashioned	1 oz	35	0.0	8.0	350	na	0.0	0.0	0	0%
(Heinz) 'Thick and Rich' original	1 oz	35	0.0	8.0	390	na	0.0	0.0	0	0%
(Hunt's) 'Bold' original	1.2 oz	46	0.3	10.8	315	.5	0.3	0.0	0	6%
(Hunt's) 'Light' original	1.1 oz	26	0.5	6.1	223	.6	0.1	0.0	0	3%
(Hunt's) original	1.2 oz	40	0.5	9.4	410	1.0	0.3	0.0	0	6%
(Kraft)	2 tbsp	45	0.0	10.0	460	na	1.0	0.0	0	18%
(Kraft) 'Thick 'n Spicy' original	2 tbsp	50	0.0	12.0	430	na	1.0	0.0	0	16%
(Open Range) original	1.2 oz	38	0.6	9.0	333	.9	0.2	0.0	0	5%
(Ott's)	1 tbsp	14	0.2	3.2	147	.1	0.1	na	<1	6%
(Skipper's)	1 tbsp	25	0.0	5.0	226	na	1.0	na	0	31%
CAJUN STYLE										
(Golden Dipt)	1 oz	90	0.0	5.0	360	na	8.0	1.0	0	78%
(Heinz)	1 tbsp	15	0.3	3.4	108	>.1 c	0.1	(tr)	na	6%
(Heinz) 'Thick and Rich'	1 oz	35	0.0	8.0	360	na	0.0	0.0	0	0%
CHUNKY										
(Heinz) 'Thick and Rich'	1 oz	30	1.0	6.0	380	na	0.0	0.0	0	0%
(Kraft) 'Thick 'n Spicy'	2 tbsp	60	0.0	13.0	420	na	1.0	0.0	0	15%
COUNTRY STYLE										
(Hunt's)	1.2 oz	39	0.4	8.8	399	.3	0.3	0.0	0	7%
(Hunt's)	1 tbsp	20	<1.0	5.0	140	<1.0	<1.0	na	0	<27%
DIJON AND HONEY										
(Estee)	1 tbsp	18	<1.0	3.0	5	na	<1.0	<1.0	0	<36%
(Lawry's)	1/2 cup	203	4.7	27.0	1768	>.4 c	1.2	na	na	8%
GARLIC (Kraft)	2 tbsp	40	0.0	9.0	420	na	0.0	0.0	0	0%
HAWAIIAN STYLE										
(Heinz)	1 tbsp	19	0.2	4.4	108	>.1 c	0.1	(tr)	na	5%
(Heinz) 'Thick and Rich'	1 oz	40	0.0	10.0	210	na	0.0	0.0	0	0%
HICKORY										
(Healthy Choice)	1.1 oz	26	0.4	5.6	229	.5	0.2	0.0	0	7%
(Heinz) 'Select'	1 oz	35	0.0	8.0	260	na	0.0	0.0	0	0%
(Hunt's)	1 tbsp	20	<1.0	5.0	160	<1.0	<1.0	na	0	<27%
(Hunt's) bold	1.2 oz	46	0.4	10.6	283	.6	0.4	0.0	0	8%
(Hunt's) 'Light'	1.1 oz	27	0.5	6.2	245	.7	0.2	0.0	0	6%
(Open Range)	1.2 oz	37	0.5	8.6	423	1.0	0.2	0.0	0	5%
HICKORY SMOKE										
(Heinz)	1 tbsp	19	0.3	4.4	56	>.1 c	0.1	(tr)	na	5%
(Heinz) 'Thick and Rich'	1 oz	35	0.0	8.0	380	na	0.0	0.0	0	0%
(Heinz) 'Thick and Rich'	1 tbsp	20	0.0	5.0	220	na	0.0	0.0	0	0%
(Kraft)	2 tbsp	45	0.0	10.0	440	na	1.0	0.0	0	18%
(Kraft) 'Thick 'n Spicy'	2 tbsp	50	0.0	12.0	430	na	1.0	0.0	0	16%
(Kraft) w/onion bits	2 tbsp	50	0.0	11.0	340	na	1.0	0.0	0	17%
HOMESTYLE (Hunt's)	1.2 oz	41	0.5	9.8	381	.5	0.1	0.0	0	2%
HONEY										
(Hain)	1 tbsp	14	0.0	1.0	120	na	1.0	na	0	69%
(Kraft) 'Thick 'n Spicy'	2 tbsp	60	0.0	13.0	340	na	1.0	0.0	0	15%
HONEY MUSTARD (Hunt's)	1.2 oz	48	0.4	11.5	450	.6	0.2	0.0	0	4%
HOT										
(Healthy Choice) and spicy	1.1 oz	25	0.3	5.7	229	.5	0.2	0.0	0	7%
(Heinz) 'Thick and Rich'	1 tbsp	20	0.0	5.0	220	na	0.0	0.0	0	0%
(Hunt's) and spicy	1.2 oz	48	0.4	11.5	450	.6	0.2	0.0	0	4%
(Kraft)	2 tbsp	45	0.0	9.0	520	na	1.0	0.0	0	20%

Food Name	Serving Size	Calories	Prot. gms	Carbs gms	Sod. mgs	Fiber gms	Fat gms	Sat. Fat gms	Chol. mgs	% Fat Cal.
(Kraft) hickory smoke	2 tbsp	45	0.0	9.0	360	na	1.0	0.0	0	20%
ITALIAN SEASONING (Kraft)	2 tbsp	50	0.0	10.0	280	na	1.0	0.0	0	18%
KANSAS CITY STYLE										
(Hunt's)	1.2 oz	43	0.4	10.0	220	.6	0.2	0.0	0	4%
(Kraft)	2 tbsp	50	0.0	11.0	270	na	1.0	0.0	0	17%
(Kraft) 'Thick 'n Spicy'	2 tbsp	60	0.0	13.0	270	na	1.0	0.0	0	15%
MESQUITE SMOKE										
(Enrico's)	1 tbsp	18	1.0	3.0	4	na	1.0	na	0	36%
(Heinz) 'Thick and Rich'	1 oz	30	0.0	7.0	380	na	0.0	0.0	0	0%
(Hunt's)	2 tbsp	40	<1.0	9.0	360	<1.0	0.0	0.0	0	0%
(Kraft)	2 tbsp	45	0.0	10.0	410	na	1.0	0.0	0	18%
(Kraft) 'Thick 'n Spicy'	2 tbsp	50	0.0	12.0	430	na	1.0	0.0	0	16%
MUSHROOM										
(Heinz)	1 tbsp	14	0.3	3.2	219	>.1 c	0.1	(tr)	na	6%
(Heinz) 'Thick and Rich'	1 oz	30	1.0	6.0	460	na	0.0	0.0	0	0%
NEW ORLEANS STYLE (Hunt's)	1.2 oz	41	0.5	9.4	383	.7	0.2	0.0	0	4%
ONION										
(Heinz)	1 tbsp	15	0.3	3.4	255	>.1 c	0.1	(tr)	na	6%
(Heinz) 'Thick and Rich'	1 oz	30	0.0	7.0	420	na	0.0	0.0	0	0%
(Kraft) w/onion bits	2 tbsp	50	0.0	11.0	340	na	1.0	0.0	0	17%
ORANGE JUICE, 'California Grill' (Lawry's)	1/4 cup	34	3.8	3.4	3846	>.1 c	0.7	na	na	18%
ORIENTAL (LaChoy)	1 tbsp	16	0.7	3.8	304	<1.0	<.1	tr	0	<5%
SALSA STYLE (Kraft)	2 tbsp	45	0.0	9.0	420	0	0.0	0.0	0	0%
SLOPPY JOE, w/beef (Libby's)	1/3 cup	110	5.0	7.0	190	na	7.0	(mq)	(mq)	57%
SMOKY										
(Cattleman's)	1 tbsp	25	0.0	5.0	300	na	0.0	0.0	0	0%
(Maull's)	1 tbsp	20	<1.0	4.0	139	>.7 c	<1.0	na	<1	<31%
(Ott's)	1 tbsp	14	0.2	3.3	149	.1	0.1	na	<1	6%
SOUTHERN STYLE (Hunt's)	1 tbsp	20	<1.0	5.0	170	<1.0	<1.0	na	0	<27%
TEXAS STYLE										
(Heinz) hot 'Thick and Rich'	1 oz	30	0.0	7.0	390	na	0.0	0.0	0	0%
(Hunt's)	1 tbsp	25	<1.0	6.0	150	<1.0	<1.0	na	0	<24%
WESTERN STYLE (Hunt's)	1 tbsp	20	<1.0	5.0	170	<1.0	<1.0	na	0	<27%
BARBECUE SPICE (Tone's)	1 tsp	9	0.3	1.4	713	.3	0.4	<.1	0	35%
BARLEY										
	1 cup	651	23.0	135.2	22	31.8	4.2	0.9	0	6%
flakes (Arrowhead Mills)	2 oz	200	5.0	45.0	1	7.2	1.0	na	0	4%
pearled, cooked	1 cup	193	3.5	44.3	5	6.0	0.7	0.2	0	3%
pearled, cooked	4 oz	139	2.6	32.0	1	4.5	0.5	0.1	0	3%
pearled, raw	1 cup	704	19.8	155.4	18	31.2	2.3	0.5	0	3%
pearled, raw	1 oz	100	2.8	22.0	3	4.4	0.3	0.1	0	3%
pearled, raw (Arrowhead Mills)	2 oz	200	5.0	45.0	1	7.2	1.0	na	0	4%
pearled, raw, medium 'Scotch Brand' 1.7 oz (Quaker)	1/4 cup	172	5.0	36.3	0	5.0	0.5	na	0	3%
pearled, raw, quick 'Scotch Brand' (Quaker)	1/3 cup	172	5.5	36.3	0	5.0	0.5	na	0	3%
raw	1 oz	100	3.5	20.8	3	4.9	0.7	0.1	0	6%
BARLEY FLOUR (Arrowhead Mills)	2 oz	200	7.0	35.0	1	7.2	1.0	na	0	5%
BARRACUDA, PACIFIC										
raw	1 lb	426	89.4	0.0	(mq)	0	5.0	(mq)	(mq)	11%
raw	100 gm	113	21.0	0.0	40	0	2.6	0.8	55	22%
raw	1 oz	27	5.6	0.0	(mq)	0	0.3	(mq)	(mq)	11%
BASELLA. See VINE SPINACH.										
BASIL										
dried (Golden Dipt)	2 grams	8	0.0	1.0	36	na	0.0	na	0	0%
dried, crumbled	1 oz	71	4.1	17.3	10	>5.0 c	1.1	(tr)	0	10%

Food Name	Serving Size	Calories	Prot. gms	Carbs gms	Sod. mgs	Fiber gms	Fat gms	Sat. Fat gms	Chol. mgs	% Fat Cal.
dried, crumbled	1 tbsp	11	0.7	2.7	2	.8	0.2	(tr)	0	tr
dried, crumbled *(Spice Islands)*	1 tsp	3	0.1	0.7	<1	>.2 c	<.1	(tr)	0	tr
dried, ground *(Durkee)*	1 tsp	5	0.0	0.0	0	0	tr	na	na	tr
dried, ground *(Laurel Leaf)*	1 tsp	5	0.0	0.0	0	0	tr	na	na	tr
fresh	2 tbsp	1	0.1	0.2	0	na	0.0	0.0	0	0%
fresh	5 leaves	1	0.1	0.1	0	na	0.0	0.0	0	0%
BASS, FRESHWATER, MIXED SPECIES										
dry-heat cooked	3 oz	124	20.6	0.0	77	0	4.0	0.9	74	30%
raw	1 lb	516	85.5	0.0	317	0	16.7	3.5	308	31%
raw	3 oz	97	16.0	0.0	59	0	3.1	0.7	58	30%
raw	1 oz	32	5.3	0.0	20	0	1.0	0.2	19	30%
BASS, SEA, MIXED SPECIES										
baked	4 oz	141	26.8	0.0	99	0	2.9	0.7	60	20%
broiled	4 oz	141	26.8	0.0	99	0	2.9	0.7	60	20%
dry-heat cooked	3 oz	105	20.1	0.0	74	0	2.2	0.6	45	20%
microwaved	4 oz	141	26.8	0.0	99	0	2.9	0.7	60	20%
raw	1 lb	439	83.6	0.0	308	0	9.1	2.3	186	20%
raw	3 oz	82	15.7	0.0	58	0	1.7	0.4	35	20%
raw	1 oz	27	5.2	0.0	19	0	0.6	0.1	12	21%
BASS, STRIPED										
dry-heat cooked	3 oz	105	19.3	0.0	75	0	2.5	0.6	88	23%
raw	1 lb	439	80.4	0.0	313	0	10.6	2.3	363	23%
raw	3 oz	82	15.1	0.0	59	0	2.0	0.4	68	23%
raw	1 oz	27	5.0	0.0	23	0	0.7	0.1	23	24%
BATTER MIX										
beer, dry mix *(Golden Dipt)*	1 oz	100	2.0	22.0	650	na	0.0	0.0	0	0%
corn dog, dry mix *(Golden Dipt)*	1 oz	100	3.0	22.0	490	(mq)	0.0	0.0	0	0%
fish and chips, dry mix *(Golden Dipt)*	1.25 oz	120	2.0	27.0	910	(mq)	0.0	0.0	0	0%
onion ring, dry mix *(Golden Dipt)*	1 oz	100	2.0	22.0	570	(mq)	0.0	0.0	0	0%
original, dry mix *(Golden Dipt)*	1 oz	100	3.0	21.0	740	(mq)	0.0	0.0	0	0%
tempura, dry mix *(Golden Dipt)*	1 oz	100	3.0	22.0	130	(mq)	0.0	0.0	0	0%
BAY LEAF										
dried, crumbled	1 oz	89	2.2	21.3	7	>7.4 c	2.4	0.6	0	19%
dried, crumbled	1 tbsp	6	0.1	1.4	0	.5	0.2	0.0	0	23%
dried, crumbled	1 tsp	2	0.1	0.5	0	.2	0.1	0.0	0	27%
dried, crumbled *(Durkee)*	1 tsp	2	0.0	0.0	0	0	tr	na	na	tr
dried, crumbled *(Laurel Leaf)*	1 tsp	2	0.0	0.0	0	0	tr	na	na	tr
dried, crumbled *(Spice Islands)*	1 tsp	5	0.1	0.3	<1	>.3 c	0.1	na	0	36%
BEAN. See individual listings.										
BEAN DINNER, W/FRANKFURTERS, FROZEN										
(Banquet)	10 oz	520	17.0	57.0	1230	(mq)	25.0	(mq)	35	43%
(Morton)	10 oz	350	11.0	46.0	1490	(mq)	13.0	(mq)	30	34%
(Swanson)	10.5 oz	440	14.0	53.0	900	(mq)	19.0	(mq)	(mq)	39%
BEAN ENTRÉE, MICROWAVE										
w/frankfurters, in sauce, 'Diner' micro cup *(Libby's)*	7.75 oz	330	15.0	38.0	930	4.3	15.0	6.0	55	39%
w/wieners, microwave cup *(Kid's Kitchen)*	7.5 oz	310	13.0	36.0	750	na	13.0	4.0	45	37%
BEAN MIX										
Cajun, w/sauce, dry *(Lipton)*	1/4 pkg	130	5.0	28.0	400	(mq)	<1.0	na	na	<6%
Cajun, w/sauce, prepared *(Lipton)*	1/2 cup	160	5.0	28.0	440	(mq)	3.0	(mq)	(mq)	17%
chicken and sauce, dry *(Lipton)*	1/4 pkg	120	6.0	26.0	470	(mq)	1.0	na	na	7%
chicken and sauce, prepared *(Lipton)*	1/2 cup	150	6.0	26.0	500	(mq)	4.0	(mq)	(mq)	22%
'Kettle Creations' bean medley with pasta, dry *(Lipton)*	1/4 cup	130	6.0	23.0	690	4.0	1.5	0.0	0	10%
BEAN SALAD, CANNED										
four-bean *(Joan of Arc)*	1/2 cup	100	3.0	23.0	660	3.3	1.0	na	0	8%

Food Name	Serving Size	Calories	Prot. gms	Carbs gms	Sod. mgs	Fiber gms	Fat gms	Sat. Fat gms	Chol. mgs	% Fat Cal.
four-bean (Read)	1/2 cup	100	3.0	23.0	660	3.3	1.0	na	0	8%
green bean, German-style (Joan of Arc)	1 cup	180	3.0	27.0	920	3.6	7.0	(mq)	na	34%
green bean, German-style (Read)	1 cup	180	3.0	27.0	920	3.6	7.0	(mq)	na	34%
three-bean (Joan of Arc)	1/2 cup	90	2.0	22.0	710	3.0	0.0	0.0	0	0%
three-bean (Read)	1/2 cup	90	2.0	22.0	710	3.0	0.0	0.0	0	0%
'Three Bean Salad' (Green Giant)	1/2 cup	70	2.0	18.0	470	3.0	<1.0	0.0	0	<10%
BEAN SPROUTS, CANNED										
(LaChoy)	2 oz	6	0.7	1.4	17	.7	0.1	na	0	10%
(LaChoy)	2.928 oz	12	1.1	2.2	20	1.1	0.1	0.0	0	6%
BEANS, BAKED. See BAKED BEANS, CANNED.										
BEANS, CANNED. See also BAKED BEANS, CANNED; BEAN SPROUTS, CANNED; BEAN SALAD, CANNED; and individual listings.										
barbecue (Open Range)	4.75 oz	185	7.1	36.4	687	7.9	3.3	1.1	1	15%
'Beans 'N' Fixins' (Big John's)	4.7 oz	127	7.1	22.6	590	6.0	3.5	1.2	3	21%
'Big John's Beans 'n Fixin's' (Hunt's)	4 oz	170	5.0	26.0	490	6.0	6.0	2.1	6	30%
'Mexe-Beans' (Old El Paso)	1/2 cup	163	10.0	31.0	627	13.0	1.0	0.0	0	5%
'Mix and Serve' (Hunt's)	4.75 oz	125	1.8	30.3	575	7.8	2.8	1.1	1	16%
mixed (Bush's Best)	1/2 cup	70	6.0	17.0	410	6.0	0.0	na	na	0%
'Pork and Beans' (Hunt's)	4.5 oz	130	6.2	27.5	516	4.3	1.2	0.4	0	7%
'Pork and Beans' (Open Range)	4.6 oz	157	6.1	26.8	621	7.4	4.8	1.7	2	25%
ranch (Open Ranch)	4.7 oz	124	6.2	22.7	628	8.3	3.2	1.0	1	20%
spiced (Gebhardt)	4.5 oz	100	7.2	19.3	654	7.6	1.6	0.6	0	12%
vegetarian, 'Deluxe' (Bush's Best)	4 oz	110	5.0	25.0	350	6.0	0.0	na	na	0%
'Vegetarian Style' (Van Camp's)	1 cup	206	10.9	42.0	950	na	0.6	na	na	3%
w/beef, 'Homestyle' (Hunt's)	9 oz	246	16.1	30.6	944	11.9	6.5	1.5	16	24%
w/franks, 'Homestyle' (Hunt's)	9 oz	319	16.5	41.0	735	12.5	9.9	3.3	23	28%
w/sausage, 'Homestyle' (Hunt's)	9 oz	306	18.7	35.7	567	11.6	9.8	3.8	18	29%
BEAR										
raw	1 lb	730	91.2	0.0	na	0	37.7	na	na	48%
raw	1 oz	45	5.6	0.0	na	0	2.3	na	na	48%
simmered	3 oz	220	27.6	0.0	na	0	11.4	na	na	48%
simmered, diced	1 cup	363	45.4	0.0	(mq)	0	18.7	(mq)	(mq)	48%
BEARNAISE. See SAUCE.										
BEAVER										
raw	1 lb	662	109.1	0.0	231	0	21.8	na	na	31%
raw	1 oz	41	6.7	0.0	14	0	1.3	na	na	30%
roasted	3 oz	180	29.6	0.0	50	0	5.9	na	103	31%
roasted, diced	1 cup	232	38.3	0.0	64	0	7.6	(mq)	(mq)	31%
BEECHNUT, DRIED										
in shell	1 lb	1595	17.2	92.7	(mq)	>10.2 c	138.4	15.8	0	74%
shelled	1 oz	164	1.8	9.5	11	>1.0 c	14.2	1.6	0	74%
BEEF										
(NOTE: TRIMMED = Lean; separable fat removed after cooking. UNTRIMMED = Separable fat not removed.)										
BRAIN										
pan-fried	3 oz	167	10.7	0.0	134	0	13.5	3.2	1696	74%
raw	4 oz	142	11.1	0.0	116	0	10.5	2.4	1889	68%

QUICK REFERENCE: BEEF CUTS AND GRADES

Beef is considerably leaner today than it was in decades past. Because of new feeding and breeding practices, beef is leaner from the beginning, and butchers trim much of the remaining fat away. When looking for low-fat beef, choose one of the leaner cuts: eye of round, top round, round tip, and top sirloin. Then check the grade. In general, the higher, more expensive grades of meat, like USDA Prime and Choice, have more fat due to a higher degree of marbling—internal fat that cannot be trimmed away. USDA Select meats have the lowest amount of fat. Finally, look for the least amount of marbling in the cut and grade you have chosen, and let appearance be the final judge.

Food Name	Serving Size	Calories	Prot. gms	Carbs gms	Sod. mgs	Fiber gms	Fat gms	Sat. Fat gms	Chol. mgs	% Fat Cal.
simmered	4 oz	181	12.6	0.0	136	0	14.2	3.3	2329	72%
BRISKET, FLAT HALF										
Trimmed										
all grades, 0-inch fat, braised	4 oz	217	35.7	0.0	71	0	7.0	2.3	108	31%
all grades, 0-inch fat, braised	3 oz	162	26.8	0.0	54	0	5.3	1.7	81	31%
all grades, 1/4-inch fat, braised	3 oz	189	26.8	0.0	54	0	8.2	2.7	81	41%
all grades, 1/2-inch fat, braised	3 oz	180	26.8	0.0	54	0	7.3	2.6	81	38%
Untrimmed										
all grades, 0-inch fat, braised	4 oz	244	34.6	0.0	70	0	10.7	3.8	108	41%
all grades, 1/4-inch fat, braised	11.5 oz	1189	81.2	0.0	183	0	93.1	36.0	310	72%
all grades, 1/4-inch fat, braised	3 oz	309	21.3	0.0	48	0	24.2	9.4	81	72%
all grades, 1/4-inch fat, raw	4 oz	328	20.2	0.0	70	0	26.7	10.6	79	75%
all grades, 1/2-inch fat, braised	3 oz	311	21.0	0.0	48	0	24.6	10.1	81	73%
all grades, 1/2-inch fat, raw	1 lb	1338	79.5	0.0	277	0	110.7	47.0	322	76%
all grades, 1/2-inch fat, raw	1 oz	84	5.0	0.0	17	0	6.9	2.9	20	76%
BRISKET, POINT HALF										
Trimmed										
all grades, 0-inch fat, braised	4 oz	277	31.8	0.0	87	0	15.6	5.9	103	53%
all grades, 0-inch fat, braised	3 oz	207	23.8	0.0	65	0	11.7	4.4	77	53%
all grades, 1/4-inch fat, braised	3 oz	222	23.8	0.0	65	0	13.3	5.0	77	56%
all grades, 1/2-inch fat, braised	3 oz	224	23.8	0.0	65	0	13.5	5.3	77	56%
all grades, 1-inch fat, braised	4 oz	296	31.8	0.0	87	0	17.8	6.7	103	56%
Untrimmed										
all grades, 0-inch fat, braised	3 oz	304	20.0	0.0	58	0	24.2	9.6	78	73%
all grades, 1/4-inch fat, braised	3 oz	343	18.8	0.0	55	0	29.1	11.5	78	78%
all grades, 1/4-inch fat, raw	1 lb	1501	73.1	0.0	295	0	131.9	53.7	345	80%
all grades, 1/4-inch fat, raw	1 oz	94	4.6	0.0	18	0	8.3	3.4	22	80%
all grades, 1/2-inch fat, braised	3 oz	347	18.7	0.0	55	0	29.6	12.3	78	78%
all grades, 1/2-inch fat, raw	1 lb	1601	71.5	0.0	290	0	143.5	61.3	345	82%
all grades, 1/2-inch fat, raw	1 oz	100	4.5	0.0	18	0	9.0	3.8	22	82%
BRISKET, WHOLE										
Trimmed										
all grades, 0-inch fat, braised	3 oz	185	25.3	0.0	59	0	8.6	3.1	79	43%
all grades, 1/4-inch fat, braised	4 oz	274	33.7	0.0	79	0	14.5	5.2	105	49%
all grades, 1/4-inch fat, braised	3 oz	206	25.3	0.0	59	0	10.9	3.9	79	49%
all grades, 1/2-inch fat, braised	3 oz	205	25.0	0.0	61	0	10.9	3.9	79	50%
Untrimmed										
all grades, 0-inch fat, braised	3 oz	247	22.8	0.0	55	0	16.6	6.4	79	62%
all grades, 0-inch fat, braised	4 oz	247	33.7	0.0	79	0	11.4	4.1	105	43%
all grades, 1/4-inch fat, braised	3 oz	327	20.0	0.0	52	0	26.8	10.5	80	75%
all grades, 1/4-inch fat, raw	1 lb	1415	76.8	0.0	290	0	120.4	48.5	331	78%
all grades, 1/4-inch fat, raw	1 oz	88	4.8	0.0	18	0	7.5	3.0	21	78%
all grades, 1/2-inch fat, braised	3 oz	332	19.5	0.0	52	0	27.6	11.2	79	76%
all grades, 1/2-inch fat, raw	1 lb	1474	75.4	0.0	281	0	127.7	53.9	336	79%
all grades, 1/2-inch fat, raw	1 oz	92	4.7	0.0	18	0	8.0	3.4	21	79%
CHUCK, ARM POT ROAST										
Trimmed										
all grades, 0-inch fat, braised	3 oz	178	28.1	0.0	56	0	6.5	2.3	86	34%
all grades, 1/4-inch fat, braised	3 oz	184	28.1	0.0	56	0	7.1	2.6	86	36%
all grades, 1/2-inch fat, braised	3 oz	196	28.1	0.0	56	0	8.5	3.2	86	41%
choice, 0-inch fat, braised	3 oz	186	28.1	0.0	56	0	7.4	2.7	86	37%
choice, 1/4-inch fat, braised	3 oz	191	28.1	0.0	56	0	7.9	2.9	86	39%
choice, 1/2-inch fat, braised	3 oz	199	28.1	0.0	56	0	8.8	3.3	86	41%
prime, 1/2-inch fat, braised	3 oz	222	28.1	0.0	56	0	11.4	4.3	86	48%

Food Name	Serving Size	Calories	Prot. gms	Carbs gms	Sod. mgs	Fiber gms	Fat gms	Sat. Fat gms	Chol. mgs	% Fat Cal.
prime, 1/2-inch fat, raw	1 lb	699	96.4	0.0	304	0	31.6	12.3	272	42%
prime, 1/2-inch fat, raw	1 oz	44	6.0	0.0	19	0	2.0	0.8	17	43%
select, 0-inch fat, braised	3 oz	168	28.1	0.0	56	0	5.3	2.0	86	30%
select, 1/4-inch fat, braised	3 oz	175	28.1	0.0	56	0	6.1	2.2	86	33%
select, 1/2-inch fat, braised	3 oz	189	28.1	0.0	56	0	7.6	2.9	86	38%
Untrimmed										
all grades, 0-inch fat, braised	3 oz	238	25.2	0.0	53	0	14.5	5.6	85	56%
all grades, 1/4-inch fat, braised	3 oz	282	23.3	0.0	51	0	20.2	8.0	84	66%
all grades, 1/4-inch fat, raw	1 lb	1111	84.0	0.0	268	0	83.3	33.8	308	69%
all grades, 1/4-inch fat, raw	1 oz	69	5.3	0.0	17	0	5.2	2.1	19	69%
all grades, 1/2-inch fat, braised	3 oz	297	23.0	0.0	51	0	22.1	9.1	84	68%
all grades, 1/2-inch fat, raw	1 lb	1166	83.1	0.0	268	0	89.8	38.4	313	71%
all grades, 1/2-inch fat, raw	1 oz	73	5.2	0.0	17	0	5.6	2.4	20	71%
choice, 0-inch fat, braised	3 oz	249	25.0	0.0	53	0	15.8	6.1	85	59%
choice, 1/4-inch fat, braised	3 oz	296	22.9	0.0	50	0	21.9	8.6	84	68%
choice, 1/4-inch fat, raw	1 lb	1157	83.4	0.0	268	0	88.8	35.9	313	71%
choice, 1/4-inch fat, raw	1 oz	72	5.2	0.0	17	0	5.6	2.3	20	71%
choice, 1/2-inch fat, braised	3 oz	301	22.9	0.0	50	0	22.5	9.3	84	69%
choice, 1/2-inch fat, raw	1 lb	1188	82.6	0.0	263	0	92.9	39.7	313	72%
choice, 1/2-inch fat, raw	1 oz	74	5.2	0.0	16	0	5.8	2.5	20	72%
prime, 1/2-inch fat, braised	3 oz	332	22.2	0.0	49	0	26.3	10.8	84	73%
prime, 1/2-inch fat, raw	1 lb	1334	80.5	0.0	259	0	109.6	46.8	318	75%
prime, 1/2-inch fat, raw	1 oz	83	5.0	0.0	16	0	6.8	2.9	20	75%
select, 0-inch fat, braised	3 oz	221	25.6	0.0	54	0	12.4	4.8	85	52%
select, 1/4-inch fat, braised	3 oz	268	23.7	0.0	51	0	18.5	7.3	85	64%
select, 1/4-inch fat, raw	1 lb	1061	84.6	0.0	268	0	77.4	31.4	308	67%
select, 1/4-inch fat, raw	1 oz	66	5.3	0.0	17	0	4.8	2.0	19	67%
select, 1/2-inch fat, braised	3 oz	286	23.3	0.0	51	0	20.8	8.5	84	67%
select, 1/2-inch fat, raw	1 lb	1075	84.8	0.0	272	0	79.2	33.8	308	68%
select, 1/2-inch fat, raw	1 oz	67	5.3	0.0	17	0	4.9	2.1	19	68%
CHUCK, BLADE ROAST										
Trimmed										
all grades, 0-inch fat, braised	3 oz	215	26.4	0.0	60	0	11.3	4.4	90	49%
all grades, 1/4-inch fat, braised	3 oz	213	26.4	0.0	60	0	11.1	4.3	90	49%
all grades, 1/2-inch fat, braised	3 oz	229	26.4	0.0	60	0	13.0	5.3	90	53%
choice, 0-inch fat, braised	3 oz	225	26.4	0.0	60	0	12.5	4.8	90	52%
choice, 1/4-inch fat, braised	3 oz	224	26.4	0.0	60	0	12.2	4.7	90	51%
choice, 1/2-inch fat, braised	3 oz	234	26.4	0.0	60	0	13.4	5.5	90	53%
prime, 1/2-inch fat, braised	3 oz	270	26.4	0.0	60	0	17.5	7.1	90	60%
prime, 1/2-inch fat, raw	1 lb	921	87.3	0.0	349	0	60.8	24.0	295	61%
prime, 1/2-inch fat, raw	1 oz	58	5.5	0.0	22	0	3.8	1.5	18	61%
select, 0-inch fat, braised	3 oz	202	26.4	0.0	60	0	9.9	3.9	90	46%
select, 1/4-inch fat, braised	3 oz	201	26.4	0.0	60	0	9.9	3.8	90	46%
select, 1/2-inch fat, braised	3 oz	218	26.4	0.0	60	0	11.6	4.7	90	50%
Untrimmed										
all grades, 0-inch fat, braised	3 oz	284	23.1	0.0	55	0	20.5	8.1	88	67%
all grades, 1/4-inch fat, braised	3 oz	293	22.6	0.0	54	0	21.8	8.7	88	69%
all grades, 1/4-inch fat, raw	1 lb	1152	77.3	0.0	304	0	91.2	36.8	327	73%
all grades, 1/4-inch fat, raw	1 oz	72	4.8	0.0	19	0	5.7	2.3	20	73%
all grades, 1/2-inch fat, braised	3 oz	326	21.6	0.0	54	0	25.8	10.8	88	73%
all grades, 1/2-inch fat, raw	1 lb	1288	75.6	0.0	299	0	107.0	45.7	331	76%
all grades, 1/2-inch fat, raw	1 oz	81	4.7	0.0	19	0	6.7	2.9	21	76%
choice, 0-inch fat, braised	3 oz	296	22.9	0.0	55	0	22.0	8.7	88	68%
choice, 1/4-inch fat, braised	3 oz	309	22.2	0.0	54	0	23.6	9.4	88	71%

Food Name	Serving Size	Calories	Prot. gms	Carbs gms	Sod. mgs	Fiber gms	Fat gms	Sat. Fat gms	Chol. mgs	% Fat Cal.
choice, 1/4-inch fat, raw	1 lb	1234	76.3	0.0	299	0	100.8	40.7	327	75%
choice, 1/4-inch fat, raw	1 oz	77	4.8	0.0	19	0	6.3	2.5	20	75%
choice, 1/2-inch fat, braised	3 oz	330	21.6	0.0	54	0	26.4	11.0	88	73%
choice, 1/2-inch fat, raw	1 lb	1320	75.2	0.0	295	0	110.7	47.3	331	77%
choice, 1/2-inch fat, raw	1 oz	83	4.7	0.0	18	0	6.9	3.0	21	77%
prime, 1/2-inch fat, braised	3 oz	354	21.7	0.0	54	0	29.0	12.1	88	75%
prime, 1/2-inch fat, raw	1 lb	1488	74.1	0.0	290	0	129.6	55.1	336	80%
prime, 1/2-inch fat, raw	1 oz	93	4.6	0.0	18	0	8.1	3.4	21	80%
select, 0-inch fat, braised	3 oz	266	23.5	0.0	56	0	18.4	7.3	88	64%
select, 1/4-inch fat, braised	3 oz	277	22.9	0.0	55	0	19.9	7.9	88	66%
select, 1/4-inch fat, raw	1 lb	1066	78.3	0.0	308	0	81.3	32.8	322	70%
select, 1/4-inch fat, raw	1 oz	67	4.9	0.0	19	0	5.1	2.0	20	70%
select, 1/2-inch fat, braised	3 oz	311	21.9	0.0	54	0	24.1	10.1	88	71%
select, 1/2-inch fat, raw	1 lb	1179	76.9	0.0	304	0	94.4	40.4	327	73%
select, 1/2-inch fat, raw	1 oz	74	4.8	0.0	19	0	5.9	2.5	20	73%
FLANK										
Trimmed										
choice, 0-inch fat, braised	3 oz	201	23.8	0.0	61	0	11.0	4.7	60	51%
choice, 0-inch fat, broiled	3 oz	176	23.0	0.0	71	0	8.6	3.7	57	46%
Untrimmed										
choice, 0-inch fat, braised	3 oz	224	22.9	0.0	59	0	14.0	5.9	61	58%
choice, 0-inch fat, broiled	3 oz	192	22.5	0.0	69	0	10.6	4.5	58	52%
choice, 0-inch fat, raw	1 oz	51	5.6	0.0	20	0	3.0	1.3	15	55%
choice, 0-inch fat, raw	4 oz	203	22.3	0.0	80	0	12.0	5.1	59	55%
HEART										
raw	4 oz	132	19.3	2.9	71	0	4.3	1.3	158	30%
simmered	3 oz	149	24.5	0.4	54	0	4.8	1.4	164	30%
KIDNEY										
raw	4 oz	121	18.8	2.5	202	0	3.5	1.1	322	27%
simmered	3 oz	122	21.7	0.8	114	0	2.9	0.9	329	23%
LEAN CUTS										
bottom round steak, 'Lite' (Heritage Lifestyle) uncooked	3 oz	108	19.0	0.0	40	na	4.0	1.0	50	33%
(Brae Beef) raw	4 oz	120	26.0	0.0	60	0	2.0	0.7	57	15%
brisket 'Lite' (Heritage Lifestyle) uncooked	3 oz	98	18.0	0.0	40	na	3.0	1.5	48	28%
burger (Lean and Free) raw	4 oz	174	22.5	0.0	64	0	9.3	(mq)	77	48%
chuck, arm pot roast, 'Lite' (Heritage Lifestyle) uncooked	3 oz	101	18.0	0.0	40	na	3.0	1.0	52	27%
chuck blade roast, 'Lite' (Heritage Lifestyle) uncooked	3 oz	128	17.0	0.0	45	na	7.0	3.0	52	49%
cube steak (Lean and Free) raw	4 oz	109	23.8	0.0	(mq)	0	1.0	(mq)	61	9%
eye round steak, 'Lite' (Heritage Lifestyle) uncooked	3 oz	111	19.0	0.0	38	na	4.0	1.0	41	32%
ground, lean, 'Lite' (Heritage Lifestyle) uncooked	3 oz	118	18.0	0.0	45	na	5.0	2.0	54	38%
lean cuts, raw (Lean and Free)	4 oz	161	21.5	0.0	(mq)	0	7.5	(mq)	67	44%
rib eye (Lean and Free) raw	4 oz	121	24.7	0.0	59	0	2.6	(mq)	71	19%
rib roast, large end, 'Lite' (Heritage Lifestyle) uncooked	3 oz	142	18.0	0.0	40	na	8.0	3.0	50	51%
rib steak, small end, 'Lite' (Heritage Lifestyle) uncooked	3 oz	118	19.0	0.0	35	na	5.0	1.0	43	38%
rolled (Lean and Free) raw	4 oz	125	25.4	0.0	60	0	2.8	(mq)	(mq)	20%
round steak (Lean and Free) raw	4 oz	111	25.7	0.0	60	0	1.1	(mq)	(mq)	9%
round tip roast, 'Lite' (Heritage Lifestyle) uncooked	3 oz	91	18.0	0.0	43	na	1.5	1.0	49	15%
sirloin steak (Lean and Free) raw	4 oz	111	24.2	0.0	67	0	1.8	(mq)	66	14%
sirloin steak, 'Lite' (Heritage Lifestyle) uncooked	3 oz	103	18.0	0.0	45	na	3.0	1.0	49	26%
sirloin tip (Lean and Free) raw	4 oz	110	23.2	0.0	62	0	1.2	(mq)	66	10%
strip loin steak (Lean and Free) raw	4 oz	113	25.2	0.0	61	0	1.8	(mq)	67	14%
T-bone (Lean and Free) raw	4 oz	125	25.5	0.0	54	0	2.7	(mq)	(mq)	19%
tenderloin fillet steak (Lean and Free) raw	4 oz	116	23.6	0.0	68	0	2.4	(mq)	61	19%
tenderloin steak, 'Lite' (Heritage Lifestyle) uncooked	3 oz	109	18.0	0.0	40	na	4.0	2.0	53	33%

Food Name	Serving Size	Calories	Prot. gms	Carbs gms	Sod. mgs	Fiber gms	Fat gms	Sat. Fat gms	Chol. mgs	% Fat Cal.
top loin steak, 'Lite' *(Heritage Lifestyle)* uncooked	3 oz	114	19.0	0.0	40	na	4.0	1.5	44	32%
top round *(Lean and Free)* raw	4 oz	134	24.6	0.0	49	0	4.5	(mq)	(mq)	29%
top round steak, 'Lite' *(Heritage Lifestyle)* uncooked	3 oz	100	19.0	0.0	40	na	3.0	1.0	48	27%
LIVER										
braised	3 oz	137	20.7	2.9	59	0	4.2	1.6	331	29%
pan-fried	3 oz	184	22.7	6.7	90	0	6.8	2.3	410	34%
pan-fried in vegetable oil	4 oz	246	30.3	8.9	120	0	9.1	3.0	547	34%
raw	4 oz	162	22.6	6.6	82	0	4.3	1.7	400	25%
LUNG										
braised	3 oz	102	17.3	0.0	86	0	3.2	1.1	235	29%
raw	4 oz	104	18.3	0.0	224	0	2.8	1.0	273	26%
PANCREAS										
braised	3 oz	230	23.0	0.0	51	0	14.6	5.0	223	59%
raw	4 oz	266	17.7	0.0	76	0	21.0	7.2	232	73%
PORTERHOUSE										
Trimmed										
choice, 1/4-inch fat, broiled	3 oz	185	23.9	0.0	56	0	9.2	3.7	68	46%
choice, 1/2-inch fat, broiled	3 oz	185	23.9	0.0	56	0	9.2	3.7	68	46%
Untrimmed										
choice, 1/4-inch fat, broiled	3 oz	259	21.1	0.0	52	0	18.8	7.6	71	67%
choice, 1/4-inch fat, raw	1 lb	1229	80.2	0.0	222	0	98.4	40.5	313	73%
choice, 1/4-inch fat, raw	1 oz	77	5.0	0.0	14	0	6.2	2.5	20	74%
choice, 1/2-inch fat, broiled	3 oz	254	21.3	0.0	52	0	18.0	7.5	71	66%
choice, 1/2-inch fat, raw	1 lb	1288	78.8	0.0	222	0	105.6	45.1	318	75%
choice, 1/2-inch fat, raw	1 oz	81	4.9	0.0	14	0	6.6	2.8	20	75%
RIB, LARGE END										
Trimmed										
all grades, ribs 6-9, 0-inch fat, roasted	3 oz	202	23.4	0.0	62	0	11.4	4.6	69	52%
all grades, ribs 6-9, 1/4-inch fat, broiled	3 oz	190	21.4	0.0	61	0	11.0	4.5	65	54%
all grades, ribs 6-9, 1/4-inch fat, roasted	3 oz	201	23.4	0.0	62	0	11.2	4.5	69	52%
all grades, ribs 6-9, 1/2-inch fat, broiled	3 oz	198	20.9	0.0	59	0	12.1	5.2	70	57%
all grades, ribs 6-9, 1/2-inch fat, roasted	3 oz	207	23.4	0.0	62	0	11.9	5.0	69	53%
choice, ribs 6-9, 0-inch fat, roasted	3 oz	215	23.4	0.0	62	0	12.7	5.1	69	55%
choice, ribs 6-9, 1/4-inch fat, broiled	3 oz	204	21.4	0.0	61	0	12.4	5.1	65	57%
choice, ribs 6-9, 1/4-inch fat, roasted	3 oz	213	23.4	0.0	62	0	12.5	5.0	69	55%
choice, ribs 6-9, 1/2-inch fat, broiled	3 oz	203	20.9	0.0	59	0	12.6	5.3	70	58%
choice, ribs 6-9, 1/2-inch fat, roasted	3 oz	211	23.4	0.0	62	0	12.3	5.2	69	54%
prime, ribs 6-9, 1/4-inch fat, broiled	3 oz	250	20.9	0.0	59	0	17.7	7.6	70	66%
prime, ribs 6-9, 1/4-inch fat, roasted	3 oz	241	23.4	0.0	62	0	15.6	6.7	69	60%
prime, ribs 6-9, 1/2-inch fat, broiled	3 oz	250	20.9	0.0	59	0	17.7	7.6	70	66%
prime, ribs 6-9, 1/2-inch fat, roasted	3 oz	241	23.4	0.0	62	0	15.6	6.7	69	60%
select, ribs 6-9, 0-inch fat, roasted	3 oz	187	23.4	0.0	62	0	9.7	3.9	69	48%
select, ribs 6-9, 1/4-inch fat, broiled	3 oz	175	21.4	0.0	61	0	9.3	3.8	65	49%
select, ribs 6-9, 1/4-inch fat, roasted	3 oz	187	23.4	0.0	62	0	9.7	3.9	69	48%
select, ribs 6-9, 1/2-inch fat, broiled	3 oz	183	20.9	0.0	59	0	10.4	4.4	70	53%
select, ribs 6-9, 1/2-inch fat, roasted	3 oz	197	23.4	0.0	62	0	10.8	4.6	69	51%
Untrimmed										
all grades, ribs 6-9, 0-inch fat, roasted	3 oz	300	19.7	0.0	55	0	24.0	9.7	72	73%
all grades, ribs 6-9, 1/4-inch fat, broiled	3 oz	295	18.1	0.0	54	0	24.2	9.8	69	75%
all grades, ribs 6-9, 1/4-inch fat, raw	1 lb	1465	73.0	0.0	249	0	127.9	52.9	322	80%
all grades, ribs 6-9, 1/4-inch fat, raw	1 oz	92	4.6	0.0	16	0	8.0	3.3	20	80%
all grades, ribs 6-9, 1/4-inch fat, roasted	3 oz	310	19.2	0.0	54	0	25.3	10.2	72	75%
all grades, ribs 6-9, 1/2-inch fat, broiled	3 oz	321	17.1	0.0	51	0	27.5	11.7	74	78%
all grades, ribs 6-9, 1/2-inch fat, raw	1 lb	1588	70.6	0.0	240	0	142.3	62.0	331	82%

Food Name	Serving Size	Calories	Prot. gms	Carbs gms	Sod. mgs	Fiber gms	Fat gms	Sat. Fat gms	Chol. mgs	% Fat Cal.
all grades, ribs 6-9, 1/2-inch fat, raw	1 oz	99	4.4	0.0	15	0	8.9	3.9	21	82%
all grades, ribs 6-9, 1/2-inch fat, roasted	3 oz	313	19.3	0.0	54	0	25.5	10.8	72	75%
choice, ribs 6-9, 0-inch fat, roasted	10.2 oz	1080	66.1	0.0	186	0	88.4	35.7	246	75%
choice, ribs 6-9, 0-inch fat, roasted	3 oz	316	19.4	0.0	54	0	25.9	10.5	72	75%
choice, ribs 6-9, 1/4-inch fat, broiled	3 oz	312	17.8	0.0	54	0	26.2	10.6	69	77%
choice, ribs 6-9, 1/4-inch fat, raw	1 lb	1565	71.4	0.0	240	0	139.8	57.9	331	82%
choice, ribs 6-9, 1/4-inch fat, raw	1 oz	98	4.5	0.0	15	0	8.7	3.6	21	81%
choice, ribs 6-9, 1/4-inch fat, roasted	3 oz	326	19.0	0.0	54	0	27.2	11.0	72	76%
choice, ribs 6-9, 1/2-inch fat, broiled	3 oz	326	17.0	0.0	51	0	28.1	11.9	74	79%
choice, ribs 6-9, 1/2-inch fat, raw	1 lb	1615	70.2	0.0	240	0	145.6	63.7	336	82%
choice, ribs 6-9, 1/2-inch fat, raw	1 oz	101	4.4	0.0	15	0	9.1	4.0	21	82%
choice, ribs 6-9, 1/2-inch fat, roasted	3 oz	316	19.3	0.0	54	0	25.9	11.0	72	75%
prime, ribs 6-9, 1/4-inch fat, broiled	3 oz	351	17.3	0.0	52	0	30.8	12.7	73	80%
prime, ribs 6-9, 1/4-inch fat, raw	1 lb	1710	70.4	0.0	240	0	156.5	65.6	331	83%
prime, ribs 6-9, 1/4-inch fat, raw	1 oz	107	4.4	0.0	15	0	9.8	4.1	21	83%
prime, ribs 6-9, 1/4-inch fat, roasted	3 oz	342	19.1	0.0	54	0	28.9	11.9	72	77%
prime, ribs 6-9, 1/2-inch fat, broiled	3 oz	361	16.9	0.0	51	0	32.1	13.6	74	81%
prime, ribs 6-9, 1/2-inch fat, raw	1 lb	1737	69.8	0.0	236	0	159.6	69.5	336	84%
prime, ribs 6-9, 1/2-inch fat, raw	1 oz	109	4.4	0.0	15	0	10.0	4.3	21	84%
prime, ribs 6-9, 1/2-inch fat, roasted	3 oz	346	18.9	0.0	54	0	29.4	12.5	72	78%
select, ribs 6-9, 0-inch fat, roasted	3 oz	281	20.0	0.0	55	0	21.7	8.8	71	71%
select, ribs 6-9, 1/4-inch fat, broiled	3 oz	275	18.3	0.0	54	0	21.9	8.9	68	73%
select, ribs 6-9, 1/4-inch fat, raw	1 lb	1379	74.0	0.0	249	0	117.7	48.7	322	78%
select, ribs 6-9, 1/4-inch fat, raw	1 oz	86	4.6	0.0	16	0	7.4	3.0	20	78%
select, ribs 6-9, 1/4-inch fat, roasted	3 oz	289	19.7	0.0	55	0	22.7	9.2	72	72%
select, ribs 6-9, 1/2-inch fat, broiled	3 oz	301	17.4	0.0	52	0	25.1	10.7	73	76%
select, ribs 6-9, 1/2-inch fat, raw	1 lb	1488	72.0	0.0	245	0	130.7	57.0	327	80%
select, ribs 6-9, 1/2-inch fat, raw	1 oz	93	4.5	0.0	15	0	8.2	3.6	20	80%
select, ribs 6-9, 1/2-inch fat, roasted	3 oz	303	19.4	0.0	54	0	24.5	10.4	72	74%
RIB, SHORTRIB										
Trimmed, choice, braised	3 oz	251	26.1	0.0	49	0	15.4	6.6	79	57%
Untrimmed										
choice, braised	3 oz	400	18.3	0.0	43	0	35.7	15.1	80	81%
choice, raw	1 lb	1760	65.3	0.0	222	0	164.3	71.5	345	85%
choice, raw	1 oz	110	4.1	0.0	14	0	10.3	4.5	22	85%
RIB, SMALL END										
Trimmed										
all grades, ribs 10-12, 0-inch fat, broiled	3 oz	181	23.8	0.0	59	0	8.8	3.5	68	45%
all grades, ribs 10-12, 1/4-inch fat, roasted	3 oz	185	22.8	0.0	60	0	9.8	3.9	67	49%
all grades, ribs 10-12, 1/2-inch fat, broiled	3 oz	188	23.8	0.0	59	0	9.5	4.0	68	47%
all grades, ribs 10-12, 1/2-inch fat, roasted	3 oz	201	22.7	0.0	64	0	11.5	4.9	68	53%
all grades, ribs 10-12, 1/4-inch fat, broiled	3 oz	188	23.8	0.0	59	0	9.5	3.8	68	47%
choice, ribs 10-12, 0-inch fat, broiled	3 oz	191	23.8	0.0	59	0	9.9	4.0	68	48%
choice, ribs 10-12, 1/4-inch fat, broiled	3 oz	198	23.8	0.0	59	0	10.7	4.3	68	50%
choice, ribs 10-12, 1/4-inch fat, roasted	3 oz	197	22.8	0.0	60	0	11.1	4.4	67	52%
choice, ribs 10-12, 1/2-inch fat, broiled	3 oz	191	23.8	0.0	59	0	9.9	4.2	68	48%
choice, ribs 10-12, 1/2-inch fat, roasted	3 oz	207	22.7	0.0	64	0	12.1	5.1	68	55%
prime, ribs 10-12, 1/4-inch fat, broiled	3 oz	221	23.8	0.0	59	0	13.2	5.6	68	56%
prime, ribs 10-12, 1/4-inch fat, roasted	3 oz	258	22.7	0.0	64	0	17.9	7.6	68	64%
prime, ribs 10-12, 1/2-inch fat, broiled	3 oz	221	23.8	0.0	59	0	13.2	5.6	68	56%
prime, ribs 10-12, 1/2-inch fat, roasted	3 oz	258	22.7	0.0	64	0	17.9	7.6	68	64%
select, ribs 10-12, 0-inch fat, broiled	3 oz	168	23.8	0.0	59	0	7.4	3.0	68	41%
select, ribs 10-12, 1/4-inch fat, broiled	3 oz	176	23.8	0.0	59	0	8.2	3.3	68	44%
select, ribs 10-12, 1/4-inch fat, roasted	3 oz	173	22.8	0.0	60	0	8.3	3.3	67	45%

Food Name	Serving Size	Calories	Prot. gms	Carbs gms	Sod. mgs	Fiber gms	Fat gms	Sat. Fat gms	Chol. mgs	% Fat Cal.
select, ribs 10-12, 1/2-inch fat, broiled	3 oz	178	23.8	0.0	59	0	8.4	3.6	68	44%
select, ribs 10-12, 1/2-inch fat, roasted	3 oz	184	22.7	0.0	64	0	9.6	4.1	68	49%
Untrimmed										
all grades, ribs 10-12, 0-inch fat, broiled	3 oz	252	21.2	0.0	54	0	17.9	7.3	71	66%
all grades, ribs 10-12, 1/4-inch fat, broiled	3 oz	286	20.1	0.0	53	0	22.1	8.9	71	71%
all grades, ribs 10-12, 1/4-inch fat, raw	1 lb	1352	76.2	0.0	240	0	113.9	46.7	318	77%
all grades, ribs 10-12, 1/4-inch fat, raw	1 oz	84	4.8	0.0	15	0	7.1	2.9	20	77%
all grades, ribs 10-12, 1/4-inch fat, roasted	3 oz	295	19.0	0.0	54	0	23.8	9.6	71	74%
all grades, ribs 10-12, 1/2-inch fat, broiled	3 oz	277	20.4	0.0	53	0	21.1	8.9	71	70%
all grades, ribs 10-12, 1/2-inch fat, raw	1 lb	1388	75.9	0.0	245	0	117.8	51.1	318	78%
all grades, ribs 10-12, 1/2-inch fat, raw	1 oz	87	4.7	0.0	15	0	7.4	3.2	20	78%
all grades, ribs 10-12, 1/2-inch fat, roasted	3 oz	305	18.9	0.0	55	0	24.9	10.5	72	75%
choice, ribs 10-12, 0-inch fat, broiled	3 oz	265	21.0	0.0	54	0	19.4	7.8	71	68%
choice, ribs 10-12, 1/4-inch fat, broiled	3 oz	297	20.0	0.0	53	0	23.5	9.5	71	73%
choice, ribs 10-12, 1/4-inch fat, raw	1 lb	1429	75.1	0.0	240	0	122.8	50.3	322	79%
choice, ribs 10-12, 1/4-inch fat, raw	1 oz	89	4.7	0.0	15	0	7.7	3.1	20	79%
choice, ribs 10-12, 1/4-inch fat, roasted	3 oz	312	18.7	0.0	53	0	25.7	10.4	71	76%
choice, ribs 10-12, 1/2-inch fat, broiled	3 oz	282	20.4	0.0	53	0	21.6	9.1	71	70%
choice, ribs 10-12, 1/2-inch fat, raw	1 lb	1415	75.5	0.0	240	0	121.2	52.5	318	78%
choice, ribs 10-12, 1/2-inch fat, raw	1 oz	88	4.7	0.0	15	0	7.6	3.3	20	78%
choice, ribs 10-12, 1/2-inch fat, roasted	3 oz	312	18.8	0.0	55	0	25.7	10.9	72	76%
prime, ribs 10-12, 1/4-inch fat, broiled	3 oz	307	20.3	0.0	53	0	24.4	10.1	71	73%
prime, ribs 10-12, 1/4-inch fat, raw	1 lb	1551	75.1	0.0	240	0	136.4	56.5	322	80%
prime, ribs 10-12, 1/4-inch fat, raw	1 oz	97	4.7	0.0	15	0	8.5	3.5	20	80%
prime, ribs 10-12, 1/4-inch fat, roasted	3 oz	354	18.6	0.0	55	0	30.5	12.6	71	79%
prime, ribs 10-12, 1/2-inch fat, broiled	3 oz	309	20.2	0.0	53	0	24.7	10.5	71	73%
prime, ribs 10-12, 1/2-inch fat, raw	1 lb	1583	74.3	0.0	240	0	140.2	60.5	322	81%
prime, ribs 10-12, 1/2-inch fat, raw	1 oz	99	4.7	0.0	15	0	8.8	3.8	20	81%
prime, ribs 10-12, 1/2-inch fat, roasted	3 oz	357	18.5	0.0	54	0	30.8	13.0	72	79%
select, ribs 10-12, 0-inch fat, broiled	3 oz	242	21.2	0.0	54	0	16.8	6.8	71	64%
select, ribs 10-12, 1/4-inch fat, broiled	3 oz	273	20.3	0.0	53	0	20.6	8.4	71	70%
select, ribs 10-12, 1/4-inch fat, raw	1 lb	1297	76.7	0.0	245	0	107.4	44.0	318	76%
select, ribs 10-12, 1/4-inch fat, raw	1 oz	81	4.8	0.0	15	0	6.7	2.8	20	76%
select, ribs 10-12, 1/4-inch fat, roasted	3 oz	281	19.1	0.0	54	0	22.2	8.9	71	72%
select, ribs 10-12, 1/2-inch fat, broiled	3 oz	263	20.7	0.0	54	0	19.4	8.2	71	68%
select, ribs 10-12, 1/2-inch fat, raw	1 lb	1288	77.2	0.0	245	0	106.4	46.2	313	76%
select, ribs 10-12, 1/2-inch fat, raw	1 oz	81	4.8	0.0	15	0	6.7	2.9	20	76%
select, ribs 10-12, 1/2-inch fat, roasted	3 oz	283	19.2	0.0	56	0	22.3	9.4	71	72%
RIB, WHOLE										
Trimmed										
all grades, ribs 6-12, 1/4-inch fat, broiled	3 oz	190	22.4	0.0	60	0	10.4	4.2	65	51%
all grades, ribs 6-12, 1/4-inch fat, roasted	3 oz	195	23.2	0.0	61	0	10.6	4.2	68	51%
all grades, ribs 6-12, 1/2-inch fat, broiled	3 oz	194	22.1	0.0	59	0	11.0	4.7	70	53%
all grades, ribs 6-12, 1/2-inch fat, roasted	3 oz	204	23.1	0.0	63	0	11.7	4.9	69	53%
choice, ribs 6-12, 1/4-inch fat, broiled	3 oz	201	22.4	0.0	60	0	11.7	4.8	65	54%
choice, ribs 6-12, 1/4-inch fat, roasted	3 oz	207	23.2	0.0	61	0	11.9	4.8	68	54%
choice, ribs 6-12, 1/2-inch fat, broiled	3 oz	198	22.1	0.0	60	0	11.5	4.8	70	51%
choice, ribs 6-12, 1/2-inch fat, roasted	3 oz	209	23.1	0.0	63	0	12.2	5.2	69	54%
prime, ribs 6-12, 1/4-inch fat, broiled	3 oz	238	22.1	0.0	59	0	15.9	6.8	69	62%
prime, ribs 6-12, 1/4-inch fat, roasted	3 oz	248	23.1	0.0	63	0	16.5	7.1	69	62%
prime, ribs 6-12, 1/2-inch fat, broiled	3 oz	238	22.1	0.0	59	0	15.9	6.8	70	62%
prime, ribs 6-12, 1/2-inch fat, roasted	3 oz	248	23.1	0.0	63	0	16.5	7.1	69	62%
select, ribs 6-12, 1/4-inch fat, broiled	3 oz	175	22.4	0.0	60	0	8.9	3.6	65	47%
select, ribs 6-12, 1/4-inch fat, roasted	3 oz	181	23.2	0.0	61	0	9.1	3.6	68	47%

Food Name	Serving Size	Calories	Prot. gms	Carbs gms	Sod. mgs	Fiber gms	Fat gms	Sat. Fat gms	Chol. mgs	% Fat Cal.
select, ribs 6-12, 1/2-inch fat, broiled	3 oz	181	22.1	0.0	59	0	9.6	4.1	70	49%
select, ribs 6-12, 1/2-inch fat, roasted	3 oz	191	23.1	0.0	63	0	10.3	4.4	69	50%
Untrimmed										
all grades, ribs 6-12, 1/4-inch fat, broiled	3 oz	291	18.9	0.0	54	0	23.3	9.5	70	74%
all grades, ribs 6-12, 1/4-inch fat, raw	1 lb	1420	74.3	0.0	245	0	122.4	50.5	322	79%
all grades, ribs 6-12, 1/4-inch fat, raw	1 oz	89	4.6	0.0	15	0	7.7	3.2	20	79%
all grades, ribs 6-12, 1/4-inch fat, roasted	3 oz	304	19.1	0.0	54	0	24.7	9.9	71	74%
all grades, ribs 6-12, 1/2-inch fat, broiled	3 oz	308	18.3	0.0	52	0	25.5	10.8	73	76%
all grades, ribs 6-12, 1/2-inch fat, raw	1 lb	1501	72.8	0.0	240	0	132.2	57.4	327	80%
all grades, ribs 6-12, 1/2-inch fat, raw	1 oz	94	4.6	0.0	15	0	8.3	3.6	20	80%
all grades, ribs 6-12, 1/2-inch fat, roasted	3 oz	324	18.6	0.0	54	0	27.0	11.4	72	77%
choice, ribs 6-12, 1/4-inch fat, broiled	3 oz	306	18.7	0.0	53	0	25.1	10.2	70	75%
choice, ribs 6-12, 1/4-inch fat, raw	1 lb	1510	72.9	0.0	240	0	133.2	54.9	327	80%
choice, ribs 6-12, 1/4-inch fat, raw	1 oz	94	4.6	0.0	15	0	8.3	3.4	20	80%
choice, ribs 6-12, 1/4-inch fat, roasted	3 oz	320	18.8	0.0	54	0	26.5	10.7	72	76%
choice, ribs 6-12, 1/2-inch fat, broiled	3 oz	313	18.2	0.0	52	0	26.1	11.0	73	76%
choice, ribs 6-12, 1/2-inch fat, raw	1 lb	1533	72.4	0.0	240	0	135.5	59.0	327	81%
choice, ribs 6-12, 1/2-inch fat, raw	1 oz	96	4.5	0.0	15	0	8.5	3.7	20	81%
choice, ribs 6-12, 1/2-inch fat, roasted	3 oz	328	18.6	0.0	54	0	27.6	11.7	72	77%
prime, ribs 6-12, 1/4-inch fat, broiled	3 oz	333	18.5	0.0	53	0	28.2	11.7	72	77%
prime, ribs 6-12, 1/4-inch fat, raw	1 lb	1651	72.2	0.0	240	0	149.0	62.2	331	82%
prime, ribs 6-12, 1/4-inch fat, raw	1 oz	103	4.5	0.0	15	0	9.3	3.9	21	82%
prime, ribs 6-12, 1/4-inch fat, roasted	3 oz	348	18.9	0.0	54	0	29.6	12.3	72	78%
prime, ribs 6-12, 1/2-inch fat, broiled	3 oz	347	17.9	0.0	51	0	29.9	12.7	73	79%
prime, ribs 6-12, 1/2-inch fat, raw	1 lb	1678	71.4	0.0	236	0	152.4	66.1	331	83%
prime, ribs 6-12, 1/2-inch fat, raw	1 oz	105	4.5	0.0	15	0	9.5	4.1	21	83%
prime, ribs 6-12, 1/2-inch fat, roasted	3 oz	361	18.3	0.0	54	0	31.4	13.3	73	79%
select, ribs 6-12, 1/4-inch fat, broiled	3 oz	275	19.1	0.0	54	0	21.4	8.7	70	72%
select, ribs 6-12, 1/4-inch fat, raw	1 lb	1347	75.1	0.0	249	0	113.7	46.9	318	77%
select, ribs 6-12, 1/4-inch fat, raw	1 oz	84	4.7	0.0	16	0	7.1	2.9	20	77%
select, ribs 6-12, 1/4-inch fat, roasted	3 oz	286	19.4	0.0	54	0	22.5	9.1	71	72%
select, ribs 6-12, 1/2-inch fat, broiled	3 oz	289	18.6	0.0	52	0	23.3	9.9	72	74%
select, ribs 6-12, 1/2-inch fat, raw	1 lb	1411	74.0	0.0	245	0	121.2	52.7	322	79%
select, ribs 6-12, 1/2-inch fat, raw	1 oz	88	4.6	0.0	15	0	7.6	3.3	20	79%
select, ribs 6-12, 1/2-inch fat, roasted	3 oz	306	19.0	0.0	54	0	24.9	10.6	72	75%
RIB EYE, SMALL END										
Trimmed										
choice, ribs 10-12, 0-inch fat, broiled	3 oz	191	23.8	0.0	59	0	9.9	4.0	68	48%
choice, ribs 10-12, 1/4-inch fat, broiled	4 oz	255	31.8	0.0	78	0	13.3	5.4	91	49%
Untrimmed										
choice, ribs 10-12, 0-inch fat, broiled	3 oz	261	21.2	0.0	54	0	18.9	7.7	71	67%
choice, ribs 10-12, 0-inch fat, raw	1 lb	1243	79.4	0.0	254	0	100.1	40.8	308	74%
choice, ribs 10-12, 0-inch fat, raw	1 oz	78	5.0	0.0	16	0	6.3	2.5	19	74%
ROUND, BOTTOM										
Trimmed										
all grades, 0-inch fat, braised	3 oz	173	26.9	0.0	43	0	6.5	2.2	82	35%
all grades, 0-inch fat, roasted	3 oz	156	24.4	0.0	56	0	5.7	1.9	66	35%
all grades, 1/4-inch fat, braised	3 oz	178	26.9	0.0	43	0	7.0	2.3	82	37%
all grades, 1/4-inch fat, roasted	3 oz	161	24.4	0.0	56	0	6.3	2.1	66	37%
all grades, 1/2-inch fat, braised	3 oz	189	26.9	0.0	43	0	8.2	2.9	82	41%
choice, 0-inch fat, braised	3 oz	181	26.9	0.0	43	0	7.4	2.5	82	38%
choice, 0-inch fat, roasted	3 oz	164	24.4	0.0	56	0	6.6	2.2	66	38%
choice, 1/4-inch fat, braised	3 oz	187	26.9	0.0	43	0	8.0	2.7	82	40%
choice, 1/4-inch fat, roasted	3 oz	168	24.4	0.0	56	0	7.1	2.4	66	40%

Food Name	Serving Size	Calories	Prot. gms	Carbs gms	Sod. mgs	Fiber gms	Fat gms	Sat. Fat gms	Chol. mgs	% Fat Cal.
choice, 1/2-inch fat, braised	3 oz	191	26.9	0.0	43	0	8.5	3.0	82	42%
prime, 1/2-inch fat, braised	3 oz	212	26.9	0.0	43	0	10.8	3.8	82	48%
prime, 1/2-inch fat, raw	1 lb	721	99.2	0.0	268	0	33.1	11.8	268	43%
prime, 1/2-inch fat, raw	1 oz	45	6.2	0.0	17	0	2.1	0.7	17	43%
select, 0-inch fat, braised	3 oz	163	26.9	0.0	43	0	5.3	1.8	82	31%
select, 0-inch fat, roasted	3 oz	145	24.4	0.0	56	0	4.6	1.5	66	30%
select, 1/4-inch fat, braised	3 oz	167	26.9	0.0	43	0	5.8	2.0	82	33%
select, 1/4-inch fat, roasted	10.5 oz	534	86.0	0.0	197	0	18.5	6.3	232.	33%
select, 1/4-inch fat, roasted	3 oz	152	24.4	0.0	56	0	5.3	1.8	66	33%
select, 1/2-inch fat, braised	3 oz	182	26.9	0.0	43	0	7.4	2.6	82	38%
Untrimmed										
all grades, 0-inch fat, braised	3 oz	181	26.5	0.0	43	0	7.5	2.6	82	39%
all grades, 0-inch fat, roasted	3 oz	160	24.3	0.0	56	0	6.3	2.1	66	37%
all grades, 1/4-inch fat, braised	3 oz	234	24.4	0.0	43	0	14.4	5.4	82	57%
all grades, 1/4-inch fat, raw	1 lb	943	91.8	0.0	249	0	60.9	23.6	290	60%
all grades, 1/4-inch fat, raw	1 oz	59	5.7	0.0	16	0	3.8	1.5	18	60%
all grades, 1/4-inch fat, roasted	3 oz	211	22.6	0.0	54	0	12.7	4.8	68	56%
all grades, 1/2-inch fat, braised	3 oz	222	25.3	0.0	43	0	12.6	4.8	82	53%
all grades, 1/2-inch fat, raw	1 lb	1021	90.2	0.0	249	0	70.5	29.3	295	64%
all grades, 1/2-inch fat, raw	1 oz	64	5.6	0.0	16	0	4.4	1.8	18	64%
choice, 0-inch fat, braised	3 oz	193	26.3	0.0	43	0	9.0	3.2	82	44%
choice, 0-inch fat, roasted	3 oz	173	24.2	0.0	55	0	7.7	2.7	66	42%
choice, 1/4-inch fat, braised	3 oz	241	24.4	0.0	43	0	15.2	5.7	82	58%
choice, 1/4-inch fat, raw	1 lb	989	91.1	0.0	249	0	66.7	25.9	290	62%
choice, 1/4-inch fat, raw	1 oz	62	5.7	0.0	16	0	4.2	1.6	18	62%
choice, 1/4-inch fat, roasted	3 oz	221	22.5	0.0	54	0	13.9	5.2	68	58%
choice, 1/2-inch fat, braised	3 oz	224	25.3	0.0	43	0	12.9	4.9	82	53%
choice, 1/2-inch fat, raw	1 lb	1030	90.1	0.0	249	0	71.5	29.7	295	64%
choice, 1/2-inch fat, raw	1 oz	64	5.6	0.0	16	0	4.5	1.9	18	64%
prime, 1/2-inch fat, braised	3 oz	252	24.9	0.0	43	0	16.2	6.2	82	59%
prime, 1/2-inch fat, raw	1 lb	1021	91.3	0.0	249	0	69.8	28.5	290	63%
prime, 1/2-inch fat, raw	1 oz	64	5.7	0.0	16	0	4.4	1.8	18	64%
select, 0-inch fat, braised	3 oz	171	26.5	0.0	43	0	6.4	2.3	82	35%
select, 0-inch fat, roasted	3 oz	150	24.3	0.0	56	0	5.1	1.7	66	32%
select, 1/4-inch fat, braised	3 oz	220	24.5	0.0	43	0	12.8	4.8	82	54%
select, 1/4-inch fat, raw	1 lb	885	92.4	0.0	254	0	54.3	21.2	286	57%
select, 1/4-inch fat, raw	1 oz	55	5.8	0.0	16	0	3.4	1.3	18	57%
select, 1/4-inch fat, roasted	3 oz	199	22.8	0.0	54	0	11.3	4.3	68	53%
select, 1/2-inch fat, braised	3 oz	215	25.4	0.0	43	0	11.8	4.5	82	51%
select, 1/2-inch fat, raw	1 lb	984	90.9	0.0	249	0	66.0	27.4	290	62%
select, 1/2-inch fat, raw	1 oz	62	5.7	0.0	16	0	4.1	1.7	18	62%
ROUND, EYE OF										
Trimmed										
all grades, 0-inch fat, roasted	3 oz	141	24.6	0.0	53	0	4.0	1.4	59	27%
all grades, 1/4-inch fat, roasted	3 oz	143	24.6	0.0	53	0	4.2	1.5	59	28%
all grades, 1/2-inch fat, roasted	3 oz	156	24.6	0.0	53	0	5.5	2.1	59	34%
choice, 0-inch fat, roasted	3 oz	149	24.6	0.0	53	0	4.8	1.8	59	31%
choice, 1/4-inch fat, roasted	3 oz	149	24.6	0.0	53	0	4.8	1.8	59	31%
choice, 1/2-inch fat, roasted	3 oz	156	24.6	0.0	53	0	5.7	2.2	59	34%
prime, 1/2-inch fat, roasted	3 oz	213	23.0	0.0	50	0	12.7	5.1	61	55%
prime, 1/2-inch fat, raw	1 lb	676	98.7	0.0	240	0	28.4	10.3	245	39%
prime, 1/2-inch fat, raw	1 oz	42	6.2	0.0	15	0	1.8	0.7	15	40%
prime, 1/2-inch fat, roasted	3 oz	168	24.6	0.0	53	0	7.0	2.7	59	39%
select, 0-inch fat, roasted	3 oz	132	24.6	0.0	53	0	3.0	1.1	59	22%

Food Name	Serving Size	Calories	Prot. gms	Carbs gms	Sod. mgs	Fiber gms	Fat gms	Sat. Fat gms	Chol. mgs	% Fat Cal.
select, 0-inch fat, roasted	10.4 oz	460	85.8	0.0	184	0	10.4	3.8	204	21%
select, 1/4-inch fat, roasted	3 oz	136	24.6	0.0	53	0	3.4	1.2	59	24%
select, 1/2-inch fat, roasted	3 oz	151	24.6	0.0	53	0	5.1	2.0	59	32%
Untrimmed										
all grades, 0-inch fat, roasted	3 oz	145	24.5	0.0	53	0	4.6	1.7	59	30%
all grades, 1/4-inch fat, raw	1 lb	966	89.4	0.0	222	0	64.8	25.8	277	62%
all grades, 1/4-inch fat, raw	1 oz	60	5.6	0.0	14	0	4.1	1.6	17	62%
choice, 0-inch fat, braised	3 oz	176	30.7	0.0	38	0	4.9	1.7	77	26%
all grades, 1/4-inch fat, roasted	3 oz	195	22.8	0.0	50	0	10.8	4.2	61	52%
all grades, 1/2-inch fat, raw	1 lb	903	91.0	0.0	227	0	57.1	24.1	272	59%
all grades, 1/2-inch fat, raw	1 oz	56	5.7	0.0	14	0	3.6	1.5	17	59%
all grades, 1/2-inch fat, roasted	3 oz	207	22.8	0.0	50	0	12.1	4.9	62	54%
choice, 0-inch fat, roasted	3 oz	153	24.5	0.0	53	0	5.4	2.0	59	33%
choice, 1/4-inch fat, raw	1 lb	989	89.4	0.0	222	0	67.1	26.5	277	63%
choice, 1/4-inch fat, raw	1 oz	62	5.6	0.0	14	0	4.2	1.7	17	63%
choice, 1/4-inch fat, roasted	3 oz	205	22.6	0.0	50	0	12.0	4.7	61	54%
choice, 1/2-inch fat, raw	1 lb	916	90.8	0.0	227	0	58.8	24.8	272	59%
choice, 1/2-inch fat, raw	1 oz	57	5.7	0.0	14	0	3.7	1.5	17	59%
choice, 1/2-inch fat, roasted	3 oz	207	22.8	0.0	50	0	12.2	5.0	62	55%
prime, 1/2-inch fat, raw	1 lb	1002	90.3	0.0	227	0	68.3	28.4	272	63%
prime, 1/2-inch fat, raw	1 oz	63	5.6	0.0	14	0	4.3	1.8	17	63%
select, 0-inch fat, roasted	3 oz	137	24.5	0.0	53	0	3.5	1.3	59	24%
select, 1/4-inch fat, raw	1 lb	916	90.0	0.0	227	0	59.1	23.5	272	60%
select, 1/4-inch fat, raw	1 oz	57	5.6	0.0	14	0	3.7	1.5	17	60%
select, 1/4-inch fat, roasted	1 oz	184	22.9	0.0	51	0	9.6	3.8	61	49%
select, 1/4-inch fat, roasted	4 oz	246	30.6	0.0	68	0	12.8	5.0	82	49%
select, 1/2-inch fat, raw	1 lb	853	91.6	0.0	227	0	51.4	21.8	268	56%
select, 1/2-inch fat, raw	1 oz	53	5.7	0.0	14	0	3.2	1.4	17	56%
select, 1/2-inch fat, roasted	3 oz	201	22.8	0.0	50	0	11.5	4.7	61	53%
ROUND, FULL CUT										
Trimmed										
choice, 1/4-inch fat, broiled	3 oz	162	24.8	0.0	54	0	6.2	2.2	66	36%
select, 1/4-inch fat, broiled	3 oz	146	24.9	0.0	54	0	4.4	1.6	66	28%
select, 1/2-inch fat, broiled	3 oz	156	24.2	0.0	54	0	5.9	2.1	70	35%
Untrimmed										
choice, 1/4-inch fat, broiled	3 oz	204	23.3	0.0	52	0	11.6	4.4	68	53%
choice, 1/4-inch fat, raw	1 lb	921	92.4	0.0	240	0	58.1	22.7	286	59%
choice, 1/4-inch fat, raw	1 oz	58	5.8	0.0	15	0	3.6	1.4	18	58%
choice, 1/2-inch fat, broiled	3 oz	233	21.7	0.0	51	0	15.5	6.2	71	62%
choice, 1/2-inch fat, raw	1 lb	1093	87.9	0.0	231	0	79.6	33.8	299	67%
choice, 1/2-inch fat, raw	1 oz	68	5.5	0.0	14	0	5.0	2.1	19	67%
select, 1/4-inch fat, broiled	3 oz	190	23.3	0.0	53	0	10.0	3.5	47	49%
select, 1/4-inch fat, raw	1 lb	866	92.4	0.0	240	0	52.6	20.8	286	56%
select, 1/4-inch fat, raw	1 oz	54	5.8	0.0	15	0	3.3	1.3	18	56%
select, 1/2-inch fat, broiled	3 oz	223	21.8	0.0	51	0	14.3	5.7	71	60%
select, 1/2-inch fat, raw	1 lb	1048	88.5	0.0	231	0	74.1	31.5	295	65%
select, 1/2-inch fat, raw	1 oz	65	5.5	0.0	14	0	4.6	2.0	18	65%
ROUND, TIP										
Trimmed										
all grades, 0-inch fat, roasted	3 oz	150	24.4	0.0	55	0	5.0	1.8	69	32%
all grades, 1/4-inch fat, roasted	3 oz	157	24.4	0.0	55	0	5.9	2.0	69	35%
all grades, 1/2-inch fat, roasted	3 oz	161	24.4	0.0	55	0	6.4	2.3	69	37%
choice, 0-inch fat, roasted	3 oz	153	24.4	0.0	55	0	5.4	1.9	69	33%
choice, 1/4-inch fat, roasted	3 oz	160	24.4	0.0	55	0	6.2	2.2	69	36%

Food Name	Serving Size	Calories	Prot. gms	Carbs gms	Sod. mgs	Fiber gms	Fat gms	Sat. Fat gms	Chol. mgs	% Fat Cal.
choice, 1/2-inch fat, roasted	3 oz	164	24.4	0.0	55	0	6.6	2.4	69	38%
prime, 1/4-inch fat, roasted	3 oz	181	24.4	0.0	55	0	8.6	3.1	69	44%
prime, 1/2-inch fat, roasted	3 oz	181	24.4	0.0	55	0	8.6	3.1	69	44%
select, 0-inch fat, roasted	3 oz	144	24.4	0.0	55	0	4.5	1.6	69	29%
select, 1/4-inch fat, roasted	3 oz	153	24.4	0.0	55	0	5.4	1.9	69	33%
select, 1/2-inch fat, roasted	3 oz	156	24.4	0.0	55	0	5.7	2.1	69	35%
Untrimmed										
all grades, 0-inch fat, roasted	3 oz	162	23.9	0.0	54	0	6.7	2.4	69	39%
all grades, 1/4-inch fat, raw	1 lb	912	87.6	0.0	259	0	59.8	23.8	295	61%
all grades, 1/4-inch fat, raw	1 oz	57	5.5	0.0	16	0	3.7	1.5	18	60%
all grades, 1/4-inch fat, roasted	3 oz	199	22.9	0.0	54	0	11.3	4.3	70	53%
all grades, 1/2-inch fat, raw	1 lb	934	87.5	0.0	259	0	62.4	26.3	295	62%
all grades, 1/2-inch fat, raw	1 oz	58	5.5	0.0	16	0	3.9	1.6	18	62%
all grades, 1/2-inch fat, roasted	3 oz	213	22.5	0.0	53	0	13.0	5.2	71	57%
choice, 0-inch fat, roasted	3 oz	170	23.8	0.0	54	0	7.6	2.8	70	42%
choice, 1/4-inch fat, raw	1 lb	962	87.0	0.0	259	0	65.2	25.8	299	63%
choice, 1/4-inch fat, raw	1 oz	60	5.4	0.0	16	0	4.1	1.6	19	63%
choice, 1/4-inch fat, roasted	3 oz	210	22.6	0.0	53	0	12.6	4.8	71	56%
choice, 1/2-inch fat, raw	1 lb	948	87.3	0.0	259	0	64.0	27.0	295	62%
choice, 1/2-inch fat, raw	1 oz	59	5.5	0.0	16	0	4.0	1.7	18	62%
choice, 1/2-inch fat, roasted	3 oz	216	22.5	0.0	53	0	13.3	5.3	71	57%
prime, 1/4-inch fat, raw	1 lb	971	88.2	0.0	263	0	66.1	26.1	295	63%
prime, 1/4-inch fat, raw	1 oz	61	5.5	0.0	16	0	4.1	1.6	18	63%
prime, 1/4-inch fat, roasted	3 oz	233	22.4	0.0	53	0	15.2	5.9	71	60%
prime, 1/2-inch fat, raw	1 lb	1012	86.8	0.0	259	0	72.9	30.4	299	65%
prime, 1/2-inch fat, raw	1 oz	63	5.4	0.0	16	0	4.6	1.9	19	66%
prime, 1/2-inch fat, roasted	3 oz	241	22.1	0.0	52	0	16.3	6.5	71	62%
select, 0-inch fat, roasted	3 oz	158	23.9	0.0	54	0	6.2	2.3	69	37%
select, 1/4-inch fat, raw	1 lb	8	0.9	0.0	3	0	0.5	0.2	3	56%
select, 1/4-inch fat, raw	1 oz	53	5.6	0.0	16	0	3.2	1.3	18	56%
select, 1/4-inch fat, roasted	3 oz	191	23.0	0.0	54	0	10.3	3.9	70	50%
select, 1/2-inch fat, raw	1 lb	875	88.4	0.0	263	0	55.7	23.6	295	59%
select, 1/2-inch fat, raw	1 oz	55	5.5	0.0	16	0	3.5	1.5	18	59%
select, 1/2-inch fat, roasted	3 oz	205	22.6	0.0	53	0	12.0	4.8	71	54%
ROUND, TOP										
Trimmed										
all grades, 0-inch fat, braised	3 oz	169	30.7	0.0	38	0	4.3	1.5	77	24%
all grades, 1/4-inch fat, braised	3 oz	174	30.7	0.0	38	0	4.8	1.6	77	26%
all grades, 1/4-inch fat, broiled	3 oz	153	26.9	0.0	52	0	4.2	1.4	71	26%
all grades, 1/2-inch fat, broiled	3 oz	162	26.9	0.0	52	0	5.3	1.8	71	31%
choice, 1/4-inch fat, braised	3 oz	181	30.7	0.0	38	0	5.5	1.9	77	29%
choice, 1/4-inch fat, broiled	3 oz	161	26.9	0.0	52	0	5.0	1.7	71	30%
choice, 1/4-inch fat, pan-fried	3 oz	193	29.8	0.0	60	0	7.3	2.1	82	36%
choice, 1/4-inch fat, pan-fried in vegetable oil	4 oz	257	39.8	0.0	81	0	9.7	2.7	110	35%
choice, 1/2-inch fat, broiled	3 oz	165	26.9	0.0	52	0	5.5	1.9	71	32%
choice, 1/2-inch fat, pan-fried	3 oz	193	29.8	0.0	60	0	7.3	2.4	82	36%
prime, 1/4-inch fat, broiled	3 oz	183	26.9	0.0	52	0	7.5	2.6	71	39%
prime, 1/2-inch fat, broiled	3 oz	183	26.9	0.0	52	0	7.5	2.6	71	39%
select, 0-inch fat, braised	3 oz	161	30.7	0.0	38	0	3.4	1.2	77	20%
select, 1/4-inch fat, braised	3 oz	167	30.7	0.0	38	0	3.9	1.3	77	22%
select, 1/4-inch fat, broiled	3 oz	144	26.9	0.0	52	0	3.2	1.1	71	21%
select, 1/2-inch fat, broiled	3 oz	156	26.9	0.0	52	0	4.6	1.6	71	28%
Untrimmed										
all grades, 0-inch fat, braised	3 oz	178	30.3	0.0	38	0	5.4	1.9	77	29%

Food Name	Serving Size	Calories	Prot. gms	Carbs gms	Sod. mgs	Fiber gms	Fat gms	Sat. Fat gms	Chol. mgs	% Fat Cal.
all grades, 1/4-inch fat, braised	3 oz	211	28.8	0.0	38	0	9.7	3.7	77	43%
all grades, 1/4-inch fat, broiled	3 oz	184	25.6	0.0	51	0	8.2	3.1	72	42%
all grades, 1/4-inch fat, raw	1 lb	798	97.4	0.0	227	0	42.5	16.7	277	50%
all grades, 1/4-inch fat, raw	1 oz	50	6.1	0.0	14	0	2.7	1.0	17	50%
all grades, 1/2-inch fat, broiled	3 oz	179	26.2	0.0	51	0	7.5	2.8	72	39%
all grades, 1/2-inch fat, raw	1 lb	780	98.7	0.0	227	0	39.7	16.5	272	48%
all grades, 1/2-inch fat, raw	1 oz	49	6.2	0.0	14	0	2.5	1.0	17	48%
choice, 0-inch fat, braised	3 oz	184	30.3	0.0	38	0	6.0	2.1	77	31%
choice, 1/4-inch fat, broiled	3 oz	190	25.6	0.0	51	0	9.0	3.3	72	44%
choice, 1/4-inch fat, pan-fried	3 oz	235	27.5	0.0	58	0	13.1	4.5	82	52%
choice, 1/4-inch fat, pan-fried in vegetable oil	4 oz	314	36.7	0.0	77	0	17.4	6.0	110	52%
choice, 1/4-inch fat, raw	1 lb	821	97.4	0.0	227	0	45.0	17.5	277	51%
choice, 1/4-inch fat, raw	1 oz	51	6.1	0.0	14	0	2.8	1.1	17	51%
choice, 1/2-inch fat, braised	3 oz	221	28.5	0.0	38	0	10.9	4.1	77	46%
choice, 1/2-inch fat, broiled	3 oz	181	26.2	0.0	51	0	7.7	2.9	72	40%
choice, 1/2-inch fat, pan-fried	3 oz	247	26.9	0.0	57	0	14.5	5.5	82	55%
choice, 1/2-inch fat, raw	1 lb	789	98.7	0.0	227	0	40.7	16.9	272	48%
choice, 1/2-inch fat, raw	1 oz	49	6.2	0.0	14	0	2.5	1.0	17	48%
prime, 1/4-inch fat, broiled	3 oz	195	26.4	0.0	51	0	9.1	3.3	71	44%
prime, 1/4-inch fat, raw	1 lb	816	100.1	0.0	231	0	42.9	16.5	268	49%
prime, 1/4-inch fat, raw	1 oz	51	6.3	0.0	14	0	2.7	1.0	17	49%
prime, 1/2-inch fat, broiled	3 oz	201	26.1	0.0	51	0	9.9	3.7	72	46%
prime, 1/2-inch fat, raw	1 lb	853	98.9	0.0	227	0	47.9	19.4	272	52%
prime, 1/2-inch fat, raw	1 oz	53	6.2	0.0	14	0	3.0	1.2	17	52%
select, 0-inch fat, braised	3 oz	170	30.3	0.0	38	0	4.5	1.6	77	25%
select, 1/4-inch fat, braised	3 oz	199	29.0	0.0	38	0	8.4	3.2	77	40%
select, 1/4-inch fat, broiled	3 oz	175	25.6	0.0	51	0	7.2	2.8	72	39%
select, 1/4-inch fat, raw	1 lb	744	98.1	0.0	227	0	36.2	14.2	272	45%
select, 1/4-inch fat, raw	1 oz	46	6.1	0.0	14	0	2.3	0.9	17	46%
select, 1/2-inch fat, broiled	3 oz	176	26.1	0.0	51	0	7.1	2.7	72	38%
select, 1/2-inch fat, raw	1 lb	748	98.8	0.0	227	0	36.3	15.2	272	45%
select, 1/2-inch fat, raw	1 oz	47	6.2	0.0	14	0	2.3	1.0	17	46%

SIRLOIN, TOP

Trimmed

Food Name	Serving Size	Calories	Prot. gms	Carbs gms	Sod. mgs	Fiber gms	Fat gms	Sat. Fat gms	Chol. mgs	% Fat Cal.
all grades, 0-inch fat, broiled	3 oz	162	25.8	0.0	56	0	5.8	2.3	76	34%
all grades, 1/4-inch fat, broiled	3 oz	166	25.8	0.0	56	0	6.1	2.4	76	35%
all grades, 1/2-Inch fat, broiled	3 oz	177	25.8	0.0	56	0	7.4	3.0	76	39%
choice, 0-inch fat, broiled	4 oz	227	34.4	0.0	75	0	8.8	3.4	101	37%
choice, 0-inch fat, broiled	3 oz	170	25.8	0.0	56	0	6.6	2.6	76	37%
choice, 1/4-inch fat, broiled	4 oz	229	34.4	0.0	75	0	9.1	3.5	101	37%
choice, 1/4-inch fat, broiled	3 oz	172	25.8	0.0	56	0	6.8	2.6	76	37%
choice, 1/4-inch fat, pan-fried	3 oz	202	27.6	0.0	65	0	9.3	3.4	84	43%
choice, 1/4-inch fat, pan-fried in vegetable oil	4 oz	270	36.8	0.0	87	0	12.4	4.6	112	43%
choice, 1/2-inch fat, broiled	3 oz	179	25.8	0.0	56	0	7.7	3.1	76	40%
choice, 1/2-inch fat, pan-fried	3 oz	202	27.6	0.0	65	0	9.3	3.5	84	43%
prime, 1/2-inch fat, broiled	3 oz	201	25.8	0.0	56	0	10.1	4.1	76	47%
prime, 1/2-inch fat, raw	1 lb	703	96.3	0.0	263	0	32.1	11.9	277	43%
prime, 1/2-inch fat, raw	1 oz	44	6.0	0.0	16	0	2.0	0.7	17	43%
select, 0-inch fat, broiled	3 oz	153	25.8	0.0	56	0	4.8	1.9	76	30%
select, 1/4-inch fat, broiled	3 oz	158	25.8	0.0	56	0	5.3	2.0	76	32%
select, 1/2-inch fat, broiled	3 oz	170	25.8	0.0	56	0	6.6	2.7	76	37%

Untrimmed

Food Name	Serving Size	Calories	Prot. gms	Carbs gms	Sod. mgs	Fiber gms	Fat gms	Sat. Fat gms	Chol. mgs	% Fat Cal.
all grades, 0-inch fat, broiled	3 oz	183	25.0	0.0	55	0	8.5	3.3	76	43%
all grades, 1/4-inch fat, broiled	3 oz	219	23.6	0.0	54	0	13.1	5.2	77	56%

Food Name	Serving Size	Calories	Prot. gms	Carbs gms	Sod. mgs	Fiber gms	Fat gms	Sat. Fat gms	Chol. mgs	% Fat Cal.
all grades, 1/4-inch fat, raw	1 lb	984	86.9	0.0	240	0	68.2	27.3	304	64%
all grades, 1/4-inch fat, raw	1 oz	62	5.4	0.0	15	0	4.3	1.7	19	64%
all grades, 1/2-inch fat, broiled	3 oz	238	23.3	0.0	54	0	15.3	6.4	77	60%
all grades, 1/2-inch fat, raw	1 lb	1179	82.7	0.0	236	0	91.5	39.2	313	71%
all grades, 1/2-inch fat, raw	1 oz	74	5.2	0.0	15	0	5.7	2.5	20	71%
choice, 0-inch fat, broiled	3 oz	195	24.8	0.0	54	0	9.8	3.9	76	47%
choice, 1/4-inch fat, broiled	3 oz	229	23.5	0.0	53	0	14.2	5.7	77	58%
choice, 1/4-inch fat, pan-fried	3 oz	277	23.9	0.0	59	0	19.4	7.6	83	65%
choice, 1/4-inch fat, pan-fried in vegetable oil	4 oz	370	31.9	0.0	79	0	25.9	10.1	111	65%
choice, 1/4-inch fat, raw	1 lb	1030	86.3	0.0	240	0	73.5	29.3	304	66%
choice, 1/4-inch fat, raw	1 oz	64	5.4	0.0	15	0	4.6	1.8	19	66%
choice, 1/2-inch fat, broiled	3 oz	241	23.3	0.0	53	0	15.7	6.5	77	60%
choice, 1/2-inch fat, pan-fried	3 oz	288	23.3	0.0	58	0	20.9	8.6	83	67%
choice, 1/2-inch fat, raw	1 lb	1198	82.5	0.0	231	0	93.8	40.1	318	72%
choice, 1/2-inch fat, raw	1 oz	75	5.2	0.0	14	0	5.9	2.5	20	72%
prime, 1/2-inch fat, broiled	3 oz	271	22.7	0.0	53	0	19.4	8.1	77	66%
prime, 1/2-inch fat, raw	1 lb	1320	80.8	0.0	231	0	108.0	45.9	322	75%
prime, 1/2-inch fat, raw	1 oz	83	5.1	0.0	14	0	6.8	2.9	20	75%
select, 0-inch fat, broiled	3 oz	166	25.2	0.0	55	0	6.4	2.5	76	36%
select, 1/4-inch fat, broiled	3 oz	208	23.8	0.0	54	0	11.8	4.7	77	53%
select, 1/4-inch fat, raw	1 lb	939	87.4	0.0	245	0	62.5	25.0	304	62%
select, 1/4-inch fat, raw	1 oz	59	5.5	0.0	15	0	3.9	1.6	19	62%
select, 1/2-inch fat, broiled	3 oz	232	23.3	0.0	53	0	14.8	6.2	77	59%
select, 1/2-inch fat, raw	1 lb	1116	83.8	0.0	236	0	84.0	36.0	313	69%
select, 1/2-inch fat, raw	1 oz	70	5.2	0.0	15	0	5.3	2.3	20	70%
SHANK CROSSCUTS										
Trimmed										
choice, 1/4-inch fat, simmered	4 oz	228	38.2	0.0	73	0	7.2	2.6	88	30%
choice, 1/4-inch fat, simmered	3 oz	171	28.6	0.0	54	0	5.4	2.0	66	30%
choice, 1/2-inch fat, simmered	3 oz	171	28.6	0.0	54	0	5.4	1.9	66	30%
Untrimmed										
choice, 1/4-inch fat, raw	1 oz	50	5.8	0.0	17	0	2.8	1.1	12	52%
choice, 1/4-inch fat, raw	3 oz	150	17.5	0.0	51	0	8.4	3.2	37	52%
choice, 1/4-inch fat, simmered	3 oz	224	26.1	0.0	52	0	12.5	4.8	68	52%
choice, 1/2-inch fat, raw	1 lb	721	95.1	0.0	277	0	35.1	14.0	195	45%
choice, 1/2-inch fat, raw	1 oz	45	5.9	0.0	17	0	2.2	0.9	12	46%
choice, 1/2-inch fat, simmered	3 oz	207	26.9	0.0	53	0	10.3	4.1	67	46%
SPLEEN										
braised	3 oz	123	21.3	0.0	48	0	3.6	1.2	295	28%
calf, raw	100 gm	104	18.3	0.0	86	0	3.0	1.0	250	27%
raw	4 oz	119	20.7	0.0	96	0	3.4	1.1	297	27%
T-BONE										
Trimmed										
choice, 1/4-inch fat, broiled	3 oz	182	23.9	0.0	56	0	8.8	3.5	68	45%
choice, 1/2-inch fat, broiled	3 oz	182	23.9	0.0	56	0	8.8	3.5	68	45%
Untrimmed										
choice, 1/4-inch fat, broiled	3 oz	253	21.2	0.0	52	0	18.0	7.3	71	66%
choice, 1/4-inch fat, raw	1 lb	1234	79.8	0.0	222	0	99.2	40.8	313	74%
choice, 1/4-inch fat, raw	1 oz	77	5.0	0.0	14	0	6.2	2.5	20	74%
choice, 1/2-inch fat, broiled	3 oz	275	20.4	0.0	51	0	20.9	8.7	71	70%
choice, 1/2-inch fat, raw	1 lb	1393	76.1	0.0	218	0	118.5	50.8	322	78%
choice, 1/2-inch fat, raw	1 oz	87	4.8	0.0	14	0	7.4	3.2	20	78%

Food Name	Serving Size	Calories	Prot. gms	Carbs gms	Sod. mgs	Fiber gms	Fat gms	Sat. Fat gms	Chol. mgs	% Fat Cal.
TENDERLOIN										
Trimmed										
all grades, 0-inch fat, broiled	3 oz	175	24.0	0.0	54	0	8.1	3.0	71	43%
all grades, 1/4-inch fat, broiled	3 oz	179	24.0	0.0	54	0	8.5	3.2	71	44%
all grades, 1/4-inch fat, roasted	3 oz	189	23.5	0.0	52	0	9.8	3.7	71	48%
all grades, 1/2-inch fat, broiled	3 oz	173	24.0	0.0	54	0	7.9	3.1	71	43%
all grades, 1/2-inch fat, roasted	3 oz	186	23.4	0.0	50	0	9.6	3.7	73	48%
choice, 0-inch fat, broiled	3 oz	180	24.0	0.0	54	0	8.6	3.2	71	45%
choice, 1/4-inch fat, broiled	3 oz	189	24.0	0.0	54	0	9.5	3.6	71	47%
choice, 1/4-inch fat, roasted	4 oz	262	31.4	0.0	82	0	14.2	5.4	94	50%
choice, 1/4-inch fat, roasted	3 oz	196	23.5	0.0	61	0	10.6	4.0	71	50%
choice, 1/2-inch fat, broiled	3 oz	176	24.0	0.0	54	0	8.1	3.2	71	43%
choice, 1/2-inch fat, roasted	3 oz	190	23.4	0.0	50	0	9.9	3.9	73	49%
prime, 1/4-inch fat, broiled	3 oz	197	24.0	0.0	54	0	10.5	4.1	71	50%
prime, 1/4-inch fat, roasted	3 oz	217	23.4	0.0	50	0	13.0	5.1	73	56%
prime, 1/2-inch fat, broiled	3 oz	197	24.0	0.0	54	0	10.5	4.1	71	50%
prime, 1/2-inch fat, roasted	3 oz	217	23.4	0.0	50	0	13.0	5.1	73	56%
select, 0-inch fat, broiled	3 oz	170	24.0	0.0	54	0	7.5	2.8	71	41%
select, 1/4-inch fat, broiled	3 oz	169	24.0	0.0	54	0	7.4	2.8	71	41%
select, 1/4-inch fat, roasted	3 oz	179	23.5	0.0	52	0	8.8	3.3	71	46%
select, 1/2-inch fat, broiled	3 oz	167	24.0	0.0	54	0	7.1	2.8	71	40%
select, 1/2-inch fat, roasted	3 oz	177	23.4	0.0	50	0	8.6	3.3	73	45%
Untrimmed										
all grades, 0-inch fat, broiled	3 oz	200	23.1	0.0	53	0	11.2	4.3	72	52%
all grades, 1/4-inch fat, broiled	3 oz	247	21.5	0.0	50	0	17.2	6.8	73	64%
all grades, 1/4-inch fat, raw	1 lb	1284	80.6	0.0	218	0	104.4	42.2	322	75%
all grades, 1/4-inch fat, raw	1 oz	80	5.0	0.0	14	0	6.5	2.6	20	75%
all grades, 1/4-inch fat, roasted	3 oz	282	20.1	0.0	48	0	21.8	8.6	73	71%
all grades, 1/2-inch fat, broiled	3 oz	226	22.1	0.0	52	0	14.6	6.0	72	60%
all grades, 1/2-inch fat, raw	1 lb	1093	84.1	0.0	222	0	81.6	34.7	313	69%
all grades, 1/2-inch fat, roasted	3 oz	258	20.8	0.0	48	0	18.7	7.7	74	67%
choice, 0-inch fat, broiled	3 oz	207	23.0	0.0	52	0	12.2	4.7	72	54%
choice, 1/4-inch fat, broiled	4 oz	356	29.4	0.0	69	0	25.6	10.0	101	66%
choice, 1/4-inch fat, broiled	3 oz	258	21.3	0.0	50	0	18.6	7.3	73	66%
choice, 1/4-inch fat, raw	1 lb	1306	80.6	0.0	218	0	106.8	43.1	322	75%
choice, 1/4-inch fat, raw	1 oz	82	5.0	0.0	14	0	6.7	2.7	20	75%
choice, 1/4-inch fat, roasted	3 oz	288	20.1	0.0	55	0	22.4	8.9	73	72%
choice, 1/2-inch fat, broiled	3 oz	230	22.0	0.0	51	0	15.1	6.2	73	61%
choice, 1/2-inch fat, raw	1 lb	1116	83.8	0.0	222	0	83.9	35.7	313	69%
choice, 1/2-inch fat, roasted	3 oz	262	20.7	0.0	48	0	19.2	7.9	74	68%
prime, 1/4-inch fat, broiled	3 oz	269	21.2	0.0	50	0	19.9	7.9	73	68%
prime, 1/4-inch fat, raw	1 lb	1288	81.2	0.0	218	0	104.6	43.0	318	74%
prime, 1/4-inch fat, raw	1 oz	81	5.1	0.0	14	0	6.5	2.7	20	74%
prime, 1/4-inch fat, roasted	3 oz	300	20.1	0.0	47	0	23.7	9.5	75	73%
prime, 1/2-inch fat, broiled	3 oz	270	21.2	0.0	50	0	19.9	8.1	73	68%
prime, 1/2-inch fat, raw	1 lb	1306	80.7	0.0	218	0	106.8	45.5	322	75%
prime, 1/2-inch fat, roasted	3 oz	304	19.9	0.0	47	0	24.4	10.0	75	73%
select, 0-inch fat, broiled	3 oz	195	23.1	0.0	53	0	10.6	4.1	72	51%
select, 1/4-inch fat, broiled	3 oz	230	21.8	0.0	51	0	15.2	6.0	73	61%
select, 1/4-inch fat, raw	1 lb	1261	80.6	0.0	218	0	101.6	41.2	322	74%
select, 1/4-inch fat, raw	1 oz	79	5.0	0.0	14	0	6.3	2.6	20	74%
select, 1/4-inch fat, roasted	3 oz	275	20.1	0.0	48	0	21.0	8.3	73	70%
select, 1/2-inch fat, broiled	3 oz	216	22.2	0.0	52	0	13.4	5.4	73	58%
select, 1/2-inch fat, raw	1 lb	1043	84.7	0.0	222	0	75.7	32.2	313	67%

Food Name	Serving Size	Calories	Prot. gms	Carbs gms	Sod. mgs	Fiber gms	Fat gms	Sat. Fat gms	Chol. mgs	% Fat Cal.
select, 1/2-inch fat, roasted	3 oz	245	21.0	0.0	48	0	17.3	7.1	74	65%
THYMUS										
braised	3 oz	271	18.6	0.0	99	0	21.2	7.3	250	72%
raw	4 oz	267	13.8	0.0	108	0	23.0	7.9	252	79%
TONGUE										
potted or deviled	100 gm	290	18.6	0.7	1430	0	23.0	9.9	110	73%
raw	4 oz	253	16.8	4.2	78	0	18.2	7.8	98	66%
simmered	3 oz	241	18.8	0.3	51	0	17.6	7.6	91	68%
smoked	100 gm	328	17.2	0.9	73	0	28.8	14.0	68	78%
whole, canned or pickled	100 gm	267	19.3	0.3	1021	0	20.3	8.7	90	70%
TOP LOIN										
Trimmed										
all grades, 0-inch fat, broiled	3 oz	168	24.3	0.0	58	0	7.1	2.7	65	40%
all grades, 1/4-inch fat, broiled	3 oz	176	24.3	0.0	58	0	8.0	3.0	65	43%
all grades, 1/2-inch fat, broiled	3 oz	173	24.3	0.0	58	0	7.6	3.0	65	41%
choice, 0-inch fat, broiled	4 oz	237	32.5	0.0	77	0	10.9	4.2	86	43%
choice, 0-inch fat, broiled	3 oz	178	24.3	0.0	58	0	8.2	3.1	65	43%
choice, 1/4-inch fat, broiled	4 oz	243	32.5	0.0	77	0	11.5	4.4	86	44%
choice, 1/4-inch fat, broiled	3 oz	182	24.3	0.0	58	0	8.6	3.3	65	44%
choice, 1/2-inch fat, broiled	3 oz	176	24.3	0.0	58	0	8.0	3.2	65	43%
prime, 1/4-inch fat, broiled	3 oz	208	24.3	0.0	58	0	11.6	4.6	65	52%
prime, 1/2-inch fat, broiled	3 oz	208	24.3	0.0	58	0	11.6	4.6	65	52%
select, 0-inch fat, broiled	3 oz	156	24.3	0.0	58	0	5.9	2.2	65	35%
select, 1/4-inch fat, broiled	3 oz	164	24.3	0.0	58	0	6.6	2.5	65	38%
select, 1/2-inch fat, broiled	3 oz	161	24.3	0.0	58	0	6.4	2.6	65	37%
Untrimmed										
all grades, 0-inch fat, broiled	3 oz	180	23.9	0.0	57	0	8.7	3.4	65	45%
all grades, 1/4-inch fat, broiled	3 oz	244	21.7	0.0	54	0	16.8	6.7	67	64%
all grades, 1/4-inch fat, raw	1 lb	1102	86.2	0.0	240	0	81.3	33.1	304	68%
all grades, 1/2-inch fat, broiled	3 oz	238	21.9	0.0	54	0	16.0	6.6	67	62%
all grades, 1/2-inch fat, raw	1 lb	1284	82.3	0.0	236	0	103.6	44.7	313	74%
choice, 0-inch fat, broiled	3 oz	194	23.7	0.0	57	0	10.2	4.0	65	49%
choice, 1/4-inch fat, broiled	3 oz	253	21.6	0.0	54	0	17.8	7.1	67	65%
choice, 1/4-inch fat, raw	1 lb	1179	85.0	0.0	240	0	90.4	36.7	304	71%
choice, 1/2-inch fat, broiled	3 oz	243	21.8	0.0	54	0	16.6	6.9	67	63%
choice, 1/2-inch fat, raw	1 lb	1311	82.0	0.0	231	0	106.7	46.1	313	75%
prime, 1/4-inch fat, broiled	3 oz	275	21.6	0.0	54	0	20.3	8.2	67	68%
prime, 1/4-inch fat, raw	1 lb	1383	83.1	0.0	236	0	114.2	46.9	313	76%
prime, 1/2-inch fat, broiled	3 oz	288	21.0	0.0	53	0	22.0	9.1	68	70%
prime, 1/2-inch fat, raw	1 lb	1461	81.1	0.0	231	0	123.7	53.0	318	77%
select, 0-inch fat, broiled	3 oz	169	23.9	0.0	57	0	7.5	2.9	65	41%
select, 1/4-inch fat, broiled	3 oz	226	22.0	0.0	54	0	14.6	5.8	67	60%
select, 1/4-inch fat, raw	1 lb	1043	86.8	0.0	245	0	74.6	30.4	299	66%
select, 1/2-inch fat, broiled	3 oz	223	22.1	0.0	54	0	14.2	5.9	67	59%
select, 1/2-inch fat, raw	1 lb	1198	83.6	0.0	236	0	93.0	40.3	308	72%
TRIPE										
canned (Armour)	6 oz	180	33.0	1.0	230	na	4.0	na	na	21%
pickled	100 gm	62	11.8	0.0	46	0	1.3	0.5	68	20%
raw	4 oz	111	16.5	0.0	52	0	4.5	2.3	107	38%
BEEF, ALTERNATIVE										
(Heartline) 'Beef Fillet Style'	2 oz	176	19.0	9.0	480	na	7.0	na	0	36%
(Heartline) 'Beef Fillet Style' lite	.5 oz	22	5.0	1.0	135	3.0	0.0	0.0	0	0%
(Heartline) 'Ground Beef Style'	2 oz	176	19.0	9.0	480	na	7.0	na	0	36%
(Heartline) 'Ground Beef Style' lite	.5 oz	22	2.0	1.0	135	3.0	0.0	0.0	0	0%

Food Name	Serving Size	Calories	Prot. gms	Carbs gms	Sod. mgs	Fiber gms	Fat gms	Sat. Fat gms	Chol. mgs	% Fat Cal.
(Heartline) 'Teriyaki Beef Style' .... 2 oz		176	19.0	9.0	450	na	7.0	na	0	36%
Canned										
(Worthington) 'Prime Stakes' .... 3.25-oz piece		160	10.0	7.0	410	(mq)	10.0	(mq)	0	57%
(Worthington) 'Savory Slices' 2-oz slices .... 2 slices		100	8.0	4.0	340	(mq)	6.0	(mq)	0	53%
(Worthington) 'Vegetable Steaks' approx 1.28-oz pieces .. 3.2 oz		110	17.0	5.0	400	(mq)	2.0	(mq)	0	17%
Frozen										
(Worthington) roll, approx 1.25-oz slices .... 2 slices		130	12.0	7.0	750	(mq)	6.0	(mq)	0	42%
(Worthington) roll, smoked, frozen, approx 2/3-oz slices .. 3 slices		120	10.0	7.0	790	(mq)	6.0	(mq)	0	44%
(Worthington) 'Stakelets' .... 2.5 oz		150	13.0	7.0	460	(mq)	8.0	1.0	0	47%
BEEF, CANNED, chopped (Armour) .... 3 oz		280	11.0	3.0	1290	na	24.0	na	na	79%
BEEF, CORNED										
(Healthy Deli) .... 1 oz		35	5.7	0.7	210	0	1.0	(mq)	11	26%
(Hillshire Farm) .... 1 oz		31	6.0	<1.0	230	0	0.4	(mq)	(mq)	11%
(Oscar Mayer) .... .6 oz		17	3.4	0.1	204	0	0.3	0.2	8	16%
brisket, cured, cooked .... 3 oz		213	15.4	0.4	964	0	16.1	5.4	83	70%
brisket, cured, raw .... 1 lb		898	66.6	0.6	553	0	67.6	21.5	245	69%
brisket, cured, raw .... 1 oz		56	4.2	0.0	35	0	4.2	1.3	15	69%
canned (Dinty Moore) .... 2 oz		130	15.0	0.0	(mq)	0	8.0	(mq)	(mq)	55%
canned, cured .... 1 oz		71	7.7	0.0	285	0	4.2	1.8	24	55%
canned, '7 oz can' (Libby's) .... 2.3 oz		160	17.0	2.0	720	0	9.0	(mq)	(mq)	52%
canned, '12 oz can' (Libby's) .... 2.4 oz		160	17.0	2.0	750	0	9.0	(mq)	(mq)	52%
'St. Paddy's' (Healthy Deli) .... 1 oz		24	3.9	1.1	290	0	0.4	(mq)	7	15%
'Slender Sliced' (Eckrich) .... 1 oz		40	6.0	1.0	270	0	1.0	(mq)	(mq)	24%
BEEF, CORNED, ALTERNATIVE										
roll, frozen (Worthington) .... 2.5 oz		150	12.0	9.0	660	(mq)	7.0	1.0	0	43%
roll, frozen (Worthington) approx .5-oz slices .... 4 slices		120	9.0	8.0	740	(mq)	6.0	1.0	0	44%
BEEF, CORNED, HASH										
canned (Armour) .... 7.5 oz		390	18.0	18.0	900	na	27.0	na	na	63%
canned, '15 oz can' (Libby's) .... 7 1/2 oz		400	18.0	20.0	1260	(mq)	27.0	(mq)	(mq)	62%
canned, '15 oz can' (Mary Kitchen) .... 7 1/2 oz		360	20.0	19.0	1386	(mq)	24.0	(mq)	(mq)	58%
canned (Mary Kitchen) .... 1 oz		47	3.0	2.0	111	na	3.0	1.0	9	57%
canned (Nalley's) .... 8 oz		420	17.0	27.0	940	(mq)	27.0	(mq)	(mq)	58%
canned, 'No Frills' (Pathmark) .... 7 1/2 oz		410	16.0	27.0	1250	(mq)	26.0	(mq)	(mq)	58%
canned, '25 oz can' (Mary Kitchen) .... 8 1/3 oz		400	22.0	19.0	1429	(mq)	27.0	(mq)	(mq)	60%
canned, '24 oz can' (Libby's) .... 8 oz		420	19.0	21.0	1330	(mq)	28.0	(mq)	(mq)	61%
canned, w/potato .... 1 cup		398	19.4	23.5	1188	>1.1 c	24.9	11.9	73	57%
microwave cup (Dinty Moore) .... 7.5 oz		350	19.0	19.0	850	na	22.0	9.0	65	57%
25% less salt, 'Premium' (Armour) .... 7.5 oz		350	19.0	21.0	790	na	21.0	na	na	54%
BEEF, CORNED, SPREAD, canned (Hormel) .... .5 oz		35	2.0	0.0	(mq)	(tr)	3.0	(mq)	(mq)	77%
BEEF, DRIED										
chipped, cooked, creamed .... 1 cup		377	20.1	17.4	1754	0	25.2	13.7	98	60%
cured .... 1 oz		47	8.3	0.4	984	0	1.1	0.5	12	22%
sliced (Armour) .... 1.1 oz		60	8.0	2.0	na	na	2.0	na	na	31%
BEEF, GROUND										
Extra lean										
baked, medium-cooked .... 3 oz		213	20.8	0.0	42	0	13.7	5.4	70	60%
baked, well-done .... 3 oz		233	25.8	0.0	54	0	13.6	5.3	91	54%
broiled, medium-cooked .... 3 oz		218	21.6	0.0	59	0	13.9	5.5	71	59%
broiled, well-done .... 3 oz		225	24.3	0.0	70	0	13.4	5.3	84	55%
pan-fried, medium-cooked .... 3 oz		217	21.2	0.0	59	0	14.0	5.5	69	60%
pan-fried, well-done .... 3 oz		224	23.8	0.0	69	0	13.6	5.3	79	56%
raw .... 1 oz		66	5.3	0.0	19	0	4.8	1.9	20	67%
raw .... 4 oz		264	21.1	0.0	75	0	19.3	7.7	78	67%

Food Name	Serving Size	Calories	Prot. gms	Carbs gms	Sod. mgs	Fiber gms	Fat gms	Sat. Fat gms	Chol. mgs	% Fat Cal.
Lean										
baked, medium-cooked	3 oz	228	20.3	0.0	48	0	15.6	6.1	66	63%
baked, well-done	3 oz	248	25.2	0.0	60	0	15.6	6.1	84	58%
broiled, medium-cooked	3 oz	231	21.0	0.0	65	0	15.7	6.2	74	63%
broiled, well-done	3 oz	238	24.0	0.0	76	0	15.0	5.9	86	58%
pan-fried, medium-cooked	3 oz	234	20.6	0.0	65	0	16.2	6.4	71	64%
pan-fried, well-done	3 oz	235	23.4	0.0	74	0	15.0	5.9	81	59%
raw	1 oz	75	5.0	0.0	20	0	5.9	2.4	21	73%
raw	4 oz	298	20.0	0.0	78	0	23.4	9.4	85	73%
Regular										
baked, medium-cooked	3 oz	244	19.6	0.0	51	0	17.8	7.0	74	67%
baked, well-done	3 oz	269	24.5	0.0	64	0	18.3	7.2	92	63%
broiled, frozen patty, medium-cooked	3 oz	240	20.8	0.0	65	0	16.7	6.6	80	64%
broiled, medium-cooked	3 oz	246	20.5	0.0	71	0	17.6	6.9	77	66%
broiled, well-done	3 oz	248	23.1	0.0	79	0	16.5	6.5	86	62%
pan-fried, medium-cooked	3 oz	260	20.3	0.0	71	0	19.2	7.5	76	68%
pan-fried, well-done	3 oz	243	23.0	0.0	79	0	16.1	6.3	83	61%
raw	1 oz	88	4.7	0.0	19	0	7.5	3.1	24	78%
raw	4 oz	350	18.8	0.0	77	0	30.0	12.2	96	78%
raw, frozen patty	3 oz	240	14.5	0.0	58	0	19.7	8.0	67	75%
BEEF DINNER, FROZEN. See also BEEF ENTRÉE, FROZEN.										
and gravy (Swanson)	11.25 oz	310	26.0	38.0	770	(mq)	6.0	(mq)	(mq)	17%
chopped (Banquet)	11 oz	420	21.0	14.0	600	(mq)	32.0	(mq)	80	67%
chopped steak, 'Hungry Man' (Swanson)	16.75 oz	640	35.0	41.0	1600	(mq)	37.0	(mq)	(mq)	52%
'Extra Helping' (Banquet)	16 oz	870	34.0	50.0	810	(mq)	61.0	(mq)	120	62%
in barbecue sauce (Swanson)	11 oz	460	30.0	51.0	860	(mq)	17.0	(mq)	(mq)	32%
Mexicana (Budget Gourmet)	12.8 oz	560	33.0	56.0	1290	(mq)	23.0	(mq)	50	37%
patty, charbroiled (Freezer Queen)	10 oz	300	17.0	20.0	1260	(mq)	17.0	(mq)	(mq)	51%
Salisbury steak (Banquet)	11 oz	500	23.0	26.0	600	(mq)	34.0	(mq)	80	61%
Salisbury steak (Freezer Queen)	10 oz	380	18.0	28.0	1260	(mq)	22.0	(mq)	(mq)	52%
Salisbury steak (Healthy Choice)	11.5 oz	300	19.0	41.0	480	na	7.0	3.0	50	21%
Salisbury steak (Le Menu)	10.5 oz	370	20.0	28.0	880	(mq)	20.0	(mq)	(mq)	48%
Salisbury steak (Morton)	10 oz	300	12.0	23.0	1420	(mq)	17.0	(mq)	40	52%
Salisbury steak (Swanson)	10.75 oz	400	18.0	43.0	880	(mq)	17.0	(mq)	(mq)	39%
Salisbury steak, charbroiled flavor 'Healthy Balance' (Banquet)	10.5 oz	270	14.0	34.0	800	na	8.0	4.0	35	27%

QUICK REFERENCE: HAMBURGERS

America has long had a love affair with the hamburger. And as any burger lover knows, the burger itself is only half the story. Usually, burgers are enveloped in a bun or sandwiched between bread slices. And, of course, many of us pile them high with a variety of toppings. The information below will give you a rough idea of how your burger fixings are adding up.

Food Name	Serving Size	Calories	Prot. gms	Carbs gms	Sod. mgs	Fiber gms	Fat gms	Sat. Fat gms	Chol. mgs	% Fat Cal.
Hamburger bun	1 bun	123	3.7	21.6	241	2.0	2.2	0.5	0	16%
White bread	1 slice	70	3.0	13.0	140	.7	1.0	na	na	12%
Whole wheat bread	1 slice	60	3.0	11.0	125	2.0	1.0	0.0	0	14%
American cheese	1 oz	110	6.0	1.0	450	0	9.0	5.0	25	74%
Catsup	1 tbsp	16	0.2	4.1	178	.2	0.1	0.0	0	5%
Mustard	1 tbsp	10	1.0	1.0	180	na	1.0	na	0	53%
Mayonnaise	1 tbsp	100	0.0	0.0	80	0	11.0	2.0	5	100%
Pickle Relish	1 tbsp	20	0.1	5.3	122	>.1 c	0.1	0.0	0	4%

Food Name	Serving Size	Calories	Prot. gms	Carbs gms	Sod. mgs	Fiber gms	Fat gms	Sat. Fat gms	Chol. mgs	% Fat Cal.
Salisbury steak 'Classics' (Armour)	11.25 oz	350	22.0	26.0	1430	(mq)	17.0	(mq)	55	44%
Salisbury steak 'Classics Lite' (Armour)	11.5 oz	300	21.0	29.0	1020	(mq)	2.0	(mq)	35	8%
Salisbury steak 'Extra Helping' (Banquet)	18 oz	910	50.0	49.0	740	(mq)	60.0	(mq)	175	58%
Salisbury steak 'Hungry Man' (Swanson)	16.5 oz	680	41.0	37.0	1730	(mq)	41.0	(mq)	(mq)	54%
Salisbury steak 'Lightstyle' (Le Menu)	10 oz	280	18.0	31.0	400	(mq)	9.0	(mq)	(mq)	29%
Salisbury steak, parmigiana 'Classics' (Armour)	11.5 oz	410	22.0	32.0	1120	(mq)	21.0	(mq)	60	47%
Salisbury steak, sirloin (Budget Gourmet)	11.5 oz	410	26.0	28.0	890	(mq)	22.0	(mq)	105	48%
Salisbury steak, w/mushroom gravy 'Extra Helping' (Banquet)	18 oz	890	51.0	48.0	685	(mq)	58.0	(mq)	169	57%
sirloin, chopped (Le Menu)	12.25 oz	430	25.0	28.0	1010	(mq)	24.0	(mq)	(mq)	51%
sirloin, chopped (Swanson)	10.75 oz	340	20.0	28.0	790	(mq)	16.0	(mq)	(mq)	43%
sirloin, roast, 'Classics' (Armour)	10.45 oz	190	19.0	21.0	970	(mq)	4.0	(mq)	55	18%
sirloin, w/barbecue sauce (Healthy Choice)	11 oz	280	17.0	44.0	240	na	4.0	2.0	25	13%
sirloin tips (Healthy Choice)	11.25 oz	270	22.0	29.0	360	na	7.0	3.0	65	24%
sliced (Morton)	10 oz	220	24.0	20.0	950	(mq)	5.0	(mq)	65	20%
sliced, 'Hungry Man' (Swanson)	15.25 oz	450	37.0	49.0	1060	(mq)	12.0	(mq)	(mq)	24%
sliced, w/gravy (Freezer Queen)	10 oz	210	18.0	18.0	1010	(mq)	7.0	(mq)	(mq)	30%
steak Diane, 'Classics Lite' (Armour)	10 oz	290	27.0	25.0	440	(mq)	9.0	(mq)	80	28%
tips (Le Menu)	11.5 oz	400	30.0	29.0	760	(mq)	18.0	(mq)	(mq)	41%
tips 'Classics' (Armour)	10.25 oz	230	22.0	20.0	820	(mq)	7.0	(mq)	70	27%
tips, in Burgundy sauce (Budget Gourmet)	11 oz	310	24.0	28.0	720	(mq)	11.0	(mq)	65	32%
BEEF ENTRÉE, ALTERNATIVE										
'Country Stew' (Worthington)	9.5 oz	220	10.0	23.0	760	(mq)	10.0	1.0	0	41%
pie, frozen (Worthington)	8 oz	360	9.0	44.0	1940	(mq)	16.0	(mq)	0	40%
BEEF ENTRÉE, CANNED										
chow mein (LaChoy)	3/4 cup	40	5.0	5.0	960	2.0	2.0	0.8	16	31%
chow mein, 'Bi-Pack' (LaChoy)	8.748 oz	83	9.3	11.1	998	3.5	0.9	0.5	12	9%
chow mein, 'Bi-Pack' (LaChoy)	3/4 cup	70	7.0	8.0	840	1.0	1.0	(mq)	20	13%
Oriental, w/noodles, 'Bi-Pack' (LaChoy)	9 oz	148	11.7	24.3	1101	3.4	1.2	0.6	13	7%
pepper, 'Bi-Pack' (LaChoy)	3/4 cup	80	7.0	10.0	950	2.0	2.0	0.6	17	21%
pepper Oriental, 'Bi-Pack' (LaChoy)	8.783 oz	101	10.1	12.7	1219	3.7	2.0	0.7	12	17%
pepper Oriental, 'Bi-Pack' (LaChoy)	3/4 cup	80	7.0	10.0	950	1.0	2.0	(mq)	18	21%
stew (Armour)	8 oz	210	11.0	16.0	1200	na	11.0	na	na	48%
stew (Dinty Moore)	8 oz	220	11.0	16.0	870	na	13.0	6.0	30	52%
stew (Estee)	7.5 oz	210	14.0	15.0	65	(mq)	11.0	5.0	30	46%
stew (Featherweight)	7.5 oz	160	17.0	17.0	400	(mq)	3.0	(mq)	35	17%
stew (Wolf Brand)	1 cup	179	9.6	10.3	1043	>.6 c	7.5	(mq)	(mq)	38%
stew, 'Big Chunk' (Nalley's)	7.5 oz	200	10.0	24.0	790	(mq)	7.0	(mq)	(mq)	32%
stew, '15-oz can' (Dinty Moore)	7.5 oz	200	10.0	15.0	810	na	12.0	6.0	30	52%
stew, '15-oz pkg' (Libby's)	7.5 oz	160	12.0	18.0	870	(mq)	5.0	(mq)	(mq)	27%
stew, 'Homestyle' (Nalley's)	8 oz	180	11.0	22.0	810	(mq)	5.0	(mq)	(mq)	25%
stew, '40-oz can' (Dinty Moore)	8 oz	210	13.0	16.0	971	(mq)	11.0	(mq)	(mq)	46%
stew, 'No Frills' (Pathmark)	8 oz	190	10.0	25.0	625	(mq)	4.0	(mq)	(mq)	21%
stew, '24-oz can' (Dinty Moore)	8 oz	220	12.0	15.0	980	(mq)	12.0	(mq)	(mq)	50%
stew, '24-oz pkg' (Libby's)	8 oz	170	12.0	19.0	930	(mq)	6.0	(mq)	(mq)	30%
pepper Oriental (LaChoy)	3/4 cup	100	7.0	12.0	1340	2.0	4.0	1.6	9	32%
BEEF ENTRÉE, DRIED										
beef and rice w/onions, prepared (Mountain House)	1 cup	330	11.0	42.0	265	(mq)	12.0	(mq)	(mq)	34%
stew, freeze-dried, prepared (Mountain House)	1 cup	260	16.0	26.0	75	(mq)	9.0	(mq)	(mq)	33%
BEEF ENTRÉE, FROZEN. See also BEEF DINNER, FROZEN.										
and broccoli, w/rice, 'Fresh & Lite' (LaChoy)	11 oz	260	17.0	42.0	1299	5.2	5.0	(mq)	51	16%
Cantonese, w/rice, 'Stir Fry' (Weight Watchers)	9 oz	200	14.0	27.0	530	na	4.0	1.0	15	18%
casserole, 'Microwave Classic' (Pillsbury)	1 pkg	430	16.0	34.0	1100	(mq)	25.0	(mq)	(mq)	53%
champignon, 'Gourmet Selection' (Tyson)	10.5 oz	370	27.0	31.0	830	(mq)	15.0	(mq)	(mq)	37%

Food Name	Serving Size	Calories	Prot. gms	Carbs gms	Sod. mgs	Fiber gms	Fat gms	Sat. Fat gms	Chol. mgs	% Fat Cal.
creamed, chipped (Myers)	3.5 oz	136	9.0	7.0	863	na	8.0	(mq)	(mq)	50%
creamed, chipped (Stouffer's)	5.5 oz	230	9.0	9.0	850	na	17.0	na	na	68%
creamed, chipped, 'Cookin' Bag' (Banquet)	4 oz	100	7.0	9.0	(mq)	na	4.0	(mq)	(mq)	36%
creamed, chipped, 'Cook-In-Pouch' (Freezer Queen)	5 oz	80	5.0	11.0	500	(mq)	2.0	(mq)	(mq)	22%
Dijon, w/pasta and vegetables (Right Course)	9.5 oz	290	20.0	31.0	580	(mq)	9.0	2.0	40	28%
fiesta, w/corn pasta (Right Course)	8 7/8 oz	270	18.0	33.0	590	(mq)	7.0	2.0	30	24%
homestyle, w/noodles, gravy, and vegetable (Stouffer's)	8 3/8 oz	230	16.0	26.0	720	na	7.0	na	na	27%
Jade garden, 'Stir Fry' (Weight Watchers)	9 oz	150	13.0	17.0	490	na	3.0	2.0	20	18%
London broil (Ultimate 200)	7.5 oz	110	17.0	4.0	320	na	3.0	1.0	25	24%
London broil, in mushroom sauce (Weight Watchers)	7.37 oz	140	18.0	9.0	510	na	3.0	1.0	40	20%
Oriental, w/vegetables and rice (Lean Cuisine)	8 5/8 oz	290	20.0	31.0	590	na	9.0	2.0	40	28%
patty, charbroiled, w/mushroom and onion gravy (Banquet)	8 oz	300	12.0	14.0	(mq)	na	21.0	(mq)	(mq)	65%
patty, charbroiled, w/ mushroom and onion gravy (Freezer Queen)	7 oz	200	13.0	10.0	960	na	12.0	(mq)	(mq)	54%
patty, charbroiled, w/mushroom gravy (Banquet)	8 oz	290	13.0	13.0	(mq)	na	21.0	(mq)	(mq)	65%
patty, charbroiled, w/mushroom gravy (Banquet)	5 oz	210	9.0	8.0	(mq)	na	15.0	(mq)	(mq)	67%
patty, charbroiled, w/ mushroom gravy (Freezer Queen)	7 oz	180	12.0	9.0	1050	na	11.0	(mq)	(mq)	54%
patty, charbroiled, w/ mushroom gravy (Freezer Queen)	5 oz	90	10.0	7.0	900	na	3.0	(mq)	(mq)	28%
pepper, Oriental (Chun King)	13 oz	310	17.0	53.0	1300	(mq)	3.0	(mq)	(mq)	9%
pie (Banquet)	7 oz	510	12.0	39.0	870	(mq)	33.0	(mq)	25	59%
pie (Myers)	3.5 oz	123	7.0	10.0	343	(mq)	6.0	(mq)	(mq)	44%
pie (Stouffer's)	10 oz	460	18.0	37.0	1130	na	27.0	na	na	53%
pie, 'Supreme Microwave' (Banquet)	7 oz	440	14.0	30.0	730	(mq)	29.0	(mq)	35	60%
'Platters' (Banquet)	10 oz	460	22.0	20.0	630	(mq)	34.0	(mq)	75	65%
pot pie (Swanson)	7 oz	370	12.0	36.0	730	(mq)	19.0	(mq)	(mq)	47%
pot pie, 'Hungry Man' (Swanson)	16 oz	610	24.0	58.0	1360	(mq)	31.0	(mq)	(mq)	46%
ragoût, w/rice pilaf (Right Course)	10 oz	300	19.0	38.0	550	(mq)	8.0	2.0	50	24%
rib, boneless, seasoned, w/barbecue sauce (Healthy Choice)	11 oz	330	28.0	40.0	530	na	6.0	2.0	70	17%
Romanoff supreme, w/pasta and vegetables (Weight Watchers)	9 oz	230	12.0	29.0	540	na	7.0	3.0	20	28%
Salisbury steak (Dining Lite)	9 oz	200	18.0	14.0	1000	na	8.0	(mq)	55	36%
Salisbury steak, charbroiled, w/vegetable medley 'Single Serve' (Freezer Queen)	9 oz	330	22.0	14.0	990	(mq)	22.0	(mq)	(mq)	58%
Salisbury steak, homestyle, w/gravy, macaroni and cheese (Stouffer's)	9 5/8 oz	350	25.0	23.0	1130	na	17.0	na	na	44%
Salisbury steak, 'Homestyle Recipe' (Swanson)	10 oz	320	21.0	22.0	980	(mq)	16.0	(mq)	(mq)	46%
Salisbury steak, supreme 'Gourmet Selection' (Tyson)	10 oz	430	16.0	34.0	810	(mq)	26.0	(mq)	(mq)	54%
Salisbury steak, w/gravy 'Cook-In-Pouch' (Freezer Queen)	5 oz	160	9.0	7.0	850	na	11.0	(mq)	(mq)	61%
Salisbury steak, w/gravy 'Cookin' Bags' (Banquet)	5 oz	190	9.0	8.0	(mq)	na	14.0	(mq)	(mq)	65%
Salisbury steak, w/gravy 'Family Entrées' (Banquet)	8 oz	300	13.0	12.0	(mq)	na	22.0	(mq)	(mq)	66%
Salisbury steak, w/gravy 'Family Suppers' (Freezer Queen)	7 oz	200	13.0	9.0	1110	na	13.0	(mq)	(mq)	57%
Salisbury steak, w/gravy and scalloped potatoes (Lean Cuisine)	9.5 oz	240	23.0	22.0	580	na	7.0	2.0	45	26%
Salisbury steak, w/mushroom gravy 'Classics' (Healthy Choice)	11 oz	280	21.0	35.0	500	na	6.0	3.0	55	19%
sirloin roast (Budget Gourmet)	9.5 oz	330	13.0	36.0	700	(mq)	14.0	(mq)	85	39%
sirloin tips (Ultimate 200)	7.5 oz	200	20.0	20.0	500	na	6.0	3.0	30	25%
sirloin tips, w/Burgundy sauce, Homestyle Recipe (Swanson)	7 oz	160	12.0	16.0	550	(mq)	5.0	(mq)	(mq)	29%
sirloin tips, w/country-style vegetables (Budget Gourmet)	10 oz	310	16.0	21.0	570	(mq)	18.0	(mq)	40	52%
sliced beef, w/barbecue sauce, 'Cookin' Bag' (Banquet)	4 oz	100	9.0	11.0	(mq)	na	2.0	(mq)	(mq)	18%
sliced beef, w/gravy, 'Cookin' Bag' (Banquet)	4 oz	100	8.0	5.0	(mq)	na	5.0	(mq)	(mq)	46%
sliced beef, w/gravy, 'Cook-In-Pouch' (Freezer Queen)	4 oz	60	9.0	4.0	500	na	1.0	(mq)	(mq)	15%

Food Name	Serving Size	Calories	Prot. gms	Carbs gms	Sod. mgs	Fiber gms	Fat gms	Sat. Fat gms	Chol. mgs	% Fat Cal.
sliced beef, w/gravy, 'Deluxe Family Suppers'										
(Freezer Queen) .... 7 oz		130	15.0	10.0	870	na	3.0	(mq)	(mq)	21%
sliced beef, w/gravy, 'Family Entrées' (Banquet) .... 8 oz		160	20.0	8.0	(mq)	(mq)	5.0	(mq)	(mq)	29%
steak, breaded (Hormel) .... 4 oz		370	14.0	13.0	(mq)	(mq)	30.0	(mq)	(mq)	71%
steak and mushroom hand-held pie, 'Aussie Pie'										
(Mrs. Paterson's) .... 5.5 oz		410	14.0	43.0	820	na	20.0	8.0	80	44%
Szechuan (Chun King) .... 13 oz		340	20.0	57.0	1810	(mq)	3.0	(mq)	(mq)	8%
teriyaki (Chun King) .... 13 oz		380	22.0	68.0	2200	(mq)	2.0	(mq)	(mq)	5%
teriyaki (Dining Lite) .... 9 oz		270	20.0	36.0	850	(mq)	5.0	(mq)	45	17%
teriyaki, w/rice and vegetables, 'Fresh & Lite' (LaChoy) ... 10 oz		240	17.0	39.9	1198	2.0	5.0	(mq)	57	17%
stew, 'Family Entrées' (Banquet) .... 7 oz		140	6.0	18.0	(mq)	(mq)	5.0	(mq)	(mq)	32%
stew, 'Family Suppers' (Freezer Queen) .... 7 oz		150	9.0	15.0	820	(mq)	6.0	(mq)	(mq)	36%
BEEF ENTRÉE, MICROWAVE										
beef and mushrooms, 'Health Selections' micro cup										
(Hormel) .... 7 oz		210	21.0	25.0	390	na	3.0	2.0	45	13%
ribs, boneless, microwave bowl (Top Shelf) ... 1 serving		440	28.0	29.0	550	(mq)	24.0	(mq)	90	49%
roast, tender, microwave bowl (Top Shelf) .... 1 serving		240	27.0	18.0	980	(mq)	7.0	(mq)	65	26%
roast beef, w/gravy and potatoes, 'American Classics'										
(Dinty Moore) .... 10 oz		260	26.0	26.0	910	na	6.0	3.0	45	21%
Salisbury steak, w/potatoes, microwave bowl (Top Shelf)	1 serving	254	29.0	22.0	1211	(mq)	6.0	(mq)	88	21%
stew (Armour) .... 7.5 oz		150	10.0	15.0	870	na	5.0	na	na	31%
stew, chunky, microwave cup (Weight Watchers) .... 7.5 oz		120	14.0	14.0	450	na	2.0	1.0	20	14%
stew, 'Diner' microwave cup (Libby's) .... 7.75 oz		240	12.0	22.0	790	0	12.0	6.0	40	44%
stew, hearty, 'Microeasy,' 1/4 pkg prepared w/1.5 lbs										
beef (Lipton) .... 1 serving		370	31.0	14.0	800	(mq)	20.0	(mq)	(mq)	50%
stew, hearty, microwave cup (Lunch Bucket) .... 7.5 oz		180	8.0	13.0	870	na	11.0	na	40	54%
stew, micro cup (Hormel) .... 7.5 oz		230	13.0	11.0	1140	na	15.0	5.0	45	58%
stew, microwave bowl (Dinty Moore) .... 10 oz		260	15.0	19.0	1180	na	14.0	6.0	45	48%
stew, microwave cup (Dinty Moore) .... 7.5 oz		180	11.0	15.0	830	na	9.0	1.0	30	44%
sukiyaki, microwave bowl (Top Shelf) .... 1 serving		330	24.0	36.0	1700	(mq)	10.0	(mq)	45	27%
w/macaroni, 'Diner' microwave cup (Libby's) .... 7.75 oz		230	10.0	34.0	670	2.5	6.0	3.0	20	24%
BEEF ENTRÉE, PACKAGED										
Salisbury steak (Top Shelf) .... 10 oz		320	25.0	22.0	910	na	15.0	7.0	70	42%
Salisbury steak, w/mushroom gravy (Ultra Slim Fast) ..... 10.5 oz		290	19.0	44.0	830	na	5.0	na	35	15%
BEEF JERKY										
'Arrowhead' (Pemmican) .... .7-oz piece		70	8.0	2.0	580	0	3.0	(mq)	(mq)	40%
'Big Jerk' (Slim Jim) .... .25-oz piece		25	3.0	1.0	220	0	1.0	(mq)	(mq)	36%
'Giant Jerk' (Slim Jim) .... .63-oz piece		60	7.0	2.0	510	0	2.0	(mq)	(mq)	33%
jalapeño (Pemmican) .... 1.3-oz piece		110	16.0	5.0	1150	0	3.0	(mq)	(mq)	24%
jalapeño (Pemmican) .... 1.1 oz		90	13.0	4.0	960	0	2.0	(mq)	(mq)	21%
jalapeño flavored steak (Pemmican) .... .25 oz		25	3.0	1.0	220	0	1.0	(mq)	(mq)	36%
'Lumberjack' (Hormel) .... 1 oz		101	5.0	0.0	304	0	9.0	(mq)	(mq)	80%
natural (Pemmican) .... 1.3-oz piece		110	16.0	5.0	1150	0	3.0	(mq)	(mq)	24%
natural (Pemmican) .... 1.1 oz		90	13.0	4.0	960	0	2.0	(mq)	(mq)	21%
natural (Pemmican) .... 1 oz		80	12.0	4.0	880	0	2.0	(mq)	(mq)	22%
natural flavored steak (Pemmican) .... .25 oz		25	3.0	1.0	220	0	1.0	(mq)	(mq)	36%
peppered (Pemmican) .... 1.3-oz piece		110	16.0	5.0	1150	0	3.0	(mq)	(mq)	24%
peppered (Pemmican) .... 1.1 oz		90	13.0	4.0	960	0	2.0	(mq)	(mq)	21%
peppered steak (Pemmican) .... .25 oz		25	3.0	1.0	220	0	1.0	(mq)	(mq)	36%
regular (Frito-Lay's) .... .21 oz		25	3.0	1.0	200	0	1.0	(mq)	10	36%
regular (Hickory Farms) .... 1 oz		100	16.0	4.0	1360	0	3.0	(mq)	73	25%
regular (Slim Jim) .... .14-oz piece		20	2.0	1.0	120	0	1.0	(mq)	(mq)	43%
regular 'Super Jerk' approx .31 oz (Slim Jim) .... 1 piece		30	4.0	1.0	250	0	1.0	(mq)	(mq)	31%
'Steakers' (Pemmican) .... 1.1-oz pouch		80	14.0	4.0	470	0	1.0	(mq)	(mq)	11%

Food Name	Serving Size	Calories	Prot. gms	Carbs gms	Sod. mgs	Fiber gms	Fat gms	Sat. Fat gms	Chol. mgs	% Fat Cal.
'Steakers' (Pemmican)	1 strip	40	5.0	2.0	160	0	1.0	(mq)	(mq)	21%
Tabasco (Pemmican)	1.3-oz piece	110	16.0	5.0	1150	0	3.0	(mq)	(mq)	24%
Tabasco (Pemmican)	1.1 oz	90	13.0	4.0	960	0	2.0	(mq)	(mq)	21%
Tabasco flavored steak (Pemmican)	.25 oz	25	3.0	1.0	220	0	1.0	(mq)	(mq)	36%
Tabasco 'Super Jerk' (Slim Jim)	.31-oz piece	30	4.0	1.0	250	0	1.0	(mq)	(mq)	31%
'Tender' (Frito-Lay's)	.7 oz	120	5.0	2.0	370	0	10.0	(mq)	25	76%
'Tender Brave' (Pemmican)	1 oz	80	14.0	2.0	830	0	2.0	(mq)	(mq)	22%
'Tender Chief' (Pemmican)	1 oz	80	14.0	2.0	830	0	2.0	(mq)	(mq)	22%
'Tender Tomahawk' (Pemmican)	.25-oz piece	20	3.0	1.0	210	0	1.0	(mq)	(mq)	36%
'Tender Trail' (Pemmican)	1 oz	80	14.0	2.0	830	0	2.0	(mq)	(mq)	22%
'Tender Tribe' (Pemmican)	1 oz	80	14.0	2.0	830	0	2.0	(mq)	(mq)	22%
teriyaki, natural style (Pemmican)	1 oz	80	12.0	4.0	800	0	2.0	(mq)	(mq)	22%
teriyaki, natural style (Pemmican)	.25-oz piece	20	3.0	1.0	200	0	1.0	(mq)	(mq)	36%
teriyaki, natural style, slab (Pemmican)	1.3 oz	100	15.0	5.0	1030	0	2.0	(mq)	(mq)	18%
BEEF JERKY, ALTERNATIVE										
'Jerquee' vegetable protein product (Stonewall's)	.5 oz	50	5.0	2.0	125	1.0	2.0	na	0	39%
'Spicy Italian Style' (Cajun Jerky)	.5 oz	50	5.0	2.0	125	1.0	2.0	na	0	39%
BEEF POT PIE. See BEEF ENTRÉE, FROZEN.										
BEEF SEASONING MIX										
(French's) dry ground, w/onions	1/4 pkg	25	1.0	6.0	440	na	0.0	0.0	0	0%
(Lawry's) marinade	1 pkg	49	1.2	10.7	7284	>.1 c	0.2	na	0	4%
(Schilling) Stroganoff	1/4 pkg	32	1.0	6.0	1078	na	0.3	na	na	9%
BEEF STEW. See BEEF ENTRÉE, CANNED; BEEF ENTRÉE, DRIED; BEEF ENTRÉE, FROZEN; BEEF ENTRÉE, MICROWAVE.										
BEEF STEW MIX, hearty, 'Microeasy' (Lipton) dry	1/4 pkg	70	2.0	14.0	730	(mq)	<1.0	na	na	<12%
BEEF STEW SEASONING MIX										
(French's) dry mix	1/6 pkg	25	0.0	5.0	770	na	0.0	0.0	0	0%
(Lawry's) 'Seasoning Blends'	1 pkg	131	5.4	25.7	3181	>1.2 c	0.7	na	0	5%
(Schilling)	1/2 pkg	33	1.3	6.0	806	na	0.3	na	na	9%
(Schilling) 'Bag'n Season'	1 pkg	87	7.5	11.0	4320	na	1.0	na	1	11%
BEEF SUET, raw	1 oz	242	0.4	0.0	2	0	26.7	14.8	19	99%
BEEF TALLOW										
	1 cup	1849	0.0	0.0	0	0	205.0	102.1	223	100%
	1 oz	256	0.0	0.0	0	0	28.4	14.1	31	100%
	1 tbsp	115	0.0	0.0	0	0	12.8	6.4	14	100%
BEEFALO										
composite of cuts, diced, roasted	1 cup	263	42.9	0.0	115	0	8.8	3.8	81	32%
composite of cuts, roasted	4 oz	213	34.8	0.0	93	0	7.2	3.0	66	32%
raw	1 lb	649	105.7	0.0	354	na	21.8	9.3	200	32%
raw	1 oz	40	6.5	0.0	22	na	1.3	0.6	12	31%
roasted	3 oz	160	26.1	0.0	70	na	5.4	2.3	49	32%
BEER. See ALCOHOLIC BEVERAGES.										
BEER, NONALCOHOLIC. See ALCOHOL-FREE BEVERAGES.										
BEER SALAMI. See LUNCHEON MEAT.										
BEERWURST										
beef	1 oz	92	3.5	0.5	264	0	8.3	3.4	16	82%
beef, 4 inch diam	1/8-inch slice	76	2.8	0.4	236	0	6.9	3.0	14	83%
beef, 2.75 inch diam	1/16-inch slice	20	0.7	0.1	62	0	1.8	0.8	4	84%
pork	1 oz	67	4.0	0.0	552	0	5.3	1.8	17	72%
pork, 4 inch diam	1/8-inch slice	55	3.3	0.5	285	0	4.3	1.4	14	72%
pork, 2.75 inch diam	1/16-inch slice	14	0.9	0.1	74	0	1.1	0.4	4	71%
pork, cured, 4 inch diam	1/8-inch slice	55	3.3	0.5	285	0	4.3	1.4	14	72%
pork, cured, 2.75 inch diam	1/16-inch slice	14	0.9	0.1	74	0	1.1	0.4	4	71%
BEET										
boiled, drained	4 oz	35	1.2	7.6	56	>1.0 c	0.1	tr	0	3%

Food Name	Serving Size	Calories	Prot. gms	Carbs gms	Sod. mgs	Fiber gms	Fat gms	Sat. Fat gms	Chol. mgs	% Fat Cal.
boiled, drained, sliced	1/2 cup	37	1.4	8.5	65	1.4	0.2	0.0	0	4%
raw, sliced	1/2 cup	29	1.1	6.5	53	1.9	0.1	0.0	0	3%
raw, trimmed	1 oz	12	0.4	2.8	20	.3	<.1	tr	0	<7%
raw, untrimmed	1 lb	133	4.5	30.4	220	3.0	0.4	0.1	0	3%
BEET, CANNED										
cut *(Stokely)*	1/2 cup	40	1.0	8.0	300	(mq)	0.0	0.0	0	0%
diced *(S&W)*	1/2 cup	40	1.0	9.0	270	(mq)	0.0	0.0	0	0%
diced *(Stokely)*	1/2 cup	35	1.0	7.0	300	(mq)	0.0	0.0	0	0%
Harvard *(Stokely)*	1/2 cup	70	1.0	18.0	135	(mq)	0.0	0.0	0	0%
Harvard, sliced, w/liquid	1/2 cup	90	1.0	22.4	199	>.8 c	0.1	0.0	0	1%
julienne *(S&W)*	1/2 cup	40	1.0	9.0	270	(mq)	0.0	0.0	0	0%
'No Salt or Sugar Added' *(Stokely)*	1/2 cup	40	1.0	8.0	40	(mq)	0.0	0.0	0	0%
pickled *(Freshlike)*	1/2 cup	40	1.0	9.0	650	na	0.0	na	na	0%
pickled *(Stokely)*	1/2 cup	100	1.0	25.0	400	(mq)	0.0	0.0	0	0%
pickled *(Veg•All)*	1/2 cup	100	1.0	25.0	650	na	0.0	na	na	0%
pickled, crinkle sliced, w/liquid *(Del Monte)*	1/2 cup	80	1.0	19.0	375	(mq)	0.0	0.0	0	0%
pickled 'Jars' *(Stokely)*	1/2 cup	90	1.0	22.0	280	(mq)	0.0	0.0	0	0%
pickled, sliced, w/liquid	1/2 cup	74	0.9	18.6	301	>.7 c	0.1	0.0	0	1%
pickled, sliced, w/red wine vinegar 'Party' *(S&W)*	1/2 cup	70	1.0	16.0	215	(mq)	0.0	0.0	0	0%
pickled, sliced, w/red wine vinegar 'Regular' *(S&W)*	1/2 cup	70	1.0	16.0	215	(mq)	0.0	0.0	0	0%
pickled, whole, extra small *(S&W)*	1/2 cup	70	1.0	16.0	215	(mq)	0.0	0.0	0	0%
regular pack, w/liquid	1/2 cup	36	1.0	8.3	323	1.4	0.1	0.0	0	2%
sliced *(A&P)*	1/2 cup	40	1.0	9.0	300	(mq)	<1.0	(tr)	0	<18%
sliced *(Featherweight)*	1/2 cup	45	1.0	10.0	55	(mq)	0.0	0.0	0	0%
sliced *(Finast)*	1/2 cup	40	1.0	9.0	390	(mq)	0.0	0.0	0	0%
sliced *(Pathmark)*	1/2 cup	45	1.0	10.0	330	(mq)	0.0	0.0	0	0%
sliced *(S&W Nutradiet)*	1/2 cup	35	1.0	9.0	40	(mq)	0.0	0.0	0	0%
sliced *(Stokely)*	1/2 cup	40	1.0	8.0	300	(mq)	0.0	0.0	0	0%
sliced, drained	1/2 cup	26	0.8	6.1	233	1.5	0.1	0.0	0	3%
sliced, 'No Salt Added' *(A&P)*	1/2 cup	35	1.0	8.0	50	(mq)	<1.0	(tr)	0	<20%
sliced, 'No Salt Added' *(Finast)*	1/2 cup	40	1.0	9.0	40	(mq)	0.0	0.0	0	0%
sliced, 'No Salt Added' *(Pathmark)*	1/2 cup	35	1.0	7.0	35	(mq)	0.0	0.0	0	0%
sliced, water packed, w/o salt *(Freshlike)*	1/2 cup	40	1.0	9.0	50	na	0.0	na	na	0%
sliced, water packed, w/o sugar or salt *(Freshlike)*	1/2 cup	40	1.0	9.0	50	na	0.0	na	na	0%
sliced, w/liquid, 'No Salt Added' *(Del Monte)*	1/2 cup	35	1.0	8.0	100	(mq)	0.0	0.0	0	0%
small, sliced *(Freshlike)*	1/2 cup	40	1.0	9.0	260	na	0.0	na	na	0%
small, sliced, 'Premium' *(S&W)*	1/2 cup	40	1.0	9.0	270	(mq)	0.0	0.0	0	0%
small, whole *(Freshlike)*	1/2 cup	40	1.0	9.0	260	na	0.0	na	na	0%
small, whole *(S&W)*	1/2 cup	40	1.0	9.0	270	(mq)	0.0	0.0	0	0%
special dietary pack, w/liquid	1/2 cup	36	1.0	8.3	57	1.4	0.1	0.0	0	2%
tiny, whole, w/liquid *(Del Monte)*	1/2 cup	35	1.0	8.0	290	(mq)	0.0	0.0	0	0%
whole *(A&P)*	1/2 cup	40	1.0	9.0	300	(mq)	<1.0	(tr)	0	<18%
whole *(IGA)*	1/2 cup	40	1.0	9.0	275	(mq)	0.0	0.0	0	0%
whole *(Stokely)*	1/2 cup	40	1.0	8.0	300	(mq)	0.0	0.0	0	0%
whole, sliced, w/liquid *(Del Monte)*	1/2 cup	35	1.0	8.0	290	(mq)	0.0	0.0	0	0%
BEET GREENS										
boiled, drained	4 oz	31	2.9	6.2	273	>1.2 c	0.2	<.1	0	5%
boiled, drained, 1-inch pieces	1/2 cup	19	1.9	3.9	174	2.1	0.1	0.0	0	4%
raw, approx 2 oz	1 leaf	6	0.6	1.3	64	1.2	<.1	tr	0	<11%
raw, 1-inch pieces	1/2 cup	4	0.4	0.8	38	.7	0.0	0.0	0	0%
raw, untrimmed	1 lb	49	4.6	10.1	510	>3.3 c	0.2	<.1	0	3%
raw, untrimmed	1 oz	5	0.5	1.1	57	>.4 c	<.1	tr	0	<12%
BEET ROOT JUICE, bottled *(Biotta)*	6 oz	75	1.8	15.9	128	(mq)	0.1	(tr)	0	1%

BELLYFISH. See MONKFISH.

Food Name	Serving Size	Calories	Prot. gms	Carbs gms	Sod. mgs	Fiber gms	Fat gms	Sat. Fat gms	Chol. mgs	% Fat Cal.
BERLINER										
beef and pork	1 oz	65	4.3	0.7	368	0	4.9	1.7	13	69%
beef and pork, 2.5 inch diam	1/4-inch slice	53	3.5	0.6	298	0	4.0	1.4	11	69%
BERRY DRINK										
'Berries & Berries' (Tropicana)	6 oz	90	<1.0	23.0	20	na	<1.0	na	na	<9%
'Berries & Berries' juice (Tropicana)	10 oz	156	(tr)	39.0	3	(tr)	0.0	0.0	0	0%
'Berry B. Wild' (Squeezit)	6.75 oz	120	0.0	29.0	5	na	0.0	na	na	0%
berry blend juice, 'Fruit Box' (Tang)	8.45 oz	140	0.0	36.0	10	na	0.0	na	0	0%
berry citrus drink, frozen, prepared (Five Alive)	6 oz	90	0.0	22.0	5	na	0.0	na	na	0%
berry juice, bottled (Juicy Juice)	6 oz	90	1.0	22.0	10	na	0.0	na	na	0%
berry juice, boxed (Juicy Juice)	8.45 oz	130	1.0	30.0	15	na	0.0	na	na	0%
berry juice, canned (Juicy Juice)	6 oz	90	0.0	22.0	10	(mq)	0.0	0.0	0	0%
berry nectar, organic (Santa Cruz Natural)	8 oz	90	<1.0	22.0	na	na	<1.0	na	na	<9%
berry punch, aseptic box or chilled (Minute Maid)	6 oz	90	0.0	23.0	20	na	0.0	na	na	0%
berry punch, frozen concentrate (Minute Maid)	6 oz	90	0.0	23.0	0	na	0.0	na	na	0%
'Bopin' Berry' (Hi-C)	6 oz	90	0.0	23.0	25	na	0.0	na	na	0%
'Great Bluedini' (Kool-Aid) 'Kool Bursts'	6.75 oz	110	0.0	28.0	10	na	0.0	na	0	0%
'Great Bluedini' (Kool-Aid) 'Koolers'	8.45 oz	110	0.0	29.0	10	na	0.0	na	0	0%
Mountain Berry Punch (Kool-Aid) 'Koolers'	8.45 oz	140	0.0	37.0	10	na	0.0	na	0	0%
'Very Berry' (Hawaiian Punch)	6 oz	90	0.0	22.0	30	(tr)	0.0	0.0	0	0%
BERRY DRINK MIX										
berry blend, sugar-free w/NutraSweet, prepared (Crystal Light)	8 oz	4	0.0	0.0	0	na	0.0	na	0	0%
'Berry Blue' sugar-free w/NutraSweet, prepared (Kool-Aid)	8 oz	4	0.0	0.0	5	na	0.0	na	0	0%
'Berry Blue' sugar-sweetened, prepared (Kool-Aid)	8 oz	80	0.0	21.0	5	na	0.0	na	0	0%
'Berry Blue' unsweetened, prepared w/sugar (Kool-Aid)	8 oz	100	0.0	25.0	0	na	0.0	na	0	0%
'Berry Blue' unsweetened, prepared w/o sugar (Kool-Aid)	8 oz	2	0.0	0.0	0	na	0.0	na	0	0%
'Great Bluedini' sugar-free w/NutraSweet, prepared (Kool-Aid)	8 oz	4	0.0	0.0	0	na	0.0	na	0	0%
'Great Bluedini' sugar-sweetened, prepared (Kool-Aid)	8 oz	70	0.0	18.0	0	na	0.0	na	0	0%
'Great Bluedini' unsweetened, prepared w/sugar (Kool-Aid)	8 oz	100	0.0	25.0	0	na	0.0	na	0	0%
'Great Bluedini' unsweetened, prepared w/o sugar (Kool-Aid)	8 oz	2	0.0	0.0	0	na	0.0	na	0	0%
Mountain Berry Punch, sugar-free w/NutraSweet, prepared (Kool-Aid)	8 oz	4	0.0	0.0	35	na	0.0	na	0	0%
Mountain Berry Punch, sugar-sweetened, prepared (Kool-Aid)	8 oz	80	0.0	20.0	15	na	0.0	na	0	0%
Mountain Berry Punch, unsweetened, prepared w/sugar (Kool-Aid)	8 oz	100	0.0	25.0	15	na	0.0	na	0	0%
Mountain Berry Punch, unsweetened, prepared w/o sugar (Kool-Aid)	8 oz	2	0.0	0.0	15	na	0.0	na	0	0%
'Surfin' Berry' sugar-free w/NutraSweet, prepared (Kool-Aid)	8 oz	4	0.0	0.0	10	na	0.0	na	0	0%
'Surfin' Berry' unsweetened, prepared w/sugar (Kool-Aid)	8 oz	100	0.0	25.0	25	na	0.0	na	0	0%
'Surfin' Berry' unsweetened, prepared w/o sugar (Kool Aid)	8 oz	2	0.0	0.0	25	na	0.0	na	0	0%

BEVERAGES. See ALCOHOL-FREE BEVERAGES; ALCOHOLIC BEVERAGES; COFFEE; DIET DRINK; MILK; SOFT DRINKS AND MIXERS; SPORTS DRINK; TEA; WATER; and individual listings.

BIBB LETTUCE. See LETTUCE.

Food Name	Serving Size	Calories	Prot. gms	Carbs gms	Sod. mgs	Fiber gms	Fat gms	Sat. Fat gms	Chol. mgs	% Fat Cal.
BISCUIT										
buttermilk, commercially baked	1 oz	103	1.8	13.8	298	na	4.7	0.7	0	40%
mixed grain, dough, baked	1 oz	86	2.0	15.6	221	na	1.8	0.5	0	19%
plain, commercially baked	1 oz	103	1.8	13.8	298	na	4.7	0.7	0	40%

Food Name	Serving Size	Calories	Prot. gms	Carbs gms	Sod. mgs	Fiber gms	Fat gms	Sat. Fat gms	Chol. mgs	% Fat Cal.
(Awrey's) country	3-inch biscuit	160	4.0	23.0	530	1.0	5.0	1.0	0	29%
(Awrey's) round	1 oz	80	2.0	12.0	260	0	3.0	1.0	0	33%
(Awrey's) sliced	2 oz	160	4.0	23.0	520	1.0	5.0	1.0	0	29%
(Awrey's) square	1 oz	80	2.0	12.0	260	0	3.0	1.0	0	33%
(Awrey's) unsliced	2 oz	160	4.0	23.0	520	1.0	5.0	1.0	0	29%
(Mrs. Winner's)	1 biscuit	245	4.0	45.0	503	na	5.0	na	na	19%
(Weight Watchers) buttermilk	1.8 oz	100	3.0	23.0	410	na	1.0	na	na	8%
(Wonder)	1 biscuit	80	2.0	14.0	140	.6	1.0	na	na	12%
BISCUIT, FROZEN (Bridgford)	2 oz	180	4.0	28.0	632	(mq)	6.0	(mq)	1	30%
BISCUIT, REFRIGERATED										
(Ballard) buttermilk, extra lights, 'Ovenready'	1 biscuit	50	1.0	10.0	180	na	0.0	0.0	0	0%
(Ballard) buttermilk, 'Ovenready'	1 biscuit	50	1.0	10.0	180	(mq)	1.0	na	na	17%
(Ballard) extra lights, 'Ovenready'	1 biscuit	50	1.0	10.0	180	na	0.0	0.0	0	0%
(Ballard) 'Ovenready'	1 biscuit	50	1.0	10.0	180	(mq)	1.0	0.0	0	17%
(Big Country) 'Butter Tastin''	1 biscuit	100	2.0	14.0	320	(mq)	4.0	<1.0	0	36%
(Big Country) buttermilk	1 biscuit	100	2.0	14.0	320	(mq)	4.0	<1.0	0	36%
(Big Country) Southern style	1 biscuit	100	2.0	14.0	320	(mq)	4.0	<1.0	0	36%
(1869 Brand) baking powder	1 biscuit	100	2.0	12.0	310	(mq)	5.0	1.0	0	45%
(1869 Brand) 'Butter Tastin'	1 biscuit	100	2.0	12.0	300	(mq)	5.0	1.0	0	45%
(1869 Brand) buttermilk	1 biscuit	100	2.0	12.0	310	(mq)	5.0	1.0	0	45%
(Good 'N Buttery) fluffy	1 biscuit	90	1.0	11.0	270	(mq)	5.0	1.0	0	48%
(Grands Inch) 'Butter Tastin'	1 biscuit	190	4.0	22.0	560	na	9.0	2.0	0	44%
(Grands Inch) cinnamon raisin	1 biscuit	190	3.0	27.0	540	na	7.0	2.0	0	34%
(Grands Inch) flaky	1 biscuit	190	4.0	23.0	530	na	8.0	2.0	0	40%
(Hungry Jack) buttermilk, 'Extra Rich'	1 biscuit	50	1.0	9.0	180	(mq)	1.0	<1.0	0	18%
(Hungry Jack) buttermilk, flaky	1 biscuit	90	2.0	12.0	300	(mq)	4.0	<1.0	0	39%
(Hungry Jack) buttermilk, fluffy	1 biscuit	90	2.0	12.0	280	(mq)	4.0	1.0	0	39%
(Hungry Jack) flaky, 'Butter Tastin''	1 biscuit	90	2.0	11.0	280	(mq)	4.0	<1.0	0	41%
(Hungry Jack) flaky	1 biscuit	80	2.0	12.0	300	(mq)	4.0	<1.0	0	39%
(Hungry Jack) honey, flaky, 'Honey Tastin''	1 biscuit	90	2.0	13.0	290	(mq)	4.0	<1.0	0	38%
(Hungry Jack) Southern style, flaky	1 biscuit	80	2.0	12.0	300	na	4.0	<1	0	39%
(Pillsbury) 'Big Premium Heat 'n Eat'	2 biscuits	280	5.0	32.0	610	(mq)	15.0	3.0	0	48%
(Pillsbury) butter	1 biscuit	50	1.0	10.0	180	(mq)	1.0	0.0	0	17%
(Pillsbury) buttermilk, 'Heat 'n Eat'	2 biscuits	170	4.0	27.0	530	(mq)	5.0	1.0	0	27%
(Pillsbury) buttermilk	1 biscuit	50	1.0	10.0	180	(mq)	1.0	1.0	0	17%
(Pillsbury) buttermilk, 'Tender Layer'	1 biscuit	50	1.0	9.0	170	(mq)	1.0	0.0	0	18%
(Pillsbury) 'Country'	1 biscuit	50	1.0	10.0	180	(mq)	1.0	0.0	0	17%
(Roman Meal) oat bran, honey nut	1 biscuit	131	2.4	19.7	278	.9	4.7	1.2	0	32%
(Roman Meal) white	2 biscuits	180	4.2	32.2	456	1.4	3.8	0.9	0	19%
(Roman Meal) white, 'Premium'	1 biscuit	127	2.4	18.8	308	(mq)	4.7	1.2	0	33%
BISCUIT, TOASTER										
(Oroweat) 'Australian'	1 biscuit	180	6.0	30.0	440	1.0	5.0	1.0	0	24%
(Oroweat) cinnamon raisin	1 biscuit	200	5.0	34.0	410	1.0	5.0	1.0	0	22%
(Oroweat) cornbread	1 biscuit	200	5.0	39.0	230	1.0	3.0	1.0	5	13%
BISCUIT MIX										
(Arrowhead Mills)	2 oz	100	4.0	19.0	96	(mq)	1.0	na	0	9%
(Bisquick)	1/2 cup	240	4.0	37.0	700	(mq)	8.0	2.0	0	31%
(Gold Medal) 'Pouch Mix,' prepared w/skim milk	1/8 recipe	90	2.0	14.0	270	(mq)	3.0	1.0	0	30%
(Health Valley) buttermilk, 'Biscuit & Pancake'	1 oz	100	4.0	20.0	170	3.3	1.0	na	0	9%
(Krusteaz) cinnamon raisin, w/glaze, prepared from mix	3-inch biscuit	200	2.0	39.0	150	1.0	4.0	na	0	18%
(Krusteaz) prepared from mix	2-inch biscuit	90	2.0	14.0	260	na	3.0	0.7	1	30%
(Martha White) prepared from mix, 'BixMix,' made w/2% milk, rolled	2-inch biscuit	90	2.0	15.0	240	na	2.0	na	2	21%
(Robin Hood) 'Pouch Mix,' prepared w/skim milk	1/8 recipe	90	2.0	14.0	270	(mq)	3.0	1.0	0	30%

Food Name	Serving Size	Calories	Prot. gms	Carbs gms	Sod. mgs	Fiber gms	Fat gms	Sat. Fat gms	Chol. mgs	% Fat Cal.
BISON. See BUFFALO, AMERICAN.										
BLACK BEAN										
boiled	4 oz	150	10.0	26.9	1	4.8	0.6	0.2	0	4%
boiled	1/2 cup	114	7.6	20.4	1	7.5	0.5	0.1	0	4%
raw	1/2 cup	331	21.0	60.5	5	14.7	1.4	0.4	0	4%
raw	1 oz	97	6.1	17.7	1	3.7	0.4	0.1	0	4%
raw *(Arrowhead Mills)*	2 oz	190	13.0	35.0	9	11.3	1.0	(tr)	0	5%
BLACK BEAN, CANNED										
(Eden Foods) organic, very low sodium, no salt added	1/2 cup	70	7.0	17.0	15	6.0	<1.0	na	0	<9%
(Green Giant)	1/2 cup	90	7.0	21.0	580	6.0	0.0	0.0	0	0%
(Joan of Arc)	1/2 cup	90	7.0	21.0	580	6.0	0.0	0.0	0	0%
(Progresso)	1/2 cup	90	9.0	19.0	350	6.5	1.0	na	0	7%
BLACK BEAN DINNER, CANNED										
Western, w/garden vegetables, 'Fast Menu' *(Health Valley)*	7.5 oz	120	13.0	14.0	170	14.5	1.0	na	0	8%
BLACK BEAN MIX, INSTANT										
prepared w/o added ingredients *(Fantastic Foods)*	1/2 cup	157	10.0	28.0	400	(mq)	2.0	(mq)	na	11%
prepared w/2 tbsp salted butter *(Fantastic Foods)*	1/2 cup	207	10.0	28.0	469	(mq)	8.0	(mq)	(mq)	32%
BLACK CHERRY DRINK MIX										
unsweetened, prepared w/sugar *(Kool-Aid)*	8 oz	100	0.0	25.0	0	na	0.0	na	0	0%
unsweetened, prepared w/o sugar *(Kool-Aid)*	8 oz	2	0.0	0.0	0	na	0.0	na	0	0%
BLACK CHERRY JUICE										
(Knudsen & Sons)	8 oz	150	2.0	38.0	na	na	0.0	na	na	0%
(Smucker's) 'Naturally 100%'	8 oz	130	0.0	31.0	10	(mq)	0.0	0.0	0	0%
BLACK PUDDING. See BLOOD SAUSAGE.										
BLACK TURTLE BEAN										
boiled	1/2 cup	120	7.5	22.4	3	4.9	0.3	0.1	0	2%
canned	1/2 cup	109	7.2	19.9	461	>1.4 c	0.4	0.1	0	3%
raw	1/2 cup	312	19.5	58.2	8	22.9	0.8	0.2	0	2%
BLACK WALNUT FLAVOR DRINK										
canned, liquid nutrition *(Ensure)*	8 oz	250	8.8	34.3	na	na	8.8	na	na	32%
BLACKBERRY										
raw	1/2 cup	37	0.5	9.2	0	3.6	0.3	na	0	7%
trimmed	1 oz	15	0.2	3.6	tr	1.3	0.1	(tr)	0	6%
untrimmed	1 lb	225	3.1	56.0	1	19.7	1.7	(tr)	0	6%
BLACKBERRY, CANNED										
in heavy syrup	4 oz	104	1.5	26.2	3	>2.9 c	0.2	(tr)	0	2%
in heavy syrup, w/liquid	1/2 cup	118	1.7	29.6	4	4.3	0.2	na	0	1%
in water *(Allens)*	1/2 cup	25	1.0	4.0	15	(mq)	<1.0	(tr)	0	<31%
BLACKBERRY, FROZEN										
unsweetened	18-oz pkg	326	6.0	79.9	5	25.5	2.2	na	0	5%
unsweetened	1 cup	97	1.8	23.7	2	7.6	0.7	na	0	6%
unsweetened	1/2 cup	49	0.9	11.8	1	>2.0 c	0.3	(tr)	0	5%
BLACKBERRY SYRUP *(Knott's Berry Farm)*	1 oz	120	0.0	30.0	0	na	0.0	na	na	0%
BLACK-EYED PEAS / cowpeas / yellow-eyed peas										
boiled, drained	1/2 cup	79	2.6	16.7	3	4.1	0.3	0.1	0	3%
boiled, drained	4 oz	110	3.6	23.1	5	5.7	0.4	0.1	0	3%
leafy tips, boiled, drained	4 oz	25	5.3	3.2	7	>3.0 c	0.1	<.1	0	3%
leafy tips, raw, chopped	1/2 cup	5	0.7	0.9	1	>.2 c	<.1	<.1	0	<12%
leafy tips, raw, trimmed	1 oz	8	1.2	1.4	2	>.4 c	0.1	<.1	0	8%
leafy tips, raw, untrimmed	1 lb	68	9.7	11.4	16	>3.1 c	0.6	0.2	0	6%
raw, in pods	1 lb	208	6.8	43.7	9	>4.2 c	0.8	0.2	0	3%
raw, trimmed	1 oz	26	0.8	5.4	1	>.5 c	0.1	<.1	0	4%
raw, trimmed	1/2 cup	65	2.1	13.6	3	>1.3 c	0.3	0.1	0	4%

Food Name	Serving Size	Calories	Prot. gms	Carbs gms	Sod. mgs	Fiber gms	Fat gms	Sat. Fat gms	Chol. mgs	% Fat Cal.
young pods w/seeds, raw, approx										
11 7/8 inches x 5/16 inch	1 pod	5	0.4	1.1	tr	>.2 c	<.1	tr	0	<13%
young pods, w/seeds, raw, trimmed	1 oz	12	0.9	2.7	1	>.5 c	0.1	<.1	0	6%
young pods, w/seeds, raw, trimmed	1/2 cup	21	1.6	4.5	2	>.8 c	0.1	<.1	0	4%
young pods, w/seeds, raw, untrimmed	1 lb	182	13.6	39.2	17	>7.0 c	1.2	0.3	0	5%
BLACK-EYED PEAS, CANNED										
(A&P) mature	7.5 oz	120	7.0	20.0	410	(mq)	1.0	(mq)	(mq)	8%
(Allens)	1/2 cup	100	7.0	18.0	370	(mq)	<1.0	(tr)	0	<8%
(Allens) mature	1/2 cup	105	5.0	18.0	300	(mq)	1.0	(mq)	(mq)	9%
(Allens) w/snaps	1/2 cup	100	5.0	20.0	370	(mq)	<1.0	(tr)	0	<8%
(Bush's Best) packed from fresh shelled	1/2 cup	70	5.0	16.0	350	3.0	0.0	na	na	0%
(Bush's Best) packed from soaked dry	1/2 cup	70	5.0	16.0	350	3.0	0.0	na	na	0%
(Bush's Best) seasoned w/bacon	1/2 cup	90	7.0	16.0	420	3.0	1.0	na	na	9%
(Green Giant) mature	1/2 cup	90	7.0	18.0	300	4.0	1.0	(tr)	0	8%
(Joan of Arc) mature	1/2 cup	90	7.0	18.0	300	4.0	1.0	(tr)	0	8%
(Luck's) mature, w/pork	1/2 cup	200	11.0	25.0	760	7.0	6.0	(mq)	(mq)	27%
BLACK-EYED PEAS, DRIED										
mature, boiled	1/2 cup	100	6.7	17.9	3	8.3	0.5	0.1	0	4%
mature, boiled	4 oz	132	8.8	23.6	5	10.9	0.6	0.2	0	4%
mature, boiled (A&P)	1 cup	230	15.0	41.0	15	(mq)	1.0	(mq)	0	4%
mature, raw	1 oz	95	6.7	17.0	5	7.7	0.4	0.1	0	4%
mature, raw	1/2 cup	283	19.8	50.4	14	22.7	1.1	0.3	0	3%
BLACK-EYED PEAS, FROZEN										
	10-oz pkg	396	25.5	71.4	17	>4.6 c	2.0	0.5	0	4%
boiled, drained	1/2 cup	112	7.2	20.2	5	>1.3 c	0.6	0.1	0	5%
boiled, drained	4 oz	150	9.6	26.9	6	>1.7 c	0.7	0.2	0	4%
(Freshlike)	3.3 oz	130	9.0	23.0	5	na	1.0	na	na	7%
(Frosty Acres)	3.3 oz	130	9.0	23.0	6	>1.0 c	1.0	(tr)	0	7%
(Seabrook)	3.3 oz	130	9.0	23.0	6	>1.0 c	1.0	(tr)	0	7%
(Southern)	3.5 oz	136	8.9	24.2	20	(mq)	0.7	(tr)	0	5%
(Veg•All)	3.3 oz	130	9.0	23.0	5	na	1.0	na	na	7%
BLINTZ										
(Golden) blueberry	1 blintz	90	2.0	18.0	150	na	1.0	0.0	10	10%
(Golden) cheese, low fat	1 blintz	80	6.0	13.0	135	na	2.0	.5	13	19%
(Golden) cherry	1 blintz	95	3.0	18.0	145	na	1.0	0.0	5	10%
(King Kold) frozen	2.5 oz	113	6.0	18.9	272	(mq)	1.6	(mq)	(mq)	13%
(King Kold) frozen 'No Salt Added'	1.5 oz	96	6.4	18.6	78	(mq)	0.5	(mq)	(mq)	4%
BLOOD PUDDING. See BLOOD SAUSAGE.										
BLOOD SAUSAGE / black pudding / blood pudding										
	1 oz	107	4.1	0.4	193	0	9.8	3.8	34	83%
approx 5 inches x 4 5/8 inches	1/16-inch slice	94	3.7	0.3	170	0	8.6	3.3	30	83%
BLOODY MARY. See ALCOHOLIC BEVERAGES.										
BLOODY MARY MIX. See ALCOHOL-FREE BEVERAGES.										
BLUEBERRY										
trimmed	1 pint	225	2.7	56.8	24	9.3	1.5	na	0	5%
trimmed	1 cup	81	1.0	20.5	9	3.3	0.6	na	0	6%
trimmed	1/2 cup	41	0.5	10.2	5	1.7	0.3	(tr)	0	6%
trimmed	1 oz	16	0.2	4.0	2	.7	0.1	(tr)	0	5%
untrimmed	1 lb	250	3.0	62.8	27	10.2	1.7	(tr)	0	6%
untrimmed	1 pint	226	2.7	56.8	24	9.2	1.5	(tr)	0	5%
BLUEBERRY, CANNED										
in heavy syrup	4 oz	100	0.7	25.0	3	1.7	0.4	(tr)	0	3%
in heavy syrup (A&P)	1/2 cup	110	<1.0	28.0	25	(mq)	<1.0	(tr)	0	<7%
in heavy syrup (S&W)	1/2 cup	111	0.0	30.0	10	(mq)	0.0	0.0	0	0%

Food Name	Serving Size	Calories	Prot. gms	Carbs gms	Sod. mgs	Fiber gms	Fat gms	Sat. Fat gms	Chol. mgs	% Fat Cal.
in heavy syrup, w/liquid	1/2 cup	113	0.8	28.2	4	1.9	0.4	na	0	3%
in water *(Lucky Leaf)*	4 oz	40	0.0	9.0	0	(mq)	0.0	0.0	0	0%
in water *(Musselman's)*	4 oz	40	0.0	9.0	0	(mq)	0.0	0.0	0	0%
BLUEBERRY, FROZEN										
sweetened	10-oz pkg	230	1.1	62.3	3	6.0	0.4	na	0	1%
sweetened	1/2 cup	94	0.5	25.2	2	2.5	0.2	(tr)	0	2%
unsweetened	20-oz pkg	289	2.4	69.0	6	15.3	3.6	na	0	10%
unsweetened	1 cup	79	0.7	18.9	2	4.2	1.0	na	0	10%
unsweetened	1/2 cup	39	0.3	9.4	1	2.5	0.5	(tr)	0	10%
BLUEBERRY NECTAR *(Knudsen & Sons)*	8 oz	135	<1.0	34.0	na	na	0.0	na	na	0%
BLUEBERRY SYRUP										
(Estee) 'Breakfast'	1 tbsp	12	0.0	3.0	10	na	0.0	0.0	0	0%
(Featherweight)	1 tbsp	16	0.0	4.0	35	(tr)	0.0	0.0	0	0%
(Knott's Berry Farm)	1 oz	120	0.0	30.0	0	na	0.0	na	na	0%
(Knott's Berry Farm) 'Light'	1 oz	50	0.0	12.0	0	na	0.0	na	na	0%
(Knudsen & Sons)	1 oz	75	<1.0	19.0	na	na	<1.0	na	na	<10%
BLUEFISH										
dry-heat cooked	3 oz	135	21.8	0.0	65	0	4.6	1.0	65	32%
raw	1 lb	562	90.9	0.0	272	0	19.2	4.2	266	32%
raw	3 oz	105	17.0	0.0	51	0	3.6	0.8	50	32%
raw	1 oz	35	5.7	0.0	17	0	1.2	0.3	17	32%
BLUEGILL										
raw	1 lb	404	88.0	0.0	368	0	3.2	0.6	304	8%
raw	1.7-oz fillet	43	9.3	0.0	38	0	0.3	0.1	32	7%
raw	1 oz	25	5.5	0.0	23	0	0.2	<.1	19	8%
BOAR, WILD										
raw	1 lb	553	97.6	0.0	na	na	15.1	4.5	na	26%
raw	1 oz	34	6.0	0.0	na	na	0.9	0.3	na	25%
roasted	3 oz	136	24.1	0.0	na	na	3.7	1.1	na	26%
roasted, diced	1 cup	224	39.6	0.0	(mq)	0	6.1	1.8	(mq)	26%
BOBWHITE. See QUAIL.										
BOCKWURST										
	1 oz	87	3.8	0.1	313	0	7.8	2.9	17	82%
7 links per lb	1 link	200	8.7	0.3	718	0	17.9	6.6	38	82%
BOK CHOY										
boiled, drained	4 oz	14	1.8	2.0	39	1.8	0.2	<.1	0	11%
boiled, drained, shredded	1/2 cup	10	1.3	1.5	29	1.4	0.1	<.1	0	7%
raw, shredded	1 cup	9	1.0	1.5	46	.7	0.1	0.0	0	8%
raw, shredded	1/2 cup	5	0.5	0.8	23	.4	0.1	tr	0	15%
raw, shredded *(Dole)*	1/2 cup	5	1.0	1.0	23	na	0.1	na	na	10%
raw, trimmed	1 oz	4	0.4	0.6	19	.3	0.1	tr	0	18%
raw, untrimmed	1 lb	52	6.0	8.7	257	4.0	0.8	0.1	0	11%
BOLOGNA. See LUNCHEON MEAT.										
BONITO. See also TUNA, SKIPJACK.										
Caribbean, raw	1 lb	626	106.6	0.0	(mq)	0	19.1	(mq)	(mq)	29%
Caribbean, raw	1 oz	39	6.7	0.0	(mq)	0	1.2	(mq)	(mq)	29%
Japanese, raw	1 lb	585	117.0	1.8	200	0	9.1	(mq)	(mq)	15%
Japanese, raw	1 oz	37	7.3	0.1	12	0	0.6	(mq)	(mq)	15%
BORAGE										
boiled, drained	4 oz	28	2.4	4.0	98	>1.2 c	0.9	(tr)	0	24%
boiled, drained	3.5 oz	25	2.1	3.5	88	>1.1 c	0.8	0.2	0	24%
raw, 1-inch pieces	1/2 cup	9	0.8	1.4	35	>.4 c	0.3	0.1	0	24%
raw, trimmed	1 oz	6	0.5	0.9	23	>.3 c	0.2	(tr)	0	24%
raw, untrimmed	1 lb	76	6.5	11.1	290	>3.3 c	2.5	na	0	24%

Food Name	Serving Size	Calories	Prot. gms	Carbs gms	Sod. mgs	Fiber gms	Fat gms	Sat. Fat gms	Chol. mgs	% Fat Cal.
BORECOLE. See KALE.										
BORLOTTI BEAN. See CRANBERRY BEAN.										
BOSTON CREAM PIE. See CAKE.										
BOTTLE GOURD. See GOURD, BOTTLE.										
BOUILLON. See SOUP.										
BOURBON. See ALCOHOLIC BEVERAGES.										
BOYSENBERRY, CANNED, in heavy syrup	1/2 cup	113	1.3	28.6	4	3.3	0.2	na	0	2%
BOYSENBERRY, FROZEN										
unsweetened, unthawed	10-oz pkg	142	3.1	34.6	3	11.1	0.7	na	0	4%
unsweetened, unthawed	1 cup	66	1.5	16.1	1	5.2	0.3	na	0	4%
BOYSENBERRY DRINK										
boysenberry juice, 'Naturally 100%' (Smucker's)	8 oz	120	0.0	30.0	10	(mq)	0.0	0.0	0	0%
boysenberry nectar (Knudsen & Sons)	8 oz	110	<1.0	33.0	na	na	0.0	na	na	0%
BOYSENBERRY SYRUP										
(Knott's Berry Farm)	1 oz	120	0.0	30.0	0	na	0.0	na	na	0%
(Knott's Berry Farm) 'Light'	1 oz	50	0.0	12.0	0	na	0.0	na	na	0%
BRAMBLE. See RASPBERRY.										
BRANDY. See ALCOHOLIC BEVERAGES.										
BRATWURST										
(Eckrich)	1 link	310	11.0	1.0	820	0	30.0	(mq)	(mq)	85%
(Hickory Farms) 'Brotwurst'	1 oz	90	4.0	1.0	277	0	8.0	(mq)	8	78%
(Hickory Farms) cheddar, 'Cheddy Brots'	1 oz	98	4.0	1.0	259	0	9.0	(mq)	7	80%
(Hillshire Farm) fresh	2 oz	190	7.0	1.0	410	0	17.0	(mq)	(mq)	83%
(Hillshire Farm) 'Fully Cooked'	2 oz	170	7.0	1.0	380	0	16.0	(mq)	(mq)	82%
(Hickory Farms) hot, 'Hot Brots'	1 oz	96	4.0	1.0	269	0	9.0	(mq)	8	80%
(Hillshire Farm) smoked	2 oz	190	8.0	1.0	540	0	17.0	(mq)	(mq)	81%
(Hillshire Farm) spicy	2 oz	180	8.0	1.0	(mq)	0	17.0	(mq)	(mq)	81%
(Kahn's)	1 link	190	7.0	2.0	490	0	17.0	(mq)	(mq)	81%
BRAUNSCHWEIGER										
(Hormel)	1 oz	80	4.0	0.0	322	0	7.0	(mq)	(mq)	80%
(JM)	1 oz	80	3.0	2.0	260	0	6.0	(mq)	(mq)	73%
(Oscar Mayer) 'German Brand'	1 oz	96	4.0	0.5	329	0	8.7	3.0	45	81%
(Oscar Mayer) liver sausage	1 oz	100	4.0	<1.0	230	na	9.0	na	50	80%
(Oscar Mayer) 'Slices'	1 oz	96	3.9	0.6	327	0	8.7	3.2	50	81%
(Oscar Mayer) 'Tube'	1 oz	97	3.9	0.7	301	0	8.7	3.0	47	81%
BRAZIL NUT/butternut/cream nut/paranut										
in shell, unblanched	1 lb	1428	31.2	27.9	3	>5.0 c	144.2	35.2	0	85%
shelled, unblanched, approx 6–8 kernels	1 oz	186	4.1	3.6	tr	>.7 c	18.8	4.6	0	85%
shelled, unblanched, approx 32 kernels	1 cup	919	20.1	17.9	2	8.0	92.7	22.6	0	85%
BREAD. See also BAGEL; BISCUIT; BUN; CROISSANT; ENGLISH MUFFIN; ROLL; MUFFIN/PASTRY, TOASTER.										
APPLE-WALNUT (Arnold)	1 slice	64	2.1	12.6	103	1.3	1.3	na	1	17%
BARBECUE, 'BBQ Loaf' (Colombo Brand)	2 oz	139	7.9	23.5	318	(mq)	1.6	na	na	10%
BRAN										
and oat, 'Light' (Oatmeal Goodness)	1 slice	40	2.0	6.0	90	(mq)	<1.0	na	0	<22%
'Bran'nola' (Brownberry)	1 slice	85	3.9	17.5	137	2.9	1.4	na	tr	13%
'Bran'nola Original' (Arnold)	1 slice	85	3.9	17.5	137	2.9	1.4	na	tr	13%
'Gold'N Bran' (Earth Grains)	1 oz	70	3.0	12.0	150	na	1.0	na	0	13%
honey bran, '1.5-lb loaf' (Pepperidge Farm)	1 slice	90	3.0	18.0	160	1.0	1.0	na	0	10%
original, natural 'Bran'nola' (Oroweat)	1 slice	100	4.0	19.0	160	2.0	1.0	0.0	0	9%
raisin (Brownberry)	1 slice	61	2.2	12.4	108	1.8	1.3	na	0	17%
BROWN										
Boston, w/white corn meal, 3.25 inch diam	1/2-inch slice	95	2.5	20.5	113	>.3 c	0.6	0.0	0	6%
Boston, w/yellow corn meal, 3.25 inch diam	1/2-inch slice	95	2.5	20.5	113	>.3 c	0.6	0.0	0	6%
canned (B&M)	1.6 oz	94	2.0	22.0	320	2.0	0.0	0.0	0	0%

Food Name	Serving Size	Calories	Prot. gms	Carbs gms	Sod. mgs	Fiber gms	Fat gms	Sat. Fat gms	Chol. mgs	% Fat Cal.
canned *(Friends)*	1.6 oz	94	2.0	22.0	320	2.0	0.0	0.0	0	0%
canned, Boston	1 oz	55	1.5	12.3	179	1.3	0.4	0.1	0	6%
canned, 'New England' *(S&W)*	2 slices	76	2.0	17.0	172	(mq)	0.0	0.0	0	0%
canned, raisin *(B&M)*	1.6 oz	92	2.0	21.0	345	2.0	0.0	0.0	0	0%
canned, raisin *(Friends)*	1.6 oz	92	2.0	21.0	345	2.0	0.0	0.0	0	0%
plain *(B&M)*	1/2-inch slice	92	2.0	21.0	345	2.0	0.0	0.0	0	0%
plain *(Friends)*	1/2-inch slice	92	2.0	21.0	345	2.0	0.0	0.0	0	0%
raisin *(B&M)*	1/2-inch slice	94	2.0	22.0	320	2.0	0.0	0.0	0	0%
raisin *(Friends)*	1/2-inch slice	94	2.0	22.0	320	2.0	0.0	0.0	0	0%
BUTTERMILK										
(Grant's Farm)	1-oz slice	70	3.0	12.0	190	na	1.0	na	0	13%
(Oroweat)	1 slice	100	4.0	20.0	210	1.0	1.0	na	0	9%
CRESCENT *(Pillsbury)*	1 serving	100	2.0	11.0	230	na	6.0	1.0	0	51%
CRISP, hard crispbread or toast	4 oz	473	15.6	80.2	278	>.2 c	9.8	2.9	10	19%
EGG	1 oz	81	2.7	13.5	139	na	1.7	0.4	14	19%
FRENCH										
enriched	1 oz	78	2.5	14.7	173	.8	0.9	0.2	0	11%
enriched, 5 inches x 2.5 inches	1 slice	101	3.2	19.4	203	>.1 c	1.0	0.2	1	9%
extra sour *(Colombo Brand)*	2 oz	150	7.7	26.9	311	(mq)	1.3	na	0	8%
extra sour, sliced *(Colombo Brand)*	2 oz	153	7.6	27.2	310	(mq)	1.6	na	0	9%
'Hearth' *(Pepperidge Farm)*	1 oz	75	2.5	14.0	160	.5	1.0	0.0	0	12%
'Parisian' *(DiCarlo)*	1 slice	70	3.0	13.0	180	.7	1.0	na	na	12%
sweet, 'French Stick' *(Colombo Brand)*	2 oz	154	7.2	27.1	331	(mq)	1.9	na	na	11%
twin *(Farm Hearth)*	1 oz	80	3.0	15.0	160	0	1.0	na	0	11%
unenriched, 5 inches x 2.5 inches	1 slice	101	3.2	19.4	203	>.1 c	1.0	0.2	1	9%
GARLIC *(Colombo Brand)*	2 oz	185	6.2	17.3	331	(mq)	10.1	(mq)	na	49%
GRAIN										
'Bran'nola' *(Arnold)*	1 slice	85	3.9	17.4	144	3.0	1.6	na	tr	15%
'Bran'nola Nutty Grains' *(Brownberry)*	1 slice	85	3.9	17.4	144	3.0	1.6	na	tr	15%
honey grain *(Grant's Farm)*	1-oz slice	70	3.0	13.0	170	na	1.0	na	0	12%
honey grain, 'Family Recipe' *(Colonial)*	1-oz slice	70	3.0	14.0	180	na	1.0	na	0	12%
honey grain, 'Family Recipe' *(Kilpatrick's)*	1-oz slice	70	3.0	14.0	180	na	1.0	na	0	12%
honey grain, 'Family Recipe' *(Rainbo)*	1-oz slice	70	3.0	14.0	180	na	1.0	na	0	12%
5-grain, organic *(BreadMill Bakery)*	1 slice	122	6.0	23.0	298	na	1.0	na	0	7%
mixed grain, 'Round Top' *(Roman Meal)*	1 slice	67	2.9	13.2	140	1.2	0.8	na	0	10%
mixed grain, 'Thin Sliced Sandwich' *(Roman Meal)*	1 slice	55	2.4	10.7	114	1.0	0.7	na	0	11%
mixed grain, toasted	1 oz	77	3.1	14.3	150	na	1.2	0.3	0	13%
mixed grain, whole grain	1 oz	71	2.8	13.1	138	2.0	1.1	0.2	0	14%
multi-grain *(Hearty Grains)*	1 slice	80	2.0	15.0	230	1.0	2.0	0.0	0	21%
multi-grain *(Weight Watchers)*	1 slice	40	2.0	9.0	100	(mq)	<1.0	na	0	<17%
9-grain, 'Light' *(Oroweat)*	1 slice	40	2.0	10.0	135	2.0	0.0	na	0	0%
7-grain *(Aunt Hattie's)*	1 slice	100	4.0	17.0	200	na	2.0	na	0	18%
7-grain *(Grant's Farm)*	1-oz slice	60	3.0	13.0	140	na	1.0	na	0	12%
7-grain, 'Hearty Slice' *(Pepperidge Farm)*	2 slices	180	5.0	36.0	340	2.0	2.0	0.0	0	10%
7-grain, 'Light' *(Grant's Farm)*	.75-oz slice	40	2.0	9.0	115	na	<1.0	na	0	<17%
'Sun Grain' *(Roman Meal)*	1 slice	68	3.2	12.3	140	1.7	1.4	na	0	17%
12-grain *(Earth Grains)*	1 oz	70	3.0	13.0	140	na	1.0	na	0	12%
12-grain *(Oroweat)*	1 slice	110	5.0	20.0	210	1.0	2.0	0.0	0	15%
GRANOLA, oat and honey *(Pepperidge Farm)*	1 slice	60	2.0	12.0	105	2.0	2.0	0.0	0	24%
HAWAIIAN *(King's Hawaiian Bread)*	2 oz	180	6.0	30.0	160	2.0	4.0	1.0	20	20%
HEALTH NUT										
(Brownberry)	1 slice	71	2.3	12.4	158	2.5	2.6	(mq)	0	29%
(Oroweat)	1 slice	110	4.0	20.0	200	2.0	2.0	0.0	0	16%

Food Name	Serving Size	Calories	Prot. gms	Carbs gms	Sod. mgs	Fiber gms	Fat gms	Sat. Fat gms	Chol. mgs	% Fat Cal.
HIGH-CALCIUM										
dark	1 oz	69	2.8	13.9	161	na	0.7	0.1	0	9%
light	1 oz	64	2.4	12.5	196	1.4	0.6	0.1	0	8%
HOLLYWOOD										
'Dark' (Hollywood)	1 slice	70	3.0	13.0	160	.8	1.0	na	na	12%
'Light' (Hollywood)	1 slice	70	3.0	13.0	150	.7	1.0	na	na	12%
HONEY NUT, and oat bran (Aunt Hattie's)	1 slice	100	5.0	16.0	180	1.0	na	na	0	0%
HONEY OAT NUT (Earth Grains)	1 oz	80	3.0	14.0	85	na	2.0	na	0	21%
HONEY WHEAT BRAN (Grant's Farm)	1-oz slice	70	3.0	14.0	120	na	1.0	na	0	12%
HONEY WHEATBERRY										
(Earth Grains)	1 oz	70	3.0	12.0	160	na	1.0	na	0	13%
(Oroweat)	1 slice	90	3.0	17.0	180	2.0	1.0	0.0	0	10%
INDIAN FRY, Navajo, 5 inch diam	1 slice	296	6.4	48.0	626	na	8.6	1.7	0	26%
ITALIAN										
'Family' (Wonder)	1 slice	70	2.0	13.0	160	.7	1.0	na	na	13%
'Francisco International' (Arnold)	1-oz slice	72	2.9	14.1	190	.8	1.1	na	0	13%
'Hearth' (Pepperidge Farm)	1 oz	80	2.0	14.0	150	0	1.0	na	0	12%
'Hi-Fibre' (Monk's)	1 slice	70	3.0	13.0	80	1.4	1.0	na	0	12%
light, 'Bakery' (Arnold)	1 slice	45	2.4	9.9	90	2.0	0.5	na	tr	8%
'Light' (Brownberry)	1 slice	44	2.3	9.9	89	2.0	0.5	na	tr	8%
thick sliced, 'Francisco International' (Arnold)	1 slice	66	2.3	13.7	111	.9	0.8	na	0	10%
OAT										
'Bran'nola Country' (Arnold)	1 slice	90	3.7	17.8	166	2.8	2.0	(mq)	tr	17%
'Bran'nola Country' (Brownberry)	1 slice	90	3.7	17.8	166	2.8	2.0	(mq)	tr	17%
country oat, 'Light' (Oroweat)	1 slice	40	2.0	10.0	135	2.0	0.0	na	0	0%
crunchy (Pepperidge Farm)	2 slices	190	8.0	34.0	290	3.0	4.0	1.0	0	18%
split top, 'Family Recipe' (Colonial)	1-oz slice	70	3.0	13.0	140	na	1.0	na	0	12%
split top, 'Family Recipe' (Kilpatrick's)	1-oz slice	70	3.0	13.0	140	na	1.0	na	0	12%
split top, 'Family Recipe' (Rainbo)	1-oz slice	70	3.0	13.0	140	na	1.0	na	0	12%
OAT BRAN										
country oat, natural, 'Bran'nola' (Oroweat)	2 slices	230	8.0	39.0	390	3.0	4.0	1.0	0	16%
honey (Roman Meal)	1 slice	71	3.2	12.7	130	.9	1.2	na	0	15%
honey (Earth Grains)	1 oz	80	3.0	13.0	105	na	1.0	na	0	12%
honey, w/whole wheat, organic (BreadMill Bakery)	1 slice	121	5.0	23.0	315	na	1.0	na	0	7%
honey nut (Roman Meal)	1 slice	72	3.3	12.1	130	1.0	1.6	na	0	19%
organic, 'Light' (BreadMill Bakery)	1 slice	113	4.0	22.0	229	na	1.0	na	0	8%
plain (Awrey's)	1 slice	50	2.0	10.0	130	1.0	0.0	0.0	0	0%
plain (Grant's Farm)	1-oz slice	70	3.0	14.0	140	na	1.0	na	0	12%
plain (Weight Watchers)	1 slice	40	1.0	10.0	100	(mq)	<1.0	na	0	<17%
'Split-Top' (Roman Meal)	1 slice	68	2.9	13.2	140	1.1	0.9	na	0	11%
OATMEAL										
cinnamon (Oatmeal Goodness)	1 slice	90	4.0	15.0	140	1.0	2.0	(mq)	0	19%
country twists (Hearty Grains)	1 slice	80	2.0	15.0	120	1.0	2.0	na	0	21%
light, 'Bakery' (Arnold)	1 slice	44	2.3	9.6	98	1.9	0.6	na	tr	10%
light, 'Light Style' (Pepperidge Farm)	1 slice	45	2.0	9.0	95	1.0	0.0	0.0	0	0%
'1.5 lb loaf' (Pepperidge Farm)	1 slice	90	3.0	17.0	200	1.0	1.0	na	0	10%
plain (Pepperidge Farm)	1 slice	70	2.0	12.0	160	1.0	1.0	na	0	14%
raisin, 'Hearty Grain' (Pillsbury)	1 slice	90	2.0	16.0	210	1.0	2.0	na	0	20%
toasted almond (Grant's Farm)	1-oz slice	80	3.0	14.0	135	na	1.0	na	0	12%
'Very Thin' (Pepperidge Farm)	1 slice	40	1.0	8.0	80	0	1.0	na	0	20%
w/bran (Oatmeal Goodness)	1 slice	90	4.0	15.0	140	1.0	2.0	(mq)	0	19%
w/sunflower seed (Oatmeal Goodness)	1 slice	90	4.0	15.0	140	1.0	2.0	(mq)	0	19%
OATNUT (Oroweat)	1 slice	100	3.0	18.0	200	1.0	2.0	0.0	0	18%

Food Name	Serving Size	Calories	Prot. gms	Carbs gms	Sod. mgs	Fiber gms	Fat gms	Sat. Fat gms	Chol. mgs	% Fat Cal.
PITA										
oat bran *(Sahara)*	1/2 pita	66	2.4	15.3	163	1.8	0.3	na	0	4%
onion, no fats, no oils, pre-sliced, 1.2 oz *(Kangaroo)*	1 pocket	75	4.0	15.0	160	na	0.0	0.0	0	0%
white *(Sahara)*	1/2 pita	79	2.9	15.6	147	(mq)	0.5	na	0	6%
white, enriched	1 oz	78	2.6	15.8	152	.5	0.3	0.1	0	4%
white, enriched	1 pita	165	5.5	33.4	322	1.0	0.7	0.1	0	4%
white, mini *(Sahara)*	1 pita	79	2.9	15.6	147	(mq)	0.5	na	0	6%
white, unenriched	1 oz	78	2.6	15.8	152	.5	0.3	0.1	0	4%
white, unenriched	1 pita	165	5.5	33.4	322	1.0	0.7	0.1	0	4%
whole-wheat	1 oz	75	2.8	15.6	151	2.1	0.7	0.1	0	8%
whole-wheat	1 pita	170	6.3	35.2	340	4.8	1.7	0.3	0	8%
whole-wheat, approx 2 oz *(Sahara)*	1 pita	150	6.0	28.0	320	>.7 c	2.0	(mq)	0	12%
PROTEIN, includes gluten	1 oz	69	3.4	12.4	155	na	0.6	0.1	0	8%
PUMPERNICKEL										
	1 oz	71	2.5	13.5	190	1.7	0.9	0.1	0	11%
'Family' *(Pepperidge Farm)*	1 slice	80	3.0	15.0	230	2.0	1.0	0.0	0	11%
plain *(Arnold)*	1 slice	70	2.7	14.7	198	1.3	0.9	na	0	10%
small, 'Party' *(Pepperidge Farm)*	4 slices	60	2.0	12.0	160	1.0	1.0	0.0	0	14%
toasted	1 oz	78	2.7	14.8	209	na	1.0	0.1	0	11%
toasted	1 slice	80	2.8	15.1	214	na	1.0	0.1	0	11%
RAISIN										
cinnamon *(Arnold)*	1 slice	67	2.1	12.9	86	.8	1.4	na	2	17%
cinnamon *(Brownberry)*	1 slice	66	2.2	12.8	107	.9	1.3	na	tr	16%
cinnamon *(Monk's)*	1 slice	70	3.0	10.0	85	(mq)	2.0	(mq)	0	26%
cinnamon *(Pepperidge Farm)*	1 slice	90	2.0	16.0	100	2.0	2.0	0.0	0	20%
cinnamon swirl *(Pepperidge Farm)*	1 slice	90	2.0	16.0	100	1.0	2.0	0.0	0	20%
orange *(Brownberry)*	1 slice	67	2.3	13.0	83	.8	1.2	na	tr	15%
unenriched	1 oz	84	2.4	16.1	120	na	1.4	0.3	0	15%
walnut *(Brownberry)*	1 slice	68	2.2	11.4	96	2.3	2.7	(mq)	tr	31%
walnut, royal *(Northridge)*	1 slice	90	2.0	16.0	90	na	2.0	na	na	20%
whole wheat, organic *(BreadMill Bakery)*	1 slice	120	5.0	24.0	327	na	1.0	na	0	7%
RICE BRAN										
golden *(Monk's)*	1 slice	70	3.0	14.0	80	1.6	1.0	na	0	12%
honey nut *(Roman Meal)*	1 slice	71	2.6	12.8	127	1.3	1.6	na	0	19%
plain *(Roman Meal)*	1 slice	70	2.8	12.4	132	1.3	1.5	na	0	18%
RYE										
caraway, 'Natural' *(Brownberry)*	1 slice	73	2.8	15.4	185	1.2	0.8	na	0	9%
Dijon *(Pepperidge Farm)*	1 slice	50	2.0	9.0	170	1.0	1.0	0.0	0	17%
Dijon, 'Hearty' *(Pepperidge Farm)*	1 slice	70	3.0	15.0	260	2.0	1.0	na	0	11%
dill *(Arnold)*	1 slice	71	2.8	14.4	187	1.3	1.0	na	0	12%
'Hearty' *(Beefsteak)*	1 slice	70	3.0	13.0	180	.7	1.0	na	na	12%
hearty rye, 'Light' *(Oroweat)*	1 slice	40	2.0	10.0	135	2.0	0.0	na	0	0%
honey cracked *(Grant's Farm)*	1-oz slice	70	3.0	13.0	190	na	1.0	na	0	12%
Jewish, seeded *(Levy's)*	1 slice	76	2.8	15.9	181	1.4	0.9	na	0	10%
Jewish, seedless *(Levy's)*	1 slice	75	2.8	16.0	178	1.3	0.8	na	0	9%
'Mild' *(Beefsteak)*	1 slice	70	3.0	13.0	180	.7	1.0	na	na	12%
'Old Allegheny' *(Braun's)*	1 slice	70	3.0	13.0	180	.7	1.0	na	0	12%
onion *(Beefsteak)*	1 slice	70	3.0	12.0	170	1.0	1.0	na	0	13%
plain *(Weight Watchers)*	1 slice	40	2.0	10.0	100	(mq)	<1.0	na	0	<16%
seeded, 'Family' *(Pepperidge Farm)*	1 slice	80	3.0	16.0	220	2.0	1.0	0.0	0	11%
seedless, 'Family' *(Pepperidge Farm)*	1 slice	80	3.0	16.0	210	2.0	1.0	0.0	0	11%
seedless, 'Natural Thin Sliced' *(Brownberry)*	1 slice	45	1.7	9.8	118	.8	0.6	na	0	11%
small, 'Party' *(Pepperidge Farm)*	4 slices	60	2.0	12.0	250	1.0	1.0	0.0	0	14%
'Soft' *(Beefsteak)*	1 slice	70	3.0	13.0	170	.9	1.0	na	0	12%

Food Name	Serving Size	Calories	Prot. gms	Carbs gms	Sod. mgs	Fiber gms	Fat gms	Sat. Fat gms	Chol. mgs	% Fat Cal.
very thin, light *(Earth Grains)*	1 oz	70	3.0	14.0	230	na	1.0	na	0	12%
wheatberry *(Beefsteak)*	1 slice	70	3.0	13.0	160	1.0	1.0	na	0	12%
SOURDOUGH										
French *(Boudin)*, approx 2-oz slices	2 slices	130	5.0	27.0	297	(mq)	1.0	na	0	7%
'Light' *(Earth Grains)*	.75 oz	40	2.0	9.0	115	na	1.0	0.2	0	17%
'Light' *(Rainbo)*	.75-oz slice	40	2.0	9.0	110	2.0	<1.0	na	0	<17%
plain *(DiCarlo)*	1 slice	70	3.0	12.0	140	.7	1.0	na	0	13%
SUNFLOWER										
and bran *(Monk's)*	1 slice	70	3.0	12.0	80	1.6	1.0	na	0	13%
'Texas Toast' *(Golden Corral)*	1 serving	170	5.0	26.0	230	na	6.0	na	0	30%
whole wheat, organic *(BreadMill Bakery)*	1 slice	129	6.0	21.0	287	na	2.0	na	0	14%
VIENNA										
light, 'Light Style' *(Pepperidge Farm)*	1 slice	45	2.0	10.0	100	1.0	0.0	0.0	0	0%
thick sliced, 'Hearth' *(Pepperidge Farm)*	1 slice	70	2.0	13.0	125	0	1.0	0.0	0	13%
WHEAT										
	1 oz	74	2.6	13.4	150	1.2	1.2	0.3	0	14%
apple honey *(Brownberry)*	1 slice	69	2.3	11.4	148	1.5	1.9	na	0	24%
'Brick Oven' *(Arnold)*	1 slice	57	2.4	10.6	104	1.7	1.5	na	tr	21%
'Butter Top' *(Home Pride)*	1 slice	70	3.0	13.0	140	.8	1.0	na	na	12%
buttertop *(Aunt Hattie's)*	1 slice	70	3.0	13.0	140	na	1.0	na	<5	12%
cracked	1 oz	74	2.5	14.0	153	1.5	1.1	0.3	0	13%
cracked *(Earth Grains)*	1 oz	70	2.0	12.0	180	na	1.0	na	0	14%
cracked *(Pepperidge Farm)*	1 slice	70	2.0	13.0	140	1.0	1.0	na	0	13%
cracked *(Wonder)*	1 slice	70	3.0	13.0	180	.8	1.0	na	na	12%
cracked wheat and honey twists *(Hearty Grains)*	1 serving	80	2.0	14.0	120	1.0	2.0	0.0	0	22%
dark, 'Bran'nola' *(Arnold)*	1 slice	83	4.1	17.6	166	2.8	1.0	na	tr	9%
'Family Recipe' *(Colonial)*	1-oz slice	70	3.0	14.0	150	na	1.0	na	0	12%
'Family Recipe' *(Kilpatrick's)*	1-oz slice	70	3.0	14.0	150	na	1.0	na	0	12%
'Family Recipe' *(Rainbo)*	1-oz slice	70	3.0	14.0	150	na	1.0	na	0	12%
'Family,' 2-lb loaf *(Pepperidge Farm)*	1 slice	70	2.0	13.0	130	2.0	1.0	0.0	0	13%
fat-free, 'Light' *(Wonder)*	1 slice	40	3.0	7.0	120	na	<1.0	na	0	<18%
'Hearth' *(Brownberry)*	1 oz	70	3.1	13.6	150	2.0	1.4	na	0	16%
'Hearty' *(Beefsteak)*	1 slice	70	3.0	11.0	160	1.4	1.0	na	0	14%
hearty, 'Bran'nola' *(Arnold)*	1 slice	88	3.8	17.1	197	2.7	1.9	na	tr	17%
hearty, 'Bran'nola' *(Brownberry)*	1 slice	88	3.8	17.1	197	2.7	1.9	na	tr	17%
honey buttered, split top, 'Family Recipe' *(Colonial)*	1-oz slice	70	3.0	14.0	140	na	1.0	na	0	12%
honey buttered, split top, 'Family Recipe' *(Kilpatrick's)*	1-oz slice	70	3.0	14.0	140	na	1.0	na	0	12%
honey buttered, split top, 'Family Recipe' *(Rainbo)*	1-oz slice	70	3.0	14.0	140	na	1.0	na	0	12%
honey wheatberry *(Arnold)*	1 slice	77	3.1	16.5	143	2.4	1.2	na	tr	12%
'Light' *(Grant's Farm)*	.75-oz slice	40	2.0	9.0	115	na	<1.0	na	0	<17%
'Light' *(Rainbo)*	.75-oz slice	40	2.0	9.0	100	2.0	<1.0	na	0	<17%
light, golden, 'Bakery' *(Arnold)*	1 slice	44	2.3	9.5	86	2.0	0.5	na	tr	9%
'Light Style' *(Pepperidge Farm)*	1 slice	45	2.0	9.0	90	1.0	0.0	0.0	0	0%
'Light 35' *(Earth Grains)*	1 oz	35	2.0	8.0	100	na	<1.0	na	0	<18%
loaf *(Pipin' Hot)*	1-inch slice	70	2.0	12.0	170	na	2.0	0.0	0	24%
multi-grain *(Beefsteak)*	1 slice	70	3.0	11.0	130	1.6	1.0	na	0	14%
'Natural' *(Brownberry)*	1 slice	80	3.0	17.0	183	2.3	1.3	na	0	13%
oatmeal *(Oatmeal Goodness)*	1 slice	90	4.0	15.0	140	1.0	2.0	(mq)	0	19%
oatmeal, 'Light' *(Oatmeal Goodness)*	1 slice	40	2.0	6.0	90	(mq)	<1.0	na	0	<22%
1.5-lb loaf *(Pepperidge Farm)*	1 slice	90	3.0	18.0	190	2.0	2.0	(mq)	0	18%
plain *(Country Grain)*	1 slice	70	3.0	12.0	160	1.3	1.0	na	na	13%
plain *(Fresh & Natural)*	1 slice	70	3.0	13.0	140	1.8	1.0	na	0	12%
plain *(Weight Watchers)*	1 slice	40	2.0	9.0	100	(mq)	<1.0	na	0	<17%
sesame, 'Hearty' *(Pepperidge Farm)*	2 slices	190	7.0	36.0	340	3.0	3.0	1.0	0	14%

Food Name	Serving Size	Calories	Prot. gms	Carbs gms	Sod. mgs	Fiber gms	Fat gms	Sat. Fat gms	Chol. mgs	% Fat Cal.
'7-Grain' *(Home Pride)*	1 slice	70	3.0	12.0	140	.8	1.0	na	na	13%
'Soft' *(Beefsteak)*	1 slice	70	3.0	12.0	160	1.6	1.0	na	0	13%
soft *(Brownberry)*	1 slice	74	2.8	13.1	127	1.0	1.8	na	tr	20%
soft, made w/buttermilk *(Aunt Hattie's)*	1 slice	70	3.0	12.0	130	na	1.0	na	na	13%
sprouted *(Pepperidge Farm)*	1 slice	70	3.0	11.0	100	2.0	2.0	(mq)	0	24%
stone ground *(Grant's Farm)*	1-oz slice	60	3.0	12.0	150	na	1.0	na	0	13%
stone ground, 'Family Recipe' *(Colonial)*	1-oz slice	70	3.0	14.0	150	na	1.0	na	0	12%
stone ground, 'Family Recipe' *(Kilpatrick's)*	1-oz slice	70	3.0	14.0	150	na	1.0	na	0	12%
stone ground, 'Family Recipe' *(Rainbo)*	1-oz slice	70	3.0	14.0	150	na	1.0	na	0	12%
'Stoneground' *(Home Pride)*	1 slice	70	3.0	12.0	140	1.9	1.0	na	0	13%
very thin *(Earth Grains)*	1 oz	70	2.0	13.0	150	na	1.0	na	0	13%
WHEAT GERM	1 oz	74	2.7	13.7	157	na	0.8	0.2	0	10%
WHEATBERRY *(Grant's Farm)*	1-oz slice	70	3.0	13.0	150	na	1.0	na	0	12%
WHITE										
	1 oz	76	2.3	14.0	153	.7	1.0	0.2	0	12%
'Brick Oven' *(Arnold)*	1 slice	61	2.2	11.3	134	.8	1.2	na	tr	17%
'Butter Top' *(Home Pride)*	1 slice	70	3.0	13.0	140	.7	1.0	na	na	12%
buttermilk *(Wonder)*	1 slice	70	2.0	13.0	160	.7	1.0	na	na	13%
buttertop, 'Homestyle' *(Aunt Hattie's)*	1 slice	70	3.0	13.0	140	na	1.0	na	0	12%
'Country White' *(Arnold)*	1 slice	98	3.4	18.6	204	1.0	1.8	na	tr	16%
enriched, 'Country Style' *(Holsum)*	1 slice	70	2.0	14.0	135	na	1.0	na	0	12%
extra fiber, 'Brick Oven' *(Arnold)*	1 slice	55	2.2	12.1	93	2.1	0.8	na	tr	11%
'Hearty Country' *(Pepperidge Farm)*	2 slices	190	7.0	38.0	340	2.0	2.0	1.0	0	9%
'High Fiber' *(Wonder)*	1 slice	40	2.0	6.0	80	2.9	0.0	0.0	0	0%
honey buttered, split top, 'Family Recipe' *(Colonial)*	1-oz slice	80	3.0	14.0	140	na	1.0	na	0	12%
honey buttered, split top, 'Family Recipe' *(Kilpatrick's)*	1-oz slice	80	3.0	14.0	140	na	1.0	na	0	12%
honey buttered, split top, 'Family Recipe' *(Rainbo)*	1-oz slice	80	3.0	14.0	140	na	1.0	na	0	12%
'Large Family,' 2-lb loaf *(Pepperidge Farm)*	1 slice	70	2.0	13.0	150	0	1.0	0.0	0	13%
'Light' *(Grant's Farm)*	.75-oz slice	40	2.0	9.0	115	na	<1.0	na	0	<17%
'Light' *(Rainbo)*	.75-oz slice	40	2.0	9.0	100	2.0	<1.0	0.0	na	<17%
'Light' *(Wonder)*	1 slice	40	3.0	7.0	110	2.0	0.0	0.0	0	0%
'Light Premium' *(Arnold)*	1 slice	42	2.3	9.6	89	2.2	0.5	na	tr	9%
'Light Premium' *(Brownberry)*	1 slice	42	2.3	9.6	89	2.2	0.5	na	tr	9%
'Light 35' *(Earth Grains)*	1 oz	35	2.0	8.0	105	na	<1.0	na	0	<18%
'Natural' *(Brownberry)*	1 slice	59	2.2	11.1	136	.6	1.1	na	tr	16%
old fashioned *(Northridge)*	1 slice	70	2.0	13.0	125	na	1.0	na	na	13%
plain *(Monk's)*	1 slice	60	3.0	10.0	95	(mq)	1.0	na	0	15%
plain *(Weight Watchers)*	1 slice	40	2.0	10.0	100	(mq)	<1.0	na	0	<16%
plain *(Wonder)*	1 slice	70	3.0	13.0	140	.7	1.0	na	na	12%
'Robust' *(Beefsteak)*	1 slice	70	3.0	13.0	140	.7	1.0	na	na	12%
sandwich *(Pepperidge Farm)*	2 slices	130	4.0	24.0	260	0	2.0	0.0	0	14%
special recipe, 'Iron Kids' *(Rainbo)*	1 slice	60	3.0	13.0	140	2.0	1.0	na	0	12%
thin *(Holsum)*	1 slice	70	2.0	14.0	160	na	1.0	na	0	12%
'Thin Sliced' *(Wonder)*	1 slice	50	2.0	10.0	120	.5	1.0	na	0	16%
'Thin Sliced,' 1-lb size *(Pepperidge Farm)*	1 slice	80	2.0	14.0	130	0	2.0	(mq)	0	22%
toasting *(Pepperidge Farm)*	1 slice	90	3.0	17.0	200	1.0	1.0	0.0	0	10%
very thin *(Earth Grains)*	1 oz	80	2.0	14.0	160	na	1.0	na	0	12%
'Very Thin' *(Pepperidge Farm)*	1 slice	40	1.0	8.0	80	0	0.0	0.0	0	0%
white loaf *(Pipin' Hot)*	1-inch slice	70	2.0	12.0	170	na	2.0	0.0	0	24%
w/buttermilk, 'Homestyle' *(Aunt Hattie's)*	1 slice	80	3.0	13.0	140	na	1.0	na	na	12%
WHOLE BRAN, 'Natural' *(Brownberry)*	1 slice	58	2.3	11.7	167	2.1	1.4	na	0	18%
WHOLE WHEAT										
	1 oz	70	2.8	13.1	149	2.0	1.2	0.3	0	15%
'Family' *(Wonder)*	1 slice	70	3.0	13.0	140	.8	1.0	na	na	12%

Food Name	Serving Size	Calories	Prot. gms	Carbs gms	Sod. mgs	Fiber gms	Fat gms	Sat. Fat gms	Chol. mgs	% Fat Cal.
'High Fiber' *(Wonder)*	1 slice	40	2.0	6.0	80	2.9	0.0	0.0	0	0%
'Light' *(Wonder)*	1 slice	40	3.0	7.0	120	2.0	0.0	0.0	0	0%
100% *(Northridge)*	1 slice	60	3.0	11.0	120	2.0	1.0	0.0	0	14%
'100% Stone Ground' *(Monk's)*	1 slice	70	3.0	13.0	110	(mq)	1.0	na	0	12%
100% whole wheat *(Earth Grains)*	1 oz	70	3.0	11.0	150	na	1.0	na	0	14%
'100%' *(Wonder)*	1 slice	70	3.0	12.0	160	1.8	1.0	na	na	13%
plain *(Aunt Hattie's)*	1 slice	90	4.0	14.0	170	na	2.0	na	0	20%
plain *(Daily)*	2-oz slice	140	6.0	26.0	0	(mq)	0.0	0.0	0	0%
'Soft 100%' *(Wonder)*	1 slice	70	4.0	10.0	140	1.8	1.0	na	0	14%
'Stoneground 100%' *(Arnold)*	1 slice	48	2.4	9.9	97	1.6	0.7	na	tr	11%
stoneground, 100% *(Oroweat)*	1 slice	60	3.0	11.0	125	2.0	1.0	0.0	0	14%
'Thin Sliced,' 1-lb loaf *(Pepperidge Farm)*	1 slice	60	2.0	12.0	110	2.0	1.0	na	0	14%
'Very Thin' *(Pepperidge Farm)*	1 slice	35	2.0	7.0	75	0	0.0	0.0	0	0%
BREAD, BROWN AND SERVE										
'Austrian' *(Du Jour)*	1 oz	70	3.0	13.0	140	.6	1.0	na	0	12%
'French' *(Du Jour)*	1 oz	70	3.0	13.0	140	.6	1.0	na	0	12%
'Italian' *(Pepperidge Farm)*	1 oz	80	2.0	14.0	150	0	1.0	na	0	12%
BREAD, QUICK, MIX										
APPLE CINNAMON										
(Pillsbury) mix only, dry	1/12 pkg	140	2.0	30.0	160	na	1.0	0.0	0	7%
(Pillsbury) prepared as directed	1/12 loaf	170	3.0	27.0	200	(mq)	6.0	(mq)	na	31%
(Pillsbury) prepared w/1/4 cup oil, 1/4 cup egg substitute	1/12 loaf	190	2.0	31.0	170	na	6.0	1.0	0	29%
(Pillsbury) prepared w/water, 1/4 cup oil, 1 egg	1/12 loaf	180	2.0	31.0	170	na	6.0	1.0	20	29%
(Pillsbury) prepared w/water, 1/4 cup oil, 1/4 cup egg substitute	1/12 loaf	190	2.0	31.0	170	na	6.0	1.0	0	29%
BANANA										
(Pillsbury) mix only, dry	1/12 pkg	120	2.0	27.0	190	na	1.0	0.0	0	7%
(Pillsbury) prepared w/water, 3 tbsp oil, 1/2 cup egg substitute	1/12 loaf	170	3.0	27.0	210	na	6.0	1.0	0	31%
(Pillsbury) prepared w/water, 3 tbsp oil, and 2 eggs	1/12 loaf	170	3.0	27.0	200	na	5.0	1.0	35	27%
BANANA NUT *(Krusteaz)* prepared as directed	3/4-inch slice	190	3.0	33.0	300	2.0	6.0	na	3	27%
BLUEBERRY NUT										
(Pillsbury) mix only, dry	1/12 pkg	130	2.0	29.0	160	na	1.0	0.0	0	7%
(Pillsbury) prepared as directed	1/12 loaf	150	2.0	26.0	150	(mq)	4.0	(mq)	na	24%
(Pillsbury) prepared w/1/4 cup oil, 1/4 cup egg substitute	1/12 loaf	180	2.0	30.0	170	na	6.0	1.0	0	30%
(Pillsbury) prepared w/water, 1/4 cup oil, 1 egg	1/12 loaf	180	2.0	30.0	160	na	6.0	1.0	20	30%
(Pillsbury) prepared w/water, 1/4 cup oil, 1/4 cup egg substitute	1/12 loaf	180	2.0	30.0	170	na	6.0	1.0	0	30%
CHERRY NUT *(Pillsbury)* prepared as directed	1/12 loaf	180	3.0	29.0	150	(mq)	5.0	(mq)	na	26%
CORNBREAD										
(Aunt Jemima) 'Easy,' prepared as directed	1 piece	196	3.5	32.7	679	1.4	6.3	1.3	13	28%
(Ballard) mix only, dry	1/16 pkg	120	2.0	24.0	560	na	2.0	<1.0	0	15%
(Ballard) prepared as directed	1/8 pan	140	3.0	25.0	570	(mq)	3.0	(mq)	na	19%
(Ballard) prepared w/1 cup milk, 1 egg	1/16 pan	150	4.0	25.0	580	na	3.0	<1.0	30	19%
(Dromedary) mix only, dry	3 tbsp	100	2.0	19.0	280	(mq)	2.0	(mq)	na	18%
(Dromedary) prepared as directed	2-inch square	130	3.0	20.0	480	(mq)	3.0	(mq)	na	23%
(Gold Medal) white, 'Pouch Mix, prepared w/egg and whole milk	1/6 pan	150	4.0	22.0	490	(mq)	5.0	(mq)	(mq)	30%
(Gold Medal) yellow, 'Pouch Mix,' prepared w/egg and whole milk	1/6 pan	150	4.0	23.0	500	(mq)	5.0	(mq)	(mq)	29%
(Krusteaz) honey, prepared as directed	1/16 pan	120	2.0	21.0	230	na	3.0	na	17	23%
(Krusteaz) Southern, prepared as directed	2-inch square	140	3.0	27.0	450	na	3.0	na	8	18%
(Martha White) buttermilk, prepared w/water	1/6 pan	110	2.0	21.0	360	na	2.0	na	0	16%
(Martha White) 'Cotton Pickin' prepared as directed	1/4 pan	170	3.0	31.0	540	(mq)	3.0	(mq)	2	17%

Food Name	Serving Size	Calories	Prot. gms	Carbs gms	Sod. mgs	Fiber gms	Fat gms	Sat. Fat gms	Chol. mgs	% Fat Cal.
(Martha White) 'Cotton Pickin' prepared w/water	1/6 pan	110	2.0	21.0	360	na	2.0	na	0	16%
(Martha White) Mexican, prepared w/2% milk	1/6 pan	140	2.0	24.0	410	na	4.0	na	25	26%
(Martha White) yellow, 'Light Crust,' prepared as directed	2 oz	140	4.0	21.0	400	(mq)	4.0	(mq)	26	27%
(Robin Hood) white, 'Pouch Mix,' prepared w/egg and whole milk	1/6 pan	150	4.0	22.0	490	(mq)	5.0	(mq)	(mq)	30%
CRANBERRY										
(Pillsbury) mix only, dry	1/12 pkg	140	2.0	30.0	150	na	1.0	0.0	0	7%
(Pillsbury) prepared as directed	1/12 loaf	160	2.0	30.0	160	(mq)	4.0	(mq)	na	22%
(Pillsbury) prepared w/water, 2 tbsp oil, 1 egg	1/12 loaf	160	2.0	30.0	150	na	4.0	1.0	20	22%
(Pillsbury) prepared w/water, 2 tbsp oil, 1/4 cup egg substitute	1/12 loaf	170	3.0	30.0	160	na	4.0	1.0	0	21%
DATE										
(Pillsbury) prepared w/water, 1 tbsp oil, 1 egg	1/12 pkg	160	2.0	32.0	150	na	3.0	1.0	0	17%
(Pillsbury) prepared w/water, 1 tbsp oil, 1/4 cup egg substitute	1/12 loaf	160	2.0	32.0	150	na	3.0	1.0	0	17%
DATE NUT										
(Dromedary) mix only, dry	1/12 pkg	166	2.0	26.0	242	(mq)	7.0	(mq)	na	36%
(Dromedary) prepared as directed	1/12 loaf	183	2.0	26.0	248	(mq)	8.0	(mq)	na	39%
GINGERBREAD										
(Betty Crocker) 'Classic' mix only, dry	1/9 pkg	200	2.0	35.0	320	na	6.0	na	0	27%
(Betty Crocker) 'Classic,' prepared w/cholesterol-free egg product	1/9 pan	210	3.0	35.0	330	(mq)	6.0	2.0	0	26%
(Betty Crocker) 'Classic,' prepared w/egg	1/9 pan	220	3.0	35.0	330	(mq)	7.0	2.0	30	29%
(Dromedary) mix only, dry	3 tbsp	100	1.0	19.0	190	(mq)	2.0	(mq)	na	18%
(Pillsbury) mix only, dry	1/9 pkg	180	2.0	32.0	300	na	5.0	1.0	0	25%
(Pillsbury) prepared as directed	3-inch square	190	2.0	36.0	310	(mq)	4.0	(mq)	na	19%
NUT										
(Pillsbury) mix only, dry	1/12 pkg	150	3.0	27.0	180	na	3.0	1.0	0	18%
(Pillsbury) prepared w/water, 2 tbsp oil, 1 egg	1/12 loaf	170	3.0	27.0	190	na	6.0	1.0	20	31%
(Pillsbury) prepared w/water, 2 tbsp oil, 1/4 cup egg substitute	1/12 loaf	170	3.0	28.0	190	na	6.0	1.0	0	30%
OATMEAL RAISIN										
(Pillsbury) mix only, dry	1/12 pkg	140	3.0	30.0	170	na	2.0	0.0	0	12%
(Pillsbury) prepared w/water, 1/4 cup oil, 1 egg	1/12 loaf	190	3.0	30.0	180	na	7.0	1.0	20	32%
(Pillsbury) prepared w/water, 1/4 cup oil, 1/4 cup egg substitute	1/12 loaf	190	3.0	30.0	180	na	7.0	1.0	0	32%
BREAD CRUMBS										
Italian style *(Devonsheer)*	1 oz	104	3.6	21.1	408	.9	1.3	na	0	11%
Italian style *(Progresso)*	2 tbsp	60	2.0	11.0	240	(mq)	<1.0	na	0	<15%
Italian style, whole-wheat *(Jaclyn's)*	.5 oz	28	4.0	13.0	5	(mq)	1.0	na	0	12%
plain	1 cup	427	13.5	78.3	931	4.5	5.8	1.4	0	12%
plain	1 oz	112	3.5	20.6	244	1.2	1.5	0.4	0	12%
plain *(Devonsheer)*	1 oz	108	3.9	21.6	272	.9	1.4	na	0	11%
plain *(Progresso)*	2 tbsp	60	2.0	11.0	110	(mq)	<1.0	na	0	<15%
seasoned	1 cup	440	17.0	84.5	3180	na	3.1	0.9	2	6%
seasoned	1 oz	104	4.0	20.0	751	na	0.7	0.2	1	6%
seasoned *(Contadina)*	1 cup	426	16.5	81.5	2970	.7	3.6	na	na	8%
seasoned *(Contadina)*	1 tbsp	35	1.0	7.0	250	.1	<1.0	na	na	<22%
BREAD DOUGH										
cornbread twists, refrigerated *(Pillsbury)*	1 twist	70	1.0	8.0	150	(mq)	4.0	<1.0	0	50%
French, crusty, refrigerated *(Pillsbury)*	1-inch slice	60	2.0	11.0	120	(mq)	<1.0	0.0	0	<15%
honey walnut, frozen *(Bridgford)*	1 oz	76	3.0	13.8	152	(mq)	0.9	na	0	11%
refrigerated *(Roman Meal)*	1 oz	85	2.3	12.6	199	.6	2.8	0.9	0	30%

Food Name	Serving Size	Calories	Prot. gms	Carbs gms	Sod. mgs	Fiber gms	Fat gms	Sat. Fat gms	Chol. mgs	% Fat Cal.
wheat, refrigerated *(Pipin' Hot)*	1-inch slice	70	0.0	12.0	170	(mq)	2.0	0.0	0	27%
white, frozen *(Bridgford)*	1 oz	76	2.5	13.8	156	(mq)	1.2	na	0	14%
white, frozen *(Rich's)*	2 slices	120	4.0	23.0	300	(mq)	1.0	na	0	8%
white, refrigerated *(Pipin' Hot)*	1-inch slice	70	3.0	12.0	170	(mq)	2.0	0.0	0	23%
BREADFRUIT										
raw	1 cup	227	2.3	59.7	4	10.8	0.5	na	0	2%
raw	1/4 small	99	1.0	26.0	2	4.7	0.2	na	0	2%
trimmed	1/2 cup	114	1.2	29.8	2	5.4	0.3	(tr)	0	2%
trimmed	1 oz	29	0.3	7.7	1	1.4	0.1	(tr)	0	3%
untrimmed	1 lb	365	3.8	96.0	6	>5.2 c	0.8	(tr)	0	2%
BREADFRUIT SEEDS										
boiled	1 oz	48	1.5	9.1	7	>.5 c	0.7	0.2	0	13%
Pacific, in soft shell, boiled	1 lb	274	8.7	52.3	na	>2.9 c	3.8	1.0	0	12%
Pacific, shelled, boiled	1 oz	48	1.5	9.1	na	>.5 c	0.7	0.2	0	13%
raw	1 oz	54	2.1	8.3	7	>.5 c	1.6	0.4	0	26%
roasted	1 oz	59	1.8	11.4	8	>.6 c	0.8	0.2	0	12%
shelled, raw	1 oz	54	2.1	8.3	na	>.5 c	1.6	0.4	0	26%
South American, in shell, raw	1 lb	590	22.8	90.2	na	>5.2 c	17.2	4.7	0	26%
South American, shelled, roasted	1 oz	59	1.8	11.4	na	>.6 c	0.8	0.2	0	12%
BREADNUT TREE SEEDS /Jamaican breadnut										
dried	1 oz	104	2.5	22.5	15	4.2	0.5	0.1	0	4%
raw	1 oz	62	1.7	13.1	9	>.7 c	0.3	0.1	0	4%
BREADSTICK										
garlic, Italian style *(Barbara's Bakery)*	1 oz	120	4.0	18.0	170	na	3.0	na	0	24%
onion *(Stella D'oro)*	1 stick	40	1.2	6.1	(mq)	(mq)	1.3	(mq)	na	29%
pizza *(Fattorie & Pandea)*	3 stick s	59	2.0	10.0	100	(mq)	1.0	na	0	16%
pizza *(Stella D'oro)*	1 stick	43	1.3	6.9	(mq)	(mq)	1.2	(mq)	na	25%
plain *(Stella D'oro)*	1 stick	41	1.0	6.5	(mq)	(mq)	1.2	(mq)	na	27%
plain, dietetic *(Stella D'oro)*	1 stick	46	1.3	7.3	10	(mq)	1.4	(mq)	na	27%
regular *(Barbara's Bakery)*	1 oz	120	4.0	18.0	170	na	3.0	na	0	24%
sesame *(Fattorie & Pandea)*	3 sticks	65	2.0	10.0	100	(mq)	2.0	(mq)	0	27%
sesame *(Stella D'oro)*	1 stick	51	1.4	6.3	(mq)	(mq)	2.2	(mq)	na	39%
sesame, dietetic *(Stella D'oro)*	1 stick	49	1.3	6.1	10	(mq)	2.1	(mq)	na	39%
sesame, Italian style *(Barbara's Bakery)*	1 oz	120	4.0	18.0	170	na	3.0	na	0	24%
soft, refrigerated *(Pillsbury)*	1 stick	100	3.0	17.0	230	(mq)	2.0	<1.0	0	18%
soft, refrigerated *(Roman Meal)*	1 stick	117	3.1	17.4	274	.8	3.9	1.2	0	30%
wheat *(Stella D'oro)*	1 stick	42	1.3	6.1	(mq)	(mq)	1.4	(mq)	na	30%
whole wheat *(Fattorie & Pandea)*	3 sticks	57	2.0	10.0	100	(mq)	1.0	na	0	16%
BREAKFAST BAR. See SNACK BAR.										
BREAKFAST DRINK MIX, INSTANT										
CHOCOLATE FLAVOR										
(Carnation) 'Instant Breakfast' dry mix	1 pouch	130	6.0	24.0	160	.2	2.0	0.7	3	13%
(Carnation) 'Instant Breakfast' dry mix, no sugar added	1 pouch	70	4.0	12.0	90	1.0	1.0	0.5	<5	23%
(Pillsbury) 'Instant Breakfast' from variety pack, dry mix	1/10 pkg	130	6.0	25.0	135	na	0.0	0.0	0	0%
(Pillsbury) 'Instant Breakfast' from variety pack, prepared w/ 8 oz 2% milk	1 cup	250	14.0	37.0	250	na	5.0	3.0	20	18%
(Pillsbury) 'Instant Breakfast' from variety pack, prepared w/ 8 oz whole milk	1 cup	290	14.0	38.0	310	(mq)	9.0	(mq)	(mq)	28%
CHOCOLATE MALT FLAVOR										
(Carnation) 'Instant Breakfast' dry mix	1 pouch	130	6.0	24.0	160	.2	2.0	0.7	3	13%
(Carnation) 'Instant Breakfast' dry mix, no sugar added	1 pouch	70	6.0	8.0	135	.2	2.0	0.8	2	24%
(Pillsbury) 'Instant Breakfast' dry mix	1 pouch	130	6.0	26.0	190	na	0.0	0.0	0	0%
COFFEE FLAVOR										
(Carnation) 'Instant Breakfast' dry mix	1 pouch	130	6.0	25.0	150	.1	0.2	0.1	3	1%

Food Name	Serving Size	Calories	Prot. gms	Carbs gms	Sod. mgs	Fiber gms	Fat gms	Sat. Fat gms	Chol. mgs	% Fat Cal.
VANILLA FLAVOR										
(Carnation) 'Instant Breakfast' dry mix	1 pouch	130	6.0	25.0	135	.1	0.2	0.1	3	1%
(Carnation) 'Instant Breakfast' dry mix, no sugar added	1 pouch	70	6.0	10.0	120	.5	0.0	0.1	3	0%
(Pillsbury) 'Instant Breakfast' dry mix	1 pouch	140	6.0	29.0	210	(mq)	0.0	0.0	na	0%
(Pillsbury) 'Instant Breakfast' prepared w/whole milk	1 cup	300	14.0	41.0	330	na	9.0	(mq)	(mq)	27%
(Pillsbury) 'Instant Breakfast' from variety pack, dry mix	1/10 pkg	130	6.0	28.0	100	na	0.0	0.0	0	0%
(Pillsbury) 'Instant Breakfast' from variety pack, prepared w/ 8 oz 2% milk	1 cup	260	14.0	40.0	220	na	5.0	2.0	20	17%
BREAKFAST JUICE. See also individual listings.										
(Health Valley)	1/2 cup	26	3.0	5.0	24	3.2	0.0	0.0	0	0%
(Knudsen & Sons) 'Natural'	8 oz	90	2.0	21.0	na	na	0.0	na	na	0%
(Smucker's) orange banana, 'Naturally 100%'	8 oz	120	0.0	30.0	10	(mq)	0.0	0.0	0	0%
BREAKFAST STRIPS. See also BACON; BACON, ALTERNATIVE.										
beef, cured, cooked	6 oz	763	53.2	2.4	3830	0	58.5	24.4	202	70%
beef, cured, cooked	3 slices	153	10.6	0.5	766	0	11.7	4.9	40	70%
beef, cured, raw	3 slices	276	8.5	0.5	649	0	26.4	10.9	56	87%
beef, cured, unheated	3 slices	276	8.5	0.5	649	0	26.4	10.9	56	87%
BREATH MINT. See CANDY, HARD.										
BROAD BEAN										
boiled, drained	4 oz	64	5.4	11.5	47	3.1	0.6	0.2	0	7%
immature, boiled, drained	100 gm	56	4.8	10.1	41	>1.9 c	0.5	0.1	0	7%
immature, raw	1 cup	78	6.1	12.7	54	4.6	0.7	0.2	0	8%
mature, boiled	1/2 cup	94	6.5	16.7	4	4.6	0.3	0.1	0	3%
mature, raw	1/2 cup	256	19.6	43.7	10	18.8	1.1	0.2	0	4%
raw, trimmed	1 oz	20	1.6	3.3	14	1.5	0.2	<.1	0	8%
raw, untrimmed	1 lb	317	24.6	51.5	220	24.0	2.6	0.6	0	7%
BROAD BEAN, DRIED										
mature, boiled	1/2 cup	93	6.5	16.7	4	4.3	0.3	0.1	0	3%
mature, boiled	4 oz	125	8.6	22.3	6	5.8	0.5	0.1	0	4%
mature, raw	1/2 cup	256	19.6	43.7	9	10.9	1.2	0.2	0	4%
mature, raw	1 oz	97	7.4	16.5	4	4.1	0.4	0.1	0	4%
BROCCOLI										
boiled, drained	4 oz	32	3.4	5.7	29	2.9	0.4	<.1	0	9%
boiled, drained, chopped	1/2 cup	22	2.3	4.0	20	2.0	0.3	0.0	0	10%
florets, raw, chopped	1/2 cup	12	1.3	2.3	12	>.5 c	0.2	0.0	0	11%
fresh (Dole)	1 med spear	40	5.0	4.0	75	5.0	1.0	na	na	20%
leaves, raw, chopped	1/2 cup	12	1.3	2.3	12	>.5 c	0.2	0.0	0	11%
raw, chopped	1/2 cup	12	1.3	2.3	12	1.2	0.2	0.0	0	11%
raw, trimmed	1 oz	8	0.8	1.5	8	.8	0.1	<.1	0	9%
raw, untrimmed	1 lb	77	8.3	14.5	73	7.7	1.0	0.2	0	9%
BROCCOLI, FROZEN. See also BROCCOLI DISHES, FROZEN; BROCCOLI ENTRÉE, FROZEN.										
chopped (A&P)	3.3 oz	25	3.0	5.0	25	(mq)	<1.0	(tr)	0	<22%
chopped (Birds Eye)	3.3 oz	25	3.0	5.0	15	3.0	0.0	0.0	0	0%
chopped (Finast)	3.3 oz	25	3.0	5.0	20	(mq)	0.0	0.0	0	0%
chopped (Frosty Acres)	3.3 oz	25	3.0	5.0	18	>1.0 c	0.0	0.0	0	0%
chopped (Seabrook)	3.3 oz	25	3.0	5.0	18	>1.0 c	0.0	0.0	0	0%
chopped (Southern)	3.5 oz	28	2.9	4.4	25	(mq)	0.3	(tr)	0	9%
chopped, boiled, drained	4 oz	32	3.5	6.1	27	2.5	0.1	<.1	0	2%
chopped, boiled, drained	1/2 cup	26	2.8	4.9	22	2.8	0.1	0.0	0	3%
chopped, unprepared	10-oz pkg	74	8.0	13.6	68	8.5	0.8	0.1	0	8%
cuts (A&P)	3.3 oz	25	3.0	5.0	25	(mq)	<1.0	(tr)	0	<22%
cuts (Birds Eye)	3.2 oz	25	3.0	5.0	25	3.0	0.0	na	0	0%
cuts (Frosty Acres)	3.3 oz	25	3.0	5.0	50	>1.0 c	0.0	0.0	0	0%
cuts (Seabrook)	3.3 oz	25	3.0	5.0	50	>1.0 c	0.0	0.0	0	0%

Food Name	Serving Size	Calories	Prot. gms	Carbs gms	Sod. mgs	Fiber gms	Fat gms	Sat. Fat gms	Chol. mgs	% Fat Cal
cuts, 'Harvest Fresh' (Green Giant)	1/2 cup	16	2.0	3.0	95	2.0	0.0	0.0	0	0%
cuts, 'Plain Polybag' (Green Giant)	1/2 cup	18	2.0	5.0	25	4.0	0.0	0.0	0	0%
cuts, 'Portion Pack' (Birds Eye)	3 oz	20	3.0	4.0	20	2.0	0.0	na	0	0%
cuts, 'Singles' (Stokely)	3 oz	25	3.0	5.0	15	(mq)	1.0	(tr)	0	22%
florets (Frosty Acres)	3.3 oz	30	3.0	5.0	14	>1.0 c	0.0	0.0	0	0%
florets, 'Deluxe' (Birds Eye)	3.3 oz	25	3.0	5.0	20	3.0	0.0	na	0	0%
spears (A&P)	3.3 oz	25	3.0	5.0	20	(mq)	<1.0	(tr)	0	<22%
spears (Birds Eye)	3.3 oz	25	3.0	5.0	20	3.0	0.0	na	0	0%
spears (Frosty Acres)	3.3 oz	25	3.0	5.0	20	>1.0 c	0.0	0.0	0	0%
spears (Seabrook)	3.3 oz	25	3.0	5.0	20	>1.0 c	0.0	0.0	0	0%
spears (Southern)	3.5 oz	30	3.0	4.8	30	(mq)	0.2	(tr)	0	6%
spears, baby (Seabrook)	3.3 oz	30	3.0	5.0	14	>1.0 c	0.0	0.0	0	0%
spears, baby, 'Deluxe' (Birds Eye)	3.3 oz	30	3.0	5.0	15	3.0	0.0	0.0	0	0%
spears, boiled, drained	4 oz	32	3.5	6.1	27	2.5	0.1	<.1	0	2%
spears, boiled, drained	10-oz pkg	70	7.8	13.4	60	7.5	0.3	0.1	0	3%
spears, boiled, drained	1/2 cup	26	2.8	4.9	22	2.7	0.1	0.0	0	3%
spears, 'Harvest Fresh' (Green Giant)	1/2 cup	20	2.0	4.0	115	2.0	0.0	0.0	0	0%
spears, mini, 2 1/2 inch x 1/4 inch, approx .6 oz (Green Giant)	1/5 pkg	18	2.0	5.0	25	3.0	0.0	0.0	0	0%
spears, unprepared	10-oz pkg	82	8.7	15.2	48	8.5	1.0	0.2	0	9%
spears, whole, 'Farm Fresh' (Birds Eye)	4 oz	30	4.0	6.0	25	3.0	0.0	0.0	0	0%
spears and florets, 'Deluxe' (Birds Eye)	3.3 oz	25	3.0	5.0	20	3.0	0.0	0.0	0	0%
BROCCOLI DISHES, FROZEN										
cuts, in butter sauce, 'One Serving' (Green Giant)	4.5 oz	45	3.0	7.0	420	3.0	2.0	<1.0	5	31%
cuts, in cheese sauce, (Finast)	3.3 oz	45	3.0	6.0	310	(mq)	0.0	0.0	0	0%
cuts, in cheese sauce, 'One Serving' (Green Giant)	5 oz	80	4.0	13.0	700	2.0	2.0	<1.0	5	21%
cuts, in cheese sauce, 'Singles' (Stokely)	4 oz	80	5.0	7.0	200	(mq)	4.0	(mq)	15	43%
fanfare, 'Valley Combinations' (Green Giant)	1/2 cup	80	3.0	14.0	340	3.0	2.0	0.0	0	21%
in cheese flavored sauce (Green Giant)	1/2 cup	60	3.0	9.0	530	2.0	2.0	<1.0	2	27%
in cheese sauce, 'Family Side Dishes' (Freezer Queen)	4.5 oz	48	2.0	8.0	280	(mq)	1.0	na	na	18%
spears, 'Butter Sauce' (Green Giant)	1/2 cup	40	2.0	6.0	350	2.0	2.0	<1.0	5	36%
spears, 'Butter Sauce Combinations' (Birds Eye)	3.3 oz	45	2.0	5.0	320	2.0	2.0	na	5	39%
w/baby carrots and water chestnuts, 'Farm Fresh' (Birds Eye)	4 oz	45	2.0	10.0	35	3.0	0.0	na	0	0%
w/cauliflower (A&P)	3.2 oz	25	2.0	4.0	20	(mq)	<1.0	(tr)	0	<27%
w/cauliflower, 'Valley Combinations' medley (Green Giant)	1/2 cup	30	2.0	10.0	80	3.0	1.0	(tr)	0	16%
w/cauliflower, 'Singles' (Stokely)	3 oz	20	2.0	4.0	15	(mq)	1.0	0.0	0	27%
w/cauliflower, 'Swiss Mix' (Frosty Acres)	3 oz	25	2.0	5.0	36	>1.0 c	0.0	0.0	0	0%
w/red peppers, 'Select' (Green Giant)	1/2 cup	25	2.0	4.0	15	2.0	0.0	0.0	0	0%
w/whole baby carrots and chestnuts, 'Singles' (Stokely)	3 oz	30	2.0	6.0	22	(mq)	1.0	0.0	0	22%
BROCCOLI ENTRÉE, FROZEN										
and baked potato wedges w/cheese sauce, 9.5-oz pkg (Healthy Choice)	1 serving	240	8.0	41.0	510	na	5.0	2.0	15	19%
au gratin w/rice, 'For One' (Birds Eye)	5.75 oz	180	6.0	27.0	430	1.0	6.0	na	5	29%
in pastry, w/cheese (Pepperidge Farm)	1 pastry	230	5.0	18.0	380	(mq)	16.0	(mq)	(mq)	61%
pot pie w/cheddar cheese, organic (Amy's Kitchen)	8 oz	390	10.0	46.0	500	3.0	18.0	na	na	42%
BROTH. See SOUP.										
BROWN BREAD. See BREAD.										
BRUSSELS SPROUTS										
boiled, drained	4 oz	44	2.9	9.8	24	4.9	0.6	0.1	0	10%
boiled, drained	1/2 cup	30	2.0	6.8	16	3.3	0.4	0.1	0	9%
boiled, drained	1 sprout	8	0.5	1.8	4	.9	0.1	0.0	0	9%
fresh (Dole)	1/2 cup	19	1.0	4.0	11	2.0	0.1	na	na	4%

Food Name	Serving Size	Calories	Prot. gms	Carbs gms	Sod. mgs	Fiber gms	Fat gms	Sat. Fat gms	Chol. mgs	% Fat Cal.
'Plain Polybag' (Green Giant)	1/2 cup	25	2.0	6.0	10	2.0	0.0	0.0	0	0%
raw	1/2 cup	19	1.5	3.9	11	1.9	0.1	0.0	0	4%
raw	1 sprout	8	0.6	1.7	5	.8	0.1	0.0	0	9%
raw, trimmed	1 oz	12	1.0	2.5	7	>.4 c	0.1	<.1	0	6%
raw, untrimmed	1 lb	174	13.8	36.6	101	>6.2 c	1.2	0.3	0	5%
BRUSSELS SPROUTS, FROZEN										
boiled, drained	4 oz	48	4.1	9.4	26	2.0	0.4	0.1	0	6%
boiled, drained	1/2 cup	33	2.8	6.5	18	>1.1 c	0.3	0.1	0	7%
(A&P)	3.3 oz	35	3.0	7.0	15	(mq)	<1.0	(tr)	0	<18%
(Birds Eye)	3.3 oz	35	3.0	7.0	15	3.0	0.0	0.0	0	0%
(Birds Eye) baby, 'Cheese Sauce Combinations'	4.5 oz	130	6.0	12.0	500	2.0	7.0	na	5	47%
(Frosty Acres)	3.3 oz	35	3.0	7.0	12	>1.0 c	0.0	0.0	0	0%
(Green Giant) in butter sauce	1/2 cup	40	3.0	8.0	280	4.0	1.0	<1.0	5	17%
(Seabrook)	3.3 oz	35	3.0	7.0	12	>1.0 c	0.0	0.0	0	0%
(Seabrook) baby	3.3 oz	40	4.0	7.0	5	>1.0 c	0.0	0.0	0	0%
(Southern)	3.5 oz	37	3.2	7.5	20	(mq)	0.0	0.0	0	0%
(Stokely) in butter sauce, 'Singles'	4 oz	50	4.0	10.0	325	(mq)	1.0	na	5	14%
(Stokely) 'Singles'	3 oz	35	4.0	7.0	10	(mq)	0.0	0.0	0	0%
BUBBLE GUM. See CANDY.										
BUCKWHEAT										
whole-grain	1/2 cup	292	11.3	60.8	1	8.5	2.9	0.6	0	8%
whole-grain	1 oz	97	3.8	20.3	<1	(mq)	1.0	0.2	0	9%
BUCKWHEAT FLOUR										
whole-grain	1 cup	402	15.1	84.7	na	(mq)	3.7	0.8	0	8%
whole-grain	1 oz	95	3.6	20.0	na	(mq)	0.9	0.2	0	8%
whole-grain (Arrowhead Mills)	2 oz	190	7.0	41.0	0	7.1	1.0	na	0	5%
whole-groat	1/2 cup	201	7.6	42.4	7	6.0	1.9	0.4	0	8%
BUCKWHEAT GROATS/kasha										
brown (Arrowhead Mills)	2 oz	190	7.0	41.0	1	7.1	1.0	na	0	5%
roasted, cooked	1/2 cup	91	3.3	19.7	4	>.5 c	0.6	0.1	0	6%
roasted, cooked	4 oz	104	3.8	22.6	5	>.6 c	0.7	0.1	0	6%
roasted, dry	1/2 cup	284	9.6	61.5	9	>1.4 c	2.2	0.5	0	7%
roasted, dry	1 oz	98	3.3	21.2	3	>.5 c	0.8	0.2	0	7%
white (Arrowhead Mills)	2 oz	190	7.0	41.0	1	7.1	1.0	na	0	5%
BUFFALO, AMERICAN/bison										
raw	1 lb	494	98.1	0.0	245	na	8.4	3.1	281	16%
raw	1 oz	31	6.1	0.0	15	0	0.5	0.2	18	16%
roasted	4 oz	162	32.3	0.0	65	0	2.7	1.0	93	16%
roasted, diced	1 cup	200	39.8	0.0	80	0	3.4	1.3	115	16%
roasted, yield from 1 lb raw	12 oz	487	96.8	0.0	193	0	8.2	3.1	279	16%
BULGUR. See also TABBOULEH MIX.										
cooked	4 oz	94	3.5	21.1	6	5.1	0.3	0.1	0	3%
cooked	1/2 cup	76	2.8	16.9	5	4.1	0.2	0.0	0	2%
dry	1/2 cup	239	8.6	53.1	12	12.8	0.9	0.2	0	3%
dry	1 oz	97	3.5	21.5	5	5.2	0.4	<.1	0	4%
BULLOCK'S HEART. See CUSTARD APPLE.										
BUN. See also BISCUIT, CROISSANT, ENGLISH MUFFIN, ROLL.										
brown and serve, partially baked	2.5-inch roll	85	2.3	14.2	146	>.1 c	2.0	0.5	2	21%
brown and serve, partially baked, unbrowned	2.5-inch roll	78	2.0	13.2	133	>.1 c	1.8	0.4	2	21%
enriched, browned	2.5-inch roll	85	2.3	14.2	146	>.1 c	2.0	0.5	2	21%
enriched, unbrowned	2.5-inch roll	84	2.2	14.2	144	>.1 c	1.9	0.5	2	21%
hard, enriched, ready to cook	3.75-inch roll	156	4.9	29.7	313	>.1 c	1.6	0.4	2	9%
hard, enriched, ready to cook	2.5-inch roll	78	2.5	14.9	156	>.1 c	0.8	0.2	1	9%
hard, unenriched, ready to cook	3.75-inch roll	156	4.9	29.7	313	>.1 c	1.6	0.4	2	9%

Food Name	Serving Size	Calories	Prot. gms	Carbs gms	Sod. mgs	Fiber gms	Fat gms	Sat. Fat gms	Chol. mgs	% Fat Cal.
hard, unenriched, ready to cook	2.5-inch roll	78	2.5	14.9	156	>.1 c	0.8	0.2	1	9%
Kaiser, 'Big' (Holsum)	1 bun	200	5.0	38.0	320	na	3.0	na	0	14%
sesame seed, 'Big BBQ Buns' (Holsum)	1 bun	200	5.0	38.0	320	na	3.0	na	0	14%
'Sof-Buns' (Holsum)	1 bun	120	3.0	23.0	190	na	2.0	na	0	15%
BUN, FRANKFURTER										
Dijon (Pepperidge Farm)	1 bun	160	5.0	23.0	230	2.0	5.0	1.0	0	29%
'Light' (Wonder)	1 bun	80	5.0	13.0	210	4.0	1.0	na	na	11%
'New England Style' (Arnold)	1 bun	108	3.7	20.9	178	1.4	2.0	(mq)	0	16%
mixed grain	1 bun	113	4.1	19.2	197	1.9	2.6	0.6	0	20%
oat bran (Awrey's)	1 bun	110	4.0	20.0	210	1.0	2.0	0.0	0	16%
'Original' (Roman Meal)	1 bun	104	4.3	19.5	210	1.8	1.9	(mq)	0	15%
plain	1 bun	123	3.7	21.6	241	na	2.2	0.5	0	16%
plain (Arnold)	1 bun	100	3.2	19.6	162	1.2	1.8	(mq)	0	15%
plain (Country Grain)	1 bun	100	4.0	18.0	230	.9	1.0	na	na	9%
plain (Pepperidge Farm)	1 bun	140	5.0	24.0	270	.5	3.0	1.0	0	19%
plain (Wonder)	1 bun	80	2.0	14.0	150	.6	1.0	na	na	12%
potato (Aunt Hattie's)	1 bun	150	5.0	23.0	260	na	4.0	na	0	24%
reduced calorie	1 bun	84	3.6	18.1	190	2.7	0.9	0.1	0	9%
reduced calorie	1 oz	56	2.3	11.9	125	1.8	0.6	0.1	0	9%
whole grain (Roman Meal)	1 bun	120	4.0	19.0	210	na	3.0	na	0	23%
BUN, HAMBURGER										
'Light' (Wonder)	1 bun	80	5.0	13.0	210	4.0	1.0	na	na	11%
mixed grain	1 bun	113	4.1	19.2	197	1.9	2.6	0.6	0	20%
mixed grain	1 oz	75	2.7	12.6	130	1.2	1.7	0.4	0	20%
'Original' (Roman Meal)	1 bun	113	4.7	21.1	228	2.0	1.9	(mq)	0	14%
plain	1 bun	123	3.7	21.6	241	na	2.2	0.5	0	16%
plain	1 oz	81	2.4	14.3	159	na	1.5	0.3	0	17%
plain (Arnold)	1 bun	115	4.3	22.0	223	1.8	2.2	(mq)	0	16%
plain (Pepperidge Farm)	1 bun	130	5.0	22.0	240	.5	2.0	1.0	0	14%
plain (Wonder)	1 bun	120	4.0	21.0	230	.9	2.0	(mq)	na	15%
potato (Aunt Hattie's)	1 bun	150	5.0	23.0	260	na	4.0	na	0	24%
reduced calorie	1 bun	84	3.6	18.1	190	2.7	0.9	0.1	0	9%
reduced calorie	1 oz	56	2.3	11.9	125	1.8	0.6	0.1	0	9%
whole grain (Roman Meal)	1 bun	130	4.0	20.0	230	na	3.0	na	0	22%
BUN, SWEET										
apple honey, multi pak, 1.5 oz (Break Cake)	1 bun	170	2.0	20.0	90	na	10.0	2.7	0	51%
cheese-topped (Entenmann's)	1 bun	240	5.0	29.0	240	na	12.0	na	na	44%
cinnamon (Entenmann's)	1 bun	230	4.0	31.0	200	na	10.0	na	na	39%
cinnamon, frozen 'Ever Fresh' 2.5 oz (Rich's)	1 bun	293	4.0	38.0	(mq)	(mq)	14.6	(mq)	na	44%
cinnamon, frozen '2/pkg' (Pepperidge Farm)	1 bun	280	4.0	34.0	190	(mq)	14.0	(mq)	na	45%
cinnamon, homestyle (Awrey's)	1 bun	240	4.0	40.0	200	1.0	7.0	1.0	5	26%
cinnamon, iced, refrigerated (Hungry Jack)	2 buns	290	3.0	37.0	570	(mq)	14.0	(mq)	na	44%
cinnamon swirl 'Grande' (Awrey's)	1 bun	340	4.0	46.0	370	1.0	16.0	3.0	10	42%
honey (Aunt Fanny's)	3 oz	360	4.0	42.0	150	na	30.0	na	10	60%
honey (Break Cake) 3 oz	1 bun	420	4.0	38.0	160	na	28.0	7.8	0	60%
honey, apple bear (Aunt Fanny's)	4 oz	460	6.0	50.0	220	na	26.0	na	5	51%
honey, birdie, jelly-filled (Aunt Fanny's)	4 oz	450	6.0	53.0	210	na	24.0	na	5	48%
honey, bogie, creme-filled (Aunt Fanny's)	4 oz	460	6.0	49.0	200	na	27.0	na	10	53%
honey, frozen, mini, 'Ever Fresh', 1.36 oz (Rich's)	1 bun	133	1.8	17.5	(mq)	(mq)	6.6	(mq)	na	44%
honey, lemon bear (Aunt Fanny's)	4 oz	440	5.0	52.0	200	na	23.0	na	5	48%
honey, multi pak (Break Cake)	1 bun	380	3.0	34.0	150	na	24.0	7.2	0	59%
honey, snow bear (Aunt Fanny's)	4 oz	480	6.0	60.0	220	na	24.0	na	5	45%
honey glazed (Tastykake)	3.25 oz	362	5.9	42.3	219	3.6	20.4	4.3	2	49%
honey glazed (Hostess)	1 bun	360	5.0	38.0	230	.8	21.0	10.0	15	52%

Food Name	Serving Size	Calories	Prot. gms	Carbs gms	Sod. mgs	Fiber gms	Fat gms	Sat. Fat gms	Chol. mgs	% Fat Cal
honey iced *(Tastykake)*	3.25 oz	348	5.0	50.0	254	1.5	14.9	3.3	2	38%
honey iced *(Hostess)*	1 bun	430	5.0	55.0	240	1.7	22.0	10.0	20	45%
pecan-caramel swirl *(Hostess)*	1 bun	240	3.0	23.0	160	1.8	15.0	7.0	10	57%
BURBOT										
dry-heat cooked	3 oz	98	21.0	0.0	105	0	0.9	0.2	65	9%
raw	1 lb	407	87.6	0.0	438	0	3.7	0.7	270	9%
raw	1 oz	26	5.5	0.0	27	0	0.2	<.1	17	8%
raw	3 oz	77	16.4	0.0	82	0	0.7	0.1	51	9%
BURDOCK ROOT / gobo										
boiled, drained	4 oz	100	2.4	24.0	5	2.1	0.2	(tr)	0	2%
boiled, drained	1 root	146	3.5	35.1	7	3.0	0.2	na	0	1%
boiled, drained	1 cup	110	2.6	26.4	5	2.3	0.2	na	0	2%
raw	1 root	112	2.4	27.1	8	5.2	0.2	na	0	2%
raw, 1-inch pieces	1 cup	85	1.8	20.5	6	3.9	0.2	na	0	2%
raw, trimmed	1 oz	20	0.4	4.9	1	.9	<.1	(tr)	0	<4%
raw, untrimmed	1 lb	245	5.2	59.0	17	>6.6 c	0.5	(tr)	0	2%
BURGER, VEGETARIAN										
canned 'Vegetarian Burger' *(Worthington)*	1/2 cup	150	19.0	9.0	780	(mq)	4.0	1.0	0	24%
canned 'Vegetarian Burger No Salt Added' *(Worthington)*	1/2 cup	160	17.0	9.0	500	(mq)	6.0	(mq)	0	34%
frozen 'FriPats' *(Worthington)*	2.25-oz piece	180	13.0	5.0	350	(mq)	12.0	2.0	0	60%
frozen 'Grillers' *(Morningstar Farms)*	2.25-oz patty	180	13.0	5.0	350	(mq)	12.0	2.0	0	60%
frozen 'Harvest Burger' original flavor *(Green Giant)*	1 burger	140	18.0	8.0	380	5.0	4.0	1.5	0	26%
frozen 'Harvest Burger' southwest style *(Green Giant)*	1 burger	140	16.0	9.0	370	5.0	4.0	1.5	0	27%
frozen, organic *(Amy's Kitchen)*	2.5 oz	173	6.0	22.0	181	1.0	4.0	na	0	24%
BURGER MIX, VEGETARIAN										
(Fantastic Foods) w/tofu, prepared, excluding cooking fat	3.4-oz burger	133	11.0	14.0	320	(mq)	5.0	(mq)	na	31%
(Love Natural Foods) 'Loveburger' prepared	4-oz burger	245	17.0	20.0	224	8.0	11.0	(mq)	0	40%
(Nature's Burger) barbecue, prepared, excluding cooking fat	3-oz burger	117	4.0	24.0	423	(mq)	0.8	na	0	6%
(Nature's Burger) 'Original' prepared, excluding cooking fat	3-oz burger	152	7.0	21.0	228	(mq)	4.0	(mq)	0	24%
(Nature's Burger) pizza, prepared, excluding cooking fat	3-oz burger	121	5.0	24.0	406	(mq)	1.0	na	0	7%
(Worthington) 'Granburger' prepared, excluding cooking fat	1 burger	110	19.9	7.0	700	(mq)	1.0	na	0	8%
BURRITO, FROZEN										
(Amy's Kitchen) bean and rice	6 oz	251	8.0	44.0	364	6.0	5.0	na	0	18%
(Don Miguel) cheese, no beans	1 burrito	410	18.0	52.0	950	3.0	14.0	4.0	45	31%
(Don Miguel) cheese and green chili	1 burrito	390	20.0	53.0	910	3.0	11.0	4.0	40	25%
(Las Campanas) bean and cheese, no lard	1 burrito	272	10.0	42.0	480	6.0	7.0	3.0	3	23%
(Las Campanas) beef and bean, no lard	1 burrito	304	10.0	39.0	504	5.0	12.0	5.0	12	36%
(Maria's) jalapeño bean and cheese	1 burrito	360	12.0	54.0	620	8.0	11.0	3.5	10	27%
(Marquez) beef, green chili, and cheese, 'Primera'	1 burrito	330	14.0	43.0	950	2.0	11.0	4.0	30	30%
(Old El Paso) bean and cheese	1 burrito	330	14.0	45.0	740	(mq)	11.0	(mq)	(mq)	30%
(Swanson) hot and spicy 'Great Starts'	1 burrito	220	9.0	30.0	490	3.0	7.0	3.0	55	29%
(Swanson) original, w/cheese and chili peppers 'Great Starts'	1 burrito	200	8.0	25.0	510	2.0	8.0	3.0	60	36%
(Swanson) w/egg, bacon, cheese 'Great Starts'	1 burrito	250	10.0	27.0	540	na	11.0	4.0	90	40%
(Swanson) w/egg, ham, cheese 'Great Starts'	1 burrito	210	9.0	29.0	350	na	6.0	2.0	60	26%
(Swanson) w/egg, pizza sauce, cheese, pepperoni 'Great Starts'	1 burrito	240	9.0	28.0	410	na	9.0	3.0	60	34%
BURRITO DINNER MIX										
(Amy's Kitchen) beans, rice, and cheese, organic	6 oz	279	10.0	43.0	370	6.0	8.0	na	9	25%
(Hormel) beef	1 burrito	205	9.0	31.0	780	(mq)	8.0	(mq)	(mq)	31%
(Old El Paso) prepared, w/filling	1 burrito	299	11.0	36.0	430	4.0	13.0	4.0	23	38%

Food Name	Serving Size	Calories	Prot. gms	Carbs gms	Sod. mgs	Fiber gms	Fat gms	Sat. Fat gms	Chol. mgs	% Fat Cal.
(Patio)	12 oz	517	18.0	74.0	1643	(mq)	16.0	(mq)	(mq)	28%
(Tio Sancho) 'Dinner Kit'	1 burrito	125	3.3	24.0	569	>.1 c	1.9	na	na	14%
BURRITO DINNER, FROZEN										
beef and bean *(Patio)*	5 oz	370	11.0	43.0	830	(mq)	16.0	(mq)	(mq)	40%
beef and bean 'Britos' *(Patio)*	3.63 oz	250	6.0	33.0	340	(mq)	10.0	(mq)	15	37%
beef and bean 'Festive Dinners' *(Old El Paso)*	11 oz	470	23.0	72.0	1180	(mq)	9.0	(mq)	(mq)	18%
beef and bean, green chili *(Patio)*	5 oz	330	12.0	43.0	770	(mq)	12.0	(mq)	(mq)	33%
beef and bean, hot *(Old El Paso)*	1 burrito	310	12.0	41.0	710	(mq)	11.0	(mq)	(mq)	32%
beef and bean, medium *(Old El Paso)*	1 burrito	330	13.0	41.0	630	(mq)	13.0	5.0	29	35%
beef and bean, mild *(Old El Paso)*	1 burrito	320	13.0	42.0	500	(mq)	11.0	(mq)	(mq)	31%
beef and bean, nacho 'Britos' *(Patio)*	3.63 oz	270	9.0	30.0	420	(mq)	13.0	(mq)	25	43%
beef and bean 'Quick Meals' 1 serving *(Healthy Choice)*	5.2 oz	270	12.0	42.0	520	na	7.0	3.0	15	23%
beef and bean, red chili *(Patio)*	5 oz	340	11.0	44.0	810	(mq)	13.0	(mq)	(mq)	35%
beef steak fajita, 'Supreme' 5-oz pkg *(Ruiz)*	1 burrito	290	11.0	42.0	240	1.0	9.0	2.0	5	28%
cheese *(Hormel)*	1 burrito	210	9.0	32.0	792	(mq)	5.0	(mq)	(mq)	22%
cheese, nacho, 'Britos' *(Patio)*	3.63 oz	250	7.0	32.0	330	(mq)	10.0	(mq)	20	37%
chicken, spicy, 'Britos' *(Patio)*	3.63 oz	250	6.0	33.0	330	(mq)	10.0	(mq)	25	37%
chicken and rice *(Hormel)*	1 burrito	200	9.0	32.0	594	(mq)	4.0	(mq)	(mq)	18%
chicken con queso 'Quick Meals' *(Healthy Choice)*	5.4 oz	280	15.0	40.0	500	na	8.0	2.0	20	25%
chicken fajita, 'Supreme', 5-oz pkg *(Ruiz)*	1 burrito	260	12.0	50.0	500	10.0	1.0	1.0	5	4%
chili, hot *(Hormel)*	1 burrito	240	9.0	33.0	619	(mq)	8.0	(mq)	(mq)	30%
green chili 'Britos' *(Patio)*	3.63 oz	250	6.0	33.0	420	(mq)	10.0	(mq)	15	37%
red chili 'Britos' *(Patio)*	3.63 oz	240	6.0	31.0	370	(mq)	10.0	(mq)	15	38%
red hot *(Patio)*	5 oz	360	12.0	43.0	800	(mq)	15.0	(mq)	(mq)	38%
BURRITO FILLING FIX, beans *(Del Monte)*	1/2 cup	110	6.0	20.0	900	na	1.0	na	na	8%
BURRITO SEASONING MIX										
(Lawry's) 'Seasoning Blends' dry mix	1 pkg	132	6.0	23.3	2516	>.9 c	1.7	na	0	12%
(Old El Paso)	1/8 pkg	17	1.0	3.0	275	1.0	0.0	0.0	0	0%
(Tio Sancho) 'Dinner Kit'	3.25 oz	265	12.3	49.3	5031	>5.5 c	2.1	na	na	7%
BUSH NUT. See MACADAMIA NUT.										
BUTTER, CLARIFIED. See GHEE.										
BUTTER, REGULAR										
lightly salted *(Breakstone's)*	1 tbsp	100	0.0	0.0	90	na	11.0	7.0	35	100%
lightly salted *(Darigold)*	1 tsp	25	0.0	0.0	25	0	3.0	1.7	7	100%
lightly salted *(Hotel Bar)*	1 tsp	35	0.0	0.0	35	0	4.0	(mq)	(mq)	100%
lightly salted *(Kellers)*	1 tsp	35	0.0	0.0	35	na	4.0	na	na	100%
lightly salted *(Land O'Lakes)*	1 tbsp	35	0.0	0.0	40	na	4.0	2.0	10	100%
salted	4-oz stick	813	1.0	0.0	937	0	92.0	57.2	248	100%
salted	1 tbsp	100	0.1	0.0	115	0	11.4	7.1	31	100%
salted	1 tsp	34	<.1	0.0	39	0	3.8	2.4	10	99%
salted *(Challenge)*	1 tbsp	100	0.0	0.0	90	na	11.0	7.0	30	100%
salted *(Darigold)*	1 tsp	35	0.0	0.0	40	0	4.0	2.5	11	100%
salted *(Hotel Bar)*	1 tsp	35	0.0	0.0	35	0	4.0	(mq)	(mq)	100%
salted *(Kellers)*	1 tsp	35	0.0	0.0	35	0	4.0	(mq)	(mq)	100%
salted *(Land O'Lakes)*	1 tsp	35	0.0	0.0	40	0	4.0	(mq)	10	100%
salted *(Seal of Arizona)*	1 tbsp	100	0.0	0.0	90	na	11.0	7.0	30	100%
salted, packed 90 pats per 1 lb	1 pat	36	<.1	0.0	41	0	4.1	2.5	11	99%
unsalted	4-oz stick	813	1.0	0.1	12	0	92.0	57.2	248	100%
unsalted	1 tbsp	100	0.1	0.0	1	0	11.4	7.1	31	100%
unsalted	1 pat	36	0.0	0.0	1	0	4.1	2.5	11	100%
unsalted	1 tsp	34	<.1	0.0	<1	0	3.8	2.4	10	99%
unsalted *(Breakstone's)*	1 tbsp	100	0.0	0.0	0	na	11.0	7.0	35	100%
unsalted *(Challenge)*	1 tbsp	100	0.0	0.0	2	na	11.0	7.0	30	100%
unsalted *(Land O'Lakes)*	1 tbsp	35	0.0	0.0	0	na	4.0	2.0	10	100%

Food Name	Serving Size	Calories	Prot. gms	Carbs gms	Sod. mgs	Fiber gms	Fat gms	Sat. Fat gms	Chol. mgs	% Fat Cal.
BUTTER, WHIPPED										
lightly salted *(Breakstone's)*	1 tbsp	70	0.0	0.0	65	na	7.0	4.0	20	100%
lightly salted *(Land O'Lakes)*	1 tbsp	25	0.0	0.0	25	na	3.0	2.0	5	100%
lightly salted *(Land O'Lakes)*	1 tbsp	25	0.0	0.0	25	na	3.0	2.0	5	100%
salted	1 tbsp	67	0.1	tr	78	0	7.6	4.7	20	99%
salted	1 tsp	23	tr	tr	26	0	2.6	1.6	7	100%
salted *(Land O'Lakes)*	1 tsp	25	0.0	0.0	25	0	3.0	(mq)	5	100%
salted, packed 120 pats per 1 lb	1 pat	27	<.1	tr	31	0	3.1	1.9	8	99%
unsalted	1 tbsp	67	0.1	tr	1	0	7.6	4.7	20	99%
unsalted	1 tsp	23	tr	tr	<1	0	2.6	1.6	7	100%
unsalted *(Breakstone's)*	1 tbsp	70	0.0	0.0	0	na	7.0	4.0	20	100%
unsalted *(Darigold)*	1 tsp	25	0.0	0.0	2	0	3.0	1.6	7	100%
unsalted *(Land O'Lakes)*	1 tbsp	25	0.0	0.0	0	na	3.0	2.0	5	100%
unsalted *(Land O'Lakes)*	1 tsp	25	0.0	0.0	0	0	3.0	(mq)	5	100%
BUTTER FLAVORED OIL *(Wesson)*	1 tbsp	122	0.0	0.0	0	0	13.6	2.0	0	100%
BUTTER FLAVORED TOPPING *(Molly McButter)*	1/2 tsp	4.0	0.0	1.0	60	na	0.0	na	0	0%
BUTTER OIL										
	1 oz	248	0.1	0.0	na	0	28.2	17.6	73	100%
anhydrous	1 cup	1796	0.6	0.0	3	0	204.0	126.9	525	100%
anhydrous	1 tbsp	112	0.0	0.0	0	0	12.7	7.9	33	100%
BUTTERBEAN. See LIMA BEAN.										
BUTTERBUR / Fuki										
boiled, drained	4 oz	9	0.3	2.4	5	>.9 c	<.1	(tr)	0	<8%
raw	1 cup	13	0.4	3.4	7	>1.2 c	0.0	na	0	0%
raw, approx .2 oz	1 stalk	1	<.1	0.2	tr	>.1 c	tr	(tr)	0	0%
raw, trimmed	1/2 cup	7	0.2	1.7	4	>.6 c	<.1	(tr)	0	<11%
raw, trimmed	1 oz	4	0.1	1.0	2	>.4 c	<.1	(tr)	0	<17%
raw, untrimmed	1 lb	57	1.6	14.4	28	>5.2 c	0.2	(tr)	0	3%
BUTTERBUR, CANNED										
	4 oz	12	0.1	0.4	5	>1.2 c	0.1	(tr)	0	31%
chopped	1 cup	4	0.1	0.5	5	>1.1 c	0.2	na	0	43%
stalks	3 stalks	1	0.1	0.2	2	>.4 c	0.1	na	0	43%
BUTTERFISH										
dry-heat cooked	3 oz	159	18.8	0.0	97	0	8.7	na	71	51%
raw	1 lb	663	78.4	0.0	401	0	36.4	(mq)	295	51%
raw	3 oz	124	14.7	0.0	76	0	6.8	2.9	55	51%
raw	1 oz	41	4.9	0.0	25	0	2.3	(mq)	18	51%
BUTTERHEAD LETTUCE . See LETTUCE.										
BUTTERMILK										
blend, cultured, dry *(Saco Foods)*	3.5 tbsp	79	7.5	10.7	168	na	0.7	na	0	8%
cultured	1 cup	99	8.1	11.7	257	0	2.2	1.3	9	20%
cultured	1 oz	11	0.9	1.4	30	0	0.2	0.1	1	16%
cultured *(A&P)*	1 cup	90	8.0	12.0	260	0	1.0	(mq)	(mq)	10%
cultured *(Crowley)*	1 cup	110	9.0	12.0	390	0	4.0	(mq)	15	30%
cultured, 1.5% 'Golden Churn' *(Borden)*	1 cup	120	8.0	11.0	250	0	4.0	(mq)	(mq)	32%
cultured, 1.5% 'Unsalted' *(Friendship)*	1 oup	120	9.0	12.0	125	0	4.0	(mq)	14	30%
cultured, 2% *(Knudsen)*	1 cup	120	8.0	12.0	140	0	5.0	(mq)	(mq)	36%
cultured, 'Unsalted' *(Crowley)*	1 cup	110	9.0	12.0	130	0	4.0	(mq)	15	30%
sweet cream, dry	1 cup	464	41.2	58.8	621	0	6.9	4.3	83	13%
sweet cream, dry	1 oz	110	9.7	13.9	147	0	1.6	1.0	20	13%
sweet cream, dry	1 tbsp	25	2.2	3.2	34	0	0.4	0.2	5	14%
BUTTERNUT. See BRAZIL NUT.										
BUTTERNUT SQUASH. See SQUASH, BUTTERNUT										

Food Name	Serving Size	Calories	Prot. gms	Carbs gms	Sod. mgs	Fiber gms	Fat gms	Sat. Fat gms	Chol. mgs	% Fat Cal.
BUTTERSCOTCH TOPPING										
....	2 tbsp	103	0.6	27.0	143	0	0.0	0.1	0	0%
(Kraft)	1 tbsp	60	0.0	13.0	70	(tr)	1.0	0.0	0	15%
(Mrs. Richardson's) caramel	2 tbsp	130	<1.0	28.0	90	na	2.0	na	5	13%
(Mrs. Richardson's) caramel fudge, microwavable	2 tbsp	130	<1.0	28.0	90	na	2.0	na	5	13%
(Smucker's)	2 tbsp	140	0.0	33.0	75	(tr)	1.0	0.0	0	6%
(Smucker's) caramel flavor 'Special Recipe'	2 tbsp	160	1.0	33.0	40	(tr)	3.0	na	na	17%

C

Food Name	Serving Size	Calories	Prot. gms	Carbs gms	Sod. mgs	Fiber gms	Fat gms	Sat. Fat gms	Chol. mgs	% Fat Cal.
CABBAGE										
boiled, drained	1 head	278	12.9	56.3	101	35.34	5.4	0.7	0	15%
boiled, drained	4 oz	24	1.1	5.4	22	>.7 c	0.3	<.1	0	9%
boiled, drained, shredded	1/2 cup	16	0.8	3.3	6	2.1	0.3	0.0	0	14%
raw, approx 2.5 lbs	1 head	227	13.1	49.3	163	20.9	2.5	0.3	0	8%
raw, medium size (Dole)	1/12 head	18	1.0	3.0	30	2.0	0.0	na	na	0%
raw, shredded	1/2 cup	9	0.5	1.9	6	.8	0.1	0.0	0	9%
raw, trimmed	1 oz	7	0.3	1.5	5	.3	0.1	tr	0	11%
raw, untrimmed	1 lb	86	4.4	19.5	65	4.0 d	0.7	0.1	0	6%
CABBAGE, DANISH										
fresh	1 head	218	11.0	48.8	163	>7.3 c	1.6	0.2	0	6%
fresh, shredded	1/2 cup	8	0.4	1.9	6	>.3 c	0.1	0.0	0	9%
CABBAGE, NAPA/Chinese cabbage										
boiled, drained	1 leaf	2	0.2	0.3	1	>.1 c	0.0	0.0	0	0%
boiled, drained, shredded	1/2 cup	10	1.3	1.5	29	>.5 c	0.1	0.0	0	7%
bok-choy, boiled, drained	4 oz	14	1.8	2.0	39	1.8	0.2	<.1	0	11%
bok-choy, boiled, drained, shredded	1/2 cup	10	1.3	1.5	29	1.4	0.1	<.1	0	7%
bok-choy, raw, shredded	1/2 cup	5	0.5	0.8	23	.4	0.1	tr	0	15%
bok-choy, raw, trimmed	1 oz	4	0.4	0.6	19	.3	0.1	tr	0	18%
bok-choy, raw, untrimmed	1 lb	52	6.0	8.7	257	4.0	0.8	0.1	0	11%
pe-tsai, boiled, drained	4 oz	16	1.7	2.7	10	1.8	0.2	<.1	0	9%
pe-tsai, boiled, drained, shredded	1/2 cup	8	0.9	1.4	6	1.0	0.1	<.1	0	9%
pe-tsai, raw, trimmed	1 oz	5	0.3	0.9	3	.3	0.1	<.1	0	16%
pe-tsai, raw, untrimmed	1 lb	68	5.1	13.6	38	4.2	0.8	0.2	0	9%
raw, shredded	1/2 cup	5	0.5	0.8	23	.4	0.1	0.0	0	15%
CABBAGE, RED										
boiled, drained	4 oz	24	1.2	5.3	9	2.7	0.2	<.1	0	7%
boiled, drained, shredded	1/2 cup	16	0.8	3.5	6	1.8	0.2	0.0	0	10%
raw, shredded	1/2 cup	9	0.5	2.1	4	.7	0.1	0.0	0	8%
raw, trimmed	1 oz	8	0.4	1.7	3	.6	0.1	tr	0	10%
CABBAGE, SAVOY										
boiled, drained	4 oz	27	2.0	6.1	27	>.8 c	0.1	<.1	0	3%
boiled, drained, shredded	1/2 cup	18	1.3	4.0	18	>.5 c	0.1	0.0	0	4%
raw, shredded	1/2 cup	9	0.7	2.1	10	1.0	0.0	0.0	0	0%
raw, trimmed	1 oz	8	0.6	1.7	8	>.2 c	<.1	tr	0	<9%
raw, untrimmed	1 lb	100	7.3	22.1	102	>2.9 c	0.4	<.1	0	3%
CABBAGE, SKUNK/swamp cabbage/water convolvulus										
boiled, drained	4 oz	23	2.4	4.2	138	>1.0 c	0.3	(tr)	0	9%
boiled, drained, chopped	1/2 cup	10	1.0	1.8	60	.9	0.1	na	0	7%
raw	1 shoot	2	0.3	0.4	15	.3	0.0	na	0	0%
raw, chopped	1/2 cup	10	1.0	1.8	60	1.2	0.1	(tr)	0	7%

Food Name	Serving Size	Calories	Prot. gms	Carbs gms	Sod. mgs	Fiber gms	Fat gms	Sat. Fat gms	Chol. mgs	% Fat Cal.
raw, trimmed, chopped	1/2 cup	6	0.7	0.9	32	.6	0.1	(tr)	0	12%
raw, untrimmed	1 lb	67	9.1	11.0	395	>3.8 c	0.7	(tr)	0	7%
CABBAGE ENTRÉE, FROZEN										
w/meat, and tomato sauce (Lean Cuisine)	9.5 oz	210	13.0	26.0	560	na	6.0	2.0	30	26%
CABBAGE TURNIP. See KOHLRABI.										
CAESAR SALAD, 'Easy Caesar Kit' (Saco).	.75 oz	98	2.0	7.0	246	na	7.0	na	4	64%
CAIMIT / star apple										
ripe, trimmed	1 oz	19	0.2	4.1	(mq)	>.3 c	0.5	na	0	21%
CAJUN SEASONING (Tone's)	1 tsp	9	0.4	2.1	215	.5	0.2	<.1	0	15%
CAJUN STYLE MARINADE, barbecue sauce (Golden Dipt)	1 oz	90	0.0	5.0	360	na	8.0	na	0	78%
CAKE. See also BREAD, QUICK.										
'Best Wishes' 6 inch (Awrey's)	1/4 cake	150	1.0	18.0	170	0	9.0	3.0	25	52%
'Four-in-One Occasion' (Awrey's)	1.3 oz	150	1.0	18.0	170	0	8.0	2.0	25	49%
Banana										
loaf (Entenmann's)	1.3 oz	90	2.0	20.0	125	na	0.0	na	0	0%
single-layer, iced, frozen (Sara Lee)	1/8 cake	170	1.0	28.0	160	(mq)	6.0	(mq)	na	32%
Black forest										
torte (Awrey's)	1/14 cake	350	3.0	38.0	330	1.0	21.0	7.0	50	54%
two-layer, frozen (Sara Lee)	1/8 cake	190	2.0	28.0	100	(mq)	8.0	(mq)	na	38%
Blueberry crunch (Entenmann's)	1 oz	70	1.0	16.0	85	(mq)	0.0	0.0	0	0%
Boston cream, 'Supreme' frozen (Pepperidge Farm)	2 7/8 oz	290	3.0	39.0	190	(mq)	14.0	6.0	50	43%
Carrot										
cream cheese icing 'Old Fashioned' frozen										
(Pepperidge Farm)	1.5 oz	150	1.0	19.0	160	(mq)	9.0	3.0	15	50%
frozen (Weight Watchers)	3 oz	170	4.0	27.0	280	(mq)	5.0	<1.0	5	27%
single-layer, iced, frozen (Sara Lee)	1/8 cake	250	3.0	30.0	240	(mq)	13.0	(mq)	25	47%
supreme, iced (Awrey's)	1 piece	210	3.0	23.0	170	0	12.0	3.0	25	51%
three-layer, cream cheese icing (Awrey's)	1/12 cake	390	5.0	44.0	310	1.0	23.0	5.0	45	51%
Cheesecake										
brownie 'Sweet Celebrations' frozen (Weight Watchers)	3.5 oz	200	9.0	34.0	260	(mq)	5.0	1.0	10	21%
cream cheese, cherry, frozen (Sara Lee)	1/6 cake	243	4.0	35.0	184	(mq)	8.0	(mq)	(mq)	32%
cream cheese, frozen (Sara Lee)	1/6 cake	230	5.0	27.0	153	(mq)	11.0	(mq)	(mq)	44%
cream cheese, strawberry, frozen (Sara Lee)	1/6 cake	222	4.0	34.0	171	(mq)	8.0	(mq)	(mq)	32%
French 'Classics' frozen (Sara Lee)	1/8 cake	250	4.0	23.0	120	(mq)	16.0	(mq)	20	57%
frozen (Weight Watchers)	3.9 oz	210	10.0	29.0	230	(mq)	7.0	2.0	20	29%
nondairy 'Better Than Cheesecake' frozen (Tofutti)	1/10 cake	160	2.0	16.0	110	(mq)	10.0	(mq)	0	56%
strawberry, French 'Classics' frozen (Sara Lee)	1/8 cake	240	3.0	28.0	125	(mq)	13.0	(mq)	20	49%
strawberry 'Sweet Celebrations' frozen (Weight Watchers)	3.9 oz	180	7.0	28.0	210	(mq)	4.0	2.0	20	21%
triple chocolate 'Sweet Celebrations' frozen										
(Weight Watchers)	1 cake	190	8.0	30.0	220	na	4.0	2.0	5	19%
Cherry, and cream, frozen (Weight Watchers)	3 oz	190	3.0	32.0	200	(mq)	6.0	1.0	5	28%
Chocolate										
(Awrey's)	.8 oz	70	1.0	11.0	110	0	3.0	1.0	15	36%
devil's food, fudge icing (Entenmann's)	1.2 oz	130	2.0	19.0	120	na	5.0	na	na	35%
devil's food, layer, frozen (Pepperidge Farm)	1 5/8 oz	180	1.0	24.0	135	(mq)	9.0	3.0	20	45%
devil's food, white icing (Awrey's)	1 piece	150	1.0	17.0	160	1.0	8.0	3.0	25	50%
double, iced (Awrey's)	1 piece	130	2.0	21.0	150	1.0	6.0	2.0	15	37%
double, three-layer (Awrey's)	1/12 cake	310	3.0	48.0	290	2.0	14.0	4.0	35	38%
double, three-layer, frozen (Sara Lee)	1/8 cake	220	3.0	26.0	130	(mq)	11.0	(mq)	20	46%
double, torte (Awrey's)	1/14 cake	340	3.0	51.0	300	2.0	15.0	4.0	35	39%
double, two-layer (Awrey's)	1/12 cake	250	3.0	38.0	260	1.0	11.0	3.0	35	38%
double, fudge, frozen (Weight Watchers)	2.75 oz	200	4.0	34.0	190	(mq)	5.0	<1.0	5	23%
'Free & Light' frozen (Sara Lee)	1/8 cake	110	2.0	26.0	140	(mq)	0.0	0.0	0	0%
frozen (Weight Watchers)	2.5 oz	180	5.0	31.0	250	(mq)	5.0	<1.0	5	24%

Food Name	Serving Size	Calories	Prot. gms	Carbs gms	Sod. mgs	Fiber gms	Fat gms	Sat. Fat gms	Chol. mgs	% Fat Cal.
fudge, layer, frozen *(Pepperidge Farm)*	1 5/8 oz	180	1.0	23.0	140	(mq)	10.0	(mq)	20	48%
fudge stripe, layer, frozen *(Pepperidge Farm)*	1 5/8 oz	170	2.0	20.0	140	(mq)	9.0	3.0	20	48%
German, frozen *(Weight Watchers)*	2.5 oz	200	4.0	31.0	220	(mq)	7.0	<1.0	5	31%
German, iced *(Awrey's)*	2-inch square	160	2.0	19.0	150	0	9.0	3.0	20	49%
German, single-layer, frozen *(Pepperidge Farm)*	1 5/8 oz	180	1.0	22.0	170	(mq)	10.0	4.0	20	50%
German, three-layer *(Awrey's)*	1/12 cake	350	3.0	46.0	300	1.0	18.0	6.0	40	45%
'Happy Birthday' *(Awrey's)*	1.4 oz	150	1.0	18.0	150	1.0	8.0	3.0	25	49%
milk, and yellow, two-layer *(Awrey's)*	1/12 cake	290	3.0	33.0	320	0	17.0	5.0	50	52%
mousse 'Classics' frozen *(Sara Lee)*	1/8 cake	260	3.0	23.0	100	(mq)	17.0	(mq)	20	60%
'Supreme' frozen *(Pepperidge Farm)*	2 7/8 oz	300	3.0	37.0	140	(mq)	16.0	7.0	25	47%
two-layer, white icing *(Awrey's)*	1/12 cake	270	3.0	34.0	290	1.0	15.0	5.0	40	48%
Cinnamon swirl, refrigerated *(Pillsbury)*	1/8 cake	180	2.0	22.0	170	(mq)	9.0	2.0	0	46%
Coconut										
butter cream *(Awrey's)*	1 piece	160	1.0	19.0	180	0	9.0	3.0	25	50%
layer, frozen *(Pepperidge Farm)*	1 5/8 oz	180	1.0	24.0	120	(mq)	8.0	3.0	20	42%
and yellow, three-layer *(Awrey's)*	1/12 cake	350	3.0	40.0	340	0	21.0	7.0	50	52%
Coffeecake										
all butter, cheese, frozen *(Sara Lee)*	1/8 cake	210	4.0	25.0	220	(mq)	11.0	(mq)	(mq)	46%
all butter, pecan, frozen *(Sara Lee)*	1/8 cake	160	3.0	19.0	180	(mq)	8.0	(mq)	(mq)	45%
all butter, streusel, frozen *(Sara Lee)*	1/8 cake	160	3.0	20.0	160	(mq)	7.0	(mq)	(mq)	41%
caramel nut *(Awrey's)*	1/12 cake	140	2.0	15.0	150	0	8.0	2.0	5	51%
cheese *(Entenmann's)*	1.6 oz	150	3.0	20.0	140	na	7.0	na	na	41%
cinnamon swirl, iced *(Pillsbury)*	1 piece	230	3.0	29.0	240	na	11.0	2.0	0	44%
crumb *(Entenmann's)*	1.3 oz	160	3.0	21.0	160	na	7.0	na	na	40%
crumb, cheese-filled *(Entenmann's)*	1.4 oz	130	3.0	18.0	140	na	6.0	na	na	39%
'Long John' *(Awrey's)*	1/12 cake	160	2.0	19.0	130	0	8.0	2.0	10	46%
pecan crumb, iced *(Pillsbury)*	1 piece	230	3.0	29.0	240	na	12.0	2.0	0	46%
French crumb, all butter *(Entenmann's)*	1.6 oz	180	2.0	26.0	220	na	8.0	na	na	39%
Golden										
layer, frozen *(Pepperidge Farm)*	1 5/8 oz	180	1.0	24.0	110	(mq)	9.0	3.0	20	45%
thick fudge icing *(Entenmann's)*	1.2 oz	130	2.0	20.0	120	na	6.0	na	na	38%
Lemon										
coconut 'Supreme' frozen *(Pepperidge Farm)*	3 oz	280	3.0	38.0	220	(mq)	13.0	6.0	30	42%
cream 'Supreme' frozen *(Pepperidge Farm)*	1 5/8 oz	170	2.0	21.0	120	(mq)	9.0	3.0	20	47%
three-layer *(Awrey's)*	1/12 cake	320	2.0	38.0	310	0	19.0	5.0	45	52%
yellow, two-layer *(Awrey's)*	1/12 cake	290	2.0	33.0	310	0	17.0	5.0	45	52%
Louisiana crunch *(Entenmann's)*	1.7 oz	180	2.0	27.0	180	na	8.0	na	na	38%
Neapolitan torte *(Awrey's)*	1/14 cake	380	3.0	43.0	370	0	22.0	7.0	55	52%
Orange										
frosty, iced *(Awrey's)*	1 piece	150	1.0	19.0	170	0	8.0	2.0	20	47%
three-layer *(Awrey's)*	1/12 cake	320	2.0	40.0	320	0	17.0	4.0	35	48%
Peanut butter torte *(Awrey's)*	1/14 cake	380	7.0	44.0	340	1.0	22.0	5.0	40	49%
Pecan streusel, refrigerated *(Pillsbury)*	1/8 cake	180	2.0	21.0	170	(mq)	9.0	2.0	0	47%
Pineapple										
cream 'Supreme' frozen *(Pepperidge Farm)*	2 oz	190	2.0	28.0	130	(mq)	7.0	2.0	20	34%
crunch *(Entenmann's)*	1 oz	70	1.0	16.0	85	(mq)	0.0	0.0	0	0%
Pistachio torte *(Awrey's)*	1/12 cake	370	3.0	41.0	370	1.0	22.0	7.0	35	53%
Pound										
(Drake's)	1/10 cake	110	2.0	16.0	70	(mq)	5.0	1.0	25	39%
all butter 'Family Size Original' frozen *(Sara Lee)*	1/15 cake	130	2.0	14.0	85	(mq)	7.0	(mq)	(mq)	50%
all butter, loaf *(Entenmann's)*	1 oz	110	2.0	15.0	150	na	5.0	na	na	40%
all butter 'Original' frozen *(Sara Lee)*	1/10 cake	130	2.0	14.0	85	(mq)	7.0	(mq)	(mq)	50%
'Free & Light' frozen *(Sara Lee)*	1/10 cake	70	1.0	17.0	105	(mq)	0.0	0.0	0	0%
golden *(Awrey's)*	1/14 loaf	130	2.0	19.0	150	0	5.0	1.0	20	35%

Food Name	Serving Size	Calories	Prot. gms	Carbs gms	Sod. mgs	Fiber gms	Fat gms	Sat. Fat gms	Chol. mgs	% Fat Cal.
'Old Fashioned Cholesterol Free' frozen										
(Pepperidge Farm)	1 oz	110	1.0	13.0	85	(mq)	6.0	1.0	0	49%
sour cream, loaf (Entenmann's)	1 oz	120	1.0	14.0	90	na	7.0	na	na	51%
Raisin spice, iced (Awrey's)	1 piece	160	1.0	21.0	120	0	8.0	2.0	20	45%
Raspberry nut (Awrey's)	1/16 cake	310	3.0	39.0	220	0	16.0	3.0	30	46%
Shortcake										
strawberry 'Dessert Lights' frozen, 3 oz										
(Pepperidge Farm)	1 piece	170	2.0	30.0	50	1.0	5.0	1.0	70	26%
strawberry, frozen (Sara Lee)	1/8 cake	190	2.0	26.0	90	(mq)	8.0	(mq)	na	39%
Sponge (Awrey's)	2-inch square	80	1.0	11.0	125	0	3.0	1.0	15	36%
Strawberry										
cream 'Supreme' frozen (Pepperidge Farm)	2 oz	190	1.0	30.0	120	(mq)	7.0	3.0	20	34%
stripe, layer, frozen (Pepperidge Farm)	1.5 oz	160	1.0	21.0	120	(mq)	8.0	3.0	20	45%
supreme, torte (Awrey's)	1/14 cake	270	3.0	38.0	310	1.0	12.0	3.0	45	40%
Vanilla, layer, frozen (Pepperidge Farm)	1 5/8 oz	190	1.0	25.0	120	(mq)	8.0	3.0	20	41%
Walnut torte (Awrey's)	1/14 cake	320	2.0	38.0	290	0	19.0	4.0	30	52%
Yellow										
(Awrey's)	.9 oz	80	1.0	12.0	135	0	3.0	1.0	20	34%
white icing (Awrey's)	2-inch square	150	1.0	18.0	180	0	9.0	3.0	25	52%
CUPCAKE										
Creme, 'Kreme Kup' (Tastykake)	1 cupcake	86	1.3	14.6	113	.6	2.8	1.0	4	28%
White (Break Cake)	1 cupcake	130	1.0	24.0	115	na	3.0	1.2	0	21%
SNACK CAKE										
bar (Sunbelt)	1.31 oz	130	1.0	28.0	130	(mq)	2.0	(mq)	<1	13%
'Be My Valentine' (Little Debbie)	2.5 oz	330	2.0	44.0	125	(mq)	17.0	(mq)	<1	45%
'Best Wishes, Miniature' (Awrey's)	3 oz	320	5.0	33.0	280	0	22.0	9.0	0	57%
'Caravella' (Little Debbie)	1.2 oz	200	2.0	26.0	95	(mq)	9.0	(mq)	<1	42%
'Christmas Tree' (Little Debbie)	1.6 oz	220	1.0	28.0	80	(mq)	11.0	(mq)	<1	46%
coconut covered 'Sno Balls' (Hostess)	1 piece	150	1.0	26.0	160	1.0	4.0	2.0	2	25%
dessert cup (Hostess)	1 piece	90	2.0	18.0	170	.4	2.0	<1.0	15	18%
dessert cup (Little Debbie)	.79 oz	80	1.0	4.0	170	(mq)	1.0	na	<1	31%
'Doodle Dandies' (Little Debbie)	2.5 oz	320	2.0	44.0	140	(mq)	16.0	(mq)	<1	44%
'Easter Bunny' (Little Debbie)	2.5 oz	320	2.0	45.0	135	(mq)	15.0	(mq)	<1	42%
fancy (Little Debbie)	2.6 oz	340	2.0	46.0	150	(mq)	16.0	(mq)	<1	43%
filled twins, 3 oz (Break Cake)	2 pieces	310	2.0	53.0	260	na	10.0	2.7	15	29%
filled twins, multi pak, 1.5 oz (Break Cake)	1 piece	150	1.0	26.0	130	na	5.0	1.3	5	29%
'Funny Bones' (Drake's)	1.25 oz	150	3.0	18.0	110	(mq)	8.0	2.0	0	46%
'Lil' Angels' (Hostess)	1 piece	90	1.0	14.0	95	(mq)	2.0	(mq)	2	23%
'Poppets' (Erewhon)	1 oz	110	2.0	24.0	10	1.0	1.0	na	na	8%
'Star Crunch' (Little Debbie)	1.08 oz	150	1.0	22.0	95	(mq)	6.0	(mq)	<1	37%
Swiss roll (Little Debbie)	2.25 oz	280	2.0	40.0	135	(mq)	12.0	(mq)	<1	39%
'Tasty Twist' (Tastykake)	1 piece	18	0.3	2.7	(mq)	(mq)	0.6	na	na	31%
'Tiger Tail' (Hostess)	1 piece	240	4.0	38.0	290	1.3	8.0	4.0	25	30%
'Zoinks' (Drake's)	1.25 oz	130	1.0	20.0	130	(mq)	5.0	1.0	10	35%
Apple streusel (Awrey's)	1 piece	160	2.0	18.0	120	0	9.0	1.0	15	50%
Banana, iced (Awrey's)	1 piece	140	1.0	17.0	120	0	8.0	2.0	20	50%
Brownie										
À la mode 'Sweet Celebrations' frozen (Weight Watchers)	1 serving	180	5.0	35.0	150	0	4.0	0.0	5	18%
chocolate 'Sweet Celebrations' frozen (Weight Watchers)	1/3 pkg	100	3.0	16.0	150	(mq)	3.0	<1.0	5	26%
chocolate chip 'Toll House Ready to Bake' frozen (Nestlé)	1.4 oz	150	2.0	19.0	60	(mq)	7.0	(mq)	na	43%
chocolate nut, mini (Break Cake)	.5 oz	70	1.0	9.0	60	na	4.0	0.6	0	47%
Dutch chocolate 'Cake' (Awrey's)	1/16 cake	340	3.0	40.0	260	1.0	20.0	4.0	35	51%
fudge (Break Cake)	2.8 oz	370	4.0	47.0	260	na	18.0	4.1	35	44%
fudge (Little Debbie)	3 oz	350	4.0	57.0	180	(mq)	12.0	(mq)	<1	31%

Food Name	Serving Size	Calories	Prot. gms	Carbs gms	Sod. mgs	Fiber gms	Fat gms	Sat. Fat gms	Chol. mgs	% Fat Cal.
fudge (Little Debbie) .... 2 oz		240	3.0	39.0	140	(mq)	8.0	(mq)	<1	30%
fudge nut (Frito-Lay's) .... 3 oz		360	3.0	56.0	225	na	14.0	na	8	35%
fudge nut, iced 'Sheet Cake' (Awrey's) .... 2.5 oz		300	3.0	36.0	210	1.0	17.0	3.0	40	50%
fudge nut 'Sheet Cake' (Awrey's) .... 1.25 oz		150	2.0	16.0	115	1.0	9.0	1.0	25	53%
fudge walnut (Tastykake) .... 3 oz		335	3.9	53.4	222	5.4	14.2	3.3	22	36%
hot fudge 'Newport' frozen (Pepperidge Farm) .... 1 ramekin		400	4.0	50.0	160	(mq)	20.0	10.0	80	46%
low-fat, fudge, chocolate icing 'Lights' (Hostess) .... 1 brownie		140	2.0	29.0	95	1.0	2.6	0.5	10	16%
mint frosting 'Sweet Celebrations' frozen										
(Weight Watchers) .... 1.23 oz		100	2.0	18.0	130	na	2.0	<1.0	5	18%
peanut butter fudge 'Sweet Celebrations' frozen										
(Weight Watchers) .... 1.23 oz		100	2.0	18.0	140	na	3.0	<1.0	5	25%
Swiss mocha fudge 'Sweet Celebrations' frozen										
(Weight Watchers) .... 1.23 oz		90	2.0	18.0	140	na	2.0	<1.0	5	18%
Caramel										
fudge, À la mode, frozen (Weight Watchers) .... 1 serving		180	4.0	35.0	170	na	3.0	<1.0	5	15%
peanut filled, chocolate coated (Little Debbie) .... 1 piece		230	3.0	28.0	120	(mq)	12.0	(mq)	<1	47%
Carrot										
(Break Cake) .... 2 pieces		370	3.0	64.0	380	na	12.0	2.2	20	29%
'Classic' frozen, 2.5 oz (Pepperidge Farm) .... 1 piece		260	2.0	32.0	280	(mq)	16.0	6.0	50	51%
'Deluxe' frozen, 1.8 oz (Sara Lee) .... 1 piece		180	3.0	26.0	200	(mq)	7.0	(mq)	na	35%
'Lights' frozen, 2.5 oz (Sara Lee) .... 1 piece		170	4.0	30.0	75	(mq)	4.0	(mq)	5	21%
multi pak, 1.2 oz (Break Cake) .... 1 piece		120	1.0	20.0	115	na	4.0	0.7	5	30%
Cheesecake										
brownie 'Sweet Celebrations' frozen (Weight Watchers) ... 3.5 oz		200	9.0	34.0	260	na	5.0	1.0	10	21%
classic, frozen, 2 oz (Sara Lee) .... 1 piece		200	4.0	16.0	150	(mq)	14.0	(mq)	na	61%
French 'Lights' frozen, 3.2 oz (Sara Lee) .... 1 piece		150	5.0	24.0	90	(mq)	4.0	(mq)	15	24%
French, strawberry 'Lights' frozen, 3.5 oz (Sara Lee) ..... 1 piece		150	3.0	29.0	65	(mq)	2.0	(mq)	5	12%
strawberry 'Manhattan' frozen (Pepperidge Farm) .... 1 piece		300	6.0	49.0	250	(mq)	9.0	5.0	150	27%
strawberry 'Sweet Celebrations' frozen (Weight Watchers) 3.9 oz		180	7.0	28.0	210	na	4.0	2.0	20	21%
Cinnamon, twirl (Aunt Fanny's) .... 1 oz		110	2.0	16.0	85	na	4.0	1.0	0	33%
Coffeecake										
(Little Debbie) .... 2.1 oz		250	3.0	39.0	210	(mq)	9.0	(mq)	<1	33%
apple cinnamon, individually wrapped, frozen (Sara Lee)	1 piece	290	4.0	40.0	270	(mq)	13.0	(mq)	na	40%
butter streusel, individually wrapped, frozen (Sara Lee) ... 1 piece		230	4.0	27.0	270	(mq)	12.0	(mq)	(mq)	47%
cinnamon crumb (Drake's) .... 1.33 oz		150	2.0	22.0	110	(mq)	6.0	1.0	10	36%
cinnamon streusel 'Microwave' frozen (Weight Watchers)	1 piece	190	3.0	28.0	250	(mq)	7.0	1.0	5	34%
cream filled 'Koffee Kake' (Tastykake) .... 1 oz		110	1.4	17.5	81	.4	4.0	0.9	16	32%
crumb (Hostess) .... 1 piece		120	1.0	19.0	80	.7	5.0	2.0	10	36%
crumb 'Light' (Hostess) .... 1 piece		80	1.0	19.0	95	.4	1.0	<1.0	0	10%
'Jr.' (Drake's) .... 1.1 oz		140	2.0	18.0	90	(mq)	6.0	1.0	10	40%
'Koffee Kake Juniors' (Tastykake) .... 2.5 oz		261	3.4	43.8	212	.9	8.5	2.1	410	29%
pecan, individually wrapped, frozen (Sara Lee) .... 1 piece		280	5.0	30.0	270	(mq)	16.0	(mq)	na	51%
'Small' (Drake's) .... 2 oz		220	3.0	33.0	160	(mq)	9.0	2.0	15	36%
Oatmeal, creme pie, individually wrapped (Little Debbie) ... 1.35 oz		170	2.0	29.0	140	na	8.0	1.0	0	37%
Shortcake										
strawberry, À la mode, frozen (Weight Watchers) .... 1 piece		170	3.0	33.0	150	na	2.0	<1.0	5	11%
strawberry 'Dessert Lights' frozen (Pepperidge Farm) .... 1 piece		170	2.0	30.0	50	1.0	5.0	1.0	70	26%
CAKE, MICROWAVE										
apple streusel, prepared (MicroRave) .... 1/12 cake		240	2.0	33.0	190	(mq)	11.0	3.0	45	41%
banana, w/vanilla frosting 'Snack' prepared (Pillsbury) ... 1/9 cake		170	1.0	26.0	160	na	7.0	2.0	10	37%
carrot, w/cream cheese frosting 'Snack' prepared										
(Pillsbury) .... 1/9 cake		170	1.0	25.0	200	na	7.0	2.0	10	38%
cinnamon pecan, prepared (MicroRave) .... 1/6 cake		290	3.0	39.0	210	(mq)	13.0	3.0	45	41%
cinnamon streusel, prepared (Streusel Swirl) .... 1/8 cake		240	2.0	33.0	180	(mq)	11.0	(mq)	na	41%

Food Name	Serving Size	Calories	Prot. gms	Carbs gms	Sod. mgs	Fiber gms	Fat gms	Sat. Fat gms	Chol. mgs	% Fat Cal
chocolate, prepared *(Pillsbury)*	1/8 cake	210	2.0	23.0	260	(mq)	13.0	(mq)	na	54%
chocolate, w/chocolate frosting, prepared *(Pillsbury)*	1/8 cake	300	2.0	35.0	310	(mq)	17.0	(mq)	na	51%
chocolate, w/vanilla frosting, prepared *(Pillsbury)*	1/8 cake	300	2.0	36.0	300	(mq)	17.0	(mq)	na	50%
chocolate supreme, double, prepared *(Pillsbury)*	1/8 cake	330	3.0	39.0	340	(mq)	19.0	(mq)	na	50%
devil's food, w/chocolate frosting, dry mix *(MicroRave)*	1/6 pkg	210	2.0	35.0	240	na	7.0	na	0	30%
German chocolate, w/coconut pecan frosting, dry mix *(MicroRave)*	1/6 pkg	230	2.0	37.0	240	na	8.0	na	0	32%
lemon, prepared *(Pillsbury)*	1/8 cake	220	2.0	23.0	180	(mq)	13.0	(mq)	na	54%
lemon, w/lemon frosting, prepared *(MicroRave)*	1/6 cake	300	2.0	37.0	250	(mq)	16.0	4.0	45	48%
lemon, w/lemon frosting, prepared *(Pillsbury)*	1/8 cake	300	2.0	37.0	220	(mq)	17.0	(mq)	na	50%
lemon supreme, double, prepared *(Pillsbury)*	1/8 cake	300	2.0	40.0	210	(mq)	15.0	(mq)	na	45%
yellow, w/chocolate frosting, prepared *(Pillsbury)*	1/8 cake	300	2.0	36.0	220	(mq)	17.0	(mq)	na	50%
yellow, w/chocolate frosting 'Singles' dry mix *(MicroRave)*	1/6 pkg	210	1.0	36.0	210	na	7.0	na	0	30%

SNACK CAKE

Brownie

Food Name	Serving Size	Calories	Prot. gms	Carbs gms	Sod. mgs	Fiber gms	Fat gms	Sat. Fat gms	Chol. mgs	% Fat Cal
caramel 'Supreme' prepared *(Betty Crocker)*	1 brownie	110	1.0	21.0	110	na	2.0	na	0	17%
caramel 'Supreme' prepared *(General Mills)*	1 brownie	110	1.0	21.0	110	na	2.0	na	0	17%
caramel fudge chunk, prepared *(Pillsbury)*	1 brownie	170	2.0	25.0	105	(mq)	7.0	(mq)	0	37%
carrot, microwave, dry mix *(Pillsbury)*	1/9 pkg	110	1.0	17.0	170	na	5.0	1.0	10	39%
chocolate chip 'Supreme' prepared *(Betty Crocker)*	1 brownie	110	1.0	20.0	85	na	3.0	na	0	24%
chocolate chip 'Supreme' prepared *(General Mills)*	1 brownie	110	1.0	20.0	85	na	3.0	na	0	24%
double chocolate, prepared *(Great Additions)*	1 brownie	140	1.0	19.0	75	na	6.0	2.0	10	40%
double fudge 'Brownies Plus' prepared *(Duncan Hines)*	1 brownie	150	2.0	22.0	105	na	6.0	na	na	36%
double fudge, prepared *(Pillsbury)*	1 brownie	160	2.0	24.0	105	(mq)	6.0	(mq)	na	34%
frosted, microwave, prepared *(MicroRave)*	1 brownie	180	2.0	27.0	130	na	7.0	na	0	35%
frosted 'Supreme' prepared *(Betty Crocker)*	1 brownie	140	1.0	26.0	100	na	3.0	na	0	20%
frosted 'Supreme' prepared *(General Mills)*	1 brownie	140	1.0	26.0	100	na	3.0	na	0	20%
fudge, mix only *(Duncan Hines)*	1 brownie	100	1.0	18.0	85	na	18.0	2.0	na	68%
fudge, 21.5-oz pkg, dry mix *(Pillsbury)*	1/24 pkg	100	1.0	20.0	85	na	2.0	1.0	0	18%
fudge, 15-oz pkg, dry mix *(Pillsbury)*	1/16 pkg	110	1.0	21.0	90	na	2.0	1.0	0	17%
fudge 'Family Size' prepared *(General Mills)*	1 brownie	110	1.0	22.0	95	na	2.0	na	0	16%
fudge 'Light' prepared *(General Mills)*	1 brownie	100	1.0	21.0	90	na	1.0	na	0	9%
fudge, microwave, prepared *(Pillsbury)*	1 brownie	190	2.0	25.0	105	(mq)	9.0	(mq)	na	43%
fudge, prepared *(Duncan Hines)*	1 brownie	130	1.0	18.0	90	na	5.0	na	na	37%
fudge, prepared *(Krusteaz)*	1 brownie	190	1.0	28.0	135	na	8.0	na	19	38%
fudge, prepared *(Lovin' Lites)*	1/24 pkg	100	1.0	19.0	80	na	2.0	1.0	10	18%
fudge 'Pouch Mix' dry mix *(Gold Medal)*	1/16 pkg	100	1.0	16.0	85	(mq)	4.0	(mq)	na	35%
fudge 'Pouch Mix' dry mix *(Robin Hood)*	1/16 pkg	100	1.0	16.0	85	(mq)	4.0	(mq)	na	35%
fudge 'Regular Size' prepared *(General Mills)*	1 brownie	110	1.0	23.0	100	na	2.0	na	0	16%
fudge 'Ultra Moist' dry mix *(Finast)*	1/16 pkg	130	2.0	20.0	120	(mq)	5.0	(mq)	na	34%
fudge, w/fudge frosting, microwave, prepared *(Pillsbury)*	1/9 pkg	240	2.0	32.0	140	na	11.0	3.0	0	42%
fudge deluxe 'Family Size' prepared *(Pillsbury)*	1 brownie	150	1.0	20.0	95	(mq)	7.0	(mq)	na	43%
fudge deluxe, prepared *(Pillsbury)*	1 brownie	150	2.0	21.0	100	(mq)	6.0	(mq)	na	37%
fudge deluxe, w/walnuts, prepared *(Pillsbury)*	1 brownie	150	2.0	19.0	90	(mq)	8.0	(mq)	na	46%
'Funfetti Frosted' prepared *(Great Additions)*	1 brownie	160	1.0	23.0	100	na	7.0	1.0	10	40%
German chocolate 'Supreme' prepared *(Betty Crocker)*	1 brownie	130	1.0	24.0	105	na	3.0	na	0	21%
German chocolate 'Supreme' prepared *(General Mills)*	1 brownie	130	1.0	24.0	105	na	3.0	na	0	21%
'Gourmet Turtle' prepared *(Duncan Hines)*	1 brownie	200	2.0	27.0	125	na	9.0	na	na	41%
milk chocolate 'Brownies Plus' prepared *(Duncan Hines)*	1 brownie	160	1.0	20.0	95	na	8.0	na	na	46%
original 'Supreme' prepared *(Betty Crocker)*	1 brownie	120	1.0	22.0	90	na	3.0	na	0	23%
original 'Supreme' prepared *(General Mills)*	1 brownie	120	1.0	22.0	90	na	3.0	na	0	23%
party 'Supreme' prepared *(Betty Crocker)*	1 brownie	140	1.0	26.0	100	na	3.0	na	0	20%
party 'Supreme' prepared *(General Mills)*	1 brownie	140	1.0	26.0	100	na	3.0	na	0	20%
peanut butter 'Brownies Plus' prepared *(Duncan Hines)*	1 brownie	150	3.0	16.0	105	na	8.0	na	na	49%

Food Name	Serving Size	Calories	Prot. gms	Carbs gms	Sod. mgs	Fiber gms	Fat gms	Sat. Fat gms	Chol. mgs	% Fat Cal.
peanut butter candies 'Supreme' prepared (Betty Crocker)	1 brownie	140	2.0	21.0	85	na	5.0	na	na	33%
prepared (Estee)	1 brownie	50	<1.0	11.0	0	na	2.0	<1.0	0	27%
rocky road, fudge (Pillsbury)	1 brownie	170	2.0	24.0	95	(mq)	8.0	(mq)	na	41%
'Singles' microwave, prepared (MicroRave)	1 brownie	250	4.0	39.0	230	na	9.0	na	0	32%
triple fudge, chunky (Pillsbury)	1 brownie	170	2.0	25.0	105	(mq)	7.0	(mq)	na	37%
walnut 'Brownies Plus' prepared (Duncan Hines)	1 brownie	150	1.0	19.0	90	na	7.0	na	na	44%
walnut, microwave, prepared (MicroRave)	1 brownie	160	2.0	21.0	95	(mq)	7.0	2.0	0	41%
walnut, prepared (Great Additions)	1 brownie	140	2.0	16.0	70	na	8.0	1.0	10	50%
walnut 'Supreme' prepared (Betty Crocker)	1 brownie	110	1.0	18.0	85	na	4.0	na	0	32%
walnut 'Supreme' prepared (General Mills)	1 brownie	110	1.0	18.0	85	na	4.0	na	0	32%
walnut 'Ultra Moist' prepared (Finast)	1 brownie	130	1.0	19.0	110	(mq)	6.0	(mq)	na	40%
w/hot fudge topping 'Singles' microwave, prepared (MicroRave)	1 brownie	340	5.0	54.0	270	na	12.0	na	0	31%
CAKE MIX										
Angel food										
chocolate, dry mix (General Mills)	1/12 pkg	150	3.0	34.0	300	(mq)	0.0	0.0	0	0%
confetti, dry mix (General Mills)	1/12 pkg	150	3.0	34.0	300	(mq)	0.0	0.0	0	0%
dry mix (Duncan Hines)	1/12 pkg	140	3.0	30.0	130	na	0.0	na	na	0%
dry mix (Lovin' Loaf)	1/8 pkg	90	2.0	20.0	210	na	0.0	0.0	0	0%
lemon custard, dry mix (General Mills)	1/12 pkg	150	3.0	34.0	300	na	0.0	na	0	0%
lemon pudding, dry mix (General Mills)	1/12 pkg	150	3.0	34.0	300	(mq)	0.0	0.0	0	0%
strawberry, dry mix (General Mills)	1/12 pkg	150	3.0	35.0	260	(mq)	0.0	0.0	0	0%
'Traditional' dry mix (Betty Crocker)	1/12 pkg	130	3.0	30.0	170	(mq)	0.0	0.0	0	0%
white, one-step, dry mix (General Mills)	1/12 pkg	150	3.0	34.0	300	na	0.0	na	0	0%
Apple cinnamon, prepared (SuperMoist)	1/12 cake	250	3.0	36.0	280	(mq)	10.0	2.0	55	37%
Banana										
dry mix (Duncan Hines)	1/12 pkg	190	2.0	36.0	280	na	4.0	11.0	0	19%
dry mix (Pillsbury Plus)	1/12 pkg	180	2.0	34.0	270	na	4.0	1.0	0	20%
Black forest										
cherry 'Bundt Ring Cake' dry mix (Pillsbury)	1/16 pkg	200	2.0	40.0	310	na	4.0	1.0	0	18%
mousse 'Tiarra' prepared (Duncan Hines)	1/12 cake	260	3.0	33.0	270	(mq)	13.0	(mq)	na	45%
Blueberry streusel, dry mix (Streusel Swirl)	1/16 pkg	210	2.0	39.0	190	na	5.0	1.0	0	22%
Boston cream, chocolate Eclair 'Bundt Ring Cake' dry mix (Pillsbury)	1/16 pkg	210	1.0	42.0	280	na	4.0	1.0	0	17%
Butter brickle, prepared (SuperMoist)	1/12 cake	250	3.0	38.0	280	(mq)	10.0	2.0	55	35%
Butter pecan, dry mix (SuperMoist)	1/12 pkg	180	1.0	35.0	300	na	4.0	na	0	20%
Butter recipe										
chocolate, dry mix (Pillsbury Plus)	1/12 pkg	170	2.0	32.0	330	na	4.0	1.0	0	21%
chocolate, dry mix (SuperMoist)	1/12 pkg	190	2.0	35.0	300	na	5.0	na	0	23%
dry mix (Pillsbury Plus)	1/12 pkg	170	2.0	35.0	270	na	3.0	1.0	0	15%
fudge, dry mix (Duncan Hines)	1/12 pkg	190	2.0	34.0	240	na	4.0	2.0	0	20%
golden, dry mix (Duncan Hines)	1/12 pkg	190	2.0	36.0	160	na	4.0	2.0	0	19%
yellow, dry mix (SuperMoist)	1/12 pkg	170	1.0	37.0	250	na	2.0	na	0	11%
Carrot										
dry mix (SuperMoist)	1/12 pkg	180	1.0	36.0	280	na	3.0	na	0	15%
'n' spice, dry mix (Pillsbury Plus)	1/12 pkg	180	2.0	33.0	280	na	5.0	1.0	0	24%
prepared (Dromedary)	1/12 cake	232	3.0	23.0	292	(mq)	15.0	(mq)	na	57%
prepared (Estee)	1/10 cake	100	1.0	18.0	65	(mq)	2.0	<1.0	0	19%
Cheesecake										
lemon 'No Bake' dry mix (Jell-O)	1 pkg	170	4.0	31.0	300	na	3.0	na	0	16%
lite 'No-Bake' prepared (Royal)	1/8 cake	210	5.0	23.0	380	(mq)	10.0	(mq)	na	45%
New York style 'No Bake' dry mix (Jell-O)	1 pkg	180	4.0	33.0	320	na	3.0	na	0	15%
'No Bake' dry mix (Jell-O)	1 pkg	160	3.0	30.0	250	na	4.0	na	0	21%
real 'No-Bake' prepared (Royal)	1/8 cake	280	5.0	31.0	370	(mq)	9.0	(mq)	na	36%

Food Name	Serving Size	Calories	Prot. gms	Carbs gms	Sod. mgs	Fiber gms	Fat gms	Sat. Fat gms	Chol. mgs	% Fat Cal.
Cherry, and cream 'Tiarra' prepared (Duncan Hines)	1/12 cake	250	4.0	34.0	265	(mq)	11.0	(mq)	na	39%
Cherry chip, dry mix (SuperMoist)	1/12 pkg	180	2.0	37.0	250	na	3.0	na	0	15%
Chocolate										
caramel 'Bundt Ring Cake' dry mix (Pillsbury)	1/16 pkg	220	2.0	43.0	350	na	5.0	1.0	5	20%
chocolate chip, dry mix (SuperMoist)	1/12 pkg	190	2.0	34.0	380	na	5.0	na	0	24%
dark, dry mix (Pillsbury Plus)	1/12 pkg	170	2.0	32.0	330	na	5.0	2.0	0	25%
devil's food, dry mix (Duncan Hines)	1/12 pkg	190	2.0	33.0	360	na	5.0	2.0	0	24%
devil's food, dry mix (Lovin' Lites)	1/12 pkg	160	3.0	32.0	370	na	2.0	1.0	0	11%
devil's food, dry mix (Pillsbury Plus)	1/12 pkg	170	2.0	32.0	330	na	4.0	1.0	0	21%
devil's food, dry mix (SuperMoist)	1/12 pkg	190	2.0	35.0	410	na	5.0	na	0	23%
devil's food 'Light' dry mix (SuperMoist)	1/12 pkg	180	2.0	36.0	330	na	3.0	na	0	15%
devil's food, prepared (Krusteaz)	1/12 cake	190	4.0	37.0	330	na	2.0	na	25	10%
devil's food 'Ultra Moist' prepared (Finast)	1/12 cake	250	3.0	33.0	360	(mq)	11.0	(mq)	na	41%
Dutch fudge, dark, dry mix (Duncan Hines)	1/12 pkg	190	2.0	33.0	455	na	5.0	2.0	0	24%
fudge, dry mix (SuperMoist)	1/12 pkg	180	2.0	35.0	430	na	4.0	na	0	20%
fudge 'Tunnel of Fudge' dry mix (Pillsbury)	1/16 pkg	210	2.0	42.0	330	na	4.0	1.0	0	17%
fudge marble, dry mix (Duncan Hines)	1/12 pkg	190	2.0	36.0	280	na	4.0	11.0	0	19%
fudge marble, dry mix (SuperMoist)	1/12 pkg	180	1.0	36.0	270	na	4.0	na	0	20%
fudge swirl, dry mix (Pillsbury Plus)	1/12 pkg	190	2.0	36.0	280	na	5.0	2.0	0	23%
German, dry mix (Pillsbury Plus)	1/12 pkg	170	2.0	33.0	270	na	4.0	1.0	0	21%
German, dry mix (SuperMoist)	1/12 pkg	180	2.0	35.0	400	na	4.0	na	0	20%
macaroon 'Bundt Ring Cake' dry mix (Pillsbury)	1/16 pkg	210	2.0	37.0	330	na	7.0	3.0	0	29%
milk, dry mix (SuperMoist)	1/12 pkg	190	2.0	34.0	320	na	5.0	na	0	24%
mousse, amaretto 'Tiarra' prepared (Duncan Hines)	1/12 cake	270	3.0	29.0	230	(mq)	16.0	(mq)	na	53%
mousse 'Bundt Ring Cake' dry mix (Pillsbury)	1/16 pkg	180	2.0	37.0	300	na	4.0	1.0	0	19%
mousse 'Tiarra' prepared (Duncan Hines)	1/12 cake	270	3.0	29.0	235	(mq)	16.0	(mq)	na	53%
prepared (Estee)	1/10 cake	100	1.0	18.0	100	(mq)	2.0	1.0	0	19%
pudding 'Classic Dessert' dry mix (Betty Crocker)	1/6 pkg	220	2.0	44.0	240	na	4.0	na	0	16%
Swiss, dry mix (Duncan Hines)	1/12 pkg	190	2.0	33.0	360	na	5.0	2.0	0	24%
Chocolate chip										
dry mix (Pillsbury Plus)	1/12 pkg	180	2.0	34.0	270	na	5.0	2.0	0	24%
dry mix (SuperMoist)	1/12 pkg	180	2.0	35.0	280	na	4.0	na	0	20%
Cinnamon streusel, dry mix (Streusel Swirl)	1/16 pkg	200	2.0	38.0	190	na	5.0	1.0	0	22%
Coffeecake										
apple cinnamon, prepared (Pillsbury)	1/8 cake	240	3.0	40.0	150	(mq)	7.0	(mq)	na	27%
'Flako' prepared (Quaker)	1 piece	156	2.1	27.1	279	.7	4.4	0.8	1	25%
prepared (Aunt Jemima)	1 piece	156	2.1	27.1	279	.7	4.4	0.8	1	25%
Lemon										
'Bundt Tunnel of Lemon' dry mix (Pillsbury)	1/16 pkg	210	1.0	44.0	270	na	4.0	1.0	0	17%
chiffon 'Classic Dessert' dry mix (Betty Crocker)	1/12 pkg	190	3.0	36.0	190	na	4.0	na	0	19%
dry mix (Pillsbury Plus)	1/12 pkg	170	2.0	34.0	260	na	3.0	1.0	0	16%
dry mix (SuperMoist)	1/12 pkg	180	1.0	36.0	260	na	4.0	na	0	20%
prepared (Estee)	1/10 cake	100	1.0	18.0	68	(mq)	2.0	<1.0	0	19%
pudding 'Classic Dessert' dry mix (Betty Crocker)	1/6 pkg	220	1.0	45.0	260	na	4.0	na	0	16%
supreme, dry mix (Duncan Hines)	1/12 pkg	190	2.0	36.0	280	na	4.0	11.0	0	19%
supreme, dry mix (Streusel Swirl)	1/16 pkg	200	2.0	37.0	290	na	6.0	1.0	0	26%
Orange, supreme, dry mix (Duncan Hines)	1/12 pkg	190	2.0	36.0	280	na	4.0	11.0	0	10%
Pineapple										
creme 'Bundt Ring Cake' dry mix (Pillsbury)	1/16 pkg	200	1.0	42.0	270	na	3.0	1.0	0	14%
supreme, dry mix (Duncan Hines)	1/12 pkg	190	2.0	36.0	280	na	4.0	11.0	0	19%
upside down 'Classic Dessert' dry mix (Betty Crocker)	1/9 pkg	240	1.0	43.0	200	na	7.0	na	0	26%
Plain, 'Funfetti' dry mix (Pillsbury Plus)	1/12 pkg	180	2.0	35.0	280	na	4.0	1.0	0	20%
Pound										
dry mix (Dromedary)	5 tbsp	130	1.0	20.0	140	(mq)	5.0	(mq)	na	35%

Food Name	Serving Size	Calories	Prot. gms	Carbs gms	Sod. mgs	Fiber gms	Fat gms	Sat. Fat gms	Chol. mgs	% Fat Cal.
golden 'Classic Dessert' dry mix (Betty Crocker)	1/12 pkg	190	1.0	28.0	150	na	8.0	na	0	38%
prepared (Estee)	1/8 cake	120	<1.5	23.0	85	na	2.5	1.0	0	19%
prepared (Martha White)	1/10 cake	120	2.0	19.0	110	(mq)	4.0	(mq)	8	30%
Rainbow chip, party cake, dry mix (SuperMoist)	1/12 pkg	180	2.0	35.0	300	na	4.0	na	0	20%
Sour cream										
chocolate, dry mix (SuperMoist)	1/12 pkg	180	2.0	35.0	410	na	4.0	na	0	20%
white, dry mix (SuperMoist)	1/12 pkg	180	2.0	36.0	280	na	3.0	na	0	15%
Spice										
dry mix (Duncan Hines)	1/12 pkg	190	2.0	36.0	280	na	4.0	11.0	0	19%
dry mix (SuperMoist)	1/12 pkg	180	1.0	36.0	300	na	4.0	na	0	20%
prepared (Estee)	1/8 cake	120	<1.0	23.0	80	na	3.0	1.0	0	22%
Strawberry										
dry mix (Pillsbury Plus)	1/12 pkg	180	2.0	35.0	290	na	4.0	1.0	0	20%
supreme, dry mix (Duncan Hines)	1/12 pkg	190	2.0	36.0	280	na	4.0	11.0	0	19%
Swirl, party cake, prepared (SuperMoist)	1/12 cake	260	3.0	36.0	280	na	11.0	na	55	39%
Vanilla										
French, dry mix (Duncan Hines)	1/12 pkg	190	2.0	36.0	280	na	4.0	11.0	0	19%
golden, dry mix (SuperMoist)	1/12 pkg	180	1.0	36.0	250	na	4.0	na	0	20%
golden, prepared (MicroRave)	1/6 cake	320	2.0	40.0	230	(mq)	17.0	5.0	35	48%
sunshine, dry mix (Pillsbury Plus)	1/12 pkg	180	2.0	34.0	280	na	5.0	2.0	0	24%
White										
dry mix (Duncan Hines)	1/12 pkg	190	2.0	36.0	250	na	4.0	2.0	0	19%
dry mix (Lovin' Lites)	1/12 pkg	170	2.0	35.0	300	na	2.0	<1.0	0	11%
dry mix (Lovin' Loaf)	1/12 pkg	170	2.0	35.0	300	na	2.0	1.0	0	11%
dry mix (Pillsbury Plus)	1/12 pkg	180	2.0	34.0	280	na	4.0	1.0	0	20%
dry mix (SuperMoist)	1/12 pkg	180	2.0	34.0	300	na	4.0	na	0	20%
'Light' dry mix (SuperMoist)	1/12 pkg	180	1.0	37.0	320	na	3.0	na	0	15%
'n fudge swirl, dry mix (Pillsbury Plus)	1/12 pkg	190	2.0	36.0	280	na	4.0	1.0	0	19%
prepared (Estee)	1/10 cake	100	1.0	18.0	68	(mq)	2.0	<1.0	0	19%
prepared (Krusteaz)	1/12 cake	190	3.0	37.0	280	na	3.0	na	2	14%
Yellow										
dry mix (Duncan Hines)	1/12 pkg	190	2.0	36.0	280	na	4.0	11.0	0	19%
dry mix (Pillsbury Plus)	1/12 pkg	180	2.0	34.0	280	na	5.0	2.0	0	24%
dry mix (SuperMoist)	1/12 pkg	180	1.0	36.0	280	na	4.0	na	0	20%
'Light' dry mix (SuperMoist)	1/12 pkg	180	1.0	37.0	290	na	3.0	na	0	15%
prepared (Krusteaz)	1/12 cake	200	3.0	36.0	330	.5	5.0	1.3	0	22%
prepared (Lovin' Loaf)	1/12 cake	180	3.0	35.0	300	na	3.0	1.0	35	15%
'Ultra Moist' prepared (Finast)	1/12 cake	240	3.0	34.0	280	(mq)	10.0	(mq)	na	38%
CALAMANSI PUNCH, 'Rain Forest' (Knudsen & Sons)	8 oz	115	<1.0	27.0	na	na	0.0	na	na	0%
CALAMARI. See SQUID, MIXED SPECIES.										
CALICO BASS. See SUNFISH.										
CALIFORNIA SHEEPSHEAD. See SHEEPSHEAD.										
CANADIAN BACON. See BACON, CANADIAN-STYLE.										
CANDLEFISH/eulachon										
dry-heat cooked	4 oz	141	25.6	0.0	87	0	3.5	0.7	102	24%
raw	1 lb	440	80.0	0.0	272	0	11.0	2.1	318	24%
raw	1 oz	27	5.0	0.0	17	0	0.7	0.1	20	24%
CANDY										
'Bridge Mix' (Brach's)	1 oz	140	2.0	17.0	30	na	7.0	na	na	45%
'Estee-ets' (Estee)	5 pieces	35	1.0	4.0	10	na	2.0	1.0	<1	47%
'Home Fashioned Favorites' (Russell Stover)	1.4 oz	170	1.0	27.0	60	1.0	7.0	4.5	5	36%
'Smoothie' 1.6 oz (Boyer)	2 pieces	250	5.0	24.0	na	na	15.0	(mq)	na	54%
'Smoothie' .5 oz (Boyer)	1 piece	75	2.5	12.5	na	na	7.5	(mq)	na	53%
'Smoothie' .275 oz (Boyer)	1 piece	38	1.3	6.3	na	na	3.8	(mq)	na	53%

Food Name	Serving Size	Calories	Prot. gms	Carbs gms	Sod. mgs	Fiber gms	Fat gms	Sat. Fat gms	Chol. mgs	% Fat Cal.
ALMOND										
'Almond Delights' (Russell Stover)	1.4 oz	210	3.0	22.0	55	1.0	12.0	5.0	10	52%
chocolate covered (Estee)	2 squares	60	1.0	4.5	10	(mq)	4.5	2.0	2	65%
chocolate covered (Featherweight)	1 section	90	1.0	6.0	20	(mq)	7.0	(mq)	na	69%
'Golden Almond Solitaires' chocolate covered (Hershey's)	1.5 oz	240	6.0	19.0	25	na	16.0	na	5	59%
'Golden Almond Solitaires' chocolate covered (Hershey's)	3 oz	455	9.9	40.0	46	>4.1 c	31.5	na	10	59%
'Jordan Almonds' candy coated (Brach's)	1 oz	120	2.0	23.0	0	(mq)	2.0	(mq)	na	15%
'Kisses w/Almonds' chocolate w/almonds, 1 oz (Hershey's)	6 pieces	160	3.0	14.0	25	na	10.0	na	na	57%
'M&M's' candy coated almonds (M&M/Mars)	1 oz	150	2.0	17.0	30	na	8.0	na	na	49%
'Solitaires' chocolate covered, 1.6 oz (Hershey's)	1/2 bar	260	6.0	20.0	25	(mq)	17.0	(mq)	5	60%
AMARETTO CHOCOLATE, 'Buffalo Ball' confection										
(Great Cakes)	1 ball	105	3.0	27.0	15	6.0	3.5	na	0	21%
BAR										
'Aero' milk chocolate, dark chocolate (Nestlé)	1 bar	210	0.0	20.0	20	na	12.0	na	na	57%
'Aero' milk chocolate, dark chocolate, bite size (Nestlé)	2 bars	85	0.0	10.0	10	na	5.0	na	na	53%
'Almond Crunch' date sweetened, carob (Carafection)	1 oz	139	2.0	17.0	26	na	7.0	na	na	45%
'Almond Joy' 1.76 oz (Hershey's)	1 bar	232	2.3	29.2	67	>.6 c	13.9	8.3	1	50%
'Almond Joy' miniatures (Hershey's)	2 pieces	120	1.0	14.0	35	na	7.0	na	na	51%
'Almond Joy' snack size (Hershey's)	1 bar	93	0.9	11.7	27	>.2 c	5.5	3.3	0	50%
'Alpine White' white chocolate w/almonds (Nestlé)	1 bar	197	3.5	17.6	4	na	12.9	6.7	26	58%
'Alpine White' white chocolate w/almonds, 2.2 oz (Nestlé)	1 bar	350	6.2	31.3	7	na	22.9	11.8	45	58%
'A-Ok' fruit juice sweetened (Natures Warehouse)	1 oz	130	3.2	16.5	32	na	6.2	na	na	42%
'Baby Ruth' chocolate w/peanuts (Nestlé)	1 bar	277	5.6	37.2	14	>2.0 c	13.3	6.8	133	41%
'Baby Ruth' chocolate w/peanuts, fun size (Nestlé)	1 bar	110	2.0	15.0	55	na	5.0	3.0	0	40%
'Bar None' 1.5 oz (Bar None)	1 bar	224	3.5	22.5	45	1.4	14.6	na	7	56%
'Bounty' dark chocolate (M&M/Mars)	1 oz	140	1.0	17.0	20	na	8.0	na	na	50%
'Bounty' milk chocolate (M&M/Mars)	1 oz	140	1.0	17.0	30	na	7.0	na	na	47%
'Brazil Nut Crunch' (Yogafection)	1 oz	180	2.0	17.0	70	0	10.0	9.0	5	54%
'Butterfinger' 2.16 oz (Nestlé)	1 bar	267	4.7	40.5	83	>.8 c	11.3	5.2	1	36%
'Butterfinger' snack size (Nestlé)	1 bar	92	1.6	13.9	29	>.3 c	3.9	1.8	0	36%
'Caramello' 5 oz (Cadbury)	1 bar	694	8.7	93.7	175	>2.1 c	35.9	na	34	44%
'Caramello' 1.6 oz (Cadbury)	1 bar	220	2.7	29.7	55	>.7 c	11.4	na	11	44%
carob (Caroby)	4 sections	150	4.0	13.0	55	(mq)	9.0	(mq)	na	54%
carob candy, plain, date sweetened (Carafection)	1 oz	139	2.0	17.0	26	na	7.0	na	na	45%
carob coated (Tiger's Milk)	1 bar	160	6.0	22.0	100	na	6.0	na	na	33%
carob coated 'Light' (Tiger's Milk)	1 bar	110	3.0	24.0	na	na	3.0	na	na	20%
'Cashew Coconut Crunch' carob candy (Carafection)	1 oz	139	2.0	17.0	26	na	7.0	na	na	45%
'Cashew Nut Crunch' (Yogafection)	1 oz	180	2.0	17.0	70	0	10.0	9.0	5	54%
'Chew!' nougat, chocolate coated, all flavors (Charleston)	1 oz	120	1.0	22.0	40	(mq)	3.0	(mq)	na	23%
chocolate tofu truffle w/pralines (Barat)	1 oz	170	4.0	12.0	10	(mq)	11.0	(mq)	0	61%
chocolate tofu w/almonds (Barat)	1 oz	170	3.0	13.0	10	(mq)	11.0	(mq)	0	61%
chocolate tofu w/almonds and raisins (Barat)	1 oz	160	3.0	14.0	10	(mq)	11.0	(mq)	0	59%
chocolate w/almonds, w/o sugar, extra thick (Fifty 50)	1 section	90	2.0	6.0	20	na	6.0	na	na	63%
chocolate w/coconut (Estee)	2 squares	60	1.0	5.0	15	na	4.0	2.5	5	60%
chocolate w/crisps and honey (Cadbury)	1 oz	150	2.0	18.0	40	(mq)	7.0	(mq)	na	44%
chocolate w/fruit and nuts (Cadbury)	1 oz	150	2.0	17.0	40	(mq)	8.0	(mq)	na	49%
chocolate w/fruit and nuts (Estee)	2 squares	60	1.0	4.5	10	(mq)	4.5	2.0	2	65%
chocolate w/fruit and nuts, w/o sugar, extra thick (Fifty 50)	1 section	80	1.0	6.0	20	na	5.0	na	na	62%
chocolate w/roasted almonds (Cadbury)	1 oz	150	3.0	15.0	40	(mq)	9.0	(mq)	na	53%
'Chunky' 1.4 oz (Nestlé)	1 bar	198	3.6	22.8	21	>1.7 c	11.7	9.3	4	50%
'Chunky' 1.25 oz (Nestlé)	1 bar	173	3.2	20.0	19	>1.5 c	10.2	8.1	4	50%
'Chunky' w/raisins, peanuts and cashews (Nestlé)	1.4 oz	170	4.0	21.0	20	na	12.0	na	na	52%
'Cookies 'N' Mint' mint chocolate, cookie pieces (Hershey's)	1 bar	220	3.0	26.0	75	na	12.0	na	na	48%

Food Name	Serving Size	Calories	Prot. gms	Carbs gms	Sod. mgs	Fiber gms	Fat gms	Sat. Fat gms	Chol. mgs	% Fat Cal.
'Crispy Crunch' carob candy, date sweetened										
(Carafection)	1 oz	139	2.0	17.0	26	na	7.0	na	na	45%
crunch (Estee)	2 squares	45	1.0	4.0	10	(mq)	3.0	2.0	2	57%
crunch, chocolate, w/o sugar, extra thick (Fifty 50)	1 section	70	1.0	6.0	20	na	5.0	na	na	62%
'Crunch' milk chocolate w/crisp rice, 1.4 oz (Nestlé)	1 bar	210	3.0	26.0	35	(mq)	10.0	(mq)	na	44%
'Crunch' milk chocolate w/crisp rice, fun size (Nestlé)	2 bars	100	1.0	13.0	15	na	5.0	3.0	na	45%
'Crunch' milk chocolate w/crisp rice, snack size (Nestlé)	1 bar	49	0.6	6.4	15	0	2.6	1.4	2	46%
'Dairy Milk' milk chocolate (Cadbury)	1 oz	150	2.0	17.0	45	(mq)	8.0	(mq)	(mq)	49%
dark chocolate, deluxe (Estee)	2 squares	50	<1.0	6.0	0	na	3.0	2.0	0	49%
'Dove' dark chocolate, miniatures (M&M/Mars)	4 pieces	130	1.0	14.0	0	na	8.0	na	na	55%
'Dove' milk chocolate, miniatures (M&M/Mars)	4 pieces	130	1.0	14.0	20	na	8.0	na	na	55%
'5th Avenue' 4.2 oz (Hershey's)	1 pkg	555	9.4	80.9	221	>1.1 c	25.2	na	5	39%
'5th Avenue' 2.1 oz (Hershey's)	1 bar	280	4.7	40.8	112	>.5 c	12.7	na	2	39%
French chocolate (Russell Stover)	1 bar	200	3.0	20.0	30	1.0	13.0	8.0	10	56%
French chocolate mint (Russell Stover)	1 bar	230	3.0	20.0	25	2.0	15.5	9.5	10	60%
'Golden Almond' chocolate w/almonds, 3 oz (Hershey's)	1 bar	466	8.9	41.3	54	>2.0 c	32.1	na	10	59%
'Golden III' 3.2 oz	1 bar	471	5.9	50.8	79	>4.9 c	30.0	na	17	54%
'Halvah' (Fantastic Foods)	1.5 oz	232	8.0	17.0	0	(mq)	10.0	(mq)	0	47%
'Hershey's Milk Chocolate Bar' (Hershey's)	1.55 oz	240	4.0	25.0	40	na	14.0	na	10	52%
'Hershey's Milk Chocolate Bar w/Almonds' (Hershey's)	1.45 oz	230	5.0	20.0	55	na	14.0	na	10	56%
'Kit Kat' chocolate covered wafer, 3.375 oz (Hershey's)	1 bar	490	6.4	59.4	97	.9	27.4	16.0	24	48%
'Kit Kat' chocolate covered wafer, 1.625 oz (Hershey's)	1 bar	235	3.1	28.5	46	.4	13.1	7.7	11	48%
'Kit Kat' chocolate covered wafer, snack size (Hershey's)	1.12 oz	170	2.0	20.0	40	na	9.0	na	na	48%
'Krackel' chocolate w/rice crisps, 2.6 oz (Hershey's)	1 bar	371	4.6	45.8	101	>.3 c	20.6	8.7	14	48%
'Krackel' chocolate w/rice crisps, 1.65 oz (Hershey's)	1 bar	236	2.9	29.1	64	>.2 c	13.1	5.6	9	48%
'Mars Almond, 1.76 oz (M&M/Mars)	1 bar	233	4.1	31.4	85	1.0	11.5	na	5	42%
milk chocolate (Estee)	2 squares	60	1.0	5.0	15	na	4.0	2.5	5	60%
milk chocolate, mini (Fifty 50)	4 pieces	90	2.0	6.0	20	na	6.0	na	na	63%
milk chocolate w/o sugar, extra thick (Fifty 50)	1 section	80	1.0	6.0	25	na	6.0	na	na	66%
'Milky Way' dark chocolate (M&M/Mars)	1.76 oz	220	1.0	36.0	115	na	8.0	na	na	33%
'Milky Way' milk chocolate, 2.1 oz (M&M/Mars)	1 bar	251	2.7	43.5	144	1.0	9.1	4.7	12	31%
'Milky Way' milk chocolate, minis (M&M/Mars)	1 piece	40	0.0	6.0	15	na	1.0	na	na	27%
'Milky Way' milk chocolate, snack size (M&M/Mars)	1 bar	75	0.8	13.1	43	.3	2.7	1.4	4	30%
mint (Estee)	2 squares	50	<1.0	6.0	0	na	3.0	2.0	0	49%
'Mint' date sweetened, carob candy (Carafection)	1 oz	139	2.0	17.0	26	na	7.0	na	na	45%
'Mint Honey Graham' carob coated (Carafection)	1 oz	139	2.0	17.0	26	na	7.0	na	na	45%
'Mounds' chocolate covered coconut, 1.9 oz (Hershey's)	1 pkg	195	1.9	31.3	68	1.7	11.7	6.2	0	44%
'Mounds' chocolate covered coconut, minis (Hershey's)	2 pieces	110	1.0	13.0	30	na	6.0	na	na	49%
'Mounds' chocolate covered coconut, snack size										
(Hershey's)	1 bar	72	0.7	11.6	25	.6	4.3	2.3	0	44%
'Mr. GoodBar' milk chocolate w/peanuts, 2.8 oz										
(Hershey's)	1 bar	406	9.9	40.5	27	3.4	25.5	14.3	16	53%
'Mr. GoodBar' milk chocolate w/peanuts, 1.75 oz										
(Hershey's)	1 bar	257	6.3	25.6	17	2.2	16.1	9.0	10	53%
'Munch' (M&M/Mars)	1.42 oz	220	6.0	19.0	110	na	14.0	na	na	56%
'My O My' fruit juice sweetened (Natures Warehouse)	1 oz	103	2.2	20.5	42	na	1.4	na	na	12%
'No How' peanut butter, fruit juice sweetened										
(Natures Warehouse)	1 oz	140	6.0	11.0	48	na	10.0	na	na	57%
'Non Stop' fruit juice sweetened (Natures Warehouse)	1 oz	122	2.0	18.2	48	na	5.0	na	na	36%
'Nut Wit' carob, caramel, and peanuts										
(Natures Warehouse)	1 oz	135	3.2	16.5	32	na	6.3	na	na	42%
'Oh Henry!' chocolate covered caramel w/peanuts, 2 oz										
(Nestlé)	1 bar	246	6.2	36.9	5	>1.5 c	9.6	3.8	135	33%
'100 Grand' 1.5 oz (Nestlé)	1 bar	195	1.5	30.9	4	>.1 c	8.5	na	80	37%

Food Name	Serving Size	Calories	Prot. gms	Carbs gms	Sod. mgs	Fiber gms	Fat gms	Sat. Fat gms	Chol. mgs	% Fat Cal.
'Original' (Cocofection)	1 oz	155	2.0	15.0	23	na	10.0	na	na	57%
'Original Honey Graham' carob coated (Carafection)	1 oz	139	2.0	17.0	26	na	7.0	na	na	45%
'Pay Day' (Pay Day)	1.85 oz	250	9.0	28.0	200	na	12.0	na	na	42%
peanut butter (Russell Stover)	1 bar	290	7.0	22.0	130	3.0	19.0	6.0	5	60%
peanut butter, carob coated (Tiger's Milk)	1 bar	160	6.0	20.0	105	na	7.0	na	na	38%
peanut butter, carob coated 'Light' (Tiger's Milk)	1 bar	110	3.0	24.0	25	4.0	3.0	na	na	20%
peanut butter and honey, carob coated (Tiger's Milk)	1 bar	160	6.0	23.0	90	na	5.0	na	na	28%
'Peanut Crunch' carob candy, date sweetened (Carafection)	1 oz	139	2.0	17.0	26	na	7.0	na	na	45%
'Protein Blast' high-energy, chocolate (Weider)	1 bar	270	18.0	40.0	110	4.0	6.0	na	na	19%
'Skor' toffee, 1.4 oz (Hershey's)	1 bar	211	1.8	22.0	92	>.1 c	13.8	na	24	57%
'Sky Bar' (Necco)	1.5 oz	196	1.9	31.5	57	0	7.1	(mq)	na	32%
'Snickers' 2.16 oz (M&M/Mars)	1 bar	278	5.9	36.8	163	1.8	13.6	7.3	7	42%
'Snickers,' minis (M&M/Mars)	1 piece	45	1.0	5.0	25	na	2.0	na	na	43%
'Snickers' snack size (M&M/Mars)	1 bar	68	1.4	9.0	40	.5	3.3	1.8	2	42%
'Soft'n Crunchy Bar' 1 3/16 oz (Heath)	2 pieces	190	1.0	19.0	85	na	12.0	(mq)	na	57%
'Special Dark' sweet chocolate bar, 2.8 oz (Hershey's)	1 bar	376	3.7	48.7	8	4.3	23.9	na	0	51%
'Special Dark' sweet chocolate bar, 1.45 oz (Hershey's)	1 bar	195	1.9	25.3	4	2.3	12.4	na	0	51%
'Symphony' milk chocolate, 2.4 oz (Hershey's)	1 bar	355	5.3	38.6	58	>.3 c	22.0	na	19	53%
'Symphony' milk chocolate, 1.4 oz (Hershey's)	1 bar	209	3.1	22.7	34	>.2 c	13.0	na	11	53%
'Symphony' milk chocolate w/almonds and toffee chips (Hershey's)	1.4 oz	220	4.0	20.0	40	na	14.0	na	na	57%
'3 Musketeers' 2.13 oz (M&M/Mars)	1 bar	250	1.9	46.1	116	1.0	7.7	3.9	7	27%
'3 Musketeers' snack size (M&M/Mars)	1 bar	75	0.6	13.8	35	.3	2.3	1.2	2	26%
'Twix' caramel, 2.0 oz (M&M/Mars)	1 pkg	272	3.1	37.5	115	1.0	13.4	na	5	43%
'Twix' cookies-n-creme (M&M/Mars)	1 bar	120	2.0	13.0	50	na	7.0	na	na	51%
'Twix' peanut butter, 1.77 oz (M&M/Mars)	1 pkg	253	5.4	28.5	148	1.6	14.5	na	6	49%
'Whatchamacallit' 1.8 oz (Hershey's)	1 bar	257	4.7	30.0	116	1.5	13.2	na	11	46%
BUBBLE GUM										
(Beechies) candy coated	1 piece	6	0.0	2.0	0	0	0.0	0.0	0	0%
(Bubble Yum)										
bananaberry split	1 piece	25	0.0	7.0	0	na	0.0	na	na	0%
checkermint	1 piece	25	0.0	7.0	0	na	0.0	na	na	0%
cherry	1 piece	25	0.0	7.0	0	na	0.0	na	na	0%
fruit	1 piece	25	0.0	7.0	0	na	0.0	na	na	0%
grape	1 piece	25	0.0	7.0	0	na	0.0	na	na	0%
Hawaiian punch	1 piece	25	0.0	7.0	0	na	0.0	na	na	0%
luscious lime	1 piece	25	0.0	7.0	0	na	0.0	na	na	0%
strawberry stripe	1 piece	25	0.0	7.0	0	na	0.0	na	na	0%
sugarless, fruit	1 piece	20	0.0	5.0	0	na	0.0	na	na	0%
sugarless, grape	1 piece	20	0.0	5.0	0	na	0.0	na	na	0%
sugarless, peppermint	1 piece	20	0.0	5.0	0	na	0.0	na	na	0%
sugarless, strawberry	1 piece	20	0.0	5.0	0	na	0.0	na	na	0%
3-flavor, grape, cherry and fruit	1 piece	25	0.0	7.0	0	na	0.0	na	na	0%
wet 'n wild watermelon	1 piece	25	0.0	7.0	0	na	0.0	na	na	0%
(Bubblicious)										
	1 piece	25	tr	6.2	0	0	tr	0.0	tr	0%
'Sugarless'	1 piece	5	tr	1.3	0	0	tr	0.0	tr	0%
(Care Free) sugarless										
fruit	1 piece	10	0.0	2.0	0	na	0.0	na	na	0%
wild cherry	1 piece	10	0.0	2.0	0	na	0.0	na	na	0%
wintergreen	1 piece	10	0.0	2.0	0	na	0.0	na	na	0%
(Chiclets)										
candy coated	1 piece	6	tr	1.5	0	0	tr	0.0	tr	0%

Food Name	Serving Size	Calories	Prot. gms	Carbs gms	Sod. mgs	Fiber gms	Fat gms	Sat. Fat gms	Chol. mgs	% Fat Cal.
'Tiny' candy coated	1 pkg	8	tr	<.1	0	0	tr	0.0	tr	0%
(Clorets) candy coated	1 piece	6	tr	1.5	0	0	tr	0.0	tr	0%
(Extra)										
classic	1 piece	6	(mq)	(mq)	0	na	(mq)	na	(mq)	0%
original	1 piece	7	(mq)	(mq)	0	na	(mq)	na	(mq)	0%
(Fruit Stripe)										
cherry	1 piece	8	0.0	2.0	0	na	0.0	na	na	0%
fruit	1 piece	8	0.0	2.0	0	na	0.0	na	na	0%
grape	1 piece	8	0.0	2.0	0	na	0.0	na	na	0%
lemon	1 piece	8	0.0	2.0	0	na	0.0	na	na	0%
(Hubba Bubba)										
all flavors except cola	1 piece	23	0.0	5.8	0	0	0.0	0.0	0	0%
cola	1 piece	23	0.0	5.3	0	0	0.0	0.0	0	0%
'Sugar-free' grape	1 piece	13	0.0	(mq)	0	0	0.0	0.0	0	0%
sugar-free, original	1 piece	14	0.0	(mq)	0	0	0.0	0.0	0	0%
BUTTERSCOTCH, squares *(Russell Stover)*	1.4 oz	180	1.0	29.0	65	1.0	6.5	5.0	5	33%
CARAMEL										
(Allen Wertz)	1 piece	37	0.0	6.0	2	na	2.0	na	1	43%
(Featherweight)	1 piece	30	0.0	5.0	10	(tr)	1.0	na	0	31%
(Kraft)	1 piece	30	0.0	6.0	25	(tr)	1.0	0.0	0	27%
butter cream, squares *(Russell Stover)*	1.4 oz	170	1.0	26.0	95	1.0	7.5	5.5	10	39%
chocolate *(Estee)*	1 piece	20	<1.0	3.0	10	(tr)	1.0	<1.0	0	36%
chocolate coated *(Pom Poms)*	1 oz	100	1.0	15.0	70	(mq)	3.0	(mq)	na	30%
marshmallow, milk chocolate, squares *(Russell Stover)*	1.4 oz	190	2.0	25.0	85	5.0	10.0	5.0	na	46%
milk chocolate coated, approx 1.93 oz *(Rolo)*	8 pieces	270	3.0	37.0	110	(tr)	12.0	(mq)	15	40%
'Milk Maid' *(Brach's)*	1 oz	110	1.0	22.0	70	(tr)	2.0	(mq)	na	16%
'Milk Maid' chocolate *(Brach's)*	1 oz	110	1.0	20.0	55	(tr)	3.0	(mq)	na	24%
'Nip' *(Pearson)*	1 oz	120	1.0	23.0	70	na	3.0	na	na	22%
nougat swirl *(Allen Wertz)*	1 piece	32	0.0	6.0	2	na	1.0	na	1	27%
pop *(Sugar Daddy)*	1 3/8 oz	150	1.0	33.0	85	(tr)	1.0	na	na	6%
'Regular' 1 5/8 oz *(Sugar Babies)*	1 pkg	180	1.0	40.0	85	(tr)	2.0	(mq)	na	10%
'Rolos' milk chocolate covered *(Hershey's)*	1.93 oz	270	3.0	37.0	110	na	12.0	na	15	40%
'Tidbits' 1 5/8 oz *(Sugar Babies)*	1 pkg	180	1.0	40.0	85	(tr)	2.0	(mq)	na	10%
vanilla *(Estee)*	1 piece	20	<1.0	3.0	10	(tr)	1.0	<1.0	0	36%
CHERRY										
'Cherry Cordials' *(Russell Stover)*	1.4 oz	170	1.0	25.0	25	2.0	7.5	4.5	5	39%
chocolate cream *(Brach's)*	1 oz	110	1.0	21.0	20	(mq)	2.0	(mq)	na	17%
dark chocolate coated *(Brach's)*	1 oz	110	1.0	22.0	20	(mq)	2.0	(mq)	na	16%
'Nibs' *(Y&S)*	1 oz	106	0.8	26.2	67	0	0.7	na	0	6%
squares *(Russell Stover)*	1.4 oz	160	1.0	28.0	40	1.0	5.5	4.5	na	30%
'Villa' milk chocolate covered *(Brach's)*	1 oz	110	1.0	22.0	20	na	2.0	na	na	16%
CHEWING GUM										
(Beech-Nut)										
cinnamon	1 piece	10	0.0	2.0	0	na	0.0	na	na	0%
fruit	1 piece	10	0.0	2.0	0	na	0.0	na	na	0%
peppermint	1 piece	10	0.0	2.0	0	na	0.0	na	na	0%
spearmint	1 piece	10	0.0	2.0	0	na	0.0	na	na	0%
(Brach's) 'Gumdinger' balls, all flavors	1 oz	110	0.0	24.0	5	0	2.0	na	0	16%
(Care Free) sugarless										
cinnamon	1 piece	8	0.0	2.0	0	na	0.0	na	na	0%
peppermint	1 piece	8	0.0	2.0	0	na	0.0	na	na	0%
spearmint	1 piece	8	0.0	2.0	0	na	0.0	na	na	0%
(Chewels) all flavors	1 piece	8	tr	2.0	0	0	tr	0.0	tr	0%
(Clorets) stick, all flavors	1 piece	9	tr	2.3	0	0	tr	0.0	tr	0%

Food Name	Serving Size	Calories	Prot. gms	Carbs gms	Sod. mgs	Fiber gms	Fat gms	Sat. Fat gms	Chol. mgs	% Fat Cal.
(Dentyne)										
all flavors	1 piece	6	tr	1.5	0	0	tr	0.0	tr	0%
'Sugarless' all flavors	1 piece	5	tr	1.1	0	0	tr	0.0	tr	0%
(Estee) gumdrops	4 pieces	25	0.0	6.0	0	na	0.0	0.0	0	0%
(Extra)										
cinnamon	1 stick	8	(mq)	(mq)	0	na	(mq)	na	(mq)	0%
peppermint	1 stick	8	(mq)	(mq)	0	na	(mq)	na	(mq)	0%
spearmint	1 stick	8	(mq)	(mq)	0	na	(mq)	na	(mq)	0%
winter fresh	1 stick	8	(mq)	(mq)	0	na	(mq)	na	(mq)	0%
(Freedent)										
cinnamon	1 stick	10	(mq)	2.0	0	na	(mq)	na	(mq)	0%
peppermint	1 stick	10	(mq)	2.0	0	na	(mq)	na	(mq)	0%
spearmint	1 stick	10	(mq)	2.0	0	na	(mq)	na	(mq)	0%
(Freshen-Up) all flavors	1 piece	13	tr	3.1	0	0	tr	0.0	tr	0%
(Fruit Stripe)										
cherry	1 piece	10	0.0	2.0	0	na	0.0	na	na	0%
lemon	1 piece	10	0.0	2.0	0	na	0.0	na	na	0%
lime	1 piece	10	0.0	2.0	0	na	0.0	na	na	0%
orange	1 piece	10	0.0	2.0	0	na	0.0	na	na	0%
(Sticklets) all flavors	1 piece	7	tr	1.9	0	0	tr	0.0	tr	0%
(Wrigley's)										
'Big Red'	1 piece	10	0.0	2.3	0	0	0.0	0.0	0	0%
'Doublemint'	1 piece	10	0.0	2.3	0	0	0.0	0.0	0	0%
'Juicy Fruit'	1 piece	10	0.0	2.3	0	0	0.0	0.0	0	0%
'Spearmint'	1 piece	10	0.0	2.3	0	0	0.0	0.0	0	0%
CHOCOLATE										
assorted, wrapped, 1-lb bag *(Brach's)*	1 oz	110	0.0	23.0	25	(mq)	2.0	(mq)	na	16%
'Bits' tofu pastilles *(Barat)*	.75 oz	120	2.0	11.0	10	(mq)	8.0	(mq)	0	58%
chewy roll *(Tootsie Roll)*	1 oz	112	0.3	22.8	6	(tr)	2.5	0.6	tr	20%
'Choc'Oh's' *(Saco Foods)*	1.5 oz	111	1.1	13.8	14	na	6.6	2.4	0	50%
chunks *(Saco Foods)*	3.5 oz	466	4.4	66.8	26	na	26.4	14.9	0	46%
coated, creme center *(Spangler)*	1 piece	80	<1.0	15.0	40	(mq)	2.0	(mq)	0	22%
coated, creme center caramel, w/nuts *(Spangler)*	1 piece	100	2.0	11.0	30	(mq)	6.0	(mq)	0	51%
coated, creme center cherry, w/nuts *(Spangler)*	1 piece	110	2.0	12.0	20	(mq)	5.0	(mq)	0	45%
coated, creme center fudge, w/nuts *(Spangler)*	1 piece	140	2.0	17.0	25	(mq)	6.0	(mq)	0	42%
coated, creme center fudge, w/pecans *(Spangler)*	1 piece	140	1.0	18.0	40	(mq)	7.0	(mq)	0	45%
coated, creme center maple, w/nuts *(Spangler)*	1 piece	110	2.0	12.0	15	(mq)	5.0	(mq)	0	45%
coated, creme center vanilla, w/nuts *(Spangler)*	1 piece	110	2.0	13.0	20	(mq)	5.0	(mq)	0	43%
cream *(Callard & Bowser)*	1 oz	120	0.3	22.3	na	(mq)	3.7	(tr)	na	27%
creamy milk, w/almonds and toffee chips *(Hershey's)*	.75 oz	280	5.0	26.0	50	(mq)	17.0	(mq)	(mq)	55%
crunch *(Featherweight)*	1 section	80	1.0	7.0	20	(mq)	6.0	(mq)	na	63%
'Gift Box' dark and milk mix *(Russell Stover)*	1.4 oz	180	2.0	26.0	45	na	8.5	4.5	5	41%
'Gourmet' assortment *(Allen Wertz)*	11.9 grams	55	1.0	9.0	13	na	2.0	na	1	31%
'Jots' *(Brach's)*	1 oz	130	1.0	21.0	30	(mq)	5.0	(mq)	na	34%
'Kisses' *(Hershey's)*	6 pieces	150	2.0	16.0	25	na	9.0	na	5	53%
'M&M's' plain *(M&M/Mars)*	10 pieces	33	0.4	4.8	7	.2	1.5	na	1	39%
'M&M'o' plain, 1.60 oz *(M&M/Mars)*	1 pkg	228	3.0	32.7	49	1.5	10.7	na	7	40%
'Malted Milk Balls' milk coated *(Brach's)*	1 oz	130	1.0	21.0	40	(mq)	5.0	(mq)	(mq)	34%
malted milk balls, milk coated *(Whoppers)*	1 oz	136	<1.0	20.0	na	na	6.0	na	na	39%
milk *(Featherweight)*	1 section	80	1.0	7.0	20	(mq)	6.0	(mq)	na	63%
milk, assortment *(Russell Stover)*	1.4 oz	190	2.0	27.0	50	na	8.5	5.0	5	40%
'Passionettes' tofu *(Barat)*	1 piece	70	1.0	6.0	5	(mq)	5.0	(mq)	0	62%
'Stars' *(Brach's)*	1 oz	150	2.0	17.0	30	(mq)	8.0	(mq)	na	49%
'Stars' approx 13 pieces *(Nabisco)*	1 oz	160	2.0	19.0	35	(mq)	8.0	(mq)	na	46%

Food Name	Serving Size	Calories	Prot. gms	Carbs gms	Sod. mgs	Fiber gms	Fat gms	Sat. Fat gms	Chol. mgs	% Fat Cal.
trail mix, premium *(Cocofection)*	1 oz	130	4.0	13.0	14	na	9.0	na	na	54%
COCONUT										
'Macaroo' chocolate coated *(Sunbelt)*	2 oz	288	3.0	33.0	75	(mq)	16.0	(mq)	<1	50%
Neapolitan *(Brach's)*	1 oz	120	1.0	24.0	40	(mq)	2.0	(mq)	na	15%
COFFEE										
(Brach's)	1 oz	120	0.0	25.0	35	0	2.0	(mq)	na	15%
'Coffee Time' *(Allen Wertz)*	1 piece	20	0.0	4.0	2	na	1.0	na	1	36%
'Coffee Time' assorted *(Allen Wertz)*	1 piece	28	0.0	5.0	2	na	1.0	na	1	31%
'Coffee Time' decaffeinated *(Allen Wertz)*	1 piece	20	0.0	4.0	2	na	1.0	na	1	36%
'Nip' *(Pearson)*	1 oz	120	1.0	23.0	70	na	3.0	na	na	22%
FONDANT, candy corn	1 cup	728	0.2	179.2	424	0	4.0	1.0	0	5%
FRUIT										
(Bonkers!) chews, all flavors	1 piece	20	0.0	5.0	0	0	0.0	0.0	0	0%
(Brach's)										
orange sticks, chocolate coated	1 oz	110	1.0	23.0	25	(mq)	2.0	(mq)	na	16%
'Orangettes'	1 oz	100	0.0	24.0	20	0	0.0	0.0	0	0%
(Featherweight)										
berry patch	1 piece	12	0.0	3.0	0	0	0.0	0.0	0	0%
drops, all flavors	.33 oz	30	0.0	8.0	15	0	0.0	0.0	0	0%
orchard	1 piece	12	0.0	3.0	0	0	0.0	0.0	0	0%
tropical blend	1 piece	12	0.0	3.0	0	0	0.0	0.0	0	0%
(Glenny's) 'Drops'										
black cherry	1 drop	6	<1.0	1.0	<1	na	<1.0	na	na	<53%
Mandarin orange	1 drop	6	<1.0	1.0	<1	na	<1.0	na	na	<53%
mixed fruit	1 drop	6	<1.0	1.0	<1	na	<1.0	na	na	<53%
twist of lemon	1 drop	6	<1.0	1.0	<1	na	<1.0	na	na	<53%
(Jujyfruits)	11 pieces	100	<1.0	25.0	0	0	<1.0	0.0	0	<8%
(Rascals) chews, all flavors	1 piece	4	tr	1.0	0	0	tr	0.0	tr	0%
(Russell Stover) lemon squares	1.4 oz	160	1.0	27.0	35	2.0	5.5	4.5	na	31%
'Skittles' *(M&M/Mars)*										
candy coated, bite size	1 oz	120	0.0	26.0	15	na	1.0	na	na	8%
candy coated, bite size, 2.3 oz	1 pkg	255	0.2	62.4	30	0	2.0	na	0	7%
'Starburst' *(M&M/Mars)*										
original fruit chews	2 oz	240	0.0	48.0	30	na	5.0	na	na	19%
tropical fruit chews	2 oz	240	0.0	48.0	30	na	5.0	na	na	19%
(Soda-Licious) all flavors	1 pouch	100	<1.0	22.0	20	na	1.0	na	na	9%
(SweeTARTS) chewy	1 oz	113	0.0	25.0	na	na	1.0	na	na	8%
'Twizzlers' *(Y&S)*										
strawberry sticks, 5 oz	1 pkg	525	4.7	131.6	393	>.1 c	2.3	na	0	4%
strawberry sticks, 2.5 oz	1 pkg	263	2.3	65.8	197	>.1 c	1.1	na	0	4%
FUDGE										
chocolate, w/walnuts *(Woodys)*	1 oz	120	2.0	18.0	25	(mq)	4.0	2.0	5	31%
'Fudgies' *(Kraft)*	1 piece	35	0.0	6.0	25	(mq)	1.0	0.0	0	27%
maple walnut *(Woodys)*	1 oz	120	1.0	19.0	25	(mq)	4.0	1.0	5	31%
mint, w/walnuts *(Woodys)*	1 oz	120	2.0	18.0	25	(mq)	4.0	2.0	5	31%
w/walnuts *(Woodys)*	1 oz	120	2.0	18.0	25	(mq)	4.0	2.0	5	31%
HARD CANDY										
(Brach's)										
'Cut Rock'	1 oz	110	0.0	27.0	10	0	0.0	0.0	0	0%
'Disks' butterscotch	1 oz	110	0.0	27.0	220	(tr)	0.0	0.0	na	0%
'Disks' cinnamon	1 oz	110	0.0	27.0	15	0	0.0	0.0	0	0%
filled, assorted	1 oz	110	0.0	27.0	15	tr	0.0	0.0	0	0%
'Imperials' cinnamon	1 oz	110	0.0	27.0	5	0	0.0	0.0	0	0%
lemon drops	1 oz	110	0.0	27.0	5	0	0.0	0.0	0	0%

Food Name	Serving Size	Calories	Prot. gms	Carbs gms	Sod. mgs	Fiber gms	Fat gms	Sat. Fat gms	Chol. mgs	% Fat Cal.
raspberry filled	1 oz	110	0.0	27.0	15	(tr)	0.0	0.0	0	0%
ribbon, crimp	1 oz	110	0.0	27.0	15	0	0.0	0.0	0	0%
'Royals'	1 oz	100	1.0	20.0	60	(mq)	2.0	(mq)	na	18%
sour balls	1 oz	110	0.0	27.0	15	0	0.0	0.0	0	0%
'Spicettes'	1 oz	100	0.0	26.0	15	0	0.0	0.0	0	0%
(Breath Savers)										
cores, mint-cinnamon	1 piece	2	0.0	<1.0	0	na	0.0	na	0	0%
cores, peppermint	1 piece	2	0.0	<1.0	0	na	0.0	na	0	0%
cores, spearmint	1 piece	2	0.0	<1.0	0	na	0.0	na	0	0%
cores, wintergreen	1 piece	2	0.0	<1.0	0	na	0.0	na	0	0%
mint-cinnamon	1 piece	8	0.0	2.0	0	na	0.0	na	0	0%
peppermint	1 piece	8	0.0	2.0	0	na	0.0	na	0	0%
spearmint	1 piece	8	0.0	2.0	0	na	0.0	na	0	0%
wintergreen	1 piece	8	0.0	2.0	0	na	0.0	na	0	0%
(Callard & Bowser) butterscotch	1 oz	115	0.0	25.2	na	(tr)	1.9	na	na	15%
(Ce De) 'Smarties'	1 roll	25	0.0	6.0	0	na	0.0	na	na	0%
(Certs)										
sugar-free, mini	1 piece	1	tr	0.4	tr	0	tr	0.0	0	0%
sugar-free, mints	1 piece	6	tr	1.6	0	0	tr	0.0	tr	0%
(Clorets)										
clear mint	1 piece	8	tr	2.1	0	0	tr	0.0	tr	0%
pressed mints	1 piece	6	tr	1.6	0	0	tr	0.0	tr	0%
(Estee)	2 pieces	25	0.0	6.0	0	na	0.0	0.0	0	0%
(Featherweight)										
butterscotch	1 piece	25	0.0	6.0	25	tr	0.0	0.0	0	0%
'Sweet Pretenders' tropical blend	1 piece	12	0.0	3.0	0	na	0.0	na	na	0%
(Fruit Juicers)										
citrus fruits	1 piece	8	0.0	2.0	0	na	0.0	na	0	0%
fruit punch	1 piece	8	0.0	2.0	0	na	0.0	na	0	0%
grape	1 piece	8	0.0	2.0	0	na	0.0	na	0	0%
mixed berries	1 piece	8	0.0	2.0	0	na	0.0	na	0	0%
strawberry	1 piece	8	0.0	2.0	0	na	0.0	na	0	0%
(Glenny's)										
fruit	1 piece	19	<1.0	4.0	<1	na	<1.0	na	na	<31%
peppermint	1 piece	19	<1.0	4.0	<1	na	<1.0	na	na	<31%
(Jolly Joes)	1 piece	9	<.1	2.1	1	0	tr	0.0	0	0%
(Jolly Rancher)										
apple	1 piece	23	na	6.0	5	na	0.0	na	na	0%
butterscotch	1 piece	25	na	6.0	37	na	<1.0	na	chol.	<27%
cherry	1 piece	23	na	6.0	3	na	0.0	na	na	0%
fire cinnamon	1 piece	23	na	6.0	5	na	0.0	na	na	0%
fruit punch	1 piece	23	na	6.0	5	na	0.0	na	na	0%
grape	1 piece	23	na	6.0	5	na	0.0	na	na	0%
lemon	1 piece	23	na	6.0	5	na	0.0	na	na	0%
orange	1 piece	23	na	6.0	4	na	0.0	na	na	0%
peach	1 piece	23	na	6.0	3	na	0.0	na	na	0%
poppermint	1 piece	23	na	6.0	3	na	0.0	na	na	0%
pink lemonade	1 piece	23	na	6.0	5	na	0.0	na	na	0%
raspberry	1 piece	23	na	6.0	5	na	0.0	na	na	0%
strawberry	1 piece	23	na	6.0	3	na	0.0	na	na	0%
watermelon	1 piece	23	na	6.0	5	na	0.0	na	na	0%
(Jurassic Park)										
'Raptor Bites' wild cherry	13 pieces	60	0.0	15.0	0	na	0.0	0.0	na	0%
'Spitters' tropical flavors	13 pieces	60	0.0	15.0	0	na	0.0	0.0	na	0%

Food Name	Serving Size	Calories	Prot. gms	Carbs gms	Sod. mgs	Fiber gms	Fat gms	Sat. Fat gms	Chol. mgs	% Fat Cal.
(Life Savers)										
butter creme mint	1 piece	8	0.0	2.0	5	0	0.0	0.0	0	0%
butter rum	1 piece	8	0.0	2.0	10	0	0.0	0.0	0	0%
butterscotch	1 piece	8	0.0	2.0	10	0	0.0	0.0	0	0%
'Cin-O-Mon'	1 piece	8	0.0	2.0	0	0	0.0	0.0	0	0%
'Cryst-O-Mint'	1 piece	8	0.0	2.0	0	na	0.0	na	0	0%
fancy fruits	1 piece	8	0.0	2.0	0	na	0.0	na	0	0%
five flavor	1 piece	8	0.0	2.0	0	na	0.0	na	0	0%
holes, butter rum	1 piece	2	0.0	<1.0	0	na	0.0	na	na	0%
holes, five flavor	1 piece	2	0.0	<1.0	0	na	0.0	na	na	0%
holes, pepomint	1 piece	2	0.0	<1.0	0	na	0.0	na	na	0%
candy coated, bite size	10 pieces	43	0.0	10.6	5	0	0.3	na	0	6%
holes, sunshine fruits	1 piece	2	0.0	<1.0	0	na	0.0	na	na	0%
holes, tangerine	1 piece	2	0.0	<1.0	0	na	0.0	na	na	0%
holes, 'Wint-O-Green'	1 piece	2	0.0	<1.0	0	na	0.0	na	na	0%
'Pep-O-Mint'	1 piece	8	0.0	2.0	0	na	0.0	na	0	0%
root beer	1 piece	8	0.0	2.0	0	0	0.0	0.0	0	0%
'Spear-O-Mint'	1 piece	8	0.0	2.0	0	na	0.0	na	0	0%
sunshine fruits	1 piece	8	0.0	2.0	0	na	0.0	na	0	0%
tropical fruits	1 piece	8	0.0	2.0	0	na	0.0	na	0	0%
wild cherry	1 piece	8	0.0	2.0	0	na	0.0	na	0	0%
'Wint-O-Green'	1 piece	8	0.0	2.0	0	na	0.0	na	0	0%
(Mike & Ike)	1 piece	9	<.1	2.1	1	0	tr	0.0	0	0%
(Pearson) 'Nip' butter rum	1 oz	120	1.0	24.0	70	na	3.0	na	na	21%
(Russell Stover) sugar-free, mix	3 pieces	70	0.0	18.0	5	na	0.0	0.0	na	0%
(Spree) fruit	1 oz	110	0.0	26.0	na	na	0.0	na	na	0%
(SweeTARTS) fruit	1 oz	110	0.0	26.0	na	na	0.0	na	na	0%
HOLIDAY										
assorted, chocolate *(Brach's)*	1 oz	110	0.0	23.0	25	(mq)	2.0	(mq)	na	16%
autumn leaves *(Brach's)*	1 oz	100	0.0	26.0	15	0	0.0	(mq)	0	0%
bell, chocolate, in foil *(Brach's)*	1 oz	150	2.0	17.0	25	(mq)	8.0	(mq)	na	49%
holiday mints *(Brach's)*	1 oz	110	0.0	26.0	0	0	1.0	na	0	8%
holiday mix *(Brach's)*	1 oz	110	0.0	27.0	10	0	0.0	0.0	0	0%
Christmas										
candy cane *(Brach's)*	1 oz	110	0.0	27.0	10	0	0.0	0.0	0	0%
candy cane *(Spangler)*	1 piece	60	<1.0	14.0	0	0	<1.0	0.0	0	<13%
jellies *(Brach's)*	1 oz	100	0.0	24.0	10	0	0.0	0.0	0	0%
jellies, snowbase *(Brach's)*	1 oz	100	0.0	24.0	5	0	0.0	0.0	0	0%
'Jots' *(Brach's)*	1 oz	130	1.0	21.0	30	na	5.0	(mq)	na	34%
nougat *(Brach's)*	1 oz	110	0.0	24.0	20	(mq)	2.0	(mq)	na	16%
ornaments *(Brach's)*	1 oz	150	2.0	17.0	50	na	8.0	(mq)	na	49%
'Pearls' mint *(Brach's)*	1 oz	110	0.0	25.0	5	0	1.0	na	0	8%
'Perkys' *(Brach's)*	1 oz	90	0.0	23.0	20	0	0.0	0.0	0	0%
Santa, chocolate, in foil *(Brach's)*	1 oz	140	2.0	18.0	40	(mq)	7.0	(mq)	na	44%
Santa, marshmallow *(Brach's)*	1 oz	120	1.0	23.0	35	0	3.0	(mq)	na	22%
snowmen, marshmallow, large pieces *(Just Born)*	1 piece	111	0.7	26.8	8	0	0.1	(tr)	na	1%
snowmen, marshmallow, small pieces *(Just Born)*	1 piece	37	0.2	8.9	3	0	<.1	(tr)	na	<2%
'Starlight' mint *(Brach's)*	1 oz	110	0.0	27.0	15	0	0.0	0.0	0	0%
trees, marshmallow, large pieces *(Just Born)*	1 piece	111	0.7	26.8	8	0	0.1	(tr)	na	1%
trees, marshmallow, small pieces *(Just Born)*	1 piece	37	0.2	8.9	3	0	<.1	(tr)	na	<2%
Easter										
'Chicks & Rabbits' assorted *(Brach's)*	1 oz	100	0.0	26.0	10	0	0.0	0.0	0	0%
corn *(Brach's)*	1 oz	100	0.0	26.0	66	0	0.0	0.0	0	0%
'Easter Fun' assorted *(Brach's)*	1 oz	100	0.0	26.0	10	0	0.0	0.0	0	0%

Food Name	Serving Size	Calories	Prot. gms	Carbs gms	Sod. mgs	Fiber gms	Fat gms	Sat. Fat gms	Chol. mgs	% Fat Cal.
eggs, chocolate, in foil (Brach's)	1 oz	150	2.0	17.0	25	(mq)	8.0	(mq)	na	49%
eggs, chocolate malted milk (Brach's)	1 oz	130	1.0	21.0	40	(mq)	5.0	(mq)	na	34%
eggs, creme (Cadbury)	1.37 oz	190	2.0	26.0	0	na	8.0	(mq)	na	39%
eggs, creme, chocolate coated buttercream (Brach's)	1 oz	120	1.0	22.0	50	(mq)	3.0	(mq)	na	23%
eggs, creme, chocolate coated cherry (Brach's)	1 oz	110	1.0	23.0	20	(mq)	2.0	(mq)	na	16%
eggs, creme, chocolate coated coconut (Brach's)	1 oz	110	0.0	22.0	40	(mq)	3.0	(mq)	na	24%
eggs, creme, chocolate coated fruit and nut (Brach's)	1 oz	110	0.0	23.0	35	(mq)	2.0	(mq)	na	16%
eggs, creme, chocolate coated maple (Brach's)	1 oz	110	0.0	23.0	30	(mq)	2.0	(mq)	na	16%
eggs, creme, chocolate coated vanilla (Brach's)	1 oz	110	0.0	23.0	25	(mq)	2.0	(mq)	na	16%
eggs, creme, mini (Cadbury)	1 oz	140	2.0	20.0	na	na	7.0	(mq)	na	42%
eggs, 'Fiesta' pastel (Brach's)	1 oz	120	1.0	23.0	25	0	3.0	(mq)	na	22%
eggs 'Hide'n Seek' (Brach's)	1 oz	110	0.0	27.0	5	0	0.0	0.0	0	0%
eggs, jelly (Brach's)	1 oz	100	0.0	24.0	15	0	0.0	0.0	0	0%
eggs, jelly, speckled (Brach's)	1 oz	110	0.0	27.0	40	0	0.0	0.0	0	0%
eggs, jelly, spiced (Brach's)	1 oz	90	0.0	22.0	10	0	0.0	0.0	0	0%
eggs, jelly 'Tiny' (Brach's)	1 oz	100	0.0	26.0	10	0	0.0	0.0	0	0%
eggs, marshmallow (Brach's)	1 oz	100	0.0	25.0	5	0	0.0	0.0	0	0%
eggs, 'Robin's Eggs' (Brach's)	1 oz	140	1.0	20.0	30	0	6.0	(mq)	na	39%
nougats (Brach's)	1 oz	100	0.0	24.0	25	(mq)	1.0	na	0	9%
peeps, marshmallow (Just Born)	1 piece	27	0.2	6.6	2	0	<.1	(tr)	0	<3%
rabbits, 'Jube' (Brach's)	1 oz	100	0.0	24.0	15	0	0.0	0.0	0	0%
rabbits, marshmallow (Brach's)	1 oz	120	1.0	22.0	55	0	3.0	(mq)	0	23%
'Starlight' mint (Brach's)	1 oz	110	0.0	27.0	15	0	0.0	0.0	0	0%

Halloween

Food Name	Serving Size	Calories	Prot. gms	Carbs gms	Sod. mgs	Fiber gms	Fat gms	Sat. Fat gms	Chol. mgs	% Fat Cal.
cats, marshmallow (Just Born)	1 piece	28	0.2	6.7	2	0	<.1	0.0	0	<3%
cats 'Scary Cats' (Brach's)	1 oz	100	0.0	26.0	85	0	0.0	0.0	0	0%
corn, Indian (Brach's)	1 oz	100	0.0	26.0	75	0	0.0	0.0	0	0%
corn, three color (Brach's)	1 oz	100	0.0	26.0	95	0	0.0	0.0	0	0%
jelly beans (Brach's)	1 oz	100	0.0	26.0	15	0	0.0	0.0	0	0%
lollipops 'Picture Pops' (Brach's)	1 oz	110	0.0	27.0	10	0	0.0	0.0	0	0%
'Mellowcremes' (Brach's)	1 oz	100	0.0	26.0	40	0	0.0	0.0	0	0%
pumpkin heads, crazy (Brach's)	1 oz	100	0.0	24.0	15	0	1.0	na	0	9%
pumpkins (Brach's)	1 oz	100	0.0	26.0	65	0	0.0	0.0	0	0%
pumpkins, marshmallow, large pieces (Just Born)	1 piece	111	0.7	26.8	8	0	0.1	0.0	0	1%
pumpkins, marshmallow, small pieces (Just Born)	1 piece	14	0.1	3.4	1	0	<.1	0.0	0	<6%
'Trick or Treat Party Pack' (Brach's)	1 oz	110	0.0	27.0	20	0	0.0	0.0	0	0%
witches teeth (Brach's)	1 oz	100	0.0	26.0	75	0	0.0	0.0	0	0%

Valentine's Day

Food Name	Serving Size	Calories	Prot. gms	Carbs gms	Sod. mgs	Fiber gms	Fat gms	Sat. Fat gms	Chol. mgs	% Fat Cal.
'Heart Box, 1-lb' (Brach's)	1 oz	110	1.0	23.0	30	na	2.0	(mq)	na	16%
'Heart Box, 1/2-lb' (Brach's)	1 oz	110	1.0	23.0	35	na	2.0	(mq)	na	16%
'Heart Box, 1/3-lb' (Brach's)	1 oz	110	1.0	23.0	25	na	2.0	(mq)	na	16%
hearts 'Conversation' large (Brach's)	1 oz	110	0.0	27.0	5	0	0.0	0.0	0	0%
hearts 'Conversation' small (Brach's)	1 oz	110	0.0	27.0	0	0	0.0	0.0	0	0%
hearts, fruity (Brach's)	1 oz	100	0.0	24.0	5	0	0.0	0.0	0	0%
hearts 'Imperial' cinnamon (Brach's)	1 oz	110	0.0	27.0	5	0	0.0	0.0	0	0%
hearts, 'Jube' cherry (Brach's)	1 oz	100	0.0	26.0	20	0	0.0	0.0	0	0%
hearts, red jelly (Brach's)	1 oz	100	0.0	24.0	10	0	0.0	0.0	0	0%
hearts 'Sassy Hearts' (Brach's)	1 oz	100	0.0	25.0	0	0	0.0	0.0	0	0%
'I Luv U' chocolate (Brach's)	1 oz	150	2.0	17.0	25	na	8.0	(mq)	na	49%
kisses, nougat (Brach's)	1 oz	110	0.0	24.0	15	na	2.0	(mq)	na	16%
lollipop, pastels (Life Savers)	1 lollipop	40	0.0	10.0	0	na	0.0	na	na	0%
'Love' (Brach's)	1 oz	150	2.0	17.0	25	na	8.0	(mq)	na	49%
'Mellowcremes' (Brach's)	1 oz	100	0.0	26.0	75	0	0.0	0.0	0	0%

Food Name	Serving Size	Calories	Prot. gms	Carbs gms	Sod. mgs	Fiber gms	Fat gms	Sat. Fat gms	Chol. mgs	% Fat Cal.
JELLIED AND GUMMED										
cinnamon bears (Brach's)	1 oz	80	0.0	21.0	10	0	0.0	0.0	0	0%
eggs (Rodda)	1 piece	7	<.1	1.7	1	0	tr	0.0	0	0%
'Fruit Bunch' (Brach's)	1 oz	100	0.0	24.0	10	na	0.0	na	na	0%
gummi bears (Brach's)	1 oz	100	2.0	22.0	15	na	0.0	na	na	0%
gummi dinosaurs, tropical (Jurassic Park)	15 pieces	140	3.0	31.0	na	0	0.0	0.0	na	0%
gummi savers (Life Savers)	1 piece	12	0.0	3.0	0	na	0.0	na	na	0%
gummi worms (Brach's)	1 oz	100	2.0	22.0	15	na	0.0	na	na	0%
gummy bears (Estee)	4 pieces	20	1.0	4.0	0	0	0.0	0.0	0	0%
gummy bears 'Amazin Fruit' approx 12 pieces (Hershey's)	1 oz	90	2.0	21.0	20	na	<1.0	na	na	<9%
gummy bears, tropical 'Amazin Fruit' (Hershey's)	1 oz	90	2.0	21.0	20	na	<1.0	na	na	<9%
hot cinnamon (Hot Tamales)	1 piece	9	<.1	2.1	1	0	tr	0.0	0	0%
jelly beans (Brach's)	1 oz	100	0.0	26.0	5	na	0.0	na	na	0%
jelly nougat (Brach's)	1 oz	100	0.0	24.0	35	(mq)	1.0	na	0	9%
'Jels' sour cherry (Brach's)	1 oz	100	0.0	26.0	10	0	0.0	0.0	0	0%
'Jube Jels' (Brach's)	1 oz	100	0.0	24.0	10	na	0.0	na	na	0%
juicy (Callard & Bowser)	1 oz	90	0.0	22.9	0	0	0.0	0.0	na	0%
mint, assorted (Brach's)	1 oz	100	0.0	26.0	0	0	0.0	0.0	0	0%
'Petite' eggs (Just Born)	1 piece	4	tr	1.1	<1	0	tr	0.0	0	0%
'Rainbow Bears' (Brach's)	1 oz	100	0.0	24.0	10	0	0.0	0.0	0	0%
'Spearmint Leaves' (Brach's)	1 oz	100	0.0	24.0	5	na	0.0	na	na	0%
spicettes (Brach's)	1 oz	100	0.0	26.0	15	na	0.0	na	na	0%
'Teenee Beanee Gourmet' (Just Born)	1 piece	4	tr	1.1	<1	0	tr	0.0	0	0%
LICORICE										
candy coated (Good & Fruity)	1 oz	106	0.6	25.7	8	0	0.1	(tr)	0	1%
candy coated (Good & Plenty)	1 oz	106	1.0	25.9	52	0	<.1	(tr)	0	<1%
'Cherry Nibs' (Y&S)	1 oz	100	1.0	23.0	80	na	<1.0	na	0	<9%
'Nip' (Pearson)	1 oz	120	1.0	23.0	70	0	3.0	na	0	22%
'Red Laces' (Brach's)	1 oz	100	2.0	22.0	10	0	0.0	0.0	0	0%
'Twin Twists' (Brach's)	1 oz	100	2.0	22.0	10	0	0.0	0.0	0	0%
'Twists' (Brach's)	1 oz	100	2.0	22.0	50	0	1.0	(tr)	0	9%
'Twizzlers Bites' cherry (Y&S)	1 oz	100	1.0	23.0	85	na	<1.0	na	0	<9%
'Twizzlers' strawberry (Y&S)	1 oz	100	1.0	23.0	95	0	1.0	(tr)	0	9%
LOLLIPOP										
all flavors (Estee)	1 lollipop	30	0.0	7.0	0	na	0.0	0.0	0	0%
all flavors (Life Savers)	1 lollipop	45	0.0	11.0	10	na	0.0	na	na	0%
all flavors bubble gum center (Spangler)	1 lollipop	57	<1.0	14.0	5	0	<1.0	(tr)	0	<13%
all flavors 'Dum Dums' (Spangler)	1 lollipop	25	<1.0	6.0	0	0	<1.0	(tr)	0	<24%
all flavors except chocolate (Tootsie Pop)	1 oz	111	0.1	26.4	1	(tr)	0.6	0.1	tr	5%
all fruit flavors (Sorbee)	1 lollipop	22	0.0	5.0	0	na	0.0	na	na	0%
all flavors 'Pops' (Brach's)	1 oz	110	0.0	27.0	10	0	0.0	0.0	0	0%
all flavors 'Saf-T-Pops' (Spangler)	1 lollipop	45	<1.0	11.0	0	0	<1.0	(tr)	0	<16%
black raspberry (Fruit Juicers)	1 lollipop	40	0.0	10.0	0	na	0.0	na	na	0%
chocolate (Tootsie Pop)	1 oz	110	0.1	26.2	2	(tr)	0.6	0.2	tr	5%
fruit (Glenny's)	1 lollipop	21	<1.0	5.0	<1	na	<1.0	na	na	<27%
fruit punch (Fruit Juicers)	1 lollipop	40	0.0	10.0	0	na	0.0	na	na	0%
pineapple (Fruit Juicers)	1 lollipop	40	0.0	10.0	0	na	0.0	na	na	0%
strawberry (Fruit Juicers)	1 lollipop	40	0.0	10.0	0	na	0.0	na	na	0%
swirled (Life Savers)	1 lollipop	45	0.0	11.0	10	na	0.0	na	na	0%
vitamin 'C' (Glenny's)	1 lollipop	35	<1.0	8.0	<1	na	<1.0	na	na	<20%
MARSHMALLOW										
'Circus Peanuts' approx 1 oz (Spangler)	4 pieces	110	<1.0	26.0	5	0	<1.0	(tr)	0	<8%
'Mallow Cup' 1.6 oz (Boyer)	2 pieces	224	2.0	30.0	na	0	11.0	(mq)	na	44%
'Mallow Cup' .5 oz (Boyer)	1 piece	71	1.0	15.0	na	0	5.0	(mq)	na	41%

Food Name	Serving Size	Calories	Prot. gms	Carbs gms	Sod. mgs	Fiber gms	Fat gms	Sat. Fat gms	Chol. mgs	% Fat Cal.
'Mallow Cup' .275 oz (Boyer)	1 piece	36	0.5	7.5	na	0	2.5	(mq)	na	41%
'Perkys Circus Peanuts' (Brach's)	1 oz	100	0.0	26.0	10	0	0.0	0.0	0	0%
toasted coconut (Just Born)	1 piece	30	0.3	6.1	6	.7	0.6	(tr)	0	17%
MINT										
'After Dinner' tofu, chocolate (Barat)	1 piece	40	1.0	4.0	0	(mq)	2.0	(mq)	0	47%
'After Eight' dark chocolate (Rowntree)	1 mint	35	0.0	6.0	0	na	1.0	na	na	27%
all flavors except cocoamint (Velamints)	1 mint	7	0.0	1.7	0	na	0.0	0.0	0	0%
'Bits' tofu, chocolate (Barat)	.75 oz	120	2.0	11.0	15	(mq)	8.0	(mq)	0	58%
butter (Kraft)	1 piece	8	0.0	2.0	0	0	0.0	0.0	0	0%
cocoamint (Velamints)	1 mint	7	4.7	1.5	0	na	0.3	na	0	10%
'Cool Blue' (Featherweight)	1 piece	25	0.0	6.0	0	0	0.0	0.0	0	0%
'Coolers/Starlight' (Brach's)	1 oz	110	0.0	27.0	15	0	0.0	0.0	0	0%
creme, chocolate covered, regular (Brach's)	1 oz	110	0.0	24.0	10	na	2.0	(mq)	na	16%
'Creme de Menthe' (Brach's)	1 oz	150	2.0	16.0	20	0	9.0	(mq)	na	53%
'Creme de Menthe' chocolate (Andes)	6 pieces	150	2.0	16.0	20	na	9.0	na	na	53%
dark chocolate coated (Spangler)	1 piece	80	<1.0	14.0	25	(mq)	2.0	(mq)	0	23%
'Dessert Mints' assorted (Brach's)	1 oz	110	0.0	27.0	0	0	0.0	0.0	na	0%
'Drops' (Glenny's)	1 drop	6	<1.0	1.0	<1	na	<1.0	na	na	<53%
filled straws (Brach's)	1 oz	110	0.0	26.0	10	0	1.0	na	0	8%
'Jots/Pearls' (Brach's)	1 oz	120	0.0	25.0	10	0	2.0	(mq)	na	15%
'Junior Mints' chocolate covered, 1 oz	12 pieces	120	1.0	24.0	10	na	3.0	(mq)	na	21%
'Kentucky Mints' (Brach's)	1 oz	110	0.0	27.0	0	0	0.0	0.0	0	0%
'Meltaway' .33 oz (Mint)	1 piece	50	0.0	5.0	10	0	3.0	(mq)	0	57%
'Nip' chocolate (Pearson)	1 oz	120	1.0	23.0	70	na	3.0	na	na	22%
'Mint Oh's' (Saco Foods)	1.5 oz	111	1.0	13.8	14	na	6.6	2.4	0	50%
parfait (Brach's)	1 oz	150	2.0	16.0	35	(tr)	9.0	(mq)	na	53%
party (Kraft)	1 piece	8	0.0	2.0	0	0	0.0	0.0	0	0%
peppermint kisses (Brach's)	1 oz	100	0.0	24.0	25	na	1.0	na	na	9%
'Peppermint Pattie' large patties (York)	1 piece	149	1.3	33.6	17	>.2 c	3.9	na	0	20%
'Peppermint Pattie' small patties (York)	1 piece	38	0.3	8.6	4	>.1 c	1.0	na	0	20%
peppermint swirls (Featherweight)	1 piece	20	0.0	5.0	0	0	0.0	0.0	0	0%
squares (Russell Stover)	1.4 oz	160	1.0	28.0	35	1.0	5.0	4.0	na	28%
thin, chocolate covered, regular (Brach's)	1 oz	110	0.0	24.0	10	na	2.0	(mq)	na	16%
NONPAREILS										
dark chocolate (Brach's)	1 oz	140	1.0	20.0	20	(mq)	6.0	(mq)	na	39%
'Sno-Caps' (Nestlé)	1 oz	140	1.0	21.0	0	(mq)	6.0	(mq)	na	38%
PEANUT										
'Bits' chocolate tofu, dipped (Barat)	1 oz	120	4.0	8.0	15	(mq)	8.0	(mq)	0	60%
candy coated (Estee)	10 pieces	70	2.0	8.0	10	na	4.0	1.0	0	47%
caramel cluster (Brach's)	1 oz	150	4.0	15.0	50	(mq)	8.0	(mq)	na	49%
chocolate coated (Cocofection)	1 oz	140	5.0	10.0	12	na	12.0	na	na	64%
chocolate coated (Estee)	2 squares	60	1.0	4.5	10	(mq)	4.5	2.0	2	65%
chocolate coated, approx 14 pieces (Nabisco)	1 oz	160	4.0	14.0	15	(mq)	9.0	(mq)	na	53%
chocolate coated 'Small' (Brach's)	1 oz	140	4.0	15.0	40	(mq)	7.0	(mq)	na	45%
filled (Brach's)	1 oz	110	1.0	25.0	20	(mq)	1.0	na	na	8%
French, burnt (Brach's)	1 oz	130	4.0	18.0	5	(mq)	5.0	(mq)	0	34%
'Goobers' chocolate covered (Nestlé)	10 pieces	51	1.4	4.9	4	>.2 c	3.3	1.2	1	54%
'Goobers' chocolate covered, 1 3/8 oz (Nestlé)	1 pkg	200	6.0	16.0	15	na	13.0	na	na	57%
'Jots' (Brach's)	1 oz	140	3.0	18.0	25	(mq)	6.0	(mq)	na	39%
'M&M's' candy coated chocolate peanuts (M&M/Mars)	10 pieces	99	2.1	11.8	19	>.3 c	5.4	na	3	47%
'M&M's' candy coated chocolate peanuts, fun size (M&M/Mars)	1 pkg	110	2.0	13.0	20	na	5.0	na	na	43%
milk chocolate coated (Brach's)	1 oz	150	3.0	15.0	30	(mq)	9.0	(mq)	(mq)	53%
'Nut Goodies' (Brach's)	1 oz	130	2.0	21.0	10	(mq)	4.0	(mq)	na	28%

Food Name	Serving Size	Calories	Prot. gms	Carbs gms	Sod. mgs	Fiber gms	Fat gms	Sat. Fat gms	Chol. mgs	% Fat Cal.
parfait *(Brach's)*	1 oz	160	3.0	14.0	60	(mq)	10.0	(mq)	na	57%
'Peanut Clusters' *(Brach's)*	1 oz	150	3.0	15.0	25	(mq)	9.0	(mq)	na	53%
'Peanut Delights' *(Russell Stover)*	1.4 oz	210	4.0	22.0	130	1.0	12.0	5.0	10	51%
PEANUT BRITTLE										
(Estee)	.5 oz	60	<1.0	10.0	20	na	2.0	<1.0	0	29%
(Estee)	.25 oz	35	<1.0	5.0	30	(mq)	1.0	<1.0	0	27%
(Kraft)	1 oz	130	3.0	20.0	135	(mq)	5.0	1.0	0	33%
(Sophie Mae)	1.4 oz	170	4.0	30.0	130	1.0	5.0	1.0	0	25%
PEANUT BUTTER										
'Bar None' *(Hershey's)*	1.5 oz	240	4.0	23.0	50	na	14.0	na	10	54%
cup *(Estee)*	1 cup	40	1.0	3.0	20	(mq)	3.0	2.5	<1	63%
cup, 1.6 oz *(Boyer)*	2 pieces	250	5.0	23.0	na	(mq)	15.0	(mq)	na	55%
cup, .5 oz *(Boyer)*	1 piece	75	2.5	12.0	na	(mq)	7.5	(mq)	na	54%
cup, .275 oz *(Boyer)*	1 piece	38	1.3	6.0	na	(mq)	3.8	(mq)	na	54%
kisses *(Brach's)*	1 oz	110	1.0	22.0	135	(mq)	2.0	(mq)	na	16%
'Kudos' chocolate covered *(M&M/Mars)*	1.3 oz	200	4.0	19.0	80	na	12.0	na	na	54%
'M&M's' candy coated *(M&M/Mars)*	1.63 oz	240	5.0	28.0	60	na	12.0	na	na	45%
'M&M's' candy coated *(M&M/Mars)*	1 oz	150	3.0	17.0	60	na	7.0	na	na	44%
'PB Max' chocolate covered cookie *(M&M/Mars)*	1 piece	240	5.0	20.0	150	na	15.0	na	na	57%
'Reese's Crunchy Peanut Butter Cups' *(Hershey's)*	1.8 oz	280	7.0	24.0	130	na	18.0	na	5	57%
'Reese's Peanut Butter Cups' *(Hershey's)*	1.6 oz	250	6.0	23.0	160	na	15.0	na	5	54%
'Reese's Peanut Butter Cups' *(Hershey's)*	1.8 oz	247	5.6	24.4	148	2.1	15.9	11.8	8	54%
'Reese's Peanut Butter Cups' miniatures *(Hershey's)*	6 cups	204	4.6	20.1	122	1.8	13.1	9.7	6	54%
'Reese's Peanut Butter Cups' snack size *(Hershey's)*	1 cup	100	2.0	9.0	60	na	6.0	na	na	55%
'Reese's Pieces' candy coated *(Hershey's)*	1.63 oz	230	7.0	28.0	80	na	10.0	na	0	39%
'Reese's Pieces' candy coated *(Hershey's)*	10 pieces	38	1.0	5.0	12	.3	1.7	na	0	39%
'Reese's Pieces' candy coated, 1.95 oz *(Hershey's)*	1 pkg	258	7.2	34.2	83	2.3	11.4	na	2	38%
toffee *(Flavor House)*	1 oz	150	4.0	17.0	90	(mq)	7.0	(mq)	na	43%
PECAN										
'Demet's Turtles' milk chocolate, pecans, caramel										
(Demet's)	1 piece	82	1.1	9.9	16	>.4 c	4.7	1.8	4	49%
'Pecan Crowns' *(Russell Stover)*	1.4 oz	200	2.0	19.0	60	1.0	13.0	4.0	5	58%
'Pecan Delights' *(Russell Stover)*	1.4 oz	220	2.0	19.0	55	1.0	14.5	5.5	5	61%
POWDER CANDY										
(Lik-m-aid Fun Dip)	1 oz	110	0.0	26.0	na	na	0.0	na	na	0%
(Pixy Stix)	1 oz	100	0.0	26.0	na	na	0.0	na	na	0%
RAISIN										
'Bits' chocolate tofu covered *(Barat)*	1 oz	120	1.0	14.0	10	(mq)	7.0	(mq)	0	51%
chocolate coated *(Brach's)*	1 oz	130	1.0	20.0	30	(mq)	5.0	(mq)	chol.	35%
chocolate coated *(Cocofection)*	1 oz	120	1.0	20.0	14	na	5.0	na	na	35%
chocolate coated *(Estee)*	8 pieces	30	<1.0	5.0	5	na	1.0	1.0	0	27%
chocolate coated, approx 29 pieces *(Nabisco)*	1 oz	130	1.0	21.0	15	(mq)	5.0	(mq)	<1	34%
'Raisinets' chocolate covered *(Nestlé)*	1 3/8 oz	180	2.0	28.0	10	na	6.0	na	0	31%
'Raisinets' chocolate covered *(Nestlé)*	10 pieces	41	0.5	7.1	4	>.1 c	1.6	0.7	0	32%
'Raisinets' chocolate covered *(Nestlé)*	1.58 oz	185	2.1	32.0	16	>.3 c	7.2	3.3	2	32%
TAFFY										
all flavors 'Salt Water Taffy' *(Brach's)*	1 oz	100	0.0	24.0	30	0	1.0	na	0	9%
apple flavor 'Laffy Taffy' 1 oz *(Beich's)*	2 pieces	110	0.0	26.0	55	0	1.0	na	0	8%
banana flavor 'Laffy Taffy' 1 oz *(Beich's)*	2 pieces	120	0.0	26.0	55	0	1.0	na	0	8%
cherry flavor 'Laffy Taffy' 1 oz *(Beich's)*	2 pieces	110	0.0	26.0	55	0	1.0	na	0	8%
grape flavor 'Laffy Taffy' 1 oz *(Beich's)*	2 pieces	110	0.0	26.0	60	0	1.0	na	0	8%
honey flavor *(Bit-O-Honey)*	1.7 oz	200	1.0	39.0	125	na	4.0	(mq)	na	18%
passion punch flavor 'Laffy Taffy' 1 oz *(Beich's)*	2 pieces	120	0.0	26.0	50	0	1.0	na	0	8%
strawberry flavor 'Laffy Taffy' 1 oz *(Beich's)*	2 pieces	110	0.0	26.0	55	0	1.0	na	0	8%

Food Name	Serving Size	Calories	Prot. gms	Carbs gms	Sod. mgs	Fiber gms	Fat gms	Sat. Fat gms	Chol. mgs	% Fat Cal.
tangy flavor *(Tangy Taffy)*	1 oz	120	0.0	23.0	na	0	2.5	2.0	na	20%
watermelon flavor 'Laffy Taffy' 1 oz *(Beich's)*	2 pieces	110	0.0	26.0	55	0	1.0	na	0	8%
TOFFEE										
(Brach's)	1 oz	110	1.0	23.0	80	0	2.0	(mq)	0	16%
(Callard & Bowser)	1 oz	135	0.5	19.2	0	0	6.5	na	na	43%
'Bits'O Brickle' *(Heath)*	3 oz	448	1.0	50.0	472	na	28.0	(mq)	na	55%
English *(Bits'O Heath)*	3.5 oz	520	3.0	62.0	390	na	31.0	(mq)	na	52%
English, 'Heath Bar' 1 3/16 oz *(Heath)*	2 pieces	180	1.0	20.0	130	(mq)	11.0	(mq)	na	54%
CANDY APPLE. See APPLE KIT.										
CANE SYRUP										
table blends	1/2 cup	397	0.0	102.4	6	0	0.0	0.0	0	0%
table blends	1 tbsp	50	0.0	12.8	tr	0	0.0	0.0	0	0%
CANNELLINI BEAN, canned, white *(Pathmark)*	1/2 cup	100	6.0	18.0	390	(mq)	0.0	0.0	0	0%
CANNELLONI, CANNED, mini *(Chef Boyardee)*	7.5 oz	230	9.0	33.0	1050	(mq)	7.0	(mq)	(mq)	27%
CANNELLONI ENTRÉE, frozen										
beef, w/tomato sauce *(Lean Cuisine)*	9 5/8 oz	200	14.0	28.0	490	na	3.0	1.0	25	14%
cheese *(Dining Lite)*	9 oz	310	19.0	38.0	650	(mq)	9.0	(mq)	70	26%
cheese, w/tomato sauce *(Lean Cuisine)*	9 1/8 oz	270	23.0	27.0	590	na	8.0	4.0	25	27%
Florentine *(Celentano)*	12 oz	350	21.0	48.0	620	(mq)	8.0	(mq)	na	21%
CANOLA AND VEGETABLE OIL, 'Best Blend' *(Wesson)*	1 tbsp	120	0.0	0.0	0	na	14.0	1.0	0	100%
CANOLA OIL										
	1/2 cup	964	0.0	0.0	0	0	109.0	7.7	0	100%
	1 oz	251	0.0	0.0	0	0	28.4	2.0	0	100%
	1 tbsp	124	0.0	0.0	0	0	14.0	1.0	na	100%
(Country Pure)	1 tbsp	120	0.0	0.0	0	na	14.0	0.0	0	100%
(Hain)	1 tbsp	120	0.0	0.0	0	0	14.0	1.0	0	100%
(Kroger)	1 tbsp	122	0.0	0.0	0	0	13.6	1.0	0	100%
(Nucoa) 'Heart Beat'	1 tbsp	120	0.0	0.0	0	0	14.0	1.0	0	100%
(Spectrum Naturals)	1 tbsp	120	0.0	0.0	0	(tr)	14.0	1.0	(tr)	100%
(Spectrum Naturals) organic	1 tbsp	120	0.0	0.0	0	(tr)	14.0	1.0	(tr)	100%
(Wesson)	1 tbsp	120	0.0	0.0	0	0	14.0	1.0	0	100%
(Wesson) 'Food Service'	1 tbsp	122	0.0	0.0	0	0	13.6	1.0	0	100%
CANOLA OIL SPRAY. See COOKING SPRAY.										
CANTALOUPE /muskmelon										
approx 5 inch diam	1/2 fruit	93	2.3	22.3	24	2.1	0.8	na	0	7%
cubed	1/2 cup	29	0.7	6.7	7	.6	0.2	(tr)	0	6%
pulp	1 oz	10	0.2	2.4	3	.3	0.1	(tr)	0	8%
untrimmed	1 lb	82	2.0	19.3	20	1.9	0.6	na	0	6%
untrimmed *(Dole)*	1/4 fruit	50	1.0	11.0	35	0	0.0	na	na	0%
CAPE GOOSEBERRY/ground cherry /poha										
in husk	1 lb	226	8.1	47.8	(mq)	>11.9 c	3.0	(mq)	0	11%
raw	1/2 cup	37	1.3	7.8	na	>2.0 c	0.5	na	0	11%
trimmed	1/2 cup	37	1.3	7.8	(mq)	>2.0 c	0.5	tr	0	11%
trimmed	1 oz	15	0.5	3.2	(mq)	>.8 c	0.2	tr	0	11%
CAPOCOLLA. See LUNCHEON MEAT.										
CAPPUCCINO. See COFFEE, FLAVORED.										
CARAMBOLA. See STAR FRUIT.										
CARAMEL TOPPING										
(Kraft)	1 tbsp	60	1.0	13.0	45	0	0.0	0.0	0	0%
(Mrs. Richardson's) fat-free	2 tbsp	130	1.0	31.0	55	na	0.0	na	0	0%
(Smucker's) hot	2 tbsp	150	1.0	28.0	75	0	4.0	(mq)	0	24%
CARAWAY SEED										
whole	1 oz	94	5.6	14.1	5	>3.6 c	4.1	0.2	0	32%
whole	1 tbsp	22	1.3	3.3	1	2.5	1.0	0.0	0	33%

Food Name	Serving Size	Calories	Prot. gms	Carbs gms	Sod. mgs	Fiber gms	Fat gms	Sat. Fat gms	Chol. mgs	% Fat Cal.
whole	1 tsp	7	0.4	1.0	0	.8	0.3	0.0	0	33%
whole *(Durkee)*	1 tsp	9	0.0	0.0	0	0	<0.1	na	na	<45%
whole *(Laurel Leaf)*	1 tsp	9	0.0	0.0	0	0	<0.1	na	na	<45%
whole *(Spice Islands)*	1 tsp	8	0.4	0.8	<1	>.2 c	0.4	tr	0	43%
CARDAMOM										
ground	1 oz	88	3.1	19.4	5	>3.2 c	1.9	0.2	0	16%
ground	1 tbsp	18	0.6	4.0	1	>.7 c	0.4	0.0	0	tr
ground	1 tsp	6	0.2	1.4	0	>.2 c	0.1	0.0	0	tr
ground *(Durkee)*	1 tsp	7	0.0	0.0	0	0	tr	na	na	tr
ground *(Laurel Leaf)*	1 tsp	7	0.0	0.0	0	0	tr	na	na	tr
CARDAMOM SEED *(Spice Islands)*	1 tsp	6	0.2	1.3	tr	>.2 c	0.1	tr	0	13%
CARDONI. See CARDOON.										
CARDOON/cardoni										
boiled, drained	4 oz	25	0.9	6.0	200	(mq)	0.1	<.1	0	3%
raw, shredded	1 cup	36	1.3	8.7	303	2.9	0.2	0.0	0	4%
raw, shredded	1/2 cup	18	0.6	4.3	151	1.4	0.1	0.0	0	4%
raw, trimmed	1 oz	6	0.2	1.4	48	(mq)	<.1	tr	0	<12%
raw, untrimmed	1 lb	44	1.6	10.9	378	(mq)	0.2	<.1	0	4%
CARIBOU										
raw	1 lb	576	102.6	0.0	259	na	15.2	5.8	376	25%
raw	1 oz	36	6.3	0.0	16	na	0.9	0.4	23	24%
roasted	4 oz	189	33.8	0.0	68	0	5.0	1.9	124	25%
roasted	3 oz	142	25.3	0.0	51	na	3.8	1.4	93	25%
roasted, diced	1 cup	234	41.7	0.0	84	0	6.2	2.4	153	25%
CARISSA/natal plum										
raw, approx .8 oz	1 med	12	0.1	2.7	1	.2	0.3	0.0	0	19%
raw, sliced	1 cup	93	0.8	20.4	5	>1.4 c	2.0	na	0	18%
raw, w/o skin and seeds, approx .8 oz	1 fruit	12	0.1	2.7	1	>.2 c	0.3	na	0	19%
trimmed	1 oz	18	0.1	3.9	1	>.3 c	0.4	0.0	0	18%
untrimmed	1 lb	240	2.0	53.2	11	>3.5 c	5.1	na	0	17%
CAROB FLAVOR DRINK										
mix, powder	1 oz	105	0.5	26.5	29	>.5 c	0.1	tr	0	1%
mix, powder	3 tsp	45	0.2	11.2	12	>.2 c	0.0	0.0	0	0%
mix, prepared w/1 cup whole milk	1 cup	195	8.2	22.6	132	>.3 c	8.2	5.1	33	38%
mix, prepared w/1 cup 2% milk	1 cup	166	8.3	22.9	134	>.2 c	4.7	2.9	18	25%
mix, prepared w/1 cup 1% milk	1 cup	147	8.2	22.9	135	>.2 c	2.6	1.6	10	16%
mix, prepared w/1 cup skim milk	1 cup	131	8.6	23.1	138	>.2 c	0.4	0.3	4	3%
CAROB FLOUR										
	1 cup	394	4.8	91.5	36	41.0	0.7	0.1	0	2%
	1 oz	51	1.3	25.2	10	3.0	0.2	tr	0	2%
	1 tbsp	31	0.4	7.1	3	3.2	0.1	0.0	0	3%
CARP										
dry-heat cooked	3 oz	138	19.4	0.0	54	0	6.1	1.2	71	41%
dry-heat cooked, approx 7.7 oz raw wt	1 fillet	275	38.9	0.0	107	0	12.2	2.4	143	41%
raw	1 lb	574	80.9	0.0	223	0	25.4	4.9	298	41%
raw	3 oz	108	15.2	0.0	42	0	4.8	0.9	56	42%
raw	1 oz	36	5.1	0.0	14	0	1.6	0.3	19	41%
raw, approx 7.7 oz	1 fillet	277	38.9	0.0	107	0	12.2	2.4	144	41%
CARROT										
baby, raw	1 large	6	0.1	1.2	5	na	0.1	0.0	0	15%
baby, raw	1 med	4	0.1	0.8	4	na	0.1	0.0	0	20%
boiled, drained	4 oz	51	1.2	11.9	75	2.2	0.2	<.1	0	3%
boiled, drained	1 med	21	0.5	4.8	30	1.6	0.1	0.0	0	4%
boiled, drained, sliced	1/2 cup	35	0.9	8.2	51	2.6	0.1	0.0	0	2%

Food Name	Serving Size	Calories	Prot. gms	Carbs gms	Sod. mgs	Fiber gms	Fat gms	Sat. Fat gms	Chol. mgs	% Fat Cal.
raw	1 med	31	0.7	7.3	25	2.3	0.1	0.0	0	3%
raw *(Dole)*	1 med	40	1.0	8.0	40	1.0	1.0	na	na	20%
raw, shredded	1/2 cup	24	0.6	5.6	19	1.7	0.1	0.0	0	4%
raw, trimmed	1 oz	12	0.3	2.9	10	.9	0.1	tr	0	7%
raw, untrimmed	1 lb	174	4.1	41.0	139	12.9	0.8	0.1	0	4%
CARROT, CANNED										
Crinkle sliced										
(A&P)	1/2 cup	30	1.0	6.0	300	(mq)	<1.0	(tr)	0	<24%
(Freshlike)	1/2 cup	30	1.0	6.0	300	na	0.0	na	na	0%
(Veg•All)	1/2 cup	30	1.0	6.0	300	na	0.0	na	na	0%
Diced										
(Allens)	1/2 cup	30	1.0	5.0	190	(mq)	<1.0	(tr)	0	<27%
'Fancy' *(S&W)*	1/2 cup	30	1.0	7.0	240	(mq)	0.0	0.0	0	0%
julienne 'Fancy' *(S&W)*	1/2 cup	30	1.0	7.0	240	(mq)	0.0	0.0	0	0%
'No Salt Added' *(A&P)*	1/2 cup	25	<1.0	6.0	40	(mq)	<1.0	(tr)	0	<24%
'No Salt or Sugar Added' *(Stokely)*	1/2 cup	35	1.0	7.0	35	(mq)	0.0	0.0	0	0%
w/liquid *(Del Monte)*	1/2 cup	30	0.0	7.0	265	(mq)	0.0	0.0	0	0%
Sliced										
(Featherweight)	1/2 cup	30	1.0	6.0	30	(mq)	0.0	0.0	0	0%
(Finast)	1/2 cup	35	1.0	8.0	370	(mq)	0.0	0.0	0	0%
(IGA)	1/2 cup	30	1.0	6.0	300	(mq)	0.0	0.0	0	0%
(Pathmark)	1/2 cup	35	1.0	7.0	310	(mq)	0.0	0.0	0	0%
(S&W Nutradiet)	1/2 cup	30	0.0	7.0	50	(mq)	0.0	0.0	0	0%
(Stokely)	1/2 cup	35	1.0	7.0	300	(mq)	0.0	0.0	0	0%
'Fancy' *(S&W)*	1/2 cup	30	1.0	7.0	240	(mq)	0.0	0.0	0	0%
large *(Allens)*	1/2 cup	30	1.0	7.0	250	(mq)	<1.0	(tr)	0	<22%
medium *(Allens)*	1/2 cup	30	1.0	7.0	250	(mq)	<1.0	(tr)	0	<22%
'No Salt Added' *(Finast)*	1/2 cup	35	1.0	8.0	30	(mq)	0.0	0.0	0	0%
'No Salt Added' *(Pathmark)*	1/2 cup	35	1.0	8.0	35	(mq)	0.0	0.0	0	0%
regular pack, drained	1/2 cup	17	0.5	4.0	176	1.1	0.1	0.0	0	5%
regular pack, w/liquid	1/2 cup	28	0.8	6.2	297	1.4	0.2	<.1	0	6%
regular pack, w/liquid, low-sodium	1/2 cup	28	0.8	6.2	48	1.4	0.2	<.1	0	6%
small *(Allens)*	1/2 cup	30	1.0	7.0	250	(mq)	<1.0	(tr)	0	<22%
special dietary pack, drained	1/2 cup	17	0.5	4.0	31	>.6 c	0.1	0.0	0	5%
special dietary pack, w/liquid	1/2 cup	28	0.8	6.2	48	>.9 c	0.2	0.0	0	6%
water-packed, w/o salt *(Freshlike)*	1/2 cup	30	1.0	6.0	40	na	0.0	na	na	0%
water-packed, w/o sugar or salt *(Freshlike)*	1/2 cup	30	1.0	6.0	40	na	0.0	na		0%
w/liquid *(Del Monte)*	1/2 cup	30	0.0	7.0	265	(mq)	0.0	0.0	0	0%
Whole										
baby *(Allens)*	1/2 cup	30	1.0	6.0	240	(mq)	<1.0	(tr)	0	<24%
tiny 'Fancy' *(S&W)*	1/2 cup	30	1.0	7.0	240	(mq)	0.0	0.0	0	0%
w/liquid	1/2 cup	26	0.7	5.7	273	1.2	0.2	<.1	0	7%
CARROT, FROZEN										
	10 oz	112	3.1	25.5	167	4.0	0.6	0.1	0	5%
(A&P)	3.3 oz	40	1.0	9.0	45	(mq)	<1.0	(tr)	0	<18%
(Seabrook)	3.3 oz	40	1.0	9.0	44	>1.0 c	0.0	0.0	0	0%
baby, whole 'Deluxe' *(Bird's Eye)*	3.3 oz	40	1.0	9.0	45	2.0	0.0	na	0	0%
baby whole, 'Harvest Fresh' *(Green Giant)*	1/2 cup	18	1.0	5.0	75	2.0	0.0	0.0	0	0%
baby, whole 'Select' *(Green Giant)*	1/2 cup	20	1.0	7.0	35	2.0	0.0	0.0	0	0%
baby whole, 'Singles' *(Stokely)*	3 oz	35	1.0	8.0	50	(mq)	0.0	0.0	0	0%
boiled, drained	4 oz	41	1.3	9.4	67	2.0	0.1	<.1	0	2%
Parisienne 'Deluxe' *(Deluxe)*	2.6 oz	30	1.0	7.0	35	2.0	0.0	na	0	0%
sliced *(Birds Eye)*	3.2 oz	35	1.0	8.0	40	1.0	0.0	na	0	0%
sliced *(Frosty Acres)*	3.3 oz	40	1.0	9.0	44	>1.0 c	0.0	0.0	0	0%

Food Name	Serving Size	Calories	Prot. gms	Carbs gms	Sod. mgs	Fiber gms	Fat gms	Sat. Fat gms	Chol. mgs	% Fat Cal.
sliced, boiled, drained	1/2 cup	26	0.9	6.0	43	>.9 c	0.1	0.0	0	3%
sliced, unprepared	1/2 cup	25	0.7	5.8	38	2.1	0.1	0.0	0	3%
whole (Southern)	3.5 oz	42	1.2	8.7	60	(mq)	0.2	0.0	0	4%
w/sweet peas, pearl onions 'Deluxe' (Birds Eye)	3.3 oz	50	2.0	10.0	60	2.0	0.0	na	0	0%
CARROT JUICE										
canned	6 oz	74	1.8	17.1	53	1.5	0.3	0.1	0	3%
canned	1/2 cup	49	1.2	11.4	36	1.0	0.2	0.0	0	3%
canned (Biotta)	6 oz	51	1.5	11.3	158	(mq)	0.1	(tr)	0	2%
canned (Hain)	6 oz	80	1.0	17.0	170	(mq)	0.0	0.0	0	0%
canned (Hollywood)	6 oz	80	1.0	17.0	170	2.0	0.0	0.0	0	0%
CASABA MELON										
cubed	1 cup	44	1.5	10.5	20	1.4	0.2	na	0	4%
1/10 of 7.75-inch melon	2-inch slice	43	1.5	10.2	20	1.3	0.2	na	0	4%
pulp	1 oz	7	0.3	1.8	3	>.1 c	<.1	(tr)	0	<10%
untrimmed	1 lb	71	2.5	16.9	33	>1.4 c	0.3	(tr)	0	3%
CASHEW /heart nut										
(Beer Nuts)	1 oz	170	5.0	8.0	65	(mq)	13.0	(mq)	0	69%
Dry roasted										
halves (Fisher)	1 oz	160	5.0	8.0	na	na	13.0	3.0	0	69%
lightly salted (Planters)	1 oz	160	5.0	9.0	115	na	13.0	2.0	0	68%
salted	1 oz	163	4.3	9.3	182	.9	13.2	2.6	0	69%
salted (Pathmark)	1 oz	170	4.0	9.0	150	(mq)	13.0	(mq)	0	69%
salted (Planters)	1 oz	160	5.0	9.0	230	(mq)	13.0	3.0	0	68%
salted, 'No Frills' (Pathmark)	1 oz	170	5.0	8.0	220	(mq)	13.0	3.0	0	69%
salted, wholes and halves	1 cup	787	21.0	44.8	877	7.8	63.5	12.5	0	69%
unsalted	1 oz	163	4.3	9.3	5	.9	13.2	2.6	0	69%
'Unsalted' (Planters)	1 oz	160	5.0	9.0	0	(mq)	13.0	3.0	0	68%
unsalted, approx 14 large or 26 small kernels	1 oz	163	4.4	9.3	4	1.7	13.2	2.6	0	68%
unsalted, wholes and halves	1 cup	787	21.0	44.8	21	7.8	63.5	12.5	0	69%
wholes (Fisher)	1 oz	160	5.0	8.0	100	na	13.0	3.0	0	69%
Honey roasted										
(Frito-Lays)	1 oz	170	4.0	9.0	115	na	14.0	na	0	71%
(Planters)	1 oz	170	4.0	11.0	170	(mq)	12.0	2.0	0	64%
halves (Fisher)	1 oz	150	4.0	7.0	na	na	13.0	3.0	0	73%
wholes (Fisher)	1 oz	150	4.0	7.0	90	na	13.0	3.0	0	73%
w/peanuts (Planters)	1 oz	170	5.0	9.0	170	(mq)	12.0	2.0	0	66%
Oil roasted										
halves (Fisher)	1 oz	170	5.0	8.0	155	na	14.0	4.0	0	71%
lightly salted (Planters)	1 oz	160	5.0	8.0	80	na	14.0	3.0	0	71%
pieces (Fisher)	1 oz	170	5.0	8.0	135	na	14.0	3.0	0	71%
salted	1 oz	164	4.6	8.1	178	1.1	13.7	2.7	0	71%
salted (Flavor House)	1 oz	180	7.0	3.0	125	(mq)	16.0	(mq)	0	78%
salted (Pathmark)	1 oz	170	5.0	8.0	150	(mq)	14.0	(mq)	0	71%
salted, approx 14 large or 18 medium kernels	1 oz	163	4.6	8.1	177	1.1	13.7	2.7	0	71%
salted, 'Fancy' (Planters)	1 oz	170	5.0	8.0	135	(mq)	14.0	3.0	0	71%
salted, halves (Planters)	1 oz	170	5.0	8.0	135	(mq)	14.0	3.0	0	71%
salted, 'No Frills' (Pathmark)	1 oz	170	5.0	8.0	150	(mq)	14.0	(mq)	0	71%
salted, wholes (Guy's)	1 oz	170	5.0	5.0	140	(mq)	14.0	(mq)	0	76%
salted, wholes and halves	1 cup	749	21.0	37.1	814	7.8	62.7	12.4	0	71%
unsalted	1 oz	164	4.6	8.1	5	1.1	13.7	2.7	0	71%
unsalted, approx 14 large or 18 medium kernels	1 oz	163	4.6	8.1	5	1.1	13.7	2.7	0	71%
unsalted, 'Fancy' (Planters)	1 oz	170	5.0	8.0	0	na	14.0	2.0	0	71%
unsalted, halves	1 cup	749	21.0	37.1	22	7.8	62.7	12.4	0	71%
'Unsalted' halves (Planters)	1 oz	170	5.0	8.0	0	(mq)	14.0	3.0	0	71%

Food Name	Serving Size	Calories	Prot. gms	Carbs gms	Sod. mgs	Fiber gms	Fat gms	Sat. Fat gms	Chol. mgs	% Fat Cal.
wholes *(Fisher)*	1 oz	170	5.0	8.0	110	na	14.0	4.0	0	71%
w/almonds *(Fisher)*	1 oz	170	5.0	6.0	95	na	15.0	2.0	0	75%
CASHEW BUTTER										
gourmet *(Roaster Fresh)*	1 oz	165	4.0	9.0	4	na	14.0	2.9	na	71%
peanut date *(Maranatha Natural)*	2 tbsp	190	8.0	8.0	8	na	14.0	na	na	66%
peanut date 'Natural' *(Westbrae)*	2 tbsp	200	6.0	8.0	2	na	15.0	na	na	71%
plain	1 oz	167	5.0	7.8	4	.6	14.0	2.8	0	71%
plain	1 tbsp	94	2.8	4.4	2	.3	7.9	1.6	0	71%
raw *(Hain)*	2 tbsp	190	6.0	8.0	(mq)	(mq)	15.0	3.0	0	71%
raw 'Natural' *(Westbrae)*	2 tbsp	300	6.0	8.0	0	na	28.0	na	na	82%
raw, unsalted *(Hain)*	2 tbsp	210	5.0	8.0	10	(mq)	19.0	3.0	0	77%
roasted *(Maranatha Natural)*	2 tbsp	190	6.0	10.0	5	na	14.0	na	na	66%
roasted 'Natural' *(Westbrae)*	2 tbsp	190	6.0	8.0	0	na	17.0	na	na	73%
toasted *(Hain)*	2 tbsp	210	7.0	7.0	15	(mq)	17.0	3.0	0	73%
CASSAVA/manioc/yuca										
trimmed	1 lb	544	14.1	122.1	36	>11.3 c	1.8	0.5	0	3%
trimmed	1 oz	34	0.9	7.6	2	>.7 c	0.1	<.1	0	3%
raw	100 gm	120	3.1	26.9	8	1.6	0.4	0.1	0	3%
CATFISH, CHANNEL										
Farmed										
dry-heat cooked	3 oz	129	15.9	0.0	68	0	6.8	1.5	54	49%
frozen, fillets *(Delta Pride)*	4 oz	132	18.0	4.8	<1	0	4.9	(mq)	62	33%
raw	3 oz	115	13.2	0.0	45	0	6.4	1.5	40	52%
raw	1 oz	33	5.2	0.0	18	0	1.2	0.3	16	34%
Wild										
dry-heat cooked	3 oz	89	15.7	0.0	43	0	2.4	0.6	61	26%
raw	3 oz	81	13.9	0.0	37	0	2.4	0.6	49	28%
CATFISH, OCEAN. See WOLF FISH.										
CATSUP/ketchup										
	1 oz	29	0.4	7.7	336	.5	0.1	<.1	0	3%
	1 tbsp	16	0.2	4.1	178	.2	0.1	0.0	0	5%
	.2-oz pkt	6	0.1	1.6	71	.1	0.0	0.0	0	0%
(Del Monte)	1/4 cup	60	1.0	16.0	675	(mq)	0.0	0.0	0	0%
(Estee)	1 tbsp	6	0.0	0.0	20	(mq)	0.0	0.0	0	0%
(Featherweight)	1 tbsp	6	0.0	1.0	5	(mq)	0.0	0.0	0	0%
(Healthy Choice)	.5 oz	9	0.3	2.0	97	.3	0.1	0.0	0	9%
(Heinz)	1 tbsp	16	0.2	3.8	213	>.2 c	0.0	0.0	0	0%
(Hunt's)	1 tbsp	16	0.3	3.7	158	.3	0.1	0.0	0	5%
(Smucker's)	1 tsp	8	0.0	2.0	45	(mq)	0.0	0.0	0	0%
(Snider's)	1 tbsp	16	0.3	3.7	158	.3	0.1	0.0	0	5%
(Stokely)	1 tbsp	20	0.0	5.0	190	(mq)	0.0	0.0	0	0%
(Weight Watchers)	2 tsp	8	0.0	2.0	110	(mq)	0.0	0.0	0	0%
'All Natural' *(Life)*	1 tbsp	17	0.0	4.0	10	(mq)	0.0	0.0	0	0%
'Food Service' *(Hunt's)*	1 tbsp	15	0.3	3.6	158	.2	0.1	0.0	0	6%
fruit-sweetened *(Westbrae)*	1 tbsp	12	0.0	2.0	110	na	0.0	na	0	0%
fruit-sweetened, no salt *(Westbrae)*	1 tbsp	12	0.0	2.0	10	na	0.0	na	0	0%
hot *(Heinz)*	1 tbsp	16	0.3	3.7	195	>.1 c	0.0	0.0	0	0%
'Lite' *(Heinz)*	1 tbsp	8	0.4	1.7	115	>.2 c	0.0	0.0	0	0%
low-sodium	1 oz	29	0.4	7.7	6	.5	0.1	<.1	0	3%
low-sodium	1 tbsp	16	0.2	4.1	3	>.2 c	0.1	0.0	0	5%
low-sodium	.2-oz pkt	6	0.1	1.6	1	>.1 c	0.0	0.0	0	0%
'Natural' *(Hain)*	1 tbsp	16	0.0	4.0	155	(mq)	0.0	0.0	0	0%
'Natural No Salt Added' *(Hain)*	1 tbsp	16	0.0	4.0	5	(mq)	0.0	0.0	0	0%
'No Salt Added' *(Del Monte)*	1/4 cup	60	1.0	16.0	25	(mq)	0.0	0.0	0	0%

Food Name	Serving Size	Calories	Prot. gms	Carbs gms	Sod. mgs	Fiber gms	Fat gms	Sat. Fat gms	Chol. mgs	% Fat Cal.
'No Salt Added' *(Hunt's)*	1 tbsp	20	0.0	5.0	0	(mq)	0.0	0.0	0	0%
organic *(Millina's Finest)*	1 oz	17	0.5	4.0	143	na	0.1	na	na	5%
portion pack *(Hunt's)*	.3175 oz	10	0.2	2.2	75	.2	0.1	0.0	0	9%
w/onions *(Heinz)*	1 tbsp	19	4.5	0.1	289	>.2 c	(tr)	0.0	0	0%
CAULIFLOWER										
boiled, drained	4 oz	27	2.1	5.2	7	2.5	0.2	<.1	0	6%
boiled, drained, approx 1.9 oz	3 flowerets	12	1.0	2.2	8	1.5	0.2	0.0	0	12%
boiled, drained, 1-inch pieces	1/2 cup	14	1.1	2.5	9	1.7	0.3	0.0	0	16%
fresh, medium size *(Dole)*	1/6 head	18	2.0	3.0	45	2.0	0.0	na	na	0%
green, fresh *(Dole)*	1/5 head	35	3.0	7.0	30	2.0	0.0	na	na	0%
raw, approx 5 oz	3 flowerets	14	1.1	2.9	17	1.4	0.1	0.0	0	5%
raw, 1-inch pieces	1/2 cup	13	1.0	2.6	15	1.3	0.1	0.0	0	6%
raw, trimmed	1 oz	7	0.6	1.4	4	.7	0.1	tr	0	10%
raw, untrimmed	1 lb	42	3.5	8.7	26	4.2	0.3	<.1	0	5%
Frozen										
	10 oz	68	5.7	13.3	68	6.5	0.8	0.1	0	9%
(A&P)	3.3 oz	25	2.0	5.0	20	(mq)	<1.0	(tr)	0	<24%
(Birds Eye)	3.3 oz	25	2.0	5.0	20	2.0	0.0	na	0	0%
(Finast)	3.3 oz	25	2.0	5.0	15	(mq)	0.0	0.0	0	0%
(Frosty Acres)	3.3 oz	25	2.0	5.0	16	>1.0 c	0.0	0.0	0	0%
(Kohl's)	3 oz	20	2.0	4.0	15	(mq)	<1.0	(tr)	0	<27%
(Seabrook)	3.3 oz	25	2.0	5.0	16	>1.0 c	0.0	0.0	0	0%
(Southern)	3.5 oz	26	2.0	4.8	30	(mq)	0.2	(tr)	0	6%
boiled, drained	4 oz	22	1.8	4.3	20	>.9 c	0.2	<.1	0	7%
boiled, drained, 1-inch pieces	1/2 cup	17	1.5	3.4	16	>.7 c	0.2	0.0	0	8%
cuts *(Green Giant)*	1/2 cup	12	1.0	3.0	25	1.0	0.0	0.0	0	0%
florets 'Plain Polybag' *(Green Giant)*	1/2 cup	12	1.0	3.0	25	2.0	0.0	0.0	0	0%
in cheddar cheese sauce 'Side Dish' *(Budget Gourmet)*	5 oz	110	6.0	10.0	300	(mq)	5.0	(mq)	25	41%
in cheese flavored sauce *(Green Giant)*	1/2 cup	60	2.0	10.0	500	2.4	2.0	(mq)	na	27%
in cheese sauce *(Finast)*	3.3 oz	40	2.0	5.0	240	(mq)	0.0	0.0	0	0%
in cheese sauce 'One Serving' *(Green Giant)*	5.5 oz	80	3.0	14.0	690	2.0	2.0	4.0	5	21%
in cheese sauce 'Singles' *(Stokely)*	4 oz	70	4.0	7.0	170	(mq)	3.0	(mq)	15	38%
'Singles' *(Stokely)*	3 oz	20	2.0	4.0	20	(mq)	0.0	0.0	0	0%
unprepared, 1-inch pieces	1/2 cup	16	1.3	3.1	16	1.5	0.2	0.0	0	9%
Pickled										
'Hot & Spicy' *(Vlasic)*	1 oz	4	0.0	1.0	435	(mq)	0.0	0.0	0	0%
sweet *(Vlasic)*	1 oz	35	0.0	9.0	225	(mq)	0.0	0.0	0	0%
CAVIAR										
black, granular	1 oz	71	6.9	1.1	420	0	5.0	1.1	165	58%
black, granular	1 tbsp	40	3.9	0.6	240	0	2.9	0.7	94	59%
red, granular	1 oz	71	6.9	1.1	420	0	5.0	1.1	165	58%
red, granular	1 tbsp	40	3.9	0.6	240	0	2.9	0.7	94	59%
CAYENNE PEPPER										
ground	1 oz	90	3.4	16.1	9	>7.1 c	4.9	0.9	0	36%
ground	1 tbsp	17	0.6	3.0	2	>1.3 c	0.9	0.2	0	36%
ground	1 tsp	6	0.2	1.0	1	>.5 c	0.3	0.1	0	36%
ground *(Spice Islands)*	1 tsp	9	0.3	1.1	<1	>.5 c	0.3	(tr)	0	33%
CECI. See GARBANZO BEAN.										
CELERIAC/celery root										
boiled, drained	4 oz	28	1.1	6.7	69	>.9 c	0.2	(tr)	0	6%
boiled, drained	100 gm	25	1.0	5.9	61	>.8 c	0.2	na	0	6%
raw	1/2 cup	30	1.2	7.2	78	1.4	0.2	na	0	5%
raw *(Frieda's)*	3.5 oz	40	1.8	8.5	100	(mq)	0.3	(tr)	0	6%
raw, trimmed	1 oz	11	0.4	2.6	28	>.4 c	0.1	(tr)	0	7%

Food Name	Serving Size	Calories	Prot. gms	Carbs gms	Sod. mgs	Fiber gms	Fat gms	Sat. Fat gms	Chol. mgs	% Fat Cal.
raw, untrimmed	1 lb	154	5.9	35.9	390	>5.1 c	1.2	na	0	0%
CELERY										
boiled, drained	4 oz	20	0.9	4.5	103	>1.0 c	0.1	<.1	0	4%
boiled, drained, diced	1/2 cup	14	0.6	3.0	68	1.2	0.1	0.0	0	6%
fresh, medium size (Dole)	2 stalks	20	1.0	4.0	140	1.4	0.0	na	na	0%
raw, diced	1/2 cup	10	0.5	2.2	52	1.0	0.1	0.0	0	8%
raw, trimmed	1 oz	5	0.2	1.0	25	.5	<.1	tr	0	<16%
raw, untrimmed	1 lb	65	3.0	14.7	352	6.5	0.6	0.1	0	7%
CELERY FLAKES (Tone's)	1 tsp	9	0.4	0.9	4	.3	0.5	<.1	0	46%
CELERY ROOT. See CELERIAC.										
CELERY ROOT JUICE, bottled (Biotta)	6 oz	67	2.7	13.1	195	(mq)	0.2	(tr)	0	3%
CELERY SALT (Tone's)	1 tsp	6	0.3	0.6	1584	.2	0.4	<.1	0	50%
CELERY SEED										
whole	1 oz	111	5.1	11.7	45	>3.4 c	7.2	0.6	0	49%
whole	1 tbsp	25	1.2	2.7	10	.8	1.6	0.1	0	48%
whole	1 tsp	8	0.4	0.8	3	.2	0.5	0.0	0	48%
whole (Durkee)	1 tsp	9	0.0	0.0	0	0	<0.1	na	na	<45%
whole (Laurel Leaf)	1 tsp	9	0.0	0.0	0	0	<0.1	na	na	<45%
whole (Spice Islands)	1 tsp	11	0.4	1.1	4	>.3 c	0.5	<.1	0	43%
CELLOPHANE NOODLES. See NOODLE, CHINESE.										
CELTUCE										
raw, approx .4 oz	1 leaf	2	0.1	0.3	1	(mq)	0.0	na	0	0%
trimmed	1 oz	6	0.2	1.0	3	>.1 c	0.1	(tr)	0	16%
untrimmed	1 lb	76	2.9	12.4	36	>1.4 c	1.0	na	0	13%
CEREAL, HOT										
(NOTE: All of the following hot cereals are dry unless otherwise noted.)										
BARLEY (Erewhon) organic plus	1 oz	110	3.0	22.0	0	1.0	1.0	na	0	8%
BRAN (H-O Brand) 'Super Bran'	1/3 cup	110	4.0	18.0	0	8.0	2.0	0.0	0	17%
BULGUR WHEAT										
(Arrowhead Mills)	2 oz	200	6.0	43.0	0	5.4	1.0	na	0	4%
(Krusteaz) 'Ala'	1/4 cup	150	4.0	33.0	0	7.0	0.0	0.0	0	0%
CORN GRITS. See GRITS.										
FARINA										
(H-O Brand) cream	3 tbsp	120	3.0	26.0	0	3.0	0.0	0.0	0	0%
(H-O Brand) instant	1 pkt	110	3.0	22.0	235	3.0	0.0	0.0	0	0%
(Krusteaz)	1 oz	100	3.0	22.0	1	1.0	0.0	0.0	0	0%
(Malt•O•Meal) 'Maple Brown Sugar' 30% formulation	1 oz	100	3.0	22.0	0	1.0	0.0	na	0	0%
GRAIN, MIXED										
(Arrowhead Mills) four grain	1 oz	94	4.0	18.0	1	7.4	1.0	na	0	9%
(Arrowhead Mills) seven grain	1 oz	100	4.0	17.0	<1	4.0	1.0	na	0	10%
(Breadshop) 'Triple Bran'	1 oz	100	6.0	15.0	5	6.0	2.0	na	0	18%
(Maltex) wheat and barley	1 oz	105	3.0	21.0	0	3.0	1.0	na	0	9%
(Malt•O•Meal) wheat and barley, chocolate flavor	1 tbsp	38	1.1	8.0	1	>.1 c	0.1	na	0	2%
(Malt•O•Meal) wheat and barley, plain	1 tbsp	38	1.1	8.0	1	>.1 c	0.1	na	0	2%
(Pritikin) hearty multi-grain, microwave instant	1 pkt	150	5.0	32.0	0	na	na	na	0	0%
(Quaker) multi-grain	1/2 cup	130	5.0	24.0	0	5.0	1.5	0.0	0	10%
(Roman Meal) multi-grain, apple, and cinnamon	2/3 cup	112	3.7	23.8	14	5.7	2.8	(mq)	<1	19%
(Roman Meal) oat and wheat, dates, raisins, and almonds	1.3 oz	140	4.0	26.0	0	3.0	0.0	(mq)	0	18%
(Roman Meal) oat and wheat, honey, coconut and almonds	1.3 oz	150	5.0	21.0	5	3.1	6.0	(mq)	0	34%
(Roman Meal) oat and wheat, rye, bran, and flax	1.2 oz	116	5.0	25.0	5	5.0	1.7	(mq)	0	11%
OAT BRAN										
(Arrowhead Mills)	1 oz	110	6.0	17.0	1	5.1 d	1.0	na	0	9%
(Breadshop) 'Oat Bran Muesli'	1 oz	100	4.0	20.0	5	3.0	2.0	na	0	16%

Food Name	Serving Size	Calories	Prot. gms	Carbs gms	Sod. mgs	Fiber gms	Fat gms	Sat. Fat gms	Chol. mgs	% Fat Cal.
(Breadshop) 'Oat Bran' 100% pure	1 oz	100	6.0	17.0	5	4.0	2.0	na	0	16%
(Erewhon) toasted wheat germ	1 oz	115	5.0	18.0	15	3.0	2.0	na	0	16%
(Health Valley) 'Natural' apple and cinnamon	1 oz	100	3.0	19.0	10	3.8	1.0	na	0	9%
(Health Valley) 'Natural' raisins and spice	1 oz	110	3.0	19.0	10	3.8	1.0	na	0	9%
(Malt•O•Meal) 'Plus 40% Oat Bran'	1.3 oz	130	6.0	25.0	0	3.0	2.0	na	0	13%
(Mother's)	1/3 cup	92	5.7	16.6	1	4.2	2.1	0.2	0	18%
(Quaker)	1 oz	92	5.7	16.6	1	4.2	2.1	0.2	0	18%
(3-Minute Brand) instant	1 oz	90	6.0	17.0	0	4.1	2.0	(mq)	0	16%
(3-Minute Brand) 'Regular'	1 oz	90	6.0	17.0	0	4.1	2.0	(mq)	0	16%
(Wholesome 'N Hearty)	1 oz	100	4.0	18.0	0	5.0	2.0	(mq)	0	17%
(Wholesome 'N Hearty) instant, apple cinnamon	1 3/8 oz	130	3.0	30.0	160	5.0	2.0	(mq)	0	12%
(Wholesome 'N Hearty) instant, honey	1.25 oz	110	3.0	26.0	160	5.0	2.0	(mq)	0	13%
OATMEAL AND OATS										
(Arrowhead Mills) instant	1 oz	100	5.8	18.0	0	4.3	2.0	(mq)	0	16%
(Arrowhead Mills) instant, apple, date, and almond	1 oz	130	5.0	23.0	3	3.7	3.0	(mq)	0	19%
(Arrowhead Mills) instant, apple spice	1 oz	130	5.0	23.0	1	3.4	2.0	(mq)	0	14%
(Arrowhead Mills) instant, cinnamon, raisin, and almond ..	1 oz	140	6.0	23.0	3	4.3	3.0	(mq)	0	19%
(Erewhon) instant, apple and cinnamon	1.25 oz	145	4.0	25.0	100	na	3.0	na	na	19%
(Erewhon) instant, apple and raisin	1.3 oz	150	4.0	27.0	100	na	3.0	na	na	18%
(Erewhon) instant, maple spice	1.2 oz	140	4.0	24.0	100	na	3.0	na	na	19%
(Erewhon) instant, oat bran	1.25 oz	125	6.0	23.0	0	4.0	3.0	na	na	19%
(Erewhon) instant, raisins, dates, and walnuts	1.2 oz	130	3.0	24.0	60	3.0	3.0	na	na	20%
(General Mills) instant, apple and cinnamon	1.5 oz	150	4.0	32.0	105	3.0	2.0	(mq)	0	11%
(General Mills) instant, cinnamon raisin	1.8 oz	170	4.0	38.0	130	3.0	2.0	(mq)	0	10%
(General Mills) 'Oatmeal Swirlers' instant, apple and cinnamon	1.7 oz	160	3.0	34.0	120	2.0	2.0	(mq)	0	11%
(General Mills) 'Oatmeal Swirlers' instant, cherry	1.7 oz	150	3.0	33.0	130	2.0	2.0	(mq)	0	11%
(General Mills) 'Oatmeal Swirlers' instant, cinnamon and spice	1.6 oz	160	3.0	35.0	100	2.0	2.0	(mq)	0	11%
(General Mills) 'Oatmeal Swirlers' instant, maple and brown sugar	1.6 oz	160	3.0	35.0	100	2.0	2.0	(mq)	0	11%
(General Mills) 'Oatmeal Swirlers' instant, milk chocolate ..	1.7 oz	170	3.0	37.0	100	2.0	2.0	(mq)	0	10%
(General Mills) 'Oatmeal Swirlers' instant, strawberry	1.6 oz	150	3.0	32.0	120	2.0	2.0	(mq)	0	11%
(H-O Brand) 'Gourmet'	1/3 cup	100	5.0	18.0	0	3.0	2.0	0.0	0	16%
(H-O Brand) instant	1 pkt	110	4.0	18.0	230	3.0	2.0	0.0	0	17%
(H-O Brand) instant, apple and cinnamon	1 pkt	130	3.0	26.0	220	3.0	2.0	0.0	0	13%
(H-O Brand) instant, box	1/2 cup	130	5.0	22.0	5	3.0	2.0	0.0	0	14%
(H-O Brand) instant, maple and brown sugar	1 pkt	160	4.0	32.0	285	3.0	2.0	0.0	0	11%
(H-O Brand) instant, raisins and spice	1 pkt	150	4.0	32.0	240	3.0	2.0	0.0	0	11%
(H-O Brand) instant, sweet 'n mellow	1 pkt	150	5.0	30.0	270	3.0	2.0	0.0	0	11%
(H-O Brand) 'Quick'	1/2 cup	130	5.0	23.0	5	3.0	2.0	0.0	0	14%
(H-O Brand) w/fiber, instant	1 pkt	110	5.0	18.0	140	3.0	2.0	0.0	0	16%
(H-O Brand) w/fiber, instant, apple and bran	1 pkt	130	3.0	26.0	140	3.0	2.0	0.0	0	13%
(H-O Brand) w/fiber, instant, box	1/3 cup	100	5.0	15.0	5	3.0	2.0	0.0	0	18%
(H-O Brand) w/fiber, instant, raisin, and bran	1 pkt	150	4.0	32.0	140	3.0	2.0	0.0	0	11%
(Maypo)	1 cup	362	12.4	67.7	18	10.1	5.0	na	0	12%
(Maypo) '30 Second' quick	1 oz	100	4.0	19.0	0	2.0	1.0	na	0	9%
(Maypo) 'Vermont Style' maple flavor	1 oz	105	4.0	20.0	0	2.0	1.0	na	0	9%
(Mother's) instant	1 oz	110	5.0	18.0	0	.3	2.0	na	0	16%
(Quaker)	1/3 cup	99	4.4	18.6	1	2.7	2.0	0.3	0	16%
(Quaker) 'Extra'	1 pkt	95	4.4	17.6	219	2.9	2.0	0.2	0	17%
(Quaker) 'Extra' apples and spice	1 pkt	133	4.3	26.7	191	3.0	1.9	0.3	0	12%
(Quaker) 'Extra' raisins and cinnamon	1 pkt	129	4.1	26.6	119	2.7	1.9	0.3	0	12%
(Quaker) instant	1 pkt	94	3.8	18.0	270	2.8	2.0	0.3	0	17%

Food Name	Serving Size	Calories	Prot. gms	Carbs gms	Sod. mgs	Fiber gms	Fat gms	Sat. Fat gms	Chol. mgs	% Fat Cal.
(Quaker) instant, apple and cinnamon	1 pkt	118	3.3	26.0	128	3.0	1.5	0.3	0	10%
(Quaker) instant, cinnamon and spice	1 pkt	164	4.5	34.9	322	3.1	2.1	0.4	0	11%
(Quaker) instant, maple and brown sugar	1 pkt	152	4.5	31.6	320	2.8	2.1	0.4	0	12%
(Quaker) instant, peaches and cream	1 pkt	129	3.4	26.3	179	2.3	2.2	0.9	0	14%
(Quaker) instant, raisins and spice	1 pkt	149	4.1	31.5	266	2.8	2.0	0.3	0	11%
(Quaker) instant, raisins, dates, and walnuts	1 pkt	141	4.0	25.1	216	2.4	3.8	0.4	0	23%
(Quaker) instant, strawberries and cream	1 pkt	129	3.4	26.6	204	2.2	2.0	1.1	0	13%
(Quaker) 'Kids' Choice' instant, cinnamon graham cookie	1 pkt	140	4.0	29.0	170	2.6	2.0	na	0	12%
(Quaker) 'Kids' Choice' instant, maple and brown sugar ..	1 pkt	140	4.0	31.0	240	2.9	2.0	na	0	11%
(Quaker) 'Kids' Choice' instant, radical raspberry	1 pkt	150	4.0	28.0	170	2.9	3.0	na	0	17%
(Quaker) 'Kids' Choice' instant, strawberries and stuff	1 pkt	140	4.0	30.0	170	2.6	2.0	na	0	12%
(Quaker) 'Old Fashioned'	1 oz	99	4.4	18.6	1	2.7	2.0	0.3	0	16%
(Quaker) plus fiber	1/2 cup	130	6.0	21.0	0	6.0	2.5	0.5	0	17%
(Quaker) plus fiber, oatmeal raisin bran	1 pkt	150	4.0	28.0	65	6.0	2.0	0.5	0	12%
(Quaker) 'Quick'	1 oz	99	4.4	18.6	1	2.7	2.0	0.3	0	16%
(Ralston)	1 cup	402	16.6	85.1	13	>2.5 c	2.5	na	0	5%
(Roman Meal)	1 cup	340	14.5	68.5	20	>2.3 c	4.0	na	0	10%
(3-Minute Brand) oat bran and raisins	1 oz	100	4.0	18.0	0	3.0	2.0	(mq)	0	17%
(3-Minute Brand) 'Old Fashioned'	1 oz	100	5.0	18.0	0	3.0	2.0	(mq)	0	16%
(3-Minute Brand) 'Quick'	1 oz	100	5.0	18.0	0	3.0	2.0	(mq)	0	16%
(3-Minute Brand) 'Quick' oat bran	1 oz	100	5.0	18.0	0	3.3	2.0	(mq)	0	16%
(3-Minute Brand) raisins	1 oz	100	5.0	18.0	0	3.0	2.0	(mq)	0	16%
(Total) instant	1.2 oz	110	4.0	22.0	220	3.0	2.0	(mq)	0	15%
(Total) instant, maple and brown sugar	1.6 oz	160	4.0	34.0	150	3.0	2.0	(mq)	0	11%
(Total) 'Quick'	1 oz	90	4.0	18.0	0	2.5	2.0	(mq)	0	17%
QUINOA (Ancient Harvest) steam-rolled flakes	1/3 cup	105	2.6	23.0	5	2.8	1.0	0.0	0	8%
RICE										
(Cream of Rice)	1 tbsp	38	0.6	8.4	1	0	0.1	na	0	2%
(Lundberg Family) 'Hot'n Creamy' cooked	1 oz	110	3.0	23.0	20	na	1.0	na	na	8%
(Lundberg Family) 'Hot'n Creamy' almonds and										
dates, cooked	1 oz	110	2.0	24.0	25	na	1.0	na	na	8%
RICE, BROWN										
(Arrowhead Mills) 'Rise & Shine'	1.5 oz	160	3.0	35.0	<1	1.6	1.0	na	0	6%
(Erewhon) cream of brown rice	1 oz	110	3.0	23.0	20	na	1.0	na	na	8%
RYE										
(Breadshop) 'Rye Date Müesli'	1 oz	100	3.0	19.0	5	4.0	2.0	na	na	17%
(Roman Meal) cream of rye	1.3 oz	110	4.0	27.0	0	5.4	<1.0	na	0	<7%
WHEAT										
(Arrowhead Mills) 'Bear Mush'	1 oz	100	3.0	21.0	<1	1.3	0.0	0.0	0	0%
(Arrowhead Mills) cracked wheat	2 oz	180	7.0	40.0	1	2.3	1.0	na	0	5%
(Cream of Wheat)	1 tbsp	39	1.1	8.1	1	0	0.2	na	0	5%
(Cream of Wheat) instant	1 oz	100	3.0	22.0	0	1.0	<1.0	<1.0	5	<8%
(Cream of Wheat) instant	1 tbsp	42	1.2	8.7	2	0	0.2	na	0	4%
(Cream of Wheat) 'Mix'n Eat' instant	1 oz	100	3.0	21.0	170	1.0	0.0	0.0	0	0%
(Cream of Wheat) 'Mix'n Eat' instant, apple and cinnamon	1 oz	130	2.0	29.0	250	1.0	0.0	0.0	0	0%
(Cream of Wheat) 'Mix'n Eat' instant, apple, banana, and										
maple	1 pkt	132	2.4	28.9	241	0	0.4	na	0	3%
(Cream of Wheat) 'Mix'n Eat' instant, brown sugar and										
cinnamon	1 oz	130	2.0	29.0	230	1.0	0.0	0.0	0	0%
(Cream of Wheat) 'Mix'n Eat' instant, maple and brown										
sugar	1 oz	130	2.0	29.0	180	1.0	0.0	0.0	0	0%
(Cream of Wheat) 'Quick'	1 tbsp	38	1.1	7.9	41	0	0.1	na	0	2%
(General Mills) 'Wheat Hearts'	1 oz	110	4.0	20.0	0	1.0	1.0	na	0	9%
(Krusteaz) 'Zoom'	1/3 cup	120	5.0	24.0	0	4.0	0.0	0.0	0	0%

Food Name	Serving Size	Calories	Prot. gms	Carbs gms	Sod. mgs	Fiber gms	Fat gms	Sat. Fat gms	Chol. mgs	% Fat Cal.
(Maltex)	1 cup	532	16.9	116.7	26	6.3	3.2	na	0	5%
(Mother's)	1/3 cup	92	2.9	20.9	1	2.2	0.6	0.1	0	5%
(Quaker)	1/3 cup	92	2.9	20.9	1	2.2	0.6	0.1	0	5%
(Wheatena)	1 oz	100	3.0	21.0	0	4.0	1.0	na	0	9%

CEREAL, READY-TO-SERVE

(NOTE: All of the following ready-to-serve cereals are in their dry form.)

Food Name	Serving Size	Calories	Prot. gms	Carbs gms	Sod. mgs	Fiber gms	Fat gms	Sat. Fat gms	Chol. mgs	% Fat Cal.
'Addam's Family' (Ralston)	1 oz	110	1.0	25.0	65	na	1.0	na	0	8%
'All Bran' extra fiber (Kellogg's)	1 oz	50	4.0	22.0	140	14.0	0.0	0.0	0	0%
'All Bran' wheat bran (Kellogg's)	1 oz	71	4.1	21.1	320	10.1	0.5	na	0	4%
'Almond Flavor O's' fat-free (Health Valley)	1 oz	90	3.0	19.0	5	5.0	0.0	na	0	0%
'Almond Raisin' low fat (Golden Temple)	1 oz	110	2.0	22.0	57	2.0	1.5	0.5	0	12%
'Almond Raisin' nectarsweet premium (Breadshop)	1 oz	120	3.5	18.0	2	2.5	4.0	0.0	0	30%
'Alpha Bits' oat and other grains (Post)	1 oz	111	2.2	24.6	180	1.2	0.7	na	0	6%
'Alpha Bits' super swirl marshmallows (Post)	1 oz	150	6.0	31.0	220	1.0	1.0	na	0	6%
'Apple Almond Müesli' (Ralston)	1.45 oz	150	4.0	31.0	140	3.0	2.0	na	0	11%
'Apple & Cinnamon Toasted Oat' (Malt•O•Meal)	1 oz	110	2.0	22.0	180	1.0	2.0	na	0	16%
'Apple Cinnamon Cheerios' (General Mills)	1 oz	110	2.0	22.0	180	1.5	2.0	na	0	16%
'Apple Cinnamon Corn Flakes' (Wonder)	1 oz	110	2.0	25.0	200	na	0.0	na	0	0%
'Apple Cinnamon' low fat (Golden Temple)	1 oz	110	2.0	22.0	59	2.0	1.5	0.5	0	12%
'Apple Cinnamon O's' fat-free (Health Valley)	1 oz	90	3.0	19.0	5	5.0	0.0	na	0	0%
'Apple Cinnamon Squares' (Kellogg's)	1 oz	90	2.0	23.0	5	2.0	0.0	0.0	0	0%
'Apple Jacks' corn and other grains (Kellogg's)	1 oz	110	1.5	25.8	125	.5	0.1	na	0	1%
'Apple Raisin Crisp' (Kellogg's)	1 oz	130	2.0	32.0	230	3.0	0.0	0.0	0	0%
'Aztec' (Erewhon)	1 oz	100	2.0	24.0	85	1.0	0.0	na	0	0%
'Banana Nut Crunch' (Post)	1 oz	120	3.0	20.0	95	2.0	3.0	na	0	23%
'Banana O's' (Erewhon)	1 oz	110	2.0	24.0	15	na	0.0	na	na	0%
'Banana Walnut Müesli' (Ralston)	1.45 oz	150	4.0	30.0	150	3.0	3.0	na	0	17%
'Basic 4' (General Mills)	3/4 cup	130	3.0	28.0	210	2.0	2.0	na	0	13%
'Batman Returns' (Ralston)	1 oz	110	1.0	26.0	190	na	0.0	na	0	0%
'Berry Berry Kix' (General Mills)	1 oz	110	1.0	25.0	170	na	1.0	na	0	8%
'Blueberry 'N Cream' nectarsweet gourmet (Breadshop) ..	1 oz	115	3.7	18.7	2	2.5	3.0	0.0	0	23%
'Blueberry Squares' (Kellogg's)	1 oz	90	2.0	23.0	5	3.0	0.0	0.0	0	0%
'Body Buddies Natural Fruit' (General Mills)	1 oz	110	2.0	24.0	280	na	1.0	na	0	8%
'Booberry' (General Mills)	1 oz	110	1.0	24.0	210	na	1.0	na	0	8%

QUICK REFERENCE: CEREAL TOPPINGS

Although it is important to know the nutrient values of the cereals we eat, it makes sense to remember that most of us do not eat our cereals as is. Instead, we add a variety of toppings—milk, sugar, or syrup, for instance. These toppings add flavor and some nutrients, but they also add fat and calories. Here is a quick look at the nutrient values of the most common cereal toppings.

Food Name	Serving Size	Calories	Prot. gms	Carbs gms	Sod. mgs	Fiber gms	Fat gms	Sat. Fat gms	Chol. mgs	% Fat Cal.
Skim milk	1 cup	86	8.4	11.9	126	0	0.4	0.3	4	4%
1% milk	1 cup	102	8.0	11.7	123	0	2.6	1.6	10	23%
2% milk	1 cup	121	8.1	11.7	122	0	4.7	2.9	18	35%
Whole milk	1 cup	150	8.0	11.0	125	0	8.0	4.9	33	49%
Soymilk, regular	8 oz	150	7.0	18.0	115	na	5.0	na	0	31%
Soymilk, light	8 oz	100	4.0	16.0	100	na	2.0	na	0	18%
White sugar	1 tsp	15	0.0	4.0	0	0	0.0	na	0	0%
Brown sugar	1 tsp	16	0.0	4.0	0	na	0.0	0.0	na	0%
Honey	1 tbsp	64	0.1	17.3	1	0	0.0	0.0	0	0%
Maple syrup	1 tbsp	52	0.0	13.4	2	0	0.0	na	0	0%

Food Name	Serving Size	Calories	Prot. gms	Carbs gms	Sod. mgs	Fiber gms	Fat gms	Sat. Fat gms	Chol. mgs	% Fat Cal.
'Bran Buds' wheat bran (Kellogg's)	1 oz	73	4.0	21.6	174	10.6	0.7	na	0	6%
'Bran Chex' wheat bran and corn (Kellogg's)	1 oz	91	2.9	22.6	264	4.6	0.8	na	0	7%
'Bran Flakes' (Arrowhead Mills)	1 oz	100	5.0	21.0	100	4.0	1.0	na	0	8%
'Bran Flakes' (Kellogg's)	1 oz	90	3.0	22.0	220	5.0	0.0	0.0	0	0%
'Bran Flakes' (Malt•O•Meal)	1 oz	90	3.0	23.0	210	5.0	1.0	na	0	8%
'Bran Flakes' (Post)	1 oz	90	3.0	23.0	210	5.0	0.0	na	0	0%
'Breakfast O's' (Barbara's Bakery)	1 oz	120	4.0	21.0	90	na	2.0	na	0	15%
Brown rice, crisp (Erewhon)	1 oz	110	2.0	24.0	185	4.0	1.0	na	na	8%
Brown rice, crisp, low sodium (Erewhon)	1 oz	110	2.0	24.0	5	4.0	1.0	na	na	8%
'Brown Rice Crisps' (Barbara's Bakery)	1 oz	120	2.0	26.0	105	na	1.0	na	0	7%
'Buñuelitos' (General Mills)	1 oz	120	1.0	25.0	120	na	2.0	na	0	15%
'C.W. Post Hearty Granola Cereal' (Post)	1 oz	130	2.0	21.0	80	(tr)	4.0	na	0	28%
'C.W. Post' oats and other grains (Post)	1 oz	126	2.6	20.3	49	2.1	4.4	3.3	0	30%
'C.W. Post' oats and other grains, raisins (Post)	1 oz	123	2.4	20.4	44	3.8	4.1	3.0	0	29%
'California Orange Crunch' honeysweet premium (Breadshop)	1 oz	130	3.5	18.0	1	2.4	5.0	0.0	0	34%
'Captain Crunch' corn and other grains (Quaker)	1 oz	120	1.5	23.0	213	.5	2.6	1.7	0	19%
'Captain Crunch Crunchberries' corn and oat (Quaker) ...	1 oz	118	1.5	23.1	198	.5	2.4	1.6	0	18%
'Captain Crunch Peanut Butter' corn (Quaker)	1 oz	125	2.0	21.5	217	.4	3.7	1.5	0	26%
'Cashew Almond Granola' (Golden Temple)	1 oz	129	4.0	19.0	3	3.5	3.5	0.5	0	26%
'Cheerios' oat and wheat (General Mills)	1 oz	111	4.3	19.6	308	2.0	1.8	0.3	0	15%
'Cinnamon & Raisin' 100% natural (Nature Valley)	1 oz	120	2.0	20.0	50	1.0	4.0	na	0	29%
'Cinnamon & Spice Crunch' psyllium and chia seed (Golden Temple)	1 oz	132	3.0	20.0	26	2.0	4.5	0.5	0	31%
'Cinnamon Apple Raisin Granola' (Golden Temple)	1 oz	125	3.0	20.0	3	2.0	3.5	0.5	0	26%
'Cinnamon Mini Buns' (Kellogg's)	1 oz	110	2.0	25.0	220	1.0	1.0	0.0	0	8%
'Cinnamon Toast Crunch' (General Mills)	1 oz	120	1.0	22.0	210	1.0	3.0	na	0	23%
'Cinnamon Toast Crunch' breakfast pack (General Mills) ..	1 oz	140	1.0	26.0	240	1.0	4.0	na	0	25%
'Cinnapple Spice' honeysweet premium (Breadshop)	1 oz	125	3.4	18.5	2	2.0	4.5	0.5	0	32%
'Clusters' (General Mills)	1 oz	110	3.0	22.0	140	2.0	2.0	na	0	15%
'Cocoa Krispies' rice (Kellogg's)	1 oz	110	1.5	25.2	217	.2	0.4	na	0	3%
'Cocoa Pebbles' rice (Post)	1 oz	116	1.3	24.4	136	.5	1.5	na	0	12%
'Cocoa Puffs' (General Mills)	1 oz	110	1.0	25.0	180	na	1.0	na	0	8%
'Coconut Almond Granola' (Golden Temple)	1 oz	145	4.0	18.0	26	3.0	7.0	2.0	0	42%
'Common Sense Oat Bran' (Kellogg's)	1 oz	100	4.0	22.0	250	3.0	1.0	0.0	0	8%
'Common Sense Oat Bran' raisins (Kellogg's)	3/4 cup	130	4.0	29.0	250	3.0	1.0	0.0	0	6%
'Complete' bran flakes, beta carotene (Kellogg's)	1 oz	90	3.0	23.0	220	5.0	<1.0	0.0	0	<8%
'Cookie-Crisp' chocolate chip and vanilla (Ralston)	1 oz	114	1.5	24.9	196	>.1 c	1.0	na	0	8%
'Corn Bran' corn bran and other grains (Ralston)	1 oz	98	1.9	23.9	244	>1.1 c	1.0	na	0	8%
'Corn Chex' (Ralston)	1 oz	111	2.0	24.9	272	>.1 c	0.1	na	0	1%
'Corn Flakes' (Arrowhead Mills)	1 oz	100	2.0	25.0	100	2.0	0.0	na	0	0%
'Corn Flakes' (Barbara's Bakery)	1 oz	110	2.0	24.0	70	na	0.0	0.0	0	0%
'Corn Flakes' (Kellogg's)	1 oz	110	2.3	24.4	291	.7	0.1	na	0	1%
'Corn Flakes' (Krusteaz)	1 oz	110	2.0	24.0	280	1.0	1.0	na	0	8%
'Corn Flakes' (Malt•O•Meal)	1 oz	110	2.0	25.0	290	1.0	0.0	na	0	0%
'Corn Flakes' (Ralston)	1 oz	111	2.2	24.6	272	>.1 c	0.1	na	0	1%
'Corn Flakes' sugar frosted (Kellogg's)	1 oz	108	1.4	25.7	230	.5	0.1	na	0	1%
'Corn Flakes' sugar frosted (Ralston)	1 oz	111	1.5	25.6	184	>.1 c	0.4	na	0	3%
'Corn Pops' (Kellogg's)	1 oz	110	1.0	26.0	90	1.0	0.0	0.0	0	0%
'Count Chocula' (General Mills)	1 oz	110	1.0	25.0	180	na	1.0	na	0	8%
'Country Corn Flakes' (General Mills)	1 oz	110	2.0	25.0	270	na	1.0	na	0	8%
'Cracklin' Bran' wheat bran and other grains (Kellogg's) ..	1 oz	108	2.6	19.5	230	4.7	4.2	na	0	30%
'Cracklin' Oat Bran' (Kellogg's)	1 oz	110	3.0	21.0	140	4.0	3.0	1.0	0	22%
'Cranberry Walnut Müesli' (Ralston)	1.45 oz	150	4.0	30.0	95	3.0	3.0	na	0	17%

Food Name	Serving Size	Calories	Prot. gms	Carbs gms	Sod. mgs	Fiber gms	Fat gms	Sat. Fat gms	Chol. mgs	% Fat Cal.
'Crisp N' Crackling Rice' (Malt•O•Meal)	1 oz	110	2.0	25.0	240	0	0.0	na	0	0%
'Crisp Rice' (Krusteaz)	1 oz	110	2.0	25.0	270	1.0	0.0	na	0	0%
'Crispix' (Kellogg's)	1 oz	110	2.0	25.0	220	0	0.0	0.0	0	0%
'Crispy Wheats 'N Raisins' wheat (General Mills)	1 oz	99	2.0	23.2	135	1.9	0.5	na	0	4%
'Crunch Graham Oat Rings' (Wonder)	1 oz	110	2.0	24.0	125	na	1.0	na	0	8%
'Crunchies' brown rice (Lundberg Family)	1 cup	171	3.0	38.0	7	na	0.8	na	na	4%
'Crunchy Oat Bran' nectarsweet gourmet (Breadshop) ..	1 oz	120	3.0	18.0	2	2.5	5.0	0.5	na	35%
'Date Almond Müesli' (Ralston)	1.45 oz	140	4.0	32.0	95	3.0	2.0	na	0	11%
'Dino Pebbles' (Post)	1 oz	110	1.0	25.0	150	tr	1.0	na	0	8%
'Double Chex' (Ralston)	1 oz	100	1.0	25.0	260	0	0.0	na	0	0%
'Double Dip Crunch' (Kellogg's)	1 oz	120	2.0	23.0	160	0	2.0	0.0	0	15%
'Fiber One' aspartame (General Mills)	1 oz	60	2.0	23.0	140	13.0	1.0	na	0	8%
'Fiberwise' (Kellogg's)	1 oz	90	3.0	23.0	140	5.0	1.0	0.0	0	8%
'Fingos' cinnamon (General Mills)	1 oz	110	1.0	22.0	170	2.0	3.0	na	0	23%
'Fingos' honey toasted oat (General Mills)	1 oz	110	2.0	21.0	210	1.5	3.0	na	0	23%
'40% Bran Flakes' wheat bran (Kellogg's)	1 oz	93	3.6	22.2	220	4.0	0.5	na	0	4%
'40% Bran Flakes' wheat bran (Post)	1 oz	92	3.2	22.5	260	5.5	0.5	na	0	4%
'40% Bran Flakes' wheat bran (Ralston)	1 oz	92	3.3	22.7	264	>1.2 c	0.4	na	0	3%
'Frankenberry' (General Mills)	1 oz	110	1.0	24.0	210	na	1.0	na	0	8%
'Froot Loops' corn and other grains (Kellogg's)	1 oz	111	1.7	25.1	145	.6	0.5	na	0	4%
'Frosted Chex Juniors' (Ralston)	1 oz	110	2.0	25.0	200	na	0.0	na	0	0%
'Frosted Flakes' (Kellogg's)	1 oz	110	1.0	26.0	200	1.0	0.0	0.0	0	0%
'Frosted Funnies' (Barbara's Bakery)	1 cup	110	2.0	27.0	100	na	0.0	na	0	0%
'Frosted Krispies' (Kellogg's)	1 oz	110	1.0	26.0	220	0	0.0	0.0	0	0%
'Frosted Mini Wheats' (Kellogg's)	1 oz	100	3.0	24.0	0	3.0	0.0	0.0	0	0%
'Frosted Mini Wheats' bite size (Kellogg's)	1 oz	100	3.0	24.0	0	3.0	0.0	0.0	0	0%
'Frosted Mini Wheats' brown sugar and cinnamon (Kellogg's)	1 oz	102	2.9	23.4	8	2.2	0.3	na	0	3%
'Frosted Rice Krinkles' rice	1 oz	109	1.4	25.9	179	.2	0.1	na	0	1%
'Frosted Rice Krispies' rice (Kellogg's)	1 oz	109	1.4	25.7	240	.2	0.1	na	0	1%
'Fruit & Fibre' oat, dates, raisins, and walnuts (Post)	1.25 oz	120	3.0	27.0	170	5.0	2.0	na	0	13%
'Fruit & Fibre' oat, peaches, raisins, and almonds (Post) ..	1.25 oz	120	3.0	26.0	170	5.0	2.0	na	0	13%
'Fruit & Fibre' oat, pineapple, banana, and coconut (Post)	1.25 oz	120	3.0	27.0	170	5.0	3.0	na	0	18%
'Fruit & Fibre' oat, tropical fruit (Post)	1.25 oz	120	3.0	27.0	170	5.0	3.0	na	0	18%
'Fruit & Frosted O's' mixed grain (Malt•O•Meal)	1 oz	110	2.0	25.0	120	1.0	1.0	na	0	8%
'Fruit & Nut' 100% natural (Nature Valley)	1 oz	130	2.0	19.0	45	1.0	5.0	na	0	35%
'Fruit 'N Nut Granola' (Golden Temple)	1 oz	129	3.0	19.0	26	2.0	4.5	0.5	0	32%
'Fruit 'n Wheat' (Erewhon)	1 oz	100	2.0	21.0	75	3.0	1.0	na	0	9%
'Fruit Wheats' apple (Nabisco)	1 oz	90	2.0	23.0	15	3.0	0.0	na	0	0%
'Fruit Whirls' (Krusteaz)	1 oz	110	1.0	25.0	120	1.0	1.0	na	0	8%
'Fruitful Bran' fruit (Kellogg's)	1 oz	120	3.0	31.0	240	5.0	0.0	0.0	0	0%
'Fruity Marshmallow Krispies' (Kellogg's)	1 1/4 cups	140	2.0	32.0	210	0	0.0	0.0	0	0%
'Fruity Pebbles' rice (Post)	1 oz	115	1.1	24.4	158	.4	1.5	na	0	12%
'Golden Crisp' (Post)	1 oz	110	2.0	26.0	45	(tr)	0.0	na	0	0%
'Golden Grahams' corn and wheat (General Mills)	1 oz	109	1.6	24.2	281	1.0	1.1	0.8	0	9%
'Golden Granola' (Golden Temple)	1 oz	138	4.0	19.0	25	2.0	6.0	1.0	0	37%
'Golden Maple Nut' honeysweet premium (Breadshop) ...	1 oz	130	3.5	17.0	2	2.0	5.0	0.8	na	35%
'Gone Nuts!' nectarsweet premium (Breadshop)	1 oz	125	3.5	17.0	2	2.5	5.0	0.5	na	35%
'Graham Chex' (Ralston)	1 oz	110	2.0	24.0	220	1.0	1.0	na	0	8%
'Graham Crackos' wheat	1 oz	103	2.1	24.5	185	1.7	0.2	na	0	2%
Granola, banana almond (Sunbelt)	1 oz	130	3.0	20.0	25	na	4.0	na	2	28%
Granola, date and almond, fat-free (Health Valley)	1 oz	90	2.0	21.0	20	2.5	0.0	na	0	0%
Granola, fruit and nut (Sunbelt)	1 oz	120	3.0	19.0	20	na	5.0	na	na	34%
Granola, raisin cinnamon, fat-free (Health Valley)	1 oz	90	2.0	21.0	20	2.5	0.0	na	0	0%

Food Name	Serving Size	Calories	Prot. gms	Carbs gms	Sod. mgs	Fiber gms	Fat gms	Sat. Fat gms	Chol. mgs	% Fat Cal.
Granola, tropical fruit, fat-free *(Health Valley)*	1 oz	90	2.0	21.0	20	2.5	0.0	na	0	0%
'Granola' toasted oat mix *(Nature Valley)*	1 oz	126	2.9	19.0	58	1.5	4.9	3.3	0	34%
'Grape-Nuts' wheat and barley *(Post)*	1 oz	101	3.3	23.3	197	2.8	0.1	na	0	1%
'Grape-Nuts Flakes' wheat and barley *(Post)*	1 oz	102	3.0	23.2	160	2.8	0.3	na	0	3%
'Great Grains' double pecan *(Post)*	1 oz	120	3.0	20.0	60	3.0	3.0	na	0	23%
'Great Grains' raisins, dates and pecans *(Post)*	1.25 oz	140	3.0	27.0	70	3.0	3.0	na	0	18%
'Hawaiian Granola' *(Golden Temple)*	1 oz	126	4.0	19.0	3	2.0	4.0	1.0	0	28%
'Hazelnut Boysenberry' organic oats *(Golden Temple)*	1 oz	135	4.0	19.0	2	3.0	5.5	0.5	0	35%
'Heritage O's' *(Natures Path)*	1 cup	165	5.0	34.0	140	4.5	<1.0	na	0	<6%
'High Fiber O's' fat-free *(Health Valley)*	1 oz	90	3.0	19.0	5	5.0	0.0	na	0	0%
'High 5' *(Barbara's Bakery)*	3/4 cup	100	3.0	23.0	180	na	0.5	na	0	4%
'High Protein Granola' *(Golden Temple)*	1 oz	124	4.0	19.0	6	2.0	3.5	0.5	0	26%
'Honey Almond Delight' *(Ralston)*	1 oz	110	2.0	23.0	200	1.0	2.0	na	0	15%
'Honey Almond Granola' *(Golden Temple)*	1 oz	130	4.0	20.0	25	3.0	3.5	0.5	0	25%
'Honey & Nut Toasted Oat' *(Malt•O•Meal)*	1 oz	110	3.0	23.0	190	2.0	1.0	na	0	8%
'Honey Apple Blueberry' honeysweet premium *(Breadshop)*	1 oz	125	3.5	18.0	1	2.5	5.0	0.5	na	34%
'Honey Blueberry Apple Granola' *(Golden Temple)*	1 oz	128	4.0	20.0	2	2.0	3.5	0.5	0	25%
'Honey Bunches of Oats' almonds *(Post)*	1 oz	120	2.0	22.0	160	1.0	3.0	na	0	22%
'Honey Bunches of Oats' honey roasted *(Post)*	1 oz	110	2.0	24.0	180	1.0	2.0	na	0	15%
'Honey Gone Nuts!' honeysweet premium *(Breadshop)*	1 oz	130	3.5	17.5	2	2.5	5.5	0.5	na	37%
'Honey Nut' toasted oatmeal *(Quaker)*	1 oz	120	3.0	20.0	110	2.0	3.0	na	0	23%
'Honey Nut Cheerios' oat and wheat *(General Mills)*	1 oz	107	3.1	22.8	257	1.3	0.7	0.1	0	6%
'Honey Nut Cheerios' oat and wheat, breakfast pack *(General Mills)*	4/5 oz	100	2.0	21.0	230	1.0	1.0	na	0	9%
'Honey Nut Crispy Rice' *(Wonder)*	1 oz	110	2.0	25.0	205	na	1.0	na	0	8%
'Honey Nut O's' *(Krusteaz)*	1 oz	110	3.0	23.0	190	2.0	1.0	na	0	8%
'HoneyComb' corn and oats *(Post)*	1 oz	111	1.6	25.3	160	.8	0.5	na	0	4%
'Just Right' fiber nuggets *(Kellogg's)*	1 oz	100	2.0	24.0	200	2.0	1.0	0.0	0	8%
'Just Right' raisins, dates, and nuts *(Kellogg's)*	3/4 cup	140	3.0	30.0	190	2.0	1.0	0.0	0	6%
'Kaboom' *(General Mills)*	1 oz	110	2.0	23.0	270	na	1.0	na	0	8%
'Kamut Flakes' *(Erewhon)*	1 oz	90	4.0	18.0	60	4.0	0.0	na	na	0%
'Kenmei Rice Bran' *(Kellogg's)*	1 oz	110	2.0	24.0	230	1.0	1.0	0.0	0	8%
'King Vitaman' corn and other grains	1 oz	115	1.5	24.1	218	.4	1.6	1.0	0	12%
'Kix' corn and other grains *(General Mills)*	1 oz	110	2.6	23.5	291	.5	0.7	0.2	0	6%
'Life' oat and other grains *(Quaker Oat)*	1 oz	105	5.2	20.3	148	1.7	0.5	na	0	4%
'Life' oat and other grains, cinnamon *(Quaker Oat)*	1 oz	105	5.2	20.3	148	>.4 c	0.5	na	0	4%
'Lite Müesli' *(Golden Temple)*	1 oz	102	3.0	20.0	60	2.0	1.0	0.0	0	9%
'Lite 'N Crunchy Granola' *(Golden Temple)*	1 oz	129	4.0	19.0	9	2.0	4.5	0.5	0	31%
'Lucky Charms' oat and other grains *(General Mills)*	1 oz	111	2.6	23.2	202	1.2	1.1	0.2	0	9%
'Lucky Charms' oat and other grains, breakfast pack *(General Mills)*	7/8 oz	110	2.0	24.0	180	na	1.0	na	0	8%
'Maple Almond Granola' *(Golden Temple)*	1 oz	129	4.0	20.0	25	2.0	3.5	0.5	0	25%
'Maple Corns' *(Arrowhead Mills)*	1 oz	100	3.0	23.0	75	3.0	1.0	na	na	8%
'Maple Frosted Corn' mini puffs *(Glenny's)*	1 oz	109	4.0	20.0	50	na	<.5	na	na	<5%
'Marshmallow Alpha Bits' *(Post)*	1 oz	110	2.0	25.0	150	1.0	1.0	na	0	8%
'Moot' wheat bran and wheat	1 oz	96	4.0	21.6	151	4.0	0.3	na	0	3%
'Müeslix Crispy Blend' *(Kellogg's)*	2/3 cup	150	3.0	32.0	150	3.0	2.0	0.0	0	11%
'Müeslix Golden Crunch' *(Kellogg's)*	1/2 cup	120	3.0	25.0	170	3.0	2.0	0.0	0	14%
'Multi Grain Cheerios' *(General Mills)*	1 oz	100	2.0	23.0	220	2.0	1.0	na	0	8%
'Multi-Bran Chex' *(Ralston)*	1 oz	90	2.0	25.0	200	4.0	1.0	na	0	8%
'Natural Blueberry Granola' *(Golden Temple)*	1 oz	132	4.0	19.0	3	2.0	5.0	1.0	0	33%
'Natural Blueberry Granola' coconut-free *(Golden Temple)*	1 oz	131	4.0	19.0	3	2.0	4.5	0.5	0	31%
'Natural Bran Flakes' *(Post)*	1 oz	90	3.0	23.0	240	5.0	0.0	na	0	0%

Food Name	Serving Size	Calories	Prot. gms	Carbs gms	Sod. mgs	Fiber gms	Fat gms	Sat. Fat gms	Chol. mgs	% Fat Cal.
'Natural Dellte Granola' (Golden Temple)	1 oz	128	3.0	20.0	26	2.0	3.5	0.5	0	26%
'Natural Foods Apple Cinnamon' low fat (Golden Temple)	1 oz	110	3.0	22.0	3	2.0	1.0	0.0	0	8%
'Natural Foods Raisin Almond' low fat (Golden Temple)	1 oz	110	3.0	22.0	3	2.0	1.0	0.0	0	8%
'Natural Foods Strawberry / Raspberry' low fat (Golden Temple)	1 oz	111	3.0	22.0	3	2.0	1.0	0.0	0	8%
'Natural' oat and wheat germ (Heartland)	1 oz	123	2.9	19.4	72	1.7	4.4	na	U	31%
'Natural' oat and wheat germ, coconut (Heartland)	1 oz	125	3.0	19.3	58	2.0	4.6	na	0	32%
'Natural' oat and wheat germ, raisins (Heartland)	1 oz	121	2.8	19.6	58	1.6	4.0	na	0	29%
'Natural Raisin Bran' (Post)	1.4 oz	120	3.0	31.0	200	6.0	1.0	na	0	6%
'Nut & Honey Crunch' (Kellogg's)	1 oz	110	2.0	24.0	200	0	1.0	0.0	0	8%
'Nut & Honey Crunch O's' (Kellogg's)	1 oz	110	2.0	22.0	190	1.0	2.0	0.0	0	16%
'Nutri-Grain' barley (Kellogg's)	1 oz	106	3.1	23.5	192	1.6	0.2	na	0	2%
'Nutri-Grain' corn (Kellogg's)	1 oz	108	2.3	24.0	187	1.8	0.7	na	0	6%
'Nutri-Grain' rye (Kellogg's)	1 oz	102	2.5	24.0	193	1.8	0.2	na	0	2%
'Nutri-Grain' wheat (Kellogg's)	1 oz	102	2.5	24.0	193	1.8	0.3	na	0	3%
'Nutri-Grain Almond Raisin' (Kellogg's)	2/3 cup	140	3.0	31.0	220	3.0	2.0	0.0	0	12%
'Nutri-Grain Raisin Bran' (Kellogg's)	1 cup	130	4.0	31.0	200	5.0	1.0	0.0	0	6%
'Oat Bran Almond' (Golden Temple)	1 oz	120	4.0	20.0	3	3.0	3.5	0.5	0	25%
'Oat Bran Apple' (Golden Temple)	1 oz	112	4.0	19.0	3	3.0	3.5	0.5	0	26%
'Oat Bran Flakes' (Arrowhead Mills)	1 oz	100	5.0	19.0	100	3.0	2.0	na	0	16%
'Oat Bran Granola' berries (Golden Temple)	1 oz	120	4.0	20.0	3	3.0	3.5	0.5	0	25%
'Oat Bran Granola' raisins and almonds (Golden Temple)	1 oz	119	3.0	19.0	3	3.0	3.5	0.5	0	26%
'Oat Bran Müesli' dates and almonds (Golden Temple)	1 oz	108	3.0	21.0	79	2.0	1.5	0.0	0	12%
'Oat Bran Müesli' raisins and hazelnuts (Golden Temple)	1 oz	102	3.0	20.0	59	3.0	1.5	0.0	0	13%
'Oat Bran Oregonberry' (Golden Temple)	1 oz	116	4.0	20.0	3	3.0	3.5	0.5	0	25%
'Oat Flakes' (Arrowhead Mills)	2 oz	220	10.0	39.0	1	8.1	4.0	(mq)	0	16%
'Oat Flakes' (Post)	1 oz	110	4.0	21.0	130	2.0	1.0	na	0	8%
'Oat Mini Puffs' (Glenny's)	1 oz	108	4.5	22.0	30	na	<.5	na	na	<4%
'Oat Mini Puffs' w/o salt, w/o sugar (Glenny's)	1 oz	108	4.5	22.0	7	na	<.5	na	na	<4%
'Oatbake Honey Bran' (Kellogg's)	1 oz	110	2.0	21.0	190	3.0	3.0	1.0	0	23%
'Oatbake Raisin Nut' (Kellogg's)	1 oz	110	2.0	21.0	190	3.0	3.0	1.0	0	23%
'Oatmeal Crisp' (General Mills)	1 oz	110	3.0	21.0	180	1.0	2.0	na	0	16%
'Oatmeal Crisp With Apples' (General Mills)	1 oz	110	2.0	23.0	180	1.0	1.0	1.0	na	8%
'Oatmeal Raisin Crisp' (General Mills)	1/2 cup	130	3.0	25.0	170	1.5	2.0	na	0	14%
'100% Bran' wheat bran and barley (Nabisco)	1 oz	76	3.5	20.7	197	>2.1 c	1.4	0.3	0	12%
'100% Natural Almond' (Golden Temple)	1 oz	123	3.0	18.0	15	2.0	4.0	1.0	0	30%
'100% Natural Apple/Cinnamon' (Golden Temple)	1 oz	120	3.0	18.0	14	2.0	4.0	1.0	0	30%
'100% Natural' mixed grain (Quaker)	1 oz	127	3.3	18.0	14	2.0	5.5	3.1	0	37%
'100% Natural' mixed grain, raisins, low fat (Quaker)	1 oz	110	3.0	21.0	15	2.1	2.0	na	0	16%
'100% Natural Oat Bran' (Golden Temple)	1 oz	70	5.0	19.0	1	5.0	2.5	0.5	0	19%
'100% Natural' oats and wheat (Quaker)	1 oz	133	3.3	17.8	12	2.4	6.1	4.1	0	39%
'100% Natural' oats and wheat, apple and cinnamon (Quaker)	1 oz	130	2.9	19.1	14	1.9	5.3	4.2	0	35%
'100% Natural' oats and wheat, raisins, low fat (Quaker)	1 oz	150	7.0	27.0	80	2.0	2.0	na	0	12%
'100% Natural' oats and wheat, raisins and dates (Quaker)	1 oz	128	2.9	18.7	12	1.9	5.3	3.5	0	36%
'100% Natural Raisin/Almond' (Golden Temple)	1 oz	120	3.0	19.0	7	2.0	4.0	1.0	0	29%
'100% Organic Blue Corn Flakes' (Health Valley)	1 oz	90	3.0	19.0	10	2.8	<1.0	na	0	<9%
'Orange Almond' nectarsweet premium (Breadshop)	1 oz	120	3.5	18.0	2	2.5	4.0	0.5	na	30%
'Orange Almond Granola' (Golden Temple)	1 oz	133	4.0	19.0	25	2.0	4.0	1.0	0	28%
'Oregon Blueberry Crunch' honeysweet gourmet (Breadshop)	1 oz	125	3.5	18.0	2	2.5	5.0	0.8	na	34%
'Organic Amaranth Flakes' (Health Valley)	1 oz	90	3.0	20.0	10	3.0	0.0	na	0	0%
'Original' toasted oatmeal (Quaker)	1 oz	100	3.0	22.0	160	2.1	1.0	na	0	8%
'Peach Pecan Müesli' (Ralston)	1.45 oz	150	4.0	30.0	150	3.0	3.0	na	0	17%

Food Name	Serving Size	Calories	Prot. gms	Carbs gms	Sod. mgs	Fiber gms	Fat gms	Sat. Fat gms	Chol. mgs	% Fat Cal.
'Peaches 'N Cream' nectarsweet gourmet (Breadshop)	1 oz	115	3.5	18.5	2	2.5	3.0	0.5	na	24%
'Post Toasties Corn Flakes' (Post)	1 oz	110	2.0	24.0	310	(tr)	0.0	na	0	0%
'Product 19' corn and other grains (Kellogg's)	1 oz	108	2.8	23.6	325	1.2	0.2	na	0	2%
'Puffed Corn' (Arrowhead Mills)	.5 oz	50	3.0	11.0	1	3.0	0.0	na	na	0%
'Puffed Kamut' (Arrowhead Mills)	.5 oz	40	2.0	10.0	0	2.0	0.0	na	na	0%
'Puffed Rice' (Arrowhead Mills)	.5 oz	50	1.0	12.0	1	3.0	0.0	na	na	0%
'Puffed Rice' (Malt•O•Meal)	.5 oz	50	1.0	12.0	0	0	0.0	na	0	0%
'Puffed Wheat' (Arrowhead Mills)	.5 oz	50	2.0	11.0	1	6.0	0.0	na	na	0%
'Puffed Wheat' (Malt•O•Meal)	.5 oz	50	2.0	10.0	0	1.0	0.0	na	0	0%
'Quisp' corn and oat	1 oz	118	1.4	23.7	228	.5	2.0	1.4	0	15%
'Raisin Apricot-Date Granola' (Golden Temple)	1 oz	127	3.0	20.0	25	2.0	3.5	0.5	0	26%
'Raisin Bran' (Barbara's Bakery)	1 oz	170	3.0	36.0	80	na	1.0	na	0	6%
'Raisin Bran' (Erewhon)	1 oz	100	3.0	22.0	80	3.0	0.0	na	0	0%
'Raisin Bran' (Krusteaz)	3/4 cup	120	3.0	30.0	210	4.0	1.0	na	0	6%
'Raisin Bran' wheat (Kellogg's)	1.3 oz	115	4.0	27.9	204	4.0	0.7	na	0	5%
'Raisin Bran' wheat (Post)	1 oz	87	2.6	21.5	185	4.0	0.5	na	0	5%
'Raisin Bran' wheat (Ralston)	1 1/3 oz	120	3.0	31.4	328	>1.1 c	0.2	na	0	1%
'Raisin Bran Flakes' (Malt•O•Meal)	1.4 oz	130	3.0	30.0	200	5.0	2.0	na	0	12%
'Raisin Grape-Nuts' (Post)	1 oz	100	3.0	23.0	140	2.0	0.0	na	0	0%
'Raisin Squares' (Kellogg's)	1 oz	90	2.0	23.0	0	2.0	0.0	0.0	0	0%
'Raspberry Almond Müesli' (Ralston)	1.45 oz	150	4.0	30.0	140	3.0	3.0	na	0	17%
'Raspberry 'N Cream' nectarsweet gourmet (Breadshop)	1 oz	115	3.8	18.5	2	2.5	3.0	0.5	na	23%
'Rice Chex' (Ralston)	1 oz	112	1.5	25.3	237	>.1 c	0.1	na	0	1%
'Rice Krispies' (Kellogg's)	1 oz	112	1.9	24.8	341	.4	0.2	na	0	2%
'Rice Krispies Treats' (Kellogg's)	1 oz	110	1.0	24.0	160	0	1.0	na	na	8%
'Rice Mini Puffs' (Glenny's)	1 oz	109	4.0	20.0	30	na	<.5	na	na	<5%
'Right Start' (Erewhon)	1 oz	90	3.0	24.0	80	5.0	0.0	na	0	0%
'Right Start With Raisins' (Erewhon)	1 oz	90	3.0	22.0	80	5.0	0.0	na	0	0%
'Ripple Crisp' (General Mills)	1 oz	110	1.0	24.0	280	1.0	<1.0	na	0	<8%
'Ripple Crisp' honey bran (General Mills)	1 oz	100	2.0	24.0	210	3.0	<1.0	na	0	<8%
'Shredded Wheat' (Barbara's Bakery)	1.4 oz	140	4.0	31.0	0	na	1.0	na	0	6%
'Shredded Wheat' (Nabisco)	1 biscuit	80	2.0	19.0	0	3.0	1.0	0.0	0	10%
'Shredded Wheat 'n Bran' (Nabisco)	1 oz	90	3.0	23.0	0	4.0	0.0	na	0	0%
'Shredded Wheat With Oat Bran' (Nabisco)	1 oz	100	3.0	22.0	0	4.0	1.0	0.0	0	8%
'6-Grain Crisp' fruit and flaxseed (Golden Temple)	1 oz	118	3.0	20.0	73	2.0	3.5	0.5	0	26%
'Smacks' (Kellogg's)	1 oz	110	2.0	25.0	70	1.0	1.0	0.0	0	8%
'Smacks' wheat (Kellogg's)	1 oz	106	2.0	24.8	75	.4	0.5	na	0	4%
'S'Mores Grahams' (General Mills)	1 oz	120	1.0	24.0	230	na	2.0	na	0	15%
'Smurf-Magic Berries' (Post)	1 oz	120	2.0	26.0	60	(tr)	1.0	na	0	7%
'Special K' rice and wheat (Kellogg's)	1 oz	111	5.6	21.3	266	.7	0.1	na	0	1%
'Spelt Flakes' (Arrowhead Mills)	1 oz	100	4.0	21.0	60	na	1.0	na	0	8%
'Spoon Size Shredded Wheat' (Nabisco)	1 oz	90	3.0	23.0	0	3.0	1.0	0.0	0	8%
'Sprinkle Spangles' corn puffs, sprinkles (General Mills)	1 oz	110	1.0	25.0	130	na	1.0	na	0	8%
'Sprouts 7' bananas and Hawaiian fruit (Health Valley)	1 oz	90	3.0	16.0	0	4.3	0.0	na	0	0%
'Sprouts 7' raisins, fat-free (Health Valley)	1 oz	90	4.0	16.0	0	4.7	0.0	na	0	0%
'Startoons' cocoa (Barbara's Bakery)	1 cup	110	2.0	26.0	140	na	0.5	na	0	4%
'Startoons' honey (Barbara's Bakery)	1 cup	110	2.0	26.0	50	na	0.0	0.0	0	0%
'Strawberry 'N Cream' nectarsweet gourmet (Breadshop)	1 oz	110	3.0	16.0	5	3.0	4.0	na	na	32%
'Strawberry Squares' (Kellogg's)	1 oz	90	2.0	23.0	5	3.0	0.0	0.0	0	0%
'Sugar Corn Pops' (Kellogg's)	1 oz	108	1.4	25.7	104	.2	0.1	na	0	1%
'Sugar Frosted Flakes' (Krusteaz)	1 oz	110	1.0	26.0	230	1.0	0.0	na	0	0%
'Sugar Frosted Flakes' (Malt•O•Meal)	1 oz	110	1.0	26.0	170	1.0	0.0	na	0	0%
'Sugar Puffs' (Malt•O•Meal)	1 oz	110	2.0	25.0	25	na	0.0	na	0	0%
'Sunflakes Multi-Grain' (Ralston)	1 oz	100	2.0	24.0	240	0	1.0	na	0	8%

Food Name	Serving Size	Calories	Prot. gms	Carbs gms	Sod. mgs	Fiber gms	Fat gms	Sat. Fat gms	Chol. mgs	% Fat Cal.
'Super Nutty Granola' *(Golden Temple)*	1 oz	135	4.0	19.0	25	3.0	5.0	1.0	0	33%
'Super O's' *(Erewhon)*	1 oz	110	3.0	24.0	5	4.0	0.0	na	0	0%
'Super Sugar Crisp' wheat *(Post)*	1 oz	106	1.9	25.6	25	.4	0.3	na	0	2%
'Supernatural' honeysweet gourmet *(Breadshop)*	1 oz	100	3.5	17.5	2	3.5	5.0	0.8	na	35%
'Supernatural New England' honeysweet gourmet *(Breadshop)*	1 oz	130	3.0	18.0	2	2.0	5.0	0.5	na	35%
'Sweet Home Farm Almond' *(Golden Temple)*	1 oz	123	3.0	18.0	14	2.0	4.0	1.0	0	30%
'Sweet Home Farm Crunchy Müesli' low fat *(Golden Temple)*	1 oz	105	3.0	21.0	98	2.0	2.0	0.5	0	16%
'Sweet Home Farm Granola' low fat *(Golden Temple)*	1 oz	110	3.0	22.0	65	2.0	2.0	0.5	0	15%
'Sweet Home Farm Raisin' *(Golden Temple)*	1 oz	120	3.0	19.0	13	2.0	4.0	1.0	0	29%
'Sweetened Puffed Wheat' *(Malt•O•Meal)*	1 oz	110	2.0	25.0	25	1.0	0.0	na	0	0%
'Swiss Style Müesli' *(Golden Temple)*	1 oz	105	3.0	19.0	15	3.0	1.5	0.0	0	13%
'Tasteeos' oat and other grains	1 oz	112	3.6	22.5	216	3.0	0.8	na	0	7%
'Team' rice and other grains *(Nabisco)*	1 oz	111	1.8	24.4	176	.4	0.5	na	0	4%
'Team Flakes' *(Nabisco)*	1 oz	110	2.0	24.0	180	na	1.0	na	0	8%
'Teenage Mutant Ninja Turtles' *(Ralston)*	1 oz	110	1.0	26.0	190	na	0.0	na	0	0%
'35% Fruit Müesli' *(Golden Temple)*	1 oz	97	3.0	19.0	16	3.0	1.0	0.0	0	9%
'Toasted Oat' 100% natural *(Nature Valley)*	1 oz	130	2.0	20.0	50	1.0	5.0	na	0	34%
'Toasted Oats' *(Krusteaz)*	1 oz	110	4.0	22.0	290	2.0	1.0	na	0	8%
'Toasted Oats' *(Malt•O•Meal)*	1 oz	110	4.0	20.0	240	2.0	2.0	na	0	16%
'Toasties' corn *(Post)*	1 oz	110	2.3	24.4	298	1.0	0.1	na	0	1%
'Tootie Fruities' *(Malt•O•Meal)*	1 oz	110	2.0	25.0	120	na	1.0	na	0	8%
'Total Corn Flakes' *(General Mills)*	1 oz	110	2.0	24.0	200	na	1.0	na	0	8%
'Total Raisin Bran' *(General Mills)*	1.5 oz	140	3.0	33.0	190	4.0	1.0	na	0	6%
'Total' wheat *(General Mills)*	1 oz	100	2.8	22.4	281	3.7	0.6	0.1	0	5%
'Triples' *(General Mills)*	1 oz	110	2.0	24.0	200	na	1.0	na	0	8%
'Triples' breakfast pack *(General Mills)*	1 oz	110	2.0	23.0	190	na	1.0	na	0	8%
'Trix' corn and other grains *(General Mills)*	1 oz	109	1.5	25.2	181	.3	0.4	na	0	3%
'Uncle Sam' *(US Mills)*	1 oz	110	4.0	20.0	65	7.0	1.0	na	0	9%
'Urkel-O's' *(Ralston)*	1 oz	110	1.0	25.0	160	na	1.0	na	0	8%
'Waffelos' wheat and other grains	1 oz	115	1.6	24.5	118	>.1 c	1.2	na	0	9%
'Wheat Chex' *(Ralston)*	1 oz	104	2.8	23.3	190	>.6 c	0.7	na	0	6%
'Wheat Flakes' *(Erewhon)*	1 oz	110	3.0	22.0	75	3.5	0.0	na	0	0%
'Wheat 'n Raisin Chex' *(Ralston)*	1 1/3 oz	130	3.5	30.1	214	>.6 c	0.3	na	0	2%
'Wheaties' *(General Mills)*	1 oz	99	2.7	22.6	270	>.5 c	0.5	0.1	0	4%
'Wheaties Honey Gold' *(General Mills)*	1 oz	100	2.0	25.0	200	1.0	1.0	na	0	8%
'Whole-Grain Shredded Wheat' *(Kellogg's)*	1 oz	90	3.0	23.0	0	4.0	0.0	0.0	0	0%
'Whole-Grain Wheat Chex' *(Ralston)*	1 oz	100	3.0	23.0	230	3.0	1.0	na	30	8%

CEREAL SNACK. See also GRANOLA AND CEREAL BAR; GRANOLA SNACK.

Food Name	Serving Size	Calories	Prot. gms	Carbs gms	Sod. mgs	Fiber gms	Fat gms	Sat. Fat gms	Chol. mgs	% Fat Cal.
'Cheerios-to-Go' *(General Mills)*	1 pouch	80	3.0	15.0	220	2.0	2.0	(mq)	0	20%
'Cheerios-to-Go' apple cinnamon *(General Mills)*	1 pouch	110	2.0	22.0	180	1.5	2.0	(mq)	0	16%
'Cheerios-to-Go' honey nut *(General Mills)*	1 pouch	110	3.0	23.0	250	1.5	1.0	na	0	8%
'Fingos' cinnamon *(General Mills)*	1 oz	110	1.0	22.0	170	2.0	3.0	na	0	23%
'Fingos' honey toasted oat *(General Mills)*	1 oz	110	2.0	21.0	210	1.5	3.0	na	0	23%

CHARD. See SWISS CHARD.

CHAYOTE

Food Name	Serving Size	Calories	Prot. gms	Carbs gms	Sod. mgs	Fiber gms	Fat gms	Sat. Fat gms	Chol. mgs	% Fat Cal.
boiled, drained	4 oz	27	0.7	5.8	1	>.7 c	0.5	(tr)	0	15%
boiled, drained, 1-inch pieces	1/2 cup	19	0.5	4.1	1	>.5 c	0.4	na	0	16%
raw, approx 7.2 oz	1 med	49	1.8	11.0	8	>1.4 c	0.6	na	0	10%
raw, 1-inch pieces	1/2 cup	16	0.6	3.6	3	>.5 c	0.2	(tr)	0	10%
raw, trimmed	1 oz	7	0.3	1.5	1	>.2 c	0.1	(tr)	0	11%
raw, untrimmed	1 lb	108	4.0	24.3	18	>3.1 c	1.4	na	0	10%

Food Name	Serving Size	Calories	Prot. gms	Carbs gms	Sod. mgs	Fiber gms	Fat gms	Sat. Fat gms	Chol. mgs	% Fat Cal.
CHEDDARWURST										
'Bun Size' *(Hillshire Farm)*	2 oz	200	8.0	1.0	480	(tr)	18.0	(mq)	(mq)	82%
'Links' *(Hillshire Farm)*	2 oz	190	8.0	1.0	480	(tr)	17.0	(mq)	(mq)	81%
CHEESE. See also CHEESE, ALTERNATIVE; CHEESE BALL; CHEESE FOOD; CHEESE LOG; CHEESE NUGGET; CHEESE NUT; CHEESE PRODUCT; CHEESE SPREAD; CHEESE STICK.										
AMERICAN										
(Borden) fat-free, low-cholesterol	1 oz	40	6.0	4.0	380	na	0.0	na	5	0%
(Borden) 'Light'	1 oz	70	6.0	1.0	420	na	4.0	na	15	56%
(Borden) 'Loaf'	1 oz	110	6.0	1.0	40	0	9.0	(mq)	(mq)	74%
(Borden) 'Slices'	1 oz	110	6.0	1.0	40	0	9.0	(mq)	(mq)	74%
(Borden) slices 'Premium'	1 oz	110	6.0	1.0	460	na	9.0	na	na	74%
(Dorman's)	1 oz	110	6.0	1.0	440	0	9.0	(mq)	(mq)	74%
(Dorman's) 'Loaf Low Sodium'	1 oz	110	6.0	1.0	140	0	9.0	(mq)	(mq)	74%
(Healthy Favorites)	2/3 oz	45	4.0	2.0	260	na	2.0	1.0	10	43%
(Hoffman's)	1 oz	110	6.0	1.0	400	0	9.0	(mq)	(mq)	74%
(Kraft) 'Deluxe Loaf'	1 oz	110	6.0	1.0	430	0	9.0	5.0	25	74%
(Kraft) 'Deluxe Slices'	1 oz	110	6.0	1.0	450	0	9.0	5.0	25	74%
(Land O'Lakes)	1 oz	110	6.0	<1.0	405	0	9.0	6.0	25	74%
(Land O'Lakes) sharp	1 oz	100	6.0	1.0	360	na	9.0	6.0	30	74%
(Old English) sharp 'Loaf'	1 oz	110	6.0	1.0	400	0	9.0	5.0	30	74%
(Old English) sharp 'Slices'	1 oz	110	6.0	1.0	440	0	9.0	5.0	30	74%
(Sargento) hot pepper	1 oz	110	6.0	0.5	410	(tr)	9.0	(mq)	27	76%
ASIAGO *(Frigo)* wheel	1 oz	110	7.0	1.0	400	0	9.0	(mq)	(mq)	72%
BABYBEL										
(Laughing Cow)	1 oz	91	7.0	tr	227	0	7.0	(mq)	22	69%
(Laughing Cow) mini	3/4 oz	74	4.7	tr	170	0	6.0	(mq)	18	74%
BLUE										
crumbled, not packed	1 cup	477	28.9	3.2	1884	0	38.8	25.2	102	73%
(Dorman's) 'Castello 70%'	1 oz	134	3.7	0.1	286	0	12.3	9.0	29	88%
(Dorman's) 'Danablu 60%'	1 oz	108	4.8	0.3	200	0	9.7	6.9	31	81%
(Dorman's) 'Danablu 50%'	1 oz	100	6.4	0.3	200	0	8.2	5.0	23	73%
(Dorman's) 'Saga 70%'	1 oz	134	3.7	0.1	286	0	12.3	9.0	29	88%
(Frigo)	1 oz	100	6.0	1.0	400	0	8.0	(mq)	(mq)	72%
(Hickory Farms) 'Domestic'	1 oz	101	6.1	0.7	396	0	8.3	(mq)	21	73%
(Kraft)	1 oz	100	6.0	1.0	330	0	9.0	5.0	30	74%
(Sargento)	1 oz	100	6.0	1.0	400	0	8.0	(mq)	21	72%
BONBEL										
(Laughing Cow)	1 oz	100	6.0	tr	227	0	8.0	(mq)	24	75%
(Laughing Cow) mini, 3/4 oz	1 oz	74	4.7	tr	170	0	6.0	(mq)	18	74%
BONBINO *(Laughing Cow)*	1 oz	103	7.0	tr	227	0	9.0	(mq)	27	74%
BRICK										
(Dorman's)	1 oz	110	7.0	1.0	180	0	8.0	(mq)	(mq)	69%
(Kraft)	1 oz	110	7.0	0.0	180	0	9.0	5.0	30	74%
(Land O'Lakes)	1 oz	110	7.0	1.0	160	0	8.0	5.0	25	69%
BRIE										
(Dorman's)	1 oz	81	5.1	0.3	229	0	6.6	4.0	20	73%
(Sargento)	1 oz	100	6.0	0.1	180	0	8.0	(mq)	28	75%
BURGER *(Sargento)*	1 oz	110	6.0	0.5	410	0	9.0	(mq)	27	76%
BUTTERNIP *(Hickory Farms)*	1 oz	110	5.2	1.1	82	0	9.4	(mq)	25	77%
CAJUN *(Sargento)*	1 oz	110	7.0	0.3	165	0	9.0	(mq)	28	74%
CALJACK *(Churny)*	1 oz	100	6.0	1.0	(mq)	0	8.0	(mq)	(mq)	72%
CAMEMBERT										
domestic	1 oz	84	5.5	0.1	236	0	6.8	4.3	20	73%
(Dorman's) '50%'	1 oz	89	5.6	0.3	285	0	7.3	4.4	23	74%

Food Name	Serving Size	Calories	Prot. gms	Carbs gms	Sod. mgs	Fiber gms	Fat gms	Sat. Fat gms	Chol. mgs	% Fat Cal.
(Dorman's) '45%'	1 oz	82	6.0	0.3	226	0	6.3	3.9	17	69%
(Hickory Farms)	1 oz	90	6.0	0.1	239	0	7.0	(mq)	26	72%
(Sargento)	1 oz	90	6.0	0.1	240	0	7.0	(mq)	20	72%
CARAWAY	1 oz	105	7.1	0.9	193	0	8.2	5.2	26	70%
CHEDDAR										
American domestic	1 oz	113	7.0	0.4	174	0	9.3	5.9	29	74%
American domestic, shredded, not packed	1 cup	455	28.1	1.5	701	0	37.5	23.8	119	74%
(Alpine Lace) 'Cheddar Flavored'	1 oz	100	7.0	1.0	95	0	8.0	5.0	25	69%
(Alpine Lace) shredded 'Ched-R-Lo' milk cheese	1 oz	80	7.0	1.0	95	na	5.0	na	20	58%
(Alta•Dena) mild	1 oz	110	7.0	1.0	200	na	9.0	na	na	72%
(Alta•Dena) sharp	1 oz	110	7.0	1.0	200	na	9.0	na	na	72%
(Axelrod) extra sharp	1 oz	110	7.0	1.0	200	0	9.0	(mq)	30	72%
(Boar's Head) sliced	1 oz	110	7.0	1.0	100	0	9.0	(mq)	18	72%
(Darigold)	1 oz	110	7.0	<1.0	170	0	9.0	5.9	29	72%
(Dorman's)	1 oz	110	7.0	1.0	200	0	9.0	(mq)	(mq)	72%
(Dorman's) 'Chedda-Delite'	1 oz	90	7.0	1.0	100	0	7.0	(mq)	(mq)	66%
(Dorman's) reduced fat 'Low Sodium'	1 oz	80	8.0	1.0	100	0	5.0	3.4	20	56%
(Dorman's) w/Monterey Jack 'Chedda-Jack'	1 oz	90	7.0	1.0	100	0	7.0	(mq)	(mq)	66%
(Featherweight) 'Low Sodium'	1 oz	110	7.0	1.0	5	0	9.0	(mq)	(mq)	72%
(Frigo)	1 oz	110	7.0	1.0	200	0	9.0	(mq)	(mq)	72%
(Golden Balance) mild, shredded 'Natural Shreds'	1 oz	90	8.0	1.0	150	na	6.0	3.0	20	60%
(Golden Balance) sharp, shredded 'Natural Shreds'	1 oz	90	8.0	1.0	130	na	6.0	3.0	20	60%
(Healthy Choice) shredded, fat-free	1 oz	40	9.0	1.0	200	na	0.0	na	5	0%
(Healthy Favorites) mild, fancy shredded	1 oz	70	8.0	0.0	220	na	4.0	2.0	15	53%
(Hickory Farms)	1 oz	110	7.0	1.0	176	0	9.0	(mq)	30	72%
(Hickory Farms) raw milk 'Light Choice Low Sodium'	1 oz	114	6.0	0.0	100	0	8.0	(mq)	30	75%
(Hoffman's) super sharp processed	1 oz	110	6.0	2.0	390	0	8.0	(mq)	(mq)	69%
(Kraft)	1 oz	110	7.0	1.0	180	0	9.0	5.0	30	72%
(Kraft) mild, finely shredded 'Light Naturals'	1 oz	80	8.0	1.0	220	na	5.0	3.0	20	56%
(Kraft) mild, reduced fat 'Light Naturals'	1 oz	80	9.0	0.0	220	0	5.0	3.0	20	56%
(Kraft) mild, shredded 'Light Naturals'	1 oz	80	9.0	0.0	220	na	5.0	3.0	20	56%
(Kraft) sharp, shredded 'Light Naturals'	1 oz	80	9.0	1.0	220	na	5.0	3.0	20	56%
(Land O'Lakes)	1 oz	110	7.0	<1.0	175	0	9.0	6.0	30	72%
(Land O'Lakes) 'Chedarella'	1 oz	100	7.0	<1.0	180	na	8.0	5.0	25	69%
(Laughing Cow)	1 oz	110	7.0	tr	227	0	9.0	(mq)	28	74%
(Sargento)	1 oz	110	7.0	0.4	176	0	9.0	(mq)	30	73%
(Sargento) mild, fancy shredded 'Preferred Light'	1 oz	90	8.0	1.0	210	na	5.0	na	15	56%
(Sargento) 'New York'	1 oz	110	7.0	0.4	180	0	9.0	(mq)	30	73%
(Weight Watchers) mild, 'Natural'	1 oz	80	8.0	1.0	150	0	5.0	3.0	15	56%
(Weight Watchers) mild, 'Natural Low Sodium'	1 oz	80	8.0	1.0	70	0	5.0	3.0	15	56%
(Weight Watchers) mild, shredded 'Natural'	1 oz	80	8.0	1.0	150	0	5.0	3.0	15	56%
CHESHIRE	1 oz	108	6.5	1.3	196	0	8.6	5.4	29	71%
CHUTTER (Hickory Farms) 'Cold Pack'	1 oz	87	6.0	2.6	213	0	5.8	(mq)	46	60%
COLBY										
(Alpine Lace) 'Colby-Lo'	1 oz	80	7.0	1.0	85	0	5.0	4.0	20	58%
(Dorman's)	1 oz	110	7.0	1.0	190	0	9.0	(mq)	(mq)	72%
(Hickory Farms) 'Light Choice Low Sodium'	1 oz	100	8.0	1.0	4	0	6.0	(mq)	20	60%
(Hickory Farms) 'Longhorn'	1 oz	112	6.7	0.7	171	0	8.6	(mq)	27	72%
(Hickory Farms) lowfat, calcium-enriched 'Light Choice'	1 oz	100	7.0	1.0	180	0	8.0	(mq)	(mq)	69%
(Kraft)	1 oz	110	7.0	1.0	180	0	9.0	5.0	30	72%
(Kraft) reduced fat 'Light Naturals'	1 oz	80	9.0	0.0	220	0	5.0	3.0	20	56%
(Kraft) w/Monterey Jack, reduced fat 'Light Naturals'	1 oz	80	8.0	1.0	220	0	5.0	3.0	20	56%
(Land O'Lakes)	1 oz	110	7.0	1.0	170	0	9.0	6.0	25	72%
(Sargento)	1 oz	110	7.0	1.0	170	0	9.0	(mq)	27	72%

Food Name	Serving Size	Calories	Prot. gms	Carbs gms	Sod. mgs	Fiber gms	Fat gms	Sat. Fat gms	Chol. mgs	% Fat Cal.
(Sargento) Jack	1 oz	110	7.0	0.5	160	0	9.0	(mq)	27	73%
(Weight Watchers) 'Natural'	1 oz	80	8.0	1.0	130	0	5.0	2.0	15	56%
COTTAGE CHEESE										
Creamed										
large curd	4 oz	117	14.1	3.0	457	0	5.1	3.2	17	40%
large curd, not packed	1 cup	217	26.2	5.6	850	0	9.5	6.0	31	40%
lowfat 1%	1 oz	20	3.5	0.8	115	0	0.3	0.2	1	14%
lowfat 2%	1 oz	25	3.9	1.0	115	0	0.5	0.3	2	19%
small curd	4 oz	117	14.1	3.0	457	0	5.1	3.2	17	40%
small curd, not packed	1 cup	217	26.2	5.6	850	0	9.5	6.0	31	40%
(Bison) chive	1/2 cup	120	14.0	4.0	420	(tr)	5.0	(mq)	20	39%
(Bison) 4% fat	1/2 cup	120	14.0	4.0	420	0	5.0	(mq)	20	39%
(Bison) garden salad	1/2 cup	110	12.0	4.0	420	(mq)	4.0	(mq)	15	36%
(Bison) lowfat 1%	1/2 cup	90	14.0	4.0	350	0	2.0	(mq)	5	20%
(Bison) w/pineapple	1/2 cup	140	10.0	18.0	340	(mq)	4.0	(mq)	15	24%
(Borden) 4% fat	1/2 cup	120	14.0	4.0	400	0	5.0	(mq)	(mq)	39%
(Borden) 4% fat, unsalted	1/2 cup	120	14.0	4.0	40	0	5.0	(mq)	(mq)	39%
(Breakstone's)	4 oz	110	13.0	3.0	370	0	5.0	3.0	25	41%
(Breakstone's) lowfat 2%	4 oz	100	14.0	4.0	510	0	2.0	1.0	15	20%
(Carnation) 4% fat, large curd	1/2 cup	115	14.0	4.0	440	na	5.0	na	na	39%
(Carnation) 4% fat, small curd	1/2 cup	115	14.0	4.0	440	na	5.0	na	na	39%
(Carnation) 4% fat, w/pineapple	1/2 cup	130	10.0	12.0	430	na	5.0	na	na	34%
(Crowley) 4% fat	1/2 cup	120	14.0	4.0	390	0	5.0	(mq)	15	39%
(Crowley) 4% fat, w/peaches	1/2 cup	140	10.0	17.0	340	(mq)	3.0	(mq)	10	20%
(Crowley) 4% fat, w/pineapple	1/2 cup	140	11.0	15.0	330	(mq)	4.0	(mq)	15	26%
(Crowley) lowfat 1%	1/2 cup	90	14.0	4.0	390	0	1.0	(mq)	5	11%
(Crowley) lowfat 1%, calcium-fortified	1/2 cup	90	14.0	4.0	390	0	1.0	(mq)	5	11%
(Crowley) lowfat 1% 'No Salt Added'	1/2 cup	90	14.0	4.0	50	0	1.0	(mq)	5	11%
(Crowley) lowfat 1%, w/pineapple	1/2 cup	110	11.0	15.0	330	(mq)	1.0	(mq)	5	8%
(Darigold) 4% fat	4 oz	120	14.0	4.0	510	0	4.2	3.2	17	34%
(Darigold) lowfat 2% 'Trim'	4 oz	100	14.0	4.0	510	0	3.2	2.0	17	29%
(Friendship) 'California Style 4%'	1/2 cup	120	14.0	4.0	380	0	5.0	(mq)	17	39%
(Friendship) 4% fat, w/pineapple	1/2 cup	140	11.0	15.0	300	(mq)	4.0	(mq)	17	26%
(Friendship) lowfat 1%	1/2 cup	90	14.0	4.0	350	0	1.0	(mq)	5	11%
(Friendship) lowfat 1%, lactose-reduced	1/2 cup	90	14.0	4.0	350	0	1.0	(mq)	5	11%
(Friendship) lowfat 1% 'No Salt Added'	1/2 cup	90	14.0	4.0	31	0	1.0	(mq)	5	11%
(Friendship) lowfat 1%, w/pineapple	1/2 cup	110	11.0	15.0	300	(mq)	1.0	(mq)	5	8%
(Friendship) lowfat 2%, pot style, large curd	1/2 cup	100	14.0	4.0	405	0	2.0	(mq)	9	20%
(Knudsen) 4% fat, large curd	4 oz	120	14.0	4.0	340	0	5.0	3.0	20	39%
(Knudsen) 4% fat, small curd	4 oz	120	14.0	4.0	370	0	5.0	3.0	20	39%
(Knudsen) 4% fat, w/pineapple	4 oz	140	10.0	14.0	260	(mq)	5.0	3.0	25	32%
(Lite-Line) lowfat 1.5%	1/2 cup	90	14.0	4.0	400	0	2.0	(mq)	(mq)	20%
(Weight Watchers) lowfat 1%	1/2 cup	90	14.0	4.0	460	0	1.0	(mq)	(mq)	11%
(Weight Watchers) lowfat 2%	1/2 cup	100	14.0	4.0	460	0	2.0	(mq)	(mq)	20%
Lowfat										
1%, not packed	1 cup	164	28.0	6.2	918	0	2.3	1.5	10	13%
2%, not packed	1 cup	203	31.0	8.2	918	0	4.4	2.8	19	20%
(Carnation) 1.5% 'Slender'	1/2 cup	90	14.0	4.0	440	na	2.0	na	na	20%
(Knudsen) 2%	4 oz	100	14.0	4.0	370	0	2.0	1.0	15	20%
(Knudsen) 2%, w/fruit cocktail	4 oz	130	11.0	16.0	330	(mq)	2.0	2.0	10	14%
(Knudsen) 2%, w/Mandarin orange	4 oz	110	11.0	11.0	320	(mq)	2.0	2.0	10	17%
(Knudsen) 2%, w/peach	6 oz	170	16.0	19.0	270	(mq)	2.0	2.0	15	11%
(Knudsen) 2%, w/pear	4 oz	110	11.0	12.0	320	(mq)	2.0	2.0	10	16%
(Knudsen) 2%, w/pineapple	6 oz	170	16.0	18.0	300	(mq)	2.0	2.0	15	12%

Food Name	Serving Size	Calories	Prot. gms	Carbs gms	Sod. mgs	Fiber gms	Fat gms	Sat. Fat gms	Chol. mgs	% Fat Cal.
(Knudsen) 2%, w/spiced apple	6 oz	180	16.0	20.0	280	(mq)	2.0	2.0	15	11%
(Knudsen) 2%, w/strawberry	6 oz	170	16.0	19.0	320	(mq)	2.0	2.0	15	11%
(Light n' Lively) 1%	4 oz	80	14.0	4.0	370	0	2.0	1.0	10	20%
(Light n' Lively) 1%, garden salad	4 oz	80	18.0	5.0	350	(mq)	2.0	1.0	10	16%
(Sealtest) 2%	4 oz	100	14.0	4.0	340	0	2.0	1.0	15	20%
Nonfat										
(Knudsen)	4 oz	70	15.0	3.0	420	0	0.0	0.0	5	0%
(Light n' Lively)	4 oz	90	14.0	7.0	400	na	0.0	0.0	10	0%
Uncreamed										
dry, large curd	4 oz	96	19.5	2.1	14	0	0.5	0.3	8	5%
dry, large curd, not packed	1 cup	123	25.0	2.7	19	0	0.6	0.4	10	5%
dry, small curd	4 oz	96	19.5	2.1	14	0	0.5	0.3	8	5%
dry, small curd, not packed	1 cup	123	25.0	2.7	19	0	0.6	0.4	10	5%
dry curd, unsalted *(Borden)*	1/2 cup	80	18.0	3.0	20	0	1.0	(mq)	(mq)	10%
dry curd, unsalted *(Darigold)*	4 oz	80	18.0	3.0	15	0	1.0	0.4	10	10%
dry curd, unsalted, nonfat *(Breakstone's)*	4 oz	90	16.0	6.0	65	0	0.0	0.0	10	0%
CREAM CHEESE										
natural	1 oz	98	2.1	0.7	83	0	9.8	6.2	31	89%
(Alta•Dena) pasteurized	1 oz	100	2.0	2.0	110	na	10.0	na	na	85%
(Crowley)	1 oz	110	2.0	1.0	100	0	9.0	(mq)	30	87%
(Darigold)	1 oz	99	2.2	0.8	84	0	9.9	6.2	31	88%
(Dorman's) '70%'	1 oz	102	2.7	0.6	200	0	9.9	6.1	30	87%
(Dorman's) '65%'	1 oz	90	3.0	0.6	200	0	8.4	5.1	26	84%
(Healthy Choice) fat-free	1 oz	30	6.0	2.0	200	na	0.0	na	5	0%
(Healthy Choice) herb and garlic, fat-free	1 oz	30	6.0	2.0	200	na	0.0	na	5	0%
(Healthy Favorites)	1 oz	60	3.0	2.0	110	na	5.0	2.0	15	69%
(Philadelphia Brand)	1 oz	100	2.0	1.0	90	0	10.0	6.0	30	88%
(Philadelphia Brand) 'Free'	1 oz	25	4.0	1.0	170	na	0.0	0.0	5	0%
(Philadelphia Brand) pasteurized process 'Light'	1 oz	60	3.0	2.0	160	na	5.0	3.0	10	69%
(Philadelphia Brand) w/chives	1 oz	90	2.0	1.0	125	(tr)	9.0	5.0	30	87%
(Philadelphia Brand) w/olive and pimento, fat-free	1 oz	90	2.0	2.0	160	na	8.0	na	na	82%
(Philadelphia Brand) w/pimento	1 oz	90	2.0	1.0	150	(tr)	9.0	5.0	30	87%
Soft										
(Friendship)	1 oz	103	1.5	0.8	70	0	10.0	(mq)	31	91%
(Philadelphia Brand)	1 oz	100	1.0	2.0	100	0	10.0	5.0	30	88%
(Philadelphia Brand) w/chives and onion	1 oz	100	2.0	2.0	100	(tr)	9.0	5.0	30	84%
(Philadelphia Brand) w/herb and garlic	1 oz	100	1.0	2.0	160	(tr)	9.0	5.0	25	87%
(Philadelphia Brand) w/olives and pimento	1 oz	90	2.0	2.0	160	(tr)	8.0	5.0	25	82%
(Philadelphia Brand) w/pineapple	1 oz	90	1.0	4.0	90	(tr)	8.0	5.0	25	78%
(Philadelphia Brand) w/smoked salmon	1 oz	90	2.0	1.0	180	0	9.0	5.0	25	87%
(Philadelphia Brand) w/strawberries	1 oz	90	1.0	4.0	75	(tr)	8.0	5.0	20	78%
Whipped										
(Philadelphia Brand)	1 oz	100	2.0	1.0	85	0	10.0	6.0	30	88%
(Philadelphia Brand) w/chives	1 oz	90	2.0	1.0	150	(tr)	8.0	5.0	30	86%
(Philadelphia Brand) w/onions	1 oz	90	2.0	2.0	170	(tr)	8.0	5.0	25	82%
(Philadelphia Brand) w/smoked salmon	1 oz	90	2.0	2.0	170	0	8.0	5.0	30	82%
(Temp-Tee)	1 oz	100	2.0	1.0	85	na	10.0	6.0	30	88%
DANBO										
(Dorman's) 20%	1 oz	62	8.9	0.3	200	0	2.8	1.7	9	41%
(Dorman's) 45%	1 oz	98	7.3	0.3	200	0	7.5	4.6	23	69%
EDAM										
(Dorman's)	1 oz	100	7.0	1.0	200	0	8.0	(mq)	(mq)	69%
(Dorman's) 45%	1 oz	91	6.7	0.3	200	0	7.0	4.3	21	69%
(Hickory Farms) 'Domestic'	1 oz	100	6.0	0.9	182	0	8.4	(mq)	24	73%

Food Name	Serving Size	Calories	Prot. gms	Carbs gms	Sod. mgs	Fiber gms	Fat gms	Sat. Fat gms	Chol. mgs	% Fat Cal.
(Kaukauna)	1 oz	100	7.0	<1.0	275	0	8.0	(mq)	25	69%
(Kraft)	1 oz	90	8.0	0.0	310	0	7.0	4.0	20	66%
(Land O'Lakes)	1 oz	100	7.0	<1.0	275	0	8.0	5.0	25	69%
(Laughing Cow)	1 oz	100	6.0	tr	227	0	8.0	(mq)	26	75%
(May-Bud)	1 oz	100	7.0	0.0	275	0	8.0	(mq)	(mq)	72%
(Sargento)	1 oz	100	7.0	0.4	270	0	8.0	(mq)	25	71%
EFORT, sheep's milk	1 oz	314	18.3	1.7	1538	0	26.0	16.4	76	75%
FARMER										
(Friendship)	1/2 cup	160	16.0	4.0	356	0	12.0	(mq)	40	57%
(Friendship) 'No Salt Added'	1/2 cup	160	16.0	4.0	8	0	12.0	(mq)	40	57%
(Hickory Farms)	1 oz	90	6.0	1.0	210	0	7.0	(mq)	20	69%
(Hickory Farms) 'Light Choice'	1 oz	90	6.0	1.0	150	0	7.0	(mq)	20	69%
(Kaukauna)	1 oz	100	7.0	<1.0	(mq)	0	8.0	(mq)	25	69%
(May-Bud)	1 oz	90	6.0	1.0	210	0	7.0	(mq)	20	69%
(Sargento)	1 oz	100	7.0	1.0	130	0	8.0	(mq)	26	69%
FETA										
sheep's milk	1 oz	75	4.0	1.2	316	0	6.0	4.2	25	72%
(Churny) 'Natural'	1 oz	75	4.7	1.2	316	0	6.5	4.2	25	71%
(Dorman's) 45%	1 oz	91	5.9	0.4	(mq)	0	7.3	(mq)	(mq)	72%
(Sargento)	1 oz	80	4.0	1.0	320	0	6.0	(mq)	25	73%
FONTINA (Sargento)	1 oz	110	7.0	0.4	(mq)	0	9.0	(mq)	33	73%
FRENCH ONION (Alouette)	1 oz	95	2.0	2.0	205	na	9.0	na	31	84%
GJETOST										
goat's milk, fresh	1 oz	82	4.5	0.9	180	0	6.8	(mq)	20	74%
(Sargento)	1 oz	130	3.0	12.0	170	0	8.0	(mq)	(mq)	55%
GOAT										
hard type	1 oz	128	8.6	0.6	98	0	10.1	7.0	30	71%
semisoft type	1 oz	103	6.1	0.7	146	0	8.5	5.8	22	74%
soft type	1 oz	76	5.3	0.3	104	0	6.0	4.1	13	71%
GOUDA										
(Dorman's)	1 oz	100	7.0	1.0	210	0	8.0	(mq)	(mq)	69%
(Kaukauna)	1 oz	100	7.0	1.0	230	0	8.0	(mq)	30	69%
(Kaukauna) w/caraway seed	1 oz	100	7.0	<1.0	230	(tr)	8.0	(mq)	30	69%
(Kaukauna) w/hickory smoke flavor	1 oz	100	7.0	<1.0	230	0	8.0	(mq)	25	69%
(Kraft)	1 oz	110	7.0	0.0	200	0	9.0	5.0	30	74%
(Land O'Lakes)	1 oz	100	7.0	1.0	230	0	8.0	5.0	30	69%
(Laughing Cow)	1 oz	110	7.0	tr	227	0	9.0	(mq)	28	74%
(Laughing Cow) mini	3/4 oz	80	5.3	tr	170	0	6.4	(mq)	21	73%
(May-Bud)	1 oz	100	7.0	1.0	230	0	8.0	(mq)	(mq)	69%
(Sargento)	1 oz	100	7.0	1.0	230	0	8.0	(mq)	32	69%
GRATED. See also PARMESAN; ROMANO.										
(Polly-O)	1 oz	130	11.0	1.0	530	0	10.0	(mq)	25	65%
(Sargento) Italian style	1 oz	110	8.0	1.0	105	0	8.0	(mq)	26	67%
GRUYERE	1 oz	116	8.4	0.1	94	0	9.1	5.3	31	71%
HAVARTI										
(Casino)	1 oz	120	6.0	0.0	140	0	11.0	7.0	35	81%
(Dorman's) 45%	1 oz	91	6.7	0.3	200	0	7.0	4.3	21	69%
(Dorman's) 60%	1 oz	118	5.4	0.3	200	0	10.6	6.5	31	81%
(Hickory Farms) 'Danish Special'	1 oz	117	5.1	0.3	198	0	10.5	(mq)	31	81%
(Sargento)	1 oz	120	5.0	0.3	200	0	11.0	(mq)	31	82%
HORSERADISH (Kaukauna) hearty, cold pack 'Cup'	1 oz	100	6.0	3.0	250	(tr)	7.0	(mq)	25	64%
HOT PEPPER (Hickory Farms)	1 oz	106	6.3	0.5	406	(tr)	8.9	(mq)	27	75%
JARLSBERG										
(Hickory Farms)	1 oz	100	7.0	1.0	130	0	7.0	(mq)	16	66%

Food Name	Serving Size	Calories	Prot. gms	Carbs gms	Sod. mgs	Fiber gms	Fat gms	Sat. Fat gms	Chol. mgs	% Fat Cal.
(Norseland) .... 1 oz		97	7.0	1.0	135	0	7.0	4.2	18	66%
LIMBURGER										
(Mohawk Valley) 'Little Gem' .... 1 oz		90	6.0	0.0	250	0	8.0	5.0	25	75%
(Sargento) .... 1 oz		90	6.0	0.1	230	0	8.0	(mq)	26	75%
MASCARPONE 'Imported' *(Galbani)* .... 1 oz		128	1.5	1.2	17	0	13.1	(mq)	39	92%
MONTEREY .... 1 oz		105	6.8	0.2	150	0	8.5	5.3	25	73%
MONTEREY JACK										
(Alpine Lace) 'Monti-Jack-Lo' .... 1 oz		80	7.0	1.0	75	0	5.0	4.0	15	58%
(Alpine Lace) 'Monti-Jack-Lo' sliced .... 1 oz		80	7.0	1.0	75	na	5.0	3.0	15	58%
(Alta•Dena) .... 1 oz		100	7.0	1.0	180	na	8.0	na	na	69%
(Alta•Dena) w/jalapeño pepper .... 1 oz		100	7.0	1.0	180	na	8.0	na	na	69%
(Axelrod) .... 1 oz		100	6.0	1.0	150	0	8.0	(mq)	30	72%
(Axelrod) w/jalapeño pepper .... 1 oz		100	6.0	1.0	220	(tr)	8.0	(mq)	30	72%
(Darigold) .... 1 oz		110	7.0	<1.0	150	0	8.0	(mq)	25	69%
(Dorman's) .... 1 oz		100	6.0	1.0	180	0	8.0	(mq)	(mq)	72%
(Dorman's) reduced fat 'Low Sodium' .... 1 oz		80	8.0	1.0	90	0	5.0	3.1	18	56%
(Hickory Farms) 'Light Choice Low Sodium' .... 1 oz		110	6.0	0.0	100	0	8.0	(mq)	30	75%
(Kaukauna) .... 1 oz		110	7.0	<1.0	150	0	9.0	(mq)	25	72%
(Kraft) .... 1 oz		110	6.0	0.0	190	0	9.0	5.0	30	77%
(Kraft) reduced fat 'Light Naturals' .... 1 oz		80	9.0	0.0	220	0	5.0	3.0	20	56%
(Kraft) reduced fat 'Light Naturals' w/peppers .... 1 oz		80	8.0	1.0	220	(tr)	5.0	3.0	20	56%
(Kraft) 'Singles' .... 1 oz		90	5.0	2.0	390	0	7.0	4.0	25	69%
(Kraft) w/caraway .... 1 oz		100	7.0	1.0	180	(tr)	8.0	5.0	30	69%
(Kraft) w/jalapeño pepper .... 1 oz		110	7.0	1.0	190	(tr)	9.0	5.0	30	72%
(Land O'Lakes) .... 1 oz		110	7.0	<1.0	150	0	9.0	5.0	20	72%
(Land O'Lakes) hot pepper .... 1 oz		110	7.0	<1.0	150	na	9.0	5.0	20	72%
(Land O'Lakes) processed 'Jalapeño Jack' .... 1 oz		90	5.0	1.0	430	na	8.0	5.0	20	75%
(May-Bud) .... 1 oz		110	7.0	0.0	150	0	9.0	(mq)	(mq)	74%
(Sargento) .... 1 oz		110	7.0	0.2	150	0	9.0	(mq)	25	74%
(Weight Watchers) 'Natural' .... 1 oz		80	8.0	1.0	120	0	5.0	2.0	15	56%
MOZZARELLA. See also CHEESE NUGGET.										
(Dorman's) .... 1 oz		90	7.0	1.0	190	0	6.0	(mq)	(mq)	63%
(Healthy Choice) fat-free, chunk .... 1 oz		40	9.0	1.0	200	na	0.0	na	5	0%
(Hickory Farms) .... 1 oz		72	6.9	0.8	132	0	4.5	(mq)	16	57%
(Hickory Farms) 'Light Choice Low Sodium' .... 1 oz		80	8.0	1.0	90	0	5.0	(mq)	15	56%
(Kraft) .... 1 oz		90	6.0	1.0	190	0	7.0	4.0	20	69%
(Polly-O) 'Fior di Latte' .... 1 oz		80	5.0	1.0	20	0	6.0	(mq)	20	69%
(Polly-O) 'Lite' .... 1 oz		70	7.0	1.0	200	0	4.0	(mq)	15	53%
(Weight Watchers) 'Natural' .... 1 oz		70	8.0	1.0	150	0	4.0	2.0	15	50%
Part skim milk										
(Alpine Lace) low moisture .... 1 oz		70	7.0	1.0	75	0	5.0	3.0	15	58%
(Crowley) .... 1 oz		70	8.0	1.0	240	0	4.0	(mq)	15	50%
(Dorman's) low moisture 'Low Sodium' .... 1 oz		80	8.0	1.0	90	0	5.0	2.6	15	56%
(Frigo) low moisture .... 1 oz		80	7.0	1.0	190	0	5.0	(mq)	10	58%
(Frigo) low moisture, reduced fat .... 1 oz		60	8.0	1.0	150	0	3.0	2.0	10	43%
(Kraft) low moisture .... 1 oz		80	8.0	1.0	200	0	5.0	3.0	15	56%
(Kraft) w/jalapeño pepper .... 1 oz		80	8.0	1.0	230	(tr)	5.0	3.0	20	56%
(Land O'Lakes) low moisture .... 1 oz		80	8.0	1.0	150	0	5.0	3.0	15	56%
(Polly-O) .... 1 oz		80	6.0	1.0	280	0	5.0	(mq)	15	62%
(Sargento) low moisture .... 1 oz		80	8.0	1.0	150	0	5.0	(mq)	15	56%
Reduced fat										
(Dorman's) 'Low Sodium' .... 1 oz		80	9.0	1.0	90	0	4.0	2.5	17	47%
(Kraft) 'Light Naturals' .... 1 oz		80	8.0	1.0	200	0	4.0	3.0	15	50%

Food Name	Serving Size	Calories	Prot. gms	Carbs gms	Sod. mgs	Fiber gms	Fat gms	Sat. Fat gms	Chol. mgs	% Fat Cal.
Shredded										
(Alpine Lace) .... 1 oz		70	7.0	1.0	75	na	5.0	na	15	58%
(Alpine Lace) sliced .... 1 oz		70	7.0	1.0	75	na	5.0	3.0	15	58%
(Healthy Choice) fat-free .... 1 oz		40	9.0	1.0	200	na	0.0	na	5	0%
(Kraft) 'Light Naturals' .... 1 oz		80	8.0	1.0	150	na	4.0	3.0	15	50%
(Sargento) fancy 'Preferred Light' .... 1 oz		60	8.0	<1.0	150	na	3.0	na	10	43%
(Weight Watchers) 'Natural' .... 1 oz		80	8.0	1.0	150	0	4.0	2.0	15	50%
Whole milk										
(Crowley) .... 1 oz		90	5.0	1.0	240	0	7.0	(mq)	25	72%
(Frigo) low moisture .... 1 oz		90	6.0	1.0	190	0	7.0	4.0	15	69%
(Sargento) .... 1 oz		90	6.0	1.0	120	0	7.0	(mq)	25	69%
(Polly-O) .... 1 oz		90	5.0	1.0	280	0	6.0	(mq)	20	69%
MOZZARELLA CHEDDAR										
(Precious) shredded 'Pizza Cheese' .... 1 oz		95	7.0	1.0	180	na	7.0	na	na	66%
MUENSTER										
(Alpine Lace) .... 1 oz		100	7.0	1.0	85	0	8.0	5.0	30	69%
(Alpine Lace) sliced 'Low Sodium' .... 1 oz		100	7.0	1.0	85	na	9.0	6.0	25	72%
(Dorman's) .... 1 oz		110	7.0	0.0	190	0	9.0	(mq)	(mq)	74%
(Dorman's) 50% .... 1 oz		100	6.4	0.3	200	0	8.2	5.0	24	73%
(Dorman's) 'Low Sodium' .... 1 oz		110	7.0	0.0	95	0	9.0	(mq)	(mq)	74%
(Dorman's) reduced fat 'Low Sodium' .... 1 oz		80	8.0	0.0	140	0	5.0	3.1	18	58%
(Hickory Farms) .... 1 oz		100	6.6	0.3	180	0	8.5	(mq)	25	74%
(Hickory Farms) 'Light Choice Low Sodium' ... 1 oz		110	7.0	0.0	95	0	9.0	(mq)	27	74%
(Kaukauna) .... 1 oz		110	7.0	<1.0	180	0	9.0	(mq)	25	72%
(Land O'Lakes) .... 1 oz		100	7.0	<1.0	180	0	9.0	5.0	25	72%
(Sargento) red rind .... 1 oz		100	7.0	0.3	180	0	9.0	(mq)	27	74%
NEUFCHATEL										
(Hickory Farms) chocolate .... 1 oz		110	2.0	8.0	90	(tr)	8.0	(mq)	33	64%
(Hickory Farms) orange .... 1 oz		100	2.0	4.0	75	(tr)	8.0	(mq)	45	75%
(Hickory Farms) peach .... 1 oz		90	2.0	3.0	85	(tr)	8.0	(mq)	39	78%
(Hickory Farms) pineapple .... 1 oz		90	2.0	2.0	60	(tr)	8.0	(mq)	33	82%
(Hickory Farms) rum date nut .... 1 oz		100	2.0	4.0	80	(tr)	8.0	(mq)	31	75%
(Hickory Farms) strawberry .... 1 oz		90	2.0	3.0	70	(tr)	8.0	(mq)	32	78%
(Kaukauna) garden vegetable .... 1 oz		80	3.0	1.0	200	(tr)	7.0	(mq)	25	80%
(Kaukauna) garlic and herbs .... 1 oz		80	3.0	1.0	150	(tr)	7.0	(mq)	25	80%
(Philadelphia Brand) 'Light' .... 1 oz		80	3.0	1.0	115	0	7.0	4.0	25	80%
NEW HOLLAND (Hickory Farms) w/herbs 'Light Choice' .... 1 oz		90	7.0	1.0	100	(tr)	8.0	(mq)	27	69%
PARMESAN										
natural, piece .... 1 oz		110	10.0	0.9	448	0	7.2	4.6	19	60%
natural, shredded .... 1 oz		116	10.6	1.0	475	0	7.7	4.9	20	60%
natural, shredded .... 1 tbsp		21	1.9	0.2	85	0	1.4	0.9	4	60%
(Churny) 'Natural' .... 1 oz		110	10.0	1.0	455	na	7.0	4.0	20	59%
(Hickory Farms) .... 1 oz		110	10.0	1.0	350	0	7.0	(mq)	(mq)	59%
(Kraft) .... 1 oz		100	9.0	1.0	290	0	7.0	4.0	20	61%
(Sargento) fresh .... 1 oz		110	10.0	1.0	450	0	7.0	(mq)	19	59%
Grated										
natural .... 1 oz		128	11.6	1.0	521	0	8.4	5.3	22	60%
natural .... 1 tbsp		23	2.1	0.2	93	0	1.5	1.0	4	60%
(Frigo) .... 1 oz		130	12.0	1.0	510	0	9.0	(mq)	(mq)	61%
(Frigo) fresh .... 1 oz		110	10.0	1.0	350	0	7.0	(mq)	(mq)	59%
(Kraft) .... 1 oz		130	12.0	1.0	430	0	9.0	5.0	30	61%
(Polly-O) .... 1 oz		130	11.0	1.0	530	0	9.0	(mq)	20	63%
(Progresso) .... 1 tbsp		23	2.0	<1.0	95	0	2.0	1.0	4	60%
(Sargento) .... 1 oz		130	12.0	2.0	530	0	9.0	(mq)	22	59%

Food Name	Serving Size	Calories	Prot. gms	Carbs gms	Sod. mgs	Fiber gms	Fat gms	Sat. Fat gms	Chol. mgs	% Fat Cal.
Hard	1 oz	111	10.1	0.9	454	0	7.3	4.7	19	60%
Wheel (Frigo)	1 oz	110	10.0	1.0	350	0	7.0	(mq)	(mq)	59%
W/Romano cheese, grated										
(Frigo)	1 oz	130	12.0	1.0	510	0	9.0	(mq)	(mq)	61%
(Sargento)	1 oz	110	10.0	1.0	400	0	7.0	(mq)	24	59%
PARMESAN REGGIANO (Galbani) 'Imported'	1 oz	105	10.1	1.0	188	0	7.1	(mq)	21	59%
PIZZA										
(Frigo) shredded	1 oz	90	6.0	1.0	190	0	7.0	(mq)	20	69%
(Frigo) shredded, lowfat	1 oz	65	9.0	1.0	150	0	3.0	(mq)	10	40%
(Healthy Choice) fancy, shredded, fat-free	1 oz	40	9.0	1.0	200	na	0.0	na	5	0%
PORT DU SALUT	1 oz	98	6.7	0.2	150	0	7.9	4.7	34	72%
PORT WINE (Hickory Farms)	1 oz	97	5.6	2.4	262	0	6.9	(mq)	18	66%
POT (Sargento)	1 oz	25	5.0	1.0	1	0	0.2	(mq)	(mq)	7%
PRIMAVERA (Bel Paese) 'Lite'	1 oz	68	6.0	2.0	165	(tr)	4.0	(mq)	14	53%
PROVOLONE										
(Alpine Lace) 'Provo-Lo'	1 oz	70	7.0	1.0	85	0	5.0	5.0	15	58%
(Dorman's)	1 oz	90	7.0	1.0	290	0	7.0	(mq)	(mq)	66%
(Frigo)	1 oz	100	7.0	1.0	230	0	7.0	(mq)	(mq)	66%
(Frigo) smoked	1 oz	100	7.0	1.0	230	0	7.0	(mq)	(mq)	66%
(Hickory Farms) 'Light Choice Low Sodium'	1 oz	90	7.0	1.0	140	0	7.0	(mq)	20	66%
(Kraft)	1 oz	100	7.0	1.0	260	0	7.0	4.0	25	66%
(Land O'Lakes)	1 oz	100	7.0	1.0	250	0	8.0	5.0	20	69%
(Sargento)	1 oz	100	7.0	1.0	250	0	8.0	(mq)	20	69%
PUB (Hickory Farms)	1 oz	94	5.6	2.4	237	0	6.9	(mq)	18	66%
QUESO BLANCO (Sargento)	1 oz	100	7.0	0.3	180	0	9.0	(mq)	27	74%
QUESO DE PAPA (Sargento)	1 oz	110	7.0	0.4	180	0	9.0	(mq)	30	73%
QUESO DE TACO (Hickory Farms)	1 oz	106	6.3	0.5	450	0	8.9	(mq)	27	75%
RICOTTA										
Light/lowfat										
(Gardenia) '95% Fat-free'	1 oz	30	3.0	2.0	130	na	1.0	na	na	31%
(Polly-O) 'Lite'	2 oz	80	7.0	3.0	65	0	4.0	(mq)	15	47%
(Precious) 'Lowfat'	1 oz	40	3.0	2.0	20	na	2.0	1.0	10	47%
(Sargento) 'Lite'	1 oz	23	3.0	1.0	20	0	1.0	(mq)	4	36%
Part skim milk										
(Crowley)	2 oz	80	7.0	3.0	50	0	4.0	(mq)	15	47%
(Frigo)	1 oz	45	3.0	1.0	100	0	3.0	(mq)	10	63%
(Frigo) 'Truly Lite' fat-free	1 oz	20	4.0	2.0	15	na	0.0	na	3	0%
(Polly-O)	2 oz	90	7.0	2.0	45	0	6.0	(mq)	20	60%
(Sargento)	1 oz	30	3.0	1.0	30	0	2.0	(mq)	10	53%
Whole milk										
(Breakstone's)	4 oz	200	12.0	6.0	95	na	15.0	8.0	55	65%
(Crowley)	2 oz	100	6.0	3.0	50	0	7.0	(mq)	25	64%
(Frigo)	1 oz	50	3.0	1.0	100	0	4.0	(mq)	15	69%
(Polly-O)	2 oz	100	7.0	2.0	45	0	7.0	(mq)	20	64%
ROMANO										
Grated										
(Frigo)	1 oz	130	12.0	1.0	510	0	9.0	(mq)	(mq)	61%
(Kraft)	1 oz	130	11.0	1.0	350	0	9.0	6.0	30	63%
(Kraft) 'Natural'	1 oz	100	8.0	1.0	250	0	7.0	4.0	20	64%
(Polly-O)	1 oz	130	11.0	1.0	530	0	10.0	(mq)	30	65%
(Progresso)	1 tbsp	23	2.0	<1.0	70	0	2.0	1.0	6	60%
(Sargento)	1 oz	110	9.0	1.0	340	0	8.0	(mq)	29	64%
Loaf (Hickory Farms)	1 oz	110	9.0	1.0	350	0	8.0	(mq)	(mq)	64%
Wedge (Frigo)	1 oz	110	9.0	1.0	350	0	8.0	(mq)	(mq)	64%

Food Name	Serving Size	Calories	Prot. gms	Carbs gms	Sod. mgs	Fiber gms	Fat gms	Sat. Fat gms	Chol. mgs	% Fat Cal.
ROQUEFORT										
....	1 oz	103	6.0	0.6	507	0	8.6	5.4	25	75%
sheep's milk	1 oz	105	6.1	0.6	513	0	8.7	5.5	26	75%
SLIM JACK *(Dorman's)*	1 oz	90	6.0	1.0	90	0	7.0	(mq)	(mq)	69%
SMOKED										
(Hickory Farms) 'Light Choice Smoky Lyte'	1 oz	80	7.0	1.0	449	0	6.0	(mq)	5	63%
(Hoffman's) sharp, processed	1 oz	110	6.0	1.0	440	0	9.0	(mq)	(mq)	74%
(Sargento) 'Smokestick'	1 oz	100	7.0	1.0	390	0	7.0	(mq)	24	66%
STRING										
(Frigo)	1 oz	80	7.0	1.0	190	0	5.0	(mq)	(mq)	58%
(Kraft) low moisture	1 oz	80	8.0	1.0	230	0	5.0	3.0	20	56%
(Polly-O)	1 oz	90	7.0	2.0	200	0	6.0	(mq)	15	60%
(Sargento)	1 oz	80	8.0	1.0	150	0	5.0	(mq)	15	56%
(Sargento) smoked	1 oz	80	8.0	1.0	150	0	5.0	(mq)	15	56%
SWISS										
domestic	1 oz	105	8.0	1.0	73	0	7.7	5.0	26	66%
domestic	1-inch cube	56	4.3	0.5	39	0	4.1	2.7	14	66%
(Boar's Head) 'Domestic'	1 oz	110	7.0	1.0	75	0	8.0	(mq)	25	69%
(Boar's Head) 'No Salt Added'	1 oz	100	8.0	<1.0	12	0	8.0	(mq)	26	67%
(Casino)	1 oz	110	8.0	1.0	35	0	8.0	5.0	30	67%
(Cracker Barrel) baby 'Natural'	1 oz	110	7.0	0.0	65	0	9.0	5.0	25	74%
(Dorman's)	1 oz	100	8.0	0.0	80	0	8.0	(mq)	(mq)	69%
(Dorman's) 'No Salt Added'	1 oz	100	8.0	0.0	8	0	8.0	(mq)	(mq)	69%
(Hickory Farms) creamy 'Cold Pack'	1 oz	92	5.6	2.5	237	0	7.2	(mq)	24	67%
(Hickory Farms) 'Domestic'	1 oz	110	8.1	1.0	75	0	7.8	(mq)	25	66%
(Hickory Farms) 'Light Choice Lorraine'	1 oz	100	8.0	0.0	35	0	7.8	(mq)	25	69%
(Hickory Farms) 'Light Choice Low Sodium'	1 oz	100	8.0	0.0	8	0	8.0	(mq)	26	69%
(Kraft)	1 oz	110	8.0	1.0	40	0	8.0	5.0	25	67%
(Kraft) aged	1 oz	110	8.0	1.0	45	0	8.0	5.0	25	67%
(Kraft) 'Light Naturals'	1 oz	90	10.0	1.0	45	0	5.0	3.0	20	51%
(Land O'Lakes)	1 oz	110	8.0	1.0	75	0	8.0	5.0	25	67%
(Sargento) 'Finland'	1 oz	110	8.0	1.0	75	0	8.0	(mq)	26	67%
(Weight Watchers) 'Natural'	1 oz	90	9.0	1.0	50	0	5.0	3.0	15	53%
Processed										
(Alpine Lace) sliced, milk cheese 'Swiss-Lo'	1 oz	90	8.0	1.0	35	na	6.0	4.0	20	60%
(Alpine Lace) 'Swiss-Lo'	1 oz	100	8.0	1.0	35	0	7.0	4.0	20	64%
(Borden)	1 oz	100	7.0	1.0	380	0	8.0	(mq)	(mq)	69%
(Borden) fat-free, low-cholesterol	1 oz	40	6.0	4.0	na	na	0.0	na	5	0%
(Dorman's) 'Reduced Fat'	1 oz	90	10.0	0.0	80	0	5.0	2.8	17	53%
(Dorman's) smoked	1 oz	100	7.0	1.0	390	0	7.0	(mq)	(mq)	66%
(Healthy Favorites) sliced, reduced fat	1 oz	80	9.0	1.0	70	na	4.0	2.0	15	47%
(Hoffman's) smoky, w/cheddar	1 oz	110	7.0	1.0	410	0	8.0	(mq)	(mq)	69%
(Kraft) 'Deluxe'	1 oz	90	7.0	1.0	420	0	7.0	4.0	25	66%
(Kraft) 'Light'	1 oz	70	6.0	2.0	350	na	3.0	2.0	15	46%
(Kraft) reduced fat 'Light Naturals'	1 oz	90	10.0	1.0	70	0	5.0	3.0	20	51%
(Kraft) '75% Very Low Sodium'	1 oz	110	8.0	1.0	10	0	8.0	5.0	25	67%
(Sargento)	1 oz	110	8.0	1.0	75	0	8.0	(mq)	26	67%
TACO										
(Frigo) shredded	1 oz	110	7.0	1.0	200	0	9.0	(mq)	(mq)	72%
(Kraft) shredded	1 oz	110	7.0	1.0	190	0	9.0	5.0	30	72%
(Sargento)	1 oz	110	7.0	0.5	160	0	9.0	(mq)	27	73%
TALEGGIO *(Tal-Fino)* 'Brand Imported'	1 oz	89	5.4	0.2	176	0	7.4	(mq)	(mq)	75%
TILSIT										
whole milk	1 oz	95	6.8	0.5	211	0	7.3	4.7	29	69%

Food Name	Serving Size	Calories	Prot. gms	Carbs gms	Sod. mgs	Fiber gms	Fat gms	Sat. Fat gms	Chol. mgs	% Fat Cal.
(Sargento)	1 oz	100	7.0	1.0	210	0	7.0	(mq)	29	66%
TYBO										
(Dorman's) 45%	1 oz	98	7.3	0.3	200	0	7.5	4.7	23	69%
(Sargento) red wax	1 oz	100	7.0	0.3	200	0	7.0	(mq)	23	68%
VERMONT (Churny)	1 oz	110	7.0	1.0	180	0	9.0	5.0	30	72%
CHEESE, ALTERNATIVE										
(Cheeztwin)	1 oz	90	5.0	3.0	400	0	6.0	(mq)	na	63%
American cheddar style (Soya Kaas)	1 oz	79	6.2	1.6	250	na	5.4	na	na	61%
American style (Delicia)	1 oz	80	6.0	1.0	300	0	6.0	(mq)	3	66%
American style (Golden Image)	1 oz	90	7.0	2.0	360	0	6.0	2.0	5	60%
American style, hickory smoked (Delicia)	1 oz	80	6.0	0.0	470	0	6.0	(mq)	1	69%
American style, lactose-free, singles (Formägg)	3/4 oz	70	5.0	<1.0	280	na	5.0	1.0	0	65%
American style, 'Low Sodium Slices' (Weight Watchers)	1 oz	50	7.0	2.0	120	0	2.0	1.0	5	33%
American style, 'Slices' (Weight Watchers)	1 oz	50	6.0	2.0	400	0	2.0	1.0	5	36%
American style, w/caraway (Delicia)	1 oz	80	6.0	1.0	275	(tr)	6.0	(mq)	3	66%
American style, w/hot pepper (Delicia)	1 oz	80	6.0	1.0	300	(tr)	6.0	(mq)	3	66%
American style, w/salami (Delicia)	1 oz	80	6.0	1.0	370	(tr)	6.0	(mq)	3	66%
California cheddar style 'AlmondRella' (Sharon's Finest)	1 oz	50	7.0	1.0	170	.4	1.4	<.2	0	28%
California cheddar style 'Zero-Fat Rella' (Sharon's Finest)	1 oz	45	8.0	3.0	170	0	0.0	0.0	0	0%
cheddar style (Frigo)	1 oz	90	5.0	1.0	280	0	7.0	1.0	0	72%
cheddar style (Sargento)	1 oz	90	7.0	<1.0	350	0	6.0	(mq)	2	63%
cheddar style, fancy shredded (Formägg)	1 oz	70	7.0	1.0	70	na	5.0	1.0	0	58%
cheddar style, shredded 'Ched-O-Mate' (Fisher)	1 oz	90	6.0	1.0	330	0	7.0	(mq)	na	69%
colby style (Golden Image)	1 oz	110	7.0	1.0	190	0	9.0	2.0	5	72%
colby style 'LoChol' (Dorman's)	1 oz	90	7.0	1.0	140	0	6.0	1.1	1	63%
colby style, Longhorn style (Delicia)	1 oz	80	6.0	1.0	550	0	6.0	(mq)	3	66%
cream cheese style (Soya Kaas)	1 oz	90	2.3	0.1	60	na	9.4	na	na	90%
cream cheese style (Weight Watchers)	1 oz	35	3.0	1.0	40	0	2.0	(mq)	na	53%
cream cheese style, all flavors 'Better than 'Cream Cheese' (Tofutti)	1 oz	80	1.0	1.0	200	(mq)	8.0	3.0	0	90%
garlic-herb style 'AlmondRella' (Sharon's Finest)	1 oz	50	7.0	1.0	170	.4	1.4	<.2	0	28%
'Heart Beat' (Nucoa)	1 oz	50	7.0	2.0	280	0	2.0	1.0	0	33%
jalapeño jack style 'Zero-Fat Rella' (Sharon's Finest)	1 oz	45	8.0	3.0	170	0	0.0	0.0	0	0%
'Jalapeño Mexi Kaas' (Soya Kaas)	1 oz	77	6.8	0.3	160	na	5.3	na	na	63%
'Low Cholesterol' (Lite-Line)	1 oz	90	5.0	2.0	430	0	7.0	(mq)	na	69%
mild cheddar style (Golden Image)	1 oz	110	7.0	0.0	190	0	9.0	2.0	5	74%
mild cheddar style 'TofuRella' (Sharon's Finest)	1 oz	80	8.0	1.0	170	na	5.0	0.8	0	56%
mild cheddar style 'TofuRella' slices (Sharon's Finest)	3/4 oz	60	5.0	1.0	280	na	4.0	0.6	0	60%
mozzarella style (Frigo)	1 oz	90	6.0	1.0	240	0	7.0	1.0	0	69%
mozzarella style (Sargento)	1 oz	80	7.0	<1.0	310	0	6.0	(mq)	2	63%
mozzarella style (Soya Kaas)	1 oz	78	6.7	1.8	155	na	5.6	na	na	60%
mozzarella style 'AlmondRella' (Sharon's Finest)	1 oz	50	7.0	1.0	170	.4	1.4	<.2	0	28%
mozzarella style, shredded 'Pizza-Mate' (Fisher)	1 oz	90	6.0	1.0	310	0	7.0	(mq)	na	69%
mozzarella style 'TofuRella' (Sharon's Finest)	1 oz	80	8.0	1.0	170	na	5.0	0.8	0	56%
mozzarella style 'TofuRella' slices (Sharon's Finest)	3/4 oz	60	5.0	1.0	280	na	4.0	0.6	0	60%
mozzarella style 'Zero-Fat Rella' (Sharon's Finest)	1 oz	45	8.0	3.0	170	0	0.0	0.0	0	0%
muenster style 'LoChol' (Dorman's)	1 oz	100	7.0	1.0	140	0	7.0	1.1	1	66%
'Sandwich-Mate' (Fisher)	1 oz	90	5.0	3.0	400	0	6.0	(mq)	na	63%
sharp cheddar style 'Slices' (Weight Watchers)	1 oz	50	6.0	2.0	400	0	2.0	1.0	5	36%
Swiss style, lactose-free, singles (Formägg)	3/4 oz	70	5.0	<1.0	280	na	5.0	1.0	0	65%
Swiss style 'LoChol' (Dorman's)	1 oz	100	7.0	1.0	140	0	7.0	1.1	1	66%
Swiss style 'Slices' (Weight Watchers)	1 oz	50	6.0	2.0	400	0	2.0	1.0	15	36%
CHEESE BALL										
cheddar, w/almonds and bacon (Kaukauna)	1 oz	100	6.0	3.0	250	(mq)	7.0	(mq)	25	64%

Food Name	Serving Size	Calories	Prot. gms	Carbs gms	Sod. mgs	Fiber gms	Fat gms	Sat. Fat gms	Chol. mgs	% Fat Cal.
green onion flavor, w/almonds (Kaukauna) .... 1 oz		100	6.0	3.0	250	(mq)	7.0	(mq)	25	64%
Port wine, w/almonds (Kaukauna) .... 1 oz		100	6.0	3.0	250	(mq)	7.0	(mq)	25	64%
sharp cheddar, w/almonds (Kaukauna) .... 1 oz		100	6.0	3.0	250	(mq)	7.0	(mq)	25	64%
CHEESE BLINTZ. See BLINTZ.										
CHEESE FLAVORED SNACKS										
(Barbara's Bakery)										
'Pinta Puffs' tangy triple cheese .... 1 oz		70	2.0	10.0	100	na	2.0	na	5	27%
puff lights .... 1 oz		40	1.0	3.0	55	na	3.0	na	na	63%
(Bearitos) puffs, cheddar, baked, original .... .5 oz		80	1.0	7.0	2	na	5.0	1.0	130	58%
(Chee•tos)										
cheddar valley .... 1 oz		160	2.0	16.0	240	1.0	9.0	na	0	53%
crunchy .... 1 oz		150	1.0	17.0	310	1.0	9.0	na	0	53%
crunchy, light .... 1 oz		140	2.0	19.0	360	(mq)	6.0	(mq)	0	39%
curls .... 1 oz		150	1.0	17.0	270	1.0	9.0	na	0	53%
flamin' hot .... 1 oz		150	2.0	16.0	240	1.0	9.0	na	0	53%
light .... 1 oz		140	2.0	19.0	280	1.0	6.0	na	0	39%
paws .... 1 oz		160	1.0	15.0	310	1.0	10.0	na	0	58%
puffed balls .... 1 oz		160	2.0	16.0	360	1.0	10.0	na	0	56%
puffs .... 1 oz		160	1.0	16.0	330	1.0	9.0	na	0	54%
(Flavor Tree) sticks, cheddar .... 1/4 cup		129	2.7	11.9	335	>.1 c	8.1	(mq)	na	56%
(Health Valley)										
'Cheddar Lite' puffs, w/organic corn, baked .... .25 oz		40	1.0	4.0	35	na	2.0	na	0	47%
puffs, fat-free .... 1 oz		100	3.0	21.0	75	.1	0.0	na	0	0%
puffs, w/chili, fat-free .... 1 oz		100	3.0	21.0	75	.1	0.0	na	0	0%
puffs, w/green onion, fat-free .... 1 oz		100	3.0	21.0	75	.1	0.0	na	0	0%
(Keebler) 'RC Ricers' zesty cheddar .... 1 oz		140	2.0	17.0	200	na	8.0	2.0	0	49%
(Planter)										
'Cheez Balls' .... 1 oz		160	2.0	14.0	270	(mq)	11.0	2.0	5	61%
'Cheez Balls' nacho .... 1 oz		160	2.0	15.0	290	na	10.0	2.0	5	57%
'Cheez Curls' .... 1 oz		160	2.0	14.0	290	(mq)	11.0	2.0	5	61%
'Cheez Curls' nacho .... 1 oz		160	2.0	15.0	290	na	10.0	2.0	5	57%
(Weight Watchers) curls, crunchy .... .5-oz pkg		70	1.0	10.0	45	na	2.0	1.0	0	29%
(Wise)										
'Cheez Doodles' baked, puffed .... 1 oz		150	2.0	16.0	360	na	9.0	na	na	53%
'Cheez Doodles' fried, crunchy .... 1 oz		160	2.0	16.0	230	na	10.0	na	na	56%
'Cheez Waffies' .... 1 oz		140	3.0	14.0	420	(mq)	8.0	(mq)	na	51%
corn spirals, nacho .... 1 oz		160	2.0	16.0	190	(mq)	10.0	(mq)	na	56%
corn twists, nacho, crispy .... 1 oz		160	2.0	16.0	190	na	10.0	na	na	56%
CHEESE FOOD										
AMERICAN										
(Darigold) .... 1 oz		80	5.0	2.0	381	0	6.0	3.8	16	66%
cold pack .... 1 oz		94	5.6	2.4	274	0	6.9	4.4	18	66%
colored *(Hoffman's)* .... 1 oz		100	5.0	3.0	490	0	7.0	(mq)	(mq)	66%
grated *(Kraft)* .... 1 oz		130	8.0	8.0	740	0	7.0	4.0	25	50%
'Light' *(Kraft)* .... 1 oz		70	6.0	2.0	420	na	4.0	3.0	15	53%
sharp, 'Singles' *(Borden)* .... 1 oz		90	5.0	2.0	470	0	7.0	(mq)	(mq)	69%
'Singles' *(Borden)* .... 1 oz		90	5.0	3.0	350	0	7.0	(mq)	(mq)	66%
'Singles' *(Kraft)* .... 1 oz		90	5.0	2.0	390	0	7.0	4.0	25	69%
'Slices' *(Borden)* .... 1 oz		100	6.0	2.0	420	0	7.0	(mq)	(mq)	66%
white, 'Singles' *(Kraft)* .... 1 oz		90	5.0	2.0	400	0	7.0	4.0	20	69%
w/Swiss cheese *(Land O'Lakes)* .... 1 oz		100	7.0	1.0	400	na	8.0	5.0	25	69%
BACON										
(Cracker Barrel) .... 1 oz		90	5.0	3.0	280	0	7.0	4.0	20	66%
'Chees'N Bacon' *(Hoffman's)* .... 1 oz		90	6.0	3.0	540	0	6.0	(mq)	(mq)	60%

Food Name	Serving Size	Calories	Prot. gms	Carbs gms	Sod. mgs	Fiber gms	Fat gms	Sat. Fat gms	Chol. mgs	% Fat Cal.
'Cheez'N Bacon' *(Kraft)*	1 oz	90	6.0	2.0	400	0	7.0	4.0	25	66%
CARAWAY, 'Swisson Rye' *(Hoffman's)*	1 oz	90	6.0	2.0	400	(tr)	7.0	(mq)	(mq)	66%
CHEDDAR										
extra sharp *(Cracker Barrel)*	1 oz	90	5.0	3.0	240	0	7.0	4.0	20	66%
extra sharp *(Land O'Lakes)*	1 oz	100	6.0	1.0	370	na	9.0	6.0	30	74%
extra sharp, cold pack 'Cup' *(Kaukauna)*	1 oz	100	6.0	3.0	250	0	7.0	(mq)	25	64%
'La Chedda' *(Land O'Lakes)*	1 oz	90	6.0	2.0	335	0	7.0	4.0	20	66%
nacho, cold pack, 'Cup' *(Kaukauna)*	1 oz	100	6.0	3.0	250	0	7.0	(mq)	25	64%
Port wine *(Cracker Barrel)*	1 oz	100	4.0	3.0	230	0	7.0	4.0	20	69%
sharp *(Cracker Barrel)*	1 oz	100	4.0	4.0	230	0	7.0	4.0	20	66%
sharp, cold pack *(Wispride)*	1 oz	100	5.0	2.0	210	0	7.0	(mq)	25	69%
sharp, cold pack 'Cup' *(Kaukauna)*	1 oz	100	6.0	3.0	250	0	7.0	(mq)	25	64%
sharp, cup 'Lite 50' *(Kaukauna)*	1 oz	70	5.0	5.0	190	na	3.0	2.0	15	40%
sharp 'Lite' *(Kaukauna)*	1 oz	70	5.0	5.0	230	0	4.0	(mq)	15	47%
smoky 'Lite' *(Kaukauna)*	1 oz	70	5.0	5.0	230	0	4.0	(mq)	15	47%
w/bacon *(Land O'Lakes)*	1 oz	110	6.0	1.0	350	na	9.0	5.0	25	74%
w/bacon and horseradish, cold pack, 'Cup' *(Kaukauna)*	1 oz	100	6.0	3.0	250	(tr)	7.0	(mq)	25	64%
GARLIC *(Kraft)*	1 oz	90	5.0	2.0	370	(tr)	7.0	4.0	20	69%
ITALIAN HERB *(Land O'Lakes)*	1 oz	90	6.0	2.0	430	na	7.0	4.0	20	66%
JALAPEÑO										
(Hoffman's)	1 oz	90	5.0	2.0	580	(tr)	7.0	(mq)	(mq)	69%
(Kraft)	1 oz	90	5.0	2.0	390	(tr)	7.0	4.0	20	69%
(Land O'Lakes)	1 oz	90	6.0	2.0	400	na	7.0	4.0	20	66%
hot, 'Mexican' *(Velveeta)*	1 oz	100	6.0	3.0	430	(tr)	7.0	4.0	25	64%
mild, 'Mexican' *(Velveeta)*	1 oz	100	6.0	3.0	420	(tr)	7.0	4.0	25	64%
'Singles' *(Kraft)*	1 oz	90	5.0	2.0	450	(tr)	7.0	4.0	25	69%
MEXICAN										
hot, shredded *(Velveeta)*	1 oz	100	6.0	3.0	430	(tr)	7.0	4.0	25	64%
mild, shredded *(Velveeta)*	1 oz	100	6.0	3.0	420	(tr)	7.0	4.0	25	64%
ONION										
(Land O'Lakes)	1 oz	90	6.0	2.0	330	(tr)	7.0	4.0	15	66%
'Chees'N Onion' *(Hoffman's)*	1 oz	100	5.0	3.0	490	(tr)	7.0	(mq)	(mq)	66%
PEPPPERONI *(Land O'Lakes)*	1 oz	90	6.0	1.0	395	0	7.0	4.0	20	69%
PIMIENTO										
'Deluxe' *(Kraft)*	1 oz	100	6.0	1.0	440	(tr)	8.0	5.0	25	72%
'Singles' *(Kraft)*	1 oz	90	5.0	2.0	390	(tr)	7.0	4.0	25	69%
PORT WINE										
cold pack *(Wispride)*	1 oz	100	5.0	3.0	210	0	7.0	(mq)	25	66%
cold pack, 'Cup' *(Kaukauna)*	1 oz	100	6.0	3.0	250	0	7.0	(mq)	25	64%
cup, 'Lite 50' *(Kaukauna)*	1 oz	70	5.0	5.0	190	na	3.0	2.0	15	40%
PROCESSED										
(Land O'Lakes)	1 oz	90	5.0	2.0	350	na	6.0	4.0	20	66%
singles, fat-free *(Healthy Choice)*	1 oz	40	6.0	3.0	390	na	0.0	na	5	0%
singles, 'Free' *(Kraft)*	1 oz	45	6.0	4.0	430	na	0.0	na	5	0%
slices *(Land O'Lakes)*	3/4 oz	70	4.0	2.0	260	na	5.0	3.0	15	65%
slices *(Land O'Lakes)*	2/3 oz	60	4.0	2.0	230	na	4.0	3.0	15	60%
SALAMI										
(Land O'Lakes)	1 oz	90	6.0	2.0	410	0	7.0	4.0	20	66%
'Chees'N Salami' *(Hoffman's)*	1 oz	90	5.0	3.0	560	0	6.0	(mq)	(mq)	63%
SHARP, 'Singles' *(Kraft)*	1 oz	100	6.0	1.0	400	0	8.0	5.0	25	72%
SHREDDED *(Velveeta)*	1 oz	100	6.0	3.0	410	0	7.0	4.0	20	64%
SMOKY, cold pack, 'Cup' *(Kaukauna)*	1 oz	100	6.0	3.0	250	0	7.0	(mq)	25	64%
SWISS										
(Velveeta)	1 oz	100	6.0	3.0	410	0	7.0	4.0	20	64%

Food Name	Serving Size	Calories	Prot. gms	Carbs gms	Sod. mgs	Fiber gms	Fat gms	Sat. Fat gms	Chol. mgs	% Fat Cal.
almond, cup, 'Lite 50' (Kaukauna)	1 oz	70	5.0	5.0	180	na	3.0	2.0	15	40%
country, cold pack,'Cup' (Kaukauna)	1 oz	100	6.0	3.0	250	0	7.0	(mq)	25	64%
country, 'Lite' (Kaukauna)	1 oz	70	6.0	5.0	200	0	4.0	(mq)	15	45%
singles (Kraft)	1 oz	90	6.0	2.0	440	0	7.0	4.0	25	66%
singles, 'Free' (Kraft)	1 oz	45	6.0	4.0	390	na	0.0	0.0	5	0%
slices, 'Singles' (Borden)	1 oz	100	6.0	2.0	420	na	7.0	na	na	66%
CHEESE LOG										
hickory smoke/white sharp cheddar, double (Kaukauna)	1 oz	100	6.0	3.0	250	(mq)	7.0	(mq)	25	64%
Port wine (Sargento)	1 oz	100	6.0	3.0	250	(mq)	7.0	(mq)	18	64%
Port wine, w/almonds (Kaukauna)	1 oz	100	6.0	3.0	250	(mq)	7.0	(mq)	25	64%
sharp cheddar (Sargento)	1 oz	100	6.0	3.0	250	(mq)	7.0	(mq)	18	64%
sharp cheddar, w/almonds (Cracker Barrel)	1 oz	90	5.0	4.0	410	(mq)	6.0	3.0	15	60%
sharp cheddar, w/almonds (Kaukauna)	1 oz	100	6.0	3.0	250	(mq)	7.0	(mq)	25	64%
smoky, w/almonds (Cracker Barrel)	1 oz	90	5.0	4.0	410	(mq)	6.0	3.0	15	60%
Swiss almond (Sargento)	1 oz	90	6.0	2.0	350	(mq)	7.0	(mq)	21	66%
Swiss almond, w/almonds (Kaukauna)	1 oz	100	6.0	3.0	250	(mq)	7.0	(mq)	25	64%
white sharp cheddar/green onion, double (Kaukauna)	1 oz	100	6.0	3.0	250	(mq)	7.0	(mq)	25	64%
CHEESE NUGGET										
mozzarella, breaded, frozen 'Hot Bites' (Banquet)	2.63 oz	240	14.0	16.0	530	(mq)	13.0	(mq)	(mq)	49%
CHEESE NUT										
Port wine (Cracker Barrel)	1 oz	90	5.0	4.0	260	(mq)	6.0	3.0	15	60%
sharp, w/bell and jalapeño peppers (Kaukauna)	1 oz	100	6.0	3.0	250	(mq)	7.0	(mq)	25	64%
sharp cheddar (Cracker Barrel)	1 oz	100	5.0	4.0	250	(mq)	7.0	3.0	20	64%
CHEESE PASTRY, pocket (Tastykake)	3 oz	325	4.4	40.8	231	1.3	16.7	3.9	11	45%
CHEESE PRODUCT										
(Alpine Lace)	1 oz	90	6.0	2.0	200	0	7.0	4.0	20	66%
'Free N' Lean' singles (Alpine Lace)	1 oz	40	8.0	1.0	260	na	0.0	0.0	5	0%
'Free Singles' (Kraft)	1 oz	45	7.0	4.0	420	0	0.0	0.0	5	0%
'Light' (Velveeta)	1 oz	70	6.0	3.0	470	0	4.0	2.0	15	50%
sandwich slices (Lunch Wagon)	1 oz	90	5.0	2.0	370	0	7.0	2.0	5	69%
'Singles' fat-free (Borden)	1 oz	40	6.0	4.0	380	na	0.0	na	5	0%
'Slices' (Velveeta)	1 oz	90	5.0	3.0	400	0	6.0	4.0	20	63%
slices, fat-free (Lite-Line)	1 slice	25	4.0	3.0	250	na	0.0	0.0	5	0%
AMERICAN FLAVOR										
(Harvest Moon)	1 oz	70	6.0	2.0	420	0	4.0	2.0	15	53%
(Lite-Line)	1 oz	50	7.0	1.0	410	0	2.0	(mq)	(mq)	36%
'Light' (Borden)	1 oz	70	6.0	1.0	420	0	5.0	(mq)	(mq)	62%
'Light Singles' (Kraft)	1 oz	70	6.0	2.0	420	0	4.0	3.0	15	53%
'Reduced Sodium' (Lite-Line)	1 oz	70	6.0	2.0	90	0	4.0	(mq)	(mq)	53%
'Singles' (Light n' Lively)	1 oz	70	6.0	2.0	420	0	4.0	3.0	15	53%
'Sodium Lite' (Lite-Line)	1 oz	70	6.0	2.0	200	0	4.0	(mq)	(mq)	53%
white 'Light Singles' (Kraft)	1 oz	70	6.0	2.0	410	0	4.0	2.0	15	53%
white 'Singles' (Light n' Lively)	1 oz	70	6.0	2.0	410	0	4.0	2.0	15	53%
CHEDDAR FLAVOR										
medium-sharp (Spreadery)	1 oz	70	5.0	3.0	250	0	4.0	2.0	15	53%
mild (Lite-Line)	1 oz	50	7.0	1.0	380	0	2.0	(mq)	(mq)	36%
sharp (Lite-Line)	1 oz	50	7.0	1.0	440	0	2.0	(mq)	(mq)	36%
sharp (Spreadery)	1 oz	70	5.0	3.0	240	0	4.0	2.0	15	53%
sharp, 'Free' (Kraft)	1 oz	45	6.0	4.0	390	0	0.0	0.0	5	0%
sharp, 'Light' (Kraft)	1 oz	70	6.0	2.0	380	0	4.0	2.0	15	53%
sharp, 'Singles' (Kraft)	1 oz	100	6.0	1.0	400	0	8.0	na	25	72%
sharp, 'Singles' (Light n' Lively)	1 oz	70	6.0	2.0	380	0	4.0	2.0	15	53%
sharp, slices (Lite-Line)	1 slice	35	4.0	1.0	300	na	2.0	na	5	47%
Vermont white (Spreadery)	1 oz	70	5.0	3.0	230	0	4.0	2.0	15	53%

Food Name	Serving Size	Calories	Prot. gms	Carbs gms	Sod. mgs	Fiber gms	Fat gms	Sat. Fat gms	Chol. mgs	% Fat Cal.
CREAM CHEESE FLAVOR 'Light' (Philadelphia Brand) ...... 1 oz		60	3.0	2.0	160	0	5.0	3.0	10	69%
MEXICAN FLAVOR mild, w/jalapeños (Spreadery) .... 1 oz		70	5.0	3.0	260	(tr)	4.0	3.0	15	53%
MOZZARELLA FLAVOR (Lite-Line) .... 1 oz		50	7.0	1.0	340	0	2.0	(mq)	(mq)	36%
MUENSTER FLAVOR (Lite-Line) .... 1 oz		50	7.0	1.0	450	0	2.0	(mq)	(mq)	36%
NACHO FLAVOR (Spreadery) .... 1 oz		70	5.0	3.0	240	0	4.0	2.0	15	53%
NEUFCHATEL										
classic ranch (Spreadery) .... 1 oz		70	2.0	1.0	190	(tr)	7.0	4.0	20	84%
French onion (Spreadery) .... 1 oz		70	2.0	2.0	135	(tr)	6.0	4.0	20	77%
garden vegetable (Spreadery) .... 1 oz		70	2.0	2.0	220	(tr)	6.0	3.0	20	77%
garlic and herb (Spreadery) .... 1 oz		70	2.0	1.0	140	(tr)	6.0	4.0	20	82%
w/strawberries (Spreadery) .... 1 oz		70	2.0	1.0	270	(tr)	5.0	3.0	15	79%
PORT WINE FLAVOR (Spreadery) .... 1 oz		70	5.0	3.0	250	0	4.0	2.0	15	53%
SWISS FLAVOR										
(Lite-Line) .... 1 oz		50	7.0	1.0	380	0	2.0	(mq)	(mq)	36%
'Free Singles' (Kraft) .... 1 oz		45	6.0	4.0	390	na	0.0	na	5	0%
'Light' (Kraft) .... 1 oz		70	6.0	2.0	350	0	3.0	2.0	15	46%
'Singles' (Light n' Lively) .... 1 oz		70	6.0	2.0	350	0	3.0	2.0	15	46%
CHEESE SPREAD										
AMERICAN										
(Kraft) .... 1 oz		80	4.0	2.0	470	0	6.0	3.0	15	69%
'Easy Cheese American' (Nabisco) .... 1 oz		80	4.0	2.0	350	na	6.0	na	na	69%
sharp 'Cracker Snacks' (Sargento) .... 1 oz		110	6.0	0.5	410	0	9.0	(mq)	27	76%
w/pimiento 'Cracker Snacks' (Sargento) .... 1 oz		110	6.0	0.5	410	(tr)	9.0	(mq)	27	76%
BACON										
(Kraft) .... 1 oz		80	5.0	1.0	560	0	7.0	4.0	20	72%
(Squeez-A-Snak) .... 1 oz		80	5.0	1.0	500	0	7.0	4.0	20	72%
BLUE (Roka) .... 1 oz		70	3.0	2.0	270	0	6.0	4.0	20	73%
BRICK 'Cracker Snacks' (Sargento) .... 1 oz		100	6.0	1.0	430	0	9.0	(mq)	25	74%
CHEDDAR										
'Easy Cheese Cheddar' (Nabisco) .... 1 oz		80	4.0	2.0	370	na	6.0	na	na	69%
'Easy Cheese Cheddar 'n Bacon' (Nabisco) .... 1 oz		80	4.0	2.0	350	na	6.0	na	na	69%
'Easy Cheese Sharp Cheddar' (Nabisco) .... 1 oz		80	4.0	2.0	320	na	6.0	na	na	69%
sharp, 'Cup' (Weight Watchers) .... 1 oz		70	4.0	7.0	190	0	3.0	2.0	10	38%
FRENCH ONION (Alouette) .... 1 oz		95	2.0	2.0	205	na	9.0	na	31	84%
GARLIC										
(Squeez-A-Snak) .... 1 oz		80	5.0	1.0	430	(tr)	7.0	4.0	20	72%
and herbs, soft 'Lite' (Rondel) .... 1 oz		70	3.0	2.0	170	na	6.0	3.0	15	73%
and spices (Alouette) .... 1 oz		95	2.0	2.0	165	na	9.0	na	31	84%
HERB										
and garlic, soft 'Light' (Alouette) .... 1 oz		60	3.0	2.0	130	na	4.5	na	15	67%
soft, 'Fines Herbes' (Rondel) .... 1 oz		90	3.0	2.0	170	na	8.0	na	na	78%
HICKORY (Squeez-A-Snak) .... 1 oz		80	5.0	1.0	440	0	7.0	4.0	20	72%
HORSERADISH, and chive (Alouette) .... 1 oz		85	2.0	1.0	130	na	8.0	na	28	86%
JALAPEÑO										
(Cheez Whiz) .... 1 oz		80	4.0	2.0	430	(tr)	6.0	4.0	20	69%
(Kraft) .... 1 oz		70	2.0	3.0	95	(tr)	5.0	3.0	15	69%
(Squeez-A-Snak) .... 1 oz		80	5.0	1.0	510	(tr)	6.0	4.0	20	69%
loaf (Kraft) .... 1 oz		80	5.0	2.0	470	(tr)	6.0	4.0	20	66%
LIMBURGER (Mohawk Valley) .... 1 oz		70	4.0	0.0	420	0	6.0	3.0	20	77%
MEXICAN										
'Easy Cheese Nacho' (Nabisco) .... 1 oz		80	4.0	2.0	340	na	6.0	na	na	69%
hot (Velveeta) .... 1 oz		80	5.0	3.0	520	(tr)	6.0	3.0	20	63%
mild (Cheez Whiz) .... 1 oz		80	4.0	2.0	430	(tr)	6.0	4.0	20	69%
mild (Velveeta) .... 1 oz		80	5.0	3.0	440	(tr)	6.0	3.0	20	63%

Food Name	Serving Size	Calories	Prot. gms	Carbs gms	Sod. mgs	Fiber gms	Fat gms	Sat. Fat gms	Chol. mgs	% Fat Cal.
OLIVE, and pimiento (Kraft)	1 oz	60	2.0	2.0	160	(tr)	5.0	3.0	15	74%
PIMIENTO										
(Kraft)	1 oz	70	2.0	3.0	120	(tr)	5.0	3.0	15	69%
(Velveeta)	1 oz	80	5.0	3.0	400	(tr)	6.0	3.0	20	63%
PINEAPPLE (Kraft)	1 oz	70	2.0	4.0	15	(tr)	5.0	3.0	75	65%
PORT WINE, 'Cup' (Weight Watchers)	1 oz	70	4.0	7.0	190	0	3.0	2.0	10	38%
SALMON (Alouette)	1 oz	70	2.0	2.0	140	na	6.0	na	20	77%
SHARP										
(Old English)	1 oz	80	5.0	1.0	480	0	7.0	4.0	20	72%
(Squeez-A-Snak)	1 oz	80	5.0	1.0	440	0	7.0	4.0	20	72%
SPINACH, creamy (Alouette)	1 oz	90	2.0	2.0	125	na	8.0	na	na	82%
SWISS, 'Cracker Snacks' (Sargento)	1 oz	100	7.0	1.0	390	0	7.0	(mq)	24	66%
VEGETABLE										
garden, soft (Rondele)	1 oz	90	3.0	3.0	160	na	8.0	na	na	75%
spring, soft 'Light' (Alouette)	1 oz	60	3.0	1.0	120	na	4.5	na	15	72%
CHEESE STICK										
cheddar, breaded, frozen (Farm Rich)	3 oz	300	10.9	19.0	740	(mq)	21.0	(mq)	(mq)	61%
cheddar, snack (Flavor Tree)	1/4 cup	129	2.7	11.9	335	>.1 c	8.1	(mq)	na	56%
hot pepper, breaded, frozen (Farm Rich)	3 oz	260	8.0	20.0	700	(mq)	17.0	(mq)	(mq)	58%
mozzarella, breaded, frozen (Farm Rich)	3 oz	240	10.0	19.0	570	(mq)	13.0	(mq)	(mq)	50%
provolone, breaded, frozen (Farm Rich)	3 oz	270	10.0	22.0	820	(mq)	16.0	(mq)	(mq)	53%
CHEESE STRAW										
made w/lard, 5 x 3/8 x 3/8 inches	10 straws	272	6.7	20.7	433	>.1 c	17.9	7.9	32	60%
made w/vegetable shortening, 5 x 3/8 x 3/8 inches	10 straws	272	6.7	20.7	433	>.1 c	17.9	6.4	19	60%
CHEESE TOPPING, cheddar, w/bacon (Tone's)	1 tsp	10	0.5	0.7	81	0	1.0	0.5	1	65%
CHEESECAKE. See CAKE.										
CHEESECAKE FILLING										
'No-Bake' lite (Royal)	1/8 pie	130	4.0	22.0	230	na	3.0	0.0	5	21%
'No-Bake' real (Royal)	1/8 pie	160	4.0	29.0	250	na	3.0	na	na	17%
CHERIMOYA. See CUSTARD APPLE.										
CHERRY										
SOUR, RED										
trimmed, w/pits	1 cup	52	1.0	12.6	3	1.2	0.3	0.1	0	5%
trimmed, w/pits	1 oz	14	0.3	3.5	1	(mq)	0.1	<.1	0	6%
trimmed, w/o pits	1 cup	78	1.5	18.9	5	1.9	0.5	0.1	0	5%
untrimmed	1 lb	203	4.1	49.7	13	(mq)	1.2	0.3	0	5%
SWEET										
trimmed, w/pits	1 cup	104	1.7	24.0	0	3.3	1.4	0.3	0	11%
trimmed, w/pits	1 oz	20	0.3	4.7	tr	.4	0.3	0.1	0	12%
trimmed, w/pits, approx 2.6 oz	10 med	49	0.8	11.3	0	1.6	0.7	0.2	0	12%
untrimmed	1 lb	293	4.9	67.6	2	6.3	3.9	1.0	0	11%
untrimmed (Dole)	1 cup	90	1.0	19.0	0	3.0	1.0	na	na	10%
CHERRY, CANNED										
SOUR, RED										
(A&P)	1/2 cup	50	<1.0	12.0	5	(mq)	<1.0	(tr)	0	<15%
in extra heavy syrup	1/2 cup	148	0.9	38.0	9	>.1 c	0.1	0.0	0	1%
in heavy syrup	1/2 cup	116	0.9	29.8	9	1.0	0.1	0.0	0	1%
in light syrup	1/2 cup	94	0.9	24.3	9	>.1 c	0.1	0.0	0	1%
in water	1/2 cup	44	0.9	10.9	9	1.0	0.1	0.0	0	2%
Pitted										
in extra heavy syrup	1/2 cup	129	0.8	33.1	8	>.1 c	0.1	<.1	0	1%
in heavy syrup	1/2 cup	103	0.8	26.4	8	>.1 c	0.1	<.1	0	1%
in light syrup	1/2 cup	85	0.8	21.9	8	>.1 c	0.1	<.1	0	1%
in water	1/2 cup	41	0.9	10.0	8	>.1 c	0.1	<.1	0	2%

Food Name	Serving Size	Calories	Prot. gms	Carbs gms	Sod. mgs	Fiber gms	Fat gms	Sat. Fat gms	Chol. mgs	% Fat Cal.
in water *(Stokely)*	1/2 cup	45	1.0	10.0	15	(mq)	0.0	0.0	0	0%
tart *(Lucky Leaf)*	4 oz	50	1.0	11.0	0	(mq)	0.0	0.0	0	0%
tart *(Musselman's)*	4 oz	50	1.0	11.0	0	(mq)	0.0	0.0	0	0%
(White House)	3.5 oz	43	0.0	11.0	5	(mq)	0.0	0.0	0	0%
SWEET										
dark *(Del Monte)*	1/2 cup	90	0.0	23.0	10	(mq)	0.0	0.0	0	0%
in extra heavy syrup	1/2 cup	116	0.7	29.7	3	>.4 c	0.2	<.1	0	2%
in heavy syrup	1/2 cup	94	0.7	24.1	3	>.4 c	0.2	<.1	0	2%
in juice	1/2 cup	61	1.0	15.7	3	>.3 c	<.1	tr	0	<1%
in light syrup	1/2 cup	76	0.7	19.6	3	>.4 c	0.2	<.1	0	2%
in light syrup *(Del Monte)*	1/2 cup	100	0.0	26.0	10	(mq)	0.0	0.0	0	0%
in water	1/2 cup	52	0.9	13.3	1	>.2 c	0.1	<.1	0	2%
Pitted										
dark *(Del Monte)*	1/2 cup	90	0.0	24.0	10	(mq)	0.0	0.0	0	0%
in extra heavy syrup	1/2 cup	133	0.8	34.1	4	>.4 c	0.2	0.0	0	1%
in heavy syrup	1/2 cup	107	0.8	27.4	4	.9	0.2	0.0	0	2%
in juice	1/2 cup	68	1.1	17.3	4	.9	0.0	0.0	0	0%
in light syrup	1/2 cup	84	0.8	21.8	4	.9	0.2	0.0	0	2%
in water	1/2 cup	57	1.0	14.6	1	.9	0.2	0.0	0	3%
CHERRY, FROZEN										
SOUR, RED										
unsweetened	4 oz	52	1.0	12.5	1	1.3	0.5	0.1	0	8%
unsweetened	1/2 cup	36	0.7	8.5	1	1.0	0.3	0.1	0	7%
SWEET										
sweetened	10-oz pkg	253	3.3	63.5	3	2.8	0.4	0.1	0	1%
sweetened	1 cup	231	3.0	57.9	3	2.6	0.3	0.1	0	1%
sweetened	4 oz	101	1.3	25.4	1	1.1	0.1	<.1	0	1%
sweetened *(Lucky Leaf)*	4 oz	130	1.0	31.0	150	(mq)	0.0	0.0	0	0%
CHERRY, MARASCHINO, in jar, w/liquid	1 oz	33	0.1	8.3	na	>.1 c	0.1	0.0	0	3%
CHERRY, PUERTO RICAN										
approx .2 oz	1 med	2	<.1	0.4	tr	>.1 c	<.1	(tr)	0	<31%
trimmed	1/2 cup	16	0.2	3.8	4	>.2 c	0.1	(tr)	0	5%
trimmed	1 oz	9	0.1	2.2	2	>.1 c	0.1	(tr)	0	9%
untrimmed	1 lb	114	1.5	27.9	26	>1.5 c	1.1	na	0	8%
CHERRY CIDER *(Knudsen & Sons)*	8 oz	100	<1.0	24.0	na	na	0.0	na	na	0%
CHERRY DRINK										
(Hi-C) aseptic box	6 oz	100	0.0	24.0	25	na	0.0	na	na	0%
(Hi-C) chilled	6 oz	100	0.0	24.0	25	na	0.0	na	na	0%
(Kool-Aid) 'Koolers'	8.45 oz	140	0.0	38.0	10	na	0.0	na	0	0%
(Squeezit) 'Chucklin Cherry'	6.75 oz	110	0.0	27.0	5	na	0.0	na	na	0%
CHERRY DRINK MIX										
(Finast) prepared	8 oz	80	0.0	21.0	15	(tr)	0.0	0.0	0	0%
(Kool-Aid) sugar-sweetened, prepared	8 oz	80	0.0	20.0	0	na	0.0	na	0	0%
(Kool-Aid) unsweetened, prepared w/sugar	8 oz	100	0.0	25.0	0	na	0.0	na	0	0%
(Kool-Aid) unsweetened, prepared w/o sugar	8 oz	2	0.0	0.0	0	na	0.0	na	0	0%
(Kool-Aid) w/NutraSweet, prepared	8 oz	4	0.0	0.0	0	na	0.0	na	0	0%
(Pathmark) 'No Frills' prepared	8 oz	90	0.0	22.0	65	(tr)	0.0	0.0	0	0%
(Wyler's) 'Fruit Slush' prepared	4 oz	157	0.0	39.3	10	(tr)	0.0	0.0	0	0%
CHERRY JUICE										
(Dole) 'Pure and Light Mountain Cherry'	6 oz	87	0.2	22.0	8	(mq)	0.1	(tr)	0	1%
(Juicy Juice) bottled	6 oz	90	1.0	23.0	10	na	0.0	na	na	0%
(Juicy Juice) boxed	8.45 oz	130	1.0	32.0	10	na	0.0	na	na	0%
(Knudsen & Sons) tart	8 oz	125	<1.0	30.0	na	na	0.0	na	na	0%
(Santa Cruz Natural) 'Cruz' organic	8 oz	125	1.0	29.0	na	na	<1.0	na	na	<7%

Food Name	Serving Size	Calories	Prot. gms	Carbs gms	Sod. mgs	Fiber gms	Fat gms	Sat. Fat gms	Chol. mgs	% Fat Cal.
(Welch's) 'Orchard'	6 oz	180	0.0	45.0	10	(tr)	0.0	0.0	0	0%
CHERRY JUICE DRINK										
(Hi-C)	8.45 oz	141	0.2	34.8	24	(tr)	0.1	(tr)	0	1%
(Hi-C)	6 oz	100	0.1	24.7	17	(tr)	0.1	(tr)	0	1%
(Tang) 'Fruit Box'	8.45 oz	130	0.0	34.0	10	na	0.0	na	0	0%
CHERRY LEMONADE										
(Knudsen & Sons)	8 oz	105	<1.0	31.0	na	na	0.0	na	na	0%
(Santa Cruz Natural) dark, sweet, organic	8 oz	60	<1.0	20.0	na	na	<1.0	na	na	<10%
CHERRY PASTRY										
(Hormel) frozen 'Cherry Dulcita'	4 oz	300	5.0	48.0	345	(mq)	9.0	(mq)	na	28%
(Tastykake) pocket	3 oz	325	4.4	40.8	231	1.3	16.7	3.9	11	45%
CHERRY PIE FILLING. See PIE FILLING.										
CHERRY STRUDEL, individual *(Aunt Fanny's)*	3 oz	320	4.0	39.0	190	na	16.0	6.5	5	46%
CHERVIL										
dried	1 oz	67	6.6	13.9	24	3.2	1.1	na	0	11%
dried	1 tbsp	4	0.4	0.9	2	.2	0.1	na	0	15%
dried	1 tsp	1	0.1	0.3	1	.1	0.0	na	0	0%
CHESTNUT, CHINESE										
boiled or steamed	1 oz	43	0.8	9.6	1	>.3 c	0.2	0.0	0	4%
dried	1 oz	103	1.9	22.6	1	>.8 c	0.5	0.1	0	4%
raw	1 oz	64	1.2	13.9	1	>.5 c	0.3	0.1	0	4%
raw, in shell	1 lb	852	16.0	187.0	13	>6.2 c	4.2	0.6	0	4%
roasted	1 oz	68	1.3	14.9	1	>.5 c	0.3	0.1	0	4%
CHESTNUT, EUROPEAN / Italian chestnut / sweet chestnut										
boiled or steamed, shelled	1 oz	37	0.8	7.9	8	>.2 c	0.4	0.1	0	9%
dried, in shell	1 lb	1357	23.2	280.5	135	>19.8 c	16.1	3.0	0	11%
dried, shelled, peeled	1 oz	105	1.4	22.3	11	>1.4 c	1.1	0.2	0	10%
dried, shelled, unpeeled	1 oz	106	1.8	22.0	11	3.3	1.3	0.2	0	11%
raw, in shell	1 lb	714	8.1	152.8	9	33.3	7.6	1.4	0	10%
raw, shelled, peeled	1 oz	56	0.5	12.5	1	>.3 c	0.4	0.1	0	7%
raw, shelled, unpeeled	1 cup	309	3.5	66.0	4	11.7	3.3	0.6	0	10%
raw, shelled, unpeeled	1 oz	60	0.7	12.9	1	2.3	0.6	0.1	0	9%
roasted, in shell	1 lb	700	9.1	151.3	6	33.4	6.3	1.2	0	8%
roasted, in shell	1 cup	350	4.5	75.7	3	18.4	3.2	0.6	0	8%
roasted, in shell	1 oz	70	0.9	15.0	1	3.7	0.6	0.1	0	8%
roasted, shelled	1 oz	70	0.9	15.0	1	3.3	0.6	0.1	0	8%
roasted, shelled, approx 17 nuts	1 cup	350	4.3	75.7	3	16.7	3.2	0.6	0	8%
CHESTNUT, ITALIAN. See CHESTNUT, EUROPEAN.										
CHESTNUT, JAPANESE										
boiled or steamed	1 oz	16	0.2	3.6	1	>.1 c	0.1	0.0	0	6%
dried, in shell	1 lb	1078	15.7	243.7	101	>6.8 c	3.7	0.5	0	3%
dried, shelled	1 oz	102	1.5	23.1	10	>.6 c	0.4	0.1	0	4%
dried, shelled	1 cup	558	8.1	126.2	53	>3.5 c	1.9	0.3	0	3%
raw, in shell	1 lb	462	6.7	104.5	43	>2.9 c	1.6	0.2	0	3%
raw, shelled	1 oz	44	0.6	9.9	4	>.3 c	0.2	0.0	0	4%
roasted	1 oz	57	0.8	12.8	5	>.3 c	0.2	0.0	0	3%
CHESTNUT, SWEET. See CHESTNUT, EUROPEAN.										
CHESTNUT FLOUR	100 gm	362	6.1	76.2	11	>2.0 c	3.7	0.0	0	9%
CHEWING GUM. See CANDY.										
CHIA SEEDS, dried	1 oz	134	4.7	13.6	11	>7.2 c	7.4	3.0	0	48%
CHICK PEA. See GARBANZO BEAN.										
CHICK PEA FLOUR. See GARBANZO FLOUR.										
CHICKEN. For fresh chicken see CHICKEN, BROILER-FRYER; CHICKEN, CAPON; CHICKEN, ROASTER; CHICKEN, STEWING.										

Food Name	Serving Size	Calories	Prot. gms	Carbs gms	Sod. mgs	Fiber gms	Fat gms	Sat. Fat gms	Chol. mgs	% Fat Cal.
CHICKEN, ALTERNATIVE										
(Heartline) 'Chicken Fillet Style'	2 oz	176	19.0	9.0	260	na	7.0	na	0	36%
(Heartline) 'Chicken Fillet Style' lite	.5 oz	22	5.0	1.0	135	3.0	0.0	0.0	0	0%
Canned										
(Worthington) diced, drained	1/4 cup	90	4.0	2.0	330	(mq)	8.0	(mq)	0	75%
(Worthington) 'FriChik' 1.6-oz pieces	2 pieces	180	11.0	4.0	610	(mq)	13.0	(mq)	0	66%
(Worthington) sliced, drained, 1.05-oz slices	2 slices	90	4.0	2.0	330	(mq)	8.0	(mq)	0	75%
Frozen										
(Morningstar Farms) nuggets, homestyle 'Country Crisps'	3 oz	250	8.0	18.0	480	(mq)	16.0	(mq)	0	58%
(Morningstar Farms) nuggets, zesty 'Country Crisps'	3 oz	280	9.0	17.0	740	(mq)	19.0	3.0	0	62%
(Morningstar Farms) patty 'Country Crisps'	2.5 oz	220	8.0	13.0	620	(mq)	15.0	2.0	0	62%
(Worthington) 'Crispy Chik'	3 oz	280	10.0	17.0	500	(mq)	19.0	(mq)	0	61%
(Worthington) diced 'Meatless Chicken'	1/2 cup	190	13.0	5.0	680	(mq)	13.0	2.0	0	62%
(Worthington) patty 'Crispy Chik'	2.5 oz	220	8.0	13.0	620	(mq)	15.0	2.0	0	62%
(Worthington) roll 'Chic-ketts'	1/2 cup	160	19.0	6.0	640	(mq)	7.0	1.0	0	39%
(Worthington) roll 'Meatless Chicken'	2.5 oz	150	11.0	4.0	570	(mq)	10.0	1.0	0	60%
(Worthington) sliced 'Meatless Chicken' 1-oz slices	2 slices	130	9.0	3.0	460	(mq)	9.0	1.0	0	63%
(Worthington) sticks 'Chik Stiks' approx 1.7-oz pieces	1 stick	110	9.0	4.0	390	(mq)	7.0	1.0	0	55%
CHICKEN, BONELESS BREAST, PREPARED										
(Hillshire Farm) smoked 'Deli Select'	1 oz	31	6.0	<1.0	290	0	0.2	(mq)	(mq)	6%
(Louis Rich) hickory-smoked	1 oz	30	5.1	0.6	356	0	0.8	0.3	14	24%
(Louis Rich) hickory-smoked, 97% fat-free	1 oz	30	5.0	<1.0	370	na	<1.0	na	15	<27%
(Louis Rich) oven-roasted 'Deluxe'	1 oz	30	4.9	0.6	332	0	0.8	0.3	14	25%
(Louis Rich) oven-roasted, 'Deluxe' 96% fat-free	1 oz	30	5.0	<1.0	330	na	1.0	na	15	27%
(Oscar Mayer) oven-roasted	1 oz	29	5.2	0.6	414	0	0.7	0.2	15	21%
(Oscar Mayer) smoked	1 oz	25	5.3	0.2	397	0	0.4	0.1	15	14%
CHICKEN, BROILER-FRYER										
BACK MEAT AND SKIN										
fried, flour-coated	4 oz	375	31.5	7.4	102	>.1 c	23.5	6.4	101	58%
raw	1 oz	90	4.0	0.0	18	0	8.1	2.4	22	82%
roasted	4 oz	340	29.4	0.0	99	0	23.8	6.6	100	65%
stewed	4 oz	293	25.2	0.0	73	0	20.6	5.7	88	65%
BACK MEAT ONLY										
raw	1 lb	624	88.0	0.0	400	0	28.8	8.0	400	41%
raw	1 oz	39	5.5	0.0	23	0	1.7	0.4	23	41%
roasted	4 oz	271	32.0	0.0	109	0	14.9	4.1	102	51%
stewed	4 oz	237	28.7	0.0	76	0	12.7	3.4	96	50%
BREAST MEAT AND SKIN										
fried, batter-dipped	4 oz	295	28.2	10.2	312	.4	15.0	4.0	96	47%
fried, flour-coated	4 oz	252	36.1	1.9	86	>.1 c	10.1	2.8	101	37%
raw	1 lb	784	94.4	0.0	288	0	41.6	12.8	288	50%
raw	1 oz	49	5.9	0.0	18	0	2.6	0.8	18	50%
roasted	4 oz	223	33.8	0.0	81	0	8.8	2.5	95	37%
stewed	4 oz	209	31.1	0.0	70	0	8.4	2.4	85	38%
BREAST MEAT ONLY										
raw	1 lb	496	104.0	0.0	288	0	6.4	1.6	256	12%
raw	1 oz	31	6.5	0.0	18	0	0.4	0.1	16	12%
roasted	4 oz	187	35.2	0.0	84	0	4.0	1.1	96	20%
stewed	4 oz	171	32.9	0.0	71	0	3.4	1.0	87	19%
DARK MEAT AND SKIN										
fried, batter-dipped	4 oz	338	24.8	10.6	335	>.1 c	21.1	5.6	101	57%
fried, flour-coated	4 oz	323	30.9	4.6	101	>.1 c	19.2	5.2	104	55%
raw	1 lb	1072	75.2	0.0	336	0	83.2	24.0	368	71%
raw	1 oz	67	4.7	0.0	21	0	5.2	1.5	23	71%

Food Name	Serving Size	Calories	Prot. gms	Carbs gms	Sod. mgs	Fiber gms	Fat gms	Sat. Fat gms	Chol. mgs	% Fat Cal.
roasted	4 oz	287	29.4	0.0	99	0	17.9	5.0	103	58%
stewed	4 oz	264	26.6	0.0	79	0	16.6	4.6	93	58%
DARK MEAT ONLY										
fried, chopped or diced	1 cup	335	40.6	3.6	136	0	16.3	4.4	134	45%
raw	1 lb	560	96.0	0.0	384	0	19.2	4.8	368	32%
raw	1 oz	35	6.0	0.0	24	0	1.2	.3	23	32%
roasted	1 cup	287	38.3	0.0	130	0	13.6	3.7	130	44%
roasted	4 oz	232	31.0	0.0	105	0	11.0	3.0	105	44%
roasted, chopped or diced	1 cup	286	38.3	0.0	130	0	13.6	3.7	130	44%
stewed	1 cup	269	36.4	0.0	104	0	12.6	3.4	123	44%
stewed	4 oz	218	29.4	0.0	84	0	10.2	2.8	100	44%
stewed, chopped or diced	1 cup	269	36.4	0.0	104	0	12.6	3.4	123	44%
DRUMSTICK MEAT AND SKIN										
fried, batter-dipped	4 oz	304	24.9	9.4	305	>.1 c	17.9	4.7	98	54%
fried, flour-coated	4 oz	278	30.6	1.8	101	>.1 c	15.6	4.2	102	52%
raw	1 lb	736	88.0	0.0	384	0	40.0	11.2	368	51%
raw	1 oz	46	5.5	0.0	24	0	2.5	.7	23	51%
roasted	4 oz	245	30.7	0.0	102	0	12.6	3.5	103	48%
stewed	4 oz	231	28.7	0.0	86	0	12.1	3.3	94	49%
DRUMSTICK MEAT ONLY										
raw	1 lb	544	92.8	0.0	400	0	16.0	3.2	352	28%
raw	1 oz	34	5.8	0.0	25	0	1.0	.2	22	28%
roasted	4 oz	195	32.1	0.0	108	0	6.4	1.7	105	31%
stewed	4 oz	192	31.2	0.0	91	0	6.5	1.7	100	32%
LEG MEAT AND SKIN										
fried, batter-dipped	4 oz	310	24.7	9.9	316	>.1 c	18.3	4.9	102	54%
fried, flour-coated	4 oz	285	30.1	2.8	99	>.1 c	16.2	4.4	105	53%
raw	1 lb	848	81.6	0.0	352	0	54.4	16.0	384	60%
raw	1 oz	53	5.1	0.0	22	0	3.4	1.0	24	60%
stewed	4 oz	249	27.4	0.0	83	0	14.7	4.0	95	55%
LEG MEAT ONLY										
raw	1 lb	544	91.2	0.0	384	0	17.6	4.8	368	30%
raw	1 oz	34	5.7	0.0	24	0	1.1	0.3	23	30%
roasted	4 oz	217	30.7	0.0	103	0	9.6	2.6	107	41%
stewed	4 oz	210	29.8	0.0	88	0	9.1	2.5	101	41%
LIGHT MEAT AND SKIN										
fried, batter-dipped	4 oz	312	26.6	10.7	324	>.1 c	17.4	4.7	94	51%
fried, flour-coated	4 oz	279	34.5	2.1	87	>.1 c	13.7	3.8	99	46%
raw	1 lb	848	91.2	0.0	288	0	49.6	14.4	304	55%
raw	1 oz	53	5.7	0.0	18	0	3.1	0.9	19	55%
roasted	4 oz	252	32.9	0.0	85	0	12.3	3.5	95	46%
stewed	4 oz	228	29.6	0.0	71	0	11.3	3.2	84	46%
LIGHT MEAT ONLY										
fried	8 oz	269	46.0	0.6	113	0	7.8	2.1	126	27%
raw	1 lb	512	105.6	0.0	304	0	8.0	1.6	256	15%
raw	1 oz	32	6.6	0.0	19	0	0.5	0.1	16	15%
roasted	1 cup	242	43.3	0.0	108	0	6.3	1.8	119	25%
roasted	4 oz	196	35.1	0.0	87	0	5.1	1.4	90	25%
roasted, chopped or diced	1 cup	242	43.3	0.0	108	0	6.3	1.8	118	25%
stewed, chopped or diced	1 cup	223	40.4	0.0	91	0	5.6	1.6	107	24%
stewed	4 oz	180	32.7	0.0	74	0	4.5	1.3	87	24%
NECK MEAT AND SKIN										
fried, batter-dipped	4 oz	374	22.5	9.9	313	>.1 c	26.7	7.1	103	65%
fried, flour-coated	4 oz	376	27.2	4.8	93	>.1 c	26.8	7.2	107	65%

Food Name	Serving Size	Calories	Prot. gms	Carbs gms	Sod. mgs	Fiber gms	Fat gms	Sat. Fat gms	Chol. mgs	% Fat Cal.
raw	1 lb	1344	64.0	0.0	288	0	118.4	33.6	448	81%
raw	1 oz	84	4.0	0.0	18	0	7.4	2.1	28	81%
simmered	4 oz	280	22.2	0.0	59	0	20.5	5.7	79	68%
NECK MEAT ONLY										
raw	1 lb	704	80.0	0.0	368	0	40.0	9.6	384	53%
raw	1 oz	44	5.0	0.0	23	0	2.5	0.6	24	53%
simmered	4 oz	203	27.9	0.0	73	0	9.3	2.4	90	43%
SKIN ONLY										
fried, batter-dipped	1 oz	112	2.9	6.6	165	>.1 c	8.2	2.2	21	66%
roasted	1 oz	129	5.8	0.0	18	0	11.5	3.2	24	82%
stewed	1 oz	103	4.3	0.0	16	0	9.4	2.6	18	83%
THIGH MEAT AND SKIN										
fried, batter-dipped	4 oz	314	24.5	10.3	327	>.1 c	18.7	5.0	105	55%
fried, flour-coated	4 oz	297	30.3	3.6	100	>.1 c	17.0	4.6	110	53%
raw	1 lb	960	78.4	0.0	352	0	68.8	19.2	384	66%
raw	1 oz	60	4.9	0.0	22	0	4.3	1.2	24	66%
roasted	4 oz	280	28.4	0.0	95	0	17.6	4.9	105	58%
stewed	4 oz	263	26.4	0.0	81	0	16.7	4.7	95	59%
THIGH MEAT ONLY										
raw	1 lb	544	89.6	0.0	384	0	17.6	4.8	384	31%
raw	1 oz	34	5.6	0.0	24	0	1.1	0.3	24	31%
roasted	4 oz	237	29.4	0.0	100	0	12.3	3.4	108	49%
stewed	4 oz	221	28.4	0.0	85	0	11.1	3.1	102	47%
WING MEAT AND SKIN										
fried, batter-dipped	4 oz	367	22.5	12.4	363	>.1 c	24.7	6.6	90	61%
fried, flour-coated	4 oz	364	29.6	2.7	87	>.1 c	25.1	6.9	92	64%
raw	1 lb	1008	83.2	0.0	336	0	72.0	20.8	352	66%
raw	1 oz	63	5.2	0.0	21	0	4.5	1.3	22	66%
roasted	4 oz	329	30.5	0.0	93	0	22.1	6.2	95	62%
stewed	4 oz	282	25.8	0.0	76	0	19.1	5.3	79	63%
WING MEAT ONLY										
raw	1 lb	576	99.2	0.0	368	0	16.0	4.8	256	27%
raw	1 oz	36	6.2	0.0	23	0	1.0	0.3	16	27%
roasted	4 oz	230	34.5	0.0	104	0	9.2	2.6	96	38%
stewed	4 oz	205	30.8	0.0	83	0	8.1	2.3	84	37%
CHICKEN, CANNED										
Chunk										
(Featherweight)	3 oz	90	16.0	0.0	60	0	3.0	(mq)	65	30%
(Hormel) breast	6.75 oz	350	41.0	0.0	855	0	20.0	(mq)	(mq)	52%
(Hormel) breast	2.5 oz	90	15.0	0.0	310	na	3.0	1.0	30	31%
(Hormel) breast, no salt	2.5 oz	90	16.0	0.0	25	na	3.0	1.0	35	30%
(Hormel) dark	6.75 oz	327	42.0	0.0	933	0	18.0	(mq)	(mq)	49%
(Hormel) white and dark	6.75 oz	340	39.0	0.0	857	0	20.0	(mq)	(mq)	54%
(Hormel) white and dark, unsalted	6.75 oz	330	42.0	0.0	75	0	18.0	(mq)	(mq)	49%
(Swanson) 'Mixin' Chicken'	2.5 oz	130	13.0	1.0	230	0	8.0	(mq)	(mq)	56%
(Swanson) white and dark	2.5 oz	100	16.0	0.0	240	0	4.0	(mq)	40	36%
Loaf (Hormel)	2 oz	130	7.0	0.0	608	0	10.0	(mq)	(mq)	76%
White (Swanson)	2.5 oz	100	15.0	0.0	235	0	4.0	(mq)	35	38%
CHICKEN, CAPON										
GIBLETS										
raw	1 lb	592	83.2	6.4	352	0	24.0	8.0	1328	38%
raw	1 oz	37	5.2	0.4	22	0	1.5	0.5	83	38%
simmered	1 cup	238	38.3	1.1	80	0	7.8	2.6	629	31%
simmered	4 oz	186	29.9	0.9	62	0	6.1	20.0	492	31%

Food Name	Serving Size	Calories	Prot. gms	Carbs gms	Sod. mgs	Fiber gms	Fat gms	Sat. Fat gms	Chol. mgs	% Fat Cal.
MEAT AND SKIN										
raw	1 lb	1056	84.8	0.0	208	0	76.8	22.4	336	67%
raw	1 oz	66	5.3	0.0	13	0	4.8	1.4	21	67%
roasted	4 oz	260	32.8	0.0	56	0	13.2	3.7	98	48%
CHICKEN, FROZEN. See also CHICKEN DINNER /ENTRÉE, FROZEN.										
BREAST										
Boneless										
(Pilgrim's Pride)	3 oz	195	15.1	10.8	450	(mq)	10.2	(mq)	26	47%
(Tyson)	3 oz	190	13.0	15.0	400	(mq)	9.0	(mq)	25	42%
(Tyson) barbecue	3 oz	110	14.0	6.0	310	na	3.0	na	35	25%
(Tyson) chunks	3 oz	240	13.0	10.0	430	(mq)	17.0	(mq)	30	62%
(Tyson) grilled	2.75 oz	100	15.0	4.0	410	na	3.0	na	45	26%
(Tyson) hot and spicy	2.75 oz	110	14.0	7.0	490	na	3.0	na	35	24%
(Tyson) skinless, Wholesale Club Item	3.5 oz	110	23.0	1.0	380	na	2.0	na	55	16%
Halves, Wholesale Club Item (Tyson)	3.5 oz	230	27.0	0.0	50	na	13.0	na	90	52%
Pieces										
(Banquet) fried	5.75 oz	220	16.0	13.0	710	(mq)	11.0	(mq)	(mq)	46%
(Tyson) mesquite, Wholesale Club Item	3.5 oz	170	27.0	1.0	540	na	7.0	na	70	36%
Portions (Swanson) fried, 'Plump & Juicy'	4.5 oz	360	23.0	21.0	800	(mq)	20.0	(mq)	(mq)	51%
Strips (Weaver)	3.3 oz	200	13.0	14.0	500	na	10.0	na	na	46%
Tenders										
(Banquet) Southern fried	2.25 oz	160	10.0	13.0	340	(mq)	7.0	(mq)	(mq)	41%
(Pilgrim's Pride)	3 oz	181	12.7	11.1	430	(mq)	9.5	(mq)	26	47%
(Tyson) blanched, Wholesale Club Item	3.5 oz	200	18.0	12.0	340	na	8.0	na	30	38%
(Tyson) breaded, Wholesale Club Item	3.5 oz	200	18.0	12.0	340	na	8.0	na	30	38%
(Tyson) Southern fried	3 oz	220	14.0	15.0	630	(mq)	11.0	(mq)	25	46%
(Tyson) unbreaded, Wholesale Club Item	3.5 oz	120	28.0	0.0	55	na	1.0	na	50	7%
Whole										
(Tyson) Wholesale Club Item	3.5 oz	210	26.0	0.0	50	na	12.0	na	80	51%
(Weaver)	4.5 oz	270	20.0	18.0	520	na	13.0	na	na	44%
(Weaver) batter-dipped	4.4 oz	310	20.0	13.0	220	na	20.0	na	na	58%
CHUNKS										
(Country Pride)	3 oz	240	10.0	15.0	560	(mq)	15.0	(mq)	(mq)	57%
(Country Pride) Southern fried	3 oz	280	10.0	14.0	690	(mq)	20.0	(mq)	(mq)	65%
(Tyson) diced	3 oz	150	26.0	0.0	50	0	5.0	(mq)	70	30%
(Tyson) mesquite flavor 'Hors D'Oeuvres'	3.5 oz	100	22.0	1.0	600	na	1.0	na	45	9%
(Tyson) microwave, boneless	3.5 oz	220	10.0	11.0	na	na	15.0	na	na	62%
LEG MEAT										
(Banquet) thighs and drumsticks, fried	6.25 oz	250	14.0	14.0	790	(mq)	14.0	(mq)	(mq)	53%
(Pilgrim's Pride) drumsters	3 oz	200	11.5	10.5	320	(mq)	12.5	(mq)	38	56%
(Tyson) drums and thighs, Wholesale Club Item	3.5 oz	270	28.0	0.0	110	na	17.0	na	130	58%
(Tyson) 'Julienne Leg Meat' Wholesale Club Item	3.5 oz	160	25.0	0.0	60	na	6.0	na	105	35%
(Tyson) thighs, skinless, Wholesale Club Item	3.5 oz	200	26.0	0.0	70	na	10.0	na	105	46%
(Weaver) batter-dipped	3 oz	210	11.0	11.0	220	na	14.0	na	na	59%
(Weaver) drums and thighs, 'Crispy Dutch Frye'	3.5 oz	290	16.0	14.0	640	na	19.0	na	na	59%
NUGGETS										
(Country Pride)	3 oz	250	11.0	14.0	460	(mq)	16.0	(mq)	(mq)	59%
(Pilgrim's Pride)	3 oz	202	12.4	10.4	370	(mq)	12.3	(mq)	31	55%
(Weaver)	2.6 oz	190	10.0	10.0	450	na	12.0	na	na	57%
(Weight Watchers)	5.9 oz	220	16.0	23.0	500	na	7.0	2.0	40	29%
PORTIONS										
(Pilgrim's Pride) fried	3 oz	255	12.0	11.9	480	(mq)	17.7	(mq)	38	63%
(Swanson) 'Homestyle Recipe'	7 oz	390	18.0	33.0	1100	(mq)	21.0	(mq)	(mq)	48%
(Swanson) 'Take-Out Pre-Fried'	3.25 oz	270	15.0	16.0	650	(mq)	16.0	(mq)	(mq)	54%

Food Name	Serving Size	Calories	Prot. gms	Carbs gms	Sod. mgs	Fiber gms	Fat gms	Sat. Fat gms	Chol. mgs	% Fat Cal.
ROASTER (Tyson) Wholesale Club Item	3.5 oz	230	27.0	0.0	80	na	13.0	na	105	52%
WINGS										
(Pilgrim's Pride) Southern fried	3 oz	228	13.3	5.1	480	(mq)	17.2	(mq)	51	68%
(Pilgrim's Pride) 'Wing Zappers'	3 oz	187	16.1	1.8	340	na	12.8	(mq)	90	62%
(Tyson) all varieties, 'Flyers'	3.5 oz	220	23.0	0.0	400	0	14.0	(mq)	(mq)	58%
(Tyson) drummettes, Wholesale Club Item	3.5 oz	260	25.0	2.0	80	na	17.0	na	135	59%
(Tyson) barbecue 'Hors D'Oeuvres' Wholesale Club Item	3.5 oz	210	24.0	3.0	430	na	12.0	na	130	50%
(Tyson) raw, hot, Wholesale Club Item	3.5 oz	280	26.0	1.0	80	na	19.0	na	135	61%
(Tyson) roaster 'Hors D'Oeuvres' Wholesale Club Item	3.5 oz	210	25.0	0.0	280	na	12.0	na	135	52%
(Weaver) batter-dipped	4 oz	400	16.0	20.0	520	na	28.0	na	na	64%
(Weaver) 'Crispy Dutch Frye'	4 oz	400	16.0	20.0	520	na	28.0	na	na	64%
(Weaver) hot	2.7 oz	170	17.0	1.0	670	na	11.0	na	na	58%
CHICKEN, ROASTER										
DARK MEAT ONLY										
raw	1 lb	512	84.8	0.0	432	0	16.0	4.8	320	30%
raw	1 oz	32	5.3	0.0	27	0	1.0	0.3	20	30%
roasted	4 oz	202	26.4	0.0	108	0	9.9	2.8	85	46%
GIBLETS, simmered	1 cup	239	38.8	1.3	87	0	7.6	2.4	518	30%
LIGHT MEAT ONLY										
raw	1 lb	496	100.8	0.0	224	0	8.0	1.6	256	15%
raw	1 oz	31	6.3	0.0	14	0	0.5	0.1	16	15%
roasted	1 cup	214	38.0	0.0	71	0	5.7	1.5	105	25%
roasted	4 oz	174	30.8	0.0	58	0	4.6	1.2	85	25%
MEAT AND SKIN										
raw	1 lb	976	78.4	0.0	304	0	72.0	20.8	336	67%
raw	1 oz	61	4.9	0.0	19	0	4.5	1.3	21	67%
roasted	4 oz	253	27.2	0.0	83	0	15.2	4.2	86	56%
CHICKEN, STEWING										
DARK MEAT ONLY										
raw	1 lb	720	89.6	0.0	464	0	36.8	9.6	352	48%
raw	1 oz	45	5.6	0.0	29	0	2.3	0.6	22	48%
stewed	1 cup	361	39.4	0.0	133	0	21.4	5.7	133	55%
stewed	4 oz	293	31.9	0.0	108	0	17.3	4.6	108	55%
GIBLETS										
raw	1 lb	560	81.6	8.0	352	0	20.8	6.4	1184	34%
raw	1 oz	35	5.1	0.5	22	0	1.3	0.4	74	34%
simmered	1 cup	281	37.3	0.2	81	0	13.5	3.9	515	45%
LIGHT MEAT ONLY										
raw	1 lb	624	104.0	0.0	240	0	19.2	4.8	208	29%
raw	1 oz	39	6.5	0.0	15	0	1.2	0.3	13	29%
stewed	1 cup	298	46.3	0.0	81	0	11.2	2.8	98	35%
stewed	4 oz	242	37.5	0.0	66	0	9.0	2.2	79	35%
MEAT AND SKIN										
raw	1 lb	1168	80.0	0.0	320	0	92.8	25.6	320	72%
raw	1 oz	73	5.0	0.0	20	0	5.8	1.6	20	72%
stewed	4 oz	323	30.5	0.0	83	0	21.4	5.8	90	61%
CHICKEN DINNER/ENTRÉE, CANNED										
(Featherweight) and dumplings	7.5 oz	160	12.0	18.0	115	(mq)	5.0	(mq)	(mq)	27%
(LaChoy)										
chow mein	3/4 cup	240	8.0	47.0	1420	1.0	2.0	0.5	19	8%
chow mein 'Bi-Pack'	8.642 oz	97	7.7	9.5	1199	3.2	3.8	1.1	17	33%
chow mein 'Bi-Pack'	3/4 cup	80	7.0	8.0	980	1.0	3.0	(mq)	18	31%
Oriental 'Bi-Pack'	3/4 cup	240	9.0	47.0	1400	1.0	2.0	(mq)	(mq)	7%
Oriental w/noodles 'Bi-Pack'	9 oz	160	10.6	23.0	1163	3.9	3.8	1.0	13	20%

Food Name	Serving Size	Calories	Prot. gms	Carbs gms	Sod. mgs	Fiber gms	Fat gms	Sat. Fat gms	Chol. mgs	% Fat Cal.
sweet and sour	3/4 cup	240	8.0	47.0	1420	1.0	2.0	0.5	19	8%
sweet and sour 'Bi-Pack'	8.959 oz	161	7.6	28.6	745	3.3	2.5	0.6	18	13%
sweet and sour 'Bi-Pack'	3/4 cup	120	7.0	18.0	440	2.0	2.0	0.5	13	15%
teriyaki 'Bi-Pack'	8.642 oz	110	7.4	14.9	1226	2.9	3.0	0.9	15	23%
teriyaki 'Bi-Pack'	3/4 cup	85	8.0	8.0	850	1.0	2.0	0.5	20	22%
(Luck's) and dumplings	7.25 oz	240	16.0	18.0	605	(mq)	11.0	(mq)	(mq)	42%
(Swanson)										
à la king	5 1/4 oz	190	10.0	9.0	690	(mq)	12.0	(mq)	(mq)	59%
and dumplings	7.5 oz	220	11.0	19.0	980	(mq)	11.0	(mq)	(mq)	45%

CHICKEN DINNER / ENTRÉE, FROZEN

(Armour)

Food Name	Serving Size	Calories	Prot. gms	Carbs gms	Sod. mgs	Fiber gms	Fat gms	Sat. Fat gms	Chol. mgs	% Fat Cal.
À la king 'Classics Lite'	11.25 oz	290	19.0	38.0	630	(mq)	7.0	(mq)	55	22%
and noodles 'Classics'	11 oz	230	19.0	23.0	660	(mq)	7.0	(mq)	50	27%
breast, Marsala 'Classics Lite'	10.5 oz	250	20.0	27.0	930	(mq)	7.0	(mq)	80	25%
Burgundy 'Classics Lite'	10 oz	210	23.0	25.0	780	(mq)	2.0	(mq)	45	9%
fettuccini 'Classics'	11 oz	260	17.0	28.0	660	(mq)	9.0	(mq)	50	31%
glazed 'Classics'	10.75 oz	300	15.0	24.0	960	(mq)	16.0	(mq)	60	48%
mesquite 'Classics'	9.5 oz	370	15.0	42.0	660	(mq)	16.0	(mq)	55	39%
Oriental 'Classics Lite'	10 oz	180	18.0	24.0	660	(mq)	1.0	(mq)	35	5%
parmigiana 'Classics'	11.5 oz	370	22.0	27.0	1060	(mq)	19.0	(mq)	75	47%
sweet and sour 'Classics Lite'	11 oz	240	18.0	39.0	820	(mq)	2.0	(mq)	35	7%
w/wine and mushroom sauce 'Classics'	10.75 oz	280	22.0	24.0	900	(mq)	11.0	(mq)	50	35%

(Banquet)

Food Name	Serving Size	Calories	Prot. gms	Carbs gms	Sod. mgs	Fiber gms	Fat gms	Sat. Fat gms	Chol. mgs	% Fat Cal.
à la king 'Cookin' Bags'	4 oz	110	8.0	9.0	na	na	5.0	(mq)	(mq)	40%
and dumplings	10 oz	430	17.0	34.0	940	(mq)	24.0	(mq)	45	51%
and dumplings 'Family Entrées'	7 oz	280	12.0	28.0	(mq)	(mq)	14.0	(mq)	(mq)	44%
drumsnackers 'Platters'	7 oz	430	20.0	49.0	690	(mq)	19.0	(mq)	(mq)	38%
fettuccini 'Healthy Balance'	11.25 oz	320	17.0	47.0	650	na	7.0	3.0	35	20%
fried	10 oz	400	15.0	45.0	1100	(mq)	22.0	(mq)	(mq)	45%
fried 'Extra Helping'	16 oz	570	20.0	70.0	1470	(mq)	28.0	(mq)	(mq)	41%
fried, white meat 'Extra Helping'	16 oz	570	20.0	70.0	1470	(mq)	28.0	(mq)	(mq)	41%
fried, white meat 'Platter'	9 oz	430	38.0	21.0	(mq)	(mq)	22.0	(mq)	105	46%
fried, white meat, hot'n spicy 'Platter'	9 oz	430	38.0	21.0	(mq)	(mq)	22.0	(mq)	105	46%
hot'n spicy 'Snack'n'	3.75 oz	140	6.0	8.0	480	(mq)	9.0	(mq)	(mq)	59%
nuggets, breast, Southern fried w/barbecue sauce	4.5 oz	370	19.0	20.0	930	(mq)	23.0	(mq)	(mq)	57%
nuggets, hot'n spicy, w/barbecue sauce	4.5 oz	360	20.0	23.0	820	(mq)	21.0	(mq)	(mq)	52%
nuggets, 'Platters'	6.4 oz	430	17.0	46.0	630	(mq)	21.0	(mq)	(mq)	43%
nuggets, Southern fried, w/barbecue sauce	4.5 oz	370	19.0	20.0	930	(mq)	23.0	(mq)	(mq)	57%
nuggets, w/barbecue sauce 'Extra Helping'	10 oz	640	29.0	56.0	1390	(mq)	36.0	(mq)	(mq)	49%
nuggets, w/sweet and sour sauce 'Extra Helping'	10 oz	650	28.1	64.0	(mq)	(mq)	34.0	(mq)	(mq)	45%
nuggets, w/sweet and sour sauce 'Microwave'	4.5 oz	360	20.0	22.0	770	(mq)	21.0	(mq)	(mq)	53%
parmesan, w/vermicelli 'Healthy Balance'	10.8 oz	290	19.0	30.0	710	na	10.0	3.0	55	32%
patties, breast, Southern fried, w/biscuit	4 oz	320	12.0	37.0	980	(mq)	14.0	(mq)	(mq)	39%
patties 'Platters'	7.5 oz	380	15.0	34.0	760	(mq)	21.0	(mq)	(mq)	49%
pie	7 oz	550	15.0	39.0	860	(mq)	36.0	(mq)	35	60%
pie 'Supreme Microwave'	7 oz	430	15.0	30.0	740	(mq)	28.0	(mq)	40	58%
primavera and vegetable 'Cookin' Bags'	4 oz	100	6.0	14.0	(mq)	(mq)	2.0	(mq)	(mq)	18%
primavera and vegetable 'Family Entrées'	7 oz	140	9.0	18.0	(mq)	(mq)	3.0	(mq)	(mq)	20%
sweet and sour 'Cookin' Bags'	4 oz	130	5.0	22.0	na	na	2.0	(mq)	(mq)	14%

(Budget Gourmet)

Food Name	Serving Size	Calories	Prot. gms	Carbs gms	Sod. mgs	Fiber gms	Fat gms	Sat. Fat gms	Chol. mgs	% Fat Cal.
and egg noodles, w/broccoli	10 oz	450	23.0	31.0	1110	(mq)	26.0	(mq)	130	52%
cacciatore	11 oz	300	20.0	27.0	810	(mq)	13.0	(mq)	60	38%
Marsala	10 oz	250	15.0	37.0	660	(mq)	5.0	(mq)	65	18%
Mexicana	12.8 oz	510	23.0	70.0	1210	(mq)	15.0	(mq)	40	27%

Food Name	Serving Size	Calories	Prot. gms	Carbs gms	Sod. mgs	Fiber gms	Fat gms	Sat. Fat gms	Chol. mgs	% Fat Cal.
Oriental, and vegetables 'Light and Healthy'	9 oz	280	19.0	44.0	690	na	6.0	1.0	20	18%
roast	11.2 oz	280	19.0	34.0	1110	(mq)	7.0	(mq)	40	23%
sweet and sour, w/rice	10 oz	350	18.0	53.0	640	(mq)	7.0	(mq)	40	18%
teriyaki	12 oz	360	20.0	44.0	610	(mq)	12.0	(mq)	55	30%
w/fettuccini	10 oz	400	23.0	29.0	740	(mq)	21.0	(mq)	100	48%
(Celentano)										
parmigiana	9 oz	330	32.0	15.0	560	(mq)	20.0	(mq)	(mq)	49%
primavera	11.5 oz	270	25.0	18.0	580	(mq)	10.0	(mq)	(mq)	34%
(Chun King)										
chow mein	13 oz	370	25.0	53.0	1560	(mq)	6.0	(mq)	(mq)	15%
Imperial	13 oz	300	17.0	54.0	1540	(mq)	1.0	(mq)	(mq)	3%
walnut, crunchy	13 oz	310	16.0	49.0	1700	(mq)	5.0	(mq)	(mq)	15%
(Country Pride) primavera sticks	3 oz	240	10.0	16.0	400	(mq)	15.0	(mq)	(mq)	57%
(Dining Lite)										
à la king	9 oz	240	14.0	30.0	780	(mq)	7.0	(mq)	40	26%
and noodles	9 oz	240	17.0	28.0	570	(mq)	7.0	(mq)	50	26%
chow mein	9 oz	180	10.0	31.0	650	(mq)	2.0	(mq)	30	10%
glazed	9 oz	220	17.0	30.0	680	(mq)	4.0	(mq)	45	16%
(Freezer Queen)										
à la king 'Cook-In-Pouch'	4 oz	70	9.0	6.0	460	na	1.0	(mq)	(mq)	13%
à la king, w/rice 'Single Serve'	9 oz	270	20.0	37.0	520	(mq)	5.0	(mq)	(mq)	17%
cacciatore 'Single Serve'	9 oz	270	20.0	33.0	710	(mq)	6.0	(mq)	(mq)	20%
croquettes, breaded, w/gravy 'Family Suppers'	7 oz	240	12.0	20.0	1000	(mq)	12.0	(mq)	(mq)	46%
nuggets 'Deluxe Family Suppers'	3 oz	270	14.0	15.0	770	(mq)	17.0	(mq)	(mq)	57%
nuggets platter	6 oz	410	14.0	36.0	950	(mq)	23.0	(mq)	(mq)	51%
pattie 'Platter'	7.5 oz	360	17.0	33.0	1160	(mq)	17.0	(mq)	(mq)	43%
primavera, sliced, w/gravy 'Cook-In-Pouch'	5 oz	80	7.0	6.0	820	na	3.0	(mq)	(mq)	34%
sweet and sour, w/rice 'Single Serve'	9 oz	300	20.0	48.0	700	(mq)	4.0	(mq)	(mq)	12%
(Green Giant) and broccoli 'Entrées'	9.5 oz	340	23.0	28.0	890	(mq)	15.0	(mq)	(mq)	40%
(Healthy Choice)										
à l'orange	9 oz	260	23.0	38.0	340	na	2.0	<1.0	40	7%
and pasta divan	11.5 oz	300	25.0	41.0	520	na	4.0	2.0	50	12%
and vegetables	11.5 oz	210	20.0	31.0	490	na	1.0	<1.0	35	4%
breast, glazed	8.5 oz	220	21.0	27.0	510	na	3.0	1.0	45	12%
cacciatore 'Classics'	12.5 oz	310	26.0	47.0	430	na	3.0	<1.0	35	9%
chow mein	9 oz	240	20.0	29.0	530	na	5.0	2.0	45	19%
chow mein, low fat, low cholesterol	9 oz	240	20.0	29.0	530	na	5.0	2.0	45	19%
Dijon	11 oz	260	22.0	38.0	420	na	3.0	1.0	45	10%
herb roasted	11 oz	380	26.0	56.0	470	na	7.0	3.0	60	16%
honey mustard, low fat, low cholesterol	9.5 oz	250	24.0	37.0	480	na	3.0	1.0	40	10%
Mandarin	10 oz	240	21.0	35.0	370	na	2.0	<1.0	45	7%
mesquite	10.5 oz	300	21.0	54.0	390	na	3.0	1.0	40	8%
Oriental	11.25 oz	200	19.0	32.0	440	na	1.0	<1.0	35	4%
parmigiana	11.5 oz	290	23.0	41.0	340	na	6.0	3.0	55	17%
roasted	12.3 oz	290	25.0	39.0	430	na	4.0	2.0	50	12%
'Salsa Chicken Dinner'	11.25 oz	240	20.0	36.0	450	na	2.0	1.0	50	7%
southwestern style, low fat, low cholesterol	12.5 oz	340	25.0	51.0	550	na	5.0	2.0	60	13%
stir fry, w/vermicelli 'Extra Portion'	12 oz	300	23.0	42.0	550	na	5.0	1.0	30	15%
sweet and sour	11.5 oz	280	20.0	52.0	320	na	2.0	<1.0	35	6%
teriyaki, low fat, low cholesterol	12.25 oz	290	24.0	39.0	560	na	4.0	1.0	55	13%
w/barbecue sauce, low fat, low cholesterol	12.75 oz	410	24.0	65.0	550	na	6.0	2.0	55	13%
(Hot Bites)										
drumsnackers	2.63 oz	220	10.0	13.0	530	(mq)	15.0	(mq)	(mq)	60%
nuggets	2.63 oz	210	11.0	11.0	550	(mq)	14.0	(mq)	(mq)	59%

Food Name	Serving Size	Calories	Prot. gms	Carbs gms	Sod. mgs	Fiber gms	Fat gms	Sat. Fat gms	Chol. mgs	% Fat Cal.
nuggets, hot'n spicy	2.63 oz	250	10.0	10.0	380	(mq)	19.0	(mq)	(mq)	68%
nuggets, Southern fried	2.63 oz	220	10.0	13.0	530	(mq)	14.0	(mq)	(mq)	58%
nuggets, w/cheddar	2.63 oz	250	11.0	11.0	560	(mq)	18.0	(mq)	(mq)	65%
primavera sticks	2.63 oz	220	10.0	11.0	350	(mq)	15.0	(mq)	(mq)	62%
tenders, breast	2.25 oz	150	11.0	12.0	280	(mq)	6.0	(mq)	(mq)	37%
tenders, breast 'Microwave'	4 oz	260	19.0	24.0	560	(mq)	10.0	(mq)	(mq)	34%
(Kid Cuisine)										
fried	7.25 oz	420	15.0	41.0	1050	(mq)	22.0	(mq)	(mq)	47%
fried 'Mega Meal'	10.8 oz	720	34.0	53.0	1400	na	41.0	na	na	52%
nuggets	6.25 oz	400	11.0	46.0	610	(mq)	19.0	(mq)	60	43%
nuggets 'Mega Meal'	8.4 oz	470	21.0	51.0	1010	na	20.0	na	na	39%
(LaChoy)										
almond, w/rice and vegetables 'Fresh & Lite'	9.75 oz	270	14.0	40.1	1092	3.0	8.0	(mq)	42	25%
Imperial, w/rice 'Fresh & Lite'	11 oz	260	13.0	45.0	1269	3.1	6.0	(mq)	46	19%
Oriental, spicy 'Fresh & Lite'	9.75 oz	270	11.0	52.0	560	4.0	4.0	(mq)	42	13%
sweet and sour, w/rice and vegetables 'Fresh & Lite'	10 oz	260	13.0	50.1	601	3.7	3.0	(mq)	53	10%
(LeMenu)										
à la king	10.25 oz	330	23.0	29.0	830	(mq)	13.0	(mq)	(mq)	36%
à la king, w/seasoned rice 'LightStyle'	8.25 oz	240	19.0	29.0	670	(mq)	5.0	1.0	30	19%
breast, glazed 'LightStyle'	10 oz	230	25.0	25.0	430	(mq)	3.0	(mq)	55	12%
breast, herb roasted, w/rice and vegetables	7.75 oz	260	22.0	29.0	500	(mq)	6.0	2.0	45	21%
Cordon Bleu	11 oz	460	23.0	47.0	850	(mq)	20.0	(mq)	(mq)	39%
Dijon, w/pasta and vegetables 'LightStyle'	8.5 oz	240	22.0	21.0	500	(mq)	7.0	2.0	40	27%
empress, w/seasoned rice 'LightStyle'	8.25 oz	210	16.0	26.0	690	(mq)	5.0	1.0	30	21%
herb-roasted 'LightStyle'	10 oz	240	27.0	18.0	400	(mq)	7.0	(mq)	70	26%
in wine sauce	10 oz	280	26.0	27.0	680	(mq)	7.0	(mq)	(mq)	23%
Kiev	8 oz	530	20.0	24.0	780	(mq)	39.0	(mq)	(mq)	67%
parmigiana	11.75 oz	410	26.0	31.0	1030	(mq)	20.0	(mq)	(mq)	44%
sweet and sour	11.25 oz	400	19.0	41.0	1020	(mq)	18.0	(mq)	(mq)	40%
sweet and sour 'LightStyle'	10 oz	250	18.0	29.0	530	(mq)	7.0	(mq)	2	25%
(Mrs. Paterson's) 'Aussie Pie'	5.5 oz	440	13.0	43.0	760	na	24.0	8.0	80	49%
(Myers)										
à la gratin	3.5 oz	129	9.0	9.0	276	(mq)	7.0	(mq)	(mq)	47%
à la king	3.5 oz	137	9.0	6.0	357	na	9.0	(mq)	(mq)	57%
and noodles	3.5 oz	136	8.0	9.0	399	(mq)	8.0	(mq)	(mq)	51%
creamed	3.5 oz	151	12.0	5.0	372	na	10.0	(mq)	(mq)	57%
croquettes	3.5 oz	168	16.0	10.0	364	na	7.0	(mq)	(mq)	38%
pie	3.5 oz	129	7.0	10.0	253	(mq)	7.0	(mq)	(mq)	48%
(Pilgrim's Pride) Cajun style	3 oz	241	13.3	8.6	480	(mq)	17.0	(mq)	51	64%
(Pillsbury)										
and cheese casserole 'Microwave Classic'	1 pkg	480	21.0	33.0	940	(mq)	29.0	(mq)	(mq)	55%
casserole 'Microwave Classic'	1 pkg	400	21.0	30.0	890	(mq)	22.0	(mq)	(mq)	49%
(Right Course)										
Italiano, w/fettuccini and vegetables	9 5/8 oz	280	24.0	29.0	560	(mq)	8.0	2.0	45	25%
sesame primavera	10 oz	320	25.0	34.0	590	(mq)	9.0	2.0	50	26%
tenderloins in barbecue sauce	8.75 oz	270	20.0	35.0	590	(mq)	6.0	1.0	40	20%
tenderloins in peanut sauce	9.25 oz	330	27.0	32.0	570	(mq)	10.0	2.0	50	28%
(Shanghai) stir fry	10.3 oz	190	22.0	19.0	1220	na	3.0	na	30	14%
(Smart Ones)										
a l'orange	8 oz	190	12.0	34.0	530	na	<1.0	<1.0	15	<5%
chow mein	9 oz	170	14.0	27.0	470	na	1.0	<1.0	20	5%
fiesta, w/Spanish rice	8 oz	210	14.0	37.0	390	na	1.0	<1.0	20	4%
Francais, w/garlic vegetables	8.5 oz	150	15.0	18.0	400	na	1.0	<1.0	5	6%
grilled, glazed, and sauce	8 oz	130	12.0	17.0	540	na	1.0	<1.0	20	7%

Food Name	Serving Size	Calories	Prot. gms	Carbs gms	Sod. mgs	Fiber gms	Fat gms	Sat. Fat gms	Chol. mgs	% Fat Cal.
honey mustard, and sauce	7.5 oz	140	11.0	20.0	220	na	1.0	<1.0	10	7%
Mirabella	9.2 oz	160	13.0	26.0	420	na	1.0	<1.0	10	6%
piccata, lemon herb	7.5 oz	160	13.0	25.0	500	na	1.0	<1.0	5	6%
(Stouffer's)										
à la king, w/rice	9.5 oz	270	18.0	38.0	800	na	5.0	na	na	17%
a l'orange, w/almond rice, 'Lean Cuisine'	8 oz	280	27.0	33.0	290	na	4.0	1.0	55	13%
and noodles, homestyle	10 oz	290	22.0	21.0	1040	na	13.0	na	na	41%
and vegetables, w/vermicelli 'Lean Cuisine'	11.75 oz	240	18.0	30.0	500	na	5.0	1.0	30	19%
breaded, baked, w/parslied potatoes and vegetables, 'Lean Cuisine'	8 oz	200	17.0	21.0	480	na	5.0	2.0	35	23%
breast, baked, in gravy, w/potato, homestyle	8 7/8 oz	250	22.0	18.0	550	na	10.0	na	na	36%
breast, fried, and whipped potatoes, homestyle	7 1/8 oz	350	17.0	30.0	900	na	18.0	na	na	46%
breast, grilled, in barbecue sauce, homestyle	7 5/8 oz	210	23.0	14.0	550	na	7.0	na	na	30%
breast, Marsala, w/vegetables, 'Lean Cuisine'	8 1/8 oz	180	22.0	13.0	430	na	4.0	1.0	55	21%
breast, Parmesan, w/rib meat, 'Lean Cuisine'	10 7/8 oz	260	24.0	25.0	580	na	7.0	2.0	60	24%
cacciatore, w/vermicelli, 'Lean Cuisine'	10 7/8 oz	280	22.0	31.0	570	na	7.0	2.0	45	23%
chow mein, w/rice	10.75 oz	250	13.0	39.0	720	na	5.0	na	na	18%
chow mein, w/rice, 'Lean Cuisine'	9 oz	240	14.0	34.0	530	na	5.0	1.0	30	19%
creamed	6.5 oz	300	19.0	8.0	690	na	21.0	(mq)	(mq)	64%
Divan	8 oz	220	24.0	11.0	610	na	10.0	na	na	39%
escalloped, and noodles	10 oz	420	21.0	30.0	840	na	24.0	na	na	51%
fettuccini, 'Lean Cuisine'	9 oz	280	23.0	33.0	500	na	6.0	3.0	35	19%
fettuccini, w/vegetable medley, homestyle	9.5 oz	350	23.0	27.0	780	na	17.0	na	na	43%
fiesta, 'Lean Cuisine'	8.5 oz	240	19.0	30.0	560	na	5.0	2.0	40	19%
glazed, w/vegetable rice, 'Lean Cuisine'	8.5 oz	250	21.0	24.0	590	na	7.0	2.0	50	26%
honey mustard, 'Lean Cuisine'	7.5 oz	230	18.0	30.0	540	na	4.0	1.0	40	16%
in barbecue sauce, w/rice pilaf, 'Lean Cuisine'	8.75 oz	260	20.0	32.0	500	na	6.0	1.0	50	21%
Italiano, w/fettuccini 'Lean Cuisine'	9 oz	270	22.0	33.0	590	na	6.0	1.0	40	20%
Oriental, w/vermicelli, 'Lean Cuisine'	9 oz	280	22.0	31.0	480	na	7.0	2.0	35	23%
parmigiana and pasta Alfredo, homestyle	9 7/8 oz	360	31.0	24.0	990	na	15.0	na	na	38%
pie	10 oz	440	16.0	32.0	750	na	27.0	na	na	56%
sweet-n-sour, w/rice, 'Lean Cuisine'	9 oz	280	17.0	39.0	490	na	6.0	1.0	50	19%
tenderloins in herb sauce, 'Lean Cuisine'	9.5 oz	240	29.0	19.0	490	na	5.0	2.0	60	19%
tenderloins in peanut sauce, 'Lean Cuisine'	9 oz	290	23.0	33.0	530	na	7.0	2.0	45	22%
tenders, breaded, w/potatoes, homestyle	8 3/8 oz	430	20.0	46.0	950	na	18.0	na	na	38%
(Swanson)										
boneless 'Hungry Man'	17.75 oz	700	48.0	65.0	1530	(mq)	28.0	(mq)	(mq)	36%
cacciatore 'Homestyle Recipe'	10.95 oz	260	15.0	33.0	1030	(mq)	8.0	(mq)	(mq)	27%
fried, barbecue flavored	10 oz	540	25.0	61.0	1160	(mq)	22.0	(mq)	(mq)	37%
fried, dark meat	9.75 oz	560	22.0	55.0	1130	(mq)	28.0	(mq)	(mq)	45%
fried, dark meat 'Hungry Man'	1 pkg	860	36.0	77.0	1660	(mq)	45.0	(mq)	(mq)	47%
fried, white meat	10.25 oz	550	22.0	60.0	1460	(mq)	25.0	(mq)	(mq)	41%
fried, white meat 'Hungry Man'	1 pkg	870	35.0	80.0	2150	(mq)	46.0	(mq)	(mq)	47%
grilled, white meat in garlic sauce, almonds	10 oz	310	17.0	39.0	630	na	9.0	na	30	27%
nibbles 'Homestyle Recipe'	4.25 oz	340	10.0	29.0	730	(mq)	20.0	(mq)	(mq)	54%
nibbles 'Plump & Juicy'	3.25 oz	300	12.0	19.0	690	(mq)	19.0	(mq)	(mq)	58%
nuggets	8.75 oz	470	19.0	47.0	650	(mq)	23.0	(mq)	(mq)	44%
nuggets 'Plump & Juicy'	3 oz	230	13.0	14.0	360	(mq)	14.0	(mq)	(mq)	54%
parmigiana 'Budget'	10 oz	300	7.0	35.0	780	na	15.0	na	na	45%
pie 'Homestyle Recipe'	8 oz	410	15.0	41.0	1030	(mq)	21.0	(mq)	(mq)	46%
pie 'Hungry Man'	16 oz	630	22.0	57.0	1600	(mq)	35.0	(mq)	(mq)	50%
thighs/drumsticks 'Plump & Juicy'	3.25 oz	290	15.0	17.0	610	(mq)	18.0	(mq)	(mq)	56%
(Swift)										
Cordon Bleu 'International'	6 oz	360	30.0	23.0	1010	(mq)	17.0	(mq)	(mq)	42%

Food Name	Serving Size	Calories	Prot. gms	Carbs gms	Sod. mgs	Fiber gms	Fat gms	Sat. Fat gms	Chol. mgs	% Fat Cal.
Kiev 'International'	6 oz	420	27.0	22.0	1030	(mq)	24.0	(mq)	(mq)	52%
(Tyson)										
a l'orange 'Gourmet Selection'	9.5 oz	300	21.0	36.0	670	(mq)	8.0	(mq)	(mq)	24%
and beef luau 'Gourmet Selection'	10.5 oz	330	18.0	42.0	1030	(mq)	10.0	(mq)	(mq)	27%
'Barbecue Chicken Meal'	12.5 oz	400	27.0	56.0	600	na	8.0	na	50	18%
breast, boneless, barbecue marinated	3.75 oz	120	22.0	5.0	400	na	3.0	(mq)	(mq)	20%
breast, boneless, butter garlic marinated	3.75 oz	160	21.0	3.0	320	na	7.0	(mq)	(mq)	40%
breast, boneless, Italian marinated	3.75 oz	130	22.0	6.0	320	na	2.0	(mq)	(mq)	14%
breast, boneless, lemon pepper marinated	3.75 oz	120	22.0	4.0	210	na	2.0	(mq)	(mq)	15%
breast, boneless, teriyaki marinated	3.75 oz	130	22.0	6.0	290	na	2.0	(mq)	(mq)	14%
breast strips, Oriental, boneless	2.75 oz	110	14.0	6.0	250	na	3.0	na	40	25%
'Chick'n Cheddar' *(Tyson)*	2.6 oz	220	11.0	11.0	310	(mq)	15.0	(mq)	40	61%
'Chick'n Chunks'	2.6 oz	220	10.0	11.0	500	(mq)	15.0	(mq)	35	62%
'Chick'n Chunks' Southern fried	2.6 oz	220	10.0	11.0	540	(mq)	15.0	(mq)	35	62%
'Chicken Marinara Meal'	13.75 oz	340	31.0	37.0	590	na	7.0	na	45	19%
'Classic Colonial' Wholesale Club Item	3.5 oz	180	13.0	11.0	190	na	9.0	na	40	46%
'Cordon Bleu' Wholesale Club Item	7 oz	480	40.0	28.0	1030	na	22.0	na	na	42%
'Cordon Bleu' Wholesale Club Item	5 oz	340	28.0	20.0	740	na	16.0	na	na	43%
Dijon 'Gourmet Selection'	8.5 oz	310	17.0	22.0	840	(mq)	17.0	(mq)	(mq)	50%
Français 'Gourmet Selection'	9.5 oz	280	19.0	20.0	1130	(mq)	14.0	(mq)	(mq)	45%
glazed, w/sauce 'Gourmet Selections'	9.25 oz	240	22.0	29.0	930	na	4.0	na	44	15%
grilled, 'Gourmet Selections'	7.75 oz	220	26.0	22.0	520	na	3.0	na	55	12%
grilled, Italian 'Gourmet Selections'	9 oz	210	28.0	19.0	420	na	3.0	na	40	13%
'Herb Chicken Meal'	13.75 oz	340	32.0	43.0	550	na	4.0	na	50	11%
'Honey Mustard Chicken Meal'	13.75 oz	390	31.0	52.0	520	na	6.0	na	50	14%
honey roasted 'Gourmet Selections'	9 oz	220	26.0	23.0	500	na	4.0	na	48	16%
'Italian Style Chicken Meal'	13.75 oz	310	30.0	38.0	600	na	4.0	na	50	12%
Kiev 'Gourmet Selection'	9.25 oz	520	16.0	40.0	1200	(mq)	33.0	(mq)	(mq)	57%
'Looney Tunes Bugs Bunny' chunks	7.7 oz	290	17.0	31.0	480	na	11.0	na	28	34%
'Looney Tunes Road Runner'	6.7 oz	300	8.0	42.0	490	na	11.0	na	24	33%
'Looney Tunes Tazmanian Devil' drummettes	8 oz	310	14.0	31.0	480	na	14.0	na	40	41%
'Looney Tunes Yosemite Sam' barbecue glazed	7.38 oz	230	12.0	28.0	510	na	8.0	na	45	31%
Marsala 'Gourmet Selection'	10.5 oz	300	19.0	26.0	900	(mq)	13.0	(mq)	(mq)	39%
mesquite breast tenders, boneless	2.75 oz	110	17.0	4.0	420	na	3.0	na	45	24%
'Mesquite Chicken Meal'	13.25 oz	330	34.0	38.0	600	na	5.0	na	45	14%
mesquite 'Gourmet Selections'	9 oz	320	23.0	39.0	660	na	8.0	na	55	23%
'Mini Cordon Bleu' Wholesale Club Item	1 piece	90	8.0	5.0	210	na	4.0	na	17	41%
nuggets 'Microwave'	3.5 oz	220	10.0	11.0	(mq)	(mq)	15.0	(mq)	(mq)	62%
Oriental 'Gourmet Selection'	10.25 oz	270	20.0	32.0	1140	(mq)	7.0	(mq)	(mq)	23%
parmigiana 'Gourmet Selection'	11.25 oz	380	19.0	37.0	1100	(mq)	17.0	(mq)	(mq)	41%
piccata 'Gourmet Selection'	9 oz	240	19.0	19.0	680	(mq)	10.0	(mq)	(mq)	37%
pie, premium	9 oz	390	16.0	36.0	1065	na	20.0	na	43	46%
pie, white meat, premium	9 oz	400	22.0	33.0	783	na	20.0	na	56	45%
roasted 'Gourmet Selections'	9 oz	200	21.0	21.0	430	na	2.0	na	42	10%
'Salsa Chicken Meal'	13.75 oz	370	34.0	52.0	470	na	6.0	na	45	14%
'Sesame Chicken Meal'	13.5 oz	400	27.0	59.0	400	na	6.0	na	45	14%
sesame 'Healthy Portions'	13.5 oz	390	27.0	58.0	410	na	5.0	1.0	45	12%
stir fry w/vegetables, Wholesale Club Item	3.5 oz	130	11.0	13.0	710	na	5.0	na	45	32%
supreme 'Gourmet Selections'	9 oz	230	21.0	23.0	480	na	6.0	na	51	24%
sweet and sour 'Gourmet Selection'	11 oz	420	22.0	50.0	850	na	15.0	(mq)	(mq)	32%
tenders 'Microwave'	3.5 oz	230	16.0	19.0	(mq)	(mq)	11.0	(mq)	(mq)	41%
'Wings of Fire' Wholesale Club Item	3.5 oz	220	26.0	2.0	390	na	12.0	na	105	49%
(Ultimate 200)										
barbecue, glazed, w/vegetables	7 oz	200	19.0	22.0	450	na	6.0	3.0	30	25%

Food Name	Serving Size	Calories	Prot. gms	Carbs gms	Sod. mgs	Fiber gms	Fat gms	Sat. Fat gms	Chol. mgs	% Fat Cal.
Cordon Bleu, w/vegetables	7.7 oz	170	19.0	15.0	560	na	5.0	1.0	40	25%
grilled, glazed	7.5 oz	150	15.0	17.0	520	na	2.0	1.0	20	12%
Imperial	8.5 oz	200	18.0	25.0	430	na	3.0	1.0	25	14%
Kiev, w/vegetables and rice	7 oz	190	14.0	22.0	470	na	5.0	2.0	15	24%
patty, Southern baked, w/vegetables	6.3 oz	170	17.0	10.0	520	na	7.0	2.0	45	37%
teriyaki	7.6 oz	150	21.0	7.0	590	na	4.0	1.0	50	24%
(Weaver)										
batter-dipped, assorted pieces	3.6 oz	290	16.0	16.0	550	na	18.0	na	na	56%
crispy, light, skinless	2.9 oz	170	14.0	9.0	320	na	9.0	na	na	47%
'Crispy Dutch Frye' assorted pieces	3.6 oz	290	16.0	16.0	550	na	18.0	na	na	56%
'Crispy Dutch Frye' breast	4.5 oz	350	22.0	17.0	520	na	22.0	na	na	56%
crispy mini drums	3 oz	210	13.0	13.0	480	na	12.0	na	na	51%
croquettes	2 pieces	280	14.0	22.0	780	na	16.0	na	na	50%
mini drums, herb and spice	3 oz	200	13.0	13.0	320	na	11.0	na	na	49%
'Rondolet, Cheese'	2.6 oz	190	11.0	12.0	520	na	11.0	na	na	52%
'Rondolet, Italian'	2.6 oz	190	11.0	11.0	560	na	11.0	na	na	53%
'Rondolet, Original'	3 oz	190	13.0	13.0	610	na	10.0	na	na	46%
'Tenders, Honey Batter'	3 oz	220	13.0	14.0	500	na	12.0	na	na	50%
'Tenders, Premium'	3 oz	170	12.0	11.0	500	na	9.0	na	na	47%
(Weight Watchers)										
fettuccini, w/parmesan sauce	8.25 oz	280	22.0	25.0	590	na	9.0	3.0	40	30%
ginger, w/vegetable, Hunan 'Stir Fry'	9 oz	160	15.0	21.0	430	na	2.0	<1.0	15	11%
grilled, Suiza, w/Spanish rice 'Mexican Style'	8.6 oz	220	21.0	18.0	590	na	7.0	2.0	60	29%
orange glazed, w/rice 'Stir Fry'	9 oz	170	14.0	25.0	360	na	2.0	<1.0	10	10%
Polynesian 'Stir Fry'	9 oz	190	12.0	34.0	240	na	1.0	<1.0	20	5%
sesame, w/lo mein noodles 'Stir Fry'	9 oz	200	19.0	23.0	420	na	4.0	2.0	10	18%
teriyaki, w/spring vegetables 'Stir Fry'	9 oz	140	13.0	16.0	470	na	3.0	2.0	20	19%
'Tex Mex' w/Spanish rice 'Mexican Style'	8.3 oz	250	18.0	33.0	590	na	5.0	2.0	35	18%
CHICKEN DINNER/ENTRÉE, PACKAGED										
(Chicken By George)										
Cajun	5 oz	180	25.0	4.0	890	na	8.0	1.0	80	38%
Caribbean grill	5 oz	200	25.0	10.0	610	na	6.0	na	80	28%
Italian bleu cheese	5 oz	180	26.0	2.0	890	na	8.0	na	85	39%
lemon herb	5 oz	170	24.0	6.0	870	na	6.0	1.0	70	31%
lemon oregano	5 oz	160	26.0	4.0	580	na	4.0	na	75	23%
mesquite barbecue	5 oz	170	25.0	6.0	790	na	6.0	1.0	70	30%
mustard dill	5 oz	180	26.0	3.0	640	na	7.0	na	80	35%
roasted	5 oz	150	26.0	2.0	710	na	4.0	na	70	24%
teriyaki	5 oz	180	25.0	9.0	740	na	5.0	1.0	70	25%
tomato herb, w/basil	5 oz	190	25.0	7.0	800	na	7.0	na	80	33%
(Chicken Helper) 'Skillet Dinner'										
cheesy broccoli, dry	1/5 pkg	160	4.0	32.0	700	na	2.0	na	5	11%
cheesy broccoli, prepared	7 oz	310	24.0	34.0	790	na	9.0	na	65	26%
creamy chicken, dry	1/5 pkg	170	6.0	26.0	720	na	5.0	na	40	26%
creamy chicken, prepared	8.25 oz	330	26.0	29.0	820	na	13.0	na	100	35%
creamy mushroom, dry	1/5 pkg	170	5.0	28.0	720	na	4.0	na	30	21%
creamy mushroom, prepared	8 oz	320	25.0	31.0	810	na	11.0	na	90	31%
fettuccini Alfredo, dry	1/5 pkg	160	6.0	25.0	690	na	4.0	na	10	23%
fettuccini Alfredo, prepared	7.5 oz	320	26.0	27.0	780	na	12.0	na	70	34%
stir fry, dry	1/5 pkg	170	4.0	36.0	800	na	<1.0	na	0	<5%
stir fry, prepared	7 oz	370	25.0	36.0	950	na	14.0	na	145	34%
(Dinty Moore) and dumplings, microwave cup	7.5 oz	190	15.0	20.0	680	na	6.0	na	30	28%
(LaChoy)										
sweet and sour, 'Dinner Classics' prepared	3/4 cup	310	32.0	30.0	860	<1.0	6.0	1.1	50	18%

Food Name	Serving Size	Calories	Prot. gms	Carbs gms	Sod. mgs	Fiber gms	Fat gms	Sat. Fat gms	Chol. mgs	% Fat Cal.
sweet and sour, w/noodles	9.383 oz	256	9.4	49.4	697	1.8	3.1	1.3	10	11%
(Libby's)										
chow mein 'Diner' microwave cup	7.75 oz	130	5.0	19.0	830	2.4	4.0	1.0	10	27%
w/pasta spirals 'Diner' microwave cup	7.75 oz	120	8.0	16.0	910	2.2	3.0	1.0	15	22%
(Lipton) 'Microeasy'										
barbecue style, dry	1/4 pkg	110	2.0	24.0	980	(mq)	<1.0	(mq)	na	<8%
barbecue style, prepared	1/4 pkg	220	16.0	24.0	1020	(mq)	6.0	(mq)	(mq)	25%
country style, dry	1/4 pkg	80	3.0	15.0	840	(mq)	<1.0	(mq)	na	<11%
country style, prepared	1/4 pkg	190	18.0	15.0	880	(mq)	6.0	(mq)	(mq)	29%
(Lunch Bucket)										
and dumplings, microwave cup	7.5 oz	140	4.0	25.0	880	na	2.0	na	na	13%
w/beans and rice 'Light'n Healthy' micro cup	7.5 oz	170	7.0	28.0	600	na	3.0	na	10	16%
(Top Shelf)										
à la king	10 oz	360	18.0	49.0	890	na	10.0	4.0	37	25%
Acapulco	1 serving	390	28.0	41.0	1320	(mq)	13.0	(mq)	55	30%
breast, glazed	10 oz	170	19.0	19.0	780	na	2.0	1.0	35	11%
breast, w/Spanish rice	10 oz	400	27.0	38.0	810	na	15.0	7.0	75	34%
'Cacciatore'	10 oz	210	21.0	25.0	810	na	3.0	na	50	13%
sweet and sour	1 serving	270	24.0	41.0	280	(mq)	1.0	(mq)	60	3%
(Ultra Slim Fast)										
and vegetables	12 oz	290	24.0	45.0	850	na	3.0	na	30	9%
chow mein	12 oz	320	25.0	43.0	580	na	6.0	na	60	17%
fettuccini	12 oz	390	31.0	38.0	980	na	12.0	na	65	28%
mesquite	12 oz	350	29.0	61.0	300	na	1.0	na	65	2%
roasted, in mushroom sauce	12 oz	280	25.0	30.0	830	na	6.0	na	55	20%
sweet and sour	12 oz	330	20.0	57.0	340	na	2.0	na	45	6%
CHICKEN ENTRÉE, ALTERNATIVE										
(Worthington) pie, frozen	8 oz	380	7.0	43.0	1200	(mq)	20.0	3.0	0	47%
CHICKEN FAT										
	1 cup	1846	0.0	0.0	0	0	204.6	61.1	174	100%
	1 oz	178	1.1	0.0	9	0	19.3	5.7	16	98%
	1 tbsp	115	0.0	0.0	0	0	12.8	3.8	11	100%
CHICKEN FRYING MIX, dry mix *(Golden Dipt)*	1 oz	90	2.0	20.0	1430	(mq)	0.0	0.0	0	0%
CHICKEN GIBLETS										
fried	1 cup	402	47.2	6.3	164	0	19.5	5.5	647	45%
simmered	1 cup	228	37.5	1.4	84	0	6.9	2.2	570	29%
CHICKEN GIZZARD										
all classes, simmered	1 cup	222	39.4	1.6	97	0	5.3	1.5	281	23%
broiler-fryer, raw, approx 1.3 oz	1 med	44	6.7	0.2	28	0	1.6	0.4	48	34%
broiler-fryer, simmered, approx .8 oz	1 med	34	6.0	0.3	15	0	0.8	0.2	43	22%
CHICKEN HEART										
all classes, simmered	1 cup	268	38.3	0.2	70	0	11.5	3.3	351	40%
broiler-fryer, raw, 1 heart	2 oz	9	1.0	<.1	5	0	0.6	0.2	8	55%
broiler-fryer, simmered	4 oz	210	29.9	0.1	54	0	9.0	2.6	275	40%
CHICKEN LIVER										
all classes, simmered	1 cup	220	34.1	1.2	71	0	7.6	2.6	883	33%
broiler-fryer, chopped, simmered	1 cup	219	34.1	1.2	71	0	7.6	2.6	883	33%
broiler-fryer, raw, approx 1.1 oz	1 liver	40	5.8	1.1	25	0	1.2	0.4	140	28%
broiler-fryer, simmered	4 oz	178	27.6	1.0	58	0	6.2	2.1	716	33%
CHICKEN POT PIE *(Swanson)*, frozen	7 oz	380	11.0	35.0	760	(mq)	22.0	(mq)	(mq)	52%
CHICKEN SALAD										
(Longacre)	1 oz	64	3.0	3.0	110	na	5.0	(mq)	15	65%
(Longacre) 'Saladfest'	1 oz	47	4.0	1.0	150	na	3.0	(mq)	15	57%
CHICKEN SALAD SPREAD, 'Spreadables' *(Libby's)*	1.9 oz	90	5.0	5.0	230	1.9	6.0	1.0	15	57%

Food Name	Serving Size	Calories	Prot. gms	Carbs gms	Sod. mgs	Fiber gms	Fat gms	Sat. Fat gms	Chol. mgs	% Fat Cal.
CHICKEN SEASONING MIX										
(Featherweight) dry mix	1/4 pkg	18	1.0	8.0	30	(mq)	0.0	0.0	0	0%
(Schilling) 'Bag 'n Season'	1 pkg	134	3.0	19.0	4771	na	5.0	na	1	34%
(Schilling) dry mix, for fried chicken	1/4 tsp	1	0.1	0.2	132	na	<.1	(tr)	na	<43%
CHICKEN SPREAD, CANNED										
(Hormel)	.5 oz	30	2.0	0.0	(mq)	0	2.0	(mq)	(mq)	69%
(Underwood) chunky	2 1/8 oz	150	10.0	2.0	440	na	9.0	3.0	40	63%
(Underwood) 'Light'	2 1/8 oz	80	11.0	2.0	330	na	3.0	1.0	30	34%
(Underwood) smoky	2 1/8 oz	150	10.0	10.0	290	na	8.0	2.0	40	47%
CHICKEN STEW										
(Dinty Moore) canned	7.5 oz	260	11.0	15.0	850	na	18.0	4.0	80	61%
(Dinty Moore) microwave cup	7.5 oz	260	11.0	15.0	850	na	18.0	4.0	80	61%
(Featherweight) w/wild rice, canned	7.5 oz	140	10.0	23.0	400	(mq)	1.0	(mq)	20	6%
(Heinz) w/dumplings, canned	7.5 oz	210	9.0	22.0	850	(mq)	9.0	(mq)	(mq)	40%
(Mountain House) freeze-dried, prepared	1 cup	230	9.0	30.0	209	(mq)	8.0	(mq)	(mq)	32%
(Swanson) canned	7 5/8 oz	160	9.0	15.0	990	(mq)	7.0	(mq)	(mq)	40%
CHICORY, WITLOOF										
raw	1/2 cup	8	0.4	1.8	1	1.4	0.0	0.0	0	0%
raw , approx 2.1 oz	1 head	9	0.5	2.1	1	1.6	0.1	0.0	0	8%
trimmed	1 oz	4	0.3	0.9	2	(mq)	<.1	tr	0	<16%
untrimmed	1 lb	61	4.0	12.9	28	(mq)	0.4	0.1	0	5%
CHICORY GREENS										
trimmed	1 oz	7	0.5	1.3	13	(mq)	0.1	<.1	0	11%
trimmed, chopped	1/2 cup	21	1.5	4.2	41	3.6	0.3	0.1	0	11%
untrimmed	1 lb	87	6.3	17.5	167	(mq)	1.1	0.3	0	9%
CHICORY ROOT										
raw, approx 2.6 oz	1 root	44	0.8	10.5	30	>1.2 c	0.1	0.0	0	2%
raw, 1-inch pieces	1/2 cup	33	0.6	7.9	23	>.9 c	0.1	0.0	0	3%
trimmed	1 oz	21	0.4	5.0	14	>.6 c	0.1	<.1	0	4%
untrimmed	1 lb	272	5.2	65.1	186	>7.3 c	0.7	0.2	0	2%
CHILI, CANNED										
beef, w/beans *(Cimmaron)*	7.5 oz	230	17.0	21.0	na	na	9.0	na	35	35%
chicken, w/beans *(Cimmaron)*	7.5 oz	180	12.0	22.0	970	na	5.0	na	60	25%
chicken, w/beans *(Stagg)*	7.5 oz	200	14.0	21.0	na	na	6.0	na	na	28%
'Chili Con Carne' *(Heinz)*	7.75 oz	350	15.0	27.0	1000	(mq)	21.0	(mq)	(mq)	53%
'Chili Mac' *(Chef Boyardee)*	7.5 oz	230	8.0	26.0	1410	(mq)	11.0	(mq)	(mq)	42%
'Chili Mac' *(Heinz)*	7.5 oz	250	10.0	26.0	860	(mq)	12.0	(mq)	(mq)	43%
country, w/beans *(Stagg)*	7.5 oz	270	14.0	25.0	na	na	12.0	na	na	41%
plain *(Gebhardt)*	1 cup	530	21.0	20.0	990	1.0	41.0	16.0	150	69%
vegetarian *(Gebhardt)*	4 oz	219	9.6	6.9	555	(mq)	17.1	(mq)	0	70%
vegetarian *(Worthington)*	2/3 cup	190	10.0	15.0	550	(mq)	10.0	1.0	0	47%
vegetarian, plain *(Gebhardt)*	4.339 oz	232	7.3	11.1	736	3.1	18.5	7.3	42	69%
vegetarian, plain *(Open Range)*	4.409 oz	176	8.8	9.4	608	2.8	12.8	5.7	24	61%
vegetarian, spicy *(Hain)*	7.5 oz	160	7.0	29.0	1060	(mq)	1.0	(mq)	0	6%
vegetarian, spicy *(Hain)* 'Reduced Sodium'	7.5 oz	170	7.0	31.0	200	(mq)	1.0	(mq)	0	6%
vegetarian, spicy *(Natural Touch)*	2/3 cup	230	12.0	19.0	890	(mq)	12.0	1.0	0	47%
vegetarian, 3-bean, mild, fat-free *(Health Valley)*	5 oz	90	10.0	12.0	180	9.0	0.0	na	0	0%
vegetarian, w/beans *(Gebhardt)*	4.444 oz	195	7.4	18.3	694	4.8	12.0	5.4	23	51%
vegetarian, w/beans *(Just Rite)*	4.55 oz	190	8.8	15.3	616	6.0	13.3	6.3	18	55%
vegetarian, w/beans *(Open Range)*	4.5 oz	136	8.6	12.6	645	5.2	8.0	3.7	13	46%
vegetarian, w/beans, 'Longhorn' *(Gebhardt)*	4.55 oz	225	9.1	16.0	545	4.1	15.7	7.2	16	59%
vegetarian, w/beans, mild *(Health Valley)*	4 oz	130	8.0	16.0	730	8.2	3.0	(mq)	0	22%
vegetarian, w/beans, mild *(Health Valley)* 'No Salt Added'	4 oz	130	8.0	16.0	25	8.2	3.0	(mq)	0	22%
vegetarian, w/beans, spicy *(Health Valley)*	4 oz	130	8.0	16.0	430	8.2	3.0	(mq)	0	22%

Food Name	Serving Size	Calories	Prot. gms	Carbs gms	Sod. mgs	Fiber gms	Fat gms	Sat. Fat gms	Chol. mgs	% Fat Cal.
vegetarian, w/beans, spicy (Health Valley) 'No Salt Added'	4 oz	130	8.0	16.0	25	8.2	0.0	(mq)	0	22%
vegetarian, w/black beans, mild, fat-free (Health Valley) ..	5 oz	140	11.0	23.0	290	12.2	0.0	na	0	0%
vegetarian, w/black beans, spicy, fat-free (Health Valley) ..	5 oz	70	7.0	9.0	180	8.0	0.0	na	0	0%
vegetarian, w/lentils, mild (Health Valley)	4 oz	130	8.0	16.0	200	8.2	3.0	(mq)	0	22%
vegetarian, w/lentils, mild (Health Valley) 'No Salt Added'	4 oz	130	8.0	16.0	50	8.2	3.0	(mq)	0	22%
vegetarian, w/tempeh, spicy (Hain)	7.5 oz	160	7.0	24.0	1350	(mq)	4.0	(mq)	0	23%
w/beans	1/2 cup	143	7.3	15.2	668	5.6	7.0	3.0	22	41%
w/beans (Armour)	6 oz	320	10.0	21.0	870	na	22.0	na	na	62%
w/beans (Armour)	7.5 oz	390	13.0	27.0	1080	na	26.0	na	na	59%
w/beans (Estee)	7.5 oz	370	16.0	27.0	125	(mq)	20.0	10.0	60	51%
w/beans (Featherweight)	7.5 oz	280	19.0	29.0	440	(mq)	10.0	(mq)	30	32%
w/beans (Gebhardt)	1 cup	495	20.0	47.0	1010	6.0	28.0	10.0	92	49%
w/beans (Just Rite)	4 oz	200	10.0	16.0	500	1.0	11.0	4.0	33	49%
w/beans (Nalley's)	7.5 oz	260	17.0	27.0	880	(mq)	9.0	(mq)	(mq)	32%
w/beans (Van Camp's)	1 cup	352	14.9	20.9	1215	>2.3 c	23.2	(mq)	(mq)	59%
w/beans (Wolf Brand)	8 oz	345	15.0	21.8	1013	>2.3 c	22.0	(mq)	(mq)	57%
w/beans '15-oz' (Dennison's)	7.5 oz	310	16.0	27.0	875	8.0	15.0	(mq)	(mq)	44%
w/beans '15-oz' (Hormel)	7.5 oz	310	17.0	23.0	1127	(mq)	17.0	(mq)	(mq)	49%
w/beans '15-oz' (Libby's)	7.5 oz	270	13.0	25.0	810	(mq)	13.0	(mq)	(mq)	44%
w/beans, 9.2 oz (Quincy's)	1 serving	346	20.0	32.0	1380	(mq)	16.0	(mq)	(mq)	41%
w/beans '24-oz' (Libby's)	8 oz	290	14.0	27.0	860	(mq)	14.0	(mq)	(mq)	43%
w/beans '25-oz' (Hormel)	8 1/3 oz	350	18.0	26.0	1202	(mq)	20.0	(mq)	(mq)	51%
w/beans '30-oz' (Dennison's)	7.5 oz	310	16.0	28.0	840	8.0	15.0	(mq)	(mq)	43%
w/beans '40-oz' (Dennison's)	8 oz	340	17.0	29.0	1050	8.0	17.0	(mq)	(mq)	45%
w/beans '40-oz' (Hormel)	8 oz	320	17.0	25.0	1135	(mq)	17.0	(mq)	(mq)	48%
w/beans, beef (Chef Boyardee)	7.5 oz	330	15.0	30.0	1005	(mq)	17.0	(mq)	(mq)	46%
w/beans, chunky (Dennison's)	7.5 oz	310	16.0	28.0	780	10.0	14.0	(mq)	(mq)	42%
w/beans, chunky (Hormel)	7.5 oz	290	15.0	25.0	780	na	14.0	na	50	44%
w/beans 'Cook-Off' (Dennison's)	7.5 oz	340	17.0	25.0	915	8.0	19.0	(mq)	(mq)	50%
w/beans, extra spicy (Wolf Brand)	7.75 oz	324	14.1	20.6	926	>2.2 c	20.6	(mq)	(mq)	57%
w/beans, hot (Armour)	7.5 oz	390	13.0	27.0	1080	na	26.0	na	na	59%
w/beans, hot (Gebhardt)	1 cup	470	16.0	47.0	1000	6.0	27.0	9.8	65	49%
w/beans, hot (Gebhardt)	4 oz	189	7.1	9.2	497	2.1	14.2	0.2	17	66%
w/beans, hot (Heinz)	7.75 oz	330	15.0	30.0	1140	(mq)	16.0	(mq)	(mq)	44%
w/beans, hot (Just Rite)	4 oz	195	11.0	16.0	495	1.0	10.0	3.5	33	46%
w/beans, hot (Nalley's)	7.5 oz	280	17.0	30.0	810	(mq)	10.0	(mq)	(mq)	32%
w/beans, hot '15 oz' (Hormel)	7.5 oz	310	16.0	24.0	1121	(mq)	16.0	(mq)	(mq)	47%
w/beans, hot '15 oz' (Dennison's)	7.5 oz	310	16.0	26.0	910	7.0	16.0	(mq)	(mq)	46%
w/beans, hot '40 oz' (Dennison's)	8 oz	350	17.0	29.0	950	7.0	19.0	(mq)	(mq)	48%
w/beans, hot, jalapeño (Nalley's)	7.5 oz	260	14.0	29.0	920	(mq)	10.0	(mq)	(mq)	34%
w/beans 'Laredo' (Stagg)	7.5 oz	260	15.0	22.0	na	na	12.0	na	na	42%
w/beans 'Micro-Cup' (Hormel)	7.5 oz	250	15.0	23.0	980	(mq)	11.0	(mq)	65	39%
w/beans 'Premium Lite' (Armour)	7.5 oz	260	16.0	27.0	1110	na	10.0	na	na	34%
w/beans 'Thick' (Nalley's)	7.5 oz	260	16.0	29.0	840	(mq)	9.0	(mq)	(mq)	31%
w/chicken, spicy (Hain)	7.5 oz	130	11.0	19.0	1030	(mq)	2.0	(mq)	40	13%
w/o beans (Armour)	7.5 oz	390	13.0	14.0	1150	na	31.0	na	na	72%
w/o beans (Hormel) ,,,,,,,,,	10.5 oz	540	24.0	19.0	1384	(mq)	41.0	(mq)	(mq)	68%
w/o beans (Just Rite)	4 oz	180	10.0	0.0	515	<1.0	11.0	3.7	41	53%
w/o beans (Libby's)	7.5 oz	390	18.0	11.0	800	(mq)	30.0	(mq)	(mq)	70%
w/o beans (Van Camp's)	1 cup	412	15.4	12.1	1499	>1.6 c	33.5	(mq)	(mq)	73%
w/o beans (Wolf Brand)	8 oz	387	20.7	16.2	1042	>2.0 c	26.6	(mq)	(mq)	62%
w/o beans 'Big Chunk' (Nalley's)	7.5 oz	270	17.0	14.0	810	(mq)	16.0	(mq)	(mq)	54%
w/o beans 'Chili-Mac' (Wolf Brand)	7.75 oz	317	11.5	22.9	854	>1.1 c	19.9	(mq)	(mq)	57%
w/o beans '15 oz' (Dennison's)	7.5 oz	300	17.0	15.0	1380	(mq)	19.0	(mq)	(mq)	57%

Food Name	Serving Size	Calories	Prot. gms	Carbs gms	Sod. mgs	Fiber gms	Fat gms	Sat. Fat gms	Chol. mgs	% Fat Cal.
w/o beans '15 oz' (Hormel)	7.5 oz	370	17.0	12.0	1012	(mq)	28.0	(mq)	(mq)	69%
w/o beans, 15 oz (Libby's)	7.5 oz	390	18.0	11.0	800	na	30.0	na	na	70%
w/o beans '19 oz' (Dennison's)	9.5 oz	380	22.0	18.0	1335	(mq)	24.0	(mq)	(mq)	57%
w/o beans 'Steak House' (Stagg)	7.5 oz	300	16.0	17.0	na	na	19.0	na	na	56%
w/o beans '25 oz' (Hormel)	8 1/3 oz	430	20.0	13.0	1070	(mq)	33.0	(mq)	(mq)	69%
w/o beans, extra spicy (Wolf Brand)	7.5 oz	363	19.4	15.3	962	>1.9 c	24.9	(mq)	(mq)	62%
w/o beans, hot '15 oz' (Hormel)	7.5 oz	370	17.0	12.0	985	(mq)	28.0	(mq)	(mq)	69%
w/o beans, w/franks 'Chilee Weenee' (Van Camp's)	1 cup	309	14.4	27.6	1057	>2.2 c	15.7	(mq)	(mq)	46%
CHILI, FREEZE-DRIED										
w/beans, prepared (Mountain House)	1 cup	390	20.0	38.0	153	(mq)	16.0	(mq)	(mq)	38%
w/beef 'Chili Mac' prepared (Mountain House)	1 cup	250	12.0	31.0	115	(mq)	8.0	(mq)	(mq)	30%
CHILI, FROZEN										
con carne 'Homestyle Recipe' (Swanson)	8.25 oz	270	20.0	26.0	740	(mq)	10.0	(mq)	(mq)	33%
con carne, w/beans (Stouffer's)	8.75 oz	260	19.0	24.0	1270	(mq)	10.0	(mq)	(mq)	34%
vegetarian (Right Course)	9.75 oz	280	9.0	45.0	590	(mq)	7.0	1.0	0	23%
CHILI, MICROWAVE										
'Chili Mac' micro cup (Hormel)	7.5 oz	192	10.0	18.0	977	na	9.0	4.0	22	42%
w/beans (Armour)	7.5 oz	300	16.0	26.0	1120	na	14.0	na	na	43%
w/beans, 'Diner' microwave cup (Libby's)	7.75 oz	280	15.0	29.0	820	4.3	12.0	6.0	40	38%
w/beans, hot, micro cup (Hormel)	7.38 oz	250	15.0	24.0	977	na	11.0	4.0	49	39%
w/beans, microwave cup (Lunch Bucket)	7.5 oz	300	16.0	26.0	1120	na	14.0	na	45	43%
w/o beans, micro cup (Hormel)	7.38 oz	290	18.0	15.0	830	na	17.0	8.0	60	54%
CHILI BEAN, CANNED. See also KIDNEY BEAN, CANNED; PINTO BEAN.										
(Gebhardt)	4.586 oz	134	7.1	30.7	630	7.2	1.0	0.4	0	6%
(Hunt's)	4 oz	102	5.7	18.1	488	(mq)	0.0	0.0	0	0%
(Hunt's)	4.48 oz	87	6.0	17.1	597	5.7	1.0	0.0	0	9%
(S&W)	1/2 cup	130	7.0	23.0	520	(mq)	1.0	na	na	7%
baked style, hot (Campbell's)	7.75 oz	180	10.0	38.0	870	(mq)	4.0	(mq)	na	16%
Caliente style (Green Giant)	1/2 cup	100	6.0	20.0	700	7.0	1.0	na	0	8%
Caliente style (Joan of Arc)	1/2 cup	100	6.0	20.0	700	7.0	1.0	na	0	8%
extra spicy (Green Giant)	1/2 cup	100	7.0	21.0	580	6.0	1.0	0.0	0	7%
extra spicy (Joan of Arc)	1/2 cup	100	7.0	21.0	580	6.0	1.0	0.0	0	7%
50% less salt (Green Giant)	1/2 cup	100	7.0	21.0	310	7.0	1.0	0.0	0	7%
50% less salt (Joan of Arc)	1/2 cup	100	7.0	21.0	310	7.0	1.0	0.0	0	7%
hot (A&P)	1/2 cup	140	8.0	24.0	440	(mq)	1.0	na	na	7%
hot (Allens)	1/2 cup	90	5.0	17.0	420	(mq)	<1.0	na	na	<9%
hot (Bush's Best)	1/2 cup	70	5.0	20.0	420	6.0	0.0	na	na	0%
in chili gravy (Dennison's)	7.5 oz	180	12.0	30.0	770	12.0	1.0	na	na	5%
in sauce (Hormel)	5 oz	130	6.0	19.0	453	(mq)	3.0	(mq)	na	21%
Mexican style (Allens)	1/2 cup	135	8.0	24.0	430	(mq)	<1.0	na	na	<7%
Mexican style (Van Camp's)	1 cup	210	11.4	39.0	730	(mq)	2.4	(mq)	na	10%
spiced (Gebhardt)	4 oz	113	7.5	19.7	590	6.7	1.1	0.1	0	8%
spicy 'Dry Beans in Sauce' (Green Giant)	1/2 cup	100	7.0	21.0	620	7.0	1.0	0.0	0	7%
spicy 'Dry Beans in Sauce' (Joan of Arc)	1/2 cup	100	7.0	21.0	620	7.0	1.0	0.0	0	7%
CHILI MIX										
'Chili Quick' dry (Gebhardt)	1.5-oz pkt	82	2.5	16.8	2784	3.0	1.1	0.1	0	11%
'Chili con Carne' prepared (Old El Paso)	1 cup	162	19.0	8.0	510	1.5	7.0	(mq)	47	37%
'Homestyle Chili Fixins' (Hunt's)	4.656 oz	84	5.6	18.5	858	6.0	1.2	0.2	0	10%
vegetarian, w/beans, prepared (Fantastic Foods)	1/2 cup	104	8.0	19.0	180	(mq)	0.8	na	0	6%
w/beans, prepared (Old El Paso)	1 cup	217	15.0	17.0	480	6.0	10.0	(mq)	32	41%
CHILI POWDER										
(Durkee)	1 tsp	11	0.0	0.0	0	0	0.01	na	na	31%
(Laurel Leaf)	1 tsp	11	0.0	0.0	0	0	0.01	na	na	31%

CHILI SAUCE. See SAUCE.

Food Name	Serving Size	Calories	Prot. gms	Carbs gms	Sod. mgs	Fiber gms	Fat gms	Sat. Fat gms	Chol. mgs	% Fat Cal.
CHILI SEASONING										
(Gebhardt)	1 tsp	6	0.0	1.0	30	(mq)	0.0	0.0	0	0%
(Gebhardt)	.0106 oz	1	0.0	0.1	0	.1	0.0	0.0	0	0%
(Gebhardt) mix 'Chili Quick'	1 tsp	10	<1.0	2.0	165	<1.0	<1.0	(mq)	0	<43%
(Hain) hot	1/4 pkg	30	1.0	5.0	370	(mq)	1.0	na	0	27%
(Hain) medium	1/4 pkg	30	1.0	5.0	300	(mq)	1.0	na	0	27%
(Hain) mild	1/2 pkg	30	1.0	5.0	330	(mq)	1.0	na	0	27%
(Lawry's) 'Seasoning Blends'	1 pkg	143	4.9	26.6	2291	>2.1 c	1.8	na	0	11%
(Old El Paso)	1/5 pkg	21	1.0	4.0	717	1.0	1.0	na	0	31%
(Schilling)	1/4 pkg	27	1.0	4.5	290	(mq)	0.5	na	na	17%
(Tio Sancho)	1.23 oz	109	4.1	6.0	832	>4.2 c	2.2	(mq)	na	33%
CHIMICHANGA										
beef 'Primera' (Marquez)	1 chimichanga	380	13.0	42.0	890	2.0	17.0	5.0	30	41%
CHIMICHANGA DINNER, FROZEN										
bean and cheese (Old El Paso)	1 pkg	380	12.0	40.0	610	(mq)	19.0	(mq)	20	45%
beef (Old El Paso)	1 piece	370	12.0	34.0	470	(mq)	21.0	(mq)	(mq)	51%
beef and cheese 'Festive Dinners' (Old El Paso)	11 oz	510	22.0	53.0	1400	(mq)	23.0	(mq)	(mq)	41%
beef and pork (Old El Paso)	1 pkg	340	13.0	35.0	700	(mq)	16.0	(mq)	(mq)	43%
beef 'Festive Dinners' (Old El Paso)	11 oz	540	23.0	65.0	1200	(mq)	21.0	(mq)	(mq)	35%
chicken (Old El Paso)	1 piece	360	13.0	33.0	470	(mq)	20.0	(mq)	(mq)	50%
CHINESE APPLE. See POMEGRANATE.										
CHINESE CABBAGE. See CABBAGE, NAPA.										
CHINESE DATE										
dried	1 oz	81	1.0	20.1	3	>.9 c	0.3	(tr)	0	3%
raw, seeded	1 oz	22	0.3	5.7	1	>.4 c	0.1	(tr)	0	4%
raw, w/seeds	1 lb	331	5.1	85.3	11	>5.9 c	0.8	na	0	2%
CHINESE FUNGUS/Jew's ear										
approx .2 oz	1 piece	2	0.0	0.4	0	0	(tr)	(tr)	0	0%
sliced	1/2 cup	13	0.2	3.3	5	0	(tr)	(tr)	0	0%
trimmed	1 oz	7	0.1	1.9	3	0	na	(tr)	0	0%
untrimmed	1 lb	111	2.1	30.0	41	0	0.2	(tr)	0	1%
CHINESE GOOSEBERRY. See KIWI FRUIT.										
CHINESE NOODLE. See NOODLE, CHINESE.										
CHINESE PARSLEY. See CORIANDER.										
CHINESE PARSLEY LEAF. See CORIANDER LEAF.										
CHINESE PARSLEY SEED. See CORIANDER SEED.										
CHINESE RADISH										
boiled, drained	4 oz	19	0.8	3.9	15	>.6 c	0.3	0.1	0	13%
boiled, drained, sliced	1/2 cup	13	0.5	2.5	10	1.2	0.2	0.1	0	13%
dried	1/2 cup	157	4.6	36.8	161	>4.9 c	0.4	0.1	0	2%
dried	1 oz	77	2.2	18.0	79	>2.4 c	0.2	0.1	0	2%
raw, 7 inches long, 2 1/4 inches diam, approx 15.1 oz	1 med	62	2.0	13.9	71	5.4	0.3	0.1	0	4%
raw, trimmed	1 oz	5	0.2	1.2	6	>.2 c	<.1	tr	0	<14%
raw, trimmed (Frieda's)	1 lb	86	4.1	19.1	(mq)	(mq)	0.5	(mq)	0	5%
raw, trimmed (Frieda's)	1 oz	5	0.3	1.2	(mq)	(mq)	<.1	tr	0	<13%
raw, trimmed, sliced	1/2 cup	8	0.3	1.8	9	.7	<.1	<.1	0	<10%
raw, untrimmed	1 lb	65	2.2	14.7	75	>2.3 c	0.4	0.1	0	5%
CHINESE WATERMELON										
boiled, drained	4 oz	15	0.5	3.4	121	>.6 c	0.2	<.1	0	10%
boiled, drained, cubes	1/2 cup	11	0.4	2.6	93	>.4 c	0.2	0.0	0	13%
raw, cubes	1 cup	17	0.5	4.0	147	>.7 c	0.3	0.0	0	13%
raw, trimmed	1 oz	4	0.1	0.9	31	.2	0.1	tr	0	18%
raw, untrimmed	1 lb	42	1.3	9.7	358	1.9	0.6	0.1	0	11%

Food Name	Serving Size	Calories	Prot. gms	Carbs gms	Sod. mgs	Fiber gms	Fat gms	Sat. Fat gms	Chol. mgs	% Fat Cal.
CHINESE YAM. See JICAMA.										
CHIVES										
....	1 oz	7	0.8	1.1	2	.9	0.2	<.1	0	19%
freeze-dried	1 tbsp	1	0.0	0.1	0	tr	0.0	0.0	0	0%
freeze-dried	1/4 cup	2	0.2	0.5	1	>.1 c	0.0	0.0	0	0%
raw, chopped	1 tbsp	1	0.1	0.1	0	.1	0.0	0.0	0	0%
raw, chopped	1 tsp	0	0.0	0.0	0	na	0.0	0.0	0	0%
CHOCOLATE, BAKING										
Bar										
semi-sweet *(Baker's)*	1 oz	140	1.0	17.0	0	na	9.0	na	0	53%
semi-sweet *(Nestlé)*	1 oz	160	2.0	16.0	0	(mq)	9.0	(mq)	na	53%
semi-sweet 'Premium' *(Hershey's)*	1 oz	140	1.0	16.0	0	(mq)	8.0	(mq)	na	51%
sweet 'German' *(Baker's)*	1 oz	140	1.0	17.0	0	(mq)	10.0	(mq)	na	56%
unsweetened *(Baker's)*	1 oz	140	3.0	9.0	0	na	15.0	na	0	74%
unsweetened *(Hershey's)*	1 oz	190	4.0	7.0	5	(mq)	16.0	(mq)	0	77%
unsweetened *(Nestlé)*	1 oz	180	4.0	9.0	0	(mq)	14.0	(mq)	na	71%
unsweetened 'Premium' *(Hershey's)*	1 oz	190	4.0	7.0	5	na	16.0	na	0	77%
white 'Premier' *(Nestlé)*	1 oz	150	2.0	18.0	15	(mq)	9.0	(mq)	na	50%
Chips										
milk chocolate *(Baker's)*	1 oz	140	2.0	18.0	25	(mq)	8.0	(mq)	5	47%
milk chocolate *(Hershey's)*	1/4 cup	220	2.0	27.0	55	na	12.0	na	10	48%
milk chocolate *(Hershey's)*	1 oz	150	2.0	27.0	55	(mq)	12.0	(mq)	10	48%
milk chocolate 'Big Chips' *(Baker's)*	1/4 cup	240	3.0	30.0	40	na	13.0	na	10	47%
mint chocolate *(Hershey's)*	1.5 oz	230	2.0	28.0	<1	(mq)	12.0	(mq)	na	47%
semi-sweet *(Baker's)*	1/4 cup	200	2.0	30.0	30	(mq)	9.0	(mq)	0	39%
semi-sweet 'Big Chips' *(Baker's)*	1/4 cup	220	2.0	31.0	0	na	13.0	na	0	47%
semi-sweet, mini, approx 1/4 cup *(Hershey's)*	1.5 oz	220	2.0	26.0	5	(mq)	12.0	(mq)	0	49%
semi-sweet, real chocolate *(Baker's)*	1/4 cup	200	2.0	28.0	0	na	11.0	na	0	45%
semi-sweet, regular *(Hershey's)*	1.5 oz	220	2.0	27.0	0	na	12.0	na	0	48%
vanilla 'White' milk *(Hershey's)*	1.5 oz	240	3.0	25.0	65	(mq)	14.0	(mq)	na	53%
Chunks										
milk chocolate, 12 pieces *(Hershey's)*	1 oz	160	2.0	16.0	25	na	9.0	na	10	53%
semi-sweet *(Hershey's)*	1 oz	140	1.0	15.0	na	(mq)	8.0	(mq)	na	53%
white 'Premier Treasures' *(Nestlé)*	1 oz	160	2.0	15.0	25	(mq)	10.0	(mq)	na	57%
Grated, bitter	1 cup	667	14.1	38.2	5	20.3	70.0	39.2	0	75%
Powder										
cocoa, 100% *(Nestlé)*	1 oz	80	7.0	5.0	5	1.0	5.0	na	na	48%
cocoa 'Premium' *(Saco Foods)*	1 tbsp	15	1.6	3.6	51	na	0.9	0.5	0	28%
Premelted, unsweetened 'Choco Bake' *(Nestlé)*	1 oz	190	4.0	7.0	na	(mq)	16.0	(mq)	0	77%
Squares										
unsweetened, grated	1 cup	689	13.6	37.4	18	20.3	73.0	43.0	0	76%
unsweetened, 1 oz	1 square	148	2.9	8.0	4	4.4	15.7	9.2	0	76%
CHOCOLATE FLAVOR DRINK. See also DIET DRINK.										
Canned										
(Frostee)	8 oz	200	2.0	30.0	160	(tr)	8.0	(mq)	na	36%
Dutch 'Lite' *(Sego)*	10 oz	150	11.0	20.0	480	(tr)	3.0	(mq)	5	18%
liquid food, nutritionally complete *(Sustacal)*	8 oz	240	14.5	33.0	220	na	5.5	na	na	21%
liquid nutrition *(Ensure)*	8 oz	250	9.3	33.8	200	na	8.8	na	5	32%
liquid nutrition 'Plus' *(Ensure)*	8 oz	355	13.5	46.8	250	na	12.6	na	5	32%
liquid nutrition, w/fiber *(Ensure)*	8 oz	260	9.9	37.8	200	na	8.8	na	5	29%
'Lite' *(Sego)*	10 oz	150	11.0	20.0	480	(tr)	3.0	(mq)	5	18%
malt 'Very Chocolate' *(Sego)*	10 oz	225	11.0	43.0	450	(tr)	1.0	na	5	4%
'Very Chocolate' *(Sego)*	10 oz	225	11.0	43.0	450	(tr)	1.0	na	5	4%

Food Name	Serving Size	Calories	Prot. gms	Carbs gms	Sod. mgs	Fiber gms	Fat gms	Sat. Fat gms	Chol. mgs	% Fat Cal.
Mix/powder										
approx 2-3 heaping tsp	.8 oz	75	0.7	19.5	45	1.3	0.7	0.4	0	7%
approx 2-3 heaping tsp, prepared w/1 cup 1% milk	1 cup	177	8.7	31.2	168	>.2 c	3.3	2.0	10	16%
approx 2-3 heaping tsp, prepared w/1 cup 2% milk	1 cup	196	8.8	31.2	167	3.8	5.4	3.3	18	23%
approx 2-3 heaping tsp, prepared w/1 cup skim milk	1 cup	161	9.1	31.4	171	>.2 c	1.1	0.7	4	6%
'Chocolate Milk Maker' (Swiss Miss)	.6702 oz	73	0.5	17.1	55	.4	0.3	0.2	0	4%
classic chocolate chip (Nestlé)	1.13 oz	90	7.0	12.0	170	6.0	2.0	na	na	19%
classic chocolate chip, prepared (Nestlé)	8 oz	180	15.0	24.0	300	6.0	2.0	na	na	10%
creamy milk chocolate (Nestlé)	1.13 oz	90	7.0	12.0	150	6.0	2.0	na	na	19%
creamy milk chocolate, prepared (Nestlé)	8 oz	180	15.0	24.0	280	6.0	2.0	na	na	10%
dairy, reduced calorie, w/aspartame	.75-oz pkt	63	5.3	10.7	166	.3	0.6	0.4	2	8%
'Hershey's Chocolate Milk Mix' (Hershey's)	3 heaping tsp	90	<1.0	22.0	40	na	<1.0	na	0	<9%
protein powder, prepared w/lowfat milk (Turbo Nutrition) ..	8 oz	330	36.0	34.0	450	na	6.0	na	na	16%
'Quik' (Nestlé)	1 heaping tsp	90	1.0	20.0	25	(mq)	1.0	(mq)	0	10%
'Quik' prepared w/skim milk (Nestlé)	1 cup	170	9.0	31.0	150	(mq)	1.0	(mq)	(mq)	5%
'Quik' prepared w/2% milk (Nestlé)	1 cup	210	9.0	31.0	150	(mq)	5.0	(mq)	(mq)	22%
'Quik' prepared w/whole milk (Nestlé)	1 cup	230	9.0	31.0	150	(mq)	9.0	(mq)	(mq)	34%
'Quik' sugar-free, approx 1 heaping tsp (Nestlé)	.2 oz	18	1.0	3.0	35	(mq)	<1.0	na	na	<36%
'Quik' sugar-free, prepared w/2% milk (Nestlé)	1 cup	140	9.0	15.0	150	(mq)	5.0	(mq)	(mq)	32%
weight gain protein powder, (Turbo Nutrition)	2 oz	210	28.0	22.0	320	na	1.0	na	na	4%
Refrigerated										
'Hershey's Genuine' (Hershey's)	8 oz	150	5.0	28.0	85	na	2.0	na	na	12%
(Yoo-Hoo)	9 oz	140	3.0	27.0	130	0	1.0	(tr)	(tr)	7%
CHOCOLATE MILK										
whole	1 cup	208	7.9	25.8	149	>.2 c	8.5	5.3	30	36%
whole	1 oz	26	1.0	3.2	19	(mq)	1.1	0.7	4	37%
whole (Hershey's)	1 cup	210	7.0	28.0	120	(mq)	9.0	(mq)	(mq)	37%
whole (Nestlé Quik)	1 cup	230	7.0	31.0	120	0.0	9.0	5.0	30	35%
3.5% fat (Hershey's)	1 cup	210	7.0	28.0	120	na	8.0	na	na	34%
2% fat	1 cup	179	8.0	26.0	150	(mq)	5.0	3.1	17	25%
2% fat (Darigold)	1 cup	190	8.0	28.0	210	(mq)	5.0	3.1	17	24%
2% fat (Lucerne)	1 cup	200	8.0	29.0	200	0.0	5.0	3.0	25	23%
2% fat (Hershey's)	1 cup	190	8.0	29.0	130	(mq)	5.0	(mq)	20	23%
2% fat 'Dutch Brand' (Borden)	1 cup	180	8.0	25.0	180	(mq)	5.0	(mq)	(mq)	25%
1% fat	1 cup	158	8.1	26.1	152	(mq)	2.5	1.5	7	14%
CHOCOLATE SAUCE. See SAUCE.										
CHOCOLATE SYRUP										
chocolate-flavored (Hershey's)	2 tbsp	103	0.9	23.9	19	<1.0	.4	.3	0	8%
'Choco-Syp' (Estee)	1 tbsp	20	0.0	5.0	5	na	0.0	0.0	0	0%
fudge-type	1 cup	1176	15.0	200.3	442	>8.2 c	45.6	19.2	41	32%
fudge type	1 oz	124	1.9	20.3	33	>.2 c	5.1	2.9	0	34%
fudge-type	1 tbsp	73	0.9	12.4	27	>.5 c	2.8	1.2	3	32%
'Quik' (Nestlé)	1.22 oz	100	1.0	22.0	45	(mq)	1.0	na	0	9%
unsweetened, 1 oz	1 pkt	134	3.4	9.6	3	>.9 c	13.5	7.2	0	70%
w/added nutrients	1 cup	735	5.4	197.4	459	5.4	3.9	2.3	0	4%
w/added nutrients	1 oz	92	0.7	24.7	57	>.2 c	0.5	0.3	0	4%
w/added nutrients	1 tbsp	46	0.3	12.4	29	.3	0.2	0.1	0	3%
w/o added nutrients	1 cup	654	5.7	170.7	399	5.4	2.7	1.6	0	3%
w/o added nutrients	1 oz	82	0.7	22.1	36	.7	0.3	0.2	0	3%
CHOCOLATE TOPPING										
(Kraft)	1 tbsp	50	1.0	11.0	15	(mq)	0.0	0.0	0	0%
(Mrs. Richardson's) dark chocolate fudge	2 tbsp	130	1.0	19.0	55	na	6.0	na	0	40%
(Mrs. Richardson's) dark, fudge, microwavable	2 tbsp	130	1.0	19.0	55	na	6.0	na	0	40%
(Nestlé) milk chocolate, w/almonds 'Candytops'	1.25 oz	230	2.0	14.0	15	(mq)	18.0	(mq)	(mq)	72%

Food Name	Serving Size	Calories	Prot. gms	Carbs gms	Sod. mgs	Fiber gms	Fat gms	Sat. Fat gms	Chol. mgs	% Fat Cal.
(Nestlé) milk chocolate, w/crisps 'Crunch Candytops'	2 tbsp	220	2.0	16.0	40	(mq)	17.0	(mq)	(mq)	68%
(Nestlé) white chocolate, w/almonds 'Candytops'	1.25 oz	230	3.0	12.0	20	(mq)	19.0	(mq)	na	74%
(Smucker's) chocolate fudge 'Magic Shell'	2 tbsp	190	1.0	16.0	50	na	15.0	na	na	67%
(Smucker's) dark chocolate 'Special Recipe'	2 tbsp	130	1.0	31.0	45	(mq)	1.0	na	na	7%
(Smucker's) flavored syrup	2 tbsp	130	1.0	27.0	35	(mq)	2.0	(mq)	na	14%
(Smucker's) 'Magic Shell'	2 tbsp	190	1.0	16.0	25	na	15.0	na	na	67%
(Smucker's) milk chocolate fudge, Swiss	2 tbsp	140	3.0	31.0	70	(mq)	1.0	na	na	6%
(Smucker's) nut 'Magic Shell'	2 tbsp	200	2.0	25.0	40	(mq)	16.0	(mq)	na	57%
CHORIZO										
....	1 oz	129	6.8	0.5	350	0	10.9	4.1	25	77%
4 inches	1 link	273	14.5	1.1	741	0	23.0	8.6	53	77%
(Carmelita) beef	2.5 oz	250	8.0	5.0	510	0	23.0	11.0	80	80%
(Carmelita) pork	2.5 oz	250	8.0	3.0	500	0	23.0	9.0	110	83%
CHOW MEIN										
chicken, w/o noodles, can	1 cup	95	6.5	17.7	725	>.8 c	0.3	0.0	8	3%
vegetarian, Mandarin, prepared w/tofu *(Tofu Classics)*	1/2 cup	110	8.0	14.0	390	(mq)	6.0	(mq)	0	38%
CHOW MEIN NOODLE										
with almonds *(Chun King)*	1/3 cup	140	4.0	15.0	380	1	7.0	1.5	0	45%
with sesame bits *(Chun King)*.	1/3 cup	140	3.0	16.0	460	1	7.0	1.0	0	45%
CHRYSANTHEMUM GARLAND										
boiled, drained	4 oz	23	1.9	4.9	60	>1.3 c	0.1	(tr)	0	3%
boiled, drained, 1-inch pieces	1/2 cup	10	0.8	2.2	27	1.2	0.1	na	0	7%
raw, 1 stem, 8.75 inches long	.5 oz	2	0.2	0.6	7	.4	<.1	(tr)	0	<22%
raw, 1-inch pieces	1 cup	4	0.4	1.1	13	.7	0.0	na	0	0%
raw, 8.75 inches long	1 stem	2	0.2	0.6	7	>.1 c	0.0	na	0	0%
raw, trimmed	1 oz	5	0.4	1.2	15	>.3 c	<.1	(tr)	0	<12%
raw, untrimmed	1 lb	76	6.8	19.0	225	>3.9 c	0.8	na	0	7%
CHUB/cisco										
raw	1 lb	446	86.1	0.0	249	0	8.7	1.9	(mq)	19%
raw	1 oz	28	5.4	0.0	16	0	0.5	0.1	(mq)	17%
smoked	1 oz	50	4.6	0.0	135	0	3.3	0.5	9	62%
smoked	1 oz	50	4.6	0.0	135	0	3.3	0.5	9	62%
CILANTRO										
approx .8 oz	9 plants	4	0.5	0.5	6	>.2 c	0.1	(tr)	0	18%
trimmed	1 oz	6	0.7	0.7	8	>.2 c	0.2	(tr)	0	24%
trimmed	1/4 cup	1	0.1	0.1	1	>.1 c	<.1	(tr)	0	<53%
untrimmed	1 lb	77	9.1	10.0	108	>3.1 c	2.3	na	0	21%
CILANTRO LEAF										
dried	1 oz	79	6.2	14.8	60	>2.9 c	1.3	na	0	12%
dried	1 tbsp	5	0.4	0.9	4	>.2 c	0.1	(tr)	0	15%
dried	1 tsp	2	0.1	0.3	1	>.1 c	<.1	(tr)	0	<36%
CILANTRO SEED										
whole	1 oz	84	3.5	15.6	10	>8.3 c	5.0	0.3	0	37%
whole	1 tbsp	15	0.6	2.8	2	>1.5 c	0.9	0.1	0	37%
whole	1 tsp	5	0.2	1.0	1	>.5 c	0.3	<.1	0	36%
whole *(Spice Islands)*	1 tsp	6	0.2	0.8	<1	>.4 c	0.3	<.1	0	40%
CINNAMON										
ground	1 oz	74	1.1	22.6	7	>6.9 c	0.9	0.2	0	8%
ground	1 tbsp	18	0.3	5.4	2	3.7	0.2	0.0	0	7%
ground	1 tsp	6	0.1	1.8	1	1.3	0.1	0.0	0	11%
ground *(Durkee)*	1 tsp	8	0.0	0.0	0	0	tr	na	na	tr
ground *(Laurel Leaf)*	1 tsp	8	0.0	0.0	0	0	tr	na	na	tr
ground *(Spice Islands)*	1 tsp	6	0.1	1.4	<1	>.3 c	<.1	(tr)	0	<13%

CISCO. See CHUB.

Food Name	Serving Size	Calories	Prot. gms	Carbs gms	Sod. mgs	Fiber gms	Fat gms	Sat. Fat gms	Chol. mgs	% Fat Cal.
CITRON, candied	1 oz	88	0.1	22.5	81	>.4 c	0.1	0.0	0	1%
CITRUS COOLER DRINK (Gatorade) 'Thirst Quencher'	8 oz	50	0.0	14.0	110	na	0.0	na	na	0%
CITRUS DRINK										
(Five Alive) chilled	6 oz	90	0.0	22.0	20	na	0.0	na	na	0%
(Fruitopia) 'Citrus Consciousness' real fruit	8 oz	120	0.0	30.0	25	na	0.0			0%
CITRUS DRINK MIX										
(Crystal Light) blend, sugar-free, w/NutraSweet	8 oz	4	0.0	0.0	0	na	0.0	na	0	0%
(Five Alive) frozen, diluted	6 oz	90	0.0	22.0	na	na	0.0	0.0	na	0%
CITRUS FRUIT JUICE DRINK										
frozen concentrate	12-oz can	685	5.1	170.5	13	>.4 c	0.4	0.0	0	1%
frozen concentrate, diluted	1 cup	114	0.7	28.5	7	0	0.0	0.0	0	0%
(Five Alive) aseptic box	8.45 oz	123	0.8	30.7	32	(tr)	0.0	0.0	0	0%
(Five Alive) chilled or frozen, berry, diluted	6 oz	88	0.2	22.1	21	(tr)	0.1	(tr)	0	1%
(Five Alive) chilled or frozen, diluted	6 oz	87	0.6	21.8	23	(tr)	0.0	(tr)	0	0%
(Five Alive) chilled or frozen, tropical, diluted	6 oz	85	0.4	21.3	19	(tr)	0.1	(tr)	0	1%
(Hi-C) 'Citrus Cooler'	6 oz	95	0.1	23.3	17	(tr)	<.1	(tr)	0	<1%
CITRUS GRILL MARINADE (Lawry's)	2 tbsp	34	3.8	3.4	3350	.1	0.4	0.1	0	11%
CITRUS JUICE (Santa Cruz Natural) organic 'Cruz'	8 oz	125	1.0	29.0	na	na	<1.0	na	na	<7%
CITRUS PUNCH										
(Minute Maid) can or bottle 'Juices To Go'	6 oz	90	0.0	23.0	20	na	0.0	na	na	0%
(Minute Maid) chilled	6 oz	90	0.0	23.0	20	na	0.0	na	na	0%
(Tampico) 2% orange, tangerine, and lemon juice	8 oz	120	<1.0	30.0	10	0	0.0	0.0	0	0%
CITRUS PUNCH DRINK										
(Sunny Delight) 'California Style'	8 oz	100	0.0	23.0	95	na	0.0	na	na	0%
(Sunny Delight) 'Florida Citrus Punch'	8 oz	120	0.0	27.0	125	na	<1.0	na	na	<8%
(Sunny Delight) 'Florida Citrus Punch' plus calcium	8 oz	130	0.0	32.0	125	na	<1.0	na	na	<7%
CITRUS PUNCH MIX (Minute Maid) frozen, concentrate	6 oz	90	0.0	22.0	0	na	0.0	na	na	0%
CITRUS SALAD (Florigold)	8 oz	120	2.7	27.2	3	(mq)	0.0	0.0	0	0%
CLAM, CANNED										
chopped (Gorton's)	3.25 oz	40	7.0	2.0	5.90	na	<1.0	na	20	<20%
chopped (Progresso)	1/2 cup	70	12.0	2.0	140	0	<1.0	(mq)	31	<14%
chopped, w/liquid (Doxsee)	6.5 oz	100	14.0	8.0	1160	0	<1.0	(mq)	(mq)	<9%
chopped, w/liquid (Orleans)	6.5 oz	100	14.0	8.0	1160	0	<1.0	(mq)	(mq)	<9%
minced (Gorton's)	3.25 oz	40	7.0	2.0	5.90	na	<1.0	na	20	<20%
minced (Progresso)	1/2 cup	70	12.0	2.0	140	0	<1.0	(mq)	31	<14%
minced, w/liquid (Doxsee)	6.5 oz	100	14.0	8.0	1160	0	<1.0	(mq)	(mq)	<9%
minced, w/liquid (Orleans)	6.5 oz	100	14.0	8.0	1160	0	<1.0	(mq)	(mq)	<9%
mixed species, drained	1 cup	237	40.9	8.2	179	0	3.1	0.3	107	12%
mixed species, drained	4 oz	168	29.0	5.8	127	0	2.2	0.2	76	13%
mixed species, drained	3 oz	126	21.7	4.4	95	0	1.7	0.2	57	13%
mixed species, liquid only	1 cup	5	1.0	0.2	516	0	0.1	0.0	7	16%
mixed species, liquid only	3 oz	2	0.3	0.1	183	0	0.0	0.0	3	0%
CLAM, MIXED SPECIES										
boiled	4 oz	168	29.0	5.8	127	0	2.2	2.1	76	13%
breaded and fried	20 small	380	26.8	19.4	684	>.3 c	21.0	5.0	115	51%
breaded and fried	4 oz	229	16.1	11.7	413	>.2 c	12.6	3.0	69	51%
breaded and fried	3 oz	172	12.1	8.8	309	>.1 c	9.5	2.3	52	51%
moist-heat cooked	20 small	133	23.0	4.6	101	0	1.8	0.2	60	13%
moist-heat cooked	3 oz	126	21.7	4.4	95	0	1.7	0.2	57	13%
poached	4 oz	168	29.0	5.8	127	0	2.2	2.1	76	13%
raw	1 lb	335	57.9	11.6	253	0	4.4	0.4	152	13%
raw	1 oz	21	3.6	0.7	16	0	0.3	<.1	10	14%
raw	20 small	133	23.0	4.6	101	0	1.8	0.2	61	13%
raw	9 large	133	23.0	4.6	101	0	1.8	0.2	61	13%

Food Name	Serving Size	Calories	Prot. gms	Carbs gms	Sod. mgs	Fiber gms	Fat gms	Sat. Fat gms	Chol. mgs	% Fat Cal.
raw	3 oz	63	10.9	2.2	48	0	0.8	0.1	29	12%
steamed	4 oz	168	29.0	5.8	127	0	2.2	2.1	76	13%
CLAM, STUFFED, New England style *(Matlaw's)*	2 clams	180	8.0	21.0	730	3.0	8.0	1.0	0	38%
CLAM JUICE										
(Doxsee)	3 oz	4	<1.0	0.0	110	0	0.0	0.0	na	0%
(Snow's)	3 oz	4	<1.0	0.0	110	0	0.0	0.0	na	0%
CLAM SAUCE. See SAUCE.										
CLAM TOMATO JUICE, canned	5.5 oz	76	1.0	18.1	664	>.2 c	0.2	0.0	0	2%
CLARIFIED BUTTER. See GHEE.										
CLEARMALT. See ALCOHOLIC BEVERAGES.										
CLOVES										
ground	1 tbsp	21	0.4	4.0	16	2.3	1.3	0.3	0	40%
ground	1 tsp	7	0.1	1.3	5	.7	0.4	0.1	0	39%
ground *(Durkee)*	1 tsp	9	0.0	0.0	0	0	<0.1	na	na	<30%
ground *(Laurel Leaf)*	1 tsp	9	0.0	0.0	0	0	<0.1	na	na	<30%
ground *(Spice Islands)*	1 tsp	7	0.1	1.2	4	.7	0.2	na	0	26%
CLUB SODA. See SOFT DRINKS AND MIXERS.										
COATING MIX. See SEASONING AND COATING MIX.										
COBBLER										
Fresh										
apple *(Stilwell)*	4 oz	200	2.0	4.0	225	(mq)	4.0	(mq)	na	60%
apple, deep dish *(Awrey's)*	1/8 pie	320	2.0	48.0	300	1.0	14.0	3.0	0	39%
blueberry, deep dish *(Awrey's)*	1/8 pie	310	2.0	45.0	360	2.0	14.0	3.0	0	40%
Frozen										
apple, 4.33 oz *(Pet-Ritz)*	1/6 pkg	290	1.0	50.0	(mq)	(mq)	9.0	(mq)	na	28%
blackberry *(Stilwell)*	4 oz	280	3.0	50.0	220	(mq)	8.0	(mq)	na	25%
blackberry, 4.33 oz *(Pet-Ritz)*	1/6 pkg	250	2.0	39.0	(mq)	(mq)	10.0	(mq)	na	35%
blueberry, 4.33 oz *(Pet-Ritz)*	1/6 pkg	370	3.0	50.0	(mq)	(mq)	12.0	(mq)	na	34%
cherry *(Stilwell)*	4 oz	250	3.0	46.0	205	(mq)	6.0	(mq)	na	22%
cherry, 4.33 oz *(Pet-Ritz)*	1/6 pkg	280	2.0	46.0	(mq)	(mq)	10.0	(mq)	na	32%
peach *(Stilwell)*	4 oz	270	2.0	55.0	200	(mq)	5.0	(mq)	na	17%
peach, 4.33 oz *(Pet-Ritz)*	1/6 pkg	260	2.0	46.0	(mq)	(mq)	10.0	(mq)	na	32%
strawberry, 4.33 oz *(Pet-Ritz)*	1/6 pkg	290	1.0	50.0	(mq)	(mq)	9.0	(mq)	na	28%
COBNUT, SHELLED. See HAZELNUT, SHELLED.										
COCKTAIL ONION. See ONION, COCKTAIL.										
COCKTAIL SAUCE. See SAUCE.										
COCOA BUTTER OIL										
	1 cup	1927	0.0	0.0	0	0	218.0	130.1	0	100%
	1 oz	251	0.0	0.0	0	0	28.4	16.9	0	100%
	1 tbsp	120	0.0	0.0	0	0	13.6	8.1	0	100%
COCOA MIX										
Amaretto creme flavor *(Swiss Miss)*	1.25 oz	150	2.0	29.0	220	(mq)	3.0	(mq)	na	18%
Bavarian chocolate, hot cocoa *(Swiss Miss)*	1 oz	110	1.0	20.0	170	0	3.0	1.3	2	24%
chocolate, w/marshmallows *(Carnation)*	1 oz	110	1.0	24.0	120	.2	1.2	1.1	2	10%
chocolate almond mocha *(Swiss Miss)*	1.235 oz	144	1.9	28.0	207	1.5	2.7	0.8	1	17%
chocolate and mint 'Cocoa Classics' *(Land O'Lakes)*	1 envelope	160	4.0	24.0	160	na	5.0	na	na	29%
chocolate and raspberry 'Cocoa Classics' *(Land O'Lakes)*	1 envelope	160	4.0	25.0	160	na	5.0	na	na	28%
chocolate Bavarian mint *(Swiss Miss)*	1.235 oz	142	1.9	28.3	231	1.5	2.3	69.0	1	15%
chocolate English toffee *(Swiss Miss)*	1.235 oz	142	1.8	28.5	223	na	2.3	0.7	1	15%
chocolate flavor *(Pathmark)*	1 oz	110	2.0	24.0	110	(mq)	1.0	(mq)	na	8%
chocolate flavor *(Swiss Miss)*	1 oz	110	1.0	24.0	125	(mq)	1.0	na	na	8%
chocolate flavor 'Sugar-free' *(Swiss Miss)*	.5 oz	50	2.0	9.0	130	(mq)	1.0	0.2	<1	17%
chocolate fudge flavor *(Carnation)*	1-oz pkt	110	1.0	24.0	135	.3	1.3	1.1	1	11%
chocolate praline and creme *(Swiss Miss)*	1.235 oz	142	2.8	28.5	223	1.5	2.3	0.7	1	14%

Food Name	Serving Size	Calories	Prot. gms	Carbs gms	Sod. mgs	Fiber gms	Fat gms	Sat. Fat gms	Chol. mgs	% Fat Cal.
chocolate raspberry truffle (Swiss Miss)	1.235 oz	144	1.8	27.8	220	1.5	2.8	0.8	1	18%
chocolate supreme 'Cocoa Classics' (Land O'Lakes)	1 envelope	160	4.0	25.0	160	na	5.0	na	na	28%
dark chocolate truffle (Swiss Miss)	1.235 oz	142	2.0	27.9	225	1.5	2.5	0.9	1	16%
diet (Swiss Miss)	.26 oz	20	2.0	3.0	180	0	<1.0	(mq)	1	<31%
diet 'Hot Cocoa Mix' (Swiss Miss)	.26 oz	22	1.9	3.8	205	.7	0.2	0.1	0	7%
double rich chocolate flavor (Swiss Miss)	1 oz	110	2.0	24.0	125	(mq)	1.0	na	0	8%
fat-free 'Hot Cocoa Mix' (Swiss Miss)	.5 oz	50	3.3	9.0	197	.7	0.3	0.0	2	5%
lite (Swiss Miss)	.75 oz	70	1.0	17.0	160	0	<1.0	(mq)	1	<11%
lite 'Hot Cocoa Mix' (Swiss Miss)	.7407 oz	74	1.5	17.1	197	1.6	0.5	0.2	0	6%
marshmallow lovers 'Hot Cocoa Mix' (Swiss Miss)	1.199 oz	132	1.6	23.6	167	.9	1.5	0.3	2	12%
milk chocolate flavor (Alba '66)	.68 oz	60	6.0	10.0	160	na	0.0	na	na	0%
milk chocolate flavor (Saco Foods)	1 oz	110	2.0	24.0	150	na	1.0	na	na	8%
milk chocolate flavor (Swiss Miss)	1-oz pkt	110	1.0	20.0	170	(mq)	3.0	1.3	<1	24%
milk chocolate flavor 'Sugar-free' (Swiss Miss)	.5 oz	60	3.0	10.0	125	(mq)	0.0	0.0	na	0%
milk chocolate flavor, w/marshmallows (Alba '66)	.68 oz	60	6.0	10.0	160	na	0.0	na	na	0%
milk chocolate 'Hot Cocoa Mix' (Swiss Miss)	1.199 oz	133	1.7	28.9	169	.9	1.5	0.3	2	10%
milk chocolate 'Hot Cocoa Mix' (Swiss Miss)	1 oz	110	1.4	23.9	139	.8	1.3	0.2	1	10%
milk chocolate w/mini marshmallows 'Hot Cocoa Mix' (Swiss Miss)	1.199 oz	132	1.8	28.5	181	.9	1.5	0.5	1	10%
milk chocolate w/mini marshmallows 'Hot Cocoa Mix' (Swiss Miss)	1 oz	109	1.5	23.5	149	.8	1.3	0.4	1	11%
milk flavor (Carnation)	1-oz pkt	110	2.0	24.0	130	.2	1.1	1.0	1	9%
mini (Pathmark)	1 oz	110	2.0	24.0	140	(mq)	1.0	(mq)	na	8%
mint flavor (Featherweight)	.44 oz	50	2.0	8.0	110	(mq)	1.0	(mq)	0	18%
mocha flavor 'Sugar-free' (Carnation)	1 pkt	50	3.0	9.0	140	.1	0.3	0.2	2	5%
reduced calorie, aspartame sweetened	1 oz	8	0.6	1.4	(mq)	(mq)	0.1	<.1	na	10%
regular (Finast)	6 oz	110	2.0	24.0	150	(mq)	1.0	(mq)	na	8%
rich, sugar-free 'Hot Cocoa Mix' (Swiss Miss)	.5 oz	50	2.6	10.0	165	.8	0.3	0.1	0	5%
rich chocolate 'Hot Cocoa Mix' (Swiss Miss)	1 oz	110	1.8	23.5	166	.8	1.2	0.4	1	10%
rich milk flavor (Carnation)	1-oz pkt	110	1.0	24.0	120	.2	1.1	1.0	1	9%
rich milk flavor 'Sugar-free' (Carnation)	1 pkt	50	4.0	8.0	160	.1	0.4	0.2	3	7%
rich milk flavor, w/marshmallows (Weight Watchers)	1 pkt	60	6.0	10.0	160	(mq)	0.0	0.0	0	0%
'70-Calorie' (Carnation)	1 pkt	70	3.0	16.0	135	>.2 c	0.3	0.2	1	3%
'Sugar-free' (Hills Bros)	3 tbsp	60	2.0	9.0	145	(mq)	2.0	(mq)	na	29%
sugar-free 'Hot Cocoa Mix' (Swiss Miss)	.7055 oz	67	3.2	13.6	242	.9	0.3	0.1	1	4%
sugar-free 'Hot Cocoa Mix' (Swiss Miss)	.5 oz	49	2.4	10.0	179	.7	0.2	0.1	0	4%
sugar-free, sweetened w/NutraSweet (Saco Foods)	1 pkt	50	3.0	9.0	150	na	1.0	na	na	16%
sugar-free, w/mini marshmallows 'Hot Cocoa Mix' (Swiss Miss)	.7055 oz	68	1.9	13.9	210	.9	0.8	0.3	2	10%
sugar-free, w/mini marshmallows 'Hot Cocoa Mix' (Swiss Miss)	.5 oz	51	1.4	10.5	159	.7	0.6	0.2	1	10%
vending 'Hot Cocoa Mix' (Swiss Miss)	1.34 oz	146	1.8	31.7	185	1.0	1.7	0.3	2	10%
white chocolate 'Hot Cocoa Mix' (Swiss Miss)	1 oz	111	3.0	21.4	130	.1	1.4	0.4	1	11%
w/added nutrients	1-oz pkt	120	1.9	24.0	201	>.2 c	3.0	1.8	1	21%
w/added nutrients, prepared	1 pkt	119	1.9	24.0	207	>.2 c	2.9	1.8	0	20%
w/aspartame	.53-oz pkt	48	3.8	8.4	104	.4	0.4	0.3	2	7%
w/aspartame, w/added calcium and potassium	.53-oz pkt	48	3.8	8.5	98	.4	0.5	0.3	1	8%
w/aspartame, w/added sodium and vitamin A	.53-oz pkt	48	3.8	8.5	168	.4	0.5	0.3	1	8%
w/marshmallows (Carnation)	1-oz pkt	110	1.0	24.0	120	.2	1.0	0.9	1	8%
w/mini marshmallows (Finast)	6 oz	110	2.0	24.0	150	(mq)	1.0	(mq)	na	8%
w/mini marshmallows (Swiss Miss)	1 oz	110	1.0	23.0	140	(mq)	1.0	na	na	9%
w/mini marshmallows 'Sugar-free' (Swiss Miss)	.5-oz pkt	50	3.0	9.0	120	(mq)	<1.0	na	na	<16%
w/o added nutrients	1-oz pkt	103	3.1	22.5	143	.3	1.1	0.7	1	9%
w/o added nutrients, prepared	3-4 heaping tsp	103	3.1	22.5	148	2.5	1.2	0.7	2	10%

Food Name	Serving Size	Calories	Prot. gms	Carbs gms	Sod. mgs	Fiber gms	Fat gms	Sat. Fat gms	Chol. mgs	% Fat Cal.
COCOA POWDER. See also CHOCOLATE, BAKING.										
(Bensdorp)	1 oz	130	6.0	8.0	5	(mq)	7.0	(mq)	<1	53%
(Hershey's) approx 1/3 cup	1 oz	120	7.0	13.0	10	(mq)	4.0	(mq)	0	31%
(Hershey's) 'European'	1 oz	90	7.0	8.0	15	(mq)	3.0	(mq)	0	31%
(Hershey's) unsweetened, European style	1 cup	170	16.6	48.8	52	>4.5 c	8.3	na	0	22%
(Hershey's) unsweetened, European style	1 tbsp	10	1.0	2.8	3	>.3 c	0.5	na	0	23%
(Nestlé)	1.5 oz	180	11.0	21.0	6	(mq)	6.0	(mq)	na	30%
COCONUT										
mature kernel, in shell	1 lb	834	7.9	35.9	47	21.2	79.0	70.0	0	80%
mature kernel, shelled	1 oz	100	0.9	4.3	6	2.6	9.5	8.4	0	80%
mature kernel, shelled, grated, packed	1 cup	460	4.3	19.8	26	11.7	43.5	38.6	0	80%
meat, raw, 2 x 2 x 1/2 inch	1 piece	159	1.5	6.8	9	4.1	15.1	13.4	0	80%
meat, raw, shredded	1 cup	283	2.7	12.2	16	7.2	26.8	23.8	0	80%
COCONUT, DRIED										
creamed	1 oz	194	1.5	6.1	11	>1.1 c	19.6	17.4	0	85%
sweetened, flaked, canned	4 oz	505	3.8	46.6	23	5.1	36.1	32.0	0	62%
sweetened, flaked, canned	1 cup	341	2.6	31.5	15	3.5	24.4	21.6	0	62%
sweetened, flaked, canned	1 oz	126	0.9	11.6	6	>.6 c	9.0	8.0	0	62%
sweetened, flaked, canned 'Angel Flake' (Baker's)	1/3 cup	110	1.0	10.0	5	(mq)	9.0	(mq)	0	65%
sweetened, flaked, packaged	7-oz pkg	943	6.5	94.7	509	8.6	64.0	56.7	0	59%
sweetened, flaked, packaged	1 cup	351	2.4	35.2	189	3.2	23.8	21.1	0	59%
sweetened, flaked, packaged	1 oz	134	0.9	13.5	73	>.6 c	9.1	8.1	0	59%
sweetened, flaked, packaged 'Angel Flake' (Baker's)	1/3 cup	120	1.0	10.0	75	(mq)	8.0	(mq)	0	62%
sweetened, flaked, packaged 'Snowflake' (Finast)	1 oz	137	1.0	12.0	<1	(mq)	9.0	(mq)	0	61%
sweetened, flaked, packaged, toasted (Baker's)	1/3 cup	200	2.0	17.0	85	(mq)	17.0	(mq)	0	67%
sweetened, shredded	7-oz pkg	997	5.7	94.9	521	9.0	70.6	62.6	0	61%
sweetened, shredded	1 cup	466	2.7	44.3	244	4.2	33.0	29.3	0	61%
sweetened, shredded	1 oz	142	0.8	13.5	74	>.6 c	10.1	8.9	0	61%
sweetened, shredded 'Premium Shred' (Baker's)	1/3 cup	140	1.0	12.0	85	(mq)	9.0	(mq)	0	61%
sweetened, shredded, toasted	1 oz	168	1.5	12.6	11	>.7 c	13.4	11.8	0	68%
sweetened, shredded, toasted 'Angel Flake' (Baker's)	1/3 cup	200	2.0	17.0	85	na	17.0	na	0	67%
unsweetened	1 oz	187	2.0	6.7	11	3.2	18.3	16.3	0	83%
COCONUT CREAM										
Canned										
liquid expressed from grated meat	1 cup	568	8.0	24.7	148	>6.9 c	52.5	46.5	0	78%
liquid expressed from grated meat	1 tbsp	36	0.5	1.6	10	>.4 c	3.4	3.0	0	79%
sweetened	1 oz	54	0.8	2.4	14	(mq)	5.0	4.5	0	78%
sweetened (Coco Lopez)	2 tbsp	120	0.0	20.0	10	(mq)	5.0	(mq)	0	36%
sweetened (Holland House)	1 oz	81	0.0	18.0	21	(mq)	(mq)	(mq)	0	0%
Raw										
liquid expressed from grated meat	1 cup	792	8.7	16.0	10	>8.9 c	83.2	73.8	0	88%
liquid expressed from grated meat	1 tbsp	49	0.5	1.0	1	>.6 c	5.2	4.6	0	89%
liquid expressed from grated meat	1 oz	94	1.0	1.9	1	(mq)	9.8	8.7	0	88%
COCONUT MILK										
canned	1 cup	445	4.6	6.3	29	>4.9 c	48.2	42.8	0	91%
canned	1 oz	56	0.6	0.8	4	(mq)	6.0	5.4	0	91%
canned	1 tbsp	30	0.3	0.4	2	>.3 c	3.2	2.8	0	91%
frozen	1 cup	485	3.9	13.4	29	>5.5 c	49.9	44.3	0	87%
frozen	1 oz	57	0.5	1.6	3	(mq)	5.9	5.2	0	86%
frozen	1 tbsp	30	0.2	0.8	2	>.3 c	3.1	2.8	0	88%
raw	1 cup	552	5.5	13.3	36	>6.3 c	57.2	50.7	0	87%
raw	1 oz	65	0.6	1.6	4	(mq)	6.8	6.0	0	87%
raw	1 tbsp	35	0.3	0.8	2	>.4 c	3.6	3.2	0	88%
COCONUT NECTAR (Knudsen & Sons)	8 oz	150	<1.0	29.0	na	na	0.0	na	na	0%

Food Name	Serving Size	Calories	Prot. gms	Carbs gms	Sod. mgs	Fiber gms	Fat gms	Sat. Fat gms	Chol. mgs	% Fat Cal.
COCONUT OIL										
....	1/2 cup	964	0.0	0.0	0	0	109.0	94.3	0	100%
....	1 oz	251	0.0	0.0	0	0	28.4	24.5	0	100%
....	1 tbsp	120	0.0	0.0	0	0	13.6	11.8	0	100%
(Hain)	1 tbsp	120	0.0	0.0	0	0	14.0	12.0	0	100%
COCONUT PINEAPPLE NECTAR, can or bottle *(Kern's)*	6 oz	140	1.0	26.0	25	na	4.0	na	na	25%
COCONUT VEGETABLE OIL										
....	1 cup	1879	0.0	0.0	0	0	218.0	188.6	0	100%
....	1 tbsp	117	0.0	0.0	0	0	13.6	11.8	0	100%
COCONUT WATER										
....	1 cup	46	1.7	8.9	252	2.6	0.5	0.4	0	10%
....	1 oz	5	0.2	1.1	30	>.1 c	0.1	<.1	0	15%
....	1 tbsp	3	0.1	0.6	16	.2	0.0	0.0	0	0%
COD, ALASKAN										
raw	1 oz	55	3.8	0.0	16	0	4.3	0.9	14	72%
raw, 6.8 oz	1/2 fillet	377	25.9	0.0	108	0	29.5	6.2	95	72%
smoked	4 oz	291	20.0	0.0	836	0	22.8	4.8	73	72%
COD, ATLANTIC										
baked	4 oz	119	25.9	0.0	88	0	1.0	0.2	62	8%
broiled	4 oz	119	25.9	0.0	88	0	1.0	0.2	62	8%
dried and salted	3 oz	247	53.4	0.0	5973	0	2.0	0.4	129	8%
dried and salted	1 oz	81	17.6	0.0	1968	0	0.7	0.1	42	8%
dry-heat cooked	3 oz	89	19.4	0.0	66	0	0.7	0.1	47	8%
microwaved	4 oz	119	25.9	0.0	88	0	1.0	0.2	62	8%
raw	1 lb	372	80.8	0.0	246	0	3.1	0.6	195	8%
raw	3 oz	70	15.1	0.0	46	0	0.6	0.1	37	8%
raw	1 oz	23	5.0	0.0	15	0	0.2	<.1	12	8%
COD, BLACK										
raw	1 lb	886	60.8	0.0	254	0	69.4	14.5	222	72%
raw	1 oz	55	3.8	0.0	16	0	4.3	0.9	14	72%
smoked	1 oz	73	5.0	0.0	209	0	5.7	1.2	18	72%
COD, FROZEN										
breaded 'Light' *(Mrs. Paul's)*	1 piece	240	15.0	22.0	430	(mq)	11.0	(mq)	(mq)	40%
breaded 'Light' *(Van de Kamp's)*	1 piece	250	17.0	20.0	510	(mq)	11.0	2.0	35	40%
breaded, lemon thyme crumb 'Select' *(Gorton's)*	1 fillet	90	12.0	5.0	240	na	2.0	<1.0	45	21%
fillet *(Booth)*	4 oz	89	20.0	0.0	350	0	1.0	(mq)	(mq)	10%
fillet *(Finast)*	4 oz	80	18.0	0.0	200	0	1.0	(mq)	(mq)	11%
fillet *(SeaPak)*	4 oz	90	20.0	0.0	135	0	1.0	(mq)	(mq)	10%
fillet 'Fishmarket Fresh' *(Gorton's)*	5 oz	110	26.0	0.0	90	0	1.0	(mq)	(mq)	8%
fillet 'Individually Wrapped' *(Booth)*	4 oz	90	20.0	0.0	80	0	1.0	(mq)	(mq)	10%
fillet, light *(Van de Kamp's)*	1 piece	250	17.0	20.0	510	na	11.0	2.0	35	40%
fillet, natural *(Van de Kamp's)*	4 oz	90	20.0	0.0	90	0	1.0	0.0	25	10%
natural *(Van de Kamp's)*	4 oz	90	20.0	0.0	90	na	1.0	0.0	25	10%
COD, PACIFIC										
dry-heat cooked	3 oz	89	19.5	0.0	77	0	0.7	0.1	40	8%
fillets, raw *(Peter Pan Seafoods)*	3.5 oz	80	17.0	na	71	na	0.6	na	37	7%
raw	1 lb	372	81.2	0.0	322	0	2.9	0.4	168	7%
raw	3 oz	70	15.2	0.0	60	0	0.5	0.1	31	7%
raw	1 oz	23	5.1	0.0	20	0	0.2	<.1	10	8%
COD CAKE, CANNED, 2 cakes *(Gorton's)*	4 oz	100	8.0	16.0	640	na	<1.0	na	15	<9%
COD ENTRÉE, FROZEN										
fillet, au gratin *(Booth)*	9.5 oz	280	27.0	18.0	1160	(mq)	11.0	(mq)	(mq)	36%
fillet, Florentine *(Booth)*	9.5 oz	244	20.0	29.0	880	(mq)	6.0	(mq)	(mq)	22%
fillet, w/lemon butter sauce and rice *(Booth)*	9.5 oz	567	22.0	27.0	1330	(mq)	38.0	(mq)	(mq)	64%

Food Name	Serving Size	Calories	Prot. gms	Carbs gms	Sod. mgs	Fiber gms	Fat gms	Sat. Fat gms	Chol. mgs	% Fat Cal.
fillet, w/mushroom sauce and rice *(Booth)*	9.5 oz	280	27.0	19.0	1010	(mq)	11.0	(mq)	(mq)	35%
COD LIVER OIL										
cherry *(Hain)*	1 tbsp	120	0.0	0.0	0	0	14.0	(mq)	75	100%
mint *(Hain)*	1 tbsp	120	0.0	0.0	0	0	14.0	(mq)	85	100%
regular	1 cup	1966	0.0	0.0	0	0	218.0	49.3	1243	100%
regular	1 tbsp	123	0.0	0.0	0	0	13.6	3.1	78	100%
regular *(Hain)*	1 tbsp	120	0.0	0.0	0	0	14.0	(mq)	85	100%
COD NUGGETS, FROZEN										
minced, crunchy 'Bunch O'Crunch' 4 oz *(Frionor)*	8 pieces	320	14.0	19.0	411	<1.0	21.0	3.0	(mq)	59%
COFFEE										
brewed	6 oz	4	0.2	0.7	2	0	0.0	0.0	0	0%
brewed 'Regular' *(Chock Full o'Nuts)*	6 oz	2	(mq)	(mq)	0	0	0.0	0.0	0	0%
freeze-dried, prepared, dark roast 'Maragor' *(Taster's Choice)*	8 oz	4	<1.0	1.0	0	0	<1.0	(tr)	0	<53%
freeze-dried, prepared 'Colombian Select' *(Taster's Choice)*	8 oz	4	<1.0	1.0	0	0	<1.0	(tr)	0	<53%
freeze-dried, prepared 'Original' *(Taster's Choice)*	8 oz	4	<1.0	1.0	0	0	<1.0	(tr)	0	<53%
COFFEE, ALTERNATIVE										
cereal grain beverage, powder *(Pero)*	1 serving	4	<1.0	<1.0	2	(tr)	0.0	0.0	0	0%
cereal grain beverage, powder *(Pionier)*	1 serving	6	0.0	1.4	0	(tr)	0.0	0.0	0	0%
cereal grain beverage, powder, dry	1 tsp	9	0.1	1.9	2	0	0.1	0.0	0	10%
cereal grain beverage, powder,'Instant,' prepared *(Postum)*	6 oz	12	0.0	3.0	0	na	0.0	0.0	0	0%
cereal grain beverage, prepared w/water	1 tsp	9	0.2	1.8	7	0	0.0	0.0	0	0%
cereal grain beverage prepared w/skim milk	6 oz	74	6.4	10.8	97	(tr)	0.4	0.2	3	5%
cereal grain beverage prepared w/1% milk	6 oz	86	6.1	10.6	94	(tr)	2.0	1.2	8	21%
cereal grain beverage prepared w/2% milk	6 oz	100	6.2	10.7	94	(tr)	3.6	2.2	14	32%
cereal grain beverage, prepared w/whole milk	6 oz	120	6.1	10.4	91	0	6.1	3.8	24	45%
cereal grain beverage, w/o added ingredients *(Kaffree Roma)*	8 oz	6	0.0	1.0	(mq)	na	0.0	0.0	0	0%
COFFEE, DECAFFEINATED										
(Chock Full o'Nuts)	6 oz	2	(mq)	(mq)	0	0	0.0	0.0	0	0%
freeze-dried, prepared, dark roast 'Maragor' *(Taster's Choice)*	8 oz	4	<1.0	1.0	0	0	<1.0	(tr)	0	<53%
freeze-dried, prepared 'Original' *(Taster's Choice)*	8 oz	4	<1.0	1.0	0	0	<1.0	(tr)	0	<53%
instant, powder	1 round tsp	4	0.2	0.8	0	0	0.0	0.0	0	0%
instant, powder, prepared	6 oz	4	0.2	0.7	5	0	0.0	0.0	0	0%
instant, prepared 'Decaf' *(Nescafé)*	8 oz	4	<1.0	1.0	0	0	<1.0	(tr)	0	<53%
instant, w/chicory, prepared *(Mountain Blend)*	8 oz	6	<1.0	1.0	0	0	<1.0	(tr)	0	<53%
'Suisse Mocha International' *(General Foods)*	6 oz	50	0.0	7.0	30	na	3.0	na	0	49%
'Suisse Mocha International' sugar-free *(General Foods)*	6 oz	30	0.0	3.0	30	na	2.0	na	0	60%
COFFEE, FLAVORED										
'Cafe Amaretto International' prepared *(General Foods)*	6 oz	50	0.0	7.0	20	(tr)	2.0	(mq)	0	39%
'Cafe Français International' prepared *(General Foods)*	6 oz	60	0.0	6.0	25	(tr)	3.0	(mq)	0	53%
'Cafe Français International' sugar-free prepared *(General Foods)*	6 oz	35	0.0	3.0	30	(tr)	2.0	(mq)	0	60%
'Cafe Irish Creme International' prepared *(General Foods)*	6 oz	50	0.0	8.0	15	(tr)	2.0	(mq)	0	36%
'Cafe Vienna International' prepared *(General Foods)*	6 oz	60	0.0	10.0	110	(tr)	2.0	(mq)	0	31%
'Cafe Vienna International' sugar-free, prepared *(General Foods)*	6 oz	30	0.0	3.0	80	(tr)	2.0	(mq)	0	60%
'Cappio Cinnamon Iced Cappuccino' *(Maxwell House)*	8 oz	130	2.0	25.0	70	na	3.0	na	15	20%

Food Name	Serving Size	Calories	Prot. gms	Carbs gms	Sod. mgs	Fiber gms	Fat gms	Sat. Fat gms	Chol. mgs	% Fat Cal.
cafe Vienna 'Cafe Coffees' prepared (Hills Bros)	6 oz	60	1.0	9.0	35	(tr)	2.0	(mq)	na	31%
'Cappio Coffee Iced Cappuccino' (Maxwell House)	8 oz	120	2.0	23.0	75	na	3.0	na	15	21%
'Cappio Mocha Iced Cappuccino' (Maxwell House)	8 oz	130	2.0	25.0	65	na	2.0	na	15	14%
'Cinnamon Hot Cappuccino' (Maxwell House)	6 oz	60	2.0	11.0	100	na	1.0	na	0	15%
'Coffee Hot Cappuccino' (Maxwell House)	6 oz	60	1.0	12.0	110	na	1.0	na	0	15%
'Double Dutch Chocolate International' prepared (General Foods)	6 oz	50	0.0	8.0	15	(tr)	2.0	(mq)	0	36%
'Dutch Chocolate Mint International' prepared (General Foods)	6 oz	50	0.0	8.0	80	(tr)	2.0	(mq)	0	36%
'French Vanilla Cafe International' prepared (General Foods)	6 oz	60	0.0	9.0	50	na	3.0	na	0	43%
'Hazelnut Belgian Cafe International' prepared (General Foods)	6 oz	60	0.0	10.0	55	na	2.0	na	0	31%
mocha, banana nut 'Sugar-free' prepared (MJB)	6 oz	39	0.8	4.9	60	(tr)	1.8	(mq)	na	42%
mocha, cherry, prepared (MJB)	6 oz	53	0.5	9.7	17	(tr)	1.4	(mq)	na	24%
mocha, fudge 'Sugar-free' prepared (MJB)	6 oz	39	1.2	4.5	88	(tr)	1.8	(mq)	na	42%
mocha, mint, prepared (MJB)	6 oz	53	0.4	9.9	16	(tr)	1.3	(mq)	na	22%
mocha, mint 'Sugar-free' prepared (MJB)	6 oz	37	0.7	5.6	43	(tr)	1.3	(mq)	na	32%
mocha, prepared (MJB)	6 oz	52	0.6	9.5	54	(tr)	1.3	(mq)	na	23%
mocha, Swiss 'Cafe Coffees' prepared (Hills Bros)	6 oz	60	1.0	8.0	10	(tr)	2.0	(mq)	na	33%
mocha, Swiss 'Cafe Coffees Sugar-free' prepared (Hills Bros)	6 oz	40	1.0	5.0	25	(tr)	2.0	(mq)	na	43%
mocha, vanilla 'Sugar-free' prepared (MJB)	6 oz	39	0.7	5.2	50	(tr)	1.7	(mq)	na	39%
'Mocha Hot Cappuccino' (Maxwell House)	6 oz	70	2.0	12.0	80	na	2.0	na	0	24%
orange, Capri 'Cafe Coffees' prepared (Hills Bros)	6 oz	60	1.0	9.0	30	(tr)	2.0	(mq)	na	31%
'Orange Cappuccino International' prepared (General Foods)	6 oz	60	0.0	10.0	100	(tr)	2.0	(mq)	0	31%
'Orange Cappuccino International sugar-free, prepared (General Foods)	6 oz	30	0.0	3.0	60	(tr)	2.0	(mq)	0	60%
COFFEE, INSTANT										
'Brava' prepared (Nescafé)	8 oz	4	<1.0	1.0	0	0	<1.0	(tr)	0	tr
Classic' prepared '(Nescafé)	8 oz	4	<1.0	1.0	0	0	<1.0	(tr)	0	tr
powder (Kava)	1 tsp	2	0.0	1.0	5	0	0.0	0.0	0	0%
prepared (Nescafé)	8 oz	4	<1.0	1.0	0	0	<1.0	(tr)	0	tr
regular powder	1 oz	68	3.5	11.7	10	0	0.1	<.1	0	2%
regular, powder	1 round tsp	4	0.2	0.7	1	0	0.0	0.0	0	0%
regular, prepared	6 oz	4	0.2	0.7	5	0	0.0	0.0	0	0%
'Silka' prepared (Nescafé)	8 oz	4	<1.0	1.0	0	0	<1.0	(tr)	0	tr
'Suisse Mocha International' prepared (General Foods)	6 oz	50	0.0	7.0	15	na	3.0	na	0	49%
'Suisse Mocha International' sugar-free, prepared (General Foods)	6 oz	30	0.0	3.0	15	na	2.0	na	0	60%
'Viennese Chocolate Cafe International' prepared (General Foods)	6 oz	50	0.0	8.0	20	na	2.0	na	0	36%
w/chicory, powder	1 round tsp	6	0.2	1.3	5	0	0.0	0.0	0	0%
w/chicory, prepared	6 oz	7	0.2	1.3	11	0	0.0	0.0	0	0%
w/chicory, prepared (Sunrise)	8 oz	6	<1.0	1.0	0	0	<1.0	(tr)	0	tr
w/chicory 'Mountain Blend' prepared (Nescafé)	8 oz	6	<1.0	1.0	0	0	<1.0	(tr)	0	tr
w/sugar, cappuccino flavor, powder	2 round tsp	62	0.4	10.7	98	0	2.1	1.8	0	00%
w/sugar, cappuccino flavor, prepared	6 oz	61	0.4	10.8	104	0	2.1	1.8	0	30%
w/sugar, French flavor, powder	2 round tsp	57	0.5	6.6	24	0	3.4	3.0	0	52%
w/sugar, French flavor, prepared	6 oz	57	0.6	6.6	30	0	3.4	3.0	0	52%
w/sugar, mocha flavor, powder	2 round tsp	51	0.5	8.4	31	.1	1.9	1.6	0	32%
w/sugar, mocha flavor, prepared	6 oz	51	0.6	8.5	36	0	1.9	1.6	0	32%
COFFEE FLAVOR DRINK, canned, liquid nutrition (Ensure)	8 oz	250	8.8	34.3	na	na	8.8	na	na	32%

Food Name	Serving Size	Calories	Prot. gms	Carbs gms	Sod. mgs	Fiber gms	Fat gms	Sat. Fat gms	Chol. mgs	% Fat Cal.
COFFEE LIQUEUR. See ALCOHOLIC BEVERAGES.										
COLA BEVERAGE. See SOFT DRINKS AND MIXERS.										
COLD CUTS. See LUNCHEON MEATS.										
COLE. See KALE.										
COLESLAW										
fresh	4 oz	78	1.5	14.1	26	>.7 c	3.0	0.4	9	30%
fresh	1/2 cup	41	0.8	7.4	14	>.4 c	1.6	0.2	5	31%
fresh	1 tbsp	6	0.1	1.0	2	>.1 c	0.2	0.0	1	29%
COLESLAW DRESSING										
(Kraft)	1 tbsp	70	0.0	4.0	200	na	6.0	1.0	10	77%
(Kraft) 'Miracle Whip'	1 tbsp	70	0.0	3.0	105	na	6.0	1.0	5	82%
(Litehouse) refrigerated	1 tbsp	80	0.0	2.0	41	na	8.0	na	na	90%
(T. Marzetti) light	1 tbsp	50	0.0	6.0	240	na	3.0	na	na	53%
(T. Marzetti) original	1 tbsp	79	<1.0	3.0	180	na	7.0	na	14	80%
(T. Marzetti) 'South Recipe'	1 tbsp	66	0.0	6.0	93	na	5.0	na	9	65%
COLEWORT. See KALE.										
COLLARDS										
boiled, drained	4 oz	31	1.5	7.0	18	>.6 c	0.2	(tr)	0	5%
boiled, drained, chopped	1/2 cup	17	0.9	3.9	161	1.3	0.1	na	0	5%
raw, chopped	1/2 cup	6	0.3	1.3	4	.7	0.0	na	0	0%
raw, trimmed	1 oz	9	0.4	2.0	6	>.2 c	0.1	(tr)	0	9%
raw, untrimmed	1 lb	80	4.1	18.4	51	>1.5 c	0.6	na	0	6%
Canned										
chopped (Allens)	1/2 cup	20	2.0	2.0	15	(mq)	<1.0	(tr)	0	<36%
chopped, greens (Bush's Best)	1/2 cup	30	2.0	5.0	320	na	0.0	na	na	0%
chopped, w/pork (Luck's)	7.5 oz	90	2.0	7.0	420	(mq)	7.0	(mq)	(mq)	64%
Frozen										
boiled, drained	4 oz	41	3.4	8.1	57	>1.2 c	0.5	(tr)	0	9%
chopped (Seabrook)	3.3 oz	25	3.0	4.0	45	>1.0 c	0.0	0.0	0	0%
chopped (Southern)	3.5 oz	30	2.7	4.6	60	(mq)	0.4	(tr)	0	11%
chopped, boiled, drained	1/2 cup	31	2.5	6.0	43	>.9 c	0.4	na	0	10%
chopped, unprepared	10-oz pkg	94	7.6	18.3	136	5.7	1.0	na	0	8%
COLORADO PINYON PINE NUT. See PINE NUT.										
CONCORD PUNCH, 'Juices To Go' (Minute Maid)	6 oz	90	0.0	23.0	20	na	0.0	na	na	0%
CONDIMENTS. See individual listings.										
COOKIE										
ALMOND										
(Health Valley) date 'Fruit Jumbos'	1 cookie	70	2.0	10.0	30	1.1	3.0	(mq)	0	36%
(Mother's) shortbread	2 cookies	120	1.0	13.0	50	na	7.0	na	na	53%
(Natures Warehouse) butter, approx 1 oz	2 cookies	122	2.0	19.2	41	na	4.1	na	na	30%
(Stella D'oro) 'Breakfast Treats'	1 cookie	101	1.6	15.4	(mq)	(mq)	3.6	(mq)	na	32%
(Stella D'oro) 'Chinese Dessert'	1 cookie	169	2.4	19.5	(mq)	(mq)	8.9	(mq)	na	48%
(Stella D'oro) toast 'Mandel'	1 cookie	58	1.3	10.2	(mq)	(mq)	1.4	na	na	22%
AMARANTH (Health Valley)	1 cookie	90	2.0	12.0	30	2.3	3.0	(mq)	0	33%
ANGEL WINGS (Stella D'oro)	1 cookie	74	1.1	7.0	(mq)	(mq)	4.7	(mq)	na	57%
ANIMAL CRACKERS										
(FFV)	1.25-oz pkg	160	2.0	26.0	150	(mq)	6.0	1.0	0	33%
(Finast) 15 pieces	1 oz	120	2.0	22.0	110	(mq)	3.0	(mq)	na	22%
(Grandma's) candied, 5 cookies	1 oz	140	1.0	20.0	80	na	6.0	na	0	39%
(Keebler) approx .5 oz	5 cookies	70	1.0	11.0	75	(mq)	2.0	<1.0	0	27%
(Mother's) circus animal	4 cookies	110	1.0	14.0	40	na	6.0	na	na	47%
(Nabisco) 'Barnum's Animals' 5 1/2 pieces	.5 oz	60	1.0	11.0	70	0	2.0	0.0	0	27%
(Sunshine)	13 cookies	130	2.0	21.0	160	(mq)	4.0	1.0	0	28%

Food Name	Serving Size	Calories	Prot. gms	Carbs gms	Sod. mgs	Fiber gms	Fat gms	Sat. Fat gms	Chol. mgs	% Fat Cal.
ANISE										
(Stella D'oro) 'Anisette Sponge'	1 cookie	51	1.1	9.9	(mq)	(mq)	0.8	na	na	14%
(Stella D'oro) 'Anisette Toast'	1 cookie	46	0.8	9.3	(mq)	(mq)	0.6	na	na	12%
(Stella D'oro) 'Anisette Toast Jumbo'	1 cookie	109	2.0	23.0	(mq)	(mq)	1.0	na	na	8%
APPLE										
(Archway) n' raisin	1 cookie	120	2.0	20.0	169	1.0	3.0	(mq)	10	24%
(Bakery Wagon) cinnamon	1 cookie	100	1.0	17.0	100	na	3.0	na	2	27%
(Bakery Wagon) filled oatmeal	1 cookie	90	1.0	14.0	115	na	4.0	na	2	38%
(Bakery Wagon) walnut raisin	1 cookie	100	2.0	17.0	110	na	3.0	na	2	26%
(Break Cake) sandwich	1 cookie	90	1.0	15.0	70	na	3.0	0.5	5	30%
(Estee) cinnamon 'Snack Crisps' new blue pkg	.66 oz	80	1.0	15.0	75	na	2.0	<1.0	0	22%
(Frookie) cinnamon oat bran	1 cookie	45	1.0	6.5	35	na	2.0	0.5	0	38%
(Frookie) 'Fruitins'	1 cookie	60	1.0	12.0	25	na	1.0	0.0	0	15%
(Frookie) spice, fat-free	1 cookie	50	1.0	11.0	80	1.0	0.0	0.0	0	0%
(Great Cakes)	4.5 oz	260	10.0	40.0	20	21.0	6.0	na	0	21%
(Health Valley) cinnamon 'Mini Fruit Centers' fat-free	3 cookies	75	2.0	17.0	60	3.0	0.0	na	0	0%
(Health Valley) 'Fruit Centers' fat-free	1 cookie	80	2.0	17.0	80	2.0	0.0	na	0	0%
(Health Valley) raisin 'Fruit Chunks'	3 cookies	85	2.0	19.0	80	3.0	0.0	na	0	0%
(Health Valley) raisin 'Jumbos' fat-free	1 cookie	80	2.0	17.0	80	3.5	0.0	na	0	0%
(Health Valley) spice, fat-free	3 cookies	80	2.0	18.0	80	3.0	0.0	na	0	0%
(Healthy Times) 'Hugga Bears' organic	1 oz	120	2.0	17.0	38	na	3.0	na	0	26%
(Nabisco) 'Newtons' 1.25 oz	1 cookie	120	1.0	24.0	110	(mq)	3.0	1.0	0	21%
(Nabisco) 'Newtons' .75 oz	1 cookie	70	1.0	15.0	70	na	2.0	0.0	0	22%
(Nabisco) 'Newtons' fat-free, .75 oz	1 cookie	70	1.0	16.0	45	0	0.0	0.0	0	0%
(Stella D'oro) bar, Dutch	1 cookie	112	1.4	18.9	(mq)	(mq)	3.3	(mq)	na	27%
(Stella D'oro) pastry, dietetic	1 cookie	86	1.0	13.0	10	(mq)	3.3	(mq)	na	35%
(Weight Watchers) fruit filled	1 cookie	80	<1.0	21.0	35	na	<1.0	na	0	<9%
(Weight Watchers) raisin bar	1 cookie	100	1.0	18.0	115	(mq)	3.0	(mq)	na	26%
APRICOT										
(Health Valley) almond 'Fancy Fruit Chunks'	2 cookies	90	2.0	14.0	45	1.8	4.0	(mq)	0	36%
(Health Valley) apple 'Fruit Chunks'	3 cookies	85	2.0	19.0	80	3.0	0.0	na	0	0%
(Health Valley) delight, fat-free	3 cookies	80	2.0	18.0	80	3.0	0.0	na	0	0%
(Health Valley) 'Fruit Centers' fat-free	1 cookie	80	2.0	17.0	80	2.0	0.0	na	0	0%
(Pepperidge Farm) raspberry 'Fruit Cookies'	2 cookies	100	1.0	15.0	50	(mq)	4.0	2.0	10	36%
(Pepperidge Farm) raspberry 'Zurich'	1 cookie	60	1.0	10.0	30	(mq)	2.0	1.0	0	29%
ARROWROOT (Nabisco) 'National Arrowroot Biscuit' 6 pieces	1 oz	130	2.0	21.0	85	0	4.0	1.0	10	28%
ASSORTED										
(Archway) 'Select Assortment'	1 cookie	50	1.0	7.0	40	(mq)	2.0	(mq)	5	36%
(Fifty 50) wafers, creme filled, w/o sugar	1 wafer	35	<1.0	4.0	10	na	2.0	na	0	47%
(Stella D'oro) 'Hostess'	1 cookie	42	0.5	5.5	(mq)	(mq)	2.0	(mq)	na	43%
(Stella D'oro) 'Lady Stella'	1 cookie	42	0.6	5.5	(mq)	(mq)	2.0	(mq)	na	43%
BANANA										
(Break Cake) creme	1 cookie	240	2.0	37.0	200	na	9.0	2.2	5	34%
(Frookie) fat-free	1 cookie	45	1.0	10.0	90	1.0	0.0	0.0	0	0%
(Health Valley) spice 'Fruit Chunks'	3 cookies	85	2.0	19.0	80	3.0	0.0	na	0	0%
(Natures Warehouse) wheat-free, fat-free	1 oz	90	1.6	20.5	84	na	0.7	0.1	0	7%
BLUEBERRY (Great Cakes)	4.5 oz	260	10.0	40.0	20	21.0	6.0	na	0	21%
BROWNIE										
(Break Cake) creme	1 cookie	240	2.0	38.0	150	na	8.0	1.8	5	31%
(Pepperidge Farm) chocolate nut 'Old Fashioned'	2 pieces	110	1.0	11.0	45	(mq)	7.0	2.0	5	57%
(Pepperidge Farm) cream sandwich 'Capri'	1 cookie	80	0.0	10.0	45	(mq)	5.0	1.0	0	53%
BUTTER										
(Barbara's Bakery) pecan bites 'Small Indulgences'	1 oz	140	2.0	16.0	95	na	8.0	na	20	50%
(Delicious) frosted, made w/Land O'Lakes butter	1 cookie	88	1.0	11.0	44	0	5.0	1.0	10	48%

Food Name	Serving Size	Calories	Prot. gms	Carbs gms	Sod. mgs	Fiber gms	Fat gms	Sat. Fat gms	Chol. mgs	% Fat Cal.
(Fifty 50) fructose sweetened, low sodium	1 cookie	40	<1.0	5.0	20	na	2.0	na	5	43%
(Keebler) flavor, chocolate coated 'Baby Bear' .5 oz	3 cookies	70	1.0	10.0	55	(mq)	2.0	<1.0	0	29%
(Keebler) flavor, chocolate coated 'E.L. Fudge' .5 oz	2 cookies	80	<1.0	10.0	40	(mq)	4.0	1.0	5	45%
(Lu) 'Little Schoolboy'	1 cookie	70	1.0	8.0	35	na	4.0	na	na	50%
(Lu) 'Petite Beurre'	1 cookie	40	1.0	7.0	45	na	1.0	na	na	22%
(Mother's) flavored	5 cookies	140	2.0	20.0	130	na	6.0	na	na	38%
(Pepperidge Farm) flavor 'Chessmen'	2 cookies	90	1.0	12.0	60	(mq)	4.0	2.0	10	41%
(Stella D'oro) 'Como Delight'	1 cookie	145	2.1	17.9	(mq)	(mq)	7.2	(mq)	na	45%
CANDY *(Oven Lovin')*	1 cookie	70	0.0	10.0	40	na	3.0	1.0	0	40%
CARAMEL										
(FFV) patties, approx 1 oz	2 cookies	150	1.0	20.0	125	(mq)	7.0	(mq)	na	43%
(Keebler) apple oatmeal 'Elfin Delights'	1 cookie	65	<1.0	12.0	55	na	2.0	<1.0	0	26%
(Natures Warehouse) crisp, wheat-free, fat-free	1 oz	90	1.6	20.5	84	na	0.7	0.1	0	7%
CAROB										
(Health Valley) 'Healthy Chips' fat-free	3 cookies	80	2.0	18.0	80	2.0	0.0	na	0	0%
(Natures Warehouse) fudge, approx 1 oz	2 cookies	116	1.4	20.5	78	na	3.1	na	na	24%
(Westbrae) 'Rice Malt Snap'	1 oz	140	2.0	18.0	70	na	7.0	na	0	44%
CARROT WALNUT 'Wholesome Choice' *(Pepperidge Farm)* . .	1 piece	60	1.0	11.0	45	(mq)	1.0	<1.0	0	16%
CHERRY										
(Great Cakes) carob	4.5 oz	280	10.0	40.0	20	21.0	8.0	na	0	27%
(Natures Warehouse) wheat-free, fat-free	1 oz	90	1.6	20.5	84	na	0.7	0.1	0	7%
CHIPS AND CREME										
(Break Cake)	1 cookie	140	1.0	21.0	130	na	6.0	1.3	2	38%
(Frookie) and vanilla sandwich 'Frookwich'	1 cookie	50	<1.0	7.0	30	na	2.0	0.0	0	36%
CHOCOLATE										
(Barbara's Bakery) raspberry 'Cookies & Creme'	2 cookies	120	2.0	18.0	80	na	5.0	na	15	36%
(Barbara's Bakery) vanilla 'Cookies & Creme'	2 cookies	120	2.0	18.0	80	na	5.0	na	15	36%
(Betty Crocker) w/peanut butter creme 'Dunkaroos'	1 tray	140	3.0	15.0	140	na	8.0	na	0	50%
(Drake's) approx 1 oz	2 cookies	130	2.0	19.0	85	(mq)	5.0	1.0	0	35%
(Estee) 'Snack Crisps'	.66 oz	80	1.0	15.0	65	na	2.0	<1.0	0	22%
(Featherweight) creme wafer	1 cookie	20	0.0	3.0	0	(mq)	1.0	na	0	43%
(Frookie) 'Animal Frackers'	6 cookies	60	1.0	9.0	70	na	2.0	0.0	0	31%
(Frookie) 'Funky Monkeys'	8 cookies	60	1.0	10.0	60	na	2.0	0.0	0	29%
(Grandma's) 'Chocolate Cookie Bits' 8 cookies	1 oz	140	2.0	19.0	180	na	6.0	na	0	39%
(Lu) 'Chocolatiers'	2 cookies	85	1.0	10.0	10	na	4.0	na	na	45%
(Lu) 'Chocolatiers' dipped	2 cookies	105	1.0	12.0	15	na	6.0	na	na	51%
(Nabisco) 'Chocolate Snap' 4 pieces	.5 oz	70	1.0	10.0	80	na	2.0	1.0	0	29%
(Nabisco) 'Pure Chocolate Middles'	.5 oz cookie	80	1.0	9.0	35	0	5.0	2.0	5	53%
(Pepperidge Farm) walnut 'Beacon Hill'	1 cookie	120	2.0	14.0	65	1.0	7.0	2.0	5	50%
(Stella D'oro) 'Castelets'	1 cookie	64	0.8	9.0	(mq)	(mq)	2.8	(mq)	na	39%
(Stella D'oro) 'Margherite'	1 cookie	72	0.9	10.2	(mq)	(mq)	3.1	(mq)	na	39%
(Tastykake) 'Soft 'n Chewy'	1.4 oz	171	2.1	26.2	111	1.1	7.0	2.1	3	36%
(Weight Watchers)	3 cookies	80	1.0	13.0	70	(mq)	3.0	(mq)	na	33%
CHOCOLATE CHIP										
(Almost Home)	.5 oz	60	1.0	8.0	45	na	3.0	1.0	2	43%
(Archway)	1 cookie	50	1.0	7.0	40	(mq)	3.0	(mq)	5	46%
(Barbara's Bakery)	1 oz	130	2.0	16.0	60	na	6.0	na	0	43%
(Barbara's Bakery) crisp 'Small Indulgences'	1 oz	140	2.0	18.0	105	na	7.0	na	15	44%
(Break Cake) approx 1 oz	5 cookies	140	2.0	20.0	115	na	6.0	1.4	5	38%
(Chips Ahoy!)	.5 oz	50	1.0	7.0	35	0	2.0	1.0	0	36%
(Chips Ahoy!) 'Chewy'	.5 oz	60	1.0	7.0	40	0	3.0	1.0	0	46%
(Chips Ahoy!) 'Mini'	.5 oz	70	1.0	9.0	50	0	3.0	1.0	0	40%
(Chips Ahoy!) pecan 'Selections'	.5 oz	100	1.0	10.0	65	0	6.0	2.0	10	55%
(Chips Ahoy!) 'Rockers'	1 cookie	60	1.0	8.0	40	na	3.0	<1.0	0	43%

Food Name	Serving Size	Calories	Prot. gms	Carbs gms	Sod. mgs	Fiber gms	Fat gms	Sat. Fat gms	Chol. mgs	% Fat Cal.
(Chips Ahoy!) 'Sprinkled'	.5 oz	60	1.0	8.0	40	0	3.0	1.0	0	43%
(Chips Ahoy!) 'Striped'	.5 oz	90	1.0	10.0	45	0	5.0	2.0	0	51%
(Chips Ahoy!) walnut 'Selections'	.5 oz	100	1.0	9.0	70	0	6.0	2.0	5	57%
(Chips Ahoy!) white fudge chunk	1 cookie	90	1.0	11.0	75	na	5.0	2.0	5	48%
(Drake's) approx 1 oz	2 cookies	140	1.0	18.0	110	(mq)	6.0	2.0	0	42%
(Duncan Hines)	2 cookies	110	1.0	15.0	85	na	5.0	<2.0	na	41%
(Entenmann's)	3 cookies	140	1.0	19.0	85	na	7.0	na	na	44%
(Estee)	3 cookies	110	1.0	13.0	20	na	5.0	2.0	0	45%
(Featherweight)	1 cookie	45	1.0	6.0	0	(mq)	2.0	(mq)	0	39%
(Fifty 50) fructose sweetened	1 cookie	35	<1.0	4.0	10	na	2.0	na	0	47%
(Finast)	1 oz	90	1.0	18.0	60	(mq)	7.0	(mq)	0	45%
(Frookie)	1 cookie	45	1.0	6.5	35	na	2.0	0.5	0	38%
(Frookie) Mandarin	1 cookie	45	1.0	6.5	35	na	2.0	0.5	0	38%
(Frookie) mint	1 cookie	45	1.0	6.5	35	na	2.0	0.5	0	38%
(Grandma's) 'Big Cookies' 2.75 oz	2 cookies	370	4.0	50.0	270	(mq)	17.0	(mq)	5	42%
(Grandma's) 'Rich'N Chewy' 3 cookies	1 oz	140	1.0	20.0	80	na	6.0	na	5	39%
(Keebler) bakery crisp 'Chips Deluxe'	1 cookie	60	1.0	7.0	45	na	3.0	1.0	0	46%
(Keebler) chewy 'Elfin Delights'	1 cookie	65	<1.0	11.0	55	na	2.0	<1.0	0	27%
(Keebler) 'Chips Deluxe' approx .5 oz	1 cookie	80	<1.0	10.0	75	(mq)	4.0	1.0	5	45%
(Keebler) 'Coconut Chocolate Drop'	1 cookie	80	1.0	10.0	60	na	5.0	2.0	0	51%
(Keebler) deluxe 'Bakery Crisp'	1 cookie	60	1.0	7.0	45	na	3.0	1.0	0	46%
(Keebler) 'Rainbow Chips Deluxe' .5 oz	1 cookie	80	1.0	11.0	45	(mq)	3.0	1.0	5	36%
(Keebler) 'Soft Batch' approx .5 oz	1 cookie	80	<1.0	10.0	70	(mq)	4.0	1.0	0	45%
(Mother's)	1 cookie	70	1.0	10.0	55	na	3.0	na	na	38%
(Mother's) angel	2 cookies	120	1.0	14.0	45	na	8.0	na	na	55%
(Nabisco) bite size 'Snack Wells'	.5 oz	60	<1.0	11.0	85	na	1.0	<1.0	0	16%
(Nabisco) 'Chocolate Chip Snaps' 3 pieces	.5 oz	70	1.0	11.0	50	0	2.0	0.0	0	27%
(Oven Lovin')	1 cookie	70	0.0	9.0	50	na	3.0	na	5	43%
(Pepperidge Farm) 'Family Request'	2 cookies	90	1.0	15.0	55	na	5.0	1.0	5	41%
(Pepperidge Farm) 'Old Fashioned'	2 cookies	100	1.0	12.0	45	(mq)	5.0	2.0	5	46%
(Pepperidge Farm) w/macadamia nuts 'Big, Soft and Chewy'	1 cookie	130	1.0	16.0	45	na	7.0	2.0	10	48%
(Pepperidge Farm) w/macadamia nuts 'Sausalito'	1 cookie	120	1.0	14.0	65	(mq)	7.0	2.0	5	51%
(Tastykake) bar, 1.5 oz	1 cookie	193	3.0	28.3	97	1.0	8.4	1.5	4	38%
(Tastykake) 'Soft 'n Chewy'	1.4 oz	174	2.3	25.5	168	.9	7.3	2.1	10	37%
(Weight Watchers)	2 cookies	90	1.0	18.0	65	na	2.0	1.0	0	19%
CHOCOLATE CHOCOLATE CHIP										
(Barbara's Bakery)	1 oz	125	2.0	17.0	50	na	5.0	na	0	37%
(Natures Warehouse) approx 1 oz	2 cookies	130	2.8	16.4	69	na	6.1	na	na	42%
(Pepperidge Farm) walnut, big, soft & chewy	1 cookie	130	1.0	17.0	45	na	6.0	2.0	5	43%
(Pillsbury's Best)	1 cookie	70	1.0	9.0	35	na	3.0	<1.0	0	40%
CHOCOLATE CHUNK										
(Chips Ahoy!) 'Chunky'	1 cookie	80	1.0	11.0	60	1.0	4.0	3.0	10	43%
(Chips Ahoy!) 'Selections'	.5 oz	90	1.0	10.0	65	0	5.0	2.0	10	51%
(Dunkin' Donuts) 1.5 oz	1 cookie	200	3.0	25.0	110	1.0	10.0	(mq)	30	45%
(Dunkin' Donuts) w/nuts, 1.5 oz	1 cookie	210	3.0	23.0	100	2.0	11.0	(mq)	30	49%
(Pepperidge Farm) 'Big, Soft and Chewy'	1 cookie	130	2.0	17.0	45	na	6.0	2.0	10	42%
CHOCOLATE-FILLED SANDWICH										
(Keebler) 'E.L. Fudge'	1 cookie	60	<1.0	8.0	35	(mq)	3.0	<1.0	5	43%
(Pepperidge Farm) 'Brussels'	2 cookies	110	1.0	13.0	65	(mq)	5.0	2.0	0	45%
(Pepperidge Farm) 'Brussels Mint'	2 cookies	130	1.0	17.0	40	(mq)	7.0	2.0	0	47%
(Pepperidge Farm) 'Double Chocolate Milano'	2 cookies	150	2.0	18.0	45	na	8.0	3.0	10	47%
(Pepperidge Farm) 'Hazelnut Milano'	2 cookies	130	2.0	15.0	30	na	8.0	2.0	5	51%
(Pepperidge Farm) 'Lido'	1 cookie	90	1.0	10.0	30	(mq)	5.0	1.0	5	51%

Food Name	Serving Size	Calories	Prot. gms	Carbs gms	Sod. mgs	Fiber gms	Fat gms	Sat. Fat gms	Chol. mgs	% Fat Cal.
(Pepperidge Farm) 'Milano'	2 cookies	120	1.0	15.0	45	(mq)	6.0	2.0	5	46%
(Pepperidge Farm) 'Mint Milano'	2 cookies	150	1.0	17.0	60	(mq)	7.0	2.0	5	47%
(Pepperidge Farm) 'Orange Milano'	2 cookies	150	1.0	17.0	60	(mq)	7.0	2.0	5	47%
(Pepperidge Farm) 'Orleans'	2 cookies	120	1.0	14.0	40	(mq)	8.0	2.0	0	55%
CHOCOLATE GRAHAM										
(Keebler) 'Thin Bits' approx .5 oz	12 cookies	70	1.0	9.0	75	(mq)	3.0	<1.0	0	40%
(Nabisco) approx .5 oz	11 cookies	60	1.0	10.0	90	(mq)	2.0	<1.0	0	29%
(Nabisco) 'Bugs Bunny'	.5 oz	60	1.0	10.0	80	na	2.0	2.0	0	29%
(Nabisco) 'Chocolate Grahams'	.5 oz	150	3.0	17.0	80	0	7.0	0.0	0	44%
(Teddy Grahams) 'Bearwichs'	.5 oz	70	1.0	10.0	60	na	3.0	1.0	0	38%
(Teddy Grahams) w/vanilla creme 'Bearwichs'	4 cookies	70	1.0	10.0	60	(mq)	3.0	<1.0	0	38%
CHOCOLATE SANDWICH										
(Estee)	1 cookie	50	<1.0	7.0	15	(mq)	2.0	1.0	0	36%
(Frookie) 'Frookwich'	1 cookie	50	<1.0	7.0	30	na	2.0	0.0	0	36%
(Keebler) 'Chocolate Creme Sandwich'	.5 oz	80	1.0	12.0	70	(mq)	4.0	1.0	0	41%
(Keebler) 'E.L. Fudge'	1 cookie	70	<1.0	9.0	50	(mq)	3.0	<1.0	0	40%
(Keebler) fudge creme 'Elfin Delights'	1 cookie	55	<1.0	10.0	50	na	2.0	<1.0	0	29%
(Keebler) peanut butter 'E.L. Fudge'	1 cookie	50	1.0	7.0	50	(mq)	3.0	<1.0	0	46%
(Little Debbie)	1.8 oz	250	3.0	35.0	260	(mq)	12.0	(mq)	<1	42%
(Oreo) 'Big Stuf'	.25 oz	200	2.0	27.0	220	1.0	9.0	3.0	5	41%
(Oreo) 'Double Stuf' 2 cookies	1 oz	70	1.0	9.0	75	na	4.0	1.0	na	47%
(Oreo) fudge covered	.75 oz	110	1.0	13.0	80	(mq)	6.0	4.0	2	49%
(Oreo) 'Halloween Treats' 1 oz	2 cookies	140	1.0	20.0	150	1.0	7.0	2.0	0	43%
(Oreo) 2 1/2 cookies	1 oz	140	1.0	20.0	170	0	6.0	0.0	0	39%
(Oreo) white fudge covered	.75 oz	110	1.0	14.0	75	(mq)	6.0	4.0	2	47%
(Weight Watchers)	2 cookies	90	1.0	15.0	90	na	3.0	1.0	0	30%
CHUNK										
(Pepperidge Farm) 'Nantucket'	1 cookie	120	1.0	15.0	60	1.0	6.0	2.0	5	46%
(Pepperidge Farm) pecan 'Chesapeake'	1 cookie	120	1.0	14.0	60	1.0	7.0	2.0	5	51%
(Pepperidge Farm) pecan 'Special Collection'	1 cookie	70	0.0	8.0	25	(mq)	4.0	1.0	10	53%
CINNAMON										
(Frookie) 'Animal Frackers'	6 cookies	60	1.0	9.0	45	na	2.0	0.0	0	31%
(Mother's) dinosaur, mini	7 cookies	70	1.0	9.0	40	na	2.0	na	na	31%
(Mother's) dinosaur grahams	1 cookie	80	1.0	12.0	50	na	3.0	na	na	34%
CINNAMON GRAHAM										
(Honey Maid) approx .5 oz	2 cookies	60	1.0	12.0	85	(mq)	1.0	<1.0	0	15%
(Keebler) 'Alpha Grahams'	6 cookies	70	1.0	10.0	55	(mq)	2.0	<1.0	0	29%
(Keebler) 'Cinnamon Crisp' .5 oz	4 cookies	70	1.0	11.0	85	(mq)	2.0	<1.0	0	27%
(Keebler) fudge covered 'Deluxe' .5 oz	2 cookies	90	<1.0	11.0	60	(mq)	4.0	1.0	0	43%
(Keebler) 'Thin Bits' approx .5 oz	12 cookies	70	1.0	10.0	50	(mq)	3.0	<1.0	0	38%
(Nabisco) 'Bugs Bunny'	.5 oz	60	1.0	11.0	80	na	2.0	2.0	0	27%
(Nabisco) fat-free 'Snack Wells'	.5 oz	50	1.0	12.0	45	na	0.0	na	0	0%
(Nabisco) w/fudge 'Cookies'N Fudge'	1 cookie	45	<1.0	6.0	35	(mq)	2.0	1.0	0	39%
(Natures Warehouse) approx 1 oz	2 cookies	113	1.2	18.8	71	na	3.6	na	na	29%
(Pepperidge Farm) sugar 'Family Request'	2 cookies	80	1.0	12.0	40	na	4.0	1.0	15	41%
(Sunshine)	1 cookie	70	1.0	11.0	95	(mq)	3.0	1.0	0	36%
(Teddy Grahams) 'Bearwichs'	.5 oz	70	1.0	10.0	60	na	3.0	1.0	0	38%
COCOA										
(Westbrae) chip 'Rice Malt Snap'	1 oz	130	2.0	18.0	60	na	7.0	na	0	44%
(Westbrae) 'Rice Malt Snap'	1 oz	140	2.0	17.0	70	na	7.0	na	0	45%
COCONUT										
(Break Cake) macaroons	2 cookies	270	2.0	34.0	160	na	14.0	12.5	0	47%
(Drake's) approx 1 oz	2 cookies	130	2.0	20.0	95	(mq)	5.0	2.0	0	34%
(Estee)	3 cookies	110	1.0	14.0	15	na	5.0	1.0	0	43%

Food Name	Serving Size	Calories	Prot. gms	Carbs gms	Sod. mgs	Fiber gms	Fat gms	Sat. Fat gms	Chol. mgs	% Fat Cal.
(Glenny's) almonds, raisins 'Nookie Bar'	1.15 oz	138	2.0	18.0	na	na	3.0	na	na	25%
(Mother's) cocadas	4 cookies	120	2.0	17.0	150	na	6.0	na	na	42%
(Mother's) macaroons	1 cookie	80	1.0	8.0	40	na	5.0	na	na	56%
(Natures Warehouse) approx 1 oz	2 cookies	130	1.4	13.9	20	na	7.6	na	na	53%
(Pepperidge Farm) chocolate-filled 'Tahiti'	1 cookie	90	0.0	9.0	25	(mq)	6.0	2.0	5	60%
(Stella D'oro) dietetic	1 cookie	52	0.8	6.8	10	(mq)	2.4	(mq)	na	42%
(Stella D'oro) macaroon	1 cookie	60	0.7	6.6	(mq)	(mq)	3.4	(mq)	na	51%
COFFEE										
(Barbara's Bakery) coffee cake crunch 'Small Indulgences'	1 oz	130	2.0	18.0	140	na	6.0	na	20	40%
(Pepperidge Farm)	1 cookie	50	0.0	6.0	20	(mq)	3.0	1.0	5	53%
CRANBERRY										
(Frookie) orange, fat-free	1 cookie	45	1.0	10.0	75	1.0	0.0	0.0	0	0%
(Nabisco) 'Newtons' fat-free	1 cookie	70	1.0	16.0	70	na	0.0	na	0	0%
(Pepperidge Farm) honey, soft 'Wholesome Choice'	1 cookie	60	1.0	11.0	50	na	2.0	<1.0	0	27%
CROKINE (Lu)	2 cookies	35	1.0	7.0	70	na	0.0	na	na	0%
DATE										
(Bakery Wagon) filled oatmeal	1 cookie	90	1.0	15.0	100	na	3.0	na	2	30%
(Break Cake) creme	1 cookie	140	1.0	21.0	140	na	5.0	1.0	2	34%
(Health Valley) delight, fat-free	3 cookies	80	2.0	18.0	80	3.0	0.0	na	0	0%
(Health Valley) 'Fruit Centers' fat-free	1 cookie	70	2.0	16.0	35	3.5	0.0	na	0	0%
(Health Valley) pecan 'Fancy Fruit Chunks'	2 cookies	90	2.0	15.0	45	1.7	4.0	(mq)	0	35%
(Pepperidge Farm) pecan 'Kitchen Hearth'	2 cookies	110	1.0	15.0	40	(mq)	5.0	2.0	10	41%
DEVIL'S FOOD										
(Break Cake) creme	1 cookie	130	1.0	20.0	120	na	5.0	1.0	0	35%
(FFV) 'Trolley Cakes' 2 oz	2 cookies	120	2.0	25.0	80	(mq)	2.0	(mq)	na	14%
(Nabisco) cakes	1 cookie	70	1.0	15.0	40	(mq)	1.0	<1.0	0	12%
DUPLEX SANDWICH (Mother's)	2 cookies	105	1.0	15.0	70	na	5.0	na	na	41%
EGG BISCUIT										
(Estee) 'Original Sandwich'	1 cookie	45	<1.0	6.0	5	(mq)	2.0	<1.0	0	39%
(FFV) 'Kreem Pilot Bread'	1 cookie	60	1.0	9.0	60	(mq)	2.0	(mq)	na	31%
(FFV) 'Royal Dainty' .7 oz	2 cookies	120	1.0	14.0	90	(mq)	6.0	(mq)	na	47%
(FFV) 'T.C. Rounds' approx 1 oz	2 cookies	160	1.0	20.0	65	(mq)	8.0	(mq)	na	46%
(FFV) 'Tango' 1.2 oz	2 cookies	160	1.0	26.0	50	(mq)	5.0	(mq)	na	29%
(Stella D'oro)	1 cookie	43	1.6	6.7	(mq)	(mq)	1.1	na	na	23%
(Stella D'oro) 'Anginetti'	1 cookie	31	0.5	4.9	(mq)	(mq)	1.0	na	na	29%
(Stella D'oro) dietetic	1 cookie	43	1.7	6.5	10	(mq)	1.1	na	na	23%
(Stella D'oro) dietetic 'Kitchen'	1 cookie	8	0.2	0.7	10	(mq)	0.5	na	na	56%
(Stella D'oro) 'Jumbo'	1 cookie	47	1.0	9.1	(mq)	(mq)	0.7	na	na	14%
(Stella D'oro) 'Roman'	1 cookie	137	2.7	20.4	(mq)	(mq)	5.0	(mq)	na	33%
(Stella D'oro) sugared	1 cookie	75	1.6	14.3	(mq)	(mq)	1.4	na	na	17%
ENGLISH TEA (Mother's) sandwich	1 cookie	100	1.0	14.0	60	na	4.0	na	na	38%
FIG										
(Estee) bar	2 cookies	90	<1.0	21.0	60	na	1.0	0.0	0	9%
(FFV) bar, vanilla	1 cookie	70	1.0	12.0	55	(mq)	1.0	<1.0	0	15%
(FFV) bar, whole wheat	1 cookie	70	1.0	11.0	50	(mq)	2.0	<1.0	0	27%
(Frookie) 'Fruitins'	1 cookie	60	1.0	12.0	25	na	1.0	0.0	0	15%
(Frookie) 'Fruitins' fat-free	2 cookies	90	1.0	21.0	75	1.0	0.0	0.0	0	0%
(Keebler) bar	1 cookie	60	1.0	11.0	70	(mq)	2.0	<1.0	0	27%
(Mother's) bar	2 cookies	110	1.0	23.0	85	na	2.0	na	na	16%
(Mother's) whole wheat	2 cookies	120	2.0	25.0	105	na	2.0	na	na	14%
(Nabisco) 'Newtons'	.5 oz	60	1.0	11.0	6	(mq)	1.0	<1.0	0	16%
(Nabisco) 'Newtons'	1.25 oz	120	1.0	24.0	110	(mq)	3.0	1.0	0	21%
(Nabisco) 'Newtons Cookie Variety'	1 oz	120	1.0	24.0	110	na	3.0	1.0	0	21%
(Nabisco) 'Newtons' fat-free, 1 piece	.75 oz	70	1.0	15.0	80	<1.0 c	0.0	0.0	0	0%

Food Name	Serving Size	Calories	Prot. gms	Carbs gms	Sod. mgs	Fiber gms	Fat gms	Sat. Fat gms	Chol. mgs	% Fat Cal.
(Natures Warehouse) bar, apple cinnamon, wheat-free ...	1 oz	98	1.0	19.0	18	na	2.0	na	na	18%
(Natures Warehouse) bar, raspberry, wheat-free	1 oz	98	1.0	19.0	18	na	2.0	na	na	18%
(Natures Warehouse) bar, wheat-free	1 oz	98	1.0	19.0	18	na	2.0	na	na	18%
(Natures Warehouse) bar, whole wheat	1 oz	98	1.0	19.0	18	na	2.0	na	na	18%
(Stella D'oro) pastry, dietetic	1 cookie	89	1.0	13.0	10	(mq)	3.7	(mq)	na	37%
FORTUNE										
(LaChoy)	1 oz	112	1.5	26.3	11	.7	0.2	0.1	0	2%
(LaChoy)	1 cookie	15	<1.0	4.0	1	<1.0	<1.0	(mq)	0	<31%
FRUIT										
(Barbara's Bakery) and nut	1 oz	140	2.0	18.0	55	na	6.0	na	0	40%
(Health Valley) 'Fruit & Fitness'	5 cookies	200	4.0	40.0	249	4.0	6.0	(mq)	0	24%
(Health Valley) Hawaiian, fat-free	3 cookies	80	2.0	18.0	80	3.0	0.0	na	0	0%
(Health Valley) tropical 'Fancy Fruit Chunks'	2 cookies	80	2.0	13.0	45	1.7	3.0	(mq)	0	31%
(Health Valley) tropical 'Fruit Centers' fat-free ...	1 cookie	80	2.0	17.0	80	2.0	0.0	na	0	0%
(Health Valley) tropical 'Fruit Jumbos'	1 cookie	70	1.0	10.0	26	1.5	2.0	(mq)	0	29%
(Stella D'oro) slices	1 cookie	60	1.1	8.7	(mq)	(mq)	2.2	(mq)	na	34%
FUDGE										
(Almost Home)	.5 oz	70	1.0	9.0	50	(mq)	3.0	<1.0	2	40%
(Almost Home) chocolate chip	.5 oz	70	1.0	9.0	50	0	3.0	1.0	2	40%
(Chips Ahoy!) mini bites 'Little Fudgies'	1 oz	230	3.0	27.0	105	0	12.0	4.0	0	47%
(Estee)	1 cookie	30	<1.0	4.0	0	(mq)	1.0	<1.0	0	31%
(Fifty 50) brownie, fructose sweetened	1 cookie	35	<1.0	5.0	0	na	2.0	na	0	43%
(Grandma's) 'Big Cookies' 2.75 oz	2 cookies	350	4.0	54.0	380	(mq)	13.0	(mq)	5	34%
(Keebler) mint 'Grasshopper' approx .5 oz	2 cookies	70	<1.0	10.0	35	(mq)	3.0	1.0	0	38%
(M&M/Mars) 'Twix'	1 bar	100	1.0	11.0	35	na	6.0	na	na	53%
(Mother's) double fudge sandwich	2 cookies	100	2.0	15.0	75	na	4.0	na	na	35%
(Mother's) wafer 'Flaky Flix'	2 cookies	130	1.0	14.0	30	na	9.0	na	30	57%
(Nabisco) caramel, peanut 'Heyday Bars' 1 piece	.75 oz	110	2.0	13.0	40	1.0	6.0	2.0	0	47%
(Nabisco) middles	.5 oz	80	1.0	9.0	35	(mq)	5.0	2.0	5	53%
(Nabisco) wafer 'Famous Wafers' 2 1/2 pieces	.5 oz	70	1.0	11.0	110	(mq)	2.0	<1.0	2	27%
(Nabisco) snaps, approx .5 oz	4 cookies	70	1.0	11.0	75	(mq)	2.0	1.0	2	27%
(Stella D'oro) 'Swiss Fudge Cookie'	1 cookie	68	0.8	8.5	(mq)	(mq)	3.4	(mq)	na	45%
(Tastykake) bar	1.8 oz	205	2.3	35.0	155	1.4	6.8	2.1	6	29%
GINGER										
(FFV) boys	1.25-oz pkg	150	2.0	26.0	210	(mq)	5.0	1.0	0	29%
(Frookie) spice	1 cookie	45	1.0	6.5	35	na	2.0	0.5	0	38%
(Pepperidge Farm) 'Gingerman'	2 cookies	70	1.0	10.0	50	(mq)	3.0	0.0	5	38%
(Westbrae) 'Rice Malt Snap'	1 oz	130	2.0	20.0	140	na	5.0	na	0	34%
GINGERSNAPS										
(Archway) '80/pkg'	1 cookie	25	1.0	4.0	20	(mq)	<1.0	na	0	<31%
(Archway) '54/pkg'	1 cookie	35	0.0	6.0	30	(mq)	1.0	na	0	27%
(Break Cake) approx 1 oz	5 cookies	130	2.0	20.0	110	na	5.0	1.2	0	34%
(Delicious)	.5 oz	64	0.8	11.3	78	na	1.7	na	<1	24%
(FFV) approx 1 oz	5 cookies	130	2.0	22.0	140	(mq)	4.0	1.0	0	27%
(Nabisco) 'Old Fashioned'	.25 oz	30	<1.0	6.0	45	(mq)	1.0	<1.0	0	24%
(Sunshine)	5 cookies	100	1.0	16.0	120	(mq)	3.0	1.0	0	28%
GRAHAM. See also HONEY GRAHAM.										
(Betty Crocker) w/chocolate frosting 'Dunkaroos'	1 tray	130	1.0	19.0	70	na	5.0	na	0	36%
(Betty Crocker) w/vanilla frosting 'Dunkaroos'	1 tray	130	<1.0	21.0	60	na	5.0	na	0	34%
(Keebler) chocolate 'Selects'	4 cookies	60	1.0	9.0	55	na	3.0	1.0	0	40%
(Keebler) honey nut 'Selects'	4 cookies	60	1.0	9.0	70	na	3.0	1.0	0	40%
(Mother's) dinosaur, original	1 cookie	70	1.0	12.0	50	na	2.0	na	na	26%
(Mother's) dinosaur, mini	7 cookies	60	1.0	9.0	40	na	1.0	na	na	18
(Nabisco) 'Bugs Bunny' 5 pieces	.5 oz	60	1.0	11.0	70	na	2.0	0.0	0	27%

Food Name	Serving Size	Calories	Prot. gms	Carbs gms	Sod. mgs	Fiber gms	Fat gms	Sat. Fat gms	Chol. mgs	% Fat Cal.
(Pepperidge Farm) cinnamon 'Goldfish'	1 oz	130	2.0	19.0	130	na	7.0	2.0	10	43%
(Pepperidge Farm) 'Goldfish'	1 oz	140	2.0	18.0	140	na	7.0	2.0	10	44%
(Teddy Grahams) snacks, chocolate	.5 oz	60	1.0	10.0	80	0	2.0	0.0	0	29%
(Teddy Grahams) snacks, cinnamon	.75-oz bag	100	1.0	16.0	120	0	3.0	1.0	0	28%
(Teddy Grahams) snacks, honey, 11 pieces	.5 oz	60	1.0	11.0	90	na	2.0	na	0	27%
(Teddy Grahams) vanilla honey 'Bearwichs'	4 cookies	70	1.0	10.0	65	(mq)	3.0	<1.0	0	38%
GRANOLA										
(Betty Crocker) chocolate filling 'Incredibites'	1 pouch	170	2.0	24.0	150	na	7.0	1.0	0	38%
(Betty Crocker) peanut butter 'Incredibites'	1 pouch	170	2.0	23.0	160	na	8.0	1.0	0	42%
(Betty Crocker) vanilla creme 'Incredibites'	1 pouch	170	2.0	24.0	180	na	7.0	1.0	0	38%
(Health Valley) 'Healthy'	3 cookies	75	2.0	17.0	60	3.0	0.0	na	0	0%
'HERMIT' (Break Cake)	1 cookie	230	3.0	38.0	280	na	7.0	1.5	10	28%
'HOB-NOBS' (Carr's)	1 cookie	72	1.1	9.6	78	(mq)	3.2	(mq)	na	40%
HONEY										
(Bakery Wagon) fruit bar	1 cookie	100	1.0	16.0	70	na	3.0	na	2	28%
(Health Valley) cinnamon, crisp 'Honey Jumbos'	1 cookie	70	1.0	10.0	35	2.6	2.0	(mq)	0	29%
(Health Valley) oat bran, fancy 'Honey Jumbos'	1 cookie	70	1.0	10.0	22	1.6	2.0	(mq)	0	29%
(Health Valley) peanut butter, crisp 'Honey Jumbos'	1 cookie	70	2.0	10.0	24	1.5	2.0	(mq)	0	27%
(Stella D'oro) 'Royal Nuggets'	1 cookie	2	0.1	0.1	na	na	0.1	na	na	53%
HONEY GRAHAM										
(Carafection) 'Original' carob coated	1 oz	139	2.0	17.0	26	na	7.0	na	na	45%
(Carr's) wheat 'Home Wheat Graham'	1 cookie	74	1.0	10.9	<1	(mq)	3.3	(mq)	na	38%
(Health Valley) 'Fancy'	7 cookies	130	3.0	21.0	89	3.5	5.0	(mq)	0	32%
(Health Valley) oat bran	7 cookies	130	3.0	25.0	47	3.4	2.0	(mq)	0	14%
(Honey Maid) .5 oz	2 pieces	60	1.0	11.0	90	(mq)	1.0	<1.0	0	16%
(Honey Maid) honey'n oat bran 'Graham Bites'	.5 oz	60	1.0	11.0	55	(mq)	2.0	<1.0	0	27%
(Keebler) approx .5 oz	4 cookies	70	1.0	12.0	85	(mq)	2.0	<1.0	0	26%
(Nabisco) vanilla, approx .5 oz	11 cookies	60	1.0	10.0	75	(mq)	2.0	<1.0	0	29%
(Pepperidge Farm) hazelnut 'Old Fashioned'	2 cookies	110	1.0	15.0	75	(mq)	6.0	2.0	0	46%
(Sunshine)	1 piece	60	1.0	10.0	90	(mq)	2.0	<1.0	0	29%
JELLY										
(Delicious) top	.8 oz	112	1.7	14.3	34	na	5.3	na	<1	43%
(FFV) tarts	1 cookie	60	<1.0	11.0	55	(mq)	2.0	<1.0	0	27%
LEMON										
(Barbara's Bakery) almond delights 'Small Indulgences'	1 oz	140	2.0	18.0	135	na	6.0	na	20	40%
(Delicious) sugar wafer	1 wafer	35	<1.0	4.0	3	na	2.0	na	0	47%
(Estee)	3 cookies	100	1.0	14.0	15	na	5.0	<1.0	0	43%
(Estee) 'Snack Crisps'	.66 oz	80	1.0	15.0	75	na	2.0	<1.0	0	22%
(Featherweight)	1 cookie	45	1.0	6.0	0	(mq)	2.0	(mq)	0	39%
(Frookie) sandwich 'Frookwich'	1 cookie	50	<1.0	7.0	30	na	2.0	0.0	0	36%
(Pepperidge Farm) nut crunch 'Old Fashioned'	2 cookies	110	1.0	13.0	50	(mq)	7.0	2.0	5	53%
(Westbrae) 'Rice Malt Snap'	1 oz	130	2.0	20.0	70	na	6.0	na	0	38%
MARSHMALLOW										
(Nabisco) cake 'Mallomars'	1 cookie	60	1.0	8.0	20	na	3.0	1.0	0	43%
(Nabisco) fudge cake 'Puffs'	.75 oz	90	1.0	14.0	45	(mq)	4.0	3.0	0	38%
(Nabisco) fudge cake 'Twirls'	1 oz	140	1.0	20.0	70	(mq)	6.0	4.0	0	39%
(Nabisco) fudge graham 'Suddenly S'Mores'	.75 oz	100	1.0	15.0	90	na	4.0	2.0	0	36%
(Nabisco) 'Pinwheels'	1 cookie	130	1.0	20.0	35	0	5.0	3.0	0	35%
(Pinwheels) chocolate cake	1 oz	130	1.0	20.0	40	(mq)	5.0	2.0	0	35%
MINI-CREME (Delicious)	1 wafer	24	<1.0	3.0	2	na	1.0	na	0	36%
MINT										
(Carafection) honey graham, carob coated	1 oz	139	2.0	17.0	26	na	7.0	na	na	45%
(FFV) sandwich, approx 1.1 oz	2 cookies	160	2.0	22.0	50	(mq)	7.0	(mq)	na	40%

Food Name	Serving Size	Calories	Prot. gms	Carbs gms	Sod. mgs	Fiber gms	Fat gms	Sat. Fat gms	Chol. mgs	% Fat Cal.
(Girl Scout Cookies) thin mints	4 cookies	160	1.0	20.0	140	2.0	9.0	6.0	0	49%
(Keebler) 'Soft Batch'	1 cookie	80	1.0	10.0	70	(mq)	4.0	1.0	0	45%
(Nabisco) sandwich 'Mystic Mint'	.5 oz	90	1.0	11.0	65	0	4.0	1.0	0	43%
MOLASSES										
(Archway)	1 cookie	100	1.0	18.0	155	2.0	2.0	(mq)	10	19%
(Bakery Wagon) iced	1 cookie	100	1.0	17.0	120	na	4.0	na	5	33%
(Grandma's) 'Old Time Big Cookies'	2 cookies	320	4.0	58.0	520	(mq)	9.0	(mq)	5	25%
(Nabisco) 'Pantry'	.5 oz	80	1.0	13.0	75	(mq)	3.0	<1.0	0	33%
(Pepperidge Farm) crisps 'Old Fashioned'	2 cookies	70	1.0	8.0	50	(mq)	3.0	0.0	0	43%
MUESLI *(Carr's)*	1 cookie	84	1.1	10.8	30	(mq)	4.1	(mq)	na	44%
OAT BRAN										
(Awrey's) raisin	1 cookie	100	1.0	14.0	115	1.0	4.0	1.0	0	38%
(Frookie) muffin	1 cookie	45	1.0	6.5	35	na	2.0	0.5	0	38%
(Health Valley) animal cookies	7 cookies	110	3.0	20.0	50	3.0	4.0	(mq)	0	28%
(Health Valley) fruit and nut	2 cookies	110	3.0	17.0	70	2.8	4.0	(mq)	0	31%
(Health Valley) fruit 'Oat Bran Fruit Jumbos'	1 cookie	70	1.0	10.0	22	1.5	2.0	(mq)	0	29%
(Health Valley) raisin 'Fancy Fruit Chunks'	2 cookies	90	2.0	15.0	95	1.6	3.0	(mq)	0	28%
(Natures Warehouse) chocolate chip, approx 1 oz	2 cookies	139	3.5	16.6	55	na	6.0	na	na	40%
(Natures Warehouse) wheat-free, approx 1 oz	2 cookies	129	2.3	16.0	54	na	6.2	na	na	43%
OATMEAL										
(Almost Home) raisin	.5 oz	70	1.0	10.0	40	1.0	3.0	1.0	2	38%
(Archway)	1 cookie	110	2.0	19.0	90	1.0	3.0	(mq)	5	24%
(Archway) apple filled	1 cookie	90	1.0	18.0	115	1.0	1.0	na	5	11%
(Archway) date filled	1 cookie	100	1.0	18.0	105	1.0	2.0	(mq)	5	19%
(Archway) iced	1 cookie	140	2.0	22.0	107	1.7	5.0	(mq)	5	32%
(Archway) 'Ruth's Golden'	1 cookie	120	2.0	20.0	122	1.2	4.0	(mq)	5	29%
(Bakers Bonus)	.5 oz	80	1.0	12.0	65	na	3.0	1.0	0	34%
(Bakery Wagon) chocolate chunk	1 cookie	100	2.0	17.0	80	na	3.0	na	2	26%
(Bakery Wagon) soft	1 cookie	100	2.0	15.0	105	na	5.0	na	2	40%
(Bakery Wagon) walnut raisin	1 cookie	100	2.0	16.0	80	na	4.0	na	2	33%
(Barbara's Bakery) raisin	1 oz	100	2.0	19.0	50	na	2.0	na	0	18%
(Break Cake) approx 1 oz	5 cookies	140	1.0	20.0	60	na	6.0	1.2	0	39%
(Chips Ahoy!) chocolate chip 'Selections'	.5 oz	90	1.0	10.0	60	na	5.0	2.0	5	51%
(Drake's) approx 1 oz	2 cookies	120	2.0	19.0	50	(mq)	4.0	1.0	0	30%
(Dunkin' Donuts) pecan, raisin	1 cookie	200	3.0	28.0	100	na	9.0	na	25	40%
(Duncan Hines) raisin	2 cookies	110	1.0	15.0	85	na	5.0	<2.0	na	41%
(Entenmann's) chocolatey chip 'Fat-Free Cholesterol-Free'	2 cookies	80	1.0	19.0	110	1.0	0.0	0.0	0	0%
(Entenmann's) raisin	2 cookies	30	1.0	17.0	120	na	0.0	na	0	0%
(Estee) raisin	3 cookies	100	2.0	14.0	15	na	4.0	<1.0	0	36%
(FFV) approx 1 oz	5 cookies	130	2.0	20.0	150	(mq)	4.0	1.0	0	29%
(Fifty 50) hearty oatmeal, fructose sweetened	1 cookie	35	<1.0	5.0	15	na	1.0	na	0	27%
(Frookie) raisin	1 cookie	45	1.0	6.5	35	na	2.0	0.5	0	38%
(Frookie) raisin, fat-free	1 cookie	50	1.0	11.0	75	1.0	0.0	0.0	0	0%
(Frookie) 7-grain oatmeal	1 cookie	45	1.0	6.5	35	na	2.0	0.5	0	38%
(Glenny's) wheat-free 'Noah 'N Friends Animal'	.5 oz	65	1.0	10.0	20	na	2.0	na	na	29%
(Grandma's) apple spice 'Big Cookies' 2.75 oz	2 cookies	330	5.0	51.0	570	(mq)	12.0	(mq)	10	33%
(Health Valley) raisin cinnamon 'Fruit Chunks'	3 cookies	85	2.0	19.0	80	3.0	0.0	na	0	0%
(Keebler) 'Old Fashion' approx .5 oz	1 cookie	80	1.0	12.0	110	(mq)	3.0	1.0	0	34%
(Keebler) w/chocolate 'Magic Middles' .5 oz	1 cookie	80	1.0	8.0	30	(mq)	5.0	1.0	0	56%
(Keebler) w/raisins, chewy 'Raisin Ruckus'	1 cookie	70	1.0	10.0	45	na	3.0	1.0	0	38%
(Little Debbie)	2.75 oz	340	5.0	52.0	440	(mq)	12.0	(mq)	2	32%
(Mother's)	1 cookie	60	1.0	8.0	80	na	3.0	na	na	43%
(Mother's) chocolate chip	1 cookie	70	1.0	10.0	85	na	3.0	na	na	38%
(Mother's) iced	1 cookie	70	1.0	10.0	70	na	3.0	na	na	38%

Food Name	Serving Size	Calories	Prot. gms	Carbs gms	Sod. mgs	Fiber gms	Fat gms	Sat. Fat gms	Chol. mgs	% Fat Cal.
(Mother's) walnut chocolate chip	1 cookie	70	1.0	9.0	60	na	3.0	na	na	40%
(Nabisco) raisin, 'Snack Wells'	1 cookie	60	1.0	10.0	65	na	1.0	<1.0	0	17%
(Natures Warehouse) raisin, approx 1 oz	2 cookies	135	2.0	17.3	44	na	6.4	na	na	43%
(Pepperidge Farm) chocolate chunk 'Dakota'	1 cookie	110	1.0	15.0	70	1.0	6.0	2.0	5	46%
(Pepperidge Farm) 'Family Request'	2 cookies	90	1.0	13.0	70	na	4.0	1.0	10	39%
(Pepperidge Farm) Irish 'Old Fashioned'	2 cookies	90	1.0	13.0	80	(mq)	5.0	1.0	5	45%
(Pepperidge Farm) raisin, soft, low-fat 'Wholesome Choice'	1 cookie	60	1.0	11.0	50	na	1.0	<1.0	0	16%
(Weight Watchers) raisin	2 cookies	90	1.0	20.0	75	na	<1.0	na	0	<10%
(Weight Watchers) spice	3 cookies	80	1.0	13.0	75	na	2.0	na	na	24%
(Westbrae) 'Rice Malt Snap'	1 oz	130	2.0	19.0	130	na	5.0	na	0	35%
ORANGE-PINEAPPLE										
(Health Valley) 'Mini Fruit Centers' fat-free	3 cookies	75	2.0	17.0	60	3.0	0.0	na	0	0%
PEACH *(Great Cakes)*	4.5 oz	260	10.0	40.0	20	21.0	6.0	na	0	21%
PEACH-APRICOT										
(FFV) bar, vanilla	1 cookie	70	<1.0	14.0	50	(mq)	1.0	<1.0	0	13%
(FFV) bar, whole wheat	1 cookie	70	<1.0	11.0	50	(mq)	2.0	<1.0	0	27%
(Health Valley) 'Mini Fruit Centers' fat-free	3 cookies	75	2.0	17.0	60	3.0	0.0	na	0	0%
(Stella D'oro) pastry	1 cookie	93	1.2	13.6	(mq)	(mq)	3.8	(mq)	na	37%
(Stella D'oro) pastry, dietetic	1 cookie	87	1.2	12.3	10	(mq)	3.7	(mq)	na	38%
PEANUT *(Health Valley)* 'Fancy Peanut Chunks'	2 cookies	100	2.0	14.0	585	2.3	3.0	(mq)	0	30%
PEANUT BUTTER										
(Bakery Wagon) oatmeal	1 cookie	110	3.0	12.0	150	na	7.0	na	2	51%
(Break Cake)	1 cookie	140	2.0	18.0	110	na	7.0	1.4	0	44%
(Break Cake) wafer	1 wafer	180	2.0	24.0	75	na	9.0	2.7	0	44%
(Delicious) and jelly sandwich 'Skippy & Welchs'	1 cookie	120	2.0	15.0	90	<1.0	6.0	1.5	0	44%
(Delicious) made w/Skippy peanut butter	1 cookie	80	2.0	7.0	65	.5	5.0	1.0	0	56%
(Estee) sandwich	1 cookie	50	1.0	5.0	35	(mq)	3.0	1.0	0	53%
(Featherweight)	1 cookie	40	1.0	5.0	10	(mq)	2.0	(mq)	0	43%
(Featherweight) creme wafer	1 cookie	25	1.0	3.0	0	(mq)	1.0	na	0	36%
(FFV) sandwich, approx 1.1 oz	2 cookies	170	2.0	21.0	110	(mq)	8.0	(mq)	na	44%
(Fifty 50) fructose sweetened	1 cookie	40	<1.0	5.0	10	na	2.0	na	0	43%
(Frookie) sandwich 'Frookwich'	1 cookie	50	<1.0	7.0	30	na	2.0	0.0	0	36%
(Glenny's) 'Noah 'N Friends Animal Cookies'	.5 oz	65	1.0	9.0	35	na	3.0	na	na	40%
(Grandma's) 'Big Cookies' 2.75 oz	2 cookies	410	7.0	43.0	410	(mq)	30.0	(mq)	10	57%
(Grandma's) cookie bits, 8 cookies	1 oz	140	3.0	19.0	125	na	6.0	na	0	38%
(Great Cakes) and jelly	4.5 oz	280	10.0	40.0	20	21.0	8.0	na	0	27%
(Keebler) chocolate chip 'Soft Batch' .5 oz	1 cookie	80	1.0	9.0	55	(mq)	5.0	1.0	0	53%
(Keebler) nut 'Soft Batch' approx .5 oz	1 cookie	80	1.0	9.0	60	(mq)	4.0	1.0	0	47%
(Mother's) sandwich 'Gaucho'	1 cookie	90	1.0	12.0	75	na	5.0	na	na	46%
(Nabisco) 'Ideal Bars'	.5 oz cookie	90	1.0	10.0	80	na	5.0	2.0	0	51%
(Nabisco) 'Nutter Butter Peanut Sandwich'	.5 oz	70	1.0	9.0	50	0	3.0	1.0	0	40%
(Natures Warehouse) approx 1 oz	2 cookies	128	3.6	18.2	29	na	6.1	na	na	39%
(Natures Warehouse) chocolate chip, approx 1 oz	2 cookies	139	4.1	13.9	50	na	8.5	na	na	52%
(Pepperidge Farm) chocolate chunk 'Cheyenne'	1 cookie	110	2.0	13.0	80	1.0	6.0	2.0	5	47%
(Pepperidge Farm) chocolate filled 'Nassau'	1 cookie	80	1.0	9.0	45	(mq)	5.0	1.0	5	53%
(Pepperidge Farm) 'Family Request'	2 cookies	80	2.0	10.0	65	na	5.0	2.0	5	48%
(Pitter Patter) cream filled, approx .5 oz	1 cookie	90	2.0	12.0	115	(mq)	4.0	<1.0	0	39%
(Planters) crispy cookie 'P.B. Crisps'	1 oz	140	3.0	17.0	125	na	7.0	2.0	0	44%
PEANUT CREME *(Nabisco)* 'Nutter Butter Patties'	.5 oz	80	2.0	8.0	45	na	4.0	1.0	0	47%
PECAN										
(Archway) crunch	1 cookie	60	1.0	8.0	45	(mq)	3.0	(mq)	5	43%
(Dunkin' Donuts) raisin cookie, 1.6 oz	1 cookie	200	3.0	28.0	100	1.0	9.0	(mq)	25	40%
PRALINE PECAN *(FFV)*	1 cookie	40	<1.0	10.0	40	(mq)	2.0	1.0	5	29%
PRUNE, pastry, dietetic *(Stella D'oro)*	1 cookie	95	1.2	15.0	10	(mq)	3.4	(mq)	na	32%

Food Name	Serving Size	Calories	Prot. gms	Carbs gms	Sod. mgs	Fiber gms	Fat gms	Sat. Fat gms	Chol. mgs	% Fat Cal.
RAISIN										
(Almost Home)	.5 oz	70	1.0	10.0	40	(mq)	3.0	<1.0	2	38%
(Archway)	1 cookie	100	2.0	18.0	107	.9	3.0	(mq)	5	25%
(Archway) bran	1 cookie	100	2.0	18.0	95	1.0 d	3.0	(mq)	5	25%
(Archway) oatmeal	1 cookie	50	1.0	7.0	20	(mq)	2.0	(mq)	0	36%
(Break Cake) creme	1 cookie	140	1.0	22.0	120	na	5.0	1.0	2	33%
(Entenmann's)	2 cookies	80	1.0	17.0	120	(mq)	0.0	0.0	0	0%
(Featherweight)	1 cookie	45	1.0	6.0	0	(mq)	2.0	(mq)	0	39%
(Grandma's) soft 'Big Cookies' approx 2.75 oz	2 cookies	320	3.0	54.0	280	(mq)	10.0	(mq)	10	28%
(Health Valley) apple 'Fruit Centers' fat-free	1 cookie	70	2.0	16.0	35	3.5	0.0	na	0	0%
(Health Valley) 'Jumbos' fat-free	1 cookie	80	2.0	17.0	80	3.5	0.0	na	0	0%
(Health Valley) nut 'Fruit Jumbos'	1 cookie	70	2.0	10.0	35	.9	3.0	(mq)	0	36%
(Health Valley) oatmeal, fat-free	3 cookies	80	2.0	18.0	80	3.0	0.0	na	0	0%
(Keebler) bar, iced	1 cookie	80	1.0	11.0	85	(mq)	4.0	1.0	0	43%
(Keebler) 'Soft Batch' approx .5 oz	1 cookie	70	1.0	10.0	65	(mq)	3.0	<1.0	0	38%
(Mother's) iced	1 cookie	80	1.0	11.0	45	na	4.0	na	na	43%
(Nabisco) nut 'Newtons'	.5 oz	60	1.0	11.0	50	(mq)	2.0	<1.0	0	27%
(Pepperidge Farm) bran 'Kitchen Hearth'	2 cookies	110	1.0	13.0	55	(mq)	5.0	2.0	5	45%
(Pepperidge Farm) 'Old Fashioned'	2 cookies	110	1.0	15.0	115	(mq)	5.0	2.0	10	41%
(Pepperidge Farm) 'Santa Fe'	1 cookie	100	1.0	16.0	70	1.0	4.0	1.0	5	35%
(Stella D'oro) 'Golden Bars'	1 cookie	109	1.6	16.0	(mq)	(mq)	4.3	(mq)	na	36%
(Sunshine)	2 cookies	110	1.0	16.0	125	(mq)	5.0	1.0	0	40%
(Tastykake) bar	1.8 oz	212	3.2	31.8	255	1.2	8.3	2.2	17	35%
(Tastykake) 'Soft'n Chewy'	1.4 oz	161	3.4	26.8	158	1.0	5.4	1.0	3	29%
(Weight Watchers) spice	3 cookies	80	1.0	13.0	75	(mq)	2.0	(mq)	na	24%
RASPBERRY										
(Bakery Wagon) filled	1 cookie	90	1.0	16.0	125	na	3.0	na	2	28%
(Frookie) 'Fruitins' fat-free	2 cookies	90	1.0	21.0	75	1.0	0.0	0.0	0	0%
(Great Cakes)	4.5 oz	260	10.0	40.0	20	21.0	6.0	na	0	21%
(Health Valley) apple 'Fruit Chunks'	3 cookies	85	2.0	19.0	80	3.0	0.0	na	0	0%
(Health Valley) apple 'Mini Fruit Centers' fat-free	3 cookies	75	2.0	17.0	60	3.0	0.0	na	0	0%
(Health Valley) 'Fruit Centers' fat-free	1 cookie	80	2.0	17.0	80	2.0	0.0	na	0	0%
(Health Valley) 'Jumbos' fat-free	1 cookie	80	2.0	17.0	80	3.5	0.0	na	0	0%
(Lu) 'Pims'	2 cookies	95	1.0	18.0	25	na	2.0	na	na	19%
(Nabisco) 'Newtons' .75 oz	1 cookie	80	1.0	15.0	70	(mq)	2.0	<1.0	0	22%
(Nabisco) 'Newtons' fat-free	1 cookie	60	1.0	16.0	75	na	0.0	na	0	0%
(Natural Nectar) swirl 'Incredible Edible Novelties'	1 cookie	220	4.0	33.0	115	na	8.0	na	20	33%
(Natures Warehouse) wheat-free, fat-free	1 oz	90	1.6	20.5	84	na	0.7	0.1	0	7%
(Pepperidge Farm) filled 'Chantilly'	1 cookie	80	1.0	14.0	35	(mq)	2.0	1.0	5	23%
(Pepperidge Farm) filled, chocolate 'Chantilly'	1 cookie	90	1.0	14.0	35	(mq)	3.0	1.0	5	31%
(Pepperidge Farm) filled 'Linzer'	1 cookie	120	2.0	20.0	55	(mq)	4.0	1.0	5	29%
(Pepperidge Farm) tart, low fat 'Wholesome Choice'	1 cookie	60	1.0	11.0	35	na	1.0	<1.0	0	16%
(Weight Watchers) fruit filled	1 cookie	80	<1.0	22.0	45	na	<1.0	na	0	<9%
REESE'S PIECES (Oven Lovin')	1 cookie	70	1.0	9.0	50	na	3.0	na	5	40%
SESAME										
(Glenny's) 'Nookie' bite size	.5 oz	60	1.0	6.0	8	na	4.0	na	na	56%
(Stella D'oro) dietetic 'Regina'	1 cookie	41	0.8	5.1	10	(mq)	2.0	(mq)	na	43%
(Stella D'oro) 'Regina'	1 cookie	48	0.9	6.1	(mq)	(mq)	2.2	(mq)	na	41%
SHORTBREAD										
(Break Cake) approx 1 oz	5 cookies	140	1.0	19.0	70	na	6.0	1.1	5	40%
(Estee)	3 cookies	100	2.0	16.0	100	na	3.0	<1.0	0	27%
(FFV) country	1 cookie	70	1.0	9.0	45	(mq)	4.0	1.0	5	47%
(Keebler) covered 'Fudge'n Caramel'	1 cookie	60	1.0	8.0	30	na	3.0	2.0	0	43%
(Keebler) fudge covered 'Toffee Toppers'	2 cookies	60	<1.0	10.0	50	na	4.0	3.0	0	45%

Food Name	Serving Size	Calories	Prot. gms	Carbs gms	Sod. mgs	Fiber gms	Fat gms	Sat. Fat gms	Chol. mgs	% Fat Cal.
(Keebler) fudge striped 'Fudge Stripes' .5 oz .... 1 cookie		50	<1.0	7.0	55	(mq)	3.0	<1.0	0	46%
(Keebler) 'Pecan Sandies' approx .5 oz .... 1 cookie		80	<1.0	9.0	75	(mq)	5.0	1.0	5	53%
(Keebler) 'Pecan Sandies' bite size .... 4 cookies		90	1.0	9.0	50	na	5.0	1.0	5	53%
(Keebler) w/chocolate center 'Magic Middles' .5 oz ...... 1 cookie		80	1.0	9.0	25	(mq)	5.0	1.0	5	53%
(Keebler) w/toffee pieces 'Toffee Sandies' .... 1 cookie		70	1.0	8.0	45	na	4.0	1.0	0	50%
(Lorna Doone) .5 oz .... 3 cookies		70	1.0	9.0	65	(mq)	4.0	<1.0	5	47%
(Mother's) striped .... 2 cookies		100	1.0	14.0	55	na	5.0	na	na	43%
(Nabisco) fudge striped 'Cookies 'n Fudge' .... .5 oz		60	1.0	7.0	50	(mq)	3.0	1.0	0	46%
(Nabisco) pecan supreme, low cholesterol .... 1 cookie		80	1.0	9.0	45	na	5.0	1.0	2	53%
(Pepperidge Farm) 'Old Fashioned' .... 2 cookies		150	1.0	17.0	85	(mq)	8.0	2.0	5	50%
(Pepperidge Farm) pecan 'Old Fashioned' .... 1 cookie		70	1.0	7.0	15	(mq)	5.0	2.0	0	58%
(Weight Watchers) .... 3 cookies		80	1.0	13.0	95	(mq)	2.0	(mq)	na	24%
SNACK, for weight control (Spicer's) .... 1 oz		100	3.0	12.0	70	9.0	4.0	na	0	38%
SPICE (Stella D'oro) 'Pfeffernusse' .... 1 piece		35	0.5	6.7	(mq)	(mq)	0.8	na	na	20%
STRAWBERRY										
(Healthy Times) 'Hugga Bears' organic .... 1 oz		120	2.0	17.0	38	na	3.0	na	0	26%
(Health Valley) 'Mini Fruit Centers' fat-free ...... 3 cookies		75	2.0	17.0	60	3.0	0.0	na	0	0%
(Nabisco) 'Newtons' .... 1.25 oz		120	1.0	24.0	110	(mq)	3.0	1.0	0	21%
(Nabisco) 'Newtons' .75 oz .... 1 cookie		70	1.0	15.0	70	na	2.0	0.0	0	22%
(Nabisco) 'Newtons' fat-free .... 1 cookie		60	1.0	16.0	80	na	0.0	na	0	0%
(Nabisco) 'Suddenly S'Mores' .... .75 oz		100	1.0	15.0	90	(mq)	4.0	2.0	0	36%
(Natural Nectar) swirl 'Incredible Edible Novelties' .... 1 cookie		220	4.0	33.0	115	na	8.0	na	20	33%
(Pepperidge Farm) 'Fruit Cookies' .... 2 cookies		100	1.0	15.0	50	(mq)	5.0	2.0	10	41%
SUGAR										
(Almost Home) .... .5 oz		70	1.0	10.0	80	na	3.0	1.0	0	38%
(Almost Home) 'Old Fashioned' .... .5 oz		70	1.0	10.0	80	(mq)	3.0	<1.0	2	38%
(Mother's) .... 1 cookie		70	1.0	8.0	35	na	4.0	na	na	50%
(Pepperidge Farm) 'Old Fashioned' .... 2 cookies		100	1.0	13.0	55	(mq)	5.0	2.0	10	45%
(Stella D'oro) 'Holiday Trinkets' .... 1 cookie		38	0.6	4.6	(mq)	(mq)	1.9	(mq)	na	45%
TAFFY (Mother's) sandwich .... 1 cookie		100	1.0	12.0	60	na	6.0	na	na	51%
TEA BISCUIT (Nabisco) 'Social Tea Biscuit' 3 pieces .... .5 oz		60	1.0	11.0	60	0	2.0	0.0	5	27%
TOFFEE										
(Chips Ahoy!) chunk, Heath 'Selections' .... 1 cookie		90	1.0	5.0	85	0	5.0	2.0	5	65%
(Delicious) w/Heath English toffee .... 1 cookie		90	1.0	10.0	45	1.0	5.0	1.0	8	51%
(Pepperidge Farm) 'Old Fashioned' .... 2 cookies		100	1.0	12.0	75	(mq)	5.0	2.0	5	46%
TOFU (Health Valley) 'The Great Tofu Cookie' .... 2 cookies		90	2.0	16.0	29	1.4	3.0	(mq)	0	27%
VANILLA										
(Barbara's Bakery) animal cookies .... 1 oz		145	2.0	18.0	85	na	7.0	na	0	44%
(Barbara's Bakery) 'Cookies & Creme' .... 2 cookies		120	1.0	18.0	75	na	5.0	na	15	37%
(Barbara's Bakery) raspberry 'Cookies & Creme' .... 2 cookies		120	1.0	18.0	75	na	5.0	na	15	37%
(Estee) .... 3 cookies		100	1.0	14.0	15	na	5.0	<1.0	0	43%
(Estee) sandwich .... 2 cookies		110	1.0	17.0	20	na	4.0	1.0	0	33%
(Featherweight) .... 1 cookie		45	1.0	6.0	0	(mq)	2.0	(mq)	0	39%
(Frookie) 'Funky Monkeys' .... 8 cookies		60	1.0	10.0	60	na	2.0	0.0	0	29%
(Frookie) sandwich 'Frookwich' .... 1 cookie		50	<1.0	7.0	30	na	2.0	0.0	0	36%
(Frookie) 'Trolls' .... 11 cookies		60	1.0	10.0	65	na	2.0	0.0	0	29%
(Glenny's) 'Noah 'N Friends Animal Cookies' .... .5 oz		65	1.0	10.0	35	na	2.0	na	na	29%
(Grandma's) cookie bits, artificially flavored .... 1 oz		140	2.0	20.0	75	na	6.0	na	5	38%
(Keebler) creme sandwich 'French' .5 oz .... 1 cookie		80	<1.0	12.0	80	(mq)	4.0	<1.0	0	41%
(Lu) 'Marie Lu' .... 1 cookie		50	1.0	8.0	45	na	2.0	na	na	33%
(Lu) 'Marie Lu' mini .... 5 cookies		50	1.0	8.0	45	na	2.0	na	na	33%
(Nabisco) creme sandwich 'Cameo' .... .5 oz		70	1.0	10.0	50	(mq)	3.0	1.0	0	38%
(Nabisco) creme sandwich 'Cookie Break' .... 1 cookie		50	1.0	7.0	35	0	2.0	0.0	0	36%
(Nabisco) creme sandwich 'Giggles' 2 pieces .... 1 oz		60	1.0	8.0	20	(mq)	3.0	<1.0	2	43%

Food Name	Serving Size	Calories	Prot. gms	Carbs gms	Sod. mgs	Fiber gms	Fat gms	Sat. Fat gms	Chol. mgs	% Fat Cal.
(Nabisco) reduced fat 'Snack Wells'	.5 oz	50	1.0	10.0	50	na	1.0	na	0	17%
(Pepperidge Farm) 'Bordeaux'	2 cookies	70	1.0	11.0	40	(mq)	3.0	1.0	0	36%
(Pepperidge Farm) chocolate coated 'Orleans'	3 cookies	90	0.0	11.0	30	(mq)	6.0	2.0	0	55%
(Pepperidge Farm) chocolate laced 'Pirouettes'	2 cookies	70	1.0	8.0	20	(mq)	4.0	1.0	5	50%
(Pepperidge Farm) chocolate nut coated 'Geneva'	2 cookies	130	1.0	14.0	50	(mq)	6.0	2.0	0	47%
(Pepperidge Farm) 'Goldfish'	1 oz	140	2.0	19.0	50	na	7.0	2.0	15	43%
(Pepperidge Farm) 'Pirouettes'	2 cookies	70	0.0	9.0	35	(mq)	4.0	1.0	5	50%
(Stella D'oro) 'Angelica Goodies'	1 cookie	106	1.7	15.7	(mq)	(mq)	4.0	(mq)	na	34%
(Stella D'oro) 'Castelets'	1 cookie	72	1.0	10.0	(mq)	(mq)	3.1	(mq)	na	39%
(Stella D'oro) 'Margherite'	1 cookie	72	1.0	10.8	(mq)	(mq)	2.8	(mq)	na	35%
(Tastykake) creme sandwich, shortbread	.4 oz	55	0.7	6.4	31	.1	3.0	0.7	0	49%
(Weight Watchers) sandwich	2 cookies	90	1.0	15.0	50	na	3.0	1.0	0	30%
WAFER										
(Archway) vanilla	1 wafer	30	0.0	6.0	30	(mq)	<1.0	na	0	<27%
(Biscos) sugar, 4 pieces	.5 oz	70	0.0	10.0	20	na	3.0	0.0	0	40%
(Biscos) waffle creme	1 wafers	45	0.0	6.0	10	0	2.0	1.0	6	43%
(Break Cake) chocolate, sugar	4 wafers	200	2.0	30.0	95	na	9.0	3.8	0	39%
(Break Cake) strawberry, sugar	4 wafers	220	1.0	28.0	100	na	11.0	3.1	0	46%
(Break Cake) 'Striper Wafer'	1 wafer	190	2.0	23.0	80	na	10.0	3.2	0	47%
(Break Cake) vanilla, sugar	4 wafers	220	1.0	28.0	105	na	11.0	3.7	0	46%
(Delicious) chocolate strawberry, sugar	1 wafer	35	<1.0	3.0	4	na	2.0	na	0	53%
(Delicious) chocolate, sugar	1 wafer	34	<1.0	2.0	5	na	2.0	na	0	60%
(Delicious) strawberry, sugar	1 wafer	35	<1.0	4.0	3	na	2.0	na	0	47%
(Delicious) sugar, assorted	.25 oz	38	<1.0	4.0	<1	na	2.0	na	2	47%
(Delicious) vanilla	.5 oz	70	0.8	10.5	41	na	2.2	na	<1	31%
(Delicious) vanilla, sugar	.25 oz	37	<1.0	4.0	<1	na	2.0	na	2	47%
(Delicious) vanilla, sugar	1 wafer	35	<1.0	4.0	3	na	2.0	na	0	47%
(Estee) chocolate creme	4 wafers	90	<1.0	11.0	0	na	5.0	<1.0	0	48%
(Estee) strawberry	3 wafers	100	<1.0	14.0	0	na	5.0	<1.0	0	43%
(Estee) vanilla	3 wafers	100	<1.0	14.0	0	na	5.0	<1.0	0	43%
(Estee) vanilla creme	4 wafers	90	<1.0	12.0	0	na	4.0	<1.0	0	41%
(Featherweight) strawberry creme	1 wafer	20	0.0	3.0	0	(mq)	1.0	na	0	43%
(Featherweight) vanilla creme	1 wafers	20	0.0	3.0	0	(mq)	1.0	na	0	43%
(FFV) vanilla, approx 1 oz	8 wafers	130	1.0	19.0	100	(mq)	5.0	1.0	5	36%
(Fifty 50) chocolate creme filled, w/o sugar	1 wafer	35	<1.0	4.0	10	na	2.0	na	0	47%
(Fifty 50) vanilla, creme filled, w/o sugar	1 wafer	35	<1.0	4.0	5	na	2.0	na	0	47%
(Keebler) vanilla, golden	4 wafers	80	<1.0	10.0	60	(mq)	3.0	1.0	0	38%
(Lu) cream	3 cookies	110	1.0	11.0	50	na	7.0	na	na	57%
(Mother's) checkerboard	5 wafers	85	1.0	13.0	15	na	4.0	na	na	39%
(Mother's) vanilla, 'Flaky Flix'	2 wafers	115	1.0	18.0	na	na	5.0	na	25	37%
(Nabisco) 'Brown Edge Wafers' 2 1/2 wafers	.5 oz	70	1.0	10.0	45	0	3.0	1.0	2	38%
(Nabisco) 'Famous Chocolate Wafers' 2 1/2 wafers	.5 oz	60	1.0	11.0	100	na	2.0	1.0	5	27%
(Nabisco) striped wafer 'Cookies 'N Fudge'	1 wafer	70	1.0	8.0	25	0	4.0	1.0	0	50%
(Nabisco) vanilla, cinnamon 'Nilla Wafers' .5 oz	3 1/2 wafers	60	1.0	11.0	45	(mq)	2.0	<1.0	5	27%
(Nabisco) vanilla, 'Nilla Wafers' approx .5 oz	3 1/2 wafers	60	1.0	11.0	45	(mq)	2.0	<1.0	5	27%
(Tastykake) vanilla, sugar	10 wafers	34	0.3	4.1	11	<.1	1.9	0.5	0	49%
(Weider) 'Victory Explosive Workout'	6 wafers	30	<1.0	6.0	60	na	0.0	na	na	0%
(Westbrae) 5-spice	4 1/2 wafers	40	1.0	8.0	30	na	0.0	na	0	0%
WALNUT										
(Keebler) 'Soft Batch' approx .5 oz	1 cookie	80	1.0	10.0	70	(mq)	4.0	1.0	0	45%
(Lu) whole wheat and cinnamon 'Marie Lu'	1 cookie	45	1.0	8.0	55	na	1.0	na	na	20%
(Mother's) fudge	1 cookie	70	1.0	8.0	50	na	4.0	na	na	50%
COOKIE DOUGH, PREPARED										
chocolate chip	1 oz	126	1.3	17.4	59	na	5.8	2.0	7	41%

Food Name	Serving Size	Calories	Prot. gms	Carbs gms	Sod. mgs	Fiber gms	Fat gms	Sat. Fat gms	Chol. mgs	% Fat Cal.
chocolate chip	1 cookie	71	0.7	9.8	33	na	3.3	1.1	4	41%
chocolate chip *(Pillsbury)*	1 cookie	70	1.0	9.0	55	(mq)	3.0	<1.0	5	40%
chocolate chip, baked	1 oz	139	1.4	19.3	66	na	6.4	2.2	8	41%
chocolate chip, baked	1 cookie	59	0.6	8.2	28	na	2.7	0.9	3	41%
chocolate chip 'Ready To Bake' *(Toll House)*	1.2 oz	150	1.0	20.0	115	(mq)	7.0	(mq)	na	43%
chocolate chip 'Ready To Bake' w/nuts *(Toll House)*	1.2 oz	160	2.0	19.0	90	(mq)	8.0	(mq)	na	46%
double chocolate chip 'Ready To Bake' 1.2 oz *(Toll House)*	2 cookies	150	2.0	19.0	60	(mq)	7.0	(mq)	na	43%
oatmeal	1 oz	120	1.5	16.7	83	na	5.4	1.4	7	40%
oatmeal	1 cookie	68	0.9	9.5	47	na	3.0	0.8	4	39%
oatmeal, baked	1 oz	134	1.7	18.6	93	na	5.9	1.5	7	40%
oatmeal, baked	1 cookie	57	0.7	7.9	39	na	2.5	0.6	3	40%
oatmeal raisin *(Pillsbury)*	1 cookie	60	1.0	9.0	55	(mq)	3.0	<1.0	0	40%
oatmeal raisin 'Ready To Bake' 2 cookies *(Toll House)*	1.2 oz	130	2.0	21.0	55	(mq)	5.0	(mq)	na	33%
peanut butter *(Pillsbury)*	1 cookie	70	1.0	9.0	75	(mq)	3.0	<1.0	5	40%
sugar	1 oz	124	1.2	16.7	120	na	5.9	1.5	8	43%
sugar	1 cookie	70	0.7	9.4	68	na	3.3	0.9	5	42%
sugar *(Pillsbury)*	1 cookie	70	1.0	9.0	70	(mq)	3.0	<1.0	5	40%
sugar, baked	1 oz	137	1.3	18.6	133	na	6.6	1.7	9	43%
COOKIE MIX										
chocolate chip *(Duncan Hines)*	2 cookies	130	1.0	20.0	85	(mq)	5.0	(mq)	na	35%
chocolate chip *(Finast)*	2 cookies	110	1.0	16.0	290	(mq)	5.0	(mq)	na	40%
chocolate chip, 2-inch diam each *(Estee)*	2 cookies	90	1.0	13.0	80	na	4.0	1.0	0	39%
chocolate chip 'Big Batch' *(Betty Crocker)*	2 cookies	120	1.0	16.0	100	(mq)	6.0	(mq)	(mq)	44%
'Deluxe' 2-inch diam *(Krusteaz)*	1 cookie	120	1.0	16.0	126	na	5.0	na	11	40%
golden sugar *(Duncan Hines)*	2 cookies	130	1.0	17.0	70	(mq)	6.0	(mq)	na	43%
oatmeal raisin *(Duncan Hines)*	2 cookies	130	2.0	18.0	70	(mq)	6.0	(mq)	na	40%
peanut butter *(Duncan Hines)*	2 cookies	140	3.0	15.0	120	(mq)	7.0	(mq)	na	47%
COOKING SPRAY										
(Mazola) corn oil 'No Stick'	2.5-sec spray	6	0.0	0.0	0	0	1.0	0.1	0	100%
(Pam) for 1/3 of 10-inch skillet	1 spray	2	0.0	0.0	0	0	1.0	na	0	100%
(Weight Watchers) 'Buttery Spray' butter flavor	1-sec spray	2	0.0	0.0	0	0	<1.0	na	0	100%
(Weight Watchers) canola oil spray	.33 grams	2	0.0	0.0	0	na	<1.0	na	0	100%
(Weight Watchers) 'Cooking Spray'	1-sec spray	2	0.0	0.0	0	0	1.0	na	0	100%
(Wesson) lite	.27 grams	<1	0.0	0.0	0	0	<1.0	na	0	100%
(Wesson) no-stick	.25 gram	2	0.0	0.0	0	0	0.3	0.0	0	100%
COOL WHIP. See CREAM TOPPING, NONDAIRY.										
CORIANDER/Chinese parsley										
raw	1 tbsp	5	0.4	0.9	4	>.2 c	0.1	na	0	15%
raw	1 tsp	2	0.1	0.3	1	>.1 c	0.0	na	0	0%
raw, approx .8 oz	9 plants	4	0.5	0.5	6	.5	0.1	na	0	18%
trimmed	1 oz	6	0.7	0.7	8	>.2 c	0.2	(tr)	0	24%
untrimmed	1 lb	77	9.1	10.0	108	>3.1 c	2.3	na	0	21%
CORIANDER LEAF/Chinese parsley leaf										
dried	1 oz	79	6.2	14.8	60	>2.9 c	1.3	na	0	12%
dried	1 tbsp	5	0.4	0.9	4	.2	0.1	(tr)	0	15%
dried	1 tsp	2	0.1	0.3	1	.1	<.1	(tr)	0	<36%
CORIANDER SEED/Chinese parsley seed										
whole	1 oz	84	3.5	15.6	10	>8.3 c	5.0	0.3	0	37%
whole	1 tbsp	15	0.6	2.8	2	>1.5 c	0.9	0.1	0	37%
whole	1 tsp	5	0.2	1.0	1	>.5 c	0.3	0.0	0	36%
whole *(Durkee)*	1 tsp	8	0.0	0.0	0	0	<0.1	na	na	<39%
whole *(Laurel Leaf)*	1 tsp	8	0.0	0.0	0	0	<0.1	na	na	<39%
whole *(Spice Islands)*	1 tsp	6	0.2	0.8	<1	>.4 c	0.3	<.1	0	40%
CORN										
cooked	1/2 cup	88	1.8	19.5	0	3.4	0.5	0.1	0	5%

Food Name	Serving Size	Calories	Prot. gms	Carbs gms	Sod. mgs	Fiber gms	Fat gms	Sat. Fat gms	Chol. mgs	% Fat Cal.
dry	1 cup	375	7.8	83.2	3	11.6	2.2	0.3	0	5%
dry	2 oz	203	4.3	45.2	2	6.3	1.2	0.2	0	5%
sweet, boiled, drained	4 oz	122	3.8	28.5	19	4.2	1.5	0.2	0	10%
sweet, raw, trimmed	1 oz	24	0.9	5.4	4	.9	0.3	0.1	0	10%
sweet, raw, untrimmed	1 lb	140	5.3	31.1	25	5.2	1.9	0.3	0	11%
sweet, white, boiled, drained, cut	1/2 cup	89	2.7	20.6	14	4.7	1.0	0.2	0	9%
sweet, white, kernels, boiled, drained	1 ear	83	2.6	19.3	13	4.4	1.0	0.2	0	9%
sweet, white, kernels from cob, raw	1 ear	77	2.9	17.1	14	2.9	1.1	0.2	0	11%
sweet, white, raw, cut	1/2 cup	66	2.5	14.7	12	2.5	0.9	0.1	0	11%
sweet, yellow, boiled, drained, cut	1/2 cup	89	2.7	20.6	14	3.0	1.0	0.2	0	9%
sweet, yellow, kernels, boiled, drained	1 ear	83	2.6	19.3	13	2.8	1.0	0.2	0	9%
sweet, yellow, kernels from cob, raw	1 ear	77	2.9	17.1	14	2.9	1.1	0.2	0	11%
sweet, yellow, raw, cut	1/2 cup	66	2.5	14.7	12	2.5	0.9	0.1	0	11%
white	1/2 cup	303	7.8	61.6	29	>2.4 c	3.9	0.6	0	11%
yellow	1/2 cup	303	7.8	61.6	29	>2.4 c	3.9	0.6	0	11%
CORN, CANNED										
cream style	1/2 cup	93	2.2	23.2	365	1.3	0.5	0.1	0	4%
cream style	4 oz	82	2.0	20.6	323	1.1	0.5	0.1	0	5%
cream style (A&P)	1/2 cup	100	2.0	25.0	330	(mq)	1.0	na	0	8%
cream style (Finast)	1/2 cup	105	2.0	25.0	350	(mq)	1.0	na	0	8%
cream style (Green Giant)	1/2 cup	100	2.0	24.0	390	2.0	<1.0	na	0	<8%
cream style (S&W Nutradiet)	1/2 cup	100	3.0	21.0	0	(mq)	1.0	na	0	9%
cream style, golden (Del Monte)	1/2 cup	80	2.0	18.0	355	(mq)	1.0	na	0	10%
cream style, golden (Pathmark)	1/2 cup	100	2.0	25.0	350	(mq)	1.0	na	0	8%
cream style, golden (Stokely)	1/2 cup	100	2.0	23.0	380	(mq)	0.0	0.0	0	0%
cream style, golden, low-sodium	4 oz	82	2.0	20.6	3	>.6 c	0.5	0.1	0	5%
cream style, golden 'No Salt Added' (Del Monte)	1/2 cup	80	2.0	20.0	10	(mq)	1.0	na	0	9%
cream style, golden, white (Stokely)	1/2 cup	100	2.0	23.0	380	(mq)	0.0	0.0	0	0%
cream style 'No Frills' (Pathmark)	1 cup	210	5.0	51.0	700	(mq)	1.0	na	0	4%
cream style 'Premium Homestyle No Starch Added' (S&W)	1/2 cup	120	3.0	24.0	285	(mq)	1.0	na	0	8%
cream style 'Premium Homestyle Starch Added' (S&W)	1/2 cup	105	2.0	25.0	435	(mq)	1.0	na	0	8%
cream style, white (Del Monte)	1/2 cup	90	2.0	21.0	355	(mq)	0.0	0.0	0	0%
'Crisp 'N Sweet' vacuum packed (Freshlike)	1/2 cup	80	2.0	18.0	5	na	1.0	na	na	10%
'Delicorn' (Green Giant)	1/2 cup	80	2.0	19.0	350	2.0	<1.0	na	0	<10%
golden (Pathmark)	1/2 cup	90	2.0	19.0	330	(mq)	1.0	na	0	10%
golden (Stokely)	1/2 cup	90	2.0	20.0	300	(mq)	0.0	0.0	0	0%
golden, cream style (Freshlike)	1/2 cup	110	2.0	25.0	290	na	1.0	na	na	8%
golden, cream style (Veg•All)	1/2 cup	110	2.0	25.0	290	na	1.0	na	na	8%
golden, cream style, no salt added (Freshlike)	1/2 cup	110	2.0	25.0	15	na	1.0	na	na	8%
golden, 50% less salt (Green Giant)	1/2 cup	70	2.0	16.0	175	2.0	<1.0	na	0	<11%
golden 'No Salt Added' (Del Monte)	1/2 cup	80	2.0	18.0	10	(mq)	1.0	na	0	10%
golden 'No Salt or Sugar Added' (Green Giant)	1/2 cup	80	3.0	18.0	0	2.0	<1.0	na	0	<10%
golden 'No Salt or Sugar Added' (Stokely)	1/2 cup	80	2.0	16.0	5	(mq)	0.0	0.0	0	0%
golden 'Pantry Express' (Green Giant)	1/2 cup	80	2.0	18.0	210	1.0	<1.0	0.0	0	<10%
golden, sweet (IGA)	1/2 cup	70	2.0	16.0	10	(mq)	1.0	na	0	11%
golden, vacuum pack (Green Giant)	1/2 cup	80	2.0	20.0	330	2.0	0.0	0.0	0	0%
golden, vacuum pack (Stokely)	1/2 cup	90	3.0	22.0	300	(mq)	0.0	0.0	0	0%
golden, whole kernel (Veg•All)	1/2 cup	80	2.0	19.0	320	na	1.0	na	na	10%
golden, whole kernel, vacuum packed (Freshlike)	1/2 cup	100	3.0	22.0	260	na	1.0	na	na	8%
golden, whole kernel, vacuum packed (Veg•All)	1/2 cup	100	3.0	22.0	260	na	1.0	na	na	8%
golden, whole kernel, water packed, w/o salt (Freshlike)	1/2 cup	80	2.0	19.0	5	na	1.0	na	na	10%
golden, whole kernel, water packed, w/o sugar and salt (Freshlike)	1/2 cup	80	2.0	19.0	5	na	1.0	na	na	10%
golden, w/liquid (Del Monte)	1/2 cup	70	2.0	17.0	355	(mq)	1.0	na	0	11%

Food Name	Serving Size	Calories	Prot. gms	Carbs gms	Sod. mgs	Fiber gms	Fat gms	Sat. Fat gms	Chol. mgs	% Fat Cal.
in brine, w/liquid (Green Giant)	1/2 cup	70	2.0	18.0	350	2.0	0.0	0.0	0	0%
kernel, w/liquid	4 oz	69	2.2	16.8	287	.9	0.5	0.1	0	6%
kernel, w/liquid (A&P)	1/2 cup	80	2.0	20.0	350	(mq)	1.0	(mq)	0	9%
kernel, w/liquid (Featherweight)	1/2 cup	80	2.0	16.0	10	(mq)	1.0	na	0	11%
kernel, w/liquid (Finast)	1/2 cup	90	2.0	20.0	390	(mq)	1.0	na	0	9%
kernel, w/liquid (Green Giant)	1/2 cup	80	2.0	18.0	280	2.7	0.0	0.0	0	0%
kernel, w/liquid (S&W Nutradiet)	1/2 cup	80	2.0	15.0	0	(mq)	1.0	na	0	12%
kernel, w/liquid, drained	4 oz	92	3.0	21.1	(mq)	1.5	1.1	0.2	0	9%
kernel, w/liquid, 50% less salt, no sugar (Green Giant)	1/2 cup	50	2.0	11.0	140	2.0	1.0	na	0	15%
kernel, w/liquid, low-sodium	4 oz	69	2.2	16.8	3	.9	0.5	0.1	0	6%
kernel, w/liquid 'No Frills' (Pathmark)	1 cup	160	5.0	38.0	550	(mq)	1.0	na	0	5%
kernel, w/liquid 'No Salt Added' (A&P)	1/2 cup	80	2.0	18.0	10	(mq)	<1.0	na	0	<10%
kernel, w/liquid 'No Salt Added' (Finast)	1/2 cup	80	3.0	19.0	10	(mq)	1.0	na	0	9%
kernel, w/liquid 'No Salt Added' (Pathmark)	1/2 cup	70	2.0	16.0	10	(mq)	1.0	na	0	11%
niblets (Green Giant)	1/2 cup	80	2.0	20.0	310	2.0	0.0	0.0	0	0%
niblets, no salt, no sugar added (Green Giant)	1/2 cup	80	2.0	18.0	0	2.0	<1.0	0.0	0	<10%
sweet, select (Green Giant)	1/2 cup	60	2.0	15.0	280	3.0	<1.0	0.0	0	<12%
sweet, white, brine pack, drained solids	1/2 cup	66	2.2	15.2	265	1.2	0.8	0.1	0	9%
sweet, white, brine pack, regular, w/liquid	1/2 cup	78	2.5	19.0	324	>.6 c	0.6	0.1	0	6%
sweet, white, brine pack, dietary, w/liquid	1/2 cup	78	2.5	19.0	4	>.6 c	0.6	0.1	0	6%
sweet, white, cream style, regular pack	1/2 cup	92	2.2	23.2	365	1.5	0.5	0.1	0	4%
sweet, white, cream style, special dietary pack	1/2 cup	92	2.2	23.2	4	>.6 c	0.5	0.1	0	4%
sweet, white, vacuum pack, regular pack	1/2 cup	83	2.5	20.4	286	>.8 c	0.5	0.1	0	5%
sweet, white, vacuum pack, special dietary pack	1/2 cup	83	2.5	20.4	3	>.8 c	0.5	0.1	0	5%
sweet, yellow, brine pack, drained solids	1/2 cup	66	2.2	15.2	265	1.1	0.8	0.1	0	9%
sweet, yellow, brine pack, regular, w/liquid	1/2 cup	78	2.5	19.0	324	1.0	0.6	0.1	0	6%
sweet, yellow, brine pack, dietary, w/liquid	1/2 cup	78	2.5	19.0	4	1.0	0.6	0.1	0	6%
sweet, yellow, cream style, regular pack	1/2 cup	92	2.2	23.2	365	1.5	0.5	0.1	0	4%
sweet, yellow, cream style, special dietary pack	1/2 cup	92	2.2	23.2	4	7.0	0.5	0.1	0	4%
sweet, yellow, vacuum pack, regular pack	1/2 cup	83	2.5	20.4	286	6.0	0.5	0.1	0	5%
sweet, yellow, vacuum pack, special dietary pack	1/2 cup	83	2.5	20.4	3	6.0	0.5	0.1	0	5%
vacuum pack, w/liquid (Del Monte)	1/2 cup	90	3.0	22.0	355	(mq)	1.0	na	0	8%
vacuum pack, w/liquid 'No Salt Added' (Del Monte)	1/2 cup	90	3.0	22.0	10	(mq)	1.0	na	0	8%
white (Green Giant)	1/2 cup	80	2.0	20.0	310	2.0	0.0	0.0	0	0%
white (Stokely)	1/2 cup	90	3.0	21.0	290	(mq)	0.0	0.0	0	0%
white, vacuum pack (A&P)	1/2 cup	100	2.0	25.0	300	(mq)	1.0	na	0	8%
white, vacuum pack (Finast)	4 oz	90	5.0	20.0	150	(mq)	1.0	na	0	8%
white, vacuum pack (Green Giant)	1/2 cup	80	2.0	20.0	290	2.0	0.0	0.0	0	0%
white, vacuum pack (Pathmark)	1/2 cup	120	3.0	25.0	350	(mq)	1.0	na	0	7%
white, vacuum pack 'Niblets' (Green Giant)	1/2 cup	80	3.0	16.0	280	1.7	1.0	na	0	11%
white, w/liquid (Del Monte)	1/2 cup	70	2.0	16.0	355	(mq)	0.0	0.0	0	0%
white, young, tender 'Premium' (S&W)	1/2 cup	90	2.0	20.0	295	(mq)	1.0	na	0	9%
whole kernel, golden, sweet (Green Giant)	1/2 cup	70	2.0	18.0	360	2.0	0.0	0.0	0	0%
whole kernel, golden, sweet, 50% less salt (Green Giant)	1/2 cup	70	2.0	16.0	180	2.0	<1.0	0.0	0	<11%
w/peppers 'Mexicorn' (Green Giant)	1/2 cup	80	2.0	19.0	450	2.0	<1.0	na	0	<10%
CORN, FROZEN										
(Health Valley)	1/3 cup	76	2.0	17.0	4	1.7	0.0	0.0	0	0%
cream style (Green Giant)	1/2 cup	110	3.0	25.0	370	2.5	1.0	0.0	0	7%
freeze-dried, prepared (Mountain House)	1/2 cup	90	2.0	18.0	<1	(mq)	1.0	na	0	10%
golden, in butter sauce (Green Giant)	1/2 cup	100	3.0	19.0	310	2.0	2.0	1.0	5	17%
in butter sauce (Finast)	1/2 cup	170	4.0	30.0	390	(mq)	4.0	(mq)	na	21%
in butter sauce 'Niblets' (Green Giant)	1/2 cup	100	2.0	18.0	280	2.0	2.0	(mq)	na	18%
in butter sauce 'Niblets One Serving' (Green Giant)	4.5 oz	120	3.0	24.0	350	3.0	2.0	<1.0	5	14%
in butter sauce 'Side Dish' (Budget Gourmet)	5.5 oz	190	4.0	31.0	310	(mq)	6.0	(mq)	15	28%

Food Name	Serving Size	Calories	Prot. gms	Carbs gms	Sod. mgs	Fiber gms	Fat gms	Sat. Fat gms	Chol. mgs	% Fat Cal.
in butter sauce 'Singles' *(Stokely)*	4 oz	110	3.0	23.0	230	(mq)	1.0	(mq)	5	8%
in sauce, country style 'Side Dish' *(Budget Gourmet)*	5.75 oz	140	4.0	19.0	290	na	5.0	(mq)	15	33%
kernel *(A&P)*	3.3 oz	80	3.0	18.0	0	(mq)	<1.0	na	0	<10%
kernel *(Finast)*	3.3 oz	80	3.0	20.0	5	(mq)	1.0	na	0	9%
kernel, cut *(Frosty Acres)*	3.3 oz	80	3.0	20.0	3	>1.0 c	1.0	na	0	9%
kernel, cut *(Seabrook)*	3.3 oz	80	3.0	20.0	3	>1.0 c	1.0	na	0	9%
kernel, cut *(Southern)*	3.5 oz	98	3.1	21.3	20	(mq)	0.7	na	0	6%
kernel, cut, petite 'Deluxe' *(Birds Eye)*	2.6 oz	70	2.0	16.0	0	2.0	1.0	na	0	11%
kernel, cut 'Portion Pack' *(Birds Eye)*	3 oz	70	3.0	18.0	0	2.0	1.0	na	0	10%
kernel, cut 'Singles' *(Stokely)*	3 oz	75	3.0	18.0	5	(mq)	1.0	na	0	10%
kernel 'Harvest Fresh Niblets' *(Green Giant)*	1/2 cup	80	2.0	17.0	40	2.0	1.0	na	0	11%
kernel 'Niblets' *(Green Giant)*	1/2 cup	90	2.0	19.0	5	2.0	<1.0	na	0	<10%
kernel 'Niblets Supersweet' *(Green Giant)*	1/2 cup	60	2.0	13.0	5	2.0	1.0	na	0	13%
kernel 'Sweet' *(Birds Eye)*	3.3 oz	80	3.0	20.0	0	2.0	1.0	na	0	9%
kernel 'Tender Sweet Deluxe' *(Birds Eye)*	3.3 oz	80	3.0	20.0	0	2.0	1.0	na	0	9%
niblets 'Butter Sauce' *(Green Giant)*	1/2 cup	100	3.0	19.0	310	2.0	2.0	1.0	5	17%
niblets 'Plain Polybag' *(Green Giant)*	1/2 cup	90	2.0	19.0	5	2.0	<1.0	0.0	0	<10%
on the cob *(A&P)*	1 ear	120	4.0	28.0	0	(mq)	1.0	na	0	7%
on the cob *(Birds Eye)*	1 ear	120	4.0	29.0	0	na	1.0	na	0	6%
on the cob *(Frosty Acres)*	1 ear	120	4.0	29.0	0	(mq)	1.0	na	0	6%
on the cob *(Seabrook)*	5-inch ear	120	4.0	29.0	4	>1.0 c	1.0	na	0	6%
on the cob *(Southern)*	5-inch ear	140	5.0	30.0	na	(mq)	1.0	na	0	6%
on the cob, baby 'Deluxe' *(Birds Eye)*	2.6 oz	25	2.0	4.0	10	2.0	0.0	na	0	0%
on the cob 'Big Ears' *(Birds Eye)*	1 ear	160	5.0	37.0	0	na	1.0	na	0	5%
on the cob, boiled, drained, kernels from ear	4 oz	59	2.0	14.1	3	>.4 c	0.5	0.1	0	7%
on the cob 'Cob Treats' *(A&P)*	2 ears	130	5.0	28.0	5	(mq)	1.0	na	0	6%
on the cob, 5.3 oz edible portion *(Ore-Ida)*	1 ear	180	5.0	39.0	40	(mq)	2.0	(mq)	0	9%
on the cob, in butter sauce 'Singles' *(Stokely)*	1 ear	70	2.0	16.0	200	(mq)	1.0	(mq)	5	11%
on the cob, kernels from ear	8 oz	123	4.1	29.4	6	>.9 c	1.0	0.2	0	6%
on the cob 'Little Ears' *(Birds Eye)*	2 ears	130	4.0	30.0	0	na	1.0	na	0	6%
on the cob, miniature 'Mini-Gold' *(Ore-Ida)*	2 ears	180	5.0	39.0	40	(mq)	2.0	(mq)	0	9%
on the cob 'Nibblers, 6-ear pkg' *(Green Giant)*	2 ears	120	4.0	27.0	10	2.0	1.0	na	0	7%
on the cob 'Nibblers Supersweet' *(Green Giant)*	2 ears	90	3.0	19.0	10	2.0	2.0	(mq)	0	17%
on the cob 'Niblet Ears' *(Green Giant)*	1 ear	120	4.0	27.0	10	2.0	1.0	na	0	7%
on the cob 'Niblet Ears Supersweet' *(Green Giant)*	1 ear	90	3.0	19.0	10	2.0	2.0	(mq)	0	17%
on the cob 'One Serving' *(Green Giant)*	2 half ears	120	4.0	26.0	10	2.0	1.0	<1.0	0	7%
on the cob 'Sweet Select' *(Green Giant)*	1 ear	90	3.0	19.0	10	2.0	2.0	0.0	0	17%
on the cob 'Sweet Select' half ears *(Green Giant)*	2 half ears	90	3.0	19.0	10	2.0	2.0	0.0	0	17%
sweet *(Birds Eye)*	3.3 oz	80	3.0	20.0	0	2.0	1.0	na	0	9%
sweet, select 'Plain Polybag' *(Green Giant)*	1/2 cup	60	2.0	13.0	5	2.0	1.0	0.0	0	13%
sweet, tender 'Butter Sauce Combination' *(Birds Eye)*	3.3 oz	90	2.0	17.0	250	2.0	2.0	na	5	19%
sweet, tender 'Deluxe' *(Birds Eye)*	3.3 oz	80	3.0	20.0	0	2.0	1.0	na	0	9%
sweet, white, kernels, boiled, drained	1 ear	59	2.0	14.1	3	3.6	0.5	0.1	0	7%
sweet, white, kernels, boiled, drained	1/2 cup	76	2.5	18.3	3	4.7	0.6	0.1	0	6%
sweet, white, kernels, unprepared	1/2 cup	72	2.5	17.1	2	4.7	0.6	0.1	0	6%
sweet, yellow, kernels, boiled, drained	1 ear	59	2.0	14.1	3	3.6	0.5	0.1	0	7%
sweet, yellow, kernels, boiled, drained	1/2 cup	76	2.5	18.3	3	>.5 c	0.6	0.1	0	6%
sweet, yellow, kernels, unprepared	1/2 cup	72	2.5	17.1	2	2.0	0.6	0.1	0	6%
white *(Green Giant)*	1/2 cup	90	2.0	19.0	5	2.0	1.0	na	0	10%
white *(Seabrook)*	3.3 oz	80	3.0	19.0	3	>1.0 c	1.0	na	0	9%
white, in butter sauce *(Green Giant)*	1/2 cup	100	2.0	20.0	280	2.3	2.0	<1.0	5	17%
white, shoepeg 'Butter Sauce' *(Green Giant)*	1/2 cup	100	2.0	20.0	280	2.0	2.0	<1.0	5	17%
white, shoepeg 'Harvest Fresh' *(Green Giant)*	1/2 cup	90	3.0	19.0	60	2.0	1.0	na	0	9%
white, shoepeg 'Select' *(Green Giant)*	1/2 cup	90	2.0	19.0	5	2.0	<1.0	0.0	0	<10%

Food Name	Serving Size	Calories	Prot. gms	Carbs gms	Sod. mgs	Fiber gms	Fat gms	Sat. Fat gms	Chol. mgs	% Fat Cal.
whole kernel, 'Portion Pack' (Birds Eye)	3 oz	70	3.0	18.0	0	2.0	1.0	na	0	10%

CORN AND BUTTERNUT SQUASH. See SQUASH, CORN AND BUTTERNUT.

CORN AND PEPPERS, CANNED

Food Name	Serving Size	Calories	Prot. gms	Carbs gms	Sod. mgs	Fiber gms	Fat gms	Sat. Fat gms	Chol. mgs	% Fat Cal.
red and green peppers, solid and liquid	1/2 cup	86	2.7	20.7	396	>.7 c	0.6	0.1	0	6%
vacuum packed (Freshlike)	1/2 cup	90	3.0	23.0	300	na	1.0	na	na	8%
vacuum packed (Veg•All)	1/2 cup	90	3.0	23.0	300	na	1.0	na	na	8%

CORN BRAN

Food Name	Serving Size	Calories	Prot. gms	Carbs gms	Sod. mgs	Fiber gms	Fat gms	Sat. Fat gms	Chol. mgs	% Fat Cal.
crude	1 cup	170	6.3	65.1	5	65.4	0.7	0.1	0	2%
crude	1 oz	64	2.4	24.3	2	24.0	0.3	<.1	0	3%

CORN CAKE

Food Name	Serving Size	Calories	Prot. gms	Carbs gms	Sod. mgs	Fiber gms	Fat gms	Sat. Fat gms	Chol. mgs	% Fat Cal.
apple cinnamon flavor (Roman Meal)	1 cake	49	<1.0	10.5	<5	na	<1.0	na	0	<1%
caramel, fat-free (Quaker)	1 cake	50	1.0	12.0	30	na	0.0	na	0	0%
caramel flavor, fat free (Roman Meal)	1 cake	50	<1.0	11.0	5	0	0.0	0	0	0%
cheddar flavor (Roman Meal)	1 cake	43	<1.0	9.0	14	na	<1.0	na	0	<1%
natural butter flavor, fat free (Roman Meal)	1 cake	40	<1.0	8.0	35	0	0.0	0	0	0%
plain	1 cake	35	0.7	7.5	44	.2	0.2	0.0	0	5%
popcorn	1 cake	38	1.0	8.0	29	.3	0.3	0.1	0	7%
popcorn, butter flavor (Chico-San)	1 cake	40	1.0	8.0	45	na	0.0	na	0	0%
popcorn, caramel (Chico-San)	1 cake	50	1.0	10.0	55	na	0.0	na	0	0%
popcorn, lightly salted (Chico-San)	1 cake	40	1.0	8.0	45	na	0.0	na	0	0%
popcorn, white cheddar cheese (Chico-San)	1 cake	50	1.0	9.0	65	na	1.0	na	0	18%
popped, butter flavor (Quaker)	1 cake	35	1.0	7.0	55	na	0.0	na	0	0%
popped, white cheddar flavor (Quaker)	1 cake	40	1.0	8.0	110	na	0.0	na	0	0%
very low sodium	1 cake	24	0.0	6.3	5	0	0.0	na	0	0%
white cheddar flavor, fat free (Roman Meal)	1 cake	45	<1.0	9.0	15	0	0.0	0	0	0%

CORN CHIPS AND SNACKS. See also TORTILLA CHIPS.

Food Name	Serving Size	Calories	Prot. gms	Carbs gms	Sod. mgs	Fiber gms	Fat gms	Sat. Fat gms	Chol. mgs	% Fat Cal.
barbecue (Bachman)	1 oz	150	<1.0	17.0	230	(mq)	9.0	(mq)	0	53%
barbecue 'Rowdy Rustlers' 34 chips (Fritos)	1 oz	150	2.0	17.0	300	1.1	9.0	na	0	52%
'Bar-B-Q Fritos' 34 pieces (Fritos)	1 oz	150	2.0	16.0	320	(mq)	9.0	(mq)	0	53%
bare bean 'Garden Vegetable Chips' (Harry's)	1 oz	144	2.7	17.0	<1	2.4	7.0	1.2	0	44%
bare bean 'Offbeat Originals' (Peddlers)	1 oz	144	2.7	17.0	<1	2.4	7.0	1.2	0	44%
beet garlic 'Garden Vegetable Chips' (Harry's)	1 oz	134	2.2	20.0	43	2.2	5.0	0.8	0	34%
beet garlic 'Offbeat Originals' (Peddlers)	1 oz	134	2.2	20.0	43	2.2	5.0	0.8	0	34%
bell pepper 'Garden Vegetable Chips' (Harry's)	1 oz	140	2.0	19.0	40	2.0	6.0	0.7	0	39%
bell pepper 'Offbeat Originals' (Peddlers)	1 oz	140	2.0	19.0	40	2.0	6.0	0.7	0	39%
blue corn 'Corn Curls' (Arrowhead Mills)	1 oz	120	3.0	22.0	54	4.0	2.0	(mq)	0	15%
blue corn 'Corn Curls Unsalted' (Arrowhead Mills)	1 oz	120	3.0	22.0	1	4.0	2.0	(mq)	0	15%
blue corn, no salt added (Barbara's Bakery)	1 oz	140	2.0	18.0	15	na	7.0	na	0	44%
blue corn, regular (Barbara's Bakery)	1 oz	140	2.0	18.0	120	na	7.0	na	0	44%
blue garlic 'Garden Vegetable Chips' (Harry's)	1 oz	129	2.6	21.0	28	3.0	4.0	0.5	0	28%
blue garlic 'Offbeat Originals' (Peddlers)	1 oz	129	2.6	21.0	28	3.0	4.0	0.5	0	28%
caramel corn puffs, apple cinnamon, fat-free (Health Valley)	1 oz	100	3.0	21.0	50	.1	0.0	na	0	0%
caramel corn puffs, original style, fat-free (Health Valley) ..	1 oz	100	3.0	21.0	45	.1	0.0	na	0	0%
caramel corn puffs, peanut flavor, fat-free (Health Valley) ..	1 oz	100	3.0	21.0	65	.1	0.0	na	0	0%
carrot caraway 'Garden Vegetable Chips' (Harry's)	1 oz	131	2.4	20.0	31	1.5	4.0	0.6	0	29%
carrot caraway 'Offbeat Originals' (Peddlers)	1 oz	131	2.4	20.0	31	1.5	4.0	0.6	0	29%
cheddar cheese (Health Valley)	1 oz	160	3.0	15.0	120	1.0	10.0	(mq)	2	56%
cheese 'Baked' (Jax)	1 oz	140	2.0	17.0	290	(mq)	7.0	(mq)	na	45%
cheese 'Baked, Corn Puffs' (Cheez Doodles)	1 oz	150	2.0	17.0	360	(mq)	8.0	(mq)	na	49%
cheese 'Cheese Curls Low Salt' (Featherweight)	1 oz	150	2.0	16.0	81	(mq)	9.0	(mq)	0	53%
cheese 'Crunchy' (Jax)	1 oz	160	2.0	14.0	250	(mq)	11.0	(mq)	na	61%
cheese curls 'Great Tasting' (Ultra Slim Fast)	1 oz	110	2.0	20.0	360	3.0	3.0	na	0	24%
cheese 'Fried Corn Puffs' (Cheez Doodles)	1 oz	160	2.0	15.0	220	(mq)	10.0	(mq)	na	57%

Food Name	Serving Size	Calories	Prot. gms	Carbs gms	Sod. mgs	Fiber gms	Fat gms	Sat. Fat gms	Chol. mgs	% Fat Cal.
chili cheese, 34 chips (Fritos)	1 oz	160	2.0	15.0	300	1.1	10.0	na	0	57%
cones, nacho-flavor	1 oz	152	1.8	16.2	270	>.1 c	9.0	7.6	1	53%
cones, plain	1 oz	145	1.6	17.8	290	>.2 c	7.6	6.4	0	47%
cool ranch (Doritos)	1 oz	140	2.0	18.0	115	0	7.0	na	0	44%
corn chips (Wise)	1 oz	160	2.0	15.0	180	(mq)	10.0	(mq)	0	57%
corn crunchies (Wise)	1 oz	160	2.0	15.0	180	(mq)	10.0	(mq)	0	57%
corn nuggets, toasted (Fritos)	1.38 oz	170	3.0	29.0	265	na	5.0	na	0	26%
corn ridgies (Wise)	1 oz	160	2.0	15.0	180	(mq)	10.0	(mq)	0	57%
corn spirals, toasted (Wise)	1 oz	160	2.0	15.0	125	(mq)	10.0	(mq)	0	57%
corn twists, crispy (Wise)	1 oz	160	2.0	15.0	125	na	10.0	na	na	57%
'Crisp 'N Thin' 18 chips (Fritos)	1 oz	160	2.0	16.0	210	1.1	10.0	na	0	56%
curls, barbecue flavored (Weight Watchers)	.5 oz	60	1.0	10.0	110	na	2.0	<1.0	0	30%
curls, pizza flavored (Weight Watchers)	.5 oz	60	1.0	10.0	130	na	2.0	<1.0	0	30%
curls, ranch flavored (Weight Watchers)	.5 oz	60	1.0	9.0	170	na	2.0	<1.0	0	30%
'Dip Size Fritos' 13 pieces (Fritos)	1 oz	150	2.0	17.0	210	(mq)	9.0	(mq)	0	52%
'Fritos' 34 pieces (Fritos)	1 oz	150	1.0	16.0	230	(mq)	9.0	(mq)	0	54%
'Low Salt' (Featherweight)	1 oz	170	2.0	15.0	3	(mq)	11.0	(mq)	0	59%
mild bean 'Garden Vegetable Chips' (Harry's)	1 oz	144	2.7	17.0	74	2.4	7.0	1.2	0	44%
mild bean 'Offbeat Originals' (Peddlers)	1 oz	144	2.7	17.0	74	2.4	7.0	1.2	0	44%
nacho cheese (Bugles)	1 oz	160	2.0	17.0	250	(mq)	9.0	(mq)	na	52%
nacho cheese (Corn Snackers)	.5-oz pkg	60	1.0	10.0	240	(mq)	2.0	(mq)	na	29%
nacho cheese flavor (Doritos)	1 oz	140	2.0	18.0	150	0	7.0	na	0	44%
nacho cheese 'Non-Stop' 34 chips (Fritos)	1 oz	150	2.0	16.0	220	1.1	9.0	na	1	53%
'No Salt Added' (Health Valley)	1 oz	160	1.0	13.0	1	1.0	11.0	(mq)	0	64%
onion-flavor	1 oz	142	2.2	18.5	278	1.1	6.4	1.2	0	41%
'Pinta Blues' picante (Barbara's Bakery)	1 oz	130	2.0	18.0	250	na	6.0	na	0	40%
'Pinta Blues' regular (Barbara's Bakery)	1 oz	140	2.0	20.0	110	na	6.0	na	0	38%
'Pinta Puffs' salsa (Barbara's Bakery)	1 oz	70	2.0	10.0	130	na	2.0	na	0	27%
'Pinta' regular (Barbara's Bakery)	1 oz	138	2.0	18.0	100	na	6.0	na	0	40%
plain	1 oz	153	1.9	16.1	179	1.4	9.5	1.3	0	54%
plain (Bachman)	1 oz	160	2.0	15.0	160	(mq)	10.0	(mq)	0	57%
plain (Bugles)	1 oz	150	2.0	18.0	290	(mq)	8.0	(mq)	0	47%
plain (Corn Snackers)	.5-oz pkg	60	1.0	10.0	190	(mq)	2.0	(mq)	0	29%
plain (Health Valley)	1 oz	160	1.0	13.0	90	1.0	11.0	(mq)	0	64%
plain (Planters)	1 oz	160	2.0	15.0	160	(mq)	10.0	2.0	0	57%
plain (Snyder's)	1 oz	160	2.0	14.0	150	(mq)	11.0	2.0	0	61%
'Potilla' chipotle chili (Barbara's Bakery)	1 oz	140	2.0	18.0	180	na	8.0	na	0	47%
'Potilla' regular (Barbara's Bakery)	1 oz	140	2.0	18.0	120	na	8.0	na	0	47%
puffs, cheese-flavor	1 oz	157	2.2	15.2	298	.3	9.8	1.9	1	56%
puffs, cheese-flavor, enriched	1 oz	110	2.3	23.6	8	>.2 c	0.7	0.1	0	6%
ranch (Bugles)	1 oz	150	2.0	16.0	290	na	9.0	na	na	53%
'Rippled Corn Chips' (Dipsy Doodles)	1 oz	160	2.0	15.0	180	(mq)	10.0	(mq)	0	57%
toasted corn, crunchy, barbecue (Cornuts)	2 oz	247	5.1	40.7	553	4.8	8.1	1.5	0	29%
toasted corn, crunchy, barbecue (Cornuts)	1 oz	124	2.5	20.3	277	2.4	4.1	0.7	0	29%
toasted corn, crunchy, chili picante (Cornuts)	1 oz	120	2.0	22.0	260	2.2	4.0	na	0	27%
toasted corn, crunchy, nacho (Cornuts)	2 oz	248	5.3	40.6	359	4.5	8.1	1.5	1	28%
toasted corn, crunchy, nacho (Cornuts)	1 oz	124	2.7	20.3	180	2.3	4.0	0.7	1	28%
toasted corn, crunchy, original (Cornuts)	2 oz	249	4.8	41.6	311	3.9	8.0	1.4	0	28%
toasted corn, crunchy, original (Cornuts)	1 oz	124	2.4	20.8	156	2.0	4.0	0.7	0	28%
toasted corn, crunchy, ranch (Cornuts)	1 oz	120	2.0	20.0	190	1.7	4.0	na	0	29%
toasted corn, crunchy, unsalted (Cornuts)	1 oz	120	2.0	19.0	30	2.7	4.0	(mq)	0	30%
'Unsalted' (Azteca)	1 oz	140	2.0	18.0	110	(mq)	7.0	(mq)	0	44%
veggie 'Garden Vegetable Chips' (Harry's)	1 oz	141	2.2	18.0	40	2.5	7.0	0.7	0	44%
veggie 'Offbeat Originals' (Peddlers)	1 oz	141	2.2	18.0	40	2.5	7.0	0.7	0	44%

Food Name	Serving Size	Calories	Prot. gms	Carbs gms	Sod. mgs	Fiber gms	Fat gms	Sat. Fat gms	Chol. mgs	% Fat Cal.
wild bean 'Garden Vegetable Chips' *(Harry's)* .... 1 oz		141	2.9	17.8	51	2.6	6.0	0.8	0	40%
wild bean 'Offbeat Originals' *(Peddlers)* .... 1 oz		141	2.9	17.8	51	2.6	6.0	0.8	0	40%
'Wild 'N Mild' 32 chips *(Fritos)* .... 1 oz		160	2.0	16.0	240	1.1	9.0	na	0	53%
yellow 'Corn Chips' *(Arrowhead Mills)* .... .75 oz		90	2.0	18.0	31	3.0	1.0	na	0	10%
yellow, w/cheese 'Corn Chips' *(Arrowhead Mills)* .... .75 oz		90	2.0	15.0	30	3.0	2.0	(mq)	na	21%
CORN FLAKE CRUMBS *(Kellogg's)* .... 1 oz		100	2.0	24.0	290	1.0	0.0	0.0	0	0%
CORN FLOUR										
masa .... 1 oz		103	2.6	21.6	1	>.5 c	1.1	0.2	0	9%
masa, enriched, white .... 1 cup		416	10.6	86.9	6	10.9	4.3	0.6	0	9%
masa, enriched, yellow .... 1 cup		416	10.6	86.9	6	>1.9 c	4.3	0.6	0	9%
'Masa Harina De Maiz' approx 1/3 cup *(Quaker)* .... 1.3 oz		137	3.5	27.4	5	2.7	1.5	na	0	10%
'Masa Trigo' approx 1/3 cup *(Quaker)* .... 1.3 oz		149	3.5	24.7	794	1.0	4.0	(mq)	0	24%
whole-grain .... 1 oz		102	2.0	21.8	1	3.8	1.1	0.2	0	9%
whole-grain, white .... 1/2 cup		209	4.0	44.6	3	5.6	2.2	0.3	0	9%
whole-grain, yellow .... 1/2 cup		209	4.0	44.6	3	7.8	2.2	0.3	0	9%
CORN FRITTER, frozen *(Mrs. Paul's)* .... 2 pieces		240	5.0	35.0	560	(mq)	9.0	(mq)	10	34%
CORN GRITS. See GRITS.										
CORN NUGGETS, FROZEN										
breaded, fried 'Quickkrisp' *(Stilwell)* .... 3 oz		210	3.0	30.0	420	(mq)	8.0	(mq)	1	35%
CORN OIL										
.... 1/2 cup		964	0.0	0.0	0	0	109.0	13.9	0	100%
.... 1 oz		251	0.0	0.0	0	0	28.4	3.6	0	100%
.... 1 tbsp		120	0.0	0.0	0	0	13.6	1.7	0	100%
(Crisco) .... 1 tbsp		120	0.0	0.0	0	0	14.0	2.0	0	100%
(Crisco) 'Puritan' .... 1 tbsp		120	0.0	0.0	0	0	14.0	1.0	0	100%
(Hain) .... 1 tbsp		120	0.0	0.0	0	0	14.0	2.0	0	100%
(Kroger) .... 1 tbsp		122	0.0	0.0	0	0	13.6	1.9	0	100%
(Mazola) .... 1 tbsp		120	0.0	0.0	0	0	14.0	2.0	0	100%
(Pathmark) .... 1 tbsp		130	0.0	0.0	0	0	14.0	2.0	0	100%
(Pathmark) 'No Frills' .... 1 tbsp		130	0.0	0.0	0	0	14.0	2.0	0	100%
(Spectrum Naturals) .... 1 tbsp		120	0.0	0.0	0	(tr)	14.0	1.5	(tr)	100%
(Wesson) .... 1 tbsp		120	0.0	0.0	0	0	14.0	2.0	0	100%
CORN OIL SPRAY. See COOKING SPRAY.										
CORN OIL SPREAD										
(Fleischmann's) 60% oil 'Light' .... 1 tbsp		80	0.0	0.0	70	na	8.0	1.0	0	100%
(Fleischmann's) 40% oil 'Extra Light' .... 1 tbsp		50	0.0	0.0	55	na	6.0	1.0	0	100%
CORN SALAD, raw .... 1/2 cup		6	0.6	1.0	1	>.2 c	0.1	na	0	12%
CORN SOUFFLÉ, FROZEN, 1 pkg *(Stouffer's)* .... 6 oz		240	7.0	27.0	760	na	11.0	na	na	42%
CORN SYRUP										
dark .... 1 cup		925	0.0	251.3	508	0	0.0	na	0	0%
dark .... 1 tbsp		56	0.0	15.3	31	0	0.0	na	0	0%
dark *(Karo)* .... 1 tbsp		60	0.0	15.0	40	0	0.0	0.0	0	0%
high-fructose .... 1 cup		871	0.0	235.6	6	0	0.0	na	0	0%
high-fructose .... 1 tbsp		53	0.0	14.4	0	0	0.0	na	0	0%
light .... 1 cup		925	0.0	251.3	397	0	0.0	na	0	0%
light .... 1 tbsp		56	0.0	15.3	24	0	0.0	na	0	0%
light *(Karo)* .... 1 tbsp		60	0.0	15.0	30	0	0.0	0.0	0	0%
table blends, refiner, and sugar .... 1 cup		1008	0.0	265.1	224	0	0.0	na	0	0%
table blends, refiner, and sugar .... 1 tbsp		64	0.0	16.8	14	0	0.0	na	0	0%
CORNBREAD. See BREAD.										
CORNMEAL										
.... 1 cup		605	15.6	123.3	58	>4.8 c	7.9	1.1	0	11%
.... 1 oz		103	2.7	21.1	10	>.8 c	1.3	0.2	0	11%
blue, whole-grain *(Arrowhead Mills)* .... 2 oz		210	6.0	41.0	1	5.6	3.0	(mq)	0	13%

Food Name	Serving Size	Calories	Prot. gms	Carbs gms	Sod. mgs	Fiber gms	Fat gms	Sat. Fat gms	Chol. mgs	% Fat Cal.
degermed	1 oz	104	8.5	22.0	1	1.5	0.5	0.1	0	4%
degermed, enriched, white	1 cup	505	11.7	107.2	4	10.2	2.3	0.3	0	4%
degermed, enriched, yellow	1 cup	505	11.7	107.2	4	10.2	2.3	0.3	0	4%
degermed, unenriched, white	1 cup	505	11.7	107.2	4	10.2	2.3	0.3	0	4%
degermed, unenriched, yellow	1 cup	505	11.7	107.2	4	10.2	2.3	0.3	0	4%
white, bolted (Aunt Jemima)	1 oz	99	2.4	20.8	337	(mq)	0.7	na	0	6%
white, bolted, enriched (Aunt Jemima)	1 oz	99	2.3	20.4	382	(mq)	0.9	na	0	8%
white, dry (Albers)	1 oz	100	2.0	22.0	0	1.5	1.0	na	0	9%
white, enriched, approx 3 tbsp (Aunt Jemima)	1 oz	102	2.4	22.2	1	1.2	0.5	na	0	4%
white, whole-grain	1 cup	442	9.9	93.8	43	8.9	4.4	0.6	0	9%
whole-grain	1 oz	103	2.3	21.8	10	3.1	1.0	0.1	0	9%
whole-grain, hi-lysine (Arrowhead Mills)	2 oz	210	4.0	43.0	1	6.8	2.0	(mq)	0	9%
yellow, dry (Albers)	1 oz	100	2.0	22.0	0	1.5	1.0	na	0	9%
yellow, enriched (Aunt Jemima)	1 oz	102	2.4	22.2	1	1.2	0.5	na	0	4%
yellow, whole-grain	1 cup	442	9.9	93.8	43	8.9	4.4	0.6	0	9%
yellow, whole-grain (Arrowhead Mills)	2 oz	210	4.0	43.0	1	6.8	2.0	(mq)	0	9%
CORNMEAL, SELF-RISING										
bolted	1 oz	95	2.3	19.9	353	>.3 c	1.0	0.1	0	9%
bolted, w/wheat flour	1 oz	99	2.4	20.8	374	>.2 c	0.8	0.1	0	7%
degermed	1 oz	101	2.4	21.2	382	>.2 c	0.5	0.1	0	5%
white (Aunt Jemima)	1 oz	98	2.3	21.1	381	>.2 c	0.5	na	0	5%
white, bolted (Aunt Jemima)	1 oz	98	2.3	21.1	381	>.2 c	0.5	na	0	5%
white, bolted, enriched (Aunt Jemima)	1 oz	99	2.3	20.4	382	(mq)	0.9	na	0	8%
white, bolted, plain, enriched	1 cup	407	10.1	85.7	1521	>1.3 c	4.2	0.6	0	9%
white, bolted, wheat flour added, enriched	1 cup	592	14.3	124.8	2242	>1.3 c	4.8	0.7	0	7%
white, buttermilk (Aunt Jemima)	3 tbsp	101	2.5	20.2	439	(mq)	1.1	na	0	10%
white, degermed, enriched	1 cup	490	11.6	103.2	1860	>.7 c	2.4	0.3	0	5%
yellow (Aunt Jemima)	3 tbsp	100	2.0	21.0	490	(mq)	1.0	na	0	9%
yellow, bolted, plain, enriched	1 cup	407	10.1	85.7	1521	>1.3 c	4.2	0.6	0	9%
yellow, bolted, wheat flour added, enriched	1 cup	592	14.3	124.8	2242	>1.3 c	4.8	0.7	0	7%
yellow, degermed, enriched	1 cup	490	11.6	103.2	1860	>.7 c	2.4	0.3	0	5%
CORNED BEEF. See BEEF, CORNED.										
CORNISH GAME HEN										
frozen (Tyson)	3.5 oz	240	28.0	0.0	70	0	14.0	(mq)	75	53%
frozen, w/skin (Tyson)	3.5 oz	250	27.0	1.0	80	na	15.0	na	155	55%
w/wild rice, Wholesale Club Item (Tyson)	3.5 oz	190	19.0	6.0	125	na	11.0	na	85	50%
CORNSTARCH										
	1 cup	488	0.3	116.8	12	1.1	0.1	0.0	0	0%
	1 oz	108	0.1	25.9	3	.3	<.1	tr	0	<1%
	1 tbsp	30	<.1	7.3	1	.1	tr	tr	0	0%
(Argo)	1 tbsp	30	0.0	7.0	0	tr	0.0	0.0	0	0%
(Cream)	1 tbsp	29	tr	7.0	tr	na	tr	na	0	0%
(Kingsford)	1 tbsp	30	0.0	7.0	0	tr	0.0	0.0	0	0%
COTTAGE CHEESE. See CHEESE.										
COTTONSEED FLOUR										
lowfat	1 oz	94	14.1	10.2	10	>.7 c	0.4	0.1	0	4%
partially defatted	1 cup	337	38.5	38.1	33	2.8	5.8	1.5	0	15%
partially defatted	1 oz	102	11.6	11.5	10	.8	1.8	0.5	0	15%
partially defatted	1 tbsp	18	2.0	2.0	2	>.1 c	0.3	0.1	0	14%
COTTONSEED KERNELS										
roasted	1 cup	754	48.6	32.6	37	8.2	54.1	14.4	0	60%
roasted	1 oz	143	9.2	6.2	7	1.6	10.3	2.7	0	60%
roasted	1 tbsp	51	3.3	2.2	3	.6	3.6	1.0	0	60%
COTTONSEED MEAL, partially defatted	1 oz	104	13.9	10.9	11	>.7 c	1.4	0.3	0	11%

Food Name	Serving Size	Calories	Prot. gms	Carbs gms	Sod. mgs	Fiber gms	Fat gms	Sat. Fat gms	Chol. mgs	% Fat Cal.
COTTONSEED OIL										
....	1 cup	1927	0.0	0.0	0	0	218.0	56.5	0	100%
....	1/2 cup	964	0.0	0.0	0	0	109.0	28.2	0	100%
....	1 tbsp	120	0.0	0.0	0	0	13.6	3.5	0	100%
(Wesson)	1 tbsp	122	0.0	0.0	0	0	13.6	3.2	0	100%
COUSCOUS										
cooked	1/2 cup	101	3.4	20.8	4.5	1.3	.1	<.1	0	1%
cooked	4 oz	127	4.3	26.3	6	1.6	0.2	<.1	0	1%
dry	1/2 cup	346	11.7	71.2	9	4.6	0.6	0.1	0	2%
dry	1 oz	107	3.6	22.0	3	1.4	0.2	<.1	0	2%
mix, dry *(Near East)*	1.25 oz	120	4.0	26.0	5	(mq)	0.0	0.0	0	0%
mix, prepared w/2 tbsp salted butter *(Fantastic Foods)* ...	1/2 cup	122	3.0	22.0	35	(mq)	3.0	(mq)	(mq)	21%
mix, prepared w/o added ingredients *(Fantastic Foods)* ..	1/2 cup	105	3.0	22.0	1	(mq)	0.0	0.0	0	0%
mix, whole-wheat *(Fantastic Foods)*	1/2 cup	94	3.5	20.0	0	(mq)	0.0	0.0	0	0%
mix, whole-wheat, prepared w/2 tbsp salted butter *(Fantastic Foods)*	1/2 cup	111	3.5	20.0	23	(mq)	2.0	(mq)	(mq)	16%
COUSCOUS PILAF MIX										
(Casbah) dry	1 oz	100	4.0	20.0	na	(mq)	0.0	0.0	0	0%
(Casbah) prepared w/o added ingredients	1/2 cup	100	4.0	20.0	na	(mq)	0.0	0.0	0	0%
(Quick Pilaf) savory, prepared w/2 tbsp salted butter	1/2 cup	124	4.0	19.0	254	(mq)	3.0	(mq)	(mq)	23%
(Quick Pilaf) savory, prepared w/o added ingredients	1/2 cup	94	4.0	19.0	215	(mq)	0.0	0.0	0	0%
COWPEA. See BLACK-EYED PEAS.										
CRAB										
ALASKAN KING										
boiled	4 oz	110	21.9	0.0	1216	0	1.7	0.2	60	15%
boiled, approx 4.7 oz	1 leg	129	25.9	0.0	1436	0	1.7	0.2	72	13%
moist-heat cooked	3 oz	82	16.5	0.0	911	0	1.3	0.1	45	15%
poached	4 oz	110	21.9	0.0	1216	0	1.7	0.2	60	15%
poached, approx 4.7 oz	1 leg	129	25.9	0.0	1436	0	1.7	0.2	72	13%
raw	1 lb	379	83.0	0.0	3792	0	2.7	(mq)	189	7%
raw	3 oz	71	15.6	0.0	711	0	0.5	0.1	36	7%
raw	1 oz	24	5.2	0.0	237	0	0.2	(mq)	12	8%
steamed	4 oz	110	21.9	0.0	1216	0	1.7	0.2	60	15%
steamed, approx 4.7 oz	1 leg	129	25.9	0.0	1436	0	1.7	0.2	72	13%
BLUE										
boiled	4 oz	116	22.9	0.0	316	0	2.0	0.3	113	16%
boiled, approx 4.75 oz	1 cup	138	27.3	0.0	376	0	2.4	0.3	135	17%
cake, fried	4 oz	176	22.9	0.5	374	>.6 c	8.5	1.7	170	45%
cake, fried, approx 2.1 oz	1 med	93	12.1	0.3	198	>.1 c	4.5	0.9	90	45%
canned	1 cup	134	27.7	0.0	450	0	1.7	0.3	120	12%
canned	4 oz	112	23.3	0.0	378	0	1.4	0.3	101	12%
canned	3 oz	84	17.4	0.0	283	0	1.0	0.2	76	12%
moist-heat cooked	1 cup	138	27.3	0.0	377	0	2.4	0.3	135	17%
moist-heat cooked	3 oz	87	17.2	0.0	237	0	1.5	0.2	85	16%
poached	4 oz	116	22.9	0.0	316	0	2.0	0.3	113	16%
poached, approx 4.75 oz	1 cup	138	27.3	0.0	376	0	2.4	0.3	135	17%
raw	1 lb	395	81.9	0.2	1329	0	4.9	1.0	355	12%
raw	3 oz	74	15.3	0.0	249	0	0.9	0.2	66	12%
raw	1 oz	25	5.1	<.1	83	0	0.3	0.1	22	12%
steamed	4 oz	116	22.9	0.0	316	0	2.0	0.3	113	16%
steamed, approx 4.75 oz	1 cup	138	27.3	0.0	376	0	2.4	0.3	135	17%
DUNGENESS										
canned *(S&W)*	3.25 oz	81	18.0	1.0	920	0	2.0	(mq)	(mq)	19%
moist-heat cooked	3 oz	94	19.0	0.8	321	0	1.0	0.1	65	10%

Food Name	Serving Size	Calories	Prot. gms	Carbs gms	Sod. mgs	Fiber gms	Fat gms	Sat. Fat gms	Chol. mgs	% Fat Cal.
raw	1 lb	391	79.0	3.3	1340	0	4.4	0.6	269	11%
raw	3 oz	73	14.8	0.6	251	0	0.8	0.1	50	11%
raw	1 oz	24	4.9	0.2	84	0	0.3	<.1	17	12%
IMPERIAL	1 cup	323	32.1	8.6	1602	0	16.7	8.8	308	48%
QUEEN										
moist-heat cooked	100 gm	115	23.7	0.0	691	0	1.5	0.2	71	13%
moist-heat cooked	3 oz	98	20.2	0.0	587	0	1.3	0.2	60	13%
raw	1 lb	407	83.9	0.0	2445	0	5.4	0.6	248	13%
raw	3 oz	77	15.7	0.0	458	0	1.0	0.1	47	13%
raw	1 oz	26	5.2	0.0	153	0	0.3	<.1	16	12%
SNOW										
frozen *(Wakefield)*	3 oz	60	13.0	0.0	270	0	1.0	(mq)	(mq)	15%
raw, Opilio, clusters *(Peter Pan Seafoods)*	3.5 oz	91	20.6	na	539	na	1.2	na	55	12%
raw, Opilio, 'Snap 'n' Eat' scored *(Peter Pan Seafoods)*	3.5 oz	91	20.6	na	539	na	1.2	na	55	12%
SOFTSHELL										
boiled	4 oz	116	22.9	0.0	316	0	2.0	0.3	113	16%
boiled, approx 4.75 oz	1 cup	138	27.3	0.0	376	0	2.4	0.3	135	17%
cake, fried	4 oz	176	22.9	0.5	374	>.6 c	8.5	1.7	170	45%
cake, fried, approx 2.1 oz	1 med	93	12.1	0.3	198	>.1 c	4.5	0.9	90	45%
poached	4 oz	116	22.9	0.0	316	0	2.0	0.3	113	16%
poached, approx 4.75 oz	1 cup	138	27.3	0.0	376	0	2.4	0.3	135	17%
raw	1 lb	395	81.9	0.2	1329	0	4.9	1.0	355	12%
raw	1 oz	25	5.1	<.1	83	0	0.3	0.1	22	12%
raw, approx .7 oz	1 crab	18	3.8	<.1	62	0	0.2	<.1	16	10%
steamed	4 oz	116	22.9	0.0	316	0	2.0	0.3	113	16%
steamed, approx 4.75 oz	1 cup	138	27.3	0.0	376	0	2.4	0.3	135	17%
CRAB, ALTERNATIVE										
	1 lb	463	54.5	46.4	3815	0	5.9	(mq)	89	12%
	1 oz	29	3.4	3.0	238	0	0.4	(mq)	6	12%
Alaskan King, made from surimi	3 oz	87	10.2	8.7	715	0	1.1	0.2	17	12%
(Icicle Brand)	3.5 oz	99	12.0	11.0	900	0	0.1	tr	10	1%
CRAB, DEVILED										
	1 cup	451	27.4	31.9	2081	0	22.6	6.5	245	46%
breaded, frozen, cake *(Mrs. Paul's)*	3 oz	180	8.0	18.0	480	(mq)	9.0	(mq)	20	44%
breaded, frozen, miniature *(Mrs. Paul's)*	3.5 oz	240	9.0	25.0	540	(mq)	12.0	(mq)	20	44%
CRAB AND SHRIMP, frozen *(Wakefield)*	3 oz	60	13.0	0.0	210	0	1.0	(mq)	(mq)	15%
CRAB CAKE										
	100 gm	147	26.2	3.9	504	0	2.1	0.4	169	14%
	1 cake	88	15.7	2.3	302	0	1.3	0.2	101	14%
blue crab	1 cake	93	12.1	0.3	198	0	4.5	0.9	90	45%
CRABAPPLE										
raw	100 gm	76	0.4	20.0	1	>.6 c	0.3	0.1	0	3%
raw, slices, w/skin	1 cup	84	0.4	21.9	1	>.7 c	0.3	0.1	0	3%
trimmed, w/skin	1 oz	22	0.1	5.7	<1	>.2 c	0.1	<.1	0	4%
trimmed, w/skin, sliced	1/2 cup	42	0.2	11.0	1	>.3 c	0.2	0.1	0	4%
untrimmed	1 lb	316	1.7	83.2	4	>2.5 c	1.3	0.2	0	3%
CRABAPPLE, CANNED										
spiced *(Lucky Leaf)*	4 oz	110	0.0	28.0	(mq)	(mq)	0.0	0.0	0	0%
spiced *(Musselman's)*	4 oz	110	0.0	28.0	(mq)	(mq)	0.0	0.0	0	0%
CRACKER										
apple cinnamon 'Orchard Crisps' *(Nabisco)*	.5 oz	60	1.0	11.0	40	na	2.0	<1.0	0	27%
bacon flavor *(Delicious)*	.5 oz	70	1.0	10.0	190	na	3.0	na	0	38%
bacon flavor 'Bacon Flavored Thins' .5 oz *(Nabisco)*	7 crackers	70	1.0	9.0	210	(mq)	4.0	1.0	0	47%
bacon flavor 'Toasteds' approx .5 oz *(Keebler)*	4 crackers	60	1.0	8.0	125	(mq)	3.0	<1.0	0	43%

Food Name	Serving Size	Calories	Prot. gms	Carbs gms	Sod. mgs	Fiber gms	Fat gms	Sat. Fat gms	Chol. mgs	% Fat Cal.
banana walnut 'Orchard Crisps' (Nabisco)	.5 oz	60	1.0	11.0	40	na	2.0	<1.0	0	27%
barbecue wheat, for weight control (Spicer's)	1 oz	100	5.0	12.0	75	9.0	5.0	na	0	40%
bar-b-que, tater crisps (Mr. Phipps)	.5 oz	60	1.0	10.0	160	na	2.0	<1.0	0	29%
bite size (Delicious)	.5 oz	70	1.0	9.0	90	na	3.0	<1.0	0	40%
bite size, low sodium (Delicious)	.5 oz	70	1.0	9.0	55	na	3.0	<1.0	0	40%
'Bits' approx .5 oz (Triscuit)	15 crackers	60	1.0	10.0	85	na	3.0	0.0	0	38%
bran (FiberRich)	1 cracker	18	1.0	6.0	10	2.8	<1.0	na	0	<24%
bran, toasted 'Bran Thins' (Nabisco)	7 crackers	60	1.0	9.0	70	(mq)	3.0	<1.0	0	40%
butter, country flavor (McCrakens)	1 oz	140	2.0	18.0	170	na	8.0	na	0	47%
butter flavor (Ritz)	4 crackers	70	1.0	9.0	140	0	4.0	1.0	0	47%
butter flavor, approx .5 oz (Escort)	3 crackers	70	1.0	9.0	115	(mq)	4.0	<1.0	0	47%
butter flavor 'Club Low Salt' approx .5 oz (Keebler)	4 crackers	60	1.0	9.0	75	(mq)	3.0	<1.0	0	40%
butter flavor, dairy, .5 oz (American Classic)	4 crackers	70	1.0	9.0	140	(mq)	3.0	<1.0	2	40%
butter flavor 'Flutters' (Pepperidge Farm)	.75 oz	100	2.0	15.0	150	(mq)	4.0	1.0	5	35%
butter flavor 'Ritz Bits' 22 pieces (Ritz)	.5 oz	70	1.0	9.0	120	(mq)	4.0	<1.0	0	47%
butter flavor 'Ritz Bits Low Salt' 22 pieces (Ritz)	.5 oz	70	1.0	9.0	60	(mq)	4.0	<1.0	0	47%
butter flavor 'Ritz Low Salt' approx .5 oz (Ritz)	4 crackers	70	1.0	9.0	60	(mq)	4.0	<1.0	0	47%
butter flavor 'Ritz' approx .5 oz (Ritz)	4 crackers	70	1.0	9.0	120	(mq)	4.0	<1.0	0	47%
butter flavor 'Toasteds Buttercrisp' .5 oz (Keebler)	4 crackers	60	1.0	8.0	125	(mq)	3.0	<1.0	0	43%
butter flavor 'Town House Low Salt' .5 oz (Keebler)	4 crackers	70	1.0	8.0	60	(mq)	4.0	<1.0	0	50%
butter flavor 'Town House' approx .5 oz (Keebler)	4 crackers	70	1.0	8.0	120	(mq)	4.0	<1.0	0	50%
butter flavor, thins 'Distinctive' (Pepperidge Farm)	4 crackers	70	1.0	10.0	115	(mq)	3.0	1.0	5	38%
cheese (Combos)	1.8 oz	240	5.0	34.0	580	(mq)	10.0	(mq)	na	37%
cheese (Delicious)	.5 oz	70	1.0	9.0	135	na	3.0	0.5	<1	40%
cheese 'Better Cheddars' (Nabisco)	.5 oz	70	2.0	8.0	130	0	4.0	1.0	0	47%
cheese 'Better Cheddars' low salt (Nabisco)	.5 oz	70	2.0	8.0	65	0	4.0	1.0	2	47%
cheese, bite size (Delicious)	.5 oz	70	1.0	9.0	135	na	3.0	0.5	<1	40%
cheese, cheddar, approx 13-16 crackers (Frito-Lay's)	.5 oz	70	1.0	8.0	150	0	4.0	na	0	50%
cheese, cheddar, baked, cracker chips 'Zings' (Nabisco)	.5 oz	70	1.0	9.0	140	na	3.0	<1.0	2	40%
cheese, cheddar 'Crackups' (Nabisco)	.5 oz	70	1.0	10.0	100	na	3.0	na	0	38%
cheese, cheddar 'Goldfish' (Pepperidge Farm)	1 oz	120	4.0	19.0	230	1.0	4.0	1.0	5	28%
cheese, cheddar 'Goldfish Thins' (Pepperidge Farm)	4 crackers	50	1.0	8.0	160	(mq)	2.0	0.0	0	33%
cheese, cheddar 'Guppies' 12 pieces (Pepperidge Farm)	.5 oz	40	1.0	5.0	95	(mq)	2.0	(mq)	na	43%
cheese, cheddar 'Original Goldfish' (Pepperidge Farm)	1 oz	130	3.0	18.0	190	1.0	5.0	1.0	0	35%
cheese, cheddar 'Snorkels' (Nabisco)	.5 oz	70	2.0	9.0	150	na	2.0	na	0	29%
cheese, cheddar, tangy (McCrakens)	1 oz	140	2.0	18.0	170	na	8.0	na	0	47%
cheese, cheddar 'Town House Jrs.' 8 pieces (Keebler)	.5 oz	80	1.0	8.0	95	(mq)	4.0	<1.0	5	50%
cheese 'Cheddar Wedges' 31 pieces (Nabisco)	.5 oz	70	1.0	9.0	150	0	3.0	1.0	0	40%
cheese 'Cheese Nips' 13 pieces (Nabisco)	.5 oz	70	1.0	9.0	130	0	3.0	1.0	0	40%
cheese 'Cheese Peanut Butter Sandwich' 4 pieces (Nabisco)	1 oz	130	3.0	15.0	320	na	7.0	1.0	0	47%
cheese 'Cheese Ritz Bits Mini Ritz' 22 pieces (Ritz)	.5 oz	70	1.0	8.0	130	0	4.0	0.0	0	50%
cheese 'Cheez-Its' (Sunshine)	12 crackers	70	2.0	7.0	135	(mq)	4.0	1.0	2	50%
cheese 'Cheez-Its Low Salt' (Sunshine)	12 crackers	70	2.0	7.0	65	(mq)	4.0	1.0	2	50%
cheese, Parmesan 'Goldfish' (Pepperidge Farm)	1 oz	120	4.0	19.0	330	1.0	4.0	1.0	5	28%
cheese, reduced fat 'Snack Wells' 18 pieces (Nabisco)	.5 oz	60	2.0	11.0	160	na	1.0	na	0	15%
cheese 'Ritz Bits Sandwiches' approx .5 oz (Ritz)	6 crackers	80	1.0	7.0	135	0	5.0	1.0	0	58%
cheese, sandwich-type w/peanut butter filling	.5 oz	68	1.8	8.1	141	.2	3.3	0.7	1	43%
cheese, Swiss 'Naturally Flavored' .5 oz (Nabisco)	7 crackers	70	1.0	9.0	170	na	3.0	1.0	0	40%
cheese 'Tid-Bits' 15 pieces (Nabisco)	.5 oz	70	1.0	8.0	200	<1.0	4.0	<1.0	5	50%
cheese, white cheddar 'Cheez-Its' (Sunshine)	.5 oz	76	1.0	9.0	160	na	4.0	<1.0	2	47%
cheese flavor (Hain)	1 oz	130	3.0	17.0	180	(mq)	6.0	(mq)	na	40%
cheese flavor, organic, fat-free (Health Valley)	.5 oz	40	1.0	9.0	80	1.9	0.0	na	0	0%
cheese flavor, 25 pieces (Rokeach)	1 oz	140	3.0	16.0	(mq)	(mq)	8.0	(mq)	na	49%

Food Name	Serving Size	Calories	Prot. gms	Carbs gms	Sod. mgs	Fiber gms	Fat gms	Sat. Fat gms	Chol. mgs	% Fat Cal.
cheese sandwich, and cheese 'Handi-Snacks' (Kraft)	1 pkg	120	4.0	9.0	360	(mq)	8.0	5.0	20	58%
cheese sandwich, and peanut butter, .5 oz (Keebler)	2 crackers	70	2.0	9.0	150	(mq)	3.0	<1.0	0	38%
cheese sandwich, cheddar 'Town House' .5 oz (Keebler)	1 cracker	70	1.0	6.0	105	(mq)	4.0	1.0	5	56%
cheese sandwich, wheat and American cheese, .5 oz (Keebler)	1 cracker	70	1.0	7.0	85	(mq)	4.0	1.0	5	53%
cheese-filled, 6 crackers (Frito-Lay's)	1.5 oz	210	4.0	24.0	470	0	10.0	na	5	45%
chicken flavor 'Chicken in a Biskit' 7 pieces (Nabisco) ...	.5 oz	80	1.0	8.0	130	(mq)	5.0	1.0	0	56%
cinnamon graham (Delicious)	.5 oz	60	1.0	11.0	50	na	2.0	0.5	0	27%
cinnamon graham, fat-free 'Snack Wells' (Nabisco)	.5 oz	50	1.0	12.0	45	na	0.0	na	0	0%
cracked pepper, fat-free 'Snack Wells' (Nabisco)	.5 oz	60	1.0	12.0	160	na	0.0	na	0	0%
cracked pepper 'Gourmet' fat-free (Frookie)	4 crackers	35	1.0	7.0	40	na	0.0	0.0	0	0%
cracked wheat, approx .5 oz (American Classic)	4 crackers	70	1.0	8.0	140	(mq)	4.0	<1.0	0	50%
cracked wheat 'Distinctive' (Pepperidge Farm)	3 crackers	100	2.0	14.0	180	1.0	4.0	1.0	0	36%
cracked wheat 'Wafers' (Hickory Farms)	8 crackers	100	2.0	17.0	290	(mq)	3.0	(mq)	na	26%
'Crackerbread' (Crisp & Light)	1 slice	17	1.0	3.0	25	(mq)	<1.0	na	0	<36%
'Crackerbread Salt Free' (Crisp & Light)	1 slice	17	1.0	3.0	<1	(mq)	<1.0	na	0	<36%
'Crackerdiles' (Delicious)	.5 oz	70	1.0	9.0	135	na	3.0	0.5	<1	40%
crispbread (Dar-Vida)	1 cracker	20	1.0	4.0	40	(mq)	<1.0	na	0	<31%
crispbread 'Breakfast' (Wasa)	1 cracker	50	2.0	8.0	65	.7	1.0	na	0	18%
crispbread, dark (Finn Crisp)	2 crackers	38	1.0	9.0	130	1.6	<1.0	na	0	<18%
crispbread 'Extra Crisp' (Wasa)	1 cracker	25	1.0	5.0	40	(mq)	0.0	0.0	0	0%
crispbread 'Fiber Plus' (Wasa)	1 cracker	35	1.0	5.0	65	2.8	1.0	na	0	27%
crispbread, garlic flavor (Weight Watchers)	2 crackers	30	<1.0	7.0	55	(mq)	0.0	0.0	0	0%
crispbread, high fiber 'Crisp Bread' (Ryvita)	1 cracker	23	0.9	4.0	10	2.0	<1.0	na	0	<32%
crispbread, high fiber 'Snackbread' (Ryvita)	1 cracker	14	0.6	3.0	25	1.0	<1.0	na	0	<39%
crispbread, regular (Finn Crisp)	2 crackers	38	1.0	9.0	130	1.6	<1.0	na	0	<18%
crispbread, thick (Kavli Norwegian)	1 slice	35	1.0	7.5	31	1.9	0.3	na	0	7%
crispbread, thin (Kavli Norwegian)	2 slices	40	1.0	8.0	32	6.0	0.3	na	0	7%
crispbread, w/caraway (Finn Crisp)	2 slices	38	1.0	9.0	130	1.6	<1.0	na	0	<18%
5-spice wafer (Westbrae)	4.5 wafers	40	1.0	8.0	30	na	0.0	na	0	0%
garlic 'Discos' (Delicious)	.5 oz	78	1.0	6.0	184	na	5.0	na	0	62%
garlic 'Garlic Tams' (Manischewitz)	10 crackers	153	2.0	19.0	165	(mq)	8.0	6.0	0	46%
garlic and herb 'Gourmet' fat-free (Frookie)	8 crackers	70	2.0	16.0	170	1.0	0.0	0.0	0	0%
graham, chocolate 'Selects' (Keebler)	4 crackers	60	1.0	9.0	55	na	3.0	1.0	0	40%
graham, honey nut 'Selects' (Keebler)	4 crackers	60	1.0	9.0	70	na	3.0	1.0	0	40%
graham cracker 'Amaranth Graham Crackers' (Health Valley)	7 crackers	110	3.0	25.0	110	3.1	3.0	(mq)	0	19%
graham cracker, apple cinnamon 'Graham Bites' (Honey Maid)	11 crackers	60	1.0	11.0	80	(mq)	2.0	<1.0	0	27%
graham cracker, approx .5 oz (Keebler)	4 crackers	70	1.0	12.0	85	(mq)	2.0	<1.0	0	26%
graham cracker, approx 1 oz (Regal)	2 crackers	140	1.0	19.0	120	(mq)	7.0	(mq)	na	44%
graham cracker, approx 1 oz (Rokeach)	8 crackers	120	2.0	21.0	(mq)	(mq)	3.0	(mq)	na	23%
graham cracker, brown sugar 'Graham Bites' .5 oz (Honey Maid)	11 crackers	60	1.0	11.0	80	(mq)	2.0	<1.0	0	27%
graham cracker 'Grahamy Bears' (Sunshine)	9 crackers	130	2.0	21.0	160	(mq)	5.0	1.0	0	33%
graham cracker, 2 pieces (Nabisco)	.5 oz	60	1.0	11.0	90	1.0	1.0	0.0	0	16%
grain, 6 pieces (Harvest Crisps)	.5 oz	60	1.0	10.0	135	1.0	2.0	0.0	0	29%
hearty wheat 'Distinctive' (Pepperidge Farm)	4 crackers	100	2.0	13.0	140	1.0	5.0	1.0	0	43%
herb, garden 'Flutters' (Pepperidge Farm)	.75 oz	100	2.0	14.0	190	(mq)	4.0	1.0	0	36%
herb, organic, fat-free (Health Valley)	.5 oz	40	1.0	9.0	80	1.9	0.0	na	0	0%
herb 'Stoned Wheat' (Health Valley)	13 crackers	120	3.0	17.0	160	3.5	6.0	(mq)	0	40%
herb 'Stoned Wheat No Salt Added' (Health Valley)	13 crackers	120	3.0	17.0	30	3.5	6.0	(mq)	0	40%
honey graham (Delicious)	.5 oz	60	1.0	11.0	50	na	2.0	0.3	0	27%
hot and spicy 'Cheez-Its' approx 12 crackers (Sunshine) ..	.5 oz	70	1.0	8.0	160	na	4.0	1.0	2	50%

Food Name	Serving Size	Calories	Prot. gms	Carbs gms	Sod. mgs	Fiber gms	Fat gms	Sat. Fat gms	Chol. mgs	% Fat Cal.
'Low Salt' (Featherweight)	2 crackers	30	0.0	5.0	1	(mq)	1.0	na	0	31%
matzo, American board (Manischewitz)	1 oz	115	2.9	22.0	na	(mq)	1.9	(mq)	0	15%
matzo 'Daily Unsalted' board (Manischewitz)	1 oz	110	3.0	24.0	1	.1	0.3	0.0	0	2%
matzo, dietetic, thin board (Manischewitz)	.8 oz	91	2.6	19.0	<1	.1	0.4	0.0	0	4%
matzo, egg	.5 oz	55	1.7	11.1	3	na	0.3	0.1	12	5%
matzo, egg, 1 oz	1 matzo	111	3.5	22.3	6	na	0.6	0.2	25	5%
matzo, egg, miniature 'Passover' approx 1 oz (Manischewitz)	10 crackers	108	3.0	20.0	10	(mq)	2.0	(mq)	20	16%
matzo, egg 'Passover' board (Manischewitz)	1.2 oz	132	4.0	27.0	5	(mq)	2.0	(mq)	25	13%
matzo, egg and onion	.5 oz	55	1.4	10.9	40	.7	0.6	0.1	8	10%
matzo, egg and onion, 1 oz	1 matzo	111	2.8	21.9	81	1.4	1.1	0.3	15	9%
matzo, egg n' onion, board (Manischewitz)	1 oz	112	3.1	23.0	180	(mq)	1.0	0.2	15	8%
matzo, miniature (Manischewitz)	10 crackers	90	2.0	20.0	10	(mq)	<1.0	na	0	<9%
matzo 'Passover' board (Manischewitz)	1.1 oz	129	3.3	27.0	5	(mq)	0.4	0.0	0	3%
matzo, plain	.5 oz	56	1.4	11.9	0	.4 ns	0.2	0.0	0	3%
matzo, plain, 1 oz	1 matzo	112	2.8	23.7	1	.9	0.4	0.1	0	3%
matzo, tea 'Daily' thin board (Manischewitz)	.9 oz	103	3.0	22.0	1	.1	0.3	0.0	0	3%
matzo, thin board (Manischewitz)	.9 oz	100	3.0	21.0	0	.1	0.3	0.0	na	3%
matzo, whole-wheat	.5 oz	50	1.9	11.2	0	1.6	0.2	0.0	0	3%
matzo, whole-wheat, 1 oz	1 matzo	100	3.7	22.4	1	3.3	0.4	0.1	0	3%
matzo, whole wheat, w/bran, board (Manischewitz)	1 oz	110	4.0	21.0	1	.6	0.6	0.0	0	5%
melba toast, bacon 'Rounds' (Old London)	.5 oz	53	2.1	10.1	126	.9	1.0	na	0	16%
melba toast, garlic 'Rounds' (Old London)	.5 oz	56	2.1	9.9	132	.6	1.2	na	0	18%
melba toast, honey bran (Devonsheer)	1 cracker	16	1.0	3.0	25	.2	0.4	0.1	0	18%
melba toast, honey bran 'Rounds' (Devonsheer)	.5 oz	52	2.1	10.2	98	.9	0.9	na	0	14%
melba toast, oat, .5 oz (Harvest Crisps)	6 crackers	60	1.0	10.0	135	(mq)	2.0	<1.0	0	29%
melba toast, onion 'Rounds' (Devonsheer)	.5 oz	51	1.9	10.7	120	.8	0.6	na	0	10%
melba toast, onion 'Rounds' (Old London)	.5 oz	52	2.0	10.2	121	.7	0.8	na	0	13%
melba toast, plain	.5 oz	55	1.7	10.9	118	.9	0.5	0.1	0	8%
melba toast, plain (Devonsheer)	1 cracker	16	1.0	3.0	30	.2	0.4	0.1	0	18%
melba toast, plain 'Rounds' (Devonsheer)	.5 oz	53	2.0	11.0	111	.8	0.6	na	0	9%
melba toast, plain 'Unsalted' (Devonsheer)	1 cracker	16	1.0	3.0	5	.2	0.4	0.1	0	18%
melba toast, plain 'Unsalted Rounds' (Devonsheer)	.5 oz	52	1.8	10.9	5	.8	0.6	na	0	10%
melba toast, plain, w/o salt	.5 oz	55	1.7	10.9	3	.9	0.5	0.1	0	8%
melba toast, pumpernickel (Old London)	.5 oz	54	1.6	11.0	156	.8	0.6	na	0	10%
melba toast, rye	.5 oz	55	1.6	11.0	127	1.1	0.5	0.1	0	8%
melba toast, rye (Devonsheer)	1 cracker	16	1.0	3.0	30	.2	0.4	0.1	0	18%
melba toast, rye (Old London)	.5 oz	52	1.8	10.9	132	.8	0.7	na	0	11%
melba toast, rye, .5 oz (Devonsheer)	1 cracker	16	1.0	3.0	30	.2	0.4	0.1	0	18%
melba toast, rye 'Rounds' (Devonsheer)	.5 oz	53	1.8	10.7	130	.9	0.6	na	0	10%
melba toast, rye 'Rounds' (Old London)	.5 oz	52	1.7	10.8	132	.9	0.7	na	0	11%
melba toast, rye 'Unsalted' (Devonsheer)	1 cracker	16	1.0	3.0	5	.2	0.4	0.1	0	18%
melba toast, sesame (Devonsheer)	1 cracker	16	1.0	3.0	25	.2	0.5	0.1	0	22%
melba toast, sesame (Old London)	.5 oz	55	2.3	8.9	148	.9	1.8	(mq)	0	27%
melba toast, sesame 'Rounds' (Devonsheer)	.5 oz	57	2.3	9.0	131	.9	1.8	(mq)	0	26%
melba toast, sesame 'Rounds' (Old London)	.5 oz	56	2.3	8.9	149	.9	1.8	(mq)	0	27%
melba toast, sesame 'Unsalted' (Old London)	.5 oz	56	2.3	8.9	5	1.0	1.8	(mq)	0	27%
melba toast, vegetable (Devonsheer)	1 cracker	16	1.0	3.0	25	.2	0.4	0.1	0	18%
melba toast, wheat	.5 oz	53	1.8	10.8	119	1.0	0.3	0.1	0	5%
melba toast, wheat (Old London)	.5 oz	51	2.1	10.5	121	.9	0.7	na	0	11%
melba toast, wheat '6-calorie' (Estee)	1 cracker	6	<1.0	1.0	5	(mq)	<1.0	<1.0	0	<53%
melba toast, wheat 'Snax' (Estee)	1 oz	100	4.0	22.0	15	(mq)	<1.0	<1.0	0	<8%
melba toast, white (Old London)	.5 oz	51	2.0	10.4	111	.8	0.6	na	0	10%
melba toast, white 'Rounds' (Old London)	.5 oz	48	2.0	9.8	111	.8	0.6	na	0	10%

Food Name	Serving Size	Calories	Prot. gms	Carbs gms	Sod. mgs	Fiber gms	Fat gms	Sat. Fat gms	Chol. mgs	% Fat Cal.
melba toast, white 'Unsalted' (Old London)	.5 oz	51	1.8	10.7	4	.8	0.6	na	0	10%
melba toast, whole grain (Old London)	.5 oz	52	2.1	10.1	116	.8	0.9	na	0	14%
melba toast, whole grain 'Rounds' (Old London)	.5 oz	54	2.1	9.9	102	.9	1.2	na	0	18%
melba toast, whole grain 'Unsalted' (Old London)	.5 oz	53	2.1	10.0	4	.9	1.0	na	0	16%
melba toast, whole wheat (Devonsheer)	1 cracker	16	1.0	3.0	30	.2	0.4	0.1	0	18%
melba toast, whole wheat 'Unsalted' (Devonsheer)	1 cracker	16	1.0	3.0	5	.2	0.4	0.1	0	18%
milk	.5 oz	65	1.1	9.9	84	na	2.2	0.4	2	31%
multi-grain (Premium)	.5 oz	60	1.0	10.0	140	na	2.0	<1.0	0	29%
multi-grain 'Wheat Thins' (Nabisco)	.5 oz	60	1.0	10.0	135	na	2.0	<1.0	0	29%
nacho cheese flavor (Delicious)	.5 oz	89	1.0	8.0	150	na	5.0	na	0	56%
natural, for weight control (Spicer's)	1 oz	100	4.0	11.0	65	9.0	4.0	na	0	38%
nutty wheat 'Wheat Thins' approx .5 oz (Nabisco)	7 crackers	70	1.0	9.0	170	(mq)	4.0	<1.0	0	47%
oat 'Oat Krisp' (Ralston)	.5 oz	50	1.0	7.0	140	3.0	2.0	0.0	0	36%
oat 'Oat Thins' approx .5 oz (Nabisco)	8 crackers	70	1.0	10.0	90	(mq)	3.0	<1.0	0	38%
oat, .5 oz (Harvest Crisps)	6 crackers	60	1.0	10.0	135	1.0	2.0	0.0	0	29%
oat bran 'Oat Bran Krisps' (Ralston)	.5 oz	60	1.0	9.0	140	3.2	3.0	(mq)	0	40%
'Old Fashioned' (Hickory Farms)	10 crackers	90	2.0	16.0	170	(mq)	3.0	(mq)	na	27%
onion (Delicious)	.5 oz	70	1.0	10.0	180	na	3.0	na	0	38%
onion 'Discos' (Delicious)	.5 oz	76	1.0	7.0	156	na	5.0	na	0	58%
onion, minced, approx .5 oz (American Classic)	4 crackers	70	1.0	10.0	120	(mq)	3.0	<1.0	0	38%
onion, organic, fat-free (Health Valley)	.5 oz	40	1.0	9.0	80	1.9	0.0	na	0	0%
onion flavor (Hain)	1 oz	130	3.0	17.0	160	(mq)	6.0	(mq)	na	40%
onion flavor 'No Salt Added' (Hain)	1 oz	130	3.0	17.0	5	(mq)	6.0	(mq)	na	40%
onion flavor 'Onion Tams' (Manischewitz)	10 crackers	150	2.0	18.0	157	(mq)	8.0	6.0	0	47%
onion flavor 'Toasteds' approx .5 oz (Keebler)	4 crackers	60	1.0	9.0	140	(mq)	3.0	<1.0	0	40%
onion garlic wafer (Westbrae)	4.5 crackers	40	1.0	8.0	50	na	0.0	na	0	0%
oyster	.5 oz	62	1.3	10.1	185	.4	1.7	0.3	0	25%
oyster (OTC)	1 cracker	25	1.0	4.0	65	(mq)	1.0	<1.0	0	31%
oyster (Premium)	20 crackers	60	1.0	10.0	210	0	1.0	0.0	0	17%
oyster (Sunshine)	16 crackers	60	1.0	11.0	190	(mq)	1.0	<1.0	0	16%
oyster, approx .5 oz (Dandy)	20 crackers	60	1.0	10.0	220	(mq)	2.0	<1.0	0	29%
oyster, low salt	.5 oz	62	1.3	10.1	90	.4	1.7	0.3	0	25%
oyster 'Oysterettes' approx .5 oz (Nabisco)	18 crackers	60	1.0	10.0	140	(mq)	1.0	<1.0	0	17%
oyster, unsalted tops	.5 oz	62	1.3	10.1	109	.4	1.7	0.3	0	25%
peanut butter (Combos)	1.8 oz	240	6.0	30.0	360	(mq)	10.0	(mq)	na	39%
peanut butter, cheese (Little Debbie)	1.4 oz	190	6.0	23.0	390	(mq)	9.0	(mq)	<1	41%
peanut butter, cheese (Little Debbie)	.93 oz	130	4.0	14.0	260	(mq)	6.0	(mq)	<1	43%
peanut butter, cheese sandwich (Handi-Snacks)	1 pkg	190	6.0	11.0	180	(mq)	14.0	4.0	0	65%
peanut butter 'Ritz Bits Sandwiches' 1 oz (Ritz)	12 crackers	80	2.0	8.0	80	na	4.0	na	0	47%
peanut butter, toast, approx .5 oz (Keebler)	2 crackers	70	2.0	9.0	120	(mq)	3.0	<1.0	0	38%
peanut butter 'Toast Sandwich' 4 pieces (Nabisco)	1 oz	130	3.0	15.0	300	na	7.0	1.0	0	47%
peanut butter, toasty (Little Debbie)	1.4 oz	200	6.0	21.0	380	(mq)	12.0	(mq)	<1	50%
peanut butter, toasty (Little Debbie)	.93 oz	140	4.0	14.0	250	(mq)	7.0	(mq)	<1	47%
peanut butter bar (Frito-Lay's)	1.75 oz	270	2.0	30.0	65	na	16.0	na	0	53%
peanut butter-filled, 6 crackers (Frito-Lay's)	1.5 oz	210	6.0	24.0	450	0	10.0	na	0	43%
pizza 'Goldfish' (Pepperidge Farm)	1 oz	130	4.0	19.0	220	1.0	5.0	1.0	5	33%
poppy, toasted, approx .5 oz (American Classic)	4 crackers	70	1.0	9.0	140	(mq)	3.0	<1.0	0	40%
pumpernickel (Delicious)	.5 oz	70	1.0	9.0	160	na	3.0	na	0	40%
pumpernickel 'Snack Sticks' (Pepperidge Farm)	8 crackers	140	3.0	20.0	330	1.0	6.0	1.0	0	37%
ranch, baked, cracker chips 'Zings' (Nabisco)	.5 oz	70	1.0	9.0	140	na	3.0	<1.0	2	40%
ranch 'Snack Crisps' (Estee)	.66 oz	80	2.0	13.0	135	na	2.0	<1.0	0	23%
'Regency' (Delicious)	.5 oz	70	1.0	9.0	100	na	<3.0	<1.0	0	<40%
rice, approx .5 oz (Harvest Crisps)	6 crackers	60	1.0	11.0	135	1.0	2.0	0.0	0	27%
rice, harvest 'Crispbread' (Weight Watchers)	2 crackers	30	<1.0	7.0	55	(mq)	0.0	0.0	0	0%

Food Name	Serving Size	Calories	Prot. gms	Carbs gms	Sod. mgs	Fiber gms	Fat gms	Sat. Fat gms	Chol. mgs	% Fat Cal.
rice bran (Health Valley)	7 crackers	130	4.0	19.0	64	1.5	4.0	(mq)	0	28%
'Rich' (Hain)	1 oz	130	3.0	18.0	160	(mq)	5.0	(mq)	na	35%
'Rich, No Salt Added' (Hain)	1 oz	130	3.0	18.0	15	(mq)	5.0	(mq)	na	35%
'Royal Lunch Milk Crackers' .5 oz (Nabisco)	1 cracker	60	1.0	10.0	80	1.0	2.0	0.0	0	29%
rusk toast	.5 oz	58	1.9	10.2	36	na	1.0	0.2	4	16%
rye	.5 oz	52	1.1	11.6	37	2.3	0.2	0.0	0	3%
rye (Hain)	1 oz	120	3.0	19.0	200	(mq)	4.0	(mq)	0	29%
rye, BBQ 'Rounds O' Rye' (Hickory Farms)	1 oz	153	2.7	13.0	60	(mq)	10.6	(mq)	na	60%
rye, dark 'Crisp Bread' (Ryvita)	1 cracker	26	0.7	6.0	35	1.3	<1.0	na	0	<25%
rye, garlic 'Rounds O' Rye' (Hickory Farms)	1 oz	147	2.7	14.5	126	(mq)	8.9	(mq)	na	54%
rye, golden 'Crispbread' (Wasa)	1 cracker	35	1.0	7.0	55	1.4	0.0	0.0	0	0%
rye, hearty 'Crispbread' (Wasa)	1 cracker	45	2.0	9.0	70	2.6	0.0	0.0	0	0%
rye, light 'Crisp Bread' (Ryvita)	1 cracker	26	0.7	6.0	20	1.3	<1.0	na	0	<25%
rye, light 'Crispbread Lite' (Wasa)	1 cracker	25	1.0	5.0	40	1.2	0.0	0.0	0	0%
rye, light 'Hi-Fiber' (Finn Crisp)	1 cracker	35	1.0	8.0	60	(mq)	1.0	na	0	20%
rye, natural 'Rounds O' Rye' (Hickory Farms)	1 oz	156	3.1	12.2	93	(mq)	10.9	(mq)	na	62%
rye 'No Salt Added' (Hain)	1 oz	120	3.0	19.0	10	(mq)	4.0	(mq)	0	29%
rye, original 'Hi-Fiber' (Finn Crisp)	1 cracker	40	1.0	10.0	95	(mq)	0.0	0.0	0	0%
rye 'RyKrisp' (Ralston)	.5 oz	40	1.0	11.0	75	na	0.0	na	0	0%
rye 'Rykrisp Twindividuals' 2 triple pieces (Ralston)	.5 oz	45	1.0	11.0	105	3.0	1.0	na	0	16%
rye 'Salt Free' (Hickory Farms)	8 crackers	90	2.0	18.0	na	(mq)	1.0	na	0	10%
rye, sandwich-type w/cheese filling	.5 oz	68	1.3	8.6	148	na	3.2	0.8	1	42%
rye, seasoned 'Rykrisp' (Ralston)	.5 oz	45	1.0	11.0	105	3.0	1.0	na	0	16%
rye, sesame 'Rykrisp' 2 triple pieces (Ralston)	.5 oz	50	1.0	10.0	105	3.0	2.0	(mq)	0	29%
rye, sesame, toasted 'Crisp Bread' (Ryvita)	1 cracker	31	1.1	5.0	10	1.4	<1.0	na	0	<27%
rye, sour cream 'Rounds O'Rye' (Hickory Farms)	1 oz	155	2.7	12.6	130	(mq)	10.7	(mq)	na	61%
rye 'Toasteds' approx .5 oz (Keebler)	4 crackers	60	1.0	8.0	140	(mq)	3.0	<1.0	0	43%
rye 'Wafers' (Hickory Farms)	8 crackers	90	2.0	17.0	250	(mq)	2.0	(mq)	na	19%
rye wafers, plain	.5 oz	47	1.4	11.4	113	na	0.1	0.0	0	2%
rye wafers, seasoned	.5 oz	54	1.3	10.5	126	na	1.3	0.2	0	20%
salsa 'Crackups' (Nabisco)	.5 oz	70	1.0	9.0	100	na	3.0	na	0	40%
salt sticks, Vienna bread type, 6.5 inches long	1 stick	106	3.3	20.3	548	>.1 c	1.1	0.2	1	10%
saltine, approx .5 oz (Zesta)	5 crackers	60	1.0	10.0	190	(mq)	2.0	<1.0	0	29%
saltine 'Bits Mini Saltine Crackers' .5 oz (Premium)	16 crackers	70	1.0	9.0	160	0	3.0	1.0	0	40%
saltine, crumbs, not packed	1 cup	303	6.3	50.0	770	>.3 c	8.4	2.0	0	25%
saltine 'Fat-Free' .5 oz (Premium)	4 crackers	50	1.0	12.0	115	0	0.0	0.0	0	0%
saltine 'Krispy' (Sunshine)	5 crackers	60	1.0	11.0	210	(mq)	1.0	<1.0	0	16%
saltine 'Krispy Unsalted Tops' (Sunshine)	5 crackers	60	1.0	11.0	120	(mq)	1.0	<1.0	0	16%
saltine, low salt	.5 oz	62	1.3	10.1	90	.4	1.7	0.3	0	25%
saltine 'Low Salt' approx .5 oz (Premium)	5 crackers	60	1.0	10.0	115	0	2.0	0.0	0	29%
saltine 'Low Salt' approx .5 oz (Zesta)	5 crackers	60	1.0	10.0	95	(mq)	2.0	<1.0	0	29%
saltine, mild cheddar 'Krispy' (Sunshine)	5 crackers	60	2.0	10.0	180	na	2.0	<1.0	2	27%
saltine, 1 7/8-inch square	10 crackers	123	2.6	20.3	312	>.1 c	3.4	0.8	0	25%
saltine, original, .5 oz (Premium)	5 crackers	60	1.0	10.0	180	0	2.0	0.0	0	29%
saltine, 10 pieces (Rokeach)	1 oz	120	2.0	20.0	na	(mq)	3.0	(mq)	0	24%
saltine, unsalted tops	.5 oz	62	1.3	10.1	109	.4	1.7	0.3	0	25%
saltine 'Unsalted' (Estee)	4 crackers	60	1.0	9.0	0	(mq)	2.0	<1.0	0	31%
saltine 'Unsalted Tops' approx .5 oz (Premium)	5 crackers	60	1.0	10.0	135	(mq)	2.0	<1.0	0	29%
saltine 'Unsalted Tops' approx .5 oz (Zesta)	5 crackers	60	1.0	10.0	85	(mq)	2.0	<1.0	0	29%
saltine, wheat, approx .5 oz (Zesta)	5 crackers	60	1.0	10.0	190	(mq)	2.0	<1.0	0	29%
saltine, wheat 'Whole Wheat Premium Plus' .5 oz (Premium)	4 crackers	60	1.0	10.0	130	1.0	2.0	0.0	0	29%
sandwich, peanut-cheese, 6 sandwiches	1 pkt	206	6.4	23.6	417	>.2 c	10.0	2.7	7	43%
sandwich, peanut-cheese, 4 sandwiches	1 pkt	137	4.3	15.7	278	>.1 c	6.7	1.8	4	43%

Food Name	Serving Size	Calories	Prot. gms	Carbs gms	Sod. mgs	Fiber gms	Fat gms	Sat. Fat gms	Chol. mgs	% Fat Cal.
sandwich, w/cheese filling	.5 oz	68	1.3	8.8	199	na	3.0	0.8	0	40%
sandwich, w/peanut butter filling	.5 oz	69	1.6	8.3	134	na	3.4	0.7	0	44%
'Schooners' 33 pieces (FFV)	.5 oz	60	1.0	10.0	130	(mq)	2.0	<1.0	0	29%
sesame (Hain)	1 oz	140	3.0	16.0	210	(mq)	7.0	(mq)	na	45%
sesame, bread wafer, approx .5 oz (Meal Mates)	3 crackers	70	1.0	9.0	160	(mq)	3.0	<1.0	0	40%
sesame 'Crisp' (FFV)	1 cracker	60	1.0	10.0	120	(mq)	2.0	<1.0	0	29%
sesame 'Crispbread' (Dar-Vida)	1 cracker	22	1.0	4.0	40	(mq)	1.0	na	0	31%
sesame 'Distinctive' (Pepperidge Farm)	4 crackers	80	2.0	12.0	140	2.0	4.0	1.0	0	39%
sesame, golden (American Classic)	4 crackers	70	1.0	9.0	120	(mq)	3.0	<1.0	0	40%
sesame, golden, .5 oz (American Classic)	4 crackers	70	1.0	9.0	120	(mq)	3.0	<1.0	0	40%
sesame, golden 'Flutters' (Pepperidge Farm)	.75 oz	110	2.0	13.0	150	(mq)	5.0	1.0	0	43%
sesame 'No Salt Added' (Hain)	1 oz	140	3.0	16.0	5	(mq)	7.0	(mq)	na	45%
sesame 'RyKrisp' (Ralston)	.5 oz	50	1.0	10.0	105	3.0	2.0	na	0	29%
sesame, savory 'Crispbread' (Wasa)	1 cracker	30	2.0	4.0	40	2.4	1.0	na	0	27%
sesame 'Snack Sticks' (Pepperidge Farm)	8 crackers	140	4.0	19.0	280	1.0	5.0	1.0	0	33%
sesame 'Toasteds' approx .5 oz (Keebler)	4 crackers	60	1.0	8.0	130	(mq)	3.0	<1.0	0	43%
sesame, wafer 'Crisp' approx .5 oz (FFV)	4 crackers	60	2.0	9.0	140	(mq)	2.0	<1.0	0	29%
sesame and cheese 'Twigs Snack Sticks' .5 oz (Nabisco)	5 crackers	70	1.0	8.0	140	(mq)	4.0	<1.0	2	50%
sesame chips (Flavor Tree)	1/4 cup	163	3.2	10.6	380	>.1 c	9.2	(mq)	0	60%
sesame wafer (Westbrae)	4.5 crackers	40	1.0	8.0	60	na	0.0	na	0	0%
sesame wheat (Delicious)	.5 oz	80	1.0	9.0	170	na	4.0	na	0	47%
sesame wheat 'Crispbread' (Wasa)	1 cracker	50	2.0	8.0	65	.6	2.0	(mq)	0	31%
sesame wheat 'Stoned Wheat' (Health Valley)	13 crackers	130	3.0	16.0	150	2.6	6.0	(mq)	0	42%
sesame wheat 'Stoned Wheat No Salt Added' (Health Valley)	13 crackers	130	3.0	17.0	20	2.6	6.0	(mq)	0	40%
seven grain 'Stoned Wheat' (Health Valley)	13 crackers	120	3.0	17.0	125	2.8	5.0	(mq)	0	36%
seven grain 'Stoned Wheat No Salt Added' (Health Valley)	13 crackers	120	3.0	17.0	20	2.8	5.0	(mq)	0	36%
seven-grain vegetable, organic, fat-free (Health Valley)	.5 oz	40	1.0	9.0	80	1.9	0.0	na	0	0%
seven-grain vegetable, organic, no salt added (Health Valley)	.5 oz	40	1.0	9.0	80	1.9	0.0	na	0	0%
snack, approx .5 oz (Finast)	12 crackers	70	1.0	9.0	135	(mq)	3.0	(mq)	na	40%
snack, approx .5 oz (Rokeach)	9 crackers	130	2.0	19.0	(mq)	(mq)	5.0	(mq)	na	35%
'Snack N' Cracker' (Delicious)	.5 oz	70	1.0	10.0	180	na	3.0	na	0	38%
'Snackers' (Delicious)	.5 oz	70	1.0	9.0	90	na	3.0	<1.0	0	40%
'Sociables' approx .5 oz (Nabisco)	6 crackers	70	1.0	9.0	135	0	4.0	1.0	0	47%
soda (Sailor Boy Pilot)	1 cracker	100	2.0	17.0	125	(mq)	3.0	<1.0	0	26%
soda 'Distinctive English Water Biscuit' (Pepperidge Farm)	4 crackers	70	2.0	13.0	100	(mq)	1.0	0.0	0	13%
soda 'English' (North Castles)	1 cracker	10	0.0	3.0	14	(mq)	0.0	0.0	0	0%
soda, .5 oz (Crown Pilot)	1 cracker	70	1.0	11.0	70	(mq)	2.0	<1.0	0	27%
soda, low salt	.5 oz	62	1.3	10.1	90	.4	1.7	0.3	0	25%
soda, 'Lunch' 1 cracker (Royal)	.5 oz	60	1.0	17.0	125	(mq)	3.0	<1.0	0	27%
soda 'Ocean Crisps' (FFV)	1 cracker	60	1.0	10.0	120	(mq)	2.0	<1.0	0	29%
soda, unsalted tops	.5 oz	62	1.3	10.1	109	.4	1.7	0.3	0	25%
soup, low salt	.5 oz	62	1.3	10.1	90	.4	1.7	0.3	0	25%
soup, unsalted tops	.5 oz	62	1.3	10.1	109	.4	1.7	0.3	0	25%
sour cream and chive (Hain)	1 oz	130	3.0	15.0	150	(mq)	6.0	(mq)	na	43%
sour cream and chive 'No Salt Added' (Hain)	1 oz	130	3.0	15.0	25	(mq)	6.0	(mq)	na	43%
sour cream and chive flavor (McCrakens)	1 oz	140	2.0	18.0	170	na	8.0	na	0	47%
sour cream and onion 'Discos' (Delicious)	.5 oz	79	1.0	6.0	162	na	5.0	na	0	62%
sour cream and onion, for weight control (Spicer's)	1 oz	100	4.0	12.0	150	6.0	4.0	0.0	0	36%
sour cream and onion 'Mr. Phipp's Tater Crisps' (Nabisco)	.5 oz	60	1.0	10.0	150	na	2.0	<1.0	0	29%
sourdough (Delicious)	.5 oz	70	1.0	9.0	160	na	3.0	na	0	40%
sourdough (Hain)	.5 oz	65	2.0	9.0	100	(mq)	3.0	(mq)	0	38%

Food Name	Serving Size	Calories	Prot. gms	Carbs gms	Sod. mgs	Fiber gms	Fat gms	Sat. Fat gms	Chol. mgs	% Fat Cal.
sourdough 'Low Salt' (Hain)	1 oz	130	3.0	18.0	10	(mq)	5.0	(mq)	0	35%
sticks 'Snack Sticks' (Pepperidge Farm)	8 crackers	130	4.0	19.0	400	1.0	5.0	2.0	0	33%
'Tam Tams' (Manischewitz)	10 crackers	147	2.0	17.0	171	(mq)	8.0	6.0	0	49%
'Tam Tams No Salt' (Manischewitz)	10 crackers	138	2.0	18.0	10	(mq)	7.0	5.0	0	44%
tamari wafer (Westbrae)	4.5 crackers	40	1.0	8.0	60	na	0.0	na	0	0%
'Uneeda Biscuits Unsalted Tops' approx .5 oz (Nabisco)	2 crackers	60	1.0	10.0	100	na	2.0	0.0	0	29%
vegetable (Hain)	1 oz	130	3.0	10.0	180	(mq)	5.0	(mq)	0	46%
vegetable, garden (Delicious)	.5 oz	70	1.0	10.0	220	na	3.0	na	0	38%
vegetable 'Garden Crisps' (Nabisco)	.5 oz	60	1.0	11.0	135	na	2.0	<1.0	0	27%
vegetable 'No Salt Added' (Hain)	1 oz	130	3.0	10.0	50	(mq)	5.0	(mq)	0	46%
'Vegetable Thins' (Nabisco)	7 crackers	70	1.0	8.0	140	(mq)	4.0	<1.0	0	50%
wafer, no salt (Westbrae)	4.5 wafers	40	1.0	8.0	0	na	0.0	na	0	0%
water (Sailor Boy Pilot)	1 cracker	100	2.0	17.0	125	(mq)	3.0	<1.0	0	26%
water 'Distinctive English Water Biscuit' (Pepperidge Farm)	4 crackers	70	2.0	13.0	100	(mq)	1.0	0.0	0	13%
water 'English' (North Castles)	1 cracker	10	0.0	3.0	14	(mq)	0.0	0.0	0	0%
water, .5 oz (Crown Pilot)	1 cracker	70	1.0	11.0	70	(mq)	2.0	<1.0	0	27%
water 'Gourmet' fat-free (Frookie)	4 crackers	35	1.0	7.0	60	na	0.0	0.0	0	0%
water, 'Lunch' 1 cracker (Royal)	.5 oz	60	1.0	17.0	125	(mq)	3.0	<1.0	0	27%
water 'Ocean Crisps' (FFV)	1 cracker	60	1.0	10.0	120	(mq)	2.0	<1.0	0	29%
water 'Table Water, Bite Size' (Carr's)	2 crackers	25	1.0	5.0	15	(mq)	1.0	na	na	27%
'Waverly Crackers' approx .5 oz (Nabisco)	4 crackers	70	1.0	10.0	160	na	3.0	na	0	38%
'Waverly Crackers Low Salt' approx .5 oz (Nabisco)	4 crackers	70	1.0	10.0	80	(mq)	3.0	<1.0	0	38%
'Waverly Wafer' approx .5 oz (Nabisco)	4 crackers	70	1.0	10.0	160	(mq)	3.0	<1.0	0	38%
wheat (Delicious)	.5 oz	70	1.0	9.0	85	na	3.0	0.5	0	40%
wheat, approx .5 oz (Sociables)	6 crackers	70	1.0	9.0	135	(mq)	3.0	<1.0	0	40%
wheat 'Bits' approx .5 oz (Triscuit)	8 crackers	60	1.0	10.0	75	(mq)	2.0	<1.0	0	29%
wheat 'Crispy Wafer' approx .5 oz (FFV)	6 crackers	70	1.0	9.0	80	(mq)	3.0	(mq)	na	40%
wheat, low salt	.5 oz	67	1.2	9.2	40	.8	2.9	0.5	0	39%
wheat 'Low Salt' approx .5 oz (Triscuit)	3 crackers	60	1.0	10.0	35	(mq)	2.0	<1.0	0	29%
'Wheat On' (Delicious)	.5 oz	68	1.0	8.0	86	na	3.0	0.5	0	43%
wheat 'Original Snackbread' (Ryvita)	1 cracker	20	0.5	4.0	20	.2	<1.0	na	0	<33%
wheat 'Original Wheat Thins' approx .5 oz (Nabisco)	8 crackers	70	1.0	9.0	120	<1.0	3.0	<1	0	40%
wheat, regular	.5 oz	67	1.2	9.2	113	.8	2.9	0.5	0	39%
wheat, sandwich, w/cheese filling	.5 oz	70	1.4	8.3	129	na	3.5	0.9	1	45%
wheat, sandwich, w/peanut butter filling	.5 oz	70	1.9	7.6	114	na	3.8	0.8	0	47%
wheat 'Snack Wells' (Nabisco)	.5 oz	50	1.0	11.0	160	na	0.0	na	0	0%
wheat 'Snacks' approx .5 oz (Finast)	7 crackers	70	1.0	9.0	85	(mq)	3.0	(mq)	na	40%
wheat 'Stone Ground' approx .5 oz (Wheatsworth)	4 crackers	70	1.0	9.0	135	(mq)	3.0	<1.0	0	40%
wheat 'Stoned Wheat' (Health Valley)	13 crackers	120	3.0	17.0	85	3.9	6.0	(mq)	0	40%
wheat 'Stoned Wheat No Salt Added' (Health Valley)	13 crackers	120	3.0	17.0	10	3.9	6.0	(mq)	0	40%
wheat 'Stoned Wheat Wafer' approx .5 oz (FFV)	4 crackers	60	1.0	10.0	170	(mq)	2.0	<1.0	0	29%
wheat 'Stoned Wheat Wafers Salt Free' (Hickory Farms)	8 crackers	100	2.0	18.0	0	(mq)	2.0	(mq)	na	18%
wheat toasted (McCrakens)	1 oz	140	2.0	18.0	170	na	8.0	na	0	47%
wheat, toasted 'Distinctive' (Pepperidge Farm)	4 crackers	80	2.0	12.0	140	(mq)	3.0	1.0	0	33%
wheat, toasted 'Flutters' (Pepperidge Farm)	.75 oz	110	2.0	13.0	170	(mq)	5.0	1.0	0	43%
wheat 'Wheat Krisp' (Ralston)	.5 oz	50	2.0	11.0	220	na	1.0	na	0	15%
wheat 'Wheat Mill Wafers Salt Free' (Hickory Farms)	4 crackers	50	1.0	9.0	na	(mq)	1.0	na	0	18%
wheat 'Wheat Tams' (Manischewitz)	10 crackers	150	2.0	18.0	180	(mq)	8.0	6.0	0	47%
wheat 'Wheat Thins' (Nabisco)	8 crackers	70	1.0	9.0	120	(mq)	3.0	<1.0	0	40%
wheat 'Wheat Thins Low Salt' approx .5 oz (Nabisco)	8 crackers	70	1.0	9.0	60	(mq)	3.0	<1.0	0	40%
wheat 'Wheats' (Sunshine)	8 crackers	70	1.0	9.0	170	(mq)	4.0	1.0	0	47%
wheat 'Whole Wheat'N Bran Wafers' (Triscuit)	3 crackers	60	1.0	10.0	75	na	2.0	na	0	29%
'Wheatine' bits (Barbara's Bakery)	.5 oz	60	2.0	9.0	132	na	2.0	na	0	29%
'Wheatines' cracked pepper (Barbara's Bakery)	.5 oz	60	2.0	9.0	132	na	2.0	na	0	29%

Food Name	Serving Size	Calories	Prot. gms	Carbs gms	Sod. mgs	Fiber gms	Fat gms	Sat. Fat gms	Chol. mgs	% Fat Cal.
'Wheatines' lightly salted tops *(Barbara's Bakery)*	.5 oz	60	2.0	9.0	132	na	2.0	na	0	29%
'Wheatines' sesame *(Barbara's Bakery)*	.5 oz	60	2.0	9.0	132	na	2.0	na	0	29%
'Wheatines' unsalted tops *(Barbara's Bakery)*	.5 oz	60	2.0	9.0	45	na	2.0	na	0	29%
wheatstone *(Delicious)*	.5 oz	70	2.0	9.0	180	na	3.0	na	0	38%
whole grain 'Crispbread' approx .35 oz *(Wasa)*	1 slice	30	2.0	4.0	40	2.4	1.0	(mq)	0	27%
whole grain 'Harvest Wheats' approx .5 oz *(Keebler)*	4 crackers	60	1.0	8.0	95	(mq)	3.0	<1.0	0	43%
whole wheat	.5 oz	63	1.3	9.7	93	1.5	2.4	0.4	0	33%
whole wheat *(Carr's)*	2 crackers	70	1.0	12.0	15	(mq)	1.0	(mq)	(mq)	15%
whole wheat *(Manischewitz)*	10 crackers	90	3.0	18.0	10	(mq)	1.0	(mq)	0	10%
whole wheat, approx .5 oz *(Ritz)*	5 crackers	70	1.0	9.0	135	0	3.0	1.0	0	40%
whole wheat 'Gourmet' fat-free *(Frookie)*	4 crackers	35	1.0	7.0	60	na	0.0	0.0	0	0%
whole wheat, low salt	.5 oz	63	1.3	9.7	35	1.5	2.4	0.4	0	33%
whole wheat, organic, fat-free *(Health Valley)*	.5 oz	40	1.0	9.0	80	1.9	0.0	na	0	0%
whole wheat 'Wheatables' approx .5 oz *(Keebler)*	12 crackers	70	1.0	9.0	140	(mq)	3.0	<1.0	0	40%
w/bacon and cheese *(Handi-Snacks)*	1 pkg	130	4.0	8.0	410	(mq)	9.0	4.0	20	63%
zesty Italian, approx 13-16 crackers *(Frito-Lay's)*	.5 oz	70	1.0	9.0	115	0	3.0	na	0	40%
zwieback	1 oz	121	2.9	21.0	66	.7	2.8	1.1	6	21%
'Zwieback Teething Toast' approx .5 oz *(Nabisco)*	2 crackers	60	2.0	10.0	20	na	1.0	na	na	16%
CRACKER CRUMBS AND MEAL										
meal	1 cup	440	10.7	93.0	32	na	2.0	0.3	0	4%
meal	1 oz	109	2.6	22.9	8	na	0.5	0.1	0	4%
(Golden Dipt) meal	1 oz	100	3.0	22.0	0	(mq)	0.0	0.0	0	0%
(Manischewitz) matzo 'Farfel'	1 cup	280	6.8	60.0	2	.2	0.8	0.0	0	3%
(Manischewitz) matzo meal 'Daily'	1 cup	514	13.0	109.0	3	.5	1.4	0.0	0	3%
(Nabisco) meal	1/4 cup	110	3.0	24.0	10	1.0	0.0	0.0	0	0%
(Premium) fat-free	2 tbsp	50	1.0	11.0	0	na	0.0	na	0	0%
CRANBERRY										
raw *(Ocean Spray)* approx 2 oz	1/2 cup	25	0.0	6.0	0	(mq)	0.0	0.0	0	0%
raw, chopped	1 cup	54	0.4	14.0	1	4.6	0.2	na	0	3%
raw, whole	1 cup	47	0.4	12.0	1	4.0	0.2	na	0	4%
trimmed	1 oz	14	0.1	3.6	<1	1.2	0.1	tr	0	6%
trimmed, chopped	1/2 cup	27	0.2	7.0	1	2.3	0.1	tr	0	3%
trimmed, whole	1/2 cup	23	0.2	6.0	1	2.0	0.1	tr	0	4%
w/stems	1 lb	210	1.7	54.6	5	18.0	0.9	na	0	4%
CRANBERRY APPLE COCKTAIL										
(Minute Maid) 'Juices To Go'	6 oz	120	0.0	30.0	20	na	0.0	na	na	0%
(Welch's) frozen, diluted	6 oz	120	0.0	30.0	0	0	0.0	0.0	0	0%
CRANBERRY APPLE DRINK										
	6 oz	123	0.2	31.5	4	0	0.0	0.0	0	0%
(A&P)	6 oz	130	<1.0	32.0	<1	(tr)	(tr)	(tr)	0	0%
(Ocean Spray) 'Cran•Apple'	6 oz	120	0.0	31.0	15	(tr)	0.0	0.0	0	0%
(Ocean Spray) 'Cran•Apple Low Calorie'	6 oz	35	0.0	9.0	15	(tr)	0.0	0.0	0	0%
(P&Q)	6 oz	130	<1.0	32.0	<1	(tr)	(tr)	(tr)	0	0%
(Pathmark)	6 oz	130	0.0	32.0	10	(tr)	0.0	0.0	0	0%
CRANBERRY APPLESAUCE, 'Cran•Fruit' *(Ocean Spray)*	2 oz	100	0.0	23.0	10	(mq)	0.0	0.0	0	0%
CRANBERRY APRICOT DRINK										
	6 oz	118	0.4	29.8	4	.2	0.0	0.0	0	0%
'Cranicot' *(Ocean Spray)*	6 oz	120	0.0	29.0	15	(tr)	0.0	0.0	0	0%
CRANBERRY BEAN/borlotti/Roman bean/rose coco										
boiled	1 cup	241	16.5	43.3	2	>1.8 c	0.8	0.2	0	3%
boiled	1/2 cup	120	8.2	21.5	1	3.0	0.4	0.1	0	3%
boiled	4 oz	154	10.6	27.7	1	3.9	0.5	0.1	0	3%
raw	1 cup	653	44.9	117.1	12	>4.9 c	2.4	0.6	0	3%
raw	1/2 cup	328	22.6	58.9	6	9.1	1.2	0.3	0	3%

Food Name	Serving Size	Calories	Prot. gms	Carbs gms	Sod. mgs	Fiber gms	Fat gms	Sat. Fat gms	Chol. mgs	% Fat Cal.
raw	1 oz	95	6.5	17.0	2	2.6	0.3	0.1	0	0%
CRANBERRY BEAN, CANNED										
	1 cup	216	14.4	39.3	863	>2.4 c	0.7	0.2	0	3%
(Progresso)	1/2 cup	110	7.0	18.0	420	12.0	<1.0	na	0	<8%
w/liquid	1/2 cup	108	7.2	19.7	431	>1.2 c	0.4	0.1	0	3%
w/liquid	4 oz	94	6.3	17.1	376	>1.0 c	0.3	0.1	0	3%
CRANBERRY BLUEBERRY JUICE *(Knudsen & Sons)*	8 oz	115	<1.0	36.0	na	na	0.0	na	na	0%
CRANBERRY COCKTAIL JUICE										
(J. Hungerford)	9.03 oz	141	0.8	35.5	0	0	0.0	0.0	0	0%
(J. Hungerford) 50% juice	9.03 oz	134	0.1	34.8	7	0	0.1	0.0	0	1%
(J. Hungerford) 100% juice	9.03 oz	133	0.0	33.0	19	0	0.0	0.0	0	0%
CRANBERRY DRINK										
(Ocean Spray) citrus 'Refreshers'	6 oz	100	0.0	26.0	15	na	0.0	na	na	0%
(Ocean Spray) 'Cran•Blueberry'	6 oz	120	0.0	31.0	10	(tr)	0.0	0.0	0	0%
(Ocean Spray) 'Cran•Raspberry'	6 oz	110	0.0	27.0	15	(tr)	0.0	0.0	0	0%
(Ocean Spray) 'Cran•Raspberry Low Calorie'	6 oz	40	0.0	9.0	15	(tr)	0.0	0.0	0	0%
(Ocean Spray) 'Cran•Strawberry'	6 oz	110	0.0	27.0	15	na	0.0	na	na	0%
(Tropicana) 'Cranberry Orchard Juice Sparkler'	8 oz	120	(tr)	30.0	20	(tr)	0.0	0.0	0	0%
CRANBERRY GRAPE COCKTAIL										
frozen, prepared *(Welch's)*	6 oz	110	0.0	27.0	0	0	0.0	0.0	0	0%
CRANBERRY GRAPE DRINK										
(Finast)	6 oz	103	0.0	26.0	5	(tr)	0.0	0.0	0	0%
(Ocean Spray) 'Cran•Grape'	6 oz	120	0.0	31.0	15	(tr)	0.0	0.0	0	0%
(Pathmark)	6 oz	103	0.0	26.0	5	(tr)	0.0	0.0	0	0%
CRANBERRY JUICE										
(Knudsen & Sons) 'Just Cranberry'	8 oz	40	<1.0	10.0	na	na	0.0	na	na	0%
(Knudsen & Sons) 'Yankee'	8 oz	125	<1.0	31.0	na	na	0.0	na	na	0%
(Lucky Leaf)	6 oz	110	0.0	26.0	10	(tr)	0.0	0.0	0	0%
(Ocean Spray) 'Cran•tastic'	6 oz	100	0.0	26.0	15	(tr)	0.0	0.0	0	0%
(Santa Cruz Natural) organic 'Sparkling'	8 oz	90	<1.0	22.0	na	na	<1.0	na	na	<9%
(Snapple) 'Cranberry Royale'	8 oz	150	0.0	37.0	25	na	0.0	0.0	0	0%
CRANBERRY JUICE COCKTAIL										
	1 cup	144	0.0	36.4	5	0	0.3	na	0	2%
	6 oz	108	0.0	27.4	4	0	0.2	0.1	0	2%
(A&P)	6 oz	100	<1.0	26.0	0	(tr)	<1.0	(tr)	0	<8%
(Ocean Spray)	6 oz	110	0.0	26.0	10	(tr)	0.0	0.0	0	0%
(Ocean Spray) 'Low Calorie'	6 oz	40	0.0	9.0	15	(tr)	0.0	0.0	0	0%
(P&Q)	6 oz	100	<1.0	24.0	0	(tr)	<1.0	(tr)	0	<8%
(Pathmark)	6 oz	100	0.0	26.0	10	(tr)	0.0	0.0	0	0%
(Pathmark) 'No Frills'	6 oz	100	0.0	26.0	10	(tr)	0.0	0.0	0	0%
(Sunkist)	6 oz	110	0.1	28.2	8	(tr)	0.1	(tr)	0	1%
(Sunkist) frozen, prepared	6 oz	110	0.1	28.2	0	(tr)	0.1	0.0	0	1%
(Veryfine)	8 oz	160	<1.0	40.0	10	(tr)	0.0	0.0	0	0%
(Welch's) frozen 'No Sugar Added' prepared	6 oz	40	0.0	10.0	5	0	0.0	0.0	0	0%
(Welch's) frozen, prepared	6 oz	100	0.0	26.0	0	0	0.0	0.0	0	0%
(Welch's) frozen, w/blueberry, prepared	6 oz	110	0.0	27.0	0	0	0.0	0.0	0	0%
(Welch's) frozen, w/raspberry, prepared	6 oz	110	0.0	28.0	0	0	0.0	0.0	0	0%
CRANBERRY JUICE DRINK										
citrus 'Refreshers' *(Ocean Spray)*	6 oz	100	0.0	26.0	15	na	0.0	na	na	0%
CRANBERRY LEMONADE										
(Knudsen & Sons)	8 oz	115	<1.0	29.0	na	na	0.0	na	na	0%
(Santa Cruz Natural) organic	8 oz	100	<1.0	24.0	na	na	<1.0	na	na	<8%
CRANBERRY NECTAR										
(Knudsen & Sons)	8 oz	110	<1.0	28.0	na	na	0.0	na	na	0%

Food Name	Serving Size	Calories	Prot. gms	Carbs gms	Sod. mgs	Fiber gms	Fat gms	Sat. Fat gms	Chol. mgs	% Fat Cal.
(Santa Cruz Natural) organic	8 oz	110	<1.0	28.0	na	na	<1.0	na	na	<7%
CRANBERRY RASPBERRY DRINK										
(Tropicana) w/strawberry 'Twister'	6 oz	110	<1.0	27.0	4	na	<1.0	na	na	<7%
(Tropicana) w/strawberry 'Twister Light' w/NutraSweet	6 oz	30	<1.0	7.0	15	na	<1.0	na	na	<22%
CRANBERRY RASPBERRY JUICE *(Knudsen & Sons)*	8 oz	100	<1.0	25.0	na	na	0.0	na	na	0%
CRANBERRY-RASPBERRY SAUCE										
'Cran•Fruit' *(Ocean Spray)*	2 oz	100	0.0	23.0	10	(mq)	0.0	0.0	0	0%
CRANBERRY SAUCE										
canned *(A&P)*	2 oz	100	<1.0	25.0	15	(mq)	<1.0	(tr)	0	<8%
canned *(Knudsen & Sons)*	1 oz	30	<1.0	8.0	na	na	<1.0	na	na	<20%
canned, sweetened	1 cup	418	0.6	107.7	80	>.8 c	0.4	na	0	1%
canned, sweetened	4 oz	171	0.2	44.1	33	>.3 c	0.2	(tr)	0	1%
jellied *(Finast)*	2 oz	90	0.0	22.0	10	(mq)	0.0	0.0	0	0%
jellied *(Ocean Spray)*	2 oz	80	0.0	22.0	10	(mq)	0.0	0.0	0	0%
jellied *(Pathmark)*	2 oz	90	0.0	22.0	10	(mq)	0.0	0.0	0	0%
jellied 'Old Fashioned' *(S&W)*	1/2 cup	90	0.0	22.0	20	(mq)	0.0	0.0	0	0%
whole berry *(Finast)*	2 oz	90	0.0	22.0	10	(mq)	0.0	0.0	0	0%
whole berry *(Ocean Spray)*	2 oz	80	0.0	21.0	10	(mq)	0.0	0.0	0	0%
whole berry 'Old Fashioned' *(S&W)*	1/2 cup	90	0.0	22.0	20	(mq)	0.0	0.0	0	0%
CRANBERRY STRAWBERRY SAUCE										
crushed, for chicken 'Cran•Fruit' *(Ocean Spray)*	2 oz	90	0.0	22.0	10	na	0.0	na	na	0%
CRAPPIE. See SUNFISH.										
CRAWFISH ENTRÉE, frozen, étouffée *(Cajun Cookin')*	12 oz	390	23.0	51.0	1110	na	10.0	(mq)	(mq)	23%
CRAYFISH, MIXED SPECIES										
farmed, moist-heat cooked	100 gm	87	17.5	0.0	97	0	1.3	0.2	137	14%
farmed, moist-heat cooked	3 oz	74	14.9	0.0	82	0	1.1	0.2	116	14%
farmed, raw	3 oz	61	12.6	0.0	53	0	0.8	0.1	91	13%
farmed, raw	8 crayfish	19	4.0	0.0	17	0	0.3	0.0	29	14%
wild, moist-heat cooked	100 gm	88	16.8	0.0	94	0	1.2	0.2	133	14%
wild, moist-heat cooked	3 oz	75	14.2	0.0	80	0	1.0	0.2	113	14%
wild, raw	3 oz	65	13.6	0.0	49	0	0.8	0.1	97	12%
wild, raw	8 crayfish	21	4.3	0.0	16	0	0.3	0.0	31	14%
CREAM										
half and half	1 cup	315	7.2	10.4	98	0	27.8	17.3	89	78%
half and half	1 oz	37	0.8	1.2	12	0	3.3	2.0	10	79%
half and half	1 tbsp	20	0.4	0.7	6	0	1.7	1.1	6	78%
half and half *(Crowley)*	1 oz	35	1.0	1.0	10	0	3.0	(mq)	15	77%
half and half *(Darigold)*	8 oz	310	8.0	11.0	120	0	27.0	17.3	89	76%
half and half *(Knudsen)*	4 oz	150	4.0	5.0	60	0	13.0	(mq)	(mq)	77%
half and half *(Rockview)*	2 tbsp	35	1.0	0.0	15	0	3.0	2.0	15	87%
heavy, whipping	1 cup	821	4.9	6.6	89	0	88.1	54.8	326	95%
heavy, whipping	1 tbsp	52	0.3	0.4	6	0	5.6	3.5	21	95%
light, whipping	1 cup	699	5.2	7.1	82	0	73.9	46.2	265	93%
light, whipping	1 tbsp	44	0.3	0.4	5	0	4.6	2.9	17	94%
light, coffee or table	1 cup	469	6.5	8.8	95	0	46.3	28.9	159	87%
light, coffee or table	1 oz	55	0.8	1.0	11	0	5.5	3.4	19	87%
light, coffee or table	1 tbsp	29	0.4	0.6	6	0	2.9	1.8	10	87%
medium, 25% fat	1 cup	583	5.9	8.3	88	0	59.7	37.2	209	90%
medium, 25% fat	1 oz	69	0.7	1.0	10	0	7.1	4.4	25	90%
medium, 25% fat	1 tbsp	37	0.4	0.5	6	0	3.8	2.3	13	91%
CREAM CHEESE. See CHEESE.										
CREAM NUT. See BRAZIL NUT.										
CREAM OF TARTAR	1 tsp	8	0.0	1.8	2	na	0.0	na	0	0%
CREAM SODA. See SOFT DRINKS AND MIXERS.										

Food Name	Serving Size	Calories	Prot. gms	Carbs gms	Sod. mgs	Fiber gms	Fat gms	Sat. Fat gms	Chol. mgs	% Fat Cal.
CREAM TOPPING										
creamy white 'Dolci Frutta Crema Bianca' (Saco Foods) ..	1 box	900	6.7	98.4	110	na	50.1	17.0	0	52%
dark chocolate 'Dolci Frutta Con Cioccolatta' (Saco Foods)	1 box	886	8.6	110.5	107	na	52.8	19.4	0	50%
frozen, whipped (La Creme)	1 tbsp	16	0.0	1.0	5	0	1.0	na	<1	69%
frozen, whipped 'Real Cream' (Kraft)	1/4 cup	30	0.0	2.0	5	0	2.0	2.0	10	69%
pressurized can, whipped	1 cup	154	1.9	7.5	78	0	13.3	8.3	46	76%
pressurized can, whipped	1 oz	73	0.9	3.5	37	0	6.3	3.9	22	76%
pressurized can, whipped	1 tbsp	8	0.1	0.4	4	0	0.7	0.4	2	76%
pressurized can, whipped (Crowley)	1 tbsp	20	<1.0	<1.0	10	0	1.0	(mq)	5	53%
whipping, heavy	1 oz	98	0.6	0.8	11	0	10.5	6.5	39	94%
whipping, heavy (Crowley)	1 oz	110	1.0	1.0	10	0	11.0	(mq)	40	93%
whipping, heavy (Darigold)	1 cup	790	6.0	8.0	90	0	81.0	50.8	290	93%
whipping, heavy 'Classic' (Darigold)	1 cup	858	5.1	6.9	77	0	90.0	23.7	334	94%
whipping, heavy 'UHT' (Darigold)	1 cup	790	6.0	8.0	90	0	81.0	50.8	290	93%
whipping, heavy, whipped	2 cups	821	4.9	6.6	89	0	90.0	54.8	326	95%
whipping, heavy, whipped	2 tbsp	52	0.3	0.4	6	0	5.6	3.5	21	95%
whipping, light	1 oz	83	0.6	0.8	10	0	8.8	5.5	31	93%
whipping, light, whipped	2 cups	699	5.2	7.1	82	0	5.6	46.2	265	51%
whipping, light, whipped	2 tbsp	44	0.3	0.4	5	0	8.8	2.9	17	97%
CREAM TOPPING, NONDAIRY										
frozen	1 cup	239	0.9	17.3	19	0	19.0	16.3	0	70%
frozen	1 oz	90	0.4	6.5	7	0	7.2	6.2	0	70%
frozen	1 tbsp	13	0.1	0.9	1	0	1.0	0.9	0	69%
frozen, chocolate 'Cool Whip' (Birds Eye)	1 tbsp	12	0.0	1.0	0	na	1.0	na	na	69%
frozen 'Cool Whip' (Birds Eye)	1 tbsp	12	0.0	1.0	0	0	1.0	(mq)	0	69%
frozen 'Cool Whip Lite' (Birds Eye)	1 tbsp	8	0.0	1.0	0	0	<1.0	(mq)	0	<69%
frozen, extra creamy 'Cool Whip Dairy Recipe' (Birds Eye)	1 tbsp	14	0.0	1.0	0	0	1.0	(mq)	0	69%
frozen, semisolid	1 cup	239	0.9	17.3	19	0	19.0	16.3	0	70%
frozen, semisolid	1 tbsp	13	0.1	0.9	1	0	1.0	0.9	0	69%
frozen 'Whip' (Pet)	1 tbsp	14	0.0	1.0	0	0	1.0	(mq)	0	69%
frozen 'Whipped Topping' (Kraft)	1/4 cup	35	0.0	2.0	10	0	3.0	3.0	0	77%
mix, dry	1.5 oz	245	2.1	22.3	52	0	17.0	15.6	0	61%
mix, prepared (D-Zerta)	1 tbsp	8	0.0	0.0	5	0	1.0	(tr)	0	100%
mix, prepared (Featherweight)	1 tbsp	4	0.0	0.0	5	0	0.0	0.0	0	0%
mix, prepared (Dream Whip)	1 tbsp	10	0.0	1.0	0	na	0.0	na	0	0%
pressurized can	1 cup	184	0.7	11.3	43	0	15.6	13.2	0	75%
pressurized can	1 oz	75	0.3	4.6	18	0	6.3	5.4	0	74%
pressurized can	1 tbsp	11	<.1	0.6	2	0	0.9	0.8	0	74%
pressurized can 'Richwhip' (Rich's)	.25 oz	20	0.0	1.0	5	0	2.0	(mq)	0	82%
prewhipped (Estee)	1 tbsp	4	<1.0	<1.0	0	0	<1.0	<1.0	0	<53%
prewhipped 'Richwhip' (Rich's)	1 tbsp	12	0.0	1.0	0	0	1.0	(mq)	0	69%
reduced calorie (D-Zerta)	1 tbsp	8	0.0	0.0	5	na	1.0	na	0	100%
unwhipped 'Richwhip' (Rich's)	.25 oz	20	0.0	1.0	10	0	2.0	(mq)	0	82%
CREAMER, NONDAIRY										
Liquid										
frozen	1/2 cup	164	1.2	13.7	95	0	12.0	11.2	0	64%
frozen	1 oz	39	0.3	3.2	22	0	2.8	0.5	0	64%
frozen	1 tbsp	20	0.2	1.7	12	0	1.5	0.3	0	64%
w/hydrogenated vegetable oil and soy protein	1/2 cup	163	1.2	13.7	95	0	12.0	2.3	0	64%
w/hydrogenated vegetable oil and soy protein	1/2 oz	20	0.2	1.7	12	0	1.5	0.3	0	64%
w/lauric acid oil and sodium caseinate	1/2 cup	164	1.2	13.7	95	0	12.0	11.2	0	64%
w/lauric acid oil and sodium caseinate	1/2 oz	20	0.2	1.7	12	0	1.5	1.4	0	64%
(Coffee-Mate)	1 tbsp	16	0.0	2.0	5	0	1.0	0.3	0	53%
(Coffee-Mate) 'Amaretto'	1 tbsp	40	0.0	5.0	5	na	2.0	na	na	47%

Food Name	Serving Size	Calories	Prot. gms	Carbs gms	Sod. mgs	Fiber gms	Fat gms	Sat. Fat gms	Chol. mgs	% Fat Cal.
(Coffee-Mate) 'Cinnamon Creme'	1 tbsp	40	0.0	5.0	5	na	2.0	na	na	47%
(Coffee-Mate) fat-free	1 tbsp	10	0.0	2.0	0	0	0.0	0.0	0	0%
(Coffee-Mate) 'Hazelnut'	1 tbsp	40	0.0	5.0	5	na	2.0	na	na	47%
(Coffee-Mate) 'Irish Creme'	1 tbsp	40	0.0	5.0	5	na	2.0	na	na	47%
(Crowley)	.5 oz	16	<1.0	1.0	5	0	1.0	na	5	53%
(Diehl)	1 tsp	10	0.0	1.0	0	0	<1.0	0.0	0	<69%
(Finast) frozen	.5 oz	20	0.0	2.0	10	0	2.0	<1.0	0	69%
(IGA)	1 tsp	10	0.0	2.0	5	0	<1.0	na	0	<53%
(N-Rich)	1 tsp	10	0.1	2.0	2	0	0.6	0.3	0	39%
(Pathmark) 'No Frills'	1 tsp	10	0.0	1.0	5	0	0.0	0.0	0	0%
(Rich's) frozen 'Coffee Rich'	.5 oz	20	0.0	2.0	10	0	2.0	<1.0	0	69%
(Rich's) frozen 'Farm Rich'	.5 oz	20	0.0	1.0	5	0	2.0	0.0	0	82%
(Rich's) frozen 'Poly Rich'	.5 oz	20	0.0	2.0	5	0	1.0	<1.0	0	53%
(Saco Foods) 'kwik kream'	1 tbsp	10	0.0	2.0	0	na	<1.0	na	0	<53%
(Westbrae)	1 tbsp	10	<1.0	2.0	10	na	<1.0	na	0	<43%
Powder										
....	1/2 cup	257	2.3	16.7	85	0	25.8	15.3	0	75%
....	1 oz	155	1.4	15.6	51	0	10.1	9.2	0	57%
....	1 tsp	11	0.1	1.1	4	0	0.7	0.7	0	57%
(Coffee-Mate)	1 tsp	10	<1.0	1.0	5	0	<1.0	0.7	0	<53%
(Coffee-Mate) 'Amaretto'	2 tsp	60	0.0	9.0	15	na	3.0	3.0	0	43%
(Coffee-Mate) 'Hazelnut'	2 tsp	60	0.0	0.0	15	na	3.0	3.0	0	100%
(Coffee-Mate) 'Irish Creme'	2 tsp	60	0.0	9.0	15	na	3.0	3.0	0	43%
(Coffee-Mate) 'Lite'	1 tsp	8	<1.0	2.0	0	0	<1.0	0.3	0	<43%
(Cremora)	1 tsp	10	0.0	1.0	5	0	<1.0	na	0	<69%
CREME DE MENTHE. See ALCOHOLIC BEVERAGES.										
CRÊPE MIX, 7-inch crêpes *(Krusteaz)*	2 crêpes	80	2.0	14.0	110	na	1.0	na	0	12%
CRESS, GARDEN										
boiled, drained	4 oz	26	2.2	4.3	9	>1.0 c	0.7	<.1	0	20%
boiled, drained	1/2 cup	16	1.3	2.6	5	.5	0.4	0.0	0	19%
raw	1/2 cup	8	0.7	1.4	4	.3	0.2	0.0	0	18%
raw, trimmed	1 oz	9	0.7	1.6	4	>.3 c	0.2	tr	0	16%
raw, untrimmed	1 lb	103	8.4	17.7	45	>3.5 c	2.3	0.1	0	17%
CROAKER, ATLANTIC										
raw	1 lb	474	80.7	0.0	252	0	14.4	4.9	277	29%
raw	3 oz	88	15.1	0.0	48	0	2.7	0.9	52	29%
raw	1 oz	29	5.0	0.0	16	0	0.9	0.3	17	29%
raw, approx 2.8 oz	1 fillet	82	14.1	0.0	44	0	2.5	0.9	48	29%
CROISSANT										
almond, 3.7 oz *(Dunkin' Donuts)*	1 croissant	420	8.0	38.0	280	3.0	27.0	(mq)	0	57%
butter *(Awrey's)*	3 oz	300	5.0	32.0	280	1.0	17.0	8.0	45	51%
butter *(Awrey's)*	2 oz	200	3.0	21.0	190	1.0	11.0	5.0	30	51%
butter *(Awrey's)*	1 oz	100	2.0	10.0	90	0	6.0	3.0	15	53%
frozen, butter, 1.5 oz *(Sara Lee)*	1 croissant	170	4.0	19.0	250	(mq)	9.0	(mq)	(mq)	47%
frozen, butter, petite *(Pepperidge Farm)*	1 croissant	140	3.0	13.0	160	(mq)	7.0	(mq)	(mq)	50%
frozen, butter, petite 1 oz *(Sara Lee)*	1 croissant	120	3.0	13.0	160	(mq)	6.0	(mq)	(mq)	46%
margarine *(Awrey's)*	2.5 oz	250	4.0	26.0	360	1.0	14.0	3.0	5	51%
margarine *(Awrey's)*	1.25 oz	120	2.0	13.0	180	0	7.0	2.0	5	51%
plain, 2.5 oz *(Dunkin' Donuts)*	1 croissant	310	7.0	27.0	240	2.0	19.0	(mq)	0	56%
'Sandwich Quartet' *(Pepperidge Farm)*	1 croissant	170	4.0	22.0	250	tr	7.0	(mq)	0	38%
wheat *(Awrey's)*	2.5 oz	240	4.0	24.0	390	1.0	14.0	3.0	5	53%
CROOKNECK SQUASH. See SQUASH, CROOKNECK.										
CROUTONS										
Caesar salad *(Brownberry)*	.5 oz	62	1.8	8.0	165	.5	2.6	(mq)	<1	37%

Food Name	Serving Size	Calories	Prot. gms	Carbs gms	Sod. mgs	Fiber gms	Fat gms	Sat. Fat gms	Chol. mgs	% Fat Cal.
Caesar salad (Reese)	.5 oz	60	2.0	9.0	130	na	2.0	na	na	29%
cheddar and Romano cheese (Pepperidge Farm)	.5 oz	60	2.0	10.0	200	(mq)	2.0	0.0	0	27%
cheddar cheese (Brownberry)	.5 oz	63	1.8	8.3	155	.3	2.8	(mq)	3	38%
cheese and garlic (Pepperidge Farm)	.5 oz	70	2.0	9.0	180	(mq)	3.0	1.0	0	38%
onion and garlic (Brownberry)	.5 oz	60	1.6	8.8	190	.4	2.2	(mq)	1	32%
onion and garlic (Pepperidge Farm)	.5 oz	70	2.0	9.0	160	(mq)	3.0	0.0	0	38%
plain	1 cup	122	3.6	22.0	209	1.5	2.0	0.5	0	15%
plain	.5 oz	58	1.7	10.4	99	.7	0.9	0.2	0	14%
seasoned	1 cup	186	4.3	25.4	495	2.0	7.3	2.0	1	36%
seasoned	.5 oz	66	1.5	9.0	175	.7	2.6	0.7	0	36%
seasoned (Brownberry)	.5 oz	59	1.6	8.5	155	.5	2.2	(mq)	<1	33%
seasoned (Pepperidge Farm)	.5 oz	70	2.0	9.0	180	(mq)	3.0	1.0	0	38%
seasoned (Weight Watchers)	1 pouch	30	1.0	5.0	120	(mq)	0.0	0.0	na	0%
sour cream and chive (Pepperidge Farm)	.5 oz	70	2.0	9.0	170	(mq)	3.0	1.0	0	38%
toasted (Brownberry)	.5 oz	56	1.7	9.7	145	.4	1.4	na	0	22%
CRUMPET										
blueberry, low-fat, cholestrol-free (Wolferman's)	1 crumpet	90	3.0	21.0	250	1.0	<1.0	na	0	<9%
brown sugar cinnamon, low-fat (Wolferman's)	1 crumpet	110	3.0	21.0	220	2.0	2.0	na	0	16%
raspberry, low-fat, cholestrol-free (Wolferman's)	1 crumpet	90	3.0	20.0	260	1.0	1.0	na	0	9%
CUCUMBER										
raw, approx 10.9 oz	1 med	39	2.1	8.3	6	2.4	0.4	0.1	0	8%
raw, slices	1/2 cup	7	0.4	1.4	1	.4	0.1	0.0	0	11%
raw, w/peel, trimmed	1 oz	4	0.2	0.8	1	.3	<.1	tr	0	<18%
raw, w/peel, untrimmed	1 lb	56	2.4	12.8	9	4.4	0.6	0.1	0	8%
CUMIN SEED										
whole	1 oz	106	5.0	12.5	48	>3.0 c	6.3	(mq)	0	45%
whole	1 tbsp	22	1.1	2.7	10	.6	1.3	na	0	44%
whole	1 tsp	8	0.4	0.9	4	.2	0.5	na	0	46%
whole (Durkee)	1 tsp	10	0.0	0.0	0	0	<0.1	na	na	<46%
whole (Laurel Leaf)	1 tsp	10	0.0	0.0	0	0	<0.1	na	na	<46%
whole (Spice Islands)	1 tsp	7	0.3	0.7	3	>.1 c	0.4	(tr)	0	47%
CUPU ASSU OIL										
	1/2 cup	964	0.0	0.0	0	0	109.0	58.0	0	100%
	1 oz	251	0.0	0.0	0	0	28.4	15.1	0	100%
	1 tbsp	120	0.0	0.0	0	0	13.6	7.2	0	100%
CUPU ASSU PUNCH, 'Rain Forest' (Knudsen & Sons)	8 oz	110	<1.0	25.0	na	na	0.0	na	na	0%
CURRANT, BLACK/European currant										
raw	1 cup	71	1.6	17.2	2	>2.7 c	0.5	0.0	0	6%
trimmed	1 oz	18	0.4	4.4	1	1.5	0.1	tr	0	5%
untrimmed	1 lb	282	6.2	68.4	8	24.1	1.8	0.2	0	5%
CURRANT, RED										
raw	1 cup	63	1.6	15.5	1	4.8	0.2	0.0	0	3%
trimmed	1 oz	16	0.4	3.9	<1	>1.0 c	0.1	tr	0	5%
untrimmed	1 lb	249	6.2	61.3	5	>15.1 c	0.9	0.1	0	3%
CURRANT, WHITE										
raw	1 cup	63	1.6	15.5	1	4.8	0.2	0.0	0	3%
trimmed	1/2 cup	31	0.8	7.7	1	>1.9 c	0.1	<.1	0	3%
trimmed	1 oz	16	0.4	3.9	<1	>1.0 c	0.1	tr	0	5%
untrimmed	1 lb	249	6.2	61.3	5	>15.1 c	0.9	0.1	0	3%
CURRANT, ZANTE										
dried	1 lb	1282	18.5	336.0	35	30.8	1.2	0.1	0	1%
dried	1 cup	408	5.9	106.7	12	9.8	0.4	0.0	0	1%
dried	1 oz	80	1.2	21.0	2	1.9	0.1	tr	0	1%
dried (Del Monte)	1/2 cup	200	2.0	53.0	10	(mq)	0.0	0.0	0	0%

Food Name	Serving Size	Calories	Prot. gms	Carbs gms	Sod. mgs	Fiber gms	Fat gms	Sat. Fat gms	Chol. mgs	% Fat Cal.
CURRY POWDER										
ground	1 oz	92	3.6	16.5	15	9.7	3.9	(mq)	0	30%
ground	1 tbsp	20	0.8	3.7	3	2.1	0.9	na	0	31%
ground	1 tsp	7	0.3	1.2	1	.7	0.3	na	0	31%
CUSK/torsk/tusk										
dry-heat cooked	3 oz	95	20.7	0.0	34	0	0.8	na	45	8%
raw	1 lb	396	86.2	0.0	143	0	3.1	(mq)	186	8%
raw	3 oz	74	16.1	0.0	26	0	0.6	0.1	35	8%
raw	1 oz	25	5.4	0.0	9	0	0.2	(mq)	12	8%
raw, approx 4.3 oz	1 fillet	106	23.2	0.0	38	0	0.8	0.2	50	7%
CUSTARD. See PUDDING MIX; PUDDING/PIE FILLING, MIX.										
CUSTARD APPLE/bullock's heart/cherimoya										
raw	100 gm	101	1.7	25.2	4	>3.4 c	0.6	na	0	5%
trimmed	1 oz	29	0.5	7.1	1	>1.0 c	0.2	(tr)	0	6%
untrimmed	1 lb	267	4.5	66.3	11	>9.0 c	1.6	na	0	5%
CUTTLEFISH, MIXED SPECIES										
moist-heat cooked	100 gm	158	32.5	1.6	744	0	1.4	0.2	224	9%
moist-heat cooked	3 oz	134	27.6	1.4	632	0	1.2	0.2	190	9%
raw	1 lb	359	73.7	3.7	1686	0	3.2	0.5	507	9%
raw	3 oz	67	13.8	0.7	316	0	0.6	0.1	95	9%
raw	1 oz	22	4.6	0.2	105	0	0.2	<.1	32	9%
CYMLING. See SQUASH, SCALLOP.										

D

Food Name	Serving Size	Calories	Prot. gms	Carbs gms	Sod. mgs	Fiber gms	Fat gms	Sat. Fat gms	Chol. mgs	% Fat Cal.
DAIKON/mullangi/Oriental radish										
boiled, drained	4 oz	19	0.8	3.9	15	>.6 c	0.3	0.1	0	13%
boiled, drained, sliced	1/2 cup	13	0.5	2.5	10	>.4 c	0.2	0.1	0	13%
dried	1/2 cup	157	4.6	36.8	161	>4.9 c	0.4	0.1	0	2%
dried	1 oz	77	2.2	18.0	79	>2.4 c	0.2	0.1	0	2%
raw, trimmed	1 oz	5	0.2	1.2	6	>.2 c	<.1	tr	0	<14%
raw, trimmed (Frieda's)	1 lb	86	4.1	19.1	(mq)	(mq)	0.5	(mq)	0	5%
raw, trimmed (Frieda's)	1 oz	5	0.3	1.2	(mq)	(mq)	<.1	tr	0	<13%
raw, trimmed, sliced	1/2 cup	8	0.3	1.8	9	>.3 c	<.1	<.1	0	<10%
raw, untrimmed	1 lb	65	2.2	14.7	75	>2.3 c	0.4	0.1	0	5%
DAIQUIRI. See ALCOHOLIC BEVERAGES.										
DANDELION GREENS										
boiled, drained	4 oz	37	2.3	7.3	50	>1.5 c	0.7	(tr)	0	14%
boiled, drained, chopped	1 cup	35	2.1	6.7	46	3.1	0.6	na	0	13%
raw, chopped	1 oz	13	0.8	2.6	22	>.5 c	0.2	(tr)	0	12%
raw, trimmed	1 lb	204	12.3	41.7	345	>7.3 c	3.2	na	0	12%
DANISH CABBAGE. See CABBAGE, DANISH.										
DANISH PASTRY										
APPLE										
(Awrey's)										
filled, 'Miniature' 1.7 oz	1 piece	160	2.0	21.0	170	0	8.0	2.0	5	44%
filled 'Round' 4.5 oz	1 piece	390	4.0	50.0	390	1.0	20.0	4.0	10	46%
filled 'Round' 2.75 oz	1 piece	270	3.0	34.0	310	1.0	14.0	3.0	5	46%
filled 'Square' 3 oz	1 piece	220	3.0	34.0	230	1.0	8.0	2.0	10	33%
(Pepperidge Farm) frozen, 2.25 oz	1 piece	220	2.0	35.0	130	(mq)	8.0	(mq)	na	33%

Food Name	Serving Size	Calories	Prot. gms	Carbs gms	Sod. mgs	Fiber gms	Fat gms	Sat. Fat gms	Chol. mgs	% Fat Cal.
(Sara Lee)										
frozen 'Free & Light'	1/8 pkg	130	2.0	30.0	120	(mq)	0.0	0.0	0	0%
frozen 'Individual' 1.3 oz	1 piece	120	2.0	15.0	120	(mq)	6.0	(mq)	na	44%
frozen twist	1/8 pkg	190	3.0	22.0	200	(mq)	10.0	(mq)	10	47%
CARAMEL *(Pillsbury)* w/nuts, refrigerated	1 piece	160	2.0	19.0	240	(mq)	8.0	2.0	0	46%
CHEESE										
(Awrey's)										
filled, 'Miniature' 1.7 oz	1 piece	170	2.0	21.0	200	4.0	9.0	2.0	5	47%
filled 'Round' 4.5 oz	1 piece	420	5.0	52.0	530	1.0	22.0	5.0	15	47%
filled 'Round' 2.75 oz	1 piece	280	3.0	34.0	350	1.0	15.0	3.0	10	48%
filled 'Square' 2.5 oz	1 piece	210	4.0	25.0	300	1.0	11.0	3.0	15	46%
(Pepperidge Farm) frozen, 2.25 oz	1 piece	240	3.0	25.0	230	(mq)	14.0	(mq)	(mq)	53%
(Sara Lee) frozen, 'Individual' 1.3 oz	1 piece	130	2.0	13.0	130	(mq)	8.0	(mq)	na	55%
CINNAMON *(Sara Lee)* twist, frozen	1/8 pkg	200	3.0	21.0	270	(mq)	12.0	(mq)	15	53%
CINNAMON-RAISIN										
(Awrey's)										
filled 'Square' 3 oz	1 piece	290	3.0	41.0	280	1.0	12.0	3.0	15	38%
filled 'Miniature' 1.5 oz	1 piece	160	2.0	21.0	150	1.0	8.0	2.0	5	44%
(Pepperidge Farm) frozen, 2.25 oz	1 piece	250	3.0	35.0	170	(mq)	11.0	(mq)	na	39%
(Pillsbury) w/icing, refrigerated	1 piece	150	2.0	20.0	230	(mq)	7.0	2.0	0	42%
(Sara Lee) frozen, 'Individual' 1.3 oz	1 piece	150	2.0	17.0	140	(mq)	8.0	(mq)	na	49%
CINNAMON-WALNUT *(Awrey's)* 'Round' 2.75 oz	1 piece	300	4.0	31.0	290	1.0	18.0	3.0	5	54%
LEMON *(Entenmann's)* twist	1.2 oz	140	2.0	17.0	140	na	7.0	na	na	45%
ORANGE *(Pillsbury)* w/icing, refrigerated	1 piece	150	2.0	19.0	250	(mq)	7.0	2.0	0	43%
PECAN RING *(Entenmann's)*	1.5 oz	190	3.0	19.0	130	na	12.0	na	na	55%
PINEAPPLE *(Awrey's)* filled, 'Miniature' 1.7 oz	1 piece	157	2.0	21.0	180	1.0	8.0	2.0	5	44%
RASPBERRY										
(Awrey's) filled 'Square' 3 oz	1 piece	260	3.0	45.0	210	1.0	8.0	2.0	10	27%
(Entenmann's) twist	1.2 oz	140	2.0	18.0	120	na	7.0	na	na	44%
(Pepperidge Farm) frozen, 2.25 oz	1 piece	220	3.0	31.0	140	(mq)	9.0	(mq)	na	37%
(Sara Lee) twist, frozen	1/8 pkg	200	3.0	25.0	220	(mq)	9.0	(mq)	15	42%
RING *(Entenmann's)*	1.5 oz	180	3.0	18.0	160	na	10.0	na	na	52%
STRAWBERRY										
(Awrey's)										
filled 'Miniature' 1.7 oz	1 piece	160	2.0	21.0	180	0	8.0	2.0	5	44%
filled 'Round' 4.5 oz	1 piece	400	4.0	53.0	410	1.0	20.0	4.0	10	44%
filled 'Round' 2.75 oz	1 piece	270	3.0	34.0	320	1.0	14.0	3.0	5	46%
WALNUT RING *(Entenmann's)*	1.5 oz	190	3.0	19.0	130	na	12.0	na	na	55%
DASHEEN										
cooked	4 oz	161	0.6	39.2	11	>1.0 c	0.1	<.1	0	1%
cooked, sliced	1/2 cup	94	0.3	22.8	10	>.6 c	0.1	<.1	0	1%
raw, sliced	1/2 cup	56	0.8	13.8	6	>.4 c	0.1	<.1	0	2%
raw, trimmed	1 oz	30	0.4	7.5	3	>.2 c	0.1	<.1	0	3%
raw, untrimmed	1 lb	419	5.9	103.2	43	>3.1 c	0.8	0.2	0	2%
DASHEEN LEAF										
raw	1/2 cup	6	0.7	0.9	1	>.3 c	0.1	<.1	0	12%
raw, trimmed	1 oz	12	1.4	1.9	1	>.6 c	0.2	<.1	0	12%
raw, untrimmed	1 lb	115	13.5	18.3	8	>5.5 c	2.0	0.4	0	12%
steamed	1/2 cup	18	2.0	3.0	2	>.4 c	0.3	0.1	0	12%
steamed	4 oz	27	3.1	4.6	2	>.6 c	0.5	0.1	0	13%
DASHEEN SHOOTS										
cooked	4 oz	16	0.8	3.6	2	>.6 c	0.1	<.1	0	5%
cooked, sliced	1/2 cup	10	0.5	2.2	1	>.4 c	0.1	<.1	0	8%
raw, sliced	1/2 cup	5	0.4	1.0	<1	>.3 c	<.1	tr	0	<14%

Food Name	Serving Size	Calories	Prot. gms	Carbs gms	Sod. mgs	Fiber gms	Fat gms	Sat. Fat gms	Chol. mgs	% Fat Cal.
raw, trimmed	1 oz	3	0.3	0.7	<1	>.2 c	<.1	tr	0	<18%
raw, untrimmed	1 lb	45	3.7	9.3	4	>2.3 c	0.4	0.1	0	7%
DATE										
Domestic, natural and dry										
chopped	1/2 cup	245	1.8	65.4	3	4.5	0.4	na	0	1%
w/pits	1 lb	1123	8.0	300.1	10	20.8	1.8	na	0	1%
w/o pits	1 oz	78	0.6	20.8	1	1.4	0.1	na	0	1%
w/o pits, 2.9 oz	10 dates	228	1.6	61.0	2	4.2	0.4	na	0	1%
w/o pits (Dole)	1/2 cup	280	5.0	62.0	0	(mq)	0.0	0.0	0	0%
Imported, pitted										
(Amport Foods) chopped	1.5 oz	135	0.0	36.0	0	5	0.0	na	0	0%
(Amport Foods) whole	1.5 oz	135	0.0	36.0	0	5	0.0	na	0	0%
(Bordo)	2 oz	204	1.2	47.2	5	>1.5 c	1.2	na	0	5%
(Bordo) diced	2 oz	203	1.0	47.5	5	>1.2 c	1.1	na	0	5%
(Dromedary) approx 1 oz	5 dates	100	1.0	23.0	0	(mq)	0.0	0.0	0	0%
(Dromedary) chopped	1/4 cup	130	1.0	31.0	0	(mq)	0.0	0.0	0	0%
DEER										
raw	1 lb	544	104.1	0.0	231	na	11.0	4.3	386	19%
raw	1 oz	34	6.4	0.0	14	na	0.7	0.3	24	20%
roasted	3 oz	134	25.7	0.0	46	na	2.7	1.1	95	19%
DIET BAR. See also SNACK BAR.										
(Figurines)										
chocolate	1 bar	100	2.0	11.0	50	1.0	5.0	1.0	0	46%
chocolate caramel	1 bar	100	2.0	11.0	65	1.0	6.0	1.0	0	51%
chocolate caramel '100'	1 bar	100	2.0	10.0	55	(mq)	6.0	(mq)	na	53%
chocolate peanut butter	1 bar	100	3.0	10.0	50	1.0	6.0	1.0	0	51%
'S'mores'	1 bar	100	2.0	11.0	55	1.0	5.0	1.0	0	46%
vanilla	1 bar	100	2.0	11.0	55	1.0	6.0	1.0	0	51%
(Nestlé)										
chewy chocolate brownie 'Sweet Success'	1 bar	120	2.0	18.0	35	3.0	4.0	na	na	31%
chewy chocolate chip 'Sweet Success'	1 bar	120	2.0	18.0	35	3.0	4.0	na	na	31%
chewy chocolate peanut butter 'Sweet Success'	1 bar	120	2.0	18.0	35	3.0	4.0	na	na	31%
(Ultra Slim Fast) chocolate chip crunch	1 bar	120	2.0	19.0	30	3.0	4.0	na	0	30%
DIET DRINK										
(Nestlé)										
chocolate mocha, ready to drink, 'Sweet Success'	10 oz	200	11.0	32.0	230	6.0	3.0	na	na	14%
chocolate raspberry truffle, powder, 'Sweet Success'	1.13 oz	90	7.0	11.0	150	6.0	2.0	na	na	20%
chocolate raspberry truffle, prepared, 'Sweet Success'	8 oz	180	15.0	23.0	na	6.0	2.0	na	280	11%
creamy milk chocolate, canned, 'Sweet Success'	10 oz	200	11.0	32.0	230	6.0	3.0	na	na	14%
dark chocolate fudge, canned, 'Sweet Success'	10 oz	200	11.0	32.0	210	6.0	3.0	na	na	14%
dark chocolate fudge, powder, 'Sweet Success'	1.13 oz	90	7.0	11.0	na	6.0	2.0	na	150	20%
dark chocolate fudge, prepared, 'Sweet Success'	8 oz	180	15.0	23.0	280	6.0	2.0	na	na	11%
rich chocolate almond, powder, 'Sweet Success'	1.13 oz	90	7.0	12.0	150	6.0	2.0	na	na	19%
rich chocolate almond, prepared, 'Sweet Success'	8 oz	180	15.0	24.0	280	6.0	2.0	na	na	10%
(Ultra Slim Fast)										
cafe mocha powder	1 scoop	100	5.0	24.0	130	6.0	<1.0	na	na	<7%
cafe mocha powder, prepared w/skim milk	8 oz	200	15.0	38.0	280	6.0	1.0	na	na	4%
chocolate fantasy 'Plus' powder	1 scoop	120	3.0	33.0	140	8.0	1.0	na	na	6%
chocolate fantasy 'Plus' powder, prepared w/skim milk	12 oz	250	15.0	50.0	330	8.0	2.0	na	na	7%
French vanilla powder	1 scoop	100	5.0	24.0	120	4.0	<1.0	na	na	<7%
French vanilla powder, prepared w/skim milk	8 oz	190	14.0	36.0	250	4.0	1.0	na	na	4%
'French Vanilla' canned	12 oz	220	13.0	38.0	240	5.0	1.0	na	na	4%
piña colada 'Plus' powder	1 scoop	90	5.0	24.0	120	6.0	<1.0	na	na	<7%
piña colada 'Plus' powder, prepared w/skim milk	8 oz	190	15.0	38.0	260	6.0	<1.0	na	na	<4%

Food Name	Serving Size	Calories	Prot. gms	Carbs gms	Sod. mgs	Fiber gms	Fat gms	Sat. Fat gms	Chol. mgs	% Fat Cal.
strawberry jubilee 'Plus' powder	1 scoop	110	3.0	32.0	140	8.0	1.0	na	na	6%
strawbery jubilee 'Plus' powder, prepared w/skim milk	12 oz	240	15.0	50.0	330	8.0	2.0	na	na	7%
DILL SEASONING, 'Parsley Patch It's a Dilly' (Schilling)	1 tsp	11	0.4	2.0	5	(tr)	0.4	na	0	27%
DILL SEED										
whole	1 oz	86	4.5	15.6	6	>6.0 c	4.1	0.2	0	32%
whole	1 tbsp	20	1.0	3.6	1	1.4	1.0	0.1	0	33%
whole	1 tsp	6	0.3	1.2	0	.4	0.3	0.0	0	31%
whole (Durkee)	1 tsp	9	0.0	0.0	0	0	<0.1	na	na	<37%
whole (Laurel Leaf)	1 tsp	9	0.0	0.0	0	0	<0.1	na	na	<37%
whole (Spice Islands)	1 tsp	9	0.3	1.2	<1	.4	0.4	na	0	38%
DILL WEED										
dried	1 oz	72	5.7	15.8	79	>3.4 c	1.2	na	0	11%
dried	1 tbsp	8	0.6	1.7	6	>.4 c	0.1	na	0	9%
dried	1 tsp	3	0.2	0.6	2	>.1 c	0.0	na	0	0%
fresh, sprigs	1 cup	4	0.3	0.6	5	na	0.1	0.0	0	20%
DIP										
ACAPULCO (Ortega)	1 oz	8	0.0	2.0	0	na	0.0	0.0	0	0%
AVOCADO (Kraft)	2 tbsp	50	1.0	3.0	210	na	4.0	2.0	0	69%
BACON AND HORSERADISH										
(Breakstone's)	2 tbsp	70	1.0	2.0	270	na	6.0	3.0	15	82%
(Kraft)	2 tbsp	60	1.0	3.0	200	na	5.0	3.0	0	74%
(Kraft) 'Premium'	2 tbsp	50	1.0	2.0	270	na	5.0	3.0	15	79%
(Sealtest)	2 tbsp	70	1.0	2.0	270	na	6.0	3.0	15	82%
BACON AND ONION										
(Breakstone's) 'Gourmet'	2 tbsp	70	1.0	2.0	210	na	6.0	3.0	15	82%
(Kraft) 'Premium'	2 tbsp	60	1.0	2.0	170	na	5.0	3.0	15	79%
BEAN										
(Chi-Chi's) 'Fiesta'	1 oz	30	1.0	4.0	126	na	1.0	na	3	31%
(Hain) hot	4 tbsp	70	4.0	10.0	250	(mq)	1.0	na	5	14%
BLACK BEAN										
(Guiltless Gourmet) barbeque, mild	1 oz	23	1.0	4.0	100	2.0	0.0	0.0	0	0%
(Guiltless Gourmet) barbeque, spicy	1 oz	23	1.0	4.0	100	2.0	0.0	0.0	0	0%
(Guiltless Gourmet) mild	1 oz	23	1.0	4.0	100	2.0	0.0	0.0	0	0%
(Guiltless Gourmet) spicy	1 oz	23	1.0	4.0	100	2.0	0.0	0.0	0	0%
(Tostitos) fat free, medium	2 tbsp	30	2.0	6.0	210	2.0	0.0	0.0	0	0%
BLUE CHEESE										
(Kraft) 'Premium'	2 tbsp	50	1.0	2.0	210	0	4.0	2.0	10	75%
(Litehouse) 'Lite' and dressing, refrigerated	1 tbsp	33	1.0	1.0	86	na	3.0	na	na	77%
(Litehouse) 'Original' and dressing, refrigerated	1 tbsp	77	1.0	0.0	82	na	8.0	na	na	95%
CAESAR (Litehouse) and dressing, refrigerated	1 tbsp	57	0.0	0.0	84	na	6.0	na	na	100%
CHEDDAR CHEESE										
(Frito-Lay's)	1 oz	45	1.0	3.0	180	na	3.0	na	1	63%
(Guiltless Gourmet) queso, mild	1 oz	20	1.0	5.0	150	0	0.0	0.0	0	0%
(Guiltless Gourmet) queso, spicy	1 oz	20	1.0	5.0	150	0	0.0	0.0	0	0%
CHEESE (Chi-Chi's) 'Fiesta'	1 oz	41	1.0	3.0	296	na	3.0	1.0	9	63%
CHILI (La Victoria)	1 tbsp	6	<1.0	1.0	90	na	<1.0	na	na	<53%
CLAM										
(Breakstone's)	2 tbsp	50	1.0	2.0	220	na	4.0	3.0	15	75%
(Breakstone's) 'Gourmet Chesapeake'	2 tbsp	50	1.0	2.0	200	na	4.0	3.0	20	75%
(Kraft)	2 tbsp	60	1.0	3.0	240	na	4.0	1.0	10	69%
(Kraft) 'Premium'	2 tbsp	45	1.0	2.0	210	na	4.0	2.0	20	75%
(Sealtest)	2 tbsp	50	1.0	2.0	220	na	4.0	3.0	15	75%
COUNTRY BLUE CHEESE										
(Litehouse) and dressing, refrigerated	1 tbsp	76	1.0	0.0	84	na	8.0	na	na	95%

Food Name	Serving Size	Calories	Prot. gms	Carbs gms	Sod. mgs	Fiber gms	Fat gms	Sat. Fat gms	Chol. mgs	% Fat Cal.
COUNTRY RANCH *(Litehouse)* and dressing, refrigerated ...	1 tbsp	61	0.0	1.0	75	na	7.0	na	na	94%
CUCUMBER *(Kraft)* creamy 'Premium'	2 tbsp	50	1.0	2.0	130	(tr)	4.0	3.0	10	75%
CUCUMBER AND ONION										
(Breakstone's)	2 tbsp	50	1.0	2.0	160	na	4.0	3.0	15	75%
(Sealtest)	2 tbsp	50	1.0	2.0	160	na	4.0	3.0	15	75%
DILL *(Nasoya)* creamy 'Vegi-Dip'	1 oz	60	2.0	4.0	100	na	4.0	(mq)	0	60%
FRENCH ONION										
(Bison)	1 oz	60	1.0	2.0	180	na	5.0	(mq)	20	79%
(Breakstone's)	2 tbsp	50	1.0	2.0	140	na	5.0	3.0	15	79%
(Frito-Lay's)	1 oz	50	1.0	3.0	180	na	3.0	na	3	63%
(Heluva Good) real sour cream	2 tbsp	50	1.0	2.0	160	0	5.0	3.0-	20	79%
(Kraft)	2 tbsp	60	1.0	3.0	140	na	4.0	2.0	0	69%
(Kraft) 'Premium'	2 tbsp	45	1.0	2.0	150	na	4.0	2.0	10	75%
(Lucerne)	2 tbsp	70	1.0	2.0	160	0	6.0	3.0	5	82%
(Nasoya) 'Vegi-Dip'	1 oz	50	2.0	4.0	100	na	3.0	(mq)	0	53%
(Sealtest)	2 tbsp	50	1.0	2.0	140	na	5.0	3.0	15	79%
GARLIC *(Life)* and dressing, w/tofu 'All Natural'	1 tbsp	70	<1.0	1.4	75	(mq)	7.1	(mq)	0	87%
GARLIC AND HERB *(Nasoya)* 'Vegi-Dip'	1 oz	50	2.0	6.0	100	(mq)	2.0	(mq)	0	36%
GUACAMOLE										
(Kraft)	2 tbsp	50	1.0	3.0	210	na	4.0	2.0	0	69%
(Lucerne)	2 tbsp	80	1.0	1.0	170	0	8.0	1.5	5	90%
HONEY MUSTARD *(Litehouse)* and dressing, refrigerated ...	1 tbsp	67	0.0	2.0	55	na	7.0	na	na	89%
HUMMUS *(Fantastic Foods)*	2 oz	111	4.0	9.5	263	(mq)	6.5	(mq)	0	52%
ITALIAN *(Litehouse)* and dressing, creamy, refrigerated	1 tbsp	60	0.0	0.0	76	na	6.0	na	na	100%
JALAPEÑO										
(Breakstone's) cheddar 'Gourmet'	2 tbsp	70	2.0	2.0	90	na	6.0	3.0	15	77%
(Frito-Lay's)	1 oz	30	1.0	4.0	115	na	1.0	na	0	31%
(Hain) medium	4 tbsp	70	4.0	10.0	150	na	1.0	na	5	14%
(Kraft)	2 tbsp	50	1.0	3.0	160	na	4.0	2.0	0	69%
(Kraft) cheese 'Premium'	2 tbsp	50	1.0	3.0	160	na	4.0	3.0	15	69%
(Litehouse) ranch, and dressing, refrigerated	1 tbsp	60	0.0	1.0	80	na	6.0	na	na	93%
(Old El Paso)	1 tbsp	14	1.0	2.0	53	1.0	0.0	0.0	0	0%
(Price's) nacho	1 oz	80	2.6	2.0	(mq)	na	7.1	(mq)	na	78%
(Wise)	2 tbsp	25	1.0	5.0	100	na	0.0	0.0	0	0%
MEXICAN BEAN *(Hain)*	4 tbsp	60	4.0	9.0	260	na	1.0	na	5	15%
MUSHROOM AND HERB *(Breakstone's)* 'Gourmet'	2 tbsp	50	1.0	2.0	150	na	4.0	3.0	10	75%
NACHO CHEESE										
(Kraft) 'Premium'	2 tbsp	55	2.0	2.0	200	0	4.0	2.0	10	69%
(Tio Sancho) 'Microwave Snacks' cheese sauce mix	3.5 oz	247	14.5	2.3	995	>.4 c	20.0	(mq)	(mq)	73%
ONION										
(Breakstone's) toasted 'Gourmet'	2 tbsp	50	1.0	2.0	170	na	5.0	3.0	10	79%
(Hain) bean	4 tbsp	70	4.0	10.0	270	(mq)	1.0	(mq)	5	14%
(Kraft) creamy 'Premium'	2 tbsp	45	1.0	2.0	160	na	4.0	2.0	10	75%
(Kraft) green	2 tbsp	60	1.0	3.0	170	na	4.0	2.0	0	69%
PEPPERCORN *(Litehouse)* and dressing, refrigerated	1 tbsp	67	0.0	0.0	66	na	7.0	na	na	100%
PICANTE SAUCE										
(Frito-Lay's)	1 oz	10	0.0	3.0	160	na	0.0	na	0	0%
(Wise)	2 tbsp	12	0.0	3.0	130	na	0.0	na	na	0%
PINTO BEAN										
(Guiltless Gourmet) barbeque, mild	1 oz	27	2.0	5.0	100	2.0	0.0	0.0	0	0%
(Guiltless Gourmet) barbeque, spicy	1 oz	27	2.0	5.0	100	2.0	0.0	0.0	0	0%
(Guiltless Gourmet) mild	1 oz	27	2.0	5.0	100	2.0	0.0	0.0	0	0%
(Guiltless Gourmet) spicy	1 oz	27	2.0	5.0	100	2.0	0.0	0.0	0	0%
POPPYSEED *(Litehouse)* and dressing, refrigerated	1 tbsp	65	0.0	3.0	83	na	6.0	na	na	82%

Food Name	Serving Size	Calories	Prot. gms	Carbs gms	Sod. mgs	Fiber gms	Fat gms	Sat. Fat gms	Chol. mgs	% Fat Cal.
RANCH										
(Heluva Good) real sour cream	2 tbsp	60	1.0	2.0	180	0	5.0	3.0	20	79%
(Litehouse) and dressing, refrigerated	1 tbsp	59	0.0	1.0	67	na	6.0	na	na	93%
(Litehouse) 'Lite' and dressing, refrigerated	1 tbsp	35	1.0	1.0	80	na	3.0	na	na	77%
(Litehouse) 'Vegi-Dip' refrigerated	1 tbsp	60	0.0	1.0	68	na	7.0	na	na	94%
(Lucerne)	2 tbsp	110	1.0	2.0	160	0	11.0	2.0	10	89%
SALSA										
(Pace) 'Chunky' medium	2 tbsp	4	<1.0	<1.0	102	na	<1.0	na	na	<53%
(Pace) 'Chunky' mild	2 tbsp	4	<1.0	<1.0	101	na	<1.0	na	na	<53%
SOUR CREAM AND CHIVES										
(Litehouse) vinaigrette, and dressing, refrigerated	1 tbsp	63	0.0	1.0	72	na	7.0	na	na	94%
TACO										
(Hain) and sauce	4 tbsp	25	1.0	5.0	350	na	1.0	na	5	27%
(Wise)	2 tbsp	12	0.0	3.0	115	na	0.0	0.0	0	0%
THOUSAND ISLAND (Litehouse) and dressing, refrigerated	1 tbsp	65	0.0	1.0	99	na	7.0	na	na	94%
VEGETABLE (T. Marzetti) and dressing	1 tbsp	88	0.0	1.0	120	na	10.0	na	2	96%
DISHCLOTH GOURD. See GOURD, DISHCLOTH.										
DOCK										
boiled, drained	4 oz	23	2.1	3.3	3	>.8 c	0.7	(tr)	0	23%
boiled, drained	100 gm	20	1.8	2.9	3	>.7 c	0.6	na	0	22%
raw, chopped	1/2 cup	15	1.3	2.1	3	1.94	0.5	na	0	25%
raw, trimmed	1 oz	6	0.6	0.9	1	>.2 c	0.2	(tr)	0	23%
raw, untrimmed	1 lb	70	6.4	10.2	13	>2.5 c	2.2	na	0	23%
DOLLARFISH										
raw	1 lb	663	78.4	0.0	401	0	36.4	(mq)	295	51%
raw	1 oz	41	4.9	0.0	25	0	2.3	(mq)	18	51%
DOLPHIN FISH. See MAHI MAHI.										
DONUT										
(Awrey's)										
crunch	1 donut	600	7.0	65.0	730	2.0	34.0	8.0	40	52%
plain	1 donut	490	6.0	48.0	650	1.0	30.0	7.0	35	56%
sugared	1 donut	610	7.0	68.0	735	2.0	35.0	8.0	40	51%
(Break Cake)										
chocolate, 1 oz	1 donut	130	1.0	14.0	115	na	8.0	2.0	5	55%
chocolate, gem, .5 oz	1 donut	70	1.0	7.0	60	na	4.0	1.0	5	53%
chocolate, gem, .5 oz	6 donuts	400	4.0	42.0	340	na	24.0	6.0	15	54%
cinnamon, 1 oz	1 donut	120	1.0	15.0	130	na	6.0	1.6	5	46%
cinnamon, gem, .5 oz	1 donut	60	1.0	8.0	70	na	3.0	0.8	5	43%
dunkin stix, .5 oz	2 stix	420	3.0	43.0	320	na	27.0	na	0	57%
powdered, 1 oz	1 donut	120	1.0	16.0	135	na	5.0	1.4	5	40%
powdered, gem, .5 oz	1 donut	60	1.0	8.0	70	na	3.0	0.7	5	43%
powdered, gem, .5 oz	6 donuts	350	4.0	47.0	400	na	16.0	4.3	15	41%
(Dunkin' Donuts)										
apple filled, w/cinnamon sugar, 2.8 oz	1 donut	250	5.0	33.0	280	1.0	11.0	(mq)	0	39%
Bavarian filled, w/chocolate frosting, 2.8 oz	1 donut	240	5.0	32.0	260	2.0	11.0	(mq)	0	40%
blueberry filled, 2.4 oz	1 donut	210	4.0	29.0	240	2.0	8.0	(mq)	0	35%
'Boston Kreme'	1 donut	240	4.0	30.0	250	na	11.0	2.0	0	42%
cinnamon, apple filled	1 donut	190	4.0	25.0	220	na	9.0	2.0	0	41%
coffee roll, glazed, 2.9 oz	1 donut	280	5.0	37.0	310	2.0	12.0	(mq)	0	39%
cruller, French, glazed, 1.3 oz	1 donut	140	2.0	16.0	130	0	8.0	(mq)	30	50%
cruller, honey dipped	1 donut	260	4.0	36.0	330	na	11.0	2.0	0	38%
jelly filled, 2.4 oz	1 donut	220	4.0	31.0	230	1.0	9.0	(mq)	0	37%
lemon filled, 2.8 oz	1 donut	260	4.0	33.0	280	1.0	12.0	(mq)	0	42%
plain, cake w/handle	1 donut	240	4.0	26.0	370	na	14.0	3.0	0	51%

Food Name	Serving Size	Calories	Prot. gms	Carbs gms	Sod. mgs	Fiber gms	Fat gms	Sat. Fat gms	Chol. mgs	% Fat Cal.
ring, buttermilk, glazed, 2.6 oz	1 donut	290	4.0	37.0	370	1.0	14.0	(mq)	10	43%
ring, chocolate, glazed, 2.5 oz	1 donut	324	3.5	34.0	383	1.9	21.0	(mq)	2	56%
ring, plain, cake	1 donut	262	3.0	23.0	330	na	18.0	4.0	0	61%
ring, plain, cake, 2.2 oz	1 donut	270	4.0	25.0	330	1.0	17.0	(mq)	10	57%
ring, powdered, cake	1 donut	270	3.0	28.0	340	na	16.0	3.0	0	54%
ring, whole wheat, glazed, 2.9 oz	1 donut	330	4.0	39.0	380	na	18.0	na	5	49%
ring, yeast, chocolate frosted, 1.9 oz	1 donut	200	4.0	25.0	190	na	10.0	2.0	0	44%
ring, yeast, glazed, 1.9 oz	1 donut	200	4.0	26.0	230	na	9.0	2.0	0	40%
(Entenmann's)										
crumb topped	1 donut	260	3.0	34.0	220	na	12.0	na	na	42%
devil's food crumb	1 donut	250	3.0	34.0	200	na	12.0	na	na	42%
rich, frosted	1 donut	280	3.0	27.0	210	na	18.0	na	na	57%
(Hostess)										
cinnamon, 'Donette Gems'	1 donut	60	1.0	7.0	70	.3	3.0	2.0	5	46%
cinnamon, 'Family Pack'	1 donut	120	2.0	14.0	140	.5	6.0	3.0	5	46%
crumb	1 donut	160	1.0	16.0	140	.9	10.0	5.0	10	57%
crumb, 'Donette Gems'	1 donut	80	1.0	8.0	70	.4	5.0	2.0	5	56%
frosted, 1.5 oz	1 donut	190	2.0	20.0	180	1.1	12.0	7.0	5	55%
frosted, 'Donette Gems'	1 donut	80	1.0	8.0	70	.4	5.0	3.0	5	56%
glazed, 'Old Fashioned'	1 donut	250	3.0	33.0	230	1.4	12.0	5.0	15	43%
glazed whirl	1 donut	190	3.0	27.0	230	.9	7.0	3.0	5	34%
honey wheat	1 donut	250	3.0	32.0	280	1.2	12.0	6.0	25	44%
plain, 'Old Fashioned'	1 donut	170	3.0	21.0	230	.9	9.0	4.0	10	46%
(Little Debbie) stick 1.67 oz	1 stick	230	2.0	26.0	180	(mq)	13.0	(mq)	<1	51%
(Rich's)										
frozen, glazed 'Ever Fresh' 1.2 oz	1 donut	141	2.4	17.2	(mq)	(mq)	7.0	(mq)	na	45%
frozen, jelly 'Ever Fresh' 2.17 oz	1 donut	213	3.6	26.0	(mq)	(mq)	9.5	(mq)	na	42%
(Tastykake)										
cinnamon, 'Assorted' 1.6 oz	1 donut	179	2.6	24.5	211	.8	8.2	2.1	11	41%
cinnamon, mini	1 donut	48	0.7	6.4	54	.3	2.4	0.6	4	43%
frosted, rich, 2 oz	1 donut	258	3.6	28.2	196	3.3	16.0	7.6	9	53%
frosted, rich, mini	1 donut	61	0.9	7.7	59	.5	3.2	1.9	4	46%
honey wheat, 2 oz	1 donut	209	2.3	33.3	190	.9	7.5	(mq)	15	32%
honey wheat, mini	1 donut	40	0.6	7.2	48	.2	1.2	0.3	3	26%
orange glazed, 2 oz	1 donut	219	2.7	32.1	178	.8	9.1	2.5	10	37%
plain, 'Assorted' 1.6 oz	1 donut	185	3.0	21.6	171	.9	10.1	2.5	12	48%
powdered sugar, 'Assorted' 1.6 oz	1 donut	188	2.6	24.4	221	.8	8.6	2.2	10	42%
powdered sugar, mini	1 donut	42	0.6	6.9	71	.2	1.3	0.3	4	28%
DRAGON'S EYE										
dried	1 oz	81	1.4	21.0	14	13.4	0.1	(tr)	0	1%
raw, approx .2 oz	1 med	2	<.1	0.5	tr	<.1	tr	(tr)	0	0%
raw, shelled and seeded	1 oz	17	0.4	4.3	tr	>.1 c	<.1	(tr)	0	<5%
raw, untrimmed	1 lb	144	3.2	36.4	1	>1.0 c	0.2	na	0	1%

DREAM WHIP. See CREAM TOPPING, NONDAIRY.

DRESSING. See SALAD DRESSING.

DRINKS. See ALCOHOL-FREE BEVERAGES; ALCOHOLIC BEVERAGES; COFFEE; DIET DRINK; MILK; SOFT DRINKS AND MIXERS; SPORTS DRINK; TEA; WATER; and individual listings.

DRINK MIX. See individual drink mix flavors.

DRUM, FRESHWATER

dry-heat cooked	3 oz	130	19.1	0.0	82	0	5.4	1.2	70	39%
raw	1 lb	541	79.5	0.0	340	0	22.4	5.1	290	39%
raw	3 oz	101	14.9	0.0	64	0	4.2	1.0	54	39%
raw	1 oz	34	5.0	0.0	21	0	1.4	0.3	18	39%

Food Name	Serving Size	Calories	Prot. gms	Carbs gms	Sod. mgs	Fiber gms	Fat gms	Sat. Fat gms	Chol. mgs	% Fat Cal.
DUCK, DOMESTICATED										
Meat and skin										
raw	1 oz	115	3.3	0.0	18	0	11.2	3.7	22	88%
roasted	4 oz	382	21.5	0.0	67	0	32.1	11.0	95	77%
Meat only										
raw	1 oz	37	5.2	0.0	21	0	1.7	0.7	22	42%
roasted	4 oz	228	26.6	0.0	74	0	12.7	4.7	101	52%
DUCK, WILD										
Breast meat, raw	1 oz	35	5.6	0.0	16	0	1.2	0.4	(mq)	33%
Meat and skin, raw	1 oz	60	4.9	0.0	16	0	4.3	1.4	23	66%
DUCK FAT										
	1 cup	1846	0.0	0.0	0	0	204.6	68.1	205	100%
	1 oz	255	0.0	0.0	0	0	28.3	9.4	28	100%
	1 tbsp	115	0.0	0.0	0	0	12.8	4.3	13	100%
DUCK LIVER, domesticated, raw	1 oz	39	5.3	1.0	(mq)	0	1.3	0.4	146	32%
DULSE, raw	100 gm	0	0.0	0.0	2085	>1.2 c	3.2	0.0	0	0%

E

Food Name	Serving Size	Calories	Prot. gms	Carbs gms	Sod. mgs	Fiber gms	Fat gms	Sat. Fat gms	Chol. mgs	% Fat Cal.
EEL, MIXED SPECIES										
broiled	4 oz	268	26.8	0.0	74	0	17.0	3.4	183	59%
dry-heat cooked	3 oz	201	20.1	0.0	55	0	12.7	2.6	137	59%
raw	1 lb	834	83.7	0.0	231	0	52.9	10.7	571	59%
raw	1 oz	52	5.2	0.0	14	0	3.3	0.7	36	59%
EGG, ALTERNATIVE										
Frozen										
(Fleischmann's) 'Egg Beaters' cheese omelet	1/2 cup	110	14.0	2.0	480	na	5.0	2.0	5	41%
(Fleischmann's) 'Egg Beaters' vegetable omelet	1/2 cup	50	7.0	5.0	170	na	0.0	0.0	0	0%
(Morningstar Farms) 'Scramblers'	1/4 cup	60	6.0	3.0	(mq)	0	3.0	(mq)	0	43%
(Tofutti) 'Egg Watchers'	2 oz	50	7.0	2.0	100	na	2.0	(mq)	0	33%
Refrigerated										
(Featherweight)	2 eggs	120	9.0	2.0	250	0	8.0	(mq)	15	62%
(Fleischmann's) 'Egg Beaters'	1/4 cup	25	5.0	1.0	80	0	0.0	0.0	0	0%
Mix										
(Healthy Choice) 'Cholesterol Free Egg Product'	1.9-oz serving	30	5.0	1.0	90	na	<1.0	0.0	0	<27%
(Tofu Scrambler) prepared w/tofu	1/2 cup	98	11.0	7.0	252	(mq)	5.0	(mq)	0	39%
EGG, CHICKEN. See also EGG WHITE, CHICKEN; EGG YOLK, CHICKEN.										
Cooked										
fried	1 large	91	6.2	0.6	162	0	6.9	1.9	211	70%
hard-boiled	1 oz	44	3.6	0.3	35	0	3.0	0.9	120	63%
hard-boiled, chopped	1 cup	211	17.1	1.5	169	0	14.4	4.4	577	64%
poached	1 large	74	6.2	0.6	140	0	5.0	1.5	212	62%
poached	1 oz	42	3.5	0.3	79	0	2.8	0.9	120	62%
scrambled	1 cup	365	24.4	4.8	616	0	26.9	8.1	774	68%
scrambled	1 large	100	6.7	1.3	168	0	7.3	2.2	211	67%
Dried										
	1 oz	168	13.0	1.4	148	0	11.9	3.6	544	65%
	1 tbsp	30	2.3	0.2	26	0	2.1	0.6	96	65%
sifted	1 cup	505	39.0	4.1	443	0	35.5	10.7	1631	65%
stabilized, glucose reduced	1 oz	174	13.7	0.7	155	0	12.5	3.7	572	66%
stabilized, glucose reduced	1 tbsp	31	2.4	0.1	27	0	2.2	0.7	101	66%

Food Name	Serving Size	Calories	Prot. gms	Carbs gms	Sod. mgs	Fiber gms	Fat gms	Sat. Fat gms	Chol. mgs	% Fat Cal.
stabilized, glucose reduced, sifted	1 cup	523	40.9	2.0	466	0	37.4	11.2	1714	66%
Pickled *(Penrose)*	1 large	80	8.0	1.0	230	0	5.0	(mq)	(mq)	56%
Raw										
fresh or frozen	1 cup	363	30.4	3.0	307	0	24.3	7.5	1033	62%
fresh or frozen	1 large	75	6.3	0.6	63	0	5.0	1.6	213	62%
fresh or frozen	1 oz	42	3.5	0.3	36	0	2.8	0.9	120	62%
EGG, DUCK										
raw	1 large	130	9.0	1.0	102	0	9.6	2.6	619	68%
raw	1 oz	52	3.6	0.4	41	0	3.9	1.0	251	69%
EGG, GOOSE										
raw	1 large	267	20.0	1.9	199	0	19.1	5.2	1227	66%
raw	1 oz	52	3.9	0.4	na	0	3.8	1.0	(mq)	67%
EGG, QUAIL										
raw	1 oz	45	3.7	0.1	na	0	3.1	1.0	239	65%
raw	1 large	14	1.2	0.0	13	0	1.0	0.3	76	65%
EGG, TURKEY										
raw	1 large	135	10.8	0.9	120	0	9.4	2.9	737	64%
raw	1 oz	48	3.9	0.3	na	0	3.4	1.0	265	65%
EGG BREAKFAST, ALTERNATIVE, FROZEN										
vegetarian, w/hash browns and links 'Scramblers'										
(Morningstar Farms)	7 oz	360	16.0	22.0	660	(mq)	23.0	(mq)	0	58%
vegetarian, w/pancakes and links 'Scramblers'										
(Morningstar Farms)	6.8 oz	380	18.0	33.0	900	(mq)	19.0	(mq)	0	46%
EGG BREAKFAST, FREEZE-DRIED										
(Mountain House)										
cheese omelet, prepared	1/2 pkg	180	13.0	8.0	207	na	9.0	(mq)	(mq)	49%
w/bacon, prepared	1/2 pkg	170	12.0	7.0	165	na	10.0	(mq)	(mq)	54%
w/butter, prepared	1/2 pkg	160	11.0	8.0	174	na	8.0	(mq)	(mq)	49%
EGG BREAKFAST, SCRAMBLED, FROZEN										
w/bacon and home fried potatoes *(Swanson)*	5.6 oz	340	11.0	16.0	690	(mq)	26.0	(mq)	(mq)	68%
w/cheddar cheese and fried potatoes *(Aunt Jemima)*	5.9 oz	250	11.0	22.0	910	(mq)	13.0	(mq)	(mq)	47%
w/ham and hash browns *(Downyflake)*	6.25 oz	360	13.0	17.0	730	(mq)	26.0	(mq)	(mq)	66%
w/ham and pecan twirl *(Downyflake)*	6.25 oz	470	15.0	40.0	670	(mq)	28.0	(mq)	(mq)	53%
w/hash browns and sausage link *(Downyflake)*	6.25 oz	420	12.0	17.0	790	(mq)	34.0	(mq)	(mq)	73%
w/home fried potatoes 'Great Starts' Budget Breakfast										
(Swanson)	4.6 oz	260	7.0	14.0	380	(mq)	19.0	(mq)	(mq)	67%
w/sausages and hash browns *(Aunt Jemima)*	5.7 oz	290	12.0	14.0	810	(mq)	20.0	(mq)	(mq)	63%
w/sausages and hash browns *(Swanson)*	6.5 oz	430	13.0	19.0	760	(mq)	34.0	(mq)	(mq)	71%
w/sausages and pancakes *(Aunt Jemima)*	5.2 oz	270	13.0	21.0	880	(mq)	14.0	(mq)	(mq)	48%
w/sausages and pecan twirl *(Downyflake)*	6.25 oz	510	16.0	39.0	710	(mq)	33.0	(mq)	(mq)	57%
EGG FOO YUNG										
(LaChoy) mix, prepared	8.8 oz	164	8.2	19.2	1250	(mq)	7.0	(mq)	na	37%
(LaChoy) packaged 'Dinner Classics' prepared	2 patties	170	8.0	20.0	1390	1.0	7.0	2.2	275	36%
EGG NOODLE. See NOODLE, EGG.										
EGG ROLL										
Frozen										
(Chun King)										
chicken	3.6 oz	220	5.0	32.0	600	(mq)	8.0	(mq)	(mq)	33%
meat and shrimp	3.6 oz	220	6.0	31.0	680	(mq)	8.0	(mq)	(mq)	33%
pork 'Restaurant Style'	3 oz	180	6.0	23.0	450	(mq)	6.0	(mq)	(mq)	32%
shrimp	3.6 oz	200	4.0	31.0	480	(mq)	6.0	(mq)	(mq)	28%
(Jeno's)										
chicken 'Snacks' approx 6 rolls	3 oz	190	5.0	21.0	350	(mq)	9.0	(mq)	(mq)	44%
meat and shrimp 'Snacks' approx 6 rolls	3 oz	200	5.0	21.0	420	(mq)	11.0	(mq)	(mq)	49%

Food Name	Serving Size	Calories	Prot. gms	Carbs gms	Sod. mgs	Fiber gms	Fat gms	Sat. Fat gms	Chol. mgs	% Fat Cal.
shrimp and cheese 'Snacks' approx 6 rolls	3 oz	190	7.0	22.0	290	(mq)	8.0	(mq)	(mq)	38%
(LaChoy)										
almond chicken	3 oz	120	5.0	19.0	290	na	3.0	na	5	22%
chicken 'Snack'	1.45 oz	90	3.0	12.0	140	na	3.0	na	<1	31%
lobster 'Snack'	1.45 oz	75	2.0	12.0	150	na	2.0	na	<1	24%
meat and shrimp 'Snack'	1.45 oz	80	3.0	11.0	115	na	3.0	na	4	33%
pork 'Restaurant Style'	3 oz	150	7.0	20.0	480	na	5.0	na	7	29%
shrimp 'Restaurant Style'	3 oz	130	5.0	19.0	260	na	4.0	na	5	27%
shrimp 'Snack'	1.45 oz	75	2.0	12.0	120	na	2.0	na	4	24%
sweet and sour chicken	3 oz	150	4.0	24.0	280	na	4.0	na	5	24%
(Worthington) vegetarian roll, frozen	3 oz	160	6.0	20.0	530	(mq)	6.0	1.0	0	34%
Refrigerated										
(Chung's)										
chicken, white meat	3 oz	150	8.0	21.0	560	4.0	6.0	1.0	9	32%
pork	3 oz	190	7.0	20.0	590	3.0	10.0	3.0	10	46%
shrimp	3 oz	170	5.0	22.0	496	10.0	7.0	1.0	11	37%
vegetable	3 oz	180	4.0	23.0	510	15.0	8.0	2.0	0	40%
EGG ROLL WRAPPER										
(Azumaya Pasta)	2 pieces	130	4.0	26.0	200	1.0	0.0	0.0	<5	0%
(Nasoya)	1 piece	23	1.0	4.5	19	(mq)	0.0	0.0	0	0%
EGG WHITE, CHICKEN										
Dried										
stabilized, glucose reduced, flakes	1 oz	100	21.8	1.2	328	0	<.1	0.0	0	<1%
stabilized, glucose reduced, powder	1 cup	402	88.2	4.8	1325	0	<.1	0.0	0	<1%
stabilized, glucose reduced, powder	1 oz	107	23.4	1.3	351	0	<.1	0.0	0	<1%
Raw										
fresh or frozen	1 cup	122	25.6	2.5	399	0	0.0	na	na	0%
fresh or frozen	1 large	17	3.5	0.3	55	0	0.0	na	na	0%
fresh or frozen	1 oz	14	3.0	0.3	46	0	0.0	0.0	0	0%
EGG WHITE STABILIZER (Tone's)	1 tsp	12	<.1	3.0	1	.1	(tr)	0.0	0	0%
EGG YOLK, CHICKEN										
Dried										
sifted	1 cup	460	20.5	0.3	61	0	41.1	12.3	1962	82%
sifted	1 oz	195	8.7	0.1	26	0	17.4	5.2	830	82%
sifted	1 tbsp	27	1.2	0.0	4	0	2.5	0.7	117	82%
Raw										
fresh	1 cup	870	40.7	4.3	104	0	75.0	23.2	3113	79%
fresh	1 oz	101	4.8	0.5	12	0	8.8	2.7	363	79%
fresh	1 large	59	2.8	0.3	7	0	5.1	1.6	213	79%
frozen, salted	100 gm	278	14.2	1.5	3932	0	23.4	7.2	973	77%
frozen, sugared	100 gm	317	14.2	11.5	56	0	23.4	7.2	973	67%
frozen, sugared	1 oz	92	3.7	2.7	16	0	7.2	2.2	328	72%
EGGNOG, NON-ALCOHOLIC										
Canned (Borden)	1/2 cup	160	3.0	16.0	80	0	9.0	(mq)	(mq)	52%
Chilled										
(Crowley)	6 oz	270	6.0	34.0	200	0	13.0	(mq)	100	42%
(Darigold)	8 oz	350	8.0	40.0	120	0	17.0	(mq)	(mq)	44%
(Darigold) 'Classic'	8 oz	390	10.0	48.0	170	0	17.0	(mq)	(mq)	40%
(Ensure) liquid nutrition	8 oz	250	8.8	34.3	na	na	8.8	na	na	32%
EGGNOG MIX										
dry, 2 heaping tsp	1 oz	111	0.1	27.7	44	0	0.3	0.1	7	2%
1 oz powder, prepared w/whole milk	1 cup	261	8.2	38.9	163	0	8.4	5.2	33	29%
1 oz powder, prepared w/2% milk	1 cup	232	8.2	39.4	166	0	5.0	3.0	18	19%
1 oz powder, prepared w/1% milk	1 cup	213	8.1	39.4	167	0	2.9	1.7	10	12%

Food Name	Serving Size	Calories	Prot. gms	Carbs gms	Sod. mgs	Fiber gms	Fat gms	Sat. Fat gms	Chol. mgs	% Fat Cal.
1 oz powder, prepared w/skim milk	1 cup	197	8.5	39.6	170	0	0.7	0.4	4	3%
EGGPLANT/aubergine										
boiled, drained	4 oz	32	0.9	7.5	3	>1.1 c	0.3	<.1	0	7%
boiled, drained, 1-inch cubes	1 cup	27	0.8	6.4	3	2.4	0.2	0.0	0	6%
raw, 1-inch pieces	1/2 cup	11	0.4	2.5	1	1.0	0.1	0.0	0	7%
raw, peeled, approx 1 lb	1 eggplant	119	4.7	27.8	14	11.5	0.8	0.2	0	5%
raw, trimmed	1 oz	7	0.3	1.8	1	.4	<.1	tr	0	<10%
raw, untrimmed	1 lb	95	4.0	23.0	13	5.5	0.4	0.1	0	3%
EGGPLANT APPETIZER, 'Caponata' (Progresso)	1/2 can	70	2.0	4.0	260	(mq)	4.0	(mq)	0	60%
EGGPLANT ENTRÉE, FROZEN										
(Celentano)										
parmigiana	10 oz	350	18.0	29.0	500	(mq)	19.0	(mq)	(mq)	48%
parmigiana	8 oz	280	14.0	23.0	400	(mq)	15.0	(mq)	(mq)	48%
parmigiana	6.25 oz	260	9.0	36.0	220	(mq)	10.0	(mq)	(mq)	33%
rollettes	11 oz	320	14.0	36.0	210	(mq)	14.0	(mq)	na	39%
(Mrs. Paul's) parmigiana	5 oz	240	6.0	18.0	600	(mq)	16.0	4.0	15	60%
ELBOW MACARONI. See PASTA.										
ELDERBERRY										
fresh	1 lb	329	3.0	83.5	na	>31.8 c	2.3	na	0	6%
fresh	1 oz	21	0.2	5.2	na	>2.0 c	0.1	(tr)	0	4%
fresh	1 cup	106	1.0	26.7	na	>10.1 c	0.7	na	0	5%
ELK										
raw	1 lb	504	104.1	0.0	263	na	6.6	2.4	249	13%
raw	1 oz	31	6.4	0.0	16	na	0.4	0.2	15	12%
roasted	3 oz	124	25.7	0.0	52	na	1.6	0.6	62	12%
roasted	4 oz	166	34.2	0.0	69	0	2.2	0.8	83	13%
roasted, diced, approx 4.9 oz	1 cup	204	42.3	0.0	85	0	2.7	1.0	102	13%
ENCHILADA (Gebhardt)	2 enchiladas	310	5.0	20.0	460	2.0	24.0	9.0	58	68%
ENCHILADA DINNER, FROZEN. See also ENCHILADA ENTRÉE, FROZEN.										
BEEF										
(Banquet)	12 oz	500	19.0	72.0	1810	(mq)	15.0	(mq)	(mq)	27%
(Banquet) chili and gravy 'Family Entrées'	7 oz	270	10.0	28.0	(mq)	(mq)	13.0	(mq)	(mq)	44%
(Healthy Choice)	13.4 oz	370	15.0	66.0	450	na	5.0	2.0	30	12%
(Old El Paso) 'Festive Dinners'	11 oz	390	24.0	56.0	1200	(mq)	8.0	(mq)	(mq)	18%
(Patio)	13.25 oz	520	16.0	59.0	1810	(mq)	24.0	(mq)	40	42%
(Swanson)	13.75 oz	480	17.0	55.0	1350	(mq)	21.0	(mq)	(mq)	40%
(Van de Kamp's) 'Mexican Dinner'	1/2 pkg	200	8.0	27.0	740	(mq)	7.0	(mq)	(mq)	31%
CHEESE										
(Banquet)	12 oz	550	22.0	71.0	2170	(mq)	19.0	(mq)	(mq)	32%
(Patio)	12.25 oz	380	14.0	59.0	2010	(mq)	10.0	(mq)	20	24%
(Old El Paso) 'Festive Dinners'	11 oz	590	24.0	51.0	1200	(mq)	31.0	(mq)	(mq)	48%
(Van de Kamp's) 'Mexican Dinner'	1/2 pkg	220	8.0	26.0	620	(mq)	9.0	(mq)	(mq)	37%
CHICKEN										
(Healthy Choice)	13.4 oz	340	14.0	61.0	470	na	5.0	2.0	30	13%
(Healthy Choice)	9.5 oz	310	14.0	44.0	480	na	9.0	3.0	35	26%
(Old El Paso) 'Festive Dinners'	11 oz	460	21.0	54.0	770	(mq)	18.0	(mq)	(mq)	35%
(Weight Watchers) nacho grande 'Mexican Style'	9 oz	280	14.0	38.0	590	na	8.0	3.0	20	26%
ENCHILADA DINNER, MIX										
(Old El Paso) prepared	1 enchilada	145	7.0	11.0	325	2.0	8.0	3.0	21	50%
(Tio Sancho) 'Dinner Kit'	1 shell	80	1.3	10.8	2	>.6 c	3.5	(mq)	na	39%
(Tio Sancho) 'Dinner Kit' and sauce mix	3 oz	278	4.5	62.0	4058	>1.8 c	1.5	(mq)	na	5%
ENCHILADA ENTRÉE, FROZEN. See also ENCHILADA DINNER, FROZEN.										
BEEF										
(Hormel)	1 enchilada	140	6.0	17.0	573	(mq)	5.0	(mq)	(mq)	33%

Food Name	Serving Size	Calories	Prot. gms	Carbs gms	Sod. mgs	Fiber gms	Fat gms	Sat. Fat gms	Chol. mgs	% Fat Cal.
(Old El Paso)	1 pkg	210	8.0	16.0	720	(mq)	13.0	(mq)	10	55%
(Ultimate 200) Ranchero	9.12 oz	190	18.0	18.0	500	na	5.0	2.0	20	24%
(Van de Kamp's) 'Mexican Entrées'	1 pkg	270	11.0	30.0	1040	(mq)	12.0	(mq)	(mq)	40%
(Van de Kamp's) 'Mexican Entrées Family Pack'	1/4 pkg	150	7.0	19.0	530	(mq)	5.0	(mq)	(mq)	30%
(Van de Kamp's) shredded, 'Mexican Entrées'	1 pkg	360	20.0	40.0	1010	(mq)	14.0	(mq)	(mq)	34%
BLACK BEAN-VEGETABLE (Amy's Kitchen)	4.75 oz	135	4.0	20.0	290	2.0	4.0	na	0	27%
CHEESE										
(Amy's Kitchen) organic	4.75 oz	210	11.0	16.0	290	2.0	9.0	na	19	43%
(Hormel)	1 enchilada	151	6.0	18.0	676	(mq)	6.0	(mq)	(mq)	36%
(Old El Paso)	1 pkg	250	10.0	24.0	830	(mq)	12.0	(mq)	(mq)	44%
(Stouffer's)	9.75 oz	490	23.0	33.0	550	na	29.0	na	na	54%
(Van de Kamp's) 'Mexican Entrées'	1 pkg	300	11.0	31.0	980	(mq)	15.0	(mq)	(mq)	45%
(Van de Kamp's) 'Mexican Entrées Family Pack'	1/4 pkg	200	7.0	19.0	460	(mq)	10.0	(mq)	(mq)	46%
CHICKEN										
(Le Menu) 'Light Style'	8 oz	280	21.0	32.0	530	(mq)	8.0	(mq)	35	25%
(Old El Paso)	1 pkg	220	8.0	20.0	740	(mq)	12.0	(mq)	(mq)	49%
(Old El Paso) w/sour cream sauce	1 pkg	280	10.0	18.0	520	(mq)	19.0	(mq)	(mq)	60%
(Stouffer's)	10 oz	490	21.0	31.0	860	na	31.0	na	na	57%
(Van de Kamp's) 'Mexican Entrées'	1 pkg	260	13.0	27.0	1010	(mq)	11.0	(mq)	(mq)	38%
(Weight Watchers) Suiza	9 oz	230	16.0	25.0	530	na	7.0	2.0	40	28%
RANCHERO (Van de Kamp's) 'Mexican Entrées'	1/2 pkg	260	11.0	26.0	630	(mq)	12.0	(mq)	(mq)	42%
SUIZA (Van de Kamp's) 'Mexican Entrées'	1 pkg	230	12.0	23.0	390	(mq)	10.0	(mq)	(mq)	39%
VEGETABLE (Legume) w/tofu and sauce	11 oz	270	14.0	36.0	390	10.3	8.0	3.0	0	27%
ENCHILADA SEASONING MIX										
(Old El Paso)	1/8 pkg	6	0.0	1.0	80	0	0.0	0.0	0	0%
(Lawry's) 'Seasoning Blends'	1 pkg	152	5.3	29.9	1723	1.2	1.2	na	na	7%
ENDIVE										
approx 1.3 lb	1 head	87	6.4	17.2	113	15.9	1.0	0.3	0	9%
chopped	1/2 cup	4	0.3	0.8	6	.8	0.1	0.0	0	17%
trimmed	1 oz	5	0.4	0.9	6	>.3 c	0.1	<.1	0	15%
untrimmed	1 lb	65	4.9	13.1	87	>3.5 c	0.8	0.2	0	9%
ENGLISH MUFFIN										
(Earth Grains)										
oat bran, 12-oz pkg	1 muffin	120	5.0	24.0	410	2.0	1.0	0.4	0	7%
plain, 12.5-oz pkg	1 muffin	130	5.0	26.0	410	1.0	1.0	0.2	0	7%
plain, 12-oz pkg	1 muffin	120	5.0	25.0	390	1.0	1.0	0.2	0	7%
raisin, 14-oz pkg	1 muffin	160	5.0	33.0	300	1.0	2.0	0.3	0	11%
raisin, 'Sun Maid' 15-oz pkg	1 muffin	160	5.0	34.0	180	2.0	1.0	0.4	0	6%
sourdough, 12.5-oz pkg	1 muffin	130	5.0	26.0	410	1.0	1.0	0.2	0	7%
sourdough, 12-oz pkg	1 muffin	120	5.0	25.0	390	1.0	1.0	0.2	0	7%
whole wheat, 15-oz pkg	1 muffin	140	6.0	28.0	450	4.0	2.0	0.4	0	12%
whole wheat, 14-oz pkg	1 muffin	130	6.0	26.0	420	4.0	1.0	0.4	0	7%
(Hi Fiber)										
cinnamon raisin	1 muffin	110	4.0	21.0	275	5.0	1.0	na	0	8%
multigrain	1 muffin	120	4.0	23.0	240	4.0	1.0	na	0	8%
plain	1 muffin	110	5.0	21.0	280	5.0	1.0	na	0	8%
(Oatmeal Goodness)										
cinnamon and raisin oatmeal	1 muffin	140	5.0	26.0	160	1.5	2.0	(mq)	0	13%
honey and oatmeal	1 muffin	140	5.0	26.0	160	1.5	2.0	(mq)	0	13%
(Oroweat)										
extra crisp	1 muffin	130	4.0	26.0	260	na	1.0	na	na	7%
health nut	1 muffin	170	6.0	29.0	220	1.0	4.0	0.0	0	21%
sourdough	1 muffin	140	4.0	27.0	370	na	1.0	na	na	7%

Food Name	Serving Size	Calories	Prot. gms	Carbs gms	Sod. mgs	Fiber gms	Fat gms	Sat. Fat gms	Chol. mgs	% Fat Cal.
(Pepperidge Farm)										
cinnamon apple	1 muffin	140	4.0	27.0	210	(mq)	1.0	0.0	0	7%
cinnamon chip	1 muffin	160	4.0	28.0	180	(mq)	3.0	0.0	0	17%
cinnamon raisin	1 muffin	150	4.0	29.0	200	(mq)	2.0	0.0	0	12%
plain	1 muffin	140	5.0	27.0	220	(mq)	1.0	0.0	0	7%
sourdough	1 muffin	135	4.0	27.0	260	(mq)	1.0	0.0	0	7%
(Roman Meal)										
honey nut and oat bran, refrigerated	1/2 muffin	81	2.5	14.7	114	1.1	1.3	0.2	0	15%
plain, 'Original'	1 muffin	146	6.4	28.5	350	2.7	1.8	(mq)	0	10%
wheatberry, 14-oz pkg	1 muffin	140	6.0	28.0	470	2.0	1.0	0.4	0	6%
(Thomas')										
honey wheat	1 muffin	129	5.0	24.0	200	>.4 c	1.1	na	0	8%
oat bran	1 muffin	116	4.2	26.0	192	2.9	1.2	na	0	8%
plain	1 muffin	130	4.3	25.4	206	(mq)	1.3	na	0	9%
raisin	1 muffin	153	4.5	30.4	200	>.2 c	1.5	(mq)	0	9%
rye	1 muffin	120	5.0	27.0	210	3.0	1.0	na	0	7%
(Wonder) plain	1 muffin	130	4.0	26.0	280	1.2	1.0	na	0	7%
ENSURE NUTRITION DRINK. See individual flavors.										
ENTRÉES. See individual entrées.										
EPPAW, raw	1/2 cup	75	2.3	15.8	6	>2.0 c	0.9	na	0	10%
EQUAL. See SUGAR SUBSTITUTE.										
EUCHALON. See CANDLEFISH.										

F

Food Name	Serving Size	Calories	Prot. gms	Carbs gms	Sod. mgs	Fiber gms	Fat gms	Sat. Fat gms	Chol. mgs	% Fat Cal.
FAJITA ENTREÉ, refrigerated *(Chicken By George)*	5 oz	170	28.0	2.0	370	na	6.0	(mq)	85	31%
FAJITA ENTREÉ, FROZEN										
beef *(Healthy Choice)*	7 oz	210	19.0	26.0	250	na	4.0	2.0	35	17%
chicken *(Healthy Choice)*	7 oz	200	17.0	25.0	310	na	3.0	1.0	35	14%
FAJITA ENTREÉ KIT										
(Tyson)	4 oz	80	7.0	2.0	240	na	2.0	na	na	33%
(Tyson) Wholesale Club Item	3.5 oz	160	10.0	18.0	420	na	5.0	na	30	29%
FAJITA MARINADE *(Old El Paso)*	1/8 jar	14	0.0	3.0	450	0	0.0	0.0	0	0%
FAJITA SAUCE. See SAUCE.										
FAJITA SEASONING MIX, 'Seasoning Blends' *(Lawry's)*	1 pkg	63	2.0	14.0	2118	>.5 c	0.4	na	na	5%
FALAFEL										
(Casbah) mix, dry	1 oz	103	7.0	15.0	na	(mq)	2.0	na	0	17%
(Fantastic Foods) mix 'Falafil' prepared	3 oz	129	8.0	20.0	188	(mq)	2.0	na	0	14%
(Near East) mix, prepared	3 patties	270	13.0	22.0	680	(mq)	15.0	(mq)	na	49%
FARINA. See CEREAL, HOT.										
FAT, ALTERNATIVE, 'Neutral Nyafat' *(Rokeach)*	1 tbsp	99	0.0	0.0	0	0	11.0	(mq)	0	100%
FATHEAD. See SHEEPSHEAD.										
FAVA BEAN /horse bean/jack bean										
boiled, drained	4 oz	64	5.4	11.5	47	>2.2 c	0.6	0.2	0	7%
mature seeds, boiled	1/2 cup	94	6.5	16.7	4	>.8 c	0.3	0.1	0	3%
mature seeds, raw	1/2 cup	256	19.6	43.7	10	18.75	1.1	0.2	0	4%
raw, trimmed	1/2 cup	40	3.1	6.4	28	>1.2 c	0.4	0.1	0	9%
raw, trimmed	1 oz	20	1.6	3.3	14	>.6 c	0.2	<.1	0	8%
raw, untrimmed	1 lb	317	24.6	51.5	220	>9.7 c	2.6	0.6	0	7%
Canned										
mature seeds	1/2 cup	91	7.0	15.9	580	>.5 c	0.3	0.1	0	3%

Food Name	Serving Size	Calories	Prot. gms	Carbs gms	Sod. mgs	Fiber gms	Fat gms	Sat. Fat gms	Chol. mgs	% Fat Cal.
mature seeds, w/liquid	4 oz	81	6.2	14.1	514	>.5 c	0.2	<.1	0	2%
Dried										
mature seeds, boiled	4 oz	125	8.6	22.3	6	5.8	0.5	0.1	0	4%
mature seeds, boiled	1/2 cup	93	6.5	16.7	4	4.3	0.3	0.1	0	3%
mature seeds, raw	1/2 cup	256	19.6	43.7	9	10.9	1.2	0.2	0	4%
mature seeds, raw	1 oz	97	7.4	16.5	4	4.1	0.4	0.1	0	4%
FEIJAO										
raw	1 fruit	25	0.6	5.3	2	na	0.4	na	0	13%
raw, purée	1 cup	119	3.0	25.8	7	na	1.9	na	0	13%
FENNEL/finocchio										
(Frieda's)	1 lb	68	5.0	11.8	408	(mq)	0.5	na	0	6%
(Frieda's)	1 oz	4	0.3	0.7	26	(mq)	<.1	(tr)	0	<18%
raw, bulb	1 bulb	73	2.9	17.1	122	na	0.5	na	0	5%
raw, leaves	100 gm	28	2.8	5.1	9	>.5 c	0.4	0.0	0	10%
raw, sliced	1 cup	27	1.1	6.3	45	na	0.2	na	0	6%
FENNEL SEED										
whole	1 oz	98	4.8	14.8	25	>4.4 c	4.2	0.1	0	33%
whole	1 tbsp	20	0.9	3.0	5	>.9 c	0.9	0.0	0	34%
whole	1 tsp	7	0.3	1.0	2	>.3 c	0.3	0.0	0	34%
whole (Durkee)	1 tsp	7	0.0	0.0	0	0	tr	na	na	tr
whole (Laurel Leaf)	1 tsp	7	0.0	0.0	0	0	tr	na	na	tr
whole (Spice Islands)	1 tsp	8	0.2	1.3	2	>.4 c	0.2	(tr)	0	23%
FENUGREEK SEED										
whole	1 oz	92	6.5	16.5	19	>2.9 c	1.8	na	0	15%
whole	1 tbsp	36	2.5	6.5	7	>1.1 c	0.7	na	0	15%
whole	1 tsp	12	0.9	2.2	2	>.4 c	0.2	na	0	13%
FETTUCCINE ENTRÉE, FROZEN										
Alfredo (Healthy Choice)	8 oz	240	10.0	36.0	370	na	7.0	2.0	45	26%
Alfredo (Lean Cuisine)	9 oz	280	14.0	41.0	570	na	7.0	3.0	15	22%
Alfredo (Weight Watchers)	8 oz	230	15.0	28.0	550	na	7.0	2.0	25	27%
Alfredo, 10-oz pkg (Stouffer's)	5 oz	245	8.0	22.0	400	na	14.0	na	na	51%
Alfredo, w/broccoli 'Lowfat' (Weight Watchers)	8 oz	230	15.0	28.0	550	na	7.0	2.0	25	27%
chicken (Healthy Choice)	8.5 oz	240	22.0	29.0	370	na	4.0	2.0	45	15%
primavera (Green Giant)	1 pkg	230	13.0	26.0	610	6.0	8.0	3.0	25	32%
primavera (Lean Cuisine)	10 oz	260	14.0	32.0	510	na	8.0	3.0	45	28%
primavera 'Microwave Garden Gourmet' (Green Giant)	1 pkg	260	17.0	25.0	640	6.0	13.0	(mq)	na	41%
w/broccoli (Dining Lite)	9 oz	290	12.0	33.0	1020	(mq)	12.0	(mq)	35	38%
w/meat sauce (Budget Gourmet)	10 oz	290	16.0	34.0	980	(mq)	10.0	(mq)	25	31%
FETTUCCINE ENTRÉE, MIX										
Alfredo 'Pasta & Cheese' prepared (Kraft)	1/2 cup	180	7.0	19.0	590	(mq)	9.0	3.0	30	44%
Alfredo 'Pasta & Sauce' (Hain)	1/4 pkg	180	5.0	27.0	420	(mq)	4.0	(mq)	na	22%
FETTUCCINE LUNCH, FROZEN,										
Alfredo sauce 'Lunch Express' w/chicken (Lean Cuisine)	10.25 oz	240	16.0	31.0	540	na	6.0	2.0	35	22%
FIELD PEAS, CANNED										
'Fresh' (Allens)	1/2 cup	100	7.0	18.0	370	(mq)	<1.0	na	0	<8%
'Fresh' w/snaps (Allens)	1/2 cup	100	5.0	20.0	370	(mq)	<1.0	na	0	<8%
tiny, 'Fresh' w/snaps (Allens)	1/2 cup	70	6.0	13.0	340	(mq)	<1.0	na	0	<11%
w/snaps (Bush's Best)	1/2 cup	80	6.0	16.0	550	3.0	0.0	na	na	0%
FIG										
candied	100 gm	299	3.5	73.7	34	>5.6 c	0.2	0.0	0	1%
raw, w/o stem	1 large	47	0.5	12.3	1	2.1	0.2	0.0	0	3%
raw, w/o stem	1 med	37	0.4	9.6	1	1.6	0.2	0.0	0	4%
trimmed	1 oz	21	0.2	5.4	<1	>.3 c	0.1	<.1	0	4%
w/stems	1 lb	333	3.4	86.1	5	>5.4 c	1.4	0.3	0	3%

Food Name	Serving Size	Calories	Prot. gms	Carbs gms	Sod. mgs	Fiber gms	Fat gms	Sat. Fat gms	Chol. mgs	% Fat Cal.
Canned										
in extra heavy syrup	4 oz	121	0.4	31.6	1	>.6 c	0.1	<.1	0	1%
in extra heavy syrup, solid and liquid	1 cup	279	1.0	72.7	3	>1.4 c	0.3	0.1	0	1%
in extra heavy syrup, w/1.75 tbsp liquid	3 fruits	91	0.3	23.7	1	>.5 c	0.1	0.0	0	1%
in heavy syrup	4 oz	100	0.4	26.0	1	>.6 c	0.1	<.1	0	1%
In heavy syrup, solid and liquid	1 cup	228	1.0	59.3	3	5.7	0.3	0.1	0	1%
in heavy syrup, whole (Del Monte)	1/2 cup	100	0.0	28.0	10	(mq)	0.0	0.0	0	0%
in heavy syrup, whole, Kadota 'Fancy' (S&W)	1/2 cup	100	0.0	28.0	10	(mq)	0.0	0.0	0	0%
in heavy syrup, w/1.75 tbsp liquid	3 fruits	75	0.3	19.5	1	1.9	0.1	0.0	0	1%
in light syrup	1/2 cup	87	0.5	22.6	2	2.2	0.1	<.1	0	1%
in light syrup	4 oz	78	0.4	20.4	1	>.6 c	0.1	<.1	0	1%
in light syrup, solid and liquid	1 cup	174	1.0	45.2	3	>1.4 c	0.3	0.1	0	1%
in light syrup, w/1.75 tbsp liquid	3 fruits	59	0.3	15.3	1	1.5	0.1	0.0	0	1%
in water	1/2 cup	65	0.5	17.3	2	>.7 c	0.1	<.1	0	1%
in water	4 oz	60	0.5	15.9	1	>.6 c	0.1	<.1	0	1%
in water, solid and liquid	1 cup	131	1.0	34.7	2	5.5	0.3	0.1	0	2%
in water, w/1.75 tbsp liquid	3 fruits	42	0.3	11.2	1	1.8	0.1	0.0	0	2%
Dried										
cooked	4 oz	122	1.5	31.3	6	>2.3 c	0.6	0.1	0	4%
stewed	1/2 cup	140	1.7	35.8	7	6.2	0.6	0.1	0	4%
uncooked	1 cup	507	6.1	130.1	22	18.5	2.3	0.5	0	4%
uncooked	4 oz	289	3.5	74.1	15	10.5	1.3	0.3	0	4%
uncooked, Calimyrna (Blue Ribbon)	1/2 cup	250	3.0	58.0	10	(mq)	2.0	(mq)	0	7%
uncooked, Calimyrna (Sun•Maid)	1/2 cup	250	3.0	58.0	10	(mq)	2.0	(mq)	0	7%
uncooked, Mission (Blue Ribbon)	1/2 cup	210	3.0	1.0	20	(mq)	(mq)	(mq)	0	0%
uncooked, Mission (Sun•Maid)	1/2 cup	210	3.0	1.0	20	(mq)	(mq)	(mq)	0	0%
uncooked, trimmed	10 fruits	477	5.7	122.2	21	17.4	2.2	0.4	0	4%
FILBERT, SHELLED. See HAZELNUT, SHELLED.										
FILBERT BUTTER, roasted (Maranatha Natural)	2 tbsp	180	5.0	6.0	5	na	16.0	na	na	77%
FILO DOUGH. See PHYLLO DOUGH.										
FINNAN HADDIE, smoked	4 oz	132	28.6	0.0	865	0	1.1	0.2	87	8%
FINOCCHIO. See FENNEL.										
FISH. See individual listings.										
FISH CAKE										
fried	1 cake	103	8.8	5.6	106	0	4.8	1.8	25	43%
fried, bite size	5 cakes	103	8.8	5.6	106	0	4.8	1.8	25	43%
frozen (Mrs. Paul's)	2 pieces	190	9.0	24.0	690	(mq)	7.0	(mq)	20	32%
FISH DINNER, FROZEN										
(Healthy Choice) lemon pepper, 10.7 oz	1 serving	300	13.0	52.0	370	na	5.0	1.0	40	15%
(Kid Cuisine) nuggets	7 oz	320	13.0	33.0	750	(mq)	15.0	(mq)	45	42%
(Morton)	9.75 oz	370	18.0	46.0	910	(mq)	13.0	(mq)	65	31%
(Swanson) n' chips	10 oz	500	20.0	60.0	960	(mq)	21.0	(mq)	(mq)	37%
FISH ENTRÉE										
Canned, Dijon 'Light' (Mrs. Paul's)	8.75 oz	200	21.0	17.0	650	(mq)	5.0	2.0	60	23%
Frozen										
fillet of, divan (Lean Cuisine)	10 3/8 oz	210	27.0	13.0	490	na	5.0	2.0	65	22%
fillet of, Florentine (Lean Cuisine)	9 5/8 oz	220	26.0	13.0	590	na	7.0	3.0	65	29%
fillet of, Florentine 'Light' (Mrs. Paul's)	8 oz	220	25.0	10.0	820	(mq)	8.0	4.0	95	34%
fish 'n fries 'Home Style Recipe' (Swanson)	6.5 oz	340	11.0	37.0	670	(mq)	16.0	(mq)	(mq)	43%
gems, fancy style (Wakefield)	4 oz	80	11.0	11.0	(mq)	(mq)	1.0	na	(mq)	9%
gems, salad style (Wakefield)	3 oz	70	10.0	8.0	(mq)	na	1.0	na	(mq)	11%
in herb sauce (Gorton's)	1 pkg	190	26.0	3.0	450	(mq)	8.0	5.0	90	38%
Mornay 'Light' (Mrs. Paul's)	9 oz	230	24.0	12.0	670	(mq)	10.0	4.0	80	39%
oven baked, w/vegetable medley (Ultimate 200)	6.64 oz	120	16.0	10.0	390	na	2.0	<1.0	0	15%

Food Name	Serving Size	Calories	Prot. gms	Carbs gms	Sod. mgs	Fiber gms	Fat gms	Sat. Fat gms	Chol. mgs	% Fat Cal.
'Platters' *(Banquet)*	8.75 oz	450	31.0	33.0	(mq)	(mq)	22.0	(mq)	95	44%
salmon, Keta *(Libby's)*	3.7 oz	130	20.0	0.0	450	na	6.0	2.0	40	40%
sticks 'Looney Tunes Sylvester' *(Tyson)*	7.5 oz	290	13.0	36.0	510	na	11.0	na	17	34%
FISH FILLET, ALTERNATIVE										
vegetarian, frozen *(Worthington)* 1.5-oz pieces	2 pieces	180	15.0	9.0	910	(mq)	9.0	2.0	0	46%
FISH FILLET, FROZEN										
battered *(Mrs. Paul's)*	2 pieces	330	16.0	28.0	650	(mq)	17.0	(mq)	60	47%
battered *(Van de Kamp's)*	1 piece	170	7.0	13.0	350	(mq)	10.0	2.0	20	53%
battered 'Crispy Batter' *(Gorton's)*	2 pieces	290	11.0	18.0	550	(mq)	19.0	8.0	35	60%
battered 'Crispy Batter' large *(Gorton's)*	1 piece	320	12.0	20.0	680	(mq)	21.0	(mq)	(mq)	60%
battered 'Crunchy' *(Gorton's)*	2 pieces	230	13.0	16.0	420	(mq)	13.0	3.0	40	50%
battered 'Crunchy' *(Mrs. Paul's)*	2 pieces	280	12.0	26.0	730	(mq)	14.0	3.0	22	45%
battered 'Crunchy Microwave' *(Gorton's)*	2 pieces	340	10.0	17.0	400	(mq)	26.0	12.0	30	68%
battered 'Crunchy Microwave' large *(Gorton's)*	1 piece	320	11.0	20.0	500	(mq)	22.0	10.0	35	62%
battered, minced 'Portions' *(Mrs. Paul's)*	2 pieces	300	11.0	21.0	540	(mq)	19.0	3.0	33	57%
battered 'Potato Crisp' *(Gorton's)*	2 pieces	300	12.0	18.0	360	(mq)	20.0	6.0	30	60%
battered, tempura 'Light Recipe' *(Gorton's)*	1 piece	200	10.0	8.0	400	(mq)	14.0	4.0	30	64%
battered 'Value Pack Portions' *(Gorton's)*	1 piece	180	7.0	13.0	490	(mq)	11.0	(mq)	(mq)	55%
breaded *(Van de Kamp's)*	2 pieces	280	11.0	18.0	280	(mq)	18.0	3.0	35	58%
breaded 'Crisp and Healthy' baked *(Van de Kamp's)*	2 pieces	150	12.0	18.0	350	na	3.0	<1.0	25	18%
breaded 'Crispy Crunchy' *(Mrs. Paul's)*	2 pieces	220	13.0	23.0	380	(mq)	9.0	2.0	22	36%
breaded, crispy 'Microwave' *(Van de Kamp's)*	1 piece	140	6.0	9.0	210	(mq)	9.0	2.0	15	57%
breaded, crispy 'Microwave' large *(Van de Kamp's)*	1 piece	290	12.0	21.0	640	(mq)	17.0	3.0	25	54%
breaded, 8 fillets *(Healthy Choice)*	2.5 oz	120	9.0	11.0	250	na	4.0	<1.0	20	31%
breaded, 4 fillets *(Healthy Choice)*	3 oz	140	10.0	14.0	300	na	4.0	<1.0	25	27%
breaded 'Light Recipe' *(Gorton's)*	1 piece	180	11.0	16.0	380	(mq)	8.0	3.0	30	40%
breaded, minced 'Crispy Crunchy Portions' *(Mrs. Paul's)*	2 pieces	230	10.0	14.0	300	(mq)	15.0	2.0	25	58%
breaded, reheated, 2 oz	1 piece	155	8.9	13.5	332	>.2 c	7.0	1.8	64	41%
breaded 'Snack Pack' *(Van de Kamp's)*	2 pieces	220	8.0	13.0	280	na	10.0	2.0	20	52%
breaded, 2 fillets *(Healthy Choice)*	3.5 oz	160	12.0	16.0	350	na	5.0	<1.0	30	29%
coated, ranch 'Specialty Microwave' *(Gorton's)*	1 piece	330	12.0	24.0	520	(mq)	21.0	(mq)	(mq)	57%
crispy, microwave *(Van de Kamp's)*	1 piece	140	6.0	9.0	210	na	9.0	2.0	15	57%
crispy, microwave large *(Van de Kamp's)*	1 piece	290	12.0	21.0	640	na	17.0	3.0	25	54%
in butter sauce 'Light' *(Mrs. Paul's)*	1 piece	140	20.0	1.0	520	na	6.0	(mq)	40	39%
marinated, Cajun style, catfish 'Select' *(Gorton's)*	1 fillet	220	22.0	3.0	560	na	13.0	3.0	90	54%
FISH LOAF, cooked	1 loaf	1507	171.3	88.7	2151	0	45.0	12.2	486	28%
FISH NUGGET, FROZEN, battered *(Van de Kamp's)*	4 pieces	130	5.0	8.0	310	na	9.0	1.0	10	61%
FISH OIL										
herring	1 cup	1966	0.0	0.0	0	0	218.0	46.4	1670	100%
herring	1 tbsp	123	0.0	0.0	0	0	13.6	2.9	104	100%
menhaden	1 cup	1966	0.0	0.0	0	0	218.0	66.3	1136	100%
menhaden	1 tbsp	123	0.0	0.0	0	0	13.6	4.1	71	100%
menhaden, fully hydrogenated	1 cup	1849	0.0	0.0	0	0	205.0	196.0	1025	100%
menhaden, fully hydrogenated	1 tbsp	113	0.0	0.0	0	0	12.5	11.9	63	100%
salmon	1 cup	1966	0.0	0.0	0	0	218.0	43.3	1057	100%
salmon	1 tbsp	123	0.0	0.0	0	0	13.6	2.7	66	100%
sardine	1 cup	1966	0.0	0.0	0	0	218.0	65.2	1548	100%
sardine	1 tbsp	123	0.0	0.0	0	0	13.6	4.1	97	100%
FISH PASTE CAKE										
Japanese, block, steamed 'Kamoboko'	4 oz	111	13.6	11.0	1134	na	1.0	(mq)	(mq)	8%
Japanese, stick, grilled 'Chikuwa'	4 oz	143	13.8	15.3	1134	na	2.4	(mq)	(mq)	16%
FISH SEASONING MIX. See SEAFOOD SEASONING MIX.										
FISH STICKS, FROZEN										
battered *(Mrs. Paul's)*	4 pieces	210	7.0	15.0	590	(mq)	12.0	(mq)	25	55%

Food Name	Serving Size	Calories	Prot. gms	Carbs gms	Sod. mgs	Fiber gms	Fat gms	Sat. Fat gms	Chol. mgs	% Fat Cal.
battered *(Van de Kamp's)*	4 pieces	160	8.0	12.0	350	(mq)	9.0	2.0	20	50%
battered 'Crispy Batter' *(Gorton's)*	4 pieces	260	9.0	16.0	480	(mq)	18.0	6.0	25	62%
battered 'Crunchy' *(Gorton's)*	4 pieces	210	7.0	15.0	240	(mq)	13.0	4.0	25	57%
battered, minced *(Mrs. Paul's)*	4 pieces	220	8.0	20.0	630	(mq)	13.0	2.0	20	51%
battered 'Potato Crisp' *(Gorton's)*	4 pieces	260	8.0	21.0	390	(mq)	16.0	5.0	25	55%
battered 'Value Pack' *(Gorton's)*	4 pieces	190	9.0	17.0	420	(mq)	9.0	(mq)	(mq)	44%
breaded *(Healthy Choice)*	2.4 oz	120	8.0	14.0	350	na	4.0	<1.0	20	29%
breaded *(Van de Kamp's)*	4 pieces	200	9.0	15.0	290	(mq)	12.0	2.0	20	53%
breaded 'Bunch o' Crunch' approx 2.7 oz *(Frionor)*	4 pieces	210	9.0	13.0	267	<.1	14.0	2.0	(mq)	59%
breaded 'Crisp and Healthy,' baked *(Van de Kamp's)*	4 pieces	120	9.0	17.0	330	na	2.0	<1.0	15	15%
breaded 'Crispy Crunchy' *(Mrs. Paul's)*	4 pieces	140	7.0	14.0	340	(mq)	6.0	(mq)	20	39%
breaded, crispy 'Microwave' *(Van de Kamp's)*	3 pieces	130	7.0	11.0	280	(mq)	7.0	1.0	15	47%
breaded, minced 'Crispy Crunchy' *(Mrs. Paul's)*	4 pieces	190	9.0	18.0	560	(mq)	8.0	(mq)	25	40%
breaded 'Snack Pack' *(Van de Kamp's)*	4 pieces	170	8.0	13.0	270	na	10.0	2.0	20	52%
breaded 'Value Pack' *(Van de Kamp's)*	4 pieces	170	8.0	13.0	270	(mq)	10.0	2.0	20	52%
breaded w/whole wheat 'Microwave' *(Booth)*	2 oz	150	6.0	14.0	210	(mq)	8.0	(mq)	(mq)	47%
FIVE-SPICE, Oriental spice *(Tone's)*	1 tsp	9	0.3	1.9	2	.5	0.3	<.1	0	24%
FLAN. See PUDDING MIX.										
FLATFISH. See FLOUNDER; HALIBUT; SOLE.										
FLAX OIL										
(Spectrum Naturals) organic 'Veg-Omega 3'	1 tbsp	120	0.0	0.0	0	(tr)	14.0	1.0	(tr)	100%
(Spectrum Naturals) organic 'Veg-Omega 3' cinnamon flavored	1 tbsp	120	0.0	0.0	0	(tr)	14.0	1.0	(tr)	100%
FLAXSEED *(Arrowhead Mills)*	1 oz	140	5.0	11.0	<1	6.0	10.0	(mq)	0	58%
FLOUNDER										
dry-heat cooked	3 oz	99	20.5	0.0	89	0	1.3	0.3	58	13%
raw	3 oz	77	16.0	0.0	69	0	1.0	0.2	41	12%
FLOUNDER, FROZEN										
(Booth) Atlantic	4 oz	90	19.0	0.0	180	0	1.0	(mq)	(mq)	11%
(Finast)	4 oz	90	19.0	0.0	150	0	1.0	(mq)	(mq)	11%
(Gorton's) crunch breaded, fillet 'Select' approx. 2.9 oz	1 fillet	190	10.0	17.0	420	na	9.0	2.0	30	43%
(Gorton's) 'Fishmarket Fresh'	5 oz	110	23.0	1.0	170	0	1.0	(mq)	(mq)	9%
(Mrs. Paul's) battered, fillets 'Crunchy'	2 pieces	220	12.0	23.0	560	(mq)	9.0	(mq)	40	37%
(Mrs. Paul's) breaded, fillets 'Light'	1 piece	240	16.0	20.0	450	(mq)	10.0	(mq)	50	39%
(SeaPak)	4 oz	90	20.0	0.0	120	0	1.0	(mq)	(mq)	10%
(Van de Kamp's) breaded fillets 'Light'	1 piece	260	18.0	21.0	480	(mq)	12.0	2.0	45	41%
(Van de Kamp's) fillet 'Light'	1 piece	260	18.0	21.0	480	na	12.0	2.0	45	41%
(Van de Kamp's) 'Natural'	4 oz	100	22.0	0.0	100	0	2.0	0.0	35	17%
FLOUNDER ENTRÉE, FROZEN										
stuffed 'Microwave Entrees' *(Gorton's)*	1 pkg	350	25.0	21.0	850	(mq)	18.0	7.0	120	47%
FLOUR. See also individual listings.										
all-purpose, 4 oz *(Gold Medal)*	1 cup	400	11.0	87.0	0	na	1.0	na	na	2%
all-purpose, 4 oz *(Red Band)*	1 cup	290	10.0	85.0	0	na	1.0	na	na	2%
all-purpose, 4 oz *(Robin Hood)*	1 cup	400	13.0	85.0	0	na	1.0	na	na	2%
'Better for Bread' 4 oz *(Gold Medal)*	1 cup	400	14.0	83.0	0	na	1.0	na	na	2%
'Drifted Snow, 4 oz *(Red Band)*	1 cup	400	11.0	87.0	0	na	1.0	na	na	2%
'La Piña' 4 oz *(Red Band)*	1 cup	400	10.0	87.0	0	na	1.0	na	na	2%
self-rising, 4 oz *(Gold Medal)*	1 cup	380	10.0	83.0	1520	na	1.0	na	na	2%
self-rising, 4 oz *(Red Band)*	1 cup	380	9.0	83.0	1520	na	1.0	na	na	2%
self-rising, 4 oz *(Robin Hood)*	1 cup	380	10.0	83.0	1520	na	1.0	na	na	2%
'Softasilk' 1 oz *(Red Band)*	1/4 cup	100	2.0	23.0	0	na	0.0	na	na	0%
unbleached, 4 oz *(Gold Medal)*	1 cup	400	11.0	87.0	0	na	1.0	na	na	2%
unbleached, 4 oz *(Robin Hood)*	1 cup	400	13.0	85.0	0	na	1.0	na	na	2%
'Wondra' 4 oz *(Red Band)*	1 cup	400	11.0	87.0	0	na	1.0	na	na	2%

Food Name	Serving Size	Calories	Prot. gms	Carbs gms	Sod. mgs	Fiber gms	Fat gms	Sat. Fat gms	Chol. mgs	% Fat Cal.
FLYING FISH										
raw	1 lb	413	95.3	0.0	(mq)	0	0.9	(mq)	(mq)	2%
raw	1 oz	26	6.0	0.0	(mq)	0	<.1	(mq)	(mq)	<4%
FON GOOT YAM. See JICAMA.										
FONDANT. See CANDY.										
FORMULA, INFANT. See BABY FOOD.										
FRANKFURTER										
beef and pork, 1 oz	1 frank	91	3.2	0.7	318	0	8.3	3.1	14	83%
cheesefurter/cheese smokie, 1 oz	1 frank	93	4.0	0.4	307	0	8.2	3.0	19	81%
cheesefurter/cheese smokie, approx 1.5 oz	1 frank	141	6.0	0.6	465	0	12.5	4.5	29	81%
chicken, 1 oz	1 frank	73	3.7	1.9	388	0	5.5	1.6	29	69%
raw, beef and pork, 2 oz	1 frank	182	6.4	1.5	638	0	16.6	6.1	28	83%
raw, w/nonfat dry milk and cereal, 2 oz	1 frank	156	8.1	0.0	627	0	12.4	5.1	37	78%
turkey, 1 oz	1 frank	64	4.1	0.4	404	0	5.0	1.7	30	71%
(Ball Park)										
beef 'Lite'	1 frank	140	7.0	1.0	na	na	12.0	na	na	77%
beef, pork and chicken 'Lite'	1 frank	140	7.0	1.0	na	na	12.0	na	na	77%
(Boar's Head)										
beef, 1 oz	1 frank	80	4.0	<1.0	(mq)	0	7.0	(mq)	15	76%
pork and beef, 1 oz	1 frank	80	4.0	<1.0	250	0	7.0	(mq)	15	76%
(Butterball) turkey	1 frank	140	7.0	2.0	610	0	11.0	(mq)	(mq)	73%
(Eckrich)										
beef 'Jumbo'	1 frank	190	6.0	2.0	520	0	17.0	(mq)	(mq)	83%
beef '1-lb pkg'	1 frank	150	5.0	2.0	400	0	14.0	(mq)	(mq)	82%
'Bunsize'	1 frank	190	6.0	2.0	500	0	17.0	(mq)	(mq)	83%
cheesefurter/cheese smokie	1 frank	180	7.0	2.0	530	0	16.0	(mq)	(mq)	80%
'Jumbo Lean Supreme'	1 frank	140	7.0	2.0	490	0	12.0	(mq)	(mq)	75%
'1-lb pkg'	1 frank	160	5.0	2.0	420	0	14.0	(mq)	(mq)	82%
(Health Valley)										
chicken 'Weiners'	1 frank	96	5.0	1.0	90	0	8.0	(mq)	49	75%
turkey 'Weiners'	1 frank	96	5.0	1.0	112	0	8.0	(mq)	35	75%
(Healthy Choice) turkey, pork, and beef 'Jumbo' lowfat	1 frank	70	8.0	5.0	570	na	2.0	1.0	20	26%
(Healthy Favorites) w/turkey, 2 oz	1 frank	57	8.5	2.1	572	0	1.6	0.6	24	25%

QUICK REFERENCE: FRANKFURTERS

The frankfurter is as American as apple pie. Unlike apple pie, though, hot dogs are rarely eaten as is. Usually, the frank is sandwiched in a bun and crowned with mustard, sauerkraut, or other condiments. These toppings do more than enhance flavor; they add fat and calories, too. The following table will give you a rough idea of how your hot dog fixings are adding up.

Food Name	Serving Size	Calories	Prot. gms	Carbs gms	Sod. mgs	Fiber gms	Fat gms	Sat. Fat gms	Chol. mgs	% Fat Cal.
Hot dog bun	1 bun	123	3.7	21.6	241	1.0	2.2	0.5	0	16%
White bread	1 slice	70	3.0	13.0	140	.7	1.0	na	na	12%
Whole wheat bread	1 slice	60	3.0	11.0	125	2.0	1.0	0.0	0	14%
American cheese	1 oz	110	0.0	1.0	450	0	0.0	5.0	26	74%
Catsup	1 tbsp	16	0.2	14.1	178	.2	0.1	0.0	0	5%
Mustard	1 tbsp	10	1.0	1.0	180	na	1.0	na	0	53%
Pickle Relish	1 tbsp	20	0.1	5.3	122	7.1	0.1	0.0	0	4%
Sauerkraut	1/2 cup	25	1.0	6.0	775	(mq)	0.0	0.0	0	0%
Chili (w/beans)	1/2 cup	143	7.3	15.2	668	5.6	7.0	3.0	22	41%

Food Name	Serving Size	Calories	Prot. gms	Carbs gms	Sod. mgs	Fiber gms	Fat gms	Sat. Fat gms	Chol. mgs	% Fat Cal
(Hebrew National) beef, 1.7 oz	1 frank	149	5.8	<1.0	497	0	14.0	(mq)	15	82%
(Hillshire Farm)										
beef 'Bun Size Wieners' 2 oz	1 frank	180	7.0	2.0	560	0	16.0	(mq)	(mq)	80%
beef 'Hot Links' 2 oz	1 frank	190	8.0	1.0	560	0	17.0	(mq)	(mq)	81%
cheesefurter/cheese smokie 'Bun Size Wieners' 2 oz	1 frank	180	7.0	2.0	530	0	16.0	(mq)	(mq)	80%
'Hot Links' 2 oz	1 frank	190	8.0	2.0	530	0	16.0	(mq)	(mq)	78%
natural casing 'Wieners' 2 oz	1 frank	180	6.0	2.0	470	0	17.0	(mq)	(mq)	83%
(Hormel)										
batter-wrapped, frozen 'Corn Dogs'	1 frank	220	7.0	21.0	656	(mq)	12.0	(mq)	(mq)	49%
batter-wrapped, frozen 'Tater Dogs'	1 frank	210	6.0	15.0	170	(mq)	14.0	(mq)	(mq)	60%
beef '1-lb pkg'	1 frank	140	5.0	1.0	463	0	13.0	(mq)	(mq)	83%
beef '12-oz pkg'	1 frank	100	4.0	1.0	362	0	10.0	(mq)	(mq)	82%
chili 'Frank 'n Stuff'	1 frank	165	7.0	2.0	517	na	15.0	(mq)	(mq)	79%
'Light & Lean 97' 1.6 oz	1 frank	45	6.0	2.0	390	na	1.0	<2.0	15	22%
Mexicali Dogs' 5 oz	1 frank	400	14.0	41.0	952	na	21.0	(mq)	(mq)	46%
'1-lb pkg'	1 frank	140	5.0	1.0	486	0	13.0	(mq)	(mq)	83%
smoked, beef 'Wranglers'	1 frank	170	7.0	2.0	619	0	15.0	(mq)	(mq)	79%
smoked 'Range Brand Wranglers'	1 frank	170	7.0	1.0	600	0	16.0	(mq)	(mq)	82%
smoked, w/cheese 'Wranglers'	1 frank	180	8.0	1.0	546	0	16.0	(mq)	(mq)	80%
'12-oz pkg'	1 frank	110	4.0	1.0	378	0	10.0	(mq)	(mq)	82%
(Hygrade) chicken 'Grillmaster'	1 frank	130	7.0	3.0	na	na	11.0	na	na	71%
(JM)										
beef, 1.2 oz	1 frank	100	4.0	1.0	350	0	9.0	(mq)	20	80%
beef 'Jumbo' 2 oz	1 frank	180	6.0	2.0	600	0	16.0	(mq)	33	82%
beef '10 per lb pkg' 1.6 oz	1 frank	140	5.0	1.0	480	0	13.0	(mq)	26	83%
cheesefurter/cheese smokie 'Cheese Franks' 1.6 oz	1 frank	140	5.0	2.0	540	0	13.0	(mq)	(mq)	81%
'German Brand' 2 oz	1 frank	160	7.0	1.0	620	0	14.0	(mq)	(mq)	80%
1.2 oz	1 frank	110	4.0	1.0	370	0	10.0	(mq)	16	82%
'10 per lb' 1.6 oz	1 frank	140	5.0	1.0	490	0	13.0	(mq)	22	83%
w/cheese 'German Brand' 2 oz	1 frank	160	8.0	2.0	620	0	14.0	(mq)	37	76%
(Kahn's)										
beef	1 frank	140	5.0	2.0	500	0	13.0	(mq)	(mq)	81%
beef 'Bun Size Franks'	1 frank	190	6.0	3.0	560	0	17.0	(mq)	(mq)	81%
beef 'Jumbo'	1 frank	190	6.0	3.0	560	0	18.0	(mq)	(mq)	82%
beef w/cheddar 'Beef n' Cheddar'	1 frank	180	7.0	2.0	640	0	16.0	(mq)	(mq)	80%
cheesefurter/cheese smokie 'Cheese Wiener'	1 frank	150	6.0	1.0	490	0	13.0	(mq)	(mq)	81%
smoked, beef 'Bun Size Beef Smokey'	1 frank	190	7.0	2.0	530	0	17.0	(mq)	(mq)	81%
smoked 'Big Red Smokey'	1 frank	170	8.0	2.0	550	0	14.0	(mq)	(mq)	76%
smoked 'Bun Size Smokey'	1 frank	180	8.0	2.0	550	0	15.0	(mq)	(mq)	77%
'Wieners'	1 frank	140	5.0	1.0	500	0	13.0	(mq)	(mq)	83%
(King Kold) beef, 2 oz	1 frank	173	9.0	1.0	815	0	16.3	(mq)	(mq)	79%
(Longacre)										
chicken	1 frank	63	4.0	1.0	230	0	5.0	(mq)	30	69%
turkey	1 frank	66	4.0	0.0	260	0	6.0	(mq)	30	77%
(Louis Rich)										
turkey 'Bun Length' 2 oz	1 frank	128	7.2	1.5	640	0	10.4	3.4	53	73%
turkey, cheese, 1.6 oz	1 frank	109	6.1	1.3	523	0	8.9	2.9	44	73%
turkey, 1.6 oz	1 frank	101	5.7	1.2	505	0	8.2	2.7	42	73%
(Mr. Turkey)										
turkey, 1.6 oz	1 frank	106	5.5	0.9	440	0	8.9	(mq)	31	76%
turkey, cheese, 1.6 oz	1 frank	109	5.9	0.9	526	0	9.1	(mq)	29	75%
(OHSE)										
beef, 1 oz	1 frank	85	3.0	1.0	280	0	8.0	(mq)	(mq)	82%
chicken, beef, and pork, 1 oz	1 frank	85	3.0	1.0	260	0	8.0	(mq)	(mq)	82%

Food Name	Serving Size	Calories	Prot. gms	Carbs gms	Sod. mgs	Fiber gms	Fat gms	Sat. Fat gms	Chol. mgs	% Fat Cal
'Wieners' 1 oz	1 frank	90	3.0	1.0	300	0	8.0	(mq)	(mq)	82%
(Oscar Mayer)										
bacon and cheddar cheese										
beef 'Bun-Length Franks' 2 oz	1 frank	182	6.3	1.4	568	0	16.8	7.3	34	83%
beef, deli 'Big & Juicy' 2.7 oz	1 frank	249	8.9	0.5	677	0	23.5	10.0	49	85%
beef 'Franks' 2 oz	1 frank	181	6.3	1.4	583	0	16.7	7.0	35	83%
beef, garlic 'Big & Juicy' 2.7 oz	1 frank	239	9.0	0.2	652	0	22.5	9.4	51	85%
beef 'Light Franks' 2 oz	1 frank	131	6.8	0.9	594	0	11.1	4.6	23	76%
beef, quarter lb, bun length 'Big & Juicy' 4 oz	1 frank	359	12.8	1.6	1146	0	33.5	14.6	64	84%
beef w/cheddar 'Franks' 2 oz	1 frank	163	7.5	1.1	655	0	14.3	6.4	36	79%
'Bun-Length Wieners' 2 oz	1 frank	184	6.3	1.4	571	0	16.9	6.2	34	83%
cheesefurter/cheese smokie 'Hot Dogs' 1.6 oz	1 frank	143	5.4	1.1	480	0	12.9	5.3	30	82%
cocktail 'Little Wieners' .3 oz	1 frank	28	1.1	0.2	92	0	2.6	1.0	5	82%
hot and spicy 'Big & Juicy' 2.7 oz	1 frank	224	9.5	0.6	773	0	20.4	7.5	46	82%
'Hot Dogs' 1.6 oz	1 frank	137	6.3	1.0	501	0	12.0	5.0	29	79%
'Light Wieners' 2 oz	1 frank	127	7.3	0.3	623	0	10.8	3.8	30	76%
97% fat free, turkey, beef 'Healthy Favorites'	1 frank	60	9.0	2.0	570	na	1.5	.5	25	23%
original 'Big & Juicy' 2.7 oz	1 frank	244	8.9	0.0	690	0	23.2	9.4	43	85%
'Wieners' 2 oz	1 frank	181	6.3	1.4	576	0	16.9	6.4	36	83%
(Pilgrim's Pride)										
'1-lb pkg' 2-oz frank	1 frank	118	7.8	1.1	456	0	8.8	(mq)	31	69%
'12-oz pkg' 1.5-oz frank	1 frank	88	5.8	0.8	342	0	6.6	(mq)	24	69%
(Quick Meal) w/chili, and cheese, 4.5 oz	1 frank	340	14.0	25.0	540	na	20.0	8.0	80	54%
(State Fair) beef, batter-wrapped, on stick 'Corn Dogs' 2.67 oz	1 frank	210	6.0	24.0	na	na	10.0	na	na	43%
(Tyson)										
chicken	1 frank	115	6.0	1.0	700	na	10.0	na	na	76%
chicken, batter-wrapped 'Corn Dogs' 3.5 oz	1 frank	280	9.0	28.0	70	(mq)	14.0	(mq)	75	46%
w/cheese	1 frank	145	7.0	1.0	680	na	11.0	na	na	76%
FRANKFURTER, ALTERNATIVE										
(Smart Dog) 'Lightlife' fat-free, 1.5 oz	1 frank	40	8.2	1.1	290	na	0.0	na	0	0%
(White Wave Soyfood) 'Healthy' 1.5 oz	1 frank	120	7.0	5.0	340	na	8.0	1.0	0	60%
(Worthington)										
canned 'Super-Links' 1.7 oz	1 frank	100	7.0	3.0	440	(mq)	7.0	1.0	0	61%
canned 'Veja-Links'	2 franks	140	8.0	4.0	330	(mq)	10.0	(mq)	0	65%
frozen 'Leanies' 1.4 oz	1 frank	100	8.0	2.0	440	(mq)	6.0	1.0	0	57%
frozen, on a stick 'Dixie Dogs' 2.5 oz	1 frank	200	8.0	21.0	640	(mq)	10.0	(mq)	0	44%
FRENCH ARTICHOKE. See ARTICHOKES, FRENCH.										
FRENCH BEAN										
boiled	4 oz	146	8.0	27.2	7	>1.6 c	0.9	0.1	0	5%
dried, boiled	1/2 cup	111	6.1	20.7	5	>1.2 c	0.7	0.1	0	6%
raw	1/2 cup	316	17.3	59.0	17	>3.4 c	1.9	0.2	0	5%
raw, dried	1 oz	97	5.3	18.2	5	>1.1 c	0.6	0.1	0	5%
FRENCH TOAST, FROZEN										
(Aunt Jemima) cinnamon swirl	3 oz	171	6.7	27.5	516	1.3	4.3	1.0	41	22%
(Aunt Jemima) 'Original'	3 oz	166	6.7	26.5	554	1.3	4.4	1.0	46	23%
(Aunt Jemima) sticks, and syrup 'Homestyle'	5.2 oz	400	7.0	48.0	640	(mq)	20.0	(mq)	(mq)	45%
(Aunt Jemima) wedges, and sausages 'Homestyle'	5.3 oz	360	13.0	40.0	780	(mq)	17.0	(mq)	(mq)	42%
(Downyflake)	2 slices	270	6.0	34.0	380	(mq)	12.0	(mq)	73	40%
(Downyflake) 'Extra Thick'	1 slice	150	5.0	11.0	340	(mq)	9.0	(mq)	(mq)	56%
(Downyflake) Texas style, and sausage	4.25 oz	400	10.0	37.0	550	(mq)	24.0	(mq)	(mq)	54%
(Krusteaz) cinnamon swirl	2 slices	270	10.0	46.0	370	na	5.0	na	120	17%
(Krusteaz) regular	2 slices	250	11.0	38.0	380	na	6.0	1.3	120	22%
(Morningstar Farms) vegetarian, cinnamon swirl, w/patties	6.5 oz	380	24.0	37.0	1220	4.0	15.0	(mq)	0	36%
(Swanson) cinnamon swirl, w/sausages 'Great Start'	5.5 oz	390	12.0	37.0	530	(mq)	21.0	(mq)	(mq)	49%

Food Name	Serving Size	Calories	Prot. gms	Carbs gms	Sod. mgs	Fiber gms	Fat gms	Sat. Fat gms	Chol. mgs	% Fat Cal.
(Swanson) mini, w/sausage 'Great Starts'	2.5 oz	190	6.0	22.0	320	(mq)	9.0	(mq)	(mq)	42%
(Swanson) oatmeal, w/lite links 'Great Starts'	4.65 oz	310	13.0	35.0	500	(mq)	13.0	(mq)	(mq)	38%
(Swanson) w/sausages 'Great Starts'	5.5 oz	380	12.0	35.0	550	(mq)	21.0	(mq)	(mq)	50%
FRENCH TOAST, STICKS										
apple cinnamon (Farm Rich)	3 oz	310	6.0	39.0	300	(mq)	15.0	(mq)	na	43%
blueberry (Farm Rich)	3 oz	310	6.0	37.0	280	(mq)	14.0	(mq)	na	42%
original (Farm Rich)	3 oz	300	5.0	37.0	280	(mq)	15.0	(mq)	na	45%
FRENCH FRY SEASONING (Tone's)	1 tsp	5	0.2	1.0	1551	.2	0.1	<.1	0	16%
FROG'S LEGS										
raw	100 gm	73	16.4	0.0	58	0	0.3	0.0	50	4%
raw	1 oz	21	4.6	0.0	(mq)	0	<1.0	(mq)	(mq)	<33%
FROGFISH. See MONKFISH.										
FROSTING MIX										
(Betty Crocker)										
cherry 'Creamy' prepared w/margarine	1/12 pkg	180	0.0	31.0	100	(tr)	6.0	3.0	0	30%
chocolate fudge 'Creamy' dry	1/12 pkg	140	<1.0	30.0	25	na	2.0	na	0	13%
chocolate fudge 'Creamy' prepared w/butter	1/12 pkg	180	<1.0	30.0	70	na	6.0	na	10	30%
chocolate fudge 'Creamy' prepared w/margarine	1/12 pkg	180	<1.0	30.0	70	na	6.0	na	0	30%
coconut pecan 'Creamy' dry	1/12 pkg	110	1.0	19.0	5	na	4.0	na	0	31%
coconut pecan 'Creamy' prepared w/butter, 2% milk	1/12 pkg	150	<1.0	19.0	50	na	8.0	na	10	47%
coconut pecan 'Creamy' prepared w/margarine, skim milk	1/12 pkg	150	<1.0	19.0	50	na	8.0	na	0	47%
milk chocolate 'Creamy' prepared w/margarine	1/12 pkg	170	1.0	29.0	40	(tr)	5.0	1.0	0	27%
rainbow chip 'Creamy' prepared w/margarine	1/12 pkg	190	<1.0	32.0	50	(tr)	7.0	2.0	0	32%
sour cream, chocolate fudge 'Creamy' prepared w/margarine	1/12 pkg	180	1.0	30.0	75	(tr)	6.0	2.0	0	30%
sour cream, white 'Creamy' prepared w/margarine	1/12 pkg	170	0.0	31.0	100	(tr)	5.0	1.0	0	27%
vanilla 'Creamy' dry	1/12 pkg	150	0.0	32.0	5	na	2.0	na	0	12%
vanilla 'Creamy' prepared w/butter	1/12 pkg	170	0.0	32.0	50	na	5.0	na	10	26%
vanilla 'Creamy' prepared w/margarine	1/12 pkg	170	0.0	32.0	50	na	5.0	na	0	26%
white 'Fluffy'	1/12 pkg	70	<1.0	16.0	40	(tr)	0.0	0.0	0	0%
(Estee)	1 tbsp	65	0.0	13.0	28	na	1.5	<1.0	0	21%
FROSTING, READY-TO-SPREAD										
(Betty Crocker)										
amaretto almond 'Creamy Deluxe'	1/12 tub	160	0.0	27.0	50	(tr)	6.0	2.0	0	33%
butter pecan 'Creamy Deluxe'	1/12 tub	170	0.0	26.0	50	na	7.0	na	0	38%
cherry 'Creamy Deluxe'	1/12 tub	160	0.0	27.0	50	na	6.0	na	0	33%
chocolate 'Creamy Deluxe'	1/12 tub	160	<1.0	24.0	60	na	7.0	na	0	39%
chocolate 'Creamy Deluxe Light'	1/12 tub	130	<1.0	28.0	60	na	2.0	na	0	13%
chocolate chip 'Creamy Deluxe'	1/12 tub	170	<1.0	27.0	30	na	7.0	na	0	36%
chocolate chip, coated 'Creamy Deluxe Party'	1/12 tub	160	<1.0	24.0	60	(tr)	7.0	2.0	0	39%
chocolate chip, double 'Creamy Deluxe'	1/12 tub	170	<1.0	24.0	60	(tr)	8.0	3.0	0	42%
chocolate coconut almond 'Creamy Deluxe'	1/12 tub	160	1.0	21.0	55	(tr)	8.0	3.0	0	45%
chocolate w/dinosaurs 'Creamy Deluxe Party'	1/12 tub	160	<1.0	24.0	60	na	7.0	na	0	39%
chocolate w/red gel 'Creamy Deluxe Party'	1/12 tub	160	<1.0	24.0	50	na	7.0	na	0	39%
chocolate w/turbo racers 'Creamy Deluxe Party'	1/12 tub	160	<1.0	24.0	50	na	7.0	na	0	39%
coconut pecan 'Creamy Deluxe'	1/12 tub	160	<1.0	20.0	60	na	9.0	na	0	49%
cream cheese 'Creamy Deluxe'	1/12 tub	170	0.0	26.0	70	na	7.0	na	0	38%
dark Dutch fudge 'Creamy Deluxe'	1/12 tub	160	1.0	22.0	70	na	7.0	na	0	41%
lemon 'Creamy Deluxe'	1/12 tub	170	0.0	28.0	70	na	6.0	na	0	33%
milk chocolate 'Creamy Deluxe'	1/12 tub	160	<1.0	25.0	55	na	6.0	na	0	34%
milk chocolate 'Creamy Deluxe Light'	1/12 tub	140	<1.0	29.0	60	na	2.0	na	0	13%
rainbow chip 'Creamy Deluxe'	1/12 tub	170	<1.0	27.0	30	na	7.0	na	0	36%
rocky road 'Creamy Deluxe'	1/12 can	150	<1.0	20.0	50	(tr)	8.0	2.0	0	46%
sour cream chocolate 'Creamy Deluxe'	1/12 tub	160	<1.0	23.0	100	na	7.0	na	0	40%

Food Name	Serving Size	Calories	Prot. gms	Carbs gms	Sod. mgs	Fiber gms	Fat gms	Sat. Fat gms	Chol. mgs	% Fat Cal.
sour cream white 'Creamy Deluxe'	1/12 tub	160	0.0	27.0	50	na	6.0	na	0	33%
vanilla 'Creamy Deluxe'	1/12 tub	160	0.0	27.0	25	na	6.0	na	0	33%
vanilla 'Creamy Deluxe Light'	1/12 tub	140	0.0	30.0	30	na	2.0	na	0	13%
vanilla w/blue gel 'Creamy Deluxe Party'	1/12 tub	160	0.0	27.0	30	na	6.0	na	0	33%
vanilla w/teddy bears 'Creamy Deluxe Party'	1/12 tub	160	0.0	27.0	25	na	6.0	na	0	33%
(Duncan Hines)										
chocolate	1/12 tub	160	0.0	24.0	90	(tr)	7.0	(mq)	na	40%
cream cheese	1/12 tub	160	0.0	24.0	120	na	8.0	2.0	na	43%
cream cheese 'Homestyle'	1/12 tub	160	0.0	26.0	75	na	6.0	2.0	0	34%
dark chocolate 'Homestyle'	1/12 tub	160	0.0	25.0	75	na	6.0	2.0	0	35%
Dutch fudge	1/12 tub	160	0.0	24.0	95	(tr)	7.0	2.0	na	40%
lemon	1/12 tub	120	0.0	18.0	60	na	6.0	2.0	na	43%
milk chocolate	1/12 tub	160	0.0	24.0	85	(tr)	7.0	2.0	na	40%
milk chocolate 'Homestyle'	1/12 tub	160	0.0	25.0	75	na	6.0	2.0	0	35%
vanilla	1/12 tub	160	0.0	24.0	80	(tr)	7.0	2.0	na	40%
vanilla 'Homestyle'	1/12 tub	160	0.0	26.0	75	na	6.0	2.0	0	34%
(Finast) milk chocolate	1/12 tub	160	0.0	25.0	105	(tr)	6.0	(mq)	na	35%
(Lovin' Lites)										
chocolate fudge	1/12 tub	130	1.0	28.0	95	1.0	2.0	1.0	0	13%
milk chocolate	1/12 tub	130	1.0	28.0	95	1.0	2.0	1.0	0	13%
vanilla	1/12 tub	130	0.0	29.0	70	0	2.0	1.0	0	13%
(Pathmark)										
chocolate, creamy	1/12 tub	160	0.0	25.0	95	(tr)	6.0	(mq)	na	35%
fudge, creamy	1/12 tub	160	0.0	25.0	100	(tr)	7.0	(mq)	na	39%
white, creamy	1/12 tub	160	0.0	25.0	95	(tr)	6.0	(mq)	na	35%
(Pillsbury)										
butter fudge 'Frosting Supreme'	1/12 tub	140	1.0	22.0	50	na	6.0	2.0	0	37%
caramel pecan 'Frosting Supreme'	1/12 tub	150	0.0	20.0	70	0	8.0	2.0	0	47%
chocolate chip 'Frosting Supreme'	1/12 tub	150	0.0	27.0	70	(tr)	5.0	(mq)	na	29%
chocolate fudge 'Frosting Supreme'	1/12 tub	150	0.0	22.0	85	na	6.0	2.0	0	38%
chocolate fudge 'Funfetti'	1/12 tub	140	0.0	23.0	80	na	6.0	2.0	0	37%
chocolate, double Dutch 'Frosting Supreme'	1/12 tub	140	1.0	22.0	45	(tr)	6.0	(mq)	na	37%
coconut almond 'Frosting Supreme'	1/12 tub	150	1.0	17.0	60	(tr)	9.0	(mq)	na	53%
coconut pecan 'Frosting Supreme'	1/12 tub	160	0.0	17.0	60	(tr)	10.0	(mq)	na	57%
cream cheese 'Frosting Supreme'	1/12 tub	160	0.0	26.0	115	(tr)	6.0	(mq)	na	34%
decorator, all flavors except chocolate	1 tbsp	70	0.0	12.0	na	(tr)	2.0	(mq)	0	27%
decorator, chocolate	1 tbsp	60	0.0	11.0	na	(tr)	2.0	(mq)	0	29%
double Dutch 'Frosting Supreme'	1/12 tub	140	1.0	22.0	50	na	6.0	2.0	0	37%
fudge 'Frosting Supreme'	1/12 tub	150	<1.0	24.0	80	(tr)	6.0	(mq)	Chol.	35%
lemon 'Frosting Supreme'	1/12 tub	160	0.0	26.0	80	(tr)	6.0	(mq)	na	34%
milk chocolate 'Frosting Supreme'	1/12 tub	150	0.0	23.0	65	na	6.0	2.0	0	37%
milk chocolate w/fudge swirl 'Frosting Supreme'	1/12 tub	150	0.0	23.0	65	na	6.0	2.0	0	37%
mint 'Frosting Supreme'	1/12 tub	150	<1.0	24.0	80	(tr)	7.0	(mq)	na	39%
mocha 'Frosting Supreme'	1/12 tub	150	<1.0	24.0	60	(tr)	6.0	(mq)	na	35%
sour cream vanilla 'Frosting Supreme'	1/12 tub	160	0.0	27.0	80	(tr)	6.0	(mq)	na	33%
strawberry 'Frosting Supreme'	1/12 tub	160	0.0	26.0	75	(tr)	6.0	(mq)	na	34%
vanilla 'Frosting Supreme'	1/12 tub	160	0.0	26.0	75	(tr)	6.0	(mq)	na	34%
vanilla 'Funfetti'	1/12 tub	150	0.0	25.0	75	0	6.0	2.0	0	35%
vanilla 'Funfetti Sunshine'	1/12 tub	150	0.0	25.0	75	0	6.0	2.0	0	35%
vanilla, pink and white 'Funfetti'	1/12 tub	150	0.0	24.0	70	(tr)	6.0	(mq)	na	36%
vanilla w/fudge swirl 'Frosting Supreme'	1/12 tub	150	0.0	25.0	75	0	6.0	2.0	0	35%
white, fluffy	1/12 tub	60	0.0	15.0	65	(tr)	0.0	0.0	0	0%
FRUCTOSE										
(Estee)	1 tsp	16	0.0	4.0	0	na	0.0	0.0	0	0%

Food Name	Serving Size	Calories	Prot. gms	Carbs gms	Sod. mgs	Fiber gms	Fat gms	Sat. Fat gms	Chol. mgs	% Fat Cal.
(Estee) packet	1 pkt	12	0.0	3.0	0	na	0.0	0.0	0	0%
(Featherweight)	1 tsp	12	0.0	3.0	0	0	0.0	0.0	0	0%

FRUIT. See individual listings.

FRUIT, MIXED

Canned

(A&P) in light syrup	1/2 cup	75	<1.0	20.0	10	(mq)	<1.0	(tr)	0	<10%
(Del Monte) chunky	1/2 cup	80	0.0	23.0	10	(mq)	0.0	0.0	0	0%
(Del Monte) chunky 'Lite'	1/2 cup	50	0.0	14.0	10	(mq)	0.0	0.0	0	0%
(Del Monte) 'Fruit Cup'	5 oz	100	0.0	27.0	10	(mq)	0.0	0.0	0	0%
(Del Monte) tropical	1/2 cup	90	0.0	26.0	10	(mq)	0.0	0.0	0	0%
(Dole) pineapple and Mandarin orange segments	1/2 cup	80	0.0	19.0	5	na	<1.0	na	na	<11%
(Dole) tropical fruit salad	1/2 cup	70	0.0	17.0	10	na	0.0	na	na	0%
(Finast) in heavy syrup, chunky	1/2 cup	70	0.0	18.0	10	(mq)	0.0	0.0	0	0%
(Kraft) salad 'Pure'	1/2 cup	80	1.0	18.0	10	(mq)	0.0	0.0	0	0%
(Libby's) in juice, chunky 'Lite'	1/2 cup	50	1.0	14.0	5	(mq)	0.0	0.0	0	0%
(Pathmark) in juice, chunky	1/2 cup	50	1.0	14.0	15	(mq)	0.0	0.0	0	0%
(Pathmark) in light syrup 'No Frills'	1 cup	150	1.0	39.0	20	(mq)	0.0	0.0	0	0%
(S&W) in juice, chunky, sweetened, clarified	1/2 cup	90	1.0	21.0	5	(mq)	0.0	0.0	0	0%
(S&W Nutradiet) chunky	1/2 cup	40	0.0	10.0	5	(mq)	0.0	0.0	0	0%
(Sun Fresh) jar, chilled, in light syrup 'Tropical Salad'	3.5 oz	88	1.2	18.7	39	2.3	0.9	0.3	1	9%

Dried

(Del Monte)	2 oz	130	1.0	34.0	10	(mq)	0.0	0.0	0	0%
(SunSweet)	2 oz	150	1.0	39.0	20	(mq)	0.0	0.0	0	0%
(SunSweet) bits	2 oz	150	2.0	40.0	50	(mq)	<1.0	(tr)	0	<5%
(Sun•Maid)	2 oz	150	1.0	39.0	20	(mq)	0.0	0.0	0	0%
(Sun•Maid) bits	2 oz	150	2.0	40.0	50	(mq)	<1.0	(tr)	0	<5%
Frozen (Birds Eye) in syrup 'Quick Thaw pouch'	5 oz	120	1.0	31.0	5	1.0	0.0	0.0	0	0%

FRUIT AND NUT MIX

(Estee)	14 pieces	70	2.0	6.0	15	na	5.0	2.0	0	58%
(Estee)	4 pieces	35	1.0	3.0	0	(mq)	2.0	2.0	<1	53%
(Planters) 'Caribbean Crunch'	1 oz	150	3.0	14.0	130	na	10.0	3.0	0	57%
(Planters) 'Fruit 'n Nut'	1 oz	150	5.0	13.0	90	(mq)	9.0	2.0	0	53%

FRUIT BAR, FROZEN. See also ICE BARS AND DESSERTS; SHERBET; SORBET.

all flavors 'Fruit Juicee' (Minute Maid)	1 bar	60	0.0	14.0	0	na	0.0	0.0	0	0%
blueberry and cream 'Fruit & Cream' (Dole)	1 bar	90	1.0	19.4	20	na	1.4	na	5	13%
cherry 'Fresh Lites' (Dole)	1 bar	25	<1.0	6.0	6	na	<1.0	na	0	<24%
cherry and yogurt 'Fruit & Yogurt' (Dole)	1 bar	80	2.0	17.0	22	na	<1.0	(mq)	(mq)	<11%
chocolate/banana and cream 'Fruit & Cream' (Dole)	1 bar	175	2.0	22.0	20	na	9.0	(mq)	na	46%
chocolate/strawberry and cream 'Fruit & Cream' (Dole)	1 bar	140	2.0	23.0	20	na	8.0	(mq)	na	42%
coconut (Sunkist)	1 bar	170	3.0	15.0	70	(mq)	10.0	(mq)	0	56%
grape 'SunTops' (Dole)	1 bar	40	<1.0	9.0	5	na	<1.0	na	0	<18%
lemon 'Fresh Lites' (Dole)	1 bar	25	<1.0	6.0	16	na	<1.0	na	0	<24%
lemonade (Sunkist)	1 bar	90	0.0	24.0	5	na	0.0	0.0	0	0%
lemonade 'SunTops' (Dole)	1 bar	40	<1.0	9.0	5	na	<1.0	na	0	<18%
orange 'Juice Bar' (Sunkist)	1 bar	100	0.0	25.0	0	na	0.0	0.0	0	0%
orange, tropical 'SunTops' (Dole)	1 bar	40	<1.0	9.0	5	na	<1.0	na	0	<18%
peach and cream 'Fruit & Cream' (Dole)	1 bar	90	1.0	19.4	19	na	1.4	na	5	13%
pineapple 'Fruit 'n Juice' (Dole)	1 bar	70	0.3	17.0	4	na	<.1	na	0	<1%
pineapple-orange 'Fresh Lites' (Dole)	1 bar	25	<1.0	6.0	7	na	<1.0	na	0	<24%
piña colada 'Fruit 'n Juice' (Dole)	1 bar	90	1.0	16.0	2	na	3.0	(mq)	0	28%
punch 'SunTops' (Dole)	1 bar	40	<1.0	9.0	5	na	<1.0	na	0	<18%
raspberry 'Fresh Lites' (Dole)	1 bar	25	<1.0	6.0	6	na	<1.0	na	0	<24%
raspberry 'Fruit 'n Juice' (Dole)	1 bar	70	0.2	16.0	14	na	<.1	na	0	<1%
raspberry and cream 'Fruit & Cream' (Dole)	1 bar	90	1.0	20.0	23	na	1.4	na	5	13%

Food Name	Serving Size	Calories	Prot. gms	Carbs gms	Sod. mgs	Fiber gms	Fat gms	Sat. Fat gms	Chol. mgs	% Fat Cal.
strawberry and cream *(Sunkist)*	1 bar	90	0.0	19.0	30	na	1.0	na	na	11%
strawberry and cream 'Fruit & Cream' *(Dole)*	1 bar	90	1.0	19.3	22	na	1.4	na	5	13%
raspberry and yogurt 'Fruit & Yogurt' *(Dole)*	1 bar	70	1.0	17.0	18	na	<1.0	(mq)	(mq)	<11%
strawberry and yogurt 'Fruit & Yogurt' *(Dole)*	1 bar	70	1.0	17.0	16	na	<1.0	(mq)	(mq)	<11%
strawberry 'Fruit 'n Juice' *(Dole)*	1 bar	70	0.2	16.0	6	na	<.1	na	0	<1%
wildberry *(Sunkist)*	1 bar	140	0.0	33.0	15	na	0.0	0.0	0	0%
FRUIT COCKTAIL, CANNED										
(Del Monte)	1/2 cup	80	0.0	23.0	10	(mq)	0.0	0.0	0	0%
(Hunt's)	4 oz	90	<1.0	23.0	7	<1.0	<1.0	na	0	<9%
fruit for salad *(Del Monte)*	1/2 cup	90	0.0	22.0	10	(mq)	0.0	0.0	0	0%
in extra heavy syrup	4 oz	98	0.4	26.0	7	>.5 c	0.1	<.1	0	1%
in extra heavy syrup, solid and liquid	1/2 cup	114	0.5	29.8	8	>.6 c	0.1	0.0	0	1%
in extra light syrup	4 oz	51	0.5	13.2	5	>.5 c	0.1	<.1	0	2%
in extra light syrup, solid and liquid	1/2 cup	55	0.5	14.3	5	>.6 c	0.1	0.0	0	2%
in heavy syrup	4 oz	83	0.4	21.4	7	>.5 c	0.1	<.1	0	1%
in heavy syrup *(A&P)*	1/2 cup	90	<1.0	24.0	15	(mq)	<1.0	(tr)	0	<8%
in heavy syrup *(Finast)*	1/2 cup	90	0.0	24.0	9	(mq)	0.0	0.0	0	0%
in heavy syrup *(Pathmark)*	1 cup	180	1.0	48.0	35	(mq)	0.0	0.0	0	0%
in heavy syrup *(S&W)*	1/2 cup	90	0.0	24.0	15	(mq)	0.0	0.0	0	0%
in heavy syrup, solid and liquid	1/2 cup	93	0.5	24.2	8	1.4	0.1	0.0	0	1%
in juice	4 oz	52	0.5	13.4	5	.7	<.1	tr	0	<2%
in juice *(Featherweight)*	1/2 cup	50	1.0	14.0	10	(mq)	0.0	0.0	0	0%
in juice *(IGA)*	1/2 cup	60	0.0	15.0	10	(mq)	0.0	0.0	0	0%
in juice *(S&W)*	1/2 cup	90	1.0	21.0	5	(mq)	0.0	0.0	0	0%
in juice 'Lite' *(Libby's)*	1/2 cup	50	0.0	13.0	10	(mq)	0.0	0.0	0	0%
in juice, solid and liquid	1/2 cup	57	0.6	14.7	5	1.4	0.0	0.0	0	0%
in light syrup	4 oz	65	0.5	16.9	7	>.5 c	0.1	<.1	0	1%
in light syrup, solid and liquid	1/2 cup	72	0.5	18.8	8	1.4	0.1	0.0	0	1%
in pear juice *(A&P)*	1/2 cup	50	1.0	14.0	15	(mq)	<1.0	(tr)	0	<13%
in water	4 oz	36	0.5	9.7	5	>.5 c	0.1	tr	0	2%
in water, solid and liquid	1/2 cup	39	0.5	10.4	5	1.3	0.1	0.0	0	2%
'Lite' *(Del Monte)*	1/2 cup	50	0.0	15.0	10	(mq)	0.0	0.0	0	0%
'No Sugar Added' *(Finast)*	1/2 cup	50	1.0	14.0	10	(mq)	0.0	0.0	0	0%
'Regulars Unsweetened' *(S&W Nutradiet)*	1/2 cup	40	0.0	10.0	5	(mq)	0.0	0.0	0	0%
FRUIT DRINK										
(Finast)	8 oz	80	0.0	21.0	15	(tr)	0.0	0.0	0	0%
(Fruitopia) 'Fruit Integration' real fruit	8 oz	120	0.0	31.0	25	na	0.0	na	na	0%
(Hi-C) 'Bubble Gum' aseptic box or chilled	6 oz	90	0.0	22.0	20	na	0.0	na	na	0%
(Hi-C) 'Double Fruit Cooler'	6 oz	93	<.1	22.9	18	(tr)	<.1	(tr)	0	<1%
(Hi-C) 'Double Fruit Cooler' aseptic box	6 oz	90	0.0	22.0	25	na	0.0	na	na	0%
(Hi-C) 'Ecto Cooler'	6 oz	95	0.1	23.3	17	(tr)	<.1	(tr)	0	<1%
(Hi-C) 'Ecto Cooler' aseptic box	6 oz	90	0.0	23.0	20	na	0.0	na	na	0%
(Hi-C) 'Hula Cooler'	6 oz	97	0.1	23.9	17	(tr)	<.1	(tr)	0	<1%
FRUIT JUICE										
(Juicy Juice) bottled	6 oz	100	1.0	23.0	10	na	0.0	na	na	0%
(Juicy Juice) boxed	8.45 oz	140	1.0	33.0	10	na	0.0	na	na	0%
(McCain) mixed fruit, 100% juice 'Junior'	4.2 oz	60	0.0	15.0	5	na	0.0	na	na	0%
FRUIT JUICE COCKTAIL										
'Orchard Harvest Blend' *(Welch's)*	6 oz	110	0.0	27.0	20	0	0.0	0.0	0	0%
'Orchard Harvest Blend' 'Cocktails-In-A-Box' *(Welch's)* ..	8.45 oz	150	0.0	38.0	20	0	0.0	0.0	0	0%
'Orchard Harvest Blend' frozen, prepared *(Welch's)*	6 oz	110	0.0	27.0	10	0	0.0	0.0	0	0%
FRUIT JUICE DRINK, mixed 'Fruit Box' *(Tang)*	8.45 oz	140	0.0	36.0	10	na	0.0	na	0	0%
FRUIT JUICE DRINK MIX										
'Mixes w/Fruit Juice' powder *(Ultra Slim Fast)*	1 scoop	90	10.0	17.0	75	6.0	0.0	na	na	0%

Food Name	Serving Size	Calories	Prot. gms	Carbs gms	Sod. mgs	Fiber gms	Fat gms	Sat. Fat gms	Chol. mgs	% Fat Cal.
'Mixes w/Fruit Juice' prepared w/orange juice										
(Ultra Slim Fast)	8 oz	200	11.0	43.0	80	6.0	<1.0	na	na	<4%
FRUIT JUICE PUNCH DRINK										
concentrate, prepared w/water	1 cup	124	0.3	30.3	12	>.3 c	0.5	0.1	0	4%
concentrate, prepared w/water	1 oz	15	0.0	3.8	2	(tr)	0.1	0.0	0	6%
concentrate, undiluted	12 oz	739	1.2	182.1	41	(tr)	3.0	0.4	0	4%
(Veryfine) can, bottle, or box '100% Juice Punch'	8 oz	122	<1.0	30.0	10	(tr)	0.0	0.0	0	0%
FRUIT PUNCH										
(Bright & Early) frozen 'Bright & Early Fruit Punch'										
prepared	6 oz	90	0.0	22.0	5	na	0.0	na	na	0%
(Juicy Juice) can, bottle, or box	6 oz	100	1.0	23.0	10	(tr)	0.0	0.0	0	0%
(Minute Maid) aseptic box, canned, or chilled	6 oz	90	0.0	22.0	20	na	0.0	na	na	0%
(Minute Maid) frozen, concentrate, prepared	6 oz	90	0.0	23.0	0	na	0.0	na	na	0%
(Pathmark) can, bottle, or box	6 oz	90	0.0	22.0	0	(tr)	0.0	0.0	0	0%
(Snapple)	8 oz	120	0.0	29.0	5	na	0.0	0.0	0	0%
FRUIT PUNCH DRINK										
(All Sport) thirst quencher, caffeine-free	8 oz	80	0.0	21.0	55	na	0.0	na	na	0%
(Bama)	8.45 oz	130	0.0	32.0	15	(tr)	0.0	0.0	0	0%
(Crowley)	8 oz	130	0.0	32.0	15	(tr)	0.0	0.0	0	0%
(Gatorade) low sodium, no caffeine	8 oz	50	0.0	14.0	110	na	0.0	0.0	0	0%
(Hawaiian Punch) island fruit	6 oz	90	0.0	22.0	30	(tr)	0.0	0.0	0	0%
(Hawaiian Punch) red 'Fruit Juicy'	6 oz	90	0.0	22.0	20	(tr)	0.0	0.0	0	0%
(Hawaiian Punch) red 'Fruit Juicy Lite'	6 oz	60	0.0	15.0	30	(tr)	0.0	0.0	0	0%
(Hawaiian Punch) tropical	6 oz	90	0.0	22.0	30	(tr)	0.0	0.0	0	0%
(Hawaiian Punch) tropical, wild fruit	6 oz	90	0.0	23.0	35	(tr)	0.0	0.0	0	0%
(Hi-C)	6 oz	96	0.1	23.7	17	(tr)	<.1	(tr)	0	<1%
(Hi-C) aseptic box or chilled	6 oz	90	0.0	23.0	20	na	0.0	na	na	0%
(Hi-C) 'Hula Punch'	6 oz	87	0.1	21.4	17	(tr)	<.1	(tr)	0	<1%
(Hi-C) 'Hula Punch Drink' aseptic box	6 oz	90	0.0	23.0	20	na	0.0	na	na	0%
(J. Hungerford) 20% juice	9.03 oz	43	0.0	11.2	32	0	0.0	0.0	0	0%
(J. Hungerford) 50% juice	9.03 oz	107	0.3	26.6	7	0	0.0	0.0	0	0%
(J. Hungerford) 100% juice	9.03 oz	116	0.5	29.5	11	0	0.0	0.0	0	0%
(Mott's)	10 oz	170	0.0	42.0	4	(tr)	0.0	0.0	0	0%
(Mott's)	9.5 oz	161	0.0	40.0	4	(tr)	0.0	0.0	0	0%
(PowerAde) thirst quencher, high energy	8 oz	70	0.0	19.0	70	na	0.0	na	na	0%
(10-K)	8 oz	60	0.0	15.0	55	na	0.0	na	na	0%
(Tropicana)	6 oz	90	<1.0	21.0	15	na	<1.0	na	na	<9%
(Tropicana) 'Single Serve'	10 oz	148	(tr)	37.0	3	(tr)	0.0	0.0	0	0%
(Welch's) 'Orchard Fruit Harvest Punch'	10 oz	180	0.0	45.0	0	0	0.0	0.0	0	0%
(Wyler's)	6 oz	84	0.0	21.3	8	(tr)	0.1	(tr)	0	1%
(Wyler's) tropical	6 oz	157	0.0	39.3	10	0	0.0	0.0	0	0%
(Wyler's) tropical 'Fruit Slush'	4 oz	157	0.0	39.3	10	(tr)	0.0	0.0	0	0%
FRUIT PUNCH DRINK MIX										
frozen concentrate, prepared	12 oz	677	0.8	173.0	33	0	0.0	0.0	0	0%
frozen, prepared w/water	1 cup	114	0.0	28.9	10	0	0.0	0.0	0	0%
frozen, prepared w/water	1 oz	14	0.0	3.6	1	0	0.0	0.0	0	0%
instant 'Thirst Quencher' prepared (Gatorade)	8 oz	60	0.0	15.0	110	na	0.0	na	na	0%
'No Frills' prepared (Pathmark)	8 oz	90	0.0	22.0	85	(tr)	0.0	0.0	0	0%
powder, w/added sodium, dry	2 rounded tbsp	97	0.0	24.8	30	0	0.0	0.0	0	0%
powder, w/added sodium, prepared	8 oz	97	0.0	24.9	37	0	0.0	0.0	0	0%
powder, w/o added sodium, dry	2 rounded tbsp	97	0.0	24.8	11	0	0.0	0.0	0	0%
powder, w/o added sodium, prepared	8 oz	97	0.0	24.9	10	0	0.0	0.0	0	0%
sugar-free, prepared (Crystal Light)	8 oz	4	0.0	0.0	0	0	0.0	0.0	0	0%
sugar-free, w/NutraSweet, prepared (Crystal Light)	8 oz	4	0.0	0.0	0	na	0.0	na	0	0%

Food Name	Serving Size	Calories	Prot. gms	Carbs gms	Sod. mgs	Fiber gms	Fat gms	Sat. Fat gms	Chol. mgs	% Fat Cal.
tropical 'Crystals' prepared *(Wyler's)*	8 oz	85	0.0	21.1	18	(tr)	0.1	(tr)	0	1%

FRUIT ROLL. See FRUIT SNACK.

FRUIT SALAD, CANNED. See FRUIT COCKTAIL, CANNED.

FRUIT SNACK

Food Name	Serving Size	Calories	Prot. gms	Carbs gms	Sod. mgs	Fiber gms	Fat gms	Sat. Fat gms	Chol. mgs	% Fat Cal.
all flavors 'Berry Bears' *(Betty Crocker)*	1 pouch	100	<1.0	22.0	20	na	<1.0	(tr)	0	<9%
all flavors 'Fruit Roll-Ups Peel-Outs' *(Betty Crocker)*	1 roll	50	<1.0	12.0	40	(mq)	<1.0	(tr)	0	<15%
all flavors 'Shark Bites' *(Betty Crocker)*	1 pouch	100	<1.0	22.0	20	na	<1.0	(tr)	0	<9%
apple *(Weight Watchers)*	1 pouch	50	<1.0	13.0	75	na	<1.0	(tr)	0	<14%
apple chips *(Weight Watchers)*	.75 oz	70	0.0	19.0	110	na	0.0	na	na	0%
apple roll *(Flavor Tree)*	1 piece	75	0.2	18.5	17	(mq)	0.0	0.0	0	0%
apricot roll *(Flavor Tree)*	1 piece	76	0.3	17.7	17	(mq)	0.5	(tr)	0	6%
assorted flavors, all shapes 'Fun Fruits' *(Sunkist)*	1 pouch	100	0.1	21.8	10	na	1.4	na	0	13%
assorted flavors 'Bugs Bunny and Friends' *(Betty Crocker)*	1 pouch	90	<1.0	21.0	30	na	1.0	na	na	9%
assorted flavors 'Chip `N Dale Rescue Rangers' *(Fruit Parade)*	1 pouch	100	0.0	22.0	10	na	1.0	na	na	9%
assorted flavors 'Darkwing Duck' *(Fruit Parade)*	1 pouch	100	0.0	22.0	10	na	1.0	na	na	9%
assorted flavors 'Dinosaurs' *(Farley's)*	1 oz	90	1.0	22.0	0	na	<1.0	na	na	<9%
assorted flavors 'Fruit Circus Fruit Bears' *(Flavor Tree)*	1.05 oz	117	0.1	25.4	12	na	1.6	na	0	12%
assorted flavors 'Tale Spin' *(Fruit Parade)*	1 pouch	100	0.0	22.0	10	na	1.0	na	na	9%
assorted flavors 'Tasmanian Devil' *(Betty Crocker)*	1 pouch	90	<1.0	21.0	30	na	1.0	na	na	9%
assorted flavors 'Teenage Mutant Ninja Turtles' *(Farley's)*	1 oz	90	1.0	22.0	0	na	<1.0	na	na	<9%
assorted flavors 'Trolls' *(Farley's)*	1 oz	90	1.0	22.0	0	na	<1.0	na	na	<9%
berry 'Fun Fruits Berry Bunch' *(Sunkist)*	1 pouch	100	0.1	21.8	10	na	1.4	na	0	13%
cherry 'Fruit by the Foot' *(Betty Crocker)*	1 roll	80	<1.0	17.0	45	na	2.0	na	na	20%
cherry 'Fruit Roll-Ups' *(Betty Crocker)*	.5-oz roll	50	<1.0	12.0	40	na	<1.0	na	na	<15%
cherry 'Fun Fruits' *(Sunkist)*	1 pouch	100	0.1	21.8	10	na	1.4	na	0	13%
cherry 'Wild Cherry Gushers' w/juicy centers *(Betty Crocker)*	1 pouch	90	<1.0	21.0	40	na	1.0	na	na	9%
cherry roll *(Flavor Tree)*	1 piece	75	0.3	18.3	18	(mq)	0.1	(tr)	0	1%
cinnamon flavor *(Weight Watchers)*	1 pouch	50	<1.0	13.0	75	na	<1.0	(tr)	0	<14%
compote *(Rokeach)*	4 oz	120	1.0	31.0	4	(mq)	1.0	na	0	7%
crazy colors 'Fruit Roll-Ups' *(Betty Crocker)*	.5-oz roll	50	<1.0	12.0	40	na	<1.0	na	na	<15%
'Fun Fruits Fantastic Fruit' *(Sunkist)*	1 pouch	100	0.1	21.8	10	na	1.4	na	0	13%
'Garfield and Friends' 'Wild Blue' *(Betty Crocker)*	1 roll	50	<1.0	12.0	20	(mq)	<1.0	(tr)	0	<15%
grape 'Fruit by the Foot' *(Betty Crocker)*	1 roll	80	<1.0	17.0	45	na	2.0	na	na	20%
grape 'Fruit Roll-Ups' *(Betty Crocker)*	.5-oz roll	50	<1.0	12.0	40	na	<1.0	na	na	<15%
grape 'Fun Fruits' *(Sunkist)*	1 pouch	100	0.1	21.8	10	na	1.4	na	0	13%
grape 'Gushin Grape Gushers' *(Betty Crocker)*	1 pouch	90	<1.0	21.0	45	na	<1.0	na	na	<9%
grape roll *(Flavor Tree)*	1 piece	76	0.2	18.5	13	(mq)	0.1	(tr)	0	1%
orange 'Fun Fruits' *(Sunkist)*	1 pouch	100	0.1	21.8	10	na	1.4	na	0	13%
peach *(Weight Watchers)*	.5 oz	50	<1.0	13.0	75	na	<1.0	na	na	<14%
raspberry 'Fruit Roll-Ups' *(Betty Crocker)*	.5-oz roll	50	<1.0	12.0	40	na	<1.0	na	na	<15%
raspberry roll *(Flavor Tree)*	1 piece	75	0.2	18.3	20	(mq)	0.1	(tr)	0	1%
strawberry *(Weight Watchers)*	1 pouch	50	<1.0	13.0	75	na	<1.0	(tr)	0	<14%
strawberry 'Fruit by the Foot' *(Betty Crocker)*	1 roll	80	<1.0	17.0	45	na	2.0	na	na	20%
strawberry 'Fruit Roll-Ups' *(Betty Crocker)*	.5-oz roll	50	<1.0	12.0	40	na	<1.0	na	na	<15%
strawberry 'Fun Fruits' *(Sunkist)*	1 pouch	100	0.1	21.0	10	na	1.4	na	0	13%
strawberry roll *(Flavor Tree)*	1 piece	74	0.2	18.0	11	(mq)	0.1	(tr)	0	1%
strawberry 'Strawberry Splash Gushers' *(Betty Crocker)*	1 pouch	90	<1.0	21.0	45	na	1.0	na	na	9%
strawberry, yogurt coated 'Creme Supremes' *(Sunkist)*	1 pouch	114	0.2	20.1	19	na	3.6	(mq)	na	29%

FRUIT SPREAD

Food Name	Serving Size	Calories	Prot. gms	Carbs gms	Sod. mgs	Fiber gms	Fat gms	Sat. Fat gms	Chol. mgs	% Fat Cal.
all flavors 'Homestyle' *(Smucker's)*	1 tsp	15	0.0	3.0	0	na	0.0	0.0	na	0%
all flavors 'Slenderella' *(Smucker's)*	1 tsp	7	0.0	2.0	0	0	0.0	0.0	0	0%
apple, no sugar added *(Fifty 50)*	1 tsp	2	0.0	<1.0	5	0	0.0	0.0	0	0%

Food Name	Serving Size	Calories	Prot. gms	Carbs gms	Sod. mgs	Fiber gms	Fat gms	Sat. Fat gms	Chol. mgs	% Fat Cal.
apricot 'All Fruit Spreadable Fruit' (Polaner)	1 tsp	14	0.0	4.0	0	na	0.0	0.0	na	0%
apricot 'Light' w/NutraSweet (Smucker's)	1 tsp	7	0.0	2.0	0	na	0.0	0.0	na	0%
apricot, low sugar (Smucker's)	1 tsp	8	0.0	2.0	10	na	0.0	0.0	na	0%
apricot 'Simply Fruit' (Smucker's)	1 tsp	16	0.0	4.0	0	na	0.0	0.0	na	0%
apricot-pineapple (Knott's Berry Farm)	1 tsp	16	0.0	4.0	0	na	0.0	na	na	0%
apricot-pineapple 'Light' w/NutraSweet (Knott's Berry Farm)	1 tsp	8	0.0	2.0	0	na	0.0	na	na	0%
apricot-pineapple, portion pack (Knott's Berry Farm)	.5 oz	35	0.0	9.0	0	na	0.0	na	na	0%
black cherry 'All Fruit Spreadable Fruit' (Polaner)	1 tsp	14	0.0	4.0	0	na	0.0	0.0	na	0%
black raspberry 'Simply Fruit' (Smucker's)	1 tsp	16	0.0	4.0	0	na	0.0	0.0	na	0%
blackberry (Knott's Berry Farm)	1 tsp	16	0.0	4.0	0	na	0.0	na	na	0%
blackberry 'Light' w/NutraSweet (Knott's Berry Farm)	1 tsp	8	0.0	2.0	0	na	0.0	na	na	0%
blackberry, low sugar (Smucker's)	1 tsp	8	0.0	2.0	10	na	0.0	na	na	0%
blackberry, portion pack (Knott's Berry Farm)	.5 oz	35	0.0	9.0	0	na	0.0	na	na	0%
blackberry 'Simply Fruit' (Smucker's)	1 tsp	16	0.0	4.0	0	na	0.0	na	na	0%
blueberry 'All Fruit Spreadable Fruit' (Polaner)	1 tsp	14	0.0	4.0	0	na	0.0	na	na	0%
blueberry 'Simply Fruit' (Smucker's)	1 tsp	16	0.0	4.0	0	na	0.0	0.0	na	0%
boysenberry (Knott's Berry Farm)	1 tsp	16	0.0	4.0	0	na	0.0	na	na	0%
boysenberry 'Light' w/NutraSweet (Knott's Berry Farm)	1 tsp	8	0.0	2.0	0	na	0.0	na	na	0%
boysenberry 'Light' w/NutraSweet (Smucker's)	1 tsp	7	0.0	2.0	0	na	0.0	0.0	na	0%
boysenberry, low sugar (Smucker's)	1 tsp	8	0.0	2.0	10	na	0.0	0.0	na	0%
boysenberry, portion pack (Knott's Berry Farm)	.5 oz	35	0.0	9.0	0	na	0.0	na	na	0%
calamansi 'Tropical Rainforest' (Knudsen & Sons)	2 tsp	35	0.0	8.0	0	na	0.0	na	na	0%
grape (Weight Watchers)	1 tsp	8	0.0	2.0	0	na	0.0	na	na	0%
grape 'All Fruit Spreadable Fruit' (Polaner)	1 tsp	14	0.0	4.0	0	na	0.0	0.0	na	0%
grape, concord, low sugar (Smucker's)	1 tsp	8	0.0	2.0	0	na	0.0	na	na	0%
grape 'Imitation' (Smucker's)	1 tsp	2	0.0	1.0	2	0	0.0	0.0	0	0%
grape, no sugar added (Fifty 50)	1 tsp	2	0.0	<1.0	5	0	0.0	0.0	0	0%
grape 'Simply Fruit' (Smucker's)	1 tsp	16	0.0	4.0	0	na	0.0	0.0	na	0%
guanabana 'Tropical Rainforest' (Knudsen & Sons)	2 tsp	35	0.0	8.0	0	na	0.0	na	na	0%
orange 'All Fruit Spreadable Fruit' (Polaner)	1 tsp	14	0.0	4.0	0	na	0.0	0.0	na	0%
orange marmalade (Knott's Berry Farm)	1 tsp	16	0.0	4.0	0	na	0.0	na	na	0%
orange marmalade 'Light' w/NutraSweet (Knott's Berry Farm)	1 tsp	8	0.0	2.0	0	na	0.0	na	na	0%
orange marmalade 'Light' w/NutraSweet (Smucker's)	1 tsp	7	0.0	2.0	0	na	0.0	0.0	na	0%
orange marmalade, low sugar (Smucker's)	1 tsp	8	0.0	2.0	10	na	0.0	0.0	na	0%
orange marmalade, no sugar added (Fifty 50)	1 tsp	2	0.0	<1.0	5	0	0.0	0.0	0	0%
orange marmalade, portion pack (Knott's Berry Farm)	.5 oz	35	0.0	9.0	0	na	0.0	na	na	0%
orange marmalade 'Simply Fruit' (Smucker's)	1 tsp	16	0.0	4.0	0	na	0.0	0.0	na	0%
peach 'Simply Fruit' (Smucker's)	1 tsp	16	0.0	4.0	0	na	0.0	0.0	na	0%
raspberry (Weight Watchers)	1 tsp	8	0.0	2.0	0	na	0.0	na	na	0%
raspberry 'All Fruit Spreadable Fruit' (Polaner)	1 tsp	14	0.0	4.0	0	na	0.0	0.0	na	0%
raspberry 'All Fruit Spreadable Fruit' seedless (Polaner)	1 tsp	14	0.0	4.0	0	na	0.0	0.0	na	0%
raspberry, no sugar added (Fifty 50)	1 tsp	2	0.0	<1.0	5	0	0.0	0.0	0	0%
red raspberry (Knott's Berry Farm)	1 tsp	16	0.0	4.0	0	na	0.0	na	na	0%
red raspberry 'Light' w/NutraSweet (Knott's Berry Farm)	1 tsp	8	0.0	2.0	0	na	0.0	na	na	0%
red raspberry 'Light' w/NutraSweet (Smucker's)	1 tsp	7	0.0	2.0	0	na	0.0	na	na	0%
red raspberry, low sugar (Smucker's)	1 tsp	8	0.0	2.0	0	na	0.0	na	na	0%
red raspberry, portion pack (Knott's Berry Farm)	.5 oz	35	0.0	9.0	0	na	0.0	na	na	0%
red raspberry 'Simply Fruit' (Smucker's)	1 tsp	16	0.0	4.0	0	na	0.0	na	na	0%
strawberry (Weight Watchers)	1 tsp	8	0.0	2.0	0	na	0.0	na	na	0%
strawberry 'All Fruit Spreadable Fruit' (Polaner)	1 tsp	14	0.0	4.0	0	na	0.0	0.0	na	0%
strawberry 'Imitation' (Smucker's)	1 tsp	2	0.0	1.0	2	na	0.0	0.0	0	0%
strawberry 'Light' w/NutraSweet (Knott's Berry Farm)	1 tsp	8	0.0	2.0	0	na	0.0	na	na	0%

Food Name	Serving Size	Calories	Prot. gms	Carbs gms	Sod. mgs	Fiber gms	Fat gms	Sat. Fat gms	Chol. mgs	% Fat Cal.
strawberry 'Light' w/NutraSweet (Smucker's) .... 1 tsp		7	0.0	2.0	0	na	0.0	na	na	0%
strawberry, low sugar (Smucker's) .... 1 tsp		8	0.0	2.0	0	na	0.0	na	na	0%
strawberry, no sugar added (Fifty 50) .... 1 tsp		2	0.0	<1.0	5	0	0.0	0.0	0	0%
strawberry 'Simply Fruit' (Smucker's) .... 1 tsp		16	0.0	4.0	0	na	0.0	na	na	0%
FRUIT SYRUP										
all flavors (Smucker's) .... 2 tbsp		100	0.0	26.0	0	na	0.0	0.0	0	0%
'Fruit 'n Maple' (Knudsen & Sons) .... 1 oz		105	<1.0	26.0	na	na	<1.0	na	na	<8%
'Fruit 'n Maple' pourable (Knudsen & Sons) .... 1 oz		105	0.0	26.0	0	na	0.0	na	na	0%
raspberry, pourable (Knudsen & Sons) .... 1 oz		75	0.0	18.0	0	na	1.0	na	na	11%
strawberry, pourable (Knudsen & Sons) .... 1 oz		75	0.0	18.0	0	na	1.0	na	na	11%
FUDGE TOPPING										
(Hershey's) .... 2 tbsp		100	1.0	14.0	30	(mq)	4.0	(mq)	5	38%
(Kraft) hot .... 1 tbsp		70	1.0	11.0	50	(mq)	2.0	1.0	0	27%
(Mrs. Richardson's) hot .... 2 tbsp		140	1.0	20.0	75	na	7.0	na	0	43%
(Mrs. Richardson's) hot, microwavable .... 2 tbsp		140	1.0	20.0	75	na	7.0	na	0	43%
(Smucker's) .... 2 tbsp		130	1.0	31.0	50	(mq)	1.0	na	na	7%
(Smucker's) hot .... 2 tbsp		110	1.0	18.0	55	(mq)	4.0	(mq)	na	32%
(Smucker's) hot 'Light' .... 2 tbsp		70	2.0	19.0	35	na	0.0	0.0	na	0%
(Smucker's) hot 'Special Recipe' .... 2 tbsp		150	2.0	23.0	60	(mq)	5.0	(mq)	na	31%
(Smucker's) 'Magic Shell' .... 2 tbsp		190	1.0	16.0	50	(mq)	15.0	(mq)	na	67%

FUKI. See BUTTERBUR.

G

Food Name	Serving Size	Calories	Prot. gms	Carbs gms	Sod. mgs	Fiber gms	Fat gms	Sat. Fat gms	Chol. mgs	% Fat Cal.
GARBANZO BEAN/ceci/chick pea										
boiled .... 4 oz		186	10.0	31.1	8	4.0	2.9	0.3	0	14%
boiled .... 1/2 cup		134	7.3	22.5	6	>2.0 c	2.1	0.2	0	14%
raw .... 1/2 cup		364	19.3	60.7	24	17.4	6.0	0.6	0	14%
raw .... 1 oz		103	5.5	17.2	7	1.8	1.7	0.2	0	14%
raw (Arrowhead Mills) .... 2 oz		200	12.0	35.0	9	7.0	3.0	(mq)	0	13%
Canned										
(A&P) .... 1/2 cup		100	6.0	17.0	270	(mq)	1.0	na	0	9%
(Allens) .... 1/2 cup		110	5.0	18.0	320	(mq)	<1.0	na	0	<9%
(Bush's Best) .... 1/2 cup		80	5.0	21.0	350	6.0	0.0	na	na	0%
(Eden Foods) organic, very low sodium, no salt added ... 1/2 cup		90	6.0	17.0	10	4.0	1.0	na	0	9%
(Eden Foods) organic, w/liquid .... 1/2 cup		110	6.0	17.0	15	4.0	2.0	na	0	16%
(Finast) .... 8 oz		210	10.0	35.0	250	(mq)	3.0	(mq)	0	13%
(Green Giant) .... 1/2 cup		90	6.0	18.0	320	5.0	2.0	na	0	16%
(Green Giant) 50% less salt .... 1/2 cup		90	6.0	18.0	160	5.0	2.0	0.0	0	16%
(Joan of Arc) 50% less salt .... 1/2 cup		90	6.0	18.0	160	5.0	2.0	0.0	0	16%
(Old El Paso) .... 1/2 cup		190	5.0	16.0	250	(mq)	<1.0	na	0	<10%
(Progresso) .... 1/2 cup		110	9.0	22.0	200	6.0	1.0	na	0	7%
(S&W) large, 50% less salt 'Lite' .... 1/2 cup		110	6.0	21.0	295	(mq)	1.0	na	0	8%
(S&W Nutradiet) .... 1/2 cup		100	5.0	19.0	5	(mq)	1.0	na	0	9%
GARBANZO FLOUR/chick pea flour										
(Arrowhead Mills) .... 2 oz		200	12.0	35.0	9	7.4	3.0	(mq)	0	13%
GARDEN SALAD										
(Joan of Arc) canned .... 1/2 cup		70	2.0	17.0	500	2.4	0.0	0.0	0	0%
(Read) canned .... 1/2 cup		70	2.0	17.0	500	2.4	0.0	0.0	0	0%
(S&W) refrigerated marinated .... 1/2 cup		60	2.0	11.0	670	(mq)	0.0	0.0	0	0%

Food Name	Serving Size	Calories	Prot. gms	Carbs gms	Sod. mgs	Fiber gms	Fat gms	Sat. Fat gms	Chol. mgs	% Fat Cal.
(Trader Joe's) refrigerated fresh vegetables, no-oil vinaigrette	1 container	90	3.0	17.0	770	2.0	1.0	0.0	5	10%
(Trader Joe's) refrigerated w/eggless egg salad, no-oil vinaigrette	1 container	140	11.0	8.0	340	2.0	7.0	1.0	0	45%
GARLIC										
trimmed	1 oz	42	1.8	9.4	5	>.4 c	0.1	<.1	0	2%
untrimmed	1 lb	587	25.1	130.5	67	>5.9 c	2.0	0.4	0	3%
GARLIC BREAD. See BREAD.										
GARLIC BREAD SEASONING										
'Garlic Bread Sprinkle' *(Schilling)*	1/4 tsp	5	<.1	0.1	25	na	0.4	na	na	82%
GARLIC BREAD SPREAD *(Lawry's)*	1/2 tbsp	47	0.2	1.0	15	>.1 c	4.6	(mq)	na	90%
GARLIC PEPPER, 'Spice Blends' *(Lawry's)*	1 tsp	11	0.2	2.0	292	.1	<.1	0.0	0	<9%
GARLIC POWDER										
dry	1 oz	94	4.8	20.6	7	.5	0.2	(tr)	0	2%
dry	1 tbsp	28	1.4	6.1	2	.2	0.1	na	0	3%
dry	1 tsp	9	0.5	2.0	1	.1	0.0	na	0	0%
dry *(Durkee)*	1 tsp	10	0.0	0.1	0	0	tr	na	na	tr
dry *(Laurel Leaf)*	1 tsp	10	0.0	0.1	0	0	tr	na	na	tr
dry *(Lawry's)* w/parsley	1 tsp	12	0.5	2.3	5	.1	0.9	na	0	42%
dry *(Spice Islands)*	1 tsp	5	0.3	1.1	<1	<.1	tr	(tr)	0	0%
GARLIC SALT										
(Lawry's)	1 tsp	4	0.1	0.8	968	<.1	<.1	(tr)	0	<20%
(Morton)	1 tsp	3	<1.0	<1.0	1300	(mq)	<.1	(tr)	0	<10%
GARLIC SEASONING										
(Gilroy) crushed	1 tsp	8	0.3	2.0	4	na	0.0	0.0	na	0%
(Gilroy) minced	1 tsp	23	0.3	2.0	4	na	1.0	na	na	50%
(Golden Dipt)	2 grams	8	0.0	1.0	87	na	0.0	na	0	0%
(Schilling) 'Parsley Patch'	1 tsp	13	0.5	2.0	1	(mq)	0.5	na	0	31%
(Schilling) 'Season All'	1/4 tsp	2	<.1	0.1	163	na	(tr)	(tr)	0	0%
GARLIC SPREAD, concentrate *(Lawry's)*	1 tbsp	15	0.0	0.2	21	0	1.6	(mq)	0	95%
GATORADE. See individual flavors.										
GEFILTE FISH										
Hors d'oeuvres *(Rokeach)*	8 balls	60	8.0	4.0	(mq)	(mq)	1.0	(mq)	(mq)	16%
In jelled broth										
(Mother's) 'Old Fashioned' 24-oz jar	1 ball	70	9.0	5.0	(mq)	(mq)	1.0	(mq)	(mq)	14%
(Mother's) 'Old Fashioned' 12-oz jar	1 ball	54	7.0	4.0	(mq)	(mq)	0.8	(mq)	(mq)	14%
(Mother's) 'Old World'	1 ball	70	8.0	7.0	(mq)	(mq)	1.0	(mq)	(mq)	13%
(Mother's) 'Unsalted'	1 ball	45	5.0	2.0	(mq)	(mq)	1.0	(mq)	(mq)	24%
(Rokeach) 'Old Vienna' 31-oz jar	3 oz	81	Prot.	9.0	(mq)	(mq)	1.0	(mq)	(mq)	11%
(Rokeach) 'Old Vienna' 24-oz jar	2.6 oz	70	8.0	8.0	(mq)	(mq)	1.0	(mq)	(mq)	12%
(Rokeach) 'Old Vienna' 12-oz jar	2 oz	54	6.0	6.0	(mq)	(mq)	1.0	(mq)	(mq)	16%
(Rokeach) 'Redi-Jelled'	4 oz	92	12.0	6.0	444	(mq)	2.0	(mq)	(mq)	20%
(Rokeach) 'Redi-Jelled'	3 oz	65	9.0	5.0	333	(mq)	1.0	(mq)	(mq)	14%
(Rokeach) 'Redi-Jelled'	2 oz	46	6.0	3.0	222	(mq)	1.0	(mq)	(mq)	20%
In liquid										
(Mother's) 'Old Fashioned' 24- or 31-oz jar	1 ball	70	9.0	7.0	(mq)	(mq)	1.0	(mq)	(mq)	12%
(Mother's) 'Old Fashioned' 12-oz jar	1 ball	54	7.0	5.0	(mq)	(mq)	0.8	(mq)	(mq)	13%
In natural broth										
(Rokeach) 24-oz jar	4 oz	60	8.0	4.0	835	(mq)	1.0	(mq)	(mq)	16%
(Rokeach) 24-oz jar	2.6 oz	50	7.0	4.0	(mq)	(mq)	1.0	(mq)	(mq)	17%
Sweet *(Mother's)* 'Old World'	1 ball	54	6.0	5.0	(mq)	(mq)	0.8	(mq)	(mq)	14%
WHITEFISH										
In jelled broth										
(Mother's) 24- or 31-oz jar	1 ball	60	9.0	4.0	(mq)	(mq)	1.0	(mq)	(mq)	15%

Food Name	Serving Size	Calories	Prot. gms	Carbs gms	Sod. mgs	Fiber gms	Fat gms	Sat. Fat gms	Chol. mgs	% Fat Cal.
(Mother's) 12-oz jar	1 ball	46	7.0	3.0	(mq)	(mq)	0.8	(mq)	(mq)	15%
In liquid										
(Mother's) 24- or 31-oz jar	1 ball	70	9.0	7.0	(mq)	(mq)	1.0	(mq)	(mq)	12%
(Mother's) 12-oz jar	1 ball	54	7.0	5.0	(mq)	(mq)	0.8	(mq)	(mq)	13%
WHITEFISH AND PIKE										
In jelled broth										
(Mother's) 24- or 31-oz jar	1 ball	60	9.0	4.0	(mq)	(mq)	1.0	(mq)	(mq)	15%
(Mother's) 12-oz jar	1 ball	46	7.0	3.0	(mq)	(mq)	0.8	(mq)	(mq)	15%
(Mother's) 'Old World'	1 ball	54	6.0	5.0	(mq)	(mq)	0.8	(mq)	(mq)	14%
(Rokeach)	2.6 oz	60	9.0	4.0	(mq)	(mq)	1.0	(mq)	(mq)	15%
(Rokeach)	2 oz	46	7.0	3.0	(mq)	(mq)	1.0	(mq)	(mq)	18%
In liquid (Mother's)	1 ball	70	9.0	7.0	(mq)	(mq)	1.0	(mq)	(mq)	12%
GELATIN, JAPANESE										
raw	1 lb	116	2.5	30.6	40	>2.0 c	0.1	<.1	0	1%
raw	1 oz	7	0.2	1.9	3	>.1 c	tr	tr	0	0%
GELATIN, UNFLAVORED (Knox)	1 pkt	25	6.0	0.0	10	0	0.0	0.0	0	0%
GELATIN DESSERT										
PREPARED FROM MIX										
(D-Zerta)										
all flavors	1/2 cup	8	2.0	0.0	0	0	0.0	0.0	0	0%
all flavors, low calorie, w/aspartame	1/2 cup	8	2.0	0.0	0	na	0.0	na	0	0%
(Featherweight)										
all flavors except lemon	1/2 cup	10	2.0	1.0	5	0	0.0	0.0	0	0%
lemon	1/2 cup	10	2.0	1.0	4	0	0.0	0.0	0	0%
(Jell-O)										
berry blue	1/2 cup	80	2.0	19.0	50	na	0.0	na	0	0%
black raspberry	1/2 cup	80	2.0	19.0	35	(tr)	0.0	0.0	0	0%
cherry	1/2 cup	80	2.0	19.0	70	(tr)	0.0	0.0	0	0%
cherry, sugar-free	1/2 cup	8	1.0	0.0	80	na	0.0	na	0	0%
concord grape	1/2 cup	80	2.0	19.0	35	(tr)	0.0	0.0	0	0%
lemon	1/2 cup	80	2.0	19.0	75	(tr)	0.0	0.0	0	0%
lemon, sugar-free	1/2 cup	8	1.0	0.0	60	na	0.0	na	0	0%
lime	1/2 cup	80	2.0	19.0	55	(tr)	0.0	0.0	0	0%
lime, sugar-free	1/2 cup	8	1.0	0.0	65	na	0.0	na	0	0%
orange, sugar-free	1/2 cup	8	1.0	0.0	55	na	0.0	na	0	0%
orange-pineapple	1/2 cup	80	2.0	19.0	65	(tr)	0.0	0.0	0	0%
raspberry, sugar-free	1/2 cup	8	1.0	0.0	55	na	0.0	na	0	0%
strawberry, sugar-free	1/2 cup	8	1.0	0.0	65	na	0.0	na	0	0%
strawberry banana, sugar-free	1/2 cup	8	1.0	0.0	55	na	0.0	na	0	0%
watermelon	1/2 cup	80	2.0	20.0	50	na	0.0	na	0	0%
wild strawberry	1/2 cup	80	2.0	19.0	75	(tr)	0.0	0.0	0	0%
(Royal)										
apple	1/2 cup	80	2.0	19.0	95	na	0.0	na	na	0%
blackberry	1/2 cup	80	2.0	19.0	95	na	0.0	na	na	0%
cherry	1/2 cup	80	2.0	19.0	95	na	0.0	na	na	0%
cherry, sugar-free	1/2 cup	8	1.0	1.0	90	na	0.0	na	na	0%
concord grape	1/2 cup	80	2.0	19.0	130	na	0.0	na	na	0%
fruit punch	1/2 cup	80	2.0	19.0	90	na	0.0	na	na	0%
lemon	1/2 cup	80	2.0	19.0	125	na	0.0	0.0	0	0%
lemon-lime	1/2 cup	80	2.0	19.0	95	na	0.0	na	na	0%
lime	1/2 cup	80	2.0	19.0	125	na	0.0	0.0	0	0%
lime, sugar-free	1/2 cup	8	1.0	1.0	100	na	0.0	na	na	0%
mixed berry	1/2 cup	80	2.0	19.0	90	na	0.0	0.0	0	0%
orange	1/2 cup	80	2.0	19.0	95	na	0.0	na	na	0%

Food Name	Serving Size	Calories	Prot. gms	Carbs gms	Sod. mgs	Fiber gms	Fat gms	Sat. Fat gms	Chol. mgs	% Fat Cal.
orange, sugar-free	1/2 cup	10	1.0	1.0	90	na	0.0	na	na	0%
peach	1/2 cup	80	2.0	19.0	95	na	0.0	na	na	0%
pineapple	1/2 cup	80	2.0	19.0	95	na	0.0	na	na	0%
raspberry	1/2 cup	80	2.0	19.0	125	na	0.0	0.0	0	0%
raspberry, sugar-free	1/2 cup	8	1.0	1.0	90	na	0.0	na	na	0%
strawberry	1/2 cup	80	2.0	19.0	105	na	0.0	0.0	0	0%
strawberry, sugar-free	1/2 cup	8	1.0	1.0	90	na	0.0	na	na	0%
strawberry banana	1/2 cup	80	2.0	19.0	105	na	0.0	0.0	0	0%
strawberry banana, sugar-free	1/2 cup	8	1.0	1.0	85	na	0.0	na	na	0%
strawberry orange	1/2 cup	80	2.0	19.0	110	na	0.0	na	na	0%
tropical fruit	1/2 cup	80	2.0	19.0	110	na	0.0	na	na	0%
READY TO SERVE										
(Estee)	1/2 cup	8	1.0	<1.0	0	(tr)	0.0	0.0	0	0%
(Jell-O) berry blue, six pack	3.5 oz	80	1.0	18.0	40	na	0.0	na	0	0%
(Jell-O) cherry, six pack	3.5 oz	80	1.0	18.0	40	na	0.0	na	0	0%
(Jell-O) strawberry, six pack	3.5 oz	80	1.0	18.0	40	na	0.0	na	0	0%
GELATIN DRINK MIX										
orange flavor	1 oz	108	10.0	17.1	47	(tr)	0.3	<.1	na	2%
orange flavor (Knox)	1 envelope	39	5.7	4.0	17	(tr)	0.1	(tr)	0	2%
GERMAN SAUSAGE. See also individual listings.										
(Hickory Farms)	1 oz	100	5.0	1.0	385	0	8.0	(mq)	20	75%
GHEE / clarified butter	1 oz	249	0.0	0.0	na	0	28.4	(mq)	(mq)	100%
GIN. See ALCOHOLIC BEVERAGES.										
GINGER										
ground	1 oz	98	2.6	20.1	9	>1.7 c	1.7	0.5	0	14%
ground	1 tbsp	19	0.5	3.8	2	.7	0.3	0.1	0	14%
ground	1 tsp	6	0.2	1.3	1	.2	0.1	0.0	0	13%
ground (Durkee)	1 tsp	7	0.0	0.0	0	0	tr	na	na	tr
ground (Laurel Leaf)	1 tsp	7	0.0	0.0	0	0	tr	na	na	tr
ground (Spice Islands)	1 tsp	6	0.1	1.2	1	.2	0.1	(mq)	0	15%
GINGER, PICKLED, Japanese	1 oz	10	0.1	2.1	105	(mq)	<.1	tr	0	<9%
GINGER ALE. See SOFT DRINKS AND MIXERS.										
GINGER ROOT										
candied, crystallized	1 lb	1544	1.4	395.4	272	>3.2 c	0.9	0.0	0	1%
candied, crystallized	1 oz	95	0.1	24.4	17	>.2 c	0.1	0.0	0	1%
raw, slices, 1-inch diam	1/4 cup	17	0.4	3.6	3	.5	0.2	0.1	0	10%
raw, slices, 1-inch diam	5 slices	8	0.2	1.7	1	.2	0.1	0.0	0	11%
trimmed	1 oz	20	0.5	4.3	4	>.3 c	0.2	0.1	0	9%
untrimmed	1 lb	291	7.4	63.6	53	>4.3 c	3.1	0.9	0	9%
GINGER TERIYAKI MARINADE (Golden Dipt)	1 oz	120	1.0	12.0	920	na	7.0	na	0	55%
GINGERBREAD. See BREAD.										
GINKGO NUT										
canned	1 cup	172	3.5	34.3	476	14.4	2.5	0.5	0	13%
canned, approx 9 large, 14 medium, or 22 small	1 oz	32	0.7	6.3	87	>.5 c	0.5	0.1	0	14%
dried	1 oz	99	2.9	20.6	4	>.3 c	0.6	0.1	0	5%
dried, in shell	1 lb	1198	35.7	249.8	46	>3.4 c	6.9	1.3	0	5%
raw	1 oz	52	1.2	10.7	2	>.1 c	0.5	0.1	0	9%
raw, in shell	1 lb	628	14.9	129.6	24	>1.7 c	5.8	1.1	0	8%
GLOBE ARTICHOKE. See ARTHICHOKES, GLOBE.										
GLUTEN. See WHEAT GLUTEN.										
GOA BEAN. See WINGED BEAN.										
GOAT										
raw	1 lb	494	93.4	0.0	372	na	10.5	3.2	259	20%
raw	1 oz	31	5.8	0.0	23	na	0.7	0.2	16	21%

Food Name	Serving Size	Calories	Prot. gms	Carbs gms	Sod. mgs	Fiber gms	Fat gms	Sat. Fat gms	Chol. mgs	% Fat Cal.
roasted	4 oz	162	30.7	0.0	98	0	3.4	1.1	85	20%
roasted, diced	1 cup	200	37.9	0.0	120	0	4.2	1.3	105	20%
GOATFISH										
raw	1 lb	435	92.5	0.0	(mq)	0	4.5	(mq)	(mq)	10%
raw	1 oz	27	5.8	0.0	(mq)	0	0.3	(mq)	(mq)	10%
GOBO. See BURDOCK ROOT.										
GOOSE, DOMESTICATED										
meat and skin, raw	1 oz	105	4.5	0.0	21	0	9.5	2.8	23	83%
meat and skin, roasted	4 oz	346	28.5	0.0	79	0	24.9	7.8	103	66%
meat only, raw	1 oz	46	6.4	0.0	25	0	2.0	0.8	24	41%
meat only, roasted	4 oz	270	32.9	0.0	86	0	14.4	5.2	109	50%
GOOSE FAT										
	1/2 cup	923	0.0	0.0	0	0	102.3	28.4	103	100%
	1 oz	255	0.0	0.0	0	0	28.3	7.9	28	100%
	1 tbsp	115	0.0	0.0	0	0	12.8	3.5	13	100%
GOOSE GIBLETS, raw	100 gm	156	21.1	0.6	70	0	7.0	2.0	350	42%
GOOSE GIZZARD, raw	100 gm	139	21.4	0.0	65	0	5.3	1.0	145	36%
GOOSE LIVER, raw	1 lb	15	1.8	0.7	15	0	0.5	0.2	57	31%
GOOSEBERRY										
whole	1 lb	202	4.0	46.2	4	>8.6 c	2.6	0.2	0	10%
whole	1 oz	12	0.2	2.9	<1	>.5 c	0.2	<.1	0	13%
whole	1 cup	66	1.3	15.3	2	6.4	0.9	0.1	0	11%
GOOSEBERRY, CANNED, in light syrup	4 oz	83	0.7	21.3	2	>1.4 c	0.2	<.1	0	2%
GOOSEFISH. See MONKFISH.										
GOURD, BOTTLE/calabash gourd/white-flowered gourd										
boiled, drained	4 oz	17	0.7	4.2	2	>.7 c	<.1	tr	0	<4%
boiled, drained, 1-inch cubes	1/2 cup	11	0.4	2.7	1	>.5 c	<.1	tr	0	<7%
raw, approx 2.4 lb	1 med	106	5.0	26.1	19	8.5	0.2	<.1	0	1%
raw, 1-inch cubes	1/2 cup	8	0.4	2.0	1	.6	<.1	tr	0	<9%
raw, trimmed	1 oz	4	0.2	1.0	1	.3	tr	tr	0	0%
raw, untrimmed	1 lb	44	2.0	10.8	8	3.5	0.1	tr	0	2%
GOURD, CALABASH. See GOURD, BOTTLE.										
GOURD, DISHCLOTH/loofah gourd/rag gourd/sponge gourd/towel gourd/vegetable sponge										
boiled, drained	4 oz	64	0.7	16.3	24	.5	0.4	<.1	0	5%
boiled, drained, 1-inch slices	1/2 cup	50	0.6	12.8	19	>.3 c	0.3	0.0	0	5%
raw, approx 8.6 oz	1 med	36	2.1	7.8	5	>.9 c	0.4	0.0	0	8%
raw, 1-inch slices	1 cup	19	1.1	4.1	3	>.5 c	0.2	0.0	0	8%
raw, trimmed	1 oz	6	0.3	1.2	1	>.1 c	0.1	tr	0	13%
raw, untrimmed	1 lb	67	4.0	14.4	11	>1.7 c	0.7	0.1	0	8%
GOURD, RAG. See GOURD, DISHCLOTH.										
GOURD, SPONGE. See GOURD, DISHCLOTH.										
GOURD, WAX										
boiled, drained	4 oz	15	0.5	3.4	121	>.6 c	0.2	<.1	0	10%
boiled, drained, cubes	1/2 cup	11	0.4	2.6	93	.9	0.2	0.0	0	13%
raw, cubes	1 cup	17	0.5	4.0	147	3.8	0.3	0.0	0	13%
raw, trimmed	1 oz	4	0.1	0.9	31	.2	0.1	tr	0	18%
raw, untrimmed	1 lb	42	1.3	9.7	358	1.9	0.6	0.1	0	11%
GOURD, WHITE/tunka										
boiled, drained	4 oz	15	0.5	3.4	121	>.6 c	0.2	<.1	0	10%
boiled, drained, cubes	1/2 cup	11	0.4	2.6	93	.9	0.2	0.0	0	13%
raw, cubes	1 cup	17	0.5	4.0	147	3.8	0.3	0.0	0	13%
raw, trimmed	1 oz	4	0.1	0.9	31	.2	0.1	tr	0	18%
raw, untrimmed	1 lb	42	1.3	9.7	358	1.9	0.6	0.1	0	11%
GOURD, WHITE-FLOWERED. See GOURD, BOTTLE.										

Food Name	Serving Size	Calories	Prot. gms	Carbs gms	Sod. mgs	Fiber gms	Fat gms	Sat. Fat gms	Chol. mgs	% Fat Cal.
GOVERNOR PLUM, trimmed .... 1 oz		31	0.1	8.4	na	>.1 c	0.0	0.0	0	0%
GRANADILLA. See PASSION FRUIT.										
GRANOLA. See CEREAL, READY-TO-SERVE.										
GRANOLA AND CEREAL BAR. See also GRANOLA SNACKS.										
(Barbara's Bakery)										
cinnamon and oats, 2 oz .... 1 bar		281	6.0	31.0	na	na	15.0	na	0	48%
coconut almond, 2 oz .... 1 bar		306	8.0	23.0	na	na	20.0	na	0	59%
peanut butter, 2 oz .... 1 bar		275	7.0	28.0	na	na	15.0	na	0	49%
(Bear Valley)										
carob-cocoa, food bar 'Pemmican' 3.75 oz .... 1 bar		440	16.0	68.0	80	7.0	12.0	na	0	24%
coconut almond, food bar 'Meal Pack' 3.75 oz .... 1 bar		400	16.0	56.0	80	6.0	12.0	na	0	27%
sesame lemon, food bar 'Meal Pack' 3.75 oz .... 1 bar		410	17.0	57.0	85	4.0	13.0	na	0	28%
fruit 'n nut, food bar 'Pemmican' 3.75 oz .... 1 bar		420	17.0	59.0	90	9.0	13.0	na	0	28%
(Glenny's)										
apple, 'Original Fruit Bar' .... 1 bar		100	2.0	15.0	15	4.0	3.0	1.0	0	28%
'Bee Pollen Sunrise' 1.5 oz .... 1 bar		190	5.0	22.0	na	na	8.0	na	na	40%
carob mint w/oat bran 'Brown Rice Treats' .... 1 bar		180	3.0	37.0	20	1.7	2.0	na	na	10%
cinnamon and raisin 'Brown Rice Treats' 1.75 oz .... 1 bar		170	2.0	38.0	30	na	1.0	na	na	5%
coconut amandine 'Moist and Chewy' 1.5 oz .... 1 bar		190	3.0	22.0	20	na	10.0	na	na	47%
'Ginseng Sunrise' 1.5 oz .... 1 bar		160	1.0	24.0	na	na	7.0	na	na	39%
oatmeal raisin 'Moist and Chewy' 1.5 oz .... 1 bar		160	3.0	30.0	25	na	3.0	na	na	17%
peanut and raisin 'Brown Rice Treats' 2 oz .... 1 bar		210	4.0	39.0	29	na	5.0	na	na	21%
peanut snack 'Moist and Chewy' 1.5 oz .... 1 bar		180	5.0	24.0	20	na	7.0	na	na	35%
plain and fancy 'Brown Rice Treats' 1.25 oz .... 1 bar		120	1.0	28.0	29	na	1.0	na	na	7%
raisin bran 'Brown Rice Treats' 1.75 oz .... 1 bar		170	2.0	38.0	17	na	1.0	na	na	5%
'Spirulina Sunrise' 1.5 oz .... 1 bar		140	3.0	21.0	na	na	5.0	na	na	32%
sunflower 'Moist and Chewy' 1.5 oz .... 1 bar		180	5.0	24.0	15	na	7.0	na	na	35%
toasted almond w/oat bran 'Brown Rice Treats' .... 1 bar		200	4.0	34.0	20	1.6	5.0	na	na	23%
(Golden Temple)										
cashew almond 'Wha Guru Chew Bar' .... 1 bar		164	3.0	15.0	63	1.0	11.0	1.0	0	58%
peanut cashew 'Wha Guru Chew Bar' .... 1 bar		167	4.0	14.0	62	1.0	11.0	1.0	0	58%
sesame almond 'Wha Guru Chew Bar' .... 1 bar		160	3.0	15.0	61	1.0	10.0	1.0	0	56%
(Health Valley)										
blueberry apple, fat-free .... 1 bar		140	3.0	33.0	10	3.7	0.0	na	0	0%
date almond flavor, fat-free .... 1 bar		140	3.0	33.0	10	3.7	0.0	na	0	0%
raspberry, fat-free .... 1 bar		140	3.0	33.0	10	3.7	0.0	na	0	0%
(Hershey's)										
chocolate chip, chocolate coated, 1.2 oz .... 1 bar		170	2.0	22.0	50	(mq)	8.0	(mq)	na	43%
cocoa creme, chocolate coated, 1.2 oz .... 1 bar		180	2.0	22.0	50	(mq)	9.0	(mq)	5	46%
cookies and creme, chocolate coated, 1.2 oz .... 1 bar		170	2.0	22.0	50	(mq)	8.0	(mq)	na	43%
peanut butter, chocolate coated, 1.2 oz .... 1 bar		180	4.0	19.0	65	(mq)	10.0	(mq)	5	50%
raspberry filled 'Common Sense Smart Start' .... 1 bar		170	2.0	28.0	160	1.0	6.0	(mq)	0	31%
(Kudo's)										
chocolate chip .... 1 bar		180	3.0	21.0	60	(mq)	9.0	na	na	46%
chocolate chunk 'Simply Kudos' .... 1 bar		100	1.0	13.0	50	na	4.0	na	na	39%
fudge, nutty .... 1 bar		190	4.0	19.0	60	(mq)	11.0	na	na	52%
honey nut 'Simply Kudos' .... 1 bar		100	2.0	13.0	55	na	4.0	na	na	38%
oatmeal raisin 'Simply Kudos' .... 1 bar		90	1.0	13.0	55	na	4.0	na	na	39%
peanut butter, chocolate coated, 1.3 oz .... 1 bar		190	4.0	18.0	70	(mq)	12.0	(mq)	na	55%
(Natural Nectar)										
almond, 'Treat Yourself Right' .... 1 bar		150	3.0	22.0	40	5.0	5.0	na	0	31%
apple-oatmeal spice, 'Fi-Bar A.M.' .... 1 bar		150	3.0	27.0	25	5.0	3.0	na	0	18%
banana nut, 'Fi-Bar A.M.' .... 1 bar		150	2.0	26.0	20	5.0	4.0	na	0	24%
cocoa almond, 'Fi-Bar Chewy & Nutty' .... 1 bar		130	3.0	21.0	20	4.0	4.0	na	0	27%

Food Name	Serving Size	Calories	Prot. gms	Carbs gms	Sod. mgs	Fiber gms	Fat gms	Sat. Fat gms	Chol. mgs	% Fat Cal.
cocoa almond crunch, 'Canadian Chewy & Nutty'	1 bar	130	3.0	21.0	20	2.0	4.0	1.0	0	27%
cocoa peanut, 'Fi-Bar Chewy & Nutty'	1 bar	130	3.0	20.0	20	4.0	1.0	na	0	9%
cocoa peanut butter crunch, 'Chewy & Nutty'	1 bar	130	3.0	20.0	20	2.0	4.0	1.0	0	28%
coconut	1 bar	120	2.0	20.0	30	6.0	4.0	1.0	0	29%
cranberry, w/wild berries 'Original Fruit Bar'	1 bar	120	2.0	23.0	15	4.0	2.0	na	0	15%
lemon 'Original Fruit Bar'	1 bar	100	2.0	15.0	15	4.0	3.0	1.0	0	28%
Mandarin orange 'Original Fruit Bar'	1 bar	100	2.0	15.0	15	4.0	3.0	1.0	0	28%
peanut butter	1 bar	130	3.0	20.0	30	6.0	4.0	1.0	0	28%
peanut butter 'Treat Yourself Right'	1 bar	150	4.0	18.0	55	5.0	5.0	na	0	34%
raisin nut bran, 'Fi-Bar A.M.'	1 bar	150	3.0	26.0	30	5.0	4.0	na	0	24%
raspberry 'Canadian'	1 bar	120	2.0	21.0	15	3.0	3.0	1.0	0	23%
raspberry 'Original Fruit Bar'	1 bar	120	2.0	23.0	15	4.0	2.0	na	0	15%
strawberry 'Canadian'	1 bar	120	2.0	21.0	15	3.0	3.0	1.0	0	23%
strawberry 'Original Fruit Bar'	1 bar	120	2.0	23.0	15	4.0	2.0	na	0	15%
strawberry-oatmeal w/almonds, 'Fi-Bar A.M.'	1 bar	150	3.0	24.0	30	5.0	4.0	na	0	25%
vanilla almond, 'Fi-Bar Chewy & Nutty'	1 bar	130	3.0	21.0	20	4.0	4.0	na	0	27%
vanilla almond crunch, 'Canadian Chewy & Nutty'	1 bar	130	3.0	21.0	20	2.0	4.0	1.0	0	27%
vanilla peanut, 'Fi-Bar Chewy & Nutty'	1 bar	130	3.0	20.0	20	4.0	4.0	na	0	28%
wild cranberry 'Canadian'	1 bar	120	2.0	21.0	15	3.0	3.0	1.0	0	23%
(Nature Valley)										
cinnamon, .8 oz	1 bar	120	2.0	17.0	70	1.0	5.0	1.0	0	37%
oat bran-honey graham, .8 oz	1 bar	110	2.0	16.0	90	1.0	4.0	<1.0	0	33%
oats and honey, .8 oz	1 bar	120	2.0	17.0	65	1.0	5.0	1.0	0	37%
peanut butter, .8 oz	1 bar	120	2.0	15.0	70	1.0	6.0	1.0	0	44%
(Nature's Choice)										
carob chip, .75 oz	1 bar	90	2.0	15.0	15	na	3.0	na	0	28%
cinnamon-raisin, .75 oz	1 bar	90	2.0	15.0	10	na	3.0	na	0	28%
oats 'n honey, .75 oz	1 bar	90	2.0	15.0	15	na	3.0	na	0	28%
peanut butter, .75 oz	1 bar	90	2.0	14.0	25	na	3.0	na	0	30%
(Nutri Grain)										
blueberry 'Smart Start' 1.5 oz	1 bar	180	2.0	26.0	170	1.0	8.0	(mq)	0	39%
corn flakes, mixed berry filled 'Smart Start'	1 bar	170	2.0	27.0	160	1.0	7.0	(mq)	0	35%
raisin bran 'Smart Start' 1.5 oz	1 bar	160	2.0	28.0	170	2.0	5.0	(mq)	0	27%
rice krispies w/almonds 'Smart Start' 1 oz	1 bar	130	2.0	18.0	65	1.0	6.0	(mq)	0	40%
strawberry 'Smart Start' 1.5 oz	1 bar	180	2.0	26.0	170	1.0	8.0	(mq)	0	39%
(Quaker)										
apple berry 'Chewy'	1 bar	120	2.0	20.0	95	na	4.0	na	0	29%
caramel nut 'Granola Dipps' 1 oz	1 bar	148	1.9	20.9	81	.7	6.4	2.8	2	39%
chocolate chip 'Chewy'	1 bar	128	2.0	19.3	90	1.4	4.7	1.5	0	33%
chocolate chip 'Granola Dipps' 1 oz	1 bar	139	1.8	18.7	78	1.0	6.3	2.8	1	41%
chocolate fudge 'Granola Dipps' 1 oz	1 bar	160	2.1	20.0	74	(mq)	7.9	(mq)	na	45%
chunky nut and raisin 'Chewy' 1 oz	1 bar	131	2.5	17.2	86	1.6	5.8	1.3	0	40%
honey and oats 'Chewy', 1 oz	1 bar	125	2.3	19.1	95	1.3	4.4	1.1	<1	32%
peanut butter 'Chewy' 1 oz	1 bar	128	3.1	17.8	116	1.2	4.9	1.3	<1	35%
peanut butter, chocolate chip 'Chewy' 1 oz	1 bar	131	3.1	17.0	112	1.2	5.7	1.5	0	39%
peanut butter, chocolate chip 'Granola Dipps'	1 bar	174	3.6	17.4	102	(mq)	10.0	(mq)	na	52%
peanut butter 'Granola Dipps' 1 oz	1 bar	170	3.0	16.5	74	1.0	9.1	3.1	?	48%
raisin and cinnamon 'Chewy' 1 oz	1 bar	128	2.2	18.6	92	1.2	5.0	1.1	<1	35%
S'mores 'Chewy' 1 oz	1 bar	126	1.9	19.7	108	1.1	4.4	1.4	0	31%
trail mix 'Chewy' 1 oz	1 bar	130	2.0	18.0	105	na	5.0	na	0	36%
(Sunbelt)										
apple bar, baked 1.31 oz	1 bar	130	1.0	28.0	130	1.0	2.0	na	na	13%
chocolate chip, chewy, 1.25 oz	1 bar	150	3.0	23.0	75	(mq)	7.0	(mq)	<1	38%
chocolate chip, fudge dipped, chewy, 1.63 oz	1 bar	220	2.0	29.0	60	(mq)	11.0	(mq)	<1	44%

Food Name	Serving Size	Calories	Prot. gms	Carbs gms	Sod. mgs	Fiber gms	Fat gms	Sat. Fat gms	Chol. mgs	% Fat Cal.
chocolate chip, fudge dipped, chewy 1.5 oz	1 bar	210	2.0	26.0	55	4.0	10.0	4.0	2	45%
oats and honey, chewy, 1 oz	1 bar	130	2.0	18.0	35	(mq)	5.0	(mq)	<1	36%
oats and honey, fudge dipped, chewy, 1.38 oz	1 bar	190	2.0	24.0	55	(mq)	10.0	(mq)	<1	46%
w/almonds, chewy, 1 oz	1 bar	120	3.0	18.0	65	(mq)	6.0	(mq)	<1	39%
w/chocolate chips, chewy 1.75 oz	1 bar	220	4.0	32.0	105	(mq)	9.0	(mq)	<1	36%
w/peanuts, fudge dipped, chewy, 2.25 oz	1 bar	300	6.0	36.0	90	(mq)	18.0	(mq)	<1	49%
w/peanuts, fudge dipped, chewy, 1.38 oz	1 bar	190	2.0	24.0	55	(mq)	10.0	(mq)	<1	46%
w/raisins, chewy, 1.25 oz	1 bar	150	2.0	24.0	65	(mq)	6.0	(mq)	<1	34%
w/raisins, fudge dipped, chewy, 1.5 oz	1 bar	200	4.0	24.0	60	(mq)	12.0	(mq)	<1	49%
GRANOLA SNACKS. See also GRANOLA AND CEREAL BAR.										
(Natural Nectar)										
almond butter crunch 'Nectar Nuggets'	1 cup	120	3.0	11.0	30	5.0	7.0	na	0	53%
almond cappuccino crunch 'Nectar Nuggets'	1 cup	110	2.0	14.0	30	5.0	5.0	na	0	41%
coconut almond crunch 'Nectar Nuggets'	1 cup	110	2.0	15.0	20	4.0	5.0	na	0	40%
peanut butter crunch 'Nectar Nuggets'	1 cup	120	4.0	11.0	30	5.0	7.0	na	0	51%
(Nature Valley)										
apple-cinnamon 'Granola Bites'	1 pkg	170	3.0	25.0	100	2.0	7.0	na	0	36%
honey nut 'Granola Bites'	1 pkg	170	3.0	24.0	120	2.0	8.0	1.0	0	40%
variety pack 'Granola Bites'	1 pkg	170	3.0	24.0	120	2.0	8.0	1.0	0	40%
(Nature's Choice)										
chocolate chip 'Grrr-Nola Treats'	.75 oz	80	1.0	15.0	5	na	2.0	na	0	22%
cinnamon toast 'Grrr-Nola Treats'	.75 oz	80	1.0	15.0	5	na	2.0	na	0	22%
peanut butter & jelly 'Grrr-Nola Treats'	.75 oz	80	1.0	14.0	5	na	3.0	na	0	31%
tutti-frutti 'Grrr-Nola Treats'	.75 oz	75	1.0	15.0	5	na	2.0	na	0	22%
GRAPE										
AMERICAN (Concord, Delaware, Niagara)								/		
(Dole)	1.5 cup	85	1.0	24.0	3	2.0	0.0	na	na	0%
Slipskin										
peeled and seeded	1 oz	18	0.2	4.9	<1	>.2 c	0.1	<.1	0	4%
trimmed	10 fruits	15	0.2	4.1	0	>.2 c	0.1	0.0	0	5%
untrimmed	1 lb	165	1.7	45.1	4	>2.0 c	0.9	0.3	0	4%
untrimmed	1 cup	58	0.6	15.8	2	>.9 c	0.3	0.1	0	4%
EUROPEAN (Muskat, Tokay, Thompson)										
Adherent skin										
trimmed	10 fruits	35	0.3	8.9	1	.5	0.3	0.1	0	7%
untrimmed	1 lb	287	2.7	72.0	7	2.8	2.3	0.8	0	7%
untrimmed	1 cup	114	1.1	28.4	3	1.6	0.9	0.3	0	6%
untrimmed w/o seeds	1 lb	309	2.9	77.4	7	3.0	2.5	0.8	0	7%
w/seeds	1/2 cup	57	0.5	14.2	2	.6	0.5	0.2	0	7%
w/seeds	1 oz	20	0.2	5.0	1	.2	0.2	0.1	0	8%
w/o seeds	1/2 cup	57	0.5	14.2	2	.6	0.5	0.2	0	7%
w/o seeds	1 oz	20	0.2	5.0	1	.2	0.2	0.1	0	8%
w/o seeds, approx 1.75 oz	10 grapes	36	0.3	8.9	1	.4	0.3	0.1	0	7%
GRAPE, CANNED										
THOMPSON, seedless										
in heavy syrup	1 cup	187	1.2	50.3	13	1.0	0.3	0.1	0	1%
in heavy syrup	4 oz	83	0.5	22.3	6	>.2 c	0.1	<.1	0	1%
in heavy syrup *(S&W)*	1/2 cup	100	0.0	25.0	5	(mq)	0.0	0.0	0	0%
in water	1 cup	98	1.2	25.2	15	2.5	0.3	0.1	0	3%
in water	4 oz	45	0.6	11.7	7	>.2 c	0.1	<.1	0	2%
GRAPE APPLE DRINK, bottle *(Mott's)*	10 oz	167	0.0	42.0	<1	0	0.0	0.0	0	0%
GRAPE DRINK										
Can, bottle, or box										
(A&P)	6 oz	100	<1.0	25.0	0	0	<1.0	(tr)	0	<8%

Food Name	Serving Size	Calories	Prot. gms	Carbs gms	Sod. mgs	Fiber gms	Fat gms	Sat. Fat gms	Chol. mgs	% Fat Cal.
(All Sport) thirst quencher, caffeine-free	8 oz	70	0.0	20.0	55	na	0.0	na	na	0%
(Bama)	8.45 oz	120	0.0	29.0	25	0	0.0	0.0	0	0%
(Bright & Early) frozen, diluted	6 oz	100	0.0	24.0	0	na	0.0	na	na	0%
(Crowley)	8 oz	130	0.0	32.0	15	0	0.0	0.0	0	0%
(Fruitopia) 'The Grape Beyond' real fruit	8 oz	130	0.0	32.0	25	na	0.0	na	na	0%
(Gatorade) low sodium, no caffeine	8 oz	50	0.0	14.0	110	na	0.0	0.0	0	0%
(Hi-C) aseptic box	6 oz	90	0.0	23.0	25	na	0.0	na	na	0%
(J. Hungerford)	9.03 oz	41	0.0	10.9	31.	0	0.0	0.0	0	0%
(Kool-Aid) 'Koolers'	8.45 oz	140	0.0	35.0	10	0	0.0	0.0	0	0%
(Pathmark)	6 oz	90	0.0	22.0	0	0	0.0	0.0	0	0%
(Squeezit) 'Grumpy Grape'	6.75 oz	120	0.0	30.0	5	na	0.0	na	na	0%
(10-K) 'Clear'	8 oz	60	0.0	15.0	55	na	0.0	na	na	0%
(Tropicana)	6 oz	90	<1.0	22.0	10	na	<1.0	na	na	<9%
(Veryfine)	8 oz	130	0.1	34.0	10	0	0.0	0.0	0	0%
(Wyler's) 'Fruit Slush'	4 oz	157	0.0	39.3	10	0	0.0	0.0	0	0%
Prepared from mix										
(Finast)	8 oz	80	0.0	21.0	15	0	0.0	0.0	0	0%
(Gatorade) instant 'Thirst Quencher'	8 oz	60	0.0	15.0	110	na	0.0	na	na	0%
(Kool-Aid) sugar-sweetened	8 oz	80	0.0	20.0	25	na	0.0	na	0	0%
(Kool-Aid) unsweetened, prepared w/sugar	8 oz	100	0.0	25.0	0	na	0.0	na	0	0%
(Kool-Aid) unsweetened, prepared w/o sugar	8 oz	2	0.0	0.0	0	na	0.0	na	0	0%
(Kool-Aid) w/NutraSweet	8 oz	4	0.0	0.0	0	na	0.0	na	0	0%
(Pathmark) 'No Frills'	8 oz	90	0.0	22.0	20	0	0.0	0.0	0	0%
(Pathmark) 'No Frills Sodium Free'	6 oz	80	0.0	22.0	0	0	0.0	0.0	0	0%
GRAPE JUICE										
Can, bottle, or box										
(IGA) 'Unsweetened'	6 oz	120	0.0	30.0	5	0	0.0	0.0	0	0%
(J. Hungerford)	9.03 oz	160	0.2	40.2	0	.1	0.0	0.0	0	0%
(J. Hungerford) 100% juice	9.03 oz	155	0.5	39.2	11	.4	0.0	0.0	0	0%
(J. Hungerford) 50% juice	9.03 oz	135	0.2	33.7	0	0	0.0	0.0	0	0%
(J. Hungerford) 20% juice	9.03 oz	41	0.0	10.9	31	0	0.0	0.0	0	0%
(Juicy Juice) blend	6 oz	100	0.0	25.0	5	0	0.0	0.0	0	0%
(Juicy Juice) bottled	6 oz	90	1.0	22.0	5	na	0.0	na	na	0%
(Juicy Juice) boxed	8.45 oz	130	1.0	31.0	10	na	0.0	na	na	0%
(Knudsen & Sons)	8 oz	130	1.0	32.0	na	na	0.0	na	na	0%
(Knudsen & Sons) Concord	8 oz	130	1.0	32.0	na	na	0.0	na	na	0%
(Kraft) 'Pure 100% Unsweetened'	6 oz	104	1.0	25.0	0	0	0.0	0.0	0	0%
(Pathmark) 'No Frills'	6 oz	113	0.0	27.0	10	0	0.0	0.0	0	0%
(Lucky Leaf)	6 oz	130	0.0	32.0	0	0	0.0	0.0	0	0%
(Minute Maid) aseptic box	6 oz	100	1.0	24.0	20	na	1.0	na	na	8%
(Pathmark) 'Unsweetened'	6 oz	120	0.0	30.0	10	0	0.0	0.0	0	0%
(S&W) Concord 'Unsweetened'	6 oz	100	1.0	25.0	9	0	0.0	0.0	0	0%
(Sippin' Pak)	8.45 oz	130	1.0	32.0	25	0	0.0	0.0	0	0%
(Squeezit 100) 'Caped Grape' 100% natural fruit juice	6.75 oz	100	0.0	24.0	20	na	0.0	na	na	0%
(Veryfine) '100%'	8 oz	153	1.0	37.0	20	0	0.0	0.0	0	0%
(Welch's) purple	6 oz	120	0.0	30.0	10	0	0.0	0.0	0	0%
(Welch's) red	8.45 oz	170	0.0	40.0	20	0	0.0	0.0	0	0%
(Welch's) red	6 oz	120	0.0	30.0	15	0	0.0	0.0	0	0%
(Welch's) sparkling red	6 oz	128	0.0	30.0	30	0	0.0	0.0	0	0%
(Welch's) sparkling white	6 oz	120	0.0	30.0	30	0	0.0	0.0	0	0%
(Welch's) 'USDA'	6 oz	120	0.0	30.0	10	0	0.0	0.0	0	0%
(Welch's) white	8.45 oz	160	0.0	39.0	20	0	0.0	0.0	0	0%
(Welch's) white	6 oz	120	0.0	30.0	15	0	0.0	0.0	0	0%

Food Name	Serving Size	Calories	Prot. gms	Carbs gms	Sod. mgs	Fiber gms	Fat gms	Sat. Fat gms	Chol. mgs	% Fat Cal.
Frozen, diluted as directed										
(Minute Maid)	6 oz	90	0.0	24.0	0	na	0.0	na	na	0%
(Sunkist)	6 oz	69	0.3	17.1	3	0	0.1	(tr)	0	1%
(Welch's) 'No Sugar Added'	6 oz	40	0.0	10.0	5	0	0.0	0.0	0	0%
(Welch's) 'Orchard'	10 oz	170	0.0	43.0	10	0	0.0	0.0	0	0%
(Welch's) 'Orchard'	6 oz	110	0.0	27.0	20	0	0.0	0.0	0	0%
(Welch's) 'Orchard Cocktails-In-A-Box'	8.45 oz	150	0.0	38.0	20	0	0.0	0.0	0	0%
(Welch's) purple	6 oz	100	0.0	25.0	0	0	0.0	0.0	0	0%
(Welch's) white	6 oz	100	0.0	25.0	0	0	0.0	0.0	0	0%
GRAPE JUICE DRINK										
(Hi-C)	8.45 oz	136	0.1	33.4	24	0	0.1	(tr)	0	1%
(Hi-C)	6 oz	96	0.1	23.7	17	0	0.1	(tr)	0	1%
(Sunkist) frozen, diluted	6 oz	69	0.3	17.0	3	0	0.1	(tr)	0	1%
(Tang) 'Fruit Box'	8.45 oz	130	0.0	34.0	10	na	0.0	na	0	0%
GRAPE PUNCH										
(Minute Maid) chilled	6 oz	90	0.0	23.0	20	na	0.0	na	na	0%
(Minute Maid) frozen concentrate	6 oz	90	0.0	23.0	0	na	0.0	na	na	0%
GRAPEFRUIT										
PINK AND RED										
Arizona/California										
fresh, 3.75 inch diam	1/2 fruit	46	0.6	11.9	1	>.3 c	0.1	0.0	0	2%
sections w/juice	1 cup	85	1.1	22.3	2	>.5 c	0.2	0.0	0	2%
trimmed	1 oz	11	0.1	2.7	<1	>.1 c	<.1	tr	0	<7%
untrimmed	1 lb	86	1.2	22.4	1	>.5 c	0.2	<.1	0	2%
Florida										
fresh (Ocean Spray)	1/2 med	50	1.0	13.0	0	(mq)	0.0	0.0	0	0%
fresh, 3.75 inch diam	1/2 fruit	37	0.7	9.2	0	1.4	0.1	0.0	0	2%
sections w/juice	1 cup	69	1.3	17.3	0	2.5	0.2	0.0	0	2%
trimmed	1 oz	9	0.2	2.1	tr	>.1 c	<.1	tr	0	<9%
untrimmed	1 lb	69	1.3	17.4	1	>.5 c	0.2	<.1	0	2%
WHITE										
California										
fresh, 3.75 inch diam	1/2 fruit	44	1.0	10.7	0	>.2 c	0.1	0.0	0	2%
sections w/juice	1 cup	85	2.0	20.9	0	>.5 c	0.2	0.0	0	2%
trimmed	1 oz	10	0.2	2.6	tr	>.1 c	<.1	tr	0	<7%
untrimmed	1 lb	81	2.0	20.2	1	>.4 c	0.2	<.1	0	2%
Florida										
fresh (Ocean Spray)	1/2 med	45	1.0	12.0	0	(mq)	0.0	0.0	0	0%
fresh, 3.75 inch diam	1/2 fruit	38	0.7	9.7	0	1.3	0.1	0.0	0	2%
sections w/juice	1 cup	74	1.5	18.8	0	2.5	0.2	0.0	0	2%
trimmed	1 oz	9	0.2	2.3	tr	<.1	<.1	tr	0	<8%
GRAPEFRUIT, CANNED										
(Featherweight) in juice	1/2 cup	40	0.0	9.0	10	(mq)	0.0	0.0	0	0%
(Finast) in light syrup	1/2 cup	80	0.0	20.0	10	(mq)	<.1	(tr)	0	<1%
(Kraft) chilled 'Pure'	1/2 cup	50	1.0	12.0	0	(mq)	0.0	0.0	0	0%
(S&W) in light syrup	1/2 cup	80	<1.0	24.0	0	(mq)	0.0	0.0	0	0%
(S&W) 'Unsweetened'	1/2 cup	40	0.0	9.0	10	(mq)	0.0	0.0	0	0%
(S&W Nutradiet)	1/2 cup	40	0.0	9.0	0	(mq)	0.0	0.0	0	0%
(Stokely) in light syrup	1/2 cup	90	1.0	23.0	5	(mq)	1.0	(tr)	0	9%
GRAPEFRUIT JUICE										
Can, bottle, or box										
(Del Monte)	6 oz	70	1.0	17.0	10	tr	0.0	0.0	0	0%
(J. Hungerford) regular	9.03 oz	120	0.3	29.8	0	.1	0.0	0.0	0	0%
(J. Hungerford) 100% juice	9.03 oz	98	0.8	24.2	6	.3	0.0	0.0	0	0%

Food Name	Serving Size	Calories	Prot. gms	Carbs gms	Sod. mgs	Fiber gms	Fat gms	Sat. Fat gms	Chol. mgs	% Fat Cal.
(J. Hungerford) 50% juice	9.03 oz	109	0.7	26.9	0	0	0.0	0.0	0	0%
(Knudsen & Sons)	8 oz	70	1.0	17.0	na	na	0.0	na	na	0%
(Knudsen & Sons) pink	8 oz	80	1.0	18.0	na	na	0.0	na	na	0%
(Kraft) '100% pure'	6 oz	70	1.0	16.0	0	tr	0.0	0.0	0	0%
(Libby's)	6 oz	70	1.0	17.0	na	na	0.0	na	0	0%
(Minute Maid)	6 oz	70	1.0	17.0	20	na	0.0	na	na	0%
(Minute Maid) 'Juices to Go'	6 oz	70	1.0	17.0	20	na	0.0	na	na	0%
(Mott's)	9.5 oz	118	1.0	29.0	5	tr	0.0	0.0	0	0%
(Mott's)	10 oz	124	1.0	30.0	5	tr	0.0	0.0	0	0%
(Ocean Spray)	6 oz	70	1.0	16.0	10	tr	0.0	0.0	0	0%
(Ocean Spray) 100%	6 oz	60	0.0	18.0	15	na	0.0	na	na	0%
(Ocean Spray) pink 'Pink Premium'	6 oz	60	1.0	15.0	10	tr	0.0	0.0	0	0%
(Ocean Spray) 'Ruby Red'	6 oz	100	0.0	24.0	15	na	0.0	na	na	0%
(S&W)	6 oz	80	1.0	18.0	10	tr	0.0	0.0	0	0%
(Snapple)	8 oz	110	0.0	25.0	45	na	0.0	0.0	0	0%
(Stokely)	6 oz	76	1.0	18.0	5	tr	1.0	(tr)	0	11%
(Sunkist) 'Fresh Squeezed'	8 oz	96	1.2	22.7	3	tr	0.2	(tr)	0	2%
(Tree Top)	6 oz	80	1.0	19.0	0	tr	0.0	0.0	0	0%
(TreeSweet) pink	6 oz	72	0.0	17.0	15	tr	0.0	0.0	0	0%
(TreeSweet) regular	6 oz	72	0.0	17.0	15	tr	0.0	0.0	0	0%
(Tropicana) 100% pure	6 oz	70	1.0	14.0	20	na	<1.0	na	na	<13%
(Tropicana) 'Ruby Red' 100% pure	6 oz	70	1.0	14.0	20	na	<1.0	na	na	<13%
(Veryfine) '100%'	8 oz	101	1.4	23.0	10	tr	0.0	0.0	0	0%
Fresh										
juice from one 3.75-inch diam fruit	6 oz	76	1.0	18.0	2	(mq)	0.2	<.1	0	2%
pink	1 cup	96	1.2	22.7	2	na	0.3	0.0	0	3%
white	1 cup	96	1.2	22.7	2	0	0.3	0.0	0	3%
Frozen, diluted as directed										
(A&P)	6 oz	80	<1.0	18.0	0	tr	<1.0	(tr)	0	<11%
(Minute Maid)	6 oz	80	1.0	18.0	0	na	0.0	na	na	0%
(Minute Maid) pink	6 oz	80	0.0	20.0	0	na	0.0	na	na	0%
(Sunkist)	6 oz	56	0.8	13.3	1	tr	0.2	(tr)	0	3%
(TreeSweet)	6 oz	78	1.0	18.0	15	tr	0.0	0.0	0	0%
GRAPEFRUIT JUICE COCKTAIL										
(IGA)	6 oz	80	0.0	20.0	15	(tr)	0.0	0.0	0	0%
(Minute Maid) 'Juices To Go'	6 oz	80	0.0	20.0	20	na	0.0	na	na	0%
(Ocean Spray)	6 oz	80	0.0	20.0	15	(tr)	0.0	0.0	0	0%
(Pathmark)	6 oz	80	0.0	20.0	15	(tr)	0.0	0.0	0	0%
(TreeSweet) 'Lite'	6 oz	40	1.0	10.0	15	(tr)	0.0	0.0	0	0%
(Tropicana) 'Twister'	8 oz	110	(tr)	28.0	1	(tr)	0.0	0.0	0	0%
(Tropicana) 'Twister Light' w/NutraSweet	6 oz	30	<1.0	6.0	20	na	<1.0	na	na	<24%
(Veryfine)	8 oz	120	<1.0	29.0	15	(tr)	0.0	0.0	0	0%
GRAPEFRUIT JUICE DRINK										
(Citrus Hill) 'Plus Calcium'	6 oz	70	<1.0	19.0	10	(tr)	<1.0	(tr)	0	<10%
(Tropicana) 'Juice Sparkler'	8 oz	110	(tr)	26.0	50	(tr)	0.0	0.0	0	0%
(Wyler's) 'Fruit Slush'	4 oz	157	0.0	39.3	10	(tr)	0.0	0.0	0	0%
GRAPESEED OIL										
	1 cup	1927	0.0	0.0	0	0	218.0	20.9	0	100%
	1 oz	251	0.0	0.0	0	0	28.4	2.7	0	100%
	1 tbsp	120	0.0	0.0	0	0	13.6	1.3	0	100%
GRAVY. See also SAUCE.										
AU JUS										
Canned or in jars										
(Franco-American)	2 oz	10	0.0	2.0	330	na	0.0	0.0	0	0%

Food Name	Serving Size	Calories	Prot. gms	Carbs gms	Sod. mgs	Fiber gms	Fat gms	Sat. Fat gms	Chol. mgs	% Fat Cal.
(Heinz) 'HomeStyle'	1/4 cup	18	0.0	2.0	350	na	1.0	na	na	53%
Prepared from mix										
(French's)	1/4 cup	10	0.0	2.0	260	na	0.0	0.0	0	0%
(Lawry's)	1 cup	84	6.3	11.1	3454	>.2 c	1.6	(mq)	na	17%
(McCormick/Schilling)	1/4 cup	20	1.0	3.5	786	na	0.3	na	na	13%
BEEF										
Canned										
(Franco-American)	2 oz	25	0.0	4.0	340	na	1.0	(mq)	(mq)	36%
(Hormel) w/chunky beef 'Great Beginnings'	5 oz	136	12.0	7.0	904	na	7.0	(mq)	(mq)	45%
BROWN										
Canned or in jars										
(Heinz) 'HomeStyle'	1/4 cup	25	1.0	3.0	320	na	1.0	na	na	36%
(Heinz) 'HomeStyle' w/onions	1/4 cup	25	1.0	3.0	330	(mq)	1.0	na	na	36%
(LaChoy)	1/2 tsp	15	<1.0	4.0	15	<1.0	<1.0	(mq)	0	<31%
Prepared from mix										
(French's)	1/4 cup	20	1.0	4.0	250	na	1.0	na	na	31%
(Lawry's)	1 cup	94	3.8	16.5	1500	>.1 c	1.4	na	na	13%
(McCormick/Schilling)	1/3 cup	30	0.7	4.7	417	na	1.0	na	na	29%
(McCormick/Schilling)	1/4 cup	23	0.5	3.5	313	na	0.8	na	na	31%
(McCormick/Schilling) 'Lite'	1/4 cup	10	<1.0	2.0	450	na	1.0	na	na	43%
(Pillsbury)	1/4 cup	15	<1.0	3.0	300	na	0.0	0.0	0	0%
(Weight Watchers)	1/4 cup	10	1.0	2.0	360	na	0.0	na	na	0%
(Weight Watchers) w/mushrooms	1/4 cup	10	1.0	2.0	270	na	0.0	na	na	0%
(Weight Watchers) w/onions	1/4 cup	10	1.0	2.0	310	na	0.0	na	na	0%
CHICKEN										
Canned or in jars										
(Franco-American)	2 oz	45	0.0	3.0	240	na	4.0	(mq)	na	75%
(Franco-American) giblet	2 oz	30	1.0	3.0	310	na	2.0	(mq)	na	53%
(Heinz) 'HomeStyle'	1/4 cup	35	1.0	3.0	350	na	2.0	(mq)	(mq)	53%
(Heinz) 'Homestyle' w/mushrooms and onions	1/4 cup	35	1.0	3.0	330	na	2.0	0.4	1	53%
(Hormel) 'Great Beginnings' w/chunky chicken	5 oz	147	14.0	5.0	567	na	8.0	(mq)	(mq)	49%
(Weight Watchers)	1/4 cup	10	1.0	2.0	410	na	0.0	na	na	0%
Prepared from mix										
(French's)	1/4 cup	25	1.0	4.0	270	na	1.0	na	na	31%
(Lawry's)	1 cup	99	2.5	15.5	980	>.1 c	2.8	(mq)	na	26%
(McCormick/Schilling)	1/4 cup	22	0.8	3.7	300	na	0.4	na	na	17%
(Pillsbury)	1/4 cup	25	<1.0	4.0	230	na	1.0	na	(mq)	31%
COUNTRY										
(Heinz) 'Homestyle' jar	2 oz	25	0.0	4.0	210	na	1.0	na	na	36%
CREAM *(Franco-American)* canned	2 oz	35	0.0	4.0	220	na	2.0	(mq)	na	53%
HERB *(McCormick/Schilling)* mix, prepared	1/4 cup	20	0.5	3.0	312	na	0.5	na	na	24%
MUSHROOM										
Canned or in jars										
(Franco-American)	2 oz	25	0.0	3.0	290	na	1.0	na	na	43%
(Heinz) 'HomeStyle'	1/4 cup	25	1.0	3.0	340	na	1.0	na	na	36%
Prepared from mix										
(French's)	1/4 cup	20	1.0	3.0	250	na	1.0	na	na	36%
(McCormick/Schilling)	1/4 cup	19	0.5	3.0	270	na	0.5	na	na	24%
ONION										
(French's) mix, prepared	1/4 cup	25	1.0	4.0	270	na	1.0	na	na	31%
(McCormick/Schilling) mix, prepared	1/4 cup	22	0.6	3.6	na	na	0.6	na	337	24%
PORK										
Canned or in jars										
(Franco-American)	1/4 cup	40	0.0	3.0	330	na	3.0	(mq)	na	69%

Food Name	Serving Size	Calories	Prot. gms	Carbs gms	Sod. mgs	Fiber gms	Fat gms	Sat. Fat gms	Chol. mgs	% Fat Cal.
(Heinz) 'HomeStyle'	1/4 cup	25	1.0	3.0	310	na	1.0	na	na	36%
(Hormel) 'Great Beginnings' w/chunky pork	5 oz	140	14.0	5.0	567	na	8.0	(mq)	(mq)	49%
Prepared from mix										
(French's)	1/4 cup	20	1.0	4.0	250	na	1.0	na	na	31%
(McCormick/Schilling)	1/4 cup	20	0.6	4.0	297	na	0.6	na	na	23%
TURKEY										
Canned or in jars										
(Franco-American)	2 oz	30	0.0	3.0	290	na	2.0	na	na	60%
(Heinz) 'HomeStyle'	1/4 cup	25	1.0	3.0	370	na	1.0	na	(mq)	36%
(Hormel) 'Great Beginnings' w/chunky turkey	5 oz	138	11.0	7.0	585	na	8.0	(mq)	(mq)	50%
Prepared from mix										
(Lawry's)	1 cup	102	2.6	13.4	1400	>.1 c	4.1	(mq)	na	37%
(McCormick/Schilling)	1/4 cup	22	0.5	4.0	353	na	0.5	na	na	20%
GREAT NORTHERN BEAN										
boiled	4 oz	134	9.4	23.9	2	6.1	0.5	0.2	0	3%
boiled, mature seeds	1/2 cup	104	7.3	18.6	2	>2.6 c	0.4	0.1	0	3%
raw	1/2 cup	308	19.9	56.8	13	36.4	1.0	0.3	0	3%
raw	1 oz	96	6.2	17.7	4	11.3	0.3	0.1	0	3%
Canned										
(A&P)	1 cup	210	14.0	38.0	0	(mq)	1.0	(mq)	0	4%
(Allens)	1/2 cup	105	5.0	17.0	440	(mq)	<1.0	(mq)	0	<9%
(Allens) w/pork	1/2 cup	100	5.0	19.0	320	(mq)	1.0	(mq)	(mq)	9%
(Bush's Best)	1/2 cup	70	5.0	16.0	380	5.0	0.0	na	na	0%
(Eden Foods) organically grown, w/liquid	1/2 cup	110	6.0	20.0	15	6.4	<1.0	na	0	<8%
(Green Giant)	1/2 cup	80	6.0	18.0	290	5.0	1.0	(mq)	0	9%
(Joan of Arc)	1/2 cup	80	6.0	18.0	290	5.0	1.0	(mq)	0	9%
(Luck's) w/pork	7.25 oz	220	12.0	32.0	645	13.0	5.0	(mq)	(mq)	20%
GREEK SALAD, w/feta cheese and pitted Kalamata										
olives, refrigerated (Trader Joe's)	1 salad	310	6.0	10.0	530	1.0	28.0	8.0	20	80%
GREEN BEAN / string bean										
boiled, drained	4 oz	40	2.1	8.9	3	2.0	0.3	0.1	0	6%
boiled, drained	1/2 cup	22	1.2	4.9	2	1.1	0.2	<.1	0	7%
raw, trimmed	1/2 cup	17	1.0	3.9	3	1.2	0.1	<.1	0	4%
raw, trimmed	1 oz	9	0.5	2.0	2	.6	<.1	tr	0	<8%
raw, untrimmed	1 lb	123	7.3	28.5	23	8.4	0.5	0.1	0	3%
GREEN BEAN, CANNED										
Cut										
(A&P)	1/2 cup	20	1.0	4.0	350	(mq)	<1.0	(tr)	0	<31%
(A&P) 'No Salt Added'	1/2 cup	20	1.0	4.0	10	(mq)	<1.0	(tr)	0	<31%
(Allens)	1/2 cup	20	1.0	4.0	350	(mq)	<1.0	(tr)	0	<31%
(Bush's Best)	1/2 cup	20	1.0	5.0	360	2.0	0.0	na	na	0%
(Del Monte) w/liquid	1/2 cup	20	1.0	4.0	355	(mq)	0.0	0.0	0	0%
(Del Monte) w/liquid 'No Salt Added'	1/2 cup	20	1.0	4.0	10	(mq)	0.0	0.0	0	0%
(Bush's Best) 'Blue Lake'	1/2 cup	20	1.0	5.0	360	2.0	0.0	na	na	0%
(Bush's Best) w/Shelly beans	1/2 cup	35	3.0	8.0	290	4.0	0.0	na	na	0%
(Featherweight)	1/2 cup	25	1.0	5.0	10	(mq)	0.0	0.0	0	0%
(Finast)	1/2 cup	20	1.0	4.0	400	(mq)	0.0	0.0	na	0%
(Finast) 'No Salt Added'	1/2 cup	20	1.0	4.0	10	(mq)	0.0	0.0	0	0%
(Finast) 'Veri-Green'	1/2 cup	20	1.0	4.0	320	(mq)	0.0	0.0	0	0%
(Freshlike)	1/2 cup	20	1.0	4.0	340	na	0.0	na	na	0%
(Freshlike) no salt added	1/2 cup	20	1.0	4.0	5	na	0.0	na	na	0%
(Freshlike) no sugar or salt, in water	1/2 cup	20	1.0	4.0	5	na	0.0	na	na	0%
(Freshlike) wax, water packed, w/o salt	1/2 cup	18	1.0	4.0	5	na	0.0	na	na	0%
(Freshlike) wax, water packed, w/o sugar or salt	1/2 cup	18	1.0	4.0	5	na	0.0	na	na	0%

Food Name	Serving Size	Calories	Prot. gms	Carbs gms	Sod. mgs	Fiber gms	Fat gms	Sat. Fat gms	Chol. mgs	% Fat Cal.
(Green Giant)	1/2 cup	16	1.0	4.0	300	1.0	0.0	0.0	0	0%
(Green Giant) 50% less salt	1/2 cup	16	<1.0	4.0	195	1.0	0.0	0.0	0	0%
(Green Giant) kitchen sliced	1/2 cup	16	<1.0	4.0	390	1.0	0.0	0.0	0	0%
(Green Giant) 'Pantry Express'	1/2 cup	12	<1.0	3.0	20	1.0	0.0	0.0	0	0%
(IGA)	1/2 cup	20	1.0	5.0	10	(mq)	0.0	0.0	0	0%
(Pathmark)	1/2 cup	20	1.0	4.0	430	(mq)	0.0	0.0	0	0%
(Pathmark) 'Blue Lake'	1/2 cup	20	1.0	4.0	430	(mq)	0.0	0.0	0	0%
(Pathmark) 'No Frills'	1 cup	35	2.0	8.0	640	(mq)	0.0	0.0	0	0%
(Pathmark) 'No Salt Added'	1/2 cup	20	1.0	5.0	10	(mq)	0.0	0.0	0	0%
(Quincy's)	4.3 oz	40	2.0	7.0	500	(mq)	1.0	na	0	20%
(S&W) 'Premium Blue Lake'	1/2 cup	20	1.0	4.0	385	(mq)	0.0	0.0	0	0%
(S&W) 'Premium Gold'	1/2 cup	20	1.0	5.0	385	(mq)	0.0	0.0	0	0%
(S&W) stringless, w/liquid	1/2 cup	20	1.0	4.0	3850	(mq)	0.0	0.0	0	0%
(S&W Nutradiet)	1/2 cup	20	1.0	4.0	5	(mq)	0.0	0.0	0	0%
(Stokely)	1/2 cup	20	1.0	4.0	360	(mq)	0.0	0.0	0	0%
(Stokely) 'No Salt or Sugar'	1/2 cup	20	1.0	4.0	5	(mq)	0.0	0.0	0	0%
(Veg•All)	1/2 cup	20	1.0	4.0	340	na	0.0	na	na	0%
French style										
(A&P)	1/2 cup	20	1.0	4.0	350	(mq)	<1.0	(tr)	0	<31%
(A&P) 'No Salt Added'	1/2 cup	20	1.0	4.0	10	(mq)	<1.0	(tr)	0	<31%
(Allens)	1/2 cup	20	1.0	4.0	350	(mq)	<1.0	(tr)	0	<31%
(Bush's Best)	1/2 cup	20	1.0	5.0	360	2.0	0.0	na	na	0%
(Del Monte) seasoned, w/liquid	1/2 cup	20	1.0	4.0	355	(mq)	0.0	0.0	0	0%
(Finast)	1/2 cup	20	1.0	4.0	400	(mq)	0.0	0.0	0	0%
(Freshlike)	1/2 cup	20	1.0	4.0	340	na	0.0	na	na	0%
(Freshlike) in water, w/o salt	1/2 cup	20	1.0	4.0	5	na	0.0	na	na	0%
(Green Giant)	1/2 cup	16	<1.0	4.0	390	1.0	0.0	0.0	0	0%
(Pathmark) 'Blue Lake'	1/2 cup	20	1.0	4.0	430	(mq)	0.0	0.0	0	0%
(Pathmark) 'No Frills'	1 cup	35	2.0	8.0	640	(mq)	0.0	0.0	0	0%
(Pathmark) 'No Salt Added'	1/2 cup	20	1.0	5.0	10	(mq)	0.0	0.0	0	0%
(S&W) 'Premium Blue Lake'	1/2 cup	20	1.0	4.0	385	(mq)	0.0	0.0	0	0%
(S&W) stringless, w/liquid	1/2 cup	20	1.0	4.0	3850	(mq)	0.0	0.0	0	0%
(Veg•All)	1/2 cup	20	1.0	4.0	340	na	0.0	na	na	0%
Italian										
(Allens)	1/2 cup	18	1.0	3.0	260	(mq)	<1.0	(tr)	0	<36%
(Del Monte) cut	1/2 cup	25	1.0	6.0	355	(mq)	0.0	0.0	0	0%
Whole										
(A&P)	1/2 cup	20	1.0	4.0	350	(mq)	<1.0	(tr)	0	<31%
(Allens) Shelly beans	1/2 cup	35	2.0	6.0	395	(mq)	<1.0	(tr)	0	<22%
(Bush's Best)	1/2 cup	20	1.0	5.0	360	2.0	0.0	na	na	0%
(Del Monte) w/liquid	1/2 cup	20	1.0	4.0	355	(mq)	0.0	0.0	0	0%
(Finast)	1/2 cup	25	1.0	4.0	400	(mq)	0.0	0.0	0	0%
(Freshlike)	1/2 cup	20	1.0	4.0	340	na	0.0	na	na	0%
(Green Giant) amandine	1/2 cup	45	2.0	5.0	300	2.0	3.0	0.0	0	49%
(IGA)	1 cup	45	2.0	8.0	640	(mq)	0.0	0.0	0	0%
(Pathmark)	1/2 cup	20	1.0	4.0	430	(mq)	0.0	0.0	0	0%
(S&W) dilled	1/2 cup	60	1.0	15.0	3850	(mq)	0.0	0.0	0	0%
(S&W) stringless, w/liquid	1/2 cup	20	1.0	4.0	3850	(mq)	0.0	0.0	0	0%
(S&W) 'Vertical Pak'	1/2 cup	20	1.0	4.0	385	(mq)	0.0	0.0	0	0%
GREEN BEAN, FREEZE-DRIED										
(Mountain House) diluted as directed	1/2 cup	35	1.0	6.0	tr	(mq)	0.0	0.0	0	0%
GREEN BEAN, FROZEN										
Cut										
(A&P)	3 oz	25	1.0	6.0	140	(mq)	<1.0	(tr)	0	<24%

Food Name	Serving Size	Calories	Prot. gms	Carbs gms	Sod. mgs	Fiber gms	Fat gms	Sat. Fat gms	Chol. mgs	% Fat Cal.
(Birds Eye)	3 oz	25	1.0	6.0	0	2.0	0.0	0.0	0	0%
(Birds Eye) 'Portion Pack'	3 oz	25	1.0	6.0	0	2.0	0.0	0.0	0	0%
(Finast)	3 oz	25	1.0	6.0	5	(mq)	0.0	0.0	0	0%
(Freshlike)	3 oz	25	1.0	6.0	5	na	0.0	na	na	0%
(Frosty Acres)	3 oz	25	1.0	6.0	3	2.0	0.0	0.0	0	0%
(Green Giant) 'Harvest Fresh'	1/2 cup	16	1.0	4.0	95	1.0	0.0	0.0	0	0%
(Green Giant) in butter sauce	1/2 cup	30	1.0	4.0	230	1.5	1.0	<1.0	5	31%
(Seabrook)	3 oz	25	1.0	6.0	3	2.0	0.0	0.0	0	0%
(Stokely) 'Singles'	3 oz	30	2.0	6.0	5	(mq)	1.0	(tr)	0	22%
French style										
(A&P)	3 oz	25	1.0	6.0	0	(mq)	<1.0	(tr)	0	<24%
(Birds Eye)	3 oz	25	1.0	6.0	0	2.0	0.0	0.0	0	0%
(Bird's Eye) w/almonds 'Combination Vegetables'	3 oz	50	3.0	8.0	340	2.0	2.0	(mq)	0	29%
(Finast)	3 oz	25	1.0	6.0	5	(mq)	0.0	0.0	0	0%
(Freshlike)	3 oz	25	1.0	6.0	5	na	0.0	na	na	0%
(Frosty Acres)	3 oz	25	1.0	6.0	3	2.0	0.0	0.0	0	0%
(Seabrook)	3 oz	25	1.0	6.0	3	2.0	0.0	0.0	0	0%
(Southern)	3.5 oz	34	1.6	6.9	20	(mq)	0.1	(tr)	0	3%
(Veg•All)	3 oz	25	1.0	6.0	5	na	0.0	na	na	0%
Italian										
(Birds Eye)	3 oz	30	2.0	7.0	0	3.0	0.0	na	0	0%
(Finast) cut	3 oz	30	2.0	7.0	5	(mq)	0.0	0.0	0	0%
(Freshlike)	3 oz	30	2.0	7.0	5	na	0.0	na	na	0%
(Frosty Acres)	3 oz	30	2.0	7.0	3	2.0	0.0	0.0	0	0%
(Seabrook)	3 oz	30	2.0	7.0	3	2.0	0.0	0.0	0	0%
(Veg•All)	3 oz	30	2.0	7.0	5	na	0.0	na	na	0%
Whole										
(Bird's Eye) Bavarian style, w/spaetzle	3.3 oz	100	2.0	11.0	350	2.0	5.0	(mq)	10	46%
(Birds Eye) 'Deluxe'	3 oz	25	1.0	5.0	0	2.0	0.0	na	0	0%
(Bird's Eye) 'Farm Fresh Whole Vegetables'	4 oz	30	2.0	7.0	0	2.0	0.0	na	0	0%
(Bird's Eye) petite 'Deluxe'	2.6 oz	20	1.0	5.0	0	2.0	0.0	na	0	0%
(Freshlike)	3 oz	25	1.0	5.0	5	na	0.0	na	na	0%
(Green Giant)	1/2 cup	14	1.0	4.0	10	1.5	0.0	0.0	0	0%
(Green Giant) and creamy mushroom 'Garden Gourmet'	1 pkg	220	6.0	29.0	860	4.0	11.0	6.0	25	41%
(Green Giant) in butter sauce 'One Serving'	5.5 oz	60	2.0	8.0	370	3.0	2.0	1.0	5	31%
(Green Giant) 'Plain Polybag'	1/2 cup	14	1.0	4.0	10	1.0	0.0	0.0	0	0%
(Seabrook)	3 oz	25	1.0	5.0	1	2.0	0.0	0.0	0	0%
(Southern)	3.5 oz	33	1.6	6.8	20	(mq)	0.1	(tr)	0	3%
(Stouffer's) mushroom casserole	4.75 oz	160	3.0	13.0	680	(mq)	11.0	(mq)	na	61%
(Veg•All)	3 oz	25	1.0	5.0	5	na	0.0	na	na	0%

GREEN ONION. See ONION, GREEN.

GRENADINE. See ALCOHOLIC BEVERAGES.

GRITS

Food Name	Serving Size	Calories	Prot. gms	Carbs gms	Sod. mgs	Fiber gms	Fat gms	Sat. Fat gms	Chol. mgs	% Fat Cal.
Dry										
white (Arrowhead Mills)	2 oz	200	5.0	43.0	1	1.5	1.0	na	0	5%
white, enriched	1 cup	579	13.7	124.2	2	2.5	1.9	0.3	0	3%
white, enriched	1 tbsp	36	0.9	7.7	0	.2	0.1	0.0	0	3%
white, enriched 'Regular/Quick' (Aunt Jemima)	3 tbsp	101	2.4	22.4	1	1.4	0.2	na	0	2%
white, unenriched	1 cup	579	13.7	124.2	2	2.5	1.9	0.3	0	3%
white, unenriched	1 tbsp	36	0.9	7.7	0	.2	0.1	0.0	0	3%
yellow (Arrowhead Mills)	2 oz	200	5.0	44.0	1	1.5	1.0	na	0	4%
yelllow, enriched	1 cup	579	13.7	124.2	2	2.5	1.9	0.3	0	3%
yellow, enriched	1 tbsp	36	0.9	7.7	0	.2	0.1	0.0	0	3%
yellow, enriched (Quick)	3 tbsp	101	2.4	22.4	1	1.2	0.2	na	0	2%

Food Name	Serving Size	Calories	Prot. gms	Carbs gms	Sod. mgs	Fiber gms	Fat gms	Sat. Fat gms	Chol. mgs	% Fat Cal.
yellow, unenriched	1 cup	579	13.7	124.2	2	2.5	1.9	0.3	0	3%
yellow, unenriched	1 tbsp	36	0.9	7.7	0	.2	0.1	0.0	0	3%
Prepared										
white, enriched, cooked w/water	1 cup	145	3.4	31.5	0	.5	0.5	0.1	0	3%
white, unenriched, cooked w/water	1 cup	145	3.4	31.5	0	.5	0.5	0.1	0	3%
yellow, enriched, cooked w/water	1 cup	145	3.4	31.5	0	.5	0.5	0.1	0	3%
yellow, unenriched, cooked w/water	1 cup	145	3.4	31.5	0	.5	0.5	0.1	0	3%
GRITS, CANNED										
golden *(Allens)*	1/2 cup	80	2.0	16.0	370	(mq)	<1.0	na	0	<11%
golden *(Bush's Best)*	1/2 cup	45	1.0	11.0	390	na	0.0	na	na	0%
golden *(Van Camp's)*	1 cup	128	2.7	27.9	701	>.8 c	0.6	na	0	4%
golden, w/red and green peppers *(Van Camp's)*	1 cup	129	2.6	28.5	685	>.7 c	0.5	na	0	4%
Mexican *(Allens)*	1/2 cup	80	2.0	16.0	330	(mq)	<1.0	na	0	<11%
white	1 cup	115	2.4	22.8	336	>.7 c	1.4	0.2	0	11%
white	4 oz	82	1.7	16.2	238	>.5 c	1.0	0.1	0	11%
white *(Allens)*	1/2 cup	70	2.0	16.0	430	(mq)	<1.0	na	0	<11%
white *(Bush's Best)*	1/2 cup	45	<1.0	11.0	450	na	0.0	na	na	0%
white *(Van Camp's)*	1 cup	138	3.0	30.0	708	>.8 c	0.7	na	0	5%
yellow	1 cup	115	2.4	22.8	336	>.7 c	1.4	0.2	0	11%
yellow	4 oz	82	1.7	16.2	238	>.5 c	1.0	0.1	0	11%
GRITS, INSTANT										
white, hominy product, dry, one packet *(Quaker)*	.8 oz	79	1.9	17.7	440	1.2	0.1	na	0	1%
w/imitation bacon bits, dry, one packet *(Quaker)*	1 oz	101	2.7	21.6	590	1.5	0.4	na	0	4%
w/imitation ham bits, dry, one packet *(Quaker)*	1 oz	99	2.7	21.3	800	1.7	0.3	na	0	3%
w/real cheddar cheese flavor, dry, one packet *(Quaker)*	1 oz	104	2.2	21.6	497	1.3	1.0	na	na	9%
GRITS, QUICK-COOKING										
Dry										
white, enriched	1 cup	579	13.7	124.2	2	2.5	1.9	0.3	0	3%
white, enriched	1 tbsp	36	0.9	7.7	0	.2	0.1	0.0	0	3%
white, unenriched	1 cup	579	13.7	124.2	2	2.5	1.9	0.3	0	3%
white, unenriched	1 tbsp	36	0.9	7.7	0	.2	0.1	0.0	0	3%
yellow, enriched	1 cup	579	13.7	124.2	2	2.5	1.9	0.3	0	3%
yellow, enriched	1 tbsp	36	0.9	7.7	0	.2	0.1	0.0	0	3%
yellow, enriched 'Quick' *(Quaker)*	3 tbsp	101	2.4	22.4	1	1.2	0.2	na	na	2%
yellow, unenriched	1 cup	579	13.7	124.2	2	2.5	1.9	0.3	0	3%
yellow, unenriched	1 tbsp	36	0.9	7.7	0	.2	0.1	0.0	0	3%
Prepared										
white, enriched, cooked w/water	1 cup	145	3.4	31.5	0	.5	0.5	0.1	0	3%
white, unenriched, cooked w/water	1 cup	145	3.4	31.5	0	.5	0.5	0.1	0	3%
yellow, enriched, cooked w/water	1 cup	145	3.4	31.5	0	.5	0.5	0.1	0	3%
yellow, unenriched, cooked w/water	1 cup	145	3.4	31.5	0	.5	0.5	0.1	0	3%
GROUND CHERRY. See CAPE GOOSEBERRY.										
GROUND HUSK TOMATO. See TOMATILLO.										
GROUPER, MIXED SPECIES										
broiled	4 oz	134	28.2	0.0	60	0	1.5	0.3	53	11%
dry-heat cooked	4 oz	134	28.2	0.0	60	0	1.5	0.3	53	11%
dry-heat cooked	3 oz	100	21.1	0.0	45	0	1.1	0.3	40	11%
microwaved	4 oz	134	28.2	0.0	60	0	1.5	0.3	53	11%
raw	1 lb	417	87.9	0.0	239	0	4.6	1.1	166	11%
raw	3 oz	78	16.5	0.0	45	0	0.9	0.2	31	11%
raw	1 oz	26	5.5	0.0	15	0	0.3	0.1	10	11%
GUACAMOLE. See DIP, AVOCADO.										
GUACAMOLE SEASONING										
(Lawry's) 'Seasoning Blend' dry mix	1 pkg	60	1.7	12.6	1495	>.8 c	0.4	(tr)	0	6%

Food Name	Serving Size	Calories	Prot. gms	Carbs gms	Sod. mgs	Fiber gms	Fat gms	Sat. Fat gms	Chol. mgs	% Fat Cal.
(Old El Paso) dry mix	1/7 pkg	7	0.0	2.0	240	0	0.0	0.0	0	0%
GUANABANA/soursop										
raw, approx 2.1 lb	1 med	416	6.3	105.3	87	>6.9 c	1.9	na	0	4%
trimmed	1 oz	19	0.3	4.8	4	>.3 c	0.1	na	0	4%
trimmed	1/2 cup	75	1.1	18.9	16	>1.2 c	0.3	na	0	3%
untrimmed	1 lb	202	3.0	51.2	42	>3.3 c	0.9	na	0	4%
GUANABANA NECTAR *(Libby's)*	6 oz	110	0.0	26.0	15	na	0.0	na	na	0%
GUANABANA PUNCH, 'Rain Forest' *(Knudsen & Sons)*	8 oz	125	<1.0	29.0	na	na	0.0	na	na	0%
GUAVA										
trimmed	1 cup	84	1.4	19.6	5	8.9	1.0	0.3	0	10%
trimmed	1 fruit	46	0.7	10.7	3	4.9	0.5	0.2	0	9%
trimmed	1 oz	15	0.2	3.4	1	>1.6 c	0.2	<.1	0	11%
untrimmed	1 lb	183	3.0	43.1	9	>20.3 c	2.2	0.6	0	10%
w/edible seeds *(Sunfresh)*	3.5 oz	70	0.0	18.0	15	6.0	0.0	0.0	7	0%
GUAVA, STRAWBERRY										
trimmed	1 cup	168	1.4	42.4	90	>15.6 c	1.5	0.4	0	7%
trimmed	1 oz	20	0.2	4.9	11	>1.8 c	0.2	<.1	0	8%
trimmed	1 fruit	4	0.0	1.0	2	>.4 c	0.0	0.0	0	0%
untrimmed	1 lb	268	2.2	66.9	141	>24.7 c	2.3	0.7	0	7%
GUAVA CRANBERRY JUICE										
organic 'Cruz' *(Santa Cruz Natural)*	8 oz	130	1.0	30.0	na	na	<1.0	na	na	<7%
GUAVA FRUIT DRINK										
Hawaiian 'Mauna La'i' *(Ocean Spray)*	6 oz	100	0.0	24.0	15	(tr)	0.0	0.0	0	0%
GUAVA JUICE										
'Orchard Tropicals' bottled, diluted *(Welch's)*	6 oz	100	0.0	25.0	20	0	0.0	0.0	0	0%
'Orchard Tropicals' frozen, diluted *(Welch's)*	6 oz	100	0.0	25.0	20	0	0.0	0.0	0	0%
GUAVA NECTAR										
(Kern's)	6 oz	110	0.0	28.0	0	na	0.0	na	na	0%
(Libby's)	6 oz	110	0.0	26.0	15	(mq)	0.0	0.0	0	0%
GUAVA PASSION DRINK										
Hawaiian 'Hawaii' *(Pathmark)*	6 oz	100	0.0	25.0	10	(tr)	0.0	0.0	0	0%
Hawaiian 'Mauna La'i' *(Ocean Spray)*	6 oz	100	0.0	25.0	10	(tr)	0.0	0.0	0	0%
GUAVA STRAWBERRY DRINK 'Refresher' *(Veryfine)*	8 oz	120	0.3	30.0	25	(tr)	0.0	0.0	0	0%
GUINEA HEN										
giblets, raw	100 gm	157	20.8	1.2	70	0	7.0	2.0	350	42%
meat and skin, raw	1 lb	567	84.0	0.0	241	0	23.2	6.3	266	38%
meat only, raw	1 oz	31	5.9	0.0	(mq)	0	0.7	(mq)	18	21%
GUMBO. See OKRA.										
GUMBO FILE POWDER *(Tone's)*	1 tsp	8	0.2	1.7	<1	.6	0.2	<.1	0	19%

H

Food Name	Serving Size	Calories	Prot. gms	Carbs gms	Sod. mgs	Fiber gms	Fat gms	Sat. Fat gms	Chol. mgs	% Fat Cal.
HADDOCK										
baked	4 oz	127	27.5	0.0	99	0	1.1	0.2	84	8%
broiled	4 oz	127	27.5	0.0	99	0	1.1	0.2	84	8%
dry-heat cooked	3 oz	95	20.6	0.0	74	0	0.8	0.1	63	8%
microwaved	4 oz	127	27.5	0.0	99	0	1.1	0.2	84	8%
raw	1 lb	396	85.8	0.0	310	0	3.3	0.6	261	8%
raw	3 oz	74	16.1	0.0	58	0	0.6	0.1	48	8%
smoked	3 oz	99	21.5	0.0	649	0	0.8	0.2	65	8%

Food Name	Serving Size	Calories	Prot. gms	Carbs gms	Sod. mgs	Fiber gms	Fat gms	Sat. Fat gms	Chol. mgs	% Fat Cal.
HADDOCK FILLET, FROZEN										
(SeaPak)	4 oz	90	18.0	0.0	120	0	1.0	(mq)	(mq)	11%
battered (Van de Kamp's)	2 pieces	250	12.0	19.0	580	na	15.0	3.0	30	52%
battered, 'Crunchy' (Mrs. Paul's)	2 pieces	190	14.0	22.0	580	(mq)	5.0	(mq)	25	24%
breaded (Van de Kamp's)	2 pieces	270	12.0	19.0	290	na	16.0	3.0	25	54%
breaded, in lemon butter, 'Microwave' (Gorton's)	1 pkg	360	23.0	19.0	730	(mq)	21.0	10.0	100	53%
breaded, 'Light' (Mrs. Paul's)	1 piece	220	17.0	15.0	350	(mq)	9.0	(mq)	45	39%
breaded, 'Light' (Van de Kamp's)	1 piece	240	15.0	21.0	380	(mq)	11.0	2.0	35	41%
'Fishmarket Fresh' (Gorton's)	5 oz	110	25.0	0.0	120	0	1.0	(mq)	(mq)	8%
natural (Van de Kamp's)	4 oz	90	21.0	0.0	125	0	1.0	0.0	20	10%
HALIBUT										
ATLANTIC										
broiled	4 oz	159	30.3	0.0	78	0	3.3	0.5	46	20%
dry-heat cooked	4 oz	159	30.3	0.0	78	0	3.3	0.5	46	20%
dry-heat cooked	3 oz	119	22.7	0.0	59	0	2.5	0.4	35	20%
microwaved	4 oz	159	30.3	0.0	78	0	3.3	0.5	46	20%
raw	1 lb	497	94.4	0.0	245	0	10.4	1.5	146	20%
raw	3 oz	94	17.7	0.0	46	0	2.0	0.3	27	20%
raw	1 oz	31	5.9	0.0	15	0	0.6	0.1	9	19%
GREENLAND										
dry-heat cooked	3 oz	203	15.7	0.0	88	0	15.1	2.6	50	68%
raw	1 lb	845	65.2	0.0	363	0	62.8	11.0	209	68%
raw	3 oz	158	12.2	0.0	68	0	11.8	2.1	39	69%
raw	1 oz	53	4.1	0.0	23	0	3.9	0.7	13	68%
PACIFIC										
broiled	4 oz	159	30.3	0.0	78	0	3.3	0.5	46	20%
dry-heat cooked	4 oz	159	30.3	0.0	78	0	3.3	0.5	46	20%
dry-heat cooked	3 oz	119	22.7	0.0	59	0	2.5	0.4	35	20%
microwaved	4 oz	159	30.3	0.0	78	0	3.3	0.5	46	20%
raw	1 lb	497	94.4	0.0	245	0	10.4	1.5	146	20%
raw	3 oz	94	17.7	0.0	46	0	2.0	0.3	27	20%
raw	1 oz	31	5.9	0.0	15	0	0.6	0.1	9	19%
raw, fillet portions, skinless (Peter Pan Seafoods)	3.5 oz	110	20.8	na	54	na	2.3	na	32	20%
HALIBUT, FROZEN										
fillet, battered (Van de Kamp's)	2 pieces	150	8.0	16.0	400	na	6.0	1.0	10	36%
steaks, w/o seasoning mix (SeaPak)	6-oz pkg	160	36.0	0.0	120	0	1.0	(mq)	(mq)	6%
HAM. See HAM, ALTERNATIVE; HAM, CANNED; HAM, CURED; HAM, FRESH; HAM PATTY.										
HAM, ALTERNATIVE										
(Worthington) frozen, roll 'Wham' approx .9-oz slices	3 slices	120	11.0	3.0	940	(mq)	7.0	1.0	0	53%
HAM, CANNED										
chopped	1 oz	68	4.6	0.1	387	0	5.3	1.8	14	72%
chopped	.75-oz slice	50	3.4	0.1	287	0	4.0	1.3	10	72%
cured, extra lean, approx 4% fat, baked	3 oz	116	18.0	0.4	965	0	4.2	1.4	25	34%
cured, extra lean, approx 4% fat, unheated	1 oz	34	5.2	0.0	356	0	1.3	0.4	11	36%
cured, extra lean and regular, baked	3 oz	142	17.8	0.4	908	0	7.2	2.4	35	47%
cured, extra lean and regular, unheated	1 oz	41	5.1	0.0	362	0	2.1	0.7	11	48%
cured, regular, approx 13% fat, baked	3 oz	192	17.5	0.4	800	0	12.9	4.3	53	62%
cured, regular, approx 13% fat, unheated	1 oz	54	4.8	0.0	352	0	3.7	1.2	11	63%
(Armour) chopped	3 oz	190	13.0	1.0	1260	na	14.0	na	na	69%
(Black Label)										
'5-lb can'	4 oz	140	20.0	0.0	1245	0	7.0	(mq)	(mq)	44%
'3-lb can'	4 oz	140	20.0	0.0	1315	0	7.0	(mq)	(mq)	44%
'1 1/2-lb can'	4 oz	150	21.0	0.0	1324	0	7.0	(mq)	(mq)	43%
(Chi-Chi's) 'Black Label'	1 oz	37	5.0	2.0	303	na	1.0	1.0	15	24%

Food Name	Serving Size	Calories	Prot. gms	Carbs gms	Sod. mgs	Fiber gms	Fat gms	Sat. Fat gms	Chol. mgs	% Fat Cal.
(EXL) 'Deli Ham' 10-lb can	4 oz	130	20.0	0.0	1368	0	6.0	(mq)	(mq)	40%
(Holiday Glaze) '3-lb can'	4 oz	130	21.0	2.0	(mq)	0	4.0	(mq)	(mq)	28%
(Hormel)										
'Bone-In'	4 oz	210	17.0	1.0	(mq)	0	15.0	(mq)	(mq)	65%
chopped, '8-lb can'	3 oz	240	12.0	1.0	1062	0	21.0	(mq)	(mq)	78%
chopped, '12-oz can'	2 oz	120	10.0	0.0	703	0	9.0	(mq)	(mq)	67%
chunk	6.75 oz	310	32.0	0.0	2241	0	20.0	(mq)	(mq)	58%
chunk	2.5 oz	110	11.0	1.0	780	na	7.0	2.0	35	57%
'Cure/81'	4 oz	160	22.0	0.0	1322	0	8.0	(mq)	(mq)	45%
'Cure/81'	1 oz	31	5.0	2.0	291	na	1.0	<2.0	15	24%
'Curemaster'	4 oz	140	22.0	1.0	1361	0	5.0	(mq)	(mq)	33%
'Curemaster'	2 oz	60	10.0	1.0	627	na	2.0	1.0	26	29%
'Light and Lean 97'	2 oz	60	10.0	1.0	450	na	2.0	1.0	26	29%
roll	4 oz	170	21.0	0.0	1338	0	10.0	(mq)	(mq)	52%
spiced	3 oz	240	13.0	1.0	1093	0	21.0	(mq)	(mq)	77%
(JM) '95% Fat-free'	2 oz	60	10.0	1.0	680	0	2.0	(mq)	(mq)	29%
(Light & Lean) 'Boneless'	2 oz	60	10.0	0.0	574	0	2.0	(mq)	(mq)	31%
(Oscar Mayer) 'Jubilee'	1 oz	29	5.0	0.1	287	0	0.9	0.4	14	28%
(Rath) hickory smoked, 'Black Hawk'	2 oz	60	10.0	1.0	720	0	2.0	(mq)	(mq)	29%

HAM, CURED
(NOTE: TRIMMED = Lean; separable fat removed. UNTRIMMED = Separable fat not removed.)
BONELESS

Food Name	Serving Size	Calories	Prot. gms	Carbs gms	Sod. mgs	Fiber gms	Fat gms	Sat. Fat gms	Chol. mgs	% Fat Cal.
center slice, country-style, trimmed, unheated	1 oz	55	7.9	0.1	764	0	2.4	0.8	20	40%
center slice, untrimmed, unheated	1 oz	58	5.7	0.0	393	0	3.7	1.3	15	59%
extra lean, approx 5% fat, baked	3 oz	123	17.8	1.3	1023	0	4.7	1.5	45	36%
extra lean, approx 5% fat, unheated	1 oz	37	5.5	0.3	405	0	1.4	0.5	13	35%
extra lean and regular, baked	3 oz	140	18.7	0.4	1177	0	6.5	2.2	48	43%
extra lean and regular, unheated	1 oz	46	5.2	0.7	362	0	2.4	0.8	15	48%
extra lean and regular, unheated, 4 x 6 1/4 inch slice	1 slice	46	5.2	0.7	362	0	2.4	0.8	15	48%
mini (JM)	3 oz	90	17.0	0.0	40	0	3.0	(mq)	(mq)	28%
regular, approx 11% fat, baked	3 oz	151	19.2	0.0	1275	0	7.7	2.7	50	47%
regular, approx 11% fat, unheated	1 oz	52	5.0	0.9	373	0	3.0	1.0	16	53%
steak, 'Jubilee' (Oscar Mayer)	2 oz	57	9.7	0.2	754	0	1.9	0.7	31	30%
steak, unheated	2 oz	69	11.1	0.0	720	0	2.4	0.8	26	33%
w/natural juices, 'EZ Cut' (JM)	2 oz	70	11.0	1.0	660	0	3.0	(mq)	(mq)	36%

WHOLE

Food Name	Serving Size	Calories	Prot. gms	Carbs gms	Sod. mgs	Fiber gms	Fat gms	Sat. Fat gms	Chol. mgs	% Fat Cal.
trimmed, fully cooked, baked	3 oz	133	21.3	0.0	1128	0	4.7	1.6	47	33%
trimmed, fully cooked, unheated	1 oz	42	6.3	0.0	430	0	1.6	0.5	15	36%
trimmed (JM)	3 oz	140	17.0	0.0	40	0	8.0	na	na	51%
untrimmed, fully cooked, baked	3 oz	207	18.3	0.0	1009	0	14.2	5.1	53	64%
untrimmed, fully cooked, unheated	1 oz	70	5.2	0.0	364	0	5.3	1.9	16	70%

HAM, FRESH. See also PORK.
(NOTE: TRIMMED = Lean; separable fat removed. UNTRIMMED = Separable fat not removed.)
LEG, RUMP HALF
Trimmed

Food Name	Serving Size	Calories	Prot. gms	Carbs gms	Sod. mgs	Fiber gms	Fat gms	Sat. Fat gms	Chol. mgs	% Fat Cal.
raw	1 lb	621	96.3	0.0	313	0	23.5	8.1	277	35%
raw	1 oz	39	6.0	0.0	20	0	1.5	0.5	17	36%
roasted	3 oz	175	26.3	0.0	55	0	6.9	2.4	82	37%
roasted, diced	1 cup	278	41.8	0.0	88	0	11.0	3.9	130	37%
Untrimmed										
raw	1 lb	1007	85.0	0.0	277	0	71.2	24.7	299	65%
raw	1 oz	63	5.3	0.0	17	0	4.4	1.5	19	65%
roasted	3 oz	214	24.5	0.0	53	0	12.1	4.5	82	53%
roasted	1.5 oz	117	11.3	0.0	26	0	7.6	2.7	40	60%

Food Name	Serving Size	Calories	Prot. gms	Carbs gms	Sod. mgs	Fiber gms	Fat gms	Sat. Fat gms	Chol. mgs	% Fat Cal.
roasted, diced . . . . 1 cup	1 cup	340	39.0	0.0	84	0	19.3	7.1	130	53%
LEG, SHANK HALF										
Trimmed										
raw . . . . 1 lb	1 lb	631	93.5	0.0	304	0	25.5	8.8	272	38%
raw . . . . 1 oz	1 oz	39	5.8	0.0	19	0	1.6	0.6	17	38%
roasted . . . . 3 oz	3 oz	183	24.0	0.0	54	0	8.9	3.1	78	46%
roasted, diced . . . . 1 cup	1 cup	290	38.1	0.0	86	0	14.2	4.9	124	46%
Untrimmed										
raw . . . . 1 lb	1 lb	1193	77.5	0.0	249	0	95.4	33.1	308	74%
raw . . . . 1 oz	1 oz	75	4.8	0.0	16	0	6.0	2.1	19	74%
roasted . . . . 3 oz	3 oz	246	21.5	0.0	50	0	17.0	6.3	78	64%
roasted . . . . 1.5 oz	1.5 oz	129	10.3	0.0	25	0	9.4	3.4	39	67%
roasted, diced . . . . 1 cup	1 cup	390	34.2	0.0	80	0	27.1	9.9	124	64%
LEG, WHOLE										
Trimmed										
raw . . . . 1 lb	1 lb	617	92.9	0.0	249	0	24.5	8.5	308	37%
raw . . . . 1 oz	1 oz	39	5.8	0.0	16	0	1.5	0.5	19	37%
roasted . . . . 3 oz	3 oz	179	25.0	0.0	54	0	8.0	2.8	80	42%
roasted . . . . 1.5 oz	1.5 oz	94	12.0	0.0	27	0	4.7	1.6	40	47%
roasted . . . . 1 cup	1 cup	285	39.7	0.0	86	0	12.7	4.5	127	42%
Untrimmed										
raw . . . . 1 lb	1 lb	1111	79.1	0.0	213	0	85.6	29.7	331	71%
raw . . . . 1 oz	1 oz	69	4.9	0.0	13	0	5.3	1.9	21	71%
roasted . . . . 3 oz	3 oz	232	22.8	0.0	51	0	15.0	5.5	80	60%
roasted . . . . 1.5 oz	1.5 oz	125	10.6	0.0	25	0	8.8	3.2	40	65%
roasted, diced . . . . 1 cup	1 cup	369	36.2	0.0	81	0	23.8	8.7	127	60%
HAM, MINCED . . . . 1 oz	1 oz	75	4.6	0.5	353	0	5.9	2.0	20	72%
HAM ENTRÉE, FROZEN										
and asparagus bake *(Stouffer's)* . . . . 9.5 oz	9.5 oz	520	18.0	32.0	1100	na	35.0	na	na	61%
and cheese casserole, 'Microwave Classic' *(Pillsbury)* . . . 1 pkg	1 pkg	470	18.0	34.0	1300	na	29.0	(mq)	(mq)	56%
dinner *(Morton)* . . . . 10 oz	10 oz	290	15.0	49.0	1400	(mq)	4.0	(mq)	45	12%
'Platters' *(Banquet)* . . . . 10 oz	10 oz	400	20.0	43.0	1180	(mq)	17.0	(mq)	50	38%
steak *(Le Menu)* . . . . 10 oz	10 oz	300	19.0	31.0	1500	(mq)	11.0	(mq)	(mq)	33%
steak 'Classics' *(Armour)* . . . . 10.75 oz	10.75 oz	270	15.0	36.0	1320	(mq)	7.0	(mq)	50	24%
w/scalloped potatoes 'Homestyle Recipe' *(Swanson)* . . . . 9 oz	9 oz	300	19.0	26.0	1080	(mq)	13.0	(mq)	(mq)	39%
HAM LUNCHEON MEAT. See LUNCHEON MEAT.										
HAM PATTY										
canned *(Hormel)* . . . . 1 patty	1 patty	180	7.0	0.0	456	0	16.0	(mq)	(mq)	84%
canned, w/cheese *(Hormel)* . . . . 1 patty	1 patty	190	7.0	0.0	468	0	18.0	(mq)	(mq)	85%
cured, boneless steak, extra lean, unheated . . . . 2-oz slice	2-oz slice	69	11.1	0.0	720	0	2.4	0.8	26	33%
cured, unheated . . . . 1 oz	1 oz	89	3.6	0.5	308	0	8.0	2.9	20	81%
grilled . . . . 4 oz	4 oz	388	15.1	1.9	1205	0	35.0	12.6	82	82%
'Premium Brown `N Serve' *(Swift)* . . . . 1 patty	1 patty	130	3.0	1.0	260	0	13.0	(mq)	(mq)	88%
HAM SPREAD										
deviled . . . . 1 cup	1 cup	790	31.3	0.0	2776	0	72.7	26.2	146	84%
deviled . . . . 4.5-oz can	4.5-oz can	449	17.8	0.0	1580	0	41.3	14.9	83	84%
deviled *(Hormel)* . . . . 1 oz	1 oz	76	4.0	1.0	214	na	6.0	2.0	19	73%
deviled *(Hormel)* . . . . 1 tbsp	1 tbsp	35	2.0	0.0	108	0	3.0	(mq)	(mq)	77%
deviled *(Underwood)* . . . . 2 1/8 oz	2 1/8 oz	220	8.0	<1.0	430	na	19.0	6.0	50	83%
deviled *(Underwood)* 'Light' . . . . 2 1/8 oz	2 1/8 oz	120	11.0	1.0	250	na	8.0	1.0	35	60%
deviled *(Underwood)* 'Smoked' . . . . 2 1/8 oz	2 1/8 oz	190	9.0	<1.0	260	na	18.0	6.0	65	80%
ham and cheese . . . . 1 oz	1 oz	69	4.6	0.6	339	0	5.3	2.4	17	70%
ham and cheese . . . . 1 tbsp	1 tbsp	37	2.4	0.3	179	0	2.8	1.3	9	70%
ham salad . . . . 1 oz	1 oz	61	2.5	3.0	259	0	4.4	1.4	10	64%

Food Name	Serving Size	Calories	Prot. gms	Carbs gms	Sod. mgs	Fiber gms	Fat gms	Sat. Fat gms	Chol. mgs	% Fat Cal.
ham salad	1 tbsp	32	1.3	1.6	137	0	2.3	0.8	6	64%
ham salad 'Spreadables' (Libby's)	1.9 oz	70	5.0	6.0	380	1.1	3.0	1.0	10	38%
HAM TACO, refrigerated, 'Border Breakfasts' (Owens)	2.17 oz	90	7.0	13.0	430	(mq)	6.0	(mq)	50	40%

HAMBURG PARSLEY. See PARSLEY ROOT.

HAMBURGER. See BEEF, GROUND.

HAMBURGER BUN. See BUN, HAMBURGER.

HAMBURGER ENTRÉE MIX

(Betty Crocker) 'Hamburger Helper'

Food Name	Serving Size	Calories	Prot. gms	Carbs gms	Sod. mgs	Fiber gms	Fat gms	Sat. Fat gms	Chol. mgs	% Fat Cal.
beef noodle, dry	1/5 pkg	140	5.0	26.0	1000	(mq)	2.0	(mq)	na	13%
beef noodle, prepared	1 cup	320	20.0	26.0	1050	(mq)	15.0	(mq)	(mq)	42%
beef Romanoff, dry	1/5 pkg	180	7.0	31.0	1030	(mq)	3.0	(mq)	na	15%
beef Romanoff, prepared	1 cup	350	22.0	31.0	1070	(mq)	16.0	(mq)	(mq)	40%
beef taco, dry	1/5 pkg	160	4.0	33.0	930	na	1.0	na	na	6%
beef taco, prepared	1 cup	330	19.0	33.0	970	na	14.0	na	na	38%
beef teriyaki, dry	1/5 pkg	180	4.0	38.0	1110	na	1.0	na	na	5%
beef teriyaki, prepared	1 cup	360	20.0	38.0	1160	na	14.0	na	na	35%
cheddar and bacon, dry	1/5 pkg	190	7.0	28.0	950	na	6.0	na	na	28%
cheddar and bacon, prepared	1 cup	400	24.0	30.0	1020	na	20.0	na	na	46%
cheeseburger macaroni, dry	1/5 pkg	190	6.0	26.0	980	(mq)	6.0	(mq)	na	30%
cheeseburger macaroni, prepared	1 cup	370	21.0	28.0	1030	(mq)	19.0	(mq)	(mq)	47%
cheesy Italian, dry	1/5 pkg	160	5.0	27.0	970	(mq)	3.0	(mq)	na	17%
cheesy Italian, prepared w/2% milk	1 cup	360	22.0	30.0	1040	(mq)	17.0	(mq)	(mq)	42%
chili macaroni, dry	1/5 pkg	150	4.0	32.0	920	na	1.0	na	na	6%
chili macaroni, prepared	1 cup	330	19.0	32.0	960	na	14.0	na	na	38%
chili tomato, dry	1/5 pkg	150	5.0	31.0	1360	(mq)	1.0	na	na	6%
chili tomato, prepared	1 cup	330	20.0	31.0	1410	(mq)	14.0	(mq)	(mq)	38%
chili w/beans, dry	1/4 pkg	130	5.0	25.0	1680	(mq)	1.0	na	na	7%
chili w/beans, prepared	1 1/4 cup	350	24.0	25.0	1740	(mq)	17.0	(mq)	(mq)	44%
creamy Stroganoff, dry	1/5 pkg	190	5.0	30.0	800	(mq)	5.0	(mq)	na	24%
creamy Stroganoff, prepared w/whole milk	1 cup	390	22.0	30.0	870	(mq)	20.0	(mq)	(mq)	46%
hamburger hash, dry	1/5 pkg	140	3.0	27.0	970	(mq)	2.0	(mq)	na	13%
hamburger hash, prepared	1 cup	320	18.0	27.0	1020	(mq)	15.0	(mq)	(mq)	43%
hamburger stew, dry	1/5 pkg	120	3.0	25.0	960	(mq)	1.0	na	na	7%
hamburger stew, prepared	1 cup	300	18.0	25.0	1010	(mq)	14.0	(mq)	(mq)	42%
lasagna, dry	1/5 pkg	160	5.0	33.0	1000	(mq)	1.0	na	na	6%
lasagna, prepared	1 cup	340	21.0	33.0	1050	(mq)	14.0	(mq)	(mq)	37%
meat loaf, dry	1/5 pkg	70	2.0	13.0	620	(mq)	1.0	na	na	13%
meat loaf, prepared	1 cup	360	27.0	14.0	710	(mq)	22.0	(mq)	(mq)	55%
mushroom and wild rice, dry	1/5 pkg	180	4.0	34.0	880	na	3.0	na	na	15%
mushroom and wild rice, prepared	1 cup	380	21.0	37.0	950	na	16.0	na	na	38%
nacho cheese, dry	1/5 pkg	160	4.0	32.0	980	na	2.0	na	na	11%
nacho cheese, prepared	1 cup	360	21.0	35.0	1050	na	15.0	na	na	38%
pizza dish, dry	1/5 pkg	180	6.0	37.0	960	(mq)	1.0	na	na	5%
pizza dish, prepared	1 cup	360	21.0	37.0	1010	(mq)	14.0	(mq)	(mq)	35%
'Pizzabake,' dry	1/6 pkg	150	4.0	29.0	800	(mq)	2.0	(mq)	na	12%
'Pizzabake,' prepared	4.5 oz	320	19.0	29.0	840	(mq)	14.0	(mq)	(mq)	40%
potato au gratin, dry	1/5 pkg	150	4.0	28.0	860	(mq)	2.0	(mq)	na	12%
potato au gratin, prepared	1 cup	320	19.0	28.0	910	(mq)	15.0	(mq)	(mq)	42%
potato Stroganoff, dry	1/5 pkg	140	3.0	28.0	900	(mq)	2.0	(mq)	na	13%
potato Stroganoff, prepared	1 cup	320	18.0	28.0	950	(mq)	15.0	(mq)	(mq)	42%
rice Oriental, dry	1/5 pkg	180	4.0	38.0	1070	(mq)	1.0	na	na	5%
rice Oriental, prepared	1 cup	340	19.0	38.0	1120	(mq)	14.0	(mq)	(mq)	36%
'Sloppy Joe Bake,' dry	1/6 pkg	180	5.0	33.0	1060	(mq)	3.0	(mq)	na	15%
'Sloppy Joe Bake,' prepared	5 oz	340	18.0	33.0	1100	(mq)	15.0	(mq)	(mq)	40%

Food Name	Serving Size	Calories	Prot. gms	Carbs gms	Sod. mgs	Fiber gms	Fat gms	Sat. Fat gms	Chol. mgs	% Fat Cal.
spaghetti, dry	1/5 pkg	170	5.0	32.0	1060	(mq)	2.0	(mq)	na	11%
spaghetti, prepared	1 cup	340	20.0	32.0	1110	(mq)	15.0	(mq)	(mq)	39%
'Tacobake,' dry	1/6 pkg	170	4.0	31.0	920	(mq)	4.0	(mq)	na	21%
'Tacobake,' prepared	5.75 oz	320	17.0	31.0	940	(mq)	15.0	(mq)	(mq)	41%
tamale pie, dry	1/5 pkg	200	4.0	39.0	890	(mq)	3.0	(mq)	na	14%
tamale pie, prepared	1 cup	380	19.0	39.0	940	(mq)	16.0	(mq)	(mq)	38%
three cheese, dry	1/5 pkg	210	7.0	30.0	910	na	7.0	na	na	30%
three cheese, prepared	1/5 pkg	400	24.0	32.0	980	na	20.0	na	na	45%
zesty Italian, dry	1/5 pkg	170	6.0	35.0	940	(mq)	1.0	na	na	5%
zesty Italian, prepared	1 cup	340	21.0	35.0	980	(mq)	13.0	(mq)	(mq)	34%
HAWAIIAN YAM. See YAM, MOUNTAIN.										
HAWS / hawthorn tree fruit										
scarlet, flesh and skin, raw	100 gm	87	2.0	20.8	0	>2.1 c	0.7	0.0	0	7%
HAZELNUT, SHELLED / cobnut / filbert										
blanched	1 oz	191	3.6	4.5	1	>.5 c	19.1	1.4	0	84%
dry-roasted, unblanched	1 oz	188	2.8	5.1	1	1.7	18.8	1.4	0	84%
dry-roasted, unblanched, w/salt	1 oz	188	2.8	5.1	221	1.7	18.8	1.4	0	84%
oil-roasted, unblanched	1 oz	187	4.1	5.4	1	1.8	18.1	1.3	0	81%
oil-roasted, unblanched, w/salt	1 oz	187	4.1	5.4	223	1.8	18.1	1.3	0	81%
unblanched	1 oz	179	3.7	4.4	1	1.7	17.8	1.3	0	83%
unblanched, chopped	1 cup	727	15.0	17.6	3	7.0	72.0	5.3	0	83%
HAZELNUT BUTTER, gourmet (Roaster Fresh)	1 oz	188	4.0	5.0	1	na	18.9	1.7	na	83%
HAZELNUT OIL										
	1 cup	1927	0.0	0.0	0	0	218.0	16.1	0	100%
	1 oz	251	0.0	0.0	0	0	28.4	2.1	0	100%
	1 tbsp	120	0.0	0.0	0	0	13.6	1.0	0	100%
HAZELNUT SPREAD, Nutella, with milk and cocoa (Ferrero)	1 tbsp	80	1.0	9.0	10	na	5.0	na	0	56%
HEART NUT. See CASHEW.										
HERB AND GARLIC MARINADE, w/lemon (Lawry's)	2 tbsp	36	3.6	3.8	3688	.4	<1.0	0.1	0	<23%
HERB SEASONING MIX										
Italian, 'Bag'n Season' (Schilling)	1 pkg	94	2.0	21.0	1367	(mq)	0.2	na	na	2%
mixed, 'Pinch of Herbs' (Lawry's)	1 tsp	9	0.3	0.9	259	>.2 c	0.5	na	0	48%
HERBAL TEA. See TEA.										
HERRING										
ATLANTIC										
broiled	4 oz	230	26.1	0.0	130	0	13.1	3.0	87	53%
dry-heat cooked	4 oz	230	26.1	0.0	130	0	13.1	3.0	87	53%
dry-heat cooked	3 oz	173	19.6	0.0	98	0	9.9	2.2	65	53%
kippered	4 oz	246	27.9	0.0	1041	0	14.0	3.2	93	53%
kippered snacks, w/smoke flavoring, drained (Beach Cliff)	3.3 oz	220	17.0	1.0	350	na	17.0	na	na	68%
microwaved	4 oz	230	26.1	0.0	130	0	13.1	3.0	87	53%
pickled	4 oz	297	16.1	10.9	987	0	20.4	2.7	15	63%
raw	1 lb	718	81.5	0.0	407	0	41.0	9.3	272	53%
raw	3 oz	134	15.3	0.0	77	0	7.7	1.7	51	53%
raw	1 oz	45	5.1	0.0	26	0	2.6	0.6	17	53%
steaks, in soybean oil, drained (Beach Cliff)	3 oz	240	16.0	0.0	350	na	20.0	na	na	74%
steaks, in water, drained (Beach Cliff)	3 oz	230	17.0	1.0	350	na	18.0	na	na	69%
steaks, w/mustard, drained (Beach Cliff)	3 oz	227	13.0	4.0	350	na	18.0	na	na	70%
steaks, w/tomato, drained (Beach Cliff)	3 oz	210	15.0	0.0	350	na	17.0	na	na	72%
LAKE										
raw	1 lb	446	86.1	0.0	249	0	8.7	1.9	(mq)	19%
raw	2.8-oz fillet	78	15.0	0.0	47	0	1.5	0.3	(mq)	18%
raw	1 oz	28	5.4	0.0	16	0	0.5	0.1	(mq)	17%
smoked	4 oz	201	18.6	0.0	545	0	13.5	2.0	36	62%

Food Name	Serving Size	Calories	Prot. gms	Carbs gms	Sod. mgs	Fiber gms	Fat gms	Sat. Fat gms	Chol. mgs	% Fat Cal.
PACIFIC										
dry-heat cooked	3 oz	213	17.9	0.0	81	0	15.1	3.5	84	66%
raw	1 lb	885	74.4	0.0	335	0	63.0	14.8	348	66%
raw	3 oz	166	13.9	0.0	63	0	11.8	2.8	65	66%
raw	1 oz	55	4.6	0.0	21	0	3.9	0.9	22	66%
HIBISCUS COOLER (Knudsen & Sons)	8 oz	95	<1.0	24.0	na	na	0.0	na	na	0%
HIBISCUS CRANBERRY JUICE (Knudsen & Sons)	8 oz	110	<1.0	28.0	na	na	0.0	na	na	0%
HICKORY NUT										
in shell	1 lb	954	18.5	26.5	1	>4.7 c	93.4	10.2	0	82%
shelled	1 oz	187	3.6	5.2	0	1.9	18.3	2.0	0	82%
HOG PLUM. See JOBO.										
HOMINY GRITS. See GRITS.										
HONEY										
extracted	1 cup	1031	1.0	279.0	17	0	0.0	0.0	0	0%
extracted	1 tbsp	64	0.1	17.3	1	0	0.0	0.0	0	0%
strained	1 cup	1031	1.0	279.0	17	0	0.0	0.0	0	0%
strained	1 tbsp	64	0.1	17.3	1	0	0.0	0.0	0	0%
(Golden Blossom)	1 tbsp	60	0.0	16.0	na	0	0.0	0.0	0	0%
(Knott's Berry Farm)	1 oz	90	0.0	23.0	0	na	0.0	na	na	0%
(Knott's Berry Farm)	1 tbsp	60	0.0	17.0	0	na	0.0	na	na	0%
(Knott's Berry Farm)	.5 oz	30	0.0	17.0	0	na	0.0	na	na	0%
(Sioux)	1 tbsp	60	0.0	16.0	na	0	0.0	0.0	0	0%
HONEY BUTTER	1 tbsp	50	<1.0	11.0	5	0	1.0	na	na	16%
HONEY ROLL SAUSAGE										
	1 oz	52	5.3	0.6	375	0	3.0	1.2	14	53%
4 inch diam	1/8-inch slice	42	4.3	0.5	304	0	2.4	0.9	11	53%
HONEYDEW MELON										
pulp	1 oz	10	0.1	2.6	3	>.2 c	<.1	(tr)	0	<8%
raw, cubed	1 cup	59	0.8	15.6	17	1.0	0.2	na	0	3%
raw, wedge	7 x 2 inches	45	0.6	11.8	13	.8	0.1	na	0	2%
untrimmed	1 lb	74	1.0	19.2	21	>1.3 c	0.2	(tr)	0	2%
untrimmed (Dole)	7 x 2 inches	50	1.0	12.0	50	>1.0 c	0.0	na	na	0%
HORSE										
roasted	3 oz	149	23.9	0.0	47	na	5.1	1.6	58	32%
roasted, diced	1 cup	245	39.4	0.0	77	0	8.5	2.7	95	33%
raw	1 lb	603	97.0	0.0	240	na	20.9	6.5	236	33%
raw	1 oz	37	6.0	0.0	15	na	1.3	0.4	15	33%
HORSE BEAN. See FAVA BEAN.										
HORSERADISH										
Prepared										
	1 tbsp	6	0.2	1.4	14	>.1 c	0.0	0.0	0	0%
	1 tsp	2	0.1	0.5	5	>.1 c	0.0	0.0	0	0%
(Crowley)	1 oz	10	<1.0	2.0	25	(mq)	<1.0	(tr)	0	<43%
(Kraft)	1 tbsp	10	0.0	1.0	140	(mq)	0.0	0.0	0	0%
(Kraft) Cream style	1 tbsp	12	0.0	1.0	85	(mq)	0.0	0.0	0	0%
(Gold's) Hot	1 tsp	4	<1.0	<1.0	60	(mq)	<1.0	(tr)	0	<53%
(Gold's) Red	1 tsp	4	<1.0	<1.0	75	(mq)	0.0	0.0	0	0%
(Gold's) White	1 tsp	4	<1.0	<1.0	55	(mq)	<1.0	(tr)	0	<53%
(Silver Spring) Cream style	1 tsp	0	0.0	0.0	10	na	0.0	na	na	0%
Raw	1 lb	288	10.6	65.3	27	>7.9 c	1.0	0.0	0	3%
HORSERADISH, JAPANESE. See WASABI.										
HORSERADISH TREE										
Leafy tips										
boiled, drained	4 oz	68	6.0	12.6	10	>2.0 c	1.1	na	0	12%

Food Name	Serving Size	Calories	Prot. gms	Carbs gms	Sod. mgs	Fiber gms	Fat gms	Sat. Fat gms	Chol. mgs	% Fat Cal.
boiled, drained, chopped .... 1 cup		25	2.2	4.7	4	.8	0.4	na	0	12%
raw, chopped .... 1 cup		13	2.0	1.7	2	.4	0.3	na	0	15%
raw, trimmed .... 1 oz		18	2.7	2.3	3	>.4 c	0.4	na	0	15%
raw, untrimmed .... 1 lb		181	26.4	23.3	26	>4.2 c	3.9	na	0	15%
Pods										
boiled, drained .... 4 oz		41	2.4	9.3	49	5.0	0.2	na	0	4%
boiled, drained, sliced .... 1 cup		42	2.5	9.6	51	5.0	0.2	na	0	4%
boiled, drained, sliced .... 1/2 cup		21	1.2	4.8	25	2.5	0.1	na	0	4%
raw, sliced .... 1 cup		37	2.1	8.5	42	3.2	0.2	na	0	4%
raw, trimmed .... 1 oz		10	0.6	2.4	12	1.2	0.1	na	0	7%
raw, untrimmed .... 1 lb		88	5.0	20.1	99	>3.1 c	0.5	na	0	4%
raw, whole, approx 15 1/3 inches long .... 1 pod		4	0.2	0.9	5	.3	0.0	na	0	0%

HOT CHOCOLATE. See COCOA MIX.

HOT DOG. See FRANKFURTER.

HOT DOG BUN. See BUN, FRANKFURTER.

HUBBARD SQUASH. See SQUASH, HUBBARD.

HUMMUS

Food Name	Serving Size	Calories	Prot. gms	Carbs gms	Sod. mgs	Fiber gms	Fat gms	Sat. Fat gms	Chol. mgs	% Fat Cal.
mix, dry (Casbah) .... 1 oz		110	5.0	10.0	na	(mq)	5.0	(mq)	0	43%
prepared .... 1/2 cup		210	6.0	24.8	300	>1.7 c	10.4	1.6	0	43%
prepared .... 1 oz		48	1.4	5.7	69	>.4 c	2.4	0.4	0	43%
HUSHPUPPY, FROZEN, 'Regular' (SeaPak) .... 4 oz		330	6.0	56.0	690	(mq)	9.0	(mq)	na	25%
HUSHPUPPY MIX										
deluxe, dry (Golden Dipt) .... 1.25 oz		120	3.0	26.0	520	(mq)	0.0	0.0	0	0%
jalapeño, dry (Golden Dipt) .... 1.25 oz		120	3.0	27.0	570	(mq)	0.0	0.0	0	0%
w/onion, dry (Golden Dipt) .... 1.25 oz		120	3.0	27.0	520	(mq)	0.0	0.0	0	0%
HYACINTH BEAN										
boiled, drained .... 4 oz		57	3.3	10.4	2	>2.0 c	0.3	0.1	0	5%
immature, boiled, drained .... 1/2 cup		22	1.3	4.1	1	>.8 c	0.1	0.1	0	4%
immature, raw .... 1/2 cup		18	0.8	3.7	1	>.5 c	0.1	0.0	0	5%
mature, boiled .... 1/2 cup		113	7.9	20.1	7	>2.4 c	0.6	0.1	0	5%
mature, raw .... 1/2 cup		361	25.1	63.8	22	>7.5 c	1.8	0.3	0	4%
raw, trimmed .... 1 oz		13	0.6	2.6	<1	>.4 c	0.1	<.1	0	7%
raw, untrimmed .... 1 lb		196	8.9	38.8	8	>5.5 c	0.8	0.4	0	4%
HYACINTH BEAN, DRIED										
mature, boiled .... 1/2 cup		114	7.9	20.1	7	>2.4 c	0.6	na	0	5%
mature, boiled .... 4 oz		133	9.2	23.5	8	>2.8 c	0.7	na	0	5%
mature, raw .... 1/2 cup		362	25.1	63.8	22	>7.5 c	1.8	na	0	4%
mature, raw .... 1 oz		98	6.8	17.2	6	>2.0 c	0.5	na	0	5%

I

Food Name	Serving Size	Calories	Prot. gms	Carbs gms	Sod. mgs	Fiber gms	Fat gms	Sat. Fat gms	Chol. mgs	% Fat Cal.
ICE BARS AND DESSERTS. See also FRUIT BAR, FROZEN; SHERBET; SORBET.										
BAR										
'All Natural' all flavors (Popsicle) .... 1 bar		60	0.0	14.0	0	(tr)	0.0	0.0	0	0%
'Ice Stripes' 1.5 oz, all flavors (Good Humor) .... 1 bar		35	0.0	8.6	0	(tr)	0.0	0.0	0	0%
'Twin Pop' all flavors (Gold Bond) .... 1 bar		60	0.0	14.0	0	(tr)	0.0	0.0	0	0%
'Water Ice' all flavors except cherry and wildberry (Popsicle) .... 1 bar		50	0.0	12.0	10	(tr)	0.0	0.0	0	0%
Cherry										
'Calippo' 4.5 oz (Good Humor) .... 1 bar		138	0.1	34.9	5	(tr)	0.1	(tr)	0	1%
'Jumbo Jet Star' 4.5 oz (Good Humor) .... 1 bar		85	0.0	19.5	0	na	0.7	na	0	8%

Food Name	Serving Size	Calories	Prot. gms	Carbs gms	Sod. mgs	Fiber gms	Fat gms	Sat. Fat gms	Chol. mgs	% Fat Cal.
'Water Ice' (Popsicle)	1 bar	70	0.0	17.0	15	(tr)	0.0	0.0	0	0%
Fruit										
and juice, 3 oz	1 bar	75	1.1	18.6	4	0	0.1	na	0	1%
and water, aspartame-sweetened	1 bar	12	0.3	3.2	3	na	0.1	na	0	6%
Lemon										
'Calippo' 4.5 oz (Good Humor)	1 bar	112	0.0	27.6	0	(tr)	0.1	(tr)	0	1%
'Great White Shark' 3 oz (Good Humor)	1 bar	68	0.0	17.0	7	na	0.1	na	(mq)	1%
Orange										
'Calippo' 4.5 oz (Good Humor)	1 bar	111	0.0	27.2	0	(tr)	0.2	(tr)	0	2%
Wildberry, 'Water Ice' (Popsicle)	1 bar	40	0.0	10.0	10	(tr)	0.0	0.0	0	0%
DESSERT										
cherry, Italian (Good Humor)	6 oz	138	0.0	34.2	0	(tr)	0.1	(tr)	0	1%
daiquiri (Baskin-Robbins)	1 scoop	140	0.0	35.0	15	na	0.0	0.0	0	0%
lime	4 oz	75	0.4	31.3	21	0	0.0	na	0	0%
pineapple-coconut	4 oz	108	0.0	22.9	34	na	2.5	na	0	20%
ICE CREAM. See also ICE CREAM, ALTERNATIVE; ICE CREAM BAR; ICE CREAM BAR, ALTERNATIVE; ICE CREAM SNACKS AND SANDWICHES; ICE MILK; ICE MILK BAR.										
ALMOND FUDGE (Baskin-Robbins) 'Jamoca'	1 scoop	270	5.0	30.0	115	na	14.0	na	32	47%
BANANA										
(Baskin-Robbins) sugar-free 'Chunky Banana'	4 oz	100	3.0	20.0	50	na	1.0	na	3	9%
(Ben & Jerry's) 'Chunky Monkey'	1/2 cup	280	4.0	29.0	50	1.0	19.0	10.0	70	61%
BORDEAUX CHERRY (Healthy Choice) 'Dairy Dessert'	4 oz	120	3.0	23.0	50	na	2.0	1.0	5	15%
BORDEAUX CHERRY CHOCOLATE CHIP										
(Healthy Choice) 'Dairy Dessert'	4 oz	120	3.0	23.0	50	na	2.0	1.0	5	15%
BOYSENBERRY (Good Humor) 'King Cone'	5 oz	340	3.9	51.6	151	(mq)	13.1	(mq)	(mq)	35%
BROWNIES 'N CREME (Weight Watchers) 'ONE-ders'	4 oz	130	4.0	20.0	115	na	4.0	na	10	27%
BUTTER ALMOND (Breyers)	4 oz	170	4.0	15.0	125	(mq)	10.0	4.0	25	54%
BUTTER CRUNCH (Sealtest)	4 oz	150	2.0	18.0	90	(tr)	7.0	4.0	25	44%
BUTTER PECAN										
(Ben & Jerry's)	1/2 cup	310	4.0	20.0	160	1.0	26.0	11.0	100	75%
(Breyers)	4 oz	180	3.0	15.0	125	(mq)	12.0	5.0	25	60%
(Frusen Glädjé)	4 oz	280	5.0	16.0	160	(mq)	21.0	(mq)	85	69%
(Häagen-Dazs)	4 oz	390	5.0	29.0	100	(mq)	24.0	9.0	110	61%
(Lady Borden)	4 oz	180	3.0	16.0	65	(mq)	12.0	(mq)	(mq)	59%
(Sealtest)	4 oz	160	3.0	16.0	125	(mq)	9.0	4.0	15	52%
BUTTER PECAN CRUNCH (Healthy Choice) 'Dairy Dessert'	4 oz	140	3.0	26.0	80	na	2.0	1.0	5	13%
CHERRY										
(Ben & Jerry's) 'Cherry Garcia'	1/2 cup	240	4.0	25.0	60	0	16.0	10.0	80	60%
(Breyers) vanilla	4 oz	150	3.0	17.0	45	(tr)	7.0	4.0	20	44%
CHOCOLATE										
(Baskin-Robbins)	1 scoop	270	5.0	32.0	160	na	14.0	na	37	46%
(Baskin-Robbins) 'World Class'	1 scoop	280	5.0	35.0	145	na	14.0	na	36	44%
(Ben & Jerry's) deep dark chocolate	1/2 cup	260	4.0	32.0	55	2.0	15.0	9.0	55	52%
(Breyers)	4 oz	160	3.0	20.0	30	(tr)	8.0	5.0	20	44%
(Darigold)	4 oz	140	2.0	17.0	70	(tr)	7.0	(mq)	(mq)	45%
(Darigold) 'Alpine'	4 oz	140	2.0	17.0	70	(tr)	7.0	(mq)	(mq)	45%
(Darigold) 'Classic'	4 oz	190	3.0	16.0	30	(tr)	13.0	(mq)	(mq)	61%
(Frusen Glädjé)	4 oz	240	5.0	17.0	65	(tr)	17.0	9.0	75	64%
(Häagen-Dazs)	4 oz	270	5.0	24.0	50	(tr)	17.0	8.0	120	57%
(Häagen-Dazs) deep	4 oz	290	5.0	26.0	70	(tr)	14.0	(mq)	(mq)	50%
(Healthy Choice) 'Dairy Dessert'	4 oz	130	3.0	24.0	70	na	2.0	1.0	5	14%
(Sealtest)	4 oz	140	2.0	18.0	50	(tr)	6.0	4.0	20	40%
CHOCOLATE, DUTCH (Borden) 'Olde Fashioned Recipe'	4 oz	130	2.0	16.0	65	(tr)	6.0	(mq)	(mq)	43%
CHOCOLATE CARAMEL NUT (Baskin-Robbins) light	4 oz	130	3.0	19.0	8	na	5.0	3.0	0	34%

Food Name	Serving Size	Calories	Prot. gms	Carbs gms	Sod. mgs	Fiber gms	Fat gms	Sat. Fat gms	Chol. mgs	% Fat Cal.
CHOCOLATE CHIP										
(Baskin-Robbins)	1 scoop	260	4.0	27.0	110	na	15.0	na	40	52%
(Breyers)	4 oz	170	3.0	18.0	45	na	10.0	na	35	52%
(Dreyer's)	4 oz	150	3.0	16.0	40	(tr)	9.0	(mq)	30	52%
(Eskimo Pie) cone 'Cookie Dough'	1 cone	280	4.0	33.0	103	na	14.0	na	14	46%
(Healthy Choice) 'Dairy Dessert'	4 oz	130	3.0	24.0	70	na	2.0	1.0	5	14%
(Sealtest)	4 oz	150	2.0	17.0	50	(tr)	8.0	(mq)	15	49%
(Weight Watchers) 'ONE-ders'	4 oz	120	3.0	19.0	80	na	4.0	na	10	29%
CHOCOLATE CHIP CHOCOLATE (Häagen-Dazs)	4 oz	290	5.0	28.0	40	(tr)	20.0	10.0	105	58%
CHOCOLATE CHIP COOKIE DOUGH (Ben & Jerry's)	1/2 cup	270	4.0	30.0	92	0	17.0	9.0	80	57%
CHOCOLATE CHOCOLATE CHIP (Frusen Glädjé)	4 oz	270	5.0	21.0	60	(tr)	18.0	9.0	55	61%
CHOCOLATE CHUNK										
(Ben & Jerry's) New York Super Fudge Chunk'	1/2 cup	290	5.0	28.0	55	2.0	20.0	11.0	50	62%
CHOCOLATE FUDGE										
(Ben & Jerry's) 'Chocolate Fudge Brownie'	1/2 cup	250	4.0	31.0	100	2.0	14.0	9.0	50	50%
(Ben & Jerry's) double chocolate fudge	1/2 cup	280	5.0	35.0	60	3.0	16.0	9.0	55	51%
(Häagen-Dazs) deep	4 oz	290	5.0	26.0	70	(tr)	14.0	(mq)	(mq)	50%
CHOCOLATE MINT (Häagen-Dazs)	4 oz	300	5.0	26.0	50	(tr)	20.0	(mq)	(mq)	59%
CHOCOLATE PEANUT BUTTER COOKIE DOUGH										
(Ben & Jerry's)	1/2 cup	300	6.0	32.0	85	2.0	20.0	9.0	55	60%
CHOCOLATE RASPBERRY TRUFFLE										
(Baskin-Robbins) 'International Creams'	1 scoop	310	4.0	35.0	115	na	17.0	na	45	50%
CHOCOLATE SWIRL (Borden)	4 oz	130	2.0	18.0	65	(tr)	6.0	(mq)	(mq)	40%
CHOCOLATE TRIPLE STRIPES (Sealtest)	4 oz	140	2.0	17.0	50	(tr)	7.0	(mq)	(mq)	45%
CHOCOLATE-PEANUT BUTTER, DEEP (Häagen-Dazs)	4 oz	330	7.0	25.0	90	(tr)	19.0	(mq)	(mq)	57%
COCONUT ALMOND FUDGE CHIP (Ben & Jerry's)	1/2 cup	320	6.0	24.0	82	2.0	28.0	15.0	75	79%
COFFEE										
(Baskin-Robbins) light 'Espresso and Cream'	4 oz	120	3.0	15.0	0	na	5.0	3.0	12	39%
(Ben & Jerry's) Aztec harvest coffee	1/2 cup	230	4.0	22.0	55	0	16.0	10.0	90	63%
(Breyers)	4 oz	150	3.0	16.0	50	0	8.0	5.0	30	49%
(Häagen-Dazs)	4 oz	270	5.0	23.0	120	0	17.0	8.0	55	58%
(Sealtest)	4 oz	140	2.0	16.0	50	0	7.0	4.0	15	47%
COFFEE ALMOND FUDGE (Ben & Jerry's)	1/2 cup	290	6.0	24.0	85	2.0	20.0	9.0	75	62%
COFFEE TOFFEE										
(Ben & Jerry's) 'Coffee Toffee Crunch'	1/2 cup	280	4.0	28.0	120	0	19.0	10.0	80	61%
(Healthy Choice) 'Dairy Dessert'	4 oz	130	3.0	25.0	80	na	2.0	1.0	5	14%
COOKIE DOUGH DYNAMO (Häagen-Dazs)	4 oz	300	4.0	31.0	110	na	18.0	na	na	54%
COOKIES 'N' CREAM										
(Breyers)	4 oz	170	3.0	19.0	60	(tr)	9.0	5.0	20	48%
(Dreyer's)	4 oz	160	3.0	18.0	80	(tr)	9.0	na	28	49%
(Healthy Choice) 'Dairy Dessert'	4 oz	130	4.0	24.0	80	na	2.0	1.0	5	14%
FUDGE, MARBLE (Dreyer's)	4 oz	150	3.0	18.0	50	(tr)	8.0	(mq)	28	46%
FUDGE BROWNIE (Healthy Choice) 'Dairy Dessert'	4 oz	130	3.0	27.0	70	na	2.0	1.0	5	13%
FUDGE ROYALE (Sealtest)	4 oz	140	3.0	19.0	55	(tr)	7.0	4.0	15	42%
FUDGE SWIRL, DOUBLE (Healthy Choice) 'Dairy Dessert' . . .	4 oz	130	3.0	24.0	70	na	2.0	1.0	5	14%
HEAVENLY HASH										
(Sealtest)	4 oz	150	2.0	19.0	50	(tr)	7.0	4.0	15	43%
(Weight Watchers) 'ONE-ders'	4 oz	130	4.0	22.0	90	na	3.0	2.0	10	21%
MACADAMIA BRITTLE (Häagen-Dazs)	4 oz	280	4.0	25.0	60	(mq)	18.0	(mq)	(mq)	58%
MAPLE WALNUT (Sealtest)	4 oz	160	3.0	17.0	40	(mq)	9.0	3.0	20	50%
MINT CHOCOLATE (Breyers)	4 oz	170	3.0	18.0	45	(tr)	10.0	6.0	25	52%
MINT CHOCOLATE CHIP (Healthy Choice) 'Dairy Dessert' . . .	4 oz	140	3.0	25.0	80	na	2.0	2.0	5	14%
MINT WITH CHOCOLATE COOKIE (Ben & Jerry's)	1/2 cup	260	4.0	27.0	120	1.0	17.0	10.0	80	59%
MOCHA ALMOND FUDGE (Breyers)	4 oz	190	4.0	20.0	60	na	10.0	na	na	48%

Food Name	Serving Size	Calories	Prot. gms	Carbs gms	Sod. mgs	Fiber gms	Fat gms	Sat. Fat gms	Chol. mgs	% Fat Cal.
MOCHA FUDGE (Ben & Jerry's)	1/2 cup	270	5.0	30.0	65	1.0	18.0	10.0	85	60%
NEAPOLITAN (Healthy Choice) 'Dairy Dessert'	4 oz	120	3.0	22.0	60	na	2.0	1.0	5	15%
PEACH										
(Baskin-Robbins) fat-free 'Just Peachy'	4 oz	100	3.0	22.0	60	na	0.0	na	0	0%
(Breyers) natural	4 oz	130	2.0	18.0	35	(tr)	6.0	3.0	15	40%
PEANUT BUTTER CUP (Ben & Jerry's)	1/2 cup	370	8.0	30.0	140	2.0	26.0	12.0	75	63%
PRALINE										
(Baskin-Robbins) light 'Praline Dream'	4 oz	130	3.0	17.0	85	na	6.0	na	11	40%
(Baskin-Robbins) pralines 'n cream	1 scoop	280	4.0	35.0	180	na	14.0	na	36	45%
(Healthy Choice) and caramel 'Dairy Dessert'	4 oz	130	3.0	26.0	70	na	2.0	1.0	5	13%
(Weight Watchers) pralines 'n creme 'ONE-ders'	4 oz	120	3.0	19.0	110	na	4.0	na	10	29%
RASPBERRY SWIRL (Healthy Choice) 'Dairy Dessert'	4 oz	120	3.0	23.0	60	na	2.0	1.0	5	15%
ROCKY ROAD										
(Baskin-Robbins)	1 scoop	300	5.0	39.0	135	na	14.0	na	32	42%
(Dreyer's)	4 oz	170	3.0	18.0	30	(tr)	10.0	(mq)	30	52%
(Healthy Choice) 'Dairy Dessert'	4 oz	160	3.0	32.0	70	na	2.0	1.0	5	11%
RUM RAISIN (Häagen-Dazs)	4 oz	250	4.0	21.0	45	(tr)	17.0	8.0	110	61%
STRAWBERRY										
(Baskin-Robbins) light 'Strawberry Royale'	4 oz	110	2.0	19.0	120	na	3.0	na	9	24%
(Baskin-Robbins) 'Very Berry'	1 scoop	220	3.0	30.0	95	na	10.0	na	30	41%
(Borden)	4 oz	130	2.0	18.0	55	(tr)	6.0	(mq)	(mq)	40%
(Borden) cream 'Olde Fashioned Recipe'	4 oz	130	2.0	19.0	55	(tr)	5.0	(mq)	(mq)	35%
(Breyers)	4 oz	130	2.0	16.0	40	(tr)	6.0	4.0	20	43%
(Frusen Glädjé)	4 oz	230	4.0	20.0	60	(tr)	15.0	10.0	65	58%
(Häagen-Dazs)	4 oz	250	4.0	23.0	40	(tr)	15.0	8.0	95	56%
(Healthy Choice) 'Dairy Dessert'	4 oz	120	2.0	23.0	50	na	2.0	1.0	5	15%
(Sealtest)	4 oz	130	2.0	18.0	40	(tr)	5.0	3.0	15	36%
SUNDAE										
(Häagen-Dazs) caramel nut	4 oz	310	5.0	26.0	100	(mq)	21.0	(mq)	(mq)	60%
(Sealtest) chocolate-marshmallow	4 oz	150	2.0	21.0	40	(tr)	6.0	4.0	20	37%
(Sealtest) peanut fudge	4 oz	140	3.0	17.0	50	(mq)	7.0	4.0	20	44%
(Weight Watchers) hot caramel fudge	4.5 oz	160	5.0	27.0	140	na	4.0	2.0	15	22%
(Weight Watchers) hot chocolate fudge	4.5 oz	160	6.0	26.0	115	na	4.0	2.0	15	22%
(Weight Watchers) hot mocha fudge	4.5 oz	160	5.0	24.0	120	na	5.0	2.0	15	28%
SWISS CHOCOLATE CANDY ALMOND (Frusen Glädjé)	4 oz	270	6.0	18.0	60	(mq)	19.0	9.0	55	64%
TOFFEE (Ben & Jerry's) 'English Toffee Crunch'	1/2 cup	310	4.0	30.0	130	0	21.0	12.0	90	61%
VANILLA										
regular, 10% fat, hardened	1 oz	57	1.0	6.8	25	0	3.1	1.9	13	47%
rich, 16% fat, hardened	1 oz	67	0.8	6.1	21	0	4.5	2.8	17	60%
(Baskin-Robbins)	1 scoop	240	4.0	24.0	115	0	14.0	(mq)	52	53%
(Ben & Jerry's)	1/2 cup	230	4.0	21.0	55	0	17.0	10.0	95	67%
(Ben & Jerry's) vanilla bean	1/2 cup	230	4.0	21.0	55	0	17.0	10.0	95	67%
(Borden) 'Olde Fashioned Recipe'	4 oz	130	2.0	15.0	55	0	7.0	(mq)	(mq)	48%
(Breyers)	4 oz	150	3.0	15.0	50	0	8.0	5.0	25	50%
(Darigold)	4 oz	130	2.0	15.0	50	0	7.0	(mq)	(mq)	48%
(Darigold) 'Alpine'	4 oz	130	2.0	15.0	50	0	7.0	(mq)	(mq)	48%
(Darigold) 'Classic'	4 oz	180	2.0	16.0	40	0	12.0	(mq)	(mq)	60%
(Dreyer's)	4 oz	160	2.0	14.0	30	0	10.0	(mq)	40	58%
(Eagle Brand) 'Homestyle'	4 oz	150	3.0	16.0	55	0	9.0	(mq)	(mq)	52%
(Frusen Glädjé)	4 oz	230	5.0	16.0	70	0	17.0	9.0	65	65%
(Good Humor) 'Cup'	3 oz	98	1.5	11.6	35	0	5.1	(mq)	(mq)	47%
(Häagen-Dazs)	4 oz	260	5.0	23.0	55	0	17.0	8.0	120	58%
(Healthy Choice) 'Dairy Dessert'	4 oz	120	4.0	21.0	60	na	2.0	1.0	5	15%
(Sealtest)	4 oz	140	2.0	16.0	50	0	7.0	4.0	20	47%

Food Name	Serving Size	Calories	Prot. gms	Carbs gms	Sod. mgs	Fiber gms	Fat gms	Sat. Fat gms	Chol. mgs	% Fat Cal.
VANILLA, FRENCH										
(Baskin-Robbins)	1 scoop	280	4.0	25.0	90	0	18.0	(mq)	90	58%
(Sealtest)	4 oz	140	2.0	16.0	50	0	7.0	(mq)	35	47%
VANILLA CARAMEL FUDGE *(Ben & Jerry's)*	1/2 cup	280	4.0	33.0	75	1.0	17.0	10.0	95	55%
VANILLA CRUNCH										
(Ben & Jerry's) 'Rainforest Crunch'	1/2 cup	300	5.0	24.0	140	0	23.0	11.0	85	69%
(Ben & Jerry's) 'Wavy Gravy'	1/2 cup	330	6.0	29.0	95	2.0	24.0	10.0	80	65%
VANILLA FUDGE *(Häagen-Dazs)*	4 oz	270	5.0	26.0	100	(tr)	17.0	(mq)	(mq)	55%
VANILLA FUDGE TWIRL *(Breyers)*	4 oz	160	3.0	19.0	55	(tr)	8.0	4.0	20	45%
VANILLA HONEY *(Häagen-Dazs)*	4 oz	250	5.0	22.0	55	0	16.0	8.0	135	57%
VANILLA SWISS ALMOND										
(Frusen Glädjé)	4 oz	270	6.0	18.0	65	(mq)	19.0	9.0	65	64%
(Häagen-Dazs)	4 oz	290	5.0	24.0	55	(mq)	19.0	(mq)	(mq)	60%
VANILLA TOFFEE CHUNK *(Frusen Glädjé)*	4 oz	270	5.0	22.0	160	0	17.0	(mq)	85	59%
VANILLA-CHOCOLATE										
(Baskin-Robbins) fat-free 'Just Chocolate Vanilla'	4 oz	100	4.0	21.0	60	na	0.0	na	0	0%
(Breyers)	4 oz	160	3.0	17.0	40	(tr)	8.0	5.0	25	47%
(Good Humor) cup 'Combo'	6 oz	201	3.8	25.6	80	(mq)	9.2	(mq)	(mq)	41%
VANILLA-CHOCOLATE-STRAWBERRY										
(Breyers)	4 oz	150	3.0	17.0	40	(tr)	8.0	4.0	20	47%
(Sealtest)	4 oz	140	2.0	18.0	50	(tr)	6.0	3.0	20	40%
(Sealtest) 'Cubic Scoops'	4 oz	130	2.0	17.0	50	(tr)	6.0	3.0	20	42%
VANILLA-PEANUT BUTTER SWIRL *(Häagen-Dazs)*	4 oz	280	5.0	19.0	120	(tr)	21.0	8.0	110	66%
WHITE RUSSIAN *(Ben & Jerry's)*	1/2 cup	240	4.0	23.0	55	0	16.0	10.0	90	60%
ICE CREAM, ALTERNATIVE										
ALL FLAVORS *(Lite Lite Tofutti)*	4 oz	90	2.0	20.0	80	na	<1.0	na	0	<9%
BLACK CHERRY *(Sealtest)* 'Free'	4 oz	100	2.0	25.0	45	(tr)	0.0	0.0	0	0%
CAPPUCCINO										
(Rice Dream)	4 oz	130	1.0	17.0	80	na	5.0	na	0	39%
(Tofutti) 'Love Drops'	4 oz	230	3.0	26.0	120	na	12.0	3.0	0	48%
CAROB *(Rice Dream)*	4 oz	130	1.0	20.0	80	na	5.0	na	0	35%
CAROB ALMOND *(Rice Dream)*	4 oz	140	1.0	20.0	80	na	6.0	na	0	39%
CAROB CHIP *(Rice Dream)*	4 oz	140	1.0	20.0	80	na	6.0	na	0	39%
CHOCOLATE										
(Lite Lite Tofutti) soft-serve	4 oz	90	2.0	20.0	80	(tr)	<1.0	na	0	<9%
(Rice Dream) 'Dream Pie'	1 pie	380	3.0	47.0	225	na	19.0	na	0	46%
(Sealtest) 'Free'	4 oz	100	3.0	23.0	50	(tr)	0.0	0.0	0	0%
(Simple Pleasures)	4 oz	140	9.0	25.0	15	0	<1.0	0.3	na	<6%
(Tofutti) 'Love Drops'	4 oz	230	3.0	26.0	100	(tr)	13.0	5.0	0	50%
(Tofutti) supreme	4 oz	210	3.0	20.0	130	(tr)	13.0	3.0	0	56%
(Weight Watchers)	4 oz	80	3.0	19.0	75	(tr)	0.0	0.0	5	0%
CHOCOLATE CHIP *(Low, Lite 'n Luscious)*	4 oz	100	3.0	19.0	80	(tr)	2.0	(mq)	4	17%
CHOCOLATE SWIRL *(Weight Watchers)*	4 oz	90	3.0	22.0	75	(tr)	0.0	0.0	5	0%
COCOA MARBLE FUDGE *(Rice Dream)*	4 oz	140	1.0	19.0	80	na	6.0	na	0	40%
COFFEE *(Simple Pleasures)*	4 oz	120	8.0	22.0	15	0	<1.0	0.3	na	<7%
COOKIES N' DREAM *(Rice Dream)*	4 oz	130	1.0	21.0	80	na	5.0	na	0	34%
JAMOCA SWISS ALMOND *(Low, Lite 'n Luscious)*	4 oz	90	3.0	19.0	100	(tr)	2.0	(mq)	4	17%
LEMON *(Rice Dream)*	4 oz	130	1.0	17.0	80	na	5.0	na	0	39%
MINT *(Rice Dream)* 'Dream Pie'	1 pie	380	3.0	47.0	225	na	19.0	na	0	46%
MINT CAROB CHIP *(Rice Dream)*	4 oz	140	1.0	20.0	80	na	6.0	na	0	39%
MOCHA *(Rice Dream)* 'Dream Pie'	1 pie	380	3.0	47.0	225	na	19.0	na	0	46%
NEAPOLITAN										
(Rice Dream)	4 oz	130	1.0	21.0	80	na	5.0	na	0	34%
(Weight Watchers)	4 oz	80	3.0	19.0	75	(tr)	0.0	0.0	5	0%

Food Name	Serving Size	Calories	Prot. gms	Carbs gms	Sod. mgs	Fiber gms	Fat gms	Sat. Fat gms	Chol. mgs	% Fat Cal.
PEACH										
(Sealtest) 'Free'	4 oz	100	2.0	23.0	45	(tr)	0.0	0.0	0	0%
(Simple Pleasures)	4 oz	135	9.0	24.0	5	0	<1.0	0.3	na	<6%
PEANUT BUTTER FUDGE (Rice Dream)	4 oz	160	3.0	19.0	100	na	7.0	na	0	42%
PINEAPPLE COCONUT (Low, Lite 'n Luscious)	4 oz	90	3.0	19.0	70	(tr)	1.0	na	3	9%
RUM RAISIN (Simple Pleasures)	4 oz	130	7.0	25.0	10	0	<1.0	0.3	na	<7%
STRAWBERRY										
(Low, Lite 'n Luscious)	4 oz	80	3.0	17.0	70	(tr)	1.0	na	3	10%
(Rice Dream)	4 oz	130	1.0	17.0	80	na	5.0	na	0	39%
(Sealtest) 'Free'	4 oz	100	2.0	23.0	40	(tr)	0.0	0.0	0	0%
(Simple Pleasures)	4 oz	120	8.0	22.0	55	0	<1.0	0.3	11	<7%
VANILLA										
(Lite Lite Tofutti) soft-serve	4 oz	90	2.0	20.0	80	na	<1.0	na	0	<9%
(Rice Dream)	4 oz	130	1.0	17.0	80	na	5.0	na	0	39%
(Rice Dream) 'Dream Pie'	1 pie	380	3.0	47.0	225	na	19.0	na	0	46%
(Sealtest) 'Free'	4 oz	100	3.0	24.0	45	0	0.0	0.0	0	0%
(Tofutti)	4 oz	200	2.0	21.0	90	na	11.0	1.5	0	52%
(Tofutti) 'Love Drops'	4 oz	220	3.0	26.0	100	na	12.0	3.0	0	48%
(Weight Watchers)	4 oz	80	3.0	20.0	75	0	0.0	0.0	5	0%
VANILLA ALMOND BARK (Tofutti)	4 oz	230	3.0	23.0	950	na	14.0	4.0	0	55%
VANILLA CHOCOLATE (Tofutti) dipped 'O's'	1 piece	40	1.0	4.0	20	na	2.0	(mq)	0	47%
VANILLA SWISS ALMOND (Rice Dream)	4 oz	140	1.0	20.0	80	na	6.0	na	0	39%
VANILLA-CHOCOLATE-STRAWBERRY (Sealtest) 'Free'	4 oz	100	3.0	23.0	40	(tr)	0.0	0.0	0	0%
VANILLA-FUDGE (Rice Dream)	4 oz	140	1.0	21.0	80	na	6.0	na	0	38%
VANILLA-FUDGE ROYALE (Sealtest) 'Free'	4 oz	100	3.0	24.0	50	(tr)	0.0	0.0	0	0%
VANILLA-STRAWBERRY ROYALE (Sealtest) 'Free'	4 oz	100	3.0	25.0	35	(tr)	0.0	0.0	0	0%
WILDBERRY										
(Rice Dream)	4 oz	130	1.0	17.0	80	na	5.0	na	0	39%
(Tofutti)	4 oz	210	2.0	22.0	100	(tr)	12.0	3.0	0	53%
ICE CREAM BAR										
ALMOND (Good Humor) toasted, 3 oz	1 bar	212	1.8	24.3	34	(mq)	11.8	(mq)	(mq)	50%
CARAMEL ALMOND (Häagen-Dazs) 'Crunch Bar'	1 bar	240	3.0	17.0	65	(mq)	18.0	7.0	40	67%
CHIP CANDY CRUNCH (Good Humor) 3 oz	1 bar	255	2.2	21.2	40	na	17.9	(mq)	(mq)	63%
CHOCOLATE										
(Häagen-Dazs) w/dark chocolate coating	1 bar	390	5.0	32.0	60	0	27.0	(mq)	(mq)	62%
(Klondike) 5 oz	1 bar	270	4.0	23.0	60	na	19.0	(mq)	(mq)	61%
(Nestlé) w/milk chocolate coating 'Quik' 3 oz	1 bar	210	3.0	19.0	40	na	14.0	(mq)	(mq)	59%
(Weight Watchers) 'Treat Bars' 2.75 oz	1 bar	100	4.0	18.0	75	(tr)	1.0	0.0	0	9%
CHOCOLATE DIP (Weight Watchers) 1.7 oz	1 bar	110	2.0	10.0	35	(tr)	7.0	3.0	5	57%
CHOCOLATE ECLAIR (Good Humor) 3 oz	1 bar	188	2.1	22.6	54	na	9.9	(mq)	(mq)	47%
CHOCOLATE FUDGE										
(Baker's) sundae, crunchy 'Fudgetastic' 4 oz	1 bar	230	3.0	24.0	40	na	14.0	(mq)	20	54%
(Baker's) sundae 'Fudgetastic' 4 oz	1 bar	220	3.0	23.0	45	na	15.0	(mq)	20	57%
(Good Humor) cake, 6.3 oz	1 bar	214	1.7	18.1	50	na	15.0	(mq)	(mq)	63%
(Weight Watchers) double, 1.75 oz	1.75 oz	60	3.0	12.0	50	(tr)	1.0	0.0	5	13%
CHOCOLATE MOUSSE										
(Weight Watchers) sugar-free, 1.75 oz	1 bar	35	2.0	9.0	30	(tr)	<1.0	0.0	5	<17%
MILK CHOCOLATE										
(Nestlé) w/almonds, milk chocolate coating, 3.7 oz	3.7 oz	350	6.0	28.0	45	na	23.0	(mq)	5	60%
ORANGE-VANILLA										
(Weight Watchers) 'Sugar-free Treat Bars'	1 bar	30	2.0	8.0	40	(tr)	<1.0	0.0	5	<18%
PEANUT BUTTER (Häagen-Dazs) 'Crunch Bar'	4 oz	270	6.0	16.0	55	(mq)	21.0	7.0	35	68%
STRAWBERRY SHORTCAKE (Good Humor) 3 oz	1 bar	176	1.7	23.8	88	na	8.2	(mq)	(mq)	42%

Food Name	Serving Size	Calories	Prot. gms	Carbs gms	Sod. mgs	Fiber gms	Fat gms	Sat. Fat gms	Chol. mgs	% Fat Cal.
VANILLA										
(Eskimo Pie) w/dark chocolate coating	1 bar	180	2.0	16.0	35	na	12.0	na	na	60%
(Eskimo Pie) w/dark chocolate coating 'Sugar-freedom'	1 bar	140	2.0	13.0	30	na	11.0	na	na	62%
(Eskimo Pie) w/milk chocolate coating	1 bar	190	5.0	18.0	16	na	12.0	na	na	54%
(Eskimo Pie) w/milk chocolate coating and almonds 'Sugar-freedom'	1 bar	140	3.0	12.0	35	na	13.0	na	na	66%
(Eskimo Pie) w/milk chocolate coating and crisp rice 'Sugar-freedom'	1 bar	150	4.0	12.0	40	na	11.0	na	na	61%
(Good Humor) w/chocolate flavor coating, 3 oz	1 bar	198	1.9	16.8	44	na	13.7	(mq)	(mq)	62%
(Häagen-Dazs) 'Crunch Bar' 4 oz	1 bar	220	3.0	16.0	55	(mq)	16.0	6.0	40	66%
(Häagen-Dazs) w/dark chocolate coating, 4 oz	1 bar	390	5.0	32.0	60	na	27.0	(mq)	(mq)	62%
(Häagen-Dazs) w/milk chocolate coating, 4 oz	1 bar	360	4.0	26.0	55	na	27.0	(mq)	(mq)	67%
(Häagen-Dazs) w/milk chocolate-almond coating, 4 oz	1 bar	370	5.0	27.0	55	(mq)	27.0	(mq)	(mq)	66%
(Häagen-Dazs) w/milk chocolate-brittle coating, 4 oz	1 bar	370	5.0	32.0	160	(tr)	25.0	(mq)	(mq)	60%
(Klondike) w/chocolate flavor coating 'Lite'	1 bar	110	3.0	14.0	50	na	6.0	5.0	5	44%
(Nestlé) w/chocolate coating and crisp rice 'Crunch' 3 oz	1 bar	180	2.0	15.0	(mq)	(mq)	13.0	(mq)	(mq)	63%
(Nestlé) w/chocolate coating and crisp rice 'Crunch Lite'	1 bar	120	2.0	16.0	50	na	5.0	na	na	39%
(Nestlé) w/white chocolate coating 'Alpine Premium' 3.7 oz	1 bar	350	6.0	25.0	5	na	25.0	(mq)	50	65%
(Oh Henry!) w/caramel peanut, milk chocolate coating, 3 oz	1 bar	320	1.0	34.0	75	(mq)	20.0	(mq)	(mq)	56%
ICE CREAM BAR, ALTERNATIVE										
(Rice Dream) chocolate	1 bar	270	1.0	33.0	115	na	16.0	na	0	51%
(Rice Dream) chocolate nutty bar	1 bar	330	5.0	29.0	110	na	23.0	na	0	60%
(Rice Dream) strawberry	1 bar	260	1.0	31.0	110	na	14.8	na	0	51%
(Rice Dream) vanilla	1 bar	275	1.0	33.0	120	na	15.8	na	0	51%
(Rice Dream) vanilla nutty bar	1 bar	330	5.0	29.0	100	na	23.0	na	0	60%
ICE CREAM CAKE (Breyers) 'Viennetta'	1 slice	190	3.0	18.0	40	0	12.0	8.0	25	56%
ICE CREAM CONE										
Cup style, wafer										
(Bozo) cake	1 cone	16	1.0	3.0	13	0	0.0	0.0	0	0%
(Keebler)	1 cone	15	1.0	4.0	20	na	1.0	1.0	0	31%
(Keebler) assorted colors	1 cone	15	1.0	4.0	20	na	1.0	1.0	0	31%
(Little Debbie)	1 cone	15	0.4	3.0	15	(mq)	0.1	0.0	<1	6%
(Nabisco) 'Comet'	1 cone	18	<1.0	4.0	5	na	<1.0	na	0	<31%
Sugar										
(Baskin-Robbins)	1 cone	60	1.0	11.0	45	(mq)	1.0	na	0	16%
(Bozo)	1 cone	53	1.0	11.0	29	.2	1.0	0.1	na	16%
(Keebler)	1 cone	45	1.0	11.0	35	na	1.0	1.0	0	16%
(Nabisco)	1 cone	50	1.0	11.0	40	na	<1.0	na	0	<16%
(Nabisco) 'Comet'	1 cone	50	1.0	11.0	40	na	<1.0	na	0	<16%
Waffle, Baskin-Robbins	1 cone	140	3.0	28.0	5	(mq)	2.0	(mq)	0	13%
ICE CREAM MIX										
Dutch chocolate, prepared (Salada)	8 oz	310	4.0	31.0	75	(tr)	19.0	(mq)	(mq)	55%
peach, prepared (Salada)	8 oz	310	4.0	32.0	60	(tr)	18.0	(mq)	(mq)	53%
vanilla, prepared (Salada)	8 oz	310	4.0	32.0	60	(tr)	18.0	(mq)	(mq)	53%
wild strawberry, prepared (Salada)	8 oz	310	4.0	32.0	60	(tr)	18.0	(mq)	(mq)	53%
ICE CREAM SNACKS AND SANDWICHES										
Nuggets										
vanilla, dark chocolate coated 'Bon Bons' (Carnation)	5 pieces	170	2.0	15.0	50	(tr)	11.0	(mq)	14	59%
vanilla, milk chocolate coated 'Bon Bons' (Carnation)	5 pieces	165	2.0	14.0	50	(tr)	11.0	(mq)	16	61%
Round novelties										
mocha, 4 oz (Natural Nectar)	1 bar	300	4.0	40.0	135	na	14.0	na	10	42%
nectar, 4 oz (Natural Nectar)	1 bar	300	4.0	38.0	120	na	15.0	na	15	45%

Food Name	Serving Size	Calories	Prot. gms	Carbs gms	Sod. mgs	Fiber gms	Fat gms	Sat. Fat gms	Chol. mgs	% Fat Cal.
Sandwich										
chocolate chip cookie, 4 oz *(Good Humor)*	1 sandwich	246	2.9	35.1	181	(mq)	10.5	(mq)	(mq)	38%
chocolate chip cookie, 2.7 oz *(Good Humor)*	1 sandwich	204	2.2	30.1	166	(mq)	8.3	(mq)	(mq)	37%
vanilla *(Weight Watchers)*	1 sandwich	150	3.0	28.0	170	(tr)	3.0	2.0	5	18%
vanilla, 5 oz *(Klondike)*	1 sandwich	230	5.0	33.0	220	(mq)	9.0	(mq)	(mq)	35%
vanilla 'Lite' *(Klondike)*	1 sandwich	100	2.0	18.0	110	na	2.0	1.0	5	18%
vanilla, 1.5 oz snacks *(Weight Watchers)*	1 sandwich	90	2.0	17.0	120	na	2.0	0.0	0	19%
vanilla, 3 oz *(Good Humor)*	1 sandwich	191	3.7	31.1	155	(mq)	5.7	(mq)	(mq)	27%
vanilla, 2.5 oz *(Good Humor)*	1 sandwich	165	3.2	26.9	134	(mq)	4.9	(mq)	(mq)	27%
vanilla 'Sugar-freedom' *(Eskimo Pie)*	1 sandwich	170	4.0	26.0	142	na	6.0	na	na	31%
Stick novelties										
banana cream *(Natural Nectar)*	1 bar	170	3.0	22.0	70	na	8.0	na	20	42%
cocoa-fudge 'n' cream *(Natural Nectar)*	1 bar	170	3.0	22.0	70	na	8.0	na	20	42%
strawberries 'n cream *(Natural Nectar)*	1 bar	120	2.0	18.0	40	na	5.0	na	15	36%
wildberry cream *(Natural Nectar)*	1 bar	120	2.0	22.0	50	na	3.0	na	15	22%
ICE CREAM TOPPING. See individual toppings.										
ICE MILK										
CARAMEL NUT *(Light n' Lively)*	4 oz	120	3.0	18.0	85	(tr)	4.0	2.0	10	30%
CHOCOLATE										
(Breyers) 'Light'	4 oz	120	3.0	18.0	55	(tr)	4.0	2.0	15	30%
(Borden)	4 oz	100	3.0	18.0	80	0	2.0	(mq)	(mq)	18%
(Darigold) 'Lite'	4 oz	110	3.0	19.0	65	(tr)	3.0	(mq)	(mq)	24%
(Weight Watchers) 'Grand Collection'	4 oz	110	4.0	18.0	75	(tr)	3.0	2.0	10	24%
CHOCOLATE CHIP										
(Light n' Lively)	4 oz	120	3.0	18.0	35	0	4.0	3.0	10	30%
(Weight Watchers) 'Grand Collection'	4 oz	120	3.0	19.0	75	(tr)	4.0	2.0	10	29%
CHOCOLATE CHOCOLATE CHIP *(Breyers)* 'Light'	4 oz	140	4.0	20.0	55	na	5.0	na	25	32%
CHOCOLATE FUDGE TWIRL *(Breyers)* 'Light'	4 oz	130	4.0	21.0	60	(tr)	4.0	2.0	10	27%
CHOCOLATE SWIRL *(Weight Watchers)* 'Grand Collection'	4 oz	120	3.0	19.0	75	(tr)	3.0	2.0	5	24%
COFFEE *(Light n' Lively)*	4 oz	100	3.0	16.0	40	0	3.0	1.0	10	26%
COOKIES N' CREAM *(Light n' Lively)*	4 oz	110	3.0	18.0	65	0	3.0	2.0	10	24%
HEAVENLY HASH										
(Breyers) 'Light'	4 oz	150	3.0	21.0	55	(tr)	5.0	3.0	10	32%
(Light n' Lively)	4 oz	120	3.0	20.0	35	(tr)	4.0	2.0	10	28%
NEAPOLITAN *(Weight Watchers)* 'Grand Collection'	4 oz	110	3.0	18.0	75	(tr)	3.0	1.0	10	24%
PECAN PRALINES 'N CREME										
(Weight Watchers) 'Grand Collection'	4 oz	120	3.0	20.0	80	(tr)	4.0	3.0	10	28%
PRALINE ALMOND *(Breyers)* 'Light'	4 oz	130	3.0	19.0	70	(tr)	5.0	2.0	10	34%
STRAWBERRY										
(Borden)	4 oz	90	2.0	17.0	65	0	2.0	(mq)	(mq)	19%
(Breyers) 'Light'	4 oz	110	3.0	18.0	50	(tr)	3.0	2.0	15	24%
SWISS ALMOND FUDGE TWIRL *(Breyers)*	4 oz	150	4.0	21.0	65	na	6.0	3.0	na	35%
TOFFEE FUDGE PARFAIT *(Breyers)* 'Light'	4 oz	140	3.0	22.0	90	(tr)	5.0	3.0	10	31%
VANILLA										
(Borden)	4 oz	90	2.0	17.0	60	0	2.0	(mq)	(mq)	19%
(Breyers) 'Light'	4 oz	120	3.0	18.0	60	0	4.0	2.0	10	30%
(Darigold)	4 oz	110	2.0	18.0	00	0	3.0	(mq)	(mq)	25%
(Light n' Lively)	4 oz	100	3.0	16.0	40	0	3.0	2.0	10	26%
(Light n' Lively) w/chocolate covered almonds	4 oz	120	3.0	17.0	45	(tr)	4.0	1.0	10	31%
(Weight Watchers) 'Grand Collection'	4 oz	100	3.0	16.0	75	0	3.0	1.0	10	26%
VANILLA-CHOCOLATE-STRAWBERRY										
(Breyers) 'Light'	4 oz	120	3.0	18.0	55	(tr)	4.0	2.0	15	30%
(Light n' Lively)	4 oz	100	2.0	17.0	35	(tr)	3.0	2.0	10	26%
VANILLA-FUDGE TWIRL *(Light n' Lively)*	4 oz	110	3.0	18.0	45	0	3.0	2.0	10	24%

Food Name	Serving Size	Calories	Prot. gms	Carbs gms	Sod. mgs	Fiber gms	Fat gms	Sat. Fat gms	Chol. mgs	% Fat Cal.
VANILLA-RASPBERRY										
(Breyers) parfait 'Light'	4 oz	130	3.0	23.0	50	(tr)	3.0	2.0	15	21%
(Light n' Lively) swirl	4 oz	110	3.0	19.0	35	0	3.0	1.0	10	24%
ICE MILK BAR										
CHOCOLATE ALMOND CRUNCH (Weight Watchers)	1 bar	120	2.0	12.0	45	na	7.0	2.0	5	53%
CHOCOLATE FUDGE, DOUBLE (Light n' Lively) nonfat	1 bar	50	2.0	11.0	45	na	0.0	na	0	0%
CHOCOLATE MOUSSE (Light n' Lively) nonfat	1 bar	50	2.0	12.0	45	na	0.0	na	0	0%
CHOCOLATE W/FUDGE SWIRL (Sealtest) nonfat 'Free'	1 bar	80	3.0	19.0	55	na	0.0	na	0	0%
ORANGE VANILLA, (Light n' Lively) nonfat	1 bar	40	1.0	10.0	15	na	0.0	na	0	0%
PRALINE (Weight Watchers) 'Crispy Praline 'N Creme'	1 bar	120	2.0	13.0	45	na	6.0	2.0	5	47%
STRAWBERRY (Light n' Lively) nonfat	1 bar	80	2.0	12.0	25	na	0.0	na	0	0%
TOFFEE (Weight Watchers) 'English Toffee Crunch'	1 bar	120	2.0	11.0	60	na	8.0	na	5	58%
VANILLA										
(Light n' Lively) chocolate dipped	1 bar	110	2.0	14.0	35	na	6.0	na	0	46%
(Sealtest) w/fudge swirl, nonfat 'Free'	1 bar	80	2.0	18.0	55	na	0.0	na	0	0%
(Sealtest) w/strawberry swirl, nonfat 'Free'	1 bar	70	2.0	17.0	60	na	0.0	na	0	0%
ICED TEA. See TEA, ICED.										
IMBU. See JOBO.										
INDIAN DATE. See TAMARIND.										
INDIAN FRY BREAD. See BREAD.										
INFANT FORMULA. See BABY FOOD.										
IRISH MOSS. See SEAWEED.										
ITALIAN SEASONING (Schilling) 'Spice Blends'	1/4 tsp	1	<.1	0.1	<1	na	na	na	0	0%
ITALIAN STONE PINE NUT. See PINE NUT.										

J

Food Name	Serving Size	Calories	Prot. gms	Carbs gms	Sod. mgs	Fiber gms	Fat gms	Sat. Fat gms	Chol. mgs	% Fat Cal.
JACK BEAN. See FAVA BEAN.										
JACKFRUIT										
trimmed	1 oz	27	0.4	6.8	1	>.3 c	0.1	(tr)	0	3%
untrimmed	1 lb	119	1.9	30.5	3	>1.3 c	0.4	na	0	3%
JALAPEÑO. See PEPPER, JALAPEÑO.										
JAM. See also FRUIT SPREAD; JELLY; PRESERVES.										
(Bama) all flavors	2 tsp	30	0.0	8.0	5	(mq)	0.0	0.0	0	0%
(Estee) all flavors	1 tsp	2	0.0	0.0	10	(mq)	0.0	0.0	0	0%
(Featherweight), all flavors	1 tsp	4	0.0	1.0	0	(mq)	0.0	0.0	0	0%
(Kraft), all flavors	1 tsp	17	0.0	4.0	0	(mq)	0.0	0.0	0	0%
(S&W Nutradiet) all flavors	1 tsp	4	0.0	1.0	0	(mq)	0.0	0.0	0	0%
APRICOT										
(Finast)	2 tsp	35	0.0	9.0	1	(mq)	0.0	0.0	0	0%
(Smucker's) natural ingredients	1 tsp	18	0.0	4.0	0	na	0.0	0.0	na	0%
APRICOT-PINEAPPLE (Smucker's) natural ingredients	1 tsp	18	0.0	4.0	0	na	0.0	0.0	na	0%
BLACK RASPBERRY (Smucker's) natural ingredients	1 tsp	18	0.0	4.0	0	na	0.0	0.0	na	0%
BLACKBERRY										
(Finast)	2 tsp	16	0.0	4.0	5	(mq)	0.0	0.0	0	0%
(Smucker's) natural ingredients	1 tsp	18	0.0	4.0	0	na	0.0	0.0	na	0%
BLUEBERRY										
(Finast)	2 tsp	16	0.0	4.0	5	(mq)	0.0	0.0	0	0%
(Smucker's) natural ingredients	1 tsp	18	0.0	4.0	0	na	0.0	0.0	na	0%
BOYSENBERRY (Smucker's) natural ingredients	1 tsp	18	0.0	4.0	0	na	0.0	0.0	na	0%

Food Name	Serving Size	Calories	Prot. gms	Carbs gms	Sod. mgs	Fiber gms	Fat gms	Sat. Fat gms	Chol. mgs	% Fat Cal.
CHERRY										
(Finast)	2 tsp	25	0.0	9.0	5	(mq)	0.0	0.0	0	0%
(Smucker's) natural ingredients	1 tsp	18	0.0	4.0	0	na	0.0	0.0	na	0%
GRAPE										
(Finast) Concord or regular	2 tsp	35	0.0	9.0	5	(tr)	0.0	0.0	0	0%
(Polaner)	2 tsp	35	0.0	9.0	5	na	0.0	0.0	na	0%
(Smucker's) Concord, natural ingredients	1 tsp	18	0.0	4.0	0	na	0.0	0.0	na	0%
(Welch's)	2 tsp	35	0.0	9.0	5	0	0.0	0.0	0	0%
ORANGE MARMALADE (Polaner)	2 tsp	35	0.0	9.0	5	na	0.0	0.0	na	0%
PEACH										
(Finast)	2 tsp	35	0.0	9.0	1	(mq)	0.0	0.0	0	0%
(Smucker's) natural ingredients	1 tsp	18	0.0	4.0	0	na	0.0	0.0	na	0%
PINEAPPLE										
(Finast)	2 tsp	35	0.0	9.0	1	(mq)	0.0	0.0	0	0%
(Smucker's) natural ingredients	1 tsp	18	0.0	4.0	0	na	0.0	0.0	na	0%
PLUM (Smucker's) natural ingredients	1 tsp	18	0.0	4.0	0	na	0.0	0.0	na	0%
RASPBERRY										
(Finast)	2 tsp	35	0.0	9.0	3	(mq)	0.0	0.0	0	0%
(Smucker's) natural ingredients, seedless	1 tsp	18	0.0	4.0	0	na	0.0	0.0	na	0%
RASPBERRY-APPLE (Welch's)	2 tsp	35	0.0	9.0	5	0	0.0	0.0	0	0%
STRAWBERRY										
(Finast)	2 tsp	35	0.0	9.0	3	(mq)	0.0	0.0	0	0%
(Kraft) 'Reduced Calorie'	1 tsp	6	0.0	2.0	5	(mq)	0.0	0.0	0	0%
(Piedmont)	2 tsp	35	0.0	9.0	10	na	0.0	na	na	0%
(Smucker's) natural ingredients, seedless	1 tsp	18	0.0	4.0	0	na	0.0	0.0	na	0%
(Welch's)	2 tsp	35	0.0	9.0	5	0	0.0	0.0	0	0%
TOMATO (Smucker's) natural ingredients	1 tsp	18	0.0	4.0	0	na	0.0	0.0	na	0%
JAMAICAN BREADNUT. See BREADNUT TREE SEEDS.										
JAMBERRY, fresh (Frieda's)	3.5 oz	25	1.4	4.2	na	(mq)	0.5	na	0	17%
JAMBOLAN. See JAVA PLUM.										
JAPANESE MEDLAR. See LOQUAT.										
JAPANESE WHITE RADISH. See RADISH, ORIENTAL.										
JAVA PLUM / jambolan										
raw	1 cup	81	1.0	21.0	19	>.4 c	0.3	na	0	3%
raw	3 fruits	5	0.1	1.4	1	(mq)	0.0	na	0	0%
w/seeds	1 lb	222	2.7	57.2	50	>1.0 c	0.9	na	0	3%
w/o seeds	1 oz	17	0.2	4.4	4	>.1 c	0.1	(tr)	0	5%
JELLY. See also JAM; FRUIT SPREAD; PRESERVES.										
(Bama) and peanut butter, spread, all flavors	2 tbsp	150	3.0	20.0	75	(mq)	7.0	(mq)	0	41%
(Estee) all flavors	1 tsp	2	0.0	0.0	10	0	0.0	0.0	0	0%
(Featherweight) all flavors, except grape	1 tsp	4	0.0	1.0	0	0	0.0	0.0	0	0%
(Kraft) all flavors	1 tsp	17	0.0	4.0	0	0	0.0	0.0	0	0%
(Smucker's) 'Slenderella,' all flavors	1 tsp	7	0.0	2.0	0	0	0.0	0.0	0	0%
APPLE										
(Bama)	2 tsp	30	0.0	8.0	5	0	0.0	0.0	0	0%
(Finast)	2 tsp	35	0.0	9.0	2	0	0.0	0.0	0	0%
(Lucky Leaf)	1 oz	80	0.0	20.0	5	0	0.0	0.0	0	0%
(Musselman's)	1 oz	80	0.0	20.0	5	0	0.0	0.0	0	0%
(Polaner)	2 tsp	35	0.0	9.0	5	na	0.0	0.0	na	0%
(Smucker's) cinnamon-flavored, natural ingredients	1 tsp	18	0.0	4.0	0	na	0.0	0.0	na	0%
(Smucker's) mint-flavored, natural ingredients	1 tsp	18	0.0	4.0	0	na	0.0	0.0	na	0%
(Smucker's) natural ingredients	1 tsp	18	0.0	4.0	0	na	0.0	0.0	na	0%
APPLE-BLACKBERRY (Musselman's)	1 oz	80	0.0	19.0	0	0	0.0	0.0	0	0%
APPLE-CHERRY (Musselman's)	1 oz	80	0.0	19.0	5	0	0.0	0.0	0	0%

Food Name	Serving Size	Calories	Prot. gms	Carbs gms	Sod. mgs	Fiber gms	Fat gms	Sat. Fat gms	Chol. mgs	% Fat Cal.
APPLE-GRAPE										
(Musselman's)	1 oz	80	0.0	20.0	5	0	0.0	0.0	0	0%
(Welch's)	2 tsp	35	0.0	9.0	5	0	0.0	0.0	0	0%
APPLE-RASPBERRY (Musselman's)	1 oz	80	0.0	19.0	0	0	0.0	0.0	0	0%
APPLE-STRAWBERRY (Musselman's)	1 oz	80	0.0	20.0	5	0	0.0	0.0	0	0%
APRICOT-PINEAPPLE										
(Knott's Berry Farm) 'Light' w/NutraSweet	1 tsp	8	0.0	2.0	0	na	0.0	na	na	0%
BLACK RASPBERRY (Smucker's) natural ingredients	1 tsp	18	0.0	4.0	0	na	0.0	0.0	na	0%
BLACKBERRY										
(Bama)	2 tsp	30	0.0	8.0	5	0	0.0	0.0	0	0%
(Knott's Berry Farm) 'Light' w/NutraSweet	1 tsp	8	0.0	2.0	0	na	0.0	na	na	0%
(Smucker's) natural ingredients	1 tsp	18	0.0	4.0	0	na	0.0	0.0	na	0%
BOYSENBERRY (Knott's Berry Farm) 'Light' w/NutraSweet	1 tsp	8	0.0	2.0	0	na	0.0	na	na	0%
CHERRY (Smucker's) natural ingredients	1 tsp	18	0.0	4.0	0	na	0.0	0.0	na	0%
CRABAPPLE (Smucker's) natural ingredients	1 tsp	18	0.0	4.0	0	na	0.0	0.0	na	0%
CURRANT										
(Finast)	2 tsp	35	0.0	9.0	2	0	0.0	0.0	0	0%
(Polaner)	2 tsp	35	0.0	9.0	5	na	0.0	0.0	na	0%
(Smucker's) natural ingredients	1 tsp	18	0.0	4.0	0	na	0.0	0.0	na	0%
ELDERBERRY (Smucker's) natural ingredients	1 tsp	18	0.0	4.0	0	na	0.0	0.0	na	0%
GRAPE										
(Bama)	2 tsp	30	0.0	8.0	5	0	0.0	0.0	0	0%
(Featherweight)	1 tsp	4	0.0	1.0	5	0	0.0	0.0	0	0%
(Finast)	2 tsp	35	0.0	9.0	5	0	0.0	0.0	0	0%
(Kraft) 'Reduced Calorie'	1 tsp	6	0.0	2.0	5	0	0.0	0.0	0	0%
(Musselman's)	1 oz	80	0.0	20.0	0	0	0.0	0.0	0	0%
(Polaner)	2 tsp	35	0.0	9.0	5	na	0.0	0.0	na	0%
(Smucker's) Concord, natural ingredients	1 tsp	18	0.0	4.0	0	na	0.0	0.0	na	0%
(Welch's)	2 tsp	35	0.0	9.0	5	0	0.0	0.0	0	0%
GREEN PEPPER (Great Impressions)	1 tbsp	50	0.0	12.6	<1	na	0.0	0.0	0	0%
GUAVA (Smucker's) natural ingredients	1 tsp	18	0.0	4.0	0	na	0.0	0.0	na	0%
JALAPEÑO										
(Great Impressions)	1 tbsp	58	0.0	14.6	51	na	0.0	0.0	0	0%
(Knott's Berry Farm)	1 oz	70	0.0	18.0	0	na	0.0	na	na	0%
(Knott's Berry Farm)	1 tsp	18	0.0	4.0	0	na	0.0	na	na	0%
MINT										
(Finast)	2 tsp	35	0.0	9.0	2	0	0.0	0.0	0	0%
(Polaner)	2 tsp	35	0.0	9.0	5	na	0.0	0.0	na	0%
MIXED FRUIT (Smucker's) natural ingredients	1 tsp	18	0.0	4.0	0	na	0.0	0.0	chol.	0%
PLUM (Smucker's) natural ingredients	1 tsp	18	0.0	4.0	0	na	0.0	0.0	na	0%
QUINCE (Smucker's) natural ingredients	1 tsp	18	0.0	4.0	0	na	0.0	0.0	na	0%
RASPBERRY										
(Knott's Berry Farm) 'Light' w/NutraSweet	1 tsp	8	0.0	2.0	0	na	0.0	na	na	0%
(Polaner)	2 tsp	35	0.0	9.0	5	na	0.0	0.0	na	0%
(Smucker's) natural ingredients	1 tsp	18	0.0	4.0	0	na	0.0	0.0	na	0%
RED PEPPER (Great Impressions)	1 tbsp	50	0.0	12.6	9	na	0.0	0.0	0	0%
STRAWBERRY										
(Finast)	2 tsp	35	0.0	9.0	2	0	0.0	0.0	0	0%
(Knott's Berry Farm) 'Light' w/NutraSweet	1 tsp	8	0.0	2.0	0	na	0.0	na	na	0%
(Polaner)	2 tsp	35	0.0	9.0	5	na	0.0	0.0	na	0%
(Smucker's) natural ingredients	1 tsp	18	0.0	4.0	0	na	0.0	0.0	na	0%
STRAWBERRY-APPLE (Polaner)	2 tsp	35	0.0	9.0	5	na	0.0	0.0	na	0%

JERKY. See BEEF JERKY.

JERUSALEM ARTICHOKE. See ARTICHOKES, JERUSALEM.

Food Name	Serving Size	Calories	Prot. gms	Carbs gms	Sod. mgs	Fiber gms	Fat gms	Sat. Fat gms	Chol. mgs	% Fat Cal.
JEW'S EAR. See CHINESE FUNGUS.										
JICAMA / Chinese yam / fon goot yam / Mexican potato / sicama / yambean tuber										
boiled, drained	4 oz	52	1.3	11.8	7	>1.3 c	0.1	(tr)	0	2%
raw, trimmed	1 oz	12	0.4	2.5	2	>.2 c	0.1	(tr)	0	7%
raw, trimmed, sliced	1/2 cup	25	0.8	5.3	4	>.4 c	0.1	(tr)	0	4%
raw, untrimmed	1 lb	170	5.8	36.5	26	>2.9 c	0.3	na	0	2%
JOBO / hog plum / imbu / yellow mombin										
seeded	1 oz	20	0.2	3.9	na	>.3 c	0.6	na	0	25%
JUICE. See individual listings.										
JUJUBE, CHINESE										
dried	100 gm	287	3.7	73.6	9	>3.0 c	1.1	na	0	3%
dried	1 oz	81	1.0	20.1	3	>.9 c	0.3	(tr)	0	3%
raw	100 gm	79	1.2	20.2	3	>1.4 c	0.2	na	0	2%
raw	1 oz	22	0.3	5.7	1	>.4 c	0.1	(tr)	0	4%
raw, w/seeds	1 lb	331	5.1	85.3	11	>5.9 c	0.8	na	0	2%
JUNKET MIX										
CHOCOLATE										
mix only, dry	2-oz pkg	207	1.4	52.2	40	>.5 c	1.9	1.1	0	7%
mix only, dry	1 tbsp	33	0.2	8.2	6	>.1 c	0.3	0.2	0	7%
prepared (Junket)	1/2 cup	120	5.0	15.0	65	na	4.0	(mq)	(mq)	31%
prepared w/2% milk	1/2 cup	110	4.3	18.4	71	>.1 c	2.9	1.7	10	22%
prepared w/whole milk	1/2 cup	125	4.3	18.1	69	>.1 c	4.5	2.8	16	31%
STRAWBERRY OR RASPBERRY										
mix only, dry	1.5-oz pkg	165	0.0	42.6	3	0	0.0	0.0	0	0%
mix only, dry	1 tbsp	38	0.0	9.9	1	0	0.0	0.0	0	0%
prepared (Junket)	1/2 cup	120	4.0	16.0	60	na	4.0	(mq)	(mq)	na
prepared w/whole milk	1 cup	238	8.0	32.0	115	0	9.0	4.9	33	34%
VANILLA										
mix only, dry	1.5-oz pkg	165	0.0	42.6	3	0	0.0	na	0	0%
mix only, dry	1 tbsp	41	0.0	10.7	1	0	0.0	na	0	0%
prepared (Junket)	1/2 cup	120	4.0	16.0	60	na	4.0	(mq)	(mq)	31%
prepared w/2% milk	1/2 cup	101	4.1	16.4	61	0	2.4	1.5	9	21%
prepared w/whole milk	1/2 cup	116	4.0	16.2	61	0	4.1	2.5	17	31%
JUTE POTHERB										
boiled, drained	4 oz	42	4.2	8.3	12	>2.2 c	0.2	<.1	0	4%
raw, trimmed	1 oz	10	1.3	1.6	2	>.3 c	0.1	<.1	0	7%
raw, untrimmed	1 lb	96	13.1	16.3	23	>3.4 c	0.7	0.1	0	5%

K

Food Name	Serving Size	Calories	Prot. gms	Carbs gms	Sod. mgs	Fiber gms	Fat gms	Sat. Fat gms	Chol. mgs	% Fat Cal.
KALE / borecole / cole / colewort										
boiled, drained	4 oz	36	2.2	6.4	26	>.9 c	0.5	0.1	0	12%
boiled, drained, chopped	1 cup	42	2.5	7.3	30	2.6	0.5	0.1	0	10%
chopped (Dole)	1/2 cup	17	1.0	0.0	16	1.3	0.6	na	na	22%
raw, chopped	1 cup	33	2.2	6.7	29	1.3	0.5	0.1	0	11%
raw, trimmed	1 oz	14	0.9	2.8	12	>.4 c	0.2	<.1	0	11%
raw, untrimmed	1 lb	137	9.1	27.7	119	>4.2 c	1.9	0.3	0	10%
Canned, chopped (Allen's)	1/2 cup	25	2.0	3.0	15	(mq)	<1.0	na	0	<31%
Frozen										
boiled, drained	4 oz	34	3.2	5.9	17	>1.1 c	0.6	0.1	0	13%
boiled, drained, chopped	1 cup	39	3.7	6.8	20	>1.2 c	0.6	0.1	0	11%

Food Name	Serving Size	Calories	Prot. gms	Carbs gms	Sod. mgs	Fiber gms	Fat gms	Sat. Fat gms	Chol. mgs	% Fat Cal.
chopped *(Frosty Acres)*	3.3 oz	25	3.0	5.0	15	>1.0 c	0.0	0.0	0	0%
chopped *(Seabrook)*	3.3 oz	25	3.0	5.0	14	>1.0 c	0.0	0.0	0	0%
chopped *(Southern)*	3.5 oz	30	2.6	4.8	30	(mq)	0.5	(tr)	0	13%
unprepared, 10-oz pkg	3.3 oz	26	2.5	4.6	14	1.88	0.4	0.1	0	11%
KALE, SCOTCH										
boiled, drained	4 oz	32	2.2	6.4	51	>1.0 c	0.5	0.1	0	12%
boiled, drained, chopped	1 cup	36	2.5	7.3	58	>1.1 c	0.5	0.1	0	10%
raw, chopped	1 cup	28	1.9	5.6	47	>.8 c	0.4	0.1	0	11%
raw, trimmed	1 oz	12	0.8	2.4	20	>.3 c	0.2	<.1	0	12%
raw, untrimmed	1 lb	115	7.8	23.0	194	>3.4 c	1.7	0.2	0	11%
KANPYO/dried gourd strips										
	1 lb	1169	38.9	295.0	68	0	2.5	0.2	0	2%
	1 oz	73	2.4	18.4	4	0	0.2	(tr)	0	2%
	1/2 cup	70	2.3	17.6	4	>2.5 c	0.2	0.0	0	2%
KANTEN										
raw	1 lb	116	2.5	30.6	40	>2.0 c	0.1	<.1	0	1%
raw	1 oz	7	0.2	1.9	3	>.1 c	tr	tr	0	0%
KASHA. See BUCKWHEAT GROATS.										
KATSUO. See TUNA, SKIPJACK.										
KATURAY/sesbania flower										
raw, approx .1 oz	1 flower	1	<.1	0.2	tr	>.1 c	tr	(tr)	0	0%
raw, trimmed	1 cup	5	0.3	1.4	3	>.3 c	<.1	(tr)	0	<12%
raw, trimmed	1 oz	8	0.4	1.9	4	>.4 c	<.1	(tr)	0	<9%
raw, untrimmed	1 lb	106	4.9	25.9	59	>5.8 c	0.2	(tr)	0	1%
steamed	4 oz	25	1.3	5.9	12	>1.8 c	0.1	(tr)	0	3%
KAUAI PUNCH, organic *(Santa Cruz Natural)*	8 oz	120	<1.0	28.0	na	na	1.0	na	na	7%
KEFIR, CULTURED										
black cherry *(Alta•Dena)*	1 cup	200	9.0	24.0	120	na	9.0	na	na	38%
boysenberry *(Alta•Dena)*	1 cup	200	9.0	24.0	120	na	9.0	na	na	38%
peach *(Alta•Dena)*	1 cup	200	9.0	24.0	120	na	9.0	na	na	38%
red raspberry *(Alta•Dena)*	1 cup	200	9.0	24.0	120	na	9.0	na	na	38%
KELP. See SEAWEED.										
KETCHUP. See CATSUP.										
KIDNEY BEAN										
California red, mature										
boiled	4 oz	141	10.4	25.4	5	>2.7 c	0.1	<.1	0	1%
boiled	1/2 cup	109	8.0	19.7	4	>2.1 c	0.1	0.0	0	1%
raw	1/2 cup	304	22.4	55.0	10	22.91	0.2	0.0	0	1%
raw	1 oz	94	6.9	17.0	3	>1.8 c	0.1	<.1	0	1%
Red, mature										
boiled	1/2 cup	112	7.6	20.1	2	6.51	0.4	0.1	0	3%
boiled	4 oz	144	9.8	25.9	2	4.1	0.6	0.1	0	4%
boiled *(A&P)*	1 cup	230	17.0	41.0	5	(mq)	1.0	na	0	4%
raw	1/2 cup	310	20.7	56.4	11	14.0	1.0	0.1	0	3%
raw	1 oz	96	6.4	17.4	3	2.9	0.1	<.1	0	1%
raw *(Arrowhead Mills)*	2 oz	190	13.0	35.0	3	11.7	1.0	na	0	5%
Royal red, mature										
boiled	4 oz	139	10.8	24.8	6	>2.6 c	0.2	<.1	0	1%
boiled	1/2 cup	108	8.4	19.2	4	>2.0 c	0.2	0.0	0	2%
raw	1/2 cup	303	23.3	53.7	12	>5.7 c	0.4	0.1	0	1%
raw	1 oz	93	7.2	16.5	4	>1.7 c	0.1	<.1	0	1%
Sprouted, mature										
boiled, drained	4 oz	37	5.5	5.4	(mq)	(mq)	0.7	0.1	0	13%
raw	1 lb	132	19.1	18.6	(mq)	(mq)	2.3	0.3	0	12%

Food Name	Serving Size	Calories	Prot. gms	Carbs gms	Sod. mgs	Fiber gms	Fat gms	Sat. Fat gms	Chol. mgs	% Fat Cal.
raw	1 cup	53	7.7	7.5	11	>1.4 c	0.9	0.1	0	12%
raw	1 oz	8	1.2	1.2	(mq)	(mq)	0.1	<.1	0	9%
KIDNEY BEAN, CANNED										
Dark red										
(Allens)	1/2 cup	105	5.0	20.0	290	(mq)	<1.0	(tr)	0	<8%
(Bush's Best)	1/2 cup	70	6.0	17.0	300	6.0	0.0	na	na	0%
(Finast)	1/2 cup	110	6.0	20.0	350	(mq)	2.0	na	0	15%
(Green Giant)	1/2 cup	90	7.0	20.0	330	5.0	<1.0	0.0	0	<8%
(Green Giant) 50% less salt	1/2 cup	90	7.0	20.0	165	5.0	<1.0	0.0	0	<8%
(Joan of Arc)	1/2 cup	90	7.0	20.0	330	5.0	<1.0	0.0	0	<8%
(Joan of Arc) 50% less salt	1/2 cup	90	7.0	20.0	165	5.0	<1.0	0.0	0	<8%
(Pathmark)	1/2 cup	110	8.0	18.0	370	(mq)	0.0	0.0	0	0%
(S&W) 50% less salt 'Lite'	1/2 cup	120	7.0	22.0	355	(mq)	1.0	(tr)	0	7%
(S&W) 'Premium'	1/2 cup	120	6.0	22.0	596	(mq)	1.0	(tr)	0	7%
(Stokely)	1/2 cup	110	7.0	20.0	360	(mq)	1.0	(tr)	0	8%
(Van Camp's)	1 cup	182	11.7	35.0	830	(mq)	0.5	(tr)	0	2%
Light red										
(Allens)	1/2 cup	105	5.0	2.0	290	(mq)	<1.0	(tr)	0	<24%
(Bush's Best)	1/2 cup	70	6.0	17.0	300	6.0	0.0	na	na	0%
(Finast)	1/2 cup	110	6.0	20.0	350	(mq)	2.0	na	0	15%
(Green Giant)	1/2 cup	90	7.0	20.0	330	5.0	<1.0	0.0	0	<8%
(Green Giant) 50% less salt	1/2 cup	90	7.0	20.0	165	5.0	<1.0	0.0	0	<8%
(Joan of Arc)	1/2 cup	90	7.0	20.0	330	5.0	<1.0	0.0	0	<8%
(Joan of Arc) 50% less salt	1/2 cup	90	7.0	20.0	165	5.0	<1.0	0.0	0	<8%
(Stokely)	1/2 cup	110	7.0	20.0	360	(mq)	1.0	(tr)	0	8%
(Van Camp's)	1 cup	184	11.5	36.0	650	(mq)	0.5	(tr)	0	2%
Red										
(A&P)	1/2 cup	110	7.0	20.0	440	(mq)	<1.0	(tr)	0	<8%
(B&M) baked	8 oz	250	15.0	42.0	640	11.0	7.0	(mq)	5	22%
(Eden Foods) organic, very low sodium, no salt added	1/2 cup	60	8.0	18.0	20	10.0	<1.0	na	0	<8%
(Friends) baked	8 oz	340	17.0	57.0	1060	11.0	4.0	2.0	4	11%
(Friends) baked, w/pork	8 oz	270	14.0	55.0	990	11.0	4.0	na	4	12%
(Green Giant)	1/2 cup	90	7.0	20.0	250	5.9	0.0	0.0	0	0%
(Hunt's)	4 oz	120	7.0	21.0	400	(mq)	0.0	0.0	0	0%
(Joan of Arc)	1/2 cup	90	7.0	20.0	250	5.9	0.0	0.0	0	0%
(Pathmark)	1/2 cup	110	8.0	18.0	370	(mq)	0.0	0.0	0	0%
(Progresso)	1/2 cup	100	9.0	21.0	210	7.0	<1.0	(tr)	0	<7%
(S&W) 50% less salt 'Lite'	1/2 cup	120	7.0	22.0	355	(mq)	1.0	(tr)	0	7%
(S&W) 'Premium'	1/2 cup	120	6.0	22.0	596	(mq)	1.0	(tr)	0	7%
(S&W Nutradiet)	1/2 cup	90	7.0	16.0	1	(mq)	1.0	(tr)	0	9%
(Stokely)	1/2 cup	110	7.0	20.0	360	(mq)	1.0	(tr)	0	8%
(Van Camp's)	1 cup	184	11.5	36.0	650	(mq)	0.5	(tr)	0	2%
(Van Camp's) 'New Orleans Style'	1 cup	178	12.1	34.0	940	(mq)	0.6	(tr)	na	3%
KIELBASA / kolbassy										
'Bun Size' (Hillshire Farm)	2 oz	180	8.0	2.0	570	0	16.0	(mq)	(mq)	78%
'Kolbase' (Hormel)	3 oz	220	12.0	1.0	904	0	19.0	(mq)	(mq)	77%
'Lean Supreme Polska' (Eckrich)	1 oz	72	4.0	1.0	224	0	6.0	(mq)	(mq)	73%
'Polska Flavorseal' (Hillshire Farm)	2 oz	190	8.0	2.0	540	0	17.0	(mq)	(mq)	79%
'Polska Flavorseal' beef (Hillshire Farm)	2 oz	190	7.0	1.0	550	0	17.0	(mq)	(mq)	83%
'Polska Flavorseal Lite' (Hillshire Farm)	2 oz	160	8.0	2.0	(mq)	0	13.0	(mq)	(mq)	75%
'Polska Flavorseal' mild (Hillshire Farm)	2 oz	190	7.0	2.0	530	0	17.0	(mq)	(mq)	81%
'Polska Links' (Hillshire Farm)	2 oz	190	7.0	2.0	530	0	17.0	(mq)	(mq)	81%
'Polska' skinless (Eckrich)	1 link	180	7.0	2.0	420	0	16.0	(mq)	(mq)	80%
skinless (Hormel)	1/2 link	180	12.0	1.0	826	0	14.0	(mq)	(mq)	71%

Food Name	Serving Size	Calories	Prot. gms	Carbs gms	Sod. mgs	Fiber gms	Fat gms	Sat. Fat gms	Chol. mgs	% Fat Cal.
KIWI FRUIT/Chinese gooseberry										
fresh, raw, w/o skin	1 large	56	0.9	13.5	5	3.1	0.4	na	0	6%
fresh, raw, w/o skin	1 med	46	0.8	11.3	4	2.6	0.3	na	0	6%
trimmed	1 oz	17	0.3	4.2	1	1.0	0.1	(tr)	0	6%
untrimmed (Dole)	2 fruit	90	1.0	18.0	0	4.0	1.0	na	na	6%
w/skin	1 lb	237	3.9	58.1	18	13.3	1.7	na	0	6%
KIWI NECTAR (Knudsen & Sons)	8 oz	60	<1.0	14.0	na	na	0.0	na	na	0%
KNACKWURST										
	4-inch link	209	8.1	1.2	687	0	18.9	6.9	39	82%
	1 oz	87	3.4	0.5	286	0	7.9	2.9	16	82%
beef (Hebrew National)	3-oz link	263	10.2	<1.0	877	0	25.0	(mq)	26	83%
'Links' (Hillshire Farm)	2 oz	180	7.0	1.0	460	0	16.0	(mq)	(mq)	82%
KOHLRABI/cabbage turnip										
boiled, drained	4 oz	33	2.0	7.6	24	>1.2 c	0.1	<.1	0	2%
boiled, drained, sliced	1/2 cup	24	1.5	5.5	17	.9	0.1	0.0	0	3%
raw, sliced	1/2 cup	19	1.2	4.3	14	2.52	0.1	0.0	0	4%
raw, trimmed	1 oz	8	0.5	1.8	6	.3	<.1	tr	0	<9%
raw, untrimmed	1 lb	57	3.6	12.9	42	2.3	0.2	<.1	0	3%
KOLBASSY. See KIELBASA										
KOOL-AID. See individual flavors.										
KOYADOFU. See TOFU.										
KUMQUAT										
raw, trimmed	1 fruit	12	0.2	3.1	1	>.7 c	0.0	na	0	0%
w/seeds	1 lb	266	3.8	69.3	25	>15.6 c	0.4	na	0	1%

L

Food Name	Serving Size	Calories	Prot. gms	Carbs gms	Sod. mgs	Fiber gms	Fat gms	Sat. Fat gms	Chol. mgs	% Fat Cal.
LAMB, DOMESTIC										
(NOTE: All USDA choice grade. TRIMMED = Lean; separable fat removed. UNTRIMMED = Separable fat not removed.)										
BRAINS										
braised	3 oz	123	10.7	0.0	114	0	8.6	2.2	1737	64%
braised, yield from 1 lb raw	12.25 oz	503	43.5	0.0	465	0	35.3	9.0	7089	65%
pan-fried	3 oz	232	14.4	0.0	133	0	18.9	4.8	2128	75%
raw	4 oz	138	11.8	0.0	127	0	9.7	2.5	1533	65%
COMPOSITE CUTS/LEG AND SHOULDER										
Trimmed										
braised, cubes	3 oz	190	28.6	0.0	59	0	7.5	2.7	92	37%
broiled, cubes	3 oz	158	23.9	0.0	65	0	6.2	2.2	77	37%
broiled, ground	3 oz	241	21.0	0.0	69	na	16.7	6.9	82	64%
raw, cubes	1 lb	608	91.7	0.0	295	0	24.0	8.6	295	37%
raw, cubes	1 oz	38	5.7	0.0	18	0	1.5	0.5	18	37%
raw, ground	1 lb	1279	75.1	0.0	268	na	106.2	46.2	331	76%
raw, ground	1 oz	79	4.6	0.0	17	na	6.6	2.8	20	76%
stewed, cubes	4 oz	253	38.2	0.0	79	0	10.0	3.6	122	37%
HEART										
braised	3 oz	157	21.2	1.6	54	0	6.7	2.7	212	40%
raw	4 oz	138	18.7	0.2	101	0	6.4	2.5	153	43%
simmered	4 oz	210	28.3	2.2	71	0	9.0	3.6	282	40%
KIDNEYS										
braised	3 oz	116	20.1	0.8	128	0	3.1	1.0	480	25%
raw	4 oz	110	17.8	0.9	177	0	3.3	1.1	382	28%

Food Name	Serving Size	Calories	Prot. gms	Carbs gms	Sod. mgs	Fiber gms	Fat gms	Sat. Fat gms	Chol. mgs	% Fat Cal.
LEG/FORESHANK										
Trimmed										
braised	3 oz	159	26.4	0.0	63	0	5.1	1.8	88	30%
braised	1 oz	53	8.8	0.0	21	0	1.7	0.6	29	30%
braised, diced	1 cup	262	43.4	0.0	104	0	8.4	3.0	146	30%
broiled, ground	1 cup	328	28.7	0.0	94	0	23.1	9.4	113	64%
broiled, ground	4 oz	321	28.1	0.0	92	0	22.3	9.2	110	64%
raw	1 lb	544	95.6	0.0	358	0	14.9	5.3	313	26%
raw	1 oz	34	5.9	0.0	22	0	0.9	0.3	19	26%
raw, ground	1 cup	637	37.4	0.0	133	0	52.9	23.0	165	76%
stewed	4 oz	212	35.2	0.0	84	0	6.8	2.4	118	30%
stewed	1 oz	53	8.8	0.0	21	0	1.7	0.6	29	30%
stewed, diced	1 cup	262	43.4	0.0	104	0	8.4	3.0	146	30%
Untrimmed										
braised	3 oz	207	24.1	0.0	61	0	11.4	4.8	90	52%
braised	1 oz	69	8.0	0.0	20	0	3.8	1.6	30	52%
braised, diced	1 cup	340	39.7	0.0	101	0	18.8	7.9	148	52%
raw	1 lb	912	85.8	0.0	327	0	60.7	26.4	327	61%
raw	1 oz	56	5.3	0.0	20	0	3.8	1.6	20	62%
stewed	1 oz	69	8.0	0.0	20	0	3.8	1.6	30	52%
stewed, diced	1 cup	340	39.7	0.0	101	0	18.8	7.9	148	52%
LEG/SHANK										
Trimmed										
raw	1 lb	567	93.1	0.0	277	0	19.0	6.8	290	32%
raw	1 oz	35	5.8	0.0	17	0	1.2	0.4	18	32%
roasted	3 oz	153	23.9	0.0	56	0	5.7	2.0	74	35%
roasted	1 oz	51	8.0	0.0	19	0	1.9	0.7	25	35%
roasted, diced	1 cup	252	39.4	0.0	92	0	9.3	3.3	122	35%
Untrimmed										
raw	1 lb	912	84.3	0.0	259	0	61.2	26.3	304	62%
raw	1 oz	56	5.2	0.0	16	0	3.8	1.6	19	62%
roasted	3 oz	191	22.5	0.0	55	0	10.6	4.3	77	52%
roasted	1 oz	64	7.5	0.0	18	0	3.5	1.4	26	51%
roasted, diced	1 cup	315	37.0	0.0	91	0	17.4	7.1	126	51%
LEG/SIRLOIN										
Trimmed										
raw	1 lb	608	93.2	0.0	290	0	23.0	8.3	299	36%
raw	1 oz	38	5.8	0.0	18	0	1.4	0.5	18	35%
roasted	3 oz	173	24.1	0.0	60	0	7.8	2.8	78	42%
roasted	1 oz	58	8.0	0.0	20	0	2.6	0.9	26	42%
roasted, diced	1 cup	286	39.7	0.0	99	0	12.8	4.6	129	42%
Untrimmed										
raw	1 lb	1234	76.8	0.0	254	0	100.3	44.1	327	75%
raw	1 oz	76	4.7	0.0	16	0	6.2	2.7	20	75%
roasted	3 oz	248	20.9	0.0	58	0	17.6	7.4	82	66%
roasted	1 oz	83	7.0	0.0	19	0	5.9	2.5	27	66%
roasted, diced	1 cup	409	34.5	0.0	95	0	28.9	12.2	136	65%
LEG/WHOLE										
Trimmed										
raw	1 lb	581	93.3	0.0	281	0	20.5	7.3	290	33%
raw	1 oz	36	5.8	0.0	17	0	1.3	0.5	18	34%
roasted	3 oz	162	24.1	0.0	58	0	6.6	2.3	76	38%
roasted	1 oz	54	8.0	0.0	19	0	2.2	0.8	25	38%
roasted, diced	1 cup	267	39.6	0.0	95	0	10.8	3.9	125	30%

Food Name	Serving Size	Calories	Prot. gms	Carbs gms	Sod. mgs	Fiber gms	Fat gms	Sat. Fat gms	Chol. mgs	% Fat Cal.
Untrimmed										
raw	1 lb	1043	81.2	0.0	254	0	77.4	33.7	313	68%
raw	1 oz	64	5.0	0.0	16	0	4.8	2.1	19	68%
roasted	3 oz	219	21.7	0.0	56	0	14.0	5.9	79	59%
roasted	1 oz	73	7.2	0.0	19	0	4.7	2.0	26	60%
roasted, diced	1 cup	361	35.8	0.0	92	0	23.0	9.6	130	59%
LIVER										
braised	3 oz	187	26.0	2.2	48	na	7.5	2.9	426	37%
pan-fried	3 oz	202	21.7	3.2	105	na	10.8	4.2	419	49%
raw	4 oz	158	23.1	2.0	79	na	5.7	2.2	421	34%
LOIN										
Trimmed										
broiled	3 oz	184	25.5	0.0	71	0	8.3	3.0	81	42%
raw	1 oz	40	5.8	0.0	19	0	1.7	0.6	18	40%
roasted	3 oz	172	22.6	0.0	56	0	8.3	3.2	74	45%
Untrimmed										
broiled	3 oz	269	21.4	0.0	65	0	19.6	8.4	85	67%
roasted	3 oz	263	19.2	0.0	54	0	20.0	8.7	81	70%
LUNGS										
braised	3 oz	96	16.9	0.0	71	0	2.6	0.9	241	26%
raw	4 oz	108	18.9	0.0	178	0	3.0	1.0	na	20%
PANCREAS										
braised	3 oz	199	19.4	0.0	44	0	12.8	5.8	340	60%
raw	4 oz	172	16.8	0.0	85	0	11.1	5.0	295	60%
RIB										
Trimmed										
broiled	3 oz	200	23.6	0.0	72	0	11.0	4.0	77	51%
raw	1 lb	767	90.6	0.0	327	0	41.9	15.0	299	51%
raw	1 oz	47	5.6	0.0	20	0	2.6	0.9	18	51%
roasted	3 oz	197	22.2	0.0	69	0	11.3	4.1	75	53%
Untrimmed										
broiled	3 oz	307	18.8	0.0	65	0	25.1	10.8	84	75%
raw	1 lb	1687	65.9	0.0	254	0	156.0	68.8	345	84%
raw	1 oz	104	4.1	0.0	16	0	9.6	4.2	21	84%
roasted	3 oz	305	18.0	0.0	62	0	25.3	10.9	82	76%
SHOULDER/ARM										
Trimmed										
braised	3 oz	237	30.2	0.0	65	0	12.0	4.3	103	47%
broiled	3 oz	170	23.5	0.0	70	0	7.7	2.9	78	42%
raw	1 oz	37	5.6	0.0	19	0	1.5	0.5	18	38%
roasted	3 oz	163	21.6	0.0	57	0	7.9	3.0	73	45%
Untrimmed										
braised	3 oz	294	25.8	0.0	61	0	20.4	8.4	102	64%
broiled	3 oz	239	20.8	0.0	65	0	16.6	7.1	82	64%
raw	1 oz	73	4.7	0.0	17	0	5.8	2.6	20	74%
roasted	3 oz	237	19.1	0.0	55	0	17.2	7.4	78	67%
SHOULDER/BLADE										
Trimmed										
braised	1 oz	81	9.1	0.0	22	0	4.7	1.8	33	54%
broiled	3 oz	179	21.7	0.0	75	0	9.6	3.4	77	50%
raw	3 oz	128	16.4	0.0	59	0	6.5	2.3	57	47%
roasted	3 oz	178	20.9	0.0	58	0	9.8	3.7	74	51%
Untrimmed										
braised	3 oz	293	24.2	0.0	64	0	21.0	8.8	99	66%

Food Name	Serving Size	Calories	Prot. gms	Carbs gms	Sod. mgs	Fiber gms	Fat gms	Sat. Fat gms	Chol. mgs	% Fat Cal.
broiled	3 oz	236	19.6	0.0	70	0	17.0	6.9	81	66%
raw	1 lb	1175	75.4	0.0	281	0	94.6	40.5	327	74%
raw	1 oz	73	4.7	0.0	17	0	5.8	2.5	20	74%
roasted	3 oz	239	18.9	0.0	56	0	17.5	7.3	78	68%
SHOULDER/WHOLE										
Trimmed										
braised	4 oz	321	37.2	0.0	90	0	10.0	7.0	133	38%
braised, diced	1 cup	396	45.9	0.0	111	0	22.2	8.6	164	52%
broiled	4 oz	238	30.8	0.0	94	0	11.9	4.4	105	47%
roasted	4 oz	231	28.3	0.0	77	0	12.2	4.6	99	49%
roasted, diced	1 cup	286	34.9	0.0	95	0	15.1	5.7	122	49%
stewed	4 oz	321	37.2	0.0	90	0	10.0	7.0	133	38%
stewed, diced	1 cup	396	45.9	0.0	111	0	22.2	8.6	164	52%
Untrimmed										
braised, diced	1 cup	482	40.2	0.0	105	0	34.4	14.5	162	66%
broiled	4 oz	315	27.7	0.0	88	0	21.8	9.1	110	64%
broiled, diced	1 cup	389	34.2	0.0	109	0	27.0	11.3	136	64%
roasted	4 oz	313	25.5	0.0	75	0	22.6	9.6	104	67%
roasted, diced	1 cup	386	31.5	0.0	92	0	28.0	11.8	129	67%
stewed	4 oz	390	32.5	0.0	85	0	27.8	11.7	132	66%
stewed, diced	1 cup	482	40.2	0.0	105	0	34.4	14.5	162	66%
SPLEEN										
braised	3 oz	133	22.5	0.0	49	0	4.1	1.3	327	29%
raw	4 oz	115	19.5	0.0	95	0	3.5	1.2	283	29%
TONGUE										
braised	3 oz	234	18.3	0.0	57	0	17.2	6.7	161	68%
raw	4 oz	252	17.8	0.0	88	0	19.5	7.5	177	71%
LAMB, NEW ZEALAND, FROZEN										
COMPOSITE CUTS										
Trimmed										
cooked	4 oz	234	33.6	0.0	57	0	10.0	4.4	124	40%
raw	1 oz	36	5.9	0.0	13	0	1.3	0.5	21	33%
Untrimmed										
raw	1 oz	182	2.0	0.0	6	0	19.2	10.0	25	96%
LEG/FORESHANK										
Trimmed										
braised	3 oz	158	26.1	0.0	42	0	5.1	2.2	86	31%
braised, diced	1 cup	260	43.1	0.0	69	0	8.5	3.7	141	31%
raw	1 lb	535	94.4	0.0	227	0	14.9	6.3	304	26%
raw	1 oz	33	5.8	0.0	14	0	0.9	0.4	19	26%
stewed	4 oz	211	34.9	0.0	56	0	6.8	3.0	115	31%
stewed, diced	1 cup	260	43.1	0.0	69	0	8.5	3.7	141	31%
Untrimmed										
braised	3 oz	219	22.9	0.0	40	0	13.5	6.7	87	57%
braised, diced	1 cup	361	37.8	0.0	66	0	22.2	10.9	143	57%
raw	1 lb	1012	81.8	0.0	204	0	73.3	37.1	322	67%
raw	1 oz	62	5.1	0.0	13	0	4.5	2.3	20	67%
stewed	4 oz	293	30.6	0.0	53	0	18.0	8.9	116	57%
stewed, diced	1 cup	361	37.8	0.0	66	0	22.2	10.9	143	57%
LEG/WHOLE										
Trimmed										
raw	1 lb	558	94.6	0.0	200	0	17.2	7.3	331	29%
raw	1 oz	34	5.8	0.0	12	0	1.1	0.5	20	30%
roasted	3 oz	154	23.5	0.0	38	0	6.0	2.6	85	37%

Food Name	Serving Size	Calories	Prot. gms	Carbs gms	Sod. mgs	Fiber gms	Fat gms	Sat. Fat gms	Chol. mgs	% Fat Cal.
roasted, diced	1 cup	253	38.8	0.0	63	0	9.8	4.3	140	36%
Untrimmed										
raw	1 lb	980	83.2	0.0	181	0	69.4	34.8	345	65%
raw	1 oz	60	5.1	0.0	11	0	4.3	2.2	21	66%
roasted	3 oz	209	21.1	0.0	37	0	13.2	6.5	86	59%
roasted, diced	1 cup	344	34.7	0.0	60	0	21.8	10.7	141	59%
LOIN										
Trimmed										
broiled	4 oz	226	33.2	0.0	62	0	9.3	4.1	129	39%
raw	1 oz	36	5.9	0.0	13	0	1.2	0.5	22	31%
roasted	3 oz	169	24.9	0.0	47	0	7.0	3.0	97	39%
Untrimmed										
broiled	3 oz	268	19.9	0.0	42	0	20.3	10.2	95	70%
raw	1 oz	85	4.6	0.0	10	0	7.3	3.7	23	78%
RIB										
Trimmed										
raw	1 lb	644	92.9	0.0	236	0	27.5	11.7	345	40%
raw	1 oz	40	5.7	0.0	15	0	1.7	0.7	21	40%
roasted	3 oz	167	20.8	0.0	41	0	8.6	3.8	80	48%
Untrimmed										
raw	1 lb	1569	67.7	0.0	181	0	142.0	72.5	367	83%
raw	1 oz	97	4.2	0.0	11	0	8.8	4.5	23	83%
roasted	3 oz	289	16.1	0.0	37	0	24.4	12.3	85	77%
SHOULDER/WHOLE										
Trimmed										
braised	3 oz	242	29.0	0.0	48	0	13.2	5.8	108	51%
braised, diced	1 cup	399	47.7	0.0	78	0	21.7	9.5	178	51%
raw	1 lb	612	91.8	0.0	213	0	24.6	10.5	322	38%
raw	1 oz	38	5.8	0.0	13	0	1.5	0.7	20	37%
stewed	6.5 oz	522	62.3	0.0	103	0	28.3	12.5	232	51%
stewed, diced	1 cup	399	47.7	0.0	78	0	21.7	9.5	178	51%
Untrimmed										
braised	3 oz	303	24.0	0.0	43	0	22.3	10.8	105	68%
braised, diced	1 cup	491	40.2	0.0	73	0	35.5	17.1	172	67%
raw	1 lb	1234	75.5	0.0	186	0	100.8	50.9	340	75%
stewed	4 oz	398	32.5	0.0	59	0	28.8	13.9	139	67%
stewed, diced	1 cup	491	40.2	0.0	73	0	35.5	17.1	172	67%
LAMB'S-QUARTER										
boiled, drained	4 oz	36	3.6	5.7	(mq)	>2.0 c	0.8	0.1	0	16%
boiled, drained, chopped	1 cup	58	5.8	9.0	52	>3.2 c	1.3	0.1	0	17%
raw	100 gm	43	4.2	7.3	43	>4.0	0.8	0.1	0	14%
raw, trimmed	1 lb	195	19.1	33.1	(mq)	>9.5 c	3.6	0.3	0	13%
raw, trimmed	1 oz	12	1.2	2.1	(mq)	>.6 c	0.2	<.1	0	12%
LARD										
pork, fresh	1 cup	1849	0.0	0.0	0	0	205.0	80.4	195	100%
pork, fresh	1 tbsp	115	0.0	0.0	0	0	12.8	5.0	12	100%
pork leaf, fresh	1 oz	243	0.5	0.0	1	0	26.7	12.8	31	99%
LASAGNA ENTRÉE, FROZEN										
(Banquet) 'Extra Helping'	16.5 oz	645	24.0	88.0	1582	(mq)	23.0	(mq)	38	32%
(Celentano)	10 oz	460	24.0	40.0	870	(mq)	24.0	(mq)	(mq)	46%
(Celentano)	8 oz	370	19.0	32.0	700	(mq)	19.0	(mq)	(mq)	46%
(Celentano)	6.25 oz	230	13.0	22.0	600	(mq)	14.0	(mq)	(mq)	47%
(Chef Boyardee)	5.97 oz	280	15.0	42.0	900	(mq)	8.0	(mq)	(mq)	24%
(Green Giant) 'Entrées'	12 oz	490	33.0	44.0	1660	(mq)	20.0	(mq)	(mq)	37%

Food Name	Serving Size	Calories	Prot. gms	Carbs gms	Sod. mgs	Fiber gms	Fat gms	Sat. Fat gms	Chol. mgs	% Fat Cal.
(Stouffer's) 96-oz tray	9.75 oz	400	30.0	37.0	940	na	14.0	na	na	32%
(Stouffer's) 21-oz pkg	10.5 oz	360	28.0	33.0	1020	na	13.0	(mq)	na	32%
(Stouffer's) 10-oz pkg	10 oz	340	18.0	40.0	840	na	12.0	na	na	32%
(Tyson) 'Gourmet Selection'	11.5 oz	380	20.0	47.0	840	(mq)	14.0	(mq)	(mq)	32%
(Weight Watchers)	10.25 oz	270	24.0	29.0	510	na	6.0	2.0	5	20%
CHEESE										
(Budget Gourmet) three cheese	10 oz	400	22.0	38.0	760	(mq)	17.0	(mq)	65	39%
(Dining Lite)	9 oz	260	14.0	36.0	800	(mq)	6.0	(mq)	30	21%
(Lean Cuisine) casserole 'Lunch Express'	9.5 oz	290	17.0	42.0	560	na	6.0	2.0	10	19%
(Weight Watchers) Italian	11 oz	290	28.0	29.0	510	na	7.0	2.0	20	22%
FLORENTINE (Smart Ones) w/spinach cheese	11 oz	220	18.0	34.0	460	na	1.0	<1.0	10	4%
IN SAUCE (Buitoni) 'Family Style'	7.3 oz	370	13.0	30.0	940	(mq)	13.0	7.0	55	41%
LOW FAT (Celentano) 'Great Choice'	10 oz	260	18.0	42.0	650	na	2.0	na	na	7%
MEAT (Buitoni) 'Single Serving'	9 oz	580	23.0	57.0	820	(mq)	19.0	12.0	110	35%
PRIMAVERA (Celentano)	11 oz	330	18.0	34.0	470	(mq)	14.0	(mq)	na	38%
SAUSAGE (Budget Gourmet) Italian	10 oz	420	20.0	38.0	950	(mq)	20.0	(mq)	80	44%
SEAFOOD (Mrs. Paul's) seafood 'Light'	9.5 oz	290	14.0	39.0	750	(mq)	8.0	3.0	57	25%
TOFU										
(Amy's Kitchen) vegetable, organic	9.5 oz	310	14.0	36.0	500	4.0	10.0	na	0	31%
(Legume) and sauce 'Classic'	8 oz	210	15.0	20.0	410	8.2	8.0	1.3	0	34%
TUNA (Lean Cuisine) w/spinach noodles	9.75 oz	240	16.0	29.0	520	na	7.0	2.0	20	26%
VEGETABLE										
(Amy's Kitchen) organic	9.5 oz	310	20.0	36.0	470	3.0	8.5	na	26	26%
(Le Menu) garden 'Light Style'	10.5 oz	260	11.0	35.0	500	(mq)	8.0	3.0	25	28%
(Legume) w/tofu and sauce	12 oz	240	14.0	26.0	520	5.8	8.0	1.7	0	31%
(Stouffer's)	10.5 oz	430	20.0	35.0	820	na	23.0	na	na	49%
(Stouffer's) 96-oz tray	9.5 oz	400	23.0	33.0	760	na	20.0	na	na	45%
(Weight Watchers) garden 'Lowfat'	11 oz	260	19.0	30.0	430	na	7.0	2.0	15	24%
W/MEAT SAUCE										
(Banquet) 'Family Entrees'	7 oz	270	15.0	30.0	(mq)	(mq)	10.0	(mq)	(mq)	33%
(Dining Lite)	9 oz	240	13.0	36.0	800	(mq)	5.0	(mq)	25	19%
(Freezer Queen) 'Deluxe Family Suppers'	7 oz	200	8.0	28.0	730	(mq)	6.0	(mq)	(mq)	27%
(Healthy Choice)	10 oz	260	18.0	37.0	420	na	5.0	2.0	20	17%
(Le Menu) 'LightStyle'	10 oz	290	19.0	36.0	510	(mq)	8.0	(mq)	30	25%
(Lean Cuisine)	10.25 oz	280	20.0	36.0	560	na	6.0	3.0	25	19%
(Swanson) 'Homestyle Recipe'	10.5 oz	400	26.0	39.0	1070	(mq)	15.0	(mq)	(mq)	34%
ZUCCHINI										
(Healthy Choice)	11.5 oz	250	14.0	41.0	400	na	3.0	2.0	15	11%
(Lean Cuisine)	11 oz	260	17.0	34.0	520	na	6.0	2.0	20	21%
LASAGNA ENTRÉE, MICROWAVE										
(Chef Boyardee)	7.5 oz	230	7.0	31.0	1080	(mq)	9.0	(mq)	18	35%
(Chef Boyardee) hearty 'Main Meals'	10.5 oz	290	13.0	41.0	na	na	8.0	na	na	25%
(Chef Boyardee) in garden vegetable sauce	7.5 oz	170	5.0	14.0	940	(mq)	1.0	<1.0	3	11%
(Hormel)	7.5 oz	250	8.0	25.0	949	na	13.0	6.0	23	47%
(Libby's) w/meat sauce 'Diner'	7.75 oz	200	9.0	29.0	790	2.4	5.0	3.0	15	23%
(Lunch Bucket) w/meat sauce	7.5 oz	220	8.0	38.0	870	na	4.0	na	30	16%
LASAGNA ENTRÉE, PACKAGED										
(Dinty Moore) w/meat sauce 'American Classics'	10 oz	320	16.0	33.0	870	na	14.0	7.0	35	39%
(Top Shelf) Italian	10 oz	350	23.0	30.0	840	na	16.0	8.0	60	40%
(Top Shelf) vegetable	10.6 oz	275	18.0	34.0	1024	(mq)	8.0	(mq)	35	26%
(Ultra Slim Fast) vegetable	12 oz	240	17.0	39.0	730	na	4.0	na	15	14%
(Ultra Slim Fast) w/meat sauce	12 oz	330	28.0	38.0	980	na	9.0	na	55	24%

LASAGNA NOODLE. See PASTA.

LAVER. See SEAWEED.

Food Name	Serving Size	Calories	Prot. gms	Carbs gms	Sod. mgs	Fiber gms	Fat gms	Sat. Fat gms	Chol. mgs	% Fat Cal.
LEEK										
boiled, drained	4 oz	35	0.9	8.6	11	>.9 c	0.2	<.1	0	5%
boiled, drained, chopped	1/4 cup	8	0.2	2.0	3	>.2 c	0.1	0.0	0	9%
raw, chopped	1/2 cup	32	0.8	7.4	10	.6	0.2	<.1	0	5%
raw, trimmed	1 oz	17	0.4	4.0	6	.3	0.1	<.1	0	5%
raw, untrimmed	1 lb	122	3.0	28.2	40	2.4	0.6	0.1	0	4%
LEEK, FREEZE-DRIED										
bulb-lower leaf portion	1 oz	91	4.3	21.2	10	>2.5 c	0.6	0.1	0	5%
bulb-lower leaf portion	1/4 cup	3	0.1	0.6	0	>.1 c	0.0	0.0	0	0%
bulb-lower leaf portion	1 tbsp	1	0.0	0.2	0	0	0.0	0.0	0	0%
LEMON										
w/peel, approx 3.9 oz	1 med	22	1.3	11.6	3	na	0.3	0.0	0	5%
w/peel, whole	1 lb	89	5.3	47.6	13	(mq)	1.3	0.2	0	5%
w/o peel, approx 3.9 oz	1 med	17	0.6	5.4	1	1.6	0.2	0.0	0	7%
w/o peel, approx 5.6 oz	1 large	24	0.9	7.8	2	2.3	0.3	0.0	0	7%
w/o peel, trimmed	1-oz wedge	5	0.3	2.9	1	na	0.1	0.0	0	7%
LEMON AND HERB SEASONING										
(Schilling) 'Spice Blends'	1/4 tsp	1	0.1	0.2	154	na	0.1	(tr)	0	43%
LEMON DILL SEASONING MIX										
(Schilling) 'Bag'n Season'	1 pkg	161	3.0	15.0	2035	(mq)	11.0	(mq)	0	58%
LEMON DRINK. See also LEMONADE.										
(Crowley) chilled	8 oz	130	0.0	32.0	15	(tr)	0.0	0.0	0	0%
(Gatorade) 'Thirst Quencher'	8 oz	50	0.0	14.0	110	na	0.0	na	na	0%
(Pathmark) 'No Frills' mix, prepared	8 oz	90	0.0	20.0	55	(tr)	0.0	0.0	0	0%
LEMON GINGER JUICE										
(Santa Cruz Natural) organic 'Cruz'	8 oz	125	1.0	29.0	na	na	<1.0	na	na	<7%
LEMON HERB MARINADE (Golden Dipt)	1 oz	130	0.0	2.0	210	na	14.0	2.0	0	94%
LEMON JUICE										
	1 cup	61	0.9	21.1	2	0	0.0	na	0	0%
	1 oz	8	0.1	2.6	<1	(tr)	0.0	0.0	0	0%
	1 tbsp	4	0.1	1.3	0	0	0.0	na	0	0%
Canned or bottled										
(A&P) reconstituted, natural strength	1 oz	6	<1.0	2.0	0	(tr)	<1.0	(tr)	0	<43%
(Lucky Leaf)	6 oz	30	1.0	6.0	35	(tr)	0.0	0.0	0	0%
(ReaLemon) reconstituted, natural strength, refrigerated	1 oz	6	0.0	2.0	10	(tr)	0.0	0.0	0	0%
(ReaLemon) reconstituted, '100%'	1 oz	6	0.0	2.0	5	(tr)	0.0	0.0	0	0%
Frozen										
single strength	1/2 cup	27	0.6	7.9	1	(tr)	0.4	0.1	0	10%
single strength	1 tbsp	3	0.1	1.0	tr	(tr)	0.1	tr	0	17%
(Minute Maid) concentrate	6 oz	8	0.0	2.0	0	na	0.0	na	na	0%
(Sunkist)	1 oz	7	0.1	2.0	<1	(tr)	0.1	(tr)	0	10%
LEMON PEEL										
candied	1 oz	88	0.1	22.6	0	>.6 c	0.1	0.0	0	1%
raw	1 tbsp	na	0.1	1.0	0	.6	0.0	0.0	0	0%
raw	1 tsp	na	0.0	0.3	0	na	0.0	0.0	0	0%
LEMON PEPPER										
Dry seasoning										
(Lawry's)	1 tsp	6	0.2	1.2	340	>.1 c	0.1	(tr)	0	14%
(Schilling) 'Parsley Patch'	1 tsp	13	0.4	1.0	2	(mq)	0.6	(tr)	0	49%
(Schilling) 'Spice Blends'	1 tsp	7	0.2	0.8	618	(mq)	0.0	0.0	0	0%
Marinade (Lawry's)	1 oz	20	0.3	2.1	800	na	1.1	na	na	51%
LEMONADE										
Can, bottle, or box										
(Fruitopia) 'Lemonade, Love & Hope,' real fruit	8 oz	110	0.0	28.0	25	na	0.0	na	na	0%

Food Name	Serving Size	Calories	Prot. gms	Carbs gms	Sod. mgs	Fiber gms	Fat gms	Sat. Fat gms	Chol. mgs	% Fat Cal
(Fruitopia) 'Pink Lemonade Euphoria,' real fruit	8 oz	120	0.0	29.0	25	na	0.0	na	na	0%
(Hi-C)	8.45 oz	109	0.1	27.2	73	(tr)	0.1	(tr)	0	1%
(J. Hungerford) pink, 20% plus juice	9.03 oz	41	0.1	10.7	39	0	0.0	0.0	0	0%
(Knudsen & Sons) 'Natural'	8 oz	100	<1.0	26.0	na	na	0.0	na	na	0%
(Minute Maid)	6 oz	80	0.0	21.0	20	na	0.0	na	na	0%
(Minute Maid) country style	6 oz	80	0.0	21.0	20	na	0.0	na	na	0%
(Minute Maid) cranberry	6 oz	90	0.0	23.0	20	na	0.0	na	na	0%
(Minute Maid) pink	6 oz	80	0.0	21.0	20	na	0.0	na	na	0%
(Minute Maid) raspberry	6 oz	90	0.0	23.0	20	na	0.0	na	na	0%
(Santa Cruz Natural) organic	8 oz	60	<1.0	21.0	na	na	<1.0	na	na	<9%
(Santa Cruz Natural) organic 'Sparkling'	8 oz	85	<1.0	20.0	na	na	<1.0	na	na	<10%
(Shasta)	12 oz	146	0.0	39.0	106	(tr)	0.0	0.0	0	0%
(Sunkist)	8 oz	141	0.0	36.0	0	(tr)	0.0	0.0	0	0%
(10-K) pink	8 oz	60	0.0	15.0	55	na	0.0	na	na	0%
(Tropicana)	6 oz	100	<1.0	22.0	35	na	<1.0	na	na	<9%
(Tropicana) 'Single Serve'	8 oz	120	(tr)	30.0	3	(tr)	0.0	0.0	0	0%
(Veryfine)	8 oz	120	0.2	30.0	25	(tr)	0.0	0.0	0	0%
(Wyler's)	6 oz	64	0.0	16.5	33	(tr)	0.0	0.0	0	0%
(Wyler's) pink 'Fruit Slush'	4 oz	157	0.0	39.3	10	(tr)	0.0	0.0	0	0%

LEMONADE DRINK MIX

Prepared from dry mix

Food Name	Serving Size	Calories	Prot. gms	Carbs gms	Sod. mgs	Fiber gms	Fat gms	Sat. Fat gms	Chol. mgs	% Fat Cal
(Country Time)	8 oz	80	0.0	20.0	20	0	0.0	0.0	0	0%
(Country Time) pink	8 oz	80	0.0	20.0	20	0	0.0	0.0	0	0%
(Country Time) pink, 'Sugar Free'	8 oz	4	0.0	0.0	0	0	0.0	0.0	0	0%
(Country Time) pink, sugar sweetened	8 oz	80	0.0	20.0	20	na	0.0	na	0	0%
(Country Time) pink, sugar-free, w/NutraSweet	8 oz	4	0.0	0.0	0	na	0.0	na	0	0%
(Country Time) 'Sugar-free'	8 oz	4	0.0	0.0	0	0	0.0	0.0	0	0%
(Crystal Light) 'Sugar-free'	8 oz	4	0.0	0.0	0	0	0.0	0.0	0	0%
(Crystal Light) sugar-free, w/NutraSweet	8 oz	4	0.0	0.0	0	na	0.0	na	0	0%
(Finast)	8 oz	80	0.0	20.0	15	0	0.0	0.0	0	0%
(Gatorade) instant 'Thirst Quencher'	8 oz	60	0.0	15.0	110	na	0.0	na	na	0%
(Kool-Aid) pink, unsweetened, prepared w/sugar	8 oz	100	0.0	25.0	0	na	0.0	na	0	0%
(Kool-Aid) pink, unsweetened, prepared w/o sugar	8 oz	2	0.0	0.0	0	na	0.0	na	0	0%
(Kool-Aid) sugar free, w/NutraSweet	8 oz	4	0.0	0.0	0	na	0.0	na	0	0%
(Kool-Aid) sugar sweetened	8 oz	80	0.0	20.0	0	na	0.0	na	0	0%
(Wyler's) 'Crystals' 32-serving pkg	8 oz	78	0.0	19.4	39	0	0.0	0.0	0	0%

Prepared from frozen concentrate

Food Name	Serving Size	Calories	Prot. gms	Carbs gms	Sod. mgs	Fiber gms	Fat gms	Sat. Fat gms	Chol. mgs	% Fat Cal
(A&P)	8 oz	110	<1.0	28.0	0	(tr)	<1.0	(tr)	0	<7%
(A&P) pink	8 oz	110	<1.0	28.0	0	(tr)	<1.0	(tr)	0	<7%
(Minute Maid)	6 oz	90	0.0	22.0	0	na	0.0	na	na	0%
(Minute Maid) country style	6 oz	90	0.0	22.0	0	na	0.0	na	na	0%
(Minute Maid) cranberry	6 oz	90	0.0	22.0	0	na	0.0	na	na	0%
(Minute Maid) pink	6 oz	90	0.0	22.0	0	na	0.0	na	na	0%
(Minute Maid) raspberry	6 oz	90	0.0	22.0	0	na	0.0	na	na	0%
(Sunkist)	8 oz	92	0.1	24.2	1	(tr)	0.0	0.0	0	0%

LEMONADE PUNCH MIX (Country Time) sugar sweetened

Food Name	Serving Size	Calories	Prot. gms	Carbs gms	Sod. mgs	Fiber gms	Fat gms	Sat. Fat gms	Chol. mgs	% Fat Cal
LEMONADE PUNCH MIX (Country Time) sugar sweetened	8 oz	80	0.0	20.0	15	na	0.0	na	0	0%

LEMON-LIME DRINK

Can, bottle, or box

Food Name	Serving Size	Calories	Prot. gms	Carbs gms	Sod. mgs	Fiber gms	Fat gms	Sat. Fat gms	Chol. mgs	% Fat Cal
(All-Sports) thirst quencher, caffeine-free	8 oz	70	0.0	19.0	55	na	0.0	na	na	0%
(Gatorade) 'Thirst Quencher'	8 oz	50	0.0	14.0	110	na	0.0	na	na	0%
(Gatorade) 'Thirst Quencher Light'	8 oz	25	0.0	7.0	80	na	0.0	na	na	0%
(PowerAde) thirst quencher, high energy	8 oz	70	0.0	19.0	70	na	0.0	na	na	0%
(10-K)	8 oz	60	0.0	15.0	55	na	0.0	na	na	0%
(Veryfine)	8 oz	120	0.1	30.0	10	(tr)	0.0	0.0	0	0%

Food Name	Serving Size	Calories	Prot. gms	Carbs gms	Sod. mgs	Fiber gms	Fat gms	Sat. Fat gms	Chol. mgs	% Fat Cal.
Prepared from dry mix										
(Crystal Light) w/NutraSweet	8 oz	4	0.0	0.0	0	na	0.0	na	0	0%
(GatorAde) instant 'Thirst Quencher'	8 oz	60	0.0	15.0	110	na	0.0	na	na	0%
(Kool-Aid) unsweetened, prepared w/sugar	8 oz	100	0.0	25.0	0	na	0.0	na	0	0%
(Kool-Aid) unsweetened, prepared w/o sugar	8 oz	2	0.0	0.0	0	na	0.0	na	0	0%
LENTIL										
boiled	1/2 cup	115	8.9	19.9	2	4.0	0.4	0.1	0	3%
boiled	4 oz	132	10.2	22.8	2	4.5	0.4	0.1	0	3%
boiled (A&P)	1 cup	210	16.0	39.0	0	(mq)	1.0	(mq)	0	4%
raw	1/2 cup	324	26.9	54.8	9	10.9	0.9	0.1	0	2%
raw	1 oz	96	8.0	16.2	3	3.2	0.3	<.1	0	3%
raw, green (Arrowhead Mills)	2 oz	190	13.0	35.0	9	8.8	1.0	(mq)	0	5%
raw, red (Arrowhead Mills)	2 oz	195	14.0	34.0	10	8.8	1.0	(mq)	0	5%
raw, sprouted	1 oz	30	2.5	6.3	3	>.9 c	0.2	<.1	0	5%
LENTIL DINNER, CANNED										
hearty, w/garden vegetables 'Fast Menu' fat-free										
(Health Valley)	7.5 oz	160	13.0	18.0	204	15.5	4.0	(mq)	0	23%
hearty, w/garden vegetables 'Fast Menu' fat-free										
(Health Valley)	5 oz	80	9.0	12.0	140	10.3	0.0	na	0	0%
LETTUCE										
BIBB, BOSTON, OR BUTTERHEAD										
raw, approx 7.75 oz, 5 inch diam	1 head	21	2.1	3.8	8	1.6	0.4	0.1	0	13%
trimmed	1 oz	4	0.4	0.7	1	.3	0.1	tr	0	17%
untrimmed	1 lb	45	4.3	7.8	18	3.4	0.7	0.1	0	12%
COS										
raw, shredded	1/2 cup	4	0.5	0.7	2	.5	0.1	0.0	0	16%
trimmed	1 oz	5	0.5	0.7	2	.5	0.1	tr	0	16%
untrimmed	1 lb	68	6.9	10.1	32	7.2	0.9	0.1	0	11%
ICEBERG										
raw, 6 inch diam	1 head	70	5.4	11.3	49	5.4	1.0	0.1	0	12%
trimmed	1 oz	4	0.3	0.6	3	.3	0.1	tr	0	20%
untrimmed	1 lb	55	4.3	9.0	39	4.3	0.8	0.1	0	12%
LEAF, shredded (Dole)	1.5 cups	12	1.0	1.0	40	1.0	0.0	na	na	0%
LOOSELEAF										
raw, shredded	1/2 cup	5	0.4	1.0	3	.53	0.1	0.0	0	14%
trimmed	1 oz	5	0.4	1.0	3	>.2 c	0.1	<.1	0	14%
untrimmed	1 lb	52	3.8	10.2	26	>2.0 c	0.9	0.1	0	13%
ROMAINE										
raw, shredded	1/2 cup	4	0.5	0.7	2	.5	0.1	0.0	0	16%
trimmed	1 oz	5	0.5	0.7	2	.5	0.1	tr	0	16%
untrimmed	1 lb	68	6.9	10.1	32	7.2	0.9	0.1	0	11%
LIMA BEAN /butterbean										
boiled, drained	4 oz	139	7.7	26.8	19	4.8	0.4	0.1	0	3%
raw, trimmed	1 oz	32	1.9	5.7	2	1.0	0.2	0.1	0	6%
raw, untrimmed	1 lb	226	13.7	40.2	16	7.4	1.7	0.4	0	7%
MATURE, DRY										
Baby										
boiled	4 oz	143	9.1	26.4	3	4.9	0.4	0.1	0	3%
boiled (A&P)	1 cup	230	16.0	40.0	15	(mq)	1.0	na	0	4%
boiled, thin-seeded	1/2 cup	115	7.3	21.2	3	7.01	0.4	0.1	0	3%
raw	1 oz	95	5.8	17.8	4	2.8	0.3	0.1	0	3%
raw, thin-seeded	1/2 cup	338	20.8	63.5	13	>5.8 c	0.9	0.2	0	2%
Large										
boiled	4 oz	130	8.8	23.7	2	8.2	0.4	0.1	0	3%

Food Name	Serving Size	Calories	Prot. gms	Carbs gms	Sod. mgs	Fiber gms	Fat gms	Sat. Fat gms	Chol. mgs	% Fat Cal.
boiled	1/2 cup	108	7.3	19.6	2	6.8	0.4	0.1	0	3%
boiled (A&P)	1 cup	230	15.0	35.0	0	(mq)	1.0	(mq)	0	4%
raw	1/2 cup	301	19.1	56.4	16	16.9	0.6	0.1	0	2%
raw	1 oz	96	6.1	18.0	5	5.4	0.2	<.1	0	2%
LIMA BEAN, CANNED										
(A&P)	1/2 cup	110	7.0	20.0	380	(mq)	<1.0	(tr)	0	<8%
(Allens) large	1/2 cup	110	5.0	18.0	370	(mq)	<1.0	(tr)	0	<9%
(Featherweight)	1/2 cup	80	5.0	16.0	25	(mq)	0.0	0.0	0	0%
(Freshlike)	1/2 cup	80	5.0	16.0	320	na	0.0	na	na	0%
(Freshlike) water packed, w/o salt	1/2 cup	80	5.0	16.0	5	na	0.0	na	na	0%
(Green Giant)	1/2 cup	80	6.0	16.0	420	3.7	0.0	0.0	0	0%
(Joan of Arc)	1/2 cup	80	6.0	16.0	420	3.7	0.0	0.0	0	0%
(S&W)	1/2 cup	100	6.0	19.0	440	(mq)	1.0	(tr)	0	8%
(Stokely)	1/2 cup	80	5.0	16.0	390	(mq)	0.0	0.0	0	0%
(Stokely) 'No Salt or Sugar Added'	1/2 cup	80	5.0	16.0	5	(mq)	0.0	0.0	0	0%
(Van Camp's)	1 cup	162	11.0	30.0	710	(mq)	0.5	(tr)	0	3%
(Veg•All)	1/2 cup	80	5.0	16.0	320	na	0.0	na	na	0%
FORDHOOK (Stokely)	1/2 cup	80	5.0	14.0	300	(mq)	0.0	0.0	0	0%
GREEN										
(A&P)	1/2 cup	80	5.0	15.0	320	(mq)	<1.0	(tr)	0	<10%
(Allens) medium	1/2 cup	90	5.0	15.0	350	(mq)	<1.0	(tr)	0	<10%
(Allens) tiny, small	1/2 cup	90	5.0	15.0	350	(mq)	<1.0	(tr)	0	<10%
(Bush's Best)	1/2 cup	90	4.0	17.0	400	4.0	0.0	na	na	0%
(Del Monte) w/liquid	1/2 cup	70	4.0	14.0	355	(mq)	0.0	0.0	0	0%
(Luck's) small, w/pork	7.5 oz	220	10.0	33.0	640	8.0	7.0	(mq)	(mq)	27%
(S&W) small 'Fancy'	1/2 cup	80	6.0	16.0	390	(mq)	0.0	0.0	0	0%
GREEN AND WHITE										
(Allens)	1/2 cup	90	5.0	15.0	370	(mq)	<1.0	(tr)	0	<10%
(Bush's Best) gem	1/2 cup	80	5.0	17.0	300	4.0	0.0	na	na	0%
W/HAM (Dennison's)	7.5 oz	250	14.0	33.0	935	9.0	7.0	(mq)	(mq)	25%
W/PORK (Luck's)	7.5 oz	230	12.0	34.0	720	9.0	7.0	(mq)	(mq)	26%
LIMA BEAN, FROZEN										
(Green Giant)	1/2 cup	100	6.0	19.0	30	5.0	0.0	0.0	0	0%
(Green Giant) 'Harvest Fresh'	1/2 cup	80	6.0	18.0	170	4.0	0.0	0.0	0	0%
(Green Giant) in butter sauce	1/2 cup	100	6.0	17.0	310	2.0	2.0	<1.0	5	16%
(Health Valley)	1/2 cup	94	6.0	18.0	26	3.4	0.0	0.0	0	0%
BABY										
boiled, drained	10-oz pkg	376	21.6	71.4	147	>6.2 c	1.3	0.3	0	3%
boiled, drained	4 oz	119	7.5	22.1	33	(mq)	0.3	0.1	0	2%
boiled, drained, immature seeds	10-oz pkg	327	20.7	60.5	90	>5.4 c	0.9	0.2	0	2%
boiled, drained, immature seeds	1/2 cup	94	6.0	17.5	26	>1.6 c	0.3	0.1	0	3%
unprepared, immature seeds	10-oz pkg	375	21.6	71.4	148	>6.2 c	1.3	0.3	0	3%
unprepared, immature seeds	1/2 cup	108	6.2	20.6	43	>1.8 c	0.4	0.1	0	3%
(A&P) green	3.3 oz	130	7.0	24.0	130	(mq)	<1.0	na	0	<7%
(Birds Eye)	3.3 oz	130	7.0	24.0	115	(mq)	0.0	0.0	0	0%
(Freshlike)	3.3 oz	130	7.0	24.0	100	na	1.0	na	na	7%
(Frosty Acres)	3.3 oz	130	7.0	24.0	125	>2.0 c	0.0	0.0	0	0%
(Seabrook)	3.3 oz	130	7.0	24.0	125	>2.0 c	0.0	0.0	0	0%
(Seabrook) butter	3.3 oz	140	7.0	26.0	213	>2.0 c	1.0	na	0	6%
(Southern)	3.5 oz	135	7.3	25.2	125	(mq)	0.5	na	0	3%
(Stokely) in butter sauce 'Singles'	4 oz	140	7.0	25.0	450	(mq)	2.0	(mq)	5	12%
(Veg•All)	3.3 oz	130	7.0	24.0	100	na	1.0	na	na	7%
FORDHOOK										
boiled, drained	10-oz pkg	301	18.2	56.3	166	>5.6 c	1.0	0.2	0	3%

Food Name	Serving Size	Calories	Prot. gms	Carbs gms	Sod. mgs	Fiber gms	Fat gms	Sat. Fat gms	Chol. mgs	% Fat Cal.
boiled, drained	4 oz	113	6.9	21.3	60	>2.1 c	0.4	0.1	0	3%
boiled, drained, immature seeds	10-oz pkg	311	18.9	58.5	165	22.4	1.1	0.2	0	3%
boiled, drained, immature seeds	1/2 cup	85	5.2	16.0	45	6.1	0.3	0.1	0	3%
unprepared, immature seeds	1/2 cup	85	5.1	15.9	46	1.6	0.3	0.1	0	3%
(A&P)	3.3 oz	100	6.0	19.0	70	(mq)	<1.0	(tr)	0	<8%
(Birds Eye)	3.3 oz	100	6.0	19.0	100	(mq)	0.0	0.0	0	0%
(Frosty Acres)	3.3 oz	100	6.0	19.0	71	>2.0 c	0.0	0.0	0	0%
(Seabrook)	3.3 oz	100	6.0	19.0	71	>2.0 c	0.0	0.0	0	0%
(Southern)	3.5 oz	105	6.4	19.1	100	(mq)	0.3	(tr)	0	3%
SPECKLED										
(Seabrook)	3.3 oz	120	7.0	23.0	19	>2.0 c	0.0	0.0	0	0%
(Southern)	3.5 oz	135	7.8	25.0	30	(mq)	0.4	(tr)	0	3%
TINY (Seabrook)	3.3 oz	110	6.0	21.0	144	>2.0 c	1.0	(tr)	0	8%
LIME										
peeled and seeded	1 oz	9	0.2	3.0	1	>.1 c	0.1	tr	0	7%
raw, 2 inch diam	1 med	20	0.5	7.1	1	1.9	0.1	0.0	0	3%
untrimmed	1 lb	115	2.7	40.2	8	>1.9 c	0.8	0.1	0	4%
LIME JUICE										
fresh	1 cup	66	1.1	22.2	2	0	0.3	0.0	0	3%
fresh	1 oz	8	0.1	2.8	<1	(tr)	<.1	tr	0	<7%
fresh	1 tbsp	4	0.1	1.4	0	0	0.0	0.0	0	0%
Canned or bottled										
	1/2 cup	26	0.3	8.2	20	(tr)	0.3	<.1	0	7%
	1 tbsp	3	<.1	1.0	2	(tr)	<.1	tr	0	<17%
unsweetened	1 cup	52	0.6	16.5	39	0	0.6	0.1	0	7%
unsweetened	1 tbsp	3	0.0	1.0	2	0	0.0	0.0	0	0%
(ReaLime) reconstituted, natural strength	1 oz	6	0.0	2.0	10	(tr)	0.0	0.0	0	0%
(Roses)	1 oz	48	0.0	12.0	6	(tr)	0.0	0.0	0	0%
(Santa Cruz Natural) organic, 'Cruz'	8 oz	120	1.0	27.0	na	na	<1.0	na	na	<7%
LIMEADE										
(Minute Maid) frozen concentrate, diluted	6 oz	70	0.0	19.0	0	na	0.0	na	na	0%
(Santa Cruz Natural) organic, 'Sparkling'	8 oz	60	<1.0	23.0	na	na	<1.0	na	na	<9%
LING										
dry-heat cooked	3 oz	94	20.7	0.0	147	0	0.7	na	43	7%
raw	1 lb	394	86.1	0.0	612	0	2.9	(mq)	(mq)	7%
raw	3 oz	74	16.1	0.0	115	0	0.5	0.1	34	7%
raw	1 oz	25	5.4	0.0	38	0	0.2	(mq)	(mq)	8%
LINGCOD										
dry-heat cooked	3 oz	93	19.2	0.0	65	0	1.2	0.2	57	12%
raw	1 lb	385	80.1	0.0	266	0	4.8	0.9	236	12%
raw	3 oz	72	15.0	0.0	50	0	0.9	0.2	44	12%
raw	1 oz	24	5.0	0.0	17	0	0.3	<.1	15	12%
LINGUINE ENTRÉE										
Frozen										
(Banquet) w/meat sauce 'Healthy Balance'	11.5 oz	290	11.0	49.0	560	na	6.0	3.0	25	18%
(Budget Gourmet) w/shrimp	10 oz	330	15.0	33.0	1250	(mq)	15.0	(mq)	75	41%
(Healthy Choice) w/shrimp	9.5 oz	230	13.0	40.0	420	na	2.0	1.0	60	8%
(Lean Cuisine) w/clam sauce	9 5/8 oz	280	17.0	36.0	560	na	8.0	2.0	30	25%
Packaged (Top Shelf) w/clam sauce	1 serving	330	12.0	30.0	1420	(mq)	18.0	(mq)	85	49%
Refrigerated										
(Contadina) egg, angel hair 'Fresh'	3 oz	260	12.0	45.0	30	na	3.0	<1.0	75	11%
(DiGiorno) herb, approx 1 1/3 cups cooked	3 oz	250	11.0	46.0	135	na	3.0	0.0	0	11%

LINGUINE NOODLE. See PASTA.

Food Name	Serving Size	Calories	Prot. gms	Carbs gms	Sod. mgs	Fiber gms	Fat gms	Sat. Fat gms	Chol. mgs	% Fat Cal.
LINSEED OIL										
edible	1/2 cup	964	0.0	0.0	0	0	109.0	10.3	0	100%
edible	1 oz	251	0.0	0.0	0	0	28.4	2.7	0	100%
edible	1 tbsp	120	0.0	0.0	0	0	13.6	1.3	0	100%
LIQUEUR. See ALCOHOLIC BEVERAGES.										
LIQUOR. See ALCOHOLIC BEVERAGES.										
LITCHI / lychee										
Dried										
	100 gm	277	3.8	70.7	3	>1.4 c	1.2	na	0	4%
	1 oz	79	1.1	20.0	1	4.6	0.3	(tr)	0	3%
Raw										
approx .6 oz	1 med	6	0.1	1.6	tr	<.1	<.1	(tr)	0	<12%
shelled and seeded	1/2 cup	63	0.8	15.7	1	>.2 c	0.4	tr	0	5%
shelled and seeded	1 oz	19	0.2	4.7	<1	>.1 c	0.1	(tr)	0	4%
untrimmed	1 lb	179	2.3	45.0	2	>.6 c	1.2	na	0	5%
LIVER. See individual animal listings.										
LIVERWURST. See LUNCHEON MEATS.										
LIVERWURST SPREAD										
(Hormel) canned	.5 oz	35	2.0	0.0	(mq)	0	3.0	(mq)	(mq)	77%
(Underwood) canned	2 1/8 oz	180	8.0	4.0	470	na	15.0	(mq)	90	74%
LOBSTER, NORTHERN										
boiled	1 cup	142	29.7	1.9	551	0	0.9	0.2	104	6%
boiled	4 oz	111	23.2	1.5	431	0	0.7	0.1	82	6%
moist-heat cooked	1 cup	142	29.7	1.9	551	0	0.9	0.2	104	6%
moist-heat cooked	3 oz	83	17.4	1.1	323	0	0.5	0.1	61	6%
poached	1 cup	142	29.7	1.9	551	0	0.9	0.2	104	6%
poached	4 oz	111	23.2	1.5	431	0	0.7	0.1	82	6%
raw	1 lb	410	85.3	2.3	(mq)	0	4.1	(mq)	432	10%
raw	3 oz	77	16.0	0.4	252	0	0.8	0.2	81	10%
raw	1 oz	26	5.3	0.1	(mq)	0	0.3	(mq)	27	11%
steamed	1 cup	142	29.7	1.9	551	0	0.9	0.2	104	6%
steamed	4 oz	111	23.2	1.5	431	0	0.7	0.1	82	6%
LOBSTER, SPINY, MIXED SPECIES										
moist-heat cooked	3 oz	122	22.5	2.7	193	0	1.6	0.3	77	13%
raw	1 lb	506	93.4	11.0	803	0	6.9	1.1	318	13%
raw	3 oz	95	17.5	2.1	150	0	1.3	0.2	59	13%
raw	1 oz	32	5.8	0.7	50	0	0.4	0.1	20	12%
LOBSTER PASTE, canned	1 tsp	13	1.5	0.1	10	0	0.7	0.4	12	50%
LOGANBERRY										
fresh, trimmed	1 lb	281	4.5	67.6	5	(mq)	2.7	(mq)	0	8%
fresh, trimmed	1 cup	89	1.4	21.5	1	>4.3 c	0.9	(mq)	0	8%
fresh, untrimmed	1 lb	267	4.3	64.2	4	(mq)	2.6	(mq)	0	8%
frozen	1 cup	81	2.2	19.1	1	7.2	0.5	na	0	5%
frozen	4 oz	62	1.7	14.8	1	(mq)	0.4	(mq)	0	5%
LONGAN										
raw, approx .2 oz	1 med	2	<.1	0.5	tr	<.1	tr	(tr)	0	0%
raw, shelled and seeded	1 oz	17	0.4	4.3	tr	>.1 c	<.1	(tr)	0	<5%
raw, untrimmed	1 lb	144	3.2	36.4	1	>1.0 c	0.2	na	0	1%
LONGAN, DRIED										
	100 gm	286	4.9	74.0	48	>2.0 c	0.4	na	0	1%
	1 oz	81	1.4	21.0	14	>.6 c	0.1	(tr)	0	1%
LONGBEAN										
boiled, drained	4 oz	53	2.9	10.4	5	>1.7 c	0.1	<.1	0	2%
boiled, drained, sliced	1/2 cup	25	1.3	4.8	2	>.8 c	0.1	<.1	0	4%

Food Name	Serving Size	Calories	Prot. gms	Carbs gms	Sod. mgs	Fiber gms	Fat gms	Sat. Fat gms	Chol. mgs	% Fat Cal.
boiled, drained, 13 1/4 inches long x 1/4 inch diam	1 pod	7	0.4	1.3	1	>.2 c	<.1	tr	0	<12%
raw, sliced	1/2 cup	22	1.3	3.8	2	(mq)	0.2	<.1	0	8%
raw, 13 1/4 inches long x 1/4 inch diam	1 pod	6	0.3	1.0	tr	(mq)	0.1	<.1	0	15%
raw, trimmed	1 oz	13	0.8	2.4	1	(mq)	0.1	<.1	0	7%
raw, untrimmed	1 lb	203	12.1	36.0	17	(mq)	1.7	0.5	0	7%
LONGBEAN, DRIED										
boiled	1/2 cup	102	7.1	18.1	4	>1.4 c	0.4	0.1	0	3%
boiled	4 oz	134	9.4	23.9	6	>1.8 c	0.5	0.1	0	3%
raw	1/2 cup	292	20.4	52.0	14	>4.0 c	1.1	0.3	0	3%
raw	1 oz	98	6.9	17.6	5	>1.4 c	0.4	0.1	0	4%
LOOFAH GOURD. See GOURD, DISHCLOTH.										
LOQUAT / Japanese medlar										
peeled and seeded	1 oz	13	0.1	3.4	<1	>.1 c	0.1	<.1	0	6%
trimmed, .6 oz	1 med	5	0.0	1.2	0	.2	0.0	0.0	0	0%
untrimmed	1 lb	132	1.2	34.1	3	>1.4 c	0.6	0.1	0	4%
LOTTE. See MONKFISH.										
LOTUS ROOT										
boiled, drained	4 oz	75	1.8	18.2	51	>1.0 c	0.1	<.1	0	1%
boiled, drained, 2.5 inch diam	10 slices	59	1.4	14.3	40	2.8	0.1	0.0	0	1%
raw, 2.5 inch diam	10 slices	45	2.1	14.0	32	4.0	0.1	0.0	0	1%
raw, 9.5 inches long	1 root	64	3.0	19.8	46	5.6	0.1	0.0	0	1%
raw, trimmed	1 oz	16	0.7	4.9	11	>.2 c	<.1	tr	0	<4%
raw, untrimmed	1 lb	201	9.3	61.8	145	>2.9 c	0.4	0.1	0	1%
LOTUS SEED										
dried	1 cup	106	4.9	20.6	2	>.8 c	0.6	0.1	0	5%
dried, approx 42 medium seeds	1 oz	94	4.4	18.3	1	>.7 c	0.6	0.1	0	6%
raw	1 oz	25	1.2	4.9	0	>.2 c	0.2	0.0	0	7%
raw, in shell	1 lb	214	9.9	41.5	3	>1.6 c	1.3	0.2	0	5%
LOX. See SALMON, CHINOOK.										
LUNCHEON MEAT										
BARBECUE LOAF (Oscar Mayer)	1 oz	46	4.5	1.7	333	0	2.3	1.0	14	46%
BOLOGNA										
(Eckrich)	1 oz	100	3.0	1.0	240	0	9.0	(mq)	(mq)	84%
(Eckrich) 'German Brand'	1 oz	80	4.0	1.0	300	0	7.0	(mq)	(mq)	76%
(Eckrich) 'Lean Supreme'	1 oz	70	4.0	1.0	240	0	6.0	(mq)	(mq)	73%
(Eckrich) 'Sandwich'	1 oz	100	3.0	1.0	240	0	9.0	(mq)	(mq)	84%
(Eckrich) 'Smorgas Pac'	1 oz	100	3.0	1.0	240	0	9.0	(mq)	(mq)	84%
(Eckrich) 'Thick Sliced, 1-lb pkg'	1.8 oz	170	5.0	2.0	430	0	15.0	(mq)	(mq)	83%
(Hillshire Farm) 'Large'	1 oz	90	3.0	<1.0	(mq)	0	8.0	(mq)	(mq)	82%
(Hillshire Farm) 'Ring'	1 oz	89	3.0	<1.0	(mq)	0	8.0	(mq)	(mq)	82%
(Hormel) 'Fine Ground, 1-lb'	2 oz	170	7.0	1.0	596	0	16.0	(mq)	(mq)	82%
(Hormel) 'Perma-Fresh'	2 slices	180	7.0	0.0	599	0	16.0	(mq)	(mq)	84%
(JM)	1 oz	90	3.0	1.0	350	0	8.0	(mq)	(mq)	82%
(JM) 'German Brand'	1 oz	70	4.0	1.0	270	0	6.0	(mq)	(mq)	73%
(Kahn's)	1 slice	90	3.0	1.0	330	0	8.0	(mq)	(mq)	82%
(Kahn's) 'Deluxe Club'	1 slice	90	3.0	1.0	290	0	8.0	(mq)	na	82%
(Kahn's) 'Deluxe Club Family Pack'	1 slice	70	2.0	1.0	220	0	6.0	(mq)	(mq)	82%
(Kahn's) 'Giant Deluxe'	1 slice	90	3.0	1.0	290	0	8.0	(mq)	(mq)	82%
(Kahn's) 'Giant Thick Deluxe'	1 slice	110	4.0	1.0	330	0	10.0	(mq)	(mq)	82%
(Kahn's) 'Thick Deluxe'	1 slice	140	5.0	1.0	450	0	13.0	(mq)	(mq)	83%
(Kahn's) 'Thin Sliced Deluxe'	1 slice	60	2.0	1.0	190	0	5.0	(mq)	(mq)	79%
(Light & Lean)	2 slices	140	6.0	2.0	(mq)	0	12.0	(mq)	(mq)	77%
(Light & Lean) 'Thin Sliced'	2 slices	70	3.0	1.0	(mq)	0	6.0	(mq)	(mq)	77%
(OHSE)	1 oz	75	3.0	3.0	280	0	6.0	(mq)	(mq)	69%

Food Name	Serving Size	Calories	Prot. gms	Carbs gms	Sod. mgs	Fiber gms	Fat gms	Sat. Fat gms	Chol. mgs	% Fat Cal.
(Oscar Mayer)	1.6 oz	144	5.0	1.1	500	0	13.3	5.1	30	83%
(Oscar Mayer)	1 oz	90	3.1	0.7	311	0	8.3	3.2	19	83%
(Oscar Mayer)	.53 oz	48	1.7	0.4	167	0	4.4	1.7	10	83%
(Oscar Mayer) 'Light'	1 oz	64	3.2	0.7	310	0	5.4	1.8	11	76%
(Oscar Mayer) Wisconsin made, ring	1 oz	90	3.0	<1.0	230	na	8.0	na	15	82%
(Oscar Mayer) w/cheese	.8 oz	74	2.7	0.6	232	0	6.8	2.6	15	82%
(Pilgrim's Pride)	1 oz	59	3.9	0.6	228	0	4.4	(mq)	16	69%
Beef										
(Boar's Head)	1 oz	74	4.0	<1.0	270	0	7.0	(mq)	17	76%
(Boar's Head) 'Premium' low cholesterol	1 oz	70	4.0	1.0	270	na	7.0	na	15	90%
(Eckrich)	1 oz	90	3.0	1.0	230	0	8.0	(mq)	(mq)	82%
(Eckrich) 'Thick Sliced'	1.5 oz	130	4.0	2.0	340	0	12.0	(mq)	(mq)	82%
(Hebrew National) 'Original Deli Style'	1 oz	90	3.0	<1.0	330	0	3.0	(mq)	15	63%
(Hormel) 'Coarse Ground, 1 lb'	2 oz	160	8.0	1.0	576	0	14.0	(mq)	(mq)	78%
(Hormel) 'Perma-Fresh'	2 slices	170	6.0	1.0	592	0	16.0	(mq)	(mq)	84%
(JM)	1 oz	90	3.0	1.0	350	0	8.0	(mq)	(JM)	82%
(Kahn's)	1 slice	90	3.0	1.0	300	0	8.0	(mq)	(mq)	82%
(Kahn's) 'Family Pack'	1 slice	70	2.0	1.0	230	0	6.0	(mq)	(mq)	82%
(Kahn's) 'Giant'	1 slice	90	3.0	1.0	300	0	8.0	(mq)	(mq)	82%
(Kahn's) 'Pounder'	1 slice	90	3.0	1.0	300	0	8.0	(mq)	(mq)	82%
(OHSE)	1 oz	85	3.0	1.0	310	0	8.0	(mq)	(mq)	82%
(Oscar Mayer)	1.6 oz	143	5.0	1.0	489	0	13.3	5.8	31	83%
(Oscar Mayer)	1 oz	89	3.1	0.6	304	0	8.2	3.7	19	83%
(Oscar Mayer)	.53 oz	48	1.7	0.3	163	0	4.4	1.9	10	83%
(Oscar Mayer) 'Light'	1 oz	64	3.5	0.9	316	0	5.3	2.1	10	73%
Beef and cheddar (Kahn's)	1 slice	90	4.0	1.0	320	0	8.0	(mq)	(mq)	78%
Beef and pork										
(Boar's Head)	1 oz	80	4.0	<1.0	250 c	0	7.0	(mq)	15	76%
(Boar's Head) 'Premium' low cholesterol	1 oz	80	4.0	1.0	250	na	7.0	na	15	79%

QUICK REFERENCE: LUNCHEON MEATS

Because of our new fat-consciousness, low-fat ham, turkey breast, and other luncheon meats are now available, with just a fraction of the fat of regular processed meats. Of course, most of us still sandwich our luncheon meats in rolls or between slices of bread, and add mustard, mayonnaise, or other toppings—toppings that add fat and calories. Here is a quick look at the nutrient values of the most common sandwich fixings.

Food Name	Serving Size	Calories	Prot. gms	Carbs gms	Sod. mgs	Fiber gms	Fat gms	Sat. Fat gms	Chol. mgs	% Fat Cal.
White bread	1 slice	70	3.0	13.0	140	.7	1.0	na	na	12%
Rye bread	1 slice	70	3.0	13.0	180	.7	1.0	na	na	12%
Whole wheat bread	1 slice	60	3.0	11.0	125	2.0	1.0	0.0	0	14%
Hoagie roll	1 roll	210	8.0	34.0	320	1.0	5.0	1.0	0	21%
Kaiser roll	1 roll	184	7.0	35.4	338	2.0	2.9	(mq)	5	13%
Sandwich roll	1 roll	123	4.5	21.6	203	1.9	3.3	(mq)	1	22%
American cheese	1 oz	110	6.0	1.0	450	0	9.0	5.0	25	74%
Cheddar cheese	1 oz	113	7.0	0.4	174	0	9.3	5.9	29	74%
Swiss cheese	1 oz	105	8.0	1.0	73	0	7.7	5.0	26	66%
Catsup	1 tbsp	16	0.2	4.1	178	.2	0.1	0.0	0	5%
Mustard	1 tbsp	10	1.0	1.0	180	na	1.0	na	0	53%
Mayonnaise	1 tbsp	100	0.0	0.0	80	0	11.0	2.0	5	100%
Pickle Relish	1 tbsp	20	0.1	5.3	122	>.1 c	0.1	0.0	0	4%

Food Name	Serving Size	Calories	Prot. gms	Carbs gms	Sod. mgs	Fiber gms	Fat gms	Sat. Fat gms	Chol. mgs	% Fat Cal.
(Healthy Deli)	1 oz	41	4.4	1.1	200	0	2.0	(mq)	9	45%
Chicken										
(Health Valley)	1 slice	85	4.0	1.0	329	0	8.0	(mq)	13	78%
(OHSE) '15% Chicken'	1 oz	90	3.0	1.0	320	0	8.0	(mq)	(mq)	82%
(Tyson)	1 slice	44	2.2	3.7	185	na	0.5	na	na	16%
Garlic										
(Eckrich)	1 oz	90	3.0	1.0	230	0	9.0	(mq)	(mq)	84%
(Eckrich) w/cheese	1 oz	90	3.0	1.0	250	0	9.0	(mq)	(mq)	84%
(JM)	1 oz	90	3.0	1.0	350	0	8.0	(mq)	(mq)	82%
(Kahn's)	1 slice	90	3.0	1.0	290	0	8.0	(mq)	(mq)	82%
Ham										
(Boar's Head)	1 oz	40	5.0	1.0	(mq)	0	2.0	(mq)	15	43%
(Oscar Mayer)	1 oz	90	3.1	0.7	301	0	8.3	3.5	18	83%
Lebanon (Oscar Mayer)	.8 oz	46	4.7	0.4	302	0	2.9	1.4	16	56%
Turkey										
(Butterball) 'Cold Cuts'	1 oz	70	4.0	2.0	370	0	6.0	(mq)	(mq)	69%
(Butterball) 'Deli/Slice 'n Serve'	1 oz	70	4.0	2.0	370	0	6.0	(mq)	(mq)	69%
(Butterball) 'Turkey Variety Pak'	.75 oz	50	3.0	1.0	280	0	4.0	(mq)	(mq)	69%
(Healthy Choice) beef and pork	.75-oz slice	25	3.0	1.0	240	na	1.0	<1.0	10	36%
(Longacre) sliced	1 oz	61	4.0	0.0	270	0	5.0	(mq)	25	74%
(Louis Rich)	1 oz	61	3.4	0.6	244	0	5.0	1.5	22	74%
(Louis Rich) mild	1 oz	59	3.8	0.7	298	0	4.5	1.5	18	69%
(Norbest) 'Blue Label' 2-2.5 lb	1 oz	68	3.5	0.5	331	0	5.6	(mq)	(mq)	76%
(Norbest) 'Blue Label' 5-lb	1 oz	57	3.8	0.3	339	0	4.4	(mq)	(mq)	71%
(OHSE)	1 oz	70	3.0	2.0	300	0	6.0	(mq)	(mq)	73%
CHICKEN										
Breast										
(Healthy Choice) deli-thin, 97% fat-free	1 slice	10	2.0	<1.0	90	na	<1.0	<1.0	5	<43%
(Healthy Choice) oven roasted, 97% fat-free	1 slice	30	6.0	1.0	300	na	<1.0	<1.0	15	<24%
(Healthy Favorites) oven roasted	.4-oz slice	12	2.0	<1.0	110	na	<1.0	na	5	<43%
(Hillshire Farm) smoked 'Deli Select'	1 oz	31	6.0	<1.0	290	0	0.2	(mq)	(mq)	6%
(Longacre) 'Premium'	1 oz	45	4.0	1.0	280	0	3.0	(mq)	20	57%
(Louis Rich) hickory smoked	1 oz	30	5.1	0.6	356	0	0.8	0.3	14	24%
(Louis Rich) oven roasted 'Deluxe'	1 oz	30	4.9	0.6	332	0	0.8	0.3	14	25%
(Louis Rich) oven roasted 'Thin Sliced'	.4-oz slice	12	1.9	0.2	130	0	0.3	0.1	6	24%
(Louis Rich) oven roasted, white meat	1-oz slice	35	4.9	0.1	301	0	1.7	0.5	16	43%
(Mr. Turkey)	1 oz	32	4.8	0.6	242	0	1.1	(mq)	9	31%
(Oscar Mayer) oven roasted	1 oz	29	5.2	0.6	414	0	0.7	0.2	15	21%
(Oscar Mayer) smoked	1 oz	25	5.3	0.2	397	0	0.4	0.2	15	14%
(Oscar Mayer) 'Thin Sliced'	.4-oz slice	13	2.1	0.3	151	0	0.4	0.1	5	27%
(Tyson) hickory smoked	1 slice	25	4.0	0.8	195	na	1.0	na	na	32%
(Tyson) honey flavored	1 slice	25	4.0	0.8	na	na	1.0	na	na	32%
(Tyson) mesquite, oven roasted	1 slice	25	4.0	0.8	na	na	1.0	na	na	32%
(Tyson) oven roasted	1 slice	25	3.7	0.8	185	na	0.5	na	na	20%
Roll										
(Longacre)	1 oz	60	4.0	1.0	210	0	5.0	(mq)	25	69%
(Pilgrim's Pride)	1-oz slice	35	5.2	0.4	260	0	1.2	(mq)	15	33%
(Tyson)	1 slice	26	3.2	1.4	153	na	0.5	na	na	20%
CHICKEN HAM										
(Healthy Favorites) smoked, w/natural juices	.4-oz slice	13	2.2	0.2	116	0	0.4	0.1	7	27%
(Pilgrim's Pride)	1-oz slice	35	4.0	0.8	430	0	1.8	(mq)	18	46%
CORNED BEEF LOAF, jellied	1 oz	43	6.5	0.0	270	0	1.7	0.7	13	37%
DUTCH BRAND LOAF										
	1-oz slice	68	3.8	1.6	354	0	5.1	1.8	13	68%

Food Name	Serving Size	Calories	Prot. gms	Carbs gms	Sod. mgs	Fiber gms	Fat gms	Sat. Fat gms	Chol. mgs	% Fat Cal.
(Eckrich)	1-oz slice	70	3.0	2.0	300	0	6.0	(mq)	(mq)	73%
(Eckrich) 'Lean Supreme'	1-oz slice	60	4.0	2.0	250	0	4.0	(mq)	(mq)	60%
(Eckrich) 'Smorgas Pac'	1-oz slice	70	3.0	2.0	300	0	6.0	(mq)	(mq)	73%
(Kahn's)	1 slice	80	3.0	1.0	280	0	7.0	(mq)	(mq)	80%
HAM										
(Boar's Head) boiled 'Deluxe'	1 oz	28	5.0	1.0	275	0	<1.0	(mq)	15	<27%
(Boar's Head) deluxe 'Deli-trition' low cholesterol	1 oz	30	5.0	1.0	280	na	1.0	na	15	30%
(Boar's Head) 'Lower Salt'	1 oz	28	5.0	<1.0	250	0	<1.0	(mq)	15	<27%
(Healthy Deli)	1 oz	33	5.9	0.2	120	0	0.8	(mq)	13	23%
(Healthy Deli) 'Deluxe'	1 oz	31	4.7	1.1	245	0	0.9	(mq)	12	26%
(Healthy Deli) 'Lessalt'	1 oz	32	4.7	1.4	190	0	0.9	(mq)	13	25%
(Healthy Deli) 'Light AM'	1 oz	27	3.9	1.4	200	0	0.6	(mq)	11	20%
(Healthy Deli) 'Taverne'	1 oz	31	5.4	0.3	210	0	0.8	(mq)	15	24%
(Healthy Favorites) boiled	.4-oz slice	12	2.0	<1.0	115	na	<1.0	na	5	<43%
(Hormel)	1 oz	29	4.0	1.0	344	na	1.0	<2.0	11	31%
(JM)	1 oz	30	4.0	1.0	360	0	1.0	(mq)	(mq)	31%
(JM) 'Slice 'n Eat' 93% Fat-free	2 oz	70	10.0	1.0	630	0	3.0	(mq)	24	38%
(JM) 'Slice 'n Eat' 95% Fat-free, presliced	2 slices	60	9.0	1.0	620	0	2.0	(mq)	30	31%
(Jones Dairy Farm) 'Farm'	1 slice	50	8.8	tr	381	0	1.1	(mq)	21	22%
(Jones Dairy Farm) 'Four Family Ham'	1 oz	35	5.8	tr	298	0	1.2	(mq)	14	32%
(Kahn's)	1 slice	30	5.0	1.0	360	0	1.0	(mq)	(mq)	27%
(Kahn's) 'Low Salt'	1 slice	30	5.0	1.0	290	0	1.0	(mq)	(mq)	27%
(Light & Lean)	2 slices	50	9.0	0.0	(mq)	0	2.0	(mq)	(mq)	33%
(OHSE)	1 oz	30	5.0	1.0	260	0	1.0	(mq)	(mq)	27%
(Oscar Mayer) boiled	.75-oz slice	23	3.9	0.3	275	0	0.7	0.1	12	27%
(Oscar Mayer) boiled 'Thin Sliced'	.4 oz	13	2.2	0.2	157	0	0.4	0.1	7	27%
(Oscar Mayer) 'Breakfast Ham'	1.5-oz slice	47	7.2	1.2	582	0	1.5	0.6	21	29%
(Oscar Mayer) 'Jubilee'	1 oz	43	5.3	0.1	365	0	2.4	0.8	15	50%
(Oscar Mayer) 'Lower Salt'	.7 oz	23	3.6	0.6	174	0	0.7	0.3	10	27%
(Swift) 'Premium Hostess'	1 oz	30	5.0	0.0	330	0	1.0	(mq)	(mq)	31%
(Swift) 'Premium Sugar Plum'	1 oz	30	5.0	1.0	280	0	1.0	(mq)	(mq)	27%
Baked										
(Healthy Deli) Virginia	1 oz	34	4.8	1.6	245	0	0.9	(mq)	12	24%
(Healthy Deli) Virginia 'Lessalt'	1 oz	32	4.7	1.4	19	0	0.9	(mq)	13	25%
(Louis Rich) 'Carving Board' cooked w/natural juices	22 grams	22	4.0	0.5	248	0	0.4	0.2	12	17%
(Oscar Mayer)	.75-oz slice	21	3.9	0.4	238	0	0.5	0.1	11	21%
Barbecue (Light & Lean)	2 slices	50	8.0	0.0	(mq)	0	2.0	(mq)	(mq)	36%
Black Forest (Healthy Deli)	1 oz	32	5.9	0.4	220	0	0.6	(mq)	16	18%
Cajun (Hillshire Farm) 'Deli Select'	1 oz	31	6.0	<1.0	350	(tr)	0.9	(mq)	(mq)	22%
Capocollo (Hormel)	1 oz	80	5.0	0.0	273	0	6.0	(mq)	(mq)	73%
Chopped										
(Eckrich)	1-oz slice	45	5.0	<1.0	350	0	2.0	(mq)	(mq)	43%
(Eckrich) 'Lean Supreme'	1-oz slice	35	10.0	<1.0	350	0	2.0	(mq)	(mq)	29%
(Hormel) 'Black Label'	1 oz	70	4.0	1.0	326	na	6.0	2.0	16	73%
(Hormel) 'Perma-Fresh'	2 slices	88	11.0	0.0	685	0	5.0	(mq)	(mq)	51%
(JM)	1-oz slice	80	4.0	1.0	370	0	7.0	(mq)	(mq)	76%
(Kahn's)	1 slice	50	5.0	1.0	000	0	3.0	(mq)	(mq)	53%
(Light & Lean)	2 slices	70	8.0	0.0	(mq)	0	4.0	(mq)	(mq)	53%
(OHSE)	1 oz	65	4.0	1.0	260	0	5.0	(mq)	(mq)	69%
(Oscar Mayer)	1-oz slice	41	4.4	0.7	303	0	2.3	0.7	14	50%
Glazed (Light & Lean)	2 slices	50	9.0	0.0	(mq)	0	2.0	(mq)	(mq)	33%
Honey										
(Boar's Head) 'Premium' low cholesterol	1 oz	35	5.0	2.0	310	na	1.0	na	15	26%
(Carl Buddig) 'Lean' smoked, chopped	1 oz	50	5.0	1.0	na	na	3.0	na	na	53%

Food Name	Serving Size	Calories	Prot. gms	Carbs gms	Sod. mgs	Fiber gms	Fat gms	Sat. Fat gms	Chol. mgs	% Fat Cal.
(Healthy Choice) 'Deli-Thin'	1 slice	10	2.0	<1.0	90	na	<1.0	<1.0	5	<43%
(Healthy Deli) 'Honey Valley'	1 oz	31	4.8	1.2	26	0	0.8	(mq)	10	23%
(Healthy Favorites)	1 slice	14	2.0	<1.0	115	na	<1.0	na	5	<43%
(Healthy Favorites) 'Breakfast' water added	1 oz	30	4.7	0.7	346	0	0.9	0.4	14	27%
(Hillshire Farm) 'Deli Select'	1 oz	31	6.0	<1.0	270	0	0.9	(mq)	(mq)	22%
(Louis Rich) 'Carving Board' w/natural juices	2.1 oz	68	10.9	1.8	761	0	1.9	0.9	33	25%
(Oscar Mayer)	.75-oz slice	23	3.8	0.5	268	0	0.6	0.3	12	24%
(Oscar Mayer) 'Thin Sliced'	.4-oz slice	13	2.2	0.3	153	0	0.4	0.2	7	27%
Jalapeño (Healthy Deli)	1 oz	25	3.7	0.8	260	(tr)	0.6	(mq)	11	23%
Peppered										
(Light & Lean) black pepper	2 slices	50	9.0	0.0	(mq)	(tr)	2.0	(mq)	(mq)	33%
(Light & Lean) red pepper	2 slices	50	9.0	0.0	(mq)	(tr)	2.0	(mq)	(mq)	33%
(Oscar Mayer) cracked black pepper	.75-oz slice	22	3.8	0.2	284	(tr)	0.8	0.3	11	31%
Prosciutto (Hormel)	1 oz	90	7.0	0.0	502	0	7.0	(mq)	(mq)	69%
Smoked										
(Carl Buddig) 'Lean' chopped	1 oz	50	5.0	1.0	na	na	3.0	na	na	53%
(Eckrich) 'Slender Sliced'	1 oz	40	5.0	1.0	360	0	2.0	(mq)	(mq)	43%
(Healthy Favorites)	.4-oz slice	14	2.0	<1.0	115	na	<1.0	na	5	<43%
(Hillshire Farm) 'Deli Select'	1 oz	31	6.0	<1.0	300	0	0.9	(mq)	(mq)	22%
(JM) golden	2 oz	80	8.0	1.0	630	0	5.0	(mq)	(mq)	56%
(JM) golden, water added	2 oz	70	8.0	4.0	810	0	2.0	(mq)	23	27%
(Light & Lean)	2 slices	50	9.0	0.0	(mq)	0	2.0	(mq)	(mq)	33%
(Louis Rich) 'Carving Board' w/natural juices	10 grams	11	1.8	0.0	124	0	0.4	0.1	5	33%
(OHSE) '95% Fat-Free'	1 oz	30	5.0	1.0	310	0	1.0	(mq)	(mq)	27%
(Oscar Mayer)	.75-oz slice	22	3.8	0.1	266	0	0.7	0.3	12	29%
HAM AND CHEESE LOAF										
(Eckrich)	1-oz slice	50	4.0	1.0	300	0	4.0	(mq)	(mq)	64%
(Hormel) '8 lb' canned	3 oz	260	13.0	1.0	1135	0	22.0	(mq)	(mq)	78%
(Hormel) 'Perma-Fresh'	2 slices	110	11.0	0.0	668	0	7.0	(mq)	(mq)	59%
(Kahn's)	1 slice	70	4.0	1.0	310	0	6.0	(mq)	(mq)	73%
(Light & Lean)	2 slices	90	8.0	0.0	(mq)	0	6.0	(mq)	(mq)	63%
(OHSE)	1 oz	65	4.0	2.0	190	0	5.0	(mq)	(mq)	65%
(Oscar Mayer)	1-oz slice	66	4.2	1.0	358	0	5.0	2.4	19	68%
HEAD CHEESE (Oscar Mayer)	1-oz slice	55	4.5	0.1	347	0	4.0	1.4	25	66%
HONEY LOAF										
(Eckrich)	1-oz slice	35	4.0	2.0	280	0	1.0	(mq)	(mq)	27%
(Eckrich) 'Smorgas Pac'	1-oz slice	35	4.0	2.0	280	0	1.0	(mq)	(mq)	27%
(Hormel) 'Perma-Fresh'	2 slices	90	1.0	0.0	584	0	5.0	(mq)	(mq)	92%
(Kahn's)	1 slice	40	4.0	1.0	320	0	2.0	(mq)	(mq)	47%
(Oscar Mayer)	1-oz slice	34	5.2	1.0	378	0	1.0	0.4	16	27%
IOWA BRAND LOAF (Hormel) 'Perma-Fresh'	2 slices	90	10.0	0.0	607	0	6.0	(mq)	(mq)	57%
JALAPEÑO LOAF (Kahn's)	1 slice	70	3.0	2.0	340	na	6.0	(mq)	(mq)	73%
LIVER CHEESE										
(JM)	1-oz slice	70	4.0	1.0	(mq)	0	6.0	(mq)	(mq)	73%
(Oscar Mayer)	1.34-oz slice	116	5.8	0.5	418	0	10.0	3.5	80	78%
LIVER LOAF										
(Hormel) 'Perma-Fresh'	2 slices	160	9.0	1.0	704	0	13.0	(mq)	(mq)	75%
(Kahn's)	1 slice	170	6.0	3.0	370	0	15.0	(mq)	(mq)	79%
LIVERWURST/liver sausage										
(Hickory Farms)	1 oz	97	4.0	1.0	249	0	9.0	(mq)	74	80%
(Jones Dairy Farm) 'Farm Club'	1 oz	80	4.5	tr	254	0	6.3	(mq)	43	76%
(Jones Dairy Farm) 'Farm Slices'	1 slice	75	3.5	tr	186	0	6.6	(mq)	43	81%
LOAF										
(Hormel) spiced, canned	3 oz	280	11.0	2.0	1110	0	26.0	(mq)	(mq)	82%

Food Name	Serving Size	Calories	Prot. gms	Carbs gms	Sod. mgs	Fiber gms	Fat gms	Sat. Fat gms	Chol. mgs	% Fat Cal.
(JM) 'P&B'	1-oz slice	70	3.0	2.0	330	0	5.0	(mq)	(mq)	69%
(Kahn's) 'P&B'	1 slice	40	5.0	1.0	270	0	2.0	(mq)	(mq)	43%
(OHSE)	1 oz	75	3.0	1.0	320	0	6.0	(mq)	(mq)	77%
MACARONI AND CHEESE LOAF										
(Eckrich)	1-oz slice	75	3.0	3.0	320	(mq)	6.0	(mq)	(mq)	69%
(OHSE)	1 oz	60	4.0	4.0	310	(mq)	3.0	(mq)	(mq)	46%
OLD-FASHIONED LOAF (Oscar Mayer)	1-oz slice	62	4.0	2.4	337	(tr)	4.0	1.6	16	58%
OLIVE LOAF										
(Eckrich)	1-oz slice	80	3.0	2.0	320	(tr)	6.0	(mq)	(mq)	73%
(Hormel) 'Perma-Fresh'	2 slices	110	7.0	5.0	810	(tr)	7.0	(mq)	(mq)	57%
(Oscar Mayer)	1-oz slice	63	2.9	3.2	392	(tr)	4.3	1.5	8	61%
PASTRAMI. See also TURKEY PASTRAMI.										
(Boar's Head) 'Round'	1 oz	40	6.0	<1.0	270	0	1.5	(mq)	16	33%
(Carl Buddig) 'Lean' smoked, chopped, sliced	1 oz	40	5.0	1.0	na	na	2.0	na	na	43%
(Healthy Deli) 'Deli Round'	1 oz	34	5.3	0.8	195	0	1.1	(mq)	14	29%
(Hillshire Farm) 'Deli Select'	1 oz	31	6.0	<1.0	290	0	0.4	(mq)	(mq)	11%
(Oscar Mayer)	.6-oz slice	16	3.4	0.1	217	0	0.3	0.2	7	16%
PEPPERED BEEF										
(Carl Buddig) 'Lean' smoked, chopped, sliced	1 oz	40	5.0	1.0	na	na	2.0	na	na	43%
(Eckrich)	1-oz slice	35	5.0	2.0	340	(tr)	1.0	(mq)	(mq)	24%
(Kahn's)	1 slice	40	5.0	1.0	340	(tr)	2.0	(mq)	(mq)	43%
(Oscar Mayer)	1-oz slice	39	5.1	1.2	367	(tr)	1.5	0.8	14	35%
PICKLE LOAF										
(Eckrich)	1-oz slice	80	3.0	2.0	270	(tr)	6.0	(mq)	(mq)	73%
(Eckrich) 'Smorgas-Pac'	1-oz slice	80	3.0	2.0	270	(tr)	6.0	(mq)	(mq)	73%
(Hormel) 'Perma-Fresh'	2 slices	102	8.0	3.0	752	(tr)	7.0	(mq)	(mq)	59%
(Kahn's)	1 slice	80	3.0	2.0	280	(tr)	7.0	(mq)	(mq)	76%
(Kahn's) 'Family-Pack'	1 slice	70	3.0	2.0	220	(tr)	6.0	(mq)	(mq)	73%
(Light & Lean)	2 slices	100	8.0	3.0	(mq)	(tr)	6.0	(mq)	(mq)	55%
(OHSE)	1 oz	60	3.0	2.0	330	(tr)	4.0	(mq)	(mq)	64%
PICKLE-PIMIENTO LOAF (Oscar Mayer)	1-oz slice	66	3.1	4.1	370	(mq)	4.1	1.5	13	56%
PORK LOAF (Eckrich) 'Slender Sliced'	1 oz	45	5.0	1.0	320	0	2.0	(mq)	(mq)	43%
ROAST BEEF										
(Healthy Deli)	1 oz	30	6.4	0.2	130	0	0.4	(mq)	13	12%
(Healthy Deli) Italian	1 oz	31	6.2	0.1	140	0	0.6	(mq)	16	18%
(Hillshire Farm) 'Deli Select' oven roasted, cured, w/o added ingredients	1 oz	31	6.0	<1.0	270	0	0.5	(mq)	(mq)	14%
(Oscar Mayer) 'Thin Sliced'	.4-oz slice	14	2.4	0.2	55	0	0.4	0.2	5	26%
SALAMI. See also TURKEY SALAMI.										
Beef										
(Boar's Head)	1 oz	60	5.0	<1.0	288	0	4.0	(mq)	20	60%
(Hebrew National) 'Original Deli-Style'	1 oz	80	7.0	<1.0	230	0	7.0	(mq)	15	66%
(Hormel) 'Party'	1 oz	90	5.0	0.0	399	0	8.0	(mq)	(mq)	78%
(Hormel) 'Perma-Fresh'	2 slices	50	3.0	0.0	219	0	5.0	(mq)	(mq)	79%
(Kahn's)	1 slice	70	3.0	1.0	250	0	6.0	(mq)	(mq)	77%
(Kahn's) 'Family-Pack'	1 slice	60	2.0	1.0	190	0	5.0	(mq)	(mq)	79%
(Oscar Mayer) 'Machiaeh Brand'	.8-oz slice	60	3.0	0.0	265	0	5.0	(mq)	15	70%
Beer										
(Eckrich)	1-oz slice	70	4.0	1.0	330	0	6.0	(mq)	(mq)	73%
(Oscar Mayer) 'Salami for Beer'	.8-oz slice	50	3.2	0.4	286	0	4.0	1.7	15	71%
(Oscar Mayer) 'Salami for Beer' beef	.8-oz slice	63	2.9	0.4	280	0	5.6	2.5	16	79%
Cooked										
(Kahn's)	1 slice	60	4.0	1.0	300	0	4.0	(mq)	(mq)	64%
(OHSE)	1 oz	65	4.0	1.0	330	0	5.0	(mq)	(mq)	69%

Food Name	Serving Size	Calories	Prot. gms	Carbs gms	Sod. mgs	Fiber gms	Fat gms	Sat. Fat gms	Chol. mgs	% Fat Cal.
Cotto										
(Eckrich)	1-oz slice	70	4.0	1.0	380	0	6.0	(mq)	(mq)	73%
(Eckrich) beef	1.3 oz	100	5.0	2.0	460	0	8.0	(mq)	(mq)	72%
(Hormel) 'Club'	1 oz	100	5.0	0.0	385	0	5.0	(mq)	(mq)	69%
(Hormel) 'Perma-Fresh'	2 slices	105	9.0	1.0	750	0	7.0	(mq)	(mq)	61%
(JM)	1-oz slice	80	4.0	2.0	270	0	6.0	(mq)	(mq)	69%
(Kahn's) 'Family Pack'	1 slice	45	3.0	1.0	230	0	3.0	(mq)	(mq)	63%
(Light & Lean)	2 slices	80	6.0	0.0	(mq)	0	6.0	(mq)	(mq)	69%
(Oscar Mayer) beef	.8-oz slice	45	3.3	0.4	296	0	3.4	1.6	19	67%
(Oscar Mayer) beef	.5-oz slice	29	2.1	0.3	193	0	2.2	1.0	12	67%
Dry or hard										
(Hickory Farms)	1 oz	120	6.0	0.0	535	0	10.0	(mq)	30	79%
(Hormel)	1 oz	110	7.0	0.0	468	0	10.0	(mq)	(mq)	76%
(Hormel) 'Homeland'	1 oz	117	6.0	2.0	448	na	10.0	4.0	29	74%
(Hormel) 'National Brand'	1 oz	120	6.0	0.0	463	0	11.0	(mq)	(mq)	81%
(Hormel) 'Perma-Fresh'	2 slices	80	4.0	0.0	339	0	7.0	(mq)	(mq)	80%
(Hormel) 'Sliced'	1 oz	110	6.0	0.0	483	0	10.0	(mq)	(mq)	79%
(JM)	1-oz slice	110	6.0	1.0	580	0	9.0	(mq)	(mq)	74%
(Oscar Mayer)	.8-oz slice	52	3.1	0.4	287	0	4.2	1.9	19	73%
(Oscar Mayer) 'Hard'	.3-oz slice	33	2.0	0.1	169	0	2.8	1.2	8	75%
Genoa										
(Hickory Farms)	1 oz	110	6.0	0.0	540	0	10.0	(mq)	20	79%
(Hormel)	1 oz	110	6.0	0.0	456	0	10.0	(mq)	(mq)	79%
(Hormel) 'DiLusso'	1 oz	100	6.0	0.0	443	0	8.0	(mq)	(mq)	75%
(Hormel) 'Gran Valore'	1 oz	110	6.0	0.0	453	0	10.0	(mq)	(mq)	79%
(Hormel) 'San Remo Brand'	1 oz	118	7.0	0.0	541	0	10.0	(mq)	(mq)	76%
(JM)	1-oz slice	100	6.0	1.0	540	0	8.0	(mq)	(mq)	72%
(Oscar Mayer)	.3-oz slice	34	1.9	0.1	162	0	2.8	1.2	9	76%
Piccolo (Hormel) 'Stick'	1 oz	120	6.0	0.0	512	0	11.0	(mq)	(mq)	81%
SOUSE LOAF (Kahn's)	1 slice	90	4.0	1.0	190	0	7.0	(mq)	(mq)	76%
SPICE LOAF										
(Hormel) canned	3 oz	280	11.0	2.0	1110	0	26.0	(mq)	(mq)	82%
(Hormel) 'Perma-Fresh'	2 slices	118	9.0	1.0	702	0	9.0	(mq)	(mq)	67%
(JM)	1-oz slice	70	4.0	1.0	370	0	6.0	(mq)	(mq)	73%
(Kahn's) 'Family Pack'	1 slice	70	3.0	1.0	180	0	6.0	(mq)	(mq)	77%
(Kahn's) 'Family Pack' beef	1 slice	60	2.0	1.0	200	0	5.0	(mq)	(mq)	79%
(Kahn's) 'Luncheon Loaf'	1 slice	80	3.0	1.0	240	0	7.0	(mq)	(mq)	80%
TURKEY. See also TURKEY LOAF / ROLL.										
(Boar's Head) 'Premium' skin on, low cholesterol	1 oz	35	6.0	1.0	200	na	1.0	na	20	26%
(Butterball) 'Cold Cuts'	1 oz	30	5.0	1.0	230	0	1.0	(mq)	(mq)	27%
(Butterball) 'Deli No Salt Added'	1 oz	45	7.0	0.0	15	0	2.0	(mq)	(mq)	39%
(Healthy Choice) 97% fat free	1 slice	30	6.0	<1.0	240	na	1.0	<1.0	10	24%
(Healthy Deli) 'Gourmet'	1 oz	28	4.9	0.5	170	0	0.6	(mq)	9	20%
(Healthy Deli) 'Lessalt'	1 oz	25	4.5	0.4	140	0	0.5	(mq)	9	19%
(Hormel) 'Perma-Fresh'	2 slices	60	9.0	0.0	484	0	2.0	(mq)	(mq)	33%
(Light & Lean)	2 slices	60	8.0	0.0	(mq)	0	2.0	(mq)	(mq)	36%
(Longacre) 'Catering'	1 oz	35	6.0	<1.0	280	0	1.0	(mq)	15	24%
(Norbest) white meat, diced	1 oz	31	4.4	1.0	318	0	0.9	(mq)	(mq)	27%
(Tyson)	1 slice	20	4.0	0.3	136	na	0.4	na	na	17%
Honey roasted (Healthy Deli)	1 oz	28	4.9	0.5	170	0	0.5	(mq)	9	17%
Honey roasted and smoked										
(Healthy Choice)	1-oz slice	35	6.0	1.0	230	na	1.0	<1.0	15	24%
(Healthy Choice) deli thin	1 slice	10	2.0	<1.0	70	na	<1.0	<1.0	5	<43%

Food Name	Serving Size	Calories	Prot. gms	Carbs gms	Sod. mgs	Fiber gms	Fat gms	Sat. Fat gms	Chol. mgs	% Fat Cal.
Oven roasted										
(Healthy Choice) deli thin	1 slice	10	2.0	<1.0	85	na	<1.0	<1.0	5	<43%
(Healthy Choice) 97% fat free	1-oz slice	30	6.0	<1.0	290	na	1.0	<1.0	10	24%
(Healthy Deli)	1 oz	26	4.7	0.4	180	0	0.2	(mq)	8	8%
(Healthy Favorites)	.4-oz slice	12	2.0	<1.0	100	na	<1.0	na	5	<43%
(Hillshire Farm) 'Deli Select'	1 oz	31	6.0	<1.0	340	0	0.2	(mq)	(mq)	6%
(Longacre)	1 oz	30	5.0	1.0	280	0	1.0	(mq)	10	27%
(Louis Rich)	1 oz	31	4.8	1.1	323	0	0.8	0.3	11	23%
(Louis Rich) 'Thin Sliced'	.4-oz slice	12	1.9	0.4	127	0	0.3	0.1	4	23%
(Oscar Mayer)	.75-oz slice	23	4.2	0.5	290	0	0.5	0.1	9	19%
(Oscar Mayer) 'Thin Sliced'	.4-oz slice	12	2.2	0.3	151	0	0.2	0.1	5	15%
Smoked										
(Butterball) 'Cold Cuts'	1 oz	35	5.0	0.0	190	0	1.0	(mq)	(mq)	31%
(Butterball) 'Turkey Variety Pak'	.75 oz	25	4.0	1.0	160	0	1.0	(mq)	(mq)	31%
(Carl Buttig) 'Lean' chopped, sliced	1 oz	50	5.0	1.0	na	na	3.0	na	na	53%
(Healthy Choice) deli thin	1 slice	10	2.0	<1.0	70	na	<1.0	<1.0	5	<43%
(Healthy Deli) '3 lb'	1 oz	29	4.8	0.5	180	0	0.5	(mq)	8	18%
(Healthy Favorites)	1 slice	12	2.0	<1.0	80	na	<1.0	na	5	<43%
(Hillshire Farm) 'Deli Select'	1 oz	31	6.0	<1.0	290	0	0.2	(mq)	(mq)	6%
(Longacre)	1 oz	26	5.0	1.0	260	0	<1.0	(mq)	10	<27%
(Louis Rich)	.74-oz slice	21	4.5	0.2	211	0	0.3	0.1	9	13%
(Louis Rich) 'Thin Sliced'	.4-oz slice	11	2.3	0.1	111	0	0.1	tr	5	9%
(Mr. Turkey)	1 oz	31	5.9	0.3	332	0	0.7	(mq)	10	20%
(Oscar Mayer)	.75-oz slice	20	4.3	0.2	300	0	0.2	0.1	9	9%
TURKEY HAM										
(Butterball) 'Cold Cuts'	1 oz	35	5.0	1.0	390	0	1.0	(mq)	(mq)	27%
(Butterball) 'Deli Thin'	1 oz	35	5.0	1.0	390	0	1.0	(mq)	(mq)	27%
(Butterball) 'Slice 'n Serve'	1 oz	35	5.0	1.0	340	0	2.0	(mq)	(mq)	43%
(Longacre)	1 oz	33	6.0	0.0	310	0	1.0	(mq)	20	27%
(Longacre) lean lite 'Deli'	1 oz	37	6.0	0.0	150	0	2.0	(mq)	25	43%
(Louis Rich) cured	1 oz	25	4.2	0.6	217	0	0.7	0.2	14	25%
Chopped										
(Louis Rich)	1 oz	46	5.2	0.2	289	0	2.8	0.7	19	54%
(Louis Rich) 92% fat-free, water added	1 oz	45	5.0	<1.0	285	na	2.0	na	25	43%
(Mr. Turkey)	1 oz	37	5.4	0.3	301	0	1.6	(mq)	17	39%
Chunk (Longacre)	1 oz	37	5.0	0.0	360	0	2.0	(mq)	25	47%
Honey cured										
(Butterball) 'Cold Cuts'	1 oz	35	5.0	1.0	380	0	1.0	(mq)	(mq)	27%
(Butterball) 'Cold Cuts' chopped	1 oz	35	5.0	2.0	290	0	1.0	(mq)	(mq)	24%
(Butterball) 'Slice 'n Serve'	1 oz	40	5.0	1.0	370	0	2.0	(mq)	(mq)	43%
(Louis Rich) 96% fat free	1 oz	25	4.0	<1.0	215	na	<1.0	na	15	<31%
(Mr. Turkey)	1 oz	32	5.4	0.3	286	0	1.0	(mq)	18	28%
(Mr. Turkey) breakfast	1 oz	33	5.0	0.4	306	0	1.3	(mq)	16	35%
(Mr. Turkey) buffet style	1 oz	32	4.7	0.4	340	0	1.3	(mq)	17	36%
(Mr. Turkey) 'Chub'	1 oz	32	4.7	0.4	340	0	1.3	(mq)	17	36%
Smoked										
(Louis Rich) 'Deli Thin' 96% fat free	1 slice	15	2.0	<1.0	110	na	<1.0	na	5	<43%
(Louis Rich) 94% fat free, water added	1 oz	35	5.0	<1.0	300	na	2.0	na	20	43%
(Louis Rich) 'Round'	1 oz	34	5.4	0.4	300	0	1.2	0.5	19	32%
(Louis Rich) 'Round' 95% fat free, water added	1-oz slice	30	5.0	<1.0	325	na	1.0	na	20	27%
(Louis Rich) 'Square'	.75-oz slice	24	4.1	0.3	213	0	0.7	0.3	14	26%
(Louis Rich) 'Square' 96% fat free	1-oz slice	25	4.0	<1.0	215	na	<1.0	na	15	<31%
(Louis Rich) 'Thin Sliced'	.4-oz slice	12	2.2	0.1	111	0	0.4	0.1	7	28%
(Louis Rich) 'Water Added'	1 oz	33	4.9	0.4	294	0	1.4	0.4	19	37%

Food Name	Serving Size	Calories	Prot. gms	Carbs gms	Sod. mgs	Fiber gms	Fat gms	Sat. Fat gms	Chol. mgs	% Fat Cal.
(Norbest) roll	1 oz	31	4.6	0.5	346	0	1.1	(mq)	(mq)	33%
(Norbest) thigh meat, Canadian style	1 oz	35	5.1	0.3	331	0	1.4	(mq)	(mq)	37%
(Norbest) thigh meat 'Gold Label'	1 oz	27	6.1	0.3	297	0	0.7	(mq)	(mq)	20%
(Norbest) thigh meat 'Tavern' 5-6 lb, whole	1 oz	27	5.4	0.3	311	0	0.8	(mq)	(mq)	24%
(Norbest) thigh meat 'Tavern' 2-2.5 lb, half	1 oz	29	4.7	0.6	312	0	0.8	(mq)	(mq)	25%
(OHSE)	1 oz	30	4.0	2.0	370	0	1.0	(mq)	(mq)	27%
TURKEY LOAF/ROLL										
(Louis Rich)	1 oz	45	4.6	0.4	270	0	2.8	0.8	16	56%
(Louis Rich) 89% fat free	1 oz	45	5.0	<1.0	270	na	3.0	na	15	53%
(Mr. Turkey) spiced	1 oz	51	4.2	0.5	292	0	3.6	(mq)	11	63%
TURKEY PASTRAMI										
(Butterball) 'Cold Cuts'	1 oz	30	5.0	0.0	290	0	1.0	(mq)	(mq)	31%
(Butterball) 'Slice 'n Serve'	1 oz	35	5.0	1.0	320	0	1.0	(mq)	(mq)	27%
(Longacre)	1 oz	32	5.0	0.0	260	0	1.0	(mq)	20	31%
(Louis Rich) 'Deli Thin' 96% fat-free	1 oz	10	2.0	<1.0	125	na	<1.0	na	5	<43%
(Louis Rich) 'Round'	1 oz	32	5.2	0.3	288	0	1.1	0.4	18	31%
(Louis Rich) 'Round' 96% fat-free	1 oz	35	5.0	<1.0	290	na	1.0	na	20	27%
(Louis Rich) 'Square'	1 oz	24	4.2	0.1	262	0	0.7	0.1	14	27%
(Louis Rich) 'Square' 96% fat-free	1 oz	25	4.0	<1.0	260	na	<1.0	na	15	<31%
(Louis Rich) Thin Sliced	1 oz	11	2.0	0.1	125	0	0.4	0.2	7	30%
(Mr. Turkey)	1 oz	28	4.8	0.1	383	0	0.9	(mq)	17	29%
(Norbest) '5-6 lb Slab'	1 oz	29	5.1	0.5	305	0	0.6	(mq)	(mq)	19%
(Norbest) '3 lb'	1 oz	29	4.8	0.3	302	0	0.8	(mq)	(mq)	26%
TURKEY SALAMI										
(Butterball) 'Cold Cuts'	1 oz	50	4.0	1.0	350	0	4.0	(mq)	(mq)	64%
(Butterball) 'Deli/Slice 'n Serve'	1 oz	50	4.0	1.0	350	0	4.0	(mq)	(mq)	64%
(Butterball) 'Turkey Variety Pak'	.75 oz	40	3.0	1.0	260	0	3.0	(mq)	(mq)	63%
(Longacre)	1 oz	52	4.0	1.0	290	0	4.0	(mq)	20	64%
(Louis Rich)	1 oz	54	4.4	0.2	263	0	4.0	1.1	20	66%
(Louis Rich) cotto	1 oz	53	4.4	0.3	271	0	3.8	1.1	21	65%
(Louis Rich) cotto, 85% fat free	1-oz slice	55	4.0	<1.0	275	na	4.0	na	25	64%
(Louis Rich) 85% fat-free	1-oz slice	55	4.0	<1.0	265	na	4.0	na	20	64%
(Mr. Turkey) cotto	1 oz	45	4.3	0.4	369	0	2.9	(mq)	16	58%
(Norbest) 'Blue Label' 5 lb	1 oz	46	4.3	0.5	270	0	2.9	(mq)	(mq)	58%
(Norbest) 'Blue Label' 2-2.5 lb	1 oz	45	4.2	0.9	314	0	2.6	(mq)	(mq)	53%
(OHSF)	1 oz	50	4.0	1.0	260	0	3.0	(mq)	(mq)	57%
LUNCHEON MEAT, ALTERNATIVE										
(Worthington) canned 'Numete' 1/2-inch slice	2.4 oz	160	8.0	6.0	570	(mq)	11.0	2.0	0	64%
(Worthington) canned 'Protose' 1/2-inch slice	2.7 oz	180	17.0	9.0	470	(mq)	8.0	1.0	0	41%
BOLOGNA TYPE										
(Worthington) frozen 'Bolono' approx .65-oz slices	2 slices	60	7.0	2.0	390	(mq)	2.0	0.0	0	33%
SALAMI TYPE										
(Worthington) frozen, roll, approx 1.5-oz slices	2 slices	90	8.0	3.0	760	(mq)	5.0	1.0	0	51%
(Worthington) frozen, sliced, approx 1.3-oz slices	2 slices	80	7.0	3.0	675	(mq)	4.0	1.0	0	47%
LUNCHEON MEAT, CANNED. See also POTTED MEAT SPREAD; SANDWICH SPREAD.										
(Armour) 'Treet'	2 oz	200	6.0	3.0	840	na	17.0	na	na	81%
(Armour) 'Treet' low salt	2 oz	190	6.0	3.0	610	na	16.0	na	na	80%
(Spam)	1 oz	86	4.0	<2.0	376	na	8.0	3.0	20	75%
(Spam) less salt	2 oz	176	8.0	1.0	550	na	15.0	5.0	38	79%
(Spam) lite	2 oz	140	8.0	1.0	560	na	12.0	4.0	43	75%
(Spam) smoke flavored	2 oz	170	8.0	0.0	774	0	15.0	(mq)	(mq)	81%
(Spam) w/cheese chunks	2 oz	170	8.0	0.0	811	0	16.0	(mq)	(mq)	82%

LUNCHEON MEAT COMBINATIONS, PACKAGED

(Eckrich) 'Lunch Makers'

Food Name	Serving Size	Calories	Prot. gms	Carbs gms	Sod. mgs	Fiber gms	Fat gms	Sat. Fat gms	Chol. mgs	% Fat Cal.
ham/Swiss cheese/crackers	1 pc each	40	2.0	2.0	170	na	2.0	na	5	53%
turkey/cheddar cheese/crackers	1 pc each	40	2.0	2.0	160	na	2.0	na	5	53%
(Hillshire Farms) 'Lunch 'n Munch'										
bologna/American cheese/crackers/Snickers	4.25 oz	490	15.0	31.0	1110	na	34.0	na	na	62%
bologna/American cheese/crackers/Snickers/6-oz drink	4.25 oz	590	15.0	55.0	1130	na	34.0	na	na	52%
chicken/Monterey jack cheese/crackers/Snickers	4.25 oz	400	19.0	31.0	1080	na	23.0	na	na	51%
ham/cheddar cheese/crackers/Snickers	4.25 oz	400	17.0	32.0	1010	na	23.0	na	na	51%
ham/cheddar cheese/crackers/Snickers/6-oz drink	4.25 oz	500	17.0	56.0	1030	na	23.0	na	na	42%
ham/Swiss cheese/crackers/Oreo	4.1 oz	370	16.0	30.0	1160	na	21.0	na	na	51%
turkey/cheddar cheese/crackers/brownie	4.5 oz	400	17.0	34.0	1240	na	22.0	na	na	49%
(Louis Rich) 'Lunch Breaks'										
turkey/cheddar cheese	1 pkg	410	22.0	23.0	1715	na	26.0	na	70	57%
turkey/Monterey jack cheese	1 pkg	400	21.0	27.0	1665	na	25.0	na	75	54%
turkey ham/Swiss cheese	1 pkg	380	24.0	25.0	1875	na	22.0	na	75	50%
turkey salami/cheddar cheese	1 pkg	430	22.0	25.0	1595	na	29.0	na	85	58%
(Oscar Mayer) 'Lunchables'										
bologna/American cheese/crackers	4.5 oz	480	18.0	20.0	1520	na	38.0	na	80	69%
chicken/Monterey jack cheese/crackers/pudding	6.2 oz	380	19.0	32.0	1200	na	21.0	na	45	48%
ham/American cheese/crackers/pudding	6.2 oz	410	19.0	33.0	1380	na	23.0	na	45	50%
ham/cheddar cheese/crackers	4.5 oz	370	21.0	18.0	1680	na	25.0	na	70	59%
ham/Swiss cheese/crackers	4.5 oz	340	22.0	18.0	1660	na	21.0	na	65	54%
ham/Swiss cheese/crackers/cookie	4.2 oz	380	18.0	29.0	1370	na	23.0	na	50	52%
turkey/cheddar cheese/crackers	4.5 oz	360	22.0	19.0	1600	na	22.0	na	70	55%
turkey/cheddar cheese/crackers/trail mix	5 oz	460	20.0	41.0	1230	na	26.0	na	40	49%
turkey/ham, deluxe variety pak	5.1 oz	370	23.0	23.0	1760	na	20.0	na	60	50%
turkey/Monterey jack cheese/wheat crackers	4.5 oz	360	21.0	18.0	1600	na	22.0	na	75	56%
LUPIN, mature seeds										
boiled	4 oz	135	17.7	11.2	5	>.8 c	3.3	0.4	0	20%
boiled	1/2 cup	99	12.9	8.2	3	2.3	2.4	0.3	0	20%
raw	1/2 cup	334	32.5	36.3	14	>12.4 c	8.8	1.0	0	22%
raw	1 oz	105	10.3	11.4	4	>3.9 c	2.8	0.3	0	23%

LYCHEE. See LITCHI.

M

Food Name	Serving Size	Calories	Prot. gms	Carbs gms	Sod. mgs	Fiber gms	Fat gms	Sat. Fat gms	Chol. mgs	% Fat Cal.
MACADAMIA NUT /bushnut										
in shell	1 lb	987	11.7	19.3	6	>7.4 c	103.7	15.5	0	88%
shelled	1 cup	941	11.1	18.4	7	12.5	98.8	14.8	0	88%
shelled	1 oz	199	2.4	3.9	1	2.6	20.9	3.1	0	88%
shelled, oil roasted, chopped	1 cup	790	8.0	14.2	8	>1.9 c	84.2	12.6	0	90%
shelled, oil roasted, kernels, 10-12	1 oz	204	2.1	3.7	2	>.5 c	21.7	3.3	0	89%
shelled, oil roasted, whole or halves	1 cup	962	9.7	17.3	9	>2.3 c	102.5	15.3	0	90%
shelled, w/salt *(Maunu Loa)*	1 oz	210	2.0	4.0	75	(mq)	21.0	(mq)	0	89%
MACADAMIA NUT BUTTER, roasted *(Maranatha Natural)*	2 tbsp	200	2.0	6.0	5	na	19.0	na	na	84%
MACARONI. See PASTA.										
MACARONI ENTRÉE, CANNED										
(Chef Boyardee) shells	7.5 oz	150	6.0	31.0	930	na	1.0	<1.0	na	6%
(Heinz)	7.5 oz	190	5.0	26.0	1105	(mq)	8.0	(mq)	(mq)	37%
W/BEEF, IN TOMATO SAUCE										
(Heinz)	7.5 oz	200	8.0	23.0	850	(mq)	8.0	(mq)	(mq)	37%
(Pathmark) 'No Frills'	7.5 oz	200	9.0	22.0	880	(mq)	8.0	(mq)	(mq)	37%

Food Name	Serving Size	Calories	Prot. gms	Carbs gms	Sod. mgs	Fiber gms	Fat gms	Sat. Fat gms	Chol. mgs	% Fat Cal.
W/CHEESE										
(Chef Boyardee)	7.5 oz	170	7.0	33.0	970	2.0	2.0	<1.0	25	10%
(Franco-American)	7 3/8 oz	170	6.0	24.0	870	(mq)	6.0	(mq)	(mq)	31%
Shells w/cheddar (Lipton) 'Hearty Ones'	11 oz	367	15.4	60.0	1406	(mq)	7.4	(mq)	14	18%
MACARONI ENTRÉE, FROZEN										
W/BEEF										
(Swanson)	12 oz	370	12.0	48.0	930	(mq)	15.0	(mq)	(mq)	36%
(Weight Watchers)	9 oz	220	14.0	31.0	510	na	4.0	2.0	10	17%
In tomato sauce (Lean Cuisine)	10 oz	250	14.0	35.0	540	na	6.0	1.0	25	22%
W/tomatoes (Stouffer's)	11.5-oz pkg	340	21.0	38.0	1440	na	12.0	na	na	31%
W/CHEESE										
(Banquet)	10 oz	420	14.0	46.0	450	(mq)	20.0	(mq)	30	43%
(Banquet) 'Casserole'	8 oz	350	11.0	36.0	930	(mq)	17.0	(mq)	(mq)	45%
(Banquet) 'Family Entrees'	8 oz	290	12.0	32.0	(mq)	(mq)	13.0	(mq)	(mq)	40%
(Budget Gourmet) 'Side Dish'	5.3 oz	210	9.0	23.0	370	(mq)	8.0	(mq)	25	36%
(Freezer Queen) 'Family Side Dish'	4 oz	110	3.0	19.0	420	(mq)	2.0	(mq)	(mq)	17%
(Green Giant)	5.7 oz	220	10.0	27.0	480	1.5	8.0	5.0	25	33%
(Green Giant) 'One Serving'	5.7 oz	230	9.0	28.0	590	(mq)	9.0	4.0	25	35%
(Healthy Choice)	9 oz	280	12.0	45.0	520	na	6.0	3.0	20	19%
(Healthy Choice)	8.5 oz	260	11.0	42.0	490	na	5.0	2.0	15	18%
(Kid Cuisine) 'Mega Meal'	12.45 oz	470	14.0	75.0	1270	na	13.0	na	na	25%
(Lean Cuisine)	9 oz	290	15.0	37.0	550	na	9.0	4.0	30	28%
(Myers)	3.5 oz	168	7.0	16.0	516	(mq)	9.0	(mq)	(mq)	47%
(Stouffer's) 76-oz pkg	9.5 oz	440	18.0	39.0	1150	na	24.0	na	na	49%
(Stouffer's) 12-oz pkg	6 oz	250	11.0	23.0	640	na	13.0	na	na	46%
(Swanson)	12.25 oz	370	13.0	43.0	1070	(mq)	15.0	(mq)	(mq)	38%
(Swanson) 'Homestyle Recipe'	10 oz	390	17.0	37.0	1150	(mq)	19.0	(mq)	(mq)	44%
Casserole (Morton)	6.5 oz	290	8.0	30.0	760	na	14.0	na	na	45%
Organic (Amy's Kitchen)	9 oz	452	22.0	58.0	434	na	18.0	na	na	34%
Pot pie (Swanson)	7 oz	200	7.0	24.0	740	(mq)	8.0	(mq)	(mq)	37%
W/broccoli (Lean Cuisine) 'Lunch Express'	9.75 oz	240	12.0	32.0	560	na	7.0	3.0	25	26%
W/cheddar and parmesan cheese (Budget Gourmet)										
'Light & Healthy'	10.5 oz	330	19.0	49.0	760	na	8.0	4.0	30	21%
W/mini franks (Kid Cuisine)	9 oz	380	9.0	55.0	1000	(mq)	14.0	(mq)	40	33%
W/soy cheese, organic (Amy's Kitchen)	9 oz	380	17.0	42.0	500	na	14.0	na	0	35%
W/3 cheeses (Weight Watchers)	9 oz	280	15.0	43.0	550	na	6.0	2.0	20	19%
MACARONI ENTRÉE, MICROWAVE										
W/BEEF										
(Chef Boyardee) 'Beefaroni'	7.5 oz	220	7.0	31.0	1145	2.0	7.0	1.0	18	29%
(Chef Boyardee) elbows in sauce	7.5 oz	210	8.0	29.0	1000	(mq)	7.0	(mq)	15	30%
(Kid's Kitchen) microwave cup	7.5 oz	200	11.0	25.0	780	na	6.0	2.0	25	27%
(Nalley's)	7.5 oz	180	9.0	29.0	900	(mq)	3.0	(mq)	(mq)	15%
W/CHEESE										
(Chef Boyardee)	7.5 oz	180	7.0	27.0	970	1.0	5.0	<1.0	20	25%
(Hormel) micro cup	7.5 oz	189	7.0	26.0	874	(mq)	6.0	(mq)	17	29%
(Kid's Kitchen) microwave cup	7.5 oz	260	12.0	28.0	650	na	11.0	6.0	45	38%
(Libby's) 'Diner' microwave cup	7.5 oz	360	14.0	27.0	1020	2.0	22.0	9.0	35	55%
(Lunch Bucket) microwave cup	7.5 oz	210	9.0	24.0	990	na	9.0	na	na	38%
MACARONI ENTRÉE, PACKAGED										
(Ultra Slim Fast) w/cheese sauce, prepared	1 cup	230	9.0	46.0	700	4.0	3.0	na	na	11%
MACARONI ENTRÉE MIX										
(Kraft) 'Dinner' spirals, prepared	3/4 cup	340	9.0	36.0	600	(mq)	18.0	4.0	10	47%
MEXICAN STYLE										
(Velveeta) 'Touch of Mexico' shells, prepared	1/2 cup	210	10.0	27.0	630	(mq)	8.0	4.0	20	33%

Food Name	Serving Size	Calories	Prot. gms	Carbs gms	Sod. mgs	Fiber gms	Fat gms	Sat. Fat gms	Chol. mgs	% Fat Cal.
W/CHEDDAR										
(Fantastic Foods) 'Traditional' prepared	1/2 cup	112	5.0	19.0	205	(mq)	2.0	(mq)	(mq)	16%
(Golden Grain) dry mix	1.81 oz	190	7.4	35.6	466	1.4	2.1	0.8	4	10%
(Golden Grain) prepared	1 serving	310	8.0	36.0	620	(mq)	15.0	(mq)	(mq)	43%
W/CHEESE										
(Kraft) 'Deluxe Dinner' prepared	3/4 cup	260	11.0	36.0	590	(mq)	8.0	4.0	20	28%
(Kraft) 'Dinner' prepared	3/4 cup	290	9.0	34.0	530	(mq)	13.0	3.0	5	41%
(Kraft) 'Dinomac Dinner' prepared	3/4 cup	310	9.0	36.0	560	(mq)	14.0	3.0	10	41%
(Kraft) 'Family Size Dinner' prepared	3/4 cup	290	9.0	34.0	490	(mq)	13.0	3.0	5	41%
(Kraft) 'Teddy Bears Dinner' prepared	3/4 cup	310	9.0	36.0	560	(mq)	14.0	3.0	10	41%
(Kraft) 'Wild Wheels Dinner' prepared	3/4 cup	310	9.0	36.0	560	(mq)	14.0	3.0	10	41%
(Velveeta) 'Bits of Bacon' shells, w/bacon, prepared	1/2 cup	240	11.0	27.0	690	(mq)	10.0	5.0	25	37%
(Velveeta) shells, prepared	1/2 cup	210	10.0	25.0	570	(mq)	8.0	4.0	20	34%
W/CURRY										
(Tofu Classics) 'Shells 'n Curry' prepared w/tofu	1/2 cup	103	8.0	15.0	275	(mq)	3.0	(mq)	na	23%
(Tofu Classics) 'Shells 'n Curry' prepared w/tofu and salted butter	1/2 cup	143	8.0	15.0	330	(mq)	7.0	(mq)	(mq)	41%
W/PARMESAN AND HERBS										
(Fantastic Foods) prepared w/whole milk	1/2 cup	109	5.0	19.0	264	(mq)	2.0	(mq)	(mq)	16%
MACE										
ground	1 oz	135	1.9	14.3	23	5.9	9.2	2.7	0	56%
ground	1 tbsp	25	0.4	2.7	4	1.1	1.7	0.5	0	55%
ground	1 tsp	8	0.1	0.9	1	.3	0.6	0.2	0	57%
ground *(Durkee)*	1 tsp	10	0.0	0.0	0	0	<0.1	na	na	<62%
ground *(Laurel Leaf)*	1 tsp	10	0.0	0.0	0	0	<0.1	na	na	<62%
ground *(Spice Islands)*	1 tsp	10	0.1	0.8	1	>.1 c	0.7	(mq)	0	64%
MACKEREL										
ATLANTIC										
baked	4 oz	297	27.0	0.0	94	0	20.2	4.7	85	63%
broiled	4 oz	297	27.0	0.0	94	0	20.2	4.7	85	63%
dry-heat cooked	3 oz	223	20.3	0.0	71	0	15.1	3.5	64	63%
microwaved	4 oz	297	27.0	0.0	94	0	20.2	4.7	85	63%
raw	1 lb	929	84.4	0.0	408	0	63.0	14.8	318	63%
raw	3 oz	174	15.8	0.0	77	0	11.8	2.8	59	63%
raw	1 oz	58	5.3	0.0	26	0	3.9	0.9	20	62%
JACK, mixed species										
canned, drained	1 cup	296	44.1	0.0	720	0	12.0	3.5	150	38%
canned, drained	4 oz	177	26.3	0.0	430	0	7.1	2.1	90	38%
dry-heat cooked	3 oz	171	21.9	0.0	94	0	8.6	2.5	51	47%
raw	1 lb	712	91.0	0.0	391	0	35.8	10.2	213	47%
raw	3 oz	134	17.1	0.0	73	0	6.7	1.9	40	47%
raw	1 oz	45	5.7	0.0	24	0	2.2	0.6	13	47%
KING										
dry-heat cooked	3 oz	114	22.1	0.0	173	0	2.2	0.4	58	18%
raw	1 lb	475	92.0	0.0	717	0	9.1	1.6	242	18%
raw	3 oz	89	17.2	0.0	134	0	1.7	0.3	45	18%
raw	1 oz	30	5.7	0.0	45	0	0.6	0.1	15	19%
PACIFIC, mixed species										
dry-heat cooked	3 oz	171	21.9	0.0	94	0	8.6	2.5	51	47%
raw	1 lb	712	91.0	0.0	391	0	35.8	10.2	213	47%
raw	3 oz	134	17.1	0.0	73	0	6.7	1.9	40	47%
raw	1 oz	45	5.7	0.0	24	0	2.2	0.6	13	47%
SPANISH										
baked	5.1-oz fillet	230	34.4	0.0	96	0	9.2	2.6	107	38%

Food Name	Serving Size	Calories	Prot. gms	Carbs gms	Sod. mgs	Fiber gms	Fat gms	Sat. Fat gms	Chol. mgs	% Fat Cal.
baked	4 oz	179	26.8	0.0	75	0	7.2	2.0	83	38%
broiled	5.1-oz fillet	230	34.4	0.0	96	0	9.2	2.6	107	38%
broiled	4 oz	179	26.8	0.0	75	0	7.2	2.0	83	38%
dry-heat cooked	3 oz	134	20.0	0.0	56	0	5.4	1.5	62	38%
microwaved	5.1-oz fillet	230	34.4	0.0	96	0	9.2	2.6	107	38%
microwaved	4 oz	179	26.8	0.0	75	0	7.2	2.0	83	38%
raw	1 lb	631	87.5	0.0	266	0	28.6	8.3	345	42%
raw	3 oz	118	16.4	0.0	50	0	5.3	1.5	65	42%
raw	1 oz	39	5.5	0.0	17	0	1.8	0.5	22	42%
MAHI MAHI/dolphin fish										
dry-heat cooked	3 oz	93	20.2	0.0	96	0	0.8	0.2	80	8%
raw	1 lb	387	83.9	0.0	397	0	3.2	0.9	331	8%
raw	3 oz	72	15.7	0.0	75	0	0.6	0.2	62	8%
raw	1 oz	24	5.2	0.0	25	0	0.2	0.1	21	8%
Fillet portions *(Peter Pan Seafoods)* raw	3.5 oz	85	18.5	na	88	na	0.7	na	73	8%
MALACCA APPLE, w/o seeds	1 oz	9	0.2	2.3	na	>.2 c	<.1	tr	0	<8%
MALT, DRY	1 oz	103	3.7	21.7	22	>1.6 c	0.5	0.0	0	4%
MALT EXTRACT, DRIED	1 oz	103	1.7	25.0	22	0	0.0	0.0	0	0%
MALT LIQUOR. See ALCOHOLIC BEVERAGES.										
MALT SYRUP										
	1 cup	1221	23.8	273.8	134	0	0.0	na	0	0%
	1 tbsp	76	1.5	17.1	8	0	0.0	na	0	0%
MALTED MILK DRINK MIX. See also BREAKFAST DRINK MIX, INSTANT.										
CHOCOLATE FLAVOR										
	1 oz	106	1.4	24.9	71	<.1	1.1	0.6	1	9%
w/added nutrients	1 oz	101	1.4	23.9	168	tr	1.0	0.6	na	8%
w/added nutrients	4-5 heap tsp	75	1.0	17.7	125	0	0.7	0.4	1	8%
(Carnation)	3 heap tsp	80	1.0	18.0	55	na	0.8	0.5	0	9%
(Kraft) 'Instant'	3 tsp	90	1.0	18.0	45	na	1.0	na	na	11%
NATURAL FLAVOR										
	1 oz	117	3.2	21.5	140	tr	2.2	1.2	6	17%
w/added nutrients	1 oz	109	2.5	23.0	115	<.1	0.8	0.4	na	7%
w/added nutrients	4-5 heap tsp	80	1.9	17.0	85	0	0.6	0.3	4	7%
w/o added nutrients	3/4 oz	87	2.3	15.9	104	0	1.7	0.9	4	17%
(Carnation) 'Original'	3 heap tsp	90	3.0	15.0	100	na	1.8	1.0	0	18%
(Kraft) 'Instant'	3 tsp	90	3.0	16.0	100	na	2.0	(mq)	na	19%
MAMMY APPLE										
peeled, w/o seeds	1 oz	14	0.1	3.5	4	.9	0.1	na	0	6%
raw	3 1/2 oz	51	0.5	12.5	15	3.0	0.5	na	0	8%
raw, trimmed, approx 3.1 lb	1 med	431	4.2	105.8	127	25.4	4.2	na	0	8%
raw, untrimmed	1 lb	139	1.4	34.0	41	>2.7 c	1.4	na	0	8%
MANDARIN ORANGE										
fresh, whole, approx 2 3/8 inch diam, 4.1 oz	1 med	37	0.5	9.4	1	1.9	0.2	<.1	0	4%
peeled, w/o seeds	1 oz	12	0.2	3.2	<1	.6	0.1	tr	0	6%
sections, w/o membrane	1/2 cup	43	0.6	10.9	2	2.3	0.2	<.1	0	4%
untrimmed	1 lb	144	2.1	36.6	4	7.4	0.6	0.1	0	3%
MANDARIN ORANGE, CANNED *(Dole)* sections	1/2 cup	70	0.0	19.0	10	na	<1.0	na	na	<11%
MANDARIN ORANGE DRINK										
w/papaya *(Tropicana)* 'Twister'	6 oz	90	<1.0	21.0	30	na	<1.0	na	na	<9%
MANGO										
peeled, w/o seed	1 oz	18	0.1	4.8	1	.3	0.1	<.1	0	4%
raw, sliced	1 cup	107	0.8	28.1	3	3.0	0.5	0.1	0	4%
raw, trimmed, approx 10.6 oz	1 med	135	1.1	35.2	4	3.7	0.6	0.1	0	4%
raw, untrimmed	1 lb	204	1.6	53.2	6	3.4	0.9	0.2	0	4%

Food Name	Serving Size	Calories	Prot. gms	Carbs gms	Sod. mgs	Fiber gms	Fat gms	Sat. Fat gms	Chol. mgs	% Fat Cal.
sliced, chilled, in jar *(Sun Fresh)* .... 3.5 oz		89	0.5	21.0	11	1.9	0.3	0.1	1	3%
MANGO DRINK										
(Arizona) 'Mucho Mango Cowboy Cocktail' .... 8 oz		100	0.0	27.0	20	na	0.0	na	na	0%
(Kern's) nectar, canned or bottled .... 6 oz		100	0.0	28.0	0	na	0.0	na	na	0%
(Libby's) nectar, canned or bottled .... 6 oz		110	0.0	26.0	0	na	0.0	na	na	0%
MANGO FLAVOR DRINK MIX *(Tang)* prepared .... 6 oz		80	0.0	20.0	0	na	0.0	na	0	0%
MANGO-PEACH JUICE *(Knudsen & Sons)* .... 8 oz		110	<1.0	29.0	na	na	0.0	na	na	0%
MANHATTAN. See ALCOHOLIC BEVERAGES.										
MANICOTTI ENTRÉE, FROZEN										
(Budget Gourmet) cheese, w/meat sauce .... 10 oz		450	20.0	33.0	920	(mq)	26.0	(mq)	50	53%
(Buitoni) 'Single Serving' .... 9 oz		470	18.0	45.0	830	(mq)	14.0	8.0	130	33%
(Celentano) .... 8 oz		300	16.0	36.0	690	(mq)	11.0	(mq)	(mq)	32%
(Celentano) cheese, w/sauce .... 10 oz		380	20.0	45.0	860	(mq)	14.0	(mq)	(mq)	33%
(Celentano) cheese, w/sauce .... 7 oz		360	21.0	35.0	580	(mq)	16.0	(mq)	(mq)	39%
(Celentano) low-fat, 'Great Choice' .... 10 oz		250	16.0	41.0	675	na	3.0	na	na	11%
(Healthy Choice) cheese .... 9.25 oz		220	15.0	34.0	310	na	3.0	2.0	30	12%
(Le Menu) three cheese .... 11.75 oz		390	19.0	44.0	870	(mq)	15.0	(mq)	(mq)	35%
(Legume) cheese, w/spinach, tofu, and sauce .... 11 oz		260	18.0	30.0	650	8.7	7.0	1.0	0	25%
(Legume) cheese, w/tofu and sauce, 'Classic' .... 8 oz		220	17.0	24.0	370	7.0	11.0	1.9	0	38%
(Weight Watchers) cheese .... 9.25 oz		260	17.0	31.0	510	na	8.0	3.0	25	27%
MANICOTTI NOODLE. See PASTA.										
MANIOC. See CASSAVA.										
MAPLE SYRUP. See also PANCAKE SYRUP.										
.... 1 cup		825	0.0	211.7	28	0	0.6	na	0	1%
.... 1 tbsp		52	0.0	13.4	2	0	0.0	na	0	0%
(Knudsen & Sons) 'Fruit 'N Maple' .... 1 oz		105	<1.0	26.0	na	na	<1.0	na	na	<8%
(Maple House) 100% pure .... 1 oz		100	0.0	61.0	4	na	0.0	na	0	0%
MARGARINE										
hydrogenated and regular corn oil .... 1 stick		815	1.0	1.0	1070	0	91.3	15.9	0	99%
hydrogenated and regular corn oil .... 1 tsp		34	0.0	0.0	44	0	3.8	0.7	0	100%
hydrogenated and regular soybean oil .... 1 stick		815	1.0	1.0	1070	0	91.3	14.9	0	99%
hydrogenated and regular soybean oil .... 1 tsp		34	0.0	0.0	44	0	3.8	0.6	0	100%
hydrogenated safflower and soybean oil .... 1 stick		815	1.0	1.0	1070	0	91.3	15.6	0	99%
hydrogenated safflower and soybean oil .... 1 tsp		34	0.0	0.0	44	0	3.8	0.7	0	100%
hydrogenated soybean and cottonseed oil .... 1 stick		815	1.0	1.0	1070	0	91.3	17.1	0	99%
hydrogenated soybean and cottonseed oil .... 1 tsp		34	0.0	0.0	44	0	3.8	0.7	0	100%
(A&P)										
'Corn Oil Quarters' .... 1 tbsp		100	<1.0	<1.0	105	0	11.0	2.0	0	93%
'Premium' .... 1 tbsp		100	<1.0	<1.0	110	0	11.0	2.0	0	93%
(Ann Page) 'Quarters' .... 1 tbsp		100	<1.0	<1.0	110	0	11.0	2.0	0	93%
(Blue Bonnet) stick .... 1 tbsp		100	0.0	0.0	95	na	11.0	2.0	0	100%
(Canoleo) 100% canola oil, all natural, dairy-free .... 1 tbsp		100	0.0	0.0	120	0	11.0	1.0	0	100%
(Fleischmann's)										
reduced calorie, 'Diet' .... 1 tbsp		50	0.0	0.0	50	na	6.0	1.0	0	100%
stick .... 1 tbsp		100	0.0	0.0	95	na	11.0	2.0	0	100%
unsalted, stick .... 1 tbsp		100	0.0	0.0	0	na	11.0	2.0	0	100%
(Hain)										
safflower oil .... 1 tbsp		100	0.0	0.0	170	0	11.0	2.0	0	100%
safflower oil, unsalted .... 1 tbsp		100	0.0	0.0	5	0	11.0	2.0	0	100%
(Hollywood)										
safflower oil .... 1 tbsp		100	0.0	0.0	130	0	11.0	5.0	0	100%
safflower oil, unsalted .... 1 tbsp		100	0.0	0.0	2	0	11.0	2.0	0	100%
(Imperial) reduced calorie, 'Diet' .... 1 tbsp		50	0.0	0.0	140	na	6.0	1.0	0	100%

Food Name	Serving Size	Calories	Prot. gms	Carbs gms	Sod. mgs	Fiber gms	Fat gms	Sat. Fat gms	Chol. mgs	% Fat Cal.
(Land O'Lakes)										
premium, corn oil, stick	1 tsp	35	0.0	0.0	35	na	4.0	1.0	0	100%
regular, soy oil, stick	1 tsp	35	0.0	0.0	35	na	4.0	1.0	0	100%
tub	1 tsp	35	0.0	0.0	35	0	4.0	(mq)	0	100%
(Mazola)										
reduced calorie, 'Diet'	1 tbsp	50	0.0	0.0	130	0	6.0	1.0	0	100%
regular	1 tbsp	100	0.0	0.0	100	0	11.0	2.0	0	100%
unsalted	1 tbsp	100	0.0	0.0	0	0	11.0	2.0	0	100%
(Nucoa)	1 tbsp	100	0.0	0.0	160	0	11.0	2.0	0	100%
(Parkay)	1 tbsp	100	0.0	0.0	105	0	11.0	2.0	0	100%
(Quincy's)	1 oz	204	<1.0	<1.0	268	0	22.0	(mq)	0	96%
(Spectrum Naturals) non-hydrogenated canola oil,										
100% dairy-free	1 tbsp	94	0.0	0.0	84	na	11.0	7.0	0	100%
MARGARINE, ALTERNATIVE										
hydrogenated and regular corn oil	1 cup	801	1.2	0.9	2226	0	90.0	14.9	0	99%
hydrogenated and regular corn oil	1 tsp	17	0.0	0.0	46	0	1.9	0.3	0	100%
hydrogenated soybean and cottonseed oil	1 cup	801	1.2	0.9	2226	0	90.0	16.7	0	99%
hydrogenated soybean and cottonseed oil	1 tsp	17	0.0	0.0	46	0	1.9	0.4	0	100%
hydrogenated soybean oil	1 cup	801	1.2	0.9	2226	0	90.0	15.1	0	99%
hydrogenated soybean oil	1 tsp	17	0.0	0.0	46	0	1.9	0.3	0	100%
MARGARINE, SOFT										
(A&P) bowl	1 tbsp	100	<1.0	<1.0	105	0	11.0	2.0	0	93%
(Blue Bonnet)	1 tbsp	100	0.0	0.0	95	na	11.0	2.0	0	100%
(Chiffon)										
cup	1 tbsp	90	0.0	0.0	95	0	10.0	1.0	0	100%
stick	1 tbsp	100	0.0	0.0	105	0	11.0	2.0	0	100%
unsalted	1 tbsp	90	0.0	0.0	0	0	10.0	2.0	0	100%
(Fleischmann's)										
lightly salted	1 tbsp	100	0.0	0.0	95	na	11.0	2.0	0	100%
unsalted	1 tbsp	100	0.0	0.0	0	na	11.0	2.0	0	100%
(Imperial)	1 tbsp	100	0.0	0.0	95	na	11.0	na	0	100%
(Nucoa)	1 tbsp	90	0.0	0.0	150	0	10.0	2.0	0	100%
(Parkay)										
reduced calorie, 'Diet'	1 tbsp	50	0.0	0.0	110	0	6.0	1.0	0	100%
regular	1 tbsp	100	0.0	0.0	105	0	11.0	2.0	0	100%
'Squeezable'	1 tbsp	90	0.0	0.0	110	0	10.0	2.0	0	100%
MARGARINE, WHIPPED										
(Blue Bonnet) stick	1 tbsp	70	0.0	0.0	70	na	7.0	1.0	0	100%
(Chiffon)	1 tbsp	70	0.0	0.0	80	0	8.0	1.0	0	100%
(Fleischmann's)										
lightly salted	1 tbsp	70	0.0	0.0	60	na	7.0	2.0	0	100%
unsalted	1 tbsp	70	0.0	0.0	0	na	7.0	2.0	0	100%
(Miracle Brand)										
cup	1 tbsp	60	0.0	0.0	70	0	7.0	1.0	0	100%
stick	1 tbsp	70	0.0	0.0	65	0	7.0	1.0	0	100%
(Parkay)										
cup	1 tbsp	70	0.0	0.0	70	0	7.0	1.0	0	100%
stick	1 tbsp	70	0.0	0.0	65	0	7.0	1.0	0	100%
MARGARINE SPREAD										
hydrogenated soybean and cottonseed oil, tub	1 cup	1236	1.4	0.0	2276	0	139.2	27.5	0	100%
hydrogenated soybean and cottonseed oil, tub	1 tsp	26	0.0	0.0	48	0	2.9	0.6	0	100%
hydrogenated soybean and hydrogenated and regular										
palm oils	1 tsp	26	0.0	0.0	48	0	2.9	0.7	0	100%

Food Name	Serving Size	Calories	Prot. gms	Carbs gms	Sod. mgs	Fiber gms	Fat gms	Sat. Fat gms	Chol. mgs	% Fat Cal.
hydrogenated soybean and hydrogenated and regular										
palm oils, tub	1 cup	1236	1.4	0.0	2276	0	139.2	30.9	0	100%
hydrogenated soybean and palm oil, stick	1 cup	1236	1.4	0.0	2276	0	139.2	32.3	0	100%
hydrogenated soybean and palm oil, stick	1 tsp	26	0.0	0.0	48	0	2.9	0.7	0	100%
60% corn oil margarine, 40% butter	1 stick	811	1.0	0.7	1014	na	91.2	32.1	99	99%
60% corn oil margarine, 40% butter	1 tsp	36	0.0	0.0	45	na	4.0	1.4	4	100%
(Blue Bonnet)										
48% vegetable oil	1 tbsp	60	<1.0	<1.0	115	na	6.0	1.0	5	87%
75% vegetable oil	1 tbsp	90	0.0	0.0	95	na	11.0	2.0	0	100%
whipped, 60% vegetable oil	1 tbsp	80	0.0	0.0	100	na	8.0	1.0	0	100%
(Blue Bonnet) 'Better Blend'										
soft	1 tbsp	90	0.0	0.0	95	na	11.0	2.0	0	100%
stick	1 tbsp	90	0.0	0.0	95	na	11.0	2.0	na	100%
unsalted	1 tbsp	90	0.0	0.0	0	na	11.0	1.0	5	100%
(Country Crock)										
'Churn style' stick	1 tbsp	80	0.0	0.0	55	na	9.0	2.0	0	100%
regular	1 tbsp	60	0.0	0.0	110	na	7.0	1.0	0	100%
(Fleischmann's) 'Move Over Butter'	1 tbsp	90	0.0	0.0	100	na	10.0	2.0	0	100%
(Hollywood) soft	1 tbsp	90	0.0	1.0	135	0	10.0	1.0	0	96%
(Imperial) 'Light'	1 tbsp	60	0.0	0.0	110	na	6.0	na	0	100%
(Kraft) 'Touch of Butter'										
bowl	1 tbsp	50	0.0	0.0	110	0	6.0	1.0	0	100%
stick	1 tbsp	90	0.0	0.0	110	0	10.0	2.0	0	100%
(Land O'Lakes) 'Country Morning Blend'										
stick	1 tsp	35	0.0	0.0	35	0	4.0	(mq)	5	100%
tub	1 tsp	30	0.0	0.0	25	0	3.0	(mq)	5	100%
unsalted, stick	1 tsp	35	0.0	0.0	0	0	4.0	(mq)	4	100%
unsalted, tub	1 tsp	30	0.0	0.0	0	0	3.0	(mq)	5	100%
(Land O'Lakes) 'Country Morning Light'										
stick	1 tsp	20	0.0	0.0	30	0	2.0	(mq)	3	100%
tub	1 tsp	20	0.0	0.0	25	0	2.0	(mq)	3	100%
(Land O'Lakes) w/sweet cream										
stick	1 tsp	30	0.0	0.0	35	0	4.0	(mq)	0	100%
tub	1 tsp	25	0.0	0.0	25	0	3.0	(mq)	0	100%
unsalted	1 tsp	30	0.0	0.0	0	0	4.0	(mq)	0	100%
(Mazola) 'Corn Oil Light'	1 tbsp	50	0.0	0.0	100	0	6.0	1.0	0	100%
(Nucoa) 'Heart Beat'										
regular	1 tbsp	25	0.0	0.0	110	0	3.0	<1.0	0	100%
unsalted	1 tbsp	24	0.0	0.0	0	0	3.0	<1.0	0	100%
(P&Q) 60% vegetable oil, stick	1 tbsp	80	<1.0	<1.0	105	0	8.0	1.0	0	90%
(Parkay) 50% vegetable oil	1 tbsp	60	0.0	0.0	110	0	7.0	1.0	0	100%
(Promise)										
'Extra Light'	1 tbsp	50	0.0	0.0	50	na	6.0	<1.0	0	100%
regular	1 tbsp	90	0.0	0.0	90	na	10.0	2.0	0	100%
'Ultra' fat-free	1 tbsp	5	0.0	0.0	90	na	0.0	0.0	0	0%
'Ultra' w/canola oil	1 tbsp	35	0.0	0.0	50	na	4.0	0.0	0	100%
(Shedd's Spread) 52% vegetable oil	1 tbsp	60	0.0	0.0	110	na	7.0	1.0	0	100%
(Van Den Bergh Foods) 'I Can't Believe It's Not Butter'										
light	1 tbsp	60	0.0	0.0	110	na	7.0	1.0	0	100%
regular	1 tbsp	90	0.0	0.0	0	0	10.0	2.0	0	100%
(Weight Watchers)										
'Country Cottage Farms' extra light, sweet, unsalted	1 tbsp	50	0.0	0.0	0	na	6.0	1.0	0	100%
'Country Cottage Farms' extra light, tub	1 tbsp	45	0.0	2.0	75	na	4.0	1.0	0	82%
'Country Cottage Farms' light	1 tbsp	50	0.0	0.0	130	0	6.0	1.0	0	100%

Food Name	Serving Size	Calories	Prot. gms	Carbs gms	Sod. mgs	Fiber gms	Fat gms	Sat. Fat gms	Chol. mgs	% Fat Cal.
light, stick	1 tbsp	60	0.0	0.0	130	0	7.0	1.0	0	100%
MARGARITA. See ALCOHOLIC BEVERAGES.										
MARINADE. See individual listings.										
MARJORAM										
dried	1 oz	77	3.6	17.2	22	5.1	2.0	na	0	18%
dried	1 tbsp	5	0.2	1.0	1	.3	0.1	na	0	16%
dried	1 tsp	2	0.1	0.4	0	.1	0.0	na	0	0%
dried (Durkee)	1 tsp	2	0.0	0.0	0	0	tr	na	na	tr
dried (Laurel Leaf)	1 tsp	2	0.0	0.0	0	0	tr	na	na	tr
dried (Spice Islands)	1 tsp	4	0.2	0.7	1	.2	0.1	(tr)	0	20%
MARMALADE, ORANGE										
(Finast)	2 tsp	35	0.0	9.0	0	(mq)	0.0	0.0	2	0%
(Knott's Berry Farm) light, w/NutraSweet	1 tsp	8	0.0	2.0	0	na	0.0	na	na	0%
(Knudsen & Sons)	2 tsp	35	<1.0	8.0	na	na	<1.0	na	na	<20%
(Smucker's)	1 tsp	18	0.0	4.0	0	(mq)	0.0	0.0	0	0%
(Smucker's) low-sugar	1 tsp	8	0.0	2.0	0	na	0.0	0.0	na	0%
(Smucker's) 'Simply Fruit'	1 tsp	16	0.0	4.0	0	na	0.0	0.0	na	0%
(Smucker's) sweet, natural ingredients	1 tsp	18	0.0	4.0	0	na	0.0	0.0	na	0%
MARMALADE PLUM. See SAPOTE.										
MARROW BEAN										
boiled	4 oz	158	11.0	28.5	7	7.2	0.4	0.1	0	2%
boiled	1/2 cup	125	8.6	22.5	6	5.7	0.3	0.1	0	2%
raw	1/2 cup	337	23.6	60.9	16	15.4	0.9	0.2	0	2%
raw	1 oz	94	6.6	17.1	5	4.3	0.2	0.1	0	2%
small, boiled	4 oz	161	10.2	29.3	2	5.0	0.7	0.2	0	4%
small, boiled	1/2 cup	127	8.1	23.2	2	3.7	0.6	0.1	0	4%
small, raw	1/2 cup	363	22.8	67.2	13	11.1	1.3	0.3	0	3%
small, raw	1 oz	95	6.0	17.6	3	2.9	0.3	0.1	0	3%
MARROW SQUASH. See SQUASH, MARROW.										
MARSHMALLOW										
(Campfire) large	2 pieces	40	0.0	10.0	10	0	0.0	0.0	0	0%
(FunMallows)	1 piece	30	0.0	7.0	15	0	0.0	0.0	0	0%
(FunMallows) miniature	10 pieces	18	0.0	5.0	5	0	0.0	0.0	0	0%
(Kraft) 'Jet Puffed'	1 piece	25	0.0	6.0	5	0	0.0	0.0	0	0%
(Kraft) miniature	10 pieces	18	0.0	5.0	5	0	0.0	0.0	0	0%
MARSHMALLOW CREME TOPPING										
(Finast)	1 oz	95	0.0	23.0	45	0	0.0	0.0	0	0%
(Kraft)	1 oz	90	0.0	23.0	20	0	0.0	0.0	0	0%
(Marshmallow Fluff)	1 tsp	59	0.0	15.0	12	0	0.0	0.0	0	0%
(Smucker's)	2 tbsp	120	0.0	29.0	0	na	0.0	0.0	na	0%
MARTINI. See ALCOHOLIC BEVERAGES.										
MASA HARINA. See CORN FLOUR.										
MATAI. See WATER CHESTNUT, CHINESE.										
MATZO. See CRACKER.										
MAYONNAISE										
(Bama)	1 tbsp	100	0.0	0.0	65	0	11.0	(mq)	(mq)	100%
(Bennett's) 'Real'	1 tbsp	110	0.0	1.0	65	0	12.0	(mq)	(mq)	96%
(Best Foods)	1 tbsp	100	0.0	0.0	80	0	11.0	2.0	5	100%
(Cains)	1 tbsp	100	0.0	0.0	80	0	11.0	2.0	10	100%
(Finast)	1 tbsp	100	0.0	0.0	80	0	11.0	2.0	10	100%
(Hain) cold processed	1 tbsp	110	0.0	0.0	70	0	12.0	2.0	5	100%
(Hellmann's)	1 tbsp	100	0.0	0.0	80	0	11.0	2.0	5	100%
(Hollywood)	1 tbsp	110	0.0	0.0	80	0	12.0	1.0	5	100%
(Kraft) 'Real'	1 tbsp	100	0.0	0.0	70	0	12.0	2.0	5	100%

Food Name	Serving Size	Calories	Prot. gms	Carbs gms	Sod. mgs	Fiber gms	Fat gms	Sat. Fat gms	Chol. mgs	% Fat Cal.
(Pathmark)	1 tbsp	100	0.0	0.0	70	0	11.0	2.0	5	100%
(Pathmark) 'No Frills'	1 tbsp	100	0.0	0.0	75	0	11.0	2.0	10	100%
(Rokeach)	1 tbsp	100	0.0	0.0	70	0	11.0	2.0	10	100%
(Westbrae)	1 tbsp	100	0.0	0.0	75	na	11.0	na	5	100%
CANOLA										
(Hain)	1 tbsp	100	0.0	<1.0	100	0	11.0	1.0	5	96%
(Hollywood)	1 tbsp	100	0.0	<1.0	100	0	11.0	1.0	5	96%
(Spectrum Naturals)	1 tbsp	100	0.0	0.0	80	(tr)	12.0	1.0	4	100%
(Spectrum Naturals) 'Lite Mayo'	1 tbsp	35	0.0	1.0	60	0.0	3.0	0.0	0	77%
(Westbrae)	1 tbsp	100	0.0	0.0	75	na	11.0	na	5	100%
LOW-SODIUM										
(Hain) 'Real No Salt Added'	1 tbsp	110	0.0	0.0	0	0	12.0	2.0	5	100%
(Weight Watchers) 'Low Sodium'	1 tbsp	50	0.0	1.0	45	0	5.0	1.0	5	92%
REDUCED CALORIE										
(Best Foods) 'Light'	1 tbsp	50	0.0	1.0	115	0	5.0	1.0	5	92%
(Estee)	1 tbsp	50	0.0	1.0	80	na	5.0	1.0	0	92%
(Featherweight)	1 tbsp	30	0.0	3.0	40	0	2.0	(mq)	10	60%
(Finast) 'Lite'	1 tbsp	40	0.0	1.0	100	0	4.0	1.0	5	90%
(Hain) 'Light Low Sodium'	1 tbsp	60	0.0	2.0	95	0	6.0	1.0	10	87%
(Hellmann's) 'Light'	1 tbsp	50	0.0	1.0	115	0	5.0	1.0	5	92%
(Janet Lee) 'Light'	1 tbsp	50	0.0	1.0	115	na	5.0	1.0	5	92%
(Kraft) 'Light'	1 tbsp	50	0.0	1.0	110	0	5.0	1.0	0	92%
(Pathmark)	1 tbsp	40	0.0	1.0	100	0	4.0	1.0	5	90%
(Smart Beat) 'Golden Corn Light'	1 tbsp	40	0.0	1.0	110	na	4.0	<1.0	0	90%
(Weight Watchers) 'Light'	1 tbsp	50	0.0	1.0	100	na	5.0	1.0	5	92%
SAFFLOWER										
(Hain)	1 tbsp	110	0.0	0.0	70	0	12.0	1.0	5	100%
(Hollywood)	1 tbsp	100	0.0	0.0	75	0	12.0	1.0	5	100%
SAFFLOWER AND SOYBEAN	1 tbsp	99	0.2	0.4	78	0	11.0	1.2	(mq)	98%
SOYBEAN										
	1 tbsp	99	0.2	0.4	78	0	11.0	1.6	8	98%
(Featherweight) 'Soyamaise'	1 tbsp	100	0.0	0.0	3	0	11.0	(mq)	5	100%
MAYONNAISE, ALTERNATIVE										
(Best Foods) 'Cholesterol Free'	1 tbsp	50	0.0	1.0	80	na	5.0	1.0	0	92%
(Hain) 'Eggless No Salt Added'	1 tbsp	110	0.0	0.0	5	0	12.0	2.0	0	100%
(Hellman's) 'Cholesterol Free'	1 tbsp	50	0.0	1.0	80	0	5.0	1.0	na	92%
(Kraft) 'Free'	1 tbsp	8	0.0	3.0	125	na	0.0	na	0	0%
(Nucoa) 'Heart Beat'	1 tbsp	40	0.0	1.0	110	0	4.0	<1.0	0	90%
(Weight Watchers) 'Cholesterol Free'	1 tbsp	50	0.0	1.0	90	0	5.0	1.0	0	92%
CANOLA (Hain) reduced calorie	1 tbsp	60	0.0	2.0	160	0	5.0	0.0	0	85%
MILK CREAM	1 tbsp	15	0.3	1.7	76	0	0.8	0.4	6	47%
SOYBEAN	1 tbsp	35	tr	2.4	75	0	2.9	0.5	4	73%
SUNFLOWER (Life) 'All Natural'	1 tbsp	71	<1.0	1.0	3	0	8.0	(mq)	0	90%
TOFU (Nasoya) 'Nayonaise'	1 tbsp	40	1.0	1.0	50	(tr)	4.0	(mq)	0	82%
MEAT. See individual listings.										
MEAT, ALTERNATIVE. See also individual listings.										
chops (Worthington) 'Choplets' canned	2 slices	100	17.0	5.0	050	(mq)	2.0	(mq)	0	17%
cutlet (Worthington) 'Multigrain' canned	2 slices	90	14.0	6.0	260	(mq)	1.0	(mq)	0	10%
unflavored (Heartline) lite	.5 oz	22	5.0	1.0	135	3.0	0.0	0.0	0	0%
MEAT EXTENDER										
soybean	1 cup	275	33.5	33.7	8	>1.5 c	2.6	0.4	0	8%
soybean	1 oz	88	10.7	10.7	3	>.5 c	0.8	0.1	0	8%
MEAT LOAF ENTRÉE, FROZEN										
(Armour) 'Classics'	11.25 oz	360	20.0	32.0	1170	(mq)	17.0	(mq)	65	42%

Food Name	Serving Size	Calories	Prot. gms	Carbs gms	Sod. mgs	Fiber gms	Fat gms	Sat. Fat gms	Chol. mgs	% Fat Cal.
(Banquet)	11 oz	440	26.0	27.0	770	(mq)	27.0	(mq)	85	53%
(Banquet) 'Cookin' Bags'	4 oz	200	10.0	8.0	(mq)	(mq)	14.0	(mq)	(mq)	64%
(Freezer Queen)	10 oz	350	19.0	26.0	910	(mq)	19.0	(mq)	(mq)	49%
(Freezer Queen) 'Family Suppers' w/tomato sauce	7 oz	230	12.0	15.0	850	(mq)	13.0	(mq)	(mq)	52%
(Healthy Choice) low-fat, low-cholesterol	12 oz	340	17.0	48.0	560	na	8.0	3.0	40	22%
(Lean Cuisine) w/macaroni and cheese	9 3/8 oz	280	26.0	26.0	540	na	8.0	3.0	55	26%
(Morton)	10 oz	310	11.0	26.0	1520	(mq)	17.0	(mq)	50	51%
(Stouffer's) homestyle, in gravy, w/whipped potatoes	9 7/8 oz	370	22.0	25.0	860	na	20.0	na	na	49%
(Swanson)	10.75 oz	360	15.0	41.0	960	(mq)	15.0	(mq)	(mq)	38%
MEAT LOAF ENTRÉE, PACKAGED										
(Dinty Moore) 'American Classics' w/mashed potatoes and gravy	10 oz	262	18.0	26.0	na	na	9.0	na	na	32%
(Ultra Slim Fast) w/tomato sauce	10.5 oz	340	19.0	52.0	780	na	9.0	na	35	22%
MEAT LOAF MIX										
(Hunt's) 'Meatloaf Fixins'	2.222 oz	23	1.5	3.9	600	.7	0.4	0.0	0	14%
(Lipton) 'Microeasy' homestyle	1/4 pkg	90	4.0	15.0	630	(mq)	1.0	na	na	11%
MEAT LOAF MIX, ALTERNATIVE										
(Natural) 'Touch Loaf Mix,' vegetarian	4 oz	180	21.0	7.0	25	(mq)	7.0	(mq)	0	36%
MEAT LOAF SEASONING										
(French's)	1/8 pkg	20	1.0	5.0	620	na	0.0	0.0	0	0%
(Lawry's) 'Seasoning Blends'	1 pkg	355	15.5	64.5	6547	>1.8 c	1.2	na	na	3%
(Schilling) 'Bag'n Season'	1 pkg	111	0.6	26.0	3090	na	0.7	na	1	6%
MEAT MARINADE MIX *(French's)*	1/8 pkg	10	0.0	2.0	540	na	0.0	0.0	0	0%
MEAT STICKS										
smoked	1 oz	156	6.1	1.5	420	na	14.1	5.9	38	81%
smoked	1 stick	109	4.3	1.1	293	na	9.8	4.1	26	80%
MEAT TENDERIZER										
(Tone's) seasoned	1 tsp	7	<.1	1.2	1650	<.1	0.2	<.1	0	26%
(Tone's) unseasoned	1 tsp	7	0.0	1.2	1760	tr	0.2	<.1	0	27%
MEATBALL, ALTERNATIVE										
vegetarian *(Worthington)* 'Non-Meat Balls'	3 pieces	100	7.0	4.0	220	(mq)	6.0	(mq)	0	55%
MEATBALL ENTRÉE										
Canned, stew										
(Chef Boyardee)	8 oz	350	9.0	24.0	1315	(mq)	24.0	(mq)	(mq)	62%
(Dinty Moore)	8 oz	240	11.0	14.0	980	na	16.0	7.0	30	59%
Frozen, BBQ homestyle *(Banquet)* 'Healthy Balance'	10.25 oz	270	14.0	43.0	680	na	5.0	3.0	25	17%
Microwave *(Dinty Moore)* microwave cup	7.5 oz	240	11.0	14.0	980	na	16.0	7.0	30	59%
MEATBALL SEASONING *(French's)* dry mix	1/4 pkg	35	1.0	7.0	830	na	0.0	0.0	0	0%
MELBA TOAST. See CRACKER.										
MELON. See individual listings.										
MELON, BITTER. See BALSAM PEAR.										
MELON BALLS, FROZEN										
cantaloupe and honeydew	1 lb	144	3.8	36.0	139	(mq)	1.1	na	0	6%
cantaloupe and honeydew	1 cup	57	1.5	13.7	54	1.2	0.4	na	0	6%
cantaloupe and honeydew	1 oz	9	0.2	2.3	9	(mq)	0.1	(tr)	0	8%
MENUDO MIX										
(Gebhardt)	1 tsp	5	<1.0	1.0	310	<1.0	<1.0	(mq)	0	<53%
(Gebhardt) spice	.0141 oz	1	0.0	0.1	45	.1	0.0	0.0	0	0%
MESQUITE MARINADE *(Lawry's)*	2 tbsp	24	3.0	3.0	4142	tr	0.4	0.1	0	13%
MESQUITE SEASONING *(Tone's)*	1 tsp	13	0.1	3.2	467	na	<.1	(tr)	0	<6%
MEXICAN FOODS. See individual listings.										
MEXICAN POTATO. See JICAMA.										
MEXICAN SEASONING *(Tone's)*	1 tsp	6	0.3	1.3	4185	.4	0.1	<.1	tr	12%

Food Name	Serving Size	Calories	Prot. gms	Carbs gms	Sod. mgs	Fiber gms	Fat gms	Sat. Fat gms	Chol. mgs	% Fat Cal.
MEXICAN STYLE DINNER, FROZEN. See also individual listings.										
(Banquet)	12 oz	490	18.0	62.0	2000	(mq)	18.0	(mq)	(mq)	34%
(Banquet) combination	12 oz	520	20.0	72.0	1980	(mq)	17.0	(mq)	(mq)	29%
(Morton)	10 oz	300	9.0	44.0	1390	(mq)	10.0	(mq)	20	30%
(Patio)	13.25 oz	540	15.0	64.0	1940	(mq)	25.0	(mq)	45	42%
(Patio) 'Fiesta'	12.25 oz	470	16.0	55.0	2040	(mq)	20.0	(mq)	30	39%
(Swanson) combination	14.25 oz	490	19.0	62.0	1760	(mq)	18.0	(mq)	(mq)	33%
(Swanson) 'Hungry Man'	20.25 oz	820	25.0	88.0	2080	(mq)	41.0	(mq)	(mq)	45%
(Van de Kamp's)	1/2 pkg	220	7.0	25.0	640	(mq)	10.0	(mq)	(mq)	41%
MILK, ALTERNATIVE. See RICE BEVERAGE; SOY BEVERAGE.										
MILK, COW'S, CANNED										
CONDENSED, SWEETENED										
	1 cup	982	24.2	166.5	389	0	26.6	16.8	104	24%
(Borden)	1/3 cup	320	7.0	54.0	115	0	8.0	(mq)	(mq)	23%
(Carnation)	1/3 cup	320	7.0	56.0	110	0	8.0	(mq)	(mq)	22%
(Diehl) 'Jerzee'	1/3 cup	320	7.0	52.0	120	0	9.0	(mq)	(mq)	26%
(Eagle)	1/2 cup	320	7.0	52.0	120	0	9.0	(mq)	(mq)	26%
EVAPORATED										
	1/2 cup	169	8.6	12.6	133	0	9.5	5.8	37	50%
(Carnation)	1/2 cup	170	8.0	12.0	135	0	10.0	(mq)	(mq)	53%
(Diehl)	1/2 cup	170	8.0	12.0	135	0	10.0	(mq)	(mq)	53%
(Finast)	1/2 cup	170	8.0	12.0	135	0	10.0	(mq)	(mq)	53%
(IGA)	1/2 cup	170	8.0	12.0	140	0	10.0	(mq)	(mq)	53%
(Pathmark)	1/2 cup	170	8.0	12.0	140	0	10.9	(mq)	(mq)	55%
(Pet)	1/2 cup	170	8.0	12.0	140	0	10.0	(mq)	36	53%
Filled (Pet)	1/2 cup	150	8.0	12.0	140	0	8.0	1.0	5	47%
Low-fat (Carnation)	1/2 cup	110	8.0	12.0	140	0	3.0	2.0	10	25%
Skim										
	1/2 cup	100	9.7	14.5	147	0	0.3	0.2	5	3%
(Carnation) 'Lite'	1/2 cup	100	9.0	14.0	150	0	<1.0	0.2	5	<9%
(Diehl)	1/2 cup	100	9.0	14.0	150	0	<1.0	(mq)	(mq)	<9%
(Finast)	1/2 cup	100	9.0	14.0	150	0	<1.0	(mq)	(mq)	<9%
(Pathmark)	1/2 cup	100	9.0	14.0	15	0	0.0	0.0	(mq)	0%
(Pet) 'Lite'	1/2 cup	100	9.0	14.0	150	0	<1.0	(mq)	10	<9%
MILK, COW'S, DRY										
LOW-FAT										
(Milkman)	1/4 pkg	90	9.0	12.0	125	na	1.0	na	na	10%
(Milkman) reconstituted	1 quart	380	35.0	48.0	500	na	5.0	na	na	12%
SKIM										
(Alba) reconstituted	8 oz	80	8.0	13.0	190	na	0.0	na	na	0%
(Carnation)	1/3 cup	80	8.0	12.0	125	na	0.0	0.0	na	0%
(Lucerne)	1/3 cup	80	8.0	12.0	125	na	0.0	0.0	na	0%
(Saco Foods)	5 tbsp	80	8.0	12.0	125	na	<1.0	na	5	<10%
(Sanalac) 'Dairy Fresh' reconstituted	8 oz	80	8.0	12.0	85	0	0.1	<.1	5	1%
(Sanalac) reconstituted	9.03 oz	80	7.5	12.3	110	0	0.1	0.0	5	1%
(Weight Watchers) 'Dairy Creamer'	1 pkt	10	1.0	1.0	15	0	0.0	0.0	na	0%
MILK, COW'S, FLUID										
WHOLE										
(A&P)	1 cup	150	8.0	11.0	120	0	8.0	(mq)	(mq)	49%
(Borden)	1 cup	150	8.0	11.0	130	0	8.0	(mq)	(mq)	49%
(Borden) 'Hi-Calcium'	1 cup	150	8.0	11.0	130	0	8.0	(mq)	(mq)	49%
(Carnation)	1 cup	150	8.0	12.0	120	0	8.0	na	33	47%
(Crowley)	1 cup	150	8.0	11.0	125	0	8.0	(mq)	30	49%
(Darigold)	1 cup	150	8.0	11.0	125	0	8.0	4.9	33	49%

Food Name	Serving Size	Calories	Prot. gms	Carbs gms	Sod. mgs	Fiber gms	Fat gms	Sat. Fat gms	Chol. mgs	% Fat Cal.
(Knudsen)	1 cup	160	9.0	12.0	180	0	8.0	(mq)	(mq)	46%
Low-sodium	1 cup	149	7.6	10.9	6	0	8.4	5.3	33	51%
3.7% fat	1 cup	157	8.0	11.4	119	0	8.9	5.6	35	51%
3.3% fat	1 cup	150	8.0	11.4	120	0	8.1	5.1	33	48%
2% FAT										
	1 cup	121	8.1	11.7	122	0	4.7	2.9	18	35%
Protein-fortified										
	1 cup	137	9.7	13.5	145	0	4.9	3.0	19	32%
(A&P)	1 cup	120	8.0	12.0	120	0	5.0	(mq)	(mq)	36%
(Borden) 'Hi-Protein'	1 cup	140	10.0	13.0	150	0	5.0	(mq)	(mq)	33%
(Crowley) 'Tone Acidophilus'	1 cup	120	8.0	11.0	125	0	5.0	(mq)	15	37%
(Darigold) 'Nutrish Acidophilus'	1 cup	120	8.0	11.0	130	0	5.0	2.9	18	37%
(Finast)	1 cup	130	9.0	12.0	130	0	5.0	(mq)	(mq)	35%
(Knudsen) 'Sweet Acidophilus'	1 cup	140	10.0	13.0	150	0	5.0	(mq)	(mq)	33%
(Viva)	1 cup	120	8.0	11.0	125	0	5.0	(mq)	(mq)	37%
W/non-fat milk solids added	1 cup	125	8.5	12.2	128	0	4.7	2.9	18	34%
1% FAT										
	1 cup	102	8.0	11.7	123	0	2.6	1.6	10	23%
(Crowley)	1 cup	100	8.0	11.0	130	0	2.0	(mq)	10	19%
Protein-fortified										
	1 cup	119	9.7	13.6	143	0	2.9	1.8	10	22%
(A&P)	1 cup	100	8.0	12.0	120	0	3.0	(mq)	(mq)	25%
(Borden)	1 cup	100	8.0	11.0	130	0	2.0	(mq)	(mq)	19%
(Crowley)	1 cup	120	10.0	14.0	150	0	2.0	(mq)	10	16%
(Crowley) 'Lactaid'	1 cup	100	8.0	11.0	125	0	2.0	(mq)	10	19%
(Darigold)	1 cup	100	8.0	13.0	130	0	2.0	1.6	10	18%
(Knudsen) 'Nice n' Light'	1 cup	130	10.0	15.0	153	0	3.0	(mq)	(mq)	21%
W/calcium added (Darigold)	1 cup	100	8.0	11.0	130	0	2.0	1.6	10	19%
W/non-fat milk solids added	1 cup	104	8.5	12.2	128	0	2.4	1.5	10	21%
SKIM										
	1 cup	86	8.4	11.9	126	0	0.4	0.3	4	4%
Protein-fortified										
(A&P)	1 cup	90	8.0	12.0	125	0	<1.0	(mq)	(mq)	<10%
(Borden)	1 cup	90	8.0	12.0	130	0	1.0	(mq)	(mq)	10%
(Borden) 'Skim-Line'	1 cup	100	10.0	13.0	150	0	1.0	(mq)	(mq)	9%
(Crowley)	1 cup	90	9.0	12.0	130	0	<1.0	(mq)	<1	<10%
(Darigold) 'Trim'	1 cup	80	8.0	11.0	130	0	1.0	0.3	4	11%
(Knudsen)	1 cup	80	9.0	12.0	130	0	(mq)	(mq)	(mq)	0%
(Weight Watchers)	1 cup	90	9.0	13.0	140	0	<1.0	(mq)	(mq)	<9%
W/non-fat milk solids added	1 cup	90	8.8	12.3	130	0	0.6	0.4	5	6%
W/vitamin A added	1 cup	86	8.4	11.9	126	0	0.4	0.3	4	4%
MILK, GOAT'S										
evaporated (Meyenberg) canned, undiluted	4 oz	143	7.9	10.0	86	na	7.9	na	na	50%
fluid, whole	1 cup	168	8.7	10.9	122	0	10.1	6.5	28	54%
fluid, whole	1 oz	20	1.0	1.3	14	0	1.2	0.8	3	54%
MILK, HUMAN										
fluid, whole	1 cup	171	2.5	17.0	42	0	10.8	4.9	34	56%
fluid, whole	1 oz	21	0.3	2.1	5	0	1.4	0.6	4	57%
fluid, whole	1 tbsp	11	0.2	1.1	3	0	0.7	0.3	2	55%
MILK, INDIA BUFFALO										
fluid, whole	1 cup	236	9.1	12.6	127	0	16.8	11.2	46	64%
fluid, whole	1 oz	27	1.1	1.5	15	0	2.0	1.3	5	63%

Food Name	Serving Size	Calories	Prot. gms	Carbs gms	Sod. mgs	Fiber gms	Fat gms	Sat. Fat gms	Chol. mgs	% Fat Cal.
MILK, LACTOSE-REDUCED										
2% FAT										
(Lactaid) 70% lactose reduced, w/vitamins A and D	1 cup	130	8.0	12.0	125	0	5.0	3.0	20	36%
(Lucerne) 70% lactose reduced, w/vitamins A and D	1 cup	120	9.0	12.0	110	0	5.0	3.0	25	35%
1% FAT										
(First Alternative) lactose free	1 cup	80	8.0	6.0	180	0	2.0	.5	0	23%
SKIM										
(Lactaid) 70% lactose reduced, w/calcium and vitamins A and D	1 cup	80	8.0	13.0	125	0	0.0	0.0	5	0%
(Lactaid) 70% lactose reduced, w/vitamins A and D	1 cup	80	8.0	13.0	125	0	0.0	0.0	5	0%
(Lactaid 100) lactose free, w/vitamins A and D	1 cup	80	8.0	13.0	125	0	0.0	0.0	5	0%
(Lucerne) 70% lactose reduced, w/vitamins A and D	1 cup	80	9.0	12.0	115	0	0.0	0.0	5	0%
MILK, REINDEER	1 cup	580	26.8	10.2	389	0	48.6	27.3	35	75%
MILK, SHEEP'S										
fluid, whole	1 cup	264	14.7	13.1	108	0	17.2	11.3	66	58%
fluid, whole	1 oz	31	1.7	1.5	12	0	2.0	1.3	(mq)	58%
MILKFISH. See AWA.										
MILKSHAKE										
chocolate, thick	10.6 oz	356	9.1	63.5	333	.9	8.1	5.0	32	20%
vanilla, thick	11 oz	350	12.1	55.6	299	0	9.5	5.9	37	24%
(MicroMagic) chocolate, frozen	11.5 oz	340	5.0	55.0	120	(tr)	8.0	(mq)	40	23%
(MicroMagic) chocolate, frozen	7 oz	200	2.0	32.0	70	(tr)	4.0	(mq)	25	21%
(MicroMagic) strawberry, frozen	11.5 oz	340	5.0	54.0	120	(tr)	9.0	(mq)	40	26%
(MicroMagic) vanilla, frozen	11.5 oz	380	8.0	60.0	150	0	13.0	(mq)	45	30%
MILKSHAKE MIX										
(Alba '77) chocolate, 'Fit'N' prepared	6 oz	346	26.1	56.0	709	>1.0 c	2.5	na	na	6%
(Alba '77) chocolate marshmallow, 'Fit'N' prepared	6 oz	346	27.5	51.5	690	>.8 c	3.6	na	na	9%
(Alba '77) double fudge, frosty, 'Fit'N' prepared	6 oz	346	28.0	52.2	728	>1.0 c	3.3	na	na	9%
(Alba '77) strawberry, 'Fit'N' prepared	6 oz	333	24.6	55.0	805	>.2 c	1.7	na	na	5%
(Alba '77) vanilla, 'Fit'N' prepared	6 oz	333	26.0	54.5	810	>.4 c	1.4	na	na	4%
(Weight Watchers) chocolate fudge	1 pkt	70	6.0	11.0	170	(tr)	1.0	na	na	12%
(Weight Watchers) orange sherbet	1 pkt	70	6.0	11.0	210	(tr)	0.0	0.0	0	0%
MILLET										
pearl, cooked	1/2 cup	143	4.2	28.4	2	1.6	1.2	0.2	0	8%
pearl, cooked	4 oz	135	4.0	26.8	2	1.5	1.1	0.2	0	7%
pearl, raw	1/2 cup	378	11.0	72.9	5	8.5	4.2	0.7	0	10%
pearl, raw	1 oz	107	3.1	20.7	1	2.4	1.2	0.2	0	10%
pearl, raw, hulled *(Arrowhead Mills)*	1 oz	90	3.0	21.0	1	1.8	1.0	(mq)	0	9%
Proso/hog millet, whole grain	3 1/2 oz	327	9.9	72.9	1	>3.2 c	2.9	1.0	0	7%
MILLET FLOUR, whole grain *(Arrowhead Mills)*	2 oz	185	6.0	41.0	1	3.7	2.0	(mq)	0	9%
MINCEMEAT. See PIE FILLING.										
MISO										
	1/2 cup	284	16.3	38.6	5033	7.4	8.4	1.2	0	26%
	1 oz	58	3.3	7.9	1034	1.5	1.7	0.2	0	26%
w/barley malt/mugi-koji	1 oz	56	2.7	8.0	1191	(mq)	1.2	(mq)	0	20%
w/rice malt, dark yellow/kome-koji	1 oz	53	3.7	5.4	1446	(mq)	1.6	(mq)	0	28%
w/rice malt, sweet/kome-koji	1 oz	62	2.7	10.4	680	(mq)	0.9	(mq)	0	13%
w/soybean malt/mame-koji	1 oz	62	4.9	3.2	1219	(mq)	3.9	(mq)	0	52%
(Eden Foods) barley/mugi, organic	1 tbsp	25	2.0	3.0	760	na	<1.0	na	na	<31%
(Eden Foods) brown rice/genmai, organic	1 tbsp	25	2.0	3.0	810	na	1.0	na	na	31%
(Eden Foods) rice/shiro, organic	1 tbsp	35	2.0	5.0	410	na	1.0	na	na	24%
(Eden Foods) soybean and rice/kome, organic	1 tbsp	25	2.0	3.0	850	na	1.0	na	na	31%
(Eden Foods) soybean/hacho, organic	1 tbsp	35	3.0	2.0	600	na	2.0	na	na	47%
(Westbrae) barley, pasteurized	1 tsp	12	<1.0	2.0	310	na	0.0	na	0	0%

Food Name	Serving Size	Calories	Prot. gms	Carbs gms	Sod. mgs	Fiber gms	Fat gms	Sat. Fat gms	Chol. mgs	% Fat Cal.
(Westbrae) brown rice, pasteurized	1 tsp	10	1.0	2.0	360	na	0.0	na	0	0%
(Westbrae) red, instant	.35 oz	35	3.0	3.0	750	na	1.0	na	na	27%
(Westbrae) red, pasteurized	1 tsp	10	1.0	1.0	375	na	0.0	na	0	0%
(Westbrae) soybean, pasteurized	1 tsp	12	1.0	1.0	265	na	0.0	na	0	0%
(Westbrae) soybean/hacho	1 tsp	14	1.0	1.0	240	na	0.0	na	0	0%
(Westbrae) white, instant	.35 oz	35	2.0	4.0	740	na	1.0	na	na	27%
MOLASSES										
	1 cup	872	0.0	225.7	121	0	0.3	na	0	0%
	1 tbsp	53	0.0	13.8	7	0	0.0	na	0	0%
Barbados	1 cup	889	0.0	229.6	49	0	0.0	0.0	0	0%
Barbados	1 oz	111	0.0	28.7	6	0	0.0	0.0	0	0%
1st extraction/light	1 cup	827	0.0	213.2	49	0	0.0	0.0	0	0%
1st extraction/light	1 oz	103	0.0	26.7	6	0	0.0	0.0	0	0%
2nd extraction/medium	1 cup	761	0.0	196.8	121	0	0.0	0.0	0	0%
2nd extraction/medium	1 oz	95	0.0	24.6	15	0	0.0	0.0	0	0%
3rd extraction/blackstrap	1 cup	771	0.0	199.4	180	0	0.0	na	0	0%
3rd extraction/blackstrap	1 tbsp	47	0.0	12.2	11	0	0.0	na	0	0%
(Br'er Rabbit) dark	1 oz	110	0.0	28.0	20	na	0.0	na	0	0%
(Br'er Rabbit) light	1 oz	110	0.0	29.0	15	na	0.0	na	0	0%
(Grandma's) mild flavor, gold	1 tbsp	70	0.0	17.0	28	0	0.0	0.0	0	0%
(Grandma's) robust flavor, green	1 tbsp	70	0.0	16.0	57	0	0.0	0.0	0	0%
(LaChoy) bead	.7055 oz	52	0.4	12.5	48	0	0.0	0.0	0	0%
(LaChoy) bead	1/2 tsp	7	<1.0	2.0	1	0	0.0	(mq)	0	0%
MONKFISH/angler fish/bellyfish/frogfish/goosefish/lotte/sea devil										
dry-heat cooked	3 oz	82	15.8	0.0	20	0	1.7	na	27	20%
raw	1 lb	343	65.7	0.0	84	0	6.9	(mq)	115	19%
raw	3 oz	65	12.3	0.0	15	0	1.3	0.3	21	19%
raw	1 oz	22	4.1	0.0	5	0	0.4	(mq)	7	18%
MONOSODIUM GLUTAMATE/MSG										
flavor enhancer (Tone's) 'MSG'	1 tsp	0	0.0	0.0	638	0	0.0	0.0	0	0%
MOOSE										
raw	1 lb	463	100.9	0.0	295	na	3.4	1.0	268	7%
raw	1 oz	29	6.2	0.0	18	na	0.2	0.1	17	7%
roasted	3 oz	114	24.9	0.0	59	na	0.8	0.3	66	7%
roasted, diced	1 cup	188	41.0	0.0	97	0	1.4	0.4	109	7%
MOSTACCIOLI. See PASTA										
MOSTACCIOLI ENTRÉE										
(Banquet) frozen, w/meat sauce, 'Family Entrees'	7 oz	170	7.0	28.0	(mq)	(mq)	3.0	(mq)	(mq)	16%
MOTH BEAN										
boiled	4 oz	133	8.9	23.8	11	>1.5 c	0.6	0.1	0	4%
boiled	1/2 cup	103	6.9	18.4	9	>1.2 c	0.5	0.1	0	4%
raw	1/2 cup	336	22.5	60.3	29	>3.9 c	1.6	0.4	0	4%
raw	1 oz	97	6.5	17.4	9	>1.1 c	0.5	0.1	0	5%
MOUNTAIN YAM. See YAM.										
MOUSSE (Estee) orange chocolate	1/2 cup	70	3.0	9.0	50	na	3.0	1.5	0	36%
MOUSSE, FROZEN										
(Weight Watchers) 'Sweet Celebrations' chocolate	2.5 oz	170	6.0	24.0	190	na	6.0	<1.0	5	31%
(Weight Watchers) 'Sweet Celebrations' praline pecan	2.75 oz	190	5.0	27.0	180	na	7.0	1.0	5	33%
(Weight Watchers) 'Sweet Celebrations' triple chocolate caramel	2.75 oz	170	4.0	31.0	120	na	4.0	1.0	5	21%
MOUSSE MIX										
(Jell-O) 'Rich & Luscious' chocolate, dry mix	1 pkg	110	3.0	18.0	45	na	3.0	na	0	24%
(Jell-O) 'Rich & Luscious' chocolate, prepared	1/2 cup	150	5.0	21.0	75	na	6.0	na	10	34%
(Jell-O) 'Rich & Luscious' chocolate fudge, dry mix	1 pkg	110	3.0	18.0	45	na	4.0	na	0	30%

Food Name	Serving Size	Calories	Prot. gms	Carbs gms	Sod. mgs	Fiber gms	Fat gms	Sat. Fat gms	Chol. mgs	% Fat Cal.
(Jell-O) 'Rich & Luscious' chocolate fudge, prepared	1/2 cup	140	5.0	20.0	75	na	6.0	na	10	35%
(Weight Watchers) chocolate, prepared w/skim milk	1/2 cup	60	3.0	9.0	45	na	3.0	(mq)	(mq)	36%
(Weight Watchers) chocolate cheesecake, prepared w/skim milk	1/2 cup	60	4.0	12.0	75	na	2.0	(mq)	(mq)	22%
(Weight Watchers) chocolate raspberry, prepared w/skim milk	1/2 cup	60	3.0	12.0	75	na	3.0	(mq)	(mq)	31%
(Weight Watchers) white chocolate almond, prepared w/skim milk	1/2 cup	60	3.0	6.0	50	na	3.0	(mq)	(mq)	43%
MSG. See MONOSODIUM GLUTAMATE.										
MUFFIN. See also ENGLISH MUFFIN.										
APPLE										
(Awrey's) 1.5-oz muffin	1 muffin	130	2.0	17.0	210	0	6.0	1.0	20	42%
(Awrey's) 2.5-oz muffin	1 muffin	220	3.0	30.0	350	1.0	10.0	2.0	35	41%
(Awrey's) w/banana nut, 'Grande' 4.2-oz muffin	1 muffin	260	3.0	27.0	160	.6	16.0	2.0	40	55%
(Hostess) w/banana walnut, mini muffin	5 muffins	160	2.0	17.0	90	(mq)	9.0	(mq)	0	52%
APPLE SPICE										
(Dunkin' Donuts) 3.5-oz muffin	1 muffin	300	6.0	52.0	360	na	8.0	na	25	24%
(Health Valley) fat-free	1 muffin	130	4.0	30.0	110	5.1	0.0	na	0	0%
APPLE STREUSEL *(Awrey's)* 'Grande' 4.2-oz muffin	1 muffin	340	6.0	50.0	540	1.0	13.0	2.0	35	34%
BANANA *(Health Valley)* fat-free	1 muffin	130	4.0	29.0	110	4.5	0.0	na	0	0%
BANANA NUT										
(Break Cake) .5-oz muffin	1 muffin	60	1.0	7.0	45	na	3.0	0.5	10	46%
(Dunkin' Donuts) 3.6-oz muffin	1 muffin	310	7.0	49.0	410	3.0	10.0	(mq)	30	29%
BLUEBERRY										
(Awrey's) 1.5-oz muffin	1 muffin	130	2.0	18.0	180	1.0	5.0	1.0	10	36%
(Awrey's) 2.5-oz muffin	1 muffin	210	3.0	31.0	280	1.0	8.0	1.0	20	35%
(Awrey's) 'Grande' 4.2-oz muffin	1 muffin	360	5.0	52.0	480	2.0	14.0	2.0	35	36%
(Break Cake)	1 muffin	60	1.0	8.0	50	na	3.0	0.5	10	43%
(Dunkin' Donuts) 3.6-oz muffin	1 muffin	280	6.0	46.0	340	na	8.0	na	30	26%
(Entenmann's)	1 muffin	200	3.0	29.0	250	na	8.0	na	na	36%
(Hostess) mini muffin	5 muffins	240	3.0	29.0	180	.7	13.0	2.0	40	48%
BLUEBERRY-APPLE *(Health Valley)* fat-free, twin pack	1 muffin	140	4.0	32.0	100	5.0	0.0	na	0	0%
BRAN *(Dunkin' Donuts)* w/raisins, 3.7-oz muffin	1 muffin	310	6.0	51.0	560	4.0	9.0	(mq)	15	26%
CARROT *(Health Valley)* fat-free, twin pack	1 muffin	130	4.0	30.0	110	5.0	0.0	na	0	0%
CINNAMON APPLE *(Hostess)* mini muffin	5 muffins	260	3.0	27.0	180	.6	16.0	2.0	45	55%
CORN										
(Awrey's) 1.5-oz muffin	1 muffin	130	2.0	20.0	270	0	5.0	1.0	15	34%
(Awrey's) 2.5-oz muffin	1 muffin	220	4.0	33.0	430	1.0	8.0	1.0	25	33%
(Dunkin' Donuts) 3.4-oz muffin	1 muffin	340	7.0	51.0	560	na	12.0	na	40	32%
CRANBERRY *(Awrey's)* 1.5-oz muffin	1 muffin	120	2.0	20.0	210	0	4.0	0.0	10	29%
CRANBERRY NUT *(Dunkin' Donuts)* 3.5-oz muffin	1 muffin	290	6.0	44.0	360	2.0	9.0	(mq)	25	29%
OAT BRAN										
(Awrey's) 2.75-oz muffin	1 muffin	180	5.0	27.0	330	2.0	7.0	1.0	0	33%
(Awrey's) pineapple raisin, 2.75-oz muffin	1 muffin	180	5.0	26.0	320	2.0	6.0	1.0	0	30%
(Dunkin' Donuts) 3.4-oz muffin	1 muffin	330	7.0	50.0	450	3.0	11.0	(mq)	0	30%
(Hostess)	1 muffin	160	2.0	21.0	150	1.5	7.0	1.0	0	41%
(Hostess) banana nut	1 muffin	140	2.0	20.0	160	1.0	5.0	1.0	0	34%
(Health Valley) almond and date	1 muffin	180	4.0	31.0	81	8.2	4.0	(mq)	0	21%
(Health Valley) blueberry	1 muffin	180	4.0	32.0	99	7.5	4.0	(mq)	0	20%
(Health Valley) 'Fancy Fruit Muffins,' raisin	1 muffin	180	4.0	31.0	90	7.8	5.0	(mq)	0	24%
RAISIN										
(Dunkin' Donuts)	1 muffin	310	6.0	51.0	560	na	9.0	na	15	26%
(Wonder) 'Raisin Rounds'	1 muffin	140	4.0	27.0	280	1.2	2.0	(mq)	0	13%

Food Name	Serving Size	Calories	Prot. gms	Carbs gms	Sod. mgs	Fiber gms	Fat gms	Sat. Fat gms	Chol. mgs	% Fat Cal.
RAISIN BRAN										
(Awrey's) 1.5-oz muffin	1 muffin	110	2.0	18.0	170	1.0	4.0	1.0	15	31%
(Awrey's) 2.5-oz muffin	1 muffin	190	3.0	30.0	280	2.0	7.0	1.0	20	32%
(Awrey's) 'Grande' 4.2-oz muffin	1 muffin	320	5.0	50.0	470	3.0	12.0	2.0	35	33%
RAISIN SPICE *(Health Valley)* fat-free	1 muffin	140	4.0	32.0	100	5.1	0.0	na	0	0%
RASPBERRY *(Health Valley)* fat-free, twin pack	1 muffin	130	4.0	30.0	110	5.0	0.0	na	0	0%
RICE BRAN-RAISIN *(Health Valley)*	1 muffin	215	5.0	35.0	124	5.5	7.0	(mq)	0	28%
SOURDOUGH *(Wonder)*	1 muffin	130	4.0	27.0	250	1.2	1.0	na	0	7%
MUFFIN, FROZEN										
APPLE SPICE										
(Healthy Choice) 2.5-oz muffin	1 muffin	190	3.0	40.0	90	na	4.0	<1.0	0	17%
(Sara Lee) 2.5-oz muffin	1 muffin	220	4.0	36.0	280	(mq)	8.0	(mq)	0	31%
(Weight Watchers) 'Microwave' 2.5-oz muffin	1 muffin	160	3.0	29.0	260	(mq)	5.0	1.0	na	26%
BANANA NUT										
(Healthy Choice) 2.5-oz muffin	1 muffin	180	3.0	32.0	80	na	6.0	<1.0	0	28%
(Weight Watchers) 'Microwave' 2.5-oz muffin	1 muffin	170	3.0	32.0	250	(mq)	5.0	1.0	10	24%
BLUEBERRY										
(Healthy Choice) 2.5-oz muffin	1 muffin	190	3.0	39.0	110	na	4.0	<1.0	0	18%
(Pepperidge Farm) 'Old Fashioned'	1 muffin	170	2.0	27.0	250	1.0	7.0	1.0	25	35%
(Sara Lee) 2.5-oz muffin	1 muffin	200	3.0	34.0	290	(mq)	8.0	(mq)	0	33%
(Sara Lee) 'Free & Light'	1 muffin	120	3.0	28.0	140	(mq)	0.0	0.0	0	0%
(Weight Watchers) 'Microwave' 2.5-oz muffin	1 muffin	170	3.0	32.0	220	(mq)	5.0	1.0	10	24%
CHEESE STREUSEL *(Sara Lee)* 2.1-oz muffin	1 muffin	220	4.0	27.0	170	(mq)	11.0	(mq)	na	44%
CHOCOLATE CHUNK *(Sara Lee)* 2.1-oz muffin	1 muffin	220	3.0	33.0	210	(mq)	8.0	(mq)	na	33%
CINNAMON SWIRL *(Pepperidge Farm)* 'Old Fashioned'	1 muffin	190	2.0	30.0	170	1.0	6.0	1.0	35	30%
CORN *(Pepperidge Farm)* 'Old Fashioned'	1 muffin	180	3.0	27.0	260	2.0	7.0	1.0	30	34%
HONEY BRAN										
(Sara Lee) golden, 2.5-oz muffin	1 muffin	250	4.0	31.0	310	(mq)	13.0	(mq)	0	46%
(Weight Watchers) 2.5-oz muffin	1 muffin	160	3.0	32.0	150	na	4.0	<1.0	5	21%
OAT BRAN										
(Pepperidge Farm) apple 'Old Fashioned Cholesterol Free'	1 muffin	190	3.0	29.0	200	2.0	7.0	1.0	0	33%
(Sara Lee) 2.5-oz muffin	1 muffin	210	4.0	35.0	320	(mq)	8.0	(mq)	0	32%
(Sara Lee) apple, 2.5-oz muffin	1 muffin	210	4.0	35.0	320	(mq)	8.0	(mq)	0	32%
RAISIN BRAN										
(Pepperidge Farm) 'Old Fashioned Cholesterol Free'	1 muffin	170	4.0	30.0	280	3.0	6.0	1.0	0	28%
(Sara Lee) 2.5-oz muffin	1 muffin	220	4.0	37.0	400	(mq)	7.0	(mq)	0	28%
MUFFIN MIX										
ALMOND *(Krusteaz)* w/poppy seed, prepared	1 muffin	160	3.0	29.0	230	2.0	4.0	1.0	27	22%
APPLE CINNAMON										
(Betty Crocker) prepared w/egg, 2% milk	1/12 recipe	120	2.0	18.0	140	(mq)	4.0	1.0	25	31%
(Betty Crocker) prepared w/egg white, skim milk	1/12 recipe	110	2.0	18.0	140	(mq)	3.0	1.0	0	25%
(General Mills) prepared	1 muffin	100	1.0	17.0	130	na	3.0	na	0	27%
(General Mills) prepared w/egg, 1/2 cup 2% milk	1 muffin	120	2.0	18.0	140	na	4.0	na	25	31%
(General Mills) prepared w/egg white, skim milk	1 muffin	110	2.0	18.0	140	na	3.0	na	0	25%
(Krusteaz) prepared	1 muffin	180	3.0	36.0	340	na	3.0	1.0	4	15%
(Martha White) prepared	1/16 recipe	140	2.0	25.0	250	(mq)	3.0	(mq)	3	20%
(Martha White) prepared w/2% milk	1 muffin	140	2.0	25.0	250	na	3.0	na	2	20%
APPLE STREUSEL										
(Betty Crocker) Dutch, prepared w/egg, whole milk	1/12 recipe	200	3.0	32.0	240	(mq)	7.0	(mq)	(mq)	31%
APPLESAUCE										
(Gold Medal) 'Pouch Mix' prepared w/egg, whole milk	1/6 recipe	160	3.0	26.0	240	(mq)	5.0	(mq)	(mq)	28%
(Robin Hood) 'Pouch Mix' prepared w/egg, whole milk	1/6 recipe	160	3.0	26.0	240	(mq)	5.0	(mq)	(mq)	28%
BANANA										
(Gold Medal) 'Pouch Mix' prepared w/egg, whole milk	1/12 recipe	150	3.0	24.0	240	(mq)	5.0	(mq)	(mq)	29%

Food Name	Serving Size	Calories	Prot. gms	Carbs gms	Sod. mgs	Fiber gms	Fat gms	Sat. Fat gms	Chol. mgs	% Fat Cal.
(Robin Hood) 'Pouch Mix' prepared w/egg, whole milk	1/12 recipe	150	3.0	24.0	240	(mq)	5.0	(mq)	(mq)	29%
BANANA NUT										
(Betty Crocker) prepared w/egg, 2% milk	1/12 recipe	120	2.0	17.0	140	(mq)	5.0	1.0	25	37%
(Betty Crocker) prepared w/egg white, skim milk	1/12 recipe	110	2.0	17.0	140	(mq)	4.0	1.0	0	32%
(General Mills) prepared	1 muffin	110	1.0	17.0	140	na	4.0	na	0	33%
(General Mills) prepared w/egg, 1/3 cup 2% milk	1 muffin	120	2.0	18.0	150	na	4.0	na	20	31%
(General Mills) prepared w/egg white, skim milk	1 muffin	120	2.0	18.0	150	na	4.0	na	0	31%
(Martha White) prepared w/2% milk	1 muffin	180	3.0	23.0	240	na	8.0	na	35	41%
BLACKBERRY										
(Martha White) prepared	1/6 recipe	140	2.0	25.0	250	(mq)	3.0	(mq)	3	20%
(Martha White) prepared w/2% milk	1 muffin	140	2.0	25.0	250	na	3.0	na	2	20%
BLUEBERRY										
(Betty Crocker) streusel 'Bake Shop' prepared	1/12 recipe	210	3.0	31.0	230	(mq)	8.0	(mq)	(mq)	35%
(Betty Crocker) wild blueberries, prepared w/egg, 2% milk	1/12 recipe	120	2.0	18.0	150	(mq)	4.0	1.0	25	31%
(Betty Crocker) wild blueberries, prepared w/egg white, skim milk	1/12 recipe	110	2.0	18.0	150	(mq)	3.0	<1.0	0	25%
(Duncan Hines) 'Bakery Style' prepared	1 muffin	190	2.0	32.0	250	na	6.0	na	na	28%
(Duncan Hines) prepared	1 muffin	120	2.0	21.0	185	na	3.0	na	na	23%
(General Mills) 'Twice the Blueberries' prepared	1 muffin	100	1.0	17.0	130	na	3.0	na	0	27%
(General Mills) 'Twice the Blueberries' prepared, no cholesterol recipe	1 muffin	110	2.0	18.0	140	na	3.0	na	0	25%
(General Mills) 'Twice the Blueberries' prepared w/egg, 1/2 cup 2% milk	1 muffin	120	2.0	18.0	140	na	4.0	na	20	31%
(Gold Medal) 'Pouch Mix' prepared w/egg, whole milk	1/6 recipe	170	3.0	26.0	240	(mq)	6.0	(mq)	(mq)	32%
(Krusteaz) prepared	1 muffin	150	3.0	27.0	260	1.0	4.0	1.0	27	23%
(Lovin' Lites) dry mix	1/12 pkg	100	2.0	21.0	150	na	1.0	0.0	0	9%
(Lovin' Lites) prepared w/egg, water	1/12 recipe	100	2.0	21.0	160	na	1.0	0.0	20	9%
(Lovin' Lites) prepared w/2 egg whites, water	1/12 recipe	100	3.0	21.0	160	na	1.0	0.0	0	9%
(Martha White) prepared	1/6 recipe	140	2.0	25.0	260	(mq)	3.0	(mq)	3	20%
(Martha White) prepared w/2% milk	1 muffin	140	2.0	25.0	260	na	3.0	na	2	20%
(Robin Hood) 'Pouch Mix' prepared w/egg, whole milk	1/6 recipe	170	3.0	26.0	240	(mq)	6.0	(mq)	(mq)	32%
BRAN										
(Duncan Hines) w/honey 'Bakery Style' prepared	1 muffin	200	2.0	32.0	220	(mq)	7.0	(mq)	na	32%
(Martha White) prepared	1/6 recipe	150	3.0	24.0	330	(mq)	5.0	(mq)	14	29%
(Martha White) prepared w/2% milk	1 muffin	150	3.0	24.0	330	na	5.0	na	35	29%
CARAMEL										
(Gold Medal) 'Pouch Mix' prepared w/egg, whole milk	1/6 recipe	150	3.0	23.0	250	(mq)	5.0	(mq)	(mq)	30%
(Robin Hood) 'Pouch Mix' prepared w/egg, whole milk	1/6 recipe	150	3.0	23.0	250	(mq)	5.0	(mq)	(mq)	30%
CARROT NUT										
(Betty Crocker) prepared w/egg, 2% milk	1/12 recipe	150	3.0	22.0	160	(mq)	5.0	1.0	25	31%
(Betty Crocker) prepared w/egg white, skim milk	1/12 recipe	150	3.0	22.0	160	(mq)	5.0	1.0	0	31%
CHOCOLATE CHIP										
(Betty Crocker) prepared	1/12 recipe	140	2.0	22.0	180	(mq)	5.0	2.0	0	32%
(Betty Crocker) prepared w/egg, 2% milk	1/12 recipe	150	2.0	22.0	180	(mq)	6.0	2.0	20	36%
(Krusteaz) prepared	1 muffin	200	3.0	35.0	340	na	5.0	1.0	11	23%
CINNAMON										
(Betty Crocker) streusel, prepared w/egg, 2% milk	1/12 recipe	200	3.0	27.0	240	(mq)	9.0	2.0	30	40%
(Duncan Hines) swirl 'Bakery Style' prepared	1 muffin	200	2.0	32.0	245	na	7.0	na	na	32%
(General Mills) streusel, prepared	1 muffin	190	2.0	27.0	220	na	8.0	na	0	38%
CORN										
(Arrowhead Mills) blue, prepared	1 muffin	110	4.0	15.0	na	2.6	4.0	(mq)	na	32%
(Dromedary) dry mix	3 1/2 tbsp	110	1.0	20.0	250	(mq)	3.0	(mq)	na	24%
(Dromedary) prepared	1 muffin	120	3.0	20.0	270	(mq)	4.0	(mq)	na	28%
(Flako) prepared	1 muffin	116	1.8	19.8	351	.7	3.3	0.6	na	26%

Food Name	Serving Size	Calories	Prot. gms	Carbs gms	Sod. mgs	Fiber gms	Fat gms	Sat. Fat gms	Chol. mgs	% Fat Cal.
(Gold Medal) prepared w/egg, whole milk	1/6 pkg	130	3.0	24.0	250	(mq)	2.0	(mq)	(mq)	14%
(Krusteaz) prepared	1 muffin	220	4.0	36.0	450	2.0	7.0	na	5	28%
(Martha White) yellow, prepared w/water	1 muffin	160	2.0	30.0	230	na	3.0	na	<1	17%
(Robin Hood) prepared w/egg, whole milk	1/6 pkg	130	3.0	24.0	250	(mq)	2.0	(mq)	(mq)	14%
CRANBERRY-ORANGE NUT										
(Duncan Hines) 'Bakery Style' prepared	1 muffin	200	2.0	30.0	215	(mq)	8.0	(mq)	na	36%
HONEY BRAN										
(Gold Medal) 'Pouch Mix' prepared w/egg, whole milk	1/6 recipe	170	5.0	25.0	240	(mq)	6.0	(mq)	(mq)	31%
(Krusteaz), prepared	1 muffin	140	3.0	23.0	290	3.0	4.0	na	0	26%
(Martha White) w/poppy seed, prepared w/2% milk	1 muffin	200	2.0	30.0	260	na	9.0	na	35	39%
(Robin Hood) 'Pouch Mix' prepared w/egg, whole milk	1/6 recipe	170	5.0	25.0	240	(mq)	6.0	(mq)	(mq)	31%
OAT										
(Gold Medal) 'Pouch Mix' prepared w/egg, 2% milk	1/6 recipe	150	4.0	23.0	220	(mq)	5.0	1.0	45	29%
(Robin Hood) 'Pouch Mix' prepared w/egg, 2% milk	1/6 recipe	150	4.0	23.0	220	(mq)	5.0	1.0	45	29%
OAT BRAN										
(Arrowhead Mills) apple spice, prepared	1 muffin	120	6.0	15.0	(mq)	5.4	4.0	(mq)	na	30%
(General Mills) prepared	1 muffin	170	3.0	26.0	230	na	6.0	na	0	32%
(Krusteaz) prepared	1 muffin	190	3.0	33.0	310	4.0	5.0	1.0	0	24%
(Hain) apple cinnamon, prepared	1 muffin	140	4.0	28.0	200	5.0	3.0	(mq)	0	17%
(Hain) banana nut, prepared	1 muffin	140	4.0	26.0	190	4.0	4.0	(mq)	0	23%
(Hain) raspberry spice, prepared	1 muffin	140	5.0	27.0	190	4.0	3.0	(mq)	0	17%
OATMEAL RAISIN										
(Arrowhead Mills) wheat-free, prepared	1 muffin	100	5.0	11.0	na	4.5	5.0	(mq)	(mq)	41%
(Betty Crocker) prepared w/egg, 2% milk	1/8 recipe	190	4.0	25.0	240	(mq)	8.0	2.0	35	38%
(Betty Crocker) prepared w/egg white, skim milk	1/8 recipe	180	4.0	25.0	240	(mq)	7.0	2.0	0	35%
(General Mills) prepared w/egg, 1/2 cup 2% milk	1 muffin	180	4.0	26.0	250	na	7.0	na	35	34%
(General Mills) prepared w/egg white, skim milk	1 muffin	170	4.0	26.0	260	na	6.0	na	0	31%
ORANGEBERRY										
(Martha White) prepared	1/6 recipe	140	2.0	25.0	220	(mq)	3.0	(mq)	2	20%
(Martha White) prepared w/2% milk	1 muffin	140	2.0	25.0	220	na	3.0	na	2	20%
PECAN CRUNCH (Duncan Hines) 'Bakery Style' prepared	1 muffin	220	3.0	27.0	250	(mq)	11.0	(mq)	na	45%
RASPBERRY										
(Martha White) prepared	1/6 recipe	140	2.0	25.0	184	(mq)	3.0	(mq)	3	20%
(Martha White) prepared w/2% milk	1 muffin	140	2.0	25.0	180	na	3.0	na	2	20%
STRAWBERRY										
(Arrowhead Mills) wheat bran, prepared	2 muffins	270	10.0	43.0	(mq)	10.5	7.0	(mq)	na	23%
(Betty Crocker) prepared w/egg, 2% milk	1/10 recipe	150	2.0	24.0	170	(mq)	5.0	2.0	25	30%
(Betty Crocker) prepared w/egg white, skim milk	1/10 recipe	140	2.0	24.0	170	(mq)	4.0	1.0	0	26%
(Martha White) prepared	1/6 recipe	140	2.0	25.0	270	(mq)	3.0	(mq)	3	20%
(Martha White) prepared w/2% milk	1 muffin	140	2.0	25.0	270	na	3.0	na	2	20%
WILD BERRY										
(General Mills) 'Light' prepared	1 muffin	90	1.0	20.0	140	na	<1.0	na	0	<10%
(General Mills) 'Light' prepared w/egg	1 muffin	90	2.0	20.0	140	na	1.0	na	20	9%
(General Mills) prepared	1 muffin	100	1.0	18.0	140	na	3.0	na	0	26%
(General Mills) prepared w/egg, 1/2 cup 2% milk	1 muffin	120	2.0	19.0	150	na	4.0	na	20	30%
(General Mills) prepared w/egg white, skim milk	1 muffin	110	2.0	19.0	150	na	3.0	na	0	24%
MUFFIN/PASTRY, TOASTER										
APPLE										
(Kellogg's) Dutch, 'Frosted Pop-Tarts' 1.8 oz each	1 pastry	210	2.0	37.0	200	0	6.0	(mq)	0	26%
(Pastry Poppers) fruit juice sweetened, low-sodium, 2 oz each	1 pastry	212	2.9	38.0	115	na	5.4	na	na	23%
(Pillsbury) 'Toaster Strudel'	1/6 pkg	200	3.0	26.0	190	na	9.0	2.0	5	41%
(Toastettes) 'Frosted Tarts' 1.5 oz each	1 pastry	190	2.0	35.0	170	1.0	5.0	1.0	0	23%
(Toastettes) 'Tarts' 1.5 oz each	1 pastry	190	2.0	36.0	170	1.0	5.0	1.0	0	23%

Food Name	Serving Size	Calories	Prot. gms	Carbs gms	Sod. mgs	Fiber gms	Fat gms	Sat. Fat gms	Chol. mgs	% Fat Cal.
APPLE SPICE, 'Muffins' *(Toaster)* .... 1 muffin		130	2.0	21.0	100	(mq)	5.0	(mq)	na	33%
APPLE-CINNAMON										
(Pepperidge Farm) 'Croissant Toaster Tarts' .... 1 pastry		170	3.0	25.0	120	(mq)	7.0	2.0	0	36%
BANANA NUT										
(Pastry Poppers) fruit juice sweetened, low-sodium,										
2 oz each .... 1 pastry		212	2.5	38.0	115	na	4.5	na	na	20%
(Thomas') 'Toast-r-Cakes' .... 1 muffin		111	1.7	16.7	192	.6	4.4	(mq)	10	35%
(Toaster) 'Muffins' .... 1 muffin		130	2.0	19.0	85	(mq)	6.0	(mq)	na	39%
(Toaster) 'Strudel Breakfast Pastries' .... 1 pastry		190	2.0	28.0	190	(mq)	8.0	(mq)	na	38%
BLUEBERRY										
(Kellogg's) 'Frosted Pop-Tarts' 1.8 oz each .... 1 pastry		210	2.0	37.0	210	0	6.0	(mq)	0	26%
(Kellogg's) 'Pop-Tarts' 1.8 oz each .... 1 pastry		210	2.0	37.0	210	0	6.0	(mq)	0	26%
(Pillsbury) 'Toaster Strudel' .... 1/6 pkg		190	3.0	26.0	210	na	9.0	2.0	5	41%
(Thomas') 'Toast-r-Cakes' .... 1 muffin		108	1.6	18.0	158	(mq)	3.3	(mq)	na	28%
(Toaster) 'Strudel Breakfast Pastries' .... 1 pastry		190	2.0	28.0	200	(mq)	8.0	(mq)	na	38%
(Toaster) wild, Maine .... 1 muffin		120	2.0	23.0	135	(mq)	3.0	(mq)	na	21%
(Toastettes) 'Frosted Tarts' 1.5 oz each .... 1 pastry		190	2.0	35.0	200	1.0	5.0	1.0	0	23%
(Toastettes) 'Tarts' 1.5 oz each .... 1 pastry		190	2.0	35.0	200	1.0	5.0	1.0	0	23%
BRAN *(Thomas')* 'Toast-r-Cakes' .... 1 muffin		103	1.7	17.6	163	(mq)	2.9	(mq)	na	25%
BROWN SUGAR-CINNAMON										
(Kellogg's) 'Frosted Pop-Tarts' .... 1 pastry		210	3.0	34.0	180	0	7.0	(mq)	0	30%
(Toastettes) 'Frosted Tarts' 1.5 oz each .... 1 pastry		190	2.0	35.0	180	1.0	5.0	1.0	0	23%
(Kellogg's) 'Pop-Tarts' 1.8 oz each .... 1 pastry		210	3.0	33.0	210	0	8.0	(mq)	0	33%
CHEESE *(Pepperidge Farm)* 'Croissant Toaster Tarts' .... 1 pastry		190	5.0	22.0	180	(mq)	10.0	3.0	10	46%
CHERRY										
(Kellogg's) 'Frosted Pop-Tarts' 1.8 oz each .... 1 pastry		200	2.0	37.0	220	0	5.0	(mq)	0	22%
(Kellogg's) 'Pop-Tarts' 1.8 oz each .... 1 pastry		210	2.0	37.0	220	0	6.0	(mq)	0	26%
(Pastry Poppers) fruit juice sweetened, low-sodium,										
2 oz each .... 1 pastry		212	2.5	38.0	115	na	4.5	na	na	20%
(Toaster) 'Strudel Breakfast Pastries' .... 1 pastry		190	2.0	26.0	200	(mq)	9.0	(mq)	na	42%
(Toastettes) 'Frosted Tarts' 1.5 oz each .... 1 pastry		190	2.0	35.0	200	1.0	5.0	1.0	0	23%
(Toastettes) 'Tarts' 1.5 oz each .... 1 pastry		190	2.0	35.0	200	1.0	5.0	1.0	0	23%
CHOCOLATE FUDGE										
(Kellogg's) 'Frosted Pop-Tarts' 1.8 oz each .... 1 pastry		200	3.0	37.0	220	0	5.0	(mq)	0	22%
CHOCOLATE-VANILLA CREME										
(Kellogg's) 'Frosted Pop-Tarts' 1.8 oz each .... 1 pastry		200	3.0	37.0	230	0	5.0	(mq)	0	22%
CINNAMON										
(Pillsbury) 'Toaster Strudel' .... 1/6 pkg		200	5.0	23.0	200	na	10.0	2.0	5	45%
(Toaster) 'Strudel Breakfast Pastries' .... 1 pastry		190	2.0	26.0	200	(mq)	8.0	(mq)	na	39%
CORN										
(Thomas') 'Toast-r-Cakes' .... 1 muffin		120	1.8	19.2	142	(mq)	4.0	(mq)	na	30%
(Toaster) 'Old Fashioned Muffins' .... 1 muffin		120	2.0	17.0	200	(mq)	5.0	(mq)	na	37%
FRUIT PUNCH *(Toastettes)* 'Frosted Tarts' 1.5 oz each ...... 1 pastry		190	2.0	35.0	200	1.0	5.0	1.0	0	23%
FUDGE *(Toastettes)* 'Frosted Tarts' 1.5 oz each .... 1 pastry		200	2.0	34.0	280	1.0	5.0	1.0	0	24%
GRAPE *(Kellogg's)* 'Frosted Pop-Tarts' 1.8 oz each .... 1 pastry		200	2.0	37.0	200	0	5.0	(mq)	200	22%
OAT BRAN *(Awrey's)* 'Toastums' w/raisins .... 1 muffin		130	3.0	17.0	310	1.0	5.0	1.0	0	36%
PEACH-APRICOT *(Pastry Poppers)* fruit juice sweetened,										
low-sodium, 2 oz each .... 1 pastry		212	2.5	38.0	115	na	4.5	na	na	20%
RAISIN BRAN *(Toaster)* 'Muffins' .... 1 muffin		120	3.0	16.0	220	(mq)	5.0	(mq)	na	37%
RASPBERRY										
(Kellogg's) 'Frosted Pop-Tarts' 1.8 oz each .... 1 pastry		200	2.0	37.0	210	0	5.0	(mq)	0	22%
(Pastry Poppers) fruit juice sweetened, low-sodium,										
2 oz each .... 1 pastry		212	2.5	38.0	115	na	4.5	na	na	20%
(Toaster) 'Strudel Breakfast Pastries' .... 1 pastry		190	2.0	27.0	200	(mq)	8.0	(mq)	na	38%

Food Name	Serving Size	Calories	Prot. gms	Carbs gms	Sod. mgs	Fiber gms	Fat gms	Sat. Fat gms	Chol. mgs	% Fat Cal.
STRAWBERRY										
(Kellogg's) 'Frosted Pop-Tarts' 1.8 oz each	1 pastry	200	2.0	37.0	190	0	5.0	(mq)	0	22%
(Kellogg's) 'Pop-Tarts' 1.8 oz each	1 pastry	210	2.0	37.0	200	0	6.0	(mq)	0	26%
(Pastry Poppers) fruit juice sweetened, low-sodium, 2 oz each	1 pastry	212	2.5	38.0	115	na	4.5	na	na	20%
(Pepperidge Farm) 'Croissant Toaster Tarts'	1 pastry	190	3.0	28.0	120	(mq)	7.0	2.0	0	34%
(Pillsbury) 'Toaster Strudel'	1/6 pkg	190	3.0	26.0	200	na	9.0	2.0	5	41%
(Toaster) 'Strudel Breakfast Pastries'	1 pastry	190	2.0	27.0	200	(mq)	8.0	(mq)	na	38%
(Toastettes) 'Frosted Tarts' 1.5 oz each	1 pastry	190	2.0	35.0	200	1.0	5.0	1.0	0	23%
(Toastettes) 'Tarts' 1.5 oz each	1 pastry	190	2.0	35.0	200	1.0	5.0	1.0	0	23%
MULBERRY										
raw	1 lb	197	6.5	44.5	46	>4.4 c	1.8	na	0	7%
raw	1 cup	60	2.0	13.7	14	2.4	0.6	na	0	8%
raw	1/2 cup	31	1.0	6.9	7	1.2	0.3	(tr)	0	8%
raw	1 oz	12	0.4	2.8	3	>.3 c	0.1	(tr)	0	7%
MULLANGI. See DAIKON.										
MULLET, STRIPED										
baked	4 oz	170	28.1	0.0	81	0	5.5	1.6	71	31%
broiled	4 oz	170	28.1	0.0	81	0	5.5	1.6	71	31%
dry-heat cooked	3 oz	127	21.1	0.0	60	0	4.1	1.2	54	30%
microwaved	4 oz	170	28.1	0.0	81	0	5.5	1.6	71	31%
raw	1 lb	530	87.8	0.0	294	0	17.2	5.1	224	31%
raw	3 oz	99	16.5	0.0	55	0	3.2	1.0	42	30%
raw	1 oz	33	5.5	0.0	18	0	1.1	0.3	14	31%
MUNG BEAN										
boiled	4 oz	119	8.0	21.7	2	2.8	0.4	0.1	0	3%
boiled	1/2 cup	106	7.1	19.3	2	7.7	0.4	0.1	0	3%
raw	1/2 cup	361	24.8	65.1	16	17.0	1.2	0.4	0	3%
raw	1 oz	98	6.8	17.8	4	2.7	0.3	0.1	0	3%
sprouted, boiled, drained	4 oz	24	2.3	4.8	11	>.6 c	0.1	<.1	0	3%
sprouted, boiled, drained	1/2 cup	13	1.3	2.6	6	.5	0.1	0.0	0	6%
sprouted, raw	1 lb	136	13.8	26.9	26	5.0	0.8	0.2	0	4%
sprouted, raw	1/2 cup	16	1.6	3.1	3	.9	0.1	0.0	0	5%
sprouted, raw	1 oz	9	0.9	1.7	2	.3	0.1	<.1	0	8%
sprouted, stir-fried	4 oz	57	4.9	12.0	(mq)	>.8 c	0.2	<.1	0	3%
sprouted, stir-fried	1/2 cup	31	2.7	6.6	6	>.4 c	0.1	0.0	0	2%
MUNG BEAN, CANNED										
drained	4 oz	14	1.6	2.4	(mq)	>.3 c	0.1	<.1	0	5%
sprouted *(LaChoy)*	2 oz	8	0.8	1.0	20	.7	0.1	na	0	11%
sprouted, drained	1/2 cup	7	0.9	1.3	87	.5	0.0	0.0	0	0%
MUNG BEAN LONG RICE										
dehydrated	1/2 cup	246	0.1	60.3	7	.4	0.0	0.0	0	0%
dehydrated	1 oz	99	<.1	24.4	3	tr	tr	tr	0	0%
MUNGO BEAN										
boiled	1/2 cup	94	6.8	16.5	6	5.8	0.5	0.0	0	5%
raw	1/2 cup	365	26.1	63.5	27	>4.6 c	1.9	0.1	0	5%
MUSHROOM, ENOKI										
raw	1 large	2	0.1	0.4	0	na	0.0	0.0	0	0%
raw	1 med	1	0.1	0.2	0	na	0.0	0.0	0	0%
MUSHROOM, JAPANESE HONEY/hon shimeji										
trimmed	1 lb	136	9.5	20.0	(mq)	(mq)	1.4	na	0	10%
trimmed	1 oz	9	0.6	1.2	(mq)	(mq)	<.1	(tr)	0	<11%
MUSHROOM, OYSTER/abalone/hiritake/shimeji/tree mushroom										
(Frieda's)	1 lb	113	9.5	20.9	18	3.6	1.8	na	0	12%

Food Name	Serving Size	Calories	Prot. gms	Carbs gms	Sod. mgs	Fiber gms	Fat gms	Sat. Fat gms	Chol. mgs	% Fat Cal.
(Frieda's)	1 oz	7	0.6	1.3	1	.2	0.1	(tr)	0	11%
MUSHROOM, SHIITAKE										
cooked	4 oz	62	1.8	16.2	5	>2.2 c	0.2	0.1	0	2%
cooked, pieces	1 cup	80	2.3	20.7	6	3.0	0.3	0.1	0	3%
dried	1 lb	1343	43.5	341.9	60	>52.2 c	4.5	1.1	0	3%
dried	1 oz	84	2.7	21.4	4	>3.3 c	0.3	0.1	0	3%
MUSHROOM, STRAW										
(Green Giant) canned	2 oz	12	1.0	2.0	290	1.0	0.0	0.0	0	0%
(Green Giant) canned, whole	1/4 cup	12	1.0	2.0	290	1.0	0.0	0.0	0	0%
MUSHROOM, WHITE										
boiled, drained	4 oz	31	2.5	5.8	2	2.5	0.5	0.1	0	12%
boiled, drained, pieces	1/2 cup	21	1.7	4.0	2	1.7	0.4	0.1	0	14%
raw, pieces	1/2 cup	9	0.7	1.6	1	.5	0.2	0.0	0	16%
raw, trimmed	1 oz	7	0.6	1.3	1	.4	0.1	<.1	0	11%
raw, untrimmed	1 lb	111	9.2	20.5	16	5.7	1.9	0.2	0	13%
Canned										
drained	4 oz	27	2.1	5.6	(mq)	(mq)	0.3	<.1	0	8%
pieces, drained	1/2 cup	19	1.5	3.9	331	1.9	0.2	0.0	0	8%
(Allens) pieces and stems	1/2 cup	20	2.0	3.0	450	(mq)	<1.0	(tr)	0	<31%
(B In B)	1/4 cup	12	1.0	2.0	240	1.0	0.0	0.0	0	0%
(B In B) w/garlic	1/4 cup	12	1.0	2.0	200	1.0	0.0	0.0	0	0%
(Empress) pieces and stems	2 oz	14	1.0	2.0	260	(mq)	na	na	0	0%
(Green Giant) in butter sauce	1/2 cup	30	2.0	4.0	330	.6	1.0	na	na	27%
(Green Giant) whole, pieces, and stems	1/4 cup	12	1.0	2.0	220	1.0	0.0	0.0	0	0%
Frozen										
(Birds Eye) whole, 'Deluxe'	2.6 oz	20	2.0	4.0	0	2.0	0.0	na	0	0%
(Freshlike)	3.5 oz	30	3.0	4.0	15	na	0.0	na	na	0%
(Green Giant) creamy 'Right for Lunch'	9.5-oz pkg	220	6.0	29.0	860	4.0	11.0	6.0	25	41%
(Stilwell) battered 'Quick Krisp'	2 oz	140	2.0	15.0	280	(mq)	8.0	(mq)	5	51%
(Veg•All)	3.5 oz	30	3.0	4.0	15	na	0.0	na	na	0%
MUSKMELON. See CANTALOUPE.										
MUSKRAT										
raw	1 lb	735	94.2	0.0	372	na	36.7	na	na	47%
raw	1 oz	45	5.8	0.0	23	na	2.3	na	na	47%
roasted	3 oz	199	25.6	0.0	81	0	10.0	na	103	47%
roasted, diced	1 cup	258	33.0	0.0	105	0	12.9	(mq)	(mq)	47%
MUSSEL, BLUE										
moist-heat cooked	4 oz	195	27.0	8.4	418	0	5.1	1.0	64	25%
moist-heat cooked	3 oz	146	20.2	6.3	314	0	3.8	0.7	48	24%
raw	1 lb	391	54.0	16.8	1296	0	10.2	1.9	127	25%
raw	1 cup	129	17.8	5.5	429	0	3.4	0.6	42	25%
raw	3 oz	73	10.1	3.1	243	0	1.9	0.4	24	25%
MUSTARD, DRY. See MUSTARD POWDER.										
MUSTARD, PREPARED										
(Featherweight)	1 tsp	5	0.0	0.0	0	0	0.0	0.0	0	0%
(French's) 'Medford'	1 tbsp	16	1.0	1.0	240	na	1.0	na	0	53%
(Grey Poupon) 'Parisian'	1 tsp	6	0.0	0.0	55	0	0.0	0.0	0	0%
(Kraft) 'Pure'	1 tbsp	11	0.0	1.0	160	0	1.0	0.0	0	69%
(Life) 'English All Natural'	1 tbsp	22	2.0	<1.0	2	na	2.0	na	0	60%
(Westbrae) 'Mt. Fuji'	1 tbsp	16	1.0	1.0	195	na	1.0	na	0	53%
DIJON										
(French's)	1 tsp	8	0.0	0.0	140	0	1.0	na	0	100%
(Grey Poupon)	1 tbsp	18	0.0	0.0	450	0	1.0	na	0	100%
(Grey Poupon) 'Country Style'	1 tsp	6	0.0	0.0	120	0	0.0	0.0	0	0%

Food Name	Serving Size	Calories	Prot. gms	Carbs gms	Sod. mgs	Fiber gms	Fat gms	Sat. Fat gms	Chol. mgs	% Fat Cal.
(Westbrae)	1 tbsp	16	1.0	1.0	195	na	1.0	na	0	53%
HORSERADISH										
(French's)	1 tbsp	16	1.0	1.0	265	na	1.0	na	0	53%
(Kraft)	1 tbsp	14	1.0	1.0	135	0	1.0	0.0	0	53%
JALAPEÑO *(Great Impressions)*	2 tsp	7	0.4	0.7	173	na	0.3	na	0	38%
ONION *(French's)*	1 tsp	8	0.0	2.0	70	na	0.0	0.0	0	0%
SPICY										
(French's) 'Bold'n Spicy'	1 tsp	6	0.0	0.0	50	na	0.0	0.0	0	0%
(Gulden's) hot, 'Diablo'	.25 oz	8	0.0	0.0	55	0	0.0	0.0	0	0%
(Gulden's) 'Spicy Brown'	.25 oz	8	0.0	0.0	45	0	0.0	0.0	0	0%
(Heinz) 'Brown'	1 tbsp	14	<1.0	1.0	115	na	1.0	0.0	0	53%
STONE GROUND										
(Hain)	1 tbsp	14	1.0	1.0	185	na	1.0	na	0	53%
(Hain) no salt added	1 tbsp	14	1.0	1.0	10	na	1.0	na	0	53%
(Westbrae)	1 tbsp	16	1.0	1.0	195	na	1.0	na	0	53%
(Westbrae) no salt added	1 tbsp	16	1.0	1.0	195	na	1.0	na	0	53%
YELLOW										
(French's)	1 tbsp	10	1.0	1.0	180	na	1.0	na	0	53%
(Gulden's) 'Creamy Mild'	.25 oz	6	0.0	0.0	60	0	0.0	0.0	0	0%
(Heinz)	1 tsp	3	0.2	0.2	55	na	0.2	na	0	53%
(Heinz) 'Mild'	1 tbsp	8	1.0	1.0	175	na	1.0	<1.0	0	53%
(Westbrae)	1 tbsp	16	1.0	1.0	195	na	1.0	na	0	53%
MUSTARD BLEND, *(Best Foods)* 'Dijonnaise'	1 tsp	12	0.0	1.0	70	na	1.0	na	0	69%
MUSTARD GREENS										
boiled, drained	4 oz	17	2.6	2.4	18	>.8 c	0.3	<.1	0	12%
boiled, drained, chopped	1/2 cup	10	1.6	1.5	11	1.4	0.2	0.0	0	13%
raw, chopped	1/2 cup	7	0.8	1.4	7	.6	0.1	0.0	0	9%
raw, untrimmed	1 lb	109	11.4	20.7	107	2.5	0.8	<.1	0	5%
Canned *(Allens)* chopped	1/2 cup	20	1.0	2.0	35	(mq)	<1.0	na	0	<43%
Frozen										
boiled, drained	10-oz pkg	40	4.8	6.6	53	>1.5 c	0.5	0.0	0	9%
boiled, drained	4 oz	22	2.6	3.5	28	>.8 c	0.3	<.1	0	10%
boiled, drained, chopped	1/2 cup	14	1.7	2.3	19	>.6 c	0.2	0.0	0	10%
chopped	1/2 cup	15	1.8	2.5	21	1.5	0.2	0.0	0	10%
unprepared	10-oz pkg	57	7.1	9.7	82	>2.3 c	0.8	0.0	0	10%
(Frosty Acres)	3.3 oz	20	2.0	3.0	20	>1.0 c	0.0	0.0	0	0%
(Seabrook) chopped	3.3 oz	20	2.0	3.0	20	>1.0 c	0.0	0.0	0	0%
(Southern) chopped	3.5 oz	25	2.5	3.6	40	(mq)	0.3	(tr)	0	10%
MUSTARD OIL										
	1 cup	1927	0.0	0.0	0	0	218.0	25.3	na	100%
	1 oz	251	0.0	0.0	0	0	28.4	3.3	0	100%
	1 tbsp	124	0.0	0.0	0	0	14.0	1.6	na	100%
MUSTARD POWDER										
ground *(Durkee)*	1 tsp	19	0.0	0.0	0	0	<0.1	na	na	<66%
ground *(Laurel Leaf)*	1 tsp	19	0.0	0.0	0	0	<0.1	na	na	<66%
ground *(Spice Islands)*	1 tsp	9	0.5	0.3	<1	<.1	0.6	na	0	63%
MUSTARD SEED, YELLOW										
whole	1 oz	133	7.1	9.9	1	>1.9 c	8.2	0.4	0	52%
whole	1 tbsp	53	2.8	3.9	1	>.7 c	3.2	0.2	0	52%
whole	1 tsp	15	0.8	1.1	0	>.2 c	1.0	0.1	0	54%
MUSTARD SPINACH / tendergreen										
boiled, drained	4 oz	18	1.9	3.2	(mq)	>.9 c	0.2	na	0	8%
boiled, drained, chopped	1/2 cup	14	1.5	2.5	13	>.7 c	0.2	na	0	10%
raw, chopped	1/2 cup	16	1.6	2.9	16	>.8 c	0.2	na	0	9%

Food Name	Serving Size	Calories	Prot. gms	Carbs gms	Sod. mgs	Fiber gms	Fat gms	Sat. Fat gms	Chol. mgs	% Fat Cal.
raw, trimmed	1 oz	6	0.6	1.1	(mq)	>.3 c	0.1	na	0	12%
raw, untrimmed	1 lb	93	9.3	16.5	(mq)	>4.2 c	1.3	na	0	10%
MUSTARD TALLOW	1 oz	256	0.0	0.0	0	0	28.4	13.4	29	100%
MUTTON TALLOW										
	1 cup	1849	0.0	0.0	0	0	205.0	97.0	209	100%
	1 tbsp	115	0.0	0.0	0	0	12.8	6.1	13	100%

MUTTONFISH. See OCEAN POUT.

N

Food Name	Serving Size	Calories	Prot. gms	Carbs gms	Sod. mgs	Fiber gms	Fat gms	Sat. Fat gms	Chol. mgs	% Fat Cal.
NACHO CHIPS. See CORN CHIPS AND SNACKS.										
NACHO SEASONING (Lawry's) 'Seasoning Blends'	1 pkg	141	6.7	15.0	2168	>1.6 c	6.8	(mq)	na	41%
NAPA CABBAGE. See CABBAGE, NAPA.										
NATAL PLUM. See CARISSA.										
NATTO. See SOYBEAN, FERMENTED.										
NAVY BEAN										
boiled	4 oz	161	9.9	29.8	1	4.1	0.6	0.2	0	3%
boiled	1/2 cup	129	7.9	23.9	1	>2.9 c	0.5	0.1	0	3%
cooked 'Michigan #1' (A&P)	1 cup	220	15.0	40.0	15	(mq)	1.0	(mq)	0	4%
raw	1/2 cup	348	23.2	63.1	15	25.0	1.3	0.3	0	3%
raw	1 oz	95	6.3	17.2	4	2.7	0.4	0.1	0	4%
NAVY BEAN, CANNED										
(Allens)	1/2 cup	160	8.0	24.0	440	(mq)	<1.0	0.1	0	<7%
(Bush's Best)	1/2 cup	60	5.0	17.0	370	7.0	0.0	na	na	0%
(Eden Foods) organic, very low sodium	1/2 cup	70	6.0	18.0	15	7.0	<1.0	na	0	<9%
(Hunt's) w/ham 'Homestyle'	9.03 oz	239	16.2	37.6	737	10.0	2.7	0.9	10	10%
NAVY BEAN, SPROUTED										
boiled, drained	4 oz	88	8.0	17.0	(mq)	>3.3 c	0.9	0.1	0	8%
raw	1 lb	306	27.9	59.2	(mq)	>11.3 c	3.2	0.4	0	8%
raw	1/2 cup	35	3.2	6.8	7	>1.3 c	0.4	0.0	0	8%
raw	1 oz	19	1.7	3.7	(mq)	>.7 c	0.2	<.1	0	8%
NECTAR. See individual flavors.										
NECTARINE										
pitted	1 oz	14	0.3	3.3	tr	.5	0.1	na	0	6%
sliced	1 cup	68	1.3	16.3	0	2.2	0.6	na	0	7%
trimmed, approx 2.5 inch diam	1 med	67	1.3	16.0	0	2.2	0.6	na	0	7%
untrimmed (Dole)	1 med	70	1.0	16.0	0	3.0	1.0	na	na	12%
whole	1 lb	204	3.9	48.6	1	6.6	1.9	na	0	8%
NEW ZEALAND SPINACH. See SPINACH, NEW ZEALAND.										
NOODLE. See NOODLE, CHINESE; NOODLE, EGG; NOODLE, JAPANESE; PASTA.										
NOODLE, CHINESE										
cellophane, dehydrated	1 lb	1594	0.7	390.6	44	>.3 c	0.3	0.1	0	0%
cellophane, dehydrated	2 oz	199	0.1	48.8	6	<.1	<.1	tr	0	<1%
chow mein	1 cup	237	3.8	25.9	198	1.8	13.8	2.0	0	51%
chow mein	1.5 oz	227	3.6	24.7	189	1.7	13.2	1.9	0	51%
long rice, dehydrated	1 lb	1594	0.7	390.6	44	>.3 c	0.3	0.1	0	0%
long rice, dehydrated	2 oz	199	0.1	48.8	6	<.1	<.1	tr	0	<1%
NOODLE, EGG										
(NOTE: All of the following egg noodles are dry unless otherwise noted.)										
DUMPLING (Creamette) w/pasteurized eggs	2 oz	220	8.0	40.0	20	na	3.0	na	70	12%

Food Name	Serving Size	Calories	Prot. gms	Carbs gms	Sod. mgs	Fiber gms	Fat gms	Sat. Fat gms	Chol. mgs	% Fat Cal.
ENRICHED										
....	2 oz	217	8.0	40.5	12	1.8	2.4	0.5	54	10%
cooked	1 cup	213	7.6	39.7	11	1.5	2.3	0.5	53	10%
EXTRA WIDE (American Beauty) enriched	2 oz	220	8.0	42.0	15	na	3.0	na	55	12%
FINE										
(American Beauty) enriched	2 oz	220	8.0	42.0	15	na	3.0	na	55	12%
(Herb's)	2 oz	230	10.0	40.0	5	na	2.0	na	60	8%
JERUSALEM ARTICHOKE										
(De Boles)	2 oz	210	9.0	41.0	0	na	1.0	na	0	4%
(De Boles) w/garlic and parsley	2 oz	210	9.0	41.0	15	na	1.0	na	0	4%
MEDIUM (American Beauty) enriched	2 oz	220	8.0	42.0	15	na	3.0	na	55	12%
PLAIN										
cooked	4 oz	151	5.4	28.2	8	2.5	1.7	0.4	37	10%
(Creamette) enriched	2 oz	221	8.0	40.0	3	.8	2.5	0.8	70	11%
(Gioia)	2 oz	220	8.0	40.0	(mq)	(mq)	3.0	(mq)	(mq)	12%
(Golden Grain)	2 oz	210	8.2	39.3	10	1.8	2.2	0.8	65	9%
(Goodman's) 'Country Style'	2 oz	220	8.0	40.0	15	(mq)	3.0	(mq)	(mq)	12%
(Mrs. Grass)	2 oz	220	8.0	40.0	200	(mq)	3.0	(mq)	(mq)	12%
(Mueller's)	2 oz	220	8.0	40.0	10	(mq)	3.0	(mq)	55	12%
(P&R)	2 oz	220	8.0	42.0	15	(mq)	3.0	(mq)	(mq)	12%
(Prince)	2 oz	210	8.0	40.0	35	(mq)	2.0	(mq)	65	9%
(San Giorgio)	2 oz	220	8.0	42.0	15	(mq)	3.0	(mq)	(mq)	12%
SPINACH										
cooked	4 oz	150	5.7	27.5	14	(mq)	1.8	0.4	37	11%
enriched	1 cup	145	5.6	26.7	27	2.6	1.7	0.4	36	11%
enriched	2 oz	218	8.3	40.1	41	3.9	2.6	0.6	54	11%
enriched, cooked	1 cup	211	8.1	38.8	19	3.7	2.5	0.6	53	11%
SUBSTITUTE (No Yolks) broad	2 oz	200	8.0	40.0	25	na	1.0	na	0	5%
UNENRICHED										
....	2 oz	74	1.5	16.1	218	.2	0.2	0.0	0	3%
cooked	1 cup	213	7.6	39.7	11	1.8	2.3	0.5	53	10%
VERY LOW SODIUM (Ronzoni) 'Egg Pastina'	2 oz	220	8.0	42.0	15	na	3.0	na	65	12%
WIDE										
(American Beauty) enriched	2 oz	220	8.0	42.0	15	na	3.0	na	55	12%
(Creamette) w/pasteurized eggs 'Fancy'	2 oz	220	8.0	40.0	20	na	3.0	na	70	12%
(Hospitality) enriched 'Valu Pack'	1 1/4 cup	235	9.0	43.0	5	2.0	2.5	0.5	80	10%
(Ronzoni) enriched 'Country Kitchen Style'	2 oz	220	8.0	42.0	15	na	3.0	na	65	12%
NOODLE, JAPANESE										
GENMAI, dry (Westbrae)	2 oz	200	5.0	41.0	411	na	1.0	na	0	5%
SOBA/BUCKWHEAT										
cooked	1 cup	113	5.8	24.4	68	>.4 c	0.1	0.0	0	1%
dry	1 lb	1526	65.2	338.5	3593	(mq)	3.2	0.6	0	2%
dry	2 oz	192	8.2	42.5	451	>.7 c	0.4	0.1	0	2%
dry (Westbrae)	2 oz	190	7.0	40.0	5	na	2.0	na	0	9%
SOMEN/WHEAT										
cooked	1 cup	231	7.0	48.5	283	>.4 c	0.3	0.0	0	1%
cooked	4 oz	149	4.5	31.2	183	>.3 c	0.2	<.1	0	1%
dry	2 oz	203	6.5	42.2	1049	2.5	0.5	0.1	0	2%
whole wheat, dry (Westbrae)	2 oz	200	7.0	41.0	375	na	1.0	na	0	5%
TRADITIONAL, dry (Westbrae)	2 oz	190	7.0	41.0	198	na	2.0	na	0	9%
UDON/WHEAT										
cooked	4 oz	115	2.8	23.0	51	(mq)	0.6	(mq)	0	5%
dry	2 oz	159	3.9	32.3	340	(mq)	0.7	(mq)	0	4%
whole wheat, organic, dry (Westbrae)	2 oz	200	7.0	41.0	375	na	1.0	na	0	5%

Food Name	Serving Size	Calories	Prot. gms	Carbs gms	Sod. mgs	Fiber gms	Fat gms	Sat. Fat gms	Chol. mgs	% Fat Cal.
NOODLE ENTRÉE/DISH										
(Dinty Moore)										
and chicken 'American Classics'	10 oz	230	17.0	24.0	1020	na	7.0	3.0	65	28%
tuna casserole 'American Classics'	10 oz	240	16.0	28.0	1280	na	7.0	4.0	65	26%
(LaChoy)										
and beef	9.03 oz	156	7.4	26.8	1332	2.9	3.5	1.5	6	19%
and chicken	8.995 oz	163	10.2	24.4	859	1.4	3.3	1.3	19	18%
and vegetables	9.383 oz	131	4.8	26.6	1311	2.9	1.3	0.6	0	9%
chow mein	2 tbsp	140	4.5	17.0	209	1.9	6.1	1.3	0	39%
chow mein, narrow	1/2 cup	150	3.0	16.0	230	<1.0	8.0	1.2	0	49%
chow mein, wide	1/2 cup	150	3.0	16.0	300	<1.0	8.0	1.2	0	49%
crispy, wide	2 tbsp	148	2.3	17.1	258	1.1	7.8	1.5	0	48%
rice	1/2 cup	130	2.0	21.0	420	<1.0	5.0	(mq)	0	33%
rice	2 tbsp	122	2.1	21.9	362	.4	3.1	0.4	0	23%
(Westbrae)										
brown rice, steamed 'Ramen'	1 oz	100	3.0	21.0	500	na	1.0	na	0	9%
buckwheat, steamed 'Ramen'	1 oz	100	3.0	20.0	500	na	0.0	na	0	0%
carrot, steamed 'Ramen'	1 oz	100	3.0	20.0	460	na	1.0	na	0	9%
curry, steamed 'Ramen'	1 oz	100	3.0	20.0	420	na	1.0	na	0	9%
5-spice, steamed 'Ramen'	1 oz	100	3.0	20.0	420	na	1.0	na	0	9%
miso, steamed 'Ramen'	1 oz	100	3.0	20.0	540	na	1.0	na	0	9%
mushroom, steamed 'Ramen'	1 oz	100	3.0	20.0	340	na	1.0	na	0	9%
onion, steamed 'Ramen'	1 oz	100	3.0	20.0	460	na	1.0	na	0	9%
seaweed, steamed 'Ramen'	1 oz	100	3.0	20.0	460	na	1.0	na	0	9%
spinach, steamed 'Ramen'	1 oz	100	3.0	20.0	460	na	1.0	na	0	9%
tofu, steamed 'Ramen'	1 oz	100	3.0	20.0	460	na	1.0	na	0	9%
whole wheat, steamed 'Ramen'	1 oz	110	3.0	22.0	480	na	1.0	na	0	8%
NOODLE ENTRÉE/DISH, CANNED										
(Heinz)										
and chicken	7.5 oz	160	6.0	19.0	930	(mq)	7.0	(mq)	(mq)	39%
w/beef, in sauce	7.5 oz	170	8.0	17.0	825	(mq)	8.0	(mq)	(mq)	42%
w/tuna	7.5 oz	170	11.0	20.0	950	(mq)	5.0	(mq)	(mq)	27%
(Nalley's)										
and chicken	7 3/8 oz	150	9.0	17.0	1000	(mq)	5.0	(mq)	(mq)	30%
and chicken w/vegetables	7 3/8 oz	160	10.0	18.0	1450	(mq)	5.0	(mq)	(mq)	29%
(Van Camp's) w/franks 'Noodle Weenee'	1 cup	245	9.3	32.9	1245	>5.0 c	8.5	(mq)	(mq)	31%
NOODLE ENTRÉE/DISH, FREEZE-DRIED										
(Mountain House) w/chicken, prepared	1 cup	270	10.0	34.0	201	(mq)	10.0	(mq)	(mq)	34%
NOODLE ENTRÉE/DISH, FROZEN										
(Banquet)										
and beef w/gravy 'Family Entrées'	8 oz	200	13.0	22.0	(mq)	(mq)	7.0	(mq)	(mq)	31%
and julienne beef w/sauce 'Family Entrées'	7 oz	170	12.0	22.0	(mq)	(mq)	3.0	(mq)	(mq)	17%
w/chicken	10 oz	350	10.0	42.0	460	(mq)	15.0	(mq)	45	39%
w/chicken 'Family Favorites'	10 oz	340	11.0	42.0	455	(mq)	15.0	(mq)	45	39%
(Stouffer's) Romanoff	6 oz	260	11.0	23.0	1260	na	14.0	na	na	48%
(Swanson) w/chicken	10.5 oz	280	7.0	45.0	740	(mq)	8.0	(mq)	(mq)	26%
NOODLE ENTRÉE/DISH, MICROWAVE										
(Hormel) and chicken 'Micro-Cup'	7.5 oz	180	7.0	18.0	1000	(mq)	8.0	(mq)	20	42%
(Kid's Kitchen) rings and chicken	7.5 oz	150	11.0	17.0	840	na	4.0	na	25	24%
(Minute)										
Alfredo, family size, prepared w/salted butter	1/2 cup	170	7.0	23.0	670	(mq)	6.0	(mq)	45	31%
Alfredo, single size, prepared w/salted butter	1/2 cup	160	7.0	23.0	660	(mq)	5.0	(mq)	40	27%
chicken or chicken flavor, family size, prepared	1/2 cup	160	6.0	23.0	570	(mq)	5.0	(mq)	35	28%
chicken or chicken flavor, single size, prepared	1/2 cup	160	6.0	25.0	610	(mq)	4.0	(mq)	35	23%

Food Name	Serving Size	Calories	Prot. gms	Carbs gms	Sod. mgs	Fiber gms	Fat gms	Sat. Fat gms	Chol. mgs	% Fat Cal.
Parmesan, family size, prepared w/salted butter	1/2 cup	170	6.0	23.0	470	(mq)	6.0	(mq)	45	32%
Parmesan, single size, prepared w/salted butter	1/2 cup	160	6.0	23.0	460	(mq)	5.0	(mq)	40	28%
w/cheddar cheese, family size, prepared w/salted butter	1/2 cup	160	6.0	20.0	530	na	7.0	na	15	38%
w/cheddar cheese, single size, prepared w/salted butter	1/2 cup	160	6.0	20.0	520	na	6.0	na	15	34%
NOODLE ENTRÉE/DISH, MIX										
(Kraft)										
cheese 'Dinner' prepared	3/4 cup	340	10.0	37.0	670	(mq)	17.0	4.0	50	45%
chicken flavor 'Dinner' prepared	3/4 cup	240	8.0	32.0	1050	(mq)	9.0	2.0	45	34%
(LaChoy)										
beef flavor 'Ramen' prepared	1 cup	225	6.0	33.0	865	4.0	8.0	1.1	0	32%
chicken flavor 'Ramen' prepared	1 cup	200	6.0	29.0	740	4.0	7.0	1.1	0	31%
(Lipton)										
Alfredo 'Noodles and Sauce' dry mix	1/4 pkg	150	6.0	22.0	510	(mq)	4.0	(mq)	(mq)	24%
beef 'Noodles and Sauce' dry mix	1/4 pkg	120	5.0	23.0	640	(mq)	2.0	(mq)	(mq)	14%
broccoli 'Noodles and Sauce' dry mix	1/4 pkg	130	5.0	22.0	430	(mq)	2.0	(mq)	(mq)	14%
butter 'Noodles and Sauce' dry mix	1/4 pkg	150	6.0	23.0	450	(mq)	4.0	(mq)	(mq)	24%
butter and herb 'Noodles and Sauce' dry mix	1/4 pkg	140	5.0	23.0	460	(mq)	3.0	(mq)	(mq)	19%
carbonara Alfredo 'Noodles and Sauce' dry mix	1/4 pkg	140	5.0	20.0	460	(mq)	4.0	(mq)	(mq)	27%
cheese 'Noodles and Sauce' dry mix	1/4 pkg	140	5.0	25.0	470	(mq)	2.0	(mq)	(mq)	13%
chicken flavor 'Noodles and Sauce' dry mix	1/4 pkg	130	5.0	23.0	390	(mq)	2.0	(mq)	(mq)	14%
Parmesan 'Noodles and Sauce' dry mix	1/4 pkg	140	6.0	21.0	410	(mq)	4.0	(mq)	(mq)	25%
sour cream and chives 'Noodles and Sauce' dry mix	1/4 pkg	150	5.0	24.0	440	(mq)	3.0	(mq)	(mq)	19%
Stroganoff 'Noodles and Sauce' dry mix	1/4 pkg	130	6.0	22.0	330	(mq)	3.0	(mq)	(mq)	19%
(Mueller's)										
Alfredo 'Chef's Series' prepared	1/2 cup	190	5.0	23.0	580	(mq)	9.0	(mq)	(mq)	42%
chicken flavor 'Chef's Series' prepared	1/2 cup	160	3.0	21.0	550	(mq)	8.0	(mq)	(mq)	43%
garlic and butter 'Chef's Series' prepared	1/2 cup	170	3.0	21.0	480	(mq)	7.0	(mq)	(mq)	40%
sour cream and chives 'Chef's Series' prepared	1/2 cup	190	4.0	22.0	470	(mq)	8.0	(mq)	(mq)	41%
Stroganoff 'Chef's Series' prepared	1/2 cup	190	5.0	22.0	620	(mq)	9.0	(mq)	(mq)	43%
(Noodle Roni)										
angel hair pasta, w/Parmesan cheese, prepared	1/2 cup	210	6.0	26.0	580	na	9.0	na	na	39%
fettuccini, prepared	1/2 cup	300	7.0	29.0	560	(mq)	18.0	(mq)	(mq)	53%
garlic, creamy, prepared	1/2 cup	300	7.0	29.0	630	(mq)	17.0	(mq)	(mq)	52%
herb and butter, prepared	1/2 cup	160	5.0	19.0	290	(mq)	7.0	(mq)	(mq)	40%
mushroom, prepared	1/2 cup	160	6.0	25.0	550	(mq)	4.0	(mq)	(mq)	23%
Parmesan, prepared	1/2 cup	240	7.0	23.0	470	(mq)	13.0	(mq)	(mq)	49%
Parmesano 'Less Fat,' prepared	1/2 cup	190	6.0	24.0	460	na	8.0	na	na	38%
Romanoff, prepared	1/2 cup	240	8.0	28.0	730	(mq)	11.0	(mq)	(mq)	41%
Stroganoff, prepared	1/2 cup	350	11.0	37.0	1190	(mq)	17.0	(mq)	(mq)	44%
(Ultra Slim Fast) w/Alfredo sauce, prepared	8 oz	240	9.0	47.0	1110	4.0	4.0	na	na	14%
NORI. See SEAWEED.										
NORWAY HADDOCK. See OCEAN PERCH, ATLANTIC.										
NUT TOPPING										
(Fisher) fancy	1 oz	170	5.0	7.0	60	na	15.0	3.0	0	74%
(Fisher) oil-roasted, w/peanuts	1 oz	160	6.0	7.0	115	na	14.0	2.0	0	71%
(Planters)	1 oz	180	5.0	6.0	0	(mq)	16.0	2.0	0	77%
(Smucker's) pecan, in syrup	2 tbsp	130	2.0	28.0	0	(mq)	1.0	na	0	7%
(Smucker's) walnut, in syrup	2 tbsp	130	2.0	27.0	0	(mq)	1.0	na	0	7%
NUTMEG										
ground	1 oz	149	1.7	14.0	5	>1.1 c	10.3	7.4	0	60%
ground	1 tbsp	37	0.4	3.5	1	1.5	2.5	1.8	0	59%
ground	1 tsp	12	0.1	1.1	0	.5	0.8	0.6	0	60%
ground *(Durkee)*	1 tsp	12	0.0	0.0	0	0	<0.1	na	na	<62%
ground *(Laurel Leaf)*	1 tsp	12	0.0	0.0	0	0	<0.1	na	na	<62%

Food Name	Serving Size	Calories	Prot. gms	Carbs gms	Sod. mgs	Fiber gms	Fat gms	Sat. Fat gms	Chol. mgs	% Fat Cal.
ground *(Spice Islands)*	1 tsp	11	0.1	0.9	<1	>.1 c	0.7	(mq)	0	61%
NUTMEG BUTTER OIL										
....	1 cup	1927	0.0	0.0	0	0	218.0	196.2	0	100%
....	1 oz	251	0.0	0.0	0	0	28.4	25.5	0	100%
....	1 tbsp	120	0.0	0.0	0	0	13.6	12.2	0	100%
NUTRASWEET. See SUGAR, ALTERNATIVE.										
NUTS, MIXED										
(Guy's) w/peanuts	1 oz	170	8.0	3.0	140	(mq)	14.0	(mq)	0	74%
(Planters) 'Select Mix' cashews, almonds, and peanuts ...	1 oz	170	5.0	7.0	100	na	14.0	2.0	0	72%
(Planters) 'Select Mix' cashews, almonds, and pecans ...	1 oz	180	4.0	6.0	85	na	16.0	2.0	0	78%
(Planters) 'Select Mix' cashews, pecans, and peanuts	1 oz	180	4.0	6.0	80	na	16.0	2.0	0	78%
Dry-roasted										
(Finast) 'No Frills' w/peanuts, salted	1 oz	180	5.0	7.0	150	(mq)	14.0	(mq)	0	72%
(Fisher) lightly salted	1 oz	170	6.0	7.0	na	na	15.0	2.0	0	72%
(Fisher) salted	1 oz	170	6.0	7.0	125	na	15.0	2.0	0	72%
(Pathmark) 'No Frills' w/peanuts, salted	1 oz	180	6.0	7.0	220	(mq)	14.0	2.0	0	71%
(Planters)	1 oz	160	5.0	7.0	250	(mq)	14.0	2.0	0	72%
(Planters) sesame nut mix	1 oz	160	5.0	8.0	330	(mq)	12.0	3.0	0	68%
(Planters) 'Unsalted'	1 oz	170	6.0	7.0	0	(mq)	15.0	2.0	0	72%
w/peanuts	1 cup	814	23.7	34.7	16	12.3	70.5	9.4	0	73%
w/peanuts	1 oz	169	4.9	7.2	3	2.6	14.6	2.0	0	73%
w/peanuts, salted	1 cup	814	23.7	34.7	917	12.3	70.5	9.4	0	73%
w/peanuts, salted	1 oz	169	4.9	7.2	190	2.6	14.6	2.0	0	73%
Honey-roasted										
(Fisher) peanuts and cashews	1 oz	150	5.0	6.0	105	na	13.0	2.0	0	73%
(Planters)	1 oz	170	5.0	9.0	140	na	13.0	2.0	0	68%
(Planters) cashews and peanuts	1 oz	170	5.0	9.0	170	(mq)	12.0	2.0	0	66%
Oil-roasted										
(Fisher) lightly salted	1 oz	170	6.0	6.0	50	na	16.0	2.0	0	75%
(Fisher) salted	1 oz	170	6.0	6.0	110	na	16.0	2.0	0	75%
(Flavor House)	1 oz	180	5.0	6.0	125	(mq)	18.0	(mq)	0	79%
(Pathmark) 'No Frills' salted	1 oz	180	4.0	7.0	150	(mq)	15.0	(mq)	0	75%
(Pathmark) 'No Frills' w/peanuts, salted	1 oz	180	6.0	5.0	150	(mq)	15.0	0.0	0	75%
(Pathmark) 'No Frills Fancy' salted	1 oz	180	4.0	7.0	150	(mq)	15.0	(mq)	0	75%
(Planters)	1 oz	180	5.0	6.0	110	na	16.0	2.0	0	77%
(Planters) 'Deluxe'	1 oz	180	4.0	6.0	110	na	17.0	3.0	0	79%
(Planters) lightly salted	1 oz	180	5.0	6.0	80	na	16.0	2.0	0	77%
(Planters) sesame nut mix	1 oz	160	5.0	8.0	200	na	13.0	2.0	0	69%
salted	1 cup	886	22.4	32.1	1008	7.9	80.9	13.1	0	77%
salted	1 oz	175	4.4	6.3	199	1.6	15.9	2.6	0	77%
w/peanuts	1 cup	876	23.8	30.4	16	14.1	80.0	12.4	0	77%
w/peanuts	1 oz	175	4.8	6.1	3	2.8	16.0	2.5	0	77%
w/peanuts, salted	1 cup	876	23.8	30.4	926	12.8	80.0	12.4	0	77%
w/peanuts, salted	1 oz	175	4.8	6.1	185	2.6	16.0	2.5	0	77%

O

Food Name	Serving Size	Calories	Prot. gms	Carbs gms	Sod. mgs	Fiber gms	Fat gms	Sat. Fat gms	Chol. mgs	% Fat Cal.
OAT. See also CEREAL, HOT.										
cooked	1 cup	87	7.0	25.1	2	3.5	1.9	0.4	0	12%
cooked	4 oz	45	3.6	13.0	1	>.4 c	1.0	0.2	0	12%
raw	1 cup	231	16.3	62.2	4	14.9	6.6	1.2	0	16%

Food Name	Serving Size	Calories	Prot. gms	Carbs gms	Sod. mgs	Fiber gms	Fat gms	Sat. Fat gms	Chol. mgs	% Fat Cal.
raw	1 oz	70	4.9	18.8	1	4.5	2.0	0.4	0	16%
steel-cut *(Arrowhead Mills)*	2 oz	220	10.0	37.0	1	2.8	4.0	(mq)	0	16%
whole grain	1 cup	607	26.3	103.4	3	(mq)	10.8	1.9	0	16%
whole grain	1 oz	110	4.8	18.8	1	(mq)	2.0	0.3	0	16%
OAT BRAN. See CEREAL, HOT.										
OAT FLOUR										
(Arrowhead Mills) whole grain	2 oz	200	7.0	43.0	1	8.3	1.0	(mq)	0	4%
(Gold Medal) blend	1 cup	390	14.0	81.0	0	4.0	3.0	(mq)	0	7%
OAT GROATS *(Arrowhead Mills)*	2 oz	220	8.0	38.0	1	5.6	4.0	(mq)	0	16%
OAT VEGETABLE OIL										
	1 cup	1927	0.0	0.0	0	0	218.0	42.8	0	100%
	1 tbsp	120	0.0	0.0	0	0	13.6	2.7	0	100%
OATMEAL. See CEREAL, HOT.										
OCEAN CATFISH. See WOLF FISH.										
OCEAN PERCH, ATLANTIC/Norway haddock/red perch/redfish/rosefish/sea perch										
baked	4 oz	137	27.1	0.0	109	0	2.4	0.4	61	17%
broiled	4 oz	137	27.1	0.0	109	0	2.4	0.4	61	17%
dry-heat cooked	3 oz	103	20.3	0.0	82	0	1.8	0.3	46	17%
microwaved	4 oz	137	27.1	0.0	109	0	2.4	0.4	61	17%
raw	1 lb	427	84.5	0.0	339	0	7.4	1.1	191	17%
raw	1 oz	27	5.3	0.0	21	0	0.5	0.1	12	18%
OCEAN PERCH, FROZEN										
(Booth)	4 oz	100	20.0	0.0	250	0	1.0	(mq)	(mq)	10%
(Gorton's) 'Fishmarket Fresh'	5 oz	140	25.0	2.0	100	0	3.0	(mq)	(mq)	20%
(Van de Kamp's) breaded 'Light'	1 piece	280	17.0	21.0	450	(mq)	14.0	3.0	35	45%
(Van de Kamp's) 'Natural'	4 oz	130	20.0	0.0	65	0	5.0	2.0	40	36%
OCEAN POUT/muttonfish										
dry-heat cooked	3 oz	87	18.1	0.0	66	0	1.0	0.4	57	11%
raw	1 lb	360	75.5	0.0	277	0	4.1	1.5	236	11%
raw	1 oz	22	4.7	0.0	17	0	0.3	0.1	15	13%
OCEANIC BONITO. See TUNA, SKIPJACK.										
OCTOBER BEAN, CANNED, w/pork *(Luck's)*	7.25 oz	230	12.0	32.0	550	10.0	6.0	(mq)	(mq)	24%
OCTOPUS										
moist-heat cooked	3 oz	139	25.3	3.7	391	0	1.8	0.4	82	12%
raw	1 lb	372	67.6	10.0	(mq)	0	4.7	1.0	219	12%
raw	1 oz	23	4.2	0.6	(mq)	0	0.3	0.1	14	12%
OHELOBERRY										
raw	1 lb	126	1.7	31.0	6	>6.0 c	1.0	na	0	6%
raw	1 cup	39	0.5	9.6	1	>1.9 c	0.3	na	0	6%
raw	1 oz	8	0.1	1.9	<1	>.4 c	0.1	(tr)	0	10%
raw, approx .4 oz	10 fruits	3	0.0	0.8	0	>.2 c	0.0	na	0	0%
OIL. See individual listings.										
OKRA/gumbo										
boiled, drained	4 oz	36	2.1	8.2	6	>1.0 c	0.2	0.1	0	4%
boiled, drained, approx 3 inches long	8 pods	27	1.6	6.1	4	2.1	0.1	0.0	0	3%
boiled, drained, sliced	1/2 cup	26	1.5	5.8	4	2.0	0.1	0.0	0	3%
raw, approx 3 inches long	8 pods	36	1.9	7.3	8	2.5	0.1	0.0	0	2%
raw, sliced	1/2 cup	19	1.0	3.8	4	1.3	0.1	0.0	0	5%
raw, trimmed	1 oz	11	0.6	2.2	2	>.3 c	<.1	tr	0	<7%
raw, untrimmed	1 lb	148	7.8	29.8	32	>3.7 c	0.4	0.1	0	2%
OKRA, FROZEN										
boiled, drained	10 oz	94	5.3	20.8	8	7.1	0.8	0.2	0	7%
boiled, drained, sliced	1/2 cup	34	1.9	7.5	3	2.6	0.3	0.1	0	7%
cut *(Freshlike)*	3.3 oz	25	1.0	6.0	5	na	0.0	na	na	0%

Food Name	Serving Size	Calories	Prot. gms	Carbs gms	Sod. mgs	Fiber gms	Fat gms	Sat. Fat gms	Chol. mgs	% Fat Cal.
cut *(Seabrook)*	3.3 oz	25	1.0	6.0	3	>1.0 c	0.0	0.0	0	0%
cut *(Southern)*	3.5 oz	31	1.6	6.5	20	(mq)	0.2	(tr)	0	5%
cut *(Veg•All)*	3.3 oz	25	1.0	6.0	5	na	0.0	na	na	0%
whole *(Freshlike)*	3.3 oz	30	2.0	7.0	5	na	0.0	na	na	0%
whole *(Seabrook)*	3.3 oz	30	2.0	7.0	2	>1.0 c	0.0	0.0	0	0%
whole *(Southern)*	3.5 oz	35	1.9	7.4	20	(mq)	0.2	(tr)	0	5%
whole *(Veg•All)*	3.3 oz	30	2.0	7.0	5	na	0.0	na	na	0%
whole, baby *(Frosty Acres)*	3.3 oz	30	2.0	7.0	2	>1.0 c	0.0	0.0	0	0%

OLD FASHIONED. See ALCOHOLIC BEVERAGES.

OLIVE

Food Name	Serving Size	Calories	Prot. gms	Carbs gms	Sod. mgs	Fiber gms	Fat gms	Sat. Fat gms	Chol. mgs	% Fat Cal.
all varieties, all sizes, pickled *(S&W)*	1 oz	46	0.0	0.0	215	(mq)	5.1	(mq)	0	100%
black, jumbo, canned	1 olive	7	0.1	0.5	75	.3	0.6	0.1	0	69%
black, large, canned	1 olive	5	0.0	0.3	38	.1	0.5	0.1	0	79%
black, small, canned	1 olive	4	0.0	0.2	28	.1	0.3	0.1	0	77%
black, super colossal, canned	1 olive	12	0.2	0.9	136	.5	1.0	0.1	0	67%
mixed varieties, chopped, pickled *(Lindsay)*	1 oz	29	0.2	1.7	249	.8	2.7	0.5	0	76%
mixed varieties, pitted, pickled *(Vlasic)*	1 oz	37	0.3	0.7	230	>.4 c	3.9	(mq)	0	90%
mixed varieties, sliced, pickled *(Lindsay)*	1/2 cup	70	0.6	4.1	598	2.0	6.5	1.1	0	76%
mixed varieties, sliced, pickled *(Lindsay)*	1 oz	29	0.2	1.7	249	.8	2.7	0.5	0	76%
salad, pickled *(Progresso)*	1/2 cup	120	1.0	1.0	2400	4.0	15.0	2.0	0	94%

OLIVE, ASCOLANO

Food Name	Serving Size	Calories	Prot. gms	Carbs gms	Sod. mgs	Fiber gms	Fat gms	Sat. Fat gms	Chol. mgs	% Fat Cal.
all sizes, pitted, pickled	1 oz	23	0.3	1.6	255	.9	1.9	0.3	0	69%
all sizes, pitted, pickled *(Lindsay)*	1 oz	23	0.3	1.6	255	.7	1.9	0.3	0	69%
colossal, pitted, pickled *(Lindsay)*	10 olives	90	1.1	6.3	1010	2.8	7.7	1.3	0	70%
jumbo, pitted, pickled	10 olives	67	0.8	4.7	745	2.5	5.7	0.8	0	70%
jumbo, pitted, pickled *(Lindsay)*	10 olives	66	0.8	4.7	745	2.1	5.7	1.0	0	70%
super colossal, pitted, pickled	10 olives	123	1.5	8.5	1365	4.6	10.4	1.4	0	70%
super colossal, pitted, pickled *(Lindsay)*	10 olives	122	1.5	8.5	1365	3.8	10.4	1.8	0	70%

OLIVE, GREEK

Food Name	Serving Size	Calories	Prot. gms	Carbs gms	Sod. mgs	Fiber gms	Fat gms	Sat. Fat gms	Chol. mgs	% Fat Cal.
all sizes, pitted, salt-cured, oil-coated, pickled	1 oz	96	0.6	2.5	932	(mq)	10.2	(mq)	0	88%
extra large, w/pits, salt-cured, oil-coated, pickled	10 olives	89	0.6	2.3	868	(mq)	9.5	(mq)	0	88%
extra large, w/pits, salt-cured, pickled	10 olives	89	0.6	2.3	868	(mq)	9.5	(mq)	0	88%
medium, w/pits, salt-cured, oil-coated, pickled	10 olives	65	0.4	1.7	631	(mq)	6.9	(mq)	0	88%
medium, w/pits, salt-cured, pickled	10 olives	65	0.4	1.7	631	(mq)	6.9	(mq)	0	88%

OLIVE, GREEN

Food Name	Serving Size	Calories	Prot. gms	Carbs gms	Sod. mgs	Fiber gms	Fat gms	Sat. Fat gms	Chol. mgs	% Fat Cal.
all sizes, pitted, pickled	1 oz	33	0.4	0.4	680	.7	3.6	(mq)	0	91%
giant, w/pits, pickled	10 olives	76	0.9	0.9	1572	1.7	8.3	(mq)	0	91%
large, w/pits, pickled	10 olives	45	0.5	0.5	926	1.0	4.9	(mq)	0	92%
small, select, w/pits, pickled	10 olives	33	0.4	0.4	686	.7	3.6	(mq)	0	91%
small, standard, w/pits, pickled	10 olives	33	0.4	0.4	686	.7	3.6	(mq)	0	91%

OLIVE, MANZANILLA

Food Name	Serving Size	Calories	Prot. gms	Carbs gms	Sod. mgs	Fiber gms	Fat gms	Sat. Fat gms	Chol. mgs	% Fat Cal.
all sizes, pitted, pickled	1 oz	33	0.2	1.8	247	.9	3.0	0.4	0	77%
all sizes, pitted, pickled *(Lindsay)*	1 oz	32	0.2	1.8	247	.9	3.0	0.5	0	77%
extra large, pitted, pickled *(Lindsay)*	10 olives	63	0.5	3.5	484	1.8	5.9	1.1	0	77%
large, pitted, pickled	10 olives	51	0.5	2.8	384	1.3	4.7	0.6	0	76%
large, pitted, pickled *(Lindsay)*	10 olives	50	0.4	2.8	388	1.4	4.8	0.8	0	77%
medium, pitted, pickled *(Lindsay)*	10 olives	44	0.3	2.4	000	1.2	4.1	0.7	0	77%
small, pitted, pickled	10 olives	37	0.3	2.0	279	1.0	3.4	0.5	0	77%
small, pitted, pickled *(Lindsay)*	10 olives	37	0.3	2.0	283	1.0	3.5	0.6	0	77%

OLIVE, MISSION

Food Name	Serving Size	Calories	Prot. gms	Carbs gms	Sod. mgs	Fiber gms	Fat gms	Sat. Fat gms	Chol. mgs	% Fat Cal.
all sizes, pitted, pickled	1 oz	33	0.2	1.8	247	.9	3.0	0.4	0	77%
all sizes, pitted, pickled *(Lindsay)*	1 oz	32	0.2	1.8	247	.9	3.0	0.5	0	77%
extra large, pitted, pickled *(Lindsay)*	10 olives	63	0.5	3.5	484	1.8	5.9	1.1	0	77%
large, pitted, pickled	10 olives	51	0.5	2.8	384	1.3	4.7	0.6	0	76%

Food Name	Serving Size	Calories	Prot. gms	Carbs gms	Sod. mgs	Fiber gms	Fat gms	Sat. Fat gms	Chol. mgs	% Fat Cal.
large, pitted, pickled *(Lindsay)*	10 olives	50	0.4	2.8	388	1.4	4.8	0.8	0	77%
medium, pitted, pickled *(Lindsay)*	10 olives	44	0.3	2.4	336	1.2	4.1	0.7	0	77%
small, pitted, pickled	10 ollives	37	0.3	2.0	279	1.0	3.4	0.5	0	77%
small, pitted, pickled *(Lindsay)*	10 olives	37	0.3	2.0	283	1.0	3.5	0.6	0	77%
OLIVE, SEVILLANO										
all sizes, pitted, pickled	1 oz	23	0.3	1.6	255	.9	1.9	0.3	0	69%
all sizes, pitted, pickled *(Lindsay)*	1 oz	23	0.3	1.6	255	.7	1.9	0.3	0	69%
colossal, pitted, pickled *(Lindsay)*	10 olives	90	1.1	6.3	1010	· 2.8	7.7	1.3	0	70%
jumbo, pitted, pickled	10 olives	67	0.8	4.7	745	2.5	5.7	0.8	0	70%
jumbo, pitted, pickled *(Lindsay)*	10 olives	66	0.8	4.7	745	2.1	5.7	1.0	0	70%
super colossal, pitted, pickled	10 olives	123	1.5	8.5	1365	4.6	10.4	1.4	0	70%
super colossal, pitted, pickled *(Lindsay)*	10 olives	122	1.5	8.5	1365	3.8	10.4	1.8	0	70%
OLIVE APPETIZER										
(Progresso)	1/2 cup	180	1.0	6.0	1600	2.5	21.0	3.0	0	87%
(Progresso) 'Condite'	1/2 cup	130	<1.0	5.0	870	2.0	14.0	2.0	0	84%
OLIVE OIL										
	1/2 cup	955	0.0	0.0	tr	0	108.0	14.6	0	100%
	1 oz	251	0.0	0.0	tr	0	28.4	3.8	0	100%
(Amore) 'Extra Virgin'	1 tbsp	130	0.0	0.0	0	0	14.0	2.0	0	100%
(Amore) 'Pure'	1 tbsp	130	0.0	0.0	0	0	14.0	2.0	0	100%
(Bertolli)	1 tbsp	120	0.0	0.0	(tr)	0	14.0	(mq)	0	100%
(Filippo Berio)	1 tbsp	120	0.0	0.0	(tr)	0	14.0	2.0	0	100%
(Hain)	1 tbsp	120	0.0	0.0	0	0	14.0	2.0	0	100%
(Pope) 100% Italian cold press, no salt	1 tbsp	120	0.0	0.0	0	na	14.0	2.0	0	100%
(Progresso) all varieties	1 tbsp	119	0.0	0.0	0	0	14.0	2.0	0	100%
(Spectrum Naturals)	1 tbsp	120	0.0	0.0	0	(tr)	14.0	2.0	(tr)	100%
(Spectrum Naturals) organic	1 tbsp	120	0.0	0.0	0	(tr)	14.0	2.0	(tr)	100%
(Wesson)	1 tbsp	120	0.0	0.0	0	0	14.0	2.0	0	100%
OMELET, FROZEN										
(Healthy Choice) turkey sausage, on English muffin	1 serving	210	16.0	30.0	470	na	4.0	2.0	20	16%
(Healthy Choice) western style, on English muffin	1 serving	200	16.0	29.0	480	na	3.0	2.0	15	13%
(Weight Watchers) ham and cheese 'Handy'	4 oz	180	14.0	18.0	420	na	5.0	3.0	10	26%
ONION										
Mature										
boiled, drained	4 oz	50	1.5	11.5	3	>.8 c	0.2	<.1	0	3%
chopped, boiled, drained	1/2 cup	46	1.4	10.7	3	1.7	0.2	0.0	0	4%
chopped, boiled, drained	1 tbsp	7	0.2	1.5	0	.2	0.0	0.0	0	0%
raw *(Dole)*	1 med	60	1.0	14.0	10	3.0	0.0	na	na	0%
raw, chopped	1/2 cup	30	0.9	6.9	2	1.3	0.1	0.0	0	3%
raw, chopped	1 tbsp	4	0.1	0.9	tr	.2	<.1	tr	0	<18%
raw, trimmed	1 oz	11	0.3	2.4	1	5	<.1	<.1	0	<8%
raw, untrimmed	1 lb	154	4.7	35.2	12	6.5	0.7	0.1	0	4%
ONION, CANNED										
sweet *(Heinz)*	1 oz	40	0.0	9.0	165	(mq)	0.0	0.0	0	0%
whole, small *(Pathmark)*	1/2 cup	35	2.0	7.0	280	(mq)	0.0	0.0	0	0%
whole, small *(S&W)*	1/2 cup	35	1.0	9.0	345	(mq)	0.0	0.0	0	0%
w/liquid	4 oz	22	1.0	4.5	421	1.2	0.1	<.1	0	4%
w/liquid, chopped	1/2 cup	21	1.0	4.5	416	1.5	0.1	0.0	0	4%
ONION, COCKTAIL, lightly spiced *(Vlasic)*	1 oz	4	0.0	1.0	365	(mq)	0.0	0.0	0	0%
ONION, DRIED										
flakes	1 oz	92	2.5	23.6	6	>1.3 c	0.1	<.1	0	1%
flakes	1/4 cup	45	1.3	11.7	3	1.3	0.1	0.0	0	2%
flakes	1 tbsp	16	0.5	4.2	1	.5	0.0	0.0	0	0%
w/green onion, minced *(Lawry's)*	1 tsp	7	0.4	1.6	1	>.6 c	0.2	(tr)	0	18%

Food Name	Serving Size	Calories	Prot. gms	Carbs gms	Sod. mgr	Fiber gms	Fat gms	Sat. Fat gms	Chol. mgs	% Fat Cal
ONION, FROZEN										
Chopped										
boiled, drained	1/2 cup	29	0.8	6.9	13	1.7	0.1	0.0	0	3%
boiled, drained	4 oz	32	0.9	7.5	14	>5.0 c	0.1	<.1	0	3%
boiled, drained	1 tbsp	4	0.1	1.0	2	.2	0.0	0.0	0	0%
unprepared	10 oz	82	2.2	19.3	34	4.5	0.3	0.1	0	3%
(Ore-Ida)	2 oz	20	0.0	4.0	10	(mq)	<1.0	(tr)	0	<36%
(Seabrook)	1 oz	8	0.0	2.0	2	0	0.0	0.0	0	0%
Diced										
(Freshlike)	3.3 oz	8	0.0	2.0	0	na	0.0	na	na	0%
(Veg•All)	3.3 oz	8	0.0	2.0	0	na	0.0	na	na	0%
Whole										
boiled, drained	4 oz	32	0.8	7.6	9	>.6 c	0.1	<.1	0	3%
(Birds Eye) small	4 oz	40	1.0	10.0	10	2.0	0.0	0.0	0	0%
(Birds Eye) small, w/cream sauce 'Combination Vegetables'	5 oz	140	2.0	12.0	400	1.0	10.0	na	0	62%
(Freshlike)	3.3 oz	35	1.0	8.0	10	na	0.0	na	na	0%
(Seabrook) small	3.3 oz	35	1.0	8.0	9	>1.0 c	0.0	0.0	0	0%
(Veg•All)	3.3 oz	35	1.0	8.0	10	na	0.0	na	na	0%
ONION, GREEN /scallion/spring onion										
chopped (Dole)	1 tbsp	2	0.1	0.3	0	tr	0.1	na	na	36%
trimmed, w/top	1 oz	19	0.5	2.1	5	.7	<.1	tr	0	<8%
trimmed, w/top, chopped	1/2 cup	16	0.9	3.7	8	1.2	0.1	<.1	0	5%
trimmed, w/top, chopped	1 tbsp	2	0.1	0.4	1	.1	<.1	tr	0	<31%
untrimmed	1 lb	140	8.0	32.0	71	10.5	0.8	0.1	0	4%
ONION, SPRING. See ONION, GREEN.										
ONION, WELSH										
trimmed	1 lb	160	8.0	28.8	na	>4.8 c	1.6	<1.6	0	10%
trimmed	1 oz	10	0.5	1.8	na	>.3 c	0.1	<.1	0	10%
ONION POWDER										
ground	1 tbsp	23	0.7	5.2	3	>.4 c	0.1	na	0	4%
ground	1 tsp	7	0.2	1.7	1	>.1 c	0.0	na	0	0%
ground (Durkee)	1 tsp	8	0.0	0.0	0	0	tr	na	na	tr
ground (Laurel Leaf)	1 tsp	8	0.0	0.0	0	0	tr	na	na	tr
ground (Spice Islands)	1 tsp	8	0.2	1.7	1	>.1 c	<.1	tr	0	<11%
ONION RINGS, FROZEN										
breaded, partially fried in vegetable oil, prepared in oven	4 oz	462	6.1	43.3	425	>.5 c	30.3	9.7	0	58%
breaded, partially fried in vegetable oil, prepared in oven	2 rings	81	1.1	7.6	75	>.1 c	5.3	1.7	0	58%
breaded, partially fried in vegetable oil, unprepared	16 oz	1171	14.3	138.6	1117	5.9	64.0	20.6	0	49%
breaded, partially fried in vegetable oil, unprepared	9 oz	658	8.0	77.8	627	3.3	36.0	11.6	0	49%
(Farm Rich) battered, precooked 'Batter Dipt'	4 oz	260	3.0	32.0	580	(mq)	13.0	(mq)	na	46%
(Farm Rich) crispy 'Onion O's'	5 rings	190	3.0	26.0	480	(mq)	9.0	(mq)	0	41%
(Mrs. Paul's) crispy	2.5 oz	190	2.0	19.0	230	(mq)	12.0	(mq)	na	56%
(Ore-Ida) 'Onion Ringers'	2 oz	140	2.0	18.0	190	(mq)	7.0	3.0	0	44%
(Stilwell) battered	3 oz	250	2.0	22.0	300	(mq)	16.0	(mq)	<1	60%
ONION SALT (Tone's)	1 tsp	1	0.1	0.4	1599	<.1	tr	tr	0	0%
OPOSSUM										
roasted	4 oz	251	34.2	0.0	(mq)	0	11.6	(mq)	(mq)	43%
roasted	3 oz	188	25.7	0.0	na	na	8.7	na	na	43%
roasted, diced	1 cup	309	42.3	0.0	(mq)	0	14.3	(mq)	(mq)	43%
ORANGE										
All commercial varieties										
approx 2 5/8 inch diam	1 med	62	1.2	15.4	0	3.1	0.2	0.0	0	3%
peeled and seeded	1 oz	13	0.3	3.3	0	.7	<.1	tr	0	<6%

Food Name	Serving Size	Calories	Prot. gms	Carbs gms	Sod. mgs	Fiber gms	Fat gms	Sat. Fat gms	Chol. mgs	% Fat Cal.
sections, w/o membrane	1 cup	85	1.7	21.1	0	4.3	0.2	0.0	0	2%
untrimmed	1 lb	156	3.1	38.9	0	7.9	0.4	0.1	0	2%
California Navel										
approx 2 7/8 inch diam	1 med	64	1.4	16.3	1	>.6 c	0.1	0.0	0	1%
peeled and seeded	1 oz	13	0.3	3.3	<1	>.1 c	<.1	tr	0	<6%
sections, w/o membrane	1 cup	76	1.7	19.2	2	>.8 c	0.2	0.0	0	2%
untrimmed	1 lb	142	3.2	35.9	2	>1.4 c	0.3	<.1	0	2%
California Valencia										
approx 2 5/8 inch diam	1 med	59	1.3	14.4	0	>.6 c	0.4	0.0	0	5%
peeled and seeded	1 oz	14	0.3	3.4	0	>.1 c	0.1	tr	0	6%
sections, w/o membrane	1 cup	88	1.9	21.4	0	>.9 c	0.5	0.1	0	5%
untrimmed	1 lb	167	3.5	40.5	0	>1.7 c	1.0	0.1	0	5%
Florida										
approx 2 5/8 inch diam	1 med	69	1.1	17.4	0	3.6	0.3	0.0	0	4%
peeled and seeded	1 oz	13	0.2	3.3	tr	>.1 c	0.1	tr	0	6%
sections, w/o membrane	1 cup	85	1.3	21.4	0	4.4	0.4	0.1	0	4%
untrimmed	1 lb	153	2.4	38.7	2	>1.2 c	0.7	0.1	0	4%
ORANGE APRICOT DRINK *(Tropicana)* 'Twister'	8 oz	115	(mq)	30.0	2	(mq)	0.0	0.0	0	0%
ORANGE APRICOT JUICE										
(Musselman's) 'Breakfast Cocktail'	6 oz	90	0.0	21.0	20	(tr)	0.0	0.0	0	0%
ORANGE APRICOT JUICE DRINK	1 oz	16	0.1	4.0	1	na	0.0	0.0	0	0%
ORANGE BANANA NECTAR *(Kern's)*	6 oz	110	1.0	25.0	0	na	0.0	na	na	0%
ORANGE CRANBERRY JUICE										
(Santa Cruz Natural) organic 'Cruz'	8 oz	125	1.0	29.0	na	na	<1.0	na	na	<7%
ORANGE CRANBERRY JUICE DRINK										
(Ocean Spray) 'Refreshers'	6 oz	100	0.0	26.0	15	na	0.0	na	na	0%
(Tropicana) 'Single Serve'	10 oz	175	(mq)	43.0	3	(mq)	0.0	0.0	0	0%
(Tropicana) 'Twister'	8 oz	115	(mq)	30.0	1	(mq)	0.0	0.0	0	0%
(Tropicana) 'Twister'	6 oz	100	<1.0	23.0	25	na	<1.0	na	na	<9%
(Tropicana) 'Twister Light' w/NutraSweet	6 oz	18	<1.0	5.0	27	na	<1.0	na	na	<27%
ORANGE DRINK										
Can, bottle, or box										
	8 oz	128	0.0	32.0	40	(tr)	tr	tr	0	0%
(Bama)	8.45 oz	120	0.0	29.0	60	(tr)	0.0	0.0	0	0%
(Crowley)	8 oz	130	0.0	32.0	15	(tr)	0.0	0.0	0	0%
(Hawaiian Punch)	6 oz	100	0.0	24.0	20	(tr)	0.0	0.0	0	0%
(Hi-C)	8.45 oz	134	0.2	32.9	24	(tr)	<.1	(tr)	0	<1%
(Hi-C)	6 oz	95	0.1	23.3	17	(tr)	<.1	(tr)	0	<1%
(Hi-C) aseptic box	6 oz	90	0.0	23.0	20	na	0.0	na	na	0%
(J. Hungerford) 20% plus juice	9.03 oz	41	0.1	10.8	23	0	0.0	0.0	0	0%
(Pathmark) 'No Frills Sodium Free'	6 oz	80	0.0	22.0	0	(tr)	0.0	0.0	0	0%
(Squeezit) 'Smarty Arty Orange'	6.75 oz	100	0.0	26.0	50	na	0.0	na	na	0%
(Sunny Delight) California style	8 oz	130	0.0	31.0	130	na	0.0	na	na	0%
(Tropicana)	6 oz	90	<1.0	22.0	35	na	<1.0	na	na	<9%
(Tropicana) 'Single Serve'	10 oz	132	(tr)	33.0	3	(tr)	0.0	0.0	0	0%
(Veryfine)	8 oz	130	<1.0	33.0	70	(tr)	0.0	0.0	0	0%
(Wyler's) 'Fruit Slush'	4 oz	157	0.0	39.3	10	(tr)	0.0	0.0	0	0%
Chilled *(Hi-C)*	6 oz	90	0.0	23.0	20	na	0.0	na	na	0%
Frozen, w/juice and pulp, diluted	6 oz	85	0.2	21.2	19	>.2 c	0.0	0.0	0	0%
Mix										
(Finast) breakfast, prepared	8 oz	80	0.0	20.0	15	(tr)	0.0	0.0	0	0%
(Kool-Aid) sugar-free, w/NutraSweet, prepared	8 oz	4	0.0	0.0	0	0	0.0	0.0	0	0%
(Kool-Aid) sugar-sweetened, prepared	8 oz	80	0.0	20.0	0	na	0.0	na	0	0%
(Kool-Aid) unsweetened, prepared w/sugar	8 oz	100	0.0	25.0	0	na	0.0	na	0	0%

Food Name	Serving Size	Calories	Prot. gms	Carbs gms	Sod. mgs	Fiber gms	Fat gms	Sat. Fat gms	Chol. mgs	% Fat Cal
(Kool-Aid) unsweetened, prepared w/o sugar	8 oz	2	0.0	0.0	0	na	0.0	na	0	0%
(Pathmark) breakfast 'No Frills' prepared	4 oz	60	0.0	15.0	0	(tr)	0.0	0.0	0	0%
ORANGE FLAVOR DRINK										
Can, bottle, or box	12 oz	729	0.3	182.0	103	.4	2.2	0.3	0	3%
Chilled (Bright & Early) diluted	6 oz	90	0.1	20.8	18	(mq)	0.2	na	0	2%
Frozen										
(Bright & Early) diluted	6 oz	90	0.1	20.8	18	(mq)	0.2	na	0	2%
w/orange pulp, diluted	1 oz	15	tr	3.8	3	(mq)	tr	tr	0	0%
Mix										
powder, unprepared	1 oz	109	<.1	28.0	5	(tr)	<.1	<.1	0	<1%
powder, unprepared	3 rounded tsp	93	tr	23.7	4	(tr)	tr	<.1	0	0%
(Tang) crystals, prepared	6 oz	90	0.0	22.0	0	(tr)	0.0	0.0	0	0%
(Tang) crystals 'Sugar-free' prepared	6 oz	6	0.0	1.0	0	(tr)	0.0	0.0	0	0%
ORANGE FRUIT JUICE BLEND										
(Mott's)	10 oz	144	1.0	35.0	6	(tr)	0.0	0.0	0	0%
(Mott's)	9.5 oz	139	1.0	34.0	6	(tr)	0.0	0.0	0	0%
ORANGE GRAPEFRUIT JUICE										
canned	8 oz	106	1.5	25.4	7	>.3 c	0.3	0.0	0	2%
canned	1 oz	13	0.2	3.2	1	0	0.0	0.0	0	0%
(Kraft) chilled 'Pure 100%'	6 oz	80	1.0	19.0	0	(mq)	0.0	0.0	0	0%
ORANGE JUICE										
fresh squeezed	8 oz	112	1.7	25.8	2	.5	0.5	0.1	0	4%
Can, bottle, or box										
	6 oz	78	1.1	18.4	5	.4	0.3	<.1	0	3%
(Del Monte) 'Unsweetened'	6 oz	80	1.0	19.0	10	(mq)	0.0	0.0	0	0%
(J. Hungerford)	9.03 oz	112	0.5	27.8	1	0	0.0	0.0	0	0%
(Minute Maid) blend 'Juices to Go'	6 oz	90	1.0	22.0	20	na	0.0	na	na	0%
(Minute Maid) 'Juices to Go'	6 oz	80	1.0	20.0	20	na	0.0	na	na	0%
(Ocean Spray)	6 oz	80	0.0	19.0	15	(mq)	0.0	(tr)	0	0%
(S&W)	6 oz	83	2.0	18.0	2	(mq)	0.0	0.0	0	0%
(Sippin' Pak)	8.45 oz	110	1.0	26.0	25	(mq)	0.0	0.0	0	0%
(Snapple)	8 oz	130	0.0	29.0	55	na	0.0	0.0	0	0%
(Stokely) 'Unsweetened'	6 oz	89	1.0	21.0	5	(mq)	1.0	(tr)	0	9%
(Sunkist)	6 oz	84	1.3	20.0	2	(mq)	0.1	(tr)	0	1%
(Tree Top)	6 oz	90	1.0	22.0	5	(mq)	0.0	0.0	0	0%
(TreeSweet)	6 oz	78	1.0	18.0	15	(mq)	0.0	0.0	0	0%
(Tropicana) '100% Pure'	8 oz	109	(mq)	24.9	3	(mq)	0.0	0.0	0	0%
(Tropicana) 'Pure Premium' 100% pure	6 oz	80	1.0	19.0	0	na	<1.0	na	na	<10%
(Tropicana) reconstituted, 100% pure	6 oz	80	1.0	16.0	20	na	<1.0	na	na	<12%
(Veryfine) blend '100%'	8 oz	120	<1.0	30.0	35	(mq)	0.0	0.0	0	0%
(Veryfine) '100%'	8 oz	121	1.5	24.0	10	(mq)	0.0	0.0	0	0%
Chilled										
	8 oz	110	2.0	25.0	2	.5	0.7	0.1	0	6%
(Citrus Hill) 'Plus Calcium'	6 oz	90	<1.0	20.0	10	(mq)	<1.0	(tr)	0	<10%
(Citrus Hill) 'Select'	6 oz	90	<1.0	20.0	10	(mq)	<1.0	(tr)	0	<10%
(Crowley)	8 oz	110	2.0	26.0	5	(mq)	0.0	0.0	0	0%
(Kraft) 'Pure 100% Unsweetened'	6 oz	80	1.0	19.0	0	(mq)	0.0	0.0	0	0%
(Minute Maid) calcium fortified	6 oz	80	1.0	20.0	20	na	0.0	na	na	0%
(Minute Maid) country style	6 oz	80	1.0	20.0	20	na	0.0	na	na	0%
(Minute Maid) country style, premium choice	6 oz	90	1.0	21.0	0	na	0.0	na	na	0%
(Minute Maid) premium choice	6 oz	90	1.0	21.0	0	na	0.0	na	na	0%
(Minute Maid) regular	6 oz	80	1.0	20.0	20	na	0.0	na	na	0%
(Sunkist)	6 oz	84	1.3	20.0	2	(mq)	0.1	(tr)	0	1%
(Sunkist) 'Fresh Squeezed'	6 oz	77	1.2	17.7	2	(mq)	0.3	(tr)	0	3%

Food Name	Serving Size	Calories	Prot. gms	Carbs gms	Sod. mgs	Fiber gms	Fat gms	Sat. Fat gms	Chol. mgs	% Fat Cal.
Frozen										
(A&P) diluted	6 oz	80	1.0	19.0	0	(mq)	<1.0	(tr)	0	<10%
(Minute Maid) calcium fortified	6 oz	80	1.0	20.0	0	na	0.0	na	na	0%
(Minute Maid) country style	6 oz	80	1.0	20.0	0	na	0.0	na	na	0%
(Minute Maid) reduced acid	6 oz	80	1.0	20.0	0	na	0.0	na	na	0%
(Minute Maid) regular	6 oz	80	1.0	20.0	0	na	0.0	na	na	0%
(Sunkist) '8-16 servings per pkg' diluted	6 oz	112	1.7	26.8	3	(mq)	0.1	(tr)	0	1%
(TreeSweet) diluted	6 oz	84	1.0	20.0	15	(mq)	0.0	0.0	0	0%
ORANGE JUICE COCKTAIL										
(Musselman's) w/grapefruit juice 'Breakfast Cocktail'	6 oz	90	1.0	22.0	20	(tr)	0.0	0.0	0	0%
(Ocean Spray)	6 oz	100	0.0	25.0	15	na	0.0	na	na	0%
(Welch's) 'Orchard'	10 oz	150	0.0	37.0	0	0	0.0	0.0	0	0%
ORANGE JUICE DRINK										
(Citrus Hill) 'Lite Premium'	6 oz	60	<1.0	14.0	10	(tr)	<1.0	(tr)	0	<13%
(Kool-Aid) 'Koolers'	8.45 oz	110	0.0	30.0	10	(tr)	0.0	0.0	0	0%
(Tang) 'Fruit Box'	8.45 oz	130	0.0	32.0	10	na	0.0	na	0	0%
(Tropicana) tropical 'Juice Sparkler'	8 oz	110	(mq)	26.0	50	(tr)	0.0	0.0	0	0%
ORANGE JUICE FLOAT (Knudsen & Sons)	8 oz	120	2.0	27.0	na	na	0.0	na	na	0%
ORANGE KIWI PASSION JUICE (Tropicana) 100% pure	6 oz	80	1.0	17.0	35	na	<1.0	na	na	<11%
ORANGE MANGO DRINK (Tropicana) 'Twister'	6 oz	90	<1.0	21.0	45	na	<1.0	na	na	<9%
ORANGE MANGO JUICE (Knudsen & Sons)	8 oz	110	<1.0	24.0	na	na	0.0	na	na	0%
ORANGE PASSION DRINK										
(Tropicana) 'Twister'	8 oz	90	(mq)	22.0	1	(mq)	0.0	0.0	0	0%
(Tropicana) 'Twister'	6 oz	80	<1.0	19.0	35	na	<1.0	na	na	<10%
ORANGE PEACH DRINK										
(Tropicana) 'Twister'	8 oz	115	(mq)	30.0	2	(mq)	0.0	0.0	0	0%
(Tropicana) 'Twister'	6 oz	90	<1.0	21.0	35	na	<1.0	na	na	<9%
ORANGE PEACH MANGO JUICE (Tropicana)100% pure	6 oz	80	1.0	19.0	20	na	<1.0	na	na	<10%
ORANGE PEEL										
candied	1 oz	88	0.1	22.6	0	>.6 c	0.1	0.0	0	1%
fresh	1 oz	na	0.4	7.1	1	(mq)	0.1	tr	0	3%
fresh	1 tbsp	na	0.1	1.5	tr	.2	<.1	tr	0	<12%
fresh	1 tsp	na	<.1	0.5	tr	.1	tr	tr	0	0%
ORANGE PINEAPPLE JUICE										
(Kraft) 'Pure 100%'	6 oz	80	1.0	19.0	0	(mq)	0.0	0.0	0	0%
(Musselman's) 'Breakfast Cocktail'	6 oz	90	1.0	23.0	15	(tr)	0.0	0.0	0	0%
(Tropicana) 100% pure	6 oz	80	1.0	19.0	15	na	<1.0	na	na	<10%
ORANGE PUNCH (Minute Maid) aseptic box	6 oz	80	0.0	20.0	20	na	0.0	na	na	0%
ORANGE RASPBERRY DRINK										
(Tropicana) 'Twister'	6 oz	80	<1.0	20.0	30	na	<1.0	na	na	<10%
(Tropicana) 'Twister Light'	6 oz	30	<1.0	6.0	30	na	<1.0	na	na	<24%
ORANGE ROUGHY / slimehead										
dry-heat cooked	3 oz	76	16.0	0.0	69	0	0.8	0.0	22	10%
raw	1 lb	571	66.7	0.0	286	0	31.8	0.6	91	52%
raw	1 oz	36	4.2	0.0	18	0	2.0	<.1	6	52%
ORANGE STRAWBERRY BANANA JUICE										
(Tropicana) 100% pure	6 oz	80	1.0	18.0	25	na	<1.0	na	na	<11%
ORANGE STRAWBERRY DRINK										
(Tropicana) w/banana 'Twister'	6 oz	80	<1.0	20.0	45	na	<1.0	na	na	<10%
(Tropicana) w/banana 'Twister Light'	6 oz	25	<1.0	6.0	20	na	<1.0	na	na	<24%
(Tropicana) w/guava 'Twister'	6 oz	80	<1.0	20.0	40	na	<1.0	na	na	<10%
ORANGEADE										
(Santa Cruz Natural) organic	8 oz	90	1.0	22.0	na	na	<1.0	na	na	<9%
(Santa Cruz Natural) organic 'Sparkling'	8 oz	90	<1.0	24.0	na	na	<1.0	na	na	<8%

Food Name	Serving Size	Calories	Prot. gms	Carbs gms	Sod. mgs	Fiber gms	Fat gms	Sat. Fat gms	Chol. mgs	% Fat Cal.
OREGANO										
dried (Golden Dipt)	2 grams	6	0.0	1.0	88	na	0.0	na	0	0%
dried (Spice Islands)	1 tsp	6	0.2	1.0	<1	>.2 c	0.1	na	0	16%
ground	1 tbsp	14	0.5	2.9	1	>.7 c	0.5	0.1	0	25%
ground	1 tsp	5	0.2	1.0	0	>.2 c	0.2	0.0	0	27%
ground (Durkee)	1 tsp	5	0.0	0.0	0	0	tr	na	na	tr
ground (Laurel Leaf)	1 tsp	5	0.0	0.0	0	0	tr	na	na	tr
ORIENTAL SEASONING MIX (Schilling) 'Bag'n Season'	1 pkg	152	5.0	31.0	1912	na	8.0	na	na	33%
OYSTER, CANNED										
Eastern	1 cup	171	17.5	9.7	278	0	6.1	1.6	136	34%
Eastern	3 oz	59	6.0	3.3	95	0	2.1	0.5	47	34%
Eastern, w/liquid	4 oz	78	8.0	4.4	127	0	2.8	0.7	62	34%
(Bumble Bee)	1 cup	218	25.4	15.4	185	0	5.3	(mq)	(mq)	23%
(S&W) mole 'Fancy'	2 oz	95	12.0	4.0	(mq)	0	3.0	(mq)	(mq)	30%
OYSTER, EASTERN										
Farmed										
dry-heat cooked	3 oz	67	5.9	6.2	139	0	1.8	0.6	32	25%
dry-heat cooked	6 med	47	4.1	4.3	96	0	1.3	0.4	22	26%
raw, approx 3 oz	6 med	50	4.4	4.7	150	0	1.3	0.4	21	24%
Wild										
dry-heat cooked	3 oz	61	7.0	4.1	207	0	1.6	0.5	42	25%
dry-heat cooked	6 med	42	4.9	2.8	144	0	1.1	0.3	29	24%
moist-heat cooked	4 oz	155	16.0	8.9	254	0	5.6	1.4	124	34%
moist-heat cooked	3 oz	116	12.0	6.7	359	0	4.2	1.3	89	34%
moist-heat cooked, approx 1.5 oz	6 med	58	5.9	3.3	177	0	2.1	0.7	44	34%
raw	1 cup	169	17.5	9.7	523	0	6.1	1.9	131	34%
raw	1 oz	20	2.0	1.1	32	0	0.7	0.2	16	34%
raw, approx 3 oz	6 med	57	5.9	3.3	177	0	2.1	0.7	45	34%
OYSTER, PACIFIC										
moist-heat cooked	3 oz	139	16.1	8.4	180	0	3.9	0.9	85	26%
moist-heat cooked	1 med	41	4.7	2.5	53	0	1.1	0.3	25	26%
raw	1 lb	370	42.9	22.5	481	0	10.4	2.3	(mq)	26%
raw	3 oz	69	8.0	4.2	90	0	2.0	0.4	43	27%
raw	1 oz	23	2.7	1.4	30	0	0.7	0.1	(mq)	28%
raw, approx 1.75 oz	1 med	41	4.7	2.5	53	0	1.1	0.3	25	26%
OYSTER PLANT. See SALSIFY.										
OYSTER STEW. See SOUP.										

P

Food Name	Serving Size	Calories	Prot. gms	Carbs gms	Sod. mgs	Fiber gms	Fat gms	Sat. Fat gms	Chol. mgs	% Fat Cal.
PALM KERNEL OIL / babassu oil										
	1 cup	1927	0.0	0.0	0	0	218.0	107.5	0	100%
	1/2 cup	964	0.0	0.0	0	0	109.0	88.7	0	100%
	1 oz	251	0.0	0.0	0	0	28.4	23.1	0	100%
	1 tbsp	120	0.0	0.0	0	0	13.6	11.1	0	100%
PALM OIL										
	1 oz	251	0.0	0.0	0	0	28.4	14.0	0	100%
	1 tbsp	120	0.0	0.0	0	0	13.6	6.7	0	100%
PAM COOKING SPRAY. See COOKING SPRAY.										
PANANG CURRY BASE (A Taste of Thai)	1 tbsp	25	0.0	2.0	180	0	2.0	1.0	0	69%

Food Name	Serving Size	Calories	Prot. gms	Carbs gms	Sod. mgs	Fiber gms	Fat gms	Sat. Fat gms	Chol. mgs	% Fat Cal.
PANCAKE, FROZEN										
(Aunt Jemima) blueberry	3.5 oz	220	6.2	42.3	826	1.7	3.7	0.7	21	15%
(Aunt Jemima) buttermilk 'Lite Microwave'	3.5 oz	140	7.0	28.0	660	(mq)	3.0	(mq)	na	16%
(Aunt Jemima) buttermilk 'Microwave'	3.5 oz	210	6.4	41.3	860	1.8	3.0	0.7	20	12%
(Aunt Jemima) 'Original Microwave'	3.5 oz	211	6.2	40.3	801	1.8	3.6	(mq)	na	15%
(Downyflake)	3 pancakes	280	5.0	45.0	920	(mq)	9.0	(mq)	na	29%
(Downyflake) blueberry	3 pancakes	290	5.0	48.0	920	(mq)	9.0	(mq)	na	28%
(Downyflake) buttermilk	3 pancakes	280	5.0	45.0	920	(mq)	9.0	(mq)	na	29%
(Krusteaz) blueberry, 4.5 oz	3 pancakes	280	8.0	49.0	710	na	5.0	1.3	14	17%
(Krusteaz) buttermilk, 4.75 oz	3 pancakes	290	8.0	53.0	900	na	5.0	1.3	14	16%
(Krusteaz) mini, microwave	6 pancakes	120	3.0	21.0	280	na	2.0	na	4	16%
(Krusteaz) whole wheat honey, 4.75 oz	3 pancakes	250	8.0	45.0	990	.7	4.0	na	12	15%
(Pillsbury) blueberry 'Microwave'	3 pancakes	250	5.0	49.0	540	(mq)	4.0	(mq)	na	14%
(Pillsbury) buttermilk 'Microwave'	3 pancakes	260	6.0	51.0	590	(mq)	4.0	(mq)	na	14%
(Pillsbury) harvest wheat 'Microwave'	3 pancakes	240	6.0	48.0	420	(mq)	4.0	(mq)	na	14%
(Pillsbury) 'Original Microwave'	3 pancakes	240	6.0	47.0	550	(mq)	4.0	(mq)	na	15%
(Weight Watchers) buttermilk 'Microwave' approx 2.5 oz	1/2 pkg	140	5.0	22.0	270	(mq)	3.0	1.0	10	20%
PANCAKE BATTER, FROZEN										
(Aunt Jemima) blueberry	3.6 oz	204	5.0	38.7	688	1.8	4.0	0.7	27	17%
(Aunt Jemima) buttermilk	3.6 oz	180	5.5	36.0	778	1.8	2.3	0.7	27	11%
(Aunt Jemima) 'Original'	3.6 oz	183	5.7	36.5	763	1.8	2.4	0.6	19	11%
PANCAKE ENTRÉE, FROZEN										
(Aunt Jemima) and sausages 'Homestyle'	6 oz	420	12.0	57.0	1140	(mq)	16.0	(mq)	(mq)	34%
(Aunt Jemima) lite, w/lite links 'Homestyle'	6 oz	310	14.0	43.0	970	(mq)	10.0	(mq)	(mq)	28%
(Aunt Jemima) lite, w/lite syrup 'Homestyle'	6 oz	260	10.0	53.0	860	(mq)	3.0	(mq)	na	10%
(Downyflake) and sausages	5.5 oz	430	11.0	47.0	1170	(mq)	23.0	(mq)	(mq)	47%
(Swanson) and sausages 'Great Starts'	6 oz	460	15.0	52.0	920	(mq)	22.0	(mq)	(mq)	43%
(Swanson) silver dollar, and sausage, Great Starts	3.75 oz	310	10.0	37.0	680	(mq)	14.0	(mq)	(mq)	40%
(Swanson) whole wheat, w/lite links 'Great Starts'	5.5 oz	350	15.0	39.0	600	(mq)	16.0	(mq)	(mq)	40%
(Swanson) w/bacon 'Great Starts'	4.5 oz	400	11.0	47.0	1000	(mq)	20.0	(mq)	(mq)	44%
PANCAKE MIX. See also PANCAKE/WAFFLE MIX.										
(NOTE: Unless otherwise stated, all pancakes are 4 inches in diameter.)										
(Hungry Jack) dry	1/14 pkg	180	4.0	33.0	650	na	3.0	1.0	0	15%
(Hungry Jack) prepared w/water	3 pancakes	180	4.0	33.0	650	na	3.0	1.0	0	15%
BLUEBERRY (Krusteaz) imitation, prepared	3 pancakes	205	5.0	39.0	660	na	4.0	na	14	17%
BLUEBERRY, WILD										
(Hungry Jack) dry	1/5 pkg	170	3.0	38.0	780	na	1.0	0.0	0	5%
(Hungry Jack) prepared w/milk/oil/egg	3 pancakes	320	6.0	41.0	820	na	14.0	3.0	45	40%
BUCKWHEAT (Krusteaz) prepared	3 pancakes	215	8.0	40.0	770	6.0	3.0	na	9	12%
BUTTERMILK										
(Health Valley) 'Biscuit & Pancake'	1 oz	100	4.0	20.0	170	3.3	1.0	na	0	9%
(Hungry Jack) 'Complete' dry	1/17 pkg	180	5.0	38.0	720	1.0	1.0	0.0	5	5%
(Hungry Jack) 'Complete' prepared w/water	3 pancakes	180	5.0	38.0	720	1.0	1.0	1.0	5	5%
(Hungry Jack) dry	1/25 pkg	120	3.0	26.0	530	.5	0.0	0.0	0	0%
(Hungry Jack) prepared w/skim milk/oil/egg whites	3 pancakes	200	6.0	28.0	570	.5	7.0	1.0	0	32%
(Hungry Jack) prepared w/2% milk/oil/egg	3 pancakes	210	6.0	28.0	560	.5	9.0	2.0	55	37%
(Krusteaz) prepared	3 pancakes	200	5.0	39.0	770	na	3.0	<1.0	10	13%
EXTRA LIGHT										
(Hungry Jack) 'Complete' dry	1/17 pkg	180	4.0	38.0	730	1.0	3.0	0.0	0	14%
(Hungry Jack) dry	1/17 pkg	180	4.0	38.0	730	1.0	3.0	0.0	0	14%
(Hungry Jack) dry	1/26 pkg	120	2.0	26.0	450	.5	0.0	0.0	0	0%
(Hungry Jack) prepared w/skim milk/oil/egg whites	3 pancakes	170	6.0	28.0	500	.5	4.0	1.0	0	21%
(Hungry Jack) prepared w/2% milk/oil/egg	3 pancakes	190	5.0	28.0	490	.5	6.0	1.0	55	29%
OAT BRAN (Krusteaz) 'Lite'	3 pancakes	130	5.0	36.0	370	10.0	1.0	na	0	5%

Food Name	Serving Size	Calories	Prot. gms	Carbs gms	Sod. mgs	Fiber gms	Fat gms	Sat. Fat gms	Chol. mgs	% Fat Cal.
WHOLE WHEAT *(Krusteaz)* honey	3 pancakes	215	8.0	42.0	630	5.0	1.0	na	9	4%
PANCAKE MIX, MICROWAVE										
(Hungry Jack) blueberry, dry	3/4 pkg	230	5.0	47.0	550	1.0	4.0	1.0	10	15%
(Hungry Jack) buttermilk, dry	3/4 pkg	260	5.0	51.0	590	1.0	4.0	1.0	10	14%
(Hungry Jack) harvest wheat, dry	3/4 pkg	230	6.0	46.0	560	3.0	4.0	1.0	10	15%
(Hungry Jack) oat bran, dry	3/4 pkg	230	6.0	45.0	580	3.0	4.0	1.0	10	15%
(Hungry Jack) original, dry	3/4 pkg	240	5.0	49.0	570	2.0	4.0	1.0	10	14%
PANCAKE SYRUP. See also MAPLE SYRUP.										
15% maple	1 cup	879	0.3	236.9	328	na	0.3	na	0	0%
15% maple	1 tbsp	56	0.0	15.0	21	na	0.0	na	0	0%
2% maple	1 cup	762	2.2	202.9	126	na	0.6	0.0	0	1%
2% maple	1 tbsp	48	0.1	12.9	8	na	0.0	0.0	0	0%
reduced calorie	100 gm	164	0.0	44.3	200	na	0.0	na	0	0%
(Aunt Jemima)										
'ButterLite'	1 oz	50	0.0	13.0	65	(tr)	0.0	0.0	0	0%
'Lite'	1 oz	54	0.1	13.1	92	.3	0.1	(tr)	0	2%
'Original,' rich maple taste	1 oz	100	0.0	26.0	60	na	0.0	na	na	0%
(Br'er Rabbit)										
dark	1 oz	120	0.0	31.0	0	na	0.0	na	0	0%
light	1 oz	120	0.0	31.0	0	na	0.0	na	0	0%
(Estee)										
	1 tbsp	4	0.0	1.0	25	(tr)	0.0	0.0	0	0%
'Breakfast'	1 tbsp	12	0.0	3.0	35	na	0.0	0.0	0	0%
(Featherweight)	1 tbsp	16	0.0	4.0	25	(tr)	0.0	0.0	0	0%
(Hungry Jack)										
'Lite'	2 tbsp	50	0.0	14.0	105	0	0.0	0.0	0	0%
regular	2 tbsp	100	0.0	26.0	25	0	0.0	0.0	0	0%
(Knott's Berry Farm)										
	1 oz	110	0.0	28.0	0	na	0.0	na	na	0%
'Country'	1 oz	110	0.0	27.0	0	na	0.0	na	na	0%
'Light' microwavable	1 oz	45	0.0	11.0	70	na	0.0	na	na	0%
w/30% real maple syrup, microwavable	1 oz	110	0.0	28.0	90	na	0.0	na	na	0%
(Log Cabin)										
'Country Kitchen'	1 oz	100	0.0	26.0	20	(tr)	0.0	0.0	0	0%
'Country Kitchen,' butter flavor	1 oz	100	0.0	27.0	100	na	0.0	na	0	0%
'Country Kitchen Lite'	1 oz	50	0.0	13.0	85	na	0.0	na	0	0%
'Lite,' reduced calorie	1 oz	50	0.0	13.0	90	na	0.0	na	0	0%
'Pancake and Waffle'	1 oz	100	0.0	26.0	35	(tr)	0.0	0.0	0	0%
(Maple Valley)										
maple syrup substitute	2 tbsp	110	0.0	27.0	50	na	0.0	na	na	0%
maple syrup substitute, 'Lite'	2 tbsp	60	0.0	16.0	60	na	0.0	na	na	0%
(Mrs. Butterworth's) thick 'n rich, 'Lite'	2 tbsp	60	0.0	15.0	65	na	0.0	na	na	0%
(Mrs. Richardson's)										
'Lite'	1 oz	50	0.0	13.0	90	na	0.0	na	na	0%
original recipe	1 oz	100	0.0	25.0	60	na	0.0	na	na	0%
(S&W) maple flavor, saccharin sweetened	1 tsp	4	0.0	1.0	25	(tr)	0.0	0.0	0	0%
(Vermont Maid)	1 tbsp	50	0.0	13.0	5	(tr)	0.0	0.0	0	0%
(Weight Watchers) 'Reduced Calorie'	1 tbsp	25	0.0	7.0	40	0	0.0	0.0	0	0%
PANCAKE/WAFFLE MIX. See also PANCAKE MIX.										
(NOTE: Unless otherwise stated, all pancakes are 4 inches in diameter.)										
(Arrowhead Mills) 'Griddle Lite' prepared	1/2 cup	260	8.0	50.0	(mq)	(mq)	3.0	(mq)	0	10%
(Aunt Jemima) 'Original' prepared	3 pancakes	116	3.4	25.4	609	1.4	0.8	0.1	0	6%
(Aunt Jemima) 'Original Complete' prepared	3 pancakes	253	7.0	50.2	1024	2.1	3.6	0.8	16	12%
(Bisquick) 'Shake 'n Pour' prepared	3 pancakes	260	6.0	48.0	850	(mq)	5.0	(mq)	0	17%

Food Name	Serving Size	Calories	Prot. gms	Carbs gms	Sod. mgs	Fiber gms	Fat gms	Sat. Fat gms	Chol. mgs	% Fat Cal.
(Estee) prepared, 3 inches each	3 pancakes	100	3.0	21.0	130	na	0.0	0.0	0	0%
(Featherweight) prepared	3 pancakes	140	6.0	24.0	90	(mq)	2.0	(mq)	5	13%
(Gold Medal) 'Pouch Mix' prepared w/egg	1/8 pouch	100	3.0	17.0	280	(mq)	2.0	(mq)	na	18%
(Hungry Jack) 'Panshakes' prepared	3 pancakes	250	7.0	43.0	880	(mq)	6.0	(mq)	na	21%
(Krusteaz) Belgian waffle, prepared, 4-inch square	1 waffle	170	5.0	22.0	350	na	7.0	na	45	37%
(Martha White) 'FlapStax' 1/4 cup batter per pancake	1 pancake	80	3.0	17.0	320	na	1.0	na	tr	10%
(Martha White) 'Light Crust' dry	2 oz	120	4.0	20.0	290	(mq)	3.0	(mq)	25	22%
(Robin Hood) 'Pouch Mix' prepared w/egg	1/8 pouch	100	3.0	17.0	280	(mq)	2.0	(mq)	na	18%
APPLE CINNAMON *(Bisquick)* 'Shake 'n Pour' prepared	3 pancakes	270	6.0	49.0	870	(mq)	5.0	(mq)	0	17%
BLUE CORN *(Arrowhead Mills)* prepared	1/2 cup	330	10.0	36.0	295	1.2	5.0	(mq)	0	20%
BLUEBERRY										
(Bisquick) 'Shake 'n Pour' prepared	3 pancakes	280	6.0	53.0	860	(mq)	5.0	(mq)	0	16%
(Hungry Jack) prepared	3 pancakes	320	6.0	41.0	820	(mq)	15.0	(mq)	na	42%
BUCKWHEAT										
(Arrowhead Mills) prepared	1/2 cup	270	11.0	53.0	(mq)	(mq)	2.0	(mq)	na	7%
(Aunt Jemima) prepared	3 pancakes	143	5.5	31.7	773	5.0	1.6	0.2	na	9%
BUTTERMILK										
(Aunt Jemima) 'Complete' prepared	3 pancakes	231	7.2	46.4	950	2.0	2.8	0.7	9	11%
(Aunt Jemima) 'Lite Complete' prepared	3 pancakes	130	7.0	25.0	570	(mq)	2.0	(mq)	na	12%
(Aunt Jemima) prepared	3 pancakes	122	4.2	26.1	698	1.3	0.7	0.1	1	5%
(Betty Crocker) complete, dry	1/2 cup	210	5.0	41.0	500	na	3.0	na	na	13%
(Betty Crocker) complete, prepared	3 pancakes	210	5.0	41.0	500	na	3.0	na	na	13%
(Betty Crocker) dry	1/2 cup	170	4.0	36.0	760	na	1.0	na	na	5%
(Betty Crocker) prepared w/milk/oil/egg	3 pancakes	280	8.0	39.0	810	na	10.0	na	na	32%
(Bisquick) 'Shake 'n Pour' prepared	3 pancakes	260	7.0	47.0	860	(mq)	5.0	(mq)	0	17%
(Hungry Jack) 'Complete' prepared	3 pancakes	180	4.0	39.0	710	(mq)	1.0	(mq)	na	5%
(Hungry Jack) 'Complete Packets' prepared	3 pancakes	180	4.0	35.0	680	(mq)	3.0	(mq)	na	15%
(Hungry Jack) prepared	3 pancakes	240	7.0	29.0	570	(mq)	11.0	(mq)	na	41%
EXTRA LIGHT *(Hungry Jack)* 'Complete' prepared w/water	3 pancakes	180	4.0	38.0	730	1.0	3.0	0.0	0	14%
MULTIGRAIN *(Arrowhead Mills)* prepared	1/2 cup	350	12.0	70.0	(mq)	.8	2.0	(mq)	na	5%
OAT BRAN										
(Arrowhead Mills) prepared	1/2 cup	200	9.0	64.0	230	1.8	2.0	(mq)	na	6%
(Bisquick) 'Shake 'n Pour' prepared	3 pancakes	240	7.0	45.0	580	1.0	4.0	(mq)	0	15%
WHOLE WHEAT *(Aunt Jemima)* prepared	3 pancakes	161	7.0	34.5	892	3.6	1.0	0.2	0	5%
PAPAYA										
peeled and seeded	1 oz	11	0.2	2.8	1	.3	<.1	<.1	0	<7%
raw *(Calavo Growers)*	1/2 med	80	0.0	19.0	15	2.7	0.0	0.0	0	0%
raw *(Del Monte)*	1/3 med	60	0.0	15.0	5	(mq)	0.0	0.0	0	0%
raw, approx 3 1/2 inch diam	1 med	119	1.9	29.8	9	5.5	0.4	0.1	0	3%
raw, cubed	1 cup	55	0.9	13.7	4	2.5	0.2	0.1	0	3%
raw, slices in light syrup *(Sunfresh)*	2/3 cup	80	<1.0	19.0	10	<1.0	0.0	0.0	0	0%
PAPAYA DRINK *(Knudsen & Sons)* concentrate	1.5 oz	90	<1.0	22.0	37	na	0.0	na	na	0%
PAPAYA JUICE *(Knudsen & Sons)* cream	2 oz	25	<1.0	6.0	na	na	0.0	na	na	0%
PAPAYA LIME JUICE *(Knudsen & Sons)*	8 oz	115	1.0	29.0	na	na	0.0	na	na	0%
PAPAYA NECTAR										
canned	1 cup	142	0.4	36.3	13	1.5	0.4	0.1	0	2%
canned	1 oz	18	0.1	4.5	2	.2	0.1	0.0	0	5%
(Kern's)	6 oz	110	0.0	27.0	5	na	0.0	na	na	0%
(Knudsen & Sons)	8 oz	100	<1.0	26.0	na	na	0.0	na	na	0%
(Knudsen & Sons) concentrate	1.5 oz	90	<1.0	22.0	na	na	0.0	na	na	0%
(Libby's)	6 oz	110	0.0	28.0	10	(mq)	0.0	0.0	0	0%
PAPAYA PUNCH *(Veryfine)*	8 oz	120	<1.0	30.0	10	(mq)	0.0	0.0	0	0%
PAPRIKA										
ground	1 oz	82	4.2	15.8	10	>5.9 c	3.7	0.6	0	29%

Food Name	Serving Size	Calories	Prot. gms	Carbs gms	Sod. mgs	Fiber gms	Fat gms	Sat. Fat gms	Chol. mgs	% Fat Cal
ground	1 tbsp	20	1.0	3.8	2	1.4	0.9	0.1	0	30%
ground	1 tsp	6	0.3	1.2	1	.4	0.3	0.0	0	31%
ground *(Durkee)*	1 tsp	8	0.0	0.0	0	0	tr	na	na	tr
ground *(Laurel Leaf)*	1 tsp	8	0.0	0.0	0	0	tr	na	na	tr
ground *(Spice Islands)*	1 tsp	7	0.3	1.1	<1	>.4 c	0.2	(tr)	0	24%
PARANUT. See BRAZIL NUT.										
PARFAIT										
chocolate *(Pearson)*	1 oz	120	1.0	23.0	70	na	3.0	na	na	22%
chocolate *(Swiss Miss)*	4 oz	170	3.0	27.0	200	0	6.0	1.4	1	31%
chocolate vanilla, fat-free *(Swiss Miss)*	4 oz	104	1.9	23.3	171	0	0.3	0.0	1	3%
peanut butter *(Pearson)*	1 oz	120	1.0	23.0	70	na	3.0	na	na	22%
vanilla *(Swiss Miss)*	4 oz	180	2.0	29.0	150	0	6.0	1.3	1	30%
vanilla chocolate *(Swiss Miss)*	4 oz	164	2.9	24.5	196	0	6.0	1.6	1	33%
vanilla chocolate 'Light' *(Swiss Miss)*	4 oz	100	2.0	20.0	110	0	1.0	0.3	0	9%
PARROT FISH / pollyfish										
raw	1 lb	390	87.5	0.0	(mq)	0	1.8	(mq)	(mq)	4%
raw	1 oz	24	5.5	0.0	(mq)	0	0.1	(mq)	(mq)	4%
PARSLEY										
dried	1 oz	78	6.4	14.6	128	>2.9 c	1.3	na	0	12%
dried	1 tbsp	4	0.3	0.7	6	.1	0.1	na	0	12%
dried	1 tsp	1	0.1	0.2	1	0	tr	na	0	0%
dried *(Durkee)*	1 tsp	1	0.0	0.0	0	0	tr	na	na	tr
dried *(Laurel Leaf)*	1 tsp	1	0.0	0.0	0	0	tr	na	na	tr
dried flakes *(Spice Islands)*	1 tsp	4	0.2	0.6	6	>.1 c	0.1	(tr)	0	12%
freeze-dried	1 oz	77	8.9	12.0	111	>2.9 c	1.5	na	0	14%
freeze-dried	1/4 cup	4	0.4	0.6	5	>.1 c	0.1	na	0	14%
freeze-dried	1 tbsp	1	0.1	0.2	2	0	tr	na	0	0%
raw	10 sprigs	4	0.3	0.6	6	na	0.1	0.0	0	20%
raw, chopped	1/2 cup	11	0.9	1.9	17	na	0.2	0.0	0	14%
raw, trimmed	1 oz	9	0.6	2.0	11	1.2	0.1	(tr)	0	8%
raw, untrimmed	1 lb	140	9.5	29.8	169	19.0	1.3	na	0	7%
PARSLEY ROOT / hamburg parsley / turnip-rooted parsley										
fresh	1 lb	50	12.7	10.4	454	5.9	2.7	na	0	21%
fresh	1 oz	3	0.8	0.7	28	.4	0.2	(tr)	0	23%
PARSLEY SEASONING										
(Schilling) all purpose 'Parsley Patch'	1 tsp	6	0.3	1.0	3	(mq)	0.0	0.0	0	0%
PARSNIP										
boiled, drained	4 oz	92	1.5	22.1	11	3.1	0.3	0.1	0	3%
boiled, drained, 9 inches long	1 parsnip	130	2.1	31.3	16	6.4	0.5	0.1	0	3%
boiled, drained, slices	1/2 cup	63	1.0	15.2	8	3.1	0.2	0.0	0	3%
raw, slices	1/2 cup	50	0.8	12.0	7	3.3	0.2	0.0	0	3%
raw, trimmed	1 oz	21	0.3	5.1	3	>.6 c	0.1	<.1	0	4%
raw, untrimmed	1 lb	289	4.6	69.4	39	>7.7 c	1.2	0.2	0	4%
PASSION FRUIT / granadilla										
purple, trimmed	1 oz	27	0.6	6.6	na	>3.1 c	0.2	(tr)	0	6%
purple, trimmed, approx 1.2 oz	1 med	17	0.4	4.2	5	1.9	0.1	na	0	5%
purple, untrimmed	1 lb	230	5.2	55.1	na	>25.8 c	1.7	na	0	6%
PASSION FRUIT BEVERAGES										
COCKTAIL										
fresh, purple	1 cup	126	1.0	33.6	15	.5	0.1	na	0	1%
fresh, purple	1 cup	16	0.1	4.2	2	tr	0.0	na	0	0%
fresh, yellow	1 cup	148	1.6	35.7	15	.5	0.4	na	0	2%
(Welch's) bottled 'Orchard Tropicals' diluted	6 oz	100	0.0	25.0	20	0	0.0	0.0	0	0%
(Welch's) frozen 'Orchard Tropicals' diluted	6 oz	100	0.0	25.0	20	0	0.0	0.0	0	0%

Food Name	Serving Size	Calories	Prot. gms	Carbs gms	Sod. mgs	Fiber gms	Fat gms	Sat. Fat gms	Chol. mgs	% Fat Cal.
(Welch's) 'Orchard Tropicals Cocktails-In-A-Box'	8.45 oz	140	0.0	34.0	20	0	0.0	0.0	0	0%
JUICE										
fresh, yellow	1 oz	19	0.2	4.5	2	.1	0.1	na	0	5%
(Knudsen & Sons) raspberry	8 oz	130	<1.0	32.0	na	na	0.0	na	na	0%
(Snapple) passion juice 'Passion Supreme'	8 oz	160	0.0	39.0	20	na	0.0	0.0	0	0%
(Veryfine) refresher, w/orange, tropical	8 oz	110	<1.0	26.0	25	na	0.0	0.0	0	0%
PASTA/macaroni. See also NOODLE, CHINESE; NOODLE, EGG; NOODLE, JAPANESE; TORTELLINI PASTA.										
(NOTE: 2 ounces uncooked pasta = approximately 1 cup cooked.)										
ACINI PEPE *(Ronzoni)* dry	2 oz	210	7.0	42.0	0	na	1.0	na	0	4%
AGNOLOTTI, refrigerated, 'Fresh' *(Contadina)*	3 oz	270	13.0	38.0	230	na	7.0	2.0	40	24%
ANGEL HAIR										
Dry										
corn *(Westbrae)*	2 oz	210	4.0	46.0	10	na	2.0	0	10	8%
Jerusalem artichoke *(De Boles)*	2 oz	210	9.0	41.0	0	na	1.0	na	0	4%
Jerusalem artichoke, garlic and parsley *(De Boles)*	2 oz	210	9.0	41.0	15	na	1.0	na	0	4%
Jerusalem artichoke, tomato and basil *(De Boles)*	2 oz	210	9.0	41.0	10	na	1.0	na	0	4%
100% durum wheat semolina *(American Beauty)*	2 oz	210	7.0	42.0	0	na	1.0	na	0	4%
wheat *(Creamette)*	2 oz	210	7.0	42.0	0	2.0	1.0	0.0	0	4%
wheat *(DiGiorno)*	3 oz	250	11.0	47.0	140	na	3.0	0.0	0	10%
whole-wheat *(De Boles)*	2 oz	210	9.0	40.0	0	na	2.0	na	0	8%
Refrigerated, fresh										
'Fresh' *(Contadina)*	3 oz	260	12.0	45.0	30	na	3.0	<1.0	75	11%
BOW TIE. See FARFELLE.										
CAPELLINI										
100% durum wheat semolina *(American Beauty)* dry	2 oz	210	7.0	42.0	0	na	1.0	na	0	4%
CURLY										
100% durum wheat semolina 'Curly-Roni'										
(American Beauty) dry	2 oz	210	7.0	42.0	0	na	1.0	na	0	4%
ELBOW										
Dry										
corn *(Westbrae)*	2 oz	210	4.0	46.0	10	na	2.0	na	0	8%
corn, wheat-free *(De Boles)*	2 oz	210	5.0	45.0	0	na	1.0	na	na	4%
Jerusalem artichoke *(De Boles)*	2 oz	210	9.0	41.0	0	na	1.0	na	0	4%
100% durum wheat semolina *(American Beauty)*	2 oz	210	7.0	42.0	0	na	1.0	na	0	4%
'Primavera' *(De Boles)*	2 oz	210	9.0	41.0	0	na	<1.0	na	0	<4%
quinoa 'Supergrain Wheat Free' *(Ancient Harvest)*	2 oz	180	5.0	36.0	5	2.5	2.0	na	0	10%
quinoa 'Supergrain Wheat Free' *(Quinoa)*	2 oz	180	5.0	36.0	5	2.5	2.0	na	0	10%
'Valu Pack' *(Hospitality)*	1/2 cup	240	8.0	48.0	0	2.0	0.5	0.0	0	2%
wheat *(Creamette)*	2 oz	210	7.0	42.0	0	.1	1.0	0.0	0	4%
whole wheat	1 cup	365	15.4	78.8	8	12.4	1.5	0.3	0	4%
whole wheat *(De Boles)*	2 oz	210	9.0	40.0	0	na	2.0	na	0	8%
FARFELLE/ bow tie										
Dry										
wheat *(De Cecco)*	2 oz	210	7.0	41.0	0	na	1.0	na	0	5%
wheat *(Ronzoni)*	2 oz	210	7.0	42.0	0	na	1.0	na	0	4%
FETTUCCINE										
Dry										
basil *(Al Dente)*	2 oz	220	8.0	40.0	20	(mq)	2.0	(mq)	(mq)	9%
curry *(Al Dente)*	2 oz	220	8.0	40.0	20	(mq)	2.0	(mq)	(mq)	9%
dill *(Al Dente)*	2 oz	220	8.0	40.0	20	(mq)	2.0	(mq)	(mq)	9%
egg noodle *(Antoine's)*	2 oz	210	7.0	41.0	0	na	1.0	na	0	5%
egg noodle, extra long *(Ronzoni)*	2 oz	220	8.0	42.0	15	na	3.0	na	65	12%
egg noodle 'Home-Style' *(De Cecco)*	2 oz	210	8.0	40.0	35	na	3.0	na	0	12%
Jerusalem artichoke *(De Boles)*	2 oz	210	9.0	41.0	0	na	1.0	na	0	4%

Food Name	Serving Size	Calories	Prot. gms	Carbs gms	Sod. mgs	Fiber gms	Fat gms	Sat. Fat gms	Chol. mgs	% Fat Cal.
spinach *(Al Dente)*	2 oz	220	8.0	40.0	20	(mq)	2.0	(mq)	(mq)	9%
spinach *(DiGiorno)*	3 oz	250	12.0	46.0	140	na	3.0	0.0	0	10%
spinach, Jerusalem artichoke *(De Boles)*	2 oz	210	9.0	41.0	5	na	<1.0	na	0	<4%
spinach and egg 'Florentine' *(American Beauty)*	2 oz	220	8.0	42.0	35	na	3.0	na	65	12%
tarragon *(Al Dente)*	2 oz	220	8.0	40.0	20	(mq)	2.0	(mq)	(mq)	9%
wheat *(DiGiorno)*	3 oz	250	11.0	47.0	140	na	3.0	0.0	0	10%
wheat, bell pepper/basil, organic *(Herb's)*	2 oz	220	10.0	40.0	5	na	2.0	na	60	8%
whole-wheat *(Al Dente)*	2 oz	210	8.0	42.0	10	(mq)	1.0	na	0	4%
Refrigerated, fresh										
spinach 'Fresh' *(Contadina)*	3 oz	260	12.0	45.0	70	na	4.0	1.0	80	14%
FUSILLI										
Dry										
rainbow *(Antoine's)*	2 oz	210	7.0	41.0	20	(mq)	1.0	na	0	5%
spinach *(De Cecco)*	2 oz	210	7.0	41.0	5	na	1.0	na	0	5%
tricolor *(Antoine's)*	2 oz	210	7.0	41.0	20	(mq)	1.0	na	0	5%
tricolor, vegetable *(Antoine's)*	2 oz	210	7.0	41.0	25	2.0	1.0	0.0	0	5%
vegetable *(Antoine's)*	2 oz	210	7.0	41.0	20	(mq)	1.0	na	0	5%
wheat *(De Cecco)*	2 oz	210	7.0	41.0	0	na	1.0	na	0	5%
GEMELLI *(Antoine's)* dry	2 oz	210	7.0	41.0	0	na	1.0	na	0	5%
LASAGNA										
Dry										
curly edge *(Ronzoni)*	2 oz	210	7.0	42.0	0	na	1.0	na	0	4%
Jerusalem artichoke *(De Boles)*	2 oz	210	9.0	41.0	0	na	1.0	na	0	4%
100% durum wheat semolina *(American Beauty)*	2 oz	210	7.0	42.0	0	na	1.0	na	0	4%
100% semolina *(Creamette)*	2 oz	210	7.0	42.0	0	na	1.0	na	0	4%
100% semolina *(De Cecco)*	2 oz	210	7.0	41.0	0	na	1.0	na	0	5%
spinach, whole-wheat, no egg *(Westbrae)*	2 oz	210	8.0	40.0	0	6.0	2.0	na	0	9%
whole-wheat *(De Boles)*	2 oz	210	9.0	40.0	0	na	2.0	na	0	8%
whole-wheat *(Health Valley)*	2 oz	170	9.0	40.0	10	7.2	1.0	na	0	4%
whole-wheat, no egg *(Westbrae)*	2 oz	210	8.0	40.0	0	7.0	2.0	na	0	9%
whole-wheat, spinach *(Health Valley)*	2 oz	170	9.0	40.0	15	7.2	1.0	na	0	4%
LINGUINE										
Dry										
Jerusalem artichoke *(De Boles)*	2 oz	210	9.0	41.0	0	na	1.0	na	0	4%
quinoa 'Supergrain Wheat Free' *(Ancient Harvest)*	2 oz	180	5.0	35.0	5	2.5	2.0	0.0	0	10%
quinoa 'Supergrain Wheat Free' *(Quinoa)*	2 oz	180	5.0	35.0	5	2.5	2.0	0.0	0	10%
wheat *(Creamette)*	2 oz	210	7.0	42.0	0	na	1.0	na	0	4%
wheat *(De Cecco)*	2 oz	210	7.0	41.0	0	na	1.0	na	0	5%
wheat *(DiGiorno)*	3 oz	250	11.0	46.0	135	na	3.0	0.0	0	11%
wheat *(Ronzoni)*	2 oz	210	7.0	42.0	0	na	1.0	na	0	4%
Refrigerated, fresh										
(DiGiorno)	3 oz	250	11.0	47.0	140	na	3.0	0.0	0	10%
MANICOTTI, extra fancy *(Ronzoni)* dry	2 oz	210	7.0	42.0	0	na	1.0	na	0	4%
MOSTACCIOLI										
Dry										
100% durum wheat semolina *(American Beauty)*	2 oz	210	7.0	42.0	0	na	1.0	na	0	4%
wheat *(Creamette)*	2 oz	210	7.0	42.0	0	2.0	1.0	0.0	0	4%
wheat *(Ronzoni)*	2 oz	210	9.0	40.0	0	2.0	1.0	0.0	0	4%
ORZO *(Ronzoni)* dry	2 oz	210	7.0	42.0	0	na	3.0	na	0	12%
PENNE RIGATI										
Dry										
(Antoine's)	2 oz	210	7.0	41.0	0	(mq)	1.0	na	0	5%
(De Cecco)	2 oz	210	7.0	41.0	0	na	1.0	na	0	5%
PENNONI *(De Cecco)* dry	2 oz	210	7.0	41.0	0	na	1.0	na	0	5%

Food Name	Serving Size	Calories	Prot. gms	Carbs gms	Sod. mgs	Fiber gms	Fat gms	Sat. Fat gms	Chol. mgs	% Fat Cal.
QUINOA										
Dry										
garden pagodas 'Supergrain Wheat Free'										
(Ancient Harvest) .... 2 oz		180	5.0	35.0	5	2.5	2.0	na	0	10%
veggie curls 'Supergrain Wheat Free' (Ancient Harvest) .. 2 oz		180	5.0	35.0	5	2.5	2.0	0.0	0	10%
veggie curls 'Supergrain Wheat Free' (Quinoa) .... 2 oz		180	5.0	35.0	5	2.5	2.0	0.0	0	10%
RADIATORE										
Dry										
tomato and spinach, tri-color (Ronzoni) .... 2 oz		210	7.0	42.0	30	na	1.0	na	0	4%
wheat (Antoine's) .... 2 oz		210	7.0	41.0	0	na	1.0	na	na	5%
RAINBOW										
100% durum wheat semolina 'Rainbo Twirl'										
(American Beauty) dry .... 2 oz		210	7.0	42.0	30	na	1.0	na	0	4%
RIBBON										
Dry										
spinach (Creamette) .... 2 oz		210	7.0	42.0	70	na	1.0	na	na	4%
wheat, mixed vegetable, organic (Herb's) .... 2 oz		220	10.0	40.0	5	na	2.0	na	60	8%
wheat, paella, w/saffron, organic (Eden Foods) .... 2 oz		228	8.0	44.0	0	na	<1.0	na	0	<4%
wheat, parsley garlic, organic (Eden Foods) .... 2 oz		228	8.0	44.0	0	na	<1.0	na	0	<4%
whole-wheat (De Boles) .... 2 oz		210	9.0	40.0	0	na	2.0	na	0	8%
yolk-free 'Pennsylvania Dutch' (Creamette) .... 2 oz		210	7.0	42.0	0	na	1.0	na	0	4%
RIGATONI										
Dry										
(Creamette) .... 2 oz		210	7.0	42.0	0	na	1.0	0.0	0	4%
(De Cecco) .... 2 oz		210	7.0	41.0	0	na	1.0	na	0	5%
(Ronzoni) .... 2 oz		210	7.0	42.0	0	na	1.0	na	0	4%
Refrigerated, fresh										
'Fresh' (Contadina) .... 2.3 oz		200	9.0	34.0	25	na	3.0	<1.0	85	14%
Jerusalem artichoke (De Boles) .... 2 oz		210	9.0	41.0	0	na	1.0	na	0	4%
ROTELLE										
Dry										
100% durum wheat semolina (American Beauty) .... 2 oz		210	7.0	42.0	30	na	1.0	na	0	4%
quinoa 'Supergrain Wheat Free' (Ancient Harvest) .... 2 oz		180	5.0	35.0	5	2.5	2.0	na	0	10%
quinoa 'Supergrain Wheat Free' (Quinoa) .... 2 oz		180	5.0	35.0	5	2.5	2.0	na	0	10%
wheat (Creamette) .... 2 oz		210	7.0	42.0	0	na	1.0	0.0	0	4%
wheat (De Cecco) .... 2 oz		210	7.0	41.0	0	na	1.0	na	0	5%
wheat (Ronzoni) .... 2 oz		210	9.0	40.0	0	2.0	1.0	0.0	0	4%
ROTINI										
Dry										
garlic and parsley (De Boles) .... 2 oz		210	9.0	41.0	15	na	1.0	na	0	4%
Jerusalem artichoke (De Boles) .... 2 oz		210	9.0	41.0	0	na	1.0	na	0	4%
100% durum wheat semolina (American Beauty) .... 2 oz		210	7.0	42.0	0	na	1.0	na	0	4%
quinoa 'Supergrain' (Ancient Harvest) .... 2 oz		210	10.0	40.0	11	8.0	1.0	na	0	4%
vegetable 'Primavera' (De Boles) .... 2 oz		210	9.0	41.0	0	na	<1.0	na	0	<4%
vegetable, tomato, and basil (De Boles) .... 2 oz		210	9.0	41.0	10	na	1.0	na	0	4%
SALAD PASTA										
100% durum wheat semolina 'Salad-Roni'										
(American Beauty) dry .... 2 oz		210	7.0	42.0	0	na	1.0	na	0	4%
SEA-SHELL										
durum wheat semolina (American Beauty) dry .... 2 oz		210	7.0	42.0	0	na	1.0	na	0	4%
SHELL										
Dry										
corn (Westbrae) .... 2 oz		210	4.0	46.0	10	na	2.0	na	0	8%
corn, wheat-free (De Boles) .... 2 oz		210	5.0	45.0	0	na	1.0	na	na	4%

Food Name	Serving Size	Calories	Prot. gms	Carbs gms	Sod. mgs	Fiber gms	Fat gms	Sat. Fat gms	Chol. mgs	% Fat Cal.
extra fancy (Ronzoni)	2 oz	210	7.0	42.0	0	na	1.0	na	0	4%
jumbo (Ronzoni)	2 oz	210	7.0	42.0	0	na	1.0	na	0	4%
medium (Creamette)	2 oz	210	7.0	42.0	0	na	1.0	0.0	0	4%
medium, 100% durum wheat semolina (American Beauty)	2 oz	210	7.0	42.0	0	na	1.0	na	0	4%
100% durum wheat semolina 'Shel-Roni' (American Beauty) dry	2 oz	210	7.0	42.0	0	na	1.0	na	0	4%
quinoa 'Supergrain Wheat Free' (Ancient Harvest)	2 oz	180	5.0	35.0	5	2.5	2.0	na	0	10%
quinoa 'Supergrain Wheat Free' (Quinoa)	2 oz	180	5.0	35.0	5	2.5	2.0	na	0	10%
'Primavera' (De Boles)	2 oz	210	9.0	41.0	0	na	<1.0	na	0	<4%
wheat (Ronzoni)	2 oz	210	7.0	42.0	0	na	1.0	na	0	4%
wheat, vegetable, no eggs, organic (Eden Foods)	2 oz	228	8.0	44.0	0	na	<1.0	na	0	<4%
whole-wheat (De Boles)	2 oz	210	9.0	40.0	0	na	2.0	na	0	8%
SPAGHETTI										
Dry										
amaranth (Health Valley)	2 oz	170	7.0	40.0	10	8.8	1.0	na	0	5%
corn (Westbrae)	2 oz	210	4.0	46.0	10	na	2.0	na	0	8%
corn, wheat-free (De Boles)	2 oz	210	5.0	45.0	0	na	1.0	na	na	4%
Jerusalem artichoke (De Boles)	2 oz	210	9.0	41.0	0	na	1.0	na	0	4%
oat bran (Health Valley)	2 oz	120	4.0	23.0	2	3.8	1.0	na	0	8%
100% durum wheat semolina (American Beauty)	2 oz	210	7.0	42.0	0	na	1.0	na	0	4%
100% semolina (Hospitality)	2 oz	210	7.0	42.0	0	2.0	0.5	0.0	0	2%
pepper 'Three Pepper Pasta' (Al Dente)	2 oz	220	8.0	40.0	20	(mq)	2.0	(mq)	(mq)	9%
protein-fortified	2 oz	213	12.4	37.4	5	>.5 c	1.3	0.2	0	6%
quinoa 'Supergrain' (Ancient Harvest)	2 oz	210	10.0	40.0	11	8.0	1.0	na	0	4%
quinoa 'Supergrain' (Quinoa)	2 oz	210	10.0	40.0	11	8.0	1.0	na	0	4%
quinoa 'Supergrain Wheat Free' (Ancient Harvest)	2 oz	180	5.0	35.0	5	2.5	2.0	0.0	0	10%
quinoa 'Supergrain Wheat Free' (Quinoa)	2 oz	180	5.0	35.0	5	2.5	2.0	0.0	0	10%
spinach	2 oz	212	7.6	42.6	21	>1.8 c	0.9	0.1	0	4%
spinach, Jerusalem artichoke (De Boles)	2 oz	210	9.0	41.0	5	na	<1.0	na	0	<4%
spinach, whole-wheat, no egg (Westbrae)	2 oz	210	8.0	40.0	0	6.0	2.0	na	0	9%
thin (Creamette)	2 oz	210	7.0	42.0	0	na	1.0	na	0	4%
thin (Ronzoni)	2 oz	210	7.0	42.0	0	na	1.0	na	0	4%
thin, 100% durum wheat semolina (American Beauty)	2 oz	210	7.0	42.0	0	na	1.0	na	0	4%
unenriched	2 oz	211	7.3	42.6	4	>.2 c	0.9	0.1	0	4%
wheat (DiGiorno)	3 oz	250	11.0	47.0	140	na	3.0	0.0	0	10%
wheat (Rummo)	2 oz	210	7.0	41.0	10	na	1.0	na	na	5%
whole-wheat	2 oz	198	8.3	42.8	5	>1.7 c	0.8	0.2	0	3%
whole-wheat (De Boles)	2 oz	210	9.0	40.0	0	na	2.0	na	0	8%
whole-wheat (Health Valley)	2 oz	170	9.0	40.0	10	7.2	1.0	na	0	4%
whole-wheat, no egg (Westbrae)	2 oz	210	8.0	40.0	0	7.0	2.0	na	0	9%
whole-wheat, spinach (Health Valley)	2 oz	170	9.0	40.0	10	7.2	1.0	na	0	4%
SPAGHETTINI (De Cecco) dry	2 oz	210	7.0	41.0	0	na	1.0	na	0	5%
SPIRAL										
Dry										
spicy (Antoine's)	2 oz	210	7.0	41.0	40	(mq)	1.0	na	0	5%
vegetable	1 cup	308	11.0	62.9	36	3.6	0.9	0.1	0	3%
wheat, sesame rice, organic (Eden Foods)	2 oz	212	10.0	40.0	0	na	1.0	na	0	4%
wheat, vegetable, no eggs, organic (Eden Foods)	2 oz	228	8.0	44.0	0	na	<1.0	na	0	<4%
TRICOLOR										
Dry										
'Primavera' (De Boles)	2 oz	200	8.0	41.0	8	(mq)	1.0	na	0	4%
spirals	1 cup	308	11.0	62.9	36	3.6	0.9	0.1	0	3%
wheat (Creamette)	2 oz	210	8.0	42.0	5	1.3	1.0	0.0	0	4%

Food Name	Serving Size	Calories	Prot. gms	Carbs gms	Sod. mgs	Fiber gms	Fat gms	Sat. Fat gms	Chol. mgs	% Fat Cal.
TRIO ITALIANO										
rotini, mostaccioli, shells *(American Beauty)* dry	2 oz	210	7.0	42.0	0	na	1.0	na	0	4%
VERMICELLI										
Dry										
extra thin *(Creamette)*	2 oz	210	7.0	42.0	0	na	1.0	na	0	4%
100% durum wheat semolina *(American Beauty)*	2 oz	210	7.0	42.0	0	na	1.0	na	0	4%
wheat *(Ronzoni)*	2 oz	210	7.0	42.0	0	na	1.0	na	0	4%
ZITI Jerusalem artichoke *(De Boles)* dry	2 oz	210	9.0	41.0	0	na	1.0	na	0	4%
ZITI RIGATI *(Ronzoni)* dry	2 oz	210	7.0	42.0	0	na	1.0	na	0	4%
PASTA DINNER, FROZEN										
penne, w/tomato sauce, Italian sausage *(Budget Gourmet)*	10 oz	320	12.0	53.0	520	na	9.0	2.0	5	24%
primavera *(Healthy Choice)*	11 oz	280	11.0	51.0	360	na	3.0	2.0	15	10%
stuffed, shells, 3-cheese 'LightStyle' *(Le Menu)*	10 oz	280	17.0	34.0	690	(mq)	8.0	(mq)	25	26%
w/chicken and herb tomato sauce *(Lean Cuisine)*	9.5 oz	270	17.0	38.0	460	na	6.0	2.0	35	20%
zesty tomato sauce over ziti 'Classics' *(Healthy Choice)* . .	12 oz	350	16.0	59.0	530	na	5.0	2.0	30	13%
PASTA DINNER MIX										
artichoke elbow 'Mac & Cheese' dry *(De Boles)*	2 oz	210	9.0	40.0	160	na	2.0	na	na	8%
artichoke elbow 'Mac & Cheese' prepared *(De Boles)*	3/4 cup	220	8.0	31.0	140	na	7.0	na	na	29%
artichoke shells and cheddar, dry *(De Boles)*	2 oz	210	9.0	40.0	160	na	2.0	na	na	8%
artichoke shells and cheddar, prepared *(De Boles)*	3/4 cup	220	8.0	31.0	140	na	7.0	na	na	29%
wheat elbow 'Mac & Cheese' dry *(De Boles)*	2 oz	210	9.0	39.0	150	na	3.0	na	na	12%
wheat elbow 'Mac & Cheese' prepared *(De Boles)*	3/4 cup	200	7.0	27.0	120	na	8.0	na	na	35%
w/beef flavored sauce, prepared *(Ultra Slim Fast)*	8 oz	230	8.0	45.0	1070	4.0	3.0	na	na	11%
w/chicken flavored sauce, prepared *(Ultra Slim Fast)*	8 oz	220	8.0	45.0	980	4.0	3.0	na	na	11%
w/tomato herb sauce, prepared *(Ultra Slim Fast)*	8 oz	220	8.0	46.0	1090	5.0	3.0	na	na	11%
w/zesty cheese sauce, prepared *(Ultra Slim Fast)*	8 oz	230	9.0	44.0	770	4.0	4.0	na	na	15%
PASTA DISH MIX. See also NOODLE ENTRÉE/DISH MIX; ROTINI ENTRÉE MIX; SPAGHETTI ENTRÉE MIX.										
Alfredo 'Pasta For One' *(Villa Lorenzo)*	2.3 oz	270	9.0	39.0	910	na	8.0	na	na	27%
butter and herbs 'Pasta For One' *(Villa Lorenzo)*	2.3 oz	270	8.0	43.0	800	na	7.0	na	na	24%
cream sauce and mushrooms 'Pasta For One'										
(Villa Lorenzo)	2.3 oz	260	8.0	42.0	800	na	6.0	na	na	21%
cream sauce and spinach 'Pasta For One' *(Villa Lorenzo)*	2.3 oz	270	9.0	43.0	900	na	6.0	na	na	21%
pesto and herbs 'Pasta For One' *(Villa Lorenzo)*	2.3 oz	260	9.0	41.0	850	na	6.0	na	na	21%
3 cheese and broccoli 'Pasta For One' *(Villa Lorenzo)*	2.3 oz	260	9.0	43.0	910	na	5.0	na	na	18%
zesty tomato 'Pasta For One' *(Villa Lorenzo)*	2.3 oz	250	8.0	47.0	680	na	3.0	na	na	11%
PASTA ENTRÉE, CANNED. See also NOODLE ENTRÉE/DISH, CANNED; RAVIOLI ENTRÉE; SPAGHETTI ENTRÉE, CANNED.										
(Chef Boyardee)										
and chicken	7.5 oz	180	10.0	30.0	850	1.0	2.0	<1.0	15	10%
in cheese sauce 'ABC's & 123's'	8.6 oz	200	6.0	42.0	1020	na	1.0	<1.0	2	5%
in cheese sauce 'Dinosaurs'	8.6 oz	200	6.0	42.0	1060	na	1.0	<1.0	2	5%
in cheese sauce 'Dinosaurs'	7.5 oz	160	4.0	33.0	790	3.0	1.0	<1.0	1	6%
in cheese sauce 'Sharks'	7.5 oz	170	5.0	34.0	780	na	1.0	<1.0	2	6%
in cheese sauce 'Smurfs'	7.5 oz	150	6.0	29.0	830	3.0	1.0	na	2	6%
in cheese sauce 'Tic Tac Toes'	8.6 oz	190	5.0	41.0	1080	na	1.0	na	na	5%
in cheese sauce 'Tic Tac Toes'	7.5 oz	160	5.0	31.0	870	3.0	1.0	<1.0	1	6%
in chicken sauce 'Pac Man'	7.5 oz	170	6.0	22.0	905	na	7.0	na	na	36%
in meat sauce, shells	7.5 oz	190	7.0	31.0	810	4.0	6.0	1.0	5	26%
in pizza sauce, spirals	7.5 oz	180	5.0	35.0	1080	3.0	3.0	<1.0	5	14%
in sauce 'ABC's & 123's'	7.5 oz	160	5.0	31.0	830	3.0	1.0	<1.0	2	6%
in sauce 'Turtles'	7.5 oz	150	4.0	31.0	830	na	1.0	na	0	6%
in tomato sauce 'Pac Man'	7.5 oz	150	6.0	30.0	830	na	1.0	<1.0	2	6%
mini bites	7.5 oz	260	8.0	30.0	1020	1.0	12.0	2.0	17	42%
'Roller Coasters'	7.5 oz	230	7.0	28.0	1070	3.0	10.0	3.0	19	39%
w/meatballs 'ABC's & 123's'	8.6 oz	280	9.0	35.0	1090	na	11.0	na	23	36%

Food Name	Serving Size	Calories	Prot. gms	Carbs gms	Sod. mgs	Fiber gms	Fat gms	Sat. Fat gms	Chol. mgs	% Fat Cal
w/meatballs 'Dinosaurs'	8.6 oz	280	9.0	36.0	1131	na	11.0	na	21	36%
w/meatballs 'Pac Man'	7.5 oz	230	7.0	32.0	880	5.0	9.0	3.0	17	34%
w/meatballs 'Sharks'	7.5 oz	230	8.0	31.0	900	na	8.0	na	15	32%
w/meatballs 'Smurfs'	7.5 oz	240	8.0	31.0	900	2.0	9.0	2.0	19	34%
w/meatballs 'Tic Tac Toes'	8.6 oz	290	8.0	39.0	1045	na	11.0	<1.0	na	35%
w/meatballs 'Tic Tac Toes'	7.5 oz	240	8.0	31.0	1000	na	9.0	na	18	34%
w/meatballs 'Turtles'	7.5 oz	220	7.0	30.0	940	na	8.0	na	20	33%
w/meatballs in sauce 'Zooroni'	7.5 oz	240	8.0	33.0	970	na	8.0	na	17	31%
w/mini meatballs 'ABC's & 123's'	7.5 oz	240	8.0	33.0	920	na	9.0	na	18	33%
w/mini meatballs 'Dinosaurs'	7.5 oz	230	7.0	32.0	960	na	8.0	na	19	32%

PASTA ENTRÉE, FROZEN. See also NOODLE ENTRÉE/DISH, FROZEN; RAVIOLI ENTRÉE; ROTINI ENTRÉE, FROZEN; SPAGHETTI ENTRÉE, FROZEN; TORTELLINI PASTA DISH/ENTRÉE, FROZEN; ZITI ENTRÉE, FROZEN.

Food Name	Serving Size	Calories	Prot. gms	Carbs gms	Sod. mgs	Fiber gms	Fat gms	Sat. Fat gms	Chol. mgs	% Fat Cal
angel hair (Smart Ones)	8.55 oz	120	8.0	18.0	290	na	<1.0	<1.0	0	<8%
angel hair pasta (Lean Cuisine)	10 oz	240	10.0	38.0	410	na	5.0	1.0	10	19%
baked, and cheese (Celentano)	6 oz	290	12.0	29.0	350	(mq)	13.0	(mq)	(mq)	42%
broccoli stuffed shells, low fat 'Great Choice' (Celentano)	10 oz	190	12.0	31.0	520	na	4.0	na	na	17%
creamy cheddar 'Pasta Accents' (Green Giant)	1/2 cup	90	4.0	14.0	280	2.0	3.0	1.0	5	27%
Dijon 'Microwave Garden Gourmet' (Green Giant)	1 pkg	300	7.0	24.0	560	3.0	20.0	(mq)	na	59%
garden herb seasoning 'Pasta Accents' (Green Giant)	1/2 cup	80	3.0	12.0	290	3.0	3.0	1.0	5	31%
garlic seasoning 'Pasta Accents' (Green Giant)	1/2 cup	100	3.0	14.0	260	2.0	4.0	2.0	5	35%
Italiano (Ultimate 200)	8 oz	190	17.0	19.0	450	na	4.0	2.0	5	20%
'Looney Tunes Bugs Bunny & Tazmanian Devil' (Tyson)	8 oz	290	13.0	41.0	420	na	8.0	na	na	25%
'Looney Tunes Daffy Duck' spaghetti & meatballs (Tyson)	8.65 oz	340	11.0	49.0	570	na	10.0	na	20	27%
'Looney Tunes Daffy Duck & Elmer Fudd' (Tyson)	8 oz	270	11.0	40.0	430	na	7.0	na	na	24%
'Looney Tunes Foghorn Leghorn & Henry Hawk' (Tyson)	8 oz	230	9.0	39.0	320	na	4.0	na	na	16%
'Looney Tunes Sylvester & Tweety' (Tyson)	8 oz	250	13.0	41.0	380	na	4.0	na	na	14%
'Looney Tunes Tweety' macaroni and cheese (Tyson)	8 oz	340	12.0	49.0	650	na	10.0	na	28	27%
Parmesan, w/sweet peas 'One Serving' (Green Giant)	5.5 oz	160	9.0	21.0	420	2.5	5.0	3.0	10	27%
Portafino, in wine sauce (Smart Ones)	9.5 oz	160	8.0	30.0	220	na	1.0	<1.0	0	6%
primavera 'Pasta Accents' (Green Giant)	1/2 cup	110	5.0	15.0	190	2.5	4.0	2.0	5	31%
Romanoff supreme (Weight Watchers)	9 oz	230	12.0	29.0	540	na	7.0	3.0	20	28%
shells, cheese, w/tomato sauce (Stouffer's)	9.25 oz	300	17.0	28.0	820	na	13.0	na	na	39%
shells, stuffed (Celentano)	8 oz	330	18.0	41.0	680	(mq)	11.0	(mq)	(mq)	30%
shells, stuffed, in tomato sauce 'Classics' (Healthy Choice)	12 oz	330	24.0	53.0	470	na	3.0	2.0	35	8%
shells, stuffed, low fat 'Great Choice' (Celentano)	10 oz	250	16.0	41.0	675	na	2.0	na	na	7%
shells, stuffed 'Single Serving' (Buitoni)	9 oz	460	18.0	46.0	840	(mq)	13.0	7.0	80	31%
shells, stuffed, w/sauce (Celentano)	10 oz	410	23.0	51.0	850	(mq)	14.0	(mq)	(mq)	30%
shells, stuffed, w/sauce (Celentano)	6.25 oz	340	17.0	31.0	420	(mq)	16.0	(mq)	(mq)	43%
shells, stuffed, w/vegetables, tofu, sauce (Legume)	11 oz	240	15.0	26.0	660	6.2	12.0	1.9	0	40%
shells and beef (Budget Gourmet)	10 oz	340	20.0	34.0	985	(mq)	14.0	(mq)	35	37%
teriyaki pasta, w/chicken 'Classics' (Healthy Choice)	12.6 oz	350	24.0	58.0	370	na	3.0	1.0	45	8%
trio 'Gourmet Selection' (Tyson)	11 oz	450	21.0	53.0	890	(mq)	17.0	(mq)	na	34%
w/shrimp 'Classics' (Healthy Choice)	12.5 oz	270	16.0	44.0	490	na	4.0	2.0	50	13%
w/turkey, Dijon sauce 'Lunch Express' (Lean Cuisine)	9 7/8 oz	290	18.0	39.0	540	na	7.0	na	35	22%

PASTA ENTRÉE, MICROWAVE. See also NOODLE ENTRÉE/DISH, MICROWAVE; RAVIOLI ENTRÉE; SPAGHETTI ENTRÉE, MICROWAVE.
(Chef Boyardee)

Food Name	Serving Size	Calories	Prot. gms	Carbs gms	Sod. mgs	Fiber gms	Fat gms	Sat. Fat gms	Chol. mgs	% Fat Cal
in cheese sauce 'ABC's & 123's'	7.5 oz	180	5.0	37.0	940	3.0	1.0	<1.0	3	5%
in cheese sauce 'Dinosaurs'	7.5 oz	180	6.0	36.0	880	3.0	1.0	<1.0	3	5%
in cheese sauce 'Tic Tac Toes'	7.5 oz	170	5.0	36.0	930	2.0	1.0	<1.0	2	5%
in sauce 'Turtles'	7.5 oz	160	5.0	33.0	870	2.0	1.0	na	3	6%
rings and franks	7.5 oz	190	7.0	31.0	980	3.0	5.0	2.0	20	23%
rings and meatballs	7.5 oz	220	8.0	33.0	990	4.0	8.0	3.0	25	31%
shells, in meat sauce	7.5 oz	210	8.0	32.0	1090	na	6.0	na	15	25%
shells, in mushroom sauce	7.5 oz	170	6.0	35.0	1080	na	1.0	<1.0	2	5%

Food Name	Serving Size	Calories	Prot. gms	Carbs gms	Sod. mgs	Fiber gms	Fat gms	Sat. Fat gms	Chol. mgs	% Fat Cal.
w/meatballs 'Dinosaurs'	7.5 oz	240	8.0	32.0	900	4.0	9.0	3.0	17	34%
w/meatballs 'Tic Tac Toes'	7.5 oz	250	7.0	32.0	1035	3.0	10.0	3.0	16	37%
w/meatballs 'Turtles'	7.5 oz	210	7.0	30.0	990	2.0	8.0	3.0	20	33%
w/mini meatballs 'ABC's & 123's'	7.5 oz	260	7.0	32.0	1005	2.0	11.0	4.0	17	39%
(Lunch Bucket)										
and garden vegetables 'Light'n Healthy'	7.5 oz	150	4.0	30.0	630	na	1.0	na	0	6%
elbows, in tomato sauce	7.5 oz	190	4.0	38.0	860	na	2.0	na	na	10%
in wine sauce, beef 'Light'n Healthy'	7.5 oz	130	5.0	21.0	600	na	3.0	na	10	21%
Italian style chicken 'Light'n Healthy'	7.5 oz	130	7.0	23.0	630	na	1.0	na	10	7%
'Pasta 'n Chicken'	7.5 oz	180	9.0	22.0	860	na	6.0	na	45	30%
PASTA SALAD MIX										
Caesar, dry *(Suddenly Salad)*	1/6 pkg	110	4.0	20.0	450	na	1.0	na	na	9%
Caesar, prepared *(Suddenly Salad)*	1/2 cup	170	4.0	20.0	450	(mq)	8.0	(mq)	na	43%
creamy macaroni, dry *(Suddenly Salad)*	1/6 pkg	100	4.0	20.0	210	na	1.0	na	na	9%
creamy macaroni, prepared *(Suddenly Salad)*	1/2 cup	200	4.0	21.0	280	(mq)	10.0	(mq)	na	47%
garden primavera, dry *(Kraft)*	1/6 box	170	5.0	21.0	490	na	7.0	2.0	0	38%
Italian 'Light,' dry *(Kraft)*	1/6 box	120	5.0	22.0	480	na	1.0	0.0	0	8%
pasta, classic, dry *(Suddenly Salad)*	1/6 pkg	120	4.0	23.0	530	na	1.0	na	na	8%
pasta, classic, prepared *(Suddenly Salad)*	1/2 cup	160	4.0	23.0	530	(mq)	6.0	(mq)	na	33%
pasta primavera, dry *(Suddenly Salad)*	1/6 pkg	90	3.0	19.0	270	na	1.0	na	na	9%
pasta primavera, prepared *(Suddonly Salad)*	1/2 cup	190	4.0	20.0	340	(mq)	10.0	(mq)	na	48%
ranch and bacon, dry *(Suddenly Salad)*	1/6 pkg	110	5.0	21.0	250	na	1.0	na	na	8%
ranch and bacon, prepared *(Suddenly Salad)*	1/2 cup	210	6.0	22.0	320	(mq)	11.0	(mq)	na	47%
tortellini, Italiano, dry *(Suddenly Salad)*	1/5 pkg	120	4.0	21.0	450	na	2.0	(mq)	na	15%
tortellini, Italiano, prepared *(Suddenly Salad)*	1/2 cup	160	4.0	21.0	450	(mq)	7.0	(mq)	na	39%
PASTA SAUCE. See SAUCE.										
PASTRAMI. See LUNCHEON MEAT.										
PASTRY. See also BREAD, SWEET; BUN, SWEET; CAKE; DANISH PASTRY; MUFFIN; PIE; ROLL, SWEET; TURNOVER.										
(Charlette Russe) w/lady fingers, whipped cream filling	1 serving	326	6.7	38.2	49	0	16.6	8.3	225	45%
(Pillsbury) pocket, refrigerated	1 piece	240	4.0	25.0	520	(mq)	13.0	3.0	0	50%
PASTRY, BAVARIAN CREAM										
(Entenmann's)	1.3 oz	80	2.0	20.0	90	na	0.0	na	0	0%
(Rich's) puff, frozen	1 piece	150	2.0	17.0	70	(mq)	8.0	(mq)	25	49%
PASTRY, CINNAMON *(Entenmann's)* filbert ring	1.5 oz	190	3.0	19.0	160	na	12.0	na	na	55%
PASTRY, DATE NUT *(Awrey's)* 1 piece	1.6 oz	230	2.0	35.0	150	1.0	10.0	2.0	15	38%
PASTRY, ÉCLAIR										
(Rich's) frozen, chocolate, 2 oz	1 piece	210	2.0	27.0	110	(mq)	10.0	(mq)	35	44%
(Weight Watchers) frozen, chocolate 'Sweet Celebrations'	2.1 oz	150	3.0	26.0	110	na	4.0	<2.0	15	24%
PATÉ, CANNED										
chicken liver	1 oz	57	3.8	1.9	109	0	3.7	1.1	111	59%
chicken liver	1 tbsp	26	1.8	0.9	50	0	1.7	0.5	51	59%
foie gras, goose liver, smoked	1 oz	131	3.2	1.3	198	0	12.4	4.1	43	86%
foie gras, goose liver, smoked	1 tbsp	60	1.5	0.6	91	0	5.7	1.9	20	86%
liver *(Sells)*	2 1/8 oz	190	8.0	4.0	470	0	16.0	(mq)	90	75%
PATTYPAN SQUASH. See SQUASH, SCALLOP.										
PEACH										
peeled, pitted	1 oz	12	0.2	3.1	tr	.5	<.1	tr	0	<6%
peeled, sliced	1/2 cup	37	0.6	9.4	1	1.4	0.1	tr	0	2%
raw, approx 4 oz	1 med	37	0.6	9.7	0	1.4	0.1	0.0	0	2%
raw, slices	1 cup	73	1.2	18.9	0	2.7	0.2	0.0	0	2%
untrimmed	1 lb	148	2.4	38.2	2	5.5	0.3	<.1	0	2%
untrimmed *(Dole)*	2 pieces	70	1.0	19.0	0	1.0	0.0	na	na	0%
PEACH, CANNED										
'Fruit Pak' *(Mott's)*	3.75 oz	75	0.0	18.0	7	(mq)	0.0	0.0	0	0%

Food Name	Serving Size	Calories	Prot. gms	Carbs gms	Sod. mgs	Fiber gms	Fat gms	Sat. Fat gms	Chol. mgs	% Fat Cal.
halves (Hunt's)	4 oz	90	<1.0	23.0	7	<1.0	<1.0	na	0	<9%
slices (Hunt's)	4 oz	90	<1.0	23.0	7	<1.0	<1.0	na	0	<9%
FREESTONE										
halves (Del Monte)	1/2 cup	90	0.0	23.0	10	(mq)	0.0	0.0	0	0%
halves (S&W Nutradiet)	1/2 cup	30	0.0	7.0	10	(mq)	0.0	0.0	0	0%
halves 'Lite' (Del Monte)	1/2 cup	60	0.0	13.0	10	(mq)	0.0	0.0	0	0%
in heavy syrup, halves (S&W)	1/2 cup	100	0.0	26.0	10	(mq)	0.0	0.0	0	0%
in heavy syrup, slices (S&W)	1/2 cup	100	0.0	26.0	10	(mq)	0.0	0.0	0	0%
slices (Del Monte)	1/2 cup	90	0.0	23.0	10	(mq)	0.0	0.0	0	0%
slices (S&W Nutradiet)	1/2 cup	30	0.0	7.0	10	(mq)	0.0	0.0	0	0%
slices 'Lite' (Del Monte)	1/2 cup	60	0.0	13.0	10	(mq)	0.0	0.0	0	0%
YELLOW CLING										
diced 'Fruit Cup' (Del Monte)	5 oz	110	0.0	28.0	10	(mq)	0.0	0.0	0	0%
halves (Del Monte)	1/2 cup	80	0.0	22.0	10	(mq)	0.0	0.0	0	0%
halves (S&W Nutradiet)	1/2 cup	30	0.0	8.0	5	(mq)	0.0	0.0	0	0%
halves 'Lite' (Del Monte)	1/2 cup	50	0.0	13.0	10	(mq)	0.0	0.0	0	0%
halves 'Lite' (Finast)	1/2 cup	50	0.0	14.0	10	(mq)	0.0	0.0	0	0%
in heavy syrup, halves (A&P)	1/2 cup	100	<1.0	25.0	10	(mq)	<1.0	na	0	<8%
in heavy syrup, halves (S&W)	1/2 cup	100	0.0	25.0	10	(mq)	0.0	0.0	0	0%
in heavy syrup, slices (A&P)	1/2 cup	100	<1.0	25.0	10	(mq)	<1.0	na	0	<8%
in heavy syrup, slices (Finast)	1/2 cup	100	0.0	25.0	6	(mq)	0.0	0.0	0	0%
in heavy syrup, slices (Pathmark)	1/2 cup	100	0.0	25.0	10	(mq)	0.0	0.0	0	0%
in heavy syrup, slices (S&W)	1/2 cup	100	0.0	25.0	10	(mq)	0.0	0.0	0	0%
in heavy syrup, whole, spiced (S&W)	1/2 cup	90	0.0	23.0	10	(mq)	0.0	0.0	0	0%
in juice (A&P)	1/2 cup	50	<1.0	12.0	10	(mq)	<1.0	tr	0	<15%
in juice, halves (A&P)	1/2 cup	50	<1.0	12.0	10	(mq)	<1.0	tr	0	<15%
in juice, halves (Featherweight)	1/2 cup	50	0.0	14.0	10	(mq)	0.0	0.0	0	0%
in juice, halves 'Lite' (Libby's)	1/2 cup	50	0.0	13.0	0	(mq)	0.0	0.0	10	0%
in juice, slices (Featherweight)	1/2 cup	50	0.0	14.0	10	(mq)	0.0	0.0	0	0%
in juice, slices (IGA)	1/2 cup	50	1.0	14.0	10	(mq)	0.0	0.0	0	0%
in juice, slices (Pathmark)	1/2 cup	50	0.0	14.0	10	(mq)	0.0	0.0	0	0%
in juice, slices 'Lite' (Libby's)	1/2 cup	50	0.0	13.0	0	(mq)	0.0	0.0	10	0%
in juice, slices, sweetened (S&W)	1/2 cup	90	0.0	20.0	10	(mq)	0.0	0.0	0	0%
in light syrup, slices 'No Frills' (Pathmark)	1/2 cup	140	1.0	36.0	15	(mq)	0.0	0.0	0	0%
slices (Del Monte)	1/2 cup	80	0.0	22.0	10	(mq)	0.0	0.0	0	0%
slices 'Lite' (Del Monte)	1/2 cup	50	0.0	13.0	10	(mq)	0.0	0.0	0	0%
slices 'Lite' (Finast)	1/2 cup	50	0.0	14.0	10	(mq)	0.0	0.0	0	0%
slices, unsweetened (S&W Nutradiet)	1/2 cup	30	0.0	8.0	5	(mq)	0.0	0.0	0	0%
spiced, w/pits (Del Monte)	3.5 oz	80	0.0	20.0	10	(mq)	0.0	0.0	0	0%
PEACH, DRIED										
sulfured, cooked, sweetened	4 oz	117	1.2	30.2	2	>1.0 c	0.2	<.1	0	1%
sulfured, cooked, sweetened, halves	1/2 cup	139	1.4	35.9	3	3.2	0.3	<.1	0	2%
sulfured, cooked, unsweetened	4 oz	87	1.3	22.3	2	>1.1 c	0.3	<.1	0	3%
sulfured, cooked, unsweetened, halves	1/2 cup	91	1.5	25.4	3	3.5	0.3	<.1	0	2%
sulfured, uncooked	4 oz	271	4.1	69.5	8	9.3	0.9	0.1	0	3%
sulfured, uncooked, approx 4.6 oz	10 halves	311	4.7	79.7	9	10.7	1.0	0.1	0	3%
sulfured, uncooked, halves	1/2 cup	192	2.9	49.1	6	6.6	0.6	0.1	0	3%
(Del Monte) uncooked	2 oz	140	2.0	35.0	10	(mq)	0.0	0.0	0	0%
(Mountain House) freeze-dried, prepared	1/4 cup	50	1.0	12.0	<1	(mq)	0.0	0.0	0	0%
(Sun•Maid)	2 oz	140	2.0	38.0	10	(mq)	0.0	0.0	0	0%
(SunSweet)	2 oz	140	2.0	38.0	10	(mq)	0.0	0.0	0	0%
PEACH, FROZEN										
slices, sweetened	10-oz pkg	267	1.8	68.1	17	4.0	0.4	0.0	0	1%
slices, sweetened	1/2 cup	118	0.8	30.0	8	1.8	0.2	<.1	0	1%

Food Name	Serving Size	Calories	Prot. gms	Carbs gms	Sod. mgs	Fiber gms	Fat gms	Sat. Fat gms	Chol. mgs	% Fat Cal.
slices, sweetened	4 oz	107	0.7	27.2	7	>.5 c	0.1	<.1	0	1%
PEACH BUTTER *(Smucker's)*	1 tsp	15	0.0	4.0	0	(mq)	0.0	0.0	0	0%
PEACH DRINK										
(Hi-C)	6 oz	101	0.1	24.8	18	(tr)	<.1	(tr)	0	<1%
(Ocean Spray) citrus 'Refreshers'	6 oz	90	0.0	23.0	15	na	0.0	na	na	0%
PEACH JUICE										
(Dole) orchard blend 'Pure & Light'	6 oz	90	0.0	24.0	10	(mq)	0.0	0.0	0	0%
(Smucker's) 'Naturally 100%'	8 oz	120	1.0	30.0	10	(mq)	0.0	0.0	0	0%
(Snapple) 'Dixie Peach'	8 oz	160	0.0	39.0	20	na	0.0	0.0	0	0%
PEACH NECTAR										
w/added ascorbic acid	1 cup	134	0.7	34.7	17	>.4 c	0.1	0.0	0	1%
w/added ascorbic acid	1 oz	17	0.1	4.3	2	0	0.0	0.0	0	0%
w/o added ascorbic acid	1 cup	134	0.7	34.7	17	1.5	0.1	0.0	0	1%
w/o added ascorbic acid	1 oz	17	0.1	4.3	2	0	0.0	0.0	0	0%
(Kern's)	6 oz	110	1.0	26.0	0	na	0.0	na	na	0%
(Knudsen & Sons)	8 oz	107	<1.0	32.0	na	na	0.0	na	na	0%
(Libby's)	6 oz	100	0.0	24.0	5	na	0.0	na	na	0%
PEANUT, SHELLED										
(Beer Nuts)	1 oz	180	7.0	7.0	60	(mq)	14.0	(mq)	0	69%
(Frito Lay) salted	1 oz	170	6.0	6.0	170	na	15.0	na	0	74%
(Little Debbie) salted	1.25 oz	230	10.0	5.0	90	(mq)	18.0	(mq)	<1	73%
(Pathmark) 'Sweet and Crunchy'	1 oz	140	4.0	15.0	30	(mq)	8.0	(mq)	0	49%
(Planters)										
hot spicy 'Heat'	1 oz	170	7.0	5.0	190	na	14.0	2.0	0	72%
mild spicy 'Heat'	1 oz	170	7.0	5.0	130	na	14.0	2.0	0	72%
'Sweet-N-Crunchy'	1 oz	140	4.0	15.0	20	na	8.0	1.0	0	49%
(Weight Watchers)	1 pouch	100	8.0	4.0	50	(mq)	7.0	(mq)	0	57%
BOILED										
salted	1/2 cup	102	4.3	6.8	240	2.82	7.0	1.0	0	59%
salted	1 oz	90	3.8	6.0	213	>.6 c	6.2	0.9	0	59%
DRY-ROASTED										
(Finast)										
lightly salted	1 oz	160	7.0	5.0	15	(mq)	14.0	(mq)	0	72%
salted	1 oz	160	8.0	6.0	120	(mq)	14.0	(mq)	0	69%
(Flavor House)										
salted	1 oz	180	8.0	5.0	200	(mq)	14.0	(mq)	0	71%
unsalted	1 oz	180	8.0	5.0	0	(mq)	14.0	(mq)	0	71%
(Frito Lay) salted	1 1/8 oz	190	7.0	7.0	300	(mq)	16.0	(mq)	0	72%
(Guy's) salted	1 oz	170	8.0	3.0	310	(mq)	14.0	(mq)	0	74%
(Pathmark)										
'No Frills' salted	1 oz	170	7.0	5.0	150	(mq)	14.0	(mq)	0	72%
'No Frills' unsalted	1 oz	180	8.0	5.0	0	(mq)	14.0	2.0	0	71%
(Planters)										
lightly salted	1 oz	170	7.0	5.0	110	na	15.0	2.0	0	74%
salted	1 oz	160	7.0	6.0	250	(mq)	14.0	2.0	0	71%
unsalted	1 oz	170	7.0	5.0	0	na	15.0	2.0	0	74%
HONEY-ROASTED										
(Eagle) 'Honey Roast'	1 oz	170	7.0	7.0	140	(mq)	13.0	(mq)	0	68%
(Fisher)										
lightly salted	1 oz	150	6.0	5.0	0	na	13.0	2.0	na	73%
salted	1 oz	150	6.0	5.0	115	na	13.0	2.0	0	73%
(Flavor House)	1 oz	160	6.0	9.0	120	(mq)	11.0	(mq)	0	62%
(Little Debbie)	1.13 oz	190	8.0	9.0	15	(mq)	13.0	(mq)	<1	63%
(Pathmark)	1 oz	170	6.0	8.0	75	(mq)	13.0	(mq)	0	68%

Food Name	Serving Size	Calories	Prot. gms	Carbs gms	Sod. mgs	Fiber gms	Fat gms	Sat. Fat gms	Chol. mgs	% Fat Cal.
(Planters)	1 oz	170	6.0	8.0	180	(mq)	13.0	2.0	0	68%
(Weight Watchers)	1 pouch	100	8.0	4.0	50	(mq)	7.0	(mq)	0	57%
OIL-ROASTED										
(Fisher) salted	1 oz	160	7.0	6.0	130	na	14.0	2.0	0	71%
(Flavor House) salted	1 oz	170	7.0	5.0	125	(mq)	15.0	(mq)	0	74%
(Pathmark) salted	1 oz	180	8.0	5.0	150	(mq)	14.0	(mq)	0	71%
(Planters)										
cocktail	1 oz	170	7.0	5.0	160	(mq)	15.0	3.0	0	74%
cocktail, unsalted	1 oz	170	7.0	5.0	0	(mq)	15.0	3.0	0	74%
lightly salted	1 oz	170	7.0	5.0	80	na	14.0	2.0	0	72%
redskin	1 oz	170	7.0	5.0	150	(mq)	15.0	5.0	0	74%
salted	1 oz	170	7.0	5.0	160	(mq)	15.0	3.0	0	74%
unsalted	1 oz	170	7.0	5.0	0	na	14.0	2.0	0	72%
PEANUT, SPANISH										
DRY-ROASTED *(Planters)*	1 oz	160	7.0	6.0	200	(mq)	14.0	3.0	0	71%
OIL-ROASTED										
salted	1/2 cup	426	20.6	12.8	319	>3.7 c	36.0	5.6	0	71%
salted	1 oz	162	7.8	4.9	121	>1.4 c	13.7	2.1	0	71%
salted *(Flavor House)*	1 oz	170	7.0	5.0	125	(mq)	15.0	(mq)	0	74%
salted *(Planters)*	1 oz	170	7.0	5.0	100	na	15.0	5.0	0	74%
shelled, salted *(Flavor House)*	1 oz	170	7.0	5.0	125	(mq)	15.0	(mq)	0	74%
shelled, salted *(Guy's)*	1 oz	170	8.0	3.0	170	(mq)	14.0	(mq)	0	74%
unsalted	1/2 cup	426	20.6	12.8	4	>3.7 c	36.0	5.6	0	71%
unsalted	1 oz	162	7.8	4.9	2	>1.4 c	13.7	2.1	0	71%
RAW										
	1 cup	832	38.2	23.1	32	13.9	72.4	11.2	0	73%
	1 oz	160	7.3	4.4	6	2.7	13.9	2.1	0	73%
(Planters)	1 oz	160	7.0	5.0	5	na	14.0	2.0	0	72%
PEANUT, VALENCIA										
oil-roasted	1 cup	848	38.9	23.5	9	>3.3 c	73.8	11.4	0	73%
oil-roasted	1/2 cup	424	19.5	11.7	4	>1.6 c	36.9	5.7	0	73%
oil-roasted	1 oz	165	7.6	4.6	2	>.6 c	14.4	2.2	0	73%
raw	1/2 cup	417	18.3	15.3	<1	>1.6 c	34.7	5.4	0	70%
raw	1 oz	160	7.0	5.8	0	>.6 c	13.3	2.0	0	70%
PEANUT, VIRGINIA										
oil-roasted, unsalted	1 cup	827	37.0	28.4	9	>7.7 c	69.5	9.1	0	71%
oil-roasted, unsalted	1 oz	162	7.2	5.6	2	>1.5 c	13.6	1.8	0	71%
raw	1 cup	822	36.8	24.2	15	>7.1 c	71.2	9.3	0	72%
raw	1 oz	158	7.1	4.6	3	>1.4 c	13.6	1.8	0	72%
PEANUT BUTTER										
(Hollywood) 'Unsalted'	1 tbsp	35	2.0	1.0	0	1.0	3.0	0.0	0	69%
(Pathmark) 'Natural'	2 tbsp	200	9.0	5.0	130	(mq)	17.0	(mq)	0	73%
(Roaster Fresh) gourmet	1 oz	166	8.0	5.0	2	na	14.0	2.4	na	71%
(S&W Nutradiet)	1 tbsp	93	3.0	2.0	10	(mq)	8.0	(mq)	0	78%
(Smucker's)										
honey sweetened	2 tbsp	200	7.0	7.0	150	na	16.0	3.0	0	72%
no salt added 'Natural'	2 tbsp	200	8.0	6.0	10	na	16.0	3.0	0	72%
CHUNKY										
(Arrowhead Mills)	2 tbsp	190	9.0	6.0	<1	4.5	16.0	(mq)	0	71%
(Bama)	2 tbsp	200	7.0	6.0	115	(mq)	17.0	(mq)	0	75%
(Estee)	2 tbsp	200	8.0	6.0	0	na	18.0	2.0	0	74%
(Featherweight)	1 tbsp	90	4.0	2.0	5	(mq)	7.0	(mq)	0	72%
(Finast) 'Crunchy'	2 tbsp	195	9.0	6.0	175	(mq)	17.0	(mq)	0	72%
(Health Valley) 'No Salt Added'	2 tbsp	180	8.0	6.0	2	2.6	14.0	(mq)	0	69%

Food Name	Serving Size	Calories	Prot. gms	Carbs gms	Sod. mgs	Fiber gms	Fat gms	Sat. Fat gms	Chol. mgs	% Fat Cal.
(Hollywood)	1 tbsp	35	2.1	1.0	25	1.0	3.0	0.0	0	69%
(Jif)										
regular	2 tbsp	190	9.0	6.0	155	(mq)	16.0	3.0	0	71%
'Simply Jif'	2 tbsp	180	9.0	5.0	50	na	16.0	3.0	0	72%
(Maranatha Natural) crunchy	2 tbsp	190	8.0	7.0	5	na	15.0	na	na	69%
(Pathmark) 'Super Chunky'	2 tbsp	200	7.0	6.0	140	(mq)	17.0	(mq)	0	75%
(Peter Pan)										
'Extra Crunchy'	2 tbsp	190	9.1	5.1	122	(mq)	16.3	2.3	0	72%
regular	2 tbsp	190	9.0	5.0	120	2.0	16.0	2.0	0	72%
'Salt Free'	2 tbsp	190	9.0	5.0	0	2.0	17.0	2.0	0	73%
(Skippy) 'Super Chunk'	2 tbsp	190	9.0	4.0	130	.6	17.0	3.0	0	75%
(Smucker's) 'Chunky Natural'	2 tbsp	200	8.0	6.0	120	(mq)	16.0	3.0	0	72%
(Westbrae)										
'Natural' w/salt	2 tbsp	190	8.0	7.0	5	na	16.0	na	0	71%
'Natural' w/o salt	2 tbsp	190	8.0	7.0	0	na	16.0	na	0	71%
SMOOTH										
(Arrowhead Mills)	2 tbsp	190	9.0	6.0	<1	4.5	16.0	(mq)	0	71%
(Bama)	2 tbsp	200	7.0	6.0	140	(mq)	17.0	(mq)	0	75%
(Estee)	1 tbsp	100	4.0	3.0	2	(mq)	8.0	1.0	0	72%
(Featherweight)	1 tbsp	90	4.0	2.0	3	(mq)	7.0	(mq)	0	72%
(Finast)	2 tbsp	195	9.0	6.0	175	(mq)	17.0	(mq)	0	72%
(Health Valley) 'No Salt Added'	2 tbsp	180	8.0	6.0	2	2.6	14.0	(mq)	0	69%
(Hollywood)	1 tbsp	35	2.1	1.0	25	1.0	3.0	0.0	0	69%
(Jif)										
regular	2 tbsp	190	9.0	6.0	155	(mq)	16.0	3.0	0	71%
'Simply Jif'	2 tbsp	180	9.0	5.0	65	na	16.0	3.0	0	72%
(Pathmark) 'No Frills Creamy'	2 tbsp	200	7.0	6.0	170	(mq)	17.0	(mq)	0	75%
(Peter Pan)										
'Creamy'	2 tbsp	190	8.6	5.7	150	(mq)	16.4	2.2	0	72%
'Creamy Salt Free'	2 tbsp	195	8.7	5.3	1	(mq)	17.1	2.4	0	73%
(Skippy) 'Creamy'	2 tbsp	190	9.0	4.0	150	.6	17.0	3.0	0	75%
(Smucker's)										
'Natural'	2 tbsp	200	8.0	6.0	120	(mq)	16.0	3.0	0	72%
'No Salt Added Natural'	2 tbsp	200	8.0	6.0	10	(mq)	17.0	1.0	0	73%
(Westbrae) 'Natural' no salt	2 tbsp	190	8.0	7.0	0	na	16.0	na	0	71%
(Woodstock) 'Old Fashioned Unsalted'	2 tbsp	200	9.0	6.0	3	(mq)	16.0	(mq)	0	71%
W/JELLY										
(Bama)	2 tbsp	150	3.0	20.0	75	(mq)	7.0	(mq)	0	41%
(Smucker's)										
'Goober Grape'	2 tbsp	180	5.0	18.0	120	na	10.0	2.0	0	50%
'Goober Strawberry'	2 tbsp	180	5.0	18.0	120	na	10.0	2.0	0	50%
PEANUT BUTTER CHIPS (Hershey's) 'Reese's'	1.5 oz	230	9.0	19.0	90	na	13.0	na	5	51%
PEANUT BUTTER TOPPING (Smucker's) caramel	2 tbsp	150	3.0	29.0	120	(mq)	2.0	(mq)	0	12%
PEANUT FLOUR										
defatted	1 cup	196	31.3	20.8	108	>2.4 c	0.3	0.0	0	1%
defatted	1 oz	92	14.6	9.7	50	>1.1 c	0.2	0.0	0	2%
low-fat	1 cup	257	20.3	18.8	1	>4.6 c	13.1	1.8	0	43%
low-fat	1 oz	120	9.5	8.8	0	>2.2 c	6.1	0.9	0	43%
PEANUT OIL										
	1/2 cup	955	0.0	0.0	0	0	108.0	18.3	0	100%
	1 oz	251	0.0	0.0	0	0	28.4	4.8	0	100%
(Hain)	1 tbsp	120	0.0	0.0	0	0	14.0	2.0	0	100%
(Planters)	1 tbsp	120	0.0	0.0	0	0	14.0	2.0	0	100%
(Spectrum Naturals)	1 tbsp	120	0.0	0.0	0	(tr)	14.0	2.0	(tr)	100%

Food Name	Serving Size	Calories	Prot. gms	Carbs gms	Sod. mgs	Fiber gms	Fat gms	Sat. Fat gms	Chol. mgs	% Fat Cal.
(Wesson)	1 tbsp	122	0.0	0.0	0	0	13.6	2.5	0	100%
PEAR										
Asian, raw	1 fruit	51	0.6	13.0	0	na	0.3	0.0	0	5%
raw, slices	1 cup	97	0.6	24.9	0	4.3	0.7	0.0	0	6%
trimmed, w/skin	1 oz	17	0.1	4.3	tr	.7	0.1	tr	0	5%
untrimmed	1 lb	247	1.6	63.1	2	10.9	1.7	0.1	0	6%
untrimmed *(Dole)*	1 fruit	100	1.0	25.0	1	4.0	1.0	na	na	8%
w/skin, sliced	1/2 cup	49	0.3	12.5	1	2.1	0.3	<.1	0	5%
PEAR, CANNED										
in extra heavy syrup	4 oz	110	0.2	28.6	6	>.7 c	0.1	tr	0	1%
in extra heavy syrup, halves	1/2 cup	127	0.3	33.0	7	>.8 c	0.2	tr	0	1%
in extra heavy syrup, solid and liquid, halves	1 cup	253	0.5	65.9	13	>1.5 c	0.3	0.0	0	1%
in extra light syrup	4 oz	53	0.3	13.8	2	>.7 c	0.1	tr	0	2%
in extra light syrup, halves	1/2 cup	58	0.4	15.1	3	>.7 c	0.1	tr	0	1%
in extra light syrup, solid and liquid, halves	1 cup	116	0.7	30.1	5	>.3 c	0.3	0.0	0	2%
in heavy syrup	4 oz	84	0.2	21.7	6	>.7 c	0.1	tr	0	1%
in heavy syrup, halves	1/2 cup	94	0.3	24.4	7	>.7 c	0.2	tr	0	2%
in heavy syrup, solid and liquid, halves	1 cup	189	0.5	48.9	13	5.1	0.3	0.0	0	1%
in juice	4 oz	57	0.4	14.7	5	1.0	0.1	tr	0	2%
in juice, halves	1/2 cup	62	0.4	16.0	5	1.1	0.1	tr	0	1%
in juice, solid and liquid, halves	1 cup	124	0.8	32.1	10	5.0	0.2	0.0	0	1%
in light syrup	4 oz	65	0.2	17.2	6	>.7 c	<.1	<.1	0	<1%
in light syrup, halves	1/2 cup	72	0.2	19.0	7	>.7 c	<.1	<.1	0	<1%
in light syrup, solid and liquid, halves	1 cup	143	0.5	38.1	13	5.0	0.1	0.0	0	1%
in water	4 oz	33	0.2	8.9	2	>.7 c	<.1	tr	0	<2%
in water, halves	1/2 cup	36	0.2	9.5	3	>.7 c	<.1	tr	0	<2%
in water, solid and liquid, halves	1 cup	71	0.5	19.1	5	4.9	0.1	0.0	0	1%
(A&P)										
in heavy syrup, halves or slices	1/2 cup	95	<1.0	25.0	10	(mq)	<1.0	(tr)	0	<8%
in juice, halves or slices	1/2 cup	60	<1.0	15.0	10	(mq)	<1.0	(tr)	0	<12%
in light syrup, halves or slices	1/2 cup	70	<1.0	20.0	10	(mq)	<1.0	(tr)	0	<10%
(Del Monte)										
Bartlett, halves 'Lite'	1/2 cup	50	0.0	14.0	10	(mq)	0.0	0.0	0	0%
Bartlett, halves or slices	1/2 cup	80	0.0	22.0	10	(mq)	0.0	0.0	0	0%
Bartlett, slices 'Lite'	1/2 cup	50	0.0	14.0	10	(mq)	0.0	0.0	0	0%
(Featherweight) in juice, halves	1/2 cup	60	0.0	15.0	10	(mq)	0.0	0.0	0	0%
(Finast)										
Bartlett, halves or slices, in heavy syrup	1/2 cup	100	0.0	25.0	10	(mq)	0.0	0.0	0	0%
Bartlett, halves or slices, 'Lite No Sugar Added'	1/2 cup	60	0.0	15.0	10	(mq)	0.0	0.0	0	0%
(Hunt's) halves	4 oz	90	1.0	23.0	6	<1.0	1.0	na	0	9%
(IGA) Bartlett, halves, unsweetened	1/2 cup	60	0.0	15.0	10	(mq)	0.0	0.0	0	0%
(Libby's) in juice, halves or slices, 'Lite'	1/2 cup	60	0.0	19.0	10	(mq)	0.0	0.0	0	0%
(Pathmark)										
Bartlett, halves, in heavy syrup	1/2 cup	90	0.0	23.0	10	(mq)	0.0	0.0	0	0%
Bartlett, halves, in juice	1/2 cup	60	0.0	15.0	10	(mq)	0.0	0.0	0	0%
Bartlett, in light syrup 'No Frills'	1 cup	140	0.0	38.0	10	(mq)	0.0	0.0	0	0%
Bartlett, slices, in heavy syrup	1 cup	180	0.0	46.0	20	(mq)	0.0	0.0	0	0%
(S&W Nutradiet)										
Bartlett, peeled, unsweetened	1/2 cup	35	0.0	10.0	10	(mq)	0.0	0.0	0	0%
in heavy syrup, halves	1/2 cup	100	0.0	25.0	10	(mq)	0.0	0.0	0	0%
in juice, slices, sweetened 'Natural Style'	1/2 cup	80	0.0	20.0	10	(mq)	0.0	0.0	0	0%
peeled, quarters	1/2 cup	35	0.0	10.0	10	(mq)	0.0	0.0	0	0%

Food Name	Serving Size	Calories	Prot. gms	Carbs gms	Sod. mgs	Fiber gms	Fat gms	Sat. Fat gms	Chol. mgs	% Fat Cal.
PEAR, DRIED										
Sulfured										
cooked, sweetened	4 oz	159	1.0	42.1	3	>3.0 c	0.3	<.1	0	2%
cooked, unsweetened	4 oz	144	1.0	38.3	3	>3.1 c	0.4	<.1	0	2%
stewed, w/added sugar, halves	1/2 cup	196	1.2	52.0	4	8.1	0.4	0.0	0	2%
stewed, w/o added sugar, halves	1/2 cup	163	1.2	43.3	4	8.2	0.4	0.0	0	2%
uncooked	10 halves	458	3.3	122.0	10	13.1	1.1	0.1	0	2%
uncooked	4 oz	297	2.1	79.0	7	>6.5 c	0.7	<.1	0	2%
PEAR JUICE										
(Knudsen & Sons)	8 oz	110	<1.0	28.0	na	na	0.0	na	na	0%
(Santa Cruz Natural) organic 'Cruz'	8 oz	135	1.0	32.0	na	na	<1.0	na	na	6%
PEAR NECTAR										
(Kern's)	6 oz	120	0.0	28.0	0	na	0.0	na	na	0%
(Libby's)	6 oz	110	0.0	28.0	0	na	0.0	na	na	0%
PEAS, CROWDER										
(Allens) canned, 'Fresh'	1/2 cup	80	5.0	15.0	370	(mq)	<1.0	na	0	<10%
(Seabrook) frozen	3 oz	130	8.0	23.0	na	>1.0 c	1.0	na	0	7%
PEAS, GREEN										
(NOTE: All peas are shelled unless otherwise noted.)										
boiled, drained	4 oz	95	6.1	17.7	3	4.2	0.2	<.1	0	2%
boiled, drained	1/2 cup	67	4.3	12.5	2	>1.9 c	0.2	0.0	0	3%
boiled, drained, in pod	4 oz	48	3.7	8.0	5	3.2	0.3	<.1	0	6%
boiled, drained, in pod	1/2 cup	34	2.6	5.6	3	2.2	0.2	<.1	0	5%
raw	1/2 cup	58	3.9	10.4	4	>1.6 c	0.3	0.1	0	5%
raw	1 oz	23	1.5	4.1	1	1.0	0.1	<.1	0	4%
raw, in pod	1 lb	140	9.3	24.9	8	5.9	0.7	0.1	0	4%
raw, trimmed	1/2 cup	30	2.0	5.4	3	1.9	0.1	<.1	0	3%
raw, trimmed	1 oz	12	0.8	2.1	1	.7	0.1	<.1	0	7%
raw, untrimmed	1 lb	180	11.9	32.2	18	11.1	0.9	0.2	0	4%
CANNED										
dietary pack, drained solids	1/2 cup	59	3.8	10.7	2	>1.7 c	0.3	0.1	0	4%
dietary pack, solids and liquid	1/2 cup	61	3.7	11.1	2	>1.8 c	0.4	0.1	0	6%
drained, low-sodium	4 oz	78	5.0	14.3	2	3.9	0.4	0.1	0	5%
regular pack, drained solids	1/2 cup	59	3.8	10.7	186	2.9	0.3	0.1	0	4%
regular pack, solids and liquid	1/2 cup	61	3.7	11.1	340	2.5	0.4	0.1	0	6%
Early/June										
(A&P)	1/2 cup	70	4.0	15.0	350	(mq)	<1.0	(tr)	0	<11%
(Allens) dry	1/2 cup	80	5.0	15.0	320	(mq)	<1.0	(tr)	0	<10%
(Del Monte) small, w/liquid	1/2 cup	50	3.0	9.0	355	(mq)	0.0	0.0	0	0%
(Green Giant)	1/2 cup	50	3.0	12.0	330	3.0	0.0	0.0	0	0%
(Green Giant) very young, small	1/2 cup	50	3.0	12.0	390	3.0	0.0	0.0	0	0%
(S&W) 'Petit Pois'	1/2 cup	70	4.0	12.0	330	(mq)	0.0	0.0	0	0%
(Stokely)	1/2 cup	60	4.0	12.0	320	(mq)	0.0	0.0	0	0%
Mixed sizes										
(A&P)	1/2 cup	60	4.0	12.0	350	(mq)	<1.0	(tr)	0	<12%
(IGA) 'No Salt or Sugar Added'	1/2 cup	50	4.0	10.0	10	(mq)	0.0	0.0	0	0%
Sweet										
wrinkled, dietary pack, drained, low sodium	1 lb	82	5.9	15.4	14	0	0.0	0.0	0	0%
wrinkled, dietary pack, drained, low sodium	1 oz	5	0.4	1.0	1	0	0.0	0.0	0	0%
wrinkled, regular pack, drained	1 lb	100	5.9	19.5	1071	0	0.0	0.0	0	0%
wrinkled, regular pack, drained	1 oz	6	0.4	1.2	66	0	0.0	0.0	0	0%
(Featherweight)	1/2 cup	70	5.0	12.0	10	(mq)	0.0	0.0	0	0%
(Finast)	1/2 cup	70	4.0	13.0	300	(mq)	1.0	(tr)	0	12%
(Finast) 'No Salt Added'	1/2 cup	60	4.0	12.0	10	(mq)	0.0	0.0	0	0%

Food Name	Serving Size	Calories	Prot. gms	Carbs gms	Sod. mgs	Fiber gms	Fat gms	Sat. Fat gms	Chol. mgs	% Fat Cal.
(Green Giant)	1/2 cup	50	4.0	11.0	320	4.0	0.0	0.0	0	0%
(Green Giant) 50% less salt	1/2 cup	50	4.0	11.0	195	3.0	0.0	0.0	0	0%
(Green Giant) mini	1/2 cup	50	4.0	12.0	340	4.0	0.0	0.0	0	0%
(Green Giant) mini, in brine	1/2 cup	60	4.0	12.0	240	4.0	<1.0	na	0	<12%
(Green Giant) very young, small	1/2 cup	50	4.0	12.0	390	4.0	0.0	0.0	0	0%
(Green Giant) very young, tender	1/2 cup	50	4.0	11.0	390	4.0	0.0	0.0	0	0%
(IGA) tiny, early/June	1/2 cup	70	4.0	12.0	340	(mq)	0.0	0.0	0	0%
(Pathmark) garden, fancy	1/2 cup	70	4.0	12.0	350	(mq)	1.0	(tr)	0	12%
(Pathmark) large, tender	1/2 cup	70	4.0	12.0	350	(mq)	1.0	(tr)	0	12%
(Pathmark) 'Little Gem'	1/2 cup	70	4.0	12.0	350	(mq)	1.0	(tr)	0	12%
(Pathmark) mixed sizes 'No Salt Added'	1/2 cup	50	4.0	10.0	10	(mq)	0.0	0.0	0	0%
(Pathmark) 'No Frills'	1 cup	120	8.0	25.0	640	(mq)	1.0	(tr)	0	6%
(Pathmark) small	1/2 cup	70	4.0	12.0	350	(mq)	1.0	(tr)	0	12%
(S&W) 'Perfection'	1/2 cup	70	4.0	12.0	330	(mq)	0.0	0.0	0	0%
(S&W Nutradiet)	1/2 cup	40	3.0	8.0	5	(mq)	0.0	0.0	0	0%
(Stokely)	1/2 cup	60	4.0	10.0	320	(mq)	0.0	0.0	0	0%
W/liquid										
low-sodium	4 oz	56	3.4	10.2	2	2.3	0.3	0.1	0	5%
(Del Monte)	1/2 cup	60	3.0	10.0	355	(mq)	0.0	0.0	0	0%
(Del Monte) 'No Salt Added'	1/2 cup	60	3.0	11.0	10	(mq)	0.0	0.0	0	0%
FREEZE-DRIED *(Mountain House)* prepared	1/2 cup	70	4.0	12.0	21	(mq)	1.0	(tr)	0	12%
FROZEN										
boiled, drained	4 oz	88	5.8	16.2	99	4.3	0.3	0.1	0	3%
boiled, drained	1/2 cup	62	4.1	11.4	70	>1.7 c	0.2	0.0	0	3%
unprepared	1/2 cup	55	3.8	9.9	81	>1.5 c	0.3	0.1	0	5%
(Birds Eye)	3.3 oz	80	5.0	13.0	130	4.0	0.0	0.0	0	0%
(Birds Eye) 'Portion Pack'	3 oz	70	5.0	12.0	120	4.0	0.0	0.0	0	0%
(Freshlike)	3.3 oz	80	5.0	13.0	75	na	0.0	na	na	0%
(Frosty Acres)	3.3 oz	80	5.0	13.0	91	>2.0 c	0.0	0.0	0	0%
(Health Valley)	1/2 cup	65	4.0	11.0	70	3.0	0.0	0.0	0	0%
(Seabrook)	3.3 oz	80	5.0	13.0	91	>2.0 c	0.0	0.0	0	0%
(Southern)	3.5 oz	79	5.5	14.0	130	(mq)	0.5	(tr)	0	6%
(Stokely) 'Singles'	3 oz	65	4.0	12.0	95	(mq)	1.0	(tr)	0	12%
(Veg•All)	3.3 oz	80	5.0	13.0	75	na	0.0	na	na	0%
Chinese										
(Chun King)	1.5 oz	20	1.0	3.0	10	(mq)	0.0	0.0	0	0%
(Seabrook)	2 oz	20	2.0	4.0	na	(mq)	0.0	0.0	0	0%
Combinations										
(Bird's Eye) w/cream sauce 'Combination Vegetables'	5 oz	180	5.0	16.0	480	3.0	11.0	na	0	54%
(Bird's Eye) w/pearl onions 'Combination Vegetables'	3.3 oz	70	5.0	13.0	440	3.0	0.0	na	0	0%
(Bird's Eye) w/potatoes, cream sauce 'Combination Vegetables'	5 oz	190	4.0	17.0	490	2.0	12.0	na	0	56%
(Budget Gourmet) and cauliflower, in cream sauce	5.75 oz	170	6.0	16.0	280	(mq)	7.0	(mq)	20	42%
(Budget Gourmet) Oriental, and water chestnuts 'Side Dish'	5 oz	120	5.0	15.0	240	(mq)	3.0	(mq)	5	25%
(Green Giant) 'LeSueur Valley'	1/2 cup	70	4.0	12.0	400	2.1	2.0	(mq)	0	22%
(Green Giant) mini, pea pods, water chestnut, butter 'LeSueur Valley'	1/2 cup	80	4.0	10.0	410	3.0	2.0	(mq)	na	24%
(Green Giant) w/onions and carrots in butter sauce 'LeSueur Valley'	1/2 cup	80	4.0	11.0	470	3.0	3.0	(mq)	na	31%
Early/June										
(Finast) in butter sauce	1/2 cup	80	8.0	15.0	400	(mq)	4.0	(mq)	na	28%
(Green Giant) 'Harvest Fresh'	1/2 cup	60	4.0	12.0	140	3.0	1.0	(tr)	0	12%
(Green Giant) in butter sauce 'One Serving'	4.5 oz	90	6.0	16.0	500	5.0	2.0	<1.0	5	17%

Food Name	Serving Size	Calories	Prot. gms	Carbs gms	Sod. mgs	Fiber gms	Fat gms	Sat. Fat gms	Chol. mgs	% Fat Cal.
(Green Giant) in butter sauce 'Select LeSueur'	1/2 cup	80	5.0	14.0	440	3.0	2.0	<1.0	5	19%
(Southern) petite	3.5 oz	64	4.7	11.0	50	(mq)	0.4	(tr)	0	5%
Sweet										
(Finast)	3.3 oz	80	5.0	13.0	125	(mq)	0.0	0.0	0	0%
(Green Giant)	1/2 cup	50	4.0	11.0	95	4.0	0.0	0.0	0	0%
(Green Giant) 'Harvest Fresh'	1/2 cup	50	4.0	12.0	135	3.0	0.0	0.0	0	0%
(Green Giant) in butter sauce	1/2 cup	80	5.0	14.0	410	4.0	2.0	<1.0	5	19%
(Stokely) in butter sauce 'Singles'	4 oz	90	5.0	16.0	335	(mq)	1.0	na	5	10%
Tiny										
(Birds Eye) tender, 'Deluxe'	3.3 oz	60	4.0	11.0	120	4.0	0.0	0.0	0	0%
(Freshlike)	3.3 oz	60	4.0	11.0	75	na	0.0	na	na	0%
(Frosty Acres)	3.3 oz	60	4.0	11.0	127	>2.0 c	0.0	0.0	0	0%
(Seabrook)	3.3 oz	60	4.0	11.0	127	>2.0 c	0.0	0.0	0	0%
(Veg•All)	3.3 oz	60	4.0	11.0	75	na	0.0	na	na	0%
PEAS, PIGEON										
immature seeds, boiled, drained	1/2 cup	85	4.6	15.0	4	na	1.0	0.3	0	10%
immature seeds, raw	10 seeds	5	0.3	1.0	0	.2	0.1	0.0	0	15%
raw, in pods	1 lb	296	15.7	52.0	11	>5.8 c	3.6	0.8	0	11%
red gram, mature seeds, boiled	1/2 cup	102	5.7	19.5	4	>.9 c	0.3	0.1	0	3%
red gram, mature seeds, raw	1/2 cup	350	22.1	64.0	17	15.3	1.5	0.3	0	4%
shelled, boiled, drained	4 oz	126	6.8	22.1	5	>3.3 c	1.5	0.1	0	11%
shelled, raw	1 oz	39	2.0	6.8	1	>.8 c	0.5	0.1	0	11%
shelled, raw, approx .1 oz	10 peas	5	0.3	1.0	tr	>.1 c	0.1	<.1	0	15%
Dried										
shelled, mature, boiled	4 oz	137	7.8	26.4	6	5.3	0.4	0.1	0	3%
shelled, mature, boiled	1/2 cup	102	5.7	19.5	5	3.9	0.3	0.1	0	3%
shelled, mature, raw	1/2 cup	350	22.1	64.0	17	13.8	1.5	0.3	0	4%
shelled, mature, raw	1 oz	97	6.2	17.8	5	3.8	0.4	0.1	0	4%
PEAS, PURPLE HULL										
(Allens) canned 'Fresh'	1/2 cup	100	6.0	16.0	370	(mq)	<1.0	(tr)	0	<9%
(Frosty Acres) frozen	3.3 oz	130	9.0	23.0	6	(mq)	0.0	0.0	0	0%
PEAS, SNAP										
(Birds Eye) carrots, water chestnuts	3.2 oz	50	2.0	11.0	20	4.0	0.0	0.0	0	0%
(Birds Eye) 'Deluxe'	2.6 oz	45	2.0	9.0	5	4.0	0.0	0.0	0	0%
(Green Giant) 'Harvest Fresh'	1/2 cup	30	2.0	8.0	100	2.0	0.0	0.0	0	0%
(Green Giant) 'Sugar Snap' frozen	1/2 cup	30	2.0	8.0	0	2.0	0.0	0.0	0	0%
PEAS, SNOW, 'Deluxe' *(Birds Eye)*	3 oz	35	2.0	6.0	0	3.0	0.0	0.0	0	0%
PEAS, WHITE ACRE, canned *(Allens)*	1/2 cup	90	7.0	14.0	440	(mq)	<1.0	(tr)	0	<10%
PEAS AND CARROTS, CANNED										
regular pack, solid and liquid	1/2 cup	49	2.8	10.9	333	4.2	0.4	0.1	0	6%
special dietary pack, solid and liquid	1/2 cup	49	2.8	10.9	5	4.2	0.4	0.1	0	6%
w/liquid	4 oz	43	2.5	9.6	295	>1.3 c	0.3	0.1	0	5%
w/liquid, low-sodium	4 oz	43	2.5	9.6	5	>1.3 c	0.3	0.1	0	5%
(A&P) early/June 'No Salt Added'	1/2 cup	60	4.0	12.0	10	(mq)	<1.0	(tr)	0	<12%
(A&P) mixed sizes	1/2 cup	60	4.0	12.0	10	(mq)	<1.0	(tr)	0	<12%
(Del Monte) w/liquid	1/2 cup	50	2.0	10.0	355	(mq)	0.0	0.0	0	0%
(Finast)	1/2 cup	55	3.0	9.0	315	(mq)	0.0	0.0	0	0%
(Freshlike)	1/2 cup	50	3.0	12.0	340	na	0.0	na	na	0%
(Freshlike) water pack, w/o salt	1/2 cup	50	3.0	12.0	30	na	0.0	na	na	0%
(Freshlike) water pack, w/o sugar, salt	1/2 cup	50	3.0	12.0	30	na	0.0	na	na	0%
(Kohl's)	1/2 cup	50	3.0	20.0	330	(mq)	<1.0	(tr)	0	<9%
(Pathmark)	1/2 cup	60	3.0	18.0	330	(mq)	1.0	(tr)	0	10%
(S&W)	1/2 cup	50	3.0	9.0	310	(mq)	0.0	0.0	0	0%
(S&W Nutradiet)	1/2 cup	35	2.0	7.0	5	(mq)	0.0	0.0	0	0%

Food Name	Serving Size	Calories	Prot. gms	Carbs gms	Sod. mgs	Fiber gms	Fat gms	Sat. Fat gms	Chol. mgs	% Fat Cal.
(Stokely)	1/2 cup	50	3.0	9.0	320	(mq)	0.0	0.0	0	0%
(Stokely) 'No Salt or Sugar Added'	1/2 cup	45	3.0	8.0	20	(mq)	0.0	0.0	0	0%
(Veg•All)	1/2 cup	50	3.0	12.0	340	na	0.0	na	na	0%
PEAS AND CARROTS, FROZEN										
boiled, drained	10-oz pkg	133	8.6	28.1	189	10.0	1.2	0.2	0	7%
boiled, drained	4 oz	54	3.5	11.5	77	>1.6 c	0.5	0.1	0	7%
boiled, drained	1/2 cup	38	2.5	8.1	54	2.9	0.3	0.1	0	6%
unprepared	10-oz pkg	151	9.7	31.7	224	9.9	1.3	0.2	0	7%
unprepared	1/2 cup	37	2.4	7.8	55	2.5	0.3	0.1	0	6%
(A&P)	3.3 oz	60	3.0	11.0	75	(mq)	<1.0	(tr)	0	<14%
(A&P) sweet peas	1/2 cup	80	5.0	13.0	90	(mq)	<1.0	(tr)	0	<11%
(Freshlike)	3.3 oz	60	3.0	11.0	60	na	0.0	na	na	0%
(Frosty Acres)	3.3 oz	60	3.0	11.0	75	>1.0 c	0.0	0.0	0	0%
(Seabrook)	3.3 oz	60	3.0	11.0	75	>1.0 c	0.0	0.0	0	0%
(Southern)	3.5 oz	64	3.2	11.7	80	(mq)	0.0	0.0	0	0%
(Veg•All)	3.3 oz	60	3.0	11.0	60	na	0.0	na	na	0%
PEAS AND ONIONS, CANNED										
solid and liquid	1/2 cup	31	2.0	5.1	265	>.7 c	0.2	0.0	0	6%
w/liquid	4 oz	58	3.7	9.7	501	>1.4 c	0.4	0.1	0	6%
(Freshlike) sweet peas, tiny onions	1/2 cup	60	4.0	12.0	440	na	0.0	na	na	0%
(Green Giant) pearl onions, w/liquid	1/2 cup	50	4.0	11.0	510	4.0	0.0	0.0	0	0%
(S&W) tiny pearl onions, w/liquid	1/2 cup	60	3.0	10.0	490	(mq)	1.0	(tr)	0	15%
PEAS AND ONIONS, FROZEN										
boiled, drained	4 oz	51	2.9	9.8	na	(mq)	0.2	<.1	0	3%
boiled, drained	1/2 cup	41	2.3	7.8	33	2.7	0.2	0.0	0	4%
unprepared	10-oz pkg	199	11.3	38.4	173	9.1	0.9	0.2	0	4%
unprepared	1/2 cup	48	2.8	9.3	42	2.2	0.2	0.0	0	4%
(Birds Eye) pearl onions 'Cheese Sauce Combinations'	5 oz	140	6.0	17.0	470	3.0	5.0	(mq)	5	33%
(Birds Eye) pearl onions 'Combination Vegetables'	3.3 oz	70	5.0	13.0	440	3.0	0.0	0.0	0	0%
(Freshlike)	3.3 oz	70	4.0	13.0	100	na	0.0	na	na	0%
(Frosty Acres) pearl onions	3.3 oz	70	4.0	13.0	80	(mq)	0.0	0.0	0	0%
(Seabrook)	3.3 oz	70	4.0	13.0	na	(mq)	0.0	0.0	0	0%
(Veg•All)	3.3 oz	70	4.0	13.0	100	na	0.0	na	na	0%
PECAN, SHELLED										
chopped (Fisher)	1 oz	190	2.0	5.0	0	na	19.0	2.0	0	86%
dried, chopped	1 cup	794	9.2	21.7	1	7.7	80.5	6.4	0	85%
dried, ground	1 cup	634	7.4	17.3	1	6.2	64.3	5.1	0	85%
dried, halves	1 cup	721	8.4	19.7	1	7.0	73.1	5.9	0	85%
dried, halves, pieces, or chips (Planters)	1 oz	190	2.0	5.0	0	(mq)	20.0	2.0	0	87%
dried, 31 large or 20 medium halves	1 oz	190	2.2	5.2	tr	1.8	19.2	1.5	0	85%
dry-roasted	1 oz	187	2.3	6.3	0	>.5 c	18.4	1.5	0	83%
ground (Fisher)	1 oz	190	2.0	5.0	0	na	19.0	2.0	0	86%
honey-roasted (Planters)	1 oz	200	2.0	8.0	0	na	18.0	2.0	80	80%
oil-roasted	1 cup	753	7.6	17.6	1	>1.8 c	78.3	6.3	0	88%
oil-roasted, 15 halves	1 oz	195	2.0	4.6	0	>.5 c	20.2	1.6	0	87%
raw (Fisher)	1 oz	190	2.0	5.0	0	na	19.0	2.0	0	86%
raw, chips (Planters)	1 oz	190	2.0	5.0	0	na	20.0	2.0	0	87%
raw, halves (Planters)	1 oz	190	2.0	5.0	0	(mq)	20.0	2.0	0	87%
raw, pieces (Planters)	1 oz	190	2.0	5.0	0	na	20.0	2.0	0	87%
PECAN FLOUR	1 oz	93	9.1	14.4	0	>.4 c	0.4	0.0	0	4%
PECTIN, unsweetened, dry mix	.5 oz	39	0.0	10.9	24	0	0.0	na	0	0%
PEPITAS										
In shell										
dried	1 lb	1817	82.4	59.8	59	>7.5 c	153.9	29.1	0	71%

Food Name	Serving Size	Calories	Prot. gms	Carbs gms	Sod. mgs	Fiber gms	Fat gms	Sat. Fat gms	Chol. mgs	% Fat Cal.
roasted, whole	1 cup	285	11.9	34.4	12	>23.0 c	12.4	2.3	0	38%
roasted, whole, approx 85 seeds	1 oz	127	5.3	15.3	5	>10.2 c	5.5	1.0	0	38%
Shelled										
dried	1 cup	747	33.9	24.6	24	>3.1 c	63.3	12.0	0	71%
dried, approx 142 kernels	1 oz	154	7.0	5.1	5	>.6 c	13.0	2.5	0	71%
roasted	1 cup	1184	74.8	30.5	40	>4.1 c	95.6	18.1	0	67%
roasted	1 oz	148	9.4	3.8	5	>.5 c	12.0	2.2	0	67%
salted	1 lb	2021	84.1	243.8	2608	>162.8 c	88.0	16.6	0	38%
salted	1 cup	285	11.9	34.4	368	>23.0 c	12.4	2.3	0	38%
salted	1 oz	127	5.3	15.3	163	>10.2 c	5.5	1.0	0	38%
PEPPER, BANANA, hot rings (Vlasic)	1 oz	4	0.0	1.0	465	(mq)	0.0	0.0	0	0%
PEPPER, BELL. See PEPPER, SWEET.										
PEPPER, CHERRY										
hot (Progresso)	1/2 cup	190	0.0	3.0	130	1.0	20.0	3.0	0	94%
hot (Vlasic)	1 oz	10	0.0	2.0	425	(mq)	0.0	0.0	0	0%
hot, pickled (Progresso)	1/2 cup	130	0.0	3.0	110	1.0	12.0	2.0	0	90%
mild (Vlasic)	1 oz	8	0.0	2.0	410	(mq)	0.0	0.0	0	0%
PEPPER, CHILI										
green, raw, approx 1.6 oz	1 med	18	0.9	4.3	3	.7	0.1	0.0	0	4%
green, raw, chopped	1/2 cup	30	1.5	7.1	5	1.1	0.2	0.0	0	5%
green, raw, trimmed	1 oz	11	0.6	2.7	2	.5	0.1	tr	0	6%
green, raw, untrimmed	1 lb	134	6.6	31.3	23	6.0	0.7	0.1	0	4%
red, raw, approx 1.6 oz	1 med	18	0.9	4.3	3	.7	0.1	0.0	0	4%
red, raw, chopped	1/2 cup	30	1.5	7.1	5	1.1	0.2	0.0	0	5%
red, raw, trimmed	1 oz	11	0.6	2.7	2	.5	0.1	tr	0	6%
red, raw, untrimmed	1 lb	134	6.6	31.3	23	6.0	0.7	0.1	0	4%
Canned										
green, chopped (Old El Paso)	2 tbsp	8	<1.0	2.0	70	(mq)	<1.0	na	0	<43%
green, diced (Rosarita)	1.058 oz	6	0.1	1.4	85	.5	0.1	0.0	0	13%
green, diced, w/liquid (Del Monte)	1/2 cup	20	0.0	5.0	690	(mq)	0.0	0.0	0	0%
green, whole (Old El Paso)	1 pepper	8	<1.0	1.0	105	(mq)	<1.0	na	0	<53%
green, whole (Rosarita)	1.235 oz	4	0.2	1.1	74	.5	0.1	0.0	0	15%
green, whole, diced, sliced, or strips (Ortega)	1 oz	10	0.0	3.0	20	(mq)	0.0	0.0	0	0%
green, whole, w/liquid (Del Monte)	1/2 cup	20	0.0	5.0	690	(mq)	0.0	0.0	0	0%
green and red, seeded, chopped, w/liquid	1/2 cup	17	0.6	4.2	(mq)	>.8 c	0.1	tr	0	5%
green and red, seeded, w/liquid	4 oz	28	1.0	6.9	(mq)	>1.4 c	0.1	<.1	0	3%
hot, green, pods, w/o seeds, solid and liquid, chopped	1/2 cup	17	0.6	4.2	798	>.8 c	0.1	0.0	0	5%
hot, green and red, seeded, w/liquid, approx 2.6 oz	1 med	18	0.7	4.5	(mq)	1.0	0.1	tr	0	4%
PEPPER, GREEN. See PEPPER, SWEET.										
PEPPER, GROUND										
black	1 oz	72	3.1	18.4	12	>3.7 c	0.9	0.4	0	8%
black	1 tbsp	16	0.7	4.2	3	1.7	0.2	0.1	0	8%
black	1 tsp	5	0.2	1.4	1	.6	0.1	0.0	0	8%
black (Durkee)	1 tsp	8	0.0	0.0	0	0	tr	na	na	tr
black (Laurel Leaf)	1 tsp	8	0.0	0.0	0	0	tr	na	na	tr
black (Spice Islands)	1 tsp	9	0.2	1.5	<1	>.2 c	0.2	(tr)	0	8%
cayenne/red	1 oz	90	3.4	16.1	9	>7.1 c	4.9	0.9	0	36%
cayenne/red	1 tbsp	17	0.6	3.0	2	>1.3 c	0.9	0.2	0	36%
cayenne/red	1 tsp	6	0.2	1.0	1	>.5 c	0.3	0.1	0	36%
cayenne/red (Durkee)	1 tsp	8	0.0	0.0	0	0	<0.1	na	na	<33%
cayenne/red (Laurel Leaf)	1 tsp	8	0.0	0.0	0	0	<0.1	na	na	<33%
cayenne/red (Spice Islands)	1 tsp	9	0.3	1.1	<1	>.5 c	0.3	(tr)	0	33%
chili (Spice Islands)	1 tsp	9	0.3	1.2	<1	>.3 c	0.3	(tr)	0	31%
pizza (Lawry's)	1 tsp	2	1.5	3.2	11	na	0.2	0.0	0	9%

Food Name	Serving Size	Calories	Prot. gms	Carbs gms	Sod. mgs	Fiber gms	Fat gms	Sat. Fat gms	Chol. mgs	% Fat Cal.
seasoned (Lawry's)	1 tsp	9	0.3	1.8	5	>.2 c	0.1	(tr)	0	<10%
seasoned 'All Pepper' (Schilling)	1/4 tsp	1	<.1	0.3	106	(mq)	0.0	0.0	0	0%
white	1 oz	84	2.9	19.5	1	>1.2 c	0.6	na	0	6%
white	1 tbsp	21	0.7	4.9	0	>.3 c	0.2	na	0	7%
white	1 tsp	7	0.3	1.6	0	>.1 c	0.1	na	0	11%
white (Durkee)	1 tsp	9	0.0	0.0	0	0	tr	na	na	tr
white (Laurel Leaf)	1 tsp	9	0.0	0.0	0	0	tr	na	na	tr
white (Spice Islands)	1 tsp	9	0.3	1.5	<1	>.1 c	0.2	(tr)	0	20%

PEPPER, JALAPEÑO

Food Name	Serving Size	Calories	Prot. gms	Carbs gms	Sod. mgs	Fiber gms	Fat gms	Sat. Fat gms	Chol. mgs	% Fat Cal.
diced (Ortega)	1 oz	10	0.0	3.0	20	(mq)	0.0	0.0	0	0%
diced (Rosarita)	1.058 oz	5	0.4	0.8	121	.6	0.2	0.0	0	27%
for nachos (La Victoria)	14 pieces	5	0.0	1.0	330	na	0.0	na	na	0%
for nachos (La Victoria)	1 tbsp	2	<1.0	1.0	335	(mq)	<1.0	(tr)	0	<53%
hot, diced (Ortega)	1 oz	8	0.0	2.0	(mq)	(mq)	0.0	0.0	0	0%
hot 'Mexican' (Vlasic)	1 oz	8	0.0	2.0	380	(mq)	0.0	0.0	0	0%
hot, tiny, Mexican (Vlasic)	1 oz	6	0.0	2.0	430	(mq)	0.0	0.0	0	0%
hot, whole (Ortega)	1 oz	8	0.0	2.0	(mq)	(mq)	0.0	0.0	0	0%
marinated (La Victoria)	1.5 pieces	10	0.0	2.0	300	na	0.0	na	na	0%
marinated (La Victoria)	1 tbsp	4	<1.0	1.0	251	(mq)	<1.0	(tr)	0	<53%
nacho sliced (Rosarita)	1.058 oz	4	0.1	1.0	448	.6	0.1	0.0	0	17%
sliced, w/liquid (Del Monte)	1/2 cup	30	1.0	6.0	1690	(mq)	1.0	(tr)	0	24%
whole (Old El Paso)	2 peppers	14	0.0	1.0	480	(mq)	1.0	(tr)	0	69%
whole (Ortega)	1 oz	10	0.0	3.0	20	(mq)	0.0	0.0	0	0%
whole (Rosarita)	1.34 oz	6	0.2	1.3	568	.7	0.2	0.0	0	23%
whole, w/escabeche (Rosarita)	1.164 oz	8	0.6	1.4	430	.9	0.2	0.0	0	18%
whole, w/liquid (Del Monte)	1/2 cup	30	1.0	6.0	1690	(mq)	1.0	(tr)	0	24%

PEPPER, PEPPERONCINI

Food Name	Serving Size	Calories	Prot. gms	Carbs gms	Sod. mgs	Fiber gms	Fat gms	Sat. Fat gms	Chol. mgs	% Fat Cal.
mild, Greek, salad (Vlasic)	1 oz	4	0.0	1.0	450	(mq)	0.0	0.0	0	0%
Tuscan (Progresso)	1/2 cup	20	0.0	7.0	5	1.0	0.0	0.0	0	0%

PEPPER, PICCALILLI (Progresso)

Food Name	Serving Size	Calories	Prot. gms	Carbs gms	Sod. mgs	Fiber gms	Fat gms	Sat. Fat gms	Chol. mgs	% Fat Cal.
PEPPER, PICCALILLI (Progresso)	1/2 cup	190	<1.0	4.0	220	1.0	20.0	3.0	0	90%

PEPPER, SWEET / bell pepper / green pepper / red pepper / yellow pepper

Food Name	Serving Size	Calories	Prot. gms	Carbs gms	Sod. mgs	Fiber gms	Fat gms	Sat. Fat gms	Chol. mgs	% Fat Cal.
boiled, drained	4 oz	32	1.0	7.6	2	>.5 c	0.2	<.1	0	5%
boiled, drained, approx 2.6 oz	1 med	20	0.7	4.9	1	>.3 c	0.2	0.0	0	7%
boiled, drained, chopped	1/2 cup	19	0.6	4.6	1	.9	0.1	0.0	0	4%
raw, approx 3.2 oz	1 med	20	0.7	4.8	1	1.5	0.1	0.0	0	4%
raw, chopped	1/2 cup	14	0.4	3.2	1	.8	0.1	0.0	0	6%
raw (Dole)	1 med	25	1.0	5.0	0	2.0	1.0	na	na	6%
raw, trimmed	1 oz	8	0.3	1.8	<1	.5	0.1	<.1	0	6%
raw, untrimmed	1 lb	99	3.3	23.9	7	6.0	0.7	0.1	0	6%

Canned

Food Name	Serving Size	Calories	Prot. gms	Carbs gms	Sod. mgs	Fiber gms	Fat gms	Sat. Fat gms	Chol. mgs	% Fat Cal.
roasted (Progresso)	1/2 cup	20	<1.0	5.0	2	1.7	<1.0	<1.0	0	<27%
solid and liquid, halves	1/2 cup	13	0.6	2.7	958	>.6 c	0.2	0.0	0	tr
'Sweet Pepper Mementos' (Heinz)	1 oz	6	0.0	1.0	320	(mq)	0.0	0.0	0	0%
w/liquid	4 oz	20	0.9	4.4	1552	>.9 c	0.3	0.1	0	tr

Freeze-dried

Food Name	Serving Size	Calories	Prot. gms	Carbs gms	Sod. mgs	Fiber gms	Fat gms	Sat. Fat gms	Chol. mgs	% Fat Cal.
....	1 oz	89	5.1	19.5	55	>4.6 c	0.9	0.1	0	8%
....	1/4 cup	5	0.3	1.1	3	>.0 c	0.1	0.0	0	14%

Frozen

Food Name	Serving Size	Calories	Prot. gms	Carbs gms	Sod. mgs	Fiber gms	Fat gms	Sat. Fat gms	Chol. mgs	% Fat Cal.
boiled, drained, chopped	4 oz	20	1.1	4.4	5	>1.0 c	0.2	<.1	0	tr
chopped, unprepared	10-oz pkg	57	3.1	12.6	14	4.5	0.6	0.1	0	tr
chopped, unprepared	1 oz	6	0.3	1.3	1	.5	0.1	0.0	0	tr
green (Seabrook)	1 oz	6	0.0	1.0	1	(mq)	0.0	0.0	0	0%
red (Seabrook)	1 oz	8	0.0	1.0	na	(mq)	0.0	0.0	0	0%

PEPPER DILL SEASONING (Golden Dipt)

Food Name	Serving Size	Calories	Prot. gms	Carbs gms	Sod. mgs	Fiber gms	Fat gms	Sat. Fat gms	Chol. mgs	% Fat Cal.
PEPPER DILL SEASONING (Golden Dipt)	2 grams	8	0.0	1.0	96	na	0.0	na	0	0%

Food Name	Serving Size	Calories	Prot. gms	Carbs gms	Sod. mgs	Fiber gms	Fat gms	Sat. Fat gms	Chol. mgs	% Fat Cal.
PEPPER STEAK DINNER										
(Armour) frozen, beef 'Classics Lite'	11.25 oz	220	17.0	29.0	970	(mq)	4.0	(mq)	35	16%
(Healthy Choice) frozen	11 oz	260	20.0	40.0	500	na	5.0	2.0	40	16%
(LaChoy)	3.81 oz	36	1.9	7.4	942	1.4	0.2	0.0	0	5%
(Le Menu) frozen	11.5 oz	370	26.0	36.0	1020	(mq)	13.0	(mq)	(mq)	32%
PEPPER STEAK DINNER MIX										
(LaChoy) 'Dinner Classics'	1/5 pkg	35	2.0	9.0	720	1.0	<1.0	(mq)	0	<17%
(LaChoy) 'Dinner Classics' prepared	3/4 cup	180	17.0	9.0	760	1.0	9.0	3.4	60	44%
PEPPER STEAK ENTRÉE										
pork and beef	1 oz	141	6.0	0.8	578	0	12.5	4.6	(mq)	81%
pork and beef, approx .2 oz	1 slice	27	1.2	0.2	112	0	2.4	0.9	(mq)	79%
(Budget Gourmet) frozen, w/rice	10 oz	300	15.0	39.0	800	(mq)	9.0	(mq)	25	27%
(Dining Lite) frozen	9 oz	260	18.0	33.0	1050	(mq)	6.0	(mq)	40	21%
(Healthy Choice) frozen	9.5 oz	250	18.0	36.0	560	na	4.0	2.0	40	14%
(LaChoy) frozen, w/rice & vegetables 'Fresh & Lite'	10 oz	280	21.0	33.0	1082	2.0	8.0	(mq)	36	25%
(Stouffer's) frozen, green, w/rice, 1 pkg	10.5 oz	310	20.0	35.0	700	na	10.0	na	na	29%
(Top Shelf) Oriental, microwave bowl	1 serving	290	25.0	25.0	1700	(mq)	10.0	(mq)	45	31%
(Tyson) frozen 'Gourmet Selection'	11.25 oz	330	20.0	38.0	1130	(mq)	11.0	(mq)	(mq)	30%
(Ultra Slim Fast) beef, and parsley rice	12 oz	270	22.0	36.0	690	na	4.0	na	45	13%
PEPPERONI										
(Hickory Farms)	1 oz	140	6.0	1.0	578	0	13.0	(mq)	23	81%
(Hormel)										
'Chunk'	1 oz	140	6.0	0.0	423	0	12.0	(mq)	(mq)	82%
'Leoni Brand'	1 oz	130	6.0	0.0	508	0	12.0	(mq)	(mq)	82%
'Perma-Fresh'	2 slices	80	3.0	0.0	281	0	7.0	(mq)	(mq)	84%
'Rosa'	1 oz	140	6.0	0.0	626	0	13.0	(mq)	(mq)	83%
'Rosa Grande'	1 oz	140	6.0	0.0	512	0	13.0	(mq)	(mq)	83%
(JM) approx .5 oz	8 slices	70	3.0	1.0	290	0	6.0	(mq)	(mq)	77%
PEPPERS AND ONIONS (Quincy's)	4 oz	80	1.0	8.0	11	(mq)	5.0	(mq)	na	56%
PERCH										
frozen (Booth)	4 oz	100	20.0	0.0	90	0	1.0	(mq)	(mq)	10%
frozen (SeaPak)	4 oz	100	19.0	0.0	80	0	2.0	(mq)	(mq)	19%
frozen, fillet, battered (Van de Kamp's)	2 pieces	310	12.0	18.0	500	na	21.0	4.0	30	61%
mixed species, dry-heat cooked	4 oz	133	28.2	0.0	90	0	1.3	0.3	130	9%
mixed species, dry-heat cooked	3 oz	99	21.1	0.0	67	0	1.0	0.2	98	10%
mixed species, raw	1 lb	413	87.9	0.0	280	0	4.2	0.8	407	10%
mixed species, raw	3 oz	77	16.5	0.0	53	0	0.8	0.2	77	10%
mixed species, raw	1 oz	26	5.5	0.0	18	0	0.3	<.1	26	11%
PERSIMMON										
Japanese , dried	1 oz	78	0.4	20.8	1	>1.0 c	0.2	(tr)	0	2%
Japanese, fresh, trimmed	1 oz	20	0.2	5.3	<1	>.4 c	0.1	(tr)	0	4%
Japanese, fresh, untrimmed	1 lb	268	2.2	70.8	6	>5.6 c	0.7	na	0	2%
Japanese, raw, 2.5 inch diam	1 med	118	1.0	31.2	2	6.1	0.3	na	0	2%
native, fresh, trimmed	1 oz	36	0.2	9.5	<1	>.4 c	0.1	(tr)	0	2%
native, fresh, untrimmed	1 lb	472	3.0	124.6	4	>5.6 c	1.5	na	0	3%
native, raw, trimmed, approx 1.1 oz	1 med	32	0.2	8.4	0	>.4 c	0.1	na	0	3%
PE-TSAI. See CABBAGE, NAPA.										
PHEASANT										
breast meat only, raw	1 oz	38	6.9	0.0	9	0	0.9	0.3	(mq)	23%
leg meat only, raw	1 oz	38	6.3	0.0	13	0	1.2	0.4	(mq)	30%
meat and skin, raw	1 oz	51	6.4	0.0	11	0	2.6	0.8	(mq)	48%
meat only, raw	1 oz	38	6.7	0.0	10	0	1.0	0.4	(mq)	25%
PHYLLO DOUGH,										
1 sheet	1 oz	85	2.0	14.9	137	na	1.7	0.3	0	19%

Food Name	Serving Size	Calories	Prot. gms	Carbs gms	Sod. mgs	Fiber gms	Fat gms	Sat. Fat gms	Chol. mgs	% Fat Cal.
1 sheet *(Apollo)*	1 oz	80	3.0	18.0	200	na	.4	0.0	0	4%
PICKLES										
BREAD AND BUTTER										
chunks 'Old-Fashion' *(Vlasic)*	1 oz	25	0.0	6.0	120	(mq)	0.0	0.0	0	0%
'Deli' *(Vlasic)*	1 oz	25	0.0	6.0	120	(mq)	0.0	0.0	0	0%
fresh	2 slices	11	0.1	2.7	101	>.1 c	0.0	0.0	0	0%
one slice *(Claussen)*	.4 oz	7	0.1	1.7	61	(mq)	tr	(tr)	0	0%
slices	1 cup	124	1.5	30.4	1144	>.9 c	0.3	0.0	0	2%
slices *(Claussen)*	1 oz	20	0.2	4.7	172	(mq)	0.1	(tr)	0	4%
slices, approx 2/3 oz *(Mrs. Fanning's)*	2 slices	16	0.0	3.0	140	(mq)	0.0	0.0	0	0%
slices 'Cucumber Slices' *(Heinz)*	1 oz	25	0.0	6.0	170	(mq)	0.0	0.0	0	0%
'Sweet Butter Chips' *(Vlasic)*	1 oz	30	0.0	7.0	160	(mq)	0.0	0.0	0	0%
'Sweet Butter Stix' *(Vlasic)*	1 oz	18	0.0	5.0	110	(mq)	0.0	0.0	0	0%
DILL										
	1 lb	81	2.8	18.7	5813	5.4	0.9	0.2	0	9%
	1 oz	5	0.2	1.2	363	.3	0.1	<.1	0	14%
baby *(Heinz)*	1 oz	4	0.0	1.0	285	(mq)	0.0	0.0	0	0%
baby *(Vlasic)*	1 oz	4	0.0	1.0	210	(mq)	0.0	0.0	0	0%
chips *(Heinz)*	1 oz	4	0.0	1.0	275	(mq)	0.0	0.0	0	0%
chunks, snack *(Vlasic)*	1 oz	4	0.0	1.0	220	(mq)	0.0	0.0	0	0%
chunks, zesty, snacks *(Vlasic)*	1 oz	4	0.0	1.0	290	(mq)	0.0	0.0	0	0%
crunchy *(Vlasic)*	1 oz	4	0.0	1.0	210	(mq)	0.0	0.0	0	0%
crunchy, half salt *(Vlasic)*	1 oz	4	0.0	1.0	125	(mq)	0.0	0.0	0	0%
crunchy, zesty *(Vlasic)*	1 oz	4	0.0	1.0	250	(mq)	0.0	0.0	0	0%
gherkins *(Vlasic)*	1 oz	4	0.0	1.0	210	(mq)	0.0	0.0	0	0%
halves 'Deli' *(Vlasic)*	1 oz	4	0.0	1.0	290	(mq)	0.0	0.0	0	0%
halves 'Deli Style' *(Heinz)*	1 oz	4	0.0	1.0	280	(mq)	0.0	0.0	0	0%
hamburger chips, half salt *(Vlasic)*	1 oz	2	0.0	1.0	175	(mq)	0.0	0.0	0	0%
hamburger slices *(Heinz)*	1 oz	2	0.0	0.0	405	(mq)	0.0	0.0	0	0%
low sodium	1 lb	81	2.8	18.7	82	5.4	0.9	0.2	0	9%
low sodium	1 oz	5	0.2	1.2	5	.3	0.1	<.1	0	14%
no garlic *(Claussen)*	1 oz	6	0.2	1.0	313	(mq)	0.1	(tr)	0	16%
no garlic, 1 piece *(Claussen)*	2.9 oz	17	0.6	2.8	895	(mq)	0.3	(tr)	0	17%
'Original' *(Vlasic)*	1 oz	4	0.0	1.0	375	(mq)	0.0	0.0	0	0%
'Polish Snack Chunks' *(Vlasic)*	1 oz	4	0.0	1.0	300	(mq)	0.0	0.0	0	0%
spears *(Claussen)*	1 oz	4	0.1	0.5	330	(mq)	0.1	(tr)	0	27%
spears, half salt *(Vlasic)*	1 oz	4	0.0	1.0	120	(mq)	0.0	0.0	0	0%
spears, kosher *(Heinz)*	1 oz	4	0.0	1.0	295	(mq)	0.0	0.0	0	0%
spears, kosher *(Vlasic)*	1 oz	4	0.0	1.0	175	(mq)	0.0	0.0	0	0%
spears, no garlic *(Vlasic)*	1 oz	4	0.0	1.0	210	(mq)	0.0	0.0	0	0%
spears, 1 piece *(Claussen)*	1.1 oz	4	0.2	0.6	373	(mq)	0.1	(tr)	0	22%
spears, Polish style *(Heinz)*	1 oz	4	0.0	1.0	285	(mq)	0.0	0.0	0	0%
spears, zesty *(Vlasic)*	1 oz	4	0.0	1.0	230	(mq)	0.0	0.0	0	0%
whole *(Featherweight)*	1 piece	4	0.0	1.0	5	(mq)	0.0	0.0	0	0%
whole 'Genuine' *(Heinz)*	1 oz	2	0.0	0.0	420	(mq)	0.0	0.0	0	0%
whole, kosher *(Heinz)*	1 oz	4	0.0	1.0	295	(mq)	0.0	0.0	0	0%
whole, Polish style *(Heinz)*	1 oz	4	0.0	1.0	285	(mq)	0.0	0.0	0	0%
whole, processed *(Heinz)*	1 oz	2	0.0	0.0	435	(mq)	0.0	0.0	0	0%
HOT AND SPICY, garden, mixed *(Vlasic)*	1 oz	4	0.0	1.0	380	(mq)	0.0	0.0	0	0%
KOSHER. See also DILL.										
chips, 'Old Fashioned' *(Heinz)*	1 oz	4	0.0	1.0	270	(mq)	0.0	0.0	0	0%
halves *(Claussen)*	1 oz	4	0.1	0.5	330	(mq)	0.1	(tr)	0	27%
halves 'Old Fashioned Deli Halves' *(Heinz)*	1 oz	4	0.0	1.0	275	(mq)	0.0	0.0	0	0%
halves, 2.3 oz *(Claussen)*	1 piece	9	0.3	1.3	769	(mq)	0.2	(tr)	0	22%

Food Name	Serving Size	Calories	Prot. gms	Carbs gms	Sod. mgs	Fiber gms	Fat gms	Sat. Fat gms	Chol. mgs	% Fat Cal.
slices *(Claussen)*	1 oz	3	0.1	0.5	319	(mq)	0.1	(tr)	0	27%
slices, .3 oz *(Claussen)*	1 piece	1	tr	0.2	107	(mq)	tr	(tr)	0	0%
SOUR										
	1 lb	48	1.5	10.2	5477	>2.8 c	0.9	0.2	0	15%
	1 oz	3	0.1	0.6	342	>.2 c	0.1	<.1	0	24%
low sodium	1 lb	48	1.5	10.2	82	>2.8 c	0.9	0.2	0	15%
low sodium	1 oz	3	0.1	0.6	5	>.2 c	0.1	<.1	0	24%
whole *(Claussen)*	1 oz	3	0.2	0.5	332	(mq)	0.1	(tr)	0	24%
whole 'Old Fashioned' *(Heinz)*	1 oz	4	0.0	1.0	280	(mq)	0.0	0.0	0	0%
whole, 1 piece *(Claussen)*	2.5 oz	9	0.4	1.3	832	(mq)	0.2	(tr)	0	21%
SWEET										
	1 lb	529	1.7	144.3	4257	5.0	1.2	0.3	0	2%
	1 oz	33	0.1	9.0	266	.3	0.1	<.1	0	2%
cubes, salad *(Heinz)*	1 oz	30	0.0	7.0	270	(mq)	0.0	0.0	0	0%
'Cucumber Stix' *(Heinz)*	1 oz	25	0.0	6.0	145	(mq)	0.0	0.0	0	0%
gherkins *(Heinz)*	1 oz	35	0.0	8.0	210	(mq)	0.0	0.0	0	0%
gherkins, midget *(Heinz)*	1 oz	35	0.0	8.0	205	(mq)	0.0	0.0	0	0%
half salt 'Sweet Butter Chips' *(Vlasic)*	1 oz	30	0.0	7.0	80	(mq)	0.0	0.0	0	0%
low sodium	1 lb	529	1.7	144.3	82	5.0	1.2	0.3	0	2%
low sodium	1 med	41	0.1	11.1	6	>.2 c	0.1	0.0	0	2%
low sodium	1 oz	33	0.1	9.0	5	.3	0.1	<.1	0	2%
low sodium	1 slice	7	0.0	1.9	1	0	0.0	0.0	0	0%
low sodium, mixed *(Heinz)*	1 oz	40	0.0	9.0	200	(mq)	0.0	0.0	0	0%
low sodium, 3 inches long, approx 1.2 oz	1 large	41	0.1	11.1	6	.4	0.1	<.1	0	2%
sliced *(Featherweight)*	3-4 slices	24	0.0	6.0	5	(mq)	0.0	0.0	0	0%
sliced *(Heinz)*	1 oz	35	0.0	8.0	205	(mq)	0.0	0.0	0	0%
sliced 'Cucumber Slices' *(Heinz)*	1 oz	20	0.0	5.0	195	(mq)	0.0	0.0	0	0%
whole, 3 inches long, approx 1.2 oz	1 large	41	0.1	11.1	328	.4	0.1	<.1	0	2%
PICKLING SPICE *(Tone's)*	1 tsp	10	0.3	1.2	1	.3	0.6	0.1	0	47%
PIE										
APPLE										
Fresh										
(Entenmann's) homestyle	2.1 oz	140	1.0	21.0	150	na	7.0	na	na	42%
(McMillin's)	4 oz	430	4.0	51.0	340	na	23.0	na	na	49%
Frozen										
(Amy's Kitchen)	8 oz	282	4.0	42.0	180	na	12.0	na	na	37%
(Banquet) 'Family Size' 3 1/3 oz	1/6 pie	250	2.0	37.0	290	(mq)	11.0	(mq)	na	39%
(Mrs. Smith's) 'Pie In Minutes' 8-inch pie	1/8 pie	210	2.0	29.0	250	(mq)	9.0	2.0	0	40%
(Pet-Ritz)	1/16 pie	330	2.0	53.0	385	(mq)	12.0	(mq)	Chol.	33%
(Sara Lee) apple streusel 'Free & Light'	1/8 pie	170	1.0	36.0	140	(mq)	2.0	(mq)	0	11%
(Sara Lee) Dutch apple 'Homestyle' 9-inch pie	1/10 pie	300	2.0	45.0	310	(mq)	12.0	(mq)	0	37%
(Sara Lee) 'Homestyle' 9-inch pie	1/10 pie	280	2.0	42.0	220	(mq)	12.0	(mq)	0	38%
(Sara Lee) 'Homestyle High' 10-inch pie	1/10 pie	400	3.0	46.0	450	(mq)	23.0	(mq)	0	51%
(Weight Watchers) 3.5 oz	1/2 pkg	200	2.0	39.0	280	(mq)	5.0	1.0	5	22%
BANANA CREAM										
Frozen										
(Banquet) 2 1/3 oz	1/6 pie	180	2.0	21.0	150	(mq)	10.0	(mq)	na	50%
(Pet-Ritz) 2 1/3 oz	1/6 pie	170	2.0	22.0	155	(mq)	9.0	(mq)	na	46%
BERRY, fresh *(McMillin's)*	4 oz	430	3.0	52.0	410	na	23.0	na	na	49%
BLACKBERRY, frozen *(Banquet)* 'Family Size' 3 1/3 oz	1/6 pie	270	3.0	40.0	350	(mq)	11.0	(mq)	na	37%
BLUEBERRY										
Frozen										
(Banquet) 'Family Size' 3 1/3 oz	1/6 pie	270	3.0	40.0	350	(mq)	11.0	(mq)	na	37%
(Mrs. Smith's) 'Pie In Minutes' 8-inch pie	1/8 pie	220	2.0	32.0	240	(mq)	9.0	2.0	0	37%

Food Name	Serving Size	Calories	Prot. gms	Carbs gms	Sod. mgs	Fiber gms	Fat gms	Sat. Fat gms	Chol. mgs	% Fat Cal.
(Pet-Ritz)	1/6 pie	370	3.0	50.0	330	(mq)	12.0	(mq)	na	34%
(Sara Lee) 'Homestyle' 9-inch pie	1/10 pie	300	2.0	45.0	210	(mq)	12.0	(mq)	0	37%
BOSTON CREAM, frozen (Weight Watchers)	3 oz	160	3.0	34.0	260	(mq)	4.0	1.0	5	20%
CHERRY										
Fresh (McMillin's)	4 oz	430	3.0	51.0	350	na	24.0	na	na	50%
Frozen										
(Banquet) 'Family Size' 3 1/3 oz	1/6 pie	250	3.0	36.0	260	(mq)	11.0	(mq)	na	39%
(Mrs. Smith's) 'Pie In Minutes' 8-inch pie	1/8 pie	220	2.0	32.0	200	(mq)	9.0	2.0	0	37%
(Pet-Ritz)	1/6 pie	300	3.0	48.0	330	(mq)	12.0	(mq)	na	35%
(Sara Lee) cherry streusel 'Free & Light'	1/10 pie	160	2.0	34.0	140	(mq)	2.0	(mq)	0	11%
(Sara Lee) 'Homestyle' 9-inch pie	1/10 pie	270	2.0	37.0	270	(mq)	13.0	(mq)	0	43%
CHOCOLATE										
Fresh (McMillin's) chocolate pudding	4 oz	420	3.0	54.0	350	na	21.0	na	na	45%
Frozen										
(Banquet) chocolate cream, 2 1/3 oz	1/6 pie	190	2.0	24.0	110	(mq)	10.0	(mq)	na	46%
(Pet Ritz) chocolate cream, 2 1/3 oz	1/6 pie	190	1.0	27.0	145	(mq)	8.0	(mq)	na	39%
(Weight Watchers) chocolate mocha 'Sweet Celebrations' 2.75 oz	1/2 pkg	160	5.0	23.0	150	(mq)	5.0	3.0	5	29%
COCONUT										
Fresh (McMillin's) coconut pudding	4 oz	450	4.0	50.0	420	na	26.0	na	na	52%
Frozen										
(Banquet) cream, 2 1/3 oz	1/6 pie	190	2.0	22.0	120	(mq)	11.0	(mq)	na	51%
(Pet Ritz) cream, 2 1/3 oz	1/6 pie	190	2.0	27.0	145	(mq)	8.0	(mq)	na	38%
COCONUT CUSTARD, fresh (Entenmann's)	1.8 oz	140	3.0	16.0	160	na	8.0	na	na	49%
EGG CUSTARD, frozen (Pet-Ritz)	1/6 pie	200	5.0	28.0	(mq)	(mq)	8.0	(mq)	(mq)	35%
LEMON										
Fresh (McMillin's)	4 oz	450	4.0	52.0	330	na	25.0	na	na	50%
Frozen										
(Banquet) cream, 2 1/3 oz	1/6 pie	170	2.0	23.0	120	(mq)	9.0	(mq)	na	45%
(Mrs. Smith's) meringue, 8-inch pie	1/8 pie	210	2.0	38.0	130	(mq)	5.0	(mq)	na	22%
(Pet Ritz) cream, 2 1/3 oz	1/6 pie	190	2.0	26.0	150	(mq)	9.0	(mq)	na	42%
MINCE										
Frozen										
(Banquet) mincemeat 'Family Size' 3 1/3 oz	1/6 pie	260	3.0	38.0	370	(mq)	11.0	(mq)	na	38%
(Pet-Ritz)	1/6 pie	280	2.0	48.0	(mq)	(mq)	9.0	(mq)	na	29%
(Sara Lee) 'Homestyle' 9-inch pie	1/10 pie	300	3.0	43.0	340	(mq)	13.0	(mq)	0	39%
NEAPOLITAN CREAM, frozen, (Pet Ritz) 2 1/3 oz	1/6 pie	180	1.0	17.0	185	(mq)	10.0	(mq)	na	56%
PEACH										
Fresh (McMillin's)	4 oz	430	4.0	52.0	370	na	24.0	na	na	49%
Frozen										
(Banquet) 'Family Size' 3 1/3 oz	1/6 pie	245	3.0	35.0	280	(mq)	11.0	(mq)	na	39%
(Mrs. Smith's) 'Pie In Minutes' 8-inch pie	1/8 pie	210	2.0	29.0	190	(mq)	9.0	2.0	0	40%
(Pet-Ritz)	1/6 pie	320	2.0	51.0	320	(mq)	12.0	(mq)	na	34%
(Sara Lee) 'Homestyle' 9-inch pie	1/10 pie	280	2.0	41.0	170	(mq)	12.0	(mq)	0	39%
PECAN										
Frozen										
(Mrs. Smith's) 'Pie In Minutes' 8-inch pie	1/8 pie	330	3.0	51.0	200	(mq)	13.0	2.0	35	35%
(Sara Lee) 'Homestyle' 9-inch pie	1/10 pie	400	4.0	56.0	290	(mq)	18.0	(mq)	55	40%
PUMPKIN										
Frozen										
(Banquet) 'Family Size' 3 1/3 oz	1/6 pie	200	3.0	29.0	350	(mq)	8.0	(mq)	na	36%
(Mrs. Smith's) 'Pie In Minutes' 8-inch pie	1/8 pie	190	3.0	30.0	230	(mq)	6.0	2.0	35	29%
(Pet Ritz) pumpkin custard	1/6 pie	250	4.0	39.0	(mq)	(mq)	9.0	(mq)	na	32%
(Sara Lee) 'Homestyle' 9-inch pie	1/10 pie	240	4.0	34.0	250	(mq)	10.0	(mq)	40	37%

Food Name	Serving Size	Calories	Prot. gms	Carbs gms	Sod. mgs	Fiber gms	Fat gms	Sat. Fat gms	Chol. mgs	% Fat Cal.
RASPBERRY, frozen *(Sara Lee)* 'Homestyle' 9-inch pie	1/10 pie	280	2.0	39.0	150	(mq)	13.0	(mq)	0	42%
STRAWBERRY										
Fresh *(McMillin's)*	4 oz	400	3.0	50.0	370	na	20.0	na	na	46%
Frozen										
(Banquet) strawberry cream, 2 1/3 oz	1/6 pie	170	2.0	22.0	120	(mq)	9.0	(mq)	na	46%
(Pet Ritz) strawberry cream, 2 1/3 oz	1/6 pie	170	2.0	20.0	145	(mq)	9.0	(mq)	na	48%
SWEET POTATO, frozen *(Pet-Ritz)*	1/6 pie	150	2.0	21.0	110	(mq)	7.0	(mq)	na	41%
PIE, SNACK										
APPLE										
(Break Cake) 'Fried Pie' 4.5 oz	2 pies	430	5.0	63.0	370	na	18.0	4.5	0	37%
(Drake's) approx 2 oz	1 piece	210	2.0	29.0	135	(mq)	10.0	2.0	0	42%
(Hostess)	1 piece	430	3.0	60.0	390	2.0	20.0	9.0	15	42%
(Hostess) French apple	1 piece	430	3.0	60.0	390	2.0	20.0	9.0	15	42%
(Little Debbie) Dutch apple, 2.17 oz	1 piece	230	2.0	42.0	150	(mq)	8.0	(mq)	<1	29%
(Little Debbie) Dutch apple, 2.5 oz	1 piece	270	2.0	48.0	170	(mq)	8.0	(mq)	<1	27%
(Tastykake) 4 oz	1 piece	296	3.0	46.0	339	2.5	12.3	2.6	0	36%
(Tastykake) French apple, 4.2 oz	1 piece	353	3.0	63.0	225	1.9	10.7	2.5	0	27%
BANANA CREAM *(Tastycake)* 4.2 oz	1 piece	382	5.2	53.9	428	1.7	16.1	5.7	26	38%
BLACKBERRY *(Hostess)*	1 piece	420	4.0	59.0	360	2.4	18.0	9.0	15	39%
BLUEBERRY										
(Hostess)	1 piece	420	4.0	59.0	360	2.4	18.0	9.0	15	39%
(Tastykake) 4 oz	1 piece	308	2.8	55.0	410	2.1	9.4	2.1	0	27%
BLUEBERRY APPLE *(Drake's)* approx 2 oz	1 piece	210	2.0	30.0	135	(mq)	10.0	2.0	0	41%
CHERRY										
(Break Cake) 'Fried Pie' 4.5 oz	2 pies	410	5.0	64.0	370	na	16.0	4.3	0	34%
(Hostess)	1 piece	460	4.0	65.0	380	2.4	20.0	9.0	15	40%
(Tastykake) 4 oz	1 piece	298	3.0	48.8	306	2.0	9.7	2.2	0	30%
CHERRY APPLE *(Drake's)* approx 2 oz	1 piece	220	2.0	30.0	135	(mq)	10.0	2.0	0	41%
CHOCOLATE PUDDING										
(Hostess) chocolate pudding	1 piece	490	5.0	76.0	439	(mq)	19.0	(mq)	21	35%
(Tastykake) chocolate pudding, 4.2 oz	1 piece	443	6.0	68.3	(mq)	(mq)	16.2	(mq)	na	33%
COCONUT CREME *(Tastykake)* 4 oz	1 piece	377	4.9	46.0	416	2.3	20.2	5.2	65	47%
LEMON										
(Break Cake) 'Fried Pie' 4.5 oz	2 pies	490	5.0	66.0	370	na	23.0	3.4	0	42%
(Drake's) approx 2 oz	1 piece	210	2.0	27.0	115	(mq)	11.0	2.0	0	46%
(Hostess)	1 piece	440	4.0	60.0	370	1.4	20.0	10.0	30	41%
(Tastykake) 4 oz	1 piece	319	3.6	48.1	375	1.7	13.2	2.9	39	37%
LEMON-LIME *(Tastykake)* 4 oz	1 piece	310	3.3	54.1	329	.2	8.8	(mq)	55	26%
MARSHMALLOW BANANA										
(Little Debbie) 3 oz	1 piece	360	3.0	60.0	180	(mq)	12.0	(mq)	<1	30%
(Little Debbie) 1.4 oz	1 piece	170	1.0	28.0	85	(mq)	6.0	(mq)	<1	32%
MARSHMALLOW CHOCOLATE										
(Little Debbie) 3 oz	1 piece	370	3.0	59.0	170	(mq)	13.0	(mq)	<1	32%
(Little Debbie) 1.4 oz	1 piece	170	1.0	28.0	85	(mq)	6.0	(mq)	<1	32%
MISSISSIPPI MUD *(Pepperidge Farm)* frozen 'American Collection'	1 ramekin	310	3.0	23.0	60	(mq)	23.0	12.0	45	67%
OATMEAL CREME										
(Little Debbie) 1.33 oz	1 piece	160	2.0	25.0	125	(mq)	6.0	(mq)	<1	33%
(Little Debbie) 2.75 oz	1 piece	350	4.0	51.0	260	(mq)	14.0	(mq)	<1	36%
PEACH										
(Hostess)	1 piece	420	4.0	60.0	360	2.0	19.0	9.0	15	40%
(Tastykake) 4 oz	1 piece	310	3.3	54.1	329	.2	8.8	(mq)	55	26%
PECAN										
(Little Debbie) 1.83 oz	1 piece	170	2.0	37.0	200	(mq)	2.0	(mq)	<1	10%

Food Name	Serving Size	Calories	Prot. gms	Carbs gms	Sod. mgs	Fiber gms	Fat gms	Sat. Fat gms	Chol. mgs	% Fat Cal.
(Little Debbie) 3 oz	1 piece	280	3.0	60.0	340	(mq)	3.0	(mq)	<1	10%
PINEAPPLE CHEESE *(Tastykake)* 4.2 oz	1 piece	343	4.5	53.9	405	2.2	13.2	3.3	19	34%
PUMPKIN *(Tastykake)* 4 oz	1 piece	324	4.5	46.5	520	1.9	14.2	4.1	28	39%
RAISIN CREME										
(Little Debbie) 2.5 oz	1 piece	290	2.0	47.0	190	(mq)	10.0	(mq)	<1	32%
(Little Debbie) 1.17 oz	1 piece	140	1.0	21.0	90	(mq)	6.0	(mq)	<1	38%
STRAWBERRY										
(Hostess)	1 piece	410	4.0	56.0	360	2.2	19.0	9.0	15	42%
(Tastykake) 4 oz	1 piece	342	3.1	57.4	303	.6	11.4	2.7	0	30%
PIE CRUST										
Mix										
(Betty Crocker) dry	1/16 pkg	120	1.0	10.0	140	(mq)	8.0	2.0	0	62%
(Flako) prepared	1 serving	247	3.7	24.4	393	1.2	15.0	4.5	9	55%
(General Mills) dry	1/16 pkg	120	1.0	10.0	150	na	8.0	na	0	62%
(Krusteaz) 9-inch pie	1/8 shell	90	1.0	10.0	120	.1	5.0	na	0	51%
(Nabisco) chocolate cookie crumbs 'Oreo' dry	2 tbsp	80	1.0	13.0	140	na	3.0	<1.0	0	33%
(Nabisco) graham crumbs 'Honey Maid' dry	2 1/2 tbsp	70	1.0	13.0	90	na	2.0	<1.0	0	24%
(Nabisco) wafer crumbs 'Nilla' dry	2 tbsp	70	1.0	12.0	55	na	2.0	<1.0	5	26%
(Pillsbury) dry	1/8 pkg	200	3.0	20.0	300	na	13.0	3.0	0	56%
Shell										
(Mrs. Smith's) 8-inch pie	1/8 shell	80	1.0	8.0	105	(mq)	5.0	1.0	0	56%
(Mrs. Smith's) '9-inch pie'	1/8 shell	90	1.0	10.0	125	(mq)	5.0	1.0	0	51%
(Mrs. Smith's) '9 5/8-inch pie'	1/8 shell	120	2.0	12.0	160	(mq)	7.0	2.0	0	53%
(Oronoque) deep dish, 9-inch pie	1/6 shell	130	2.0	11.0	130	na	9.0	2.0	0	61%
(Oronoque) regular, 9-inch pie	1/6 shell	120	2.0	9.0	115	na	8.0	2.0	0	62%
(Pet-Ritz)	1/6 shell	110	1.0	11.0	110	(mq)	7.0	(mq)	7	57%
(Pet-Ritz) all vegetable shortening	1/6 shell	110	2.0	10.0	60	(mq)	8.0	2.0	0	60%
(Pet-Ritz) deep dish, 1 oz	1/6 shell	130	1.0	12.0	120	(mq)	8.0	(mq)	7	58%
(Pet-Ritz) deep dish, whole-grain	1/6 shell	130	1.0	14.0	125	(mq)	8.0	(mq)	na	55%
(Pet-Ritz) graham cracker	1/6 shell	110	1.0	8.0	80	(mq)	6.0	(mq)	7	60%
(Pet-Ritz) 9 5/8-inch pie	1/6 shell	170	2.0	15.0	180	(mq)	11.0	(mq)	7	59%
(Pet-Ritz) tart	3-inch shell	150	3.0	12.0	150	(mq)	10.0	(mq)	7	60%
(Pet-Ritz) vegetable shortening, deep dish	1/6 shell	140	2.0	12.0	75	(mq)	9.0	2.0	0	59%
(Pillsbury) 'All Ready' 2-crust pie	1/8 shell	240	2.0	24.0	210	(mq)	15.0	(mq)	15	57%
Stick *(Betty Crocker)*	1/8 stick	120	1.0	10.0	140	(mq)	8.0	2.0	0	62%
PIE FILLING										
(NOTE: All pie fillings are canned unless otherwise noted.)										
APPLE										
(Comstock)	3.5 oz	120	0.0	30.0	15	.4	0.0	0.0	0	0%
(Comstock) 'Lite'	3.5 oz	80	0.0	20.0	10	.4	0.0	0.0	0	0%
(Lucky Leaf)	4 oz	120	0.0	30.0	60	(mq)	0.0	0.0	0	0%
(Lucky Leaf) apple turnover, diced	4 oz	120	0.0	30.0	60	(mq)	0.0	0.0	0	0%
(Lucky Leaf) 'Deluxe'	4 oz	120	0.0	35.0	40	(mq)	0.0	0.0	0	0%
(Lucky Leaf) 'Plus'	4 oz	121	0.3	30.2	24	(mq)	0.0	0.0	0	0%
(Musselman's)	4 oz	120	0.0	30.0	60	(mq)	0.0	0.0	0	0%
(Musselman's) apple turnover, diced	4 oz	120	0.0	30.0	60	(mq)	0.0	0.0	0	0%
(Musselman's) 'Deluxe'	4 oz	120	0.0	35.0	40	(mq)	0.0	0.0	0	0%
(Musselman's) 'Plus'	4 oz	121	0.3	30.2	24	(mq)	0.0	0.0	0	0%
(Pathmark) 'No Frills'	4 oz	130	0.0	33.0	60	(mq)	0.0	0.0	0	0%
(White House)	3.5 oz	121	0.0	29.0	44	(mq)	1.0	(tr)	0	7%
APRICOT										
(Comstock)	3.5 oz	110	0.0	29.0	100	.4	0.0	0.0	0	0%
(Lucky Leaf)	4 oz	150	0.0	39.0	90	(mq)	0.0	0.0	0	0%
(Musselman's)	4 oz	150	0.0	39.0	90	(mq)	0.0	0.0	0	0%

Food Name	Serving Size	Calories	Prot. gms	Carbs gms	Sod. mgs	Fiber gms	Fat gms	Sat. Fat gms	Chol. mgs	% Fat Cal.
BANANA *(Comstock)*	3.5 oz	110	1.0	22.0	300	.5	2.0	(tr)	0	16%
BLACKBERRY										
(Lucky Leaf)	4 oz	120	1.0	31.0	140	(mq)	0.0	0.0	0	0%
(Lucky Leaf) 'Plus'	4 oz	121	0.9	30.1	20	(mq)	0.0	0.0	0	0%
(Musselman's)	4 oz	120	1.0	31.0	140	(mq)	0.0	0.0	0	0%
(Musselman's) 'Plus'	4 oz	121	0.9	30.1	20	(mq)	0.0	0.0	0	0%
BLUEBERRY										
(Comstock)	3.5 oz	110	0.0	28.0	15	.5	0.0	0.0	0	0%
(Comstock) 'Lite'	3.5 oz	75	0.0	17.0	15	.6	0.0	0.0	0	0%
(Lucky Leaf) cultivated	4 oz	120	1.0	31.0	150	(mq)	0.0	0.0	0	0%
(Lucky Leaf) 'Plus'	4 oz	145	0.3	35.2	17	(mq)	0.0	0.0	0	0%
(Musselman's) cultivated	4 oz	120	1.0	31.0	150	(mq)	0.0	0.0	0	0%
(Musselman's) 'Plus'	4 oz	145	0.3	35.2	17	(mq)	0.0	0.0	0	0%
(White House)	3.5 oz	118	0.0	28.0	48	(mq)	1.0	(tr)	0	7%
BOYSENBERRY										
(Lucky Leaf)	4 oz	120	1.0	31.0	140	(mq)	0.0	0.0	0	0%
(Musselman's)	4 oz	120	1.0	31.0	140	(mq)	0.0	0.0	0	0%
CHERRY										
(Comstock)	3.5 oz	110	0.0	28.0	15	.3	0.0	0.0	0	0%
(Comstock) 'Lite'	3.5 oz	75	0.0	19.0	15	.3	0.0	0.0	0	0%
(Lucky Leaf)	4 oz	120	1.0	29.0	50	(mq)	0.0	0.0	0	0%
(Musselman's)	4 oz	120	1.0	29.0	50	(mq)	0.0	0.0	0	0%
(Musselman's) 'Plus'	4 oz	108	0.8	26.0	10	(mq)	0.2	(tr)	0	2%
(Pathmark) 'No Frills'	4 oz	130	0.0	33.0	60	(mq)	0.0	0.0	0	0%
(White House)	3.5 oz	141	0.0	33.0	54	(mq)	1.0	(tr)	0	6%
CHOCOLATE *(Comstock)*	3.5 oz	130	1.0	26.0	240	.2	3.0	(mq)	0	20%
COCONUT *(Comstock)*	3.5 oz	120	1.0	22.0	290	.2	3.0	(mq)	0	23%
GOOSEBERRY										
(Lucky Leaf)	4 oz	180	0.0	45.0	30	(mq)	0.0	0.0	0	0%
(Musselman's)	4 oz	180	0.0	45.0	30	(mq)	0.0	0.0	0	0%
LEMON										
(Comstock)	3.5 oz	140	0.0	34.0	110	.1	1.0	(tr)	0	6%
(Lucky Leaf)	4 oz	200	0.0	48.0	235	(mq)	2.0	(mq)	na	9%
(Lucky Leaf) 'French'	4 oz	180	0.0	42.0	140	(mq)	1.0	(tr)	na	5%
(Musselman's)	4 oz	200	0.0	48.0	235	(mq)	2.0	(mq)	na	9%
(Musselman's) 'French'	4 oz	180	0.0	42.0	140	(mq)	1.0	(tr)	na	5%
MINCEMEAT										
(Comstock)	3.5 oz	150	0.0	39.0	180	.7	1.0	(tr)	0	6%
(Lucky Leaf)	4 oz	190	0.0	48.0	145	(mq)	1.0	(tr)	na	5%
(Musselman's)	4 oz	190	0.0	48.0	145	(mq)	1.0	(tr)	na	5%
(None Such)	1/3 cup	200	1.0	48.0	280	(mq)	1.0	(tr)	na	4%
(None Such) condensed	1/4 pkg	220	1.0	50.0	310	(mq)	2.0	(mq)	na	8%
(None Such) w/brandy and rum	1/3 cup	220	1.0	48.0	260	(mq)	2.0	(mq)	na	8%
(S&W) w/brandy, 'Old Fashioned'	4 oz	234	1.1	55.6	234	(mq)	2.3	(mq)	na	8%
PEACH										
(Comstock)	3.5 oz	110	0.0	26.0	20	.2	0.0	0.0	0	0%
(Lucky Leaf)	4 oz	150	0.0	37.0	65	(mq)	0.0	0.0	0	0%
(Lucky Leaf) 'Plus'	4 oz	113	0.7	27.4	16	(mq)	0.0	0.0	0	0%
(Musselman's)	4 oz	150	0.0	37.0	65	(mq)	0.0	0.0	0	0%
(Musselman's) 'Plus'	4 oz	113	0.7	27.4	16	(mq)	0.0	0.0	0	0%
(White House)	3.5 oz	117	0.0	28.0	30	(mq)	1.0	(tr)	0	7%
PINEAPPLE										
(Comstock)	3.5 oz	100	0.0	28.0	65	.4	0.0	0.0	0	0%
(Lucky Leaf)	4 oz	110	0.0	30.0	65	(mq)	0.0	0.0	0	0%

Food Name	Serving Size	Calories	Prot. gms	Carbs gms	Sod. mgs	Fiber gms	Fat gms	Sat. Fat gms	Chol. mgs	% Fat Cal.
(Musselman's)	4 oz	110	0.0	30.0	65	(mq)	0.0	0.0	0	0%
PUMPKIN										
(Comstock)	3.5 oz	100	0.0	24.0	180	(mq)	0.0	0.0	0	0%
(Libby's)	1 cup	260	2.0	64.0	0	(mq)	0.3	0.0	440	1%
(Lucky Leaf)	4 oz	170	1.0	33.0	200	(mq)	4.0	(mq)	na	21%
(Musselman's)	4 oz	170	1.0	33.0	200	(mq)	4.0	(mq)	na	21%
(Stokely)	1/2 cup	170	1.0	44.0	420	(mq)	0.0	0.0	0	0%
RAISIN										
(Comstock)	3.5 oz	120	0.0	32.0	80	(mq)	0.0	0.0	0	0%
(Lucky Leaf)	4 oz	130	1.0	34.0	120	(mq)	1.0	(tr)	na	6%
(Musselman's)	4 oz	130	1.0	34.0	120	(mq)	1.0	(tr)	na	6%
RASPBERRY, BLACK										
(Lucky Leaf)	4 oz	190	0.0	43.0	50	(mq)	0.0	0.0	0	0%
(Musselman's)	4 oz	190	0.0	43.0	50	(mq)	0.0	0.0	0	0%
RASPBERRY, RED										
(Lucky Leaf)	4 oz	190	0.0	46.0	80	(mq)	0.0	0.0	0	0%
(Musselman's)	4 oz	190	0.0	46.0	80	(mq)	0.0	0.0	0	0%
STRAWBERRY										
(Comstock)	3.5 oz	100	0.0	25.0	20	.6	0.0	0.0	0	0%
(Lucky Leaf)	4 oz	120	0.0	30.0	75	(mq)	0.0	0.0	0	0%
(Lucky Leaf) 'Plus'	4 oz	138	0.9	33.5	17	(mq)	0.0	0.0	0	0%
(Musselman's)	4 oz	120	0.0	30.0	75	(mq)	0.0	0.0	0	0%
(Musselman's) 'Plus'	4 oz	138	0.9	33.5	17	(mq)	0.0	0.0	0	0%
STRAWBERRY-RHUBARB										
(Lucky Leaf) strawberry-rhubarb	4 oz	120	0.0	31.0	95	(mq)	0.0	0.0	0	0%
(Musselman's) strawberry-rhubarb	4 oz	120	0.0	31.0	95	(mq)	0.0	0.0	0	0%
PIE MIX										
BANANA CREAM										
(Jell-O) 'No Bake' dry	1 pkg	140	1.0	25.0	190	na	5.0	na	0	30%
(Jell-O) 'No Bake' prepared	1/8 pie	240	3.0	27.0	300	(mq)	14.0	(mq)	30	51%
BOSTON CREAM										
(Betty Crocker) 'Classic' dry	1/8 pkg	230	1.0	48.0	370	na	4.0	na	0	16%
(Betty Crocker) 'Classic' prepared w/egg and 2% milk	1/8 pkg	270	4.0	50.0	390	na	6.0	na	30	20%
(Jell-O) mousse 'No Bake' dry	1 pkg	160	2.0	22.0	320	na	7.0	na	0	40%
(Jell-O) mousse 'No Bake' prepared	1/8 pie	260	4.0	25.0	430	(mq)	17.0	(mq)	30	57%
CHOCOLATE										
(Royal) chocolate mint 'No-Bake' prepared	1/8 pie	260	5.0	25.0	280	(mq)	15.0	(mq)	na	53%
(Royal) mousse 'No-Bake' prepared	1/8 pie	230	4.0	27.0	260	(mq)	12.0	(mq)	na	47%
COCONUT CREAM										
(Jell-O) 'No Bake' dry	1 pkg	160	1.0	25.0	200	na	7.0	na	0	38%
(Jell-O) 'No Bake' prepared	1/8 pie	260	3.0	27.0	300	(mq)	16.0	(mq)	30	55%
KEY LIME (Royal) dry	1 serving	50	0.0	13.0	120	na	0.0	0.0	0	0%
LEMON										
(Royal) dry	1 serving	50	0.0	13.0	120	0	0.0	0.0	0	0%
(Royal) lemon meringue 'No Bake' prepared	1/8 pie	310	3.0	50.0	250	(mq)	11.0	(mq)	na	32%
PUMPKIN										
(Jell-O) 'No Bake' dry	1 pkg	140	1.0	28.0	330	na	3.0	na	0	10%
(Jell-O) 'No Bake' prepared	1/8 pie	250	4.0	31.0	450	(mq)	13.0	(mq)	30	46%
(Libby's) prepared	1/6 pie	390	7.0	53.0	70	(mq)	17.0	5.0	380	39%
VANILLA CREME										
(Lucky Leaf) prepared	4 oz	150	0.0	32.0	145	(mq)	3.0	(mq)	na	17%
(Musselman's) prepared	4 oz	150	0.0	32.0	145	(mq)	3.0	(mq)	na	17%
PIEROGIES, FROZEN										
pasta pocket, potato and American cheese filled (Mrs. T's)	1 pocket	70	3.0	10.0	180	na	2.0	na	5	26%

Food Name	Serving Size	Calories	Prot. gms	Carbs gms	Sod. mgs	Fiber gms	Fat gms	Sat. Fat gms	Chol. mgs	% Fat Cal.
pasta pocket, potato and cheddar cheese filled *(Mrs. T's)*	1 pocket	60	2.0	11.0	170	8.0	<1.0	na	2	<15%
pasta pocket, potato and onion filled *(Mrs. T's)*	1 pocket	50	2.0	10.0	140	na	<1.0	na	2	<16%
pasta pocket, sauerkraut filled *(Mrs. T's)*	1 pocket	50	2.0	9.0	220	na	<1.0	na	0	<17%
PIGEON. See SQUAB.										
PIGNOLIA. See PINE NUT.										
PIG'S EAR										
frozen, raw	1 oz	66	6.4	0.0	54	0	4.3	(mq)	23	60%
frozen, simmered	4 oz	188	18.1	0.0	189	0	12.2	(mq)	102	60%
PIG'S FEET										
pickled *(Penrose)*	6 oz	220	19.0	2.0	2890	0	15.0	(mq)	(mq)	62%
pickled, cured	1 lb	921	61.3	0.1	4187	0	73.2	25.3	417	73%
pickled, cured	1 oz	58	3.8	0.0	262	0	4.6	1.6	26	73%
raw	1 oz	75	6.3	0.0	18	0	5.3	1.8	30	65%
simmered	5 oz	275	27.3	0.0	43	0	17.6	6.1	142	59%
PIG'S HEART										
braised	1 cup	215	34.2	0.6	51	0	7.3	1.9	320	32%
braised	4 oz	168	26.8	0.5	40	0	5.7	1.5	251	32%
raw	1 oz	33	4.9	0.4	16	0	1.2	0.3	37	34%
PIG'S JOWL, raw	1 oz	186	1.8	0.0	7	0	19.7	7.2	26	96%
PIG'S KNUCKLES, pickled *(Penrose)*	6 oz	290	23.0	1.0	2380	0	21.0	(mq)	(mq)	66%
PIG'S TAIL										
raw	1 oz	107	5.0	0.0	18	0	9.5	3.3	28	81%
simmered	3 oz	337	14.4	0.0	21	0	30.4	10.6	110	83%
PIG'S TONGUE										
braised	3 oz	230	20.5	0.0	93	0	15.8	5.5	124	63%
cured, '8-lb can' *(Hormel)*	3 oz	190	17.0	0.0	966	0	13.0	(mq)	(mq)	63%
raw	1 oz	64	4.6	0.0	31	0	4.9	1.7	29	71%
PIKE, NORTHERN										
dry-heat cooked	3 oz	96	21.0	0.0	42	0	0.8	0.1	43	8%
raw	1 lb	401	87.3	0.0	177	0	3.1	0.5	177	7%
raw	3 oz	75	16.4	0.0	33	0	0.6	0.1	33	8%
raw	1 oz	25	5.5	0.0	11	0	0.2	<.1	11	8%
PIKE, WALLEYE										
dry-heat cooked	3 oz	101	20.9	0.0	55	0	1.3	0.3	94	12%
raw	1 lb	420	86.8	0.0	230	0	5.5	1.1	390	13%
raw	3 oz	79	16.3	0.0	43	0	1.0	0.2	73	12%
raw	1 oz	26	5.4	0.0	14	0	0.3	<.1	24	11%
PILAF DINNER, CANNED										
oat bran, w/garden vegetables 'Fast Menu' *(Health Valley)*	7.5 oz	210	8.0	31.0	445	5.8	7.0	(mq)	0	29%
PILAF MIX										
lentil, approx 1/2 cup cooked or 1 oz dry *(Casbah)*	1 serving	100	5.0	20.0	(mq)	(mq)	0.0	0.0	0	0%
three-grain, w/herbs, prepared w/salted butter										
(Quick Pilaf)	1/2 cup	142	3.0	24.0	324	(mq)	4.0	(mq)	(mq)	25%
three-grain, w/herbs, prepared w/o butter *(Quick Pilaf)* ...	1/2 cup	110	3.0	24.0	278	(mq)	0.6	na	0	5%
PILI NUT, CANARY TREE										
dried	1 cup	863	13.0	4.8	4	>3.4 c	95.5	37.4	0	92%
dried, 15 kernels	1 oz	204	3.1	1.1	1	>.8 c	22.6	8.9	0	92%
dried, in shell	1 lb	619	9.3	3.4	3	>2.4 c	68.5	26.8	0	92%
PIMIENTO, CAN OR JAR										
....	2 oz	13	0.6	2.9	8	>.6 c	0.2	<.1	0	11%
....	1 tbsp	3	0.1	0.6	2	>.1 c	<.1	tr	0	<24%
all varieties, drained *(Dromedary)*	1 oz	10	0.0	2.0	5	(mq)	0.0	0.0	0	0%
PIMIENTO SPREAD *(Price's)*	1 oz	80	3.0	2.0	na	na	6.0	(mq)	(mq)	73%
PIÑA COLADA. See ALCOHOLIC BEVERAGES.										

Food Name	Serving Size	Calories	Prot. gms	Carbs gms	Sod. mgs	Fiber gms	Fat gms	Sat. Fat gms	Chol. mgs	% Fat Cal.
PINE NUT/Colorado pinyon pine nut/Italian stone pine nut/pignolia/pinocchio/piñon										
whole	1 oz	161	3.3	5.5	20	3.0	17.3	2.7	0	82%
whole	1 tbsp	52	2.4	1.4	0	.4	5.1	0.8	0	75%
whole	10 kernels	6	0.1	0.2	1	.1	0.6	0.1	0	82%
PINEAPPLE										
candied, approx 1/2 cup	4-oz container	357	0.9	90.4	7	>.9 c	0.5	0.0	0	1%
raw, diced pieces	1 cup	76	0.6	19.2	2	1.9	0.7	0.1	0	7%
raw, 3 1/2 inch diam	1 slice	41	0.3	10.4	1	1.0	0.4	0.0	0	8%
raw, 3 1/2 inch diam, 3/4 inch thick (Del Monte)	2 slices	90	1.0	24.0	5	(mq)	0.0	0.0	0	0%
trimmed	1 oz	14	0.1	3.5	<1	.3	0.1	tr	0	6%
untrimmed	1 lb	117	0.9	29.2	2	2.8	1.0	0.1	0	7%
untrimmed (Dole)	2 slices	90	1.0	21.0	10	2.0	1.0	na	na	9%
PINEAPPLE, CANNED										
chunks	1/2 cup	75	0.5	19.6	2	.9	0.1	tr	0	1%
chunks (A&P)	1/2 cup	70	<1.0	18.0	10	(mq)	<1.0	(tr)	0	<11%
chunks, unsweetened 'Hawaiian' (Pathmark)	1/2 cup	70	0.0	18.0	10	(mq)	0.0	0.0	0	0%
crushed (A&P)	1/2 cup	70	<1.0	18.0	10	(mq)	<1.0	(tr)	0	<11%
crushed (Empress)	1/2 cup	70	0.0	18.0	10	(mq)	0.0	0.0	0	0%
crushed, unsweetened 'Hawaiian' (Pathmark)	1/2 cup	70	0.0	18.0	10	(mq)	0.0	0.0	0	0%
'Fruit Pak' (Mott's)	3.75 oz	86	0.0	21.0	2	(mq)	0.0	0.0	0	0%
in extra heavy syrup	4 oz	94	0.4	24.4	1	>.5 c	0.1	<.1	0	1%
in extra heavy syrup, chunks	1/2 cup	109	0.4	28.0	2	>.6 c	0.1	<.1	0	1%
in extra heavy syrup, chunks, w/liquid	1 cup	216	0.9	55.9	3	>1.1 c	0.3	0.0	0	1%
in extra heavy syrup, crushed	1/2 cup	109	0.4	28.0	2	>.6 c	0.1	<.1	0	1%
in extra heavy syrup, w/1.25 tbsp liquid	1 slice	48	0.2	12.5	1	>.3 c	0.1	0.0	0	2%
in heavy syrup	4 oz	88	0.4	22.9	1	>.5 c	0.1	<.1	0	1%
in heavy syrup, chunks (A&P)	1/2 cup	90	<1.0	23.0	10	(mq)	<1.0	(tr)	0	<9%
in heavy syrup, chunks 'Hawaiian' (Pathmark)	1/2 cup	90	0.0	23.0	10	(mq)	0.0	0.0	0	0%
in heavy syrup, chunks, tidbits, or crushed	1/2 cup	100	0.5	25.8	2	>.6 c	0.1	<.1	0	1%
in heavy syrup, chunks or crushed, w/liquid	1 cup	199	0.9	51.5	3	1.8	0.3	0.0	0	1%
in heavy syrup, crushed (A&P)	1/2 cup	90	<1.0	23.0	10	(mq)	<1.0	(tr)	0	<9%
in heavy syrup, slices (A&P)	2 slices	90	<1.0	23.0	10	(mq)	<1.0	(tr)	0	<9%
in heavy syrup, slices 'Hawaiian' (Pathmark)	1/2 cup	90	0.0	23.0	10	(mq)	0.0	0.0	0	0%
in heavy syrup, slices '100% Hawaiian' (S&W)	2 slices	90	0.0	23.0	0	(mq)	0.0	0.0	0	0%
in heavy syrup, w/1.25 tbsp liquid	1 slice	45	0.2	11.7	1	.4	0.1	0.0	0	2%
in juice	4 oz	68	0.5	17.8	1	.9	0.1	tr	0	1%
in juice, all cuts (Dole)	1/2 cup	70	0.5	17.5	1	(mq)	0.5	(tr)	0	6%
in juice, chunks (Del Monte)	1/2 cup	70	0.0	18.0	10	(mq)	0.0	0.0	0	0%
in juice, chunks or tidbits, w/liquid	1 cup	150	1.0	39.2	3	1.8	0.2	0.0	0	1%
in juice, crushed (Del Monte)	1/2 cup	70	0.0	18.0	10	(mq)	0.0	0.0	0	0%
in juice, slices (A&P)	2 slices	70	<1.0	18.0	10	(mq)	<1.0	(tr)	0	<11%
in juice, slices (Del Monte)	1/2 cup	70	0.0	18.0	10	(mq)	0.0	0.0	0	0%
in juice, slices (Featherweight)	1/2 cup	70	0.0	18.0	10	(mq)	0.0	0.0	0	0%
in juice, slices '100% Hawaiian' (S&W)	1/2 cup	70	0.0	17.0	10	(mq)	0.0	0.0	0	0%
in juice, tidbits (Del Monte)	1/2 cup	70	0.0	18.0	10	(mq)	0.0	0.0	0	0%
in juice, w/1.25 tbsp liquid	1 slice	35	0.2	9.1	1	.4	0.1	0.0	0	2%
in light syrup	1/2 cup	66	0.5	16.9	2	>.6 c	0.1	<.1	0	1%
in light syrup	4 oz	59	0.4	15.3	1	>.5 c	0.1	<.1	0	1%
in light syrup, w/liquid	1 cup	131	0.9	33.9	3	1.8	0.3	0.0	0	2%
in light syrup, w/1.75 tbsp liquid	1 slice	30	0.2	7.8	1	.4	0.1	0.0	0	3%
in pineapple juice (Dole)	1/2 cup	70	0.0	18.0	10	na	<1.0	na	na	<11%
in pineapple syrup (Dole)	1/2 cup	90	0.0	23.0	10	na	0.0	na	na	0%
in syrup, all cuts (Del Monte)	1/2 cup	90	0.0	23.0	10	(mq)	0.0	0.0	0	0%
in syrup, all cuts (Dole)	1/2 cup	95	0.4	24.8	2	(mq)	0.2	(tr)	0	2%

Food Name	Serving Size	Calories	Prot. gms	Carbs gms	Sod. mgs	Fiber gms	Fat gms	Sat. Fat gms	Chol. mgs	% Fat Cal.
in water	4 oz	36	0.5	9.4	1	>.5 c	0.1	tr	0	2%
in water, tidbits	1/2 cup	40	0.5	10.2	2	>.6 c	0.1	tr	0	2%
in water, tidbits, w/liquid	1 cup	79	1.1	20.4	2	1.7	0.2	0.0	0	2%
in water, w/1.25 tbsp liquid	1 slice	19	0.3	4.8	1	.4	0.1	0.0	0	4%
spears, approx 3.1 oz (Del Monte)	2 spears	50	0.0	14.0	10	(mq)	0.0	0.0	0	0%
spears or slices, unsweetened 'Hawaiian' (Pathmark)	1/2 cup	70	0.0	18.0	10	(mq)	0.0	0.0	0	0%
tidbits	1/2 cup	75	0.5	19.6	2	.9	0.1	tr	0	1%
unsweetened, slices (S&W Nutradiet)	1/2 cup	60	0.0	15.0	10	(mq)	0.0	0.0	0	0%
PINEAPPLE, FROZEN										
sweetened, chunks	1/2 cup	104	0.5	27.1	2	1.3	0.1	0.0	0	1%
sweetened, chunks	4 oz	96	0.5	25.2	2	>.3 c	0.1	tr	0	1%
PINEAPPLE CITRUS DRINK										
'Thirst Quencher Light' (Gatorade)	8 oz	25	0.0	7.0	80	na	0.0	na	na	0%
PINEAPPLE COCKTAIL JUICE										
w/banana 'Orchard Tropicals' (Welch's) bottled	6 oz	100	0.0	24.0	20	0	0.0	0.0	0	0%
w/banana 'Orchard Tropicals' (Welch's) boxed	8.45 oz	140	0.0	34.0	20	0	0.0	0.0	0	0%
w/banana 'Orchard Tropicals' (Welch's) frozen	6 oz	100	0.0	24.0	20	0	0.0	0.0	0	0%
w/grapefruit juice (Ocean Spray)	6 oz	110	0.0	26.0	5	(mq)	0.0	0.0	0	0%
PINEAPPLE COCONUT JUICE (Knudsen & Sons)	8 oz	110	<1.0	24.0	na	na	0.0	na	na	0%
PINEAPPLE DRINK										
frozen 'Bright & Early Pineapple' prepared (Bright & Early)	6 oz	90	0.0	23.0	0	na	0.0	na	na	0%
w/grapefruit (Tropicana)	6 oz	100	<1.0	24.0	10	na	<1.0	na	na	<8%
w/grapefruit juice	6 oz	90	0.6	21.6	24	tr	0.2	<.1	0	2%
w/grapefruit juice (Del Monte)	6 oz	90	0.0	24.0	50	(mq)	0.0	0.0	0	0%
w/grapefruit juice (Pathmark)	6 oz	80	0.0	21.0	0	(mq)	0.0	0.0	0	0%
w/grapefruit juice 'Single Serve' (Tropicana)	10 oz	159	(tr)	39.0	3	(mq)	0.0	0.0	0	0%
w/grapefruit juice 'Twister' (Tropicana)	8 oz	125	(tr)	32.0	2	(mq)	0.0	0.0	0	0%
w/pink grapefruit juice (Del Monte)	6 oz	90	0.0	24.0	50	(mq)	0.0	0.0	0	0%
PINEAPPLE GRAPEFRUIT JUICE										
canned	1 cup	117	0.5	29.0	35	.3	0.3	0.0	0	2%
canned	1 oz	15	0.1	3.6	4	tr	0.0	0.0	0	0%
PINEAPPLE JUICE										
Can, bottle, or box										
	6 oz	104	0.6	25.8	2	>.2 c	0.2	<.1	0	2%
(Dole)	6 oz	103	0.8	25.4	2	(mq)	0.2	(tr)	0	2%
(Knudsen & Sons)	8 oz	110	<1.0	25.0	na	na	0.0	na	na	0%
(Minute Maid)	6 oz	90	1.0	23.0	20	na	0.0	na	na	0%
(Mott's)	9.5 oz	169	0.0	42.0	0	(mq)	0.0	0.0	0	0%
50% juice (J. Hungerford)	9.03 oz	123	0.4	30.8	0	0	0.0	0.0	0	0%
float (Knudsen & Sons)	8 oz	130	2.0	31.0	na	na	0.0	na	na	0%
'Hawaiian' (Pathmark)	6 oz	100	0.0	25.0	10	(mq)	0.0	0.0	0	0%
'No Frills Unsweetened' (Pathmark)	6 oz	100	0.0	25.0	0	(mq)	0.0	0.0	0	0%
'100%' (Veryfine)	8 oz	125	0.7	31.0	10	(mq)	0.0	0.0	0	0%
100% juice (J. Hungerford)	9.03 oz	124	0.6	31.3	9	.3	0.0	0.0	0	0%
regular (J. Hungerford)	9.03 oz	114	0.4	28.6	0	0	0.0	0.0	0	0%
'Unsweetened' (Del Monte)	6 oz	100	0.0	25.0	10	(mq)	0.0	0.0	0	0%
'Unsweetened' (IGA)	6 oz	100	0.0	25.0	10	(mq)	0.0	0.0	0	0%
'Unsweetened' (S&W)	6 oz	100	0.0	25.0	0	(mq)	0.0	0.0	0	0%
unsweetened, w/added ascorbic acid	1 cup	140	0.8	34.4	3	.3	0.2	0.0	0	1%
unsweetened, w/added ascorbic acid	1 oz	18	0.1	4.3	0	0	0.0	0.0	0	0%
unsweetened, w/o added ascorbic acid	1 cup	140	0.8	34.4	3	.3	0.2	0.0	0	1%
unsweetened, w/o added ascorbic acid	1 oz	18	0.1	4.3	0	0	0.0	0.0	0	0%
Frozen or chilled										
(Dole)	6 oz	90	0.0	22.0	5	na	0.0	na	na	0%

Food Name	Serving Size	Calories	Prot. gms	Carbs gms	Sod. mgs	Fiber gms	Fat gms	Sat. Fat gms	Chol. mgs	% Fat Cal.
(Minute Maid)	6 oz	90	1.0	23.0	0	na	0.0	na	na	0%
concentrate (Dole) diluted	6 oz	100	0.0	25.0	7	(mq)	na	na	0	0%
unsweetened concentrate, diluted	1 cup	130	1.0	31.9	3	.3	0.1	0.0	0	1%
unsweetened concentrate, diluted	1 oz	16	0.1	4.0	0	0	0.0	0.0	0	0%
unsweetened concentrate, undiluted	6 oz	387	2.8	95.7	6	.7	0.2	0.0	0	1%
w/grapefruit (Dole)	6 oz	90	1.0	23.0	8	(mq)	na	na	0	0%
w/grapefruit '100% Pure' (Tropicana)	8 oz	120	(mq)	29.3	3	(mq)	0.0	0.0	0	0%
w/pink grapefruit (Dole)	6 oz	101	0.4	25.4	tr	(mq)	0.1	(tr)	0	1%
PINEAPPLE NECTAR (Libby's)	6 oz	110	0.0	27.0	na	na	0.0	na	30	0%
PINEAPPLE ORANGE DRINK										
	6 oz	96	2.4	22.2	6	0	0.0	0.0	0	0%
(Del Monte)	6 oz	90	0.0	24.0	20	0	0.0	0.0	0	0%
(Veryfine)	8 oz	130	0.0	32.0	10	(mq)	0.0	0.0	0	0%
PINEAPPLE ORANGE JUICE										
(Dole)	6 oz	100	1.0	23.0	8	(mq)	na	na	0	0%
chilled, carton (Dole)	6 oz	90	0.0	22.0	10	na	0.0	na	na	0%
chilled, w/banana, carton (Dole)	6 oz	100	0.0	23.0	10	na	0.0	na	na	0%
chilled, w/guava, carton (Dole)	6 oz	100	<1.0	21.0	10	na	0.0	na	na	0%
frozen, can (Dole)	6 oz	90	1.0	22.0	10	na	0.0	na	na	0%
frozen, w/banana, can (Dole)	6 oz	90	1.0	21.0	5	na	0.0	na	na	0%
frozen, w/guava, can (Dole)	6 oz	100	<1.0	22.0	10	na	0.0	na	na	0%
frozen or chilled (Minute Maid)	6 oz	90	1.0	23.0	0	na	0.0	na	na	0%
w/banana (Dole)	6 oz	90	0.8	23.0	5	(mq)	0.1	(tr)	0	1%
PINEAPPLE PASSION JUICE										
frozen, can, w/banana (Dole)	6 oz	100	<1.0	21.0	10	na	0.0	na	na	0%
frozen, carton, w/banana (Dole)	6 oz	100	<1.0	21.0	10	na	0.0	na	na	0%
PINEAPPLE TOPPING										
	1 cup	860	0.3	225.8	214	3.4	0.3	na	0	0%
	2 tbsp	106	0.0	27.9	26	.4	0.0	na	0	0%
(Kraft)	1 tbsp	50	0.0	13.0	0	(mq)	0.0	0.0	0	0%
(Smucker's)	2 tbsp	130	0.0	32.0	0	(mq)	0.0	0.0	0	0%
PINK BEAN										
boiled	4 oz	169	10.3	31.6	2	5.0	0.6	0.1	0	3%
mature seeds, boiled	1/2 cup	125	7.6	23.4	2	4.5	0.4	0.1	0	3%
mature seeds, raw	1/2 cup	360	22.0	67.4	8	13.3	1.2	0.3	0	3%
raw	1 oz	97	5.9	18.2	2	2.5	0.3	0.1	0	3%
PINOCCHIO. See PINE NUT.										
PIÑON. See PINE NUT.										
PINTO BEAN										
(Allens)	1/2 cup	105	5.0	18.0	480	(mq)	<1.0	na	0	<9%
boiled	4 oz	155	9.3	29.1	2	4.5	0.6	0.1	0	3%
boiled (A&P)	1 cup	230	17.0	42.0	5	na	1.0	na	0	4%
mature seeds, boiled	1/2 cup	116	7.0	21.8	2	7.3	0.4	0.1	0	3%
mature seeds, raw	1/2 cup	326	20.0	60.9	10	23.4	1.1	0.2	0	3%
raw	1 oz	96	5.9	18.0	3	3.4	0.3	0.1	0	3%
raw (Arrowhead Mills)	2 oz	200	13.0	36.0	3	11.2	1.0	na	0	4%
raw, dry (Evans)	1 cup	660	43.0	121.0	19	na	2.0	na	na	3%
sprouted, mature seeds, boiled, drained	4 oz	25	2.1	4.6	58	>1.1 c	0.4	<.1	0	12%
sprouted, mature seeds, raw	1 lb	280	23.8	52.6	694	>12.3 c	4.1	0.5	0	11%
sprouted, mature seeds, raw	1 oz	18	1.5	3.3	43	>.8 c	0.3	<.1	0	12%
Canned										
(Bush's Best)	1/2 cup	60	5.0	15.0	350	5.0	0.0	na	na	0%
(Gebhardt)	4 oz	197	12.8	35.7	608	(mq)	0.5	na	0	2%
(Green Giant)	1/2 cup	90	6.0	20.0	280	5.0	1.0	0.0	0	8%

Food Name	Serving Size	Calories	Prot. gms	Carbs gms	Sod. mgs	Fiber gms	Fat gms	Sat. Fat gms	Chol. mgs	% Fat Cal.
(Joan of Arc)	1/2 cup	90	6.0	20.0	280	5.2	1.0	na	0	8%
(Old El Paso)	1/2 cup	100	6.0	19.0	320	8.0	0.0	0.0	0	0%
(Progresso)	1/2 cup	110	8.0	21.0	410	6.5	<1.0	na	0	<7%
baked style, and Great Northern, w/pork *(Luck's)*	7.25 oz	200	12.0	29.0	822	(mq)	5.0	(mq)	(mq)	22%
baked style, w/pork, 15-oz can *(Luck's)*	7.5 oz	220	12.0	30.0	787	7.0	6.0	(mq)	(mq)	24%
baked style, w/pork, 29-oz can *(Luck's)*	7.25 oz	220	11.0	30.0	520	11.0	6.0	(mq)	(mq)	25%
mature seeds	1/2 cup	94	5.5	17.5	499	4.2	0.4	0.1	0	4%
organic, very low sodium, no salt added *(Eden Foods)*	1/2 cup	70	6.0	17.0	15	6.0	<1.0	na	0	<9%
organic, w/liquid *(Eden Foods)*	1/2 cup	110	6.0	20.0	20	6.4	<1.0	na	0	<8%
picante style *(Green Giant)*	1/2 cup	100	7.0	21.0	580	6.6	1.0	na	0	7%
picante style *(Joan of Arc)*	1/2 cup	100	7.0	21.0	580	6.6	1.0	na	0	7%
w/liquid	4 oz	88	5.2	16.5	472	>1.4 c	0.4	0.1	0	4%
Frozen										
	10-oz pkg	484	27.8	92.3	na	(mq)	1.4	0.2	0	3%
(Seabrook)	3.2 oz	160	9.0	29.0	na	(mq)	0.0	0.0	0	0%
boiled, drained	4 oz	184	10.6	35.0	na	(mq)	0.5	0.1	0	2%
immature seeds, boiled, drained, 10-oz pkg	1/3 pkg	152	8.8	29.0	78	>2.8 c	0.5	0.1	0	3%
immature seeds, unprepared, 10-oz pkg	1/3 pkg	160	9.2	30.6	86	5.4	0.5	0.1	0	3%
PISTACHIO BUTTER, roasted *(Maranatha Natural)*	2 tbsp	170	6.0	7.0	5	na	13.0	na	na	69%
PISTACHIO NUT										
In shell										
dried	1 lb	1309	46.7	56.3	13	24.5	109.7	13.9	0	71%
dried *(Dole)*	1 oz	90	3.0	3.0	250	na	7.0	na	na	72%
dried *(Fisher)*	1 oz	170	5.0	7.0	85	na	14.0	2.0	0	72%
dried *(Fisher)* red tint	1 oz	170	5.0	7.0	85	na	14.0	2.0	0	72%
dry-roasted	1 lb	1429	35.2	64.9	14	>4.3 c	124.5	15.8	0	74%
dry-roasted, salted	1 lb	1429	35.2	64.9	1840	>4.3 c	124.5	15.8	0	74%
Shelled										
dried	1 cup	739	26.3	31.8	8	13.8	61.9	7.8	0	71%
dried, approx 47 kernels	1 oz	164	5.8	7.1	2	3.1	13.7	1.7	0	71%
dry-roasted	1 cup	776	19.1	35.2	8	13.8	67.6	8.6	0	74%
dry-roasted	1 oz	172	4.2	7.8	2	3.1	15.0	1.9	0	74%
dry-roasted *(Dole)*	1 oz	163	6.0	7.0	2	(mq)	14.0	(mq)	0	71%
dry-roasted *(Planters)*	1 oz	170	5.0	6.0	250	(mq)	15.0	2.0	0	75%
dry-roasted, natural *(Planters)*	1 oz	170	6.0	6.0	250	na	14.0	2.0	0	72%
dry-roasted, red tint *(Planters)*	1 oz	170	6.0	6.0	250	na	14.0	2.0	0	72%
PITA BREAD. See BREAD.										
PITANGA / Surinam cherry										
raw	1 cup	57	1.4	13.0	5	>1.0 c	0.7	na	0	10%
raw, trimmed	1/2 cup	29	0.7	6.5	3	>.5 c	0.3	(tr)	0	9%
raw, trimmed	1 oz	9	0.2	2.1	1	>.2 c	0.1	(tr)	0	9%
raw, trimmed, approx .3 oz	1 med	2	0.1	0.5	0	tr	0.0	na	0	0%
raw, untrimmed	1 lb	132	3.2	29.9	11	>2.4 c	1.6	na	0	10%
PIZZA, FRENCH BREAD, FROZEN										
Canadian style bacon, 1 pkg *(Stouffer's)*	5.5 oz	370	18.0	40.0	1070	na	15.0	na	na	37%
cheese *(Healthy Choice)*	5.6 oz	300	21.0	48.0	500	na	3.0	2.0	20	9%
cheese *(Lean Cuisine)*	5 1/8 oz	300	17.0	38.0	310	na	9.0	3.0	15	27%
cheese *(Pappalo's)*	1 piece	360	16.0	40.0	830	(mq)	15.0	(mq)	(mq)	38%
cheese, microwave *(Oven Lovin')*	1 serving	350	17.0	40.0	700	na	14.0	5.0	15	36%
cheese 'Microwave' *(Pillsbury)*	1 piece	370	18.0	41.0	680	(mq)	15.0	(mq)	(mq)	36%
cheese, 1 pkg *(Stouffer's)*	5 1/8 oz	350	16.0	40.0	630	na	14.0	na	na	36%
cheese 'Zap' *(Banquet)*	4.5 oz	310	14.0	41.0	800	(mq)	10.0	(mq)	35	29%
combination *(Pappalo's)*	1 piece	430	19.0	41.0	1120	(mq)	21.0	(mq)	(mq)	44%
combination, microwave *(Oven Lovin')*	1 serving	420	18.0	41.0	910	na	21.0	10.0	30	45%

Food Name	Serving Size	Calories	Prot. gms	Carbs gms	Sod. mgs	Fiber gms	Fat gms	Sat. Fat gms	Chol. mgs	% Fat Cal.
deluxe (Healthy Choice)	6.25 oz	330	23.0	41.0	490	na	8.0	3.0	35	22%
deluxe (Lean Cuisine)	6 1/8 oz	350	22.0	40.0	580	na	11.0	4.0	30	29%
deluxe, 1 pkg (Stouffer's)	6 1/8 oz	420	21.0	40.0	950	na	19.0	na	na	41%
deluxe 'Zap' (Banquet)	4.8 oz	330	13.0	39.0	890	(mq)	13.0	(mq)	25	36%
double cheese, 1 pkg (Stouffer's)	5 7/8 oz	420	22.0	43.0	850	na	18.0	na	na	38%
hamburger, 1 pkg (Stouffer's)	6 oz	410	23.0	39.0	650	na	18.0	na	na	40%
Italian turkey sausage (Healthy Choice)	6.45 oz	320	23.0	42.0	440	na	7.0	3.0	30	20%
pepperoni (Healthy Choice)	6.25 oz	320	22.0	41.0	490	na	8.0	3.0	30	22%
pepperoni (Lean Cuisine)	5 1/4 oz	340	19.0	41.0	580	na	11.0	5.0	25	29%
pepperoni (Pappalo's)	1 piece	410	16.0	41.0	1130	(mq)	20.0	(mq)	(mq)	44%
pepperoni, microwave (Oven Lovin')	1 serving	410	18.0	40.0	980	na	21.0	8.0	35	45%
pepperoni 'Microwave' (Pillsbury)	1 piece	430	19.0	45.0	940	(mq)	19.0	(mq)	(mq)	40%
pepperoni, 1 pkg (Stouffer's)	5 3/4 oz	400	19.0	39.0	880	na	19.0	na	na	42%
pepperoni 'Zap' (Banquet)	4.5 oz	350	15.0	36.0	1060	(mq)	16.0	(mq)	40	41%
pepperoni and mushroom (Stouffer's)	6 oz	410	19.0	40.0	920	na	19.0	na	na	42%
sausage (Lean Cuisine)	6 oz	350	22.0	42.0	600	na	10.0	4.0	35	26%
sausage (Pappalo's)	1 piece	410	18.0	41.0	1000	(mq)	18.0	(mq)	(mq)	41%
sausage (Stouffer's)	6 oz	430	20.0	40.0	840	na	21.0	na	na	44%
sausage, microwave (Oven Lovin')	1 serving	400	18.0	41.0	830	na	20.0	10.0	25	43%
sausage 'Microwave' (Pillsbury)	1 piece	410	18.0	48.0	860	(mq)	16.0	(mq)	(mq)	35%
sausage and pepperoni (Stouffer's)	6.25 oz	460	23.0	41.0	920	na	23.0	na	na	45%
sausage combo, and pepperoni 'Microwave' (Pillsbury)	1 piece	450	19.0	47.0	950	(mq)	21.0	(mq)	(mq)	42%
three cheese (Lean Cuisine)	5.5 oz	330	23.0	38.0	350	na	10.0	3.0	20	27%
vegetable deluxe (Stouffer's)	6.5 oz	420	18.0	41.0	830	na	20.0	na	na	43%
PIZZA, FROZEN										
(Banquet)										
pepperoni 'Pizza Pie'	6-oz pie	470	11.0	45.0	970	na	27.0	na	35	52%
sausage 'Pizza Pie'	6-oz pie	500	11.0	48.0	860	na	29.0	na	35	53%
sausage and pepperoni 'Pizza Pie'	6-oz pie	470	12.0	43.0	930	na	27.0	na	40	53%
(Celeste)										
cheese	1/4 pie	315	14.0	28.0	690	2.2	17.0	7.0	20	48%
cheese 'Pizza for One'	1 pie	500	21.0	48.0	1070	3.6	25.0	11.0	40	45%
deluxe	1/4 pie	380	16.0	29.0	870	3.1	22.0	7.0	20	52%
deluxe 'Pizza for One'	1 pie	580	23.0	51.0	1290	4.4	32.0	10.0	20	49%
four cheese, original 'Pizza for One'	1 pie	540	25.0	47.0	1500	na	30.0	na	50	48%
four cheese, zesty 'Pizza for One'	1 pie	550	24.0	45.0	1500	na	31.0	na	50	50%
pepperoni	1/4 pie	370	15.0	29.0	940	2.4	21.0	7.0	15	52%
pepperoni 'Pizza for One'	1 pie	545	20.0	50.0	1290	3.9	30.0	9.0	20	49%
sausage	1/4 pie	375	16.0	30.0	900	3.3	22.0	7.0	15	52%
sausage 'Pizza for One'	1 pie	570	23.0	49.0	1300	4.2	32.0	10.0	20	50%
suprema	1/4 pie	380	17.0	29.0	970	3.0	24.0	7.0	15	54%
suprema 'Pizza for One'	1 pie	680	27.0	54.0	1590	4.5	39.0	12.0	20	52%
vegetable 'Pizza for One'	1 pie	490	20.0	44.0	1200	na	26.0	na	na	48%
(Jeno's)										
combination 'Crisp 'N Tasty'	1/2 pizza	280	10.0	27.0	680	1.0	15.0	4.0	15	48%
pepperoni 'Crisp 'N Tasty'	1/2 pizza	280	10.0	28.0	710	1.0	15.0	4.0	15	47%
pepperoni 'Pizza Pocket'	1 serving	370	12.0	35.0	700	na	20.0	6.0	25	49%
sausage 'Crisp 'N Tasty'	1/2 pizza	280	10.0	27.0	640	1.0	15.0	3.0	10	48%
sausage 'Pizza Pocket'	1 serving	360	11.0	35.0	660	na	19.0	7.0	15	48%
sausage and pepperoni 'Pizza Pocket'	1 serving	360	12.0	35.0	710	na	20.0	7.0	20	49%
supreme 'Pizza Pocket'	1 serving	370	12.0	36.0	720	na	19.0	7.0	20	47%
(Oven Lovin')										
cheese, microwave	1/2 pie	250	11.0	24.0	430	na	12.0	4.0	10	44%
combination, microwave	1/2 pie	310	13.0	26.0	580	na	18.0	7.0	20	51%

Food Name	Serving Size	Calories	Prot. gms	Carbs gms	Sod. mgs	Fiber gms	Fat gms	Sat. Fat gms	Chol. mgs	% Fat Cal.
pepperoni, microwave	1/2 pie	300	13.0	25.0	620	na	17.0	6.0	25	50%
sausage, microwave	1/2 pie	290	12.0	26.0	510	na	16.0	7.0	15	49%
supreme, microwave	1/2 pie	310	13.0	27.0	570	na	18.0	7.0	20	50%
(Pappalo's)										
pepperoni, 9 inch, traditional crust	1/2 pie	390	23.0	47.0	870	4.0	14.0	6.0	45	31%
pepperoni, 12 inch, traditional crust	1/4 pie	350	22.0	40.0	700	4.0	11.0	5.0	45	29%
pepperoni, pan pizza	1/6 pie	350	22.0	40.0	720	3.0	11.0	6.0	50	29%
sausage, 9 inch, traditional crust	1/2 pie	380	22.0	47.0	680	4.0	13.0	6.0	40	30%
sausage, 12 inch, traditional crust	1/4 pie	350	22.0	39.0	600	4.0	12.0	6.0	40	31%
sausage, pan pizza	1/5 pie	350	22.0	39.0	530	3.0	11.0	5.0	40	29%
sausage and pepperoni, 9 inch, traditional crust	1/2 pie	390	23.0	45.0	650	4.0	15.0	7.0	45	33%
sausage and pepperoni, 12 inch, traditional crust	1/4 pie	360	23.0	40.0	730	4.0	12.0	6.0	45	30%
sausage and pepperoni, pan pizza	1/5 pie	360	22.0	40.0	630	3.0	12.0	6.0	45	30%
supreme, 9 inch, traditional crust	1/2 pie	400	25.0	46.0	700	4.0	16.0	7.0	45	34%
supreme, 12 inch, traditional crust	1/4 pie	350	22.0	38.0	640	4.0	12.0	6.0	45	31%
supreme, pan pizza	1/5 pie	340	22.0	37.0	610	3.0	12.0	6.0	45	31%
three cheese, 9 inch, traditional crust	1/2 pie	350	21.0	47.0	640	4.0	11.0	6.0	30	27%
three cheese, 12 inch, traditional crust	1/4 pie	310	20.0	41.0	440	4.0	7.0	4.0	30	21%
three cheese, pan pizza	1/5 pie	310	20.0	39.0	490	3.0	8.0	5.0	30	23%
(Pepperidge Farm)										
cheese, croissant pastry	1 pie	430	15.0	41.0	640	(mq)	23.0	(mq)	(mq)	48%
deluxe, croissant pastry	1 pie	440	16.0	43.0	790	(mq)	23.0	(mq)	(mq)	47%
pepperoni, croissant pastry	1 pie	420	14.0	43.0	690	(mq)	22.0	(mq)	(mq)	47%
(Tombstone)										
bacon, Canadian style, 'Original' 12 inch	3.6 oz	230	12.0	23.0	580	na	10.0	4.0	25	39%
bacon cheeseburger, 'Special Order' 12 inch	4.7 oz	330	17.0	29.0	730	na	16.0	7.0	40	44%
cheese, microwave, 7 inch	7.7 oz	500	25.0	45.0	940	na	24.0	8.0	40	44%
cheese, original, 9 inch	5.6 oz	380	18.0	40.0	730	na	17.0	7.0	35	40%
cheese, 'Original' 12 inch	3.4 oz	230	11.0	23.0	460	na	10.0	4.0	25	40%
cheese, w/hamburger, 'Original', 12 inch	3.7 oz	250	13.0	23.0	570	na	12.0	5.0	30	43%
cheese, w/Italian sausage 'Italian Style Thincrust'	3.2 oz	220	11.0	15.0	490	na	13.0	5.0	30	53%
cheese, w/pepperoni 'Italian Style Thincrust'	3 oz	230	11.0	15.0	540	na	14.0	5.0	25	55%
cheese, w/pepperoni, 'Original' 12 inch	3.6 oz	260	12.0	23.0	620	na	14.0	5.0	30	47%
cheese, w/sausage, mushrooms, 'Original' 12 inch	3.8 oz	240	13.0	23.0	570	na	11.0	4.0	30	41%
cheese, w/sausage, 'Original' 12 inch	3.7 oz	240	13.0	23.0	590	na	11.0	4.0	30	41%
cheese and hamburger, original, 9 inch	6.3 oz	440	22.0	41.0	960	na	21.0	8.0	50	43%
cheese and pepperoni, microwave, 7 inch	7.5 oz	550	27.0	38.0	1240	na	32.0	11.0	55	53%
cheese and pepperoni, original, 9 inch	6.3 oz	480	21.0	40.0	1100	na	26.0	10.0	50	49%
cheese and sausage, original, 9 inch	6.3 oz	420	22.0	41.0	1000	na	19.0	7.0	50	40%
chicken, 'Light' 8 inch	4.5 oz	240	17.0	28.0	450	na	8.0	3.0	25	29%
chicken deluxe 'Light' approx 1/2 pizza	3.7 oz	180	13.0	23.0	440	2.0	4.0	1.0	15	20%
deluxe, original, 9 inch	7.0 oz	440	24.0	41.0	1010	na	20.0	7.0	55	41%
deluxe, 'Original' 12 inch	3.9 oz	240	13.0	23.0	570	na	11.0	4.0	30	41%
four cheese 'Special Order'	4.3 oz	300	15.0	28.0	630	na	14.0	6.0	35	42%
four meat 'Special Order'	4.6 oz	320	17.0	28.0	810	na	15.0	6.0	40	43%
four meat, 'Special Order' 9 inch	3.9 oz	280	14.0	24.0	670	na	14.0	6.0	35	45%
Italian sausage, microwave, 7 inch	8.0 oz	550	28.0	38.0	1210	na	32.0	10.0	65	52%
Italian sausage 'Special Order'	4.5 oz	300	17.0	28.0	740	na	13.0	6.0	40	39%
pepperoni, 'Double Top' w/double cheese , 12 inch	4.8 oz	360	20.0	24.0	920	na	20.0	8.0	50	51%
pepperoni 'Light' 8 inch	4.0 oz	250	16.0	27.0	630	na	10.0	4.0	20	34%
pepperoni 'Special Order'	4.4 oz	320	16.0	28.0	780	na	16.0	7.0	40	45%
pepperoni 'Special Order' 9 inch	3.7 oz	280	13.0	24.0	650	na	14.0	6.0	30	46%
pepperoni and sausage, original, 9 inch	6.6 oz	490	24.0	40.0	1230	na	26.0	10.0	60	48%
ranchero deluxe 'Mexican Style Thincrust'	3.4 oz	230	11.0	16.0	530	na	13.0	5.0	40	52%

Food Name	Serving Size	Calories	Prot. gms	Carbs gms	Sod. mgs	Fiber gms	Fat gms	Sat. Fat gms	Chol. mgs	% Fat Cal.
sausage, 'Double Top' w/double cheese, 12 inch	4.8 oz	330	21.0	24.0	860	na	16.0	6.0	50	44%
sausage, w/pepperoni, 'Original' 12 inch	3.7 oz	260	13.0	23.0	640	na	13.0	5.0	30	45%
sausage and pepperoni, 'Double Top' w/double cheese, 12 inch	4.8 oz	340	21.0	24.0	910	na	18.0	7.0	50	47%
sausage and pepperoni, microwave, 7 inch	8 oz	570	32.0	39.0	1430	na	32.0	11.0	70	50%
supreme 'Italian Style Thincrust'	3.38 oz	230	11.0	16.0	520	na	14.0	5.0	30	54%
supreme, 'Light' 8 inch	4.6 oz	250	17.0	26.0	660	na	9.0	3.0	20	32%
supreme, 'Light' 12 inch	4.5 oz	250	15.0	29.0	630	na	9.0	na	35	32%
supreme, microwave, 7 inch	8.5 oz	550	27.0	40.0	1260	na	31.0	10.0	55	51%
supreme, 'Original' 12 inch	3.8 oz	270	12.0	24.0	630	na	14.0	5.0	30	47%
supreme 'Special Order'	4.4 oz	320	17.0	29.0	800	na	15.0	6.0	40	42%
supreme, 'Special Order' 9 inch	4.0 oz	280	13.0	24.0	640	na	14.0	6.0	35	46%
taco, microwave, 7 inch	8.4 oz	590	28.0	41.0	1460	na	34.0	13.0	100	53%
three sausage, 'Special Order' 9 inch	3.8 oz	260	14.0	24.0	600	na	12.0	5.0	35	42%
vegetable, 'Light' 8 inch	4.4 oz	240	14.0	30.0	500	na	8.0	3.0	10	29%
vegetable, 'Light' 12 inch	4.3 oz	230	12.0	30.0	420	na	7.0	3.0	10	27%
(Totino's)										
Canadian bacon 'Party Pizza'	1/2 pie	330	15.0	42.0	860	3.0	13.0	2.0	10	34%
cheese 'Pan Pizza'	1/6 pie	290	15.0	35.0	440	na	10.0	4.0	20	31%
cheese 'Party Pizza'	1/2 pie	290	13.0	40.0	530	2.0	10.0	3.0	15	30%
cheese 'Party Pizza Family Size'	1/3 pie	320	14.0	43.0	580	2.0	11.0	3.0	15	30%
combination 'Party Pizza'	1/2 pie	370	15.0	43.0	920	3.0	17.0	4.0	20	40%
combination 'Party Pizza Family Size'	1/3 pie	400	17.0	47.0	990	3.0	18.0	4.0	20	39%
hamburger 'Party Pizza'	1/2 pie	350	16.0	37.0	780	3.0	17.0	4.0	15	42%
pepperoni 'Pan Pizza'	1/6 pie	330	16.0	35.0	620	na	15.0	6.0	30	40%
pepperoni 'Party Pizza'	1/2 pie	380	14.0	41.0	980	3.0	19.0	4.0	15	44%
pepperoni 'Party Pizza Family Size'	1/3 pie	410	16.0	44.0	1060	3.0	20.0	4.0	20	43%
sausage 'Pan Pizza'	1/6 pie	320	16.0	35.0	500	na	13.0	7.0	20	36%
sausage 'Party Pizza'	1/2 pie	370	15.0	44.0	800	3.0	17.0	4.0	10	39%
sausage 'Party Pizza Family Size'	1/3 pie	410	16.0	48.0	870	4.0	18.0	4.0	15	39%
sausage and pepperoni 'Pan Pizza'	1/6 pie	330	16.0	35.0	560	na	15.0	7.0	25	40%
PIZZA CRUST, 'All Ready' (Pillsbury)	1/8 crust	90	3.0	16.0	170	(mq)	1.0	0.0	0	11%
PIZZA CRUST MIX										
deep dish, prepared w/water, crust only (Martha White) ..	1 slice	110	3.0	23.0	110	na	<1.0	na	0	<8%
'Pouch Mix' (Gold Medal)	1/6 pkg	110	3.0	22.0	220	(mq)	1.0	(mq)	na	8%
'Pouch Mix' (Robin Hood)	1/6 pkg	110	3.0	22.0	220	(mq)	1.0	(mq)	na	8%
'Quick & Easy' (Chef Boyardee)	1/6 pkg	150	6.0	26.0	300	(mq)	2.0	(mq)	na	12%
regular, prepared w/water, crust only (Martha White)	1 slice	100	2.0	19.0	125	na	2.0	na	0	18%
PIZZA DINNER, FROZEN										
cheese (Kid Cuisine)	6.85 oz	380	11.0	57.0	390	na	12.0	na	25	28%
cheese 'Mega Meal' (Kid Cuisine)	9.7 oz	430	17.0	75.0	700	na	7.0	na	na	15%
hamburger (Kid Cuisine)	6.85 oz	330	11.0	50.0	700	na	10.0	na	15	27%
PIZZA ENTRÉE, FROZEN										
cheese (Weight Watchers)	6.03 oz	300	24.0	36.0	310	na	7.0	2.0	10	21%
deluxe combination 'Lowfat' (Weight Watchers)	7.32 oz	320	25.0	36.0	370	na	9.0	2.0	10	25%
hamburger 'Looney Tunes Wile E. Coyote' (Tyson)	6 oz	310	12.0	40.0	630	na	11.0	na	13	32%
pepperoni 'Looney Tunes Foghorn Leghorn' (Tyson)	6.35 oz	400	13.0	57.0	610	na	13.0	na	18	30%
pepperoni 'Lowfat' (Weight Watchers)	6.08 oz	320	25.0	36.0	550	na	8.0	2.0	15	23%
supreme, hand held 'Aussie Pie' (Mrs. Paterson's)	5.5 oz	470	12.0	44.0	880	na	27.0	10.0	75	52%
PIZZA MIX										
cheese 'Complete' (Chef Boyardee)	1/4 pkg	230	9.0	36.0	740	(mq)	6.0	(mq)	na	23%
cheese, kit (Contadina)	4.94 oz	320	16.0	41.0	850	na	10.0	4.0	20	28%
cheese '2 Complete' (Chef Boyardee)	1/8 pkg	210	10.0	31.0	650	(mq)	5.0	(mq)	(mq)	22%
pepperoni 'Complete' (Chef Boyardee)	1/4 pkg	250	13.0	31.0	870	(mq)	9.0	(mq)	(mq)	32%

Food Name	Serving Size	Calories	Prot. gms	Carbs gms	Sod. mgs	Fiber gms	Fat gms	Sat. Fat gms	Chol. mgs	% Fat Cal.
pepperoni, kit *(Contadina)*	4.94 oz	370	18.0	38.0	980	na	16.0	6.0	30	39%
pepperoni '2 Complete' *(Chef Boyardee)*	1/8 pkg	210	10.0	31.0	595	(mq)	7.0	(mq)	(mq)	28%
plain *(Chef Boyardee)*	1/4 pkg	180	6.0	32.0	640	(mq)	3.0	(mq)	na	15%
sausage *(Chef Boyardee)*	1/4 pkg	270	14.0	34.0	930	(mq)	10.0	(mq)	(mq)	32%
PIZZA ROLL, FROZEN										
cheese, approx 6 rolls *(Jeno's)*	3 oz	240	8.0	23.0	350	(mq)	12.0	(mq)	(mq)	47%
combination *(Jeno's)*	3 oz	220	10.0	26.0	230	1.9	9.0	3.0	15	36%
hamburger, approx 6 rolls *(Jeno's)*	3 oz	240	9.0	21.0	280	(mq)	13.0	(mq)	(mq)	49%
pepperoni, approx 6 rolls *(Jeno's)*	3 oz	220	9.0	26.0	350	1.8	9.0	3.0	20	37%
pepperoni and cheese, approx 6 rolls *(Jeno's)*	3 oz	230	7.0	22.0	390	(mq)	13.0	(mq)	(mq)	50%
pepperoni and cheese 'Microwave' 6 rolls *(Jeno's)*	3 oz	240	7.0	23.0	440	(mq)	13.0	(mq)	(mq)	49%
sausage *(Jeno's)*	3 oz	210	9.0	26.0	340	1.6	7.0	2.0	15	31%
sausage and cheese 'Microwave' approx 6 rolls *(Jeno's)*	3 oz	250	8.0	24.0	440	(mq)	13.0	(mq)	(mq)	48%
sausage and pepperoni, approx 6 rolls *(Jeno's)*	3 oz	230	7.0	22.0	380	(mq)	13.0	(mq)	(mq)	50%
PLANTAIN										
cooked	4 oz	132	0.9	35.3	6	(mq)	0.2	na	0	1%
cooked, sliced	1 cup	179	1.2	48.0	8	3.5	0.3	na	0	1%
raw, approx 9.7 oz	1 med	218	2.3	57.1	7	>.9 c	0.7	na	0	3%
raw, sliced	1 cup	181	1.9	47.2	6	3.4	0.6	na	0	3%
raw, trimmed	1 oz	35	0.4	9.0	1	>.1 c	0.1	na	0	2%
raw, trimmed, approx 9.7 oz	1 med	218	2.3	57.1	7	4.1	0.7	na	0	3%
raw, untrimmed	1 lb	360	3.8	94.0	12	>1.5 c	1.1	na	0	3%
PLUM										
pitted	1 oz	16	0.2	3.7	tr	>.2 c	0.2	<.1	0	10%
raw, sliced	1 cup	91	1.3	21.5	0	2.5	1.0	0.1	0	9%
raw, 2 1/8 inch diam	1 med	36	0.5	8.6	0	1.0	0.4	0.0	0	9%
untrimmed *(Dole)*	2 pieces	70	1.0	17.0	0	1.0	1.0	na	na	11%
w/pits	1 lb	235	3.4	55.5	2	>2.6 c	2.6	0.2	0	9%
PLUM, JAPANESE										
peeled and seeded	1 oz	13	0.1	3.4	<1	>.1 c	0.1	<.1	0	6%
raw, approx .6 oz	1 med	5	<.1	1.2	tr	>.1 c	<.1	tr	0	<15%
untrimmed	1 lb	132	1.2	34.1	3	>1.4 c	0.6	0.1	0	4%
PLUM, PURPLE, CANNED										
halves or whole, unpeeled *(S&W Nutradiet)*	1/2 cup	52	0.0	13.0	0	(mq)	0.0	0.0	0	0%
in extra heavy syrup	1/2 cup	133	0.5	34.3	25	>.4 c	0.1	<.1	0	1%
in extra heavy syrup, pitted	4 oz	115	0.4	29.8	22	>.4 c	0.1	tr	0	1%
in extra heavy syrup, unpeeled, halves *(S&W)*	1/2 cup	135	0.0	35.0	25	(mq)	0.0	0.0	0	0%
in extra heavy syrup, unpeeled, whole *(S&W)*	1/2 cup	135	0.0	35.0	25	(mq)	0.0	0.0	0	0%
in extra heavy syrup, w/liquid	1 cup	264	0.9	68.7	50	>.8 c	0.3	0.0	0	1%
in extra heavy syrup, w/2.75 tbsp liquid	3 plums	134	0.5	35.0	25	>.4 c	0.1	0.0	0	1%
in heavy syrup	1/2 cup	115	0.5	30.0	25	>.4 c	0.1	<.1	0	1%
in heavy syrup *(Stokely)*	1/2 cup	130	0.0	30.0	25	(mq)	0.0	0.0	0	0%
in heavy syrup, pitted	4 oz	101	0.4	26.4	22	>.4 c	0.1	tr	0	1%
in heavy syrup, w/liquid	1 cup	230	0.9	60.0	49	2.6	0.3	0.0	0	1%
in heavy syrup, w/2.75 tbsp liquid	3 plums	118	0.5	30.9	25	1.3	0.1	0.0	0	1%
in juice	1/2 cup	73	0.7	19.1	2	.5	<.1	tr	0	<1%
in juice, pitted	4 oz	66	0.6	17.2	1	.4	<.1	tr	0	<1%
in juice, whole *(Featherweight)*	1/2 cup	80	1.0	18.0	10	(mq)	0.0	0.0	0	0%
in light syrup	1/2 cup	79	0.5	20.5	25	>.4 c	0.1	<.1	0	1%
in light syrup *(Stokely)*	1/2 cup	100	0.0	16.0	20	(mq)	0.0	0.0	0	0%
in light syrup, pitted	4 oz	71	0.4	18.5	23	>.4 c	0.1	tr	0	1%
in water	1/2 cup	51	0.5	13.7	1	>.3 c	<.1	tr	0	<1%
in water, pitted	4 oz	46	0.4	12.5	1	>.3 c	<.1	tr	0	<1%

POHA. See CAPE GOOSEBERRY.

Food Name	Serving Size	Calories	Prot. gms	Carbs gms	Sod. mgs	Fiber gms	Fat gms	Sat. Fat gms	Chol. mgs	% Fat Cal.
POI										
fresh	1/2 cup	134	0.5	32.7	14	.5	0.2	0.0	0	1%
fresh	1 oz	32	0.1	7.7	3	.1	<.1	tr	0	<3%
POKEBERRY SHOOTS										
boiled, drained	4 oz	23	2.6	3.5	na	(mq)	0.5	na	0	16%
boiled, drained	1/2 cup	16	1.9	2.5	15	1.2	0.3	na	0	13%
raw	1/2 cup	18	2.1	3.0	18	1.4	0.3	na	0	12%
raw, trimmed	4 oz	26	2.9	4.2	na	(mq)	0.5	na	0	14%
POLENTA MIX, prepared *(Fantastic Foods)*	1/2 cup	106	3.0	18.0	246	(mq)	2.0	(mq)	na	18%
POLISH SAUSAGE										
	1 oz	92	4.0	0.5	248	0	8.1	2.9	20	80%
link, 10 inches long x 1 1/4 inch diam, 8 oz	1 large	739	32.0	3.7	1989	0	65.2	23.4	158	80%
(Hillshire Farm) 'Links'	2 oz	190	7.0	2.0	520	0	17.0	(mq)	(mq)	81%
(Hormel)	2 links	170	9.0	0.0	574	0	14.0	(mq)	(mq)	78%
(OHSE)	1 oz	80	4.0	1.0	290	0	7.0	(mq)	(mq)	76%
(OHSE) hot	1 oz	70	4.0	3.0	270	0	5.0	(mq)	(mq)	62%
(Pilgrim's Pride)	3 oz	131	13.2	2.3	780	0	7.7	(mq)	72	53%
POLLACK, ALASKAN										
baked	4 oz	128	26.7	0.0	132	0	1.3	0.3	109	10%
broiled	4 oz	128	26.7	0.0	132	0	1.3	0.3	109	10%
microwaved	4 oz	128	26.7	0.0	132	0	1.3	0.3	109	10%
raw	1 lb	365	77.9	0.0	449	0	3.6	0.7	323	9%
raw	1 oz	23	4.9	0.0	28	0	0.2	<.1	20	8%
POLLACK, ATLANTIC										
raw	1 lb	416	88.2	0.0	391	0	4.4	0.6	320	10%
raw	3 oz	78	16.5	0.0	73	0	0.8	0.1	60	10%
raw	1 oz	26	5.5	0.0	24	0	0.3	<.1	20	11%
POLLACK, WALLEYE										
baked	4 oz	128	26.7	0.0	132	0	1.3	0.3	109	10%
broiled	4 oz	128	26.7	0.0	132	0	1.3	0.3	109	10%
dry-heat cooked	3 oz	96	20.0	0.0	99	0	1.0	0.2	82	10%
microwaved	4 oz	128	26.7	0.0	132	0	1.3	0.3	109	10%
raw	1 lb	365	77.9	0.0	449	0	3.6	0.7	323	9%
raw	3 oz	69	14.6	0.0	84	0	0.7	0.1	60	10%
raw	1 oz	23	4.9	0.0	28	0	0.2	<.1	20	8%
POLLYFISH. See PARROTFISH.										
POMEGRANATE / Chinese apple										
raw, approx 3 3/8 inch diam	1 med	105	1.5	26.4	5	.9	0.5	na	0	4%
trimmed	1 oz	19	0.3	4.9	1	>.1 c	0.1	na	0	4%
untrimmed	1 lb	172	2.4	43.6	8	>.5 c	0.8	na	0	4%
POMEGRANATE JUICE *(Knudsen & Sons)*	8 oz	85	<1.0	21.0	na	na	0.0	na	na	0%
POMELO / pumelo										
raw, approx 5 1/2 inches diam, 2.4 lbs	1 med	228	4.6	58.6	7	6.1	0.2	(tr)	0	1%
sections	1/2 cup	36	0.7	9.1	1	1.0	<.1	(tr)	0	<1%
trimmed	1 oz	11	0.2	2.7	1	>.1 c	<.1	(tr)	0	<1%
untrimmed	1 lb	95	1.9	24.4	3	>.5 c	0.1	(tr)	0	1%
POMFRET										
raw	1 lb	663	78.4	0.0	401	0	36.4	(mq)	295	51%
raw	1 oz	41	4.9	0.0	25	0	2.3	(mq)	18	51%
POMPANO, FLORIDA										
baked	4 oz	239	26.4	0.0	86	0	13.8	5.1	73	54%
broiled	4 oz	239	26.4	0.0	86	0	13.8	5.1	73	54%
dry-heat cooked	3 oz	179	20.1	0.0	65	0	10.3	3.8	54	54%
microwaved	4 oz	239	26.4	0.0	86	0	13.8	5.1	73	54%

Food Name	Serving Size	Calories	Prot. gms	Carbs gms	Sod. mgs	Fiber gms	Fat gms	Sat. Fat gms	Chol. mgs	% Fat Cal.
raw	1 lb	745	83.8	0.0	294	0	42.9	15.9	227	54%
raw	1 oz	46	5.2	0.0	18	0	2.7	1.0	14	54%

POPCORN
(NOTE: All popcorn is popped unless otherwise noted.)

(Bachman)

Food Name	Serving Size	Calories	Prot. gms	Carbs gms	Sod. mgs	Fiber gms	Fat gms	Sat. Fat gms	Chol. mgs	% Fat Cal.
cheese flavor	.5 oz	90	1.0	7.0	165	(mq)	6.0	(mq)	na	63%
'Lite'	.5 oz	50	1.0	10.0	35	2.0	1.0	(mq)	0	17%
regular	.5 oz	80	1.0	7.0	160	(mq)	6.0	(mq)	0	63%
white cheddar cheese flavor	.5 oz	70	1.0	7.0	150	(mq)	4.0	(mq)	na	53%

(Bearitos)

Food Name	Serving Size	Calories	Prot. gms	Carbs gms	Sod. mgs	Fiber gms	Fat gms	Sat. Fat gms	Chol. mgs	% Fat Cal.
cheese flavor 'Organic'	1 oz	137	3.1	13.2	122	2.0	8.0	(mq)	na	53%
'Organic 50% Less Oil'	.5 oz	70	2.0	9.0	70	na	3.0	na	0	38%
'Organic Lite'	1 oz	132	2.8	14.7	39	2.7	6.9	(mq)	0	47%
'Organic No Salt'	1 oz	108	3.6	21.7	1	.7	0.8	na	0	7%
'Organic Traditional'	1 oz	140	2.4	12.0	85	3.0	9.2	(mq)	0	59%

(Bonnie Lee)

Food Name	Serving Size	Calories	Prot. gms	Carbs gms	Sod. mgs	Fiber gms	Fat gms	Sat. Fat gms	Chol. mgs	% Fat Cal.
w/oil and salt	1 oz	172	3.0	20.0	230	(mq)	8.0	(mq)	na	44%
w/o oil and salt	1 oz	109	3.0	20.0	<1	(mq)	1.0	na	0	9%
(Cape Cod) white cheddar cheese flavor	.5 oz	80	2.0	6.0	150	(mq)	5.0	(mq)	na	58%
(Clover Club) white cheddar cheese flavor	.5 oz	70	1.0	6.0	140	(mq)	5.0	(mq)	na	62%
(Cracker Jack) caramel coated, w/peanuts	1 oz	120	2.0	22.0	85	(mq)	3.0	(mq)	80	22%
(Estee) caramel coated	1 oz	140	3.0	25.0	55	(mq)	3.0	1.5	5	19%

(Frito Lay)

Food Name	Serving Size	Calories	Prot. gms	Carbs gms	Sod. mgs	Fiber gms	Fat gms	Sat. Fat gms	Chol. mgs	% Fat Cal.
cheese flavor	.5 oz	80	1.0	7.0	180	(mq)	5.0	(mq)	0	58%
regular	.5 oz	70	1.0	9.0	200	(mq)	3.0	(mq)	0	40%

(Jiffy Pop)

Food Name	Serving Size	Calories	Prot. gms	Carbs gms	Sod. mgs	Fiber gms	Fat gms	Sat. Fat gms	Chol. mgs	% Fat Cal.
butter flavor 'Pan Popcorn'	4 cups	130	3.0	16.0	270	2.0	6.0	(mq)	0	42%
'Pan Popcorn'	4 cups	130	3.0	16.0	270	2.0	6.0	(mq)	0	42%

(Jolly Time)

Food Name	Serving Size	Calories	Prot. gms	Carbs gms	Sod. mgs	Fiber gms	Fat gms	Sat. Fat gms	Chol. mgs	% Fat Cal.
white, air-popped	3 cups	60	2.0	15.0	2	4.0	<1.0	na	0	<12%
white, w/o salt	4 cups	75	3.0	20.0	2	5.0	1.0	na	0	9%
yellow, air-popped	3 cups	60	2.0	14.0	2	4.0	<1.0	na	0	<12%
yellow, w/o salt	4 cups	75	3.0	19.0	2	5.0	1.0	na	0	9%

(Keebler)

Food Name	Serving Size	Calories	Prot. gms	Carbs gms	Sod. mgs	Fiber gms	Fat gms	Sat. Fat gms	Chol. mgs	% Fat Cal.
honey caramel 'Pop Deluxe'	1 oz	120	<1.0	22.0	180	(mq)	3.0	1.0	0	23%
white cheddar cheese flavor	1 oz	140	1.0	13.0	270	(mq)	10.0	2.0	5	62%

(Kettle Poppins)

Food Name	Serving Size	Calories	Prot. gms	Carbs gms	Sod. mgs	Fiber gms	Fat gms	Sat. Fat gms	Chol. mgs	% Fat Cal.
lightly salted	.5 oz	70	2.0	9.0	40	1.0	2.5	0.5	0	34%
white cheddar	.5 oz	70	2.0	9.0	120	1.0	2.5	0.5	1	34%

(Laura Scudder)

Food Name	Serving Size	Calories	Prot. gms	Carbs gms	Sod. mgs	Fiber gms	Fat gms	Sat. Fat gms	Chol. mgs	% Fat Cal.
'Tender Baby White Corn'	.5 oz	80	1.0	6.0	140	(mq)	6.0	(mq)	0	66%
white cheddar cheese flavor	.5 oz	70	1.0	6.0	140	(mq)	5.0	(mq)	na	62%

(Nature's Choice)

Food Name	Serving Size	Calories	Prot. gms	Carbs gms	Sod. mgs	Fiber gms	Fat gms	Sat. Fat gms	Chol. mgs	% Fat Cal.
caramel, original	1 oz	108	1.0	25.0	na	na	1.0	na	0	8%
caramel, w/peanuts	1 oz	114	1.0	23.0	na	na	1.0	na	0	9%

(Orville Redenbacher)

Food Name	Serving Size	Calories	Prot. gms	Carbs gms	Sod. mgs	Fiber gms	Fat gms	Sat. Fat gms	Chol. mgs	% Fat Cal.
caramel 'Ready-to-Eat'	1 oz	112	0.9	22.4	65	3.2	3.5	0.7	1	25%
hot air 'Gourmet' prepared	3 cups	40	1.0	10.0	0	3.0	<1.0	(mq)	0	<17%
original 'Gourmet' prepared	3 cups	80	1.0	10.0	0	3.0	4.0	na	0	45%
white 'Gourmet'	3 cups	80	1.0	10.0	0	3.0	4.0	na	0	45%
white cheddar cheese 'Ready-to-Eat'	1.058 oz	139	3.4	16.5	285	4.4	8.6	1.2	1	49%

(Pops-Rite)

Food Name	Serving Size	Calories	Prot. gms	Carbs gms	Sod. mgs	Fiber gms	Fat gms	Sat. Fat gms	Chol. mgs	% Fat Cal.
white, w/o salt, air popped	1 oz	100	3.0	20.0	na	.6	2.0	(mq)	0	16%
white, w/o salt, oil popped	1 oz	220	3.0	20.0	na	.6	15.0	(mq)	0	60%

Food Name	Serving Size	Calories	Prot. gms	Carbs gms	Sod. mgs	Fiber gms	Fat gms	Sat. Fat gms	Chol. mgs	% Fat Cal.
yellow, w/o salt, air popped	1 oz	100	2.0	21.0	na	.6	2.0	(mq)	0	16%
yellow, w/o salt, oil popped	1 oz	220	2.0	21.0	na	.6	15.0	(mq)	0	60%
(Smartfood) white cheddar cheese flavor	.5 oz	80	2.0	7.0	150	(mq)	5.0	(mq)	na	56%
(Ultra Slim Fast) butter flavor 'Lite 'N Tasty'	.5 oz	60	2.0	10.0	150	2.0	2.0	na	0	27%
(Vic's)										
caramel, lite 'Gourmet'	1/2 cup	60	1.0	10.0	50	na	2.0	na	0	29%
white, lite 'Gourmet'	1 cup	35	1.0	6.0	15	na	2.0	na	0	39%
white cheddar cheese, lite 'Gourmet'	2/3 cup	40	1.0	4.0	50	na	2.0	na	1	47%
yellow cheddar cheese, lite 'Gourmet'	2/3 cup	40	1.0	4.0	60	na	2.0	na	1	47%
(Weight Watchers)										
butter	.66-oz pkg	90	2.0	13.0	100	na	3.0	na	na	31%
caramel	.9-oz pkg	100	1.0	23.0	45	na	1.0	0.0	0	9%
'Lightly Salted'	.66-oz pkg	80	2.0	12.0	65	(mq)	4.0	(mq)	0	39%
white cheddar cheese flavor	.66-oz pkg	100	2.0	10.0	85	(mq)	6.0	(mq)	na	53%
(Wise)										
butter flavor, 1 cup	.5 oz	80	1.0	7.0	140	(mq)	5.0	(mq)	0	58%
'Tender Baby White Corn'	.5 oz	80	1.0	6.0	140	(mq)	6.0	(mq)	0	66%
'Tender Eating Baby Popcorn'	.5 oz	70	1.0	4.0	120	(mq)	6.0	(mq)	0	73%
white cheddar cheese flavor	.5 oz	70	1.0	6.0	140	(mq)	5.0	(mq)	na	62%
POPCORN, FROZEN										
(Orville Redenbacher)										
butter flavor 'Gourmet' microwave	3 cups	100	2.0	11.0	240	3.0	6.0	1.3	0	51%
natural 'Gourmet' microwave	3 cups	100	2.0	11.0	200	3.0	6.0	1.3	0	51%
(Pillsbury)										
butter flavor	3 cups	210	3.0	20.0	480	(mq)	13.0	(mq)	na	56%
'Original'	3 cups	210	3.0	20.0	420	(mq)	13.0	(mq)	na	56%
'Salt-Free'	3 cups	170	3.0	23.0	na	(mq)	7.0	(mq)	0	38%
POPCORN, MICROWAVE										
(NOTE: All microwave popcorn is popped unless otherwise noted.)										
(Betty Crocker)										
butter flavor 'Pop•Secret'	1/4 bag	120	2.0	13.0	250	2.0	8.0	na	0	55%
butter flavor 'Pop•Secret By Request'	1/3 bag	60	2.0	12.0	160	na	1.0	na	0	14%
butter flavor 'Pop•Secret Light'	1/4 bag	90	2.0	13.0	160	2.0	4.0	na	0	38%
butter flavor 'Pop•Secret Pop Qwiz'	1 bag	110	2.0	11.0	210	2.0	7.0	na	0	55%
butter flavor, salt-free 'Pop•Secret'	1/4 bag	120	2.0	13.0	5	2.0	7.0	na	0	51%
butter flavor, singles 'Pop•Secret'	1 bag	250	4.0	27.0	460	4.0	16.0	na	0	54%
butter flavor, singles 'Pop•Secret Light'	1 bag	180	4.0	28.0	310	4.0	8.0	na	0	36%
cheese flavor 'Pop•Secret'	1/3 bag	170	3.0	15.0	260	2.0	11.0	(mq)	0	58%
natural 'Pop•Secret'	1/4 bag	120	2.0	13.0	250	2.0	8.0	na	0	55%
natural 'Pop•Secret By Request'	1/3 bag	60	2.0	12.0	170	na	1.0	na	0	14%
natural 'Pop•Secret Light'	1/4 bag	90	2.0	13.0	200	2.0	4.0	na	0	38%
natural 'Pop•Secret Pop Qwiz'	1 bag	110	2.0	11.0	220	2.0	7.0	na	0	55%
natural, singles 'Pop•Secret Light'	1 bag	170	4.0	26.0	440	4.0	7.0	na	0	34%
(Featherweight)										
butter flavor 'Low Salt'	3 cups	100	3.0	14.0	70	(mq)	3.0	(mq)	0	28%
'Natural Low Salt'	3 cups	80	3.0	14.0	0	(mq)	1.0	na	0	12%
(Jiffy Pop)										
butter flavor	4 cups	140	3.0	17.0	270	3.0	7.0	(mq)	0	44%
natural	4 cups	140	3.0	17.0	270	3.0	7.0	(mq)	0	44%
(Jolly Time)										
butter flavor	3 cups	90	2.0	13.0	95	3.0	5.0	1.0	0	43%
butter flavor, light	3 cups	60	2.0	12.0	105	3.0	2.0	0.5	0	24%
cheddar flavor	3 cups	155	3.0	17.0	220	4.0	10.0	1.0	0	53%
natural	3 cups	120	2.0	15.0	125	3.0	7.0	1.5	0	48%

Food Name	Serving Size	Calories	Prot. gms	Carbs gms	Sod. mgs	Fiber gms	Fat gms	Sat. Fat gms	Chol. mgs	% Fat Cal.
natural, light	3 cups	70	2.0	13.0	110	3.0	2.0	0.6	0	23%
(Orville Redenbacher)										
butter flavor 'Gourmet'	3 cups	100	2.0	11.0	240	3.0	6.0	1.3	0	51%
butter flavor, light 'Gourmet'	3 cups	70	2.0	8.0	110	3.0	3.0	<1.0	0	40%
butter flavor, light, snack size	3 cups	70	2.0	11.0	90	na	3.0	na	0	34%
butter flavor, salt-free 'Gourmet'	3 cups	100	2.0	11.0	0	3.0	6.0	1.3	0	51%
butter flavor 'Smart•Pop'	3 cups	50	2.0	11.0	100	na	1.0	na	0	15%
butter flavor, snack size	3 cups	100	2.0	11.0	140	na	6.0	na	0	51%
butter toffee flavor 'Gourmet'	2 1/2 cups	210	2.0	26.0	85	2.0	12.0	3.0	<1	49%
caramel flavor 'Gourmet'	2 1/2 cups	240	2.0	29.0	90	2.0	14.0	3.4	<1	50%
cheddar cheese flavor 'Gourmet'	3 cups	130	2.0	14.0	280	3.0	8.0	1.8	2	53%
natural 'Gourmet'	3 cups	100	2.0	11.0	200	3.0	6.0	1.3	0	51%
natural, light 'Gourmet'	3 cups	70	2.0	8.0	115	3.0	3.0	<1.0	0	40%
natural, salt-free 'Gourmet'	3 cups	100	2.0	11.0	0	3.0	6.0	1.3	0	51%
red herb and garlic flavor, 2 tbsp unpopped	1.27 oz	150	1.9	15.4	366	4.0	10.7	2.6	0	58%
sour cream 'n onion flavor 'Gourmet'	3 cups	160	2.0	12.0	270	3.0	12.0	2.7	0	66%
zesty butter flavor 'Reddenbutter' 2 tbsp unpopped	1.27 oz	148	2.1	15.9	259	4.0	10.2	2.5	0	56%
(Pillsbury)										
butter flavor	3 cups	210	3.0	20.0	410	(mq)	13.0	(mq)	na	56%
'Original'	3 cups	210	3.0	20.0	410	(mq)	13.0	(mq)	0	56%
(Planters)										
butter flavor	3 cups	140	2.0	13.0	0	(mq)	10.0	1.0	560	60%
natural	3 cups	140	2.0	14.0	0	(mq)	9.0	1.0	560	56%
(Pop Weavers)										
butter flavor	4 cups	140	3.0	20.0	230	4.0	8.0	(mq)	0	44%
'Natural'	4 cups	140	3.0	20.0	230	4.0	8.0	(mq)	0	44%
(Pops-Rite)										
butter flavor	3 cups	90	2.0	13.0	140	(mq)	5.0	(mq)	0	43%
'Natural'	3 cups	90	2.0	13.0	190	(mq)	5.0	(mq)	0	43%
(Weight Watchers)	1-oz pkg	100	4.0	22.0	5	(mq)	1.0	na	0	8%
POPCORN OIL										
(Orville Redenbacher) popping	1 tbsp	120	0.0	0.0	0	0	14.0	2.0	0	100%
(Planters)	1 tbsp	120	0.0	0.0	0	na	14.0	2.0	0	100%
(Wesson) buttery flavor popping oil	1 tbsp	120	0.0	0.0	0	0	13.5	2.0	0	100%
(Wesson) popping and topping oil 'Food Service'	1 tbsp	122	0.0	0.0	0	0	13.5	2.0	0	100%
POPCORN SEASONING										
(McCormick/Schilling) 'Parsley Patch'	1 tsp	10	0.6	3.0	4	na	0.1	(tr)	0	6%
POPPY SEED										
whole	1 oz	151	5.1	6.7	6	>1.8 c	12.6	1.4	0	71%
whole	1 tbsp	47	1.6	2.1	2	2.6	3.9	0.4	0	70%
whole	1 tsp	15	0.5	0.7	1	.8	1.3	0.1	0	71%
whole *(Durkee)*	1 tsp	15	0.0	0.0	0	0	<0.1	na	na	<60%
whole *(Laurel Leaf)*	1 tsp	15	0.0	0.0	0	0	<0.1	na	na	<60%
whole *(Spice Islands)*	1 tsp	13	0.6	0.8	<1	>.2 c	0.9	na	0	59%
POPPY SEED OIL										
	1 cup	1927	0.0	0.0	0	0	218.0	29.4	0	100%
	1 oz	251	0.0	0.0	0	0	28.4	3.8	0	100%
	1 tbsp	120	0.0	0.0	0	0	13.6	1.8	0	100%

PORK. See also HAM, CANNED; HAM, CURED; HAM, FRESH; HAM PATTY.

(NOTE: TRIMMED = Lean; separable fat removed. UNTRIMMED = Separable fat not removed.)

BACKFAT

wholesale cuts, raw	1 lb	3683	13.3	0.0	50	0	402.3	146.1	259	99%
wholesale cuts, raw	1 oz	230	0.8	0.0	3	0	25.1	9.1	16	99%

Food Name	Serving Size	Calories	Prot. gms	Carbs gms	Sod. mgs	Fiber gms	Fat gms	Sat. Fat gms	Chol. mgs	% Fat Cal.
BACKRIB										
Untrimmed										
raw	1 lb	1279	73.1	0.0	340	0	107.0	39.6	367	77%
raw	1 oz	80	4.6	0.0	21	0	6.7	2.5	23	77%
raw 'Gourmet' *(JM)*	5.5 oz	220	15.0	0.0	50	0	18.0	(mq)	(mq)	73%
roasted	3 oz	315	20.6	0.0	86	0	25.1	9.3	100	73%
BELLY										
wholesale cuts, raw	1 lb	2350	42.4	0.0	145	0	240.5	87.7	327	93%
wholesale cuts, raw	1 oz	147	2.7	0.0	9	0	15.0	5.5	20	93%
BOSTON BUTT										
Trimmed										
cured, medium fat, chopped, roasted	1 cup	340	38.9	0.0	1393	0	19.3	7.0	123	53%
cured, medium fat, roasted	9.8 oz	678	77.6	0.0	2777	0	38.5	13.9	246	53%
BRAINS										
braised	3 oz	117	10.3	0.0	77	0	8.1	1.8	2169	64%
in milk gravy *(Armour)*	2.75 oz	110	7.0	1.0	400	na	8.0	na	na	69%
raw	1 oz	36	2.9	0.0	34	0	2.6	0.6	622	67%
CENTER LOIN										
Trimmed										
braised	3 oz	172	25.3	0.0	53	0	7.1	2.6	72	39%
broiled	3 oz	172	25.7	0.0	51	0	6.9	2.5	70	38%
chopped, braised	1 cup	381	48.7	0.0	77	0	19.2	6.6	155	47%
chopped, broiled	1 cup	323	44.8	0.0	109	0	14.7	5.1	137	43%
chopped, roasted	1 cup	336	39.9	0.0	97	0	18.3	6.3	127	51%
pan-fried	3 oz	197	27.4	0.0	73	0	8.9	3.1	78	42%
pan-fried in vegetable oil	4 oz	302	32.6	0.0	96	0	14.0	6.2	121	49%
raw	1 oz	45	6.2	0.0	19	0	2.0	0.7	18	42%
roasted	3 oz	169	23.4	0.0	56	0	7.7	2.8	67	43%
Untrimmed										
braised	3 oz	210	23.8	0.0	50	0	12.0	4.5	73	53%
broiled	3 oz	204	24.4	0.0	49	0	11.1	4.1	70	51%
chopped, braised	1 cup	496	41.2	0.0	71	0	35.5	12.8	150	66%
chopped, broiled	1 cup	442	38.4	0.0	98	0	30.9	11.3	136	64%
chopped, pan-fried in vegetable oil	1 cup	372	40.3	0.0	119	0	22.3	7.6	150	56%
chopped, roasted	1 cup	427	35.6	0.0	90	0	30.5	11.0	127	66%
pan-fried	3 oz	235	25.4	0.0	68	0	14.1	5.1	78	56%
pan-fried in vegetable oil	4 oz	425	26.4	0.0	82	0	34.6	12.0	117	75%
raw	1 oz	80	5.2	0.0	16	0	6.2	2.2	20	73%
roasted	3 oz	199	22.4	0.0	54	0	11.4	4.3	68	53%
CENTER RIB										
Trimmed										
braised	3 oz	175	24.1	0.0	35	0	8.0	3.1	60	43%
broiled	3 oz	186	26.1	0.0	55	0	8.3	2.9	69	42%
chopped, braised	1 cup	388	48.2	0.0	73	0	20.2	7.0	136	49%

QUICK REFERENCE: PORK CUTS AND GRADES

Pork is considerably leaner today than it was in decades past. Because of new feeding and breeding practice, pork is leaner from the beginning, and butchers trim much of the remaining fat away. When looking for low-fat pork, choose one of the leaner cuts: tenderloin, ham (95% lean), boneless sirloin chops, boneless loin roast, and boneless loin chops. Then check the grade. In general, the higher, more expensive grades of meat, like USDA Prime and Choice, have more fat due to a higher degree of marbling—internal fat that cannot be trimmed away. USDA Select meats have the lowest amount of fat. Finally, look for the least amount of marbling in the cut and grade you have chosen, and let appearance be the final judge.

Food Name	Serving Size	Calories	Prot. gms	Carbs gms	Sod. mgs	Fiber gms	Fat gms	Sat. Fat gms	Chol. mgs	% Fat Cal.
chopped, broiled	1 cup	361	40.3	0.0	94	0	20.9	7.2	132	54%
chopped, pan-fried in vegetable oil	1 cup	360	39.1	0.0	70	0	21.4	7.4	113	55%
chopped, roasted	1 cup	343	39.5	0.0	64	0	19.3	6.7	111	52%
pan-fried	3 oz	185	23.9	0.0	44	0	9.2	3.4	59	46%
pan-fried in vegetable oil	4 oz	291	31.7	0.0	57	0	17.4	6.0	92	55%
raw	1 lb	676	100.3	0.0	204	0	27.3	9.4	249	38%
roasted	3 oz	190	24.4	0.0	40	0	9.5	3.7	60	47%
Untrimmed										
braised	3 oz	213	22.7	0.0	34	0	12.8	5.0	62	56%
broiled	3 oz	224	24.5	0.0	53	0	13.2	4.8	70	55%
chopped, braised	1 cup	514	40.0	0.0	67	0	38.0	13.7	133	68%
chopped, broiled	1 cup	480	34.4	0.0	85	0	36.9	13.3	130	71%
chopped, pan-fried in vegetable oil	1 cup	546	30.3	0.0	63	0	46.2	16.7	118	77%
chopped, roasted	1 cup	445	34.6	0.0	62	0	33.0	11.9	113	68%
pan-fried	3 oz	225	22.3	0.0	43	0	14.4	5.4	62	59%
pan-fried in vegetable oil	4 oz	442	24.5	0.0	51	0	37.4	13.5	95	78%
raw	1 oz	82	5.1	0.0	11	0	6.6	2.4	18	74%
roasted	3 oz	217	23.3	0.0	39	0	13.0	5.0	62	56%
CHITTERLINGS										
raw	1 oz	71	2.8	0.1	10	0	6.5	2.3	45	84%
simmered	3 oz	258	8.7	0.0	33	0	24.4	8.6	122	86%
CHOP, BONELESS, 'America's Cut' (JM)	6 oz	330	38.0	0.0	90	0	20.0	(mq)	(mq)	54%
COMPOSITE CUTS										
Trimmed										
loin and shoulder, cooked	3 oz	179	25.0	0.0	48	0	8.0	2.8	72	42%
loin and shoulder, raw	1 lb	653	96.3	0.0	245	0	26.7	9.2	272	38%
loin and shoulder, raw	1 oz	41	6.0	0.0	15	0	1.7	0.6	17	39%
retail cuts, cooked	3 oz	232	23.4	0.0	53	0	14.6	5.3	77	58%
retail cuts, raw	1 lb	980	86.0	0.0	249	0	67.8	24.0	304	64%
retail cuts, raw	1 oz	61	5.4	0.0	16	0	4.2	1.5	19	64%
roasted	3 oz	180	24.9	0.0	50	0	8.2	2.9	73	43%
Untrimmed										
loin and shoulder, cooked	3 oz	214	23.6	0.0	48	0	12.6	4.5	73	55%
loin and shoulder, raw	1 lb	907	88.6	0.0	231	0	58.5	20.3	290	60%
loin and shoulder, raw	1 oz	57	5.5	0.0	14	0	3.7	1.3	18	60%
raw	1 lb	1030	82.8	0.0	245	0	74.8	26.2	313	67%
raw	1 oz	64	5.2	0.0	15	0	4.7	1.6	20	67%
KIDNEYS										
braised	1 cup	211	35.6	0.0	112	0	6.6	2.1	672	29%
braised	3 oz	128	21.6	0.0	68	0	4.0	1.3	408	29%
raw	1 oz	28	4.7	0.0	34	0	0.9	0.3	90	30%
LIVER										
braised	3 oz	140	22.1	3.2	42	0	3.7	1.2	302	25%
fried	3 oz	205	25.4	2.1	94	0	9.8	2.9	372	45%
raw	1 oz	38	6.1	0.7	25	0	1.0	0.3	85	25%
LOIN										
Trimmed										
blade, braised	3 oz	191	21.3	0.0	53	0	11.1	4.0	71	54%
blade, broiled	3 oz	199	21.6	0.0	68	0	11.8	4.3	71	55%
blade, chopped, braised	1 cup	438	41.6	0.0	113	0	28.8	9.9	158	61%
blade, chopped, broiled	1 cup	420	34.9	0.0	108	0	30.1	10.4	140	66%
blade, chopped, roasted	1 cup	391	34.6	0.0	95	0	27.0	9.3	125	64%
blade, pan-fried	3 oz	205	21.0	0.0	66	0	12.8	4.4	70	58%
blade, pan-fried in vegetable oil	4 oz	321	27.6	0.0	84	0	22.5	7.7	110	65%

Food Name	Serving Size	Calories	Prot. gms	Carbs gms	Sod. mgs	Fiber gms	Fat gms	Sat. Fat gms	Chol. mgs	% Fat Cal.
blade, raw	1 lb	712	87.4	0.0	304	0	37.4	12.9	290	49%
blade, roasted	3 oz	210	22.6	0.0	25	0	12.6	4.5	79	56%
country-style ribs, braised	3 oz	199	22.1	0.0	54	0	11.6	4.2	73	54%
country-style ribs, raw	1 lb	712	87.4	0.0	304	0	37.4	12.9	290	49%
country-style ribs, raw	1 oz	45	5.5	0.0	19	0	2.3	0.8	18	49%
country-style ribs, roasted	3 oz	210	22.6	0.0	25	0	12.6	4.5	79	56%
whole, braised	3 oz	173	24.3	0.0	43	0	7.8	2.9	67	42%
whole, broiled	3 oz	178	24.3	0.0	54	0	8.3	3.1	67	44%
whole, chopped, braised	1 cup	382	46.2	0.0	105	0	20.4	7.1	147	50%
whole, chopped, broiled	1 cup	360	39.0	0.0	105	0	21.4	7.4	133	55%
whole, chopped, roasted	1 cup	336	37.7	0.0	97	0	19.5	6.7	126	54%
whole, raw	1 oz	44	5.9	0.0	18	0	2.1	0.7	17	45%
whole, roasted	3 oz	178	24.3	0.0	49	0	8.2	3.0	69	43%
whole or half, center cut, boneless (JM)	3 oz	190	16.0	0.0	50	0	13.0	(mq)	(mq)	65%
Untrimmed										
blade, braised	3 oz	275	18.6	0.0	47	0	21.6	8.1	72	72%
blade, broiled	3 oz	272	19.1	0.0	59	0	21.1	7.9	73	71%
blade, chopped, braised	1 cup	574	33.5	0.0	97	0	47.7	17.2	151	76%
blade, chopped, broiled	1 cup	550	28.9	0.0	94	0	47.4	17.0	137	79%
blade, chopped, roasted	1 cup	510	29.5	0.0	85	0	42.6	15.3	126	77%
blade, pan-fried	3 oz	291	18.3	0.0	57	0	23.6	8.6	72	74%
blade, pan-fried in vegetable oil	4 oz	469	21.3	0.0	69	0	41.9	15.1	108	82%
blade, raw	1 lb	1293	71.8	0.0	245	0	109.4	38.0	327	77%
blade, roasted	3 oz	275	20.2	0.0	25	0	20.9	7.8	79	70%
country-style ribs, braised	3 oz	252	20.3	0.0	50	0	18.3	6.8	74	67%
country-style ribs, raw	1 lb	1093	77.1	0.0	263	0	84.9	29.4	313	71%
country-style ribs, raw	1 oz	68	4.8	0.0	16	0	5.3	1.8	20	71%
country-style ribs, roasted	3 oz	279	19.9	0.0	44	0	21.5	7.8	78	71%
whole, braised	4 oz	417	30.8	0.0	74	0	31.6	11.4	116	70%
whole, broiled	3 oz	206	23.2	0.0	53	0	11.8	4.4	68	53%
whole, chopped, braised	1 cup	515	38.0	0.0	91	0	39.1	14.1	143	70%
whole, chopped, broiled	1 cup	484	33.0	0.0	92	0	38.1	13.8	132	72%
whole, chopped, roasted	1 cup	447	32.8	0.0	88	0	34.0	12.3	126	70%
whole, raw	1 lb	898	89.5	0.0	227	0	57.1	19.8	286	59%
whole, roasted	3 oz	211	23.0	0.0	50	0	12.4	4.6	70	55%
LUNGS										
braised	3 oz	84	14.1	0.0	69	0	2.6	0.9	329	29%
raw	1 oz	24	4.0	0.0	43	0	0.8	0.3	91	31%
PANCREAS										
braised	3 oz	186	24.2	0.0	36	0	9.2	3.2	268	46%
raw	1 oz	56	5.3	0.0	12	0	3.8	1.3	55	62%
SHOULDER										
Trimmed										
arm picnic, braised	3 oz	211	27.4	0.0	87	0	10.4	3.5	97	46%
arm picnic, chopped, braised	1 cup	347	45.2	0.0	143	0	17.1	5.9	160	46%
arm picnic, chopped, roasted	1 cup	319	37.4	0.0	112	0	17.7	6.1	133	52%
arm picnic, raw	1 lb	635	89.6	0.0	372	0	27.9	9.7	295	41%
arm picnic, raw	1 oz	40	5.6	0.0	23	0	1.8	0.6	18	42%
arm picnic, roasted	3 oz	194	22.7	0.0	68	0	10.7	3.7	81	52%
Boston blade, braised	3 oz	232	26.4	0.0	64	0	13.2	4.7	99	53%
Boston blade, broiled	3 oz	193	22.7	0.0	63	0	10.7	3.8	80	52%
Boston blade, chopped, braised	1 cup	412	43.6	0.0	105	0	24.6	8.5	162	56%
Boston blade, chopped, broiled	1 cup	384	35.2	0.0	118	0	25.8	8.9	147	62%
Boston blade, chopped, roasted	1 cup	358	34.1	0.0	102	0	23.6	8.1	137	61%

Food Name	Serving Size	Calories	Prot. gms	Carbs gms	Sod. mgs	Fiber gms	Fat gms	Sat. Fat gms	Chol. mgs	% Fat Cal.
Boston blade, raw	1 oz	47	5.4	0.0	20	0	2.6	0.9	19	52%
Boston blade, roasted	3 oz	197	20.6	0.0	75	0	12.2	4.4	72	57%
whole, chopped, roasted	1 cup	341	35.5	0.0	107	0	21.0	7.2	135	57%
whole, raw	1 lb	671	88.7	0.0	345	0	32.4	11.2	304	45%
whole, raw	1 oz	42	5.5	0.0	22	0	2.0	0.7	19	45%
whole, roasted	3 oz	195	21.5	0.0	64	0	11.5	4.1	77	55%
whole, roasted, diced	1 cup	310	34.2	0.0	101	0	18.3	6.5	122	55%
Untrimmed										
arm picnic, roasted	3 oz	269	20.0	0.0	59	0	20.4	7.5	80	70%
Boston blade, braised	3 oz	271	24.4	0.0	59	0	18.5	6.8	96	63%
Boston blade, broiled	3 oz	220	21.7	0.0	59	0	14.1	5.1	81	59%
Boston blade, chopped, braised	1 cup	519	37.0	0.0	94	0	40.1	14.4	155	71%
Boston blade, chopped, broiled	1 cup	490	30.6	0.0	105	0	39.8	14.3	144	75%
Boston blade, raw	1 lb	989	80.1	0.0	286	0	71.8	24.9	322	67%
Boston blade, roasted	3 oz	229	19.6	0.0	57	0	16.0	5.9	73	65%
whole, chopped, roasted	1 cup	456	30.8	0.0	96	0	36.0	13.0	134	73%
whole, diced, roasted	1 cup	394	31.4	0.0	92	0	28.9	10.6	122	67%
whole, raw	1 lb	1070	77.9	0.0	295	0	81.6	28.3	322	70%
whole, raw	1 oz	67	4.9	0.0	18	0	5.1	1.8	20	70%
whole, roasted	3 oz	248	19.8	0.0	58	0	18.2	6.7	77	67%
SIRLOIN										
Trimmed										
boneless, braised	3 oz	149	23.0	0.0	39	0	5.6	2.0	69	35%
boneless, broiled	3 oz	164	26.5	0.0	48	0	5.7	1.9	78	33%
boneless, raw	1 lb	581	95.5	0.0	231	0	19.1	6.6	286	31%
boneless, roasted	3 oz	168	24.5	0.0	48	0	7.0	2.5	73	39%
braised	3 oz	167	23.0	0.0	45	0	7.7	2.7	69	43%
broiled	3 oz	181	24.2	0.0	61	0	8.6	3.1	72	44%
chopped, braised	1 cup	365	46.9	0.0	83	0	18.2	6.3	154	47%
chopped, broiled	1 cup	340	39.6	0.0	84	0	19.0	6.6	137	52%
chopped, roasted	1 cup	330	38.5	0.0	87	0	18.4	6.4	126	52%
raw	1 oz	43	6.0	0.0	14	0	1.9	0.7	18	42%
raw, approx 3.1 oz	1 chop	133	19.8	0.0	48	0	5.4	1.9	59	38%
roasted	3 oz	184	24.5	0.0	54	0	8.8	3.1	73	45%
Untrimmed										
boneless, braised	3 oz	161	22.6	0.0	39	0	7.1	2.6	69	41%
boneless, broiled	3 oz	177	25.9	0.0	48	0	7.3	2.5	77	39%
boneless, raw	1 lb	658	93.3	0.0	227	0	28.6	9.9	290	41%
boneless, roasted	3 oz	176	24.2	0.0	48	0	8.0	2.9	73	43%
braised	3 oz	208	21.6	0.0	43	0	12.8	4.7	70	57%
broiled	3 oz	220	22.6	0.0	58	0	13.7	5.0	73	58%
chopped, braised	1 cup	493	39.2	0.0	76	0	36.0	13.0	148	67%
chopped, broiled	1 cup	463	33.8	0.0	77	0	35.4	12.8	136	70%
chopped, roasted	1 cup	407	35.1	0.0	83	0	28.6	10.3	127	65%
raw	1 oz	78	4.9	0.0	12	0	6.3	2.3	20	74%
roasted	3 oz	222	23.1	0.0	51	0	13.6	4.8	74	57%
SPARERIBS										
Untrimmed										
braised	3 oz	337	24.7	0.0	79	0	25.8	9.4	103	70%
raw	1 lb	1297	77.5	0.0	345	0	107.0	40.5	354	76%
raw	1 oz	81	4.8	0.0	22	0	6.7	2.5	22	76%
raw 'Gourmet' *(JM)*	4.5 oz	250	14.0	0.0	70	0	22.0	(mq)	(mq)	78%
SPLEEN										
braised	3 oz	127	24.0	0.0	91	0	2.7	0.9	420	20%

Food Name	Serving Size	Calories	Prot. gms	Carbs gms	Sod. mgs	Fiber gms	Fat gms	Sat. Fat gms	Chol. mgs	% Fat Cal.
raw	1 oz	28	5.1	0.0	28	0	0.7	0.2	103	24%
STOMACH, raw	1 oz	45	4.7	0.0	15	0	2.7	na	55	56%
TENDERLOIN										
Trimmed										
boneless *(JM)*	3 oz	120	17.0	0.0	40	0	5.0	(mq)	(mq)	40%
broiled	3 oz	159	25.9	0.0	55	0	5.4	1.9	80	32%
chopped or diced, roasted	1 cup	232	40.3	0.0	94	0	6.7	2.3	130	27%
raw	1 lb	544	95.2	0.0	227	0	15.5	5.3	295	27%
raw	1 oz	34	5.9	0.0	14	0	1.0	0.3	18	28%
roasted	3 oz	139	23.9	0.0	48	0	4.1	1.4	67	28%
Untrimmed										
broiled	3 oz	171	25.4	0.0	54	0	6.9	2.5	80	38%
raw	1 lb	617	93.2	0.0	222	0	24.5	8.5	299	37%
raw	1 oz	39	5.8	0.0	14	0	1.5	0.5	19	37%
roasted	3 oz	147	23.6	0.0	47	0	5.1	1.8	67	33%
TOP LOIN										
Trimmed										
braised	3 oz	172	24.7	0.0	36	0	7.3	2.7	62	40%
broiled	3 oz	173	26.5	0.0	55	0	6.6	2.3	68	36%
chopped, braised	1 cup	388	48.2	0.0	73	0	20.2	7.0	136	49%
chopped, broiled	1 cup	361	40.3	0.0	94	0	20.9	7.2	132	54%
chopped, pan-fried in vegetable oil	1 cup	360	39.1	0.0	70	0	21.4	7.4	113	55%
chopped, roasted	1 cup	343	39.5	0.0	64	0	19.3	6.7	111	52%
pan-fried	3 oz	191	25.9	0.0	48	0	8.9	3.1	65	44%
pan-fried in vegetable oil	4 oz	291	31.7	0.0	57	0	17.4	6.0	92	55%
raw	1 oz	46	6.2	0.0	13	0	2.1	0.7	16	43%
roast, boneless, raw	1 lb	640	98.9	0.0	204	0	24.0	8.3	249	35%
roast, boneless, raw	1 oz	40	6.2	0.0	13	0	1.5	0.5	16	35%
roasted	3 oz	165	25.7	0.0	38	0	6.1	2.2	66	35%
Untrimmed										
braised	3 oz	198	23.6	0.0	36	0	10.8	4.0	64	51%
broiled	3 oz	195	25.5	0.0	54	0	9.6	3.4	69	46%
chopped, braised	1 cup	533	38.7	0.0	66	0	40.8	14.8	133	70%
chopped, broiled	1 cup	504	33.2	0.0	83	0	40.1	14.5	130	73%
chopped, pan-fried in vegetable oil	1 cup	549	30.1	0.0	63	0	46.5	16.8	118	78%
chopped, roasted	1 cup	462	33.9	0.0	62	0	35.2	12.7	115	70%
pan-fried	3 oz	218	24.7	0.0	47	0	12.6	4.5	66	53%
pan-fried in vegetable oil	3 oz	337	18.5	0.0	39	0	28.6	10.3	72	78%
raw	1 oz	86	4.9	0.0	11	0	7.3	2.6	18	77%
roast, boneless, raw	1 lb	866	91.8	0.0	195	0	52.7	18.2	268	56%
roast, boneless, raw	1 oz	54	5.7	0.0	12	0	3.3	1.1	17	57%
roasted	3 oz	192	24.5	0.0	37	0	9.7	3.5	66	47%
PORK, CANNED										
	1 oz	95	3.5	0.6	365	0	8.6	3.1	18	83%
approx .75 oz	1 slice	70	2.6	0.4	271	0	6.4	2.3	13	83%
(Hormel)	3 oz	240	11.0	2.0	1056	0	21.0	(mq)	(mq)	78%
(Hormel) chopped	3 oz	200	12.0	2.0	1073	0	16.0	(mq)	(mq)	72%
PORK, CURED										
blade roll, untrimmed, diced, roasted	1 cup	402	24.2	0.5	1362	0	32.9	11.7	94	75%
blade roll, untrimmed, diced, unheated	1 cup	377	23.1	0.0	1750	0	30.8	11.1	74	75%
blade roll, untrimmed, roasted	4 oz	325	19.6	0.4	1103	0	26.6	9.5	76	75%
blade roll, untrimmed, unheated	1 oz	76	4.7	0.0	354	0	6.2	2.3	15	75%
boneless, blade roll, untrimmed, roasted	3 oz	244	14.7	0.3	827	0	20.0	7.1	57	75%
boneless, blade roll, untrimmed, unheated	1 oz	76	4.7	0.0	354	0	6.2	2.3	15	75%

Food Name	Serving Size	Calories	Prot. gms	Carbs gms	Sod. mgs	Fiber gms	Fat gms	Sat. Fat gms	Chol. mgs	% Fat Cal.
PORK, GROUND										
cooked	3 oz	252	21.8	0.0	62	0	17.6	6.6	80	65%
raw	1 oz	75	4.8	0.0	16	0	6.0	2.2	20	74%
(JM)	3 oz	190	15.0	0.0	40	0	14.0	(mq)	(mq)	68%
PORK, SALT, cured, raw	1 oz	212	1.4	0.0	404	0	22.8	8.3	24	97%
PORK DINNER, FROZEN, chow mein 'Bi-Pack' (LaChoy)	8.642 oz	87	5.6	10.3	1218	2.9	3.2	1.2	10	31%
PORK ENTRÉE										
Canned										
chow mein 'Bi-Pack' (LaChoy)	3/4 cup	80	6.0	7.0	970	2.0	3.0	(mq)	14	34%
sweet and sour (LaChoy)	3/4 cup	250	6.0	48.0	1540	1.0	4.0	1.4	18	14%
Frozen										
barbecued back ribs 'Pork Classics' (John Morrell)	4.75 oz	240	12.0	8.0	480	0	17.0	(mq)	62	66%
barbecued chops, center cut 'Pork Classics' (John Morrell)	4.5 oz	230	29.0	7.0	410	0	9.0	(mq)	90	36%
barbecued loin, thin sliced 'Pork Classics' (John Morrell)	3 oz	150	17.0	5.0	440	0	6.0	(mq)	52	38%
barbecued spare ribs 'Pork Classics' (John Morrell)	4.5 oz	250	12.0	7.0	470	0	18.0	(mq)	51	68%
barbecued tenderloin 'Pork Classics' (John Morrell)	3 oz	130	18.0	3.0	220	0	5.0	(mq)	53	35%
breaded, steak (Hormel)	3 oz	220	12.0	11.0	(mq)	(mq)	15.0	(mq)	(mq)	60%
pattie deluxe 'Looney Tunes Porky Pig' (Tyson)	6.5 oz	370	14.0	48.0	490	na	14.0	na	35	34%
sweet and sour (Chun King)	13 oz	400	11.0	78.0	1460	na	5.0	(mq)	(mq)	11%
PORK FAT										
separable fat from fully cooked ham, roasted	1 oz	167	2.2	0.0	177	0	17.5	6.4	24	95%
separable fat from fully cooked ham, unheated	1 oz	164	1.6	<.1	143	0	17.4	6.4	19	96%
separable fat from ham and arm picnic, roasted	3 oz	502	6.5	0.0	530	0	52.6	19.3	73	95%
separable fat from ham and arm picnic, roasted	1 oz	168	2.2	0.0	177	0	17.5	6.4	24	95%
separable fat from ham and arm picnic, unheated	1 oz	164	1.6	0.0	143	0	17.4	6.4	19	96%
PORK RIND SNACK										
(Baken-ets)	1 oz	160	12.0	2.0	850	na	10.0	(mq)	25	62%
(Baken-ets) hot 'n spicy	1 oz	150	17.0	1.0	750	na	9.0	na	25	53%
PORK SEASONING AND COATING MIX										
'Bag'n Season' (Schilling)	1 pkg	103	1.1	23.6	3126	(mq)	0.4	na	0	4%
POT ROAST DINNER/ENTRÉE, FROZEN										
homestyle (Right Course)	9.25 oz	220	17.0	22.0	550	(mq)	7.0	2.0	35	29%
homestyle, w/browned potatoes (Stouffer's)	8 7/8 oz	280	20.0	24.0	690	na	11.0	na	na	36%
Yankee (Budget Gourmet)	11 oz	380	27.0	22.0	690	(mq)	21.0	(mq)	70	49%
Yankee (Healthy Choice)	11 oz	260	19.0	36.0	400	na	4.0	2.0	55	14%
Yankee (Le Menu)	10 oz	330	26.0	27.0	700	(mq)	13.0	(mq)	(mq)	36%
Yankee 'Classics' (Armour)	10 oz	310	25.0	26.0	670	(mq)	12.0	(mq)	85	35%
POT ROAST SEASONING MIX										
'Bag'n Season' (Schilling)	1 pkg	55	3.9	8.5	3030	na	0.6	na	0	10%
'Seasoning Blends' (Lawry's)	1 pkg	122	3.7	25.0	4008	>.5 c	0.7	na	0	5%
POTATO										
Baked										
in skin	4 oz	124	2.6	28.6	9	>.7 c	0.1	<.1	0	1%
in skin, pulp only	4 oz	105	2.2	24.4	6	1.7	0.1	<.1	0	1%
in skin, skin only	2 oz	112	2.4	26.1	12	2.3	0.1	<.1	0	1%
pulp	1/2 cup	57	1.2	13.1	3	.9	0.1	0.0	0	2%
Boiled										
in skin	2 oz	44	1.6	9.8	8	>2.1 c	0.1	<.1	0	2%
in skin, pulp only	4 oz	99	2.1	22.8	5	1.7	0.1	<.1	0	1%
in skin, pulp only	1/2 cup	68	1.5	15.7	3	1.4	0.1	0.0	0	1%
in skin, pulp only, approx 2.5 inch diam	1 potato	118	2.5	27.4	5	2.5	0.1	0.0	0	1%
pulp only	4 oz	98	1.9	22.7	6	>.4 c	0.1	<.1	0	1%
pulp only	1/2 cup	67	1.3	15.6	4	1.4	0.1	0.0	0	1%

Food Name	Serving Size	Calories	Prot. gms	Carbs gms	Sod. mgs	Fiber gms	Fat gms	Sat. Fat gms	Chol. mgs	% Fat Cal.
pulp only, approx 2.5 inch diam	1 potato	116	2.3	27.0	7	2.4	0.1	0.0	0	1%
Hash brown, cooked in vegetable oil	4 oz	237	2.7	24.2	27	>.5 c	15.8	6.2	0	57%
Microwaved										
in skin	4 oz	119	2.8	27.4	9	>.9 c	0.1	<.1	0	1%
in skin, pulp only	4 oz	113	2.4	26.4	8	>.5 c	0.1	<.1	0	1%
in skin, pulp only	1/2 cup	78	1.6	18.2	5	>.3 c	0.1	0.0	0	1%
in skin, skin only	2 oz	75	2.5	16.8	9	>1.8 c	0.1	<.1	0	1%
Raw										
peeled	1 oz	22	0.6	5.1	2	.5	<.1	tr	0	<4%
pulp only, diced	1/2 cup	59	1.5	13.5	5	1.2	0.1	0.0	0	2%
skin only	2 oz	33	1.5	7.1	6	>1.0 c	0.1	<.1	0	3%
unpeeled	1 lb	269	7.1	61.2	21	5.4	0.3	0.1	0	1%
POTATO, CANNED										
(Stokely)	1/2 cup	50	2.0	11.0	360	(mq)	0.0	0.0	0	0%
(Veg•All)	1/2 cup	60	1.0	13.0	260	na	0.0	na	na	0%
approx 1.2 oz	1 potato	21	0.5	4.8	(mq)	>.1 c	0.1	<.1	0	4%
diced (Bush's Best)	1/2 cup	40	1.0	8.0	340	na	0.0	na	na	0%
diced (Taylor's Brand)	1 cup	90	3.0	25.0	292	(mq)	0.0	0.0	0	0%
drained	4 oz	68	1.6	15.4	(mq)	>.3 c	0.2	0.1	0	3%
drained	1/2 cup	54	1.3	12.3	234	>.2 c	0.2	0.1	0	3%
drained, approx 1 inch diam	1 potato	21	0.5	4.8	91	>.1 c	0.1	0.0	0	4%
new, extra small, whole (S&W)	1/2 cup	45	2.0	9.0	310	na	0.0	0.0	0	0%
new, small, whole (IGA)	1/2 cup	45	2.0	9.0	300	na	0.0	0.0	0	0%
new, whole, drained (Hunt's)	4 oz	70	2.0	15.0	230	<1.0	<1.0	na	0	<12%
sliced (Bush's Best)	1/2 cup	40	1.0	8.0	340	na	0.0	na	na	0%
sliced (Taylor's Brand)	1 cup	90	3.0	25.0	292	(mq)	0.0	0.0	0	0%
sliced, w/liquid (Del Monte)	1/2 cup	45	1.0	10.0	355	(mq)	0.0	0.0	0	0%
white, diced (Allens)	1/2 cup	45	2.0	10.0	360	(mq)	<1.0	(tr)	0	<16%
white, double diced (Allens)	1/2 cup	45	2.0	10.0	540	(mq)	<1.0	(tr)	0	<16%
white, sliced (A&P)	1/2 cup	45	2.0	11.0	320	(mq)	<1.0	(tr)	0	<15%
white, sliced (Allens)	1/2 cup	45	2.0	10.0	360	(mq)	<1.0	(tr)	0	<16%
white, sliced 'No Salt Added' (Pathmark)	1 cup	100	3.0	20.0	15	(mq)	0.0	0.0	0	0%
white, small, sliced (Finast)	1/2 cup	55	1.0	13.0	375	(mq)	0.0	0.0	0	0%
white, small, whole (Finast)	1/2 cup	55	1.0	13.0	375	(mq)	0.0	0.0	0	0%
white, whole (A&P)	1/2 cup	45	2.0	11.0	320	(mq)	<1.0	(tr)	0	<15%
white, whole 'No Salt Added' (Pathmark)	1 cup	100	3.0	20.0	15	(mq)	0.0	0.0	0	0%
whole (Bush's Best)	1/2 cup	40	1.0	8.0	340	na	0.0	na	na	0%
whole, w/liquid	1 cup	120	4.1	26.0	903	4.8	0.5	0.1	0	4%
whole, w/liquid	1/2 cup	60	2.0	13.0	452	>.4 c	0.2	0.1	0	3%
whole, w/liquid (Del Monte)	1/2 cup	45	1.0	10.0	355	(mq)	0.0	0.0	0	0%
w/liquid	4 oz	45	1.5	9.8	341	>.3 c	0.2	<.1	0	4%
POTATO, FINNISH YELLOW, raw (Frieda's)	3.5 oz	100	3.3	22.0	na	(mq)	na	na	0	0%
POTATO, FREEZE-DRIED										
hash brown, prepared (Mountain House)	1 cup	150	2.0	36.0	(mq)	(mq)	0.0	0.0	na	0%
POTATO, FROZEN										
fried	9 oz	419	6.5	63.8	58	>1.3 c	16.5	7.8	0	35%
fried, cottage cut, heated in oven	4 oz	247	3.9	38.6	51	>.8 c	9.3	4.4	0	33%
fried, partially fried in oil, heated in oven	4 oz	252	3.9	38.4	35	4.8	9.9	4.7	0	35%
fried, partially fried in oil, heated in oven	1.75 oz	111	1.7	17.0	15	2.1	4.4	2.1	0	35%
hash brown, prepared in vegetable oil	4 oz	247	3.6	31.9	39	2.3	13.0	5.1	0	45%
hash brown, w/butter sauce, prepared	4 oz	202	2.8	27.4	115	(mq)	10.0	3.8	26	43%
puffs, partially fried in oil, prepared	4 oz	252	3.8	34.6	846	>.7 c	12.2	5.8	0	42%
whole, peeled	10 oz	221	6.7	49.6	71	>1.1 c	0.5	0.1	0	2%
whole, peeled, boiled, drained	4 oz	74	2.2	16.5	23	>.4 c	0.1	<.1	0	1%

Food Name	Serving Size	Calories	Prot. gms	Carbs gms	Sod. mgs	Fiber gms	Fat gms	Sat. Fat gms	Chol. mgs	% Fat Cal.
(A&P)										
fried, crinkle cut	3.5 oz	140	2.0	25.0	25	(mq)	4.0	(mq)	0	25%
fried, regular	3.5 oz	140	2.0	25.0	25	(mq)	4.0	(mq)	0	25%
fried, shoestring	3.5 oz	170	2.0	24.0	50	(mq)	6.0	(mq)	0	34%
fried, steak fries	3.5 oz	140	2.0	24.0	30	(mq)	4.0	(mq)	0	26%
hash brown	3.5 oz	80	2.0	17.0	20	(mq)	0.0	0.0	0	0%
morsels	3.5 oz	140	2.0	23.0	30	(mq)	4.0	(mq)	0	27%
(Heinz)										
fried, crinkle cut 'Deep Fries'	3 oz	150	2.0	22.0	30	(mq)	6.0	3.0	0	36%
fried 'Deep Fries'	3 oz	160	2.0	23.0	20	(mq)	6.0	3.0	0	35%
fried, shoestring 'Deep Fries'	3 oz	200	2.0	25.0	20	(mq)	10.0	5.0	0	46%
hash brown, w/butter and onions 'Deep Fries'	3 oz	110	1.0	14.0	80	(mq)	7.0	4.0	5	51%
(MicroMagic)										
fried	3 oz	290	3.0	40.0	30	(mq)	13.0	(mq)	na	41%
fried, skinny	3 oz	350	4.0	49.0	40	(mq)	15.0	(mq)	na	39%
sticks 'Tater Sticks'	4 oz	390	2.0	43.0	620	(mq)	22.0	(mq)	na	52%
(Ore-Ida)										
fried, cottage cut	3 oz	120	2.0	19.0	25	(mq)	5.0	2.0	0	35%
fried 'Country Style Dinner Fries'	3 oz	110	2.0	19.0	30	(mq)	3.0	2.0	0	24%
fried, crinkle cut 'Golden Crinkles'	3 oz	120	2.0	19.0	35	(mq)	4.0	2.0	0	30%
fried, crinkle cut 'Lites'	3 oz	90	1.0	16.0	35	(mq)	2.0	(mq)	0	21%
fried, crinkle cut, microwave	3.5 oz	180	2.0	26.0	35	(mq)	8.0	4.0	0	39%
fried, crinkle cut 'Pixie Crinkles'	3 oz	140	2.0	21.0	40	(mq)	6.0	3.0	0	37%
fried 'Crisp Crowns'	3 oz	160	2.0	20.0	525	(mq)	9.0	4.0	0	48%
fried 'Crispers!'	3 oz	230	2.0	25.0	545	(mq)	15.0	8.0	0	56%
fried, French, extra crispy 'Nacho Crispers'	3 oz	180	2.0	21.0	280	na	10.0	na	0	50%
fried, French 'Fast Fries'	3 oz	150	2.0	23.0	230	na	7.0	na	0	39%
fried 'Golden Fries'	3 oz	120	2.0	19.0	35	(mq)	4.0	2.0	0	30%
fried 'Lites'	3 oz	90	2.0	16.0	30	(mq)	2.0	<1.0	0	20%
fried, shoestring	3 oz	140	2.0	21.0	30	(mq)	6.0	3.0	0	37%
fried, shoestring 'Lites'	3 oz	90	1.0	15.0	25	(mq)	4.0	2.0	0	36%
fried, wedges 'Home Style Potato Wedges'	3 oz	100	2.0	17.0	45	(mq)	3.0	1.0	0	26%
fried, w/onions 'Crispy Crowns'	3 oz	170	1.0	20.0	570	(mq)	9.0	5.0	0	49%
hash brown 'Golden Patties'	2.5 oz	140	1.0	15.0	295	(mq)	8.0	4.0	0	53%
hash brown, microwave	2 oz	130	1.0	12.0	170	(mq)	8.0	4.0	0	58%
hash brown, shredded	3 oz	70	1.0	15.0	40	(mq)	<1.0	na	0	<12%
hash brown 'Southern Style'	3 oz	70	1.0	16.0	35	(mq)	<1.0	na	0	<12%
hash brown, w/cheddar 'Cheddar Browns'	3 oz	90	2.0	13.0	415	(mq)	2.0	1.0	10	23%
mashed, natural butter flavor, prepared w/2% milk	1/2 cup	170	4.0	23.0	230	na	5.0	na	5	29%
mashed, natural butter flavor, unprepared	2.25 oz	100	1.0	14.0	140	na	3.0	na	5	31%
puffs, bacon flavored 'Tater Tots'	3 oz	140	2.0	19.0	625	(mq)	6.0	3.0	0	39%
puffs 'Tater Tots'	3 oz	140	1.0	19.0	550	(mq)	7.0	3.0	0	44%
puffs 'Tater Tots' microwave	4 oz	200	2.0	29.0	670	(mq)	9.0	4.0	0	40%
puffs, w/onion 'Tater Tots'	3 oz	140	2.0	19.0	715	(mq)	6.0	3.0	0	39%
whole, small	3 oz	70	2.0	16.0	45	(mq)	<1.0	(tr)	0	<11%
(Quick 'n Crispy)										
fried, crinkle cut	4 oz	370	3.0	44.0	50	(mq)	19.0	(mq)	na	48%
fried, shoestring	4 oz	390	3.0	48.0	50	(mq)	20.0	(mq)	na	47%
fried, thin cuts	4 oz	370	3.0	44.0	50	(mq)	19.0	(mq)	na	48%
wedges	4 oz	280	3.0	36.0	40	(mq)	13.0	(mq)	na	43%
(Seabrook)										
diced and hash-shred	4 oz	80	2.0	19.0	41	(mq)	0.0	0.0	0	0%
fried	3 oz	120	2.0	20.0	25	(mq)	4.0	(mq)	na	29%
fried, cottage cut	2.8 oz	110	1.0	17.0	14	(mq)	4.0	(mq)	na	33%

Food Name	Serving Size	Calories	Prot. gms	Carbs gms	Sod. mgs	Fiber gms	Fat gms	Sat. Fat gms	Chol. mgs	% Fat Cal.
fried, crinkle cut	3 oz	120	2.0	20.0	24	(mq)	4.0	(mq)	na	29%
fried, shoestring	3 oz	140	2.0	20.0	45	(mq)	6.0	(mq)	na	38%
white, whole, boiled	3.2 oz	60	2.0	13.0	5	(mq)	0.0	0.0	0	0%
(Southern) white, whole	3.5 oz	69	2.0	15.0	20	(mq)	0.1	(tr)	0	1%
POTATO CHIPS AND SNACKS										
(Allens)										
barbecue flavor	1 oz	150	2.0	14.0	280	(mq)	9.0	(mq)	0	56%
hot flavor	1 oz	150	2.0	14.0	200	(mq)	9.0	(mq)	0	56%
potato sticks, shoestring, canned	1 oz	140	2.0	16.0	190	(mq)	8.0	(mq)	na	50%
potato sticks, shoestring, canned 'No Salt'	1 oz	140	1.0	16.0	10	(mq)	8.0	(mq)	na	51%
regular flavor	1 oz	160	2.0	14.0	270	(mq)	10.0	(mq)	0	58%
(Bachman)										
'Kettle Cooked'	1 oz	140	2.0	16.0	115	(mq)	8.0	(mq)	0	50%
pasta snack chip 'Pastapazazz'	1 oz	150	2.0	15.0	340	(mq)	9.0	(mq)	na	54%
'Ridge'	1 oz	160	2.0	14.0	260	(mq)	10.0	(mq)	0	58%
'Ruffled'	1 oz	160	2.0	14.0	260	(mq)	10.0	(mq)	0	58%
Saratoga-style 'Kettle Cooked'	1 oz	140	2.0	16.0	115	(mq)	8.0	(mq)	0	50%
sour cream and onion flavor	1 oz	150	2.0	14.0	200	(mq)	9.0	(mq)	0	56%
'Unsalted'	1 oz	160	2.0	14.0	5	(mq)	10.0	(mq)	0	58%
vinegar flavor	1 oz	150	2.0	15.0	610	(mq)	9.0	(mq)	0	54%
(Barbara's Bakery)										
herb and garlic flavor 'True Blues'	1 oz	140	2.0	15.0	120	na	9.0	na	0	54%
ripple	1 oz	150	2.0	14.0	250	na	10.0	na	0	58%
'True Blues'	1 oz	150	2.0	15.0	120	na	10.0	na	0	57%
(Barrel O'Fun)	1 oz	150	2.0	14.0	160	.4	10.0	(mq)	0	58%
(Cape Cod)										
dill and sour cream flavor	1 oz	150	2.0	16.0	160	(mq)	8.0	(mq)	0	50%
dill and sour cream flavor 'No Salt'	1 oz	150	2.0	16.0	15	(mq)	8.0	(mq)	0	50%
'No Salt Added'	1 oz	150	2.0	16.0	0	(mq)	8.0	(mq)	0	50%
regular flavor	1 oz	150	2.0	16.0	120	(mq)	8.0	(mq)	0	50%
'Waves'	1 oz	150	2.0	16.0	120	(mq)	8.0	(mq)	0	50%
(Cottage Fries) 'No Salt Added'	1 oz	160	2.0	14.0	5	(mq)	11.0	(mq)	0	61%
(Eagle)										
barbecue flavor 'Extra Crunchy'	1 oz	150	2.0	16.0	220	(mq)	8.0	(mq)	0	50%
barbecue flavor 'Extra Crunchy Louisiana'	1 oz	150	2.0	16.0	140	(mq)	8.0	(mq)	0	50%
barbecue flavor 'Thins'	1 oz	150	2.0	15.0	220	(mq)	10.0	(mq)	0	57%
'Eagle Thins'	1 oz	150	2.0	15.0	220	(mq)	10.0	(mq)	0	57%
'Extra Crunchy'	1 oz	150	2.0	16.0	180	(mq)	8.0	(mq)	0	50%
'Idaho Russet'	1 oz	150	2.0	16.0	180	(mq)	8.0	(mq)	0	50%
'Ridged Thins'	1 oz	150	2.0	15.0	220	(mq)	10.0	(mq)	0	57%
sour cream and onion flavor 'Ridged'	1 oz	150	2.0	15.0	280	(mq)	10.0	(mq)	0	57%
(Eden Foods)										
brown rice chips	1 oz	130	2.0	19.0	197	na	5.0	na	na	35%
sea vegetable chips	1 oz	130	1.0	22.0	200	na	5.0	na	na	33%
wasabi snack chips	1 oz	130	1.0	22.0	200	(mq)	4.0	(mq)	0	28%
(Featherweight) 'Low Salt'	1 oz	160	2.0	14.0	4	(mq)	11.0	(mq)	0	61%
(Flavor Tree) sour cream and onion flavor potato sticks	1/4 cup	127	3.0	12.5	360	>.1 c	8.3	(mq)	na	55%
(Funyuns) rings, onion flavor, approx 11 rings	1 oz	140	2.0	18.0	275	(mq)	6.0	(mq)	0	40%
(Great Snackers)										
barbecue flavor	1 serving	60	1.0	8.0	170	(mq)	3.0	(mq)	0	43%
cheddar cheese flavor	1 serving	60	1.0	8.0	170	(mq)	3.0	(mq)	0	43%
sour cream and onion flavor	.5 oz	70	1.0	10.0	140	na	3.0	1.0	0	38%
toasted onion flavor	1 serving	60	1.0	8.0	120	(mq)	3.0	(mq)	0	43%

Food Name	Serving Size	Calories	Prot. gms	Carbs gms	Sod. mgs	Fiber gms	Fat gms	Sat. Fat gms	Chol. mgs	% Fat Cal.
(Hain)										
carrot chip	1 oz	150	2.0	16.0	160	(mq)	9.0	(mq)	0	53%
carrot chip, barbecue	1 oz	140	2.0	16.0	160	(mq)	8.0	(mq)	0	50%
carrot chip 'No Salt Added'	1 oz	150	2.0	16.0	30	(mq)	7.0	(mq)	0	47%
(Health Valley)										
'Country'	1 oz	160	2.0	15.0	60	.9	10.0	(mq)	0	57%
'Country Dip'	1 oz	160	2.0	15.0	60	.9	10.0	(mq)	0	57%
'Country Dip No Salt Added'	1 oz	160	2.0	15.0	1	.9	10.0	(mq)	0	57%
'Country Natural No Salt Added'	1 oz	160	2.0	15.0	1	.9	10.0	(mq)	0	57%
'Country No Salt Added'	1 oz	160	2.0	15.0	1	.9	10.0	(mq)	0	57%
'Country Ripple'	1 oz	160	2.0	15.0	60	.9	10.0	(mq)	0	57%
'Country Ripple No Salt Added'	1 oz	160	2.0	15.0	1	.9	10.0	(mq)	0	57%
'Natural'	1 oz	160	2.0	15.0	60	.9	10.0	(mq)	0	57%
(Keebler)										
original flavor, lightly seasoned	1 oz	140	1.0	18.0	190	na	7.0	1.0	0	45%
sour cream and onion flavor	1 oz	140	2.0	17.0	260	na	7.0	1.0	0	45%
(Kettle Chips)										
jalapeño jack flavor	1 oz	150	2.0	15.0	110	na	9.0	1.0	0	54%
lightly salted	1 oz	150	2.0	15.0	80	na	9.0	1.0	0	54%
New York cheddar flavor	1 oz	150	2.0	15.0	100	na	9.0	1.0	0	54%
no salt	1 oz	150	2.0	15.0	10	na	9.0	1.0	0	54%
organically grown, w/sea salt	1 oz	150	2.0	15.0	80	na	9.0	1.0	0	54%
salsa w/mesquite flavor	1 oz	150	2.0	15.0	120	na	9.0	1.0	0	54%
sea salt and vinegar flavor	1 oz	150	2.0	15.0	120	na	9.0	1.0	0	54%
yogurt and green onion flavor	1 oz	150	2.0	15.0	120	na	9.0	1.0	0	54%
(King Kold)										
au gratin flavor	1 oz	150	2.0	15.0	220	(mq)	8.0	(mq)	na	51%
barbecue flavor 'BBQ'	1 oz	140	2.0	16.0	360	(mq)	8.0	(mq)	na	50%
dill flavor	1 oz	150	2.0	16.0	340	(mq)	8.0	(mq)	na	50%
onion-garlic flavor	1 oz	150	2.0	15.0	420	(mq)	9.0	(mq)	na	54%
regular flavor	1 oz	150	2.0	16.0	160	(mq)	9.0	(mq)	0	53%
'Rip-L'	1 oz	150	2.0	16.0	150	(mq)	9.0	(mq)	0	53%
sour cream and onion flavor	1 oz	150	2.0	15.0	220	(mq)	10.0	(mq)	na	57%
(Lay's)										
barbecue flavor, approx 15-20 chips	1 oz	150	1.0	15.0	270	1.1	9.0	na	0	56%
barbecue flavor 'Kansas City Style' approx 15-20 chips	1 oz	150	2.0	15.0	270	1.1	9.0	na	0	54%
Cajun flavor 'Crunch Tators Amazin Cajun'	1 oz	150	2.0	17.0	150	1.1	8.0	na	0	49%
cheddar cheese flavor, approx 15-20 chips	1 oz	150	2.0	14.0	1	1.1	10.0	na	0	58%
'Flamin' Hot' approx 15-20 chips	1 oz	150	2.0	15.0	190	1.1	9.0	na	0	54%
jalapeño flavor 'Crunch Tators Hoppin' Jalapeño'	1 oz	140	1.0	18.0	200	1.1	7.0	na	0	45%
mesquite flavor 'Crunch Tators Mighty Mesquite'	1 oz	150	2.0	17.0	135	1.1	8.0	na	0	49%
original flavor, approx 15-20 chips	1 oz	150	1.0	15.0	170	1.1	10.0	na	0	58%
original flavor 'Crunch Tators' approx 16 chips	1 oz	150	2.0	17.0	120	1.1	8.0	na	0	49%
salt and vinegar flavor, approx 15-20 chips	1 oz	150	1.0	14.0	390	1.1	10.0	na	0	60%
sour cream and onion flavor, approx 15-20 chips	1 oz	160	2.0	15.0	220	1.1	10.0	na	1	57%
tangy ranch flavor, approx 15-20 chips	1 oz	160	2.0	15.0	210	1.1	10.0	na	0	57%
'Unsalted'	1 oz	150	2.0	15.0	10	(mq)	10.0	(mq)	0	57%
(Louise's)										
mesquite barbecue flavor, fat-free	1 oz	100	2.0	23.0	200	na	<1.0	na	0	<8%
original flavor, fat-free	1 oz	100	2.0	23.0	200	na	<1.0	na	0	<8%
vinegar and salt flavor, fat-free	1 oz	100	2.0	23.0	200	na	<1.0	na	0	<8%
(Mr. Phipps)										
tater crisps, bar-b-que flavor	.5 oz	60	1.0	10.0	160	na	2.0	<1.0	0	29%
tater crisps, sour cream 'n onion flavor	.5 oz	60	1.0	10.0	150	na	2.0	<1.0	0	29%

Food Name	Serving Size	Calories	Prot. gms	Carbs gms	Sod. mgs	Fiber gms	Fat gms	Sat. Fat gms	Chol. mgs	% Fat Cal.
(Munchos) plain, approx 16 chips	1 oz	160	1.0	15.0	230	na	10.0	na	0	58%
(Nabisco)										
baked, cheddar cheese flavor, cracker chips 'Zings'	.5 oz	70	1.0	9.0	140	na	3.0	<1.0	2	40%
baked, ranch flavor, cracker chips 'Zings'	.5 oz	70	1.0	9.0	140	na	3.0	<1.0	2	40%
cracker chips, baked 'Zings'	.5 oz	70	1.0	10.0	115	na	3.0	<1.0	0	38%
(O'Boisies)										
regular flavor	1 oz	150	1.0	16.0	180	(mq)	9.0	2.0	0	54%
sour cream and onion flavor	1 oz	150	2.0	15.0	190	(mq)	9.0	2.0	0	54%
(Planters)										
potato sticks	1 oz	160	1.0	15.0	0	na	10.0	2.0	170	58%
potato sticks, barbecue flavor	1 oz	160	1.0	15.0	0	na	10.0	2.0	220	58%
(Poore Brothers)										
barbecue flavor	1 oz	150	2.0	15.0	0	2.0	10.0	2.0	60	57%
Cajun flavor	1 oz	140	2.0	16.0	0	2.0	8.0	1.0	55	50%
dill pickle flavor	1 oz	140	2.0	16.0	0	2.0	8.0	1.0	95	50%
grilled steak and onion flavor	1 oz	140	2.0	15.0	0	2.0	8.0	1.0	110	51%
jalapeño flavor	1 oz	140	2.0	16.0	0	2.0	9.0	2.0	100	53%
Parmesan and garlic flavor	1 oz	140	2.0	16.0	0	2.0	9.0	2.0	80	53%
regular flavor	1 oz	140	2.0	17.0	0	2.0	8.0	1.0	40	49%
salt and vinegar flavor	1 oz	140	2.0	15.0	0	1.0	9.0	2.0	125	54%
unsalted	1 oz	140	2.0	17.0	0	2.0	8.0	1.0	5	49%
(Pringle's)										
barbecue flavor 'Light'	1 oz	150	2.0	17.0	125	(mq)	8.0	(mq)	na	49%
cheese flavor 'Cheez-ums'	1 oz	170	2.0	12.0	200	(mq)	13.0	(mq)	na	68%
French onion flavor 'Idaho Rippled'	1 oz	170	2.0	13.0	175	(mq)	12.0	(mq)	na	64%
'Idaho Rippled'	1 oz	170	2.0	13.0	150	(mq)	12.0	(mq)	na	64%
'Light'	1 oz	150	2.0	17.0	120	(mq)	8.0	(mq)	na	49%
ranch flavor 'Light'	1 oz	150	2.0	17.0	135	(mq)	8.0	(mq)	na	49%
'Regular'	1 oz	170	2.0	12.0	170	(mq)	13.0	(mq)	na	68%
sour cream and onion flavor	1 oz	170	2.0	13.0	135	(mq)	12.0	(mq)	na	64%
taco and cheddar flavor 'Idaho Rippled'	1 oz	170	2.0	13.0	160	(mq)	12.0	(mq)	na	64%
(Ray's)										
taro chips, salted	1 oz	139	2.0	20.0	167	na	6.0	na	0	38%
taro chips, unsalted	1 oz	139	2.0	20.0	15	na	6.0	na	0	38%
(Ruffles)										
barbecue flavor	1 oz	150	1.0	16.0	320	(mq)	9.0	(mq)	0	54%
Cajun flavor 'Cajun Spice'	1 oz	150	1.0	15.0	240	(mq)	10.0	(mq)	0	58%
cheddar and sour cream flavor	1 oz	150	2.0	16.0	260	(mq)	9.0	(mq)	0	53%
'Choice' 40% less fat, approx 16 chips	1 oz	130	2.0	18.0	130	1.0	6.0	1.0	0	40%
'Light Choice' 1/3 less fat	1 oz	130	2.0	19.0	140	na	6.0	na	0	39%
mesquite barbecue flavor 'Mesquite Grille'	1 oz	160	2.0	14.0	260	(mq)	10.0	(mq)	0	58%
ranch flavor	1 oz	160	2.0	15.0	240	(mq)	10.0	(mq)	0	57%
regular flavor	1 oz	150	1.0	15.0	190	(mq)	10.0	(mq)	0	58%
sour cream and onion flavor	1 oz	150	2.0	15.0	240	(mq)	9.0	(mq)	0	54%
(Schlotzsky's) barbecue, deli style	1 oz	150	2.0	17.0	115	na	6.0	na	0	42%
(Snacktime)										
jalapeño flavor 'Krunchers!'	1 oz	150	2.0	16.0	270	(mq)	9.0	(mq)	0	53%
'Krunchers!'	1 oz	150	2.0	16.0	170	(mq)	9.0	(mq)	0	53%
mesquite barbecue flavor 'Krunchers!'	1 oz	150	2.0	16.0	200	(mq)	9.0	(mq)	0	53%
(Spicer's)										
barbecue wheat flavor, for weight control	1 oz	100	5.0	12.0	75	9.0	5.0	na	0	40%
natural flavor, for weight control	1 oz	100	4.0	11.0	65	9.0	4.0	na	0	38%
sour cream and onion flavor, for weight control	1 oz	100	4.0	12.0	150	6.0	4.0	0.0	0	36%

Food Name	Serving Size	Calories	Prot. gms	Carbs gms	Sod. mgs	Fiber gms	Fat gms	Sat. Fat gms	Chol. mgs	% Fat Cal.
(Sun Chips)										
multi-grain snacks, French onion flavor	1 oz	140	3.0	18.0	120	na	7.0	na	0	43%
multi-grain snacks, harvest cheddar flavor	1 oz	140	2.0	18.0	125	na	7.0	na	0	44%
multi-grain snacks, original flavor	1 oz	150	2.0	18.0	100	na	8.0	na	0	47%
(Tato Skins)										
potato skins, baked	1 oz	150	1.0	17.0	160	(mq)	8.0	1.0	0	50%
potato skins, cheese n' bacon flavor,	1 oz	150	1.0	17.0	180	(mq)	8.0	1.0	0	50%
potato skins, sour cream n' chives flavor	1 oz	150	1.0	17.0	180	(mq)	8.0	1.0	0	50%
(Westbrae)										
no salt	1 oz	150	2.0	16.0	10	na	8.0	na	0	50%
'Ripple'	1 oz	150	2.0	16.0	100	na	8.0	na	0	50%
salted	1 oz	160	2.0	15.0	100	na	10.0	na	0	57%
(Wise)										
barbecue flavor	1 oz	150	2.0	14.0	240	(mq)	10.0	(mq)	0	58%
barbecue flavor 'Ridgies'	1 oz	150	2.0	14.0	240	(mq)	10.0	(mq)	0	58%
hot flavor	1 oz	160	2.0	14.0	290	(mq)	11.0	(mq)	0	61%
'New York Deli'	1 oz	160	2.0	14.0	120	(mq)	11.0	(mq)	0	61%
onion-garlic flavor	1 oz	150	2.0	14.0	250	(mq)	10.0	(mq)	0	58%
'Plain'	1 oz	150	2.0	14.0	190	(mq)	10.0	(mq)	0	58%
'Ridgies'	1 oz	150	2.0	14.0	190	(mq)	10.0	(mq)	0	58%
'Ridgies Super Crispy'	1 oz	150	2.0	14.0	220	(mq)	10.0	(mq)	0	58%
rings, onion flavor	1 oz	130	<1.0	21.0	360	(mq)	5.0	(mq)	0	34%
'Rippled'	1 oz	150	2.0	14.0	190	(mq)	10.0	(mq)	0	58%
sour cream and onion flavor 'Ridgies'	1 oz	160	2.0	14.0	240	(mq)	11.0	(mq)	na	61%
(Zapp's)										
Cajun flavor 'Lite Kettle'	1 oz	150	2.0	16.0	94	(mq)	8.0	(mq)	0	50%
Cajun flavor 'Original Kettle'	1 oz	150	2.0	16.0	94	(mq)	8.0	(mq)	0	50%
jalapeño flavor 'Original Kettle'	1 oz	150	2.0	16.0	85	(mq)	8.0	(mq)	na	50%
'Lite Kettle'	1 oz	150	2.0	16.0	45	(mq)	8.0	(mq)	0	50%
'Lite Kettle No Salt Added'	1 oz	150	2.0	16.0	<1	(mq)	8.0	(mq)	0	50%
mesquite barbecue flavor 'Lite Kettle'	1 oz	150	2.0	16.0	87	(mq)	8.0	(mq)	0	50%
mesquite barbecue flavor 'Original Kettle'	1 oz	150	2.0	16.0	87	(mq)	8.0	(mq)	0	50%
'Original Kettle'	1 oz	150	2.0	16.0	45	(mq)	8.0	(mq)	0	50%
'Original Kettle No Salt Added'	1 oz	150	2.0	16.0	<1	(mq)	8.0	(mq)	0	50%
sour cream and onion flavor 'Lite Kettle'	1 oz	150	2.0	16.0	79	(mq)	8.0	(mq)	na	50%
POTATO DISH, CANNED, au gratin *(Pantry Express)*	1/2 cup	120	3.0	17.0	430	1.5	5.0	2.0	5	38%
POTATO DISH, FROZEN										
au gratin 'Family Side Dish' *(Freezer Queen)*	4 oz	100	2.0	19.0	440	(mq)	2.0	(mq)	na	18%
au gratin 'For One' *(Birds Eye)*	5.5 oz	240	8.0	24.0	590	1.0	13.0	(mq)	30	48%
au gratin 'One Serving' *(Green Giant)*	5.5 oz	200	7.0	20.0	560	(mq)	10.0	4.0	20	46%
au gratin, side dish *(Stouffer's)*	5.75 oz	170	5.0	17.0	670	na	9.0	na	na	48%
baked, butter 'Twice Baked' *(Ore-Ida)*	5 oz	200	4.0	27.0	350	na	9.0	na	0	40%
baked, cheddar cheese 'Twice Baked' *(Ore-Ida)*	5 oz	190	4.0	28.0	420	na	7.0	na	0	33%
baked, ranch 'Twice Baked' *(Ore-Ida)*	5 oz	180	5.0	28.0	320	na	6.0	na	0	29%
baked, sour cream and chives 'Twice Baked' *(Ore-Ida)*	5 oz	180	4.0	28.0	360	na	6.0	na	0	30%
baked, stuffed w/cheddar cheese *(Oh Boy!)*	6 oz	142	4.0	23.0	612	(mq)	4.0	(mq)	6	25%
baked, stuffed w/cheese flavored topping *(Green Giant)*	5 oz	200	4.0	33.0	520	(mq)	6.0	(mq)	na	27%
baked, stuffed w/real bacon *(Oh Boy!)*	6 oz	116	4.0	18.0	641	(mq)	3.0	(mq)	5	24%
baked, stuffed w/sour cream and chives *(Green Giant)*	5 oz	230	5.0	31.0	580	(mq)	10.0	(mq)	na	39%
baked, stuffed w/sour cream and chives *(Oh Boy!)*	6 oz	129	3.0	18.0	418	(mq)	5.0	(mq)	2	35%
baked, topped w/salsa and cheese *(Ore-Ida)*	5.6 oz	160	5.0	25.0	350	na	4.0	na	10	23%
cheddared, 'Side Dish' *(Budget Gourmet)*	5.5 oz	230	7.0	22.0	450	(mq)	13.0	(mq)	35	50%
cheddared, w/broccoli 'Side Dish' *(Budget Gourmet)*	5 oz	130	6.0	18.0	340	(mq)	4.0	(mq)	25	27%
fried, 'Country Style Dinner Fries' *(Ore-Ida)*	3 oz	110	2.0	19.0	30	(mq)	3.0	2.0	0	24%

Food Name	Serving Size	Calories	Prot. gms	Carbs gms	Sod. mgs	Fiber gms	Fat gms	Sat. Fat gms	Chol. mgs	% Fat Cal.
fried, w/onions 'Crispy Crowns' (Ore-Ida)	3 oz	170	1.0	20.0	570	(mq)	9.0	5.0	0	49%
garden casserole, low-fat, 'Quick Meals' (Healthy Choice)	9.25 oz	180	12.0	23.0	360	na	4.0	2.0	20	21%
hash brown, w/butter and onions, 'Deep Fries' (Heinz)	3 oz	110	1.0	14.0	80	(mq)	7.0	4.0	5	51%
hash brown, w/cheddar, 'Cheddar Browns' (Ore-Ida)	3 oz	90	2.0	13.0	415	(mq)	2.0	1.0	10	23%
nacho, 'Side Dish' (Budget Gourmet)	5 oz	180	10.0	14.0	360	(mq)	10.0	(mq)	30	48%
new, in sour cream sauce, 'Side Dish' (Budget Gourmet)	5 oz	120	3.0	15.0	300	(mq)	6.0	(mq)	20	43%
'O'Brien' (Ore-Ida)	3 oz	60	1.0	14.0	25	(mq)	<1.0	na	0	<13%
puffs, w/bacon-flavored vegetable protein, 'Tater Tots' (Ore-Ida)	3 oz	140	2.0	19.0	625	(mq)	6.0	3.0	0	39%
puffs, w/onion, 'Tater Tots' (Ore-Ida)	3 oz	140	2.0	19.0	715	(mq)	6.0	3.0	0	39%
scalloped, side dish (Stouffer's)	5.75 oz	130	4.0	16.0	610	na	6.0	na	na	40%
shredded, w/cheese sauce and vegetables, 'Singles' (Stokely)	4.5 oz	130	5.0	15.0	480	(mq)	6.0	(mq)	15	40%
sliced, w/cheddar cheese sauce and bacon, 'Singles' (Stokely)	4.5 oz	150	3.0	24.0	460	(mq)	5.0	(mq)	10	29%
three cheese, 'Side Dish' (Budget Gourmet)	5.75 oz	230	8.0	25.0	410	(mq)	11.0	(mq)	30	43%
wedges, hot and spicy, 'Texas Crispers' (Ore-Ida)	3 oz	180	2.0	19.0	250	na	10.0	na	0	52%
w/broccoli and cheese flavor sauce, 'One Serving' (Green Giant)	5.5 oz	130	4.0	19.0	720	(mq)	5.0	1.0	5	33%
w/broccoli and cheese sauce, 'Family Side Dish' (Freezer Queen)	5.5 oz	140	3.0	25.0	79	(mq)	3.0	(mq)	na	19%
POTATO DISH, MICROWAVE										
au gratin, 'Microwave Shelf Pack' (Green Giant)	1/2 cup	120	3.0	17.0	430	1.5	5.0	2.0	5	36%
scalloped, microwave cup (Lunch Bucket)	7.5 oz	160	4.0	20.0	770	na	7.0	na	35	40%
scalloped, w/ham, micro cup (Hormel)	7.5 oz	260	8.0	21.0	810	(mq)	16.0	(mq)	25	55%
POTATO DISH MIX										
and cheese, au gratin, 'Potatoes & Cheese' (Kraft) prepared	1/2 cup	130	4.0	19.0	570	(mq)	5.0	2.0	40	33%
and cheese, broccoli au gratin (Kraft) prepared	1/2 cup	150	5.0	20.0	530	(mq)	5.0	2.0	40	31%
broccoli au gratin 'Potato Medleys' (Betty Crocker) dry	1/5 pkg	110	2.0	22.0	550	(mq)	1.0	na	na	9%
broccoli au gratin 'Potato Medleys' (Betty Crocker) prepared w/margarine and 2% milk	1/2 cup	140	3.0	23.0	590	(mq)	4.0	(mq)	(mq)	26%
cheddar, w/mushrooms 'Potato Medleys' (Betty Crocker) dry	1/5 pkg	110	2.0	22.0	490	(mq)	1.0	na	na	9%
cheddar, w/mushrooms 'Potato Medleys' (Betty Crocker) prepared w/margarine and whole milk	1/2 cup	140	3.0	23.0	530	(mq)	4.0	(mq)	(mq)	26%
scalloped, w/broccoli 'Potato Medleys' (Betty Crocker) dry	1/5 pkg	100	2.0	19.0	460	(mq)	2.0	(mq)	na	18%
scalloped, w/broccoli 'Potato Medleys' (Betty Crocker) prepared	1/2 cup	140	3.0	21.0	500	(mq)	5.0	(mq)	(mq)	32%
scalloped, w/green beans and mushrooms (Betty Crocker) dry	1/5 pkg	110	2.0	20.0	460	(mq)	2.0	(mq)	na	17%
scalloped, w/green beans and mushrooms (Betty Crocker) prepared	1/2 cup	140	3.0	21.0	500	(mq)	5.0	(mq)	(mq)	32%
'SpudFlakes' (Martha White) prepared w/2% milk	1/3 cup	120	2.0	15.0	345	na	6.0	na	18	44%
w/cheese, scalloped, and ham (Kraft) prepared	1/2 cup	150	5.0	20.0	510	(mq)	5.0	2.0	15	31%
w/cheese, scalloped 'Potatoes & Cheese' (Kraft) prepared	1/2 cup	140	4.0	20.0	500	(mq)	5.0	2.0	25	32%
w/cheese, sour cream and chive (Kraft) prepared	1/2 cup	150	5.0	20.0	610	(mq)	5.0	2.0	10	31%
w/two cheeses 'Potatoes & Cheese' (Kraft) prepared	1/2 cup	130	4.0	19.0	540	(mq)	4.0	2.0	10	28%
POTATO ENTRÉE, FROZEN										
baked, chicken divan (Weight Watchers)	11.25 oz	280	17.0	38.0	480	na	7.0	2.0	30	22%
baked, homestyle turkey (Weight Watchers)	11.25 oz	230	17.0	27.0	510	na	7.0	3.0	45	26%
baked, vegetable primavera (Weight Watchers)	11.15 oz	320	11.0	49.0	500	na	9.0	2.0	5	25%
baked, w/broccoli and cheddar (Lean Cuisine)	10 3/8 oz	290	14.0	37.0	590	na	9.0	4.0	20	28%

Food Name	Serving Size	Calories	Prot. gms	Carbs gms	Sod. mgs	Fiber gms	Fat gms	Sat. Fat gms	Chol. mgs	% Fat Cal.
baked, w/broccoli and cheese *(Weight Watchers)*	10.5 oz	270	10.0	43.0	570	na	6.0	6.0	5	20%
baked, w/broccoli and ham *(Weight Watchers)*	11.5 oz	240	19.0	30.0	520	na	5.0	3.0	15	19%
baked, w/cheese sauce and broccoli 'Light & Healthy' *(Budget Gourmet)*	10.5 oz	300	13.0	40.0	740	na	10.0	4.0	30	30%
baked, w/sour cream *(Lean Cuisine)*	10 3/8 oz	230	9.0	38.0	570	na	5.0	2.0	15	19%
POTATO FLOUR										
	1/2 cup	316	7.2	71.9	31	5.5	0.7	0.2	0	2%
	1 oz	100	2.3	22.7	10	1.8	0.2	0.1	0	2%
POTATO MIX										
AU GRATIN										
(Betty Crocker) prepared w/margarine and skim milk	1/2 cup	150	4.0	21.0	600	(mq)	5.0	(mq)	(mq)	31%
(Fantastic Foods) prepared w/whole milk	1/2 cup	156	6.0	25.0	440	(mq)	4.0	(mq)	(mq)	23%
(Fantastic Foods) prepared w/whole milk and salted butter	1/2 cup	196	6.0	25.0	495	(mq)	8.0	(mq)	(mq)	37%
(French's) tangy, prepared	1/2 cup	130	4.0	20.0	480	(mq)	5.0	(mq)	na	32%
(General Mills) dry	1/6 pkg	100	2.0	20.0	520	na	1.0	na	na	9%
(General Mills) homestyle, w/broccoli, dry	1/6 pkg	90	2.0	18.0	490	na	1.0	na	na	10%
(General Mills) homestyle, w/broccoli, prepared w/margarine and 2% milk	1/2 cup	140	3.0	19.0	550	na	6.0	na	na	38%
(General Mills) prepared w/margarine and 2% milk	1/2 cup	150	3.0	21.0	580	na	6.0	na	na	36%
(Idahoan) prepared	1/2 cup	130	3.0	18.0	475	(mq)	5.0	(mq)	(mq)	35%
(Pillsbury) 'Specialty' tangy, dry	1/6 pkg	90	2.0	19.0	470	1.0	1.0	0.0	0	10%
(Pillsbury) tangy, prepared w/butter and whole milk	1/2 cup	140	3.0	20.0	520	1.0	6.0	3.0	15	37%
CASSEROLE *(French's)* cheddar and bacon, prepared	1/2 cup	130	4.0	18.0	390	(mq)	5.0	(mq)	na	34%
COUNTRY STYLE										
(Fantastic Foods) prepared	1/2 cup	85	3.0	19.0	316	(mq)	0.3	na	na	3%
(Fantastic Foods) prepared w/salted butter	1/2 cup	118	3.0	19.0	362	(mq)	4.0	(mq)	(mq)	29%
HASH BROWN										
(Betty Crocker) w/onions, prepared	1/6 pkg	110	2.0	24.0	40	(mq)	1.0	na	na	8%
(Betty Crocker) w/onions, prepared w/margarine	1/2 cup	160	2.0	24.0	100	(mq)	6.0	(mq)	na	34%
(General Mills)	1/6 pkg	110	2.0	24.0	25	na	<1.0	na	na	<8%
(General Mills) prepared w/margarine	1/2 cup	160	2.0	24.0	100	na	6.0	na	na	34%
(Idahoan) herb and butter, dry	1/6 pkg	90	2.0	16.0	425	(mq)	2.0	(mq)	na	20%
(Idahoan) prepared w/unsalted butter	1/2 cup	140	2.0	18.0	50	(mq)	7.0	(mq)	na	44%
(Idahoan) 'Quick One-Pan' prepared	1/2 cup	140	2.0	18.0	400	(mq)	7.0	(mq)	na	44%
JULIENNE										
(General Mills) dry	1/6 pkg	90	2.0	17.0	520	na	1.0	na	na	11%
(General Mills) prepared w/margarine and 2% milk	1/2 cup	130	3.0	19.0	580	na	5.0	na	na	34%
MASHED										
(Betty Crocker) bacon and cheddar 'Twice Baked' dry	1/6 pkg	110	3.0	19.0	500	(mq)	2.0	(mq)	na	17%
(Betty Crocker) bacon and cheddar 'Twice Baked' prepared	1/2 cup	210	6.0	21.0	600	(mq)	11.0	(mq)	(mq)	48%
(Betty Crocker) butter, herbed 'Twice Baked' dry	1/6 pkg	100	2.0	18.0	440	(mq)	2.0	(mq)	na	18%
(Betty Crocker) butter, herbed 'Twice Baked' prepared	1/2 cup	220	5.0	20.0	540	(mq)	13.0	(mq)	(mq)	54%
(Betty Crocker) cheddar, mild, w/onion 'Twice Baked' dry	1/6 pkg	100	2.0	18.0	540	(mq)	2.0	(mq)	na	18%
(Betty Crocker) cheddar, mild, w/onion 'Twice Baked' prepared	1/2 cup	190	5.0	19.0	640	(mq)	11.0	(mq)	(mq)	51%
(Betty Crocker) cheddar cheese 'Potato Buds' dry	1/12 pkg	110	2.0	20.0	440	na	2.0	na	na	17%
(Betty Crocker) cheddar cheese 'Potato Buds' prepared	1/2 cup	180	3.0	21.0	510	na	9.0	na	na	46%
(Betty Crocker) cheddar cheese 'Potato Buds' reduced fat recipe, dry	1/12 pkg	140	3.0	21.0	480	na	5.0	na	na	32%
(Betty Crocker) 'Potato Buds' prepared	1/2 cup	130	3.0	17.0	360	(mq)	6.0	(mq)	(mq)	40%
(Betty Crocker) 'Potato Buds' prepared w/o added salt	1/2 cup	130	3.0	17.0	90	(mq)	6.0	(mq)	(mq)	40%
(Country Store) prepared	1/3 cup	70	1.0	16.0	10	(mq)	0.0	0.0	0	0%

Food Name	Serving Size	Calories	Prot. gms	Carbs gms	Sod. mgs	Fiber gms	Fat gms	Sat. Fat gms	Chol. mgs	% Fat Cal.
(General Mills) American cheese, homestyle, dry	1/6 pkg	100	2.0	20.0	560	na	1.0	na	na	9%
(General Mills) American cheese, homestyle, prepared w/margarine and 2% milk	1/2 cup	150	3.0	21.0	620	na	6.0	na	na	36%
(General Mills) cheddar and bacon, dry	1/6 pkg	100	2.0	20.0	480	na	1.0	na	na	9%
(General Mills) cheddar and bacon, prepared w/margarine and 2% milk	1/2 cup	150	3.0	21.0	540	na	6.0	na	na	36%
(General Mills) cheddar cheese, homestyle, dry	1/6 pkg	90	2.0	19.0	470	na	1.0	na	na	10%
(General Mills) cheddar cheese, homestyle, prepared w/margarine and 2% milk	1/2 cup	150	3.0	21.0	530	na	6.0	na	na	36%
(Hungry Jack) 'Flakes' prepared	1/2 cup	140	3.0	17.0	380	(mq)	7.0	(mq)	na	44%
(Idahoan) cheddar, spicy, dry	1/6 pkg	90	2.0	17.0	450	(mq)	1.0	na	na	11%
(Idahoan) cheddar, spicy, prepared	1/2 cup	140	3.0	21.0	500	(mq)	5.0	(mq)	(mq)	32%
(Pillsbury) cheddar and bacon 'Specialty' dry	1/6 pkg	90	2.0	18.0	430	1.0	1.0	0.0	0	10%
(Pillsbury) cheddar and bacon 'Specialty' prepared w/butter and whole milk	1/2 cup	140	3.0	19.0	480	1.0	6.0	3.0	15	38%
SCALLOPED										
(Betty Crocker) cheesy, dry	1/6 pkg	90	2.0	19.0	500	(mq)	1.0	na	na	10%
(Betty Crocker) cheesy, prepared	1/2 cup	140	3.0	20.0	560	(mq)	5.0	(mq)	(mq)	33%
(Betty Crocker) dry	1/6 pkg	90	2.0	19.0	520	(mq)	1.0	na	na	10%
(Betty Crocker) prepared	1/2 cup	140	3.0	20.0	580	(mq)	5.0	(mq)	(mq)	33%
(Betty Crocker) sour cream and chives, dry	1/6 pkg	100	2.0	19.0	460	(mq)	2.0	(mq)	na	18%
(Betty Crocker) sour cream and chives, prepared	1/2 cup	140	3.0	21.0	520	(mq)	5.0	(mq)	(mq)	32%
(Betty Crocker) w/ham, dry	1/5 pkg	100	2.0	20.0	470	(mq)	1.0	(mq)	(mq)	9%
(Betty Crocker) w/ham, prepared	1/2 cup	160	4.0	22.0	540	(mq)	6.0	(mq)	(mq)	34%
(French's) creamy Italian, prepared	1/2 cup	120	4.0	19.0	430	(mq)	3.0	(mq)	na	23%
(French's) crispy top, w/savory onion mix, prepared	1/2 cup	140	3.0	20.0	430	na	5.0	(mq)	na	33%
(French's) real cheese, prepared	1/2 cup	140	4.0	19.0	380	(mq)	5.0	(mq)	na	33%
(French's) sour cream and chives, prepared	1/2 cup	150	3.0	19.0	550	(mq)	7.0	(mq)	na	42%
(General Mills) dry	1/6 pkg	90	2.0	19.0	510	na	1.0	na	na	10%
(General Mills) prepared w/margarine and 2% milk	1/2 cup	140	3.0	20.0	570	na	5.0	na	na	33%
(General Mills) smoky cheddar, dry	1/6 pkg	100	2.0	20.0	520	na	1.0	na	na	9%
(General Mills) smoky cheddar, prepared w/margarine and 2% milk	1/2 cup	140	3.0	21.0	580	na	5.0	na	na	32%
(General Mills) sour cream 'n chive	1/6 pkg	100	2.0	19.0	460	na	2.0	na	na	18%
(General Mills) sour cream 'n chive, prepared w/margarine and 2% milk	1/2 cup	150	3.0	20.0	520	na	6.0	na	na	37%
(General Mills) w/ham, dry	1/5 pkg	100	2.0	20.0	550	na	1.0	na	na	9%
(General Mills) w/ham, prepared w/margarine and 2% milk	1/2 cup	170	4.0	22.0	620	na	7.0	na	na	38%
(Idahoan) prepared	1/2 cup	140	3.0	20.0	425	(mq)	5.0	(mq)	(mq)	33%
(Idahoan) prepared w/o added salt, w/unsalted butter	1/2 cup	140	3.0	16.0	55	(mq)	7.0	(mq)	(mq)	45%
(Idahoan) sour cream and chives, dry	1/6 pkg	90	2.0	15.0	340	(mq)	2.0	(mq)	na	21%
(Idahoan) sour cream and chives, prepared	1/2 cup	130	2.0	18.0	400	(mq)	5.0	(mq)	(mq)	36%
(Pillsbury) sour cream and chives 'Specialty,' dry	1/6 pkg	100	2.0	18.0	450	1.0	2.0	1.0	0	18%
(Pillsbury) sour cream and chives, 'Specialty,' prepared w/butter and whole milk	1/2 cup	150	3.0	20.0	500	1.0	6.0	4.0	15	37%
STUFFED										
(Betty Crocker) sour cream and chives 'Twice Baked,' dry	1/6 pkg	90	2.0	17.0	480	(mq)	2.0	(mq)	na	19%
(Betty Crocker) sour cream and chives 'Twice Baked' prepared	1/2 cup	200	5.0	19.0	570	(mq)	11.0	(mq)	(mq)	51%
WESTERN										
(Arrowhead Mills) flakes	2 oz	140	5.0	44.0	24	na	0.0	0.0	0	0%
(Barbara's Bakery) dry	4 oz	389	7.0	89.0	63	na	1.0	na	1	2%
(French's) creamy, prepared	1/2 cup	130	3.0	20.0	520	(mq)	4.0	(mq)	na	28%
(General Mills) cheesy homestyle, dry	1/6 pkg	100	2.0	19.0	500	na	2.0	na	na	18%

Food Name	Serving Size	Calories	Prot. gms	Carbs gms	Sod. mgs	Fiber gms	Fat gms	Sat. Fat gms	Chol. mgs	% Fat Cal.
(General Mills) cheesy homestyle, prepared w/margarine and 2% milk	1/2 cup	150	3.0	20.0	560	na	6.0	na	na	37%
(General Mills) potato buds, dry	1/8 pkg	70	2.0	16.0	20	na	0.0	na	na	0%
(General Mills) potato buds, prepared	1/2 cup	130	3.0	17.0	360	na	6.0	na	na	40%
(General Mills) potato buds, prepared w/o salt	1/2 cup	130	3.0	17.0	90	na	6.0	na	na	40%
(Hungry Jack) flakes	13.3 oz	70	1.0	16.0	25	1.0	0.0	0.0	0	0%
(Hungry Jack) flakes, prepared w/margarine, 2% milk, and water	1/2 cup	130	2.0	17.0	85	1.0	6.0	1.0	0	42%
(Hungry Jack) flakes, prepared w/margarine, 2% milk, salt, and water	1/2 cup	130	2.0	17.0	260	1.0	6.0	1.0	0	42%
(Idaho) granules	13.3 oz	60	1.0	14.0	30	1.0	0.0	0.0	0	0%
(Idaho) granules, prepared	1/2 cup	130	2.0	16.0	320	(mq)	6.0	(mq)	na	43%
(Idaho) granules, prepared w/margarine, 2% milk, and water	1/2 cup	120	2.0	16.0	85	1.0	5.0	0.0	0	39%
(Idaho) granules, prepared w/margarine, 2% milk, salt, and water	1/2 cup	120	2.0	16.0	190	1.0	5.0	0.0	0	39%
(Idaho Spuds) flakes	13.3 oz	70	1.0	15.0	40	1.0	0.0	0.0	0	0%
(Idaho Spuds) flakes, prepared	1/2 cup	140	3.0	17.0	380	(mq)	7.0	(mq)	na	44%
(Idaho Spuds) flakes, prepared w/margarine, 2% milk, and water	1/2 cup	130	3.0	16.0	105	1.0	6.0	1.0	0	42%
(Idaho Spuds) flakes, prepared w/margarine, 2% milk, salt, and water	1/2 cup	130	3.0	16.0	370	1.0	6.0	1.0	0	42%
(Idahoan) dry	1/3 cup	80	2.0	18.0	15	2.0	0.0	0.0	0	0%
(Idahoan) 'Complete' dry	1/3 cup	100	2.0	19.0	310	2.0	2.0	.5	0	18%
(Pillsbury) cheesy 'Specialty' dry	1/6 pkg	100	2.0	19.0	490	1.0	2.0	0.0	0	18%
(Pillsbury) cheesy 'Specialty,' prepared w/butter and whole milk	1/2 cup	150	3.0	20.0	540	1.0	6.0	3.0	15	37%
(Pillsbury) creamy white sauce, 'Specialty,' dry	1/6 pkg	100	2.0	19.0	410	1.0	2.0	0.0	0	18%
POTATO PANCAKE										
(Idaho) 3 inch diam each, prepared	3 cakes	90	3.0	16.0	420	(mq)	2.0	(mq)	na	19%
(Kosher Empire) frozen, triangle, latkes w/onions	2 oz	77	1.0	13.0	108	na	2.4	na	na	28%
(Pillsbury) 'Specialty'	1/8 pkg	70	2.0	16.0	400	1.0	0.0	0.0	0	0%
(Pillsbury) 'Specialty' prepared w/water and egg, 3 inch diam each	3 cakes	90	3.0	16.0	420	1.0	2.0	0.0	55	19%
POTATO SALAD, CANNED										
(Joan of Arc) German	1/2 cup	120	2.0	23.0	550	1.6	3.0	(mq)	na	21%
(Joan of Arc) homestyle	1/2 cup	340	4.0	32.0	1070	3.0	22.0	(mq)	na	58%
(Read) German	1/2 cup	120	2.0	23.0	550	1.6	3.0	(mq)	na	21%
(Read) homestyle	1/2 cup	340	4.0	32.0	1070	3.0	22.0	(mq)	na	58%
POTATO SALAD SEASONING *(Tone's)*	1 tsp	5	0.2	0.3	1498	.1	0.2	<.1	0	47%
POTATO STARCH *(Featherweight)*	1 cup	620	0.0	154.0	51	na	1.0	na	0	1%
POTATO STICKS. See POTATO CHIPS AND SNACKS.										
POTTED MEAT SPREAD. See also LUNCHEON MEAT, CANNED; SANDWICH SPREAD.										
beef	1 cup	558	39.4	0.0	2925	0	43.2	20.3	175	71%
chicken	1 cup	558	39.4	0.0	2925	0	43.2	20.3	175	71%
turkey	1 cup	558	39.4	0.0	2925	0	43.2	20.3	175	71%
(Hormel)	1 oz	53	4.0	2.0	280	na	4.0	2.0	23	60%
(Hormel)	1 tbsp	30	2.0	0.0	145	0	2.0	(mq)	(mq)	69%
(Libby's)	1.83 oz	110	7.0	0.0	320	0	9.0	(mq)	(mq)	74%
POULTRY SEASONING										
dry	1 oz	87	2.7	18.6	8	3.2	2.1	na	0	18%
dry	1 tbsp	11	0.4	2.4	1	.4	0.3	na	0	19%
dry	1 tsp	5	0.1	1.0	0	.2	0.1	na	0	17%

Food Name	Serving Size	Calories	Prot. gms	Carbs gms	Sod. mgs	Fiber gms	Fat gms	Sat. Fat gms	Chol. mgs	% Fat Cal.
PRESERVES. See also FRUIT SPREAD; JAM; JELLY; MARMALADE.										
APPLE BUTTER										
(Bama)	2 tsp	25	0.0	6.0	5	na	0.0	na	na	0%
(Knudsen & Sons) organic	2 tbsp	25	0.0	6.0	0	na	0.0	na	na	0%
(Lucky Leaf)	4 oz	200	0.0	49.0	15	na	1.0	na	0	4%
(Musselman's)	4 oz	200	0.0	49.0	15	na	1.0	na	0	4%
(Smucker's) 'Autumn Harvest'	1 tsp	12	0.0	3.0	0	(mq)	0.0	0.0	0	0%
(Smucker's) cider	1 tsp	12	0.0	3.0	0	(mq)	0.0	0.0	0	0%
(Smucker's) natural	1 tsp	12	0.0	3.0	0	(mq)	0.0	0.0	0	0%
(Smucker's) 'Simply Fruit'	1 tsp	16	0.0	4.0	0	(mq)	0.0	0.0	0	0%
(Smucker's) spiced	1 tsp	12	0.0	3.0	0	na	0.0	0.0	na	0%
(Tap'n Apple)	1 oz	45	<1.0	13.2	<1	.5	<.1	0.0	0	<2%
(White House)	1 oz	50	0.0	12.0	5	(mq)	0.0	0.0	0	0%
APRICOT										
(Knott's Berry Farm)	1 tsp	18	0.0	4.0	0	na	0.0	na	na	0%
(Polaner)	2 tsp	35	0.0	9.0	5	na	0.0	0.0	na	0%
APRICOT-PINEAPPLE										
(Knott's Berry Farm)	1 tsp	18	0.0	4.0	0	na	0.0	na	na	0%
(Knudsen & Sons)	2 tsp	35	<1.0	8.0	na	na	<1.0	na	na	<20%
BING CHERRY (Knott's Berry Farm)	1 tsp	18	0.0	4.0	0	na	0.0	na	na	0%
BLACK CHERRY (Knudsen & Sons)	2 tsp	35	<1.0	8.0	na	na	<1.0	na	na	<20%
BLACKBERRY										
(Knott's Berry Farm) seedless	1 tsp	18	0.0	4.0	0	na	0.0	na	na	0%
(Knudsen & Sons)	2 tsp	35	<1.0	8.0	na	na	<1.0	na	na	<20%
(Knudsen & Sons) organic	2 tsp	25	<1.0	7.0	na	na	<1.0	na	na	<22%
(Polaner) seedless	2 tsp	35	0.0	9.0	5	na	0.0	0.0	na	0%
BLUEBERRY										
(Knott's Berry Farm)	1 tsp	18	0.0	4.0	0	na	0.0	na	na	0%
(Knudsen & Sons)	2 tsp	35	<1.0	8.0	na	na	<1.0	na	na	<20%
(Knudsen & Sons) organic	2 tsp	25	<1.0	7.0	na	na	<1.0	na	na	<22%
(Polaner)	2 tsp	35	0.0	9.0	5	na	0.0	0.0	na	0%
BOYSENBERRY										
(Knott's Berry Farm)	1 tsp	18	0.0	4.0	0	na	0.0	na	na	0%
(Knudsen & Sons)	2 tsp	35	<1.0	8.0	na	na	<1.0	na	na	<20%
CONCORD GRAPE (Knudsen & Sons)	2 tsp	35	<1.0	8.0	na	na	<1.0	na	na	<20%
KADOTA FIG (Knott's Berry Farm)	1 tsp	18	0.0	4.0	0	na	0.0	na	na	0%
PEACH										
(Bama)	2 tsp	30	0.0	8.0	5	na	0.0	na	na	0%
(Knudsen & Sons)	2 tsp	35	<1.0	8.0	na	na	<1.0	na	chol.	<20%
(Polaner)	2 tsp	35	0.0	9.0	5	na	0.0	0.0	na	0%
PINEAPPLE (Polaner)	2 tsp	35	0.0	9.0	5	na	0.0	0.0	na	0%
RED CHERRY (Knott's Berry Farm)	1 tsp	18	0.0	4.0	0	na	0.0	na	na	0%
RED RASPBERRY										
(Knott's Berry Farm) seedless	1 tsp	18	0.0	4.0	0	na	0.0	na	na	0%
(Knudsen & Sons)	2 tsp	35	<1.0	8.0	na	na	<1.0	na	na	<20%
(Knudsen & Sons) organic	2 tsp	25	<1.0	7.0	na	na	<1.0	na	na	<22%
(Polaner)	2 tsp	35	0.0	0.0	5	na	0.0	0.0	na	0%
(Polaner) seedless	2 tsp	35	0.0	9.0	5	na	0.0	0.0	na	0%
(Smucker's) natural ingredients	1 tsp	18	0.0	4.0	0	na	0.0	0.0	na	0%
STRAWBERRY										
(Bama)	2 tsp	30	0.0	8.0	5	na	0.0	na	na	0%
(Knott's Berry Farm) pure, seedless	1 tsp	18	0.0	4.0	0	na	0.0	na	na	0%
(Knudsen & Sons)	2 tsp	35	<1.0	8.0	na	na	<1.0	na	na	<20%
(Knudsen & Sons) organic	2 tsp	25	<1.0	7.0	na	na	<1.0	na	na	<22%

Food Name	Serving Size	Calories	Prot. gms	Carbs gms	Sod. mgs	Fiber gms	Fat gms	Sat. Fat gms	Chol. mgs	% Fat Cal.
(Polaner)	2 tsp	35	0.0	9.0	5	na	0.0	0.0	na	0%
(Smucker's) natural ingredients	1 tsp	18	0.0	4.0	0	na	0.0	0.0	na	0%
PRETZELS										
(A & Eagle)	1 oz	110	3.0	22.0	570	(mq)	2.0	(mq)	0	15%
(Bachman) 'Nutzels'	1 oz	110	3.0	21.0	470	(mq)	2.0	(mq)	0	16%
(Bachman) 'Petite'	1 oz	110	3.0	21.0	410	(mq)	2.0	(mq)	0	16%
(Bachman) 'Petite Sodium Free'	1 oz	110	3.0	21.0	2	(mq)	2.0	(mq)	0	16%
(Estee) 'Unsalted'	5 pretzels	25	<1.0	5.0	5	<1.0	<1.0	<1.0	0	<27%
(Featherweight) 'Low Salt'	20 pretzels	110	3.0	23.0	30	(mq)	1.0	na	0	8%
(Mister Salty) 'Juniors'	1 oz	110	2.0	22.0	500	(mq)	2.0	(mq)	na	16%
(Pepperidge Farm) 'Goldfish'	1 oz	110	3.0	20.0	160	1.0	3.0	0.0	0	23%
(Rokeach) 'Baldies Unsalted'	1 oz	110	2.0	20.0	30	(mq)	0.0	0.0	0	0%
(Rold Gold) 'Tiny Tim'	1 oz	110	2.0	23.0	610	(mq)	1.0	na	0	8%
BAVARIAN										
(Barbara's Bakery) 1 oz	2 pretzels	110	4.0	21.0	200	na	<1.0	na	0	<8%
(Barbara's Bakery) no salt added, 1 oz	2 pretzels	110	4.0	21.0	10	na	<1.0	na	0	<8%
(Rold Gold) 1 oz	3 pretzels	120	3.0	22.0	430	na	2.0	na	0	15%
BEER (Quinlan)	1 oz	110	2.6	21.6	446	.1	1.4	na	0	12%
BRAIDS (Keebler) 'Butter Pretzels'	1 oz	110	3.0	21.0	620	(mq)	1.0	<1.0	0	9%
CHEDDAR (Combos)	10 nuggets	143	2.9	19.5	335	>.1 c	5.8	na	3	37%
CHIPS										
'Mr. Phipps' (Nabisco) lightly salted, .5 oz	8 chips	60	1.0	11.0	200	0	1.0	0.0	0	16%
'Mr. Phipps' (Nabisco) original, .5 oz	8 chips	60	1.0	10.0	310	0	1.0	0.0	0	17%
'Mr. Phipps' (Nabisco) sesame, .5 oz	8 chips	60	1.0	10.0	250	na	2.0	0.0	0	29%
DUTCH STYLE										
	7.5-oz pkg	831	20.9	161.7	3578	>.6 c	9.6	2.1	0	11%
	1 pretzel	62	1.6	12.1	269	>.1 c	0.7	0.2	0	10%
(Estee) 'Unsalted'	2 pretzels	110	3.0	23.0	30	na	<1.0	<1.0	0	<8%
(Mister Salty) 1 oz	2 pretzels	110	3.0	22.0	440	(mq)	1.0	0.0	5	8%
(Rokeach)	1 oz	110	3.0	24.0	na	(mq)	0.0	0.0	na	0%
(Rokeach) 'Unsalted'	1 oz	110	2.0	20.0	30	(mq)	0.0	0.0	0	0%
HARD										
(Bachman)	1 oz	110	3.0	23.0	290	(mq)	<1.0	na	0	<8%
(Bachman) unsalted	1 oz	110	3.0	23.0	50	(mq)	<1.0	na	0	<8%
plain, made w/unenriched flour, salted	10 twists	322	4.2	31.7	5	>1.0 c	20.8	6.6	0	57%
plain, made w/unenriched flour, unsalted	10 twists	229	5.5	47.5	1029	1.9	2.1	0.5	0	8%
plain, salted	10 twists	229	5.5	47.5	1029	1.9	2.1	0.5	0	8%
plain, unsalted	10 twists	229	5.5	47.5	173	1.9	2.1	0.5	0	8%
whole wheat	2 oz	205	6.3	46.0	115	>1.0 c	1.5	0.3	0	6%
HONEYSWEET (Barbara's Bakery) 1 oz	2 pretzels	110	3.0	21.0	200	na	<1.0	na	0	<9%
KNOTS (Keebler) 'Butter Pretzels'	1 oz	110	3.0	21.0	530	(mq)	1.0	<1.0	0	9%
LOGS										
(Bachman)	1 oz	110	3.0	21.0	470	(mq)	2.0	(mq)	0	16%
(Quinlan)	1 oz	103	2.7	21.5	388	.3	0.8	na	0	7%
MINIS										
(Barbara's Bakery) 1 oz	17 pretzels	110	4.0	21.0	290	na	<1.0	na	0	<8%
(Barbara's Bakery) no salt added, 1 oz	17 pretzels	110	4.0	21.0	10	na	<1.0	na	0	<8%
(Mister Salty) 1 oz	22 pretzels	110	3.0	21.0	450	na	1.0	0.0	0	9%
NINE-GRAIN (Barbara's Bakery) 1 oz	2 pretzels	110	4.0	21.0	200	na	<1.0	na	0	<8%
OAT BRAN (Quinlan)	1 oz	115	3.5	21.8	156	.3	1.5	na	0	12%
PARTY										
(Delicious)	1 oz	110	3.0	23.0	500	na	1.0	na	0	8%
(Rokeach) 'Party Cannister'	1 oz	110	2.0	23.0	na	(mq)	1.0	na	0	8%
RICE BRAN, 'No-Salt' (Quinlan)	1 oz	101	2.6	19.5	52	2.0	2.3	(mq)	0	19%

Food Name	Serving Size	Calories	Prot. gms	Carbs gms	Sod. mgs	Fiber gms	Fat gms	Sat. Fat gms	Chol. mgs	% Fat Cal.
RINGS										
(Bachman)	1 oz	110	3.0	21.0	410	(mq)	2.0	(mq)	0	16%
(Mister Salty)	1 oz	110	3.0	21.0	510	(mq)	2.0	(mq)	na	16%
(Mister Salty) butter flavor	1 oz	110	3.0	21.0	570	(mq)	2.0	(mq)	na	16%
RODS										
(Bachman)	1 oz	110	3.0	21.0	240	(mq)	2.0	(mq)	0	16%
(Rold Gold)	1 oz	110	3.0	22.0	550	(mq)	2.0	(mq)	0	15%
(Seyfert's) butter flavor	1 oz	110	3.0	21.0	530	(mq)	1.0	na	na	9%
STICKS										
(Delicious)	1 oz	110	3.0	23.0	500	na	1.0	na	1	8%
(Mister Salty)	1 oz	110	3.0	22.0	620	(mq)	1.0	na	na	8%
(Mister Salty) butter flavor	1 oz	110	3.0	22.0	620	(mq)	1.0	na	na	8%
(Mister Salty) fat-free	1 oz	110	3.0	23.0	380	<1.0	<1.0	<1.0	5	<8%
(Mister Salty) very thin, 1 oz	92 sticks	110	3.0	22.0	600	1.0	3.0	0.0	0	21%
(Pepperidge Farm) 'Snack Sticks'	8 sticks	120	3.0	23.0	430	1.0	3.0	0.0	0	21%
(Quinlan)	1 oz	105	2.7	22.3	538	.3	0.6	na	0	5%
(Rold Gold)	1 oz	110	2.0	23.0	760	(mq)	1.0	na	0	8%
THINS										
(Bachman)	1 oz	110	3.0	21.0	410	(mq)	2.0	(mq)	0	16%
(Bachman) 'Thin'n Light'	1 oz	110	3.0	21.0	410	(mq)	2.0	(mq)	0	16%
(Quinlan)	1 oz	104	2.8	22.0	765	.1	0.6	na	0	5%
(Quinlan) tiny	1 oz	109	2.6	21.2	601	.2	1.5	na	0	12%
(Quinlan) tiny 'No-Salt'	1 oz	115	2.7	22.4	10	.2	1.6	na	0	13%
(Quinlan) 'Ultra Thins'	1 oz	106	2.7	22.5	618	.1	0.6	na	0	5%
(Rold Gold) baked, 33% less sodium 'Fat Free'	1 oz	110	3.0	23.0	340	1.0	0.0	0.0	0	0%
TREATS (Bachman)	1 oz	110	3.0	21.0	410	(mq)	2.0	(mq)	0	16%
TWISTS										
(Bachman)	1 oz	110	3.0	21.0	410	(mq)	2.0	(mq)	0	16%
(Delicious)	1 oz	110	3.0	23.0	500	na	1.0	na	0	8%
(Mister Salty) .5 oz	5 twists	110	3.0	21.0	580	1.0	2.0	0.0	0	16%
(Mister Salty) fat-free, 1 oz	9 twists	110	3.0	23.0	380	<1.0	<1.0	<1.0	5	<8%
(Rold Gold) thin, 1 oz	10 twists	110	2.0	23.0	470	(mq)	1.0	na	0	8%
(Rold Gold) tiny, 1 oz	15 twists	110	2.0	23.0	420	na	1.0	na	0	8%
(Ultra Slim Fast)	1 oz	100	2.0	21.0	460	3.0	1.0	na	0	9%
PRICKLY PEAR										
raw, trimmed	1 oz	12	0.2	2.7	1	>.5 c	0.1	na	0	7%
raw, trimmed, approx 4.8 oz	1 fruit	42	0.8	9.9	5	3.7	0.5	na	0	10%
raw, untrimmed	1 lb	140	2.5	32.6	18	>6.2 c	1.7	na	0	10%
PROSCIUTTO. See LUNCHEON MEAT, HAM.										
PRUNE										
dehydrated	4 oz	384	4.2	101.0	6	>3.3 c	0.8	0.1	0	2%
dehydrated, cooked	4 oz	128	1.4	33.7	2	>1.1 c	0.3	<.1	0	2%
Canned										
in heavy syrup, w/liquid	1 cup	246	2.0	65.1	7	8.9	0.5	0.0	0	2%
in heavy syrup, w/liquid	1/2 cup	123	1.0	32.5	3	4.5	0.2	<.1	0	1%
in heavy syrup, w/2 tbsp liquid	5 fruits	90	0.8	23.9	3	3.3	0.2	0.0	0	2%
pitted, in heavy syrup, w/liquid	4 oz	119	1.0	31.5	3	4.4	0.2	<.1	0	1%
PRUNE, DRIED										
pitted	1 cup	385	4.2	101.0	6	11.6	0.8	0.1	0	2%
pitted	4 oz	271	3.0	71.1	5	8.2	0.6	<.1	0	2%
pitted, approx 3 oz	10 fruits	201	2.2	52.7	3	6.1	0.4	0.0	0	2%
pitted, cooked, stewed, sweetened	4 oz	141	1.2	37.3	2	4.5	0.2	<.1	0	1%
pitted, cooked, stewed, unsweetened	4 oz	121	1.3	31.8	2	7.5	0.3	<.1	0	2%
(Del Monte)	2 oz	120	1.0	31.0	10	(mq)	0.0	0.0	0	0%

Food Name	Serving Size	Calories	Prot. gms	Carbs gms	Sod. mgs	Fiber gms	Fat gms	Sat. Fat gms	Chol. mgs	% Fat Cal.
(Del Monte) 'Moist Pak'	2 oz	120	1.0	30.0	10	(mq)	0.0	0.0	0	0%
(Del Monte) pitted	2 oz	140	1.0	35.0	10	(mq)	0.0	0.0	0	0%
(Dole)	2 oz	140	1.0	36.0	10	na	1.0	na	na	6%
(Mariani) pitted, premium	1/4 cup	140	1.0	36.0	10	4.0	0.0	na	0	0%
(SunSweet)	2 oz	120	1.0	32.0	10	(mq)	0.0	0.0	0	0%
(SunSweet) pitted	2 oz	140	1.0	36.0	10	(mq)	0.0	0.0	0	0%
PRUNE JUICE										
	6 oz	136	1.2	33.5	8	1.9	0.1	<.1	0	1%
(Del Monte) 'Unsweetened'	6 oz	120	1.0	33.0	10	(mq)	0.0	0.0	0	0%
(J. Hungerford) 100% juice	9.03 oz	178	1.5	43.9	10	2.5	0.0	0.0	0	0%
(Knudsen & Sons) organic	8 oz	170	1.0	42.0	na	na	0.0	na	na	0%
(Lucky Leaf)	6 oz	150	0.0	36.0	0	(mq)	0.0	0.0	0	0%
(Mott's)	6 oz	130	1.0	32.0	8	(mq)	0.0	0.0	0	0%
(Mott's) country style	6 oz	130	1.0	32.0	7	(mq)	0.0	0.0	0	0%
(Pathmark) 'All Natural'	6 oz	120	1.0	30.0	10	(mq)	0.0	0.0	0	0%
(Pathmark) w/prune pulp 'Homestyle'	6 oz	130	1.0	32.0	10	(mq)	0.0	0.0	0	0%
(S&W) 'Unsweetened'	6 oz	120	1.0	31.0	20	(mq)	0.0	0.0	0	0%
(SunSweet)	6 oz	130	1.0	33.0	20	(mq)	0.0	0.0	0	0%
PRUNE WHIP										
cold	1 cup	203	5.7	48.0	213	>.8 c	0.3	0.0	0	1%
hot	1 cup	140	4.0	33.2	148	>.5 c	0.2	0.0	0	1%
PUDDING, FROZEN										
butterscotch (Rich's)	3 oz	130	2.0	18.0	130	na	6.0	(mq)	0	40%
chocolate (Rich's)	3 oz	140	2.0	18.0	135	na	7.0	(mq)	0	44%
vanilla (Rich's)	3 oz	130	2.0	18.0	160	na	6.0	(mq)	0	40%
PUDDING, READY-TO-SERVE										
ALMOND (Rice Dream) 'Dream Pudding,' non-dairy, low fat	4 oz	150	1.0	31.0	30	na	2.0	na	0	12%
BANANA										
(Del Monte) 'Pudding Cup'	5 oz	180	3.0	30.0	285	na	5.0	(mq)	na	25%
(Lucky Leaf)	4 oz	150	2.0	24.0	110	na	5.0	(mq)	na	30%
(Musselman's)	4 oz	150	2.0	24.0	110	na	5.0	(mq)	na	30%
(Rice Dream) 'Dream Pudding,' non-dairy, fat-free	4 oz	120	1.0	30.0	5	na	0.0	na	0	0%
(Snack Pack)	4.25 oz	145	2.0	22.0	180	0	6.0	1.3	1	36%
(Snack Pack)	4 oz	158	1.5	25.0	163	0	5.7	1.7	0	33%
BUTTERSCOTCH										
(Crowley)	4.5 oz	150	3.0	27.0	210	na	3.0	(mq)	10	18%
(Del Monte) 'Pudding Cup'	5 oz	180	3.0	31.0	285	na	5.0	(mq)	na	25%
(Featherweight)	1/2 cup	100	0.0	21.0	160	na	1.0	na	0	10%
(Lucky Leaf)	4 oz	170	2.0	26.0	135	na	7.0	(mq)	chol.	36%
(Musselman's)	4 oz	170	2.0	26.0	135	na	7.0	(mq)	na	36%
(Rice Dream) 'Dream Pudding,' non-dairy, fat-free	4 oz	120	1.0	30.0	5	na	0.0	na	0	0%
(Snack Pack)	4.25 oz	170	2.0	27.0	210	0	6.0	1.4	1	32%
(Snack Pack)	4 oz	153	1.7	23.6	211	0	5.7	1.7	1	34%
(Swiss Miss)	4 oz	156	2.5	24.1	182	0	5.6	1.4	1	32%
(Ultra Slim Fast) 'Lite 'N Tasty'	4 oz	100	2.0	21.0	230	2.0	<1.0	na	0	<9%
(White House)	3.5 oz	113	1.0	20.0	195	na	3.0	(mq)	na	24%
BUTTERSCOTCH-CHOCOLATE-VANILLA SWIRL (Jell-O)	4 oz	180	3.0	28.0	140	na	5.0	(mq)	0	27%
CARAMELLO (Hershey's)	4 oz	180	3.0	28.0	170	na	6.0	na	0	30%
CAROB (Rice Dream) 'Dream Pudding' non-dairy, fat-free	4 oz	130	1.0	31.0	30	na	0.0	na	0	0%
CHOCOLATE										
(Crowley)	4.5 oz	190	4.0	29.0	100	na	3.0	(mq)	10	17%
(Del Monte) 'Pudding Cup'	5 oz	190	4.0	31.0	280	na	6.0	(mq)	na	28%
(Del Monte) 'Pudding Snack Light'	4.25 oz	100	2.0	19.0	85	na	1.0	0.0	0	10%
(Estee)	1/2 cup	70	5.0	12.0	85	na	<1.0	<1.0	2	<12%

Food Name	Serving Size	Calories	Prot. gms	Carbs gms	Sod. mgs	Fiber gms	Fat gms	Sat. Fat gms	Chol. mgs	% Fat Cal.
(Featherweight)	1/2 cup	100	1.0	21.0	110	na	1.0	na	0	9%
(Hershey's)	4 oz	180	3.0	29.0	260	na	5.0	na	0	26%
(Jell-O) 'Free'	4 oz	100	3.0	24.0	200	na	0.0	na	0	0%
(Jell-O) 'Light Pudding Snacks'	4 oz	100	3.0	21.0	125	na	2.0	(mq)	5	16%
(Jell-O) 'Pudding Snacks'	5.5 oz	230	4.0	38.0	170	na	8.0	(mq)	0	30%
(Jell-O) 'Pudding Snacks'	4 oz	170	3.0	28.0	130	na	6.0	(mq)	0	30%
(Lucky Leaf)	4 oz	180	2.0	27.0	100	na	7.0	(mq)	na	35%
(Musselman's)	4 oz	180	2.0	27.0	100	na	7.0	(mq)	na	35%
(Pathmark) 'No Frills'	5 oz	200	2.0	30.0	140	na	8.0	(mq)	na	36%
(Rice Dream) 'Dream Pudding,' non-dairy, fat-free	4 oz	170	1.0	39.0	30	na	0.0	na	0	0%
(Snack Pack)	4.25 oz	160	2.0	28.0	125	na	5.0	(mq)	0	27%
(Snack Pack)	4 oz	161	2.3	24.6	178	0	5.9	1.5	0	33%
(Snack Pack) fat-free	4 oz	96	2.0	21.2	212	0	0.4	0.0	0	4%
(Snack Pack) 'Light'	4 oz	100	3.0	20.1	120	na	2.0	(mq)	0	16%
(Swiss Miss)	4 oz	166	3.1	25.8	177	0	5.7	1.5	1	31%
(Swiss Miss) fat-free	4 oz	99	1.8	22.3	154	0	0.4	0.0	1	4%
(Swiss Miss) 'Light'	4 oz	100	3.0	20.1	120	na	(mq)	na	0	0%
(Swiss Miss) sundae	4 oz	220	2.0	36.0	140	0	7.0	1.7	5	29%
(White House)	3.5 oz	120	2.0	22.0	130	na	4.0	(mq)	na	27%
CHOCOLATE FUDGE										
(Del Monte) 'Pudding Cup'	5 oz	190	4.0	31.0	260	na	6.0	(mq)	na	28%
(Jell-O) 'Light Pudding Snacks'	4 oz	100	3.0	22.0	125	na	1.0	na	5	8%
(Jell-O) 'Pudding Snacks'	4 oz	170	3.0	28.0	130	na	6.0	(mq)	0	30%
(Lucky Leaf)	4 oz	180	2.0	25.0	105	na	8.0	(mq)	na	40%
(Musselman's)	4 oz	180	2.0	25.0	105	na	8.0	(mq)	na	40%
(Snack Pack)	4.25 oz	165	2.0	27.0	125	0	6.0	1.2	1	32%
(Snack Pack)	4 oz	158	2.3	23.9	178	0	5.9	1.7	0	34%
(Swiss Miss)	4 oz	175	3.3	27.9	207	0	5.6	1.6	1	29%
(Swiss Miss) fat-free	4 oz	103	1.8	23.3	151	0	0.3	0.0	1	3%
(Swiss Miss) 'Light'	4 oz	100	3.0	20.0	120	0	1.0	0.3	0	9%
CHOCOLATE FUDGE-MILK CHOCOLATE SWIRL (Jell-O)	4 oz	170	3.0	28.0	135	na	6.0	(mq)	0	30%
CHOCOLATE-ALMOND (Hershey's)	4 oz	180	3.0	29.0	210	na	6.0	na	0	30%
CHOCOLATE-CARAMEL SWIRL										
(Jell-O) 'Pudding Snacks'	4 oz	170	3.0	28.0	130	na	6.0	(mq)	0	30%
(Snack Pack)	4 oz	165	2.5	25.3	178	0	5.9	1.5	1	32%
(Snack Pack) 4 pack	4 oz	170	2.0	27.0	180	na	6.0	na	0	32%
(Swiss Miss)	4 oz	165	2.5	25.3	178	0	5.9	1.5	1	32%
CHOCOLATE-MARSHMALLOW										
(Snack Pack)	4.25 oz	165	2.0	26.0	125	0	6.0	1.3	1	33%
(Snack Pack)	4 oz	155	1.9	23.4	124	0	5.9	1.9	0	34%
CHOCOLATE-MINT SWIRL (Jell-O) 'Free'	4 oz	100	3.0	24.0	220	na	0.0	na	0	0%
CHOCOLATE-PEANUT BUTTER SWIRL										
(Snack Pack)	4 oz	169	2.4	25.7	173	0	6.3	1.6	1	34%
(Snack Pack) 4 pack	4 oz	170	3.0	26.0	180	na	7.0	na	0	35%
CHOCOLATE-VANILLA SWIRL										
(Hershey's) 'Kisses'	4 oz	180	3.0	29.0	210	na	6.0	na	0	30%
(Hershey's) 'Kisses Free'	4 oz	100	2.0	22.0	180	na	0.0	na	0	0%
(Jell-O) combo 'Light Pudding Snacks'	4 oz	100	3.0	21.0	125	na	2.0	(mq)	5	16%
(Jell-O) 'Free'	4 oz	100	3.0	24.0	220	na	0.0	na	0	0%
(Jell-O) 'Pudding Snacks'	5.5 oz	240	4.0	39.0	180	na	8.0	(mq)	0	30%
(Jell-O) 'Pudding Snacks'	4 oz	170	3.0	28.0	135	na	6.0	(mq)	0	30%
CHOCOLATE-VANILLA-CHOCOLATE SWIRL (Swiss Miss)	4 oz	172	2.8	26.6	163	0	6.0	1.6	1	32%
COCONUT										
(Rice Dream) 'Dream Pudding,' non-dairy, low fat	4 oz	150	1.0	32.0	10	na	2.0	na	0	12%

Food Name	Serving Size	Calories	Prot. gms	Carbs gms	Sod. mgs	Fiber gms	Fat gms	Sat. Fat gms	Chol. mgs	% Fat Cal.
LEMON										
(Rice Dream) 'Dream Pudding,' non-dairy, fat-free	4 oz	120	1.0	30.0	5	na	0.0	na	0	0%
(Snack Pack)	4.25 oz	150	<1.0	30.0	75	<1.0	4.0	0.8	0	23%
(Snack Pack)	4 oz	138	0.1	28.0	85	0	2.8	0.8	0	18%
(White House)	3.5 oz	152	0.0	37.0	65	na	1.0	na	na	6%
MILK CHOCOLATE										
(Jell-O) 'Pudding Snacks'	4 oz	170	4.0	29.0	135	na	6.0	(mq)	0	29%
(Snack Pack)	4 oz	166	1.8	26.4	166	0	5.9	1.5	1	32%
(Snack Pack) 4 pack	4 oz	160	2.0	26.0	170	na	6.0	na	0	33%
(Swiss Miss)	4 oz	166	1.8	26.4	166	0	2.9	1.5	1	19%
MILK CHOCOLATE-CHOCOLATE FUDGE SWIRL (Jell-O)	4 oz	170	3.0	28.0	135	na	6.0	na	0	30%
RICE										
(Crowley)	4.5 oz	125	4.0	22.0	80	na	2.0	(mq)	10	15%
(Lucky Leaf)	4 oz	120	3.0	20.0	95	na	3.0	(mq)	na	23%
(Musselman's)	4 oz	120	3.0	20.0	95	na	3.0	(mq)	na	23%
(White House)	3.5 oz	111	1.0	20.0	135	na	3.0	(mq)	na	24%
S'MORES SWIRL										
(Snack Pack)	4 oz	154	1.4	24.7	129	0	5.6	1.5	1	33%
(Snack Pack) 4 pack	4 oz	150	2.0	25.0	125	na	6.0	na	0	33%
TAPIOCA										
(Crowley)	4.5 oz	135	4.0	27.0	70	na	1.0	na	5	7%
(Del Monte) 'Pudding Cup'	5 oz	180	3.0	30.0	250	na	4.0	(mq)	na	21%
(Jell-O) 'Pudding Snacks'	4 oz	170	3.0	27.0	140	na	4.0	(mq)	0	23%
(Lucky Leaf)	4 oz	140	1.0	20.0	95	na	6.0	(mq)	na	39%
(Musselman's)	4 oz	140	1.0	20.0	95	na	6.0	(mq)	na	39%
(Snack Pack)	4.25 oz	160	2.0	28.0	200	na	4.0	1.1	0	23%
(Snack Pack)	4 oz	151	2.0	22.9	134	0	5.7	1.1	1	34%
(Snack Pack) fat-free	4 oz	94	2.1	20.7	185	0	0.4	0.0	0	4%
(Snack Pack) 'Light'	4 oz	100	2.0	18.1	105	na	2.0	(mq)	0	18%
(Swiss Miss)	4 oz	138	2.1	23.6	180	0	3.9	0.9	1	26%
(Swiss Miss) fat-free	4 oz	99	2.0	22.0	151	0	0.3	0.0	1	3%
(Swiss Miss) 'Light'	4 oz	100	2.0	18.1	105	na	2.0	(mq)	0	18%
(White House)	3.5 oz	131	1.0	19.0	105	na	6.0	(mq)	na	40%
VANILLA										
(Crowley)	4.5 oz	140	3.0	26.0	130	na	3.0	(mq)	10	19%
(Del Monte) 'Pudding Cup'	5 oz	180	3.0	32.0	285	na	5.0	(mq)	na	24%
(Del Monte) 'Pudding Snack Light'	4.25 oz	100	1.0	19.0	200	na	1.0	0.0	0	10%
(Estee)	1/2 cup	70	4.0	12.0	65	na	<1.0	<1.0	2	<12%
(Featherweight)	1/2 cup	100	0.0	20.0	150	na	2.0	(mq)	0	18%
(Jell-O) 'Free'	4 oz	100	3.0	23.0	250	na	0.0	na	0	0%
(Jell-O) 'Light Pudding Snacks'	4 oz	100	3.0	20.0	130	na	2.0	(mq)	5	16%
(Jell-O) 'Pudding Snacks'	5.5 oz	250	4.0	38.0	190	na	9.0	(mq)	0	33%
(Jell-O) 'Pudding Snacks'	4 oz	180	3.0	28.0	140	na	7.0	(mq)	0	34%
(Lucky Leaf)	4 oz	170	2.0	25.0	135	na	7.0	(mq)	na	37%
(Musselman's)	4 oz	170	2.0	25.0	135	na	7.0	(mq)	na	37%
(Pathmark) 'No Frills'	5 oz	200	2.0	28.0	150	na	8.0	(mq)	na	38%
(Snack Pack)	4.25 oz	170	1.0	28.0	180	na	6.0	1.6	0	32%
(Snack Pack)	4 oz	158	1.5	25.0	141	0	5.7	1.5	0	33%
(Snack Pack) fat-free	4 oz	93	1.8	20.8	167	0	0.4	0.0	1	4%
(Swiss Miss)	4 oz	156	2.5	24.1	181	0	5.6	1.4	1	32%
(Swiss Miss) fat-free	4 oz	98	1.6	22.1	162	0	0.4	0.0	1	4%
(Swiss Miss) 'Light'	4 oz	100	2.0	18.1	110	na	2.0	(mq)	0	18%
(Swiss Miss) sundae	4 oz	175	2.0	26.5	174	0	6.8	1.7	1	35%
(Ultra Slim Fast) 'Lite 'N Tasty'	4 oz	100	2.0	21.0	230	2.0	<1.0	na	0	<9%

Food Name	Serving Size	Calories	Prot. gms	Carbs gms	Sod. mgs	Fiber gms	Fat gms	Sat. Fat gms	Chol. mgs	% Fat Cal.
(White House) .... 3.5 oz	3.5 oz	111	1.0	20.0	135	na	3.0	(mq)	na	24%
VANILLA-CHOCOLATE SWIRL *(Jell-O)* 'Pudding Snacks' ... 4 oz	4 oz	180	3.0	28.0	140	na	6.0	(mq)	0	30%
PUDDING MIX. See also PUDDING/PIE FILLING MIX.										
BANANA										
(Jell-O) 'Instant' prepared .... 1/2 cup	1/2 cup	160	4.0	28.0	410	na	4.0	(mq)	15	22%
(Jell-O) 'Instant Sugar-free' prepared w/2% milk .... 1/2 cup	1/2 cup	80	4.0	11.0	390	na	2.0	(mq)	10	23%
BANANA CREAM										
(Jell-O) 'Microwave' prepared .... 1/2 cup	1/2 cup	150	4.0	25.0	220	na	4.0	(mq)	15	24%
(Royal) 'Instant' prepared .... 1/2 cup	1/2 cup	180	4.0	29.0	390	na	5.0	(mq)	(mq)	25%
(Royal) prepared .... 1/2 cup	1/2 cup	160	4.0	27.0	210	na	4.0	(mq)	(mq)	23%
BUTTER ALMOND *(Royal)* toasted 'Instant' prepared .... 1/2 cup	1/2 cup	170	4.0	30.0	350	na	4.0	(mq)	(mq)	21%
BUTTER PECAN *(Jell-O)* 'Instant' prepared ... 1/2 cup	1/2 cup	170	4.0	28.0	410	na	5.0	(mq)	15	26%
BUTTERSCOTCH										
(D-Zerta) low calorie, prepared w/skim milk .... 1/2 cup	1/2 cup	70	4.0	12.0	65	na	0.0	na	0	0%
(Featherweight) 'Instant' prepared .... 1/2 cup	1/2 cup	100	4.0	19.0	190	na	0.0	0.0	5	0%
(Featherweight) prepared .... 1/2 cup	1/2 cup	12	0.0	3.0	6	na	0.0	0.0	0	0%
(Jell-O) 'Instant' prepared .... 1/2 cup	1/2 cup	160	4.0	28.0	450	na	4.0	(mq)	15	22%
(Jell-O) 'Instant Sugar-free' prepared w/2% milk .... 1/2 cup	1/2 cup	90	4.0	12.0	390	na	2.0	(mq)	10	22%
(Jell-O) 'Microwave' prepared .... 1/2 cup	1/2 cup	170	4.0	28.0	180	na	4.0	(mq)	15	22%
(Jell-O) prepared .... 1/2 cup	1/2 cup	170	4.0	30.0	190	na	4.0	(mq)	15	21%
(Royal) 'Instant' prepared .... 1/2 cup	1/2 cup	180	4.0	29.0	390	na	5.0	(mq)	(mq)	25%
(Royal) 'Instant Sugar-free' prepared w/2% milk .... 1/2 cup	1/2 cup	100	4.0	16.0	470	na	2.0	(mq)	(mq)	18%
(Royal) prepared .... 1/2 cup	1/2 cup	160	4.0	27.0	210	na	4.0	(mq)	(mq)	23%
CHOCOLATE										
(D-Zerta) low calorie, prepared w/skim milk .... 1/2 cup	1/2 cup	60	5.0	11.0	70	na	0.0	na	0	0%
(Featherweight) 'Instant' prepared .... 1/2 cup	1/2 cup	110	5.0	22.0	190	na	0.0	0.0	5	0%
(Featherweight) prepared .... 1/2 cup	1/2 cup	12	0.0	3.0	0	na	0.0	0.0	15	0%
(Jell-O) 'Cook 'n Serve Sugar-free' prepared w/skim milk .. 1/2 cup	1/2 cup	70	5.0	13.0	160	na	3.0	na	na	27%
(Jell-O) 'Cook 'n Serve Sugar-free' prepared w/2% milk ... 1/2 cup	1/2 cup	90	5.0	13.0	160	na	3.0	(mq)	10	27%
(Jell-O) 'Instant' prepared .... 1/2 cup	1/2 cup	180	4.0	31.0	480	na	4.0	(mq)	15	21%
(Jell-O) 'Instant Sugar-free' prepared w/2% milk .... 1/2 cup	1/2 cup	90	4.0	13.0	380	na	3.0	(mq)	10	28%
(Jell-O) 'Microwave' prepared .... 1/2 cup	1/2 cup	170	5.0	28.0	190	na	5.0	(mq)	15	25%
(Jell-O) prepared .... 1/2 cup	1/2 cup	160	5.0	28.0	170	na	4.0	(mq)	15	21%
(Royal) dark and sweet, prepared .... 1/2 cup	1/2 cup	180	5.0	33.0	150	na	4.0	(mq)	(mq)	19%
(Royal) 'Instant' prepared .... 1/2 cup	1/2 cup	190	4.0	35.0	390	na	4.0	(mq)	(mq)	19%
(Royal) 'Instant Sugar-free' prepared w/2% milk .... 1/2 cup	1/2 cup	110	5.0	17.0	480	na	3.0	(mq)	(mq)	24%
(Royal) prepared .... 1/2 cup	1/2 cup	180	5.0	33.0	150	na	4.0	(mq)	(mq)	19%
(Weight Watchers) 'Instant' prepared w/skim milk .... 1/2 cup	1/2 cup	90	6.0	18.0	420	na	1.0	na	na	9%
CHOCOLATE FUDGE										
(Jell-O) 'Instant' prepared .... 1/2 cup	1/2 cup	180	5.0	31.0	440	na	5.0	(mq)	15	24%
(Jell-O) 'Instant Sugar-free' prepared w/2% milk .... 1/2 cup	1/2 cup	100	5.0	14.0	330	na	3.0	(mq)	10	26%
(Jell-O) prepared .... 1/2 cup	1/2 cup	160	5.0	28.0	170	na	4.0	(mq)	15	21%
CHOCOLATE-CHOCOLATE CHIP *(Royal)* prepared .... 1/2 cup	1/2 cup	190	4.0	35.0	390	na	4.0	(mq)	(mq)	19%
CHOCOLATE-MINT *(Royal)* 'Instant' prepared .... 1/2 cup	1/2 cup	190	4.0	35.0	390	na	4.0	(mq)	(mq)	19%
COCONUT, TOASTED *(Royal)* 'Instant' prepared .... 1/2 cup	1/2 cup	170	4.0	30.0	350	na	4.0	(mq)	(mq)	21%
COCONUT CREAM *(Jell-O)* 'Instant' prepared .... 1/2 cup	1/2 cup	180	4.0	27.0	320	na	6.0	(mq)	15	30%
EGG										
(Jell-O) custard 'Americana' prepared .... 1/2 cup	1/2 cup	160	5.0	23.0	200	na	5.0	(mq)	80	29%
(Royal) custard, prepared .... 1/2 cup	1/2 cup	150	4.0	22.0	115	na	5.0	(mq)	(mq)	30%
FLAN										
(Jell-O) prepared .... 1/2 cup	1/2 cup	150	4.0	26.0	65	na	4.0	(mq)	15	23%
(Royal) w/caramel sauce, prepared .... 1/2 cup	1/2 cup	150	4.0	22.0	115	na	5.0	(mq)	(mq)	30%
FRENCH VANILLA										
(Jell-O) 'Instant' prepared .... 1/2 cup	1/2 cup	160	4.0	28.0	400	na	4.0	(mq)	15	22%

Food Name	Serving Size	Calories	Prot. gms	Carbs gms	Sod. mgs	Fiber gms	Fat gms	Sat. Fat gms	Chol. mgs	% Fat Cal.
(Jell-O) prepared	1/2 cup	170	4.0	30.0	190	na	4.0	(mq)	15	21%
KEY LIME (Royal) prepared	1/2 cup	160	1.0	30.0	120	na	3.0	(mq)	(mq)	18%
LEMON										
(Featherweight) custard, prepared	1/2 cup	40	1.0	8.0	40	na	0.0	0.0	0	0%
(French's) prepared	1/2 cup	110	1.0	22.0	110	na	1.0	na	na	8%
(Jell-O) 'Instant' prepared	1/2 cup	170	4.0	29.0	360	na	4.0	(mq)	15	21%
(Royal) 'Instant' prepared	1/2 cup	180	1.0	29.0	350	na	5.0	(mq)	(mq)	27%
(Royal) prepared	1/2 cup	160	1.0	30.0	120	na	3.0	(mq)	(mq)	na
MILK CHOCOLATE										
(Jell-O) 'Instant' prepared	1/2 cup	180	5.0	31.0	470	na	5.0	(mq)	15	24%
(Jell-O) 'Microwave' prepared	1/2 cup	160	4.0	27.0	190	na	5.0	(mq)	15	27%
(Jell-O) prepared	1/2 cup	160	4.0	28.0	170	na	4.0	(mq)	15	22%
PISTACHIO										
(Jell-O) 'Instant' prepared	1/2 cup	170	4.0	28.0	410	na	5.0	(mq)	15	26%
(Jell-O) 'Instant Sugar-free' prepared w/2% milk	1/2 cup	90	4.0	12.0	390	na	3.0	(mq)	10	30%
(Royal) nut 'Instant' prepared	1/2 cup	170	4.0	30.0	350	na	4.0	(mq)	(mq)	21%
RASPBERRY (Salada) pudding and pie glaze, prepared	1/2 cup	130	0.0	32.0	5	na	0.0	0.0	0	0%
RICE (Jell-O) 'Americana' prepared	1/2 cup	170	5.0	30.0	160	na	4.0	na	15	21%
STRAWBERRY (Salada) pudding and pie glaze, prepared ...	1/2 cup	130	0.0	32.0	5	na	0.0	0.0	0	0%
VANILLA										
(D-Zerta) low calorie, prepared w/skim milk	1/2 cup	70	4.0	12.0	65	na	0.0	na	0	0%
(Featherweight) custard, prepared	1/2 cup	40	1.0	8.0	40	na	0.0	0.0	0	0%
(Featherweight) 'Instant' prepared	1/2 cup	100	4.0	19.0	190	na	0.0	0.0	5	0%
(Featherweight) prepared	1/2 cup	12	0.0	3.0	6	na	0.0	0.0	0	0%
(Jell-O) 'Cook 'n Serve Sugar-free' prepared w/skim milk ..	1/2 cup	60	4.0	11.0	200	na	2.0	na	na	23%
(Jell-O) 'Cook 'n Serve Sugar-free' prepared w/2% milk ...	1/2 cup	80	4.0	11.0	200	na	2.0	(mq)	10	23%
(Jell-O) 'Instant' prepared	1/2 cup	170	4.0	29.0	410	na	4.0	(mq)	15	21%
(Jell-O) 'Instant Sugar-free' prepared w/2% milk	1/2 cup	90	4.0	12.0	390	na	2.0	(mq)	10	22%
(Jell-O) 'Microwave' prepared	1/2 cup	160	4.0	26.0	180	na	4.0	(mq)	15	23%
(Jell-O) prepared	1/2 cup	160	4.0	26.0	200	na	4.0	(mq)	15	23%
(Jell-O) tapioca 'Americana' prepared	1/2 cup	160	4.0	27.0	170	na	4.0	(mq)	15	23%
(Royal) 'Instant' prepared	1/2 cup	180	4.0	29.0	390	na	5.0	(mq)	(mq)	25%
(Royal) 'Instant Sugar-free' prepared w/2% milk	1/2 cup	100	4.0	16.0	470	na	2.0	(mq)	na	18%
(Royal) prepared	1/2 cup	160	4.0	27.0	210	na	4.0	(mq)	(mq)	23%
(Royal) tapioca, prepared	1/2 cup	160	4.0	27.0	150	na	4.0	(mq)	(mq)	23%
PUDDING / PIE FILLING MIX. See also PUDDING MIX.										
BANANA (Jell-O) instant, sugar-free, prepared w/2% milk ...	1/2 cup	80	4.0	11.0	390	na	2.0	na	10	23%
BANANA CREAM										
(Jell-O) instant, prepared	1/2 cup	160	4.0	28.0	410	na	4.0	na	15	22%
(Jell-O) microwave, prepared	1/2 cup	150	4.0	25.0	220	na	4.0	na	15	24%
(Jell-O) prepared, w/o crust	1/6 pie	100	3.0	17.0	160	na	3.0	na	10	25%
(Royal) dry	1 serving	80	0.0	20.0	110	0	0.0	0.0	0	0%
(Royal) instant, dry	1 serving	90	0.0	22.0	390	na	0.0	0.0	0	0%
BUTTER PECAN (Jell-O) instant, prepared	1/2 cup	170	4.0	28.0	410	na	5.0	na	15	26%
BUTTERSCOTCH										
(D-Zerta) reduced calorie, prepared	1/2 cup	70	4.0	12.0	65	na	0.0	na	0	0%
(Jell-O) instant, prepared	1/2 cup	160	4.0	28.0	450	na	4.0	na	15	22%
(Jell-O) instant, sugar-free, prepared w/2% milk	1/2 cup	90	4.0	12.0	390	na	2.0	na	10	22%
(Jell-O) microwave, prepared	1/2 cup	170	4.0	28.0	180	na	4.0	na	15	22%
(Jell-O) prepared	1/2 cup	170	4.0	30.0	190	na	4.0	na	15	21%
(Nabisco) 'My•T•Fine' prepared	1/2 cup	90	0.0	22.0	190	na	0.0	0.0	na	0%
(Royal) instant, dry	1 serving	90	0.0	22.0	400	na	0.0	0.0	0	0%
(Royal) prepared	1/2 cup	90	0.0	23.0	180	0	0.0	0.0	0	0%
CHERRY-VANILLA (Royal) instant, dry	1 serving	90	0.0	23.0	300	0	0.0	0.0	0	0%

Food Name	Serving Size	Calories	Prot. gms	Carbs gms	Sod. mgs	Fiber gms	Fat gms	Sat. Fat gms	Chol. mgs	% Fat Cal.
CHOCOLATE										
(D-Zerta) reduced calorie, prepared	1/2 cup	60	5.0	11.0	70	na	0.0	na	0	0%
(Jell-O) instant, prepared	1/2 cup	180	4.0	31.0	480	na	4.0	na	15	21%
(Jell-O) instant, sugar-free, prepared w/2% milk	1/2 cup	90	4.0	13.0	380	na	3.0	na	10	28%
(Jell-O) microwave, prepared	1/2 cup	170	5.0	28.0	190	na	5.0	na	15	25%
(Jell-O) prepared	1/2 cup	160	5.0	28.0	170	na	4.0	na	15	21%
(Jell-O) sugar-free, prepared w/2% milk	1/2 cup	90	5.0	13.0	160	na	3.0	na	10	27%
(Nabisco) 'My•T•Fine' prepared	1/2 cup	100	1.0	23.0	135	0	0.0	0.0	0	0%
(Royal) dark and sweet, instant, dry	1 serving	110	1.0	25.0	460	0	0.0	0.0	0	0%
(Royal) dark and sweet, prepared	1/2 cup	90	1.0	22.0	95	1.0	0.0	0.0	0	0%
(Royal) instant, dry	1 serving	110	1.0	27.0	450	0	0.0	0.0	0	0%
(Royal) instant, sugar-free, prepared	1/2 cup	50	0.0	11.0	420	na	0.0	na	na	0%
(Royal) prepared	1/2 cup	90	1.0	22.0	90	0	0.0	0.0	0	0%
CHOCOLATE FUDGE										
(Jell-O) instant, prepared	1/2 cup	180	5.0	31.0	440	na	5.0	na	15	24%
(Jell-O) instant, sugar-free, prepared w/2% milk	1/2 cup	100	5.0	14.0	330	na	3.0	na	10	26%
(Jell-O) prepared	1/2 cup	160	5.0	28.0	170	na	4.0	na	15	21%
(Nabisco) 'My•T•Fine' prepared	1/2 cup	100	1.0	24.0	140	1.0	0.0	0.0	na	0%
CHOCOLATE-ALMOND										
(Nabisco) 'My•T•Fine' prepared	1/2 cup	100	1.0	23.0	135	na	1.0	0.0	0	9%
(Royal) instant, prepared	1/2 cup	120	0.0	26.0	440	na	1.0	na	na	8%
CHOCOLATE-CHOCOLATE CHIP (Royal) instant, dry	1 serving	110	1.0	26.0	390	0	1.0	0.0	0	8%
CHOCOLATE-PEANUT BUTTER CHIP (Royal) instant, dry	1 serving	110	1.0	26.0	480	0	1.0	0.0	0	8%
COCONUT, TOASTED (Royal) instant, prepared	1/2 cup	100	0.0	20.0	450	na	2.0	na	na	18%
COCONUT CREAM										
(Jell-O) instant, prepared	1/2 cup	180	4.0	27.0	320	na	6.0	na	15	30%
(Jell-O) prepared, w/o crust	1/6 pie	110	3.0	16.0	140	na	4.0	na	10	32%
EGG (Royal) custard, prepared	1/2 cup	60	0.0	16.0	75	na	0.0	na	na	0%
FLAN										
(Jell-O) prepared	1/2 cup	150	4.0	26.0	65	na	4.0	na	15	23%
(Royal) caramel custard, prepared	1/2 cup	60	0.0	15.0	55	na	0.0	na	na	0%
FRENCH VANILLA										
(Jell-O) instant, prepared	1/2 cup	160	4.0	28.0	400	na	4.0	na	15	22%
(Jell-O) prepared	1/2 cup	170	4.0	30.0	190	na	4.0	na	15	21%
LEMON										
(Jell-O) instant, prepared	1/2 cup	170	4.0	29.0	360	na	4.0	na	15	21%
(Nabisco) 'My•T•Fine' dry	1 serving	90	0.0	22.0	170	na	0.0	0.0	0	0%
(Royal) instant, dry	1 serving	90	0.0	23.0	320	na	0.0	0.0	0	0%
MILK CHOCOLATE										
(Jell-O) instant, prepared	1/2 cup	180	5.0	31.0	470	na	5.0	na	15	24%
(Jell-O) microwave, prepared	1/2 cup	160	4.0	27.0	190	na	5.0	na	15	27%
(Jell-O) prepared	1/2 cup	160	4.0	28.0	170	na	4.0	na	15	22%
PISTACHIO										
(Jell-O) instant, prepared	1/2 cup	170	4.0	28.0	410	na	5.0	na	15	26%
(Jell-O) instant, sugar-free, prepared w/2% milk	1/2 cup	90	4.0	12.0	390	na	3.0	na	10	30%
(Royal) instant, dry	1 serving	90	0.0	22.0	360	0	1.0	0.0	0	9%
STRAWBERRY (Royal) instant, dry	1 serving	100	0.0	24.0	330	na	0.0	0.0	0	0%
TAPIOCA (Nabisco) 'My•T•Fine' dry	1 serving	80	0.0	19.0	160	na	0.0	0.0	0	0%
VANILLA										
(D-Zerta) reduced calorie, w/aspartame, prepared	1/2 cup	70	4.0	12.0	65	na	0.0	na	0	0%
(Jell-O) instant, prepared	1/2 cup	170	4.0	29.0	410	na	4.0	na	15	21%
(Jell-O) instant, sugar-free, prepared w/2% milk	1/2 cup	90	4.0	12.0	390	na	2.0	na	10	22%
(Jell-O) microwave, prepared	1/2 cup	160	4.0	26.0	180	na	4.0	na	15	23%

Food Name	Serving Size	Calories	Prot. gms	Carbs gms	Sod. mgs	Fiber gms	Fat gms	Sat. Fat gms	Chol. mgs	% Fat Cal.
(Jell-O) prepared	1/2 cup	160	4.0	26.0	200	na	4.0	na	15	23%
(Jell-O) sugar-free, w/aspartame, prepared w/2% milk	1/2 cup	80	4.0	11.0	200	na	2.0	na	10	23%
(Nabisco) 'My•T•Fine' prepared	1/2 cup	90	0.0	22.0	120	0	0.0	0.0	0	0%
(Royal) instant, dry	1 serving	90	0.0	23.0	325	na	0.0	0.0	0	0%
VANILLA-CHOCOLATE CHIP (Royal) instant, dry	1 serving	90	0.0	22.0	350	0	1.0	0.0	0	9%

PUERTO RICAN CHERRY. See CHERRY, PUERTO RICAN.

PUFF PASTRY, FROZEN

Food Name	Serving Size	Calories	Prot. gms	Carbs gms	Sod. mgs	Fiber gms	Fat gms	Sat. Fat gms	Chol. mgs	% Fat Cal.
sheet (Pepperidge Farm)	1/4 sheet	260	4.0	22.0	290	(mq)	17.0	(mq)	na	60%
shell, mini (Pepperidge Farm)	1 shell	50	1.0	4.0	40	(mq)	4.0	(mq)	na	64%
shell, patty (Pepperidge Farm)	1 shell	210	3.0	16.0	180	(mq)	15.0	(mq)	na	64%
shell, ready to bake	1 shell	259	3.4	21.2	117	na	17.9	2.5	0	62%
shell, ready to bake	1 oz	156	2.1	12.8	71	na	10.8	1.5	0	62%

PUMELO. See POMELO.

PUMPKIN

Food Name	Serving Size	Calories	Prot. gms	Carbs gms	Sod. mgs	Fiber gms	Fat gms	Sat. Fat gms	Chol. mgs	% Fat Cal.
boiled, drained	4 oz	23	0.8	5.5	1	>.9 c	0.1	<.1	0	3%
boiled, drained, mashed	1/2 cup	24	0.9	6.0	1	>1.0 c	0.1	0.1	0	3%
raw, 1-inch cubes	1/2 cup	15	0.6	3.8	1	1.0	0.1	0.0	0	5%
raw, trimmed	1 oz	7	0.3	1.8	<1	>.3 c	<.1	<.1	0	<10%
raw, untrimmed	1 lb	83	3.2	20.6	3	>3.5 c	0.3	0.2	0	3%

PUMPKIN, CANNED

Food Name	Serving Size	Calories	Prot. gms	Carbs gms	Sod. mgs	Fiber gms	Fat gms	Sat. Fat gms	Chol. mgs	% Fat Cal.
	1/2 cup	41	1.3	9.9	6	3.4	0.3	0.2	0	6%
w/winter squash	4 oz	39	1.2	9.2	6	>1.8 c	0.3	0.2	0	6%
(Del Monte)	1/2 cup	35	1.0	9.0	10	(mq)	0.0	0.0	0	0%
(Libby's)	1/2 cup	42	1.4	10.1	6	3.8	0.4	na	0	7%
(Libby's) solid pack	1/2 cup	42	1.4	10.1	6	3.8	0.4	na	na	7%
(Stokely)	1/2 cup	40	2.0	10.0	15	(mq)	0.0	0.0	0	0%

PUMPKIN FLOWER

Food Name	Serving Size	Calories	Prot. gms	Carbs gms	Sod. mgs	Fiber gms	Fat gms	Sat. Fat gms	Chol. mgs	% Fat Cal.
boiled, drained	4 oz	17	1.2	3.7	7	>1.0 c	0.1	<.1	0	4%
boiled, drained	1/2 cup	10	0.7	2.2	4	.6	0.1	0.0	0	7%
raw	1 cup	5	0.3	1.1	2	>.2 c	0.0	0.0	0	0%
raw, trimmed	1 oz	4	0.3	0.9	1	>.2 c	<.1	<.1	0	<16%
raw, trimmed	1/2 cup	3	0.2	0.5	1	>.1 c	<.1	tr	0	<24%
raw, untrimmed	1 lb	23	1.6	5.2	7	>1.0 c	0.1	0.1	0	3%

PUMPKIN LEAF

Food Name	Serving Size	Calories	Prot. gms	Carbs gms	Sod. mgs	Fiber gms	Fat gms	Sat. Fat gms	Chol. mgs	% Fat Cal.
boiled, drained	4 oz	24	3.1	3.8	9	>1.2 c	0.2	0.1	0	6%
boiled, drained	1/2 cup	7	1.0	1.2	3	1.0	0.1	0.0	0	9%
raw	1/2 cup	4	0.6	0.5	2	>.2 c	0.1	0.0	0	17%
raw, trimmed	1 oz	5	0.9	0.7	3	>.3 c	0.1	0.1	0	12%
raw, untrimmed	1 lb	36	5.9	4.3	20	>1.9 c	0.7	0.4	0	13%

PUMPKIN PIE SPICE

Food Name	Serving Size	Calories	Prot. gms	Carbs gms	Sod. mgs	Fiber gms	Fat gms	Sat. Fat gms	Chol. mgs	% Fat Cal.
dried	1 tbsp	19	0.3	3.9	3	.8	0.7	na	0	27%
dried	1 tsp	6	0.1	1.2	1	.3	0.2	na	0	26%

PUMPKIN SEED

Food Name	Serving Size	Calories	Prot. gms	Carbs gms	Sod. mgs	Fiber gms	Fat gms	Sat. Fat gms	Chol. mgs	% Fat Cal.
dried	1 lb	1817	82.4	59.8	59	>7.5 c	153.9	29.1	0	71%
roasted	1 lb	2021	84.1	243.8	82	>162.8 c	88.0	16.6	0	38%
roasted	1 cup	285	11.9	34.4	12	>23.0 c	12.4	2.3	0	38%
roasted, approx 85 seeds	1 oz	127	5.3	15.3	5	>10.2 c	5.5	1.0	0	38%
w/squash seeds, roasted	1 cup	285	11.9	34.4	12	>23.0 c	12.4	2.3	0	38%
w/squash seeds, roasted	1 oz	127	5.3	15.3	5	>10.2 c	5.5	1.0	0	38%

PUMPKIN SEED, SHELLED

Food Name	Serving Size	Calories	Prot. gms	Carbs gms	Sod. mgs	Fiber gms	Fat gms	Sat. Fat gms	Chol. mgs	% Fat Cal.
dried	1 cup	747	33.9	24.6	24	19.0	63.3	12.0	0	71%
dried, approx 142 kernels	1 oz	154	7.0	5.1	5	3.9	13.0	2.5	0	71%
roasted	1 cup	1184	74.8	30.5	40	14.7	95.6	18.1	0	67%
roasted	1 oz	148	9.4	3.8	5	1.9	12.0	2.2	0	67%

Food Name	Serving Size	Calories	Prot. gms	Carbs gms	Sod. mgs	Fiber gms	Fat gms	Sat. Fat gms	Chol. mgs	% Fat Cal.
w/squash seed kernels, dried	1 cup	747	33.9	24.6	25	19.0	63.3	12.0	0	71%
w/squash seed kernels, dried, approx 142 kernels	1 oz	154	7.0	5.1	5	3.9	13.0	2.5	0	71%
w/squash seed kernels, roasted	1 cup	1185	74.8	30.5	41	14.7	95.6	18.1	0	67%
w/squash seed kernels, roasted	1 oz	149	9.4	3.8	6	1.9	12.0	2.2	0	67%
PUNCH. See also FRUIT PUNCH; and individual listings.										
(J. Hungerford)	9.03 oz	133	0.0	33.4	2	0	0.0	0.0	0	0%
(Squeezit) 'Mean Green Puncher'	6.75 oz	100	0.0	25.0	5	na	0.0	na	na	0%
(Squeezit) 'Rockin Red Puncher'	6.75 oz	110	0.0	28.0	5	na	0.0	na	na	0%
PURPLESAURUS REX DRINK MIX										
(Kool-Aid) sugar-free, w/NutraSweet, prepared	8 oz	4	0.0	0.0	5	na	0.0	na	0	0%
(Kool-Aid) sugar-sweetened, prepared	8 oz	80	0.0	21.0	5	na	0.0	na	0	0%
(Kool-Aid) unsweetened, prepared w/sugar	8 oz	100	0.0	25.0	5	na	0.0	na	0	0%
(Kool-Aid) unsweetened, prepared w/o sugar	8 oz	2	0.0	0.0	5	na	0.0	na	0	0%
PURSLANE /pussley										
boiled, drained	4 oz	20	1.7	4.0	50	>.9 c	0.2	(tr)	0	7%
boiled, drained	1/2 cup	10	0.9	2.1	26	>.5 c	0.1	na	0	7%
raw	1 cup	7	0.6	1.5	19	>.3 c	0.0	na	0	0%
raw, trimmed	1 oz	5	0.4	1.0	13	>.2 c	<.1	(tr)	0	<14%
raw, trimmed	1/2 cup	4	0.3	0.7	10	>.2 c	<.1	(tr)	0	<18%
raw, untrimmed	1 lb	56	4.5	11.8	156	>2.8 c	0.3	(tr)	0	4%

Q

Food Name	Serving Size	Calories	Prot. gms	Carbs gms	Sod. mgs	Fiber gms	Fat gms	Sat. Fat gms	Chol. mgs	% Fat Cal.
QUAIL /bobwhite										
breast meat only, raw	1 oz	35	6.4	0.0	16	0	0.8	0.2	(mq)	22%
meat and skin, raw	1 oz	54	5.6	0.0	15	0	3.4	1.0	(mq)	58%
raw	1 oz	34	6.0	0.0	29	0	0.9	0.1	24	25%
QUAIL GIBLETS, raw	3.5 oz	176	21.8	6.7	70	0	6.2	2.0	350	33%
QUICHE										
(Nancy's) Classic French, Montery jack and swiss, w/bacon	1 quiche	520	21.0	30.0	670	1.0	37.0	18.0	210	62%
(Nancy's) French baked, broccoli, cheddar	1 quiche	490	17.0	33.0	750	2.0	33.0	16.0	165	60%
QUINCE										
raw, trimmed	1 med	52	0.4	14.1	4	1.8	0.1	0.0	0	2%
raw, trimmed	1 oz	16	0.1	4.3	1	>.5 c	<.1	tr	0	<5%
raw, untrimmed	1 lb	158	1.1	42.3	11	>4.7 c	0.3	<.1	0	2%
QUINOA, WHOLE GRAIN										
dry	1/2 cup	318	11.1	58.6	18	5.0	4.9	0.5	0	14%
dry	1 oz	106	3.7	19.5	na	(mq)	1.6	0.2	0	13%
dry (Ancient Harvest)	1/4 cup	159	5.0	28.0	8	5.7	2.0	na	0	12%
dry (Eden Foods)	2 oz	200	8.0	38.0	30	4.3	4.0	na	0	16%
dry (Quinoa)	1/4 cup	159	5.0	28.0	8	5.7	2.0	na	0	12%
steam-rolled, flakes (Ancient Harvest)	1/3 cup	105	2.6	23.0	5	2.8	1.0	0.0	0	8%
steam-rolled, flakes (Quinoa)	1/3 cup	105	2.6	23.0	5	2.8	1.0	0.0	0	8%
QUINOA FLOUR, WHOLE GRAIN										
non-gluten (Ancient Harvest)	1/4 cup	132	4.0	24.0	10	4.7	2.0	na	0	14%
non-gluten (Quinoa)	1/4 cup	132	4.0	24.0	10	4.7	2.0	na	0	14%
QUINOA PASTA. See PASTA.										
QUINOA SEED (Arrowhead Mills)	2 oz	200	9.0	35.0	3	5.3	3.0	na	0	13%

R

Food Name	Serving Size	Calories	Prot. gms	Carbs gms	Sod. mgs	Fiber gms	Fat gms	Sat. Fat gms	Chol. mgs	% Fat Cal.
RABBIT										
Domesticated										
raw	1 lb	617	91.0	0.0	186	na	25.2	7.5	259	38%
raw	1 oz	38	5.6	0.0	11	na	1.5	0.5	16	38%
roasted	3 oz	167	24.7	0.0	40	na	6.8	2.0	70	38%
roasted, diced	1 cup	216	31.9	0.0	52	0	8.8	2.6	90	38%
stewed	3 oz	175	25.8	0.0	31	na	7.2	2.1	73	39%
stewed, diced	1 cup	288	42.5	0.0	52	0	11.8	3.5	120	39%
Wild										
raw	1 lb	517	98.8	0.0	227	na	10.5	3.1	367	19%
raw	1 oz	32	6.1	0.0	14	na	0.7	0.2	23	21%
stewed	3 oz	147	28.1	0.0	38	na	3.0	0.9	105	19%
stewed, diced	1 cup	242	46.2	0.0	63	0	4.9	1.5	172	19%
RACCOON										
roasted	3 oz	217	24.8	0.0	na	na	12.3	na	na	53%
roasted, diced	1 cup	357	40.9	0.0	(mq)	0	20.3	(mq)	(mq)	53%
RADICCHIO										
raw	1 med	2	0.1	0.4	2	na	0.0	na	0	0%
raw, shredded	1/2 cup	5	0.3	0.9	4	na	0.1	na	0	16%
RADISH										
fresh (Dole)	7 med	20	0.0	3.0	35	(mq)	0.0	na	na	0%
raw, sliced	1/2 cup	10	0.4	2.1	14	.9	0.3	0.0	0	21%
raw, 1 inch long, 3/4 inch diam	10 radishes	8	0.3	1.6	11	.7	0.2	0.0	0	19%
raw, trimmed	1 oz	5	0.2	1.0	7	.7	0.2	tr	0	27%
raw, untrimmed	1 lb	68	2.5	14.6	98	>2.2 c	2.2	0.1	0	22%
RADISH, BLACK/winter radish										
raw, trimmed	1 lb	77	4.5	16.3	82	(mq)	0.5	(mq)	0	5%
raw, trimmed	1 oz	5	0.3	1.0	5	(mq)	<.1	tr	0	<15%
RADISH, ORIENTAL. See DAIKON.										
RADISH, WHITE ICICLE										
raw	1 med	2	0.2	0.5	3	>.1 c	0.0	0.0	0	0%
raw, sliced	1/2 cup	7	0.6	1.3	8	>.4 c	0.1	0.0	0	11%
raw, trimmed	1 oz	4	0.3	0.7	5	>.2 c	<.1	tr	0	<18%
raw, untrimmed	1 lb	41	3.2	7.7	47	>2.1 c	0.3	0.1	0	6%
RADISH, WINTER. See RADISH, BLACK.										
RADISH LEAVES, trimmed	1 oz	15	0.8	2.8	(mq)	>.4 c	0.1	tr	0	6%
RADISH SEED										
sprouted	1 lb	186	17.3	13.9	28	(mq)	11.5	3.5	0	45%
sprouted	1 oz	12	1.1	0.9	2	(mq)	0.7	0.2	0	44%
sprouted, raw	1/2 cup	8	0.7	0.7	1	>.4 c	0.5	0.2	0	45%
RAG GOURD. See GOURD, DISHCLOTH.										
RAINBOW PUNCH (Kool-Aid) 'Koolers'	8.45 oz	130	0.0	36.0	10	na	0.0	na	0	0%
RAINBOW PUNCH MIX										
(Kool-Aid) sugar-sweetened	8 oz	80	0.0	21.0	20	na	0.0	na	0	0%
(Kool-Aid) unsweetened, prepared w/sugar	8 oz	100	0.0	25.0	0	na	0.0	na	0	0%
(Kool-Aid) unsweetened, prepared w/o sugar	8 oz	2	0.0	0.0	0	na	0.0	na	0	0%
RAINBOW SMELT. See SMELT, RAINBOW.										
RAISIN										
Dark										
seedless	1 cup packed	495	5.3	130.6	20	8.8	0.8	0.3	0	1%
seedless	1 cup	435	4.7	114.7	17	7.7	0.7	0.2	0	1%

Food Name	Serving Size	Calories	Prot. gms	Carbs gms	Sod. mgs	Fiber gms	Fat gms	Sat. Fat gms	Chol. mgs	% Fat Cal.
seedless	1 oz	85	0.9	22.4	3	1.5	0.1	<.1	0	1%
seedless (Cinderella) Thompson	1/2 cup	250	3.0	66.0	15	5.8	0.0	0.0	0	0%
seedless (Dole)	1/2 cup	260	3.0	63.0	25	(mq)	0.0	0.0	0	0%
seedless (Finast)	.5 oz	45	0.0	11.0	5	(mq)	0.0	0.0	0	0%
seedless (Sun•Maid)	1/2 cup	290	3.0	69.0	15	(mq)	0.0	0.0	0	0%
seedless (Sun•Maid) California sun-dried, 100% natural	1/2 cup	250	3.0	68.0	10	4.5	0.0	na	na	0%
w/seeds	1 cup packed	488	4.2	129.5	46	11.2	0.9	0.3	0	2%
w/seeds	1 cup	429	3.7	113.8	41	9.9	0.8	0.3	0	2%
w/seeds	1 oz	84	0.7	22.2	8	.2	0.2	0.1	0	2%
w/seeds (Sun•Maid) Muscat	1/2 cup	270	2.0	67.0	25	na	1.0	na	na	3%
Golden										
seedless	1 lb	1368	15.4	360.7	54	15.9	2.1	0.7	0	1%
seedless	1 cup packed	498	5.6	131.2	20	5.8	0.8	0.3	0	1%
seedless	1 cup	438	4.9	115.3	17	>2.1 c	0.7	0.2	0	1%
seedless	1 oz	86	1.0	22.5	3	>.4 c	0.1	<.1	0	1%
seedless (Del Monte) natural	3 oz	250	3.0	68.0	15	(mq)	0.0	0.0	0	0%
seedless (Dole)	1/2 cup	260	3.0	63.0	25	(mq)	0.0	0.0	0	0%
w/seed (Del Monte)	3 oz	260	3.0	68.0	10	(mq)	0.0	0.0	0	0%
w/seed (Dole)	1/2 cup	250	3.0	66.0	25	na	0.0	na	na	0%
w/seed (Sun•Maid) California	1/2 cup	250	3.0	68.0	10	4.5	0.0	na	na	0%
RASPBERRY / bramble										
trimmed	1 pint	153	2.8	36.1	0	21.2	1.7	0.1	0	9%
trimmed	1 cup	60	1.1	14.2	0	8.4	0.7	0.0	0	9%
trimmed	1 oz	14	0.3	3.3	tr	1.3	0.2	tr	0	11%
untrimmed	1 lb	215	4.0	50.4	1	20.5	2.4	0.1	0	9%
untrimmed	1 pint	154	2.8	36.1	tr	15.3	1.7	0.1	0	9%
Canned										
red, in heavy syrup	4 oz	103	0.9	26.5	3	(mq)	0.1	tr	0	1%
red, in heavy syrup, solid and liquid	1/2 cup	116	1.1	29.9	4	4.2	0.2	0.0	0	1%
Frozen										
red, in light syrup (Birds Eye) 'Quick Thaw Pouch'	5 oz	100	1.0	25.0	0	4.0	1.0	tr	0	8%
red, sweetened, unthawed	10 oz	293	2.0	74.3	3	12.5	0.5	0.0	0	2%
red, sweetened, unthawed	1 cup	258	1.8	65.4	3	11.0	0.4	0.0	0	1%
sweetened	10 oz	291	2.0	74.3	1	12.5	0.5	<.1	0	2%
sweetened	1/2 cup	128	0.9	32.7	1	6.3	0.2	tr	0	1%
sweetened	4 oz	117	0.8	29.7	1	5.0	0.2	tr	0	2%
RASPBERRY DRINK, W/CRANBERRY										
(A&P)	6 oz	110	<1.0	27.0	0	(tr)	<1.0	(tr)	0	<7%
(Finast)	6 oz	110	0.0	27.0	10	(tr)	0.0	0.0	0	0%
(Pathmark)	6 oz	110	0.0	27.0	10	(tr)	0.0	0.0	0	0%
(Pathmark) 'Sodium Free'	6 oz	110	0.0	27.0	0	(tr)	0.0	0.0	0	0%
RASPBERRY JUICE										
(Apple & Eve) w/cranberry	6 oz	90	0.0	21.0	10	(mq)	0.0	0.0	0	0%
(Dole) blend 'Pure & Light Country Raspberry'	6 oz	87	0.3	24.0	15	(tr)	0.2	(tr)	0	2%
(Santa Cruz Natural) red, organic	8 oz	120	1.0	28.0	na	na	<1.0	na	na	<7%
(Smucker's) red 'Naturally 100%'	8 oz	120	0.0	30.0	10	(tr)	0.0	0.0	0	0%
RASPBERRY JUICE COCKTAIL										
(Welch's) 'Orchard,' bottled	10 oz	160	0.0	40.0	10	0	0.0	0.0	0	0%
RASPBERRY JUICE FLOAT (Knudsen & Sons)	8 oz	130	2.0	31.0	na	na	0.0	na	na	0%
RASPBERRY LEMONADE										
(Knudsen & Sons)	8 oz	110	<1.0	28.0	na	na	0.0	na	na	0%
(Santa Cruz Natural) organic	8 oz	60	<1.0	20.0	na	na	<1.0	na	na	<10%
(Santa Cruz Natural) 'Sparkling' organic	8 oz	85	<1.0	20.0	na	na	<1.0	na	na	<10%
RASPBERRY NECTAR (Knudsen & Sons)	8 oz	120	<1.0	30.0	na	na	0.0	na	na	0%

Food Name	Serving Size	Calories	Prot. gms	Carbs gms	Sod. mgs	Fiber gms	Fat gms	Sat. Fat gms	Chol. mgs	% Fat Cal.
RASPBERRY-PEACH JUICE (Knudsen & Sons)	8 oz	115	<1.0	28.0	na	na	0.0	na	na	0%
RASPBERRY PUNCH MIX										
(Kool-Aid) sugar-sweetened, prepared	8 oz	80	0.0	20.0	25	na	0.0	na	0	0%
(Kool-Aid) unsweetened, prepared w/sugar	8 oz	100	0.0	25.0	25	na	0.0	na	0	0%
(Kool-Aid) unsweetened, prepared w/o sugar	8 oz	2	0.0	0.0	25	na	0.0	na	0	0%
RASPBERRY SYRUP (Knudsen & Sons)	1 oz	75	<1.0	18.0	na	na	<1.0	na	na	<11%
RASPBERRY TOPPING, fat-free (Smucker's) 'Light'	2 tbsp	55	0.0	14.0	0	na	0.0	0.0	na	0%
RAVIOLI ENTRÉE										
CANNED										
Beef										
(Chef Boyardee) 'Sir Chomps'	7.5 oz	170	7.0	32.0	690	4.0	3.0	1.0	15	15%
(Chef Boyardee) w/meat sauce 'Smurfs'	7.5 oz	230	9.0	38.0	1160	na	5.0	na	11	19%
(Estee)	7.5 oz	230	8.0	25.0	100	(mq)	11.0	4.0	10	43%
(Finast) w/sauce	7.5 oz	250	7.0	33.0	1165	(mq)	10.0	(mq)	(mq)	36%
(Franco-American) w/meat sauce 'RavioliO's'	7.5 oz	250	10.0	35.0	920	(mq)	8.0	(mq)	(mq)	29%
(Nalley's)	7.5 oz	180	8.0	30.0	1040	(mq)	3.0	(mq)	(mq)	15%
(Pathmark) bite size, w/tomato sauce 'No Frills'	7.5 oz	180	7.0	28.0	890	(mq)	4.0	(mq)	(mq)	21%
(Pathmark) w/tomato sauce 'No Frills'	7.5 oz	180	7.0	28.0	890	(mq)	4.0	(mq)	(mq)	21%
Cheese										
(Buitoni) w/sauce	7.5 oz	190	7.0	27.0	790	(mq)	6.0	2.0	5	28%
(Chef Boyardee) 'Sir Chomps'	7.5 oz	170	6.0	38.0	740	6.0	1.0	<1.0	5	5%
(Pathmark) w/tomato sauce 'No Frills'	7.5 oz	185	7.0	27.0	790	(mq)	6.0	(mq)	(mq)	28%
Chicken										
(Buitoni) meat, w/sauce	7.5 oz	180	7.0	28.0	890	(mq)	4.0	1.0	5	21%
(Chef Boyardee)	7.5 oz	180	7.0	29.0	1100	na	4.0	na	13	20%
(Chef Boyardee) mini	7.5 oz	220	7.0	29.0	1090	na	8.0	na	na	33%
FROZEN										
(Celentano)	6.5 oz	380	21.0	50.0	510	(mq)	11.0	(mq)	(mq)	26%
(Celentano) mini	4 oz	250	13.0	39.0	210	(mq)	5.0	(mq)	(mq)	18%
Cheese										
(Amy's Kitchen) organic	1 cup	215	12.0	26.0	346	3.0	5.0	na	7	23%
(Buitoni)	4 oz	360	12.0	31.0	220	(mq)	8.0	5.0	65	30%
(Healthy Choice) baked	9 oz	250	14.0	44.0	420	na	2.0	1.0	20	7%
(Kid Cuisine) mini	8.75 oz	250	6.0	52.0	730	(mq)	2.0	(mq)	20	7%
(Lean Cuisine) w/tomato sauce	8.5 oz	240	13.0	30.0	590	na	8.0	3.0	55	30%
(Smart Ones) Florentine	8.5 oz	130	8.0	22.0	540	na	1.0	<1.0	5	7%
(Ultra Slim Fast)	12 oz	330	21.0	60.0	770	na	3.0	na	40	8%
(Weight Watchers) baked	9 oz	240	18.0	27.0	370	na	6.0	2.0	30	23%
MICROWAVE										
(Kid's Kitchen) mini microwave cup	7.5 oz	230	10.0	34.0	870	na	6.0	3.0	15	24%
Beef										
(Chef Boyardee)	7.5 oz	190	7.0	31.0	1160	2.0	4.0	2.0	11	19%
(Chef Boyardee) 'Main Meals' microwave cup	10.5 oz	290	12.0	52.0	na	na	4.0	na	na	12%
(Hormel) w/tomato sauce micro cup	7.5 oz	247	8.0	28.0	951	(mq)	11.0	(mq)	21	41%
(Libby's) w/sauce 'Diner' microwave cup	7.75 oz	240	13.0	35.0	890	2.2	5.0	4.0	15	19%
Cheese, w/meat sauce (Chef Boyardee)	7.5 oz	200	6.0	37.0	1010	(mq)	3.0	(mq)	10	14%
REFRIGERATED										
(Contadina) w/beef 'Fresh'	3 oz	270	13.0	30.0	250	na	11.0	3.0	75	37%
(Contadina) w/cheese 'Fresh'	3 oz	270	13.0	30.0	360	na	11.0	6.0	75	37%
(DiGiorno) w/Italian herb cheese, cooked	1 cup	280	12.0	35.0	490	na	10.0	4.0	35	32%
(DiGiorno) w/Italian sausage, cooked	1 cup	270	13.0	34.0	520	na	9.0	4.0	40	30%
RAZZLEBERRY JUICE (Knudsen & Sons)	8 oz	90	<1.0	21.0	na	na	0.0	na	na	0%
RED BEAN, CANNED										
(A&P)	1/2 cup	120	7.0	23.0	400	(mq)	<1.0	tr	0	<7%

Food Name	Serving Size	Calories	Prot. gms	Carbs gms	Sod. mgs	Fiber gms	Fat gms	Sat. Fat gms	Chol. mgs	% Fat Cal.
(Allens)	1/2 cup	115	7.0	20.0	350	(mq)	<1.0	tr	0	<8%
(Bush's Best)	1/2 cup	70	5.0	17.0	350	6.0	0.0	na	na	0%
(Green Giant)	1/2 cup	90	6.0	19.0	340	5.0	1.0	tr	0	8%
(Joan of Arc)	1/2 cup	90	6.0	19.0	340	5.0	1.0	tr	0	8%
(Van Camp's)	1 cup	194	11.0	38.0	928	(mq)	0.6	tr	0	3%
Small										
(B&M) baked style	8 oz	223	9.0	36.0	725	11.0	5.0	2.0	5	20%
(Hunt's)	4.48 oz	89	6.2	18.9	713	5.5	0.5	0.0	0	4%
RED CABBAGE. See CABBAGE, RED.										
RED CURRY BASE (A Taste of Thai)	1 tbsp	20	0.0	1.0	430	0	1.5	0.5	0	77%
RED PERCH. See OCEAN PERCH, ATLANTIC.										
REDFISH. See OCEAN PERCH, ATLANTIC.										
REDHEAD. See SHEEPSHEAD.										
REFRIED BEANS, CANNED										
	1/2 cup	135	7.8	23.3	534	6.7	1.4	0.5	0	9%
	4 oz	121	7.1	21.0	481	6.0	1.2	0.5	na	9%
(Del Monte)	1/2 cup	130	6.0	20.0	530	(mq)	2.0	(mq)	na	15%
(Gebhardt)	4 oz	130	7.0	20.0	490	(mq)	2.0	(mq)	na	14%
(Little Pancho)	1/2 cup	80	6.0	15.0	330	(mq)	0.0	0.0	na	0%
(Old El Paso)	1/4 cup	55	3.0	8.0	200	2.5	<1.0	(mq)	1	<17%
(Rosarita)	4.5 oz	109	6.1	19.8	497	6.2	2.8	1.3	1	20%
NO-FAT (Rosarita)	4.5 oz	92	7.3	19.5	481	6.2	0.5	0.0	0	4%
ORGANIC										
(Bearitos)	1 oz	30	1.7	4.8	61	.3	0.5	(mq)	0	15%
(Bearitos) no salt	1 oz	29	1.7	4.7	2	.2	0.5	(mq)	0	15%
(Bearitos) spicy	1 oz	31	1.6	4.9	56	.5	0.6	(mq)	0	17%
SPICY										
(Del Monte)	1/2 cup	130	6.0	20.0	480	(mq)	2.0	(mq)	na	15%
(Old El Paso)	1/4 cup	35	1.0	5.0	280	2.0	1.0	0.0	1	27%
(Rosarita)	4.5 oz	109	6.4	19.9	530	6.2	2.6	1.3	1	18%
VEGETARIAN										
(Old El Paso) spicy	1/4 cup	70	6.0	15.0	730	5.0	1.0	na	0	10%
(Rosarita)	4.5 oz	118	7.7	20.9	550	6.0	2.3	0.4	0	15%
(Rosarita) spicy	4 oz	120	7.0	19.0	470	(mq)	2.0	(mq)	0	15%
(Rosarita) w/canola oil	4 oz	100	7.0	18.0	480	6.0	2.0	<1.0	0	15%
(Rosarita) w/soybean oil	4 oz	100	7.0	18.0	480	6.0	2.0	0.5	0	15%
W/BACON (Rosarita)	4.5 oz	116	8.2	18.7	489	8.2	3.1	1.2	1	21%
W/CHEESE (Old El Paso)	1/4 cup	36	2.0	4.0	280	2.0	1.0	1.0	2	27%
W/GREEN CHILIES										
(Little Pancho)	1/2 cup	80	6.0	15.0	330	(mq)	0.0	0.0	na	0%
(Old El Paso)	1/4 cup	49	3.0	8.0	252	2.5	<1.0	(mq)	na	<17%
(Rosarita)	4.5 oz	110	6.1	19.7	495	6.0	2.9	1.8	1	20%
W/JALAPEÑO (Gebhardt)	4.5 oz	106	6.8	19.0	380	6.0	3.0	1.4	1	21%
W/NACHO CHEESE (Rosarita)	4.5 oz	122	7.9	20.6	482	6.2	3.1	1.0	1	20%
W/ONION (Rosarita)	4.5 oz	114	6.4	20.8	508	6.2	2.8	1.3	1	19%
W/SAUSAGE (Old El Paso)	1/4 cup	180	6.0	8.0	300	(mq)	8.0	(mq)	(mq)	56%
REFRIED BEANS, DRIED (Rosarita)	1/3 cup	123	7.2	20.5	469	6.9	4.5	1.0	0	27%
REFRIED BEANS ENTRÉE (Chi-Chi's)	7.5 oz	250	9.0	29.0	930	na	11.0	2.0	5	39%
REFRIED BEANS MIX										
(Fantastic Foods) instant, prepared w/o added ingredients	1/2 cup	157	10.0	28.0	400	(mq)	2.0	(mq)	0	11%
(Fantastic Foods) instant, prepared w/2 tbsp salted butter	1/2 cup	207	10.0	28.0	469	(mq)	8.0	(mq)	na	32%
RELISH. See also specific listings.										
CHOWCHOW										
sour, w/cauliflower, onion, mustard	1 cup	70	3.4	9.8	3211	>1.4 c	3.1	0.0	0	35%

Food Name	Serving Size	Calories	Prot. gms	Carbs gms	Sod. mgs	Fiber gms	Fat gms	Sat. Fat gms	Chol. mgs	% Fat Cal.
sweet, w/cauliflower, onion, mustard	1 cup	284	3.7	66.2	1291	>2.2 c	2.2	0.0	0	7%
CRANBERRY-ORANGE										
canned	1/2 cup	246	0.4	63.8	44	>.8 c	0.1	na	0	0%
canned	4 oz	202	0.3	52.4	36	>.7 c	0.1	(tr)	0	0%
DILL *(Vlasic)*	1 oz	2	0.0	1.0	415	(mq)	0.0	0.0	0	0%
HAMBURGER										
pickle	1/2 cup	157	0.8	42.1	1337	>1.1 c	0.7	0.1	0	4%
pickle	1 tbsp	19	0.1	5.2	164	>.1 c	0.1	0.0	0	4%
(Heinz)	1 oz	40	0.0	9.0	255	(mq)	0.0	0.0	0	0%
HOT DOG										
pickle	1/2 cup	111	1.8	28.5	1331	>1.1 c	0.6	0.1	0	4%
pickle	1 tbsp	14	0.2	3.5	164	>.1 c	0.1	0.0	0	6%
(Heinz)	1 oz	35	0.0	8.0	200	(mq)	0.0	0.0	0	0%
(Vlasic)	1 oz	40	0.0	8.0	255	(mq)	1.0	(tr)	0	22%
INDIA										
(Heinz)	1 oz	35	0.0	9.0	215	(mq)	0.0	0.0	0	0%
(Vlasic)	1 oz	30	0.0	8.0	205	(mq)	0.0	0.0	0	0%
JALAPEÑO *(Old El Paso)*	2 tbsp	16	1.0	4.0	100	1.0	0.0	0.0	0	0%
PICCALILLI										
(Claussen)	1 oz	26	0.3	5.6	170	(mq)	0.3	(tr)	0	10%
(Heinz)	1 oz	30	0.0	7.0	145	(mq)	0.0	0.0	0	0%
(Vlasic) hot	1 oz	35	0.0	8.0	165	(mq)	0.0	0.0	0	0%
PICKLE										
sweet	1/2 cup	159	0.5	42.8	989	>1.1 c	0.6	0.1	0	3%
sweet	1 tbsp	20	0.1	5.3	122	>.1 c	0.1	0.0	0	4%
(Claussen)	1 tbsp	14	0.2	2.9	90	(mq)	0.2	(tr)	0	13%
SWEET										
	1 tbsp	21	0.1	5.1	107	(mq)	0.1	(tr)	0	4%
chopped	1 cup	338	1.2	83.3	1744	>2.0 c	1.5	0.0	0	4%
chopped	1 tbsp	21	0.1	5.1	107	>.1 c	0.1	0.0	0	4%
finely cut	1 cup	338	1.2	83.3	1744	>2.0 c	1.5	0.0	0	4%
finely cut	1 tbsp	21	0.1	5.1	107	>.1 c	0.1	0.0	0	4%
(Heinz)	1 oz	35	0.0	9.0	205	(mq)	0.0	0.0	0	0%
(Vlasic)	1 oz	30	0.0	8.0	220	(mq)	0.0	0.0	0	0%
RENNIN, enzyme tablet, unsweetened	1 tablet	1	0.0	0.2	234	0	0.0	na	0	0%
RHUBARB										
frozen	1/2 cup	14	0.4	3.5	1	(mq)	0.1	(tr)	0	6%
frozen	4 oz	24	0.6	5.8	2	(mq)	0.1	(tr)	0	3%
frozen, sweetened, cooked	4 oz	132	0.4	35.4	1	2.3	0.1	(tr)	0	1%
frozen, sweetened, cooked	1/2 cup	139	0.5	37.4	1	2.4	0.1	na	0	1%
raw, diced	1/2 cup	13	0.6	2.8	2	1.1	0.1	na	0	6%
raw, trimmed	1 oz	6	0.3	1.3	1	>.2 c	0.1	(tr)	0	12%
raw, untrimmed	1 lb	71	3.0	15.4	14	>2.4 c	0.7	na	0	8%
RICE, ARBORIO, dry *(Colavita)*	1 oz	100	2.0	22.0	5	(mq)	0.0	0.0	0	0%
RICE, BASMATI										
BROWN										
(Arrowhead Mills) long grain, dry	2 oz	200	4.0	44.0	3	3.1	1.0	na	0	5%
(Fantastic Foods) cooked	1/2 cup	102	3.0	22.0	3	(mq)	0.5	na	0	4%
(Fantastic Foods) cooked, prepared w/1 tbsp salted butter	1/2 cup	115	3.0	22.0	20	(mq)	2.0	(mq)	(mq)	15%
WHITE										
(Fantastic Foods) cooked	1/2 cup	103	2.0	23.0	1	(mq)	0.0	0.0	0	0%
(Fantastic Foods) cooked, prepared w/1 tbsp salted butter	1/2 cup	116	2.0	23.0	18	(mq)	1.0	(mq)	(mq)	8%
(Texmati) long grain, cooked	1/2 cup	82	3.0	31.0	0	(mq)	0.0	0.0	0	0%

Food Name	Serving Size	Calories	Prot. gms	Carbs gms	Sod. mgs	Fiber gms	Fat gms	Sat. Fat gms	Chol. mgs	% Fat Cal.
RICE, BROWN										
(Lundberg Family) cooked	1 cup	232	4.9	49.7	0	3.3	1.2	na	na	5%
(Minute) instant	1/2 cup	120	3.0	25.0	5	na	1.0	na	0	7%
(Uncle Ben's) precooked, prepared	1/2 cup	90	2.0	21.0	11	1.0	1.0	na	0	9%
LONG GRAIN										
cooked	1/2 cup	109	2.5	22.5	5	1.8	0.9	0.2	0	8%
cooked	4 oz	126	2.9	26.0	6	1.9	1.0	0.2	0	7%
cooked (Carolina)	1/2 cup	110	2.0	23.0	0	(mq)	0.0	0.0	0	0%
cooked (Mahatma)	1/2 cup	110	2.0	23.0	10	(mq)	0.0	0.0	0	0%
cooked (River)	1/2 cup	110	2.0	23.0	na	(mq)	0.0	0.0	0	0%
cooked (S&W)	3.5 oz	119	3.0	26.0	0	(mq)	0.0	0.0	0	0%
cooked (Uncle Ben's)	2/3 cup	130	3.0	27.0	0	(mq)	1.0	na	0	7%
dry	1 oz	105	2.3	21.9	2	1.0	0.8	0.2	0	7%
dry	1/2 cup	340	7.3	71.1	6	3.2	2.7	0.5	0	7%
dry (Arrowhead Mills)	2 oz	200	4.0	44.0	3	3.1	1.0	na	0	5%
quick-cooked (S&W)	3.5 oz	110	2.0	25.0	0	(mq)	0.0	0.0	0	0%
MEDIUM GRAIN										
cooked	4 oz	127	2.6	26.7	1	>.3 c	0.9	0.2	0	7%
cooked	1/2 cup	110	2.3	23.0	1	>.3 c	0.8	0.2	0	7%
dry	1/2 cup	344	7.1	72.4	4	>.9 c	2.5	0.5	0	7%
dry	1 oz	103	2.1	21.6	1	>.3 c	0.8	0.2	0	7%
dry (Arrowhead Mills)	2 oz	200	4.0	44.0	3	3.4	1.0	na	0	5%
SHORT GRAIN (Arrowhead Mills) dry	2 oz	200	4.0	44.0	3	3.4	1.0	na	0	5%
RICE, GLUTINOUS										
cooked	1/2 cup	116	2.4	25.3	6	1.2	0.2	0.1	0	2%
cooked	4 oz	110	2.3	23.9	6	1.1	0.2	<.1	0	2%
dry	1/2 cup	120	2.2	26.4	0	2.6	0.2	0.1	0	2%
dry	1 oz	105	1.9	23.2	2	.8	0.2	<.1	0	2%
RICE, WHITE										
LONG GRAIN										
cooked	1/2 cup	194	13.7	52.3	3	.3	5.6	1.0	0	16%
cooked	4 oz	111	2.3	24.1	3	.9	0.2	<.1	0	2%
cooked (Carolina)	1/2 cup	100	2.0	22.0	10	(mq)	0.0	0.0	0	0%
cooked (Finast)	1/2 cup	115	2.0	26.0	0	(mq)	0.0	0.0	0	0%
cooked (Mahatma)	1/2 cup	110	2.0	23.0	na	(mq)	0.0	0.0	0	0%
cooked (River)	1/2 cup	100	2.0	22.0	10	(mq)	0.0	0.0	0	0%
cooked (S&W)	3.5 oz	106	2.0	23.0	0	(mq)	0.0	0.0	0	0%
cooked (Uncle Ben's)	2/3 cup	130	3.0	28.0	0	(mq)	1.0	na	0	7%
cooked (Water Maid)	1/2 cup	100	2.0	22.0	10	(mq)	0.0	0.0	0	0%
raw, enriched	1/2 cup	336	6.6	73.6	5	1.2	0.6	0.2	0	2%
raw, unenriched	1 oz	103	2.0	22.7	1	.3	0.2	<.1	0	2%
In cooking bag										
(Minute)	1/2 cup	90	2.0	20.0	0	(mq)	0.0	0.0	0	0%
(Success) enriched, cooked	1/2 cup	100	2.0	21.0	0	(mq)	0.0	0.0	0	0%
(Uncle Ben's)	1/2 cup	90	2.0	20.0	10	(mq)	<1.0	na	0	<9%
Parboiled										
cooked	1/2 cup	100	2.0	21.8	3	.4	0.2	0.1	0	2%
cooked	4 oz	129	2.6	28.0	3	.6	3.1	0.1	0	19%
enriched, cooked	1/2 cup	100	2.0	21.8	3	.4	0.2	0.1	0	2%
unenriched, dry	1/2 cup	341	6.3	75.2	5	>.3 c	0.5	0.1	0	1%
(Uncle Ben's) 'Converted'	2/3 cup	120	2.0	28.0	0	(mq)	<1.0	na	0	<7%
Precooked or instant										
cooked (Carolina) 'Instant'	1/2 cup	110	2.0	23.0	na	(mq)	0.0	0.0	0	0%
cooked (Minute) 'Original'	2/3 cup	120	3.0	27.0	5	na	0.0	na	0	0%

Food Name	Serving Size	Calories	Prot. gms	Carbs gms	Sod. mgs	Fiber gms	Fat gms	Sat. Fat gms	Chol. mgs	% Fat Cal.
cooked *(Minute)* 'Premium'	2/3 cup	120	3.0	27.0	0	(mq)	0.0	0.0	0	0%
cooked *(Uncle Ben's)*	2/3 cup	120	3.0	27.0	10	(mq)	<1.0	na	0	<7%
dry	1/2 cup	182	3.7	40.1	3	>.2 c	0.1	0.0	0	1%
dry	1 oz	107	2.2	23.7	2	.5	0.1	<.1	0	1%
enriched, cooked	1/2 cup	80	1.7	17.4	2	>.1 c	0.1	0.0	0	1%
MEDIUM GRAIN										
cooked	1/2 cup	345	6.3	76.0	5	.3	0.5	0.1	0	1%
cooked	4 oz	147	2.7	32.4	tr	.1	0.2	0.1	0	1%
dry	1 oz	102	1.9	22.5	<1	.4	0.2	<.1	0	2%
enriched, dry	1/2 cup	353	6.5	77.8	1	1.4	0.6	0.2	0	2%
unenriched, cooked	1/2 cup	133	2.4	29.2	0	>.1 c	0.2	0.1	0	1%
unenriched, dry	1/2 cup	353	6.5	77.8	1	>.3 c	0.6	0.2	0	2%
SHORT GRAIN										
cooked	1/2 cup	333	6.1	73.6	1	>.3 c	0.5	0.1	0	1%
cooked	4 oz	147	2.7	32.6	tr	>.1 c	0.2	0.1	0	1%
dry	1/2 cup	130	2.4	28.6	0	2.8	0.2	0.1	0	1%
dry	1 oz	101	1.8	22.4	<1	2.2	0.1	<.1	0	1%
unenriched, cooked	1/2 cup	133	2.4	29.3	0	>.1 c	0.2	0.1	0	1%
unenriched, dry	1/2 cup	358	6.5	79.2	1	>.3 c	0.5	0.1	0	1%
RICE, WILD										
cooked	4 oz	115	4.5	24.2	3	2.1	0.4	0.1	0	3%
cooked	1/2 cup	83	3.3	17.5	2	1.5	0.3	0.0	0	3%
cooked *(Fantastic Foods)*	1/2 cup	83	3.0	18.0	0	(mq)	0.0	0.0	0	0%
dry	1/2 cup	286	11.8	59.9	6	5.0	0.9	0.1	0	3%
dry	1 oz	101	4.2	21.2	2	1.5	0.3	<.1	0	3%
RICE BEVERAGE										
almond 'Amazake' *(Grainaissance)*	8 oz	198	4.0	37.0	20	na	4.0	na	na	18%
apricot 'Amazake' *(Grainaissance)*	8 oz	158	3.0	36.0	20	na	0.0	0.0	na	0%
carob 'Lite' *(Rice Dream)*	8 oz	150	1.0	32.0	80	na	3.0	na	0	17%
chocolate flavored *(Rice Dream)*	8 oz	190	1.0	44.0	80	na	3.0	na	0	13%
cocoa-almond 'Amazake' *(Grainaissance)*	8 oz	198	4.0	36.0	20	na	4.0	na	na	18%
mocha java 'Amazake' *(Grainaissance)*	8 oz	178	3.0	37.0	20	na	2.0	na	na	10%
original flavor 'Amazake' *(Grainaissance)*	8 oz	148	2.0	34.0	20	na	0.0	0.0	na	0%
original flavor 'Horchata' *(Don José)*	8 oz	70	<1.0	6.0	95	na	4.0	na	0	56%
sesame 'Amazake' *(Grainaissance)*	8 oz	198	4.0	37.0	20	na	1.0	na	na	5%
strawberry 'Horchata' *(Don José)*	8 oz	70	<1.0	7.0	95	na	3.5	na	0	50%
vanilla 'Lite' *(Rice Dream)*	8 oz	120	1.0	28.0	80	na	2.0	na	0	13%
vanilla pecan 'Amazake' *(Grainaissance)*	8 oz	198	4.0	37.0	20	na	4.0	na	na	18%
RICE BRAN										
crude	1 oz	90	3.8	14.1	1	6.2	5.9	1.2	0	43%
crude	1/3 cup	88	3.7	13.9	1	5.9	5.8	1.2	0	43%
RICE BRAN OIL										
	1 cup	1927	0.0	0.0	0	0	218.0	42.9	0	100%
	1 oz	251	0.0	0.0	0	0	28.4	5.6	0	100%
	1 tbsp	120	0.0	0.0	0	0	13.6	2.7	0	100%
(Hain)	1 tbsp	120	0.0	0.0	0	0	14.0	3.0	0	100%
RICE CAKE										
(Lundberg Family) sodium-free, all flavors	1 cake	60	1.4	14.0	3	na	0.5	na	na	7%
(Lundberg Family) very low sodium, all flavors	1 cake	60	1.4	14.0	30	na	0.5	na	na	7%
APPLE CINNAMON										
(Hain) mini	1/2 cup	60	1.0	12.0	10	0	<1.0	(tr)	0	<15%
(Quaker)	1 cake	40	1.0	9.0	0	na	0.0	na	0	0%
(Quaker) mini	5 cakes	50	1.0	12.0	0	na	0.0	na	0	0%
BARBEQUE *(Hain)* mini	.5 oz	70	1.0	10.0	50	0	3.0	na	0	38%

Food Name	Serving Size	Calories	Prot. gms	Carbs gms	Sod. mgs	Fiber gms	Fat gms	Sat. Fat gms	Chol. mgs	% Fat Cal.
BROWN RICE										
buckwheat	1 cake	34	0.8	7.2	10	.3	0.3	0.1	0	8%
buckwheat, unsalted	1 cake	35	0.7	7.3	2	>.2 c	0.3	0.1	0	8%
corn	1 cake	35	0.8	7.3	26	.3	0.3	0.1	0	8%
multi-grain	1 cake	35	0.8	7.2	23	.3	0.3	0.1	0	8%
multi-grain, unsalted	1 cake	34	0.8	7.2	0	>.1 c	0.3	0.1	0	8%
plain	1 cake	35	0.7	7.3	29	.4	0.3	0.1	0	8%
rye	1 cake	35	0.7	7.2	10	.4	0.3	0.1	0	8%
sesame seed	1 cake	35	0.7	7.3	20	>.2 c	0.3	0.1	0	8%
sesame seed, unsalted	1 cake	35	0.8	7.2	0	>.2 c	0.3	0.1	0	8%
unsalted	1 cake	34	0.8	7.1	26	0	0.3	0.1	0	8%
CARAMEL CORN (Quaker) mini	5 cakes	50	1.0	12.0	35	na	0.0	na	0	0%
CAROB COATED										
(Carafection) 'Mint Rice Crisps'	1 oz	139	2.0	17.0	26	na	7.0	na	na	45%
(Carafection) 'Rice Crisps'	1 oz	139	2.0	17.0	26	na	7.0	na	na	45%
CHEESE (Hain) mini	5 cakes	60	1.0	10.0	80	0	2.0	na	0	29%
CINNAMON										
(Chico-San) sugar, mini	5 cakes	50	1.0	12.0	0	na	0.0	na	0	0%
(Quaker) crunch, fat-free	1 cake	50	1.0	11.0	25	na	0.0	0.0	0	0%
CORN (Quaker)	1 cake	35	0.7	7.4	53	.2	0.2	na	na	5%
DILL (Lundberg Family) creamy, mini	5 cakes	60	1.0	13.0	57	na	<1.0	na	2	<14%
FIVE-GRAIN (Hain)	1 cake	40	<1.0	8.0	10	(mq)	<1.0	(tr)	0	<20%
HONEY NUT										
(Chico-San) unglazed, mini	4 cakes	60	1.0	2.0	35	na	1.0	na	0	43%
(Hain) mini	.5 oz	60	1.0	11.0	30	0	<1.0	(tr)	0	<16%
MUGWORT (Grainaissance) bake & serve 'Mochi'	2 oz	140	3.0	29.0	2	na	1.3	na	na	8%
MULTI-GRAIN										
(Chico-San) very low sodium	1 cake	35	1.0	8.0	30	na	0.0	na	0	0%
(Pritikin) sodium-free	1 cake	35	1.0	7.0	0	na	0.0	na	0	0%
(Pritikin) very low sodium	1 cake	35	1.0	7.0	30	na	0.0	na	0	0%
(Quaker)	.32 oz	34	0.9	6.9	29	.4	0.4	0.1	0	10%
NACHO CHEESE										
(Hain) mini	.5 oz	70	1.0	10.0	90	0	2.0	na	5	29%
(Lundberg Family) mini	5 cakes	57	1.0	13.0	116	na	<1.0	na	<1	14%
PLAIN										
(Chico-San) original	1 cake	35	1.0	8.0	30	na	0.0	na	0	0%
(Grainaissance) organic bake & serve 'Mochi'	2 oz	140	3.0	29.0	2	na	1.3	na	na	8%
(Hain)	1 cake	40	<1.0	8.0	10	(mq)	<1.0	(tr)	0	<20%
(Hain) mini	.5 oz	60	1.0	12.0	20	0	<1.0	(tr)	0	<15%
(Hain) mini, unsalted	.5 oz	60	1.0	12.0	5	0	<1.0	(tr)	0	<15%
(Hain) unsalted	1 cake	40	<1.0	8.0	5	(mq)	<1.0	(tr)	0	<20%
(Konriko) 'Original Unsalted'	1 cake	30	0.0	7.0	<1	(mq)	0.0	0.0	0	0%
(Pritikin) sodium-free	1 cake	35	1.0	7.0	0	na	0.0	na	0	0%
(Pritikin) very low sodium	1 cake	35	1.0	7.0	35	na	0.0	na	0	0%
(Quaker)	.32 oz	35	0.8	7.1	36	.3	0.3	0.1	0	8%
(Quaker) lightly salted	1 cake	35	1.0	7.0	35	na	0.0	na	0	0%
(Quaker) unsalted	.32 oz	35	0.8	7.2	0	.3	0.3	0.1	0	8%
RAISIN-CINNAMON (Grainaissance) bake & serve 'Mochi'	2 oz	143	2.9	30.0	77	na	1.2	na	na	8%
RANCH										
(Hain) mini	.5 oz	70	1.0	9.0	90	(mq)	3.0	na	0	40%
(Quaker)	1 cake	35	1.4	6.5	52	.8	0.3	0.0	0	8%
SESAME										
(Chico-San) original	1 cake	35	1.0	8.0	0	na	0.0	na	0	0%
(Hain)	1 cake	40	<1.0	8.0	10	(mq)	<1.0	(tr)	0	<20%

Food Name	Serving Size	Calories	Prot. gms	Carbs gms	Sod. mgs	Fiber gms	Fat gms	Sat. Fat gms	Chol. mgs	% Fat Cal.
(Hain) unsalted	1 cake	40	<1.0	8.0	5	(mq)	<1.0	(tr)	0	<20%
(Pritikin) sodium-free	1 cake	35	1.0	7.0	0	na	0.0	na	0	0%
(Pritikin) very low sodium	1 cake	35	1.0	7.0	35	na	0.0	na	0	0%
(Quaker)	.32 oz	35	0.8	7.1	36	.3	0.3	0.1	0	8%
(Westbrae) 'Double Sesame'	.28 oz	30	<1.0	6.0	65	na	<1.0	na	0	<24%
SESAME-GARLIC										
(Grainaissance) bake & serve 'Mochi'	2 oz	143	3.2	28.0	25	na	1.9	na	na	12%
(Westbrae)	.28 oz	30	<1.0	6.0	55	na	<1.0	na	0	<24%
TERIYAKI										
(Hain) mini	.5 oz	50	1.0	12.0	75	0	<1.0	(tr)	0	<15%
(Westbrae)	.28 oz	30	<1.0	6.0	45	na	<1.0	na	0	<24%
WHEAT *(Quaker)*	1 cake	34	1.4	6.7	52	.8	0.3	0.1	0	8%
RICE DISH										
CANNED										
Fried *(LaChoy)*	4.903 oz	236	5.1	53.4	1024	1.9	1.1	0.2	0	4%
Spanish										
(Featherweight)	7.5 oz	140	4.0	30.0	32	(mq)	0.0	0.0	0	0%
(Heinz)	7.25 oz	150	3.0	26.0	1045	(mq)	5.0	(mq)	na	28%
(Old El Paso)	1/2 cup	70	1.0	15.0	400	1.0	1.0	0.0	0	12%
(Van Camp's)	1 cup	160	3.1	27.0	1270	(mq)	4.0	(mq)	na	23%
DRIED, w/chicken, freeze-dried *(Mountain House)*	1 cup	400	13.0	41.0	241	(mq)	13.0	(mq)	(mq)	35%
FROZEN										
Country style *(Birds Eye)* 'International Rice Recipes'	3.3 oz	90	2.0	19.0	380	1.0	0.0	0.0	0	0%
Florentine *(Green Giant)* 'Rice Originals'	1/2 cup	140	4.0	22.0	400	na	4.0	2.0	10	26%
French style *(Birds Eye)* 'International Rice Recipes'	3.3 oz	110	3.0	23.0	610	(mq)	0.0	0.0	0	0%
Fried										
w/chicken *(Chun King)*	8 oz	260	14.0	41.0	1460	(mq)	4.0	(mq)	(mq)	14%
w/pork *(Chun King)*	8 oz	270	10.0	44.0	1210	(mq)	6.0	(mq)	(mq)	20%
Medley *(Green Giant)* 'Rice Originals'	1/2 cup	100	3.0	19.0	310	(mq)	1.0	<1.0	5	9%
Mexican style, w/chicken *(Lean Cuisine)* 'Lunch Express'	9 1/8 oz	270	12.0	43.0	580	na	5.0	1.0	20	17%
Oriental, w/vegetables *(Budget Gourmet)* 'Side Dish'	5.75 oz	210	4.0	27.0	310	(mq)	10.0	(mq)	20	42%
Pilaf										
'Rice Originals' *(Green Giant)*	1/2 cup	110	2.0	21.0	530	(mq)	1.0	<1.0	2	9%
w/green beans *(Budget Gourmet)* 'Side Dish'	5.5 oz	240	4.0	35.0	350	(mq)	9.0	(mq)	10	34%
Spanish style *(Birds Eye)* 'International Rice Recipes'	3.3 oz	110	3.0	24.0	540	(mq)	0.0	0.0	0	0%
White and wild *(Green Giant)* 'Rice Originals'	1/2 cup	130	3.0	24.0	540	(mq)	2.0	<1.0	0	14%
Wild, w/sherry *(Green Giant)* 'Microwave Garden Gourmet'	1 pkg	210	6.0	40.0	580	3.0	4.0	2.0	10	16%
W/broccoli										
au gratin *(Birds Eye)* 'For One'	5.75 oz	180	6.0	27.0	430	1.0	6.0	(mq)	5	29%
in cheese flavored sauce *(Green Giant)*	1/2 cup	120	3.0	18.0	510	>.2 c	4.0	(mq)	na	30%
in cheese sauce *(Green Giant)* 'One Serving'	5.5 oz	180	5.0	25.0	550	(mq)	6.0	2.0	5	31%
'Rice Originals' *(Green Giant)*	1/2 cup	120	3.0	18.0	510	na	4.0	1.0	5	30%
W/peas and mushrooms in sauce, *(Green Giant)* 'One Serving'	5.5 oz	130	4.0	27.0	410	(mq)	2.0	<1.0	5	13%
W/spinach in cheese sauce *(Green Giant)* 'Italian Blend'	1/2 cup	140	4.0	22.0	400	(mq)	4.0	2.0	10	26%
RICE DISH MIX										
(Arrowhead Mills)	2 oz	200	4.0	43.0	0	na	1.0	na	na	5%
ALFREDO *(Country Inn)* prepared	1/2 cup	140	4.0	23.0	570	(mq)	4.0	(mq)	na	25%
AMANDINE *(Hain)* '3-Grain Goodness' prepared	1/2 cup	130	3.0	17.0	260	(mq)	5.0	(mq)	0	36%
BEEF BROCCOLI										
(Rice-A-Roni) 'Rice & Sauce'	1/4 pkg	120	3.0	24.0	530	na	0.0	na	na	0%
(Rice-A-Roni) 'Rice & Sauce' prepared	1/2 cup	140	3.0	24.0	550	na	3.0	na	na	20%
BEEF FLAVOR										
(Finast) dry mix	1.3 oz	130	4.0	26.0	780	(mq)	1.0	na	na	7%

Food Name	Serving Size	Calories	Prot. gms	Carbs gms	Sod. mgs	Fiber gms	Fat gms	Sat. Fat gms	Chol. mgs	% Fat Cal.
(Lipton) 'Rice and Sauce' dry mix	1/2 pkg	120	3.0	26.0	570	(mq)	<1.0	na	na	<7%
(Lipton) 'Rice and Sauce' prepared w/1 tbsp butter	1/2 cup	150	3.0	26.0	600	(mq)	3.0	(mq)	(mq)	19%
(Mahatma) prepared	1/2 cup	100	2.0	20.0	340	(mq)	0.0	0.0	0	0%
(Minute) microwave, family size, dry mix	1 pkg	140	4.0	28.0	530	na	0.0	na	0	0%
(Minute) microwave, family size, prepared w/salted butter	1/2 cup	160	4.0	28.0	560	na	3.0	na	10	17%
(Minute) microwave, single size, dry mix	1 pkg	140	4.0	28.0	530	na	0.0	na	0	0%
(Minute) microwave, single size, prepared w/salted butter	1/2 cup	150	4.0	28.0	550	na	2.0	na	5	12%
(Rice-A-Roni) dry mix	1.13 oz	110	3.0	24.0	560	(mq)	1.0	na	na	8%
(Rice-A-Roni) prepared	1/2 cup	140	4.0	24.0	610	(mq)	4.0	(mq)	na	24%
(Success) prepared	1/2 cup	100	2.0	19.0	370	(mq)	0.0	0.0	0	0%
W/mushrooms										
(Rice-A-Roni) dry mix	1.27 oz	120	4.0	26.0	710	(mq)	<1.0	na	na	<7%
(Rice-A-Roni) prepared	1/2 cup	150	4.0	26.0	740	(mq)	3.0	(mq)	na	18%
W/vermicelli (Make-It-Easy) dry mix	1.3 oz	130	3.0	28.0	(mq)	(mq)	1.0	na	0	7%
BROWN AND WILD										
(Success) prepared	1/2 cup	120	3.0	23.0	500	(mq)	0.0	0.0	0	0%
(Uncle Ben's) prepared	1/2 cup	130	4.0	27.0	500	(mq)	1.0	na	0	7%
Herb (Arrowhead Mills) 'Quick'	2 oz	140	4.0	28.0	128	4.0	1.0	na	0	7%
Spanish style (Arrowhead Mills) 'Quick'	2 oz	150	4.0	30.0	145	2.8	1.0	na	0	6%
Vegetable herb (Arrowhead Mills) 'Quick'	2 oz	150	4.0	30.0	85	4.0	1.0	na	0	6%
W/mushrooms (Uncle Ben's) prepared	1/2 cup	130	4.0	27.0	500	(mq)	1.0	na	na	7%
CAJUN										
(Lipton) 'Rice and Sauce' dry mix	1/4 pkg	120	4.0	26.0	600	(mq)	<1.0	na	0	<7%
(Lipton 'Rice and Sauce' prepared w/1 tbsp butter	1/2 cup	150	4.0	26.0	630	(mq)	3.0	(mq)	(mq)	18%
CHICKEN FLAVOR										
(Finast) dry mix	1.6 oz	160	4.0	31.0	950	(mq)	2.0	(mq)	na	11%
(Lipton) 'Rice and Sauce' dry mix	1/4 pkg	130	3.0	25.0	440	(mq)	1.0	na	na	7%
(Lipton) 'Rice and Sauce' prepared w/1 tbsp butter	1/2 cup	150	3.0	25.0	470	(mq)	4.0	(mq)	(mq)	24%
(Mahatma) prepared	1/2 cup	100	2.0	20.0	620	(mq)	0.0	0.0	0	0%
(Minute) microwave, family size, dry mix	1 pkg	130	3.0	27.0	640	na	1.0	na	0	7%
(Minute) microwave, family size prepared w/salted butter	1/2 cup	160	3.0	27.0	670	na	4.0	na	10	23%
(Minute) microwave, single size, dry mix	1 pkg	130	3.0	27.0	640	na	1.0	na	0	7%
(Minute) microwave, single size, prepared w/salted butter	1/2 cup	150	3.0	27.0	660	na	3.0	na	5	18%
(Rice-A-Roni) dry mix	1.13 oz	110	3.0	24.0	520	(mq)	1.0	na	na	8%
(Rice-A-Roni) prepared	1/2 cup	150	3.0	24.0	560	(mq)	4.0	(mq)	na	25%
(Success) prepared	1/2 cup	110	3.0	18.0	420	(mq)	2.0	(mq)	na	18%
Florentine										
(Rice-A-Roni) 'Savory Classics' dry mix	1.12 oz	108	3.7	21.7	874	1.2	0.8	0.1	1	7%
(Rice-A-Roni) 'Savory Classics' prepared	1/2 cup	130	4.0	22.0	910	(mq)	4.0	(mq)	(mq)	26%
Honey-lemon, w/broccoli (Suzi Wan) prepared	7.5 oz	370	23.0	45.0	640	(mq)	11.0	(mq)	na	27%
W/broccoli										
(Rice-A-Roni) dry mix	1.23 oz	120	3.0	25.0	670	(mq)	1.0	na	na	7%
(Rice-A-Roni) prepared	1/2 cup	150	3.0	25.0	710	(mq)	3.0	(mq)	na	19%
(Suzi Wan) prepared	1/2 cup	120	4.0	23.0	500	(mq)	1.0	na	na	8%
W/creamy mushroom (Country Inn) prepared	1/2 cup	140	3.0	25.0	510	(mq)	3.0	(mq)	na	19%
W/homestyle vegetables (Country Inn) prepared	1/2 cup	140	4.0	25.0	490	(mq)	3.0	(mq)	na	19%
W/mushroom										
(Country Inn) 'Mushroom Royale' prepared	1/2 cup	120	4.0	25.0	560	(mq)	1.0	na	na	7%
(Rice-A-Roni) dry mix	1.17 oz	130	4.0	26.0	790	(mq)	1.0	na	na	7%
(Rice-A-Roni) prepared	1/2 cup	180	4.0	26.0	840	(mq)	7.0	(mq)	na	34%
W/mushroom stock (Country Inn) prepared	1/2 cup	130	4.0	25.0	560	(mq)	1.0	na	na	7%
W/vegetables										
(Rice-A-Roni) dry mix	1.2 oz	120	3.0	25.0	760	(mq)	<1.0	na	na	<7%
(Rice-A-Roni) prepared	1/2 cup	140	3.0	25.0	790	(mq)	3.0	(mq)	na	19%

Food Name	Serving Size	Calories	Prot. gms	Carbs gms	Sod. mgs	Fiber gms	Fat gms	Sat. Fat gms	Chol. mgs	% Fat Cal.
(Suzi Wan) prepared	1/2 cup	120	3.0	24.0	550	(mq)	1.0	na	na	8%
W/vegetables and vermicelli *(Make-It-Easy)* dry mix	1.3 oz	130	3.0	28.0	(mq)	(mq)	1.0	na	na	7%
DRUMSTICK										
(Minute) dry mix	1 pkg	120	3.0	25.0	650	na	0.0	na	0	0%
(Minute) prepared w/salted butter	1/2 cup	150	3.0	25.0	690	na	4.0	na	10	24%
FLORENTINE *(Country Inn)* prepared	1/2 cup	140	4.0	24.0	380	(mq)	3.0	na	na	19%
FRIED										
(Minute) dry mix	1 pkg	120	3.0	25.0	550	na	0.0	na	0	0%
(Minute) prepared w/oil, w/o salt or butter	1/2 cup	160	3.0	25.0	550	na	5.0	na	0	29%
(Rice-A-Roni) dry mix	1 oz	110	3.0	21.0	670	(mq)	1.0	na	na	9%
(Rice-A-Roni) prepared	1/2 cup	110	3.0	21.0	700	(mq)	5.0	(mq)	na	32%
W/almonds										
(Rice-A-Roni) '1/2 less salt' dry mix	1/5 pkg	120	3.0	26.0	460	na	1.0	na	0	7%
(Rice-A-Roni) '1/2 less salt' prepared	1/2 cup	130	3.0	26.0	470	na	2.0	na	0	13%
JASMINE, soft *(A Taste of Thai)*	1/4 cup	160	3.0	36.0	0	0	0.0	0.0	0	0%
HERB										
And butter										
(Lipton) 'Rice and Sauce' prepared w/1 tbsp butter	1/2 cup	150	3.0	24.0	470	(mq)	5.0	(mq)	(mq)	29%
(Rice-A-Roni) dry mix	1 oz	110	2.0	22.0	760	(mq)	1.0	na	na	9%
(Rice-A-Roni) prepared	1/2 cup	130	2.0	22.0	790	(mq)	4.0	(mq)	na	27%
Au gratin										
(Country Inn) prepared	1/2 cup	140	4.0	25.0	450	(mq)	3.0	(mq)	na	19%
(Success) prepared	1/2 cup	100	2.0	20.0	260	(mq)	0.0	0.0	0	0%
Wild rice and herbs *(Arrowhead Mills)*	1/4 pkg	140	4.0	28.0	220	3.0	1.0	na	na	7%
LONG GRAIN AND WILD										
(Lipton) 'Rice and Sauce Original' dry mix	1/4 pkg	120	4.0	26.0	530	(mq)	<1.0	na	na	<7%
(Lipton) 'Rice and Sauce Original' prepared w/1 tbsp butter	1/2 cup	150	4.0	26.0	560	(mq)	3.0	(mq)	(mq)	18%
(Mahatma) prepared	1/2 cup	100	2.0	20.0	480	(mq)	0.0	0.0	0	0%
(Minute) dry mix	1 pkg	120	3.0	25.0	530	na	0.0	na	0	0%
(Minute) prepared w/salted butter	1/2 cup	150	3.0	25.0	570	na	4.0	na	10	24%
(Minute) prepared w/o salt or butter	2/3 cup	120	3.0	27.0	0	na	0.0	na	0	0%
(Near East) prepared	1/2 cup	130	3.0	21.0	430	(mq)	4.0	(mq)	na	27%
(Rice-A-Roni) 'Original' dry mix	1.1 oz	110	3.0	23.0	620	(mq)	0.0	0.0	na	0%
(Rice-A-Roni) 'Original' prepared	1/2 cup	130	3.0	23.0	660	(mq)	3.0	(mq)	na	21%
(Uncle Ben's) 'Fast Cooking' prepared	1/2 cup	100	3.0	21.0	410	(mq)	<1.0	na	0	<9%
(Uncle Ben's) 'Fast Cooking' prepared w/salt and butter	1/2 cup	130	3.0	21.0	450	(mq)	4.0	(mq)	(mq)	27%
(Uncle Ben's) 'Original' prepared w/salt and butter	1/2 cup	120	3.0	22.0	520	(mq)	2.0	(mq)	(mq)	15%
(Uncle Ben's) 'Original' prepared w/o salt or butter	1/2 cup	100	3.0	22.0	500	(mq)	<1.0	na	0	<8%
Mexican *(Old El Paso)* prepared	1/2 cup	140	2.0	28.0	370	(mq)	2.0	(mq)	0	13%
Pilaf										
(Rice-A-Roni) dry mix	1 oz	100	2.0	23.0	510	(mq)	0.0	0.0	na	0%
(Rice-A-Roni) prepared	1/2 cup	130	3.0	23.0	550	(mq)	3.0	(mq)	na	21%
W/chicken and almonds										
(Rice-A-Roni) dry mix	1.2 oz	120	3.0	23.0	660	(mq)	1.0	na	na	8%
(Rice-A-Roni) prepared	1/2 cup	140	3.0	24.0	690	(mq)	4.0	(mq)	na	25%
W/chicken sauce										
(Uncle Ben's) prepared w/salt and butter	1/2 cup	160	4.0	27.0	680	(mq)	5.0	(mq)	(mq)	27%
(Uncle Ben's) prepared w/o salt or butter	1/2 cup	140	4.0	27.0	650	(mq)	2.0	(mq)	0	13%
ORIENTAL										
(Hain) '3-Grain Goodness' prepared	1/2 cup	120	4.0	15.0	300	(mq)	5.0	(mq)	na	37%
(Lipton) dry mix	1/4 pkg	120	4.0	26.0	330	(mq)	<1.0	na	na	<7%
(Lipton) prepared w/1 tbsp butter	1/2 cup	150	4.0	26.0	360	(mq)	3.0	(mq)	(mq)	18%

Food Name	Serving Size	Calories	Prot. gms	Carbs gms	Sod. mgs	Fiber gms	Fat gms	Sat. Fat gms	Chol. mgs	% Fat Cal.
PILAF										
(Casbah) dry mix	1 oz	90	2.0	20.0	(mq)	(mq)	0.0	0.0	0	0%
(Casbah) prepared	1/2 cup	90	2.0	20.0	(mq)	(mq)	0.0	0.0	0	0%
(Lipton) 'Rice and Sauce'	1/4 pkg	120	3.0	25.0	400	(mq)	<1.0	na	na	<7%
(Lipton) 'Rice and Sauce' prepared w/1 tbsp margarine	1/2 cup	140	3.0	25.0	440	(mq)	3.0	(mq)	na	19%
(Lipton) 'Rice and Sauce' prepared w/2 tbsp butter	1/2 cup	170	3.0	25.0	470	(mq)	6.0	(mq)	(mq)	33%
(Near East) prepared	1/2 cup	140	3.0	21.0	450	(mq)	5.0	(mq)	na	32%
(Rice-A-Roni) dry mix	1.2 oz	120	4.0	25.0	570	(mq)	0.0	0.0	0	0%
(Rice-A-Roni) prepared	1/2 cup	150	4.0	25.0	550	(mq)	4.0	(mq)	na	24%
(Success) prepared	1/2 cup	120	2.0	24.0	410	(mq)	0.0	0.0	0	0%
Beef flavored (Near East) prepared	1/2 cup	140	3.0	21.0	470	(mq)	5.0	(mq)	na	32%
Brown rice										
(Quick Pilaf) Spanish, prepared w/o salt or butter	1/2 cup	98	2.0	21.0	314	(mq)	0.7	na	na	6%
(Quick Pilaf) Spanish, prepared w/2 tbsp salted butter	1/2 cup	136	2.0	21.0	369	(mq)	5.0	(mq)	(mq)	33%
(Quick Pilaf) w/miso, prepared w/o salt or butter	1/2 cup	105	3.0	21.0	240	(mq)	1.0	na	na	9%
(Quick Pilaf) w/miso, prepared w/2 tbsp salted butter	1/2 cup	145	3.0	21.0	295	(mq)	5.5	(mq)	(mq)	34%
Chicken flavored (Near East) prepared	1/2 cup	140	3.0	21.0	420	(mq)	5.0	(mq)	na	32%
French										
(Minute) microwave, family size, dry mix	1 pkg	110	2.0	24.0	390	na	0.0	na	0	0%
(Minute) microwave, family size, prepared w/salted butter	1/2 cup	130	2.0	24.0	420	na	3.0	na	10	21%
(Minute) microwave, single size, dry mix	1 pkg	110	2.0	24.0	390	na	0.0	na	0	0%
(Minute) microwave, single size, prepared w/salted butter	1/2 cup	120	2.0	24.0	410	na	2.0	na	5	15%
Garden										
(Rice-A-Roni) 'Savory Classics' dry mix	1.12 oz	113	3.6	22.9	964	1.1	0.8	0.2	1	6%
(Rice-A-Roni) 'Savory Classics' prepared	1/2 cup	140	4.0	23.0	1000	(mq)	4.0	(mq)	(mq)	25%
Lentil (Near East) prepared	1/2 cup	170	6.0	21.0	430	(mq)	7.0	(mq)	na	37%
Nutted										
(Casbah) dry mix	1 oz	160	4.0	30.0	(mq)	(mq)	2.0	(mq)	0	12%
(Casbah) prepared	1/2 cup	160	4.0	30.0	(mq)	(mq)	2.0	(mq)	0	12%
Spanish										
(Casbah) dry mix	1 oz	90	2.0	20.0	(mq)	(mq)	0.0	0.0	0	0%
(Casbah) prepared	1/2 cup	90	2.0	20.0	(mq)	(mq)	0.0	0.0	0	0%
(Country Inn) w/vegetables, prepared	1/2 cup	120	3.0	25.0	280	(mq)	1.0	na	na	7%
Wheat (Near East) Spanish, prepared	1/2 cup	150	3.0	21.0	380	(mq)	6.0	(mq)	na	36%
RIB ROAST										
(Minute) dry mix	1 pkg	120	3.0	25.0	680	na	0.0	na	0	0%
(Minute) prepared w/salted butter	1/2 cup	150	3.0	25.0	720	na	4.0	na	10	24%
RISOTTO										
(Rice-A-Roni) dry mix	1.5 oz	160	4.0	32.0	1070	(mq)	1.0	na	na	6%
(Rice-A-Roni) prepared	1/2 cup	200	4.0	32.0	1130	(mq)	6.0	(mq)	na	27%
Chicken and cheese (Country Inn) prepared	1/2 cup	120	3.0	23.0	410	(mq)	2.0	(mq)	na	15%
SPANISH STYLE										
(Arrowhead Mills) quick, dry mix	1/4 pkg	150	4.0	30.0	255	2.0	1.0	na	na	6%
(Lipton) 'Rice and Sauce' dry mix	1/4 pkg	120	3.0	26.0	540	(mq)	<1.0	na	na	<7%
(Lipton) 'Rice and Sauce' prepared w/1 tbsp butter	1/2 cup	140	3.0	26.0	570	(mq)	3.0	(mq)	(mq)	19%
(Mahatma) prepared	1/2 cup	100	2.0	20.0	190	(mq)	0.0	0.0	0	0%
(Near East) prepared	1/2 cup	170	3.0	24.0	540	(mq)	7.0	(mq)	na	37%
(Rice-A-Roni) dry mix	.97 oz	110	3.0	22.0	950	(mq)	1.0	na	na	8%
(Rice-A-Roni) prepared	1/2 cup	150	4.0	25.0	1090	(mq)	4.0	(mq)	na	24%
STROGANOFF										
(Rice-A-Roni) dry mix	1.35 oz	150	4.0	27.0	770	(mq)	3.0	(mq)	na	18%
(Rice-A-Roni) prepared	1/2 cup	200	4.0	27.0	810	(mq)	8.0	(mq)	na	37%
SWEET AND SOUR										
(Suzi Wan) 'Dinner Recipe' prepared	7.5 oz	220	4.0	48.0	240	(mq)	1.0	na	na	4%

Food Name	Serving Size	Calories	Prot. gms	Carbs gms	Sod. mgs	Fiber gms	Fat gms	Sat. Fat gms	Chol. mgs	% Fat Cal.
(Suzi Wan) 'Dinner Recipe' prepared w/o butter	1/2 cup	130	3.0	28.0	460	(mq)	1.0	na	na	7%
(Suzi Wan) 'Dinner Recipe' prepared w/o butter or salt ...	7.5 oz	340	24.0	49.0	290	(mq)	5.0	(mq)	(mq)	13%
TERIYAKI										
(Suzi Wan) 'Dinner Recipe' prepared	7.5 oz	180	5.0	39.0	910	(mq)	1.0	na	na	5%
(Suzi Wan) 'Dinner Recipe' prepared w/o butter	1/2 cup	120	3.0	25.0	690	(mq)	1.0	na	na	7%
(Suzi Wan) 'Dinner Recipe' prepared w/o butter or salt ...	7.5 oz	360	22.0	39.0	970	(mq)	12.0	(mq)	(mq)	31%
THREE-FLAVOR *(Suzi Wan)* prepared	1/2 cup	120	4.0	24.0	570	(mq)	1.0	na	na	7%
W/ASPARAGUS										
Au gratin *(Country Inn)* prepared	1/2 cup	130	4.0	22.0	310	(mq)	3.0	(mq)	na	21%
W/hollandaise sauce										
(Lipton) w/hollandaise sauce 'Rice & Sauce' dry mix	1/4 pkg	120	4.0	25.0	460	(mq)	1.0	na	na	7%
(Lipton) w/hollandaise sauce 'Rice and Sauce' prepared										
w/butter	1/2 cup	170	4.0	25.0	530	(mq)	7.0	(mq)	(mq)	35%
(Lipton) w/hollandaise sauce 'Rice and Sauce' prepared										
w/margarine	1/2 cup	150	4.0	25.0	500	(mq)	4.0	(mq)	(mq)	24%
W/BROCCOLI										
Amandine *(Country Inn)* prepared	1/2 cup	130	4.0	23.0	600	(mq)	2.0	(mq)	na	14%
Au gratin										
(Country Inn) prepared	1/2 cup	130	4.0	22.0	300	(mq)	3.0	(mq)	na	21%
(Rice-A-Roni) 'Savory Classics' dry mix	1.12 oz	129	3.6	20.9	372	1.1	3.4	1.1	4	24%
(Rice-A-Roni) 'Savory Classics' prepared	1/2 cup	180	4.0	21.0	440	(mq)	9.0	(mq)	(mq)	45%
Stir-fry										
(Suzi Wan) prepared w/salt and butter	7.5 oz	370	22.0	37.0	800	(mq)	15.0	(mq)	na	36%
(Suzi Wan) prepared w/o salt or butter	7.5 oz	200	5.0	37.0	750	(mq)	3.0	(mq)	na	14%
W/cheddar cheese										
(Minute) microwave, dry mix	1 pkg	140	4.0	26.0	500	na	2.0	na	5	13%
(Minute) microwave, prepared w/salted butter	1/2 cup	160	4.0	26.0	530	na	5.0	na	10	27%
W/CAULIFLOWER, AU GRATIN										
(Country Inn) prepared	1/2 cup	130	4.0	23.0	570	(mq)	3.0	(mq)	na	20%
(Rice-A-Roni) 'Savory Classics' dry mix	.5 oz	141	4.4	22.7	372	1.1	3.6	1.1	5	23%
(Rice-A-Roni) 'Savory Classics' prepared	1/2 cup	170	4.0	23.0	410	(mq)	7.0	(mq)	(mq)	37%
W/CHEESE										
Cheddar										
(Rice-A-Roni) white, w/herbs, prepared	1 cup	130	7.0	52.0	940	1.0	5.0	2.0	10	16%
(Rice-A-Roni) zesty 'Savory Classics' dry mix	1.3 oz	151	4.6	24.7	541	.9	3.8	1.3	6	23%
(Rice-A-Roni) zesty 'Savory Classics' prepared	1/2 cup	180	5.0	25.0	580	(mq)	7.0	(mq)	(mq)	34%
Parmesan										
(Rice-A-Roni) creamy, w/herbs 'Savory Classics' dry mix ..	1.22 oz	145	4.8	22.0	432	.8	4.2	1.4	7	26%
(Rice-A-Roni) creamy, w/herbs 'Savory Classics' prepared	1/2 cup	170	5.0	22.0	470	(mq)	7.0	(mq)	(mq)	37%
(Ultra Slim Fast) w/chicken flavored sauce, prepared	8 oz	240	5.0	56.0	1080	4.0	1.0	na	na	4%
W/GREEN BEANS, AMANDINE										
(Country Inn) casserole, prepared	1/2 cup	120	3.0	23.0	370	(mq)	2.0	na	na	15%
(Rice-A-Roni) 'Savory Classics' dry mix	1.25 oz	152	4.8	22.3	416	1.0	4.8	1.4	6	29%
(Rice-A-Roni) 'Savory Classics' prepared	1/2 cup	210	5.0	22.0	490	(mq)	11.0	(mq)	(mq)	48%
W/MUSHROOMS										
(Country Inn) creamy, w/wild rice, prepared	1/2 cup	140	3.0	24.0	310	(mq)	3.0	(mq)	na	20%
(Lipton) 'Rice and Sauce' dry mix	1/4 pkg	120	3.0	26.0	550	(mq)	<1.0	na	na	<7%
(Lipton) 'Rice and Sauce' prepared w/1 tbsp butter	1/2 cup	150	3.0	26.0	580	(mq)	3.0	(mq)	(mq)	19%
W/ORIENTAL STYLE SAUCE *(Ultra Slim Fast)* prepared	8 oz	240	5.0	58.0	900	4.0	1.0	na	na	3%
W/VEGETABLES										
And cheddar										
(Lipton) dry mix	1/4 pkg	130	3.0	26.0	420	(mq)	2.0	(mq)	na	13%
(Lipton) prepared w/1 tbsp margarine	1/2 cup	160	3.0	26.0	450	(mq)	5.0	(mq)	na	28%
(Lipton) prepared w/2 tbsp butter	1/2 cup	180	3.0	26.0	490	(mq)	7.0	(mq)	(mq)	35%

Food Name	Serving Size	Calories	Prot. gms	Carbs gms	Sod. mgs	Fiber gms	Fat gms	Sat. Fat gms	Chol. mgs	% Fat Cal.
Medley (Country Inn) prepared	1/2 cup	140	4.0	28.0	390	(mq)	1.0	na	na	7%
Spring vegetable and cheese										
(Arrowhead Mills) vegetable herb, dry mix	1/4 pkg	150	4.0	30.0	150	3.0	1.0	na	na	6%
(Rice-A-Roni) 'Savory Classics' dry mix	1.22 oz	141	4.4	22.8	388	1.2	3.5	1.2	6	23%
(Rice-A-Roni) 'Savory Classics' prepared	1/2 cup	170	4.0	23.0	420	(mq)	7.0	(mq)	(mq)	37%
YELLOW										
(Mahatma) prepared	1/2 cup	100	2.0	21.0	480	(mq)	0.0	0.0	0	0%
(Rice-A-Roni) dry mix	1.16 oz	110	2.0	25.0	730	(mq)	0.0	0.0	0	0%
(Rice-A-Roni) prepared	1/2 cup	140	2.0	25.0	780	(mq)	4.0	(mq)	na	25%
(Success) prepared	1/2 cup	100	2.0	21.0	480	(mq)	0.0	0.0	0	0%
RICE FLOUR										
brown	1/2 cup	287	5.7	60.4	6	3.6	2.2	0.4	0	7%
brown	1 oz	103	2.0	21.7	2	1.3	0.8	0.2	0	7%
brown (Arrowhead Mills)	2 oz	200	4.0	44.0	3	3.1	1.0	na	0	5%
brown (Featherweight)	1 cup	500	11.0	113.0	7	(mq)	1.0	na	0	2%
white	1/2 cup	289	4.7	63.3	0	1.9	1.1	0.3	0	4%
white	1 oz	104	1.7	22.7	tr	.7	0.4	0.1	0	4%
RICE SEASONING (Lawry's) Mexican 'Seasoning Blends'	1 pkg	94	3.9	17.0	3246	>2.1 c	2.0	(mq)	na	18%
RICE SYRUP (Lundberg Family) organic 'Sweet Dreams'	1 tbsp	42	<1.0	10.0	2	na	<1.0	na	na	<17%
RIGATONI. See PASTA.										
RIGATONI ENTRÉE										
(Budget Gourmet) w/broccoli and chicken, in cream sauce,										
frozen	10.8 oz	290	19.0	44.0	710	na	7.0	3.0	30	20%
(Chef Boyardee) microwave	7.5 oz	210	8.0	31.0	1080	na	6.0	na	17	26%
(Chef Boyardee) 'Special Recipe,' canned	7.5 oz	210	9.0	33.0	1040	4.0	6.0	2.0	20	24%
(Healthy Choice) w/chicken 'Classics' frozen	12.5 oz	360	31.0	50.0	430	na	4.0	2.0	60	10%
(Healthy Choice) w/meat sauce, frozen	9.5 oz	260	16.0	34.0	540	na	6.0	2.0	30	21%
(Lean Cuisine) baked w/meat sauce and cheese, frozen	9.75 oz	250	18.0	27.0	430	na	8.0	3.0	25	29%
(Stouffer's) w/meat sauce, homestyle, frozen	12 oz	400	21.0	49.0	860	na	13.0	na	na	30%
ROAST BEEF ENTRÉE										
(Libby's) canned, w/gravy	6 oz	210	27.3	6.5	1030	na	8.0	na	na	35%
(Top Shelf) frozen, tender	10 oz	240	28.0	19.0	880	na	6.0	2.0	60	22%
ROAST BEEF HASH										
(Armour) canned	7.5 oz	350	19.0	20.0	1310	na	21.0	na	na	55%
(Mary Kitchen) canned	7.5 oz	350	20.0	18.0	1142	(mq)	22.0	(mq)	(mq)	57%
(Stouffer's) frozen	10 oz	380	30.0	16.0	1340	(mq)	22.0	(mq)	(mq)	52%
ROAST BEEF LUNCHEON MEAT. See LUNCHEON MEAT.										
ROAST BEEF SPREAD, CANNED										
(Hormel)	.5 oz	31	2.0	0.0	(mq)	0	2.0	(mq)	(mq)	69%
(Underwood)	2 1/8 oz	140	9.0	<1.0	360	na	11.0	5.0	45	71%
(Underwood) 'Light'	2 1/8 oz	90	9.0	2.0	210	na	6.0	2.0	30	55%
(Underwood) mesquite-smoked	2 1/8 oz	126	9.0	<1.0	300	na	11.0	5.0	45	71%
ROCK-A-DILE RED DRINK										
(Kool-Aid) 'Kool Bursts'	6.75 oz	110	0.0	30.0	10	na	0.0	na	0	0%
(Kool-Aid) 'Koolers'	8.45 oz	130	0.0	34.0	10	na	0.0	na	0	0%
ROCK-A-DILE RED DRINK MIX										
(Kool-Aid) sugar-free w/NutraSweet, prepared	8 oz	4	0.0	0.0	0	na	0.0	na	0	0%
(Kool-Aid) sugar-sweetened, prepared	8 oz	70	0.0	18.0	0	na	0.0	na	0	0%
(Kool-Aid) unsweetened, prepared w/sugar	8 oz	100	0.0	25.0	0	na	0.0	na	0	0%
(Kool-Aid) unsweetened, prepared w/o sugar	8 oz	2	0.0	0.0	0	na	0.0	na	0	0%
ROCKET. See ARUGULA.										
ROCKFISH, PACIFIC, MIXED SPECIES										
baked, broiled, or microwaved	4 oz	137	27.3	0.0	87	0	2.3	0.5	50	16%
baked, broiled, or microwaved	3 oz	103	20.4	0.0	65	0	1.7	0.4	37	16%

Food Name	Serving Size	Calories	Prot. gms	Carbs gms	Sod. mgs	Fiber gms	Fat gms	Sat. Fat gms	Chol. mgs	% Fat Cal.
raw	1 lb	427	85.1	0.0	272	0	7.1	1.7	156	16%
raw	3 oz	80	15.9	0.0	51	0	1.3	0.3	30	16%
raw	1 oz	27	5.3	0.0	17	0	0.4	0.1	10	15%
ROE, MIXED SPECIES										
dry-heat cooked	3 oz	173	24.3	1.6	99	0	7.0	1.6	407	38%
dry-heat cooked	1 oz	58	8.1	0.5	33	0	2.3	0.5	136	38%
raw	1 lb	635	101.2	6.8	(mq)	0	29.1	6.6	1696	38%
raw	3 oz	119	19.0	1.3	77	0	5.5	1.2	318	38%
raw	1 oz	39	6.3	0.4	25	0	1.8	0.4	105	38%
raw	1 tbsp	22	3.6	0.2	(mq)	0	1.0	0.2	60	37%
ROLL. See also BREAD; BUN; CROISSANT; ENGLISH MUFFIN.										
BUTTER *(Pillsbury)* 'Butterflake' refrigerated	1 roll	140	3.0	20.0	530	(mq)	5.0	1.0	0	33%
BUTTERMILK *(Wonder)* brown and serve	1 roll	80	2.0	13.0	140	.6	2.0	(mq)	na	23%
CRESCENT										
(Pepperidge Farm) 'Deli Classic'	1 roll	110	2.0	13.0	150	tr	6.0	3.0	15	47%
(Pillsbury) refrigerated	1 roll	100	2.0	11.0	230	(mq)	6.0	2.0	5	51%
CLUB *(Pepperidge Farm)* 'Deli Classic' brown and serve	1 roll	100	3.0	19.0	190	.5	1.0	0.0	0	9%
DINNER										
egg	1-oz roll	87	2.7	14.7	155	1.1	1.8	0.5	14	19%
oat bran	1-oz roll	67	2.7	11.4	117	1.2	1.3	0.2	0	17%
rye	1-oz roll	81	2.9	15.1	253	na	1.0	0.2	0	11%
wheat	1-oz roll	77	2.4	13.0	96	na	1.8	0.4	0	21%
whole wheat	1-oz roll	75	2.5	14.5	136	na	1.3	0.2	0	15%
(Arnold) 'Dinner Party' 24 per pkg	1 roll	51	1.9	9.4	81	.8	1.2	(mq)	1	19%
(Awrey's)	1 roll	60	2.0	11.0	115	0	1.0	0.0	0	15%
(Awrey's) 'Black Forest'	1 roll	50	2.0	10.0	110	0	1.0	0.0	0	16%
(Awrey's) cracked wheat	1 roll	50	2.0	10.0	120	0	1.0	0.0	0	16%
(Awrey's) crusty	1 roll	70	2.0	12.0	150	0	1.0	0.0	0	14%
(Awrey's) poppy seed	1 roll	59	2.0	11.0	115	0	1.0	0.0	0	15%
(Awrey's) sesame seed	1 roll	60	2.0	11.0	115	0	1.0	0.0	0	15%
(Home Pride) wheat	1 roll	70	3.0	12.0	140	.6	1.0	na	0	13%
(Home Pride) white	1 roll	80	2.0	14.0	170	.6	2.0	(mq)	0	22%
(Pepperidge Farm) country style 'Classic'	1 roll	50	2.0	9.0	90	0	1.0	0.0	0	17%
(Pepperidge Farm) 'Old Fashioned'	1 roll	50	2.0	7.0	85	tr	2.0	1.0	5	33%
(Pepperidge Farm) 'Party'	1 roll	30	1.0	5.0	50	tr	1.0	na	0	27%
(Roman Meal)	1 roll	69	2.9	13.0	140	1.2	1.2	(mq)	0	15%
(Wonder)	1 roll	80	2.0	14.0	140	.6	1.0	na	na	12%
EGG *(Levy's)* 'Old Country Deli'	1-oz roll	146	5.3	28.1	431	2.0	2.8	(mq)	11	16%
FINGER *(Pepperidge Farm)* w/poppy seeds	1 roll	50	2.0	8.0	80	tr	2.0	0.0	5	31%
49ER										
(Colombo Brand) sour	1.2-oz roll	90	4.8	16.4	189	(mq)	0.6	na	na	6%
(Colombo Brand) sweet	1.2-oz roll	96	4.5	15.4	196	(mq)	1.8	(mq)	na	17%
FRENCH STYLE										
	1 oz	79	2.4	14.2	173	na	1.2	0.3	0	14%
(Du Jour) petite, brown and serve	1 roll	230	9.0	45.0	490	1.8	2.0	(mq)	0	8%
(Francisco) 'International'	1 roll	108	4.2	21.3	285	1.2	1.5	na	0	12%
(Pepperidge Farm) 'Deli Classic' brown and serve, 3 per pkg	1/2 roll	120	4.0	24.0	250	.5	1.0	0.0	0	7%
(Pepperidge Farm) 'Deli Classic' 9 per pkg	1 roll	100	4.0	20.0	230	.5	1.0	0.0	0	9%
GEM STYLE *(Wonder)* brown and serve	1 roll	80	2.0	13.0	140	.6	2.0	(mq)	na	23%
HARD	1 oz	83	2.8	14.9	154	na	1.2	0.2	0	13%
HEARTH										
(Brownberry) 'Hearth' assorted	1 roll	124	4.4	23.7	247	1.5	2.3	(mq)	7	16%
(Pepperidge Farm) 'Hearth' brown and serve	1 roll	50	2.0	10.0	100	tr	1.0	0.0	0	16%

Food Name	Serving Size	Calories	Prot. gms	Carbs gms	Sod. mgs	Fiber gms	Fat gms	Sat. Fat gms	Chol. mgs	% Fat Cal.
HOAGIE										
(Pepperidge Farm) soft 'Deli Classic'	1 roll	210	8.0	34.0	320	1.0	5.0	1.0	0	21%
(Wonder)	1 roll	400	13.0	73.0	800	3.0	7.0	(mq)	na	16%
ITALIAN (Du Jour) crusty, brown and serve	1 roll	80	3.0	16.0	200	.6	1.0	na	0	11%
KAISER										
	1 oz	83	2.8	14.9	154	na	1.2	0.2	0	13%
(Arnold) 'Francisco'	1 roll	184	7.0	35.4	338	2.0	2.9	(mq)	5	13%
(Brownberry) 'Hearth'	1 roll	152	5.4	29.3	318	1.9	2.8	(mq)	9	15%
LUIGI (Colombo Brand) 'Twin Pack'	2-oz roll	146	7.6	25.4	334	(mq)	1.6	(mq)	na	10%
ONION (Levy's) 'Old Country Deli'	1-oz roll	153	6.1	30.8	380	1.8	1.9	(mq)	11	10%
PAN (Wonder)	1 roll	80	2.0	14.0	140	.6	1.0	na	na	12%
PARKER HOUSE										
(Bridgford)	1-oz roll	85	2.5	15.8	172	(mq)	1.3	na	0	14%
(Pepperidge Farm)	1 roll	60	2.0	9.0	80	tr	1.0	0.0	5	17%
POTATO (Pepperidge Farm) 'Hearty Classic'	1 roll	90	2.0	14.0	125	tr	3.0	(mq)	0	30%
SANDWICH										
(Arnold) egg 'Dutch'	1 roll	123	4.5	21.6	203	1.9	3.3	(mq)	1	22%
(Awrey's) oat bran	1 roll	120	4.0	22.0	250	1.0	2.0	0.0	0	15%
(Pepperidge Farm) onion, w/poppy seeds	1 roll	150	5.0	26.0	260	.5	3.0	1.0	0	18%
(Pepperidge Farm) potato	1 roll	160	4.0	28.0	260	1.0	4.0	1.0	0	22%
(Pepperidge Farm) salad 'Deli Classic'	1 roll	110	4.0	16.0	150	(mq)	4.0	(mq)	10	31%
(Pepperidge Farm) soft 'Family'	1 roll	100	4.0	18.0	190	.5	2.0	1.0	0	17%
(Pepperidge Farm) w/sesame seeds	1 roll	140	5.0	23.0	230	.5	3.0	1.0	0	19%
SOURDOUGH (Pepperidge Farm) French style	1 roll	100	4.0	19.0	240	.5	1.0	na	0	9%
STEAK										
(Colombo Brand) sour	2.6-oz roll	200	10.1	35.1	413	(mq)	2.2	(mq)	na	10%
(Colombo Brand) sweet	2.6-oz roll	206	10.0	34.2	439	(mq)	3.3	(mq)	0	14%
TWIST (Pepperidge Farm) golden 'Heat 'n Serve'	1 roll	110	2.0	14.0	150	tr	5.0	2.0	5	41%
ROLL, MIX										
(Dromedary) dry mix	1/8 pkg	209	6.0	41.0	363	(mq)	2.0	(mq)	na	9%
(Dromedary) prepared	2 rolls	239	6.0	41.0	410	(mq)	5.0	(mq)	na	19%
(Krusteaz) prepared	1 roll	150	3.0	28.0	190	na	3.0	na	0	18%
(Pillsbury) prepared	2 rolls	270	4.0	25.0	420	(mq)	17.0	(mq)	na	57%
(Pillsbury) 'Hot Roll Mix' dry mix	1/16 pkg	100	3.0	21.0	200	na	0.0	0.0	0	0%
(Pillsbury) 'Hot Roll Mix' prepared	1 roll	120	4.0	21.0	210	na	2.0	0.0	15	15%
ROLL, SWEET. See also BUN, SWEET; DANISH PASTRY.										
APPLE										
(Break Cake) 4.5 oz	2 rolls	380	8.0	75.0	460	na	5.0	1.6	0	12%
(Break Cake) multi-pak, 1.4 oz	1 roll	120	2.0	24.0	150	na	2.0	0.5	0	15%
APPLE CINNAMON, old fashioned (Aunt Fanny's) individual	2 oz	180	4.0	34.0	125	1.5	1.0	1.5	5	6%
CARAMEL NUT (Aunt Fanny's) individual	2 oz	190	4.0	33.0	125	1.0	6.0	2.0	5	27%
CHEESE	1 oz	102	2.0	12.4	101	na	5.2	1.6	16	45%
CHERRY										
(Break Cake) 4.5 oz	2 rolls	400	8.0	79.0	390	na	3.0	1.8	0	7%
(Break Cake) multi-pak, 1.4 oz	1 roll	130	2.0	25.0	125	na	2.0	0.6	0	14%
CINNAMON										
(Aunt Fanny's) duos, individual	1.9 oz	180	4.0	32.0	150	1.0	5.0	1.5	5	24%
(Aunt Fanny's) individual	2 oz	190	4.0	34.0	160	1.0	5.0	2.0	5	23%
(Aunt Fanny's) rectangular 11-oz size	2 oz	181	3.0	33.0	64	na	4.0	<1.0	6	20%
(Awrey's) homestyle	1 roll	240	4.0	40.0	200	1.0	7.0	1.0	5	26%
(Awrey's) swirl 'Grande'	1 roll	340	4.0	46.0	370	1.0	16.0	3.0	10	42%
(Break Cake) 4.5 oz	2 rolls	420	9.0	73.0	430	na	10.0	2.5	0	22%
(Break Cake) multi-pak, 1.3 oz	1 roll	120	3.0	22.0	125	na	3.0	0.8	0	21%
(Hungry Jack) refrigerated dough w/icing, prepared	2 rolls	290	3.0	37.0	570	(mq)	14.0	(mq)	na	44%

Food Name	Serving Size	Calories	Prot. gms	Carbs gms	Sod. mgs	Fiber gms	Fat gms	Sat. Fat gms	Chol. mgs	% Fat Cal.
(Pillsbury) refrigerated dough w/icing, prepared	1 roll	110	1.0	17.0	260	(mq)	5.0	1.0	0	39%
CINNAMON NUT *(Break Cake)* 3 oz	2 rolls	330	5.0	52.0	220	na	11.0	na	na	30%
CINNAMON RAISIN *(Aunt Fanny's)* rectangular 11-oz size	2 oz	181	4.0	34.0	83	na	3.0	<1.0	8	15%
DIXIE FRUIT ROLL *(Aunt Fanny's)* individual	2 oz	180	3.0	34.0	120	1.0	4.0	1.5	5	20%
PECAN										
(Aunt Fanny's) rectangular 11-oz size	2 oz	184	4.0	32.0	79	na	4.0	<1.0	8	20%
(Break Cake) multi-pak, 1.3 oz	1 roll	120	2.0	22.0	120	na	3.0	0.6	0	22%
RAISIN CINNAMON *(Break Cake)* multi-pak, 1.25 oz	1 roll	120	2.0	21.0	110	na	3.0	0.7	0	23%
STRAWBERRY *(Aunt Fanny's)* rectangular 11-oz size	2 oz	190	4.0	35.0	140	na	4.0	na	5	19%
ROLL, SWEET, FROZEN										
APPLE *(Weight Watchers)* sweet 'Microwave'	1/2 pkg	160	3.0	27.0	100	(mq)	4.0	<1.0	5	23%
CHEESE *(Weight Watchers)* 'Microwave'	1/2 pkg	180	5.0	32.0	210	(mq)	4.0	<1.0	5	20%
CINNAMON										
(Pepperidge Farm) 2 per pkg	1 roll	280	4.0	34.0	190	(mq)	14.0	(mq)	na	45%
(Sara Lee) all butter	2-oz roll	230	3.0	31.0	220	(mq)	11.0	(mq)	na	42%
(Sara Lee) all butter, w/icing packet	.5-oz pkt	50	0.0	12.0	0	(mq)	0.0	0.0	0	0%
(Weight Watchers) glazed	2.1 oz	180	4.0	31.0	170	na	5.0	<1.0	5	24%
STRAWBERRY *(Weight Watchers)* 'Microwave'	1/2 pkg	170	3.0	29.0	90	(mq)	5.0	1.0	20	26%
ROLL DOUGH, FROZEN										
unraised, enriched, 2 x 2 3/8 inches	1 roll	75	2.1	13.3	135	>.1 c	1.4	0.3	1	17%
unraised, unenriched, 2 x 2 3/8 inches	1 roll	75	2.1	13.3	135	>.1 c	1.4	0.3	1	17%
ROMAN BEAN. See CRANBERRY BEAN.										
ROOT BEER. See SOFT DRINKS AND MIXERS.										
ROOT BEER FLOAT *(Skipper's)*	1 serving	302	3.0	33.0	66	na	10.0	(mq)	10	39%
ROQUETTE. See ARUGULA.										
ROSE APPLE										
raw	100 gm	25	0.6	5.7	0	>1.1 c	0.3	na	0	10%
trimmed	1 oz	7	0.2	1.6	tr	>.3 c	0.1	(tr)	0	11%
untrimmed	1 lb	76	1.8	17.3	1	>3.3 c	0.9	na	0	10%
ROSE COCO BEAN. See CRANBERRY BEAN.										
ROSEFISH. See OCEAN PERCH, ATLANTIC.										
ROSELLE										
raw, trimmed	1 cup	28	0.6	6.4	3	>.7 c	0.4	na	0	11%
trimmed	1 oz	14	0.3	3.2	2	>.3 c	0.2	(tr)	0	11%
untrimmed	1 lb	136	2.7	31.3	16	>3.2 c	1.8	na	0	11%
ROSEMARY										
dried	1 oz	94	1.4	18.2	14	>5.0 c	4.3	na	0	33%
dried	1 tbsp	11	0.2	2.1	2	>.6 c	0.5	na	0	33%
dried	1 tsp	4	0.1	0.8	1	>.2 c	0.2	na	0	33%
dried *(Durkee)*	1 tsp	5	0.0	0.0	0	0	tr	na	na	tr
dried *(Laurel Leaf)*	1 tsp	5	0.0	0.0	0	0	tr	na	na	tr
dried *(Spice Islands)*	1 tsp	5	0.1	0.8	1	>.2 c	0.2	(tr)	0	33%
ROTINI. See PASTA.										
ROTINI ENTRÉE, FROZEN										
(Green Giant) cheddar 'Microwave Garden Gourmet'	1 pkg	230	9.0	32.0	570	4.5	10.0	6.0	20	35%
(Mrs. Paul's) seafood 'Light'	9 oz	240	12.0	34.0	570	(mq)	6.0	2.0	25	23%
(Weight Watchers) three cheese, w/vegetables	9 oz	270	14.0	34.0	500	na	8.0	3.0	5	27%
ROTINI ENTRÉE MIX										
(Velveeta) w/cheese and broccoli, dry mix	1/4 box	210	1.0	24.0	730	na	8.0	5.0	25	42%
(Velveeta) w/cheese and broccoli, prepared	1/2 cup	210	10.0	24.0	730	na	8.0	5.0	25	35%
RUCULO. See ARUGULA.										
RUGULA. See ARUGULA.										
RUM. See ALCOHOLIC BEVERAGES.										

Food Name	Serving Size	Calories	Prot. gms	Carbs gms	Sod. mgs	Fiber gms	Fat gms	Sat. Fat gms	Chol. mgs	% Fat Cal.
RUTABAGA										
boiled, drained	4 oz	39	1.2	8.8	20	1.8	0.2	<.1	0	4%
boiled, drained, cubed	1/2 cup	33	1.1	7.4	17	1.5	0.2	0.0	0	5%
boiled, drained, mashed	1/2 cup	47	1.5	10.5	24	2.2	0.3	0.0	0	5%
raw, cubed	1/2 cup	25	0.8	5.7	14	1.8	0.1	0.0	0	3%
raw, trimmed	1 oz	10	0.3	2.3	6	>.3 c	0.1	tr	0	8%
raw, untrimmed	1 lb	140	4.6	31.4	77	>4.2 c	0.8	0.1	0	5%
RUTABAGA, CANNED (Allens) diced	1/2 cup	20	1.0	4.0	260	(mq)	<1.0	(tr)	0	<31%
RYE										
flakes	1/2 cup	281	12.4	58.6	5	>1.3 c	2.1	0.2	0	6%
flakes (Arrowhead Mills)	2 oz	190	7.0	42.0	1	7.6	1.0	(mq)	0	4%
whole grain	1 cup	567	25.0	117.9	10	>2.5 c	4.2	0.5	0	6%
whole grain	1 oz	95	4.2	19.8	2	>.4 c	0.7	0.1	0	6%
whole grain (Arrowhead Mills)	2 oz	190	7.0	42.0	1	7.6	1.0	(mq)	0	4%
RYE CAKE (Quaker) 'Grain Cakes'	.32-oz piece	35	1.4	6.5	52	.8	0.3	0.0	0	8%
RYE FLOUR										
dark	1/2 cup	207	9.0	44.0	1	14.5	1.7	0.2	0	7%
dark	1 oz	92	4.0	19.5	<1	(mq)	0.8	0.1	0	7%
light	1/2 cup	187	4.3	40.9	1	7.4	0.7	0.1	0	3%
light	1 oz	104	2.4	22.7	<1	4.1	0.4	<.1	0	4%
medium	1/2 cup	181	4.8	39.5	2	7.4	0.9	0.1	0	4%
medium	1 oz	100	2.7	22.0	1	4.1	0.5	0.1	0	4%
(Arrowhead Mills) whole grain	2 oz	190	9.0	39.0	1	7.6	1.0	(mq)	0	5%
(Krusteaz)	1 cup	351	11.0	73.0	1	3.0	2.0	<1.0	0	5%
(Pillsbury) 'Bohemian Style' w/wheat flour	1 cup	400	11.0	86.0	0	(mq)	1.0	(mq)	0	2%
(Pillsbury's Best)	1 cup	400	12.0	83.0	0	(mq)	2.0	(mq)	0	5%
(Robin Hood) stone ground	1 cup	360	13.0	86.0	10	13.0	2.0	(mq)	0	4%

RYE WHISKEY. See ALCOHOLIC BEVERAGES.

S

Food Name	Serving Size	Calories	Prot. gms	Carbs gms	Sod. mgs	Fiber gms	Fat gms	Sat. Fat gms	Chol. mgs	% Fat Cal.
SABLEFISH / skil										
cooked	3 oz	213	14.6	0.0	61	0	16.7	3.5	54	72%
raw	1 lb	886	60.8	0.0	254	0	69.4	14.5	222	72%
raw	3 oz	166	11.4	0.0	48	0	13.0	2.7	42	72%
raw	1 oz	55	3.8	0.0	16	0	4.3	0.9	14	72%
raw, approx 6.8 oz	1/2 fillet	376	25.9	0.0	108	0	29.5	6.2	95	72%
smoked	4 oz	291	20.0	0.0	836	0	22.8	4.8	73	72%
smoked	3 oz	218	15.0	0.0	626	0	17.1	3.6	54	72%
SACCHARIN. See SUGAR, ALTERNATIVE.										
SAFFLOWER OIL										
'Hi-Oleic' (Hain)	1 tbsp	120	0.0	0.0	0	0	14.0	1.0	0	100%
high oleic (Spectrum Naturals)	1 tbsp	120	0.0	0.0	0	(tr)	14.0	1.0	(tr)	100%
high oleic, unrefined (Spectrum Naturals)	1 tbsp	120	0.0	0.0	0	(tr)	14.0	1.0	(tr)	100%
linoleic	1/2 cup	964	0.0	0.0	0	0	109.0	0.0	0	100%
linoleic	1 tbsp	120	0.0	0.0	0	0	13.6	1.2	0	100%
oleic	1/2 cup	964	0.0	0.0	0	0	109.0	6.7	0	100%
oleic	1 tbsp	120	0.0	0.0	0	0	13.6	0.8	0	100%
organic, unrefined (Spectrum Naturals)	1 tbsp	120	0.0	0.0	0	(tr)	14.0	1.0	(tr)	100%
over 70% oleic	1 cup	1927	0.0	0.0	0	0	218.0	21.3	na	100%
over 70% oleic	1 tbsp	124	0.0	0.0	0	0	14.0	1.4	na	100%

Food Name	Serving Size	Calories	Prot. gms	Carbs gms	Sod. mgs	Fiber gms	Fat gms	Sat. Fat gms	Chol. mgs	% Fat Cal.
SAFFLOWER SEED, dried, kernels .... 1 oz		147	4.6	9.7	1	>.7 c	10.9	1.0	0	63%
SAFFLOWER SEED MEAL, partially defatted .... 1 oz		97	10.1	13.8	1	>2.2 c	0.7	0.1	0	6%
SAFFRON										
dried .... 1 oz		88	3.2	18.5	42	>1.0 c	1.7	na	0	15%
dried .... 1 tbsp		7	0.2	1.4	3	.1	0.1	na	0	12%
dried .... 1 tsp		2	0.1	0.5	1	tr	0.0	na	0	0%
SAGE										
ground .... 1 oz		89	3.0	17.2	3	5.1	3.6	2.0	0	29%
ground .... 1 tbsp		6	0.2	1.2	0	.4	0.3	0.1	0	33%
ground .... 1 tsp		2	0.1	0.4	0	.1	0.1	0.1	0	31%
ground (*Durkee*) .... 1 tsp		3	0.0	0.0	0	0	tr	na	na	tr
ground (*Laurel Leaf*) .... 1 tsp		3	0.0	0.0	0	0	tr	na	na	tr
ground (*Spice Islands*) .... 1 tsp		4	0.1	0.6	<1	.1	0.1	<.1	0	24%
SALAD DRESSING										
BACON (*Kraft*) creamy 'Reduced Calorie' .... 1 tbsp		30	0.0	2.0	150	na	2.0	0.0	0	69%
BACON AND TOMATO										
(*Estee*) .... 1 tbsp		8	<1.0	1.0	35	na	<1.0	<1.0	5	<53%
(*Kraft*) .... 1 tbsp		70	0.0	1.0	130	na	7.0	1.0	0	94%
(*Kraft*) 'Reduced Calorie' .... 1 tbsp		30	0.0	2.0	150	na	2.0	0.0	0	69%
BLUE CHEESE										
.... 1 cup		1235	11.8	18.1	2680	na	128.1	24.2	42	91%
.... 1 tbsp		77	0.7	1.1	167	na	8.0	1.5	3	91%
(*Ayla's Organics*) fat free .... 2 tbsp		30	1.0	4.0	140	0	0.0	0.0	0	0%
(*Estee*) .... 1 tbsp		8	<1.0	1.0	50	na	<1.0	<1.0	0	<53%
(*Featherweight*) 'Neu Bleu' .... 1 tbsp		4	0.0	1.0	110	na	0.0	0.0	0	0%
(*Hidden Valley Ranch*) 'Lowfat' .... 1 tbsp		10	0.0	3.0	140	na	0.0	na	0	0%
(*Kraft*) chunky .... 1 tbsp		60	1.0	2.0	230	na	6.0	1.0	5	82%
(*Kraft*) chunky 'Reduced Calorie' .... 1 tbsp		30	0.0	2.0	240	na	2.0	1.0	5	69%
(*Kraft*) 'Free' .... 1 tbsp		16	0.0	4.0	120	na	0.0	na	0	0%
(*Lawry's*) 'Classic' .... 1 tbsp		186	0.1	1.9	385	>.1 c	2.0	(mq)	na	69%
(*Litehouse*) country, dressing and dip, refrigerated ...... 1 tbsp		76	1.0	0.0	84	na	8.0	na	na	95%
(*Litehouse*) 'Lite' dressing and dip, refrigerated .... 1 tbsp		33	1.0	1.0	86	na	3.0	na	na	77%
(*Litehouse*) 'Original' dressing and dip, refrigerated ..... 1 tbsp		77	1.0	0.0	82	na	8.0	na	na	95%
(*Roka*) .... 1 tbsp		60	1.0	1.0	170	na	6.0	1.0	10	87%
(*Roka*) 'Reduced Calorie' .... 1 tbsp		16	1.0	1.0	280	na	1.0	1.0	5	53%
(*S&W Nutradiet*) .... 1 tbsp		25	0.0	2.0	200	na	2.0	na	0	69%
(*Skipper's*) premium .... 1 pouch		222	1.0	4.0	240	na	23.0	(mq)	8	91%
(*T. Marzetti*) .... 1 tbsp		90	1.0	1.0	180	na	9.0	na	2	91%
(*T. Marzetti*) chunky, refrigerated ...... 1 tbsp		78	1.0	1.0	159	na	8.0	na	14	90%
(*T. Marzetti*) 'Lite' refrigerated .... 1 tbsp		45	0.0	0.0	150	na	5.0	na	5	100%
(*Wish-Bone*) chunky .... 1 tbsp		75	0.4	0.7	149	na	7.9	1.2	1	94%
(*Wish-Bone*) chunky 'Lite' .... 1 tbsp		40	0.3	1.5	197	na	3.7	0.8	1	82%
(*Wish-Bone*) chunky, lite 'Food Service' .... .5 oz		40	0.0	1.0	200	na	4.0	<1.0	0	90%
(*Wish-Bone*) 'Healthy Sensation!' .... .5 oz		20	na	4.0	140	na	na	na	0	0%
BUTTERMILK										
(*Hain*) 'Old Fashioned' .... 1 tbsp		70	(mq)	(mq)	100	na	7.0	(mq)	0	90%
(*Hollywood*) 'Old Fashion' .... 1 tbsp		75	0.0	1.0	40	0	8.0	1.0	0	95%
(*Kraft*) creamy .... 1 tbsp		80	0.0	1.0	120	0	8.0	1.0	5	90%
(*Kraft*) creamy 'Reduced Calorie' .... 1 tbsp		30	0.0	1.0	125	na	3.0	0.0	5	90%
(*Seven Seas*) 'Buttermilk Recipe' .... 1 tbsp		80	0.0	1.0	130	na	8.0	1.0	5	90%
(*T. Marzetti*) and herbs .... 1 tbsp		95	0.0	0.0	150	na	10.0	na	3	95%
(*T. Marzetti*) bacon, refrigerated .... 1 tbsp		93	0.0	0.0	127	na	10.0	na	2	97%
(*T. Marzetti*) blue cheese, refrigerated ...... 1 tbsp		90	1.0	1.0	161	na	10.0	na	5	92%

Food Name	Serving Size	Calories	Prot. gms	Carbs gms	Sod. mgs	Fiber gms	Fat gms	Sat. Fat gms	Chol. mgs	% Fat Cal.
CAESAR										
(Estee)	2 tbsp	8	<1.0	<1.0	130	na	<1.0	0.0	2	<53%
(Hain) creamy	1 tbsp	60	0.0	1.0	220	na	6.0	(mq)	5	93%
(Hain) creamy 'Low Salt'	1 tbsp	60	0.0	1.0	15	na	6.0	(mq)	5	93%
(Hollywood)	1 tbsp	70	1.0	2.0	65	0	7.0	1.0	0	90%
(Kraft) golden	1 tbsp	70	0.0	1.0	180	na	7.0	1.0	0	94%
(Lawry's) 'Classic'	1 tbsp	130	0.8	1.0	337	>.1 c	13.5	1.8	na	94%
(Litehouse) dressing and dip, refrigerated	1 tbsp	57	0.0	0.0	84	na	6.0	na	na	95%
(T. Marzetti)	1 tbsp	80	0.0	1.0	170	na	8.0	na	2	90%
(T. Marzetti) house	1 tbsp	75	<1.0	<1.0	180	na	8.0	na	1	96%
(T. Marzetti) refrigerated	1 tbsp	75	0.0	0.0	178	na	8.0	na	0	96%
(Weight Watchers)	1 tbsp	4	0.0	1.0	200	na	0.0	0.0	0	0%
(Wish-Bone)	1 tbsp	77	0.4	0.9	248	na	8.0	1.2	1	93%
(Wish-Bone) w/olive oil 'Lite'	.5 oz	30	0.0	1.0	170	na	3.0	na	0	90%
CALIFORNIA FRENCH										
(Catalina) nonfat 'Free'	1 tbsp	16	0.0	3.0	120	na	0.0	0.0	0	0%
(T. Marzetti)	1 tbsp	90	1.0	5.0	100	na	6.0	na	4	60%
(T. Marzetti) 'Fat-Free'	1 tbsp	16	<1.0	4.0	140	na	0.0	na	0	0%
(T. Marzetti) 'Light'	1 tbsp	40	0.0	3.0	180	na	3.0	na	2	69%
CELERY SEED										
(T. Marzetti) and onion	1 tbsp	75	0.0	9.0	90	na	6.0	na	0	60%
(T. Marzetti) refrigerated	1 tbsp	72	0.0	5.0	101	na	5.0	na	0	63%
CHEESE										
(Featherweight)	1 tbsp	20	0.0	1.0	70	na	2.0	(mq)	0	90%
(Hain) vinaigrette	1 tbsp	55	0.0	0.0	130	na	6.0	(mq)	5	98%
(Hollywood)	1 tbsp	80	0.0	2.0	60	0	8.0	1.0	0	90%
CHINESE VINEGAR										
(Lawry's) w/sesame and ginger 'Classic'	1 tbsp	145	0.2	2.4	325	0	15.0	2.1	0	93%
CITRUS (Hain) tangy 'Canola'	1 tbsp	50	0.0	1.0	75	na	5.0	(mq)	0	90%
CREAMY										
(Estee)	1 tbsp	4	0.0	1.0	13	na	0.0	0.0	0	0%
(Hain)	1 tbsp	80	0.0	0.0	100	na	8.0	(mq)	0	90%
(Hain) 'No Salt Added'	1 tbsp	80	0.0	1.0	25	na	8.0	(mq)	0	90%
(Hollywood)	1 tbsp	90	0.0	2.0	140	0	9.0	1.0	0	90%
(Kraft) no oil 'Reduced Calorie'	1 tbsp	4	0.0	1.0	220	na	0.0	0.0	0	0%
(Kraft) 'Reduced Calorie'	1 tbsp	25	0.0	1.0	120	na	2.0	0.0	0	72%
(Kraft) w/real sour cream	1 tbsp	50	0.0	1.0	120	na	5.0	1.0	0	90%
(Kraft) zesty	1 tbsp	50	0.0	1.0	260	na	5.0	1.0	0	90%
(Kraft) zesty 'Reduced Calorie'	1 tbsp	20	0.0	1.0	230	na	2.0	0.0	0	90%
(Lawry's) w/Parmesan cheese 'Classic'	1 oz	156	0.0	4.5	178	>.1 c	15.1	2.1	na	88%
(Life) egg-free 'All Natural'	1 tbsp	39	<1.0	2.0	4	na	4.0	(mq)	0	92%
(Pathmark)	1 tbsp	70	0.0	1.0	260	na	7.0	1.0	0	90%
(Pathmark) zesty	1 tbsp	70	0.0	1.0	370	na	8.0	1.0	0	95%
(Pathmark) zesty 'Reduced Calorie'	1 tbsp	6	0.0	1.0	190	na	0.0	0.0	0	0%
(Rancher's Choice)	1 tbsp	90	0.0	1.0	140	na	10.0	1.0	5	96%
(Rancher's Choice) 'Reduced Calorie'	1 tbsp	30	0.0	1.0	150	na	3.0	0.0	5	90%
(S&W Nutradiet)	1 tbsp	10	0.0	1.0	180	na	1.0	na	na	90%
(S&W Nutradiet) no oil	1 tbsp	2	0.0	0.0	290	na	0.0	0.0	0	0%
(Seven Seas)	1 tbsp	70	0.0	1.0	240	na	7.0	1.0	0	90%
(Wish-Bone)	1 tbsp	56	0.1	1.5	149	na	5.5	0.9	<1	89%
(Wish-Bone) 'Lite'	1 tbsp	26	0.1	2.0	148	na	2.0	0.4	<1	68%
(Weight Watchers) 'Single Serve' 1 packet	1 tbsp	9	0.0	2.0	430	na	0.0	0.0	0	0%
CUCUMBER										
(Featherweight) creamy	1 tbsp	4	0.0	1.0	80	na	0.0	0.0	0	0%

Food Name	Serving Size	Calories	Prot. gms	Carbs gms	Sod. mgs	Fiber gms	Fat gms	Sat. Fat gms	Chol. mgs	% Fat Cal.
(Hain) dill, creamy	1 tbsp	80	0.0	0.0	210	na	8.0	(mq)	5	90%
(Kraft) creamy	1 tbsp	70	0.0	1.0	190	na	8.0	1.0	0	95%
(Kraft) creamy 'Reduced Calorie'	1 tbsp	25	0.0	1.0	220	na	2.0	0.0	0	72%
(Weight Watchers) creamy	1 tbsp	18	(mq)	4.0	85	na	0.0	0.0	na	0%
DIJON										
(Estee) creamy	1 tbsp	8	<1.0	<1.0	100	na	<1.0	<1.0	5	<53%
(Featherweight) creamy	1 tbsp	20	0.0	1.0	80	na	2.0	(mq)	0	90%
(Great Impressions) mustard	1 tbsp	57	0.4	0.3	103	na	6.1	(mq)	18	95%
(Hain) vinaigrette	1 tbsp	50	0.0	0.0	180	na	5.0	(mq)	5	90%
(Hollywood) vinaigrette	1 tbsp	60	0.0	2.0	40	0	6.0	1.0	0	90%
(Wish-Bone) vinaigrette 'Classic'	1 tbsp	60	0.2	1.0	171	na	6.1	0.9	<1	92%
(Wish-Bone) vinaigrette 'Lite Classic'	1 tbsp	30	0.1	1.1	176	na	2.8	(mq)	0	84%
DILL										
(Ayla's Organics) creamy, fat free	2 tbsp	15	0.0	3.0	140	0.0	0.0	0.0	0	0%
(Nasoya) creamy 'Vegi-Dressing'	1 tbsp	40	1.0	1.0	50	na	3.0	(mq)	0	68%
FRENCH										
(Ayla's Organics) fat free	2 tbsp	10	0.0	3.0	150	0.0	0.0	0.0	0	0%
(Catalina)	1 tbsp	60	0.0	4.0	180	na	5.0	1.0	0	74%
(Catalina) 'Reduced Calorie'	1 tbsp	18	0.0	3.0	120	na	1.0	0.0	0	50%
(Estee)	1 tbsp	4	0.0	1.0	10	na	0.0	0.0	0	0%
(Estee) creamy	2 tbsp	10	0.0	2.0	130	na	0.0	0.0	0	0%
(Featherweight)	1 tbsp	14	0.0	3.0	15	na	0.0	0.0	0	0%
(Great Impressions) w/green pepper, low calorie	1 tbsp	64	0.2	4.1	188	na	5.2	(mq)	0	73%
(Hain) creamy	1 tbsp	60	0.0	1.0	80	na	6.0	(mq)	0	90%
(Hain) spicy mustard 'Canola'	1 tbsp	50	1.0	1.0	190	na	5.0	(mq)	5	90%
(Hollywood) creamy	1 tbsp	70	0.0	2.0	45	0	7.0	1.0	0	89%
(Kraft)	1 tbsp	60	0.0	2.0	125	na	6.0	1.0	0	90%
(Kraft) 'Miracle'	1 tbsp	70	0.0	3.0	240	na	6.0	1.0	0	77%
(Kraft) nonfat 'Free'	1 tbsp	20	0.0	4.0	120	na	0.0	0.0	0	0%
(Kraft) 'Reduced Calorie'	1 tbsp	20	0.0	3.0	120	na	1.0	0.0	0	43%
(Litehouse) country herb, dressing and marinade, refrigerated	1 tbsp	54	0.0	2.0	196	na	5.0	na	na	85%
(Pathmark) creamy	1 tbsp	60	0.0	2.0	90	na	5.0	1.0	0	75%
(Pathmark) 'Reduced Calorie'	1 tbsp	20	0.0	3.0	160	na	1.0	0.0	0	43%
(Pritikin) style, fat-free, sodium-free	1 tbsp	10	0.0	3.0	0	na	0.0	0.0	0	0%
(S&W Nutradiet)	1 tbsp	18	0.0	3.0	120	na	0.0	0.0	0	0%
(Seven Seas) creamy	1 tbsp	60	0.0	2.0	240	na	6.0	1.0	0	90%
(Seven Seas) 'French! Light'	1 tbsp	35	0.0	2.0	210	na	3.0	0.0	0	77%
(T. Marzetti) country	1 tbsp	72	0.0	4.0	110	na	6.0	na	6	77%
(T. Marzetti) 'Frenchette'	1 tbsp	10	0.0	3.0	140	na	0.0	na	0	0%
(T. Marzetti) honey, refrigerated	1 tbsp	74	0.0	5.0	115	na	6.0	na	0	73%
(T. Marzetti) honey blue, refrigerated	1 tbsp	70	0.0	5.0	122	na	6.0	na	1	77%
(T. Marzetti) honey 'Lite' refrigerated	1 tbsp	48	0.0	5.0	118	na	3.0	na	0	57%
(T. Marzetti) 'Light'	1 tbsp	16	0.0	3.0	160	na	1.0	na	0	56%
(Ultra Slim Fast) 'Cholesterol Free'	1 tbsp	20	0.0	4.0	105	na	<1.0	na	0	<36%
(Weight Watchers) low-calorie	1 tbsp	10	0.0	2.0	170	na	0.0	0.0	0	0%
(Wish-Bone) creamy, garlic	1 tbsp	55	0.1	1.8	158	>.1 c	5.3	(mq)	0	86%
(Wish-Bone) 'Deluxe'	1 tbsp	60	0.1	2.3	83	na	5.4	0.8	0	81%
(Wish-Bone) 'Deluxe Food Service'	1 tbsp	61	0.1	2.4	86	0	5.6	(mq)	0	83%
(Wish-Bone) garlic	1 tbsp	55	0.1	1.8	158	>.1 c	5.3	(mq)	0	86%
(Wish-Bone) 'Healthy Sensation!'	.5 oz	20	0.0	4.0	120	na	na	na	0	0%
(Wish-Bone) 'Lite'	1 tbsp	31	0.0	2.1	70	0	2.5	(mq)	0	73%
(Wish-Bone) 'Lite Sweet 'n Spicy'	1 tbsp	18	0.0	3.2	110	na	0.5	na	0	26%
(Wish-Bone) low-calorie 'Lite'	1 tbsp	30	0.1	1.9	67	na	2.5	0.1	0	74%

Food Name	Serving Size	Calories	Prot. gms	Carbs gms	Sod. mgs	Fiber gms	Fat gms	Sat. Fat gms	Chol. mgs	% Fat Cal.
(Wish-Bone) red, low-calorie 'Lite'	1 tbsp	17	0.2	3.2	155	na	0.4	na	0	21%
(Wish-Bone) style 'Lite'	.5 oz	18	0.0	3.0	140	na	na	na	0	0%
(Wish-Bone) style, lite 'Food Service'	.5 oz	30	0.0	2.0	75	na	3.0	na	0	90%
(Wish-Bone) sweet 'n spicy	.5 oz	70	0.0	3.0	160	na	6.0	<1.0	0	77%
(Wish-Bone) sweet 'n spicy 'Lite'	.5 oz	18	0.0	4.0	130	na	na	na	0	0%
FRUIT SALAD										
(Great Impressions) orange marmalade	1 tbsp	87	0.2	5.4	48	na	7.1	(mq)	11	74%
(Knott's Berry Farm)	1 tbsp	50	2.0	3.0	75	na	5.0	na	na	69%
GARLIC										
(Ayla's Organics) and onion, fat free	2 tbsp	10	0.0	2.0	140	0	0.0	0.0	0	0%
(Ayla's Organics) creamy, fat free	2 tbsp	30	1.0	4.0	140	0	0.0	0.0	0	0%
(Estee) creamy	1 tbsp	2	0.0	0.0	10	na	0.0	0.0	0	0%
(Hain) and sour cream	1 tbsp	70	0.0	0.0	100	na	7.0	(mq)	0	90%
(Kraft) creamy	1 tbsp	50	0.0	1.0	170	na	5.0	1.0	0	92%
(Life) w/tofu 'All Natural' dressing and dip	1 tbsp	70	<1.0	1.4	0	(mq)	7.1	(mq)	75	91%
(Nasoya) herb 'Vegi-Dressing'	1 tbsp	40	1.0	1.0	50	na	3.0	(mq)	0	77%
(Pritikin) and herb, fat-free, sodium-free	1 tbsp	6	0.0	2.0	0	na	0.0	0.0	0	0%
(T. Marzetti) Italian, refrigerated	1 tbsp	81	0.0	1.0	73	na	9.0	na	9	95%
(Wish-Bone) creamy	1 tbsp	74	0.1	0.5	158	>.6 c	8.0	(mq)	0	97%
(Wish-Bone) Sierra	.5 oz	80	0.0	1.0	125	na	8.0	na	na	90%
GINGER PLUM VINAIGRETTE										
(Simply Delicious) 'Un-Dressing'	1 tbsp	36	0.0	1.0	199	na	4.0	na	0	90%
HERB										
(Featherweight)	1 tbsp	6	0.0	1.0	5	na	0.0	0.0	0	0%
(Featherweight) garden	1 tbsp	25	0.0	2.0	65	na	2.0	(mq)	0	72%
(Hain) savory 'No Salt Added'	1 tbsp	90	0.0	0.0	25	na	10.0	(mq)	0	100%
(Marie's) vinaigrette, fat-free 'Lite & Zesty'	1 tbsp	16	0.0	4.0	130	na	0.0	na	0	0%
(Pritikin) vinaigrette, fat-free, sodium-free	1 tbsp	8	0.0	2.0	0	na	0.0	na	0	0%
(Seven Seas) and spice 'Viva'	1 tbsp	60	0.0	1.0	170	na	6.0	1.0	0	90%
(Seven Seas) and spice 'Viva Herbs & Spices! Light'	1 tbsp	30	0.0	1.0	200	na	3.0	0.0	0	90%
(Simply Delicious) garlic vinaigrette 'Un-Dressing'	1 tbsp	43	0.0	1.0	132	na	4.0	na	0	90%
(Wish-Bone) creamy 'Classics'	1 tbsp	70	0.0	1.2	228	na	7.3	(mq)	0	93%
HOMESTYLE										
(Dorothy Lynch)	1 tbsp	55	0.1	5.0	85	na	3.8	0.5	0	63%
(Dorothy Lynch) 'Reduced Calorie'	1 tbsp	30	0.0	7.0	80	na	<1.0	(mq)	0	<24%
HONEY AND SESAME (Hain)	1 tbsp	60	0.0	2.0	210	na	5.0	(mq)	0	75%
HONEY MUSTARD										
(Knott's Berry Farm) 'Peggy Jane's'	1 tbsp	60	0.0	2.0	40	na	6.0	na	na	90%
(Litehouse) dressing and dip, refrigerated	1 tbsp	67	0.0	2.0	55	na	7.0	na	na	94%
(Simply Delicious) vinaigrette 'Un-Dressing'	1 tbsp	41	0.0	2.0	122	na	4.0	na	0	87%
(T. Marzetti) Dijon	1 tbsp	67	0.0	3.0	51	na	6.0	na	7	82%
(T. Marzetti) Dijon, refrigerated	1 tbsp	68	0.0	3.0	103	na	6.0	na	9	82%
(Wish-Bone) Dijon 'Healthy Sensation!'	1 tbsp	25	0.0	5.0	140	na	0.0	na	0	0%
ITALIAN										
(Ayla's Organics) fat free	2 tbsp	10	0.0	2.0	140	0	0.0	0.0	0	0%
(Estee)	2 tbsp	4	0.0	1.0	130	na	0.0	0.0	0	0%
(Featherweight)	1 tbsp	4	0.0	1.0	120	na	0.0	0.0	0	0%
(Hain) 'Canola'	1 tbsp	50	0.0	1.0	150	na	5.0	(mq)	0	92%
(Hain) 'Traditional'	1 tbsp	80	0.0	0.0	330	na	8.0	(mq)	0	90%
(Hain) 'Traditional No Salt Added'	1 tbsp	60	0.0	1.0	20	na	6.0	(mq)	0	93%
(Hollywood)	1 tbsp	90	0.0	1.0	300	0	9.0	1.0	0	90%
(Kraft) 'Deliciously Light'	1 tbsp	35	0.0	1.0	115	na	3.0	na	0	77%
(Kraft) house	1 tbsp	60	0.0	1.0	115	na	6.0	1.0	0	90%
(Kraft) house 'Reduced Calorie'	1 tbsp	30	0.0	1.0	115	na	2.0	0.0	0	60%

Food Name	Serving Size	Calories	Prot. gms	Carbs gms	Sod. mgs	Fiber gms	Fat gms	Sat. Fat gms	Chol. mgs	% Fat Cal.
(Kraft) nonfat 'Free'	1 tbsp	6	0.0	1.0	210	na	0.0	0.0	0	0%
(Kraft) oil-free 'Reduced Calorie'	1 tbsp	4	0.0	1.0	220	na	0.0	0.0	0	0%
(Kraft) 'Presto'	1 tbsp	70	0.0	1.0	150	na	7.0	1.0	0	90%
(Kraft) zesty	1 tbsp	50	0.0	1.0	260	na	5.0	1.0	0	92%
(Kraft) zesty 'Reduced Calorie'	1 tbsp	20	0.0	1.0	230	na	2.0	0.0	0	90%
(Marie's) vinaigrette, fat-free 'Lite & Zesty'	1 tbsp	16	0.0	4.0	135	na	0.0	na	0	0%
(Nasoya) 'Vegi-Dressing'	1 tbsp	40	1.0	1.0	50	na	3.0	(mq)	0	77%
(Ott's)	1 tbsp	80	<.1	0.2	87	tr	9.1	(mq)	<1	99%
(Pritikin) fat-free, sodium-free	1 tbsp	8	0.0	2.0	0	na	0.0	na	0	0%
(Seven Seas) 'Free Viva'	1 tbsp	4	0.0	1.0	220	na	0.0	0.0	0	0%
(Seven Seas) 'Viva'	1 tbsp	50	0.0	1.0	240	na	5.0	1.0	0	92%
(Seven Seas) 'Viva Italian! Light'	1 tbsp	30	0.0	1.0	230	na	3.0	0.0	0	90%
(Skipper's) gourmet	1 pouch	140	0.0	2.0	200	na	15.0	(mq)	0	94%
(Skipper's) lo-cal	1 pouch	17	0.0	2.0	680	na	1.0	na	0	53%
(T. Marzetti) 'Fat-Free'	1 tbsp	5	0.0	1.0	270	na	0.0	na	0	0%
(T. Marzetti) 'Frenchette'	1 tbsp	6	0.0	2.0	280	na	0.0	na	0	0%
(T. Marzetti) gusto	1 tbsp	58	0.0	0.0	204	na	8.0	na	0	100%
(T. Marzetti) 'Light'	1 tbsp	35	0.0	1.0	300	na	3.0	na	0	77%
(T. Marzetti) w/olive oil	1 tbsp	60	0.0	1.0	220	na	7.0	na	0	94%
(Ultra Slim Fast) 'Cholesterol Free'	1 tbsp	6	0.0	1.0	105	na	<1.0	na	0	<69%
(Wish-Bone)	1 tbsp	46	0.0	1.5	280	na	4.5	0.6	0	87%
(Wish-Bone) blended	.5 oz	35	0.0	1.0	210	na	4.0	<1.0	0	90%
(Wish-Bone) 'Food Service'	.5 oz	45	0.0	2.0	290	na	5.0	<1.0	0	85%
(Wish-Bone) 'Healthy Sensation!'	1 tbsp	6	0.0	1.0	140	na	0.0	na	0	0%
(Wish-Bone) 'Lite'	1 tbsp	7	0.2	0.9	212	na	0.3	na	0	38%
(Wish-Bone) lite 'Food Service'	.5 oz	6	0.0	1.0	250	na	na	na	0	0%
(Wish-Bone) 'Robusto'	1 tbsp	47	0.1	1.8	288	na	4.5	0.6	0	84%
(Weight Watchers) style	1 tbsp	6	0.0	1.0	200	na	0.0	na	na	0%
(Weight Watchers) style 'Single Serve' 1 packet	.75 oz	8	0.0	2.0	270	na	0.0	na	na	0%
ITALIAN, CREAMY										
(Estee)	2 tbsp	14	<1.0	2.0	130	na	<1.0	0.0	0	<43%
(Kraft)	1 tbsp	60	0.0	1.0	115	na	6.0	1.0	0	93%
(Kraft) 'Deliciously Light'	1 tbsp	25	0.0	1.0	120	na	2.0	na	0	72%
(Kraft) 'Reduced Calorie'	1 tbsp	25	0.0	1.0	120	na	2.0	0.0	0	72%
(Kraft) w/real sour cream	1 tbsp	50	0.0	1.0	120	na	5.0	1.0	0	92%
(Litehouse) dressing and dip, refrigerated	1 tbsp	60	0.0	0.0	76	na	6.0	na	na	90%
(Seven Seas) 'Viva Creamy Italian! Light'	1 tbsp	45	0.0	1.0	230	na	4.0	1.0	0	80%
(T. Marzetti)	1 tbsp	80	0.0	1.0	100	na	8.0	na	4	90%
(Weight Watchers)	1 tbsp	12	0.0	3.0	85	na	0.0	na	na	0%
(Weight Watchers) whipped	1 tbsp	50	0.0	2.0	80	na	5.0	5.0	5	90%
(Wish-Bone)	.5 oz	60	0.0	1.0	150	na	6.0	<1.0	0	93%
(Wish-Bone) 'Food Service'	.5 oz	25	0.0	4.0	140	na	na	na	0	0%
(Wish-Bone) 'Lite'	.5 oz	25	0.0	4.0	140	na	na	na	0	0%
LEMON TAHINI VINAIGRETTE										
(Simply Delicious) 'Un-Dressing'	1 tbsp	43	0.0	1.0	170	na	4.0	na	9	83%
LIME CILANTRO VINAIGRETTE										
(Simply Delicious) 'Un-Dressing'	1 tbsp	41	0.0	1.0	116	na	4.0	na	0	88%
MAYONNAISE TYPE. See also MAYONNAISE.										
(A&P)	1 tbsp	70	<1.0	2.0	100	na	7.0	1.0	0	90%
(Bama)	1 tbsp	50	0.0	3.0	105	0	4.0	(mq)	na	75%
(Finast)	1 tbsp	70	0.0	2.0	90	0	7.0	(mq)	na	89%
(Kraft) 'Miracle Whip'	1 tbsp	70	0.0	2.0	85	0	7.0	1.0	5	89%
(Kraft) 'Miracle Whip Light'	1 tbsp	40	0.0	3.0	120	0	3.0	na	0	67%
(Kraft) nonfat 'Miracle Whip Free'	1 tbsp	15	0.0	3.0	105	0	0.0	0.0	0	0%

Food Name	Serving Size	Calories	Prot. gms	Carbs gms	Sod. mgs	Fiber gms	Fat gms	Sat. Fat gms	Chol. mgs	% Fat Cal.
(P&Q)	1 tbsp	50	<1.0	3.0	110	0	5.0	1.0	8	90%
(Pathmark) 'No Frills'	1 tbsp	50	0.0	3.0	120	0	5.0	1.0	5	90%
(Spin Blend)	1 tbsp	60	0.0	3.0	110	0	5.0	1.0	10	75%
(Spin Blend) cholesterol free	1 tbsp	40	0.0	2.0	110	0	4.0	1.0	0	90%
(Weight Watchers) whipped	1 tbsp	45	0.0	3.0	100	0	4.0	1.0	0	80%
(Weight Watchers) whipped, fat-free	1 tbsp	12	0.0	4.0	125	na	0.0	0.0	0	0%
(Weight Watchers) whipped, light	1 tbsp	50	0.0	1.0	100	na	5.0	1.0	5	92%
(Weight Watchers) whipped, low-sodium	1 tbsp	50	0.0	1.0	45	na	5.0	1.0	5	92%
OIL AND VINEGAR										
W/balsamic vinegar (Great Impressions)	1 tbsp	67	<1.0	2.3	367	na	6.5	(mq)	0	87%
W/olive oil										
(Kraft)	1 tbsp	70	0.0	1.0	210	0	8.0	1.0	0	95%
(Wish-Bone) Italian 'Classic'	1 tbsp	34	0.0	1.7	190	0	3.0	0.4	0	80%
(Wish-Bone) 'Lite Classic'	.5 oz	20	0.0	2.0	170	na	2.0	na	0	90%
(Wish-Bone) vinaigrette	1 tbsp	28	0.0	1.8	111	0	2.3	(mq)	0	74%
(Wish-Bone) vinaigrette 'Lite'	1 tbsp	16	0.1	1.9	111	0	0.9	0.1	0	50%
W/red wine vinegar										
(Estee)	1 tbsp	2	0.0	0.0	10	0	0.0	0.0	0	0%
(Featherweight)	1 tbsp	6	0.0	1.0	100	0	0.0	0.0	0	0%
(Great Impressions)	1 tbsp	64	<1.0	2.5	277	na	6.1	(mq)	0	86%
(Kraft)	1 tbsp	60	0.0	4.0	200	na	4.0	1.0	0	60%
(Pathmark)	1 tbsp	70	0.0	2.0	235	na	7.0	1.0	0	89%
(Seven Seas) 'Free'	1 tbsp	6	0.0	1.0	190	na	0.0	0.0	0	0%
(Seven Seas) 'Viva'	1 tbsp	70	0.0	1.0	290	na	7.0	1.0	0	90%
(Seven Seas) 'Viva Red Wine!'	1 tbsp	45	0.0	1.0	190	na	4.0	1.0	0	80%
W/Cabernet (Lawry's) 'Classics'	1 tbsp	138	0.0	4.9	178	0	13.7	1.0	na	86%
W/white wine vinegar (Great Impressions)	1 tbsp	63	<1.0	0.8	242	na	6.6	(mq)	0	94%
ONION AND CHIVES										
(Kraft) creamy	1 tbsp	70	0.0	1.0	150	na	7.0	1.0	0	90%
(Wish-Bone) 'Lite'	1 tbsp	37	0.2	1.6	164	na	3.3	(mq)	0	81%
ORIENTAL STYLE (Featherweight)	1 tbsp	20	0.0	1.0	75	na	2.0	(mq)	0	90%
PARMESAN (Hidden Valley Ranch) Italian 'Lowfat'	1 tbsp	16	0.0	3.0	140	na	1.0	na	0	56%
PARMESAN PEPPERCORN										
(T. Marzetti)	1 tbsp	81	<1.0	<1.0	129	na	9.0	na	6	98%
(T. Marzetti) refrigerated	1 tbsp	85	0.0	1.0	154	na	9.0	2.0	5	95%
PEPPERCORN										
(Litehouse) dressing and dip, refrigerated	1 tbsp	67	0.0	0.0	66	na	7.0	na	na	94%
(Simply Delicious) pink, vinaigrette 'Un-Dressing'	1 tbsp	40	0.0	1.0	148	na	4.0	na	0	90%
(T. Marzetti) cracked, refrigerated	1 tbsp	62	0.0	0.0	135	na	7.0	na	13	100%
(Weight Watchers) creamy	1 tbsp	8	0.0	2.0	85	na	0.0	0.0	na	0%
POPPYSEED										
(Great Impressions)	1 tbsp	131	0.1	8.0	130	na	11.0	(mq)	0	75%
(Hain) 'Rancher's'	1 tbsp	60	0.0	0.0	105	na	7.0	(mq)	5	100%
(Knott's Berry Farm) 'Peggy Jane's'	1 tbsp	60	0.0	4.0	90	na	5.0	na	na	74%
(Litehouse) dressing and dip, refrigerated	1 tbsp	65	0.0	3.0	83	na	6.0	na	na	82%
(T. Marzetti)	1 tbsp	72	<1.0	5.0	146	na	6.0	na	8	75%
(T. Marzetti) refrigerated	1 tbsp	65	0.0	5.0	97	na	5.0	na	5	69%
POTATO SALAD (T. Marzetti)	1 tbsp	80	0.0	3.0	170	na	7.0	na	9	79%
RANCH										
(Hidden Valley Ranch) honey Dijon 'Lowfat'	1 tbsp	20	0.0	3.0	140	na	1.0	na	0	43%
(Hidden Valley Ranch) original 'Light'	1 tbsp	40	0.0	2.0	140	na	4.0	na	5	90%
(Kraft) nonfat 'Free'	1 tbsp	16	0.0	3.0	150	na	0.0	0.0	0	0%
(Litehouse) country, dressing and dip, refrigerated	1 tbsp	61	0.0	1.0	75	na	7.0	na	na	94%
(Litehouse) dressing and dip, refrigerated	1 tbsp	59	0.0	1.0	67	na	6.0	na	na	93%

Food Name	Serving Size	Calories	Prot. gms	Carbs gms	Sod. mgs	Fiber gms	Fat gms	Sat. Fat gms	Chol. mgs	% Fat Cal.
(Litehouse) jalapeño, dressing and dip, refrigerated ..... 1 tbsp		60	0.0	1.0	80	na	6.0	na	na	90%
(Litehouse) 'Lite' dressing and dip, refrigerated .... 1 tbsp		35	1.0	1.0	80	na	3.0	na	na	77%
(Pritikin) fat-free, sodium-free .... 1 tbsp		16	0.0	4.0	0	na	0.0	0.0	0	0%
(Seven Seas) 'Buttermilk Recipe Ranch! Light' .... 1 tbsp		50	0.0	1.0	135	na	5.0	1.0	0	92%
(Seven Seas) 'Free' .... 1 tbsp		16	0.0	4.0	120	na	0.0	0.0	0	0%
(Seven Seas) 'Viva' .... 1 tbsp		80	0.0	1.0	135	na	8.0	1.0	5	90%
(Seven Seas) 'Viva Ranch! Light' .... 1 tbsp		50	0.0	2.0	125	na	5.0	1.0	5	90%
(Skipper's) house .... 1 pouch		188	1.0	2.0	302	na	20.0	(mq)	0	94%
(T. Marzetti) .... 1 tbsp		90	0.0	0.0	92	na	2.0	na	3	100%
(T. Marzetti) buttermilk, refrigerated .... 1 tbsp		93	0.0	0.0	127	na	10.0	na	2	97%
(T. Marzetti) buttermilk 'Lite' refrigerated .... 1 tbsp		45	0.0	1.0	135	na	5.0	na	3	100%
(T. Marzetti) Caesar .... 1 tbsp		95	<1.0	1.0	150	na	10.0	na	3	95%
(T. Marzetti) 'Fat-Free' .... 1 tbsp		12	<1.0	3.0	220	na	0.0	na	0	0%
(T. Marzetti) garden .... 1 tbsp		100	0.0	1.0	165	na	10.0	na	2	90%
(T. Marzetti) honey Dijon .... 1 tbsp		89	<1.0	1.0	100	na	9.0	na	14	91%
(T. Marzetti) honey Dijon, refrigerated .... 1 tbsp		79	<1.0	1.0	101	na	8.0	na	14	90%
(T. Marzetti) 'Light' .... 1 tbsp		40	0.0	2.0	166	na	4.0	na	2	90%
(T. Marzetti) Parmesan, refrigerated .... 1 tbsp		86	0.0	1.0	120	na	9.0	na	6	95%
(T. Marzetti) peppercorn .... 1 tbsp		85	0.0	1.0	13	na	9.0	na	4	95%
(T. Marzetti) peppercorn 'Fat-Free' .... 1 tbsp		14	0.0	3.0	173	na	0.0	0.0	0	0%
(T. Marzetti) style .... 1 tbsp		90	1.0	5.0	100	na	6.0	na	4	60%
(Weight Watchers) creamy .... 1 tbsp		25	0.0	6.0	80	na	0.0	0.0	0	0%
(Weight Watchers) creamy 'Single Serve' .... 1 pkt		35	0.0	8.0	140	na	0.0	0.0	0	0%
(Wish-Bone) .... 1 tbsp		78	0.1	1.1	156	na	8.3	1.2	4	94%
(Wish-Bone) 'Food Service' .... .5 oz		80	0.0	1.0	105	na	8.0	1.0	5	90%
(Wish-Bone) 'Healthy Sensation!' .... 1 tbsp		16	0.0	3.0	140	na	0.0	na	0	0%
(Wish-Bone) 'Lite' .... 1 tbsp		42	0.2	2.5	148	na	3.5	0.7	5	75%
RED WINE VINAIGRETTE										
(Wish-Bone) .... 1 tbsp		51	0.0	4.2	216	(tr)	3.8	0.5	0	67%
(Wish-Bone) 'Lite' .... .5 oz		20	0.0	2.0	140	na	2.0	na	0	90%
ROMANO										
(T. Marzetti) cheese Italian .... 1 tbsp		80	0.0	0.0	135	na	8.0	na	2	90%
(T. Marzetti) cheese Italian, refrigerated .... 1 tbsp		77	<1.0	<1.0	183	na	8.0	na	3	94%
RUSSIAN										
(Ayla's Organics) fat free .... 2 tbsp		10	0.0	3.0	140	0	0.0	0.0	0	0%
(Featherweight) .... 1 tbsp		6	0.0	1.0	125	(mq)	0.0	0.0	0	0%
(Kraft) .... 1 tbsp		60	0.0	4.0	130	(mq)	5.0	1.0	0	74%
(Kraft) creamy .... 1 tbsp		60	0.0	2.0	150	(mq)	5.0	1.0	5	75%
(Kraft) 'Reduced Calorie' .... 1 tbsp		30	0.0	4.0	130	(mq)	1.0	0.0	0	30%
(Kraft) w/pure honey, low-calorie .... 1 tbsp		60	0.0	4.0	130	(mq)	5.0	1.0	0	74%
(S&W Nutradiet) .... 1 tbsp		25	0.0	4.0	120	(mq)	1.0	(mq)	0	36%
(Weight Watchers) whipped .... 1 tbsp		50	0.0	2.0	80	na	5.0	1.0	5	90%
(Wish-Bone) .... 1 tbsp		46	0.1	6.0	147	(mq)	2.5	0.4	0	48%
(Wish-Bone) 'Food Service' .... 1 tbsp		47	0.1	6.0	147	(mq)	2.5	(mq)	0	48%
(Wish-Bone) 'Lite' .... 1 tbsp		22	0.1	3.9	126	(mq)	0.6	0.1	0	25%
SAN FRANCISCO (Lawry's) w/Romano cheese 'Classic' .... 1 oz		136	0.6	2.0	547	>.1 c	14.0	1.9	na	92%
SANTA FE (Wish-Bone) .... .5 oz		70	0.0	1.0	105	na	7.0	1.0	5	90%
SESAME SEED										
(Ayla's Organics) toasted, fat free .... 2 tbsp		20	0.0	3.0	190	0	0.0	0.0	0	0%
(Nasoya) garlic 'Vegi-Dressing' .... 1 tbsp		40	1.0	1.0	50	(mq)	3.0	(mq)	0	68%
(Wish-Bone) vinaigrette 'Food Service' .... .5 oz		35	0.0	3.0	260	na	2.0	na	0	51%
SOUR CREAM										
(Crowley) nondairy .... 1 oz		40	1.0	1.0	5	0	4.0	(mq)	0	90%
(Friendship) 'Sour Treat' .... 1 oz		36	1.0	2.0	15	na	3.0	(mq)	0	75%

Food Name	Serving Size	Calories	Prot. gms	Carbs gms	Sod. mgs	Fiber gms	Fat gms	Sat. Fat gms	Chol. mgs	% Fat Cal
SOUR CREAM AND CHIVES										
(Litehouse) vinaigrette, refrigerated	1 tbsp	63	0.0	1.0	72	na	7.0	na	na	100%
SPINACH SALAD (T. Marzetti) refrigerated	1 tbsp	35	0.0	2.0	100	na	3.0	na	0	92%
SWEET AND SAUCY (T. Marzetti)	1 tbsp	65	0.0	4.0	180	na	5.0	na	0	69%
SWEET AND SOUR										
(T. Marzetti)	1 tbsp	72	0.0	5.0	100	na	6.0	na	0	73%
(T. Marzetti) 'Fat-Free'	1 tbsp	20	0.0	5.0	130	na	0.0	0.0	0	0%
(T. Marzetti) 'Light'	1 tbsp	45	0.0	5.0	105	na	3.0	na	0	60%
(T. Marzetti) refrigerated	1 tbsp	72	0.0	5.0	99	na	6.0	na	0	73%
SWISS CHEESE VINAIGRETTE (Hain)	1 tbsp	60	0.0	0.0	160	na	7.0	(mq)	5	100%
THOUSAND ISLAND										
(Estee)	1 tbsp	8	0.0	2.0	30	(mq)	0.0	0.0	0	0%
(Featherweight)	1 tbsp	18	0.0	3.0	70	(mq)	0.0	0.0	0	0%
(Hain)	1 tbsp	50	0.0	0.0	85	(mq)	5.0	(mq)	0	90%
(Hollywood)	1 tbsp	60	0.0	3.0	15	0	6.0	1.0	5	90%
(Kraft)	1 tbsp	60	0.0	2.0	150	(mq)	5.0	1.0	5	75%
(Kraft) and bacon	1 tbsp	60	0.0	2.0	100	(mq)	6.0	1.0	0	90%
(Kraft) nonfat 'Free'	1 tbsp	20	0.0	5.0	135	(mq)	0.0	0.0	0	0%
(Kraft) 'Reduced Calorie'	1 tbsp	20	0.0	3.0	135	(mq)	1.0	0.0	0	43%
(Litehouse) dressing and dip, refrigerated	1 tbsp	65	0.0	1.0	99	na	7.0	na	na	97%
(S&W Nutradiet)	1 tbsp	25	0.0	2.0	105	(mq)	2.0	(mq)	na	72%
(Seven Seas) creamy	1 tbsp	50	0.0	2.0	150	(mq)	5.0	1.0	5	90%
(Seven Seas) 'Thousand Island! Light'	1 tbsp	30	0.0	3.0	160	(mq)	2.0	0.0	5	60%
(Skipper's)	1 pouch	160	0.0	8.0	415	na	14.0	(mq)	6	80%
(T. Marzetti)	1 tbsp	74	0.0	2.0	120	na	7.0	na	5	85%
(T. Marzetti) 'Fat-Free'	1 tbsp	17	0.0	4.0	172	na	0.0	0.0	0	0%
(T. Marzetti) 'Frenchette'	1 tbsp	20	0.0	3.0	155	na	0.0	0.0	4	0%
(T. Marzetti) 'Light'	1 tbsp	35	0.0	3.0	155	na	3.0	na	4	77%
(T. Marzetti) refrigerated	1 tbsp	82	0.0	6.0	93	na	5.0	na	0	55%
(Ultra Slim Fast) 'Cholesterol Free'	1 tbsp	18	0.0	4.0	95	na	<1.0	na	0	<36%
(Weight Watchers) whipped	1 tbsp	50	0.0	2.0	80	na	5.0	1.0	5	90%
(Wish-Bone)	1 tbsp	63	0.1	3.1	158	(mq)	5.6	0.8	7	80%
(Wish-Bone) 'Food Service'	1 tbsp	40	0.2	2.6	107	0	3.2	(mq)	9	72%
(Wish-Bone) 'Healthy Sensation!'	.5 oz	20	0.0	4.0	135	na	na	na	0	0%
(Wish-Bone) 'Lite'	1 tbsp	36	0.2	1.9	99	(mq)	3.0	0.4	9	76%
(Wish-Bone) lite 'Food Service'	.5 oz	20	na	4.0	140	na	na	na	0	0%
TOMATO										
(Featherweight) zesty	1 tbsp	2	0.0	0.0	5	0	0.0	0.0	0	0%
(Hain) vinaigrette, garden 'Canola'	1 tbsp	60	0.0	1.0	150	na	6.0	(mq)	0	90%
(Weight Watchers) vinaigrette	1 tbsp	8	0.0	2.0	150	na	0.0	0.0	0	0%
VEGETABLE (T. Marzetti) dressing and dip, refrigerated	1 tbsp	88	0.0	1.0	120	na	10.0	na	2	96%
VINTAGE (Lawry's) w/sherry wine 'Classic'	1 tbsp	110	4.3	2.5	415	>.1 c	10.5	2.1	0	86%
WHITE WINE										
(Lawry's) w/Chardonnay 'Classic'	1 tbsp	153	0.0	2.7	178	>.1 c	15.7	2.0	0	93%
(Marie's) fat-free 'Lite & Zesty'	1 tbsp	20	0.0	5.0	135	na	0.0	na	0	0%
SALAD DRESSING MIX										
BACON (Lawry's) dry mix	1 pkg	65	5.2	9.1	1820	>.5 c	0.8	na	na	11%
BLUE CHEESE										
(Hain) 'No Oil' prepared	1 tbsp	14	1.0	1.0	180	na	1.0	na	5	53%
(Hidden Valley Ranch) dry mix	1 pkg	112	4.0	19.0	1931	na	2.0	na	0	16%
(Weight Watchers) dry mix	1 tbsp	8	0.0	1.0	110	na	0.0	na	na	0%
BLUE CHEESE AND HERBS (Good Seasons) dry mix	1 pkg	4	0.0	1.0	150	na	0.0	na	0	0%
BUTTERMILK										
(Hain) 'No Oil' prepared	1 tbsp	11	1.0	1.0	150	na	<1.0	na	0	<53%

Food Name	Serving Size	Calories	Prot. gms	Carbs gms	Sod. mgs	Fiber gms	Fat gms	Sat. Fat gms	Chol. mgs	% Fat Cal.
(Hidden Valley Ranch) original recipe, dry mix, .4 oz	1 pkg	25	3.0	na	2167	na	0.0	na	0	0%
(Good Seasons) 'Farm Style' dry mix	1 pkg	4	0.0	1.0	95	na	0.0	na	0	0%
CAESAR										
(Lawry's) dry mix	1 pkg	75	3.4	8.7	1962	>.3 c	3.1	(mq)	na	37%
(Hain) 'No Oil' prepared	1 tbsp	6	0.0	1.0	200	na	<1.0	na	0	<69%
CHEESE AND GARLIC										
(Good Seasons) dry mix	1 pkg	4	0.0	1.0	170	na	0.0	na	0	0%
(Hain) 'No Oil' prepared	1 tbsp	6	<1.0	1.0	180	na	<1.0	na	0	<53%
DILL (Good Seasons) 'Classic' dry mix	1 tbsp	2	0.0	0.0	150	na	0.0	na	0	0%
FRENCH										
(Hain) 'No Oil' prepared	1 tbsp	12	0.0	3.0	340	na	0.0	0.0	0	0%
(Weight Watchers) style, dry mix	1 tbsp	3	0.0	1.0	150	na	0.0	na	na	0%
GARLIC AND HERBS (Good Seasons) dry mix	1 pkg	4	0.0	1.0	190	na	0.0	na	0	0%
HERB										
(Good Seasons) 'Classic' dry mix	1 pkg	2	0.0	0.0	150	na	0.0	na	0	0%
(Hain) 'No Oil' prepared	1 tbsp	2	0.0	1.0	140	na	0.0	0.0	0	0%
(Hidden Valley Ranch) creamy, dry mix	1 pkg	76	3.0	16.0	1931	na	0.0	na	0	0%
HONEY MUSTARD (Good Seasons) dry mix	1 tbsp	6	0.0	1.0	125	na	0.0	na	0	0%
ITALIAN										
(Good Seasons) dry mix	1 pkg	2	0.0	1.0	170	na	0.0	na	0	0%
(Good Seasons) 'Lite' prepared	1 tbsp	25	0.0	1.0	180	na	3.0	(mq)	0	87%
(Good Seasons) mild	1 tbsp	70	0.0	1.0	190	na	8.0	(mq)	0	95%
(Good Seasons) 'No Oil' prepared	1 tbsp	6	0.0	2.0	30	na	0.0	na	0	0%
(Good Seasons) zesty, dry mix	1 pkg	2	0.0	1.0	120	na	0.0	na	0	0%
(Good Seasons) zesty 'Lite' prepared	1 tbsp	25	0.0	1.0	135	na	3.0	(mq)	0	87%
(Hain) 'No Oil' prepared	1 tbsp	2	0.0	1.0	170	na	0.0	0.0	0	0%
(Lawry's) dry mix	1 pkg	45	1.6	9.3	2255	>.3 c	0.2	na	na	4%
(Lawry's) w/cheese, dry mix	1 pkg	74	2.2	11.6	1624	>.2 c	2.1	(mq)	na	26%
(Weight Watchers) dry mix	1 tbsp	2	0.0	0.0	140	na	0.0	na	na	0%
ITALIAN, CREAMY (Weight Watchers) dry mix	1 tbsp	3	0.0	1.0	180	na	0.0	na	na	0%
ITALIAN CHEESE										
(Good Seasons) dry mix	1 pkg	4	0.0	1.0	130	na	0.0	na	0	0%
(Good Seasons) 'Lite' prepared	1 tbsp	25	0.0	1.0	135	na	3.0	(mq)	0	87%
LEMON AND HERBS (Good Seasons) dry mix	1 pkg	2	0.0	1.0	140	na	0.0	na	0	0%
PEPPERCORN										
(Hidden Valley Ranch) original recipe, prepared	1 tbsp	58	0.0	1.0	110	na	3.0	na	4	87%
RANCH										
(Good Seasons) dry mix	1 pkg	4	0.0	1.0	70	na	0.0	na	0	0%
(Good Seasons) 'Lite' prepared	1 tbsp	30	1.0	2.0	115	na	2.0	(mq)	5	60%
(Hidden Valley Ranch) 'Original' dry mix	1 pkg	93	3.0	18.0	2211	na	1.0	na	0	10%
(Hidden Valley Ranch) reduced calorie, dry mix	1 pkg	98	3.0	17.0	2301	na	2.0	na	0	18%
(Hidden Valley Ranch) w/bacon, dry mix	1.2 oz	118	7.0	1.0	1953	na	2.0	na	0	36%
RUSSIAN (Weight Watchers) dry mix	1 tbsp	4	0.0	1.0	120	na	0.0	na	na	0%
SPICY PEANUT (A Taste of Thai) dry mix	1 tbsp	40	1.0	6.0	360	1.0	1.5	0.5	0	33%
THOUSAND ISLAND										
(Hain) 'No Oil' prepared	1 tbsp	12	0.0	3.0	150	na	0.0	0.0	<1	0%
(Weight Watchers) dry mix	1 tbsp	4	0.0	1.0	140	na	0.0	na	na	0%
SALAD MIX. See also PASTA DISH MIX; PASTA SALAD MIX.										
(Saco Foods) 'Easy Caesar' unprepared	.75 oz	98	2.0	7.0	246	na	7.0	na	4	64%
SALAD SEASONING (Schilling) 'Salad Supreme'	1 tsp	11	0.7	0.5	2807	(mq)	0.1	na	0	16%
SALAD TOPPING										
(Salad Nibbler) crouton topping, buttermilk ranch	1 oz	128	7.0	13.0	241	na	5.0	na	2.0	36%
(Salad Nibbler) crouton topping, seasoned cheddar	1 oz	129	6.0	13.0	224	na	6.0	na	2.0	42%
(Special Edition) sesame salad nuggets	1 tbsp	35	<1.0	3.0	115	na	2.5	na	na	58%

Food Name	Serving Size	Calories	Prot. gms	Carbs gms	Sod. mgs	Fiber gms	Fat gms	Sat. Fat gms	Chol. mgs	% Fat Cal
(Special Edition) sesame salad nuggets, garlic and cheese	1 tbsp	40	<1.0	3.0	130	na	2.5	na	na	58%
SALAMI. See LUNCHEON MEAT.										
SALISBURY STEAK DINNER. See BEEF DINNER, FROZEN.										
SALISBURY STEAK ENTRÉE. See BEEF ENTRÉE, FROZEN; BEEF ENTRÉE, PACKAGED.										
SALMON, ALTERNATIVE, smoked *(Mox Lox)*	1.5 oz	25	2.0	3.0	380	na	<1.0	na	5	<31%
SALMON, ATLANTIC										
Farmed										
dry-heat cooked	3 oz	175	18.8	0.0	52	0	10.5	2.1	54	56%
raw	3 oz	156	16.9	0.0	50	0	9.2	1.9	50	55%
Wild										
dry-heat cooked	3 oz	155	21.6	0.0	48	0	6.9	1.1	60	42%
raw	3 oz	121	16.9	0.0	37	0	5.4	0.8	47	42%
SALMON, CANNED										
CHUM										
(Bumble Bee)	1 cup	306	47.3	0.0	(mq)	0	11.4	(mq)	(mq)	35%
(Bumble Bee) w/liquid	3.5 oz	160	20.0	0.0	490	na	8.0	2.0	60	47%
COHO *(Deming's)* boiled	1/2 cup	140	22.0	0.0	450	0	5.0	(mq)	(mq)	34%
MIXED *(Libby's)* skinless, boneless	3.25 oz	110	16.0	1.0	420	na	4.0	1.0	50	35%
PINK										
Alaska, w/liquid *(Deming's)*	1/2 cup	140	20.0	0.0	450	0	6.0	1.0	65	40%
chunk, skinless, boneless, in spring water										
(Chicken of the Sea)	2 oz	60	10.0	0.0	280	na	2.0	na	na	31%
chunk, skinless, boneless, w/liquid *(Deming's)*	3.25 oz	120	17.0	0.0	420	0	5.0	(mq)	(mq)	40%
skinless, boneless, w/liquid *(Bumble Bee)*	3.5 oz	120	17.0	0.0	420	na	5.0	1.0	25	40%
solids, w/bone and liquid	3 oz	118	16.8	0.0	64	0	5.1	1.3	47	41%
w/liquid	4 oz	158	22.4	0.0	628	0	6.9	1.7	(mq)	41%
w/liquid *(Bumble Bee)*	1 cup	310	45.1	0.0	851	0	13.0	(mq)	(mq)	39%
w/liquid *(Bumble Bee)*	3.5 oz	160	20.0	0.0	490	na	8.0	2.0	50	47%
w/liquid *(Del Monte)*	1/2 cup	160	22.0	0.0	660	0	7.0	(mq)	(mq)	42%
w/liquid *(Featherweight)*	2 oz	70	11.0	0.0	45	0	3.0	(mq)	20	38%
w/liquid *(Libby's)*	7.75 oz	310	45.0	0.0	790	0	13.0	(mq)	(mq)	39%
SOCKEYE										
(Bumble Bee)	1 cup	376	44.7	0.0	1148	0	20.5	(mq)	(mq)	51%
(Libby's)	7.75 oz	380	45.0	0.0	760	0	21.0	(mq)	(mq)	51%
Alaska *(Deming's)*	1/2 cup	170	20.0	0.0	450	0	9.0	2.0	65	50%
Alaska, med *(Deming's)*	1/2 cup	150	21.0	0.0	450	0	7.0	2.0	65	43%
blueback *(Rubinstein's)*	1/2 cup	170	20.0	0.0	450	0	9.0	(mq)	(mq)	50%
blueback *(S&W Nutradiet)*	1/2 cup	188	22.0	0.0	45	0	11.0	(mq)	(mq)	53%
blueback 'Fancy' *(S&W)*	1/2 cup	190	25.0	0.0	590	0	10.0	(mq)	(mq)	47%
skinless, boneless, w/liquid *(Bumble Bee)*	3.5 oz	130	17.0	0.0	420	na	6.0	1.0	30	44%
solids, w/bone, drained	3 oz	130	17.4	0.0	457	0	6.2	1.4	37	45%
solids, w/bone, drained, w/o salt	3 oz	130	17.4	0.0	64	0	6.2	1.4	37	45%
w/liquid *(Bumble Bee)*	3.5 oz	180	20.0	0.0	490	na	10.0	2.0	60	53%
w/liquid *(Del Monte)*	1/2 cup	180	23.0	0.0	660	0	9.0	(mq)	(mq)	47%
SALMON, CHINOOK/king/lox/smoked										
dry-heat cooked	3 oz	196	21.9	0.0	51	0	11.4	2.7	72	54%
raw	1 lb	816	91.0	0.0	213	0	47.4	11.4	299	54%
raw	3 oz	153	17.0	0.0	40	0	8.9	2.1	56	54%
raw, approx 7 oz	1/2 fillet	356	39.7	0.0	93	0	20.7	5.0	131	54%
smoked	3 oz	99	15.5	0.0	666	0	3.7	0.8	20	35%
smoked, lox	4 oz	133	20.7	0.0	2268	0	4.9	1.1	26	35%
smoked, lox	3 oz	99	15.5	0.0	1700	0	3.7	0.8	20	35%
SALMON, CHUM/dog/keta										
dry-heat cooked	3 oz	131	21.9	0.0	54	0	4.1	0.9	81	30%

Food Name	Serving Size	Calories	Prot. gms	Carbs gms	Sod. mgs	Fiber gms	Fat gms	Sat. Fat gms	Chol. mgs	% Fat Cal.
raw	1 lb	544	91.3	0.0	449	0	17.1	3.8	336	30%
raw	3 oz	102	17.1	0.0	43	0	3.2	0.7	63	30%
raw	1 oz	34	5.7	0.0	14	0	1.1	0.2	21	30%
raw, approx 7 oz	1/2 fillet	238	39.9	0.0	99	0	7.5	1.7	147	30%
raw, fillet portions (Peter Pan Seafoods)	3.5 oz	120	20.1	na	50	na	3.8	na	74	30%
raw, sides, w/pinbone, (Peter Pan Seafoods)	3.5 oz	120	20.1	na	50	na	3.8	na	74	30%
raw, solids, w/bone, drained, w/o salt	3 oz	120	18.2	0.0	64	0	4.7	1.3	33	37%
raw, steaks (Peter Pan Seafoods)	3.5 oz	120	20.1	na	50	na	3.8	na	74	30%
SALMON, COHO / silver										
Farmed										
dry-heat cooked	3 oz	151	20.7	0.0	44	0	7.0	1.6	54	43%
raw	3 oz	136	18.1	0.0	40	0	6.5	1.5	43	45%
Wild										
dry-heat cooked	3 oz	118	19.9	0.0	49	0	3.7	0.9	47	30%
moist-heat cooked	3 oz	156	23.3	0.0	45	0	6.4	1.4	48	38%
raw	1 lb	662	98.1	0.0	211	0	27.0	5.0	177	38%
raw	3 oz	124	18.4	0.0	39	0	5.0	1.1	38	38%
raw	1 oz	41	7.6	0.0	13	0	1.7	0.3	11	34%
raw, approx 7 oz	1/2 fillet	289	42.8	0.0	91	0	11.7	2.5	89	38%
SALMON, DOG. See SALMON, CHUM.										
SALMON, FROZEN, steak, w/o seasoning mix (SeaPak)	8-oz pkg	270	46.0	0.0	115	0	9.0	(mq)	170	31%
SALMON, HUMPBACK. See SALMON, PINK.										
SALMON, KETA. See SALMON, CHUM.										
SALMON, KING. See SALMON, CHINOOK.										
SALMON, PINK / humpback										
dry-heat cooked	3 oz	127	21.7	0.0	73	0	3.8	0.6	57	28%
raw	1 lb	527	90.4	0.0	302	0	15.6	2.5	236	28%
raw	3 oz	99	17.0	0.0	57	0	2.9	0.5	44	28%
raw	1 oz	33	5.7	0.0	19	0	1.0	0.2	15	28%
SALMON, RED. See SALMON, SOCKEYE.										
SALMON, REDEYE. See SALMON, SOCKEYE.										
SALMON, SILVER. See SALMON, COHO.										
SALMON, SMOKED. See SALMON, CHINOOK.										
SALMON, SOCKEYE / red / redeye										
dry-heat cooked	4 oz	245	31.0	0.0	75	0	12.4	2.2	99	47%
dry-heat cooked	3 oz	184	23.2	0.0	56	0	9.3	1.6	74	47%
raw	1 lb	763	96.6	0.0	211	0	38.8	6.8	283	48%
raw	3 oz	143	18.1	0.0	40	0	7.3	1.3	53	48%
raw	1 oz	48	6.0	0.0	13	0	2.4	0.4	18	47%
raw, approx 7 oz	1/2 fillet	333	42.2	0.0	93	0	17.0	3.0	123	48%
SALSA. See also SAUCE.										
(Hot Cha Cha) 'Texas'	1 oz	6	0.3	2.5	2	.4	0.0	0.0	0	0%
(La Victoria) 'Brava'	1 tbsp	6	<1.0	1.0	100	(mq)	<1.0	(tr)	0	<53%
(La Victoria) 'Casera'	1 tbsp	4	<1.0	1.0	80	(mq)	<1.0	(tr)	0	<53%
(La Victoria) 'Supreme'	2 tbsp	10	0.0	2.0	220	na	0.0	na	na	0%
(La Victoria) 'Victoria'	1 tbsp	4	<1.0	1.0	80	(mq)	<1.0	(tr)	0	<53%
BURRITO (Del Monte)	1/4 cup	20	0.0	4.0	355	(mq)	0.0	0.0	0	0%
EXTRA CHUNKY (Rosarita) 'de Mexico Style'	2 tbsp	30	1.0	7.0	280	na	<1.0	na	0	<22%
GREEN CHILI										
(Del Monte) mild	1/4 cup	20	0.0	3.0	590	(mq)	0.0	0.0	0	0%
(Hain) hot	1/4 cup	22	1.0	4.0	480	(mq)	0.0	0.0	0	0%
(La Victoria)	2 tbsp	10	0.0	2.0	150	na	0.0	na	na	0%
(Nabisco) hot	1 tbsp	6	0.0	2.0	190	na	0.0	0.0	0	0%
(Nabisco) medium 'Green Chile Salsa'	1 tbsp	6	0.0	1.0	190	na	0.0	0.0	0	0%

Food Name	Serving Size	Calories	Prot. gms	Carbs gms	Sod. mgs	Fiber gms	Fat gms	Sat. Fat gms	Chol. mgs	% Fat Cal.
(Nabisco) mild 'Green Chile Salsa'	1 tbsp	8	0.0	2.0	190	na	0.0	0.0	0	0%
(Old El Paso) 'Thick 'n Chunky'	2 tbsp	3	0.0	1.0	270	(mq)	0.0	0.0	0	0%
(Ortega) hot	1 oz	10	0.0	2.0	180	(mq)	0.0	0.0	0	0%
(Ortega) medium	1 oz	8	0.0	2.0	180	(mq)	0.0	0.0	0	0%
(Ortega) mild	1 oz	8	0.0	2.0	180	(mq)	0.0	0.0	0	0%
(Rosarita) mild	1.093 oz	7	0.3	1.5	167	.3	0.1	0.0	0	11%
(Territorial House)	.5 oz	4	<1.0	<1.0	80	na	<1.0	na	na	<53%
HOT										
(Chi-Chi's)	1 oz	8	2.0	2.0	153	na	2.0	2.0	2	53%
(Enrico's) 'Chunky Style'	2 tbsp	8	1.0	2.0	34	(mq)	0.0	0.0	0	0%
(Enrico's) 'Chunky Style No Salt Added'	2 tbsp	8	1.0	2.0	10	(mq)	0.0	0.0	0	0%
(Old El Paso) 'Thick 'n Chunky'	2 tbsp	6	<1.0	1.0	170	(mq)	<1.0	(tr)	0	<53%
(Pablo's) 'Deli Style'	1 oz	10	1.0	2.0	250	na	0.0	0.0	0	0%
(Rosarita) chunky	3 tbsp	25	1.0	6.0	300	<1.0	<1.0	(mq)	0	<24%
JALAPEÑO										
(La Victoria) green	1 tbsp	4	<1.0	1.0	105	(mq)	<1.0	(tr)	0	<53%
(La Victoria) red	1 tbsp	6	<1.0	1.0	95	(mq)	<1.0	(tr)	0	<53%
MEDIUM										
(Chi-Chi's)	1 oz	7	2.0	2.0	135	na	2.0	2.0	2	53%
(Litehouse) 'Zesty'	1 tbsp	4	0.0	1.0	110	na	0.0	0.0	na	0%
(Old El Paso) 'Thick 'n Chunky'	2 tbsp	6	<1.0	1.0	170	(mq)	<1.0	(tr)	0	<53%
(Ortega) thick and chunky	1 tbsp	4	0.0	1.0	150	na	0.0	0.0	0	0%
(Pace) 'Thick & Chunky'	2 tbsp	4	<1.0	<1.0	101	na	<1.0	na	na	<53%
(Rosarita) chunky	3 tbsp	25	1.0	6.0	350	<1.0	<1.0	(mq)	0	<24%
(Rosarita) 'Traditional'	1.093 oz	7	0.3	1.6	234	.5	0.1	0.0	0	11%
MILD										
(Chi-Chi's)	1 oz	7	2.0	2.0	116	na	2.0	2.0	2	53%
(Enrico's) 'Chunky Style'	2 tbsp	8	1.0	2.0	34	(mq)	0.0	0.0	0	0%
(Enrico's) 'Chunky Style No Salt Added'	2 tbsp	8	1.0	2.0	10	(mq)	0.0	0.0	0	0%
(Hain)	1/2 cup	20	1.0	4.0	410	(mq)	0.0	0.0	0	0%
(Hunt's) 'Homestyle'	1.093 oz	27	0.5	6.2	236	.6	0.2	0.0	0	6%
(Old El Paso) 'Thick 'n Chunky'	2 tbsp	6	<1.0	1.0	170	(mq)	<1.0	(tr)	0	<53%
(Pablo's) 'Deli Style'	1 oz	10	1.0	2.0	250	na	0.0	0.0	0	0%
(Pace) and dip, mild 'Chunky'	2 tbsp	4	<1.0	<1.0	101	na	<1.0	na	na	<53%
(Pace) 'Thick & Chunky'	2 tbsp	4	<1.0	<1.0	101	na	<1.0	na	na	<53%
(Rosarita) 'Casa Mamita'	1.129 oz	7	0.4	1.2	170	.4	0.1	0.0	0	12%
(Rosarita) chunky	3 tbsp	25	1.0	6.0	340	<1.0	<1.0	(mq)	0	<24%
(Rosarita) roasted	1.093 oz	10	0.5	1.7	233	.6	0.3	0.0	0	24%
(Rosarita) 'Traditional'	1.093 oz	7	0.6	1.4	247	.5	0.1	0.0	0	10%
OMELETTE *(La Victoria)*	1 tbsp	6	<1.0	1.0	95	(mq)	<1.0	(tr)	0	<53%
PICANTE										
(Del Monte) hot	1/2 cup	20	0.0	4.0	385	(mq)	0.0	0.0	0	0%
(Del Monte) hot and chunky	1/4 cup	15	0.0	3.0	405	(mq)	0.0	0.0	0	0%
(La Victoria) medium	2 tbsp	5	0.0	1.0	180	na	0.0	na	na	0%
(La Victoria) mild	2 tbsp	10	1.0	2.0	230	na	0.0	na	na	0%
(LàCasita) mild, chunky	2 oz	16	<1.0	4.0	226	na	0.0	0.0	0	0%
(Old El Paso) hot	2 tbsp	10	<1.0	2.0	160	na	<1.0	na	0	<43%
(Old El Paso) medium	2 tbsp	10	<1.0	2.0	160	na	<1.0	na	0	<43%
(Old El Paso) mild	2 tbsp	10	<1.0	2.0	160	na	<1.0	na	0	<43%
(Ortega)	1 oz	10	0.0	2.0	300	(mq)	0.0	0.0	0	0%
(Rosarita)	1.093 oz	7	0.4	1.3	247	.2	0.1	0.0	0	12%
RANCHERA										
(La Victoria)	1 tbsp	6	<1.0	1.0	85	(mq)	<1.0	(tr)	0	<53%
(Ortega)	1 oz	12	0.0	3.0	250	(mq)	0.0	0.0	0	0%

Food Name	Serving Size	Calories	Prot. gms	Carbs gms	Sod. mgs	Fiber gms	Fat gms	Sat. Fat gms	Chol. mgs	% Fat Cal.
ROJA *(Del Monte)* mild	1/4 cup	20	0.0	4.0	510	(mq)	0.0	0.0	0	0%
TACO										
(Nabisco) 'Hot Thick and Smooth'	1 tbsp	8	0.0	2.0	105	0	0.0	0.0	0	0%
(Nabisco) 'Medium Thick and Smooth'	1 tbsp	8	0.0	2.0	105	0	0.0	0.0	0	0%
(Nabisco) 'Mild Thick and Smooth'	1 tbsp	8	0.0	2.0	115	0	0.0	0.0	0	0%
(Ortega) hot	1 oz	10	0.0	2.0	300	(mq)	0.0	0.0	0	0%
(Ortega) mild	1 oz	10	0.0	2.0	290	(mq)	0.0	0.0	0	0%
(Rosarita) medium, chunky	3 tbsp	25	1.0	6.0	310	<1.0	<1.0	(mq)	0	<24%
(Rosarita) mild	2 oz	27	1.0	6.1	304	.1	0.1	tr	<1	3%
(Rosarita) mild, chunky	3 tbsp	25	1.0	6.0	300	<1.0	<1.0	(mq)	0	<24%
TOMATILLO										
(Rosarita) green 'de Mexico Style'	2 tbsp	20	1.0	4.0	190	na	<1.0	na	0	<31%
(Rosarita) medium	1.093 oz	8	0.1	1.8	188	.5	0.2	0.0	0	19%
TRADITIONAL *(Rosarita)* 'de Mexico Style'	2 tbsp	12	1.0	3.0	350	na	0.0	na	0	0%
VERDE *(Old El Paso)* Thick `n Chunky'	2 tbsp	10	<1.0	2.0	135	(mq)	<1.0	0.0	0	<43%
VERY LOW SODIUM *(Pritikin)*	1/4 cup	25	1.0	5.0	15	na	0.0	na	0	0%
SALSIFY / oyster plant / vegetable oyster										
boiled, drained	4 oz	77	3.1	17.4	18	3.5	0.2	(tr)	0	2%
boiled, drained, sliced	1/2 cup	46	1.9	10.5	11	2.1	0.1	na	0	2%
raw, sliced	1/2 cup	55	2.2	12.5	13	2.2	0.1	na	0	2%
raw, trimmed	1 oz	23	0.9	5.3	6	>.5 c	0.1	(tr)	0	4%
raw, untrimmed	1 lb	325	13.0	73.4	79	>7.1 c	0.8	na	0	2%
SALSIFY, BLACK /scorzonera										
raw	1 lb	372	15.0	84.4	91	(mq)	0.1	(tr)	0	0%
raw	1 oz	23	0.9	5.3	6	(mq)	tr	(tr)	0	0%
SALT										
iodized *(Morton)*	1 tsp	0	0.0	0.0	2300	0	0.0	0.0	0	0%
kosher *(Morton)*	1 tsp	0	0.0	0.0	1880	0	0.0	0.0	0	0%
mixture 'Lite Salt' *(Morton)*	1 tsp	<1	0.0	tr	1100	0	0.0	0.0	0	0%
non-iodized *(Morton)*	1 tsp	0	0.0	0.0	2300	0	0.0	0.0	0	0%
plain	1 cup	0	0.0	0.0	112398	0	0.0	0.0	0	0%
plain	1 tbsp	0	0.0	0.0	6976	0	0.0	0.0	0	0%
plain	1 tsp	0	0.0	0.0	2325	0	0.0	0.0	0	0%
sea *(Hain)*	1 tsp	0	0.0	0.0	2255	0	0.0	0.0	0	0%
SALT, ALTERNATIVE										
Plain										
(Estee) 'Salt-It'	1/8 tsp	0	0.0	0.0	0	0	0.0	0.0	0	0%
(Featherweight)	1/4 tsp	0	0.0	0.0	0	0	0.0	0.0	0	0%
(Lawry's) 'Salt-Free'	1 tsp	10	0.3	1.8	2	>.4 c	0.2	(tr)	0	18%
(Morton)	1 tsp	<1	0.0	0.1	<1	na	0.0	0.0	0	0%
Seasoned										
(Estee) 'Seasoned Salt-It'	1/8 tsp	0	0.0	0.0	0	na	0.0	0.0	0	0%
(Featherweight)	1/4 tsp	0	0.0	0.0	0	0	0.0	0.0	0	0%
(Health Valley) all-purpose 'Instead of Salt'	1 tsp	11	0.5	1.5	3	0	0.5	(tr)	0	36%
(Lawry's) 'Salt-Free'	1 tsp	3	0.1	0.6	7	>.1 c	<.1	(tr)	0	<24%
(Morton)	1 tsp	2	<.1	0.5	<1	na	<.1	(tr)	0	<27%
SALT PORK, cured *(Hormel)*	2 oz	320	4.0	0.0	1800	0	33.0	10.0	40	95%
SALT SEASONING										
(Lawry's)	1 tsp	4	0.1	0.6	1367	>.1 c	0.1	(tr)	0	24%
(Lawry's) 'Hot 'n Spicy'	1 tsp	3	0.1	1.5	79	>.1 c	0.1	(tr)	0	12%
(Lawry's) 'Lite'	1 tsp	8	0.3	1.7	357	>.1 c	<.1	(tr)	0	<10%
(Morton)	1 tsp	4	<1.0	<1.0	1300	na	<.1	(tr)	0	<10%
(Morton) 'Nature's Seasons'	1 tsp	3	<.1	<1.0	1400	na	<.1	(tr)	0	<17%
(Schilling)	1 tsp	4	0.2	0.6	980	na	na	(tr)	0	0%

Food Name	Serving Size	Calories	Prot. gms	Carbs gms	Sod. mgs	Fiber gms	Fat gms	Sat. Fat gms	Chol. mgs	% Fat Cal.
(Schilling) 'Salt 'n Spice'	1 tsp	3	0.2	0.6	939	na	na	(tr)	0	0%
SANDWICH										
BEEF										
(Hot Pockets) frozen, pocket, and cheddar	5 oz	370	17.0	36.0	1390	(mq)	17.0	(mq)	60	42%
(Lean Pockets) frozen, pocket, and broccoli	1 pkg	250	11.0	30.0	760	(mq)	8.0	(mq)	(mq)	31%
(Manwich) extra thick and chunky, prepared	1 sandwich	330	17.0	36.0	870	3.0	13.0	4.7	50	36%
(Manwich) Mexican, prepared	1 sandwich	310	17.0	30.0	690	2.0	13.0	4.7	50	38%
(Manwich) original, prepared	1 sandwich	320	17.0	31.0	590	2.0	13.0	4.7	50	38%
(Manwich) 'Sloppy Joe' prepared	1 sandwich	310	17.0	31.0	620	1.0	13.0	4.7	50	38%
(Tyson) frozen, barbecue, microwave	1 sandwich	200	15.0	29.0	600	na	2.7	na	30	12%
CANADIAN BACON										
(Quick Meal) muffin, w/egg and cheese	4.5 oz	250	16.0	29.0	680	na	8.0	4.0	115	29%
CHEESEBURGER										
(Kid Cuisine) frozen	6.25 oz	400	12.0	47.0	550	(mq)	19.0	(mq)	40	42%
(Kid Cuisine) frozen, double 'Mega Meal'	9.1 oz	480	20.0	55.0	1040	na	20.0	na	na	38%
(MicroMagic) frozen	4.75 oz	450	17.0	29.0	790	(mq)	25.0	(mq)	80	55%
CHICKEN										
(Banquet) patties, breast meat 'Microwave'	4 oz	310	16.0	31.0	664	(mq)	14.0	(mq)	(mq)	40%
(BestFresh) breast, teriyaki, charbroiled	1 sandwich	490	34.0	45.0	1030	6.0	20.0	4.0	60	36%
(BestFresh) w/cucumber yogurt dressing	1 sandwich	390	24.0	38.0	960	1.0	15.0	4.0	70	35%
(Hot Pockets) frozen, pocket, and cheddar	5 oz	310	16.0	38.0	720	(mq)	11.0	(mq)	(mq)	31%
(Kid Cuisine)	8.2 oz	470	16.0	61.0	830	na	17.0	na	40	33%
(Lean Pockets) frozen, pocket, Oriental	1 pkg	250	14.0	35.0	840	(mq)	6.0	(mq)	(mq)	22%
(Lean Pockets) frozen, pocket, Parmesan	1 pkg	270	19.0	35.0	750	(mq)	6.0	(mq)	(mq)	20%
(Lean Pockets) frozen, pocket, white meat only 'Fajita' ...	1 sandwich	250	13.0	36.0	810	na	6.0	2.0	30	22%
(Lean Pockets) frozen, pocket, white meat only, glazed 'Supreme'	1 sandwich	240	10.0	35.0	630	na	7.0	3.0	30	26%
(MicroMagic) frozen	4.5 oz	390	13.0	42.0	650	(mq)	16.0	(mq)	35	40%
(Quick Meal)	4.3 oz	320	16.0	40.0	640	na	11.0	2.0	65	31%
(Quick Meal) biscuit	4.2 oz	310	13.0	36.0	900	na	13.0	na	50	37%
(Quick Meal) grilled	4.7 oz	300	21.0	35.0	620	na	9.0	na	60	27%
(Tyson) boneless, grilled	3.5 oz	200	15.0	25.0	470	na	5.0	na	32	22%
(Tyson) breast, boneless, grilled	3.5 oz	150	17.0	2.0	400	na	8.0	na	44	49%
(Tyson) frozen, barbecue 'Microwave'	4 oz	230	16.0	27.0	510	(mq)	6.0	(mq)	(mq)	24%
(Tyson) frozen, breast 'Microwave'	3.5 oz	275	14.0	27.0	(mq)	(mq)	12.0	(mq)	(mq)	40%
(Tyson) frozen, mini 'Microwave'	3.5 oz	230	12.0	39.0	(mq)	(mq)	5.0	(mq)	(mq)	18%
(Ultimate 200) grilled	4 oz	200	18.0	22.0	420	na	5.0	2.0	20	22%
EGG										
(Jimmy Dean) frozen, w/egg and cheese	1 biscuit	300	11.0	28.0	890	2.0	16.0	6.0	95	48%
(Jimmy Dean) frozen, w/ham and cheese	1 biscuit	240	13.0	26.0	720	1.0	10.0	3.0	100	38%
(Jimmy Dean) w/sausage and cheese	1 biscuit	390	14.0	28.0	1040	2.0	27.0	10.0	115	62%
(Swanson) frozen, w/beefsteak and cheese 'Great Starts'	4.9 oz	360	17.0	27.0	730	(mq)	20.0	(mq)	(mq)	51%
(Swanson) frozen, w/Canadian bacon and cheese 'Great Starts'	5.2 oz	420	16.0	37.0	1845	(mq)	22.0	(mq)	(mq)	48%
(Swanson) frozen, w/Canadian bacon and cheese 'Great Starts'	4.1 oz	290	15.0	25.0	770	(mq)	15.0	(mq)	(mq)	46%
(Swanson) frozen, w/sausage and cheese 'Great Starts'	5.5 oz	460	18.0	35.0	1310	(mq)	28.0	(mq)	(mq)	54%
ENGLISH MUFFIN *(Weight Watchers)*	4 oz	240	14.0	29.0	540	na	8.0	2.0	15	30%
FISH FILLET *(Quick Meal)*	5.2 oz	430	16.0	56.0	910	na	16.0	4.0	68	33%
HAM AND CHEESE										
(Hot Pockets) frozen, pocket	5 oz	360	19.0	36.0	1320	(mq)	16.0	(mq)	90	40%
(Owens) refrigerated 'Border Breakfasts'	2 oz	150	7.0	14.0	600	(mq)	6.0	(mq)	(mq)	39%
(Swanson) refrigerated, bagel 'Great Starts'	3 oz	240	12.0	28.0	600	(mq)	8.0	(mq)	(mq)	31%

Food Name	Serving Size	Calories	Prot. gms	Carbs gms	Sod. mgs	Fiber gms	Fat gms	Sat. Fat gms	Chol. mgs	% Fat Cal.
(Ultimate 200) frozen, pocket	4 oz	200	14.0	24.0	490	na	6.0	2.0	5	26%
(Weight Watchers) bagel	3 oz	210	13.0	28.0	460	na	6.0	2.0	15	25%
HAMBURGER (MicroMagic) frozen	4 oz	350	13.0	26.0	500	(mq)	18.0	(mq)	55	51%
HOT DOG										
(Kid Cuisine)	6.7 oz	450	13.0	27.0	880	na	19.0	na	40	52%
(Kid Cuisine) 'Mega Meal'	8.25 oz	500	16.0	52.0	1260	na	25.0	na	na	45%
OMELET										
(Weight Watchers) 'Classic'	3.84 oz	210	14.0	22.0	410	na	7.0	4.0	30	30%
(Weight Watchers) 'Garden'	3.60 oz	210	9.0	28.0	480	na	6.0	2.0	15	27%
PIZZA										
(Amy's Kitchen) frozen, pocket, cheese calzone, organic	4.5 oz	313	15.0	41.0	272	4.0	9.0	na	24	27%
(Hot Pockets) frozen, pocket, pepperoni	5 oz	380	17.0	40.0	1240	(mq)	17.0	(mq)	45	40%
(Hot Pockets) frozen, pocket, sausage	5 oz	360	15.0	40.0	590	(mq)	16.0	(mq)	65	40%
(Lean Pockets) frozen, pocket 'Deluxe'	1 pkg	280	14.0	34.0	500	(mq)	9.0	(mq)	na	30%
(Lean Pockets) frozen, pocket, sausage and pepperoni 'Deluxe'	1 sandwich	300	13.0	37.0	670	na	11.0	5.0	35	33%
(Ultimate 200) pocket 'Deluxe'	4 oz	200	15.0	25.0	400	na	5.0	3.0	5	22%
PORK (Quick Meal) barbecue	4.3 oz	350	16.0	40.0	550	na	14.0	5.0	65	36%
RIB (Swanson) hot, smothered	10.25 oz	340	13.0	50.0	690	na	10.0	na	25	26%
SAUSAGE										
(Jimmy Dean) refrigerated, microwave	1 sandwich	160	5.0	10.0	360	na	11.0	na	na	62%
(Owens) refrigerated, biscuit 'Border Breakfasts'	2 oz	210	6.0	14.0	400	(mq)	14.0	(mq)	(mq)	61%
(Owens) refrigerated, biscuit, smoked 'Border Breakfasts'	2 oz	200	4.0	15.0	786	(mq)	6.0	(mq)	(mq)	42%
(Owens) refrigerated, biscuit, w/egg and cheese 'Border Breakfasts'	2.5 oz	250	8.0	15.0	500	(mq)	15.0	(mq)	(mq)	60%
(Quick Meal) biscuit	3.7 oz	350	10.0	29.0	870	na	22.0	na	40	56%
(Quick Meal) biscuit, w/cheese	4.3 oz	420	13.0	31.0	1060	na	27.0	10.0	60	58%
(Quick Meal) biscuit, w/egg	4.5 oz	350	11.0	30.0	780	na	21.0	na	110	54%
(Quick Meal) muffin, w/egg and cheese	5.1 oz	76	3.0	5.0	143	na	4.0	na	26	53%
(Swanson) frozen, biscuit, w/egg 'Great Starts'	4.7 oz	410	14.0	36.0	1180	(mq)	22.0	(mq)	(mq)	50%
(Weight Watchers) frozen, biscuit 'Microwave'	3 oz	220	11.0	19.0	560	na	11.0	2.0	70	45%
SUBMARINE (BestFresh) 'Deluxe'	1 sandwich	790	39.0	59.0	2070	8.0	44.0	17.0	105	50%
TURKEY										
(BestFresh) smoked	1 sandwich	580	39.0	49.0	1770	7.0	26.0	10.0	80	40%
(Healthy Deli) w/corned beef 'Doubledecker'	1 oz	30	5.1	0.6	195	0	0.7	(mq)	12	22%
(Healthy Deli) w/ham 'Doubledecker'	1 oz	30	4.8	0.8	185	0	0.9	(mq)	11	27%
(Hot Pockets) pocket, frozen, w/ham and cheese	5 oz	320	17.0	37.0	780	(mq)	11.0	(mq)	(mq)	31%
(Lean Pockets) pocket, frozen, w/broccoli and cheese	1 sandwich	260	13.0	32.0	680	na	9.0	3.0	30	31%
VEGETABLE										
(Ken & Robert's) pocket, barbecue style 'Truly Amazing'	5 oz	320	11.0	50.0	560	1.5	10.0	0.6	0	27%
(Ken & Robert's) pocket, broccoli cheddar 'Truly Amazing'	5 oz	275	11.0	37.0	540	.1	9.0	0.7	0	30%
(Ken & Robert's) pocket, Greek style 'Truly Amazing'	5 oz	270	11.0	35.0	500	tr	10.0	1.0	0	33%
(Ken & Robert's) pocket, Indian style 'Truly Amazing'	5 oz	300	9.6	41.0	500	.9	12.0	1.0	0	35%
(Ken & Robert's) pocket, Oriental style 'Truly Amazing'	5 oz	295	9.6	40.8	572	.9	12.0	0.9	0	35%
(Ken & Robert's) pocket, pizza style 'Truly Amazing'	5 oz	315	12.0	42.0	620	1.2	12.0	1.0	0	33%
(Ken & Robert's) pocket, Tex Mex style 'Truly Amazing'	5 oz	310	11.0	43.0	595	.3	11.0	1.0	0	31%
SANDWICH SEASONING MIX, dry (Manwich)	.25 oz	20	<1.0	5.0	350	<1.0	<1.0	na	0	<27%
SANDWICH SPREAD. See also LUNCHEON MEAT, CANNED; POTTED MEAT SPREAD.										
'Chub' (Oscar Mayer)	1 oz	67	2.0	4.3	273	0	4.7	1.8	10	63%
pork and beef	1 oz	67	2.2	3.4	287	0	4.9	1.7	11	66%
pork and beef	1 tbsp	35	1.1	1.8	152	0	2.6	0.9	6	67%
SAPODILLA										
approx 7.5 oz	1 med	141	0.8	33.9	20	9.0	1.9	na	0	11%
pulp	1 cup	200	1.1	48.1	29	12.7	2.7	na	0	11%

Food Name	Serving Size	Calories	Prot. gms	Carbs gms	Sod. mgs	Fiber gms	Fat gms	Sat. Fat gms	Chol. mgs	% Fat Cal
trimmed	1 oz	24	0.1	5.7	3	1.5	0.3	na	0	10%
untrimmed	1 lb	300	1.6	72.5	44	19.2	4.0	na	0	11%
SAPOTE/marmalade plum										
trimmed	1 oz	38	0.6	9.6	3	>.5 c	0.2	na	0	4%
trimmed, approx 11.2 oz	1 med	301	4.8	76.0	23	5.8	1.4	na	0	4%
untrimmed	1 lb	431	6.8	108.7	31	>6.1 c	1.9	na	0	4%
SARDINE										
ATLANTIC										
in soybean oil, drained	3.75-oz can	191	22.6	0.0	465	0	10.5	1.4	131	51%
in soybean oil, drained	2 oz	118	14.8	0.0	286	0	6.5	0.9	81	50%
in soybean oil, drained, approx .8 oz	2 med	50	5.9	0.0	121	0	2.8	0.4	34	52%
BRISLING, w/liquid (Underwood)	3.75-oz can	260	19.0	1.0	450	0	20.0	(mq)	(mq)	69%
MAINE										
in mustard sauce, drained (Beach Cliff)	3 oz	227	13.0	4.0	350	na	18.0	na	na	70%
in soybean oil, drained (Beach Cliff)	3 oz	240	16.0	0.0	20	na	20.0	na	na	74%
in tomato sauce, drained (Beach Cliff)	3 oz	210	15.0	0.0	350	na	17.0	na	na	72%
in water, drained (Beach Cliff)	3 oz	230	17.0	1.0	350	na	18.0	na	na	69%
MIXED										
'Kippered Snacks' (Brunswick)	3.5 oz	185	16.0	1.0	610	0	14.0	(mq)	(mq)	65%
in mustard sauce (Underwood)	3.75 oz	220	16.0	2.0	650	na	16.0	(mq)	(mq)	67%
in oil (Featherweight)	1 7/8 oz	130	19.0	1.0	65	0	10.0	(mq)	45	53%
in soya oil, drained (Underwood)	3.75 oz	230	16.0	1.0	400	na	18.0	na	na	70%
in Tabasco sauce, drained (Underwood)	3 oz	220	16.0	1.0	400	na	16.0	(mq)	(mq)	68%
in tomato sauce (Del Monte)	1/2 cup	360	19.0	45.0	540	(mq)	12.0	(mq)	(mq)	30%
in tomato sauce (Underwood)	3.75 oz	220	16.0	2.0	500	na	16.0	(mq)	(mq)	67%
in water (Featherweight)	1 7/8 oz	95	9.0	1.0	65	0	7.0	(mq)	20	61%
NORWAY										
in mild sardine oil, drained (Empress)	3.75-oz can	260	19.0	1.0	(mq)	0	20.0	(mq)	(mq)	69%
in mild sardine oil, w/liquid (Empress)	3.75-oz can	460	19.0	1.0	(mq)	0	42.0	(mq)	(mq)	83%
NORWEGIAN BRISLING (S&W)	1.5 oz	130	10.0	0.0	220	0	10.0	(mq)	(mq)	69%
PACIFIC										
in tomato sauce, drained	13 oz	659	60.5	0.0	1532	.3	44.3	11.4	226	62%
in tomato sauce, drained	2 oz	101	9.3	1.0	235	2.2	6.8	1.8	35	60%
in tomato sauce, drained, approx 1.3 oz	1 med	68	6.2	0.0	157	.2	4.6	1.2	23	63%
SAUCE. See also APPLESAUCE; BARBECUE SAUCE; CRANBERRY SAUCE; SALSA; TOMATO SAUCE.										
ALFREDO SAUCE										
(Betty Crocker) 'Recipe Sauces'	4 oz	190	1.0	8.0	650	na	17.0	6.0	20	81%
(Contadina)	4 oz	350	6.0	6.0	500	na	34.0	20.0	100	86%
(Contadina) 'Fresh' refrigerated	6 oz	540	9.0	10.0	620	na	53.0	(mq)	85	86%
(Contadina) 'Light' refrigerated	3.33 oz	150	7.0	7.0	460	na	10.0	na	40	62%
(DiGiorno) reduced fat 'Lighter Varieties'	1/4 cup	180	5.0	15.0	580	na	11.0	6.0	35	55%
(DiGiorno) refrigerated	2 oz	200	4.0	2.0	490	na	20.0	12.0	55	88%
(Progresso) 'Authentic Pasta Sauces'	1/2 cup	340	13.0	6.0	1080	na	30.0	19.0	95	78%
APPLE-APRICOT SAUCE										
(Lucky Leaf/ Musselman's) 'Fruit n' Sauce'	4 oz	90	0.0	22.0	20	(mq)	0.0	0.0	0	0%
APPLE-CHERRY SAUCE										
(Lucky Leaf/ Musselman's) 'Fruit n' Sauce'	4 oz	100	0.0	24.0	20	(mq)	0.0	0.0	0	0%
APPLE-CRANBERRY SAUCE										
(Lucky Leaf/Musselman's) 'Fruit n' Sauce'	4 oz	80	0.0	19.0	15	(tr)	0.0	0.0	0	0%
APPLE-PEACH SAUCE										
(Lucky Leaf/ Musselman's) 'Fruit n' Sauce'	4 oz	90	0.0	22.0	20	(mq)	0.0	0.0	0	0%
APPLE-PINEAPPLE SAUCE										
(Lucky Leaf/ Musselman's) 'Fruit n' Sauce'	4 oz	110	0.0	26.0	20	(mq)	0.0	0.0	0	0%

Food Name	Serving Size	Calories	Prot. gms	Carbs gms	Sod. mgs	Fiber gms	Fat gms	Sat. Fat gms	Chol. mgs	% Fat Cal.
APPLE-STRAWBERRY SAUCE										
(Lucky Leaf/ Musselman's) 'Fruit n' Sauce'	4 oz	100	0.0	24.0	20	(mq)	0.0	0.0	0	0%
BASIL-HERB SAUCE (Golden Dipt) 'Nature Bay'	2 grams	8	0.0	1.0	36	na	0.0	na	0	0%
BEARNAISE SAUCE (Great Impressions)	2 tbsp	192	0.5	0.2	148	na	21.0	(mq)	48	99%
BEEF SAUCE										
(Ragu) barbecue 'Beef Tonight'	4 oz	70	2.0	15.0	580	na	<1.0	na	0	<12%
(Ragu) skillet lasagna 'Beef Tonight'	4 oz	60	3.0	9.0	630	na	1.0	na	5	16%
(Ragu) Stroganoff 'Beef Tonight'	4 oz	130	1.0	6.0	770	na	12.0	na	10	83%
BOLOGNESE SAUCE										
(Contadina)	5 oz	130	8.0	0.0	500	na	7.0	1.0	25	66%
(Contadina) 'Fresh' refrigerated	7.5 oz	230	22.0	12.0	600	(mq)	11.0	(mq)	50	42%
(Progresso) 'Authentic Pasta Sauces'	1/2 cup	150	10.0	12.0	520	2.6	8.0	2.0	20	45%
BROWN GRAVY SAUCE (LaChoy)	3.139 oz	284	2.2	68.5	400	0	0.1	0.0	0	0%
BROWNING SAUCE (Gravymaster)	1 tsp	12	0.5	2.4	<1	tr	tr	(tr)	0	0%
CACCIATORE SAUCE (Recipe Sauces)	3.9 oz	40	1.0	9.0	570	na	<1.0	na	0	<18%
CARBONARA SAUCE (DiGiorno) refrigerated	2 oz	200	4.0	3.0	380	na	19.0	9.0	40	86%
CHARDONNAY SAUCE (Golden Dipt) 'Nature Bay'	1 oz	60	0.0	1.0	160	na	6.0	na	0	93%
CHEDDAR CHEESE SAUCE										
(J. Hungerford) 'Stadium'	2.011 oz	80	1.0	6.0	500	0	5.0	1.5	4	62%
(Lucky Leaf/Musselman's)	4 oz	220	3.0	12.0	1000	0	18.0	(mq)	(mq)	73%
(Lucky Leaf/Musselman's) aged	4 oz	240	5.0	11.0	920	0	20.0	(mq)	(mq)	74%
(Lucky Leaf/Musselman's) aged, mild	4 oz	200	5.0	9.0	790	0	18.0	(mq)	(mq)	74%
(Lucky Leaf/Musselman's) aged, sharp	4 oz	230	9.0	6.0	850	0	17.0	(mq)	(mq)	72%
CHEESE SAUCE										
(Snow's) Welsh rarebit	1/2 cup	170	9.0	10.0	460	na	11.0	na	na	57%
(White House) aged	3.5 oz	213	4.0	10.0	810	0	18.0	(mq)	(mq)	74%
CHICKEN SAUCE										
(Ragu) cacciatore 'Chicken Tonight'	4 oz	70	1.0	12.0	490	na	2.0	na	0	26%
(Ragu) country French 'Chicken Tonight'	4 oz	140	1.0	6.0	730	na	12.0	na	5	79%
(Ragu) creamy, primavera 'Chicken Tonight'	4 oz	90	1.0	9.0	650	na	6.0	na	5	57%
(Ragu) creamy, w/mushrooms 'Chicken Tonight'	4 oz	110	1.0	5.0	650	na	10.0	na	5	79%
(Ragu) herbed, w/wine 'Chicken Tonight'	4 oz	100	2.0	13.0	610	na	4.0	na	5	38%
(Ragu) honey mustard, light 'Chicken Tonight'	4 oz	50	1.0	12.0	420	na	<1.0	0.0	0	<15%
(Ragu) sweet and sour 'Chicken Tonight'	4 oz	80	0.0	19.0	280	na	0.0	na	0	0%
(Ragu) sweet and spicy, light 'Chicken Tonight'	4 oz	50	2.0	10.0	390	na	<1.0	0.0	0	<16%
CHILI SAUCE										
(Chef Boyardee) hot dog, w/beef	1 oz	30	1.0	4.0	140	(mq)	1.0	na	na	31%
(Del Monte) tomato	1/4 cup	70	1.0	17.0	835	(mq)	0.0	0.0	0	0%
(El Molino) green, mild	2 tbsp	10	0.0	2.0	210	(mq)	0.0	0.0	0	0%
(Featherweight)	1 tbsp	8	0.0	2.0	10	(mq)	0.0	0.0	0	0%
(Gebhardt) hot dog	2 tbsp	20	1.0	2.0	150	(mq)	1.0	na	na	43%
(Heinz)	1 oz	30	0.0	7.0	430	0	0.0	0.0	0	0%
(Hunt's)	1.199 oz	35	0.3	8.0	393	.7	0.1	0.0	0	3%
(Las Palmas) red	1/2 cup	25	1.0	3.0	670	0	1.0	na	0	36%
(Manwich) 'Chili Fixin's'	5.3 oz	110	6.0	20.0	900	5.0	<1.0	na	0	<8%
(S&W) 'Chili Makin's'	1/2 cup	100	5.0	20.0	782	(mq)	1.0	na	0	8%
(Wolf Brand) hot dog	1.25 oz	44	1.5	4.4	199	>.4 c	2.3	(mq)	na	47%
CHOCOLATE SAUCE (Chocolate Mountain)	2 tbsp	120	1.0	20.0	80	na	4.0	na	4	30%
CLAM SAUCE										
Red										
(Buitoni)	5 oz	190	8.0	28.0	560	(mq)	6.0	1.0	20	27%
(Contadina) 'Fresh' refrigerated	7.5 oz	120	7.0	15.0	800	(mq)	4.0	(mq)	35	29%
(Ferrara)	4 oz	70	5.0	8.0	320	(mq)	2.0	0.0	10	26%
(Progresso)	1/2 cup	70	5.0	7.0	560	(mq)	3.0	(mq)	(mq)	36%

Food Name	Serving Size	Calories	Prot, gms	Carbs gms	Sod. mgs	Fiber gms	Fat gms	Sat. Fat gms	Chol. mgs	% Fat Cal.
White										
(Contadina) 'Fresh' refrigerated	6 oz	290	8.0	13.0	800	(mq)	23.0	(mq)	94	71%
(Ferrara)	4 oz	80	5.0	4.0	570	(mq)	5.0	1.0	10	56%
(Progresso)	1/2 cup	110	9.0	1.0	280	(mq)	8.0	(mq)	(mq)	64%
COCKTAIL SAUCE										
(Del Monte)	1/4 cup	70	1.0	17.0	765	na	0.0	0.0	0	0%
(Estee)	1 tbsp	10	<1.0	2.0	35	na	<1.0	<1.0	0	<43%
(Golden Dipt) extra hot	1 tbsp	20	0.0	5.0	210	na	0.0	0.0	0	0%
(Golden Dipt) regular	1 tbsp	20	0.0	5.0	210	na	0.0	0.0	0	0%
(Great Impressions)	1 tbsp	21	0.2	4.7	182	na	0.1	(tr)	0	4%
(Great Impressions) 'Brandy Glow'	1 tbsp	68	0.2	1.6	106	na	6.7	(mq)	10	89%
(Great Impressions) 'Low Salt'	1 tbsp	21	0.2	4.8	6	na	0.1	(tr)	0	4%
(Sauceworks)	1 tbsp	14	0.0	3.0	170	na	0.0	0.0	0	0%
(Skipper's)	1 tbsp	20	0.0	5.0	216	na	0.0	0.0	0	0%
(Stokely)	1 tbsp	18	0.0	5.0	90	na	0.0	0.0	0	0%
CRANBERRY-ORANGE SAUCE										
(Ocean Spray) crushed, for chicken 'Cran•Fruit'	2 oz	90	0.0	23.0	10	na	0.0	na	na	0%
CRANBERRY-RASPBERRY SAUCE										
(Ocean Spray) crushed, for chicken 'Cran•Fruit'	2 oz	90	0.0	23.0	10	na	0.0	na	na	0%
CREOLE SAUCE										
(Enrico's) Cajun 'Light'	4 oz	76	2.0	9.0	284	na	2.8	(mq)	0	36%
(Golden Dipt) cooking sauce	1 oz	20	0.0	2.0	190	na	1.0	na	0	53%
DIABLO SAUCE *(Escoffier)*	1 tbsp	20	0.0	4.0	160	na	0.0	0.0	0	0%
DIJONAISSE SAUCE *(Golden Dipt)* cooking sauce	1 oz	52	0.0	2.0	130	na	4.0	na	0	82%
ENCHILADA SAUCE										
(Gebhardt)	3 tbsp	25	<1.0	3.0	170	<1.0	1.0	0.7	<1	36%
(La Victoria)	1 cup	80	1.0	10.0	1520	(tr)	5.0	(mq)	0	51%
(Rosarita)	3 oz	20	0.0	4.0	430	(tr)	0.0	0.0	0	0%
Green *(Old El Paso)*	2 tbsp	11	<1.0	3.0	200	0	0.0	0.0	0	0%
Hot										
(Del Monte)	1/2 cup	45	1.0	11.0	1090	(tr)	0.0	0.0	0	0%
(El Molino)	2 tbsp	16	0.0	2.0	100	(tr)	1.0	na	0	53%
(Las Palmas)	1/2 cup	25	1.0	3.0	670	0	1.0	na	0	36%
(Old El Paso)	1/4 cup	30	<1.0	4.0	250	(tr)	1.0	na	0	31%
(Ortega)	1 oz	12	0.0	3.0	280	(tr)	0.0	0.0	0	0%
Mild										
(Del Monte)	1/2 cup	45	1.0	11.0	1150	(tr)	0.0	0.0	0	0%
(Old El Paso)	1/4 cup	25	<1.0	4.0	250	(tr)	1.0	na	0	31%
(Ortega)	1 oz	12	0.0	3.0	280	(tr)	0.0	0.0	0	0%
(Rosarita)	2.5 oz	25	<1.0	3.0	230	<1.0	1.0	<1.0	0	36%
FAJITA SAUCE *(Tio Sancho)* 'Skillet Sauce'	1 oz	14	0.5	1.8	590	>.1 c	0.5	(tr)	0	33%
FORESTIERA SAUCE *(Contadina)* 'Fresh' refrigerated	7.5 oz	270	6.0	15.0	830	na	9.0	(mq)	15	49%
FOUR CHEESE SAUCE										
(Contadina)	4 oz	300	8.0	7.0	400	na	27.0	14.0	80	80%
(Contadina) 'Fresh' refrigerated	6 oz	470	12.0	8.0	500	0	45.0	(mq)	147	84%
(DiGiorno) refrigerated	2 oz	170	4.0	3.0	340	na	16.0	9.0	45	84%
FRENCH WHITE SAUCE *(Golden Dipt)* cooking sauce	1 oz	55	0.0	3.0	210	na	4.0	na	0	75%
GARLIC-CHILI PEPPER SAUCE *(A Taste of Thai)*	1 tbsp	10	0.0	2.0	220	0	0.0	0.0	0	0%
GARLIC-HERB SAUCE *(Golden Dipt)* 'Nature Bay'	2 grams	8	0.0	1.0	87	na	0.0	na	0	0%
GUAVA SAUCE cooked	1/2 cup	43	0.4	11.3	5	4.3	0.2	0.1	0	4%
HERB AND GARLIC SAUCE *(Lawry's)* w/lemon juice	1/4 cup	36	3.6	3.8	3688	<.1	0.4	na	na	11%
HOLLANDAISE SAUCE *(Great Impressions)*	2 tbsp	192	0.5	0.3	107	(mq)	21.0	(mq)	48	98%
HONEY SOY SAUCE										
(Golden Dipt) cooking sauce	1 oz	90	0.0	5.0	250	na	8.0	na	0	78%

Food Name	Serving Size	Calories	Prot. gms	Carbs gms	Sod. mgs	Fiber gms	Fat gms	Sat. Fat gms	Chol. mgs	% Fat Cal.
(Golden Dipt) 'Nature Bay'	1 oz	90	0.0	5.0	250	na	8.0	na	0	78%
HORSERADISH SAUCE										
(Great Impressions)	1 tbsp	74	0.0	1.4	199	(mq)	7.6	(mq)	1	92%
(Heinz)	1 tbsp	74	0.2	2.0	113	(mq)	7.4	(mq)	na	88%
(Life) strong 'All Natural'	1/2 tbsp	7	<1.0	<1.0	2	(mq)	<1.0	(tr)	0	<53%
(Sauceworks)	1 tbsp	50	0.0	2.0	105	(mq)	5.0	1.0	5	85%
HOT DOG SAUCE (Just Rite)	2 oz	60	2.0	6.0	220	<1.0	3.0	1.1	7	46%
HOT PEPPER SAUCE										
(Gebhardt) 'Louisiana Style'	1/2 tsp	0	0.0	(tr)	45	(tr)	0.0	0.0	0	0%
(Tabasco)	1/4 tsp	<1	tr	<1.0	9	(tr)	tr	(tr)	0	0%
HOT SAUCE (Gebhardt)	1/2 tsp	<1	<1.0	<1.0	55	<1.0	<1.0	(mq)	0	<53%
JALAPEÑO CHEESE SAUCE										
(Pablo's) 'Deli Style'	1 oz	59	2.0	4.0	470	na	4.0	<1.0	5	60%
(White House)	3.5 oz	193	3.0	10.0	890	(tr)	16.0	(mq)	(mq)	74%
LEMON BUTTER-DILL SAUCE										
(Golden Dipt) cooking sauce	1 oz	110	0.0	5.0	180	na	10.0	1.0	0	82%
LEMON-DILL SAUCE (Golden Dipt) 'Nature Bay'	1 oz	110	0.0	3.0	150	na	11.0	na	0	89%
LOBSTER SAUCE (Progresso) rock	1/2 cup	120	4.0	11.0	430	2.0	8.0	1.0	10	55%
MARINARA SAUCE										
(Angela Mia)	4.400 oz	47	1.9	9.0	503	3.1	1.5	0.3	0	24%
(Buitoni)	1/2 cup	70	1.0	11.0	570	(mq)	3.0	<1.0	0	36%
(DiGiorno) refrigerated	5 oz	110	3.0	12.0	680	na	6.0	1.0	5	47%
(Millina's Finest) organic, fat-free	4 oz	48	2.0	9.0	210	na	0.5	na	na	9%
(Millina's Finest) Zinfandel, organic, fat-free	4 oz	44	2.0	9.0	215	na	0.5	na	na	9%
(Pathmark) 'All Natural'	1/2 cup	80	2.0	12.0	710	(mq)	2.0	(mq)	0	24%
(Pathmark) 'No Frills'	1/2 cup	80	1.0	12.0	620	(mq)	3.0	(mq)	0	34%
(Prego)	4 oz	100	1.0	10.0	620	(mq)	6.0	(mq)	0	55%
(Progresso)	1/2 cup	90	4.0	9.0	520	(mq)	5.0	1.0	1	46%
(Progresso) 'Authentic Pasta Sauces'	1/2 cup	110	4.0	10.0	250	2.4	6.0	1.5	4	49%
(Rokeach)	3 oz	60	1.0	9.0	257	(mq)	2.0	(mq)	0	31%
(Westbrae)	4 oz	40	2.0	7.0	370	na	<1.0	na	0	<20%
(Westbrae) w/mushrooms	4 oz	50	2.0	7.0	380	na	29.0	na	0	88%
MESQUITE SAUCE (Lawry's) w/lime juice	1/4 cup	24	3.0	3.0	4142	>.1 c	0.4	(tr)	0	13%
MUSHROOM SAUCE (Quincy's)	3 oz	27	1.0	5.0	366	na	<1.0	na	na	<27%
NACHO CHEESE SAUCE										
(J. Hungerford)	2.011 oz	120	2.0	7.0	440	0	9.0	2.0	5	69%
(J. Hungerford) 'Stadium'	2.011 oz	80	1.0	6.0	410	0	5.0	1.5	4	62%
(Kaukauna)	1 oz	80	3.0	4.0	330	0	6.0	(mq)	8	66%
(Lucky Leaf)	4 oz	220	4.0	11.0	1010	0	18.0	(mq)	(mq)	73%
(Musselman's)	4 oz	220	4.0	11.0	1010	0	18.0	(mq)	(mq)	73%
(Pablo's) 'Deli Style'	1 oz	59	2.0	4.0	470	na	4.0	<1.0	5	60%
(White House)	3.5 oz	193	3.0	10.0	890	0	16.0	(mq)	(mq)	74%
NEWBURG SAUCE (Snow's) w/sherry	1/3 cup	120	3.0	10.0	520	na	8.0	(mq)	na	58%
ORANGE SAUCE (LaChoy) Mandarin	1 tbsp	24	<.1	6.1	38	.1	tr	0.0	0	0%
ORANGE-DIJON SAUCE (Golden Dipt) 'Nature Bay'	1 oz	110	0.0	6.0	200	na	9.0	na	0	77%
OREGANO-HERB SAUCE (Golden Dipt) 'Nature Bay'	2 grams	6	0.0	1.0	88	na	0.0	na	0	0%
PARMIGIANA SAUCE (Betty Crocker) 'Recipe Sauces'	3.9 oz	50	2.0	9.0	430	na	1.0	<1.0	0	17%
PASTA SAUCE/spaghetti sauce										
(Angela Mia)	4.409 oz	49	1.5	10.6	607	2.5	0.5	0.0	0	9%
(Campbell's) 'Homestyle'	4 oz	40	2.0	10.0	360	2.0	0.0	na	0	0%
(Enrico's) 'All Natural'	4 oz	60	2.0	9.0	345	(mq)	1.0	na	0	17%
(Hunt's) 'Homestyle'	4 oz	60	2.0	10.0	530	2.0	2.0	0.3	0	27%
(Hunt's) 'Olde Country'	4 oz	60	2.0	8.0	560	na	2.0	na	0	31%
(Progresso)	1/2 cup	110	3.0	13.0	660	(mq)	5.0	1.0	2	41%

Food Name	Serving Size	Calories	Prot gms	Carbs gms	Sod mgs	Fiber gms	Fat gms	Sat Fat gms	Chol mgs	% Fat Cal.
(Ragu) 'Old World Style'	4 oz	80	2.0	9.0	740	na	4.0	na	0	45%
(Ragu) 'Slow Cooked Homestyle'	4 oz	110	2.0	15.0	510	na	5.0	na	0	40%
(Ragu) 'Thick & Hearty'	4 oz	100	2.0	15.0	460	(mq)	3.0	(mq)	0	28%
Garden										
(Prego) combination	4 oz	80	2.0	14.0	420	(mq)	2.0	(mq)	na	22%
(Pritikin) chunky	1/2 cup	50	2.0	11.0	30	na	0.0	na	0	0%
(Ragu) harvest 'Todays Recipe'	4 oz	50	2.0	8.0	370	na	1.0	0.0	0	18%
Garlic and herb										
(Healthy Choice)	4 oz	40	2.0	9.0	350	na	<1.0	na	0	<17%
(Hunt's) 'Classic'	4.409 oz	58	1.9	9.5	598	1.8	2.1	0.3	0	29%
(Hunt's) 'Light'	4.409 oz	39	2.2	7.3	379	2.6	0.8	0.1	0	16%
(Hunt's) 'Olde Country'	4.409 oz	63	2.3	8.9	522	3.3	2.7	0.4	0	35%
Garlic and onion										
(Campbell's) extra	4 oz	50	2.0	12.0	320	2.0	<1.0	na	0	<14%
(Del Monte)	1/2 cup	70	1.0	10.0	430	na	2.0	na	na	29%
(Healthy Choice) chunky	4 oz	40	2.0	10.0	350	na	0.0	na	0	0%
(Prego)	4 oz	110	1.0	16.0	510	(mq)	4.0	(mq)	na	35%
Italian										
(Campbell's)	4 oz	50	2.0	12.0	360	2.0	0.0	na	0	0%
(Healthy Choice) vegetable, chunky	4 oz	40	1.0	9.0	350	na	0.0	0.0	0	0%
(Hunt's) vegetable 'Olde Country'	4.409 oz	64	2.5	9.0	616	2.8	2.6	0.4	0	34%
(Pastorelli) 'Italian Chef'	4 oz	81	3.0	11.0	430	>1.1 c	3.0	(mq)	na	33%
(Ragu) 'Fresh Italian'	4 oz	90	2.0	13.0	490	(mq)	3.0	(mq)	0	31%
(Ragu) garden combination 'Chunky Gardenstyle'	4 oz	110	2.0	15.0	500	na	5.0	na	0	40%
Meat										
(Chef Boyardee) w/ground beef 'Jars'	4 oz	90	2.0	14.0	605	(mq)	3.0	(mq)	(mq)	30%
(Hunt's)	4.444 oz	65	1.9	10.9	604	1.9	2.3	0.6	3	29%
(Hunt's) 'Homestyle'	4.409 oz	56	2.2	6.9	596	1.6	2.6	1.2	2	39%
(Hunt's) 'Light'	4.409 oz	45	2.1	7.9	437	2.9	1.2	0.6	2	21%
(Hunt's) 'Olde Country'	4.409 oz	56	2.5	7.2	474	2.7	2.6	0.6	0	38%
(Ragu) 'Homestyle'	4 oz	110	2.0	15.0	510	na	5.0	na	2	40%
Meat flavor										
(Chef Boyardee)	3.75 oz	80	2.0	11.0	650	(mq)	3.0	(mq)	na	34%
(Chef Boyardee) 'Original'	3.75 oz	120	3.0	13.0	650	(mq)	6.0	(mq)	na	46%
(Contadina) 'Original Recipe'	1/2 cup	100	2.7	17.2	430	na	3.2	1.1	2	27%
(Del Monte)	1/2 cup	70	2.0	9.0	440	na	2.0	na	na	29%
(Hunt's)	4 oz	70	2.0	12.0	570	(mq)	2.0	(mq)	na	24%
(P&Q)	1/2 cup	70	1.0	11.0	510	(mq)	2.0	(mq)	na	27%
(Pathmark) 'All Natural'	1/2 cup	80	2.0	11.0	790	(mq)	3.0	(mq)	na	34%
(Pathmark) 'No Frills'	1/2 cup	90	2.0	11.0	620	(mq)	5.0	(mq)	na	46%
(Prego)	4 oz	140	2.0	20.0	660	(mq)	6.0	(mq)	na	38%
(Progresso)	1/2 cup	110	4.0	13.0	660	(mq)	5.0	1.0	5	40%
(Weight Watchers)	1/3 cup	50	2.0	9.0	440	(mq)	1.0	(mq)	na	17%
Meatless										
(Chef Boyardee) 'Jars'	4 oz	60	1.0	11.0	790	(mq)	1.0	na	na	16%
(P&Q)	1/2 cup	70	1.0	14.0	540	(mq)	1.0	na	na	13%
(Pathmark) 'All Natural'	1/2 cup	70	2.0	11.0	710	(mq)	2.0	(mq)	na	26%
(Pathmark) 'No Frills'	1/2 cup	80	1.0	11.0	583	(mq)	3.0	(mq)	na	36%
Mushroom										
(Campbell's)	4 oz	50	2.0	11.0	330	2.0	<1.0	na	0	<15%
(Campbell's) 'Healthy Request'	4 oz	50	2.0	11.0	330	2.0	<1.0	na	0	<15%
(Contadina) 'Original Recipe'	1/2 cup	90	2.1	17.5	430	na	2.3	0.4	0	21%
(Del Monte)	1/2 cup	70	1.0	11.0	440	na	2.0	na	na	27%
(Healthy Choice) chunky	4 oz	45	2.0	10.0	350	na	0.0	na	0	0%

Food Name	Serving Size	Calories	Prot. gms	Carbs gms	Sod. mgs	Fiber gms	Fat gms	Sat. Fat gms	Chol. mgs	% Fat Cal.
(Hunt's)	4.444 oz	65	1.9	10.9	604	1.9	2.3	0.3	0	29%
(Hunt's) 'Homestyle'	4.409 oz	56	2.2	6.9	586	1.6	2.6	0.4	0	39%
(Hunt's) 'Light'	4.409 oz	39	2.2	7.3	379	2.6	0.8	0.1	0	16%
(Hunt's) 'Olde Country'	4.409 oz	53	2.1	7.0	542	2.7	2.7	0.4	0	40%
(Prego) w/extra spice 'Extra Chunky'	4 oz	100	2.0	17.0	450	(mq)	3.0	(mq)	na	26%
(Ragu) chunky 'Todays Recipe'	4 oz	50	2.0	8.0	370	na	1.0	0.0	0	18%
(Ragu) 'Homestyle'	4 oz	110	2.0	15.0	530	na	2.0	na	0	21%
(Ragu) super 'Chunky Gardenstyle'	4 oz	110	2.0	15.0	500	na	5.0	na	0	40%
(Ragu) 'Thick & Hearty'	4 oz	100	2.0	15.0	460	na	3.0	na	0	28%
Mushroom and green pepper										
(Enrico's) 'All Natural'	4 oz	60	2.0	9.0	345	(mq)	1.0	na	0	17%
(Enrico's) 'All Natural No Salt Added'	4 oz	60	2.0	9.0	30	(mq)	1.0	na	0	17%
(Prego) 'Extra Chunky'	4 oz	100	2.0	14.0	410	(mq)	4.0	(mq)	na	36%
(Ragu) 'Chunky Gardenstyle'	4 oz	110	2.0	15.0	500	na	5.0	na	0	40%
Mushroom and onion										
(Prego) 'Extra Chunky'	4 oz	100	2.0	13.0	490	(mq)	4.0	(mq)	na	38%
(Ragu) 'Chunky Gardenstyle'	4 oz	110	2.0	15.0	560	na	5.0	na	0	40%
Mushroom and tomato										
(DiGiorno) w/plum tomatoes, refrigerated	5 oz	100	3.0	20.0	240	na	1.0	0.0	0	9%
(Millina's Finest) organic, fat-free	4 oz	45	2.0	9.0	198	na	0.5	na	na	9%
(Prego) 'Extra Chunky'	4 oz	110	1.0	14.0	500	(mq)	5.0	(mq)	na	43%
Mushroom flavor										
(Chef Boyardee)	3.75 oz	60	1.0	11.0	790	(mq)	1.0	na	na	16%
(Chef Boyardee) 'Jars'	4 oz	70	1.0	11.0	655	(mq)	2.0	(mq)	na	27%
(Chef Boyardee) 'Original'	3.75 oz	80	1.0	13.0	680	(mq)	3.0	(mq)	na	33%
(Enrico's)	4 oz	60	2.0	9.0	(mq)	(mq)	1.0	na	0	17%
(Enrico's) w/fresh mushrooms	4 oz	60	2.0	9.0	336	(mq)	1.0	na	0	17%
(Featherweight)	4 oz	60	2.0	11.0	310	(mq)	1.0	na	0	15%
(Hunt's)	4 oz	70	2.0	12.0	560	(mq)	2.0	(mq)	0	24%
(P&Q)	1/2 cup	70	1.0	14.0	580	(mq)	1.0	na	na	13%
(Pathmark) 'All Natural'	1/2 cup	70	2.0	11.0	730	(mq)	2.0	(mq)	na	26%
(Prego)	4 oz	130	2.0	20.0	630	(mq)	5.0	(mq)	na	34%
(Progresso)	1/2 cup	110	3.0	13.0	630	(mq)	5.0	1.0	5	41%
(Weight Watchers)	1/3 cup	40	1.0	9.0	430	(mq)	0.0	0.0	0	0%
No salt added										
(Eden Foods) organic	4 oz	80	3.0	14.0	0	na	2.0	na	na	21%
(Enrico's) 'All Natural No Salt Added'	4 oz	60	2.0	9.0	30	(mq)	1.0	na	0	17%
(Prego) 'No Salt Added'	4 oz	110	2.0	11.0	25	(mq)	6.0	(mq)	na	51%
Original (Pritikin)	1/2 cup	60	2.0	14.0	35	na	1.0	na	0	12%
Parmesan, 'Classic' (Hunt's)	4.409 oz	50	1.8	7.8	634	1.8	2.1	0.3	0	33%
Primavera										
(Progresso) creamy 'Authentic Pasta Sauces'	1/2 cup	190	5.0	8.0	410	1.0	17.0	10.0	54	75%
(Westbrae)	4 oz	60	2.0	7.0	490	na	3.0	na	0	43%
(Westbrae) no salt	4 oz	40	2.0	7.0	105	na	0.0	na	0	0%
Sausage and green pepper (Prego) 'Extra Chunky'	4 oz	160	3.0	19.0	500	(mq)	8.0	(mq)	(mq)	45%
Sicilian (Progresso) 'Authentic Pasta Sauces'	1/2 cup	30	<1.0	2.0	660	<1.0	2.5	<1.0	0	65%
Sweet pepper and onion (Millina's Finest) organic, fat-free	4 oz	41	2.0	7.0	305	na	0.5	na	na	11%
Three cheese (Prego)	4 oz	100	3.0	17.0	410	na	2.0	(mq)	(mq)	18%
Tomato and basil										
(Hunt's) 'Classic'	4.409 oz	48	1.8	7.5	613	3.9	2.1	0.3	0	34%
(Millina's Finest) organic, fat-free	4 oz	46	2.0	9.0	232	na	0.5	na	na	9%
Tomato and herb										
(Ragu) 'Homestyle'	4 oz	110	2.0	15.0	510	na	5.0	na	0	40%
(Ragu) 'Ragu Fine Italian'	4 oz	90	2.0	13.0	490	na	3.0	na	0	31%

Food Name	Serving Size	Calories	Prot. gms	Carbs gms	Sod. mgs	Fiber gms	Fat gms	Sat. Fat gms	Chol. mgs	% Fat Cal.
(Ragu) 'Today's Recipe'	4 oz	50	2.0	8.0	370	na	1.0	0.0	0	18%
Tomato chunks (Hunt's) 'Chunky Style'	4 oz	50	1.0	12.0	470	na	<1.0	na	0	<15%
Tomato-based										
(Prego) and basil	4 oz	100	2.0	18.0	370	(mq)	2.0	(mq)	na	18%
(Prego) and onion 'Extra Chunky'	4 oz	110	2.0	14.0	490	(mq)	5.0	(mq)	na	41%
Tomatoes, garlic, and onion (Ragu) 'Chunky Gardenstyle'	4 oz	110	2.0	15.0	500	na	5.0	na	0	40%
Traditional										
(Contadina) 'Original Recipe'	1/2 cup	90	2.0	17.0	440	na	2.3	0.4	0	21%
(Del Monte)	1/2 cup	70	1.0	11.0	430	na	2.0	na	na	27%
(Healthy Choice)	4 oz	40	2.0	9.0	380	na	<1.0	na	0	<17%
(Hunt's) 'Homestyle'	4.409 oz	56	2.2	3.9	596	1.6	2.6	0.4	0	49%
(Hunt's) 'Light'	4.409 oz	39	2.2	7.3	421	2.6	0.8	0.1	0	16%
(Hunt's) 'Olde Country'	4.409 oz	53	2.1	7.0	542	2.7	2.7	0.4	0	40%
(Hunt's) 'Traditional'	4 oz	70	2.0	12.0	530	(mq)	2.0	(mq)	0	24%
Zinfandel wine (Sutter Home)	1/2 cup	100	2.0	11.0	520	na	5.0	na	0	46%
PEPPER STEAK SAUCE (Betty Crocker) 'Recipe Sauces'	3.8 oz	50	1.0	8.0	270	na	2.0	na	0	33%
PEPPER-DILL SAUCE (Golden Dipt) 'Nature Bay'	2 grams	8	0.0	1.0	96	na	0.0	na	0	0%
PESTO SAUCE										
(Contadina) refrigerated 'Fresh'	2.33 oz	350	6.0	6.0	420	(mq)	34.0	(mq)	10	86%
(DiGiorno) refrigerated	2.3 oz	340	8.0	5.0	430	na	32.0	6.0	20	85%
PICANTE SAUCE										
(Estee)	2 tbsp	8	<1.0	2.0	60	(mq)	0.0	0.0	0	0%
(Gebhardt)	1 tbsp	4	0.0	1.0	120	(mq)	0.0	0.0	0	0%
(Wise)	2 tbsp	12	0.0	3.0	130	(mq)	0.0	0.0	0	0%
All varieties										
(Old El Paso)	2 tbsp	8	<1.0	2.0	310	(mq)	<1.0	na	0	<43%
(Old El Paso) 'Chunky'	2 tbsp	7	0.0	2.0	270	(mq)	0.0	0.0	0	0%
Extra mild (Pace) 'Thick & Chunky'	2 tsp	3	0.3	0.5	111	na	0.1	na	na	22%
Hot										
(Chi-Chi's)	1 oz	10	2.0	2.0	268	na	2.0	2.0	2	53%
(Guiltless Gourmet)	1 oz	8	0.0	1.0	133	<1.0	0.0	0.0	0	0%
(Pace) 'Thick & Chunky'	2 tsp	3	0.3	0.5	111	na	0.1	na	na	22%
(Rosarita) chunky	3 tbsp	18	<1.0	4.0	515	<1.0	<1.0	(mq)	0	<31%
(Rosarita) zesty jalapeño	1.093 oz	8	0.4	1.7	246	.7	0.2	0.0	0	18%
Medium										
(Chi-Chi's)	1 oz	8	2.0	2.0	192	na	2.0	2.0	2	53%
(Guiltless Gourmet)	1 oz	8	0.0	1.0	133	<1.0	0.0	0.0	0	0%
(Pace) 'Thick & Chunky'	2 tsp	3	0.3	0.5	111	na	0.1	na	na	22%
(Rosarita) chunky	3 tbsp	16	<1.0	4.0	650	<1.0	(mq)	(mq)	0	0%
(Rosarita) zesty jalapeño	1.093 oz	9	0.4	1.7	254	.6	0.2	0.0	0	18%
Mild										
(Azteca)	1 tbsp	4	0.0	1.0	85	(mq)	0.0	0.0	0	0%
(Chi-Chi's)	1 oz	9	2.0	2.0	198	na	2.0	2.0	2	53%
(Guiltless Gourmet)	1 oz	8	0.0	1.0	133	<1.0	0.0	0.0	0	0%
(Hunt's) 'Homestyle'	1.093 oz	11	0.5	2.1	256	.5	0.2	0.0	0	15%
(Pace) 'Thick & Chunky'	2 tsp	3	0.3	0.5	111	na	0.1	na	na	22%
(Rosarita)	3.5 oz	45	2.0	9.0	1015	(mq)	<1.0	na	0	<17%
(Rosarita) chunky	3 tbsp	25	1.0	5.0	630	<1.0	<1.0	(mq)	0	<27%
(Rosarita) zesty jalapeño	1.093 oz	8	0.5	1.7	239	.5	0.1	0.0	0	9%
PIZZA SAUCE										
(Angela Mia)	2.222 oz	27	1.4	5.2	190	1.8	0.6	0.0	0	17%
(Angela Mia) super heavy 'Premium Choice'	2.258 oz	28	2.5	5.8	36	2.9	0.5	0.0	0	12%
(Chef Boyardee) w/cheese	2.63 oz	70	1.0	7.0	385	(mq)	4.0	(mq)	(mq)	53%
(Chef Boyardee) w/cheese 'Jars'	3.88 oz	90	1.0	10.0	565	(mq)	6.0	(mq)	(mq)	55%

Food Name	Serving Size	Calories	Prot. gms	Carbs gms	Sod. mgs	Fiber gms	Fat gms	Sat. Fat gms	Chol. mgs	% Fat Cal.
(Contadina) original 'Quick & Easy'	1/4 cup	30	1.0	5.0	330	(mq)	1.0	na	na	27%
(Contadina) 'Pizza Squeeze'	1/4 cup	30	1.0	5.0	330	(mq)	1.0	na	na	27%
(Contadina) w/Italian cheese	1/4 cup	30	1.0	5.0	380	(mq)	1.0	(mq)	(mq)	27%
(Contadina) w/pepperoni	1/4 cup	40	1.0	5.0	360	(mq)	2.0	(mq)	(mq)	43%
(Eden Foods) and pasta sauce, organic	4 oz	80	3.0	10.0	320	na	3.0	na	na	34%
(Enrico's) 'Homemade Style All Natural'	4 oz	60	2.0	9.0	(mq)	(mq)	1.0	na	0	17%
(Enrico's) 'Homemade Style All Natural No Salt'	4 oz	60	2.0	9.0	30	(mq)	1.0	na	0	17%
(Hunt's)	2.363 oz	32	1.8	4.9	416	1.5	1.1	0.0	0	27%
(Hunt's)	2.222 oz	21	1.3	3.8	251	1.6	0.5	0.0	0	18%
(Pastorelli) 'Italian Chef'	4 oz	90	3.0	12.0	430	(mq)	3.0	na	na	31%
(Pizza Quick)	3 tbsp	35	1.0	3.0	330	(mq)	2.0	na	0	53%
(Pizza Quick) traditional	1.7 oz	35	1.0	3.0	330	na	2.0	na	0	53%
PLUM SAUCE *(LaChoy)* tangy	1 oz	45	0.1	10.8	17	(mq)	0.1	(tr)	0	2%
RIB SAUCE *(Dip n' Joy)* 'Saucy Rib'	1 oz	60	0.0	14.0	250	na	0.0	0.0	0	0%
RIGOLLETO SAUCE *(DiGiorno)* refrigerated	5 oz	110	2.0	9.0	660	na	8.0	1.0	0	62%
ROBERT SAUCE *(Escoffier)* 'Sauce Robert'	1 tbsp	20	0.0	5.0	70	tr	0.0	0.0	0	0%
SANDWICH SAUCE										
(Hormel) 'Not-so-Sloppy Sloppy Joe'	2.24 oz	70	1.0	16.0	730	na	1.0	0.0	5	12%
(Libby's) 'Sloppy Joe'	2.5 oz	45	1.0	10.0	na	na	<1.0	na	440	<17%
(Manwich)	2.5 oz	40	1.0	10.0	390	na	0.0	0.0	na	0%
(Manwich) bold	2.222 oz	62	0.5	13.1	802	.8	1.1	0.0	0	15%
(Manwich) extra thick and chunky	2.5 oz	60	1.0	15.0	640	na	<1.0	na	na	<12%
(Manwich) Mexican	2.258 oz	26	1.2	5.0	552	.8	0.2	0.0	0	7%
(Manwich) Mexican 'Sloppy Joe'	2.5 oz	35	1.0	9.0	460	na	<1.0	na	na	<18%
(Manwich) thick and chunky	2.293 oz	44	1.4	8.6	737	.8	0.5	0.0	0	10%
SEAFOOD COCKTAIL SAUCE *(Heinz)*	1/4 cup	60	1.0	13.0	680	na	0.0	0.0	0	0%
SEAFOOD SAUCE										
(Great Impressions) Creole	1 tbsp	21	0.2	4.7	182	na	0.1	na	0	4%
(Great Impressions) dipping	1 tbsp	17	0.6	2.2	129	na	0.7	na	0	36%
(Great Impressions) dipping, Polynesian	1 tbsp	38	<1.0	9.5	127	na	<1.0	na	0	<18%
SEASONING SAUCE *(A Taste of Thai)*	1 tbsp	15	2.0	1.0	1760	0	0.0	0.0	0	0%
SHOYU. See SOY SAUCE.										
SHRIMP SAUCE *(Tone's)* 'Craboil'	1 tsp	10	0.3	1.2	1	.3	0.6	0.1	1	47%
SOY SAUCE										
shoyu	1 tbsp	9	0.9	1.5	3314	0	tr	tr	0	0%
shoyu, low-sodium	1 tbsp	9	0.9	1.5	600	0	tr	tr	0	0%
tamari	1 tbsp	11	1.9	1.0	1005	0	<.1	tr	0	<7%
(Eden Foods) shoyu, organic	1/2 tsp	2	0.0	0.0	140	na	0.0	na	na	0%
(Eden Foods) shoyu, organic, reduced sodium	1/2 tsp	2	0.0	0.0	80	na	0.0	na	na	0%
(Kikkoman)	1 tbsp	10	na	0.9	892	0	tr	(tr)	0	0%
(Kikkoman) 'Lite'	1 tbsp	11	na	1.3	600	0	tr	(tr)	0	0%
(LaChoy)	1 tsp	<1	0.2	0.3	429	0	0.0	0.0	0	0%
(LaChoy) 'Lite'	1 tsp	<1	0.2	0.3	220	0	0.0	0.0	0	0%
(Westbrae) mild	1/2 tsp	2	1.0	1.0	85	na	0.0	na	0	0%
(Westbrae) organic	1/2 tsp	2	1.0	1.0	105	na	0.0	na	0	0%
(Westbrae) tamari	1/2 tsp	2	1.0	1.0	170	na	0.0	na	0	0%
(Westbrae) wheat-free	1/2 tsp	3	1.0	1.0	140	na	0.0	na	0	0%
SPAGHETTI SAUCE. See PASTA SAUCE.										
STEAK SAUCE										
(A.1.)	1 tbsp	18	0.0	4.0	160	na	0.0	na	0	0%
(A.1.) bold	1 tbsp	18	0.0	4.0	160	na	0.0	na	0	0%
(Heinz) '57'	1 tbsp	16	0.0	4.0	190	0	0.0	0.0	0	0%
(Heinz) hickory smoke '57'	1 tbsp	16	0.0	4.0	180	0	0.0	0.0	0	0%
(Heinz) traditional	1 tbsp	12	0.2	2.6	200	na	0.0	0.0	0	0%

Food Name	Serving Size	Calories	Prot. gms	Carbs gms	Sod. mgs	Fiber gms	Fat gms	Sat. Fat gms	Chol. mgs	% Fat Cal
(Hunt's)	1 tbsp	10	0.3	2.3	256	.3	0.1	0.0	0	8%
(Lea & Perrins)	1 oz	40	<1.0	10.0	220	na	<1.0	na	na	<17%
STIR-FRY SAUCE										
(Kikkoman)	1 tsp	6	0.3	2.3	120	tr	tr	(tr)	0	0%
(LaChoy) Mandarin	4.48 oz	71	2.3	15.6	851	1.3	0.2	0.0	0	3%
(LaChoy) sweet and sour	4.797 oz	146	2.2	34.8	821	1.5	0.1	0.0	0	1%
(LaChoy) Szechwan	4.55 oz	73	2.8	16.0	612	2.1	0.2	0.0	0	2%
(Lawry's)	1/4 cup	120	1.9	19.6	1128	>.2 c	3.8	(mq)	na	29%
STROGANOFF SAUCE (Betty Crocker) 'Recipe Sauces'	4 oz	60	1.0	6.0	540	na	4.0	na	10	56%
SWEET AND SOUR SAUCE										
(A Taste of Thai) tangy, hot	2 tbsp	30	0.0	8.0	95	0	0.0	0.0	0	0%
(Betty Crocker) 'Recipe Sauces'	4.1 oz	130	<1.0	32.0	360	na	0.0	na	0	0%
(Contadina)	1/2 cup	150	<1.0	32.0	430	.1	3.0	1.0	0	17%
(Great Impressions) Hawaiian	2 tbsp	102	0.0	25.5	<1	na	0.0	0.0	0	0%
(Great Impressions) hot	2 tbsp	102	0.0	25.5	<1	na	0.0	0.0	0	0%
(Great Impressions) regular	2 tbsp	102	0.0	25.5	<1	na	0.0	0.0	0	0%
(Hickory Farms) Hawaiian	2 tbsp	102	0.0	25.5	2	na	0.0	0.0	0	0%
(Hickory Farms) regular	2 tbsp	102	0.0	25.5	<1	na	0.0	0.0	0	0%
(Kikkoman)	1 tbsp	18	na	4.0	63	na	0.0	0.0	0	0%
(LaChoy)	1 tbsp	30	na	7.0	320	na	na	na	0	0%
(LaChoy) duck sauce	1 tbsp	26	<.1	6.9	59	0	tr	0.0	0	0%
(Lawry's)	1/4 cup	549	3.4	11.7	4056	>.4 c	7.5	(mq)	na	53%
(Sauceworks)	1 tbsp	25	0.0	5.0	50	na	0.0	0.0	0	0%
SZECHUAN SAUCE (LaChoy) hot and spicy	1 oz	48	0.1	12.0	141	0	0.2	0.0	0	4%
TACO SAUCE										
(Estee)	2 tbsp	14	<1.0	3.0	25	(mq)	0.0	0.0	0	0%
(Hain) and dip	4 tbsp	25	1.0	5.0	350	na	1.0	na	5	27%
(Lawry's) 'Sauce'n Seasoner'	1/4 cup	40	0.7	7.6	636	0	0.6	(tr)	0	14%
(Old El Paso)	2 tbsp	15	1.0	3.0	300	1.0	0.0	0.0	0	0%
(Rosarita)	.1764 oz	2	0.1	0.4	40	.1	0.0	0.0	0	0%
Chunky (Lawry's)	1/4 cup	22	0.9	4.0	549	>.4 c	0.4	(tr)	0	16%
Green (La Victoria)	1 tbsp	0	0.0	1.0	90	na	0.0	na	na	0%
Hot										
(Chi-Chi's)	1 oz	18	2.0	4.0	254	na	2.0	2.0	1	43%
(Del Monte)	1/4 cup	15	0.0	4.0	440	(mq)	0.0	0.0	0	0%
(Old El Paso)	2 tbsp	10	<1.0	2.0	130	(mq)	<1.0	na	na	<43%
(Ortega)	1 oz	12	0.0	3.0	210	(mq)	0.0	0.0	0	0%
Medium										
(Heinz)	1 tbsp	6	0.0	1.0	(mq)	(mq)	0.0	0.0	0	0%
(Old El Paso)	2 tbsp	10	<1.0	2.0	130	(mq)	<1.0	na	na	<43%
Mild										
(Del Monte)	1/2 cup	15	0.0	4.0	480	(mq)	0.0	0.0	0	0%
(Enrico's) 'No Salt Added'	2 tbsp	14	1.0	3.0	25	(mq)	0.0	0.0	0	0%
(Heinz)	1 tbsp	6	0.0	1.0	(mq)	(mq)	0.0	0.0	0	0%
(Old El Paso)	2 tbsp	10	<1.0	2.0	130	(mq)	<1.0	na	na	<43%
(Ortega)	1 oz	12	0.0	3.0	220	(mq)	0.0	0.0	0	0%
Red										
(El Molino) mild	2 tbsp	10	0.0	2.0	170	(mq)	0.0	0.0	0	0%
(La Victoria)	1 tbsp	5	0.0	1.0	80	na	0.0	na	na	0%
Thick, chunky (Chi-Chi's)	1 oz	12	2.0	3.0	140	na	2.0	2.0	2	47%
Western style (Ortega)	1 oz	8	0.0	2.0	180	(mq)	0.0	0.0	0	0%
TAMARI SAUCE. See SOY SAUCE.										
TARTAR SAUCE										
(Best Foods)	1 tbsp	70	0.0	0.0	220	na	8.0	1.0	5	100%

Food Name	Serving Size	Calories	Prot. gms	Carbs gms	Sod. mgs	Fiber gms	Fat gms	Sat. Fat gms	Chol. mgs	% Fat Cal.
(Best Foods) reduced fat	1 tbsp	30	0.0	3.0	210	na	2.0	0.0	0	60%
(Golden Dipt)	1 tbsp	70	0.0	2.0	100	na	7.0	1.0	10	89%
(Golden Dipt) 'Lite'	1 tbsp	50	0.0	4.0	40	na	4.0	1.0	5	69%
(Great Impressions)	1 tbsp	86	0.2	1.2	76	na	9.0	(mq)	10	94%
(Heinz)	2 tbsp	140	0.0	4.0	240	na	14.0	2.0	5	89%
(Hellmann's)	1 tbsp	70	0.0	0.0	220	na	8.0	1.0	5	100%
(Kraft) nonfat 'Free'	1 tbsp	10	0.0	3.0	120	na	0.0	0.0	0	0%
(Life) egg-free 'All Natural'	1 tbsp	38	<1.0	<1.0	2	na	4.0	(mq)	0	82%
(Sauceworks)	1 tbsp	50	0.0	2.0	85	na	5.0	1.0	5	85%
(Sauceworks) natural lemon and herb flavor	1 tbsp	70	0.0	0.0	85	na	8.0	1.0	5	100%
(Skipper's)	1 tbsp	65	0.0	0.0	102	na	7.0	(mq)	4	100%
(Weight Watchers)	1 tbsp	35	0.0	3.0	80	na	3.0	1.0	5	69%
TERIYAKI SAUCE										
(Betty Crocker) 'Recipe Sauces'	3.9 oz	60	2.0	13.0	860	na	<1.0	na	0	<13%
(Golden Dipt) ginger marinade	1 oz	120	1.0	12.0	920	na	7.0	1.0	0	55%
(Kikkoman)	1 tbsp	15	na	2.7	630	na	tr	(tr)	tr	0%
(Kikkoman) 'Baste & Glaze'	1 tbsp	27	na	6.0	420	na	tr	(tr)	0	0%
(LaChoy)	1/2 tsp	5	<1.0	1.0	290	<1.0	<1.0	(mq)	0	<53%
(LaChoy) basting sauce	1/2 tsp	2	<1.0	<1.0	110	<1.0	<1.0	(mq)	0	<53%
(LaChoy) 'Lite'	1/2 tsp	5	<1.0	1.0	85	<1.0	<1.0	(mq)	0	<53%
(LaChoy) 'Sauce and Marinade'	1 oz	30	1.0	5.0	1640	na	0.0	0.0	na	0%
(LaChoy) stir-fry sauce	4.621 oz	105	2.3	24.3	1152	1.6	0.1	0.0	0	1%
(LaChoy) thick and rich	1 oz	41	0.7	9.4	509	<.1.0	0.1	<.1	<1	2%
(Lawry's) barbecue marinade	1/8 cup	82	4.1	13.7	6115	>.1 c	1.1	(mq)	na	12%
(Lawry's) w/pineapple juice	1/4 cup	72	6.4	11.0	7100	>.1 c	0.4	(tr)	na	5%
VEGETABLE SAUCE										
(Contadina) refrigerated, garden 'Light'	.5 oz	50	2.0	10.0	620	na	0.0	na	0	0%
WORCESTERSHIRE SAUCE										
(French's) regular	1 tbsp	10	0.0	2.0	160	na	0.0	0.0	0	0%
(French's) smoky	1 tbsp	10	0.0	2.0	160	na	0.0	0.0	0	0%
(Heinz)	1 tsp	0	0.0	0.0	55	na	0.0	0.0	0	0%
(Lea & Perrins)	1 tsp	5	<1.0	1.0	55	na	<1.0	na	0	<53%
(Lea & Perrins) white wine	1 tsp	4	<1.0	1.0	40	na	<1.0	na	0	<53%
(Life) 'All Natural'	1/2 tbsp	5	<1.0	1.0	2	na	<1.0	na	0	<53%
SAUCE MIX										
ALFREDO SAUCE										
(French's) 'Pasta Toss' dry mix	2 tsp	25	1.0	2.0	310	na	2.0	na	na	60%
(Lawry's) 'Pasta Alfredo' dry mix	1 pkg	226	8.0	19.2	3222	>.6 c	13.3	(mq)	na	52%
BEARNAISE SAUCE dry mix	.9-oz pkg	90	3.5	14.8	841	>.1 c	2.2	0.3	tr	21%
BEEF SAUTÉ SAUCE (Lipton) golden, dry mix	1/6 pkg	120	3.0	24.0	520	na	2.0	na	na	14%
CHEESE SAUCE										
(French's) prepared	1/4 cup	80	3.0	7.0	430	na	4.0	(mq)	(mq)	47%
(McCormick/Schilling) dry mix	1/4 pkg	35	2.0	3.5	477	na	1.5	na	na	38%
(McCormick/Schilling) nacho, dry mix	1/4 pkg	42	3.0	4.5	409	na	1.5	na	na	31%
CHICKEN SAUCE										
(Lawry's) southwest 'Seasoning Blends' dry mix	1 pkg	71	1.1	16.0	3947	na	0.3	0.0	na	4%
(McCormick/Schilling) cacciatore 'Sauce Blends' dry mix	1 pkg	132	3.6	28.0	1092	(mq)	4.8	(mq)	na	26%
(McCormick/Schilling) Creole 'Sauce Blends' dry mix	1 pkg	140	2.0	24.0	1084	(mq)	4.8	(mq)	na	29%
(McCormick/Schilling) curry 'Sauce Blends' dry mix	1 pkg	152	2.4	24.0	1288	(mq)	5.6	(mq)	na	32%
(McCormick/Schilling) Dijon 'Sauce Blends' dry mix	1 pkg	156	3.2	20.0	1414	(mq)	6.8	(mq)	na	40%
(McCormick/Schilling) mesquite marinade 'Sauce Blends' dry mix	1 pkg	132	1.6	24.0	2068	(mq)	3.0	(mq)	na	21%
(McCormick/Schilling) teriyaki 'Sauce Blends' dry mix	1 pkg	172	6.8	28.0	1380	(mq)	3.6	(mq)	na	19%
CURRY SAUCE, prepared	1/2 cup	135	5.3	12.9	638	>.2 c	7.4	3.0	18	48%

Food Name	Serving Size	Calories	Prot. gms	Carbs gms	Sod. mg	Fiber gm	Fat gms	Sat. Fat gms	Chol. mgs	% Fat Cal.
HOLLANDAISE SAUCE *(McCormick/Schilling)* dry mix	1/4 pkg	51	1.0	3.5	170	(mq)	3.8	(mq)	na	66%
LEMON BUTTER SAUCE *(Weight Watchers)* dry mix	1 tbsp	6	1.0	1.0	90	na	0.0	na	na	0%
MUSHROOM SAUCE dry mix	1-oz pkg	99	4.1	15.5	1766	>.3 c	2.7	0.4	0	24%
PASTA SAUCE										
(Estee) prepared w/margarine and skim milk	4 oz	60	2.0	9.0	30	(mq)	1.0	<1.0	0	17%
(Featherweight) prepared w/margarine and skim milk	4 oz	60	2.0	11.0	310	(mq)	1.0	na	0	15%
(French's) cheese and garlic 'Pasta Toss' dry mix	2 tsp	25	1.0	2.0	320	(mq)	2.0	(mq)	na	60%
(French's) Italian 'Pasta Toss' dry mix	2 tsp	25	1.0	2.0	340	(mq)	2.0	(mq)	na	60%
(French's) Italian style, prepared	5/8 cup	100	2.0	15.0	790	(mq)	4.0	(mq)	na	35%
(French's) Romanoff 'Pasta Toss' dry mix	2 tsp	30	1.0	1.0	310	(mq)	2.0	(mq)	na	69%
(French's) w/mushrooms, prepared	5/8 cup	100	2.0	13.0	1050	(mq)	4.0	(mq)	na	38%
(Lawry's) 'Rich & Thick' dry mix	1 pkg	147	3.5	28.1	2172	>.5 c	2.2	(mq)	na	14%
(Lawry's) w/imported mushrooms, dry mix	1 pkg	143	5.2	26.0	2015	>2.1 c	1.5	(mq)	na	10%
(McCormick/Schilling) dry mix	1/4 pkg	32	1.0	6.0	615	(mq)	0.3	na	na	9%
(Prego) prepared w/margarine and skim milk	4 oz	130	2.0	20.0	630	(mq)	5.0	(mq)	na	34%
(Ragu) prepared w/margarine and skim milk	4 oz	80	2.0	9.0	740	(mq)	4.0	(mq)	0	45%
PEANUT SAUCE *(A Taste of Thai)* dry mix	2 tbsp	25	1.0	4.0	115	(mq)	0.5	0.0	0	18%
PESTO SAUCE *(French's)* 'Pasta Toss' dry mix	2 tsp	20	1.0	1.0	280	(mq)	1.0	na	na	53%
SANDWICH SAUCE *(Manwich)* dry mix	.2469 oz	22	0.2	5.3	351	.3	0.1	0.0	0	4%
SEAFOOD SAUCE *(Progresso)* prepared	1/2 cup	110	5.0	12.0	445	2.3	6.0	<1.0	11	44%
SOUR CREAM SAUCE *(McCormick/Schilling)* dry mix	1/4 pkg	44	1.3	4.0	272	na	2.8	(mq)	na	54%
STROGANOFF SAUCE										
(Lawry's) dry mix	1 pkg	123	4.5	25.5	2814	>.8 c	0.3	na	na	2%
(Natural Touch) prepared	4 oz	90	4.0	10.0	na	na	3.0	(mq)	na	33%
SWEET AND SOUR SAUCE, dry mix	2-oz pkg	220	0.6	54.5	584	na	0.1	<.1	0	0%
TACO SAUCE *(Tio Sancho)* 'Dinner Kit' dry mix	2-oz pkg	62	1.6	13.4	750	>.5 c	0.2	na	na	3%
TERIYAKI SAUCE dry mix	1.6-oz pkg	130	4.1	27.6	4784	na	0.9	0.1	0	6%
WHITE SAUCE prepared	1/2 cup	121	5.1	10.7	398	>.1 c	6.7	3.2	17	49%
SAUERKRAUT, CANNED										
(A&P)	1/2 cup	20	1.0	5.0	800	(mq)	<1.0	(tr)	0	tr
(Allens) w/liquid, shredded	1/2 cup	21	1.0	5.0	880	(mq)	<1.0	(tr)	0	tr
(Bush's Best) 'Bavarian Kraut'	1/2 cup	60	1.0	15.0	400	3.0	0.0	na	na	0%
(Bush's Best) 'Kraut' deli style	1/2 cup	20	1.0	5.0	680	na	0.0	na	na	0%
(Bush's Best) 'Kraut' shredded	1/2 cup	20	1.0	5.0	680	na	0.0	na	na	0%
(Claussen)	1/2 cup	17	0.6	3.2	517	(mq)	0.2	(tr)	0	tr
(Del Monte)	1/2 cup	25	1.0	6.0	775	(mq)	0.0	0.0	0	0%
(Eden Foods) organic	1/2 cup	25	2.0	4.0	580	2.8	<1.0	na	na	tr
(Finast)	1/2 cup	30	1.0	6.0	800	(mq)	0.0	0.0	0	0%
(Pathmark)	1/2 cup	20	0.0	4.0	880	(mq)	0.0	0.0	0	0%
(Snow Floss)	1/2 cup	28	1.0	4.0	780	1.0	0.0	0.0	0	0%
(Stokely) 'Bavarian'	1/2 cup	30	1.0	7.0	780	(mq)	0.0	0.0	0	0%
(Stokely) w/liquid, shredded and chopped	1/2 cup	20	1.0	4.0	810	(mq)	0.0	0.0	0	0%
(Vlasic) 'Old Fashioned'	1 oz	4	0.0	1.0	280	(mq)	0.0	0.0	0	0%
SAUERKRAUT JUICE										
canned	1 cup	24	1.7	5.6	1905	0	0.0	0.0	0	0%
canned or bottled *(Biotta)*	6 oz	21	1.1	4.0	1482	(mq)	0.1	(tr)	0	tr
canned or bottled *(S&W)*	5 oz	14	1.0	3.0	1120	(mq)	0.0	0.0	0	0%
SAUSAGE. See also individual listings.										
(Hickory Farms) 'Safari'	1 oz	98	5.0	1.0	343	0	9.0	(mq)	14	77%
(Hillshire Farm) 'Country Recipe'	2 oz	180	7.0	2.0	490	0	16.0	(mq)	(mq)	80%
(Hormel)	3 oz	290	12.0	1.0	(mq)	0	27.0	(mq)	(mq)	82%
(JM) .5-oz patties, cooked	1 patty	70	2.0	1.0	170	0	6.0	(mq)	(mq)	82%
(JM) raw	1 oz	130	3.0	1.0	180	0	14.0	(mq)	(mq)	89%
(Jones Dairy Farm)	1 patty	155	5.5	tr	281	0	14.4	(mq)	36	86%

Food Name	Serving Size	Calories	Prot. gms	Carbs gms	Sod. mgs	Fiber gms	Fat gms	Sat. Fat gms	Chol. mgs	% Fat Cal.
(Jones Dairy Farm) 'Golden Brown'	1 patty	155	4.6	tr	250	0	14.7	(mq)	29	88%
(Jones Dairy Farm) 'Golden Brown' mild	1 link	100	2.6	tr	150	0	9.8	(mq)	18	90%
(Jones Dairy Farm) 'Golden Brown' spicy	1 link	100	2.8	tr	159	0	9.5	(mq)	18	88%
Brown and serve										
(Eckrich) 'Lean Supreme Heat 'n Serve'	2 links	120	7.0	1.0	440	0	10.0	(mq)	(mq)	74%
(Hormel)	2 links	140	6.0	0.0	430	0	13.0	(mq)	(mq)	83%
(Hormel) uncooked	2 links	180	7.0	0.0	411	0	17.0	(mq)	(mq)	85%
(Jones Dairy Farm) 'Light'	1 link	60	3.5	1.0	150	0	4.1	(mq)	16	67%
(Swift) 'Country Recipe'	1 link	130	4.0	1.0	240	0	12.0	(mq)	(mq)	84%
(Swift) 'Country Recipe'	1 patty	130	4.0	1.0	240	0	12.0	(mq)	(mq)	84%
(Swift) microwave	1 link	120	4.0	1.0	270	0	12.0	(mq)	(mq)	84%
(Swift) 'Premium Original'	1 link	130	3.0	1.0	260	0	12.0	(mq)	(mq)	87%
(Swift) 'Premium Original'	1 patty	120	4.0	1.0	270	0	12.0	(mq)	(mq)	84%
(Swift) smoked flavor	1 link	120	4.0	1.0	280	0	11.0	(mq)	(mq)	83%
Roll										
(Eckrich) minced	1-oz slice	80	4.0	1.0	300	0	7.0	(mq)	(mq)	76%
(Jones Dairy Farm) 'Cello Roll'	1 slice	105	3.7	tr	200	0	9.6	(mq)	24	85%
BEEF										
(Eckrich)	1 oz	100	3.0	<1.0	270	0	9.0	(mq)	(mq)	84%
(Eckrich) 'Lean Supreme'	1 oz	80	4.0	1.0	230	0	7.0	(mq)	(mq)	76%
(Eckrich) 'Smok-Y-Links'	2 links	160	6.0	2.0	350	0	14.0	(mq)	(mq)	80%
(Hillshire Farm) 'Bun Size'	2 oz	180	8.0	2.0	570	0	16.0	(mq)	(mq)	78%
(Hillshire Farm) 'Flavorseal'	2 oz	180	7.0	2.0	490	0	16.0	(mq)	(mq)	80%
(Jones Dairy Farm) 'Golden Brown'	1 link	75	3.8	tr	159	0	6.1	(mq)	18	78%
(Oscar Mayer) 'Smokies' 1.5-oz links	1 link	124	5.4	0.7	429	0	11.0	4.7	27	80%
(Swift) 'Premium Brown 'N Serve'	1 link	120	4.0	1.0	250	0	12.0	(mq)	(mq)	84%
BEEF AND CHEDDAR *(Hillshire Farms)* 'Flavorseal'	2 oz	190	8.0	1.0	500	0	15.0	(mq)	(mq)	79%
CHEESE										
(Hormel) 'Smokie Cheezers'	2 links	168	9.0	1.0	623	0	15.0	(mq)	(mq)	77%
(Oscar Mayer) 'Smokies'	1.5 oz	126	5.7	0.7	452	0	11.2	4.4	28	80%
Hot										
(Eckrich) 'Smok-Y-Links'	2 links	150	6.0	1.0	360	0	14.0	(mq)	(mq)	82%
(Hillshire Farm) 'Flavorseal'	2 oz	180	7.0	2.0	510	0	16.0	(mq)	(mq)	80%
Maple-flavored *(Eckrich)* 'Smok-Y-Links'	2 links	160	6.0	2.0	390	0	14.0	(mq)	(mq)	80%
W/ham *(Eckrich)* 'Smok-Y-Links'	2 links	160	6.0	2.0	500	0	15.0	(mq)	(mq)	81%
HOT										
(JM) .5-oz patties, cooked	1 patty	70	2.0	1.0	170	0	6.0	(mq)	(mq)	82%
(JM) patties, raw	1 oz	130	3.0	1.0	180	0	14.0	(mq)	(mq)	89%
(OHSE) 'Hot Links'	1 oz	80	4.0	4.0	310	0	3.0	(mq)	(mq)	46%
ITALIAN STYLE										
cooked	3 oz	268	16.6	1.3	765	0	21.3	7.5	65	73%
cooked	2.4 oz	216	13.4	1.0	618	0	17.2	6.1	52	73%
pork, cooked	1 oz	92	5.7	0.4	261	0	7.3	2.6	22	73%
pork, raw	1 oz	98	4.0	0.2	207	0	8.9	3.2	22	83%
raw	4 oz	391	16.1	0.7	826	0	35.4	12.7	86	83%
raw	3.2 oz	315	13.0	0.6	665	0	28.5	10.2	69	83%
Hot *(Hillshire Farm)* 'Links'	2 oz	180	7.0	1.0	(mq)	0	17.0	(mq)	(mq)	83%
Mild *(Hillshire Farm)* 'Links'	2 oz	190	7.0	1.0	(mq)	0	17.0	(mq)	(mq)	83%
Smoked *(Hillshire Farm)* 'Flavorseal'	2 oz	200	7.0	1.0	500	0	18.0	(mq)	(mq)	84%
MAPLE-FLAVORED *(Swift)* brown and serve	1 link	120	3.0	1.0	260	0	12.0	(mq)	(mq)	87%
NEW ENGLAND STYLE										
(Eckrich)	1 oz	35	5.0	1.0	370	(tr)	1.0	(mq)	(mq)	27%
(Light & Lean)	2 slices	90	10.0	0.0	(mq)	0	6.0	(mq)	(mq)	57%
(Oscar Mayer) .8-oz slices	1 slice	29	3.9	0.4	291	(tr)	1.3	0.6	14	41%

Food Name	Serving Size	Calories	Prot. gms	Carbs gms	Sod. mgs	Fiber gms	Fat gms	Sat. Fat gms	Chol. mgs	% Fat Cal.
PICKLED										
(Penrose) beer, .5-oz links	1 link	40	2.0	1.0	220	0	3.0	(mq)	(mq)	69%
(Penrose) firecracker, 1.5-oz links	1 link	120	6.0	1.0	620	0	10.0	(mq)	(mq)	76%
(Penrose) firecracker, .5-oz links	1 link	40	2.0	1.0	220	0	3.0	(mq)	(mq)	69%
(Penrose) firecracker, giant, 2.1-oz links	1 link	170	9.0	1.0	870	0	14.0	(mq)	(mq)	76%
(Penrose) hot, .5-oz links	1 link	40	2.0	1.0	220	0	3.0	(mq)	(mq)	69%
(Penrose) Polish, .5-oz links	1 link	40	2.0	1.0	220	0	3.0	(mq)	(mq)	69%
(Penrose) red hot, .5-oz links	1 link	40	2.0	1.0	220	0	3.0	(mq)	(mq)	69%
POLISH STYLE										
	1 oz	92	4.0	0.5	248	0	8.1	2.9	20	80%
10-inch sausage	1 link	740	32.0	3.7	1989	0	65.2	23.5	159	80%
PORK										
4-inch links, cooked	1 link	48	2.5	0.1	168	0	4.1	1.4	11	78%
4-inch links, raw	1 link	117	3.3	0.3	187	0	11.3	4.1	19	88%
fresh, cooked	1 oz	105	5.6	0.3	367	0	8.8	3.1	24	77%
fresh, raw	2 oz	238	6.7	0.6	380	0	23.0	8.3	39	88%
patties, 1/4 inch x 3 7/8 inch diam, cooked	1 patty	100	5.3	0.3	349	0	8.4	2.9	22	77%
patties, 1/4 inch x 3 7/8 inch diam, raw	1 patty	238	6.7	0.6	380	0	23.0	8.3	39	88%
(Hormel) 'Little Sizzlers'	2 links	103	6.0	0.0	172	0	9.0	(mq)	(mq)	77%
(Hormel) 'Little Sizzlers'	1 oz	130	3.0	2.0	192	na	13.0	5.0	19	85%
(Hormel) 'Midget Links'	2 links	143	7.0	0.0	327	0	13.0	(mq)	(mq)	81%
(Jimmy Dean) cooked	1 oz	120	4.0	<1.0	240	na	11.0	na	na	83%
(Jimmy Dean) links	2 links	180	7.0	<1.0	380	na	17.0	na	na	83%
(Jimmy Dean) 'Light'	1.2 oz	80	6.0	<1.0	230	na	7.0	na	25	69%
(Jimmy Dean) patties	1 patty	140	5.0	<1.0	300	na	13.0	na	na	83%
(JM) 'Tasty Link' cooked	1.4 oz	190	6.0	1.0	290	0	18.0	(mq)	(mq)	85%
(JM) 'Tasty Link' raw	1.8 oz	260	6.0	1.0	380	0	26.0	(mq)	(mq)	89%
(Jones Dairy Farm)	1 link	140	2.9	tr	176	0	13.7	(mq)	24	91%
(Jones Dairy Farm) 'Golden Brown Light'	1 link	55	3.3	0.5	132	0	4.2	(mq)	16	71%
(Jones Dairy Farm) 'Light'	1 link	70	4.2	1.0	232	0	5.0	(mq)	21	68%
(Oscar Mayer) 'Little Friers' cooked	8.9 oz	989	40.7	2.8	2641	0	90.3	33.4	210	82%
(Oscar Mayer) 'Little Friers' cooked	1 link	82	3.4	0.2	219	0	7.5	2.7	17	82%
(Tyson) country, whole hog	3.5 oz	320	13.0	1.0	905	na	29.0	na	49	82%
PORK AND BACON *(JM)* 'Tasty Link' raw	1.8 oz	220	6.0	1.0	340	0	21.0	(mq)	(mq)	87%
PORK AND BEEF										
fresh, cooked	1 oz	112	3.9	0.8	228	0	10.3	3.7	(mq)	83%
fresh, 1/4 inch x 3 7/8-inch diam patties, cooked	1 patty	107	3.7	0.7	217	0	9.8	3.5	19	83%
fresh, 2 inch x 3/4-inch diam links, cooked	1 link	51	1.8	0.4	105	0	4.7	1.7	9	83%
smoked, 4 inch x 1 1/8-inch diam links	1 link	228	9.1	1.0	643	0	20.6	7.2	48	82%
smoked, 2 inch x 3/4-inch diam links	1 link	54	2.1	0.2	151	0	4.8	1.7	11	82%
smoked, w/flour and nonfat dry milk added, 4 inch x 1 1/8-inch diam links	1 link	182	9.5	2.7	741	0	14.6	5.3	59	73%
smoked, w/flour and nonfat dry milk added, 2 inch x 3/4-inch diam links	1 link	43	2.2	0.6	174	0	3.4	1.3	14	73%
smoked, w/nonfat dry milk added, 4 inch x 1 1/8-inch diam links	1 link	213	9.0	1.3	798	0	18.8	6.6	44	80%
smoked, w/nonfat dry milk added, 2 inch x 3/4-inch diam links	1 link	50	2.1	0.3	188	0	4.4	1.6	10	81%
SAGE *(Jimmy Dean)* cooked	1 oz	120	4.0	<1.0	240	na	11.0	na	na	83%
SMOKED										
(Eckrich) 'Lean Supreme'	1 oz	70	4.0	1.0	230	0	6.0	(mq)	(mq)	73%
(Eckrich) 'Skinless'	1 link	180	7.0	2.0	420	0	16.0	(mq)	(mq)	80%
(Hillshire Farm) 'Bun Size'	2 oz	180	8.0	2.0	570	0	16.0	(mq)	(mq)	78%
(Hillshire Farm) 'Flavorseal'	2 oz	190	7.0	1.0	500	0	17.0	(mq)	(mq)	83%

Food Name	Serving Size	Calories	Prot. gms	Carbs gms	Sod. mgs	Fiber gms	Fat gms	Sat. Fat gms	Chol. mgs	% Fat Cal.
(Hillshire Farm) 'Links'	2 oz	190	8.0	1.0	520	0	18.0	(mq)	(mq)	82%
(Hillshire Farm) 'Lite'	2 oz	160	8.0	2.0	(mq)	0	13.0	(mq)	(mq)	75%
(Hormel) 'Smokies'	2 links	160	9.0	2.0	597	0	14.0	(mq)	(mq)	74%
(OHSE)	1 oz	80	4.0	1.0	320	0	7.0	(mq)	(mq)	76%
(Oscar Mayer) 'Big & Juicy Smokie Links' 2.7-oz links	1 link	227	9.3	1.2	757	0	20.5	7.0	48	82%
(Oscar Mayer) 'Little Smokies' .3-oz links	1 link	27	1.2	0.1	92	0	2.5	0.9	6	81%
(Oscar Mayer) 'Smokie Links' 1.5-oz links	1 link	126	5.4	0.6	426	0	11.3	4.2	28	81%
(Pilgrim's Pride)	3 oz	144	13.1	2.5	890	0	9.1	(mq)	64	57%
SWEDISH STYLE *(Hickory Farms)*	1 oz	100	5.0	0.0	380	0	9.0	(mq)	20	80%
TURKEY										
(Butterball)	1 oz	50	4.0	<1.0	250	0	4.0	(mq)	(mq)	64%
(Jimmy Dean) 'Light'	1.2 oz	80	6.0	<1.0	230	na	7.0	na	25	69%
(Louis Rich) cooked	1 link	46	5.4	0.1	234	0	2.7	1.5	18	53%
(Louis Rich) 85% fat-free, cooked	24 gm	45	6.0	<1.0	235	na	3.0	na	20	49%
(Norbest) 'Tasti-Lean' chub or links	1 oz	53	4.6	0.3	179	0	2.8	(mq)	(mq)	56%
Breakfast type										
(Hudson's) ground	1 oz	65	4.3	0.0	180	0	5.3	(mq)	(mq)	74%
(Louis Rich) 85% fat-free	1 oz	55	6.0	<1.0	230	na	3.0	na	25	49%
(Louis Rich) ground, cooked	1 oz	56	5.9	0.2	215	0	3.5	1.5	22	56%
(Mr. Turkey)	1 oz	58	4.6	0.4	181	0	4.3	(mq)	16	66%
Smoked										
(Louis Rich)	1 oz	43	4.5	0.7	249	0	2.4	0.6	19	51%
(Louis Rich) 90% fat-free	1 oz	40	5.0	<1.0	250	na	2.0	na	20	43%
(Louis Rich) w/cheese	1 oz	47	4.7	0.7	269	0	2.8	0.8	18	54%
(Louis Rich) w/cheddar, 90% fat-free	1 oz	45	5.0	<1.0	270	na	3.0	na	20	53%
(Mr. Turkey)	1 oz	47	4.5	0.5	230	0	3.4	(mq)	19	61%
TURKEY AND PORK *(Jimmy Dean)* 'Light'	1.2 oz	80	6.0	<1.0	230	na	7.0	na	25	69%
W/BACON *(Swift)* brown and serve	1 link	120	4.0	1.0	270	0	11.0	(mq)	(mq)	83%
W/HAM *(Swift)* brown and serve	1 link	130	3.0	1.0	260	0	13.0	(mq)	(mq)	88%
SAUSAGE, ALTERNATIVE										
(Heartline) 'Italian Sausage Style'	2 oz	176	19.0	9.0	680	na	7.0	na	0	36%
(Heartline) 'Pepperoni Style' lite	.5 oz	22	5.0	1.0	135	3.0	0.0	0.0	0	0%
Canned *(Worthington)* 'Saucettes'	2 links	140	10.0	5.0	350	(mq)	9.0	1.0	0	57%
Frozen										
(Morningstar Farms) links, 'Breakfast Links'	3 links	190	12.0	3.0	500	(mq)	14.0	2.0	0	68%
(Morningstar Farms) patties, 'Breakfast Patties'	2 patties	190	15.0	7.0	710	(mq)	12.0	2.0	0	55%
(Worthington) links, 'Prosage'	3 links	190	13.0	4.0	570	(mq)	14.0	2.0	0	65%
(Worthington) patties, 'Prosage'	2 patties	210	18.0	4.0	780	(mq)	14.0	3.0	0	59%
(Worthington) roll, 'Prosage' 3/8-inch slice	2 slices	180	13.0	4.0	570	(mq)	12.0	2.0	0	61%
SAUSAGE, CANNED										
(Hormel) hot	1 patty	150	7.0	0.0	549	0	13.0	(mq)	(mq)	81%
(Hormel) mild	1 patty	150	7.0	0.0	541	0	13.0	(mq)	(mq)	81%
SAUSAGE SEASONING, pork *(Tone's)*	1 tsp	12	0.4	2.7	1	.7	0.3	0.2	0	18%
SAUSAGE STICK										
(Hickory Farms) 'Sportsman Stick'	1 oz	138	9.0	4.0	1075	0	10.0	(mq)	40	63%
BEEF										
(Pemmican) Pepperoni	1.1 oz	170	8.0	2.0	500	0	14.0	(mq)	(mq)	76%
(Pemmican) Tabasco	1.1 oz	120	5.0	2.0	410	0	10.0	(mq)	(mq)	76%
(Pemmican) Teriyaki	1.1 oz	150	8.0	5.0	410	0	11.0	(mq)	(mq)	66%
SMOKED										
(Slim Jim) 'Big Slim'	.52 oz	80	3.0	1.0	220	0	7.0	(mq)	(mq)	80%
(Slim Jim) 'Giant Slim'	1.1 oz	180	7.0	2.0	470	0	16.0	(mq)	(mq)	80%
(Slim Jim) 'Jumbo Jim'	1 oz	150	8.0	2.0	430	0	12.0	(mq)	(mq)	73%
(Slim Jim) 'Super Slim'	.7 oz	110	4.0	1.0	300	0	10.0	(mq)	(mq)	82%

Food Name	Serving Size	Calories	Prot. gms	Carbs gms	Sod. mgs	Fiber gms	Fat gms	Sat. Fat gms	Chol. mgs	% Fat Cal.
Mild *(Slim Jim)* 'Handi-Paks'	.31 oz	50	2.0	1.0	130	0	4.0	(mq)	(mq)	75%
Nacho *(Slim Jim)* 'Super Slim'	.31 oz	40	2.0	1.0	160	0	3.0	(mq)	(mq)	69%
Pepperoni *(Slim Jim)* 'Handi-Paks'	.31 oz	50	2.0	1.0	130	0	4.0	(mq)	(mq)	75%
Spicy										
(Slim Jim) 'Handi-Paks'	.31 oz	50	2.0	1.0	130	0	4.0	(mq)	(mq)	75%
(Pemmican)	.8 oz	110	5.0	1.0	410	0	10.0	(mq)	(mq)	79%
Tabasco *(Slim Jim)* 'Handi-Paks'	.31 oz	50	2.0	1.0	130	0	4.0	(mq)	(mq)	75%
SUMMER SAUSAGE										
Beef *(Hickory Farms)*	1 oz	100	5.0	1.0	345	0	8.0	(mq)	20	75%
Smoked *(Slim Jim)*	.5 oz	80	3.0	1.0	200	0	7.0	(mq)	(mq)	80%
Teriyaki *(Pemmican)*	.8 oz	110	5.0	1.0	410	0	10.0	(mq)	(mq)	79%
SAUSAGE TACO										
refrigerated *(Owens)* 'Border Breakfasts'	2.17 oz	190	7.0	11.0	345	(mq)	12.0	(mq)	65	60%
SAVORY										
ground	1 oz	77	1.9	19.5	7	>4.3 c	1.7	na	0	15%
ground	1 tbsp	12	0.3	3.0	1	>.7 c	0.3	na	0	17%
ground	1 tsp	4	0.1	1.0	0	>.2 c	0.1	na	0	17%
ground *(Durkee)*	1 tsp	5	0.0	0.0	0	0	tr	na	na	tr
ground *(Laurel Leaf)*	1 tsp	5	0.0	0.0	0	0	tr	na	na	tr
ground *(Spice Islands)*	1 tsp	5	0.1	1.0	<1	>.2 c	0.1	(tr)	0	17%
SAVOY CABBAGE. See CABBAGE, SAVOY.										
SCALLION. See ONION, GREEN.										
SCALLOP, ALTERNATIVE										
canned *(Worthington)* 'Vegetable Skallops'	1/2 cup	90	15.0	4.0	430	(mq)	2.0	(mq)	0	19%
canned *(Worthington)* 'Vegetable Skallops' no salt	1/2 cup	80	13.0	4.0	80	(mq)	1.0	na	0	12%
mixed species, made from surimi	3 oz	84	10.9	9.0	676	0	0.4	0.1	19	4%
SCALLOP, MIXED SPECIES										
breaded, fried	4 oz	244	20.5	11.5	526	>.2 c	12.4	3.0	69	47%
fried, frozen *(Mrs. Paul's)*	3 oz	200	9.0	22.0	410	(mq)	8.0	(mq)	(mq)	37%
raw	1 lb	400	76.1	10.7	730	0	3.4	0.4	152	8%
raw	3 oz	75	14.3	2.0	137	0	0.7	0.1	28	9%
raw	1 oz	25	4.8	0.7	46	0	0.2	<.1	9	8%
SCALLOP SQUASH. See SQUASH, SCALLOP.										
SCORZONERA. See SALSIFY, BLACK.										
SCRAPPLE										
....	1 oz	60	2.5	4.1	268	0	3.8	1.4	12	56%
(Jones Dairy Farm)	1 slice	65	2.7	4.2	165	0	3.7	(mq)	24	55%
SCOTCH. See ALCOHOLIC BEVERAGES.										
SCHAV. See SOUP.										
SCREWDRIVER. See ALCOHOLIC BEVERAGES.										
SCROD ENTRÉE, FROZEN										
baked 'Microwave Entrees' *(Gorton's)*	1 pkg	320	22.0	17.0	420	(mq)	18.0	4.0	80	51%
SCUP/sea bream										
dry-heat cooked	3 oz	115	20.6	0.0	46	0	3.0	na	57	25%
raw	1 lb	477	85.6	0.0	191	0	12.4	(mq)	(mq)	25%
raw	3 oz	89	16.0	0.0	36	0	2.3	0.5	44	24%
raw	1 oz	30	5.4	0.0	12	0	0.8	(mq)	(mq)	25%
SEA BASS. See BASS, SEA, MIXED SPECIES.										
SEA BREAM. See SCUP.										
SEA DEVIL. See MONKFISH.										
SEA PERCH. See OCEAN PERCH, ATLANTIC.										
SEA TROUT. See TROUT, SEA, MIXED SPECIES.										
SEAFOOD ENTRÉE, CANNED. See individual listings.										

Food Name	Serving Size	Calories	Prot. gms	Carbs gms	Sod. mgs	Fiber gms	Fat gms	Sat. Fat gms	Chol. mgs	% Fat Cal.
SEAFOOD ENTRÉE, FROZEN. See also individual listings.										
(Armour) w/natural herbs 'Classics Lite'	10 oz	190	13.0	29.0	1020	(mq)	2.0	(mq)	35	10%
(Budget Gourmet) Newburg	10 oz	350	17.0	43.0	660	(mq)	12.0	(mq)	70	31%
(Budget Gourmet) scallop and shrimp 'Mariner'	11.5 oz	320	16.0	43.0	690	na	9.0	(mq)	70	26%
(Cajun Cookin') gumbo	17 oz	330	16.0	51.0	1330	(mq)	7.0	(mq)	(mq)	19%
(Gorton's) clam 'Crunchy Clam Strips' microwave, 5.8-oz pkg	2.9 oz	270	8.0	20.0	350	na	17.0	na	20	58%
(Pillsbury) casserole 'Microwave Classic'	1 pkg	420	15.0	37.0	950	(mq)	24.0	(mq)	(mq)	51%
(Swanson) Creole, w/rice 'Homestyle Recipe'	9 oz	240	7.0	40.0	810	(mq)	6.0	(mq)	(mq)	22%
SEAFOOD FRYING MIX										
(Golden Dipt)	2/3 oz	60	1.0	14.0	600	(mq)	0.0	0.0	0	0%
(Golden Dipt) fish fry	2/3 oz	60	2.0	14.0	430	(mq)	0.0	0.0	0	0%
(Golden Dipt) fish fry, Cajun style	2/3 oz	60	2.0	14.0	470	(mq)	0.0	0.0	0	0%
SEAFOOD SALAD. See also individual listings.										
(Longacre) w/crabmeat 'Saladfest'	1 oz	45	1.0	3.0	130	na	3.0	(mq)	5	63%
SEAFOOD SEASONING MIX										
(Featherweight)	1/4 pkg	18	1.0	8.0	10	(mq)	0.0	0.0	0	0%
(Golden Dipt) all-purpose	1/4 tsp	2	0.0	0.0	85	na	0.0	0.0	0	0%
(Golden Dipt) blackened redfish	1/4 tsp	2	0.0	0.0	140	na	0.0	0.0	0	0%
(Golden Dipt) fish, broiled	1/4 tcp	2	0.0	0.0	125	na	0.0	0.0	0	0%
(Golden Dipt) lemon pepper	1/4 tsp	8	1.0	1.0	115	na	0.0	0.0	0	0%
(Golden Dipt) shrimp and crab, Cajun style	1/4 tsp	2	0.0	0.0	200	na	0.0	0.0	0	0%
(Schilling) Chesapeake Bay	1/2 tsp	2	0.1	0.2	202	na	0.1	na	0	43%
SEASONING AND COATING MIX. See also individual listings.										
(Golden Dipt) breading	1 oz	90	3.0	20.0	630	(mq)	0.0	0.0	0	0%
(Shake 'N Bake) country mild recipe	1/4 pkt	80	1.0	10.0	500	na	4.0	na	0	45%
(Shake 'N Bake) Italian herb recipe	1/4 pkt	80	2.0	14.0	610	na	1.0	na	0	12%
For chicken										
(Oven Fry) 'Extra Crispy'	1/4 pkt	120	3.0	21.0	840	na	2.0	na	0	16%
(Oven Fry) 'Home Style Flour Recipe'	1/4 pkt	90	1.0	15.0	980	na	2.0	na	0	22%
(Shake 'N Bake) hot and spicy	1/4 pkt	80	2.0	15.0	380	na	2.0	na	0	21%
(Shake 'N Bake) 'Original Barbecue Recipe'	1/4 pkt	90	1.0	18.0	840	na	2.0	na	0	19%
(Shake 'N Bake) 'Original Recipe'	1/4 pkt	80	2.0	14.0	450	na	2.0	na	0	22%
For fish (Shake 'N Bake) 'Original Recipe'	1/4 pkt	70	1.0	14.0	410	na	1.0	na	0	13%
For pork										
(Oven Fry) 'Extra Crispy'	1/8 pkt	60	2.0	10.0	350	na	1.0	na	0	16%
(Shake 'N Bake) hot and spicy	1/8 pkt	45	1.0	8.0	220	na	1.0	na	0	20%
(Shake 'N Bake) 'Original Barbecue Recipe'	1/8 pkt	35	0.0	8.0	260	na	0.0	na	0	0%
(Shake 'N Bake) 'Original Recipe'	1/8 pkt	40	1.0	8.0	310	na	1.0	na	0	20%
SEAWEED										
Dried										
agar	1 oz	87	1.8	22.9	29	2.2	0.1	<.1	0	1%
nori	1 lb	158	26.4	23.2	217	>1.2 c	1.3	0.3	0	6%
nori	1 oz	10	1.6	1.4	14	>.1 c	0.1	<.1	0	7%
spirulina	1 oz	82	16.3	6.8	297	>1.0 c	2.2	0.8	0	18%
Raw										
agar	1 lb	116	2.5	30.6	40	2.2	0.1	<.1	0	1%
agar	1 oz	7	0.2	1.9	3	.1	tr	tr	0	0%
Irish moss	1 lb	222	6.9	55.8	303	(mq)	0.7	0.2	0	3%
Irish moss	1 oz	14	0.4	3.5	19	(mq)	<.1	tr	0	<6%
kelp	1 lb	195	7.6	43.4	1056	6.0	2.5	1.1	0	10%
kelp	100 gm	43	1.7	9.6	233	1.3	0.6	0.3	0	11%
kelp	1 oz	12	0.5	2.7	66	.4	0.2	0.1	0	12%
laver	1 lb	158	26.4	23.2	217	1.2	1.3	0.3	0	6%

Food Name	Serving Size	Calories	Prot. gms	Carbs gms	Sod. mgs	Fiber gms	Fat gms	Sat. Fat gms	Chol. mgs	% Fat Cal.
laver	100 gm	35	5.8	5.1	48	.3	0.3	0.1	0	6%
laver	1 oz	10	1.6	1.4	14	.1	0.1	<.1	0	7%
spirulina	1 lb	120	26.9	11.0	444	1.5	1.8	0.6	0	10%
spirulina	1 oz	8	1.7	0.7	28	.1	0.1	<.1	0	9%
wakame	1 lb	206	13.7	41.5	3957	2.5	2.9	0.6	0	11%
wakame	1 oz	13	0.9	2.6	247	.2	0.2	<.1	0	11%
SELTZER. See SOFT DRINKS AND MIXERS.										
SEMOLINA										
enriched	1/2 cup	311	5.7	68.6	6	3.3	0.5	0.1	0	2%
unenriched	1/2 cup	109	2.3	23.7	1	.3	0.2	0.1	0	2%
whole grain	1 cup	602	21.2	121.6	2	6.5	1.8	0.3	0	3%
whole grain	1 oz	102	3.6	20.6	<1	1.1	0.3	<.1	0	3%
SESAME BUTTER. See also TAHINI. MIX										
gourmet *(Roaster Fresh)*	1 oz	168	5.0	6.0	3	na	15.0	2.2	na	75%
made from raw and stone ground kernels	1 oz	162	5.1	7.4	21	2.6	13.6	1.9	0	71%
made from raw and stone ground kernels	1 tbsp	86	2.7	3.9	11	1.4	7.2	1.0	0	71%
made from roasted kernels	1 oz	169	4.8	6.0	33	2.6	15.3	2.1	0	76%
made from roasted kernels	1 tbsp	89	2.5	3.2	17	1.4	8.1	1.1	0	76%
made from unroasted kernels	1 oz	172	5.1	5.1	0	2.6	16.0	2.2	0	78%
made from unroasted kernels	1 tbsp	85	2.5	2.5	0	1.3	7.9	1.1	0	78%
organic *(Arrowhead Mills)*	1 oz	170	6.0	4.0	<1	2.6	17.0	(mq)	0	79%
organic, Mid-Eastern *(Westbrae)*	2 tbsp	220	9.0	3.0	na	na	20.0	na	0	79%
organic 'Natural' *(Westbrae)*	2 tbsp	220	6.0	6.0	35	na	19.0	na	0	78%
paste	1 oz	169	5.1	7.2	3	1.5	14.4	2.0	0	73%
paste	1 tbsp	95	2.9	4.1	2	.9	8.1	1.1	0	72%
SESAME FLOUR										
high-fat	1 oz	149	8.7	7.6	12	>1.8 c	10.5	1.5	0	59%
low-fat	1 oz	95	14.2	10.1	11	>1.4 c	0.5	0.1	0	4%
partially defatted	1 oz	108	11.5	10.0	12	>1.7 c	3.4	0.5	0	26%
SESAME MEAL, partially defatted	1 oz	161	4.8	7.4	11	>1.1 c	13.6	1.9	0	72%
SESAME OIL										
	1/2 cup	964	0.0	0.0	0	0	109.0	15.5	0	100%
	1 oz	251	0.0	0.0	0	0	28.4	4.0	0	100%
	1 tbsp	120	0.0	0.0	0	0	13.6	1.9	0	100%
(Eden Foods) hot pepper	1 tbsp	120	0.0	0.0	0	na	14.0	2.0	na	100%
(Eden Foods) toasted	1 tbsp	120	0.0	0.0	0	na	14.0	2.0	na	100%
(Eden Foods) unrefined	1 tbsp	120	0.0	0.0	0	na	14.0	2.0	0	100%
(Hain)	1 tbsp	120	0.0	0.0	0	0	14.0	2.0	0	100%
(Spectrum Naturals)	1 tbsp	120	0.0	0.0	0	(tr)	14.0	2.0	(tr)	100%
(Spectrum Naturals) unrefined	1 tbsp	120	0.0	0.0	0	(tr)	14.0	2.0	(tr)	100%
SESAME SEASONING										
(Schilling) all-purpose 'Parsley Patch'	1 tsp	15	0.6	1.0	2	na	1.0	na	0	58%
SESAME SEED/sim sim										
Decorticated										
dried	1 tbsp	47	2.1	0.8	3	.2	4.4	na	0	77%
dried	1 tsp	16	.7	.3	1	.1	1.5	na	0	77%
Kernels										
dried	1 cup	882	39.6	14.1	59	>4.4 c	82.2	11.5	0	78%
dried	1 oz	167	7.5	2.7	11	>.8 c	15.5	2.2	0	77%
dried	1 tbsp	47	2.1	0.8	3	.2	4.4	0.6	0	77%
dried	1 tsp	16	0.7	0.3	1	.1	1.5	0.2	0	77%
dried *(Arrowhead Mills)*	1 oz	160	6.0	4.0	3	3.7	14.0	(mq)	0	76%
dried, toasted	1 oz	161	4.8	7.4	11	4.8	13.6	1.9	0	72%

Food Name	Serving Size	Calories	Prot. gms	Carbs gms	Sod. mgs	Fiber gms	Fat gms	Sat. Fat gms	Chol. mgs	% Fat Cal.
Whole										
dried	1 lb	2598	80.4	106.4	51	53.5	225.3	31.6	0	73%
dried	1 cup	825	25.5	33.8	16	17.0	71.5	10.0	0	73%
dried	1 oz	162	5.0	6.6	3	3.3	14.1	2.0	0	73%
dried	1 tbsp	52	1.6	2.1	1	1.1	4.5	0.6	0	73%
dried (Arrowhead Mills)	1 oz	160	5.0	6.0	4	3.1	14.0	(mq)	0	74%
dried (Durkee)	1 tsp	13	0.0	0.0	0	0	<0.1	na	na	<41%
dried (Laurel Leaf)	1 tsp	13	0.0	0.0	0	0	<0.1	na	na	<41%
roasted	1 oz	160	4.8	7.3	3	4.0	13.6	1.9	0	72%
SESAME STICKS										
(Barbara's Bakery)	1 oz	130	3.0	20.0	255	na	4.0	na	na	28%
(Flavor Tree)	1/4 cup	133	3.1	10.6	358	>.1 c	9.1	(mq)	0	60%
(Flavor Tree) 'No Salt'	1/4 cup	131	3.2	13.4	7	>.1 c	8.1	(mq)	0	52%
SESBANIA FLOWER. See KATURAY.										
SHAD, AMERICAN										
dry-heat cooked	3 oz	214	18.5	0.0	55	0	15.0	na	82	65%
raw	1 lb	891	76.8	0.0	233	0	62.5	(mq)	(mq)	65%
raw	3 oz	167	14.4	0.0	43	0	11.7	3.8	64	65%
raw	1 oz	56	4.8	0.0	14	0	3.9	(mq)	(mq)	65%
SHAKE 'N BAKE. See SEASONING AND COATING MIX.										
SHALLOT										
freeze-dried	1 oz	99	3.5	22.9	17	>1.3 c	0.1	<.1	0	1%
freeze-dried	1/4 cup	13	0.4	2.9	2	>.2 c	0.0	0.0	0	0%
freeze-dried	1 tbsp	3	0.1	0.7	1	tr	0.0	0.0	0	0%
raw	100 gm	72	2.5	16.8	12	>.7 c	0.1	0.0	0	1%
raw	1 tbsp	7	0.3	1.7	1	>.1 c	0.0	0.0	0	0%
raw, trimmed	1 oz	20	0.7	4.8	3	>.2 c	<.1	tr	0	<4%
raw, untrimmed	1 lb	287	10.0	67.1	48	>2.8 c	0.4	0.1	0	1%
SHARK										
Mako, boneless steak, raw (Peter Pan Seafoods)	3.5 oz	87	19.1	na	79	na	1.2	na	51	12%
Mixed species										
batter-dipped, fried	3 oz	194	15.8	5.4	104	na	11.7	2.7	50	55%
raw	1 lb	591	95.2	0.0	360	0	20.5	4.2	232	33%
raw	3 oz	110	17.8	0.0	67	0	3.8	0.8	43	32%
raw	1 oz	37	5.9	0.0	22	0	1.3	0.3	14	33%
SHEANUT OIL										
	1/2 cup	964	0.0	0.0	0	0	109.0	50.8	0	100%
	1 oz	251	0.0	0.0	0	0	28.4	13.2	0	100%
	1 tbsp	120	0.0	0.0	0	0	13.6	6.3	0	100%
SHEEPSHEAD/California sheepshead/fathead/redhead										
baked	6.6-oz fillet	234	48.4	0.0	136	0	3.0	0.7	(mq)	12%
baked	4 oz	143	29.5	0.0	83	0	1.8	0.4	(mq)	12%
baked	3 oz	107	22.1	0.0	62	0	1.4	0.3	54	13%
broiled	6.6-oz fillet	234	48.4	0.0	136	0	3.0	0.7	(mq)	12%
broiled	4 oz	143	29.5	0.0	83	0	1.8	0.4	(mq)	12%
microwaved	6.6-oz fillet	234	48.4	0.0	136	0	3.0	0.7	(mq)	12%
microwaved	4 oz	143	29.5	0.0	83	0	1.8	0.4	(mq)	12%
raw	1 lb	490	91.7	0.0	324	0	10.9	2.8	(mq)	21%
raw	3 oz	92	17.2	0.0	60	0	2.0	0.5	43	21%
raw	1 oz	31	5.7	0.0	20	0	0.7	0.2	(mq)	22%
roasted	4 oz	143	29.5	0.0	83	0	1.8	0.4	(mq)	12%
SHELLIE BEAN, CANNED										
w/liquid	1/2 cup	37	2.2	7.6	407	4.2	0.2	0.0	0	4%
w/liquid	4 oz	34	2.0	7.0	379	3.9	0.2	<.1	0	5%

Food Name	Serving Size	Calories	Prot. gms	Carbs gms	Sod. mgs	Fiber gms	Fat gms	Sat. Fat gms	Chol. mgs	% Fat Cal.
(Stokely)	1/2 cup	35	2.0	7.0	470	(mq)	0.0	0.0	0	0%
SHERBET. See also FRUIT BAR, FROZEN; ICE BARS AND DESSERTS; SORBET.										
all flavors *(Sealtest)*	1/2 cup	130	1.0	28.0	30	na	1.0	0.0	5	7%
orange	1/2 cup	132	1.1	29.2	44	>.3 c	1.9	1.1	5	12%
orange	1 oz	40	0.3	8.6	13	tr	0.6	0.3	2	13%
orange *(Borden)*	1/2 cup	110	1.0	25.0	40	na	1.0	(mq)	(mq)	8%
orange *(Darigold)*	1/2 cup	120	1.0	26.0	25	na	1.0	(mq)	(mq)	8%
vanilla-orange 'Cubic Scoops' *(Sealtest)*	4 oz	130	2.0	22.0	40	(tr)	4.0	2.0	15	27%
vanilla-red raspberry 'Cubic Scoops' *(Sealtest)*	4 oz	130	2.0	22.0	40	(tr)	4.0	2.0	15	27%
SHERBET BAR										
all flavors 'Fat-Free' *(Fudgsicle)*	1 bar	70	2.0	14.0	45	na	0.0	0.0	0	0%
all flavors 'Sugar-Free' *(Fudgsicle)*	1 bar	35	2.0	6.0	50	na	1.0	na	5	22%
chocolate *(Fudgsicle)*	1 bar	70	2.0	12.0	70	na	1.0	na	na	14%
chocolate, w/nuts 'Sugar-Free Fudge Nut Dip' *(Fudgsicle)*	1 bar	130	2.0	12.0	40	(mq)	8.0	(mq)	5	56%
orange	2.75-oz bar	91	0.7	20.1	30	>.2 c	1.3	0.8	3	12%
w/cream, all flavors 'Sugar-Free' *(Creamsicle)*	1 bar	25	1.0	5.0	20	na	1.0	na	na	27%
SHORT RIBS ENTRÉE, FROZEN										
(Armour) boneless 'Classics'	9.75 oz	380	24.0	34.0	790	(mq)	16.0	(mq)	90	38%
(Stouffer's) in gravy	9 oz	350	30.0	12.0	900	na	20.0	(mq)	(mq)	52%
(Tyson) 'Gourmet Selection'	11 oz	470	25.0	38.0	950	(mq)	24.0	(mq)	(mq)	46%
SHORTENING										
COMMERCIAL										
hydrogenated soybean oil and cottonseed oil	1 cup	1812	0.0	0.0	0	0	205.0	52.5	0	100%
hydrogenated soybean oil and cottonseed oil	1 tbsp	113	0.0	0.0	0	0	12.8	3.3	0	100%
lard and vegetable oil	1 cup	1845	0.0	0.0	0	0	205.0	73.2	115	100%
lard and vegetable oil	1 tbsp	115	0.0	0.0	0	0	12.8	4.6	7	100%
(Wesson) 'Crystal'	1 tbsp	122	0.0	0.0	0	0	13.5	2.0	0	100%
(Wesson) 'Lo-Melt'	1 tbsp	122	0.0	0.0	0	0	13.5	3.8	0	100%
(Wesson) 'Super'	1 tbsp	122	0.0	0.0	0	0	13.5	3.6	0	100%
(Wesson) 'Wesgold'	1 tbsp	122	0.0	0.0	0	0	13.5	2.6	0	100%
(Wesson) 'Wespour'	1 tbsp	122	0.0	0.0	0	0	13.5	2.5	0	100%
For baking										
hydrogenated soybean, palm, and cottonseed oils	1 cup	1812	0.0	0.0	0	0	205.0	59.1	0	100%
hydrogenated soybean, palm, and cottonseed oils	1 tbsp	113	0.0	0.0	0	0	12.8	3.7	0	100%
For bread										
hydrogenated soybean oil and cottonseed oil	1 cup	1812	0.0	0.0	0	0	205.0	45.1	0	100%
hydrogenated soybean oil and cottonseed oil	1 tbsp	113	0.0	0.0	0	0	12.8	2.8	0	100%
For cakes and frostings										
hydrogenated soybean and cottonseed oils	1 cup	1812	0.0	0.0	0	0	205.0	55.8	0	100%
hydrogenated soybean and cottonseed oils	1 tbsp	113	0.0	0.0	0	0	12.8	3.5	0	100%
hydrogenated soybean oil	1 cup	1812	0.0	0.0	0	0	205.0	41.0	0	100%
hydrogenated soybean oil	1 tbsp	113	0.0	0.0	0	0	12.8	2.6	0	100%
For confectionery										
fractionated palm oil	1 cup	1927	0.0	0.0	0	0	218.0	142.8	0	100%
fractionated palm oil	1 tbsp	120	0.0	0.0	0	0	13.6	8.9	0	100%
hydrogenated coconut and/or palm kernel oil	1 cup	1812	0.0	0.0	0	0	205.0	187.2	0	100%
hydrogenated coconut and/or palm kernel oil	1 tbsp	113	0.0	0.0	0	0	12.8	11.7	0	100%
Heavy duty, for frying										
beef tallow and cottonseed oil	1 cup	1845	0.0	0.0	0	0	205.0	92.1	205	100%
beef tallow and cottonseed oil	1 tbsp	115	0.0	0.0	0	0	12.8	5.8	13	100%
hydrogenated palm oil	1 cup	1812	0.0	0.0	0	0	205.0	97.4	0	100%
hydrogenated palm oil	1 tbsp	113	0.0	0.0	0	0	12.8	6.1	0	100%
hydrogenated soybean and cottonseed oils	1 cup	1812	0.0	0.0	0	0	205.0	31.6	0	100%
hydrogenated soybean and cottonseed oils	1 tbsp	113	0.0	0.0	0	0	12.8	2.0	0	100%

Food Name	Serving Size	Calories	Prot. gms	Carbs gms	Sod. mgs	Fiber gms	Fat gms	Sat. Fat gms	Chol. mgs	% Fat Cal.
hydrogenated soybean oil, 30% linoleic	1 cup	1812	0.0	0.0	0	0	205.0	37.7	0	100%
hydrogenated soybean oil, 30% linoleic	1 tbsp	113	0.0	0.0	0	0	12.8	2.4	0	100%
hydrogenated soybean oil, under 1% linoleic	1 cup	1812	0.0	0.0	0	0	205.0	43.2	0	100%
hydrogenated soybean oil, under 1% linoleic	1 tbsp	113	0.0	0.0	0	0	12.8	2.7	0	100%
Multi-purpose										
hydrogenated soybean and palm oils	1 cup	1812	0.0	0.0	0	0	205.0	62.4	0	100%
hydrogenated soybean and palm oils	1 tbsp	113	0.0	0.0	0	0	12.8	3.9	0	100%
HOUSEHOLD										
hydrogenated soybean and cottonseed oils	1 cup	1812	0.0	0.0	0	0	205.0	51.3	0	100%
hydrogenated soybean and cottonseed oils	1 tbsp	113	0.0	0.0	0	0	12.8	3.2	0	100%
hydrogenated soybean oil and palm oil	1 cup	1812	0.0	0.0	0	0	205.0	62.7	0	100%
hydrogenated soybean oil and palm oil	1 tbsp	113	0.0	0.0	0	0	12.8	3.9	0	100%
lard and vegetable oil	1 cup	1845	0.0	0.0	0	0	205.0	82.6	115	100%
lard and vegetable oil	1 tbsp	115	0.0	0.0	0	0	12.8	5.2	7	100%
(Crisco) vegetable	1 tbsp	110	0.0	0.0	0	0	12.0	3.0	0	100%
(Crisco) vegetable, butter flavor	1 tbsp	110	0.0	0.0	0	0	12.0	3.0	0	100%
(Finast) vegetable	1 tbsp	110	0.0	0.0	0	0	13.0	(mq)	0	100%
(Finast) vegetable, butter flavor	1 tbsp	110	0.0	0.0	0	0	12.0	3.0	0	100%
(Wesson)	1 tbsp	100	0.0	0.0	0	0	12.0	4.0	0	100%
SHOYU. See SAUCE, SOY.										
SHRIMP, ALTERNATIVE										
made from surimi	1 lb	458	56.2	41.4	3198	0	6.7	(mq)	163	13%
made from surimi	1 oz	29	3.5	2.6	200	0	0.4	na	10	13%
made from surimi	3 oz	86	10.5	7.8	599	0	1.3	0.3	31	14%
SHRIMP, MIXED SPECIES										
boiled	4 oz	112	23.7	(mq)	254	0	1.2	0.3	221	10%
boiled, .8-oz size	4 shrimp	22	4.6	(mq)	49	0	0.2	0.1	43	9%
breaded, fried	3 oz	206	18.2	9.8	292	>.1 c	10.4	1.8	150	46%
breaded, fried	1.1 oz	73	6.4	3.4	103	<.1	3.7	0.6	53	46%
breaded, fried, .8-oz size	4 shrimp	73	6.4	3.4	103	0	3.7	0.6	53	46%
fried	4 oz	274	24.3	13.0	390	>.2 c	13.9	2.4	201	46%
moist-heat cooked	3 oz	84	17.8	0.0	190	0	0.9	0.3	166	10%
moist-heat cooked, .8-oz size	4 shrimp	22	4.6	0.0	49	0	0.2	0.1	43	9%
poached	4 oz	112	23.7	(mq)	254	0	1.2	0.3	221	10%
poached, .8-oz size	4 shrimp	22	4.6	(mq)	49	0	0.2	0.1	43	9%
raw	1 lb	481	92.1	4.1	673	0	7.8	1.5	692	15%
raw	3 oz	90	17.3	0.8	126	0	1.5	0.3	129	16%
raw, .8-oz size	4 shrimp	30	5.7	0.3	41	0	0.5	0.1	43	16%
steamed	4 oz	112	23.7	(mq)	254	0	1.2	0.3	221	10%
steamed, .8-oz size	4 shrimp	22	4.6	(mq)	49	0	0.2	0.1	43	9%
Canned										
drained	1 cup	154	29.5	1.3	216	0	2.5	0.5	221	15%
drained	3 oz	102	19.6	0.9	144	0	1.7	0.3	147	16%
drained	4 oz	136	26.2	1.2	192	0	2.2	0.4	196	15%
drained (Louisiana Brand)	2 oz	58	12.0	0.0	(mq)	0	1.0	(mq)	(mq)	16%
large, drained (ShopRite)	2 oz	50	10.0	0.0	720	0	1.0	(mq)	(mq)	18%
SHRIMP CHOW MEIN, canned										
(LaChoy)	3/4 cup	35	4.0	4.0	940	2.0	1.0	0.3	50	22%
(LaChoy) 'Bi-Pack'	8.536 oz	60	3.9	10.2	935	2.9	1.0	0.0	30	14%
(LaChoy) 'Bi-Pack'	3/4 cup	50	3.0	7.0	860	2.0	1.0	(mq)	19	18%
SHRIMP COCKTAIL										
(Booth) w/garlic butter sauce and vegetable rice	10 oz	400	13.0	40.0	750	(mq)	25.0	(mq)	(mq)	52%
(Budget Gourmet) w/fettuccine	9.5 oz	375	10.0	38.0	660	(mq)	20.0	(mq)	145	48%
(LaChoy) w/lobster sauce 'Fresh & Lite'	10 oz	240	12.0	36.4	946	2.8	6.2	(mq)	118	22%

Food Name	Serving Size	Calories	Prot. gms	Carbs gms	Sod. mgs	Fiber gms	Fat gms	Sat. Fat gms	Chol. mgs	% Fat Cal.
(Mrs. Paul's) w/clams and linguini 'Light'	10 oz	240	12.0	36.0	750	(mq)	5.0	2.0	40	19%
(Sau-Sea)	4 oz	113	7.0	19.0	1020	na	1.0	(mq)	102	8%
(SeaPak) 'Super Valu' heat and serve	4 oz	210	12.0	30.0	730	(mq)	4.0	(mq)	80	18%
SHRIMP ENTRÉE, FROZEN										
BAY, BABY (Armour) 'Classics Lite'	9.75 oz	220	12.0	31.0	890	(mq)	6.0	(mq)	105	24%
BATTERED										
(SeaPak) 'Shrimp 'n Batter'	4 oz	260	11.0	20.0	470	(mq)	15.0	(mq)	20	52%
(SeaPak) w/crabmeat stuffing	4 oz	260	8.0	27.0	780	(mq)	13.0	(mq)	(mq)	46%
BREADED										
(Gorton's) original seasoning	2.7 oz	200	9.0	15.0	450	na	12.0	na	50	53%
(Gorton's) popcorn style	2.7 oz	220	8.0	16.0	450	na	14.0	na	50	57%
(Gorton's) scampi seasoning	2.7 oz	210	9.0	16.0	440	na	12.0	na	50	52%
(Mrs. Paul's) fried	3 oz	200	9.0	16.0	430	(mq)	11.0	(mq)	(mq)	50%
BUTTERFLY										
(Gorton's) 'Specialty'	4 oz	160	19.0	16.0	540	na	<1.0	na	(mq)	<6%
(SeaPak) breaded 'Mikado'	4 oz	160	12.0	26.0	170	(mq)	1.0	(mq)	110	6%
BUTTERFLY/ROUND (SeaPak) breaded	4 oz	150	14.0	20.0	(mq)	(mq)	1.0	(mq)	(mq)	6%
CAJUN STYLE (Mrs. Paul's) 'Light'	9 oz	230	9.0	37.0	740	(mq)	5.0	1.0	60	20%
CREOLE										
(Armour) 'Classics Lite'	11.25 oz	260	6.0	53.0	900	(mq)	2.0	(mq)	45	7%
(Cajun Cookin')	12 oz	390	17.0	55.0	1130	(mq)	11.0	(mq)	(mq)	26%
(Healthy Choice)	11.25 oz	230	8.0	45.0	430	na	2.0	<1.0	60	8%
CRISP (Gorton's) 'Specialty'	4 oz	280	9.0	26.0	740	(mq)	15.0	(mq)	(mq)	49%
CRUNCHY										
(Gorton's) 'Crunchy Shrimp' microwave	2 oz	160	7.0	12.0	380	na	9.0	na	40	52%
(Gorton's) whole 'Microwave Specialty'	5 oz	380	14.0	35.0	870	(mq)	20.0	3.0	65	48%
ETOUFFEE (Cajun Cookin')	17 oz	360	19.0	52.0	1170	(mq)	9.0	(mq)	(mq)	22%
FETTUCCINE ALFREDO (Booth)	10 oz	260	19.0	28.0	620	(mq)	8.0	(mq)	(mq)	28%
JAMBALAYA (Cajun Cookin')	12 oz	450	20.0	43.0	800	(mq)	20.0	(mq)	(mq)	42%
MARINARA										
(Healthy Choice)	10.5 oz	260	10.0	51.0	320	na	1.0	<1.0	60	4%
(Smart Ones) w/linguini	8 oz	150	8.0	26.0	390	na	<1.0	<1.0	60	<6%
NEW ORLEANS, w/wild rice (Booth)	10 oz	230	13.0	35.0	950	(mq)	5.0	(mq)	(mq)	19%
ORIENTAL, w/pineapple rice (Booth)	10 oz	190	11.0	30.0	950	(mq)	3.0	(mq)	(mq)	14%
PRIMAVERA										
(Booth) w/fettucini	10 oz	200	16.0	28.0	760	(mq)	3.0	(mq)	(mq)	13%
(Mrs. Paul's) 'Light'	9.5 oz	180	11.0	28.0	840	(mq)	3.0	1.0	125	15%
(Right Course)	9 5/8 oz	240	12.0	32.0	590	(mq)	7.0	1.0	50	26%
SCAMPI (Gorton's) 'Microwave Entrées'	1 pkg	390	10.0	21.0	470	(mq)	30.0	(mq)	(mq)	69%
STIR-FRY (Shanghai)	10.3 oz	170	18.0	19.0	1200	na	2.0	na	55	11%
SHRIMP ENTRÉE, PACKAGED										
(Ultra Slim Fast) creole	12 oz	240	12.0	45.0	730	na	4.0	na	80	14%
(Ultra Slim Fast) marinara	12 oz	290	17.0	53.0	880	na	3.0	na	70	9%
SHRIMP PASTE, canned	1 tsp	13	1.5	0.1	10	0	0.7	0.4	12	50%
SHRIMP SALAD										
(Longacre) 'Saladfest'	1 oz	45	2.0	2.0	150	na	3.0	(mq)	25	63%
(Longacre) 'Saladfest' w/seafood	1 oz	42	2.0	2.0	160	na	3.0	(mq)	15	63%
SICAMA. See JICAMA.										
SILVER HAKE. See WHITING, MIXED SPECIES.										
SIM SIM. See SESAME SEED.										
SISYMBRIUM SEED										
whole, dried	1 cup	235	9.0	43.1	68	>22.0 c	3.4	0.7	0	13%
whole, dried	1 oz	90	3.5	16.5	26	>8.4 c	1.3	0.3	0	13%
SKIL. See SABLEFISH.										

Food Name	Serving Size	Calories	Prot. gms	Carbs gms	Sod. mgs	Fiber gms	Fat gms	Sat. Fat gms	Chol. mgs	% Fat Cal.
SKUNK CABBAGE. See CABBAGE, SKUNK.										
SLIMEHEAD. See ORANGE ROUGHY.										
SLOPPY JOE SEASONING MIX										
(French's)	1/8 pkg	16	0.0	4.0	390	(mq)	0.0	0.0	0	0%
(Lawry's) 'Seasoning Blends'	1 pkg	126	2.8	27.7	3442	>.8 c	0.4	na	0	3%
(Schilling)	1/4 pkg	26	0.5	6.0	750	(mq)	0.5	na	0	15%
SMELT, RAINBOW										
broiled	4 oz	141	25.6	0.0	87	0	3.5	0.7	102	24%
dry-heat cooked	4 oz	141	25.6	0.0	87	0	3.5	0.7	102	24%
dry-heat cooked	3 oz	105	19.2	0.0	65	0	2.6	0.5	77	23%
microwaved	4 oz	141	25.6	0.0	87	0	3.5	0.7	102	24%
raw	1 lb	440	80.0	0.0	272	0	11.0	2.1	318	24%
raw	3 oz	82	15.0	0.0	51	0	2.1	0.4	59	24%
raw	1 oz	27	5.0	0.0	17	0	0.7	0.1	20	24%
SNACK. See CORN CHIPS AND SNACKS; SNACK BAR; SNACK MIX.										
SNACK BAR. See also DIET BAR.										
(Barbara's Bakery)										
apple, real fruit, .5 oz	1 bar	50	0.0	11.0	0	na	0.0	0.0	0	0%
apricot, real fruit, .5 oz	1 bar	50	0.0	11.0	0	na	0.0	0.0	0	0%
cherry, real fruit, .5 oz	1 bar	50	0.0	11.0	0	na	0.0	0.0	0	0%
grape, real fruit, .5 oz	1 bar	50	0.0	11.0	0	na	0.0	0.0	0	0%
raspberry, real fruit, .5 oz	1 bar	50	0.0	11.0	1	na	0.0	0.0	0	0%
(Bear Valley)										
carob-cocoa, food bar 'Pemmican'	3.75 oz	440	16.0	68.0	80	7.0	12.0	na	0	24%
coconut almond, food bar 'Meal Pack'	3.75 oz	400	13.0	56.0	80	6.0	12.0	na	0	28%
fruit 'n nut, food bar 'Pemmican'	3.75 oz	420	17.0	59.0	90	9.0	13.0	na	0	28%
sesame lemon, food bar 'Meal Pack'	3.75 oz	410	17.0	57.0	85	4.0	13.0	na	0	28%
(Carnation)										
chocolate chip, breakfast bar	1 bar	200	6.0	20.0	180	1.4	11.0	4.2	<1	49%
chocolate crunch, breakfast bar	1 bar	190	6.0	20.0	150	1.2	10.0	3.9	<1	46%
peanut butter chocolate chip, breakfast bar	1 bar	200	6.0	20.0	170	1.4	11.0	3.0	<1	49%
peanut butter crunch, breakfast bar	1 bar	190	6.0	20.0	180	1.0	10.0	2.8	<1	46%
(Earth Grains)										
banana apple walnut 'Bagel Power Bar'	1 bar	270	12.0	45.0	280	na	6.0	na	0	19%
citrus almond w/mixed fruit 'Bagel Power Bar'	1 bar	260	12.0	45.0	280	na	4.0	na	0	14%
fruit and nut 'Bagel Power Bar'	1 bar	240	9.0	48.0	280	na	3.0	na	0	11%
(Glenny's)										
apple-cinnamon	1.25 oz	120	1.0	28.0	15	na	<1.0	na	na	<7%
caramel	1.25 oz	120	1.0	29.0	65	na	<1.0	na	na	<7%
chocolate	1.25 oz	120	1.0	28.0	20	na	<1.0	na	na	<7%
raspberry	1.25 oz	120	1.0	29.0	15	na	<1.0	na	na	<7%
(Health Valley)										
apple, fat-free	1 bar	140	3.0	33.0	10	3.7	0.0	na	0	0%
'Apple Bakes'	1 bar	100	2.0	16.0	27	2.8	3.0	(mq)	0	27%
apricot, fat-free	1 bar	140	3.0	33.0	10	3.7	0.0	na	0	0%
date, fat-free	1 bar	140	3.0	33.0	10	3.7	0.0	na	0	0%
'Date Bakes'	1 bar	100	3.0	16.0	25	2.8	3.0	(mq)	0	26%
'Fruit & Fitness'	1 bar	200	4.0	39.0	234	4.8	3.0	(mq)	0	14%
'Oat Bran, Fig & Nut Bakes'	1 bar	110	2.0	19.0	18	3.1	3.0	(mq)	0	24%
oat bran, raisin, and cinnamon	1 bar	140	3.0	32.0	12	6.3	2.0	(mq)	0	11%
'Oat Bran Apricot Bakes'	1 bar	100	2.0	19.0	18	2.9	2.0	(mq)	0	18%
'Oat Bran Jumbo Fruit and Nut Bars'	1 bar	150	4.0	29.0	11	8.4	4.0	(mq)	0	21%
'Oat Bran Jumbo Fruit Bars'	1 bar	170	4.0	28.0	9	6.7	5.0	(mq)	0	26%
raisin, fat-free	1 bar	140	3.0	33.0	10	3.7	0.0	na	0	0%

Food Name	Serving Size	Calories	Prot. gms	Carbs gms	Sod. mgs	Fiber gms	Fat gms	Sat. Fat gms	Chol. mgs	% Fat Cal.
'Raisin Bakes'	1 bar	100	2.0	16.0	19	2.8	3.0	(mq)	0	27%
rice bran, almond, and date	1 bar	190	4.0	29.0	6	5.6	6.0	(mq)	0	29%
(Kudos)										
peaches and cream 'Pan Squares'	1 square	150	2.0	22.0	105	2.0	6.0	na	na	36%
peanut butter and chocolate chip 'Pan Squares'	1 square	170	3.0	20.0	105	2.0	9.0	na	na	47%
strawberry and cream cheese 'Pan Squares'	1 square	150	2.0	22.0	105	2.0	6.0	na	na	36%
(Tiger's Milk) peanut butter and honey, carob coated	1 bar	160	6.0	23.0	90	na	5.0	na	na	28%
(Weider)										
'Sportsfood Enerquench Bar'	1 bar	200	6.0	44.0	80	na	1.0	na	na	4%
'Sportsfood Protein Bar'	1 bar	160	10.0	21.0	140	na	4.0	na	na	23%
SNACK BAR MIX, PREPARED										
(Betty Crocker)										
caramel oatmeal 'Supreme Dessert'	1 bar	110	1.0	15.0	65	na	5.0	na	0	41%
chocolate and toffee 'Supreme Dessert'	1 bar	110	1.0	17.0	55	na	4.0	na	10	33%
chocolate peanut butter 'Supreme Dessert'	1 bar	110	1.0	14.0	100	na	5.0	na	10	43%
date 'Classic'	1 bar	60	1.0	9.0	35	(mq)	2.0	1.0	0	31%
lemon-Sunkist 'Supreme Dessert' prepared w/4 eggs	1 bar	110	1.0	17.0	65	na	4.0	na	30	33%
M&M cookie bars 'Supreme Dessert'	1 bar	110	1.0	16.0	80	na	5.0	1.0	10	40%
raspberry 'Supreme Dessert'	1 bar	100	1.0	16.0	95	na	4.0	1.0	0	35%
SNACK MIX										
(Doo Dads) original recipe, 1 oz	1/2 cup	129	2.9	18.2	360	1.9	5.2	na	0	36%
(Flavor Tree)										
'Party Mix'	1/4 cup	163	3.4	12.3	407	>.1 c	11.0	(mq)	0	61%
'Party Mix No Salt'	1 1/2 cup	163	3.9	13.2	8	>.1 c	10.8	(mq)	0	59%
(Pepperidge Farm)										
cheese, super cheddar 'Goldfish Party Mix'	1 oz	140	4.0	15.0	330	na	7.0	1.0	15	45%
'Classic'	1 oz	140	4.0	14.0	360	1.0	8.0	1.0	0	50%
lightly smoked	1 oz	150	4.0	13.0	350	1.0	9.0	1.0	0	54%
nutty deluxe, cashews and almonds 'Goldfish'	1/2 cup	180	5.0	20.0	330	2.0	9.0	1.5	25	45%
original, honey roasted peanuts 'Goldfish'	1/2 cup	170	5.0	21.0	360	2.0	8.0	1.5	5	41%
spicy	1 oz	140	4.0	14.0	340	1.0	8.0	2.0	5	50%
(Ralston)										
barbecue 'Chex' 2/3 cup	1 oz	130	3.0	18.0	380	na	5.0	na	0	35%
'Chex Traditional' 2/3 cup	1 oz	120	3.1	18.5	288	>.5 c	4.9	na	0	34%
cool sour cream and onion 'Chex' 2/3 cup	1 oz	130	3.0	19.0	300	(mq)	5.0	(mq)	na	34%
golden cheddar 'Chex' 2/3 cup	1 oz	130	3.0	19.0	300	(mq)	5.0	(mq)	na	34%
nacho cheese 'Chex' 2/3 cup	1 oz	130	3.0	19.0	430	(mq)	5.0	(mq)	na	34%
(Ritz) traditional, baked	1 oz	130	2.0	18.0	310	na	6.0	1.0	0	40%
SNAPPER, RED, MIXED SPECIES										
broiled	4 oz	145	3.0	0.0	65	0	2.0	0.1	53	60%
dry-heat cooked	4 oz	145	3.0	0.0	65	0	2.0	0.1	53	60%
dry-heat cooked	3 oz	109	22.4	0.0	48	0	1.5	0.3	40	13%
microwaved	4 oz	145	3.0	0.0	65	0	2.0	0.1	53	60%
raw	1 lb	452	93.0	0.0	291	0	6.1	1.3	168	13%
raw	3 oz	85	17.4	0.0	54	0	1.1	0.2	31	13%
raw	1 oz	28	5.8	0.0	18	0	0.4	0.1	10	13%

SNOW PEAS. See PEAS, SNOW.

SOBA NOODLE. See NOODLE, JAPANESE.

SODA. See SOFT DRINKS AND MIXERS.

SODA, CLUB. See SOFT DRINKS AND MIXERS.

SOFT DRINKS AND MIXERS. See also WATER, SPARKLING, FLAVORED.

Food Name	Serving Size	Calories	Prot. gms	Carbs gms	Sod. mgs	Fiber gms	Fat gms	Sat. Fat gms	Chol. mgs	% Fat Cal.
(A&W)										
cream soda	1 oz	14	0.1	3.6	2	0	tr	0.0	0	0%
cream soda, 'Diet'	1 oz	<1	0.1	0.0	4	0	<.1	0.0	0	<69%

Food Name	Serving Size	Calories	Prot. gms	Carbs gms	Sod. mgs	Fiber gms	Fat gms	Sat. Fat gms	Chol. mgs	% Fat Cal.
root beer	1 oz	15	<.1	3.5	5	0	<.1	0.0	0	<6%
root beer, 'Diet'	1 oz	<1	0.1	0.0	4	0	tr	0.0	0	0%
(Canada Dry)										
collins mixer	8 oz	80	0.0	20.0	17	0	0.0	0.0	0	0%
ginger ale	8 oz	90	0.0	21.0	7	0	0.0	0.0	0	0%
ginger ale, 'Golden'	8 oz	100	0.0	24.0	24	0	0.0	0.0	0	0%
grape, 'Concord'	8 oz	130	0.0	32.0	21	0	0.0	0.0	0	0%
half and half	8 oz	110	0.0	26.0	17	0	0.0	0.0	0	0%
tonic	8 oz	90	0.0	22.0	7	0	0.0	0.0	0	0%
whiskey sour mixer	8 oz	90	0.0	22.0	17	0	0.0	0.0	0	0%
(Coca Cola)										
cherry cola	6 oz	76	0.0	20.0	4	0	0.0	0.0	0	0%
cherry cola, 'Diet'	6 oz	<1	0.0	0.2	4	0	0.0	0.0	0	0%
cola, caffeine-free	6 oz	77	0.0	20.0	4	0	0.0	0.0	0	0%
cola, 'Classic'	6 oz	72	0.0	19.0	7	0	0.0	0.0	0	0%
cola, diet, caffeine-free	6 oz	<1	0.0	0.2	4	0	0.0	0.0	0	0%
cola, diet, w/caffeine	6 oz	<1	0.0	0.2	4	0	0.0	0.0	0	0%
cola, w/caffeine	6 oz	77	0.0	20.0	4	0	0.0	0.0	0	0%
(Dr. Diablo) cola	12 oz	140	0.0	38.0	14	0	0.0	0.0	0	0%
(Dr. Pepper)										
cola	12 oz	150	0.0	38.4	18	0	0.0	0.0	0	0%
cola, caffeine-free	12 oz	150	0.0	38.4	18	0	0.0	0.0	0	0%
diet	12 oz	3	0.0	0.2	18	0	0.0	0.0	0	0%
diet, caffeine-free	12 oz	3	0.0	0.2	18	0	0.0	0.0	0	0%
(Fanta)										
ginger ale	6 oz	63	0.0	16.0	14	0	0.0	0.0	0	0%
grape	6 oz	86	0.0	22.0	7	0	0.0	0.0	0	0%
orange	6 oz	88	0.0	23.0	7	0	0.0	0.0	0	0%
root beer	6 oz	78	0.0	20.0	10	0	0.0	0.0	0	0%
(Fresca) citrus	6 oz	2	0.0	0.2	tr	0	0.0	0.0	0	0%
(Health Valley)										
ginger ale	12 oz	153	1.0	35.0	30	0	1.0	0.0	0	6%
root beer, 'Old Fashioned'	12 oz	120	1.0	26.0	12	0	1.0	0.0	0	8%
root beer, sarsaparilla	12 oz	153	1.0	35.0	27	0	1.0	0.0	0	6%
wild berry	12 oz	142	1.0	33.0	27	0	1.0	(tr)	0	6%
(Hires)										
cream soda, caffeine-free	6 oz	90	<1.0	24.0	40	0	<1.0	na	na	<8%
cream soda, 'Diet' caffeine-free	6 oz	2	<1.0	<1.0	45	0	<1.0	na	na	<53%
root beer, caffeine-free	6 oz	90	<1.0	23.0	55	0	<1.0	na	na	<9%
root beer, 'Diet' caffeine-free, w/NutraSweet	6 oz	2	<1.0	<1.0	70	0	<1.0	na	na	<53%
(Jolt) cola	6 oz	85	0.0	20.7	10	0	0.0	0.0	0	0%
(Mello Yello)										
citrus	6 oz	87	0.0	22.0	14	0	0.0	0.0	0	0%
citrus, diet	6 oz	3	0.0	0.2	<1	0	0.0	0.0	0	0%
(Mountain Dew)										
citrus	12 oz	179	0.0	44.4	31	0	0.0	0.0	0	0%
citrus, diet	12 oz	4	0.0	0.7	<1	0	0.0	0.0	0	0%
(Mr. Pibb) cola	6 oz	71	0.0	19.0	10	0	0.0	0.0	0	0%
(Mug)										
root beer	12 oz	168	0.0	42.0	39	0	0.0	0.0	0	0%
root beer, 'Diet'	12 oz	4	0.0	1.2	39	0	0.0	0.0	0	0%
(Natural 90 Diet) all flavors	6 oz	2	0.0	<1.0	10	0	0.0	0.0	0	0%
(Pathmark) cola, 'No Frills Sugar-free'	8 oz	0	0.0	tr	(mq)	0	0.0	0.0	0	0%

Food Name	Serving Size	Calories	Prot. gms	Carbs gms	Sod. mgs	Fiber gms	Fat gms	Sat. Fat gms	Chol. mgs	% Fat Cal.
(Pepsi)										
cherry cola, 'Diet Wild Cherry'	12 oz	1	0.0	na	2	0	0.0	0.0	0	0%
cherry cola, 'Wild Cherry'	12 oz	163	0.0	43.2	2	0	0.0	0.0	0	0%
cola, caffeine-free	12 oz	160	0.0	39.6	2	0	0.0	0.0	0	0%
cola, clear 'Diet Crystal' w/NutraSweet	6 oz	0	0.0	0.0	35	0	0.0	na	na	0%
cola, diet, caffeine-free	12 oz	<1	0.0	0.2	2	0	0.0	0.0	0	0%
cola, diet, w/caffeine	12 oz	<1	0.0	0.2	2	0	0.0	0.0	0	0%
cola, 'Light'	12 oz	<1	0.0	0.1	2	0	0.0	0.0	0	0%
cola, w/caffeine	12 oz	160	0.0	39.6	2	0	0.0	0.0	0	0%
(Santa Cruz Naturals) ginger ale, organic 'Sparkling'	8 oz	155	<1.0	36.0	na	0	<1.0	na	na	<6%
(Schweppes)										
blackberry, 'Royal'	6 oz	35	0.0	8.0	5	0	0.0	0.0	0	0%
citrus, tropical 'Royal'	6 oz	35	0.0	8.0	5	0	0.0	0.0	0	0%
club soda	6 oz	0	0.0	0.0	25	0	0.0	0.0	0	0%
collins mixer	6 oz	75	0.0	18.0	51	0	0.0	0.0	0	0%
ginger ale	6 oz	65	0.0	16.0	10	0	0.0	0.0	0	0%
ginger ale, raspberry	6 oz	65	0.0	16.0	10	0	0.0	0.0	0	0%
ginger ale, raspberry 'Diet'	6 oz	2	0.0	<1.0	55	0	0.0	0.0	0	0%
ginger ale, 'Sugar-free'	6 oz	2	0.0	<1.0	39	0	0.0	0.0	0	0%
ginger beer	6 oz	70	0.0	17.0	30	0	0.0	0.0	0	0%
grape	6 oz	95	0.0	23.0	15	0	0.0	0.0	0	0%
grapefruit	6 oz	80	0.0	20.0	28	0	0.0	0.0	0	0%
kiwi-passion fruit, 'Royal'	6 oz	35	0.0	8.0	5	0	0.0	0.0	0	0%
lemon, bitter	6 oz	82	0.0	20.0	13	0	0.0	0.0	0	0%
lemon, sour	6 oz	79	0.0	19.0	12	0	0.0	0.0	0	0%
lemon-lime	6 oz	72	0.0	18.0	30	0	0.0	0.0	0	0%
orange, sparkling	6 oz	88	0.0	22.0	17	0	0.0	0.0	0	0%
peaches 'n cream, 'Royal'	6 oz	35	0.0	8.0	5	0	0.0	0.0	0	0%
root beer	6 oz	76	0.0	19.0	17	0	0.0	0.0	0	0%
seltzer, all flavors	6 oz	0	0.0	0.0	5	0	0.0	0.0	0	0%
seltzer, 'Low Sodium'	6 oz	0	0.0	0.0	7	0	0.0	0.0	0	0%
seltzer, 'Sodium-free'	6 oz	0	0.0	0.0	5	0	0.0	0.0	0	0%
strawberry-banana, 'Royal'	6 oz	35	0.0	8.0	5	0	0.0	0.0	0	0%
tonic	6 oz	64	0.0	16.0	8	0	0.0	0.0	0	0%
tonic, 'Diet'	6 oz	2	0.0	<1.0	45	0	0.0	0.0	0	0%
vanilla bean, 'Royal'	6 oz	35	0.0	8.0	5	0	0.0	0.0	0	0%
Vichy water	6 oz	0	0.0	0.0	76	0	0.0	0.0	0	0%
wild cherry, 'Royal'	6 oz	35	0.0	8.0	5	0	0.0	0.0	0	0%
wild raspberry, 'Royal'	6 oz	35	0.0	8.0	5	0	0.0	0.0	0	0%
(7•Up)										
cherry citrus	12 oz	148	0.0	38.7	32	0	0.0	0.0	0	0%
cherry citrus, diet	12 oz	4	0.0	tr	32	0	0.0	0.0	0	0%
lemon-lime	12 oz	144	0.0	36.2	32	0	0.0	0.0	0	0%
lemon-lime, diet	12 oz	4	0.0	0.0	32	0	0.0	0.0	0	0%
(Shasta)										
apple, 'Yoshi Apple'	8 oz	130	0.0	31.0	30	0	0.0	0.0	na	0%
berry, 'Luigi Berry'	8 oz	130	0.0	32.0	30	0	0.0	0.0	na	0%
black cherry	12 oz	162	0.0	44.0	29	0	0.0	0.0	0	0%
cherry, 'Princess Toadstool Cherry'	8 oz	130	0.0	31.0	30	0	0.0	0.0	na	0%
cherry cola	12 oz	140	0.0	38.0	22	0	0.0	0.0	0	0%
citrus mist	12 oz	170	0.0	46.0	19	0	0.0	0.0	0	0%
club soda	12 oz	0	0.0	0.0	46	0	0.0	0.0	0	0%
cola	12 oz	147	0.0	40.0	3	0	0.0	0.0	0	0%
cola, 'Free'	12 oz	151	0.0	41.0	2	0	0.0	0.0	0	0%

Food Name	Serving Size	Calories	Prot. gms	Carbs gms	Sod. mgs	Fiber gms	Fat gms	Sat. Fat gms	Chol. mgs	% Fat Cal.
collins mixer	12 oz	118	0.0	32.0	23	0	0.0	0.0	0	0%
cream soda, 'Creme'	12 oz	154	0.0	42.0	23	0	0.0	0.0	0	0%
ginger ale	12 oz	120	0.0	33.0	23	0	0.0	0.0	0	0%
grape	12 oz	177	0.0	48.0	34	0	0.0	0.0	0	0%
lemon-lime	12 oz	146	0.0	39.0	19	0	0.0	0.0	0	0%
orange	12 oz	177	0.0	48.0	28	0	0.0	0.0	0	0%
red berry	12 oz	158	0.0	43.0	20	0	0.0	0.0	0	0%
root beer	12 oz	154	0.0	42.0	31	0	0.0	0.0	0	0%
strawberry	12 oz	147	0.0	40.0	36	0	0.0	0.0	0	0%
tonic	12 oz	121	0.0	33.0	17	0	0.0	0.0	0	0%
(Slice)										
lemon-lime	12 oz	150	0.0	38.4	69	0	0.0	0.0	0	0%
lemon-lime, 'Diet'	12 oz	16	0.0	2.4	69	0	0.0	0.0	0	0%
orange, 'Diet'	12 oz	12	0.0	2.3	2	0	0.0	0.0	0	0%
orange, Mandarin	12 oz	193	0.0	50.4	<1	0	0.0	0.0	0	0%
(Snapple)										
'Amazin' Grape'	8 oz	120	0.0	28.0	5	0	0.0	0.0	0	0%
'Cherry Lime Rickey'	8 oz	110	0.0	27.0	0	0	0.0	0.0	0	0%
'Creme D'Vanilla'	8 oz	130	0.0	33.0	0	0	0.0	0.0	0	0%
'French Cherry'	8 oz	120	0.0	29.0	0	0	0.0	0.0	0	0%
'Kiwi Peach'	8 oz	120	0.0	29.0	0	0	0.0	0.0	0	0%
'Kiwi Strawberry'	8 oz	130	0.0	33.0	5	0	0.0	0.0	0	0%
'Mango Madness'	8 oz	130	0.0	33.0	5	0	0.0	0.0	0	0%
'Passion Supreme'	8 oz	120	0.0	29.0	0	0	0.0	0.0	0	0%
'Peach Melba'	8 oz	120	0.0	31.0	0	0	0.0	0.0	0	0%
'Raspberry'	8 oz	120	0.0	31.0	0	0	0.0	0.0	0	0%
'Tru Root Beer'	8 oz	110	0.0	29.0	0	0	0.0	0.0	0	0%
(Spree)										
cherry-lime	12 oz	158	0.0	43.0	2	0	0.0	0.0	0	0%
cola	12 oz	147	0.0	40.0	1	0	0.0	0.0	0	0%
ginger ale	12 oz	120	0.0	33.0	1	0	0.0	0.0	0	0%
grapefruit	12 oz	154	0.0	42.0	1	0	0.0	0.0	0	0%
lemon-lime	12 oz	154	0.0	42.0	1	0	0.0	0.0	0	0%
lemon-tangerine	12 oz	165	0.0	45.0	1	0	0.0	0.0	0	0%
lime, Mandarin	12 oz	154	0.0	42.0	1	0	0.0	0.0	0	0%
root beer	12 oz	154	0.0	42.0	2	0	0.0	0.0	0	0%
tropical blend	12 oz	146	0.0	41.0	2	0	0.0	0.0	0	0%
(Sprite)										
lemon-lime	6 oz	71	0.0	18.0	23	0	0.0	0.0	0	0%
lemon-lime, diet	6 oz	2	0.0	0.0	tr	0	0.0	0.0	0	0%
(Squirt)										
citrus	1 oz	13	tr	3.2	2	0	tr	na	na	0%
citrus, 'Diet'	1 oz	<1	tr	0.1	1	0	tr	na	na	0%
citrus berry, 'Ruby Red'	8 oz	120	0.0	30.0	25	0	0.0	na	na	0%
(Tab)										
cola, caffeine-free	6 oz	<1	0.0	0.2	4	0	0.0	0.0	0	0%
cola, w/caffeine	6 oz	<1	0.0	0.2	4	0	0.0	0.0	0	0%
(Vernor's)										
ginger	3.5 oz	40	0.1	10.0	4	0	0.1	na	na	2%
ginger, 'Diet'	3.5 oz	<1	0.1	0.1	7	0	0.1	na	na	53%
(Wink) grapefruit	8 oz	120	0.0	30.0	19	0	0.0	0.0	0	0%
(Yoo-Hoo) chocolate	9 oz	140	3.0	27.0	130	0	1.0	(tr)	(tr)	7%
SOLE										
dry-heat cooked	3 oz	99	20.5	0.0	89	0	1.3	0.3	58	13%

Food Name	Serving Size	Calories	Prot. gms	Carbs gms	Sod. mgs	Fiber gms	Fat gms	Sat. Fat gms	Chol. mgs	% Fat Cal.
raw	3 oz	77	16.0	0.0	69	0	1.0	0.2	41	12%
SOLE, FROZEN										
Dinner *(Healthy Choice)* au gratin	11 oz	270	16.0	40.0	470	na	5.0	3.0	55	17%
Entrée										
(Gorton's) in lemon butter 'Microwave Entrees'	1 pkg	380	25.0	17.0	560	(mq)	24.0	11.0	120	56%
(Gorton's) seafood stuffed 'Select' approx 5 oz	1 fillet	160	16.0	18.0	730	na	3.0	<1.0	50	17%
(Healthy Choice) w/lemon butter sauce	8.25 oz	230	16.0	33.0	430	na	4.0	2.0	45	16%
Fillet										
(Booth) Atlantic	4 oz	90	19.0	0.0	180	0	1.0	(mq)	(mq)	11%
(Gorton's) 'Fishmarket Fresh'	5 oz	110	24.0	1.0	140	0	1.0	(mq)	(mq)	8%
(Mrs. Paul's) breaded 'Light'	1 fillet	240	16.0	20.0	450	(mq)	10.0	(mq)	50	39%
(SeaPak)	4 oz	90	20.0	0.0	135	0	1.0	(mq)	(mq)	10%
(Van de Kamp's) breaded 'Light'	1 fillet	250	17.0	18.0	480	(mq)	12.0	2.0	45	44%
(Van de Kamp's) 'Natural'	4 oz	100	22.0	0.0	105	0	2.0	1.0	35	17%
SOMEN NOODLE. See NOODLE, JAPANESE.										
SORBET. See also FRUIT BARS, FROZEN; ICE BARS AND DESSERTS; SHERBET.										
(Baskin-Robbins)										
fruit whip	1 scoop	80	0.0	24.0	20	na	0.0	0.0	0	0%
red raspberry	1 scoop	140	0.0	34.0	25	na	0.0	0.0	(mq)	0%
(Cascadian Farms)										
blackberry	1 oz	25	0.6	21.2	na	na	0.1	na	na	1%
raspberry	1 oz	28	0.7	20.9	na	na	0.2	na	na	2%
strawberry	1 oz	26	0.6	22.0	na	na	0.1	na	na	1%
(Dole)										
orange, Mandarin	4 oz	110	0.5	28.0	9	na	0.1	(tr)	0	1%
peach	4 oz	120	0.6	28.0	11	na	0.6	na	0	5%
pineapple	4 oz	120	0.5	28.0	11	na	0.1	(tr)	0	1%
raspberry	4 oz	110	0.4	28.0	12	na	<.1	na	0	<1%
strawberry	4 oz	110	0.5	28.0	1	na	0.1	(tr)	0	1%
(Frusen Glädjé) raspberry	1/2 cup	140	0.0	36.0	10	na	0.0	0.0	0	0%
(Häagen Dazs)										
blueberry, and vanilla ice cream	1/2 cup	190	3.0	25.0	35	na	8.0	(mq)	(mq)	39%
Key lime, and vanilla ice cream	1/2 cup	200	2.0	29.0	30	na	7.0	(mq)	(mq)	34%
lemon 'Ice Cream Shop'	4 oz	140	1.0	34.0	5	na	0.0	0.0	na	0%
orange, and vanilla ice cream	1/2 cup	190	3.0	27.0	35	na	8.0	(mq)	(mq)	38%
orange 'Ice Cream Shop'	4 oz	113	1.0	30.0	7	na	0.0	0.0	na	0%
raspberry, and vanilla ice cream	1/2 cup	180	2.0	23.0	35	na	8.0	(mq)	(mq)	42%
raspberry 'Ice Cream Shop'	4 oz	93	0.0	22.0	7	na	0.0	0.0	na	0%
SORGHUM										
broomcorn, whole grain	100 gm	327	9.9	72.9	1	>3.2 c	2.9	1.0	0	7%
whole grain	1 cup	650	21.7	143.3	na	>4.6 c	6.3	0.9	0	8%
whole grain	1 oz	96	3.2	21.2	na	>.7 c	0.9	0.1	0	8%
SORGHUM SYRUP										
	1/2 cup	424	0.0	112.2	na	0	0.0	0.0	0	0%
	1 tbsp	53	0.0	4.0	na	0	0.0	0.0	0	0%
SORREL										
boiled, drained	4 oz	23	2.1	3.3	3	>.8 c	0.7	(tr)	0	23%
raw, trimmed	1 oz	6	0.6	0.9	1	>.2 c	0.2	(tr)	0	23%
raw, trimmed, chopped	1/2 cup	15	1.3	2.1	3	1.9	0.5	(tr)	0	25%
raw, untrimmed	1 lb	70	6.4	10.2	13	>2.5 c	2.2	na	0	23%
SOUP, CANNED, CONDENSED										
(NOTE: Unless otherwise specified, PREPARED = prepared as directed w/water.)										
ASPARAGUS, CREAM OF										
prepared	1 cup	87	2.3	10.7	981	.7	4.1	1.0	5	42%

Food Name	Serving Size	Calories	Prot. gms	Carbs gms	Sod. mgs	Fiber gms	Fat gms	Sat. Fat gms	Chol. mgs	% Fat Cal.
prepared w/whole milk	8 oz	161	6.3	16.4	1042	.7	8.2	3.3	22	45%
unprepared	10.75 oz	210	5.6	26.0	2385	1.2	9.9	2.5	12	41%
(Campbell's) prepared	8 oz	80	2.0	10.0	820	(mq)	4.0	(mq)	5	43%
BEAN										
(Campbell's) 'Homestyle' prepared	8 oz	130	6.0	25.0	700	(mq)	1.0	(mq)	na	7%
W/bacon										
(Campbell's) 'Healthy Request'	4 oz	140	6.0	22.0	470	6.0	4.0	na	5	24%
(Campbell's) 'Healthy Request' prepared	8 oz	140	6.0	21.0	470	(mq)	4.0	(mq)	5	25%
(Campbell's) prepared	8 oz	140	6.0	21.0	840	(mq)	4.0	(mq)	5	25%
W/frankfurters										
prepared	1 cup	188	10.0	22.0	1093	>1.5 c	7.0	2.1	13	33%
unprepared	11.25 oz	455	24.2	53.4	2653	>3.6 c	16.9	5.2	30	33%
W/pork										
prepared	1 cup	172	7.9	22.8	951	8.6	5.9	1.5	3	30%
unprepared	11.5 oz	418	19.2	55.3	2309	20.9	14.4	3.7	6	30%
BEEF										
(Campbell's) prepared	8 oz	80	5.0	10.0	830	(mq)	2.0	(mq)	10	23%
W/bouillon (Campbell's) prepared	8 oz	16	3.0	1.0	820	na	0.0	0.0	0	0%
W/broth (Campbell's) prepared	8 oz	16	3.0	1.0	820	na	0.0	0.0	0	0%
W/vegetables (Campbell's) 'Healthy Request'	4 oz	70	5.0	9.0	490	na	2.0	na	5	24%
BEEF MUSHROOM										
prepared	1 cup	73	5.8	6.3	942	>.5 c	3.0	1.5	7	36%
unprepared	10.75 oz	186	14.0	15.9	2358	>.9 c	7.3	3.7	15	36%
BEEF NOODLE										
prepared	1 cup	83	4.8	9.0	952	0	3.1	1.1	5	34%
unprepared	10.75 oz	204	11.7	21.8	2315	1.8	7.5	2.8	12	34%
(Campbell's) prepared	8 oz	70	4.0	7.0	830	(mq)	3.0	(mq)	15	38%
(Campbell's) 'Homestyle' prepared	8 oz	80	5.0	7.0	810	(mq)	4.0	(mq)	20	43%
W/ground beef (Campbell's) prepared	8 oz	90	4.0	10.0	820	(mq)	4.0	(mq)	25	39%
BLACK BEAN										
prepared	1 cup	116	5.6	19.8	1198	4.5	1.5	0.4	0	12%
unprepared	11 oz	282	13.7	48.1	2910	21.2	3.7	1.0	0	12%
BROCCOLI, CREAM OF										
(Campbell's) prepared	8 oz	80	1.0	8.0	790	(mq)	5.0	(mq)	na	56%
(Campbell's) prepared w/whole milk	8 oz	140	5.0	14.0	850	(mq)	7.0	(mq)	(mq)	45%
CELERY, CREAM OF										
prepared	1 cup	90	1.7	8.8	949	.7	5.6	1.4	15	55%
prepared w/whole milk	1 cup	164	5.7	14.5	1009	.7	9.7	3.9	32	52%
unprepared	10.75 oz	220	4.0	21.4	2309	1.8	13.6	3.4	34	55%
(Campbell's) prepared	8 oz	100	2.0	8.0	820	(mq)	7.0	(mq)	5	61%
CHEESE										
prepared	1 cup	156	5.4	10.5	958	0	10.5	6.7	30	60%
prepared w/whole milk	1 cup	231	9.5	16.2	1019	0	14.6	9.1	48	56%
unprepared	11 oz	378	13.2	25.6	2331	2.5	25.4	16.2	72	60%
Cheddar (Campbell's) prepared	8 oz	110	4.0	10.0	810	na	6.0	(mq)	10	49%
Nacho										
(Campbell's) prepared	8 oz	110	4.0	8.0	740	na	8.0	(mq)	na	60%
(Campbell's) prepared w/whole milk	8 oz	180	8.0	13.0	800	na	12.0	(mq)	(mq)	56%
CHICKEN										
W/barley (Campbell's) prepared	8 oz	70	3.0	10.0	850	(mq)	2.0	(mq)	(mq)	26%
W/dumplings										
prepared	1 cup	96	5.6	6.1	860	.7	5.5	1.3	34	51%
unprepared	10.5 oz	235	13.6	14.7	2095	1.8	13.4	3.2	80	52%
(Campbell's) 'Chicken 'n Dumplings' prepared	8 oz	80	4.0	9.0	960	(mq)	3.0	(mq)	25	34%

Food Name	Serving Size	Calories	Prot. gms	Carbs gms	Sod. mgs	Fiber gms	Fat gms	Sat. Fat gms	Chol. mgs	% Fat Cal.
W/rice										
prepared	1 cup	60	3.5	7.2	815	0	1.9	0.5	7	29%
unprepared	10.5 oz	146	8.6	17.4	1982	1.5	4.7	1.1	15	29%
(Campbell's) prepared	8 oz	60	2.0	7.0	790	(mq)	3.0	(mq)	10	43%
(Campbell's) 'Healthy Request'	4 oz	60	2.0	7.0	480	na	2.0	na	10	33%
(Campbell's) 'Healthy Request' prepared	8 oz	60	2.0	7.0	480	(mq)	3.0	(mq)	10	43%
CHICKEN, CREAM OF										
prepared	1 cup	117	3.4	9.3	986	.2	7.4	2.1	10	57%
unprepared	10.75 oz	284	8.3	22.5	2397	.6	17.9	5.1	24	57%
(Campbell's) prepared	8 oz	110	2.0	9.0	810	na	7.0	(mq)	10	59%
(Campbell's) 'Healthy Request'	4 oz	70	2.0	11.0	490	na	2.0	na	10	26%
(Campbell's) 'Healthy Request' prepared	8 oz	70	2.0	11.0	490	na	2.0	na	10	26%
W/broccoli										
(Campbell's)	4 oz	110	3.0	9.0	710	na	7.0	na	10	57%
(Campbell's) prepared	8 oz	110	3.0	9.0	710	na	7.0	na	10	57%
CHICKEN BROTH										
prepared	1 cup	39	4.9	0.9	776	0	1.4	0.4	0	35%
unprepared	10.75 oz	95	13.5	2.3	1909	0	3.2	1.0	3	31%
(Campbell's) prepared	8 oz	30	1.0	2.0	710	na	2.0	(mq)	0	60%
CHICKEN GUMBO										
prepared	1 cup	56	2.6	8.4	954	2.0	1.4	0.3	5	22%
unprepared	10.75 oz	137	6.4	20.3	2321	4.7	3.5	0.8	9	23%
CHICKEN MUSHROOM										
prepared	1 cup	132	4.4	9.3	942	>.2 c	9.1	2.4	10	60%
unprepared	10.75 oz	332	10.7	23.2	2358	.6	22.3	5.9	24	60%
Creamy (Campbell's) prepared	8 oz	120	3.0	8.0	920	(mq)	8.0	(mq)	15	62%
CHICKEN NOODLE										
prepared	1 cup	75	4.1	9.4	1106	.7	2.5	0.7	7	29%
unprepared	10.5 oz	182	9.6	22.7	2256	1.8	5.5	1.5	15	28%
(Campbell's) prepared	8 oz	60	3.0	8.0	900	(mq)	2.0	(mq)	15	29%
(Campbell's) 'Healthy Request'	4 oz	60	3.0	8.0	460	na	2.0	na	15	29%
(Campbell's) 'Healthy Request' prepared	8 oz	60	3.0	8.0	440	(mq)	2.0	(mq)	15	29%
(Campbell's) 'Homestyle' prepared	8 oz	70	3.0	8.0	880	(mq)	3.0	(mq)	15	38%
Broth and noodles (Campbell's) prepared	8 oz	45	1.0	8.0	860	(mq)	1.0	(mq)	10	20%
Creamy										
(Campbell's)	4 oz	120	4.0	10.0	800	na	7.0	na	na	53%
(Campbell's) prepared	8 oz	120	4.0	10.0	800	na	7.0	na	10	53%
(Campbell's) prepared w/2% milk	8 oz	180	8.0	16.0	850	na	9.0	na	na	46%
Curly noodle (Campbell's) prepared	8 oz	80	3.0	11.0	800	(mq)	3.0	(mq)	15	33%
Double noodle in broth										
(Campbell's)	4 oz	90	4.0	13.0	700	na	2.0	na	na	21%
(Campbell's) prepared	8 oz	90	4.0	13.0	700	na	2.0	na	na	21%
Ring noodle (Campbell's) 'Noodle-O's' prepared	8 oz	70	3.0	9.0	820	(mq)	2.0	(mq)	20	27%
CHICKEN VEGETABLE										
prepared	1 cup	75	3.6	8.6	945	1.0	2.8	0.8	10	34%
unprepared	10.5 oz	182	8.8	20.9	2298	>.3 c	6.9	2.1	21	34%
(Campbell's) prepared	8 oz	70	3.0	8.0	850	(mq)	3.0	(mq)	10	38%
CHILI BEEF										
prepared	1 cup	170	6.7	21.5	1035	9.5	6.6	3.3	13	35%
unprepared	11.25 oz	412	16.2	52.1	2514	>3.5 c	16.0	8.0	32	35%
(Campbell's) prepared	8 oz	140	5.0	20.0	840	(mq)	5.0	(mq)	10	31%
CLAM CHOWDER										
Manhattan style										
prepared	1 cup	78	2.2	12.2	578	1.5	2.2	0.4	2	26%

Food Name	Serving Size	Calories	Prot. gms	Carbs gms	Sod. mgs	Fiber gms	Fat gms	Sat. Fat gms	Chol. mgs	% Fat Cal.
unprepared	10.75 oz	186	5.3	29.7	1394	3.7	5.4	0.9	6	26%
(Campbell's) prepared	8 oz	70	2.0	10.0	820	(mq)	2.0	(mq)	0	27%
(Campbell's) 'Seashore Soups'	4 oz	70	2.0	10.0	820	na	2.0	na	5	27%
(Doxsee) prepared	7.5 oz	70	3.0	11.0	780	(mq)	2.0	(mq)	(mq)	24%
(Snow's)	3.75 oz	70	3.0	9.0	630	na	2.0	na	na	27%
(Snow's) prepared	7.5 oz	70	3.0	11.0	780	(mq)	2.0	(mq)	(mq)	24%
New England style										
prepared	8 oz	95	4.8	12.4	915	1.5	2.9	0.4	5	28%
prepared w/whole milk	8 oz	164	9.5	16.6	992	1.5	6.6	3.0	22	36%
(Campbell's) prepared	8 oz	80	3.0	12.0	870	(mq)	3.0	(mq)	5	31%
(Campbell's) prepared w/whole milk	8 oz	150	7.0	17.0	930	(mq)	7.0	(mq)	(mq)	40%
(Campbell's) 'Seashore Soups'	4 oz	80	3.0	12.0	870	na	3.0	na	5	31%
(Gorton's) prepared w/whole milk	1/4 can	140	7.0	17.0	740	(mq)	5.0	(mq)	15	32%
(Snow's)	3.75 oz	70	5.0	8.0	620	na	2.0	na	na	26%
(Snow's) prepared w/whole milk	7.5 oz	140	8.0	13.0	670	(mq)	6.0	(mq)	(mq)	39%
CONSOMMÉ										
Beef	10.5 oz	72	13.0	4.3	1550	0	0.0	na	0	0%
Beef, w/gelatin										
prepared	1 cup	29	5.4	1.8	637	na	0.0	0.0	0	0%
unprepared	10.5 oz	71	13.0	4.3	1550	na	0.0	0.0	0	0%
(Campbell's) prepared	8 oz	25	4.0	2.0	750	na	0.0	0.0	0	0%
CORN, CREAM OF, GOLDEN										
(Campbell's)	4 oz	110	2.0	18.0	700	na	3.0	na	5	25%
(Campbell's) prepared	8 oz	110	2.0	18.0	700	na	3.0	na	5	25%
(Campbell's) prepared w/2% milk	8 oz	160	6.0	23.0	760	na	5.0	na	10	28%
CORN CHOWDER, NEW ENGLAND										
(Snow's)	3.75 oz	80	2.0	13.0	590	na	2.0	na	na	23%
(Snow's) prepared w/whole milk	7.5 oz	150	5.0	18.0	640	na	6.0	na	na	37%
FISH CHOWDER, NEW ENGLAND										
(Snow's)	3.75 oz	60	5.0	6.0	560	na	2.0	na	na	29%
(Snow's) prepared w/whole milk	7.5 oz	130	9.0	11.0	620	(mq)	6.0	(mq)	(mq)	40%
GREEN PEA										
prepared	1 cup	165	8.6	26.5	988	2.8	2.9	1.4	0	16%
prepared w/whole milk	1 cup	239	12.6	32.2	1046	2.8	7.0	4.0	18	26%
unprepared	11.25 oz	399	20.9	64.4	2399	7.0	7.1	3.4	0	16%
(Campbell's) prepared	8 oz	160	8.0	25.0	820	(mq)	3.0	(mq)	5	17%
MINESTRONE										
prepared	1 cup	82	4.3	11.2	911	1.0	2.5	0.6	2	27%
unprepared	10.5 oz	203	10.4	27.3	2217	2.4	6.1	1.3	3	27%
(Campbell's) prepared	8 oz	80	3.0	13.0	900	(mq)	2.0	(mq)	0	22%
MUSHROOM										
Beefy (Campbell's) prepared	8 oz	60	4.0	5.0	960	(mq)	3.0	(mq)	10	43%
Golden (Campbell's) prepared	8 oz	70	2.0	9.0	870	(mq)	3.0	(mq)	5	38%
W/beef stock										
prepared	1 cup	85	3.2	9.3	969	.7	4.0	1.6	7	42%
unprepared	10.75 oz	207	7.7	22.6	2358	.3	9.8	3.8	18	42%
MUSHROOM, CREAM OF										
prepared	1 cup	129	2.3	9.3	1032	.5	9.0	2.4	2	64%
prepared w/whole milk	1 cup	203	6.1	15.0	1076	.5	13.6	5.1	20	59%
unprepared	10.75 oz	314	4.9	22.6	2470	.9	23.1	6.3	3	65%
(Campbell's) prepared	8 oz	100	2.0	8.0	820	(mq)	7.0	(mq)	0	61%
(Campbell's) 'Healthy Request'	4 oz	60	1.0	9.0	480	na	2.0	na	5	31%
(Campbell's) 'Healthy Request' prepared	8 oz	60	1.0	9.0	480	(mq)	2.0	na	5	31%

Food Name	Serving Size	Calories	Prot. gms	Carbs gms	Sod. mgs	Fiber gms	Fat gms	Sat. Fat gms	Chol. mgs	% Fat Cal.
MUSHROOM BARLEY										
prepared	1 cup	73	1.9	11.7	891	.7	2.3	0.4	0	28%
unprepared	10.75 oz	186	4.6	29.3	2227	1.8	5.5	1.1	0	27%
(Rokeach) prepared	1 cup	85	3.4	17.3	904	(mq)	0.2	na	na	2%
ONION										
prepared	1 cup	58	3.8	8.2	1053	1.0	1.7	0.3	0	24%
unprepared	10.5 oz	137	9.1	19.9	2563	2.1	4.2	0.6	0	25%
unprepared	8 oz	113	7.5	16.4	2116	1.7	3.5	0.5	0	25%
French (Campbell's) prepared	8 oz	60	2.0	9.0	900	(mq)	2.0	(mq)	5	29%
ONION, CREAM OF										
prepared	1 cup	107	2.8	12.7	927	>.5 c	5.3	1.5	15	44%
prepared w/whole milk	1 cup	186	6.8	18.4	1004	.7	9.4	4.0	32	46%
unprepared	10.75 oz	268	6.7	31.7	2318	1.2	12.8	3.6	37	43%
(Campbell's) prepared	8 oz	100	2.0	12.0	830	(mq)	5.0	(mq)	15	45%
(Campbell's) prepared w/half water, half milk	8 oz	140	4.0	15.0	860	(mq)	7.0	(mq)	(mq)	45%
OYSTER STEW										
prepared	1 cup	58	2.1	4.1	981	0	3.8	2.5	14	58%
prepared w/whole milk	1 cup	135	6.2	9.8	1041	0	7.9	5.1	32	53%
unprepared	10.5 oz	143	5.1	9.9	2384	0	9.3	6.1	33	58%
(Campbell's) prepared	8 oz	70	2.0	5.0	840	(mq)	5.0	(mq)	25	62%
(Campbell's) prepared w/whole milk	8 oz	140	6.0	10.0	890	(mq)	9.0	(mq)	(mq)	56%
PASTA										
Alphabet (Campbell's) prepared	8 oz	80	3.0	10.0	800	(mq)	3.0	(mq)	10	34%
Chicken and stars (Campbell's) prepared	8 oz	60	3.0	7.0	870	(mq)	2.0	(mq)	10	31%
Teddy bears in chicken broth										
(Campbell's)	4 oz	60	2.0	11.0	770	na	1.0	na	5	15%
(Campbell's) prepared	8 oz	60	2.0	11.0	770	na	1.0	na	5	15%
PEPPER POT										
prepared	1 cup	104	6.4	9.4	971	.5	4.6	2.0	10	40%
unprepared	10.5 oz	250	15.5	22.8	2360	>1.2 c	11.3	5.0	24	40%
(Campbell's) prepared	8 oz	90	5.0	9.0	970	(mq)	4.0	(mq)	40	39%
POTATO, CREAM OF										
prepared	1 cup	73	1.8	11.5	1000	.5	2.4	1.2	5	29%
prepared w/whole milk	1 cup	149	5.8	17.2	1061	.5	6.4	3.8	22	39%
unprepared	10.75 oz	180	4.2	27.9	2431	1.2	5.7	3.0	15	29%
(Campbell's) prepared	8 oz	80	1.0	12.0	870	(mq)	3.0	(mq)	5	34%
(Campbell's) prepared w/tofu, 1 tbsp oil	8 oz	120	3.0	15.0	900	(mq)	4.0	(mq)	(mq)	33%
SCOTCH BROTH										
prepared	1 cup	80	5.0	9.5	1012	1.2	2.6	1.1	5	29%
unprepared	10.5 oz	197	12.1	23.0	2461	>.9 c	6.4	2.7	12	29%
(Campbell's) prepared	8 oz	80	4.0	9.0	870	na	3.0	(mq)	10	34%
SEAFOOD CHOWDER, NEW ENGLAND										
(Snow's)	3.75 oz	60	4.0	6.0	640	na	2.0	na	na	31%
(Snow's) prepared w/whole milk	7.5 oz	140	8.0	14.0	670	na	6.0	(mq)	(mq)	38%
SHRIMP, CREAM OF										
prepared	1 cup	90	2.8	8.2	976	.2	5.2	3.3	17	52%
prepared w/whole milk	1 cup	164	6.8	13.9	1037	.3	9.3	5.8	35	50%
unprepared	10.75 oz	220	6.8	19.9	2373	.6	12.6	7.9	40	52%
(Campbell's) prepared	8 oz	90	2.0	8.0	810	na	6.0	(mq)	20	57%
(Campbell's) prepared w/whole milk	8 oz	160	5.0	13.0	860	na	10.0	(mq)	(mq)	56%
(Campbell's) 'Seashore Soups'	4 oz	90	2.0	8.0	810	na	6.0	2.0	20	57%
(Campbell's) 'Seashore Soups' prepared w/2% milk	4 oz	140	5.0	13.0	810	na	10.0	3.0	20	56%
SPLIT PEA										
W/egg barley (Rokeach) prepared	1 cup	132	8.2	23.6	757	(mq)	0.5	na	na	3%

Food Name	Serving Size	Calories	Prot. gms	Carbs gms	Sod. mgs	Fiber gms	Fat gms	Sat. Fat gms	Chol. mgs	% Fat Cal.
W/ham										
prepared	1 cup	190	10.3	28.0	1007	>.7 c	4.4	1.8	8	21%
unprepared	11.5 oz	460	25.0	67.8	2445	>1.6 c	10.7	4.3	20	21%
W/ham and bacon (Campbell's) prepared	8 oz	160	9.0	24.0	780	(mq)	4.0	(mq)	5	21%
STOCKPOT										
prepared	1 cup	99	4.9	11.5	1047	>.5 c	3.9	0.9	5	35%
unprepared	11 oz	243	11.8	27.9	2546	>1.3 c	9.5	2.1	9	35%
TOMATO										
prepared	1 cup	85	2.0	16.6	871	.5	1.9	0.4	0	19%
prepared w/whole milk	1 cup	161	6.1	22.3	932	.5	6.0	2.9	17	32%
unprepared	10.75 oz	207	5.0	40.3	2120	1.2	4.7	0.9	0	19%
(Campbell's) prepared	8 oz	90	1.0	17.0	680	(mq)	2.0	(mq)	0	20%
(Campbell's) prepared w/whole milk	8 oz	150	5.0	22.0	740	(mq)	4.0	(mq)	(mq)	25%
(Campbell's) 'Healthy Request'	4 oz	90	1.0	17.0	430	na	2.0	na	0	20%
(Campbell's) 'Healthy Request' prepared	8 oz	90	1.0	17.0	430	(mq)	2.0	(mq)	0	20%
(Campbell's) 'Healthy Request' prepared w/half 2% milk, half water	8 oz	140	5.0	22.0	490	na	3.0	na	5	20%
(Campbell's) 'Healthy Request' prepared w/skim milk	4 oz	130	5.0	22.0	490	na	2.0	na	5	14%
(Campbell's) 'Healthy Request' prepared w/whole milk	8 oz	150	5.0	22.0	490	(mq)	4.0	na	10	25%
Italian, w/basil and oregano										
(Campbell's)	4 oz	90	1.0	21.0	740	na	0.0	na	0	0%
(Campbell's) prepared	8 oz	90	1.0	21.0	740	na	0.0	na	0	0%
Zesty (Campbell's) prepared	8 oz	100	1.0	20.0	760	(mq)	2.0	na	na	18%
TOMATO, CREAM OF										
(Campbell's) 'Homestyle' prepared	8 oz	110	1.0	20.0	810	(mq)	3.0	(mq)	5	24%
(Campbell's) 'Homestyle' prepared w/whole milk	8 oz	180	5.0	25.0	860	(mq)	7.0	(mq)	(mq)	34%
TOMATO BEEF W/NOODLES										
prepared	1 cup	139	4.5	21.1	917	1.5	4.3	1.6	5	27%
unprepared	10.75 oz	342	10.8	51.5	2230	>.3 c	10.4	3.9	9	27%
TOMATO BISQUE										
prepared w/milk	1 cup	198	6.3	29.4	1109	>.8 c	6.6	3.1	23	29%
unprepared	11 oz	300	5.5	57.6	2546	2.5	6.1	1.3	12	18%
(Campbell's) prepared	8 oz	120	2.0	22.0	820	(mq)	3.0	(mq)	5	22%
TOMATO RICE										
prepared	1 cup	119	2.1	21.9	815	1.5	2.7	0.5	2	20%
unprepared	11 oz	290	5.1	53.3	1981	4.1	6.6	1.3	3	20%
(Campbell's) 'Old Fashioned' prepared	8 oz	110	1.0	22.0	730	(mq)	2.0	(mq)	0	16%
TURKEY NOODLE										
prepared	1 cup	68	3.9	8.6	815	.7	2.0	0.6	5	27%
unprepared	10.75 oz	168	9.5	21.0	1983	1.8	4.8	1.3	12	26%
(Campbell's) prepared	8 oz	70	3.0	9.0	880	(mq)	2.0	(mq)	15	27%
TURKEY VEGETABLE										
prepared	1 cup	72	3.1	8.6	906	.5	3.0	0.9	2	37%
unprepared	10.5 oz	179	7.5	21.0	2202	1.5	7.4	2.2	3	37%
(Campbell's) prepared	8 oz	70	2.0	8.0	710	(mq)	3.0	(mq)	10	40%
VEGETABLE										
(Campbell's) prepared	8 oz	90	3.0	14.0	830	(mq)	2.0	(mq)	0	21%
(Campbell's) 'Homestyle' prepared	8 oz	60	2.0	9.0	880	(mq)	2.0	(mq)	0	29%
(Campbell's) 'Old Fashioned' prepared	8 oz	60	2.0	9.0	880	(mq)	2.0	(mq)	0	29%
Hearty, w/pasta										
(Campbell's)	4 oz	70	3.0	15.0	800	na	<1.0	na	0	<11%
(Campbell's) prepared	8 oz	70	3.0	15.0	800	na	<1.0	na	0	<11%
Vegetarian										
prepared	1 cup	72	2.1	12.0	822	.5	1.9	0.3	0	23%

Food Name	Serving Size	Calories	Prot. gms	Carbs gms	Sod. mgs	Fiber gms	Fat gms	Sat. Fat gms	Chol. mgs	% Fat Cal.
unprepared	10.5 oz	176	5.1	29.1	2003	1.3	4.7	0.7	0	24%
(Campbell's) prepared	8 oz	80	2.0	13.0	790	(mq)	2.0	(mq)	0	23%
W/beef broth										
prepared	1 cup	82	3.0	13.1	810	.5	1.9	0.4	2	21%
unprepared	10.5 oz	197	7.2	31.9	1970	3.7	4.7	1.1	3	21%
W/beef stock										
(Campbell's) 'Healthy Request'	4 oz	90	3.0	14.0	500	na	2.0	na	5	21%
(Campbell's) 'Healthy Request' prepared	8 oz	90	3.0	14.0	500	(mq)	2.0	(mq)	5	21%
VEGETABLE BEEF										
prepared	1 cup	78	5.6	10.2	956	.5	1.9	0.9	5	21%
unprepared	10.75 oz	192	13.6	24.7	2327	4.9	4.6	2.1	12	21%
(Campbell's) prepared	8 oz	70	4.0	10.0	780	(mq)	2.0	(mq)	10	24%
(Campbell's) 'Healthy Request' prepared	8 oz	70	4.0	10.0	470	(mq)	2.0	(mq)	10	24%
WON TON *(Campbell's)* prepared	8 oz	40	2.0	5.0	850	(mq)	1.0	na	10	24%
SOUP, CANNED, READY-TO-SERVE										
BEAN										
(Grandma Brown's)	1 cup	190	9.0	30.9	700	9.8	3.4	(mq)	<1	16%
W/ham										
(Campbell's) 'Chunky Old Fashioned'	11 oz	290	14.0	38.0	1110	(mq)	9.0	(mq)	na	28%
(Campbell's) 'Chunky Old Fashioned'	9 5/8 oz	250	12.0	33.0	960	(mq)	8.0	(mq)	na	29%
(Campbell's) 'Home Cookin'	9.5 oz	180	12.0	25.0	890	(mq)	4.0	(mq)	(mq)	20%
(Campbell's) 'Home Cookin'	10.75 oz	210	14.0	29.0	1000	(mq)	4.0	(mq)	(mq)	17%
(Healthy Choice)	7.5 oz	220	12.0	35.0	480	na	4.0	1.0	5	16%
(Hormel) 'Hearty Soup'	7.5 oz	190	9.0	29.0	640	na	4.0	1.0	23	19%
BEEF										
(Progresso)	10.5 oz	180	15.0	17.0	840	(mq)	6.0	(mq)	35	30%
(Progresso)	9.5 oz	160	13.0	15.0	760	(mq)	5.0	(mq)	35	29%
Bouillon	8 oz	17	2.7	0.1	782	0	0.5	0.3	0	29%
Broth *(College Inn)*	7 oz	16	3.0	1.0	960	na	0.0	0.0	0	0%
Chunky										
(Campbell's) 'Chunky'	10.75 oz	200	15.0	24.0	1100	(mq)	5.0	(mq)	(mq)	22%
(Campbell's) 'Chunky'	9.5 oz	170	13.0	21.0	970	(mq)	4.0	(mq)	(mq)	21%
Fat-free *(Health Valley)*	6.9 oz	10	1.0	2.0	290	0	0.0	na	0	0%
Fat-free, no salt added *(Health Valley)*	6.9 oz	10	1.0	2.0	5	0	0.0	na	0	0%
Hearty										
(Healthy Choice) 'Hearty Beef'	7.5 oz	120	9.0	17.0	580	na	2.0	1.0	20	15%
(Progresso)	9.5 oz	160	15.0	15.0	820	(mq)	4.0	2.0	35	23%
Stroganoff style *(Campbell's)* 'Chunky'	10.75 oz	320	15.0	28.0	1230	(mq)	16.0	(mq)	(mq)	46%
W/barley										
(Progresso)	10.5 oz	150	13.0	16.0	870	3.0	5.0	(mq)	30	28%
(Progresso)	9.5 oz	140	12.0	16.0	780	3.0	4.0	(mq)	30	24%
W/broth										
(College Inn)	1 cup	18	2.0	1.0	1280	0	0.0	0.0	(mq)	0%
(Health Valley)	7.5 oz	17	1.0	2.0	420	0	1.0	na	1	43%
(Health Valley) 'No Salt Added'	7.5 oz	17	1.0	2.0	0	0	1.0	na	1	43%
(Progresso) seasoned	4 oz	10	2.0	<1.0	380	0	<1.0	na	0	<43%
(Swanson)	7.25 oz	18	2.0	0.0	750	0	1.0	na	(mq)	53%
W/minestrone										
(Progresso)	10.5 oz	180	15.0	18.0	1000	(mq)	6.0	(mq)	35	29%
(Progresso)	9.5 oz	170	13.0	16.0	910	(mq)	5.0	(mq)	30	28%
W/noodles *(Progresso)*	9.5 oz	170	15.0	18.0	1030	(mq)	4.0	(mq)	40	21%
W/tomato juice	1 oz	11	0.2	2.6	40	0	0.0	0.0	0	0%
W/vegetables										
(Lipton) 'Hearty Ones'	11 oz	229	10.4	40.0	921	(mq)	3.0	(mq)	29	12%

Food Name	Serving Size	Calories	Prot. gms	Carbs gms	Sod. mgs	Fiber gms	Fat gms	Sat. Fat gms	Chol. mgs	% Fat Cal.
(Progresso)	10.5 oz	170	17.0	18.0	880	(mq)	3.0	(mq)	40	16%
(Progresso)	9.5 oz	150	15.0	16.0	790	(mq)	3.0	(mq)	35	18%
W/vegetables and pasta										
(Campbell's) 'Home Cookin'	10.75 oz	140	12.0	18.0	1060	(mq)	2.0	(mq)	(mq)	13%
(Campbell's) 'Home Cookin'	9.5 oz	120	10.0	16.0	940	(mq)	2.0	(mq)	(mq)	15%
BERRY										
Blueberry (Great Impressions)	6 oz	95	0.4	22.5	92	(mq)	0.3	na	0	3%
Three berry (Great Impressions)	6 oz	107	0.5	25.8	90	(mq)	0.2	na	0	2%
BLACK BEAN										
(Health Valley)	7.5 oz	160	7.0	24.0	285	17.0	3.0	(mq)	0	18%
(Health Valley) 'No Salt Added'	7.5 oz	160	7.0	24.0	20	17.0	3.0	(mq)	0	18%
(Health Valley) w/vegetables, fat-free ...	7.5 oz	70	9.0	9.0	290	17.0	0.0	na	0	0%
BORSCHT										
(Gold's)	8 oz	100	4.0	21.0	1280	(mq)	0.0	0.0	0	0%
(Rokeach)	1 cup	96	0.8	23.0	985	>.3 c	0.3	(tr)	0	3%
(Rokeach) 'Unsalted'	1 cup	103	0.8	23.0	50	>.5 c	0.3	(tr)	0	3%
Low-calorie										
(Gold's)	8 oz	20	1.0	5.0	1160	(mq)	<1.0	0.0	0	<27%
(Manischewitz)	1 cup	20	1.0	4.0	725	(mq)	0.0	0.0	0	0%
(Rokeach) 'Diet'	1 cup	29	0.8	5.8	897	>.8 c	0.2	(tr)	0	6%
W/beets (Manischewitz)	1 cup	80	1.0	20.0	660	(mq)	0.0	0.0	0	0%
BROCCOLI, CREAM OF (Andersen's) ...	7.5 oz	170	5.0	20.0	670	na	8.0	na	na	42%
CHERRY (Great Impressions)	6 oz	123	0.6	29.6	88	(mq)	0.2	na	0	2%
CHICKEN										
(Progresso) 'Homestyle'	9.5 oz	110	11.0	12.0	740	na	3.0	(mq)	20	23%
Broth										
(Campbell's) 'Healthy Request'	8 oz	16	3.0	1.0	470	na	0.0	na	0	0%
(Campbell's) 'Low Sodium'	10.5 oz	30	3.0	2.0	85	0	1.0	na	(mq)	31%
(College Inn)	1 cup	35	1.0	0.0	1320	0	3.0	(mq)	(mq)	87%
(College Inn)	7 oz	35	1.0	0.0	990	0	3.0	1.0	5	87%
(College Inn) lower salt	7 oz	20	1.0	0.0	550	0	2.0	1.0	5	82%
(Hain)	8.75 oz	70	2.0	0.0	870	0	6.0	(mq)	5	87%
(Health Valley) fat-free	6.9 oz	20	4.0	1.0	290	0	0.0	na	0	0%
(Hain) 'No Salt Added'	8.75 oz	60	3.0	0.0	75	0	5.0	(mq)	5	79%
(Health Valley)	7.5 oz	35	4.0	1.0	410	0	2.0	(mq)	2	47%
(Health Valley) 'No Salt Added'	7.5 oz	35	4.0	1.0	0	0	2.0	(mq)	2	47%
(Pritikin) defatted	1 cup	18	3.0	1.0	160	0	1.0	0.0	0	36%
(Progresso)	4 oz	8	2.0	0.0	360	0	0.0	0.0	5	0%
(Swanson)	7.25 oz	30	2.0	2.0	900	0	2.0	(mq)	(mq)	53%
(Swanson) 'Natural Goodness'	7.25 oz	20	2.0	1.0	580	0	1.0	na	(mq)	43%
Chunky										
(Campbell's) 'Chunky Old Fashioned'	10.75 oz	180	12.0	21.0	1220	na	5.0	(mq)	(mq)	25%
(Campbell's) 'Chunky Old Fashioned'	9.5 oz	150	10.0	18.0	1070	na	4.0	(mq)	(mq)	24%
(Healthy Choice) 'Hearty Chicken'	7.5 oz	150	9.0	17.0	530	na	5.0	1.0	35	30%
Hearty										
(Progresso)	10.5 oz	130	14.0	9.0	960	na	4.0	(mq)	30	28%
(Progresso)	9.5 oz	130	13.0	11.0	900	na	4.0	(mq)	25	27%
Nuggets, w/vegetables and noodles										
(Campbell's) 'Chunky'	10.75 oz	190	11.0	24.0	1060	(mq)	6.0	(mq)	(mq)	28%
(Campbell's) 'Chunky'	9.5 oz	170	9.0	21.0	940	(mq)	6.0	(mq)	(mq)	31%
W/meatballs (Progresso) 'Chickarina'	9.5 oz	130	8.0	13.0	820	(mq)	5.0	(mq)	20	35%
W/noodles										
(Campbell's) 'Home Cookin'	10.75 oz	140	13.0	12.0	1150	(mq)	4.0	(mq)	(mq)	27%
(Campbell's) 'Home Cookin'	9.5 oz	110	11.0	10.0	1020	(mq)	3.0	(mq)	(mq)	24%

Food Name	Serving Size	Calories	Prot. gms	Carbs gms	Sod. mgs	Fiber gms	Fat gms	Sat. Fat gms	Chol. mgs	% Fat Cal.
(Campbell's) 'Low Sodium'	10.75 oz	170	13.0	17.0	90	(mq)	5.0	(mq)	(mq)	27%
W/ribbon pasta *(Pritikin)*	1 cup	80	6.0	13.0	180	1.0	1.0	0.0	5	11%
W/rice										
(Campbell's) 'Chunky'	9.5 oz	140	10.0	16.0	1060	(mq)	4.0	(mq)	30	26%
(Healthy Choice)	7.5 oz	140	5.0	18.0	510	na	4.0	1.0	15	28%
(Hormel) 'Hearty Soup'	7.5 oz	110	5.0	17.0	890	na	2.0	1.0	6	17%
W/wild rice *(Progresso)*	9.5 oz	120	6.0	17.0	850	na	3.0	<1.0	20	23%
CHICKEN, CREAM OF *(Progresso)*	9.5 oz	190	10.0	12.0	970	(mq)	11.0	(mq)	35	53%
CHICKEN BARLEY *(Progresso)*	9.25 oz	100	10.0	12.0	740	3.5	2.0	(mq)	20	17%
CHICKEN GUMBO, w/sausage										
(Campbell's) 'Home Cookin'	10.75 oz	140	11.0	15.0	1090	(mq)	4.0	(mq)	(mq)	26%
(Campbell's) 'Home Cookin'	9.5 oz	120	9.0	13.0	960	(mq)	3.0	(mq)	(mq)	24%
CHICKEN MINESTRONE										
(Campbell's) 'Home Cookin'	10.75 oz	180	15.0	17.0	950	(mq)	6.0	(mq)	(mq)	30%
(Campbell's) 'Home Cookin'	9.5 oz	160	13.0	15.0	840	(mq)	5.0	(mq)	(mq)	29%
(Progresso)	10.5 oz	140	12.0	14.0	1060	(mq)	4.0	(mq)	20	26%
(Progresso)	9.5 oz	130	12.0	12.0	870	(mq)	3.0	(mq)	20	22%
CHICKEN MUSHROOM, CREAMY										
(Campbell's) 'Chunky'	10.5 oz	270	12.0	13.0	1280	(mq)	19.0	(mq)	(mq)	63%
(Campbell's) 'Chunky'	9 3/8 oz	240	10.0	12.0	1140	(mq)	17.0	(mq)	(mq)	64%
CHICKEN NOODLE										
(Hain)	9.5 oz	120	9.0	11.0	980	(mq)	4.0	(mq)	20	31%
(Hain) 'No Salt Added'	9.5 oz	120	9.0	12.0	90	(mq)	4.0	(mq)	25	30%
(Healthy Choice) 'Old Fashioned Chicken Noodle'	7.5 oz	90	5.0	9.0	520	na	3.0	1.0	20	33%
(Hormel) 'Hearty Soup'	7.5 oz	110	7.0	14.0	690	na	3.0	1.0	18	24%
(Lipton) 'Hearty Ones Homestyle'	11 oz	227	10.1	37.4	989	(mq)	4.0	(mq)	37	16%
(Progresso)	10.5 oz	120	12.0	8.0	970	(mq)	4.0	(mq)	40	31%
(Progresso)	9.5 oz	120	11.0	10.0	920	(mq)	4.0	(mq)	40	30%
(Progresso) 'Healthy Classics'	8 oz	80	7.0	10.0	460	na	2.0	<1.0	15	21%
(Weight Watchers)	10.5 oz	80	6.0	9.0	1230	(mq)	2.0	(mq)	(mq)	23%
Chunky										
(Campbell's) 'Chunky'	10.75 oz	200	14.0	20.0	1140	(mq)	7.0	(mq)	(mq)	32%
(Campbell's) 'Chunky'	9.5 oz	180	12.0	18.0	1000	(mq)	7.0	(mq)	(mq)	34%
Hearty *(Campbell's)* 'Healthy Request'	8 oz	80	9.0	7.0	470	na	2.0	na	25	22%
CHICKEN RICE										
(Campbell's) 'Home Cookin'	10.75 oz	150	14.0	10.0	1090	(mq)	6.0	(mq)	(mq)	36%
(Campbell's) 'Home Cookin'	9.5 oz	130	12.0	9.0	960	(mq)	5.0	(mq)	(mq)	35%
(Progresso)	10.5 oz	120	9.0	12.0	990	(mq)	4.0	(mq)	25	30%
(Progresso)	9.5 oz	130	9.0	16.0	750	(mq)	3.0	(mq)	25	21%
Chunky	8 oz	127	12.3	13.0	888	1.0	3.2	1.0	12	22%
Hearty *(Campbell's)* 'Healthy Request'	8 oz	110	5.0	15.0	480	na	3.0	na	10	25%
W/vegetables *(Progresso)* 'Healthy Classics'	8 oz	80	7.0	11.0	440	na	2.0	<1.0	10	20%
CHICKEN VEGETABLE										
(Hain)	9.5 oz	120	8.0	14.0	930	(mq)	4.0	(mq)	15	29%
(Hain) 'No Salt Added'	9.5 oz	130	8.0	14.0	100	(mq)	4.0	(mq)	20	29%
(Campbell's) 'Chunky'	9.5 oz	170	10.0	19.0	1080	(mq)	6.0	(mq)	25	32%
(Campbell's) 'Chunky Low Sodium'	10.75 oz	240	15.0	21.0	95	(mq)	11.0	(mq)	10	41%
(Campbell's) 'Home Cookin'	10.75 oz	180	11.0	25.0	970	na	4.0	na	na	20%
(Pritikin)	1 cup	70	5.0	12.0	150	2.0	1.0	<1.0	5	12%
(Progresso)	9.5 oz	140	9.0	17.0	800	(mq)	4.0	(mq)	25	26%
Chunky										
(Health Valley)	7.5 oz	125	7.0	20.0	425	4.0	2.0	(mq)	11	14%
(Health Valley) 'No Salt Added'	7.5 oz	125	7.0	20.0	60	4.0	2.0	(mq)	11	14%
Hearty *(Campbell's)* 'Healthy Request'	8 oz	120	7.0	16.0	420	na	3.0	na	10	23%

Food Name	Serving Size	Calories	Prot. gms	Carbs gms	Sod. mgs	Fiber gms	Fat gms	Sat. Fat gms	Chol. mgs	% Fat Cal.
CHILI BEEF										
(Campbell's) 'Chunky'	11 oz	290	21.0	37.0	1120	(mq)	7.0	(mq)	(mq)	21%
(Campbell's) 'Chunky'	9.75 oz	260	18.0	33.0	990	(mq)	6.0	(mq)	(mq)	21%
(Healthy Choice) Thick and hearty	7.5 oz	150	11.0	22.0	560	na	1.0	<1.0	15	6%
CLAM CHOWDER										
Manhattan style										
(Campbell's) 'Chunky'	10.75 oz	160	7.0	24.0	1110	(mq)	4.0	(mq)	(mq)	23%
(Campbell's) 'Chunky'	9.5 oz	150	7.0	21.0	980	(mq)	4.0	(mq)	(mq)	24%
(Health Valley)	7.5 oz	110	6.0	15.0	510	13.4	2.0	(mq)	15	18%
(Health Valley) 'No Salt Added'	7.5 oz	110	6.0	15.0	60	13.4	2.0	(mq)	15	18%
(Progresso)	9.5 oz	120	13.0	13.0	800	(mq)	2.0	(mq)	10	15%
New England style										
(Campbell's) 'Chunky'	10.75 oz	290	9.0	26.0	1200	(mq)	17.0	(mq)	(mq)	52%
(Campbell's) 'Chunky'	9.5 oz	260	8.0	23.0	1060	(mq)	15.0	(mq)	(mq)	52%
(Campbell's) 'Healthy Request'	8 oz	100	4.0	14.0	490	na	3.0	na	10	27%
(Campbell's) 'Home Cookin'	10.75 oz	260	8.0	15.0	1240	na	18.0	na	na	64%
(Gorton's) 'New England Style'	7.5 oz	140	7.0	17.0	720	na	5.0	na	20	32%
(Hain)	9.25 oz	180	8.0	26.0	780	(mq)	4.0	(mq)	25	21%
(Hormel) 'Hearty Soup'	7.5 oz	130	5.0	16.0	790	na	5.0	2.0	30	35%
(Progresso)	10.5 oz	220	7.0	21.0	1050	(mq)	12.0	(mq)	20	49%
(Progresso)	9.25 oz	220	8.0	20.0	950	(mq)	12.0	(mq)	(mq)	49%
(Weight Watchers)	7.5 oz	90	5.0	16.0	450	na	0.0	na	5	0%
CORN AND VEGETABLE, fat-free (Health Valley)	7.5 oz	70	4.0	13.0	290	3.0	0.0	na	0	0%
CORN CHOWDER										
(Campbell's) 'Chunky'	10.75 oz	340	14.0	23.0	1200	(mq)	21.0	(mq)	(mq)	56%
(Campbell's) 'Chunky'	9.5 oz	300	12.0	21.0	1060	(mq)	19.0	(mq)	(mq)	56%
(Progresso)	9.25 oz	200	5.0	22.0	840	(mq)	10.0	(mq)	10	46%
CRAB	8 oz	76	5.5	10.3	1235	.7	1.5	0.4	10	18%
CREOLE										
(Campbell's) 'Chunky'	10.75 oz	240	11.0	31.0	910	na	8.0	(mq)	na	30%
(Campbell's) 'Chunky'	9.5 oz	220	10.0	28.0	800	na	7.0	(mq)	na	29%
ESCAROLE, in chicken broth (Progresso)	9.25 oz	30	2.0	2.0	1100	(mq)	1.0	na	5	36%
GAZPACHO	8 oz	56	8.7	0.8	1183	3.7	2.2	0.3	0	34%
HAM AND BEAN										
(Campbell's) w/butterbeans 'Chunky'	10.75 oz	280	12.0	34.0	1180	(mq)	10.0	(mq)	(mq)	33%
(Progresso)	9.5 oz	140	11.0	28.0	950	8.0	2.0	(mq)	10	10%
LEMON (Great Impressions)	6 oz	90	0.2	22.1	109	(mq)	<1.0	na	0	<9%
LENTIL										
(Health Valley)	7.5 oz	170	9.0	28.0	435	17.0	2.0	(mq)	0	11%
(Health Valley) 'No Salt Added'	7.5 oz	170	9.0	28.0	25	17.0	2.0	(mq)	0	11%
(Progresso)	10.5 oz	140	10.0	24.0	1000	6.5	4.0	(mq)	0	21%
(Progresso)	9.5 oz	140	10.0	25.0	840	6.5	4.0	(mq)	0	21%
(Progresso) 'Healthy Classics'	8 oz	120	7.0	19.0	420	na	1.0	<1.0	0	8%
Hearty										
(Campbell's) 'Home Cookin'	10.75 oz	170	11.0	28.0	930	(mq)	2.0	(mq)	na	10%
(Campbell's) 'Home Cookin'	9.5 oz	140	9.0	24.0	820	(mq)	1.0	na	na	6%
Vegetarian										
(Hain)	9.5 oz	160	9.0	25.0	690	(mq)	3.0	(mq)	5	17%
(Hain) 'No Salt Added'	9.5 oz	160	9.0	24.0	65	(mq)	3.0	(mq)	5	17%
W/carrots, fat-free (Health Valley)	7.5 oz	70	8.0	10.0	290	15.0	0.0	na	0	0%
W/ham	8 oz	139	9.3	20.2	1319	>1.4 c	2.8	1.1	7	18%
W/sausage (Progresso)	9.5 oz	170	8.0	21.0	840	5.0	8.0	(mq)	20	38%
MACARONI AND BEAN										
(Progresso)	10.5 oz	150	9.0	27.0	1020	8.0	4.0	(mq)	0	20%

Food Name	Serving Size	Calories	Prot. gms	Carbs gms	Sod. mgs	Fiber gms	Fat gms	Sat. Fat gms	Chol. mgs	% Fat Cal.
(Progresso)	9.5 oz	140	8.0	25.0	920	(mq)	5.0	(mq)	0	25%
MENUDO (Old El Paso)	1/2 can	476	15.0	14.0	770	2.0	52.0	21.0	176	80%
MINESTRONE										
(Campbell's) 'Chunky'	9.5 oz	160	6.0	24.0	870	(mq)	4.0	(mq)	0	23%
(Campbell's) 'Healthy Request'	8 oz	90	4.0	13.0	420	na	2.0	na	2	21%
(Campbell's) 'Home Cookin'	10.75 oz	140	4.0	22.0	1220	(mq)	3.0	(mq)	na	21%
(Campbell's) 'Home Cookin'	9.5 oz	120	4.0	20.0	1080	(mq)	3.0	(mq)	na	22%
(Hain)	9.5 oz	170	8.0	27.0	1060	(mq)	2.0	(mq)	0	11%
(Hain) 'No Salt Added'	9.5 oz	160	7.0	28.0	35	(mq)	4.0	(mq)	0	21%
(Health Valley)	7.5 oz	130	6.0	19.0	637	12.5	3.0	(mq)	0	21%
(Health Valley) 'No Salt Added'	7.5 oz	130	6.0	19.0	80	12.5	3.0	(mq)	0	21%
(Health Valley) 'Real Italian Fat-Free' .	7.5 oz	80	8.0	12.0	290	4.0	0.0	0.0	0	0%
(Healthy Choice)	7.5 oz	160	6.0	30.0	520	na	2.0	<1.0	0	11%
(Hormel) 'Hearty Soup'	7.5 oz	100	5.0	17.0	460	na	1.0	<2.0	5	9%
(Lipton) 'Hearty Ones'	11 oz	189	8.0	36.1	821	(mq)	3.2	(mq)	6	14%
(Progresso)	10.5 oz	120	7.0	25.0	930	7.0	3.0	(mq)	0	17%
(Progresso)	9.5 oz	130	7.0	22.0	1010	6.0	4.0	(mq)	0	24%
(Progresso) chunky, hearty	9.25 oz	110	7.0	16.0	740	(mq)	2.0	(mq)	5	16%
(Progresso) chunky, zesty	9.5 oz	150	7.0	19.0	1130	4.0	8.0	(mq)	10	41%
(Progresso) 'Healthy Classics'	8 oz	120	4.0	19.0	490	na	2.0	<1.0	0	16%
MUSHROOM, CREAM OF										
(Campbell's) 'Low Sodium'	10.5 oz	210	3.0	18.0	55	(mq)	14.0	(mq)	(mq)	60%
(Hain)	9.25 oz	110	4.0	16.0	740	(mq)	4.0	(mq)	15	31%
(Progresso)	9.25 oz	160	4.0	14.0	1120	(mq)	10.0	(mq)	15	56%
(Weight Watchers)	10.5 oz	90	3.0	14.0	1250	(mq)	2.0	(mq)	na	21%
MUSHROOM BARLEY										
(Hain)	9.5 oz	100	4.0	17.0	600	(mq)	2.0	(mq)	10	18%
(Health Valley)	7.5 oz	100	5.0	16.0	394	8.5	2.0	(mq)	0	18%
(Health Valley) 'No Salt Added'	7.5 oz	100	5.0	16.0	20	8.5	2.0	(mq)	0	18%
PEPPER STEAK										
(Campbell's) 'Chunky'	9.5 oz	160	12.0	21.0	920	(mq)	3.0	(mq)	(mq)	17%
(Campbell's) 'Chunky'	10.75 oz	180	14.0	24.0	1050	(mq)	3.0	(mq)	(mq)	15%
POTATO, CREAM OF (Andersen's)	7.5 oz	200	4.0	25.0	630	na	10.0	na	na	44%
POTATO LEEK										
(Health Valley)	7.5 oz	130	4.0	23.0	360	7.4	2.0	(mq)	0	14%
(Health Valley) 'No Salt Added'	7.5 oz	130	4.0	23.0	20	7.4	2.0	(mq)	0	14%
SCHAV (Gold's)	8 oz	25	2.0	4.0	1380	na	0.0	0.0	15	0%
SIRLOIN BURGER										
(Campbell's) 'Chunky'	10.75 oz	220	12.0	23.0	1240	na	9.0	(mq)	(mq)	37%
(Campbell's) 'Chunky'	9.5 oz	200	11.0	20.0	1090	na	8.0	(mq)	(mq)	37%
SPLIT PEA										
(Andersen's)	7.5 oz	130	9.0	24.0	770	na	0.0	na	na	0%
(Campbell's) 'Low Sodium'	10.75 oz	230	12.0	37.0	30	(mq)	4.0	(mq)	(mq)	16%
(Grandma Brown's)	1 cup	208	11.7	31.0	522	5.8	4.1	(mq)	<1	18%
(Hain)	9.5 oz	170	11.0	28.0	970	(mq)	1.0	na	0	6%
(Hain) 'No Salt Added'	9.5 oz	170	11.0	29.0	40	(mq)	1.0	na	0	5%
(Progresso)	9.5 oz	160	11.0	27.0	1050	4.5	3.0	(mq)	5	15%
Green										
(Health Valley)	7.5 oz	190	11.0	34.0	276	14.7	0.3	na	0	2%
(Health Valley) 'No Salt Added'	7.5 oz	190	11.0	34.0	25	14.7	0.3	na	0	2%
(Hain) vegetarian	9.5 oz	170	11.0	28.0	970	(mq)	1.0	na	0	6%
(Hain) vegetarian 'No Salt Added'	9.5 oz	170	13.0	27.0	70	(mq)	1.0	na	0	5%
(Progresso)	10.5 oz	201	12.0	31.0	920	(mq)	3.0	(mq)	na	14%
W/ ham										

Food Name	Serving Size	Calories	Prot. gms	Carbs gms	Sod. mgs	Fiber gms	Fat gms	Sat. Fat gms	Chol. mgs	% Fat Cal.
(Campbell's) 'Chunky'	10.5 oz	230	12.0	33.0	1080	(mq)	6.0	(mq)	(mq)	23%
(Campbell's) 'Chunky'	9.5 oz	210	11.0	30.0	950	(mq)	5.0	(mq)	(mq)	22%
(Campbell's) 'Home Cookin'	10.75 oz	230	16.0	38.0	1310	(mq)	1.0	na	(mq)	4%
(Campbell's) 'Home Cookin'	9.5 oz	200	14.0	34.0	1150	(mq)	1.0	na	(mq)	5%
(Healthy Choice)	7.5 oz	170	10.0	25.0	460	na	3.0	1.0	10	16%
(Progresso)	10.5 oz	160	11.0	24.0	980	6.0	5.0	(mq)	15	24%
(Progresso)	9.5 oz	150	11.0	23.0	880	5.0	5.0	(mq)	15	25%
STEAK AND POTATO										
(Campbell's) 'Chunky'	10.75 oz	200	14.0	24.0	1140	(mq)	5.0	(mq)	(mq)	23%
(Campbell's) 'Chunky'	9.5 oz	170	12.0	21.0	1000	(mq)	4.0	(mq)	(mq)	21%
TOMATO										
(Health Valley)	7.5 oz	100	2.0	17.0	450	1.2	3.0	(mq)	0	26%
(Health Valley) 'No Salt Added'	7.5 oz	100	2.0	17.0	40	1.2	3.0	(mq)	0	26%
(Healthy Choice) 'Tomato Garden'	7.5 oz	130	4.0	22.0	510	na	3.0	1.0	5	21%
(Progresso)	9.5 oz	120	4.0	20.0	1100	(mq)	3.0	(mq)	0	22%
Beef, w/rotini (Progresso)	9.5 oz	170	12.0	18.0	930	(mq)	6.0	(mq)	30	31%
Garden										
(Campbell's) 'Home Cookin'	10.75 oz	150	2.0	29.0	930	(mq)	3.0	(mq)	na	18%
(Campbell's) 'Home Cookin'	9.5 oz	130	2.0	25.0	820	(mq)	2.0	(mq)	na	14%
W/tomato pieces (Campbell's) 'Low Sodium'	10.5 oz	190	4.0	30.0	45	(mq)	6.0	(mq)	(mq)	28%
W/tortellini (Progresso)	9.25 oz	130	5.0	16.0	1040	(mq)	5.0	(mq)	10	35%
TOMATO VEGETABLE, fat-free (Health Valley)	7.5 oz	50	5.0	8.0	290	3.0	0.0	na	0	0%
TORTELLINI										
(Progresso)	9.5 oz	90	5.0	11.0	930	(mq)	3.0	(mq)	10	30%
(Progresso) Creamy	9.25 oz	240	5.0	17.0	910	(mq)	16.0	8.5	35	62%
TURKEY	8 oz	135	10.2	14.1	923	>.9 c	4.4	1.2	9	29%
TURKEY RICE										
(Hain)	9.5 oz	100	8.0	10.0	970	(mq)	3.0	(mq)	20	27%
(Hain) 'No Salt Added'	9.5 oz	120	7.0	13.0	85	(mq)	4.0	(mq)	15	31%
TURKEY VEGETABLE										
(Campbell's) 'Chunky'	9 3/8 oz	150	9.0	16.0	1060	(mq)	6.0	(mq)	(mq)	35%
(Weight Watchers)	10.5 oz	70	4.0	10.0	1020	(mq)	2.0	(mq)	(mq)	24%
VEGETABLE										
(Campbell's) 'Chunky'	10.75 oz	160	4.0	28.0	1100	(mq)	4.0	(mq)	0	22%
(Campbell's) 'Chunky'	9.5 oz	150	4.0	25.0	970	(mq)	4.0	(mq)	0	24%
(Health Valley)	7.5 oz	110	4.0	20.0	296	4.0	1.0	na	0	9%
(Health Valley) 'No Salt Added'	7.5 oz	110	4.0	20.0	40	4.0	1.0	na	0	9%
(Healthy Choice) 'Country Vegetable'	7.5 oz	120	3.0	23.0	540	na	1.0	<1.0	0	8%
(Progresso)	9.5 oz	80	4.0	15.0	1190	3.5	2.0	(mq)	5	19%
(Progresso) 'Healthy Classics'	8 oz	80	4.0	13.0	450	na	1.0	<1.0	5	12%
Country										
(Campbell's) 'Home Cookin'	10.75 oz	120	4.0	20.0	1070	(mq)	2.0	(mq)	na	16%
(Campbell's) 'Home Cookin'	9.5 oz	100	3.0	18.0	940	(mq)	2.0	(mq)	na	18%
(Hormel) 'Hearty Soup'	7.5 oz	90	4.0	14.0	730	na	2.0	<2.0	2	20%
5 bean, chunky										
(Health Valley)	7.5 oz	110	4.0	21.0	448	10.6	2.0	(mq)	0	15%
(Health Valley) 'No Salt Added'	7.5 oz	110	4.0	21.0	56	10.6	2.0	(mq)	0	15%
14 garden vegetables, fat-free (Health Valley)	7.5 oz	50	4.0	9.0	260	3.0	0.0	na	0	0%
Hearty (Campbell's) 'Healthy Request'	8 oz	90	3.0	17.0	480	na	1.0	na	0	10%
Italian, w/pasta										
(Hain)	9.5 oz	160	4.0	25.0	910	(mq)	5.0	(mq)	20	28%
(Hain) 'Low Sodium'	9.5 oz	140	4.0	22.0	90	(mq)	6.0	(mq)	20	34%
Mediterranean (Campbell's) 'Chunky'	9.5 oz	170	4.0	24.0	1010	(mq)	6.0	(mq)	na	33%
Vegetarian										

Food Name	Serving Size	Calories	Prot. gms	Carbs gms	Sod. mgs	Fiber gms	Fat gms	Sat. Fat gms	Chol. mgs	% Fat Cal.
chunky *(Weight Watchers)*	10.5 oz	100	3.0	18.0	1250	(mq)	2.0	(mq)	0	18%
(Hain)	9.5 oz	140	4.0	22.0	920	(mq)	4.0	(mq)	0	26%
(Hain) 'No Salt Added'	9.5 oz	150	5.0	23.0	45	(mq)	5.0	(mq)	0	29%
W/barley, fat-free *(Health Valley)*	7.5 oz	60	4.0	11.0	270	4.0	0.0	na	0	0%
W/beef stock *(Weight Watchers)*	10.5 oz	90	4.0	13.0	1370	(mq)	2.0	(mq)	(mq)	21%
VEGETABLE BEEF										
(Campbell's) 'Chunky Low Sodium'	10.75 oz	180	14.0	19.0	90	(mq)	5.0	(mq)	(mq)	25%
(Campbell's) 'Chunky Old Fashioned'	10.75 oz	190	13.0	20.0	1100	(mq)	6.0	(mq)	25	29%
(Campbell's) 'Chunky Old Fashioned'	9.5 oz	160	12.0	17.0	970	(mq)	5.0	(mq)	25	28%
(Campbell's) hearty	8 oz	120	8.0	17.0	460	na	2.0	na	15	15%
(Campbell's) 'Home Cookin'	10.75 oz	140	13.0	17.0	1160	(mq)	3.0	(mq)	(mq)	18%
(Campbell's) 'Home Cookin'	9.5 oz	120	11.0	15.0	1020	(mq)	2.0	(mq)	(mq)	15%
(Hormel) 'Hearty Soup'	7.5 oz	90	6.0	15.0	730	na	1.0	<2.0	5	10%
(Healthy Choice) 'Vegetable Beef'	7.5 oz	130	8.0	21.0	530	na	1.0	<1.0	15	7%
VEGETABLE BROTH										
(Hain)	9.5 oz	45	1.0	10.0	1180	na	0.0	0.0	0	0%
(Hain) 'Low Sodium'	9.5 oz	40	1.0	8.0	85	na	<1.0	na	0	<20%
SOUP, FROZEN										
ASPARAGUS, CREAM OF										
(Kettle Ready)	6 oz	62	0.8	5.1	406	(mq)	4.3	1.5	na	62%
(Myers)	9.75 oz	152	11.0	10.0	992	(mq)	8.0	(mq)	na	46%
BARLEY BEAN *(Tabatchnick)*	7.5 oz	130	6.0	22.0	217	(mq)	2.0	(mq)	0	14%
BEAN										
Northern bean *(Tabatchnick)*	7.5 oz	164	8.0	29.0	240	(mq)	2.0	(mq)	0	11%
Savory, w/ham *(Kettle Ready)*	6 oz	113	6.8	20.2	459	(mq)	3.6	1.0	(mq)	23%
W/beef and vegetables, hearty *(Kettle Ready)*	6 oz	85	4.2	10.7	448	(mq)	3.0	0.6	(mq)	31%
BLACK BEAN, w/ham *(Kettle Ready)*	6 oz	154	8.1	23.0	613	(mq)	6.2	1.3	(mq)	31%
BROCCOLI, CREAM OF										
(Kettle Ready)	6 oz	94	0.9	6.4	417	(mq)	7.2	2.6	na	69%
(Myers)	9.75 oz	174	8.0	11.0	905	(mq)	11.0	(mq)	na	57%
(Tabatchnick)	7.5 oz	90	4.0	10.0	285	(mq)	4.0	(mq)	4	39%
CABBAGE *(Tabatchnick)*	7.5 oz	110	2.0	21.0	185	(mq)	2.0	(mq)	0	16%
CAULIFLOWER, CREAM OF *(Kettle Ready)*	6 oz	93	2.3	5.5	445	(mq)	7.0	3.1	na	67%
CHEDDAR CHEESE, CREAM OF										
(Kettle Ready)	6 oz	158	4.1	7.3	616	>.1 c	12.5	6.1	na	71%
(Kettle Ready) w/broccoli	6 oz	137	4.0	4.7	533	na	11.3	5.2	na	75%
CHEESE, w/broccoli *(Myers)*	9.75 oz	325	12.0	19.0	1257	(mq)	23.0	(mq)	na	63%
CHICKEN *(Tabatchnick)*	7.5 oz	65	2.0	10.0	255	na	2.0	(mq)	0	27%
CHICKEN, CREAM OF *(Kettle Ready)*	6 oz	98	5.7	5.0	668	na	6.2	2.3	(mq)	57%
CHICKEN GUMBO *(Kettle Ready)*	6 oz	94	3.5	12.1	473	(mq)	3.5	0.7	(mq)	34%
CHICKEN NOODLE										
(Kettle Ready)	6 oz	94	5.0	12.0	569	(mq)	3.0	0.6	(mq)	28%
(Myers)	9.75 oz	87	8.0	5.0	1046	(mq)	5.0	(mq)	(mq)	46%
CHILI										
(Kettle Ready)	6 oz	161	11.7	14.0	454	(mq)	6.5	2.0	na	36%
(Kettle Ready) jalapeño	6 oz	173	11.0	14.7	531	(mq)	8.0	2.1	na	41%
CLAM CHOWDER										
Boston *(Kettle Ready)*	6 oz	131	3.5	13.0	417	(mq)	7.3	1.5	(mq)	50%
Manhattan style *(Kettle Ready)*	6 oz	69	3.6	8.0	549	(mq)	2.6	0.5	(mq)	34%
New England style										
(Kettle Ready)	6 oz	116	3.0	11.4	373	(mq)	6.5	2.4	(mq)	50%
(Myers)	9.75 oz	152	7.0	21.0	910	(mq)	5.0	(mq)	(mq)	29%
(Stouffer's)	8 oz	180	8.0	16.0	790	(mq)	9.0	(mq)	(mq)	46%
(Tabatchnick)	7.5 oz	98	6.0	14.0	255	(mq)	2.0	(mq)	0	18%

Food Name	Serving Size	Calories	Prot. gms	Carbs gms	Sod. mgs	Fiber gms	Fat gms	Sat. Fat gms	Chol. mgs	% Fat Cal.
CORN CHOWDER w/broccoli (Kettle Ready)	6 oz	102	1.4	13.0	323	(mq)	5.0	1.8	na	44%
LENTIL (Tabatchnick)	7.5 oz	170	11.0	27.0	240	(mq)	2.0	(mq)	0	11%
MINESTRONE										
(Kettle Ready) hearty	6 oz	104	3.3	15.2	577	(mq)	4.4	1.1	na	35%
(Tabatchnick)	7.5 oz	137	8.0	24.0	265	(mq)	2.0	(mq)	0	12%
MUSHROOM, CREAM OF										
(Kettle Ready)	6 oz	85	0.6	6.2	371	(mq)	6.4	2.4	na	68%
(Tabatchnick)	6 oz	75	3.0	11.0	325	(mq)	2.0	(mq)	3	24%
MUSHROOM BARLEY										
(Tabatchnick)	7.5 oz	92	2.0	16.0	234	(mq)	2.0	(mq)	0	20%
(Tabatchnick) 'No Salt'	7.5 oz	97	4.0	18.0	77	(mq)	1.0	na	0	9%
ONION, French (Kettle Ready)	6 oz	42	0.7	5.0	562	(mq)	2.2	0.4	na	47%
PEA										
(Tabatchnick)	7.5 oz	175	10.0	31.0	290	(mq)	1.0	na	0	5%
(Tabatchnick) 'No Salt'	7.5 oz	175	10.0	31.0	79	(mq)	1.0	na	0	5%
SEAFOOD BISQUE (Myers)	9.75 oz	163	9.0	13.0	1393	na	8.0	(mq)	(mq)	45%
SPINACH, CREAM OF										
(Myers)	9.75 oz	174	9.0	10.0	905	(mq)	11.0	(mq)	na	57%
(Stouffer's)	8 oz	210	7.0	12.0	1020	(mq)	15.0	(mq)	na	64%
(Tabatchnick)	7.5 oz	85	5.0	12.0	200	(mq)	2.0	(mq)	4	21%
SPLIT PEA W/HAM (Kettle Ready)	6 oz	155	11.1	25.3	483	(mq)	4.4	1.3	(mq)	21%
TOMATO RICE (Tabatchnick)	6 oz	73	2.0	14.0	300	(mq)	1.0	na	0	12%
TOMATO TORTELLINI (Kettle Ready)	6 oz	122	3.5	15.0	447	(mq)	5.4	1.3	na	40%
VEGETABLE										
(Kettle Ready) garden	6 oz	85	2.6	12.3	296	(mq)	3.0	0.5	na	31%
(Tabatchnick)	7.5 oz	97	4.0	18.0	190	(mq)	1.0	na	0	9%
(Tabatchnick) 'No Salt'	7.5 oz	92	2.0	16.0	77	(mq)	2.0	(mq)	0	20%
VEGETABLE BEEF (Myers)	9.75 oz	120	9.0	8.0	1030	(mq)	6.0	(mq)	(mq)	44%
ZUCCHINI (Tabatchnick)	6 oz	80	3.0	12.0	285	(mq)	2.0	(mq)	3	23%
SOUP, MICROWAVE										
BEAN										
W/bacon and ham (Campbell's)	7.5 oz	230	8.0	38.0	830	(mq)	5.0	(mq)	(mq)	20%
W/ham, chowder (Hormel) 'Micro-Cup Hearty Soups'	1 pkg	191	10.0	31.0	664	(mq)	3.0	(mq)	30	14%
BEEF, w/vegetable (Hormel) 'Micro-Cup Hearty Soups'	1 pkg	71	5.0	12.0	811	(mq)	1.0	(mq)	9	12%
CHICKEN										
W/rice (Campbell's) 'Microwave'	7.5 oz	100	3.0	14.0	820	(mq)	4.0	(mq)	(mq)	35%
W/vegetables and rice (Hormel) 'Micro-Cup Hearty Soups'	1 pkg	114	5.0	16.0	1025	(mq)	3.0	(mq)	7	24%
CHICKEN NOODLE										
(Campbell's) 'Microwave'	7.5 oz	100	5.0	11.0	870	(mq)	4.0	(mq)	(mq)	36%
(Hormel) 'Micro-Cup Hearty Soups'	1 pkg	108	7.0	14.0	686	(mq)	3.0	(mq)	22	24%
(Lunch Bucket) microwave cup	7.25 oz	90	4.0	13.0	810	na	2.0	na	25	21%
(Weight Watchers) microwave cup	7.5 oz	90	8.0	13.0	450	na	1.0	na	15	10%
CHILI BEEF (Campbell's) 'Microwave'	7.5 oz	190	7.0	32.0	870	(mq)	4.0	(mq)	(mq)	19%
CLAM CHOWDER										
New England (Hormel) 'Micro-Cup Hearty Soups'	1 pkg	118	5.0	15.0	882	(mq)	5.0	(mq)	30	36%
MINESTRONE (Hormel) 'Micro-Cup Hearty Soups'	1 pkg	104	7.0	15.0	903	(mq)	2.0	(mq)	10	17%
NOODLE										
Beef flavor (Campbell's) 'Cup Microwave'	1.35 oz	130	6.0	23.0	1270	(mq)	2.0	(mq)	(mq)	13%
Chicken flavor (Campbell's) 'Cup Microwave'	1.35 oz	140	7.0	22.0	1340	(mq)	3.0	(mq)	na	19%
Pork flavor, w/vegetables (Campbell's) 'Hearty Microwave'	1.7 oz	180	7.0	32.0	1320	(mq)	2.0	(mq)	na	10%
W/chicken broth (Campbell's) 'Cup Microwave'	1.35 oz	130	6.0	23.0	1360	(mq)	2.0	(mq)	na	13%
VEGETABLE, country										
(Hormel) 'Micro-Cup Hearty Soups'	1 pkg	89	5.0	13.0	865	(mq)	2.0	(mq)	1	20%
(Lunch Bucket) microwave cup	7.25 oz	70	1.0	15.0	740	na	1.0	na	0	12%

Food Name	Serving Size	Calories	Prot. gms	Carbs gms	Sod. mgs	Fiber gms	Fat gms	Sat. Fat gms	Chol. mgs	% Fat Cal.
VEGETABLE BEEF										
(Campbell's) 'Microwave' .... 7.5 oz		100	5.0	16.0	830	(mq)	2.0	(mq)	(mq)	18%
(Weight Watchers) microwave cup .... 7.5 oz		90	8.0	13.0	450	na	1.0	na	10	10%
SOUP MIX										
(NOTE: Unless otherwise specified, PREPARED = prepared as directed w/water.)										
ASPARAGUS, prepared .... 8 oz		52	2.0	7.9	707	.3	1.5	0.2	0	25%
ASPARAGUS, CREAM OF, prepared .... 8 oz		58	2.2	8.9	800	na	1.7	0.1	0	26%
BEAN W/BACON, prepared .... 1 cup		106	5.5	16.4	927	9.0	2.2	1.0	3	18%
BEEF										
Beef flavor, w/noodles										
(Campbell's) 'Ramen Noodle' prepared .... 6 oz		160	5.0	32.0	890	(mq)	1.0	na	na	6%
(Estee) prepared .... 6 oz		20	1.0	3.0	140	(mq)	<1.0	<1.0	<1	<36%
(Lipton) 'Cup-A-Soup' prepared .... 6 oz		44	1.7	7.6	746	na	0.7	na	na	15%
(Lipton) 'Hearty' prepared .... 6 oz		107	3.5	20.2	698	>.2 c	1.4	na	na	12%
Beef flavor, w/noodles and vegetables										
(Campbell's) prepared .... 6 oz		220	7.0	44.0	1600	(mq)	2.0	(mq)	na	8%
Broth										
cubed .... 1 cube		6	0.6	0.6	864	0	0.1	0.1	0	16%
cubed, prepared .... 6 oz		5	0.6	0.6	869	0	0.1	0.1	0	16%
powder, prepared .... 8 oz		20	1.3	1.9	1362	0	0.7	0.3	0	33%
Hearty (Soup Starter) 'Homestyle' .... 27 gm/.945 oz		90	2.0	20.0	740	na	<1.0	na	na	<9%
Vegetable (Soup Starter) 'Homestyle' .... 26 gm/.91 oz		90	3.0	18.0	790	na	<1.0	na	0	<10%
W/noodles (Ultra Slim Fast) 1 envelope, prepared .... 6 oz		45	5.0	7.0	700	2.0	<1.0	na	5	<16%
BEEF NOODLE, prepared .... 8 oz		40	2.2	6.0	1042	.8	0.8	0.3	3	18%
BLACK BEAN										
(Fantastic Foods) 'Jumpin' black beans, prepared ...... 10 oz		170	12.0	40.0	490	13.0	1.0	na	0	4%
BROCCOLI										
Creamy										
(Lipton) 'Cup-A-Soup' prepared .... 6 oz		62	1.1	9.1	610	>.3 c	2.4	(mq)	na	35%
(Lipton) 'Cup-A-Soup Food Service' prepared .... 6 oz		62	1.7	8.9	658	(mq)	2.3	(mq)	na	33%
(Ultra Slim Fast) 1 envelope, prepared .... 6 oz		75	5.0	14.0	800	2.0	<1.0	na	0	<11%
Golden (Lipton) 'Cup-A-Soup Lite' prepared .... 6 oz		42	1.3	16.3	427	(mq)	1.2	na	1	13%
W/cheese (Lipton) 'Cup-A-Soup' prepared .... 6 oz		70	1.7	9.8	595	(mq)	3.4	(mq)	na	40%
BOUILLON										
Beef flavor										
cubed .... 1 cube		6	0.6	0.6	864	(tr)	0.1	0.1	tr	16%
cubed (Steero) .... 1 cube		6	<1.0	1.0	930	(tr)	<1.0	na	na	<53%
cubed (Wyler's) .... 1 cube		6	<1.0	1.0	930	(tr)	<1.0	na	na	<53%
instant (Featherweight) .... 1 tsp		18	0.0	2.0	10	(tr)	1.0	na	5	53%
instant (Lite-Line) 'Low Sodium' .... 1 tsp		12	<1.0	2.0	5	(tr)	<1.0	na	na	<43%
instant (Steero) .... 1 tsp		6	<1.0	1.0	930	(tr)	<1.0	na	na	<53%
instant (Weight Watchers) 'Broth Mix' .... 1 pkt		8	1.0	1.0	930	(tr)	0.0	0.0	0	0%
instant (Wyler's) .... 1 tsp		6	<1.0	1.0	930	(tr)	<1.0	na	na	<53%
powder .... 1 pkt		14	1.0	1.4	1019	0	0.5	0.3	1	32%
powder, prepared .... 8 oz		19	1.3	1.9	1359	0	0.7	0.4	1	33%
Brown										
(G. Washington's) 'Seasoning & Broth' .... .14 oz		6	0.0	1.0	1015	(tr)	0.0	0.0	0	0%
(G. Washington's) 'Seasoning & Broth' kosher .... .14 oz		6	0.0	1.0	1110	(tr)	0.0	0.0	0	0%
Chicken flavor										
cubed .... 1 cube		9	0.7	1.1	1152	(tr)	0.2	0.1	1	20%
cubed (Steero) .... 1 cube		8	<1.0	1.0	990	(tr)	<1.0	na	na	<53%
cubed (Wyler's) .... 1 cube		8	<1.0	1.0	900	(tr)	<1.0	na	na	<53%
instant (Featherweight) .... 1 tsp		18	0.0	2.0	5	(tr)	1.0	na	5	53%
instant (Lite-Line) 'Low Sodium' .... 1 tsp		12	<1.0	2.0	5	(tr)	<1.0	na	na	<43%

Food Name	Serving Size	Calories	Prot. gms	Carbs gms	Sod. mgs	Fiber gms	Fat gms	Sat. Fat gms	Chol. mgs	% Fat Cal.
instant *(Steero)*	1 tsp	8	<1.0	1.0	990	(tr)	<1.0	na	na	<53%
instant *(Weight Watchers)* 'Broth Mix'	1 pkt	8	1.0	1.0	990	(tr)	0.0	0.0	0	0%
instant *(Wyler's)*	1 tsp	8	<1.0	1.0	900	(tr)	<1.0	na	na	<53%
Golden										
(G. Washington's) 'Seasoning & Broth'	.13 oz	6	0.0	1.0	935	(tr)	0.0	0.0	0	0%
(G. Washington's) 'Seasoning & Broth' kosher	.13 oz	6	0.0	1.0	1015	(tr)	0.0	0.0	0	0%
Onion flavor										
(G. Washington's) 'Seasoning and Broth'	.18 oz	12	1.0	2.0	695	(tr)	0.0	0.0	0	0%
(Wyler's) instant	1 tsp	10	<1.0	1.0	670	(tr)	<1.0	na	0	<53%
Vegetable flavor										
(G. Washington's) 'Seasoning & Broth'	.18 oz	12	1.0	2.0	715	(tr)	0.0	0.0	0	0%
(Wyler's) instant	1 tsp	6	<1.0	1.0	910	(tr)	<1.0	(tr)	0	<53%
CAULIFLOWER, prepared	8 oz	69	2.9	10.7	843	>.2 c	1.7	0.3	0	22%
CELERY, prepared	8 oz	63	2.6	9.8	838	>.2 c	1.6	0.3	0	23%
CHEESE										
(Fantastic Noodles) creamy cheddar w/noodles, prepared	7 oz	178	7.0	21.0	578	(mq)	8.0	(mq)	na	39%
(Hain) cheese and broccoli, prepared	6 oz	310	7.0	19.0	980	(mq)	22.0	(mq)	na	66%
(Hain) 'Savory Soup & Sauce Mix' prepared	6 oz	250	6.0	20.0	890	na	16.0	(mq)	na	58%
CHICKEN										
prepared	8 oz	107	1.8	13.3	1185	.3	5.3	3.4	3	44%
(Soup Starter) 'Homestyle'	.735 oz	70	2.0	15.0	770	na	<1.0	na	10	<12%
Broth										
cubed	1 cube	10	0.7	1.1	1152	0	0.2	0.1	1	20%
cubed, prepared	6 oz	9	0.7	1.1	593	0	0.2	0.1	0	20%
(Lipton) 'Cup-A-Soup' prepared	6 oz	20	0.4	3.3	605	na	0.6	na	1	27%
Creamy, w/vegetables *(Lipton)* prepared	6 oz	93	1.7	14.4	708	(mq)	3.1	(mq)	na	30%
Creamy, w/white meat *(Campbell's)* prepared	6 oz	90	3.0	12.0	1020	na	4.0	(mq)	(mq)	38%
Florentine *(Lipton)* 'Lite'	6 oz	42	10.0	7.6	481	na	0.5	na	6	6%
Hearty										
(Lipton) 'Country Style'	6 oz	69	3.8	11.1	688	na	1.1	na	na	14%
(Lipton) 'Supreme' prepared	6 oz	107	2.0	11.4	848	na	5.9	(mq)	na	50%
Lemon *(Lipton)* 'Cup-A-Soup Lite' prepared	6 oz	48	2.0	9.1	419	na	0.4	na	4	8%
W/corn *(Lipton)* 'Country' prepared	6 oz	133	3.3	17.5	704	>.2 c	5.5	(mq)	na	37%
W/noodles *(Ultra Slim Fast)* 1 envelope, prepared	6 oz	45	5.0	6.0	970	2.0	<1.0	na	5	<17%
CHICKEN, CREAM OF										
(Lipton) 'Cup-A-Soup' prepared	6 oz	84	1.4	9.7	757	na	4.4	(mq)	na	47%
(Lipton) 'Food Service' prepared	6 oz	84	1.7	9.4	840	na	4.4	(mq)	na	47%
CHICKEN LEEK										
creamy *(Ultra Slim Fast)* 1 envelope, prepared	6 oz	50	5.0	7.0	1070	2.0	<1.0	na	2	<16%
CHICKEN NOODLE										
prepared	1 cup	53	3.0	7.4	1284	.8	1.2	0.3	3	21%
(Campbell's) 'Lowfat Block' prepared	1 cup	160	5.0	32.0	940	(mq)	1.0	na	na	6%
(Campbell's) 'Quality Recipe' prepared	1 cup	100	5.0	16.0	710	(mq)	2.0	(mq)	na	18%
(Campbell's) 'Ramen Noodle' prepared	1 cup	190	5.0	26.0	970	(mq)	8.0	(mq)	na	37%
(Estee) 'Instant' prepared	6 oz	25	1.0	4.0	135	(mq)	<1.0	<1.0	<1	<31%
(Lipton) 'Cup-A-Soup' prepared	6 oz	48	3.0	6.6	635	(mq)	1.1	na	na	21%
(Lipton) 'Supreme' prepared	6 oz	107	1.7	11.8	757	(mq)	5.9	(mq)	na	50%
(Mrs. Grass) 'Chickeny Rich'	1/4 pkg	70	2.0	10.0	900	(mq)	2.0	(mq)	na	27%
Creamy, hearty *(Lipton)* prepared	7 oz	179	5.1	21.4	639	(mq)	8.2	(mq)	na	41%
Hearty										
(Lipton) prepared	1 cup	83	4.4	13.3	753	(mq)	1.3	na	na	14%
(Lipton) prepared	7 oz	118	4.8	21.2	655	(mq)	1.5	na	na	12%
W/ meat										
(Campbell's) white meat	6 oz	90	6.0	12.0	770	(mq)	2.0	(mq)	(mq)	20%

Food Name	Serving Size	Calories	Prot. gms	Carbs gms	Sod. mgs	Fiber gms	Fat gms	Sat. Fat gms	Chol. mgs	% Fat Cal.
(Lipton) 'Cup' prepared	6 oz	46	2.6	6.6	660	(mq)	1.0	na	(mq)	20%
(Lipton) 'Value Pack' prepared	6 oz	46	2.6	6.6	660	(mq)	1.0	na	(mq)	20%
(Lipton) white meat, diced, prepared	1 cup	81	4.3	12.1	795	(mq)	1.8	(mq)	(mq)	20%
W/rice (Lipton) prepared	6 oz	47	2.2	7.7	667	(mq)	0.8	na	na	15%
W/vegetables										
(Campbell's) prepared	1 cup	270	6.0	38.0	1470	(mq)	10.0	(mq)	na	34%
(Campbell's) lowfat, prepared	1 cup	220	7.0	44.0	1500	(mq)	2.0	(mq)	na	8%
(Lipton) 'Cup' prepared	6 oz	47	2.5	7.8	566	>.2 c	0.6	na	8	12%
(Lipton) hearty, prepared	1 cup	75	3.0	12.3	687	(mq)	1.6	na	na	19%
CHICKEN RICE, prepared	8 oz	61	2.5	9.3	981	0	1.4	0.3	3	21%
CHICKEN VEGETABLE, prepared	8 oz	50	2.7	7.8	807	>.3 c	0.8	0.2	3	15%
CHILI PEPPER (A Taste of Thai) hot and sour, prepared	1 cup	40	0.0	5.0	1330	0	2.0	1.0	0	47%
CLAM CHOWDER										
Manhattan style (Golden Dipt)	1/4 pkg	80	2.0	13.0	700	(mq)	2.0	1.0	3	23%
New England style (Golden Dipt)	1/4 pkg	70	2.0	12.0	680	(mq)	2.0	1.0	2	24%
CONSOMMÉ, w/gelatin, prepared	1 cup	17	2.2	2.1	3299	0	0.0	na	0	0%
GINGER (A Taste of Thai) tangy coconut, prepared	1 cup	250	3.0	3.0	1050	0	1.5	0.5	0	36%
GREEN PEA										
(Lipton) 'Cup-A-Soup' prepared	6 oz	113	4.2	14.4	553	>.2 c	4.2	(mq)	na	34%
(Lipton) 'Cup-A-Soup Food Service' prepared	6 oz	115	3.5	15.1	635	>.7 c	4.5	(mq)	na	35%
HERB (Lipton) savory, w/garlic 'Recipe Secrets' prepared ...	8 oz	35	<1.0	7.0	490	na	<1.0	na	na	<22%
LEEK										
Creamy (Ultra Slim Fast) 1 envelope prepared	6 oz	80	5.0	15.0	780	2.0	<1.0	na	0	<10%
LENTIL (Hain) 'Savory Soup Mix' prepared	6 oz	130	4.0	20.0	810	(mq)	2.0	(mq)	na	16%
LOBSTER BISQUE (Golden Dipt) prepared	1/4 pkg	30	1.0	5.0	560	na	1.0	na	2	27%
MINESTRONE										
(Hain) 'Savory Soup Mix' prepared	6 oz	110	4.0	20.0	870	(mq)	1.0	na	na	9%
(Manischewitz) prepared	6 oz	50	3.0	9.0	160	(mq)	<1.0	na	na	<16%
MUSHROOM										
(Estee) 'Instant' prepared	6 oz	40	1.0	3.0	115	(mq)	2.0	1.0	10	53%
(Hain) 'Savory Soup & Recipe Mix' prepared	6 oz	210	4.0	11.0	710	(mq)	15.0	(mq)	na	69%
(Hain) 'Savory Soup & Recipe Mix No Salt Added' prepared	6 oz	250	5.0	15.0	180	(mq)	20.0	(mq)	na	69%
Beef flavor (Lipton) prepared	1 cup	38	1.7	6.7	763	(mq)	0.5	na	na	12%
MUSHROOM, CREAM OF (Lipton) 'Cup-A-Soup' prepared	6 oz	71	1.3	9.1	756	(mq)	3.2	(mq)	na	41%
NOODLE										
(Campbell's) 'Quality Soup & Recipe' prepared	1 cup	110	5.0	19.0	700	(mq)	2.0	(mq)	na	16%
(Lipton) 'Cup-A-Soup Ring Noodle' prepared	6 oz	47	2.7	7.6	650	(mq)	0.7	na	na	13%
(Lipton) 'Giggle Noodle' prepared	1 cup	77	2.9	11.4	784	(mq)	2.1	(mq)	na	25%
(Lipton) 'Ring-O-Noodle' prepared	1 cup	71	2.7	10.4	784	(mq)	2.0	(mq)	na	26%
Beef flavor										
(Cup O'Noodles) prepared	1 cup	290	8.0	33.0	1490	(mq)	14.0	(mq)	na	43%
(Oodles of Noodles) prepared	1 cup	390	9.0	49.0	1810	(mq)	18.0	(mq)	na	41%
(Top Ramen) prepared	1 cup	390	9.0	49.0	1810	(mq)	18.0	(mq)	na	41%
Beefy, w/vegetables (Lipton) prepared	1 cup	85	2.5	16.7	810	(mq)	0.9	na	na	10%
Chicken flavor										
(Cup O'Noodles) prepared	1 cup	300	9.0	32.0	1790	(mq)	16.0	(mq)	na	47%
(Cup O'Noodles) 'Hearty' prepared	1 cup	300	8.0	35.0	1210	(mq)	14.0	(mq)	na	42%
(Oodles of Noodles) prepared	1 cup	400	10.0	48.0	1910	(mq)	18.0	(mq)	na	41%
(Top Ramen) prepared	1 cup	400	10.0	48.0	1910	(mq)	18.0	(mq)	na	41%
Hearty (Campbell's) 'Quality Soup & Recipe' prepared	1 cup	90	4.0	15.0	840	(mq)	1.0	na	na	11%
Hearty, w/vegetables (Lipton) prepared	1 cup	75	3.0	12.3	687	(mq)	1.6	na	na	19%
Oriental										
(Campbell's) 'Ramen Noodle' prepared	1 cup	190	5.0	26.0	930	(mq)	8.0	(mq)	na	37%

Food Name	Serving Size	Calories	Prot. gms	Carbs gms	Sod. mgs	Fiber gms	Fat gms	Sat. Fat gms	Chol. mgs	% Fat Cal.
(Campbell's) 'Ramen Noodle Lowfat Block' prepared	1 cup	150	5.0	31.0	940	(mq)	1.0	na	na	6%
(Oodles of Noodles) prepared	1 cup	390	10.0	49.0	1660	(mq)	18.0	(mq)	na	41%
(Top Ramen) prepared	1 cup	390	10.0	49.0	1660	(mq)	18.0	(mq)	na	41%
Oriental, w/vegetables										
(Campbell's) 'Cup-A-Ramen' prepared	1 cup	270	6.0	38.0	1210	(mq)	10.0	(mq)	na	34%
(Campbell's) 'Cup-A-Ramen Lowfat' prepared	1 cup	220	7.0	44.0	1400	(mq)	2.0	(mq)	na	8%
Pork flavor										
(Campbell's) 'Ramen Noodle' prepared	1 cup	200	5.0	26.0	860	(mq)	8.0	(mq)	na	37%
(Campbell's) 'Ramen Noodle Lowfat Block' prepared	1 cup	150	4.0	31.0	1140	(mq)	1.0	na	na	6%
(Oodles of Noodles) prepared	1 cup	390	10.0	51.0	2060	(mq)	20.0	(mq)	na	43%
(Top Ramen) prepared	1 cup	390	10.0	51.0	2060	(mq)	20.0	(mq)	na	43%
Pork flavor, w/old fashioned vegetables										
(Cup O'Noodles) 'Hearty' prepared	6 oz	290	6.0	34.0	1250	(mq)	15.0	(mq)	na	46%
Pork flavor, w/seafood (Cup O'Noodles) 'Hearty' prepared ..	1 cup	300	7.0	34.0	1170	(mq)	15.0	(mq)	na	45%
Pork flavor, w/shrimp (Cup O'Noodles) prepared	1 cup	300	10.0	32.0	1480	(mq)	14.0	(mq)	na	43%
W/chicken broth										
(Campbell's) 'Cup 2 Minute Soup' prepared	6 oz	90	4.0	15.0	910	(mq)	2.0	(mq)	na	19%
(Campbell's) 'Double Noodle'	1.78 oz	200	8.0	36.0	770	na	2.0	na	na	9%
(Campbell's) 'Double Noodle' prepared	8 oz	200	8.0	36.0	770	na	2.0	na	na	9%
ONION										
(Campbell's) 'Quality Soup & Recipe' prepared	1 cup	30	1.0	7.0	700	(mq)	0.0	0.0	0	0%
(Estee) prepared	6 oz	25	1.0	4.0	140	(mq)	<1.0	<1.0	0	<31%
(Hain) 'Savory Soup, Dip & Recipe Mix' prepared	6 oz	50	2.0	6.0	900	(mq)	2.0	(mq)	na	36%
(Hain) 'Savory Soup, Dip & Recipe Mix' no salt, prepared .	6 oz	50	1.0	9.0	470	(mq)	1.0	na	na	18%
(Lipton) prepared	1 cup	20	0.7	4.3	632	(mq)	0.2	na	na	8%
(Lipton) 'Cup-A-Soup' prepared	6 oz	27	0.9	4.7	665	>.1 c	0.5	na	na	17%
(Mrs. Grass) 'Soup & Dip Mix' prepared	1/4 pkg	35	1.0	6.0	1070	(mq)	<1.0	na	0	<24%
Beefy (Lipton) prepared	1 cup	29	0.8	4.2	803	(mq)	1.0	na	na	31%
Creamy										
(Lipton) 'Cup-A-Soup' prepared	6 oz	70	1.2	9.5	678	>.2 c	3.2	(mq)	na	40%
(Ultra Slim Fast) 1 envelope, prepared	6 oz	45	5.0	7.0	1180	2.0	<1.0	na	0	<16%
Golden, w/chicken broth (Lipton) prepared	1 cup	62	1.1	11.0	716	(mq)	1.5	na	na	22%
Mushroom (Lipton) prepared	1 cup	41	1.4	6.8	684	(mq)	0.9	na	na	20%
ORIENTAL (Lipton) 'Cup-A-Soup Lite' prepared	6 oz	45	1.5	5.8	457	na	1.7	na	3	34%
OXTAIL prepared	8 oz	71	2.8	9.0	1210	.5	2.6	1.3	3	33%
POTATO LEEK (Hain) 'Savory Soup Mix' prepared	6 oz	260	4.0	20.0	690	(mq)	18.0	(mq)	na	63%
SPLIT PEA										
Green										
(Hain) 'Savory Soup Mix' prepared	6 oz	310	4.0	16.0	940	(mq)	10.0	(mq)	na	53%
(Manischewitz) prepared	6 oz	45	3.0	9.0	320	(mq)	<1.0	na	0	<16%
Fat-free, thick and creamy (Fantastic Foods) 'Splittin Pea'	10 oz	145	13.0	31.0	490	3.0	1.0	na	0	5%
W/carrots (Health Valley)	7.5 oz	80	9.0	17.0	290	12.5	0.0	na	0	0%
SEAFOOD CHOWDER (Golden Dipt)	1/4 pkg	70	2.0	12.0	730	na	2.0	1.0	2	24%
SHRIMP										
Bisque (Golden Dipt) dry mix	1/4 pkg	30	1.0	5.0	570	na	1.0	na	2	27%
W/vegetables										
(Campbell's) 'Cup-A-Ramen' prepared	1 cup	280	6.0	40.0	1190	(mq)	10.0	(mq)	na	33%
(Campbell's) 'Lowfat' prepared	1 cup	230	7.0	45.0	1290	(mq)	2.0	(mq)	na	8%
TOMATO										
(Estee) 'Instant' prepared	6 oz	40	1.0	5.0	95	(mq)	<1.0	<1.0	0	<27%
(Hain) 'Savory Soup & Recipe Mix' prepared	6 oz	220	3.0	19.0	770	(mq)	14.0	(mq)	na	59%
(Lipton) 'Cup-A-Soup' prepared	6 oz	103	2.5	21.2	524	(mq)	0.9	na	na	8%
(Lipton) 'Cup-A-Soup Food Service' prepared	6 oz	100	2.8	20.1	563	(mq)	0.9	na	na	8%
Creamy (Ultra Slim Fast) 1 envelope, prepared	6 oz	60	5.0	10.0	990	2.0	<1.0	na	0	<13%

Food Name	Serving Size	Calories	Prot. gms	Carbs gms	Sod. mgs	Fiber gms	Fat gms	Sat. Fat gms	Chol. mgs	% Fat Cal.
Creamy, w/herb (Lipton) 'Cup-A-Soup Lite' prepared	6 oz	66	1.6	14.1	305	(mq)	0.3	na	2	4%
Minestrone (Cous•cous)	10 oz	200	9.0	41.0	590	na	0.0	na	na	0%
TOMATO VEGETABLE										
prepared	8 oz	56	2.0	10.2	1146	.5	0.9	0.4	0	14%
W/noodles (Fantastic Noodles) prepared	7 oz	158	5.0	20.0	434	(mq)	8.0	(mq)	na	42%
VEGETABLE										
(Campbell's) 'Quality Soup & Recipe' prepared	1 cup	40	1.0	8.0	710	(mq)	0.0	0.0	0	0%
(Hain) 'Savory Soup Mix' prepared	6 oz	80	2.0	13.0	730	(mq)	1.0	na	na	13%
(Hain) 'Savory Soup Mix No Salt Added' prepared	6 oz	80	2.0	13.0	330	(mq)	1.0	na	na	13%
(Lipton) prepared	1 cup	39	1.6	6.9	640	>.4 c	0.5	na	na	12%
(Manischewitz) prepared	6 oz	50	3.0	9.0	65	(mq)	<1.0	na	0	<16%
Country (Lipton) prepared	1 cup	80	2.6	15.7	803	(mq)	0.7	na	na	8%
Curry, w/noodles (Fantastic Noodles) prepared	7 oz	150	5.0	18.0	472	(mq)	7.0	(mq)	na	41%
Garden (Lipton) 'Lots-A-Noodles Cup-A-Soup' prepared ...	7 oz	123	4.3	23.1	720	(mq)	1.5	na	na	11%
Harvest										
(Lipton) 'Country Style' prepared	6 oz	95	2.0	18.9	569	>.5 c	1.2	na	na	11%
(Lipton) 'Cup-A-Soup Country Style' prepared	6 oz	91	1.7	18.8	459	>.5 c	1.2	na	na	12%
Hearty (Ultra Slim Fast) 1 envelope, prepared	6 oz	45	5.0	5.0	850	2.0	<1.0	na	0	<18%
Miso, w/noodles (Fantastic Noodles) prepared	7 oz	152	5.0	19.0	434	(mq)	7.0	(mq)	na	40%
Noodle, w/meatballs (Lipton) 'Country Style' prepared	6 oz	95	4.9	15.4	764	>.5 c	1.6	na	na	15%
Parmesan (Cous•cous)	10 oz	200	9.0	35.0	550	na	3.0	na	na	13%
Spring (Lipton) 'Cup-A-Soup' prepared	6 oz	33	1.1	5.9	746	>.3 c	0.8	na	6	21%
VEGETABLE BEEF, prepared	8 oz	53	2.9	8.0	1002	.5	1.1	0.6	0	19%
VIRGINIA PEA										
(Lipton) prepared	6 oz	113	4.7	14.6	664	>.4 c	4.1	(mq)	<1	32%
(Lipton) 'Country Style' prepared	6 oz	148	5.3	17.3	828	>.8 c	6.4	(mq)	na	39%
SOUR CREAM										
....	1 cup	493	7.3	9.8	123	0	48.2	30.0	102	86%
....	1 oz	61	0.9	1.2	15	0	5.9	3.7	13	86%
....	1 tbsp	26	0.4	0.5	6	0	2.5	1.6	5	86%
(Bison)	1 oz	50	1.0	1.0	15	0	5.0	(mq)	20	85%
(Breakstone's)	1 tbsp	30	0.0	1.0	5	0	3.0	2.0	10	87%
(Crowley)	1 oz	50	1.0	1.0	15	0	5.0	(mq)	20	85%
(Darigold)	1 tbsp	23	0.9	1.1	5	0	2.8	1.8	5	76%
(Friendship)	2 tbsp	55	1.0	1.0	15	0	5.0	(mq)	42	85%
(Knudsen) 'Hampshire'	1 oz	60	1.0	1.0	10	0	6.0	3.0	20	87%
(Sealtest)	1 tbsp	30	0.0	1.0	5	0	3.0	2.0	10	87%
French onion (Crowley)	1 oz	50	1.0	1.0	130	0	5.0	(mq)	20	85%
Pasteurized, 100% natural (Alta•Dena)	1 oz	60	1.0	1.0	15	0	6.0	na	na	87%
W/acidophilus, cultured (Alta•Dena) 'Kefir'	1 oz	70	1.0	1.0	40	0	6.0	na	na	87%
W/chives (Land O'Lakes) 'Light'	2 tbsp	40	2.0	4.0	150	na	2.0	1.0	5	43%
HALF AND HALF										
(Breakstone's) 'Light Choice'	1 tbsp	25	1.0	1.0	10	0	2.0	1.0	5	69%
(Sealtest) 'Light'	1 tbsp	25	1.0	1.0	10	0	2.0	1.0	5	69%
Cultured	1 tbsp	20	0.4	0.6	6	0	1.8	1.1	6	80%
LIGHT / LOW-FAT										
(Crowley)	1 oz	30	1.0	2.0	25	0	2.0	(mq)	5	60%
(Friendship) 'Lite Delite'	2 tbsp	35	1.0	2.0	25	0	2.0	(mq)	8	60%
(Knudsen)	1 oz	40	1.0	2.0	20	0	3.0	2.0	10	69%
(Land O'Lakes) 'Light'	2 tbsp	40	2.0	4.0	35	na	2.0	1.0	5	43%
(Naturally Yours) 'Real•Dairy' no fat	2 tbsp	15	3.0	1.0	15	na	0.0	0.0	0	0%
(Weight Watchers)	2 tbsp	35	2.0	2.0	40	0	2.0	(mq)	(mq)	53%
SOUR CREAM, ALTERNATIVE / NONDAIRY										
....	1 cup	479	5.5	15.3	235	0	44.9	40.9	0	83%

Food Name	Serving Size	Calories	Prot. gms	Carbs gms	Sod. mgs	Fiber gms	Fat gms	Sat. Fat gms	Chol. mgs	% Fat Cal.
.... 1 oz		59	0.7	1.9	29	0	5.5	5.0	0	83%
(Crowley) dressing .... 1 oz		40	1.0	1.0	5	0	4.0	(mq)	0	82%
(Pet) .... 1 tbsp		25	<1.0	<1.0	25	0	2.0	(mq)	<1	69%
Cultured										
.... 1 cup		479	5.5	15.2	235	0	44.9	40.9	0	83%
.... 1 oz		58	0.7	1.9	29	0	5.5	5.0	0	83%
(Light n' Lively) nonfat .... 1 tbsp		10	1.0	1.0	30	na	0.0	0.0	10	0%
SOURSOP. See GUANABANA.										
SOY BEVERAGE										
(Edensoy) 'Extra' original .... 8.45 oz		140	10.0	14.0	110	na	4.0	0.6	na	27%
(Edensoy) original .... 8.45 oz		140	10.0	14.0	120	na	4.0	0.6	0	27%
(Health Valley) fat-free 'Soy Moo' ..... 1 cup		110	7.0	19.0	25	0	0.0	na	0	0%
(Soyamel) powdered mix, prepared .... 8 oz		130	7.0	10.0	210	na	7.0	1.0	0	48%
(WestSoy) 'Lite' plain .... 8 oz		100	4.0	16.0	100	na	2.0	na	0	18%
(WestSoy) 'Natural' original .... 8 oz		150	7.0	18.0	115	na	5.0	na	0	31%
(WestSoy) 'Natural' unsweetened .... 8 oz		100	7.0	5.0	40	na	5.0	na	0	48%
(WestSoy) 'Plus' plain .... 8 oz		150	6.0	18.0	140	na	5.0	na	0	32%
ALMOND FLAVOR										
(WestSoy) 'Lite' .... 6 oz		160	5.0	26.0	140	na	4.0	na	0	23%
(WestSoy) 'Natural' .... 6 oz		250	7.0	31.0	140	(mq)	11.0	(mq)	0	39%
BANANA FLAVOR (WestSoy) 'Lite' creamy banana .... 6 oz		160	5.0	26.0	140	na	3.0	na	0	18%
CAROB FLAVOR										
(Ah Soy) .... 6 oz		160	4.0	30.0	120	(mq)	3.0	(mq)	0	17%
(Edensoy) .... 8.45 oz		160	6.0	30.0	125	na	5.0	na	0	24%
(WestSoy) 'Plus' .... 8 oz		160	6.0	21.0	80	na	5.0	na	0	29%
Malted										
(WestSoy) 'Lite' .... 6 oz		160	5.0	27.0	140	na	3.0	na	0	17%
(WestSoy) 'Natural' .... 6 oz		270	7.0	37.0	120	(mq)	11.0	(mq)	0	36%
CHOCOLATE FLAVOR (Ah Soy) .... 6 oz		160	4.0	29.0	120	(mq)	3.0	(mq)	0	17%
COCOA FLAVOR										
(WestSoy) 'Lite' .... 8 oz		140	3.0	27.0	95	na	2.0	na	10	13%
(WestSoy) 'Lite' w/mint .... 6 oz		160	5.0	26.0	140	na	3.0	na	0	18%
COFFEE FLAVOR (WestSoy) 'Natural' java malted .... 6 oz		270	7.0	37.0	140	(mq)	11.0	(mq)	0	36%
VANILLA FLAVOR										
(Ah Soy) .... 6 oz		160	5.0	23.0	140	(mq)	5.0	(mq)	0	29%
(Edensoy) 'Extra' .... 8.45 oz		150	8.0	25.0	95	3.0	3.0	0.4	na	17%
(Edensoy) 'Natural Vanilla' .... 8.45 oz		150	8.0	25.0	140	na	3.0	0.4	0	17%
(WestSoy) 'Lite' .... 8 oz		110	3.0	20.0	80	na	2.0	na	0	16%
(WestSoy) 'Lite' vanilla royale .... 6 oz		160	5.0	26.0	140	na	3.0	na	0	18%
(WestSoy) 'Plus' .... 8 oz		150	6.0	20.0	120	na	5.0	na	0	30%
All natural (WestSoy) .... 8 oz		120	4.0	22.0	140	na	2.5	0.5	0	18%
Malted (WestSoy) 'Natural' .... 6 oz		250	7.0	31.0	140	(mq)	11.0	(mq)	0	39%
SOY FLOUR										
defatted .... 1 oz		93	13.3	10.9	6	>1.2 c	0.3	<.1	0	3%
defatted, stirred .... 1/2 cup		165	23.5	19.2	10	8.8	0.6	0.1	0	3%
full-fat .... 1 oz		124	9.8	10.0	4	>1.3 c	5.9	0.8	0	40%
full-fat (Arrowhead Mills) .... 2 oz		250	20.0	18.0	1	8.1	11.0	(mq)	0	39%
full-fat, roasted .... 1 oz		125	9.9	9.5	3	>.6 c	6.2	0.9	0	42%
full-fat, roasted, stirred .... 1/2 cup		185	14.6	14.1	5	>.9 c	9.2	1.3	0	42%
full-fat, stirred .... 1/2 cup		183	14.5	14.8	5	4.0	8.7	1.3	0	40%
low-fat .... 1 oz		92	13.2	10.8	5	>1.2 c	1.9	0.3	0	15%
low-fat, stirred .... 1/2 cup		143	20.5	16.7	8	4.5	3.0	0.4	0	15%
SOY MEAL										
defatted, raw .... 1/2 cup		207	27.4	24.5	2	>3.5 c	1.5	0.2	0	6%

Food Name	Serving Size	Calories	Prot. gms	Carbs gms	Sod. mgs	Fiber gms	Fat gms	Sat. Fat gms	Chol. mgs	% Fat Cal.
defatted, raw	1 oz	96	12.7	11.4	1	0.0	0.7	0.1	0	6%
SOY MILK. See SOY BEVERAGE.										
SOY PROTEIN CONCENTRATE										
acid wash extracted	1 oz	93	16.3	8.7	252	>1.1 c	0.1	0.0	0	1%
acid/water wash extracted	1 oz	94	16.5	8.8	255	>1.1 c	0.1	0.1	0	1%
alcohol extracted	1 oz	93	16.3	8.7	1	>1.1 c	0.1	0.0	0	1%
SOY PROTEIN ISOLATE										
	1 oz	95	22.6	2.1	281	1.6	1.0	0.1	0	8%
potassium type	1 oz	91	22.6	2.9	14	>.1 c	0.2	0.1	0	2%
w/potassium	1 oz	96	22.9	0.2	14	>.1 c	1.0	0.1	0	9%
w/sodium	1 oz	96	22.9	0.2	281	>.1 c	1.0	0.1	0	9%
SOYBEAN										
Dried										
boiled	4 oz	196	18.9	11.2	1	>2.3 c	10.2	1.5	0	43%
boiled	1/2 cup	149	14.3	8.5	1	5.2	7.7	1.1	0	43%
dry-roasted	1/2 cup	387	34.0	28.1	2	7.0	18.6	2.7	0	40%
dry-roasted	1 oz	128	11.2	9.3	1	>1.5 c	6.1	0.9	0	40%
raw	1/2 cup	387	33.9	28.1	2	11.6	18.5	2.7	0	40%
raw	1 oz	118	10.3	8.6	1	3.5	5.7	0.8	0	40%
raw (Arrowhead Mills)	2 oz	230	19.0	19.0	2	13.2	10.0	na	0	37%
roasted	1/2 cup	405	30.3	28.9	140	>4.0 c	21.8	3.2	0	45%
roasted	1 oz	134	10.0	9.5	46	>1.3 c	7.2	1.0	0	45%
Green										
boiled, drained	4 oz	160	14.0	12.5	na	>2.1 c	7.3	0.8	0	38%
boiled, drained	1/2 cup	127	11.1	9.9	13	3.8	5.8	0.7	0	38%
raw	1/2 cup	188	16.6	14.1	19	5.4	8.7	1.0	0	39%
raw, in pods	1 lb	353	31.1	26.6	na	>4.0 c	16.4	1.8	0	39%
raw, shelled	1 oz	42	3.7	3.1	na	>.6 c	1.9	0.2	0	39%
Kernels, roasted/toasted										
whole	1 cup	489	40.0	33.0	4	3.9	25.9	3.4	0	44%
whole	1 oz	129	10.5	8.7	1	1.0	6.8	0.9	0	44%
Mature										
boiled	1/2 cup	149	14.3	8.5	1	5.2	7.7	1.1	0	43%
dry-roasted	1/2 cup	387	34.0	28.1	2	7.0	18.6	2.7	0	40%
raw	1/2 cup	387	33.9	28.1	2	8.7	18.5	2.7	0	40%
roasted	1/2 cup	405	30.3	28.9	140	>4.0 c	21.8	3.2	0	45%
Mature, sprouted										
boiled, drained	1 cup	48	6.6	4.6	5	>1.0 c	1.8	0.0	0	27%
raw	1 lb	580	59.4	50.7	62	>10.4 c	30.4	3.3	0	38%
raw	1/2 cup	43	4.6	3.3	5	>.8 c	2.3	0.3	0	40%
steamed	1/2 cup	38	4.0	3.1	5	.4	2.1	0.3	0	40%
stir-fried	3.5 oz	125	13.1	9.4	14	>2.5 c	7.1	1.0	0	42%
SOYBEAN, FERMENTED. See also MISO.										
natto	1/2 cup	187	15.6	12.6	6	>1.4 c	9.7	1.4	0	44%
natto	1 oz	60	5.0	4.1	2	0	3.1	0.5	0	43%
SOYBEAN CURD CAKE. See TOFU.										
SOYBEAN FLAKES (Arrowhead Mills)	2 oz	250	20.0	18.0	2	8.1	11.0	(mq)	0	39%
SOYBEAN LECITHIN OIL										
	1/2 cup	964	0.0	0.0	0	0	109.0	16.7	0	100%
	1 oz	251	0.0	0.0	0	0	28.4	4.3	0	100%
	1 tbsp	120	0.0	0.0	0	0	13.6	2.1	0	100%
SOYBEAN OIL										
	1 cup	1927	0.0	0.0	0	0	218.0	31.4	0	100%
hydrogenated	1 cup	1927	0.0	0.0	0	0	218.0	32.5	0	100%

Food Name	Serving Size	Calories	Prot. gms	Carbs gms	Sod. mgs	Fiber gms	Fat gms	Sat. Fat gms	Chol. mgs	% Fat Cal.
hydrogenated	1 oz	251	0.0	0.0	0	0	28.4	4.2	0	100%
hydrogenated	1 tbsp	120	0.0	0.0	0	0	13.6	2.0	0	100%
(Hain)	1 tbsp	120	0.0	0.0	0	0	14.0	2.0	0	100%
(IGA)	1 tbsp	120	0.0	0.0	0	0	14.0	2.0	0	100%
SOYBEAN-COTTONSEED OIL										
hydrogenated	1/2 cup	964	0.0	0.0	0	0	109.0	19.6	0	100%
hydrogenated	1 oz	251	0.0	0.0	0	0	28.4	5.1	0	100%
hydrogenated	1 tbsp	120	0.0	0.0	0	0	13.6	2.4	0	100%
SPAGHETTI. See PASTA.										
SPAGHETTI ENTRÉE, CANNED										
W/beef (Chef Boyardee) 'Beef-O-Getti'	7.5 oz	220	7.0	27.0	1240	(mq)	9.0	(mq)	(mq)	37%
W/beef, in tomato sauce (Chef Boyardee)	7.5 oz	240	7.0	30.0	1120	(mq)	9.0	(mq)	(mq)	35%
W/frankfurters (Van Camp's) 'Spaghettee Weenee'	1 cup	243	9.4	34.7	1128	>.5 c	7.4	(mq)	(mq)	27%
W/frankfurters, in tomato sauce (Franco-American)										
'SpaghettiOs'	7.5 oz	220	8.0	26.0	1000	(mq)	9.0	(mq)	(mq)	37%
W/meatballs										
(Estee)	7.5 oz	240	9.0	19.0	130	(mq)	14.0	6.0	30	53%
(Featherweight)	7.5 oz	160	12.0	23.0	400	(mq)	3.0	(mq)	20	16%
(Nalley's)	7.5 oz	190	10.0	29.0	950	(mq)	4.0	(mq)	(mq)	19%
W/meatballs, in sauce (Buitoni)	7.5 oz	190	9.0	21.0	940	(mq)	8.0	6.0	20	38%
W/meatballs, in tomato sauce										
(Chef Boyardee)	7.5 oz	230	8.0	30.0	970	(mq)	9.0	(mq)	(mq)	35%
(Franco-American)	7 3/8 oz	220	10.0	28.0	870	(mq)	8.0	(mq)	(mq)	32%
(Franco-American) 'SpaghettiOs'	7 3/8 oz	220	9.0	25.0	950	(mq)	9.0	(mq)	(mq)	37%
(Pathmark) 'No Frills'	7.5 oz	200	9.0	22.0	860	(mq)	8.0	(mq)	(mq)	37%
W/tomato and cheese sauce (Franco-American)										
'SpaghettiOs'	7.5 oz	170	5.0	33.0	860	(mq)	2.0	(mq)	na	11%
W/tomato sauce, rings (Finast)	7.5 oz	150	4.0	31.0	480	(mq)	1.0	na	na	6%
SPAGHETTI ENTRÉE, FREEZE-DRIED										
(Mountain House) w/meat and sauce, prepared	1 cup	260	12.0	41.0	(mq)	(mq)	5.0	(mq)	(mq)	18%
SPAGHETTI ENTRÉE, FROZEN										
Parmesan, w/Italian-style green beans (Stouffer's)	10.25 oz	240	10.0	30.0	810	na	9.0	na	na	34%
W/beef (Dining Lite)	9 oz	220	12.0	25.0	440	(mq)	8.0	(mq)	20	33%
W/beef sauce and mushrooms (Le Menu) 'LightStyle'	9 oz	280	12.0	45.0	450	(mq)	6.0	1.0	15	19%
W/Italian-style meatballs (Swanson) 'Homestyle Recipe'	13 oz	490	23.0	60.0	940	(mq)	18.0	(mq)	(mq)	33%
W/meat sauce										
(Banquet) 'Casserole'	8 oz	270	14.0	35.0	1250	(mq)	8.0	(mq)	(mq)	27%
(Freezer Queen) 'Single Serve'	10 oz	350	14.0	47.0	610	(mq)	12.0	(mq)	(mq)	31%
(Kid Cuisine)	9.25 oz	310	9.0	43.0	690	(mq)	12.0	(mq)	35	34%
(Lean Cuisine)	11.5 oz	290	15.0	45.0	500	na	6.0	2.0	20	18%
(Stouffer's)	12 7/8 oz	320	16.0	38.0	560	na	12.0	na	na	33%
(Weight Watchers)	10 oz	240	16.0	28.0	490	na	7.0	1.0	5	26%
W/meatballs										
(Banquet)	10 oz	290	11.0	44.0	580	(mq)	10.0	(mq)	30	29%
(Morton)	10 oz	200	6.0	39.0	1090	(mq)	3.0	(mq)	10	13%
(Stouffer's) 19.5-oz pkg	1/2 pkg	290	14.0	37.0	790	na	9.0	na	na	28%
(Stouffer's) 12 5/8-oz pkg	1 pkg	440	22.0	53.0	960	na	16.0	na	na	32%
(Swanson)	12.5 oz	390	14.0	46.0	1100	(mq)	17.0	(mq)	(mq)	39%
W/meatballs and sauce (Lean Cuisine)	9.5 oz	290	20.0	36.0	550	na	7.0	2.0	30	22%
SPAGHETTI ENTRÉE, MICROWAVE										
(Lunch Bucket) 'Spaghetti 'n Meatsauce' microwave cup	7.5 oz	240	9.0	39.0	870	na	5.0	na	30	19%
Rings (Kid's Kitchen) microwave cup	7.5 oz	180	8.0	35.0	930	na	1.0	1.0	10	5%
Rings and franks in tomato sauce (Kid's Kitchen)										
microwave cup	7.5 oz	290	12.0	33.0	960	na	12.0	na	30	38%

Food Name	Serving Size	Calories	Prot. gms	Carbs gms	Sod. mgs	Fiber gms	Fat gms	Sat. Fat gms	Chol. mgs	% Fat Cal.
W/meatballs										
(Chef Boyardee) 'Microwave'	7.5 oz	230	7.0	29.0	1060	(mq)	10.0	(mq)	20	39%
(Hormel) micro cup	7.5 oz	210	10.0	27.0	930	na	7.0	3.0	20	30%
(Kid's Kitchen) microwave cup	7.5 oz	220	11.0	26.0	880	na	8.0	4.0	20	33%
W/meatballs, in sauce (Libby's) 'Diner'	7.75 oz	190	10.0	31.0	870	2.2	3.0	1.0	15	14%
SPAGHETTI ENTRÉE, PACKAGED										
Spaghettini (Top Shelf)	1 serving	240	13.0	35.0	1020	(mq)	5.0	(mq)	5	19%
W/beef and mushroom sauce (Ultra Slim Fast)	12 oz	370	20.0	49.0	990	na	10.0	na	25	25%
W/meat sauce (Top Shelf)	10 oz	260	14.0	37.0	980	na	6.0	2.0	20	21%
SPAGHETTI ENTRÉE MIX										
(Kraft) 'Mild American Dinner' prepared	1 cup	300	10.0	50.0	630	(mq)	7.0	2.0	0	21%
(Kraft) 'Tangy Italian Style Dinner' prepared	1 cup	310	11.0	49.0	670	(mq)	8.0	2.0	5	23%
Low-fat, w/whole wheat noodles (Fantastic Foods)										
'All-O-Round'	10 oz	211	10.0	45.0	275	na	2.0	na	4	8%
W/condensed meat sauce (Chef Boyardee)										
'Dinner' prepared	3.25 oz	250	12.0	37.0	595	(mq)	6.0	(mq)	(mq)	22%
W/meat sauce										
(Chef Boyardee) 'Dinner' prepared	7.9 oz	240	12.0	42.0	1155	(mq)	3.0	(mq)	(mq)	11%
(Kraft) 'Dinner' prepared	1 cup	360	12.0	47.0	880	(mq)	14.0	4.0	15	35%
W/mushroom sauce (Chef Boyardee) 'Dinner' prepared	7.9 oz	210	11.0	41.0	1085	(mq)	1.0	na	na	4%
SPAGHETTI SEASONING (Tone's)	1 tsp	11	0.2	2.5	469	.1	<.1	tr	tr	<8%
SPAGHETTI SQUASH. See SQUASH, SPAGHETTI.										
SPAM. See LUNCHEON MEAT, CANNED.										
SPARE RIB SEASONING MIX, 'Bag'n Season' (Schilling)	1 pkg	185	0.3	42.0	3690	na	1.5	na	2	7%
SPINACH										
boiled, drained	4 oz	26	3.4	4.3	79	2.5	0.3	<.1	0	11%
boiled, drained	1/2 cup	21	2.7	3.4	63	2.0	0.2	0.0	0	11%
raw	10-oz pkg	62	8.1	9.9	224	7.4	1.0	0.2	0	11%
raw (Dole)	3 oz	9	3.0	0.1	107	8.0	0.3	na	na	18%
raw, chopped	1/2 cup	6	0.8	1.0	22	.7	0.1	0.0	0	11%
raw, chopped	1 oz	6	0.8	1.0	22	.7	0.1	<.1	0	11%
raw, untrimmed	1 lb	73	9.3	11.4	257	8.5	1.1	0.2	0	11%
SPINACH, CANNED										
drained solids	1/2 cup	25	3.0	3.6	29	>.9 c	0.5	0.1	0	15%
drained solids, no salt added	4 oz	26	3.2	3.9	31	3.2	0.6	0.1	0	16%
w/liquid	4 oz	22	2.4	3.3	362	1.0	0.4	0.1	0	14%
w/liquid, low-sodium	4 oz	22	2.4	3.3	85	1.0	0.4	0.1	0	14%
(Allens)	1/2 cup	28	2.0	3.0	35	(mq)	<1.0	(tr)	0	<31%
(Allens) chopped	1/2 cup	28	2.0	3.0	330	(mq)	<1.0	(tr)	0	<31%
(Allens) sliced	1/2 cup	28	2.0	3.0	330	(mq)	<1.0	(tr)	0	<31%
(Allens) whole	1/2 cup	28	2.0	3.0	330	(mq)	<1.0	(tr)	0	<31%
(Bush's Best) chopped	1/2 cup	25	2.0	4.0	330	na	0.0	na	na	0%
(Del Monte) chopped, w/liquid	1/2 cup	25	2.0	4.0	355	(mq)	0.0	0.0	0	0%
(Del Monte) whole, w/liquid	1/2 cup	25	2.0	4.0	355	(mq)	0.0	0.0	0	0%
(Del Monte) whole, w/liquid, 'No Salt Added'	1/2 cup	25	2.0	4.0	35	(mq)	0.0	0.0	0	0%
(Featherweight)	1/2 cup	35	2.0	4.0	30	(mq)	1.0	(tr)	0	27%
(Finast)	1/2 cup	25	3.0	4.0	360	(mq)	0.0	0.0	0	0%
(Finast) 'No Salt Added'	1/2 cup	25	3.0	4.0	110	(mq)	0.0	0.0	0	0%
(Freshlike) cut	1/2 cup	20	2.0	4.0	340	na	0.0	na	na	0%
(Freshlike) cut, water-packed, w/o salt	1/2 cup	20	2.0	4.0	20	na	0.0	na	na	0%
(Freshlike) cut, water packed, w/o sugar or salt	1/2 cup	20	2.0	4.0	20	na	0.0	na	na	0%
(Pathmark) 'No Frills'	1 cup	45	5.0	8.0	700	(mq)	1.0	(tr)	0	15%
(Pathmark) 'No Salt Added'	1/2 cup	30	2.0	4.0	35	(mq)	1.0	(tr)	0	27%
(Pathmark) whole	1/2 cup	30	2.0	4.0	370	(mq)	1.0	(tr)	0	15%

Food Name	Serving Size	Calories	Prot. gms	Carbs gms	Sod. mgs	Fiber gms	Fat gms	Sat. Fat gms	Chol. mgs	% Fat Cal.
(S&W) 'Premium Northwest'	1/2 cup	25	2.0	3.0	395	(mq)	0.0	0.0	0	0%
(Stokely)	1/2 cup	30	2.0	3.0	420	(mq)	0.0	0.0	0	0%
(Veg•All) cut	1/2 cup	20	2.0	4.0	340	na	0.0	na	na	0%
SPINACH, FROZEN										
Chopped										
boiled, drained	10-oz pkg	62	6.9	11.7	189	>2.4 c	0.5	0.1	0	5%
boiled, drained	1/2 cup	27	3.0	5.1	82	>1.0 c	0.2	0.0	0	5%
unprepared	10-oz pkg	68	8.3	11.4	210	8.5	0.9	0.1	0	9%
unprepared	1 cup	37	4.6	6.2	115	4.7	0.5	0.1	0	9%
(A&P)	3.3 oz	20	3.0	4.0	90	(mq)	<1.0	(tr)	0	<24%
(Birds Eye)	3.3 oz	20	3.0	3.0	90	3.0	0.0	0.0	0	0%
(Finast)	3.3 oz	20	3.0	3.0	70	(mq)	0.0	0.0	0	0%
(Frosty Acres)	3.3 oz	20	3.0	3.0	70	>1.0 c	0.0	0.0	0	0%
(Seabrook)	3.3 oz	20	3.0	3.0	70	>1.0 c	0.0	0.0	0	0%
(Southern)	3.5 oz	25	3.0	3.5	100	(mq)	0.3	(tr)	0	9%
Creamed										
(Birds Eye) 'Combination Vegetables'	3 oz	60	2.0	5.0	310	1.0	4.0	na	0	56%
(Green Giant)	1/2 cup	70	3.0	10.0	480	(mq)	3.0	<1.0	2	34%
(Stouffer's)	4.5 oz	170	4.0	7.0	380	(mq)	14.0	(mq)	na	74%
Leaf										
boiled, drained	10-oz pkg	62	6.9	11.7	189	6.6	0.5	0.1	0	6%
boiled, drained	4 oz	32	3.6	6.1	98	2.4	0.2	<.1	0	4%
unprepared	10-oz pkg	68	8.3	11.4	210	8.5	0.9	0.1	0	9%
unprepared	1 cup	37	4.6	6.2	115	4.7	0.5	0.1	0	9%
(A&P)	3.3 oz	25	3.0	4.0	100	(mq)	<1.0	(tr)	0	<24%
(Birds Eye) 'Portion Pack'	3.2 oz	20	3.0	3.0	70	2.0	0.0	0.0	0	0%
(Birds Eye) whole leaf	3.3 oz	20	3.0	4.0	90	3.0	0.0	na	0	0%
(Finast)	3.3 oz	20	3.0	4.0	75	(mq)	0.0	0.0	0	0%
(Freshlike) cut	3.3 oz	20	3.0	4.0	75	na	0.0	na	na	0%
(Frosty Acres)	3.3 oz	20	3.0	4.0	75	>1.0 c	0.0	0.0	0	0%
(Green Giant) cut, in butter sauce	1/2 cup	40	3.0	6.0	380	3.5	2.0	<1.0	5	33%
(Green Giant) 'Harvest Fresh'	1/2 cup	25	4.0	5.0	170	3.0	0.0	0.0	0	0%
(Green Giant) 'Plain Polybag'	1/2 cup	25	3.0	6.0	100	5.0	0.0	0.0	0	0%
(Seabrook) cut	3.3 oz	20	3.0	4.0	77	>1.0 c	0.0	0.0	0	0%
(Southern) whole	3.5 oz	25	2.9	3.6	100	(mq)	0.3	(tr)	0	9%
(Veg•All) cut	3.3 oz	20	3.0	4.0	75	na	0.0	na	na	0%
SPINACH, NEW ZEALAND										
boiled, drained	4 oz	14	1.5	2.5	121	>.7 c	0.2	<.1	0	10%
boiled, drained, chopped	1/2 cup	11	1.2	2.0	96	>.6 c	0.2	0.0	0	12%
raw, chopped	1/2 cup	4	0.4	0.7	36	>.2 c	0.1	0.0	0	17%
raw, untrimmed	1 lb	47	4.9	8.2	425	>2.3 c	0.7	0.1	0	11%
SPINACH ENTRÉE, FROZEN										
au gratin (Budget Gourmet)	6 oz	120	5.0	14.0	410	(mq)	5.0	(mq)	40	37%
creamed (Stouffer's)	4.5 oz	190	4.0	8.0	400	na	16.0	na	na	75%
soufflé (Stouffer's)	6 oz	220	9.0	11.0	820	na	15.0	na	na	63%
SPINACH SALAD, 'Sassy Spinach Kit' (Saco)	1/2 cup	157	2.0	14.0	437	1.0	11.0	2.0	3	63%
SPIRULINA										
dried	100 gm	290	57.5	23.9	1048	3.6	7.7	2.7	0	18%
dried	1 oz	82	16.3	6.8	297	>1.0 c	2.2	0.8	0	18%
raw	100 gm	26	5.9	2.4	98	>.3 c	0.4	0.1	0	10%
SPLIT PEAS										
boiled	4 oz	134	9.5	23.9	2	2.6	0.4	0.1	0	3%
boiled (A&P)	1 cup	220	16.0	40.0	15	(mq)	<1.0	(tr)	0	<4%
boiled, mature seeds	1/2 cup	116	8.2	20.7	2	8.1	0.4	0.1	0	3%

Food Name	Serving Size	Calories	Prot. gms	Carbs gms	Sod. mgs	Fiber gms	Fat gms	Sat. Fat gms	Chol. mgs	% Fat Cal.
raw	1 oz	97	7.0	17.1	4	1.6	0.3	<.1	0	3%
raw, green (Arrowhead Mills)	2 oz	200	14.0	35.0	14	7.5	1.0	na	0	4%
raw, mature seeds	1/2 cup	334	24.1	59.2	15	25.0	1.1	0.2	0	3%

SPONGE GOURD. See GOURD, DISHCLOTH.

SPORTS DRINK

CHOCOLATE

Food Name	Serving Size	Calories	Prot. gms	Carbs gms	Sod. mgs	Fiber gms	Fat gms	Sat. Fat gms	Chol. mgs	% Fat Cal.
(Weider) 'Dynamic Muscle Builder'	11 oz	220	18.0	36.0	260	na	<1.0	na	na	<4%
(Weider) 'Dynamic Weight Gainer'	11 oz	280	18.0	48.0	320	na	2.0	na	na	6%
(Weider) high-energy 'Protein Blast'	11.5 oz	270	22.0	44.0	240	na	<1.0	na	na	<3%
(Weider) 'Sports Line Power Shake' Dutch chocolate	11 oz	220	15.0	37.0	150	na	<1.0	na	na	<4%

FRUIT PUNCH (Pro-formance) ... 8 oz | 99 | 0.0 | 26.0 | 0 | na | 0.0 | na | na | 0%

GRAPE

Food Name	Serving Size	Calories	Prot. gms	Carbs gms	Sod. mgs	Fiber gms	Fat gms	Sat. Fat gms	Chol. mgs	% Fat Cal.
(Opti-Carb 140)	16 oz	140	0.0	35.0	9	na	0.0	0.0	na	0%
(Pro-formance)	8 oz	99	0.0	26.0	0	na	0.0	na	na	0%

LEMON

Food Name	Serving Size	Calories	Prot. gms	Carbs gms	Sod. mgs	Fiber gms	Fat gms	Sat. Fat gms	Chol. mgs	% Fat Cal.
(Knudsen & Sons) 'Isotonic Sports Beverage'	8 oz	60	0.0	21.0	35	na	0.0	na	na	0%
(Pro-formance)	8 oz	99	0.0	26.0	0	na	0.0	na	na	0%

LEMONADE

Food Name	Serving Size	Calories	Prot. gms	Carbs gms	Sod. mgs	Fiber gms	Fat gms	Sat. Fat gms	Chol. mgs	% Fat Cal.
(Power Burst) advanced performance beverage	8 oz	50	0.0	14.0	25	na	0.0	na	na	0%

LEMON-LIME (Shasta) caffeine-free, 'Body Works' ... 8 oz | 60 | 0.0 | 15.0 | 95 | na | 0.0 | 0.0 | na | 0%

ORANGE

Food Name	Serving Size	Calories	Prot. gms	Carbs gms	Sod. mgs	Fiber gms	Fat gms	Sat. Fat gms	Chol. mgs	% Fat Cal.
(All Sport) caffeine-free	8 oz	70	0.0	19.0	55	na	0.0	na	na	0%
(Gatorade)	8 oz	50	0.0	14.0	110	na	0.0	na	na	0%
(Opti-Carb 140)	16 oz	140	0.0	35.0	9	na	0.0	0.0	na	0%
(PowerAde)	8 oz	70	0.0	19.0	70	na	0.0	na	na	0%
(Pro-formance)	8 oz	99	0.0	26.0	0	na	0.0	na	na	0%
(Shasta) caffeine-free, 'Body Works'	8 oz	60	0.0	15.0	95	na	0.0	0.0	na	0%
(10-K)	8 oz	60	0.0	15.0	55	na	0.0	na	na	0%

SPORTS DRINK MIX

(Tiger's Milk)

Food Name	Serving Size	Calories	Prot. gms	Carbs gms	Sod. mgs	Fiber gms	Fat gms	Sat. Fat gms	Chol. mgs	% Fat Cal.
'Breakfast Booster' dry	2 level tbsp	70	2.0	14.0	20	na	<1.0	na	na	<12%
'Energy Booster' dry	3 heap tbsp	120	0.0	28.0	10	na	<1.0	na	na	<7%
'Protein Booster' Dutch chocolate, dry	3 heap tbsp	90	8.0	12.0	140	na	<1.0	na	na	<10%
'Protein Booster' vanilla-orange creme, dry	3 heap tbsp	90	8.0	12.0	140	na	<1.0	na	na	<10%

(Weider)

Food Name	Serving Size	Calories	Prot. gms	Carbs gms	Sod. mgs	Fiber gms	Fat gms	Sat. Fat gms	Chol. mgs	% Fat Cal.
'Big' chocolate malt, sugar-free, dry	4 scoops	320	18.0	58.0	370	na	2.0	na	na	6%
'Carbo Energizer' orange, dry	4 scoops	230	0.0	58.0	40	na	0.0	na	na	0%
'Crash Weight Gain No. 7' vanilla, dry	4 heap tbsp	300	6.0	61.0	84	na	3.0	na	0	9%
'Dynamic Body Shaper' Dutch chocolate, dry	2 scoops	110	13.0	12.0	170	na	<1.0	na	na	<8%
'Dynamic Muscle Builder' dry	3 heap tbsp	100	18.0	6.0	116	na	0.0	na	na	0%
'Dynamic Muscle Builder' natural chocolate, dry	2 scoops	120	18.0	9.0	170	na	1.0	na	na	8%
'Dynamic Muscle Builder' natural vanilla, dry	2 scoops	120	18.0	9.0	180	na	<1.0	na	na	<8%
'Dynamic Weight Gainer' Dutch chocolate, dry	4 scoops	320	18.0	61.0	400	na	<1.0	na	na	<3%
'Dynamic Weight Gainer' peanut butter, dry	4 scoops	330	18.0	61.0	390	na	2.0	na	na	5%
'90 Plus' vanilla, sugar-free, dry	2 scoops	100	25.0	1.0	150	na	0.0	na	na	0%
'N2itro-Fire' protein blend, dry	2 tbsp	110	8.0	17.0	100	na	1.0	na	na	8%
'Victory Explosive Workout' citrus, dry	4 tbsp	190	0.0	48.0	50	na	0.0	na	na	0%

SPOT

Food Name	Serving Size	Calories	Prot. gms	Carbs gms	Sod. mgs	Fiber gms	Fat gms	Sat. Fat gms	Chol. mgs	% Fat Cal.
dry-heat cooked	3 oz	134	20.2	0.0	31	0	5.3	1.6	65	37%
raw	1 lb	559	84.0	0.0	130	0	22.2	6.7	(mq)	37%
raw	1 oz	35	5.2	0.0	8	0	1.4	0.4	(mq)	38%

SPREAD, VEGETARIAN

Food Name	Serving Size	Calories	Prot. gms	Carbs gms	Sod. mgs	Fiber gms	Fat gms	Sat. Fat gms	Chol. mgs	% Fat Cal.
	1 cup	953	2.3	54.9	(mq)	(mq)	83.2	12.4	187	77%
	1 oz	110	0.3	6.4	(mq)	(mq)	9.6	1.4	22	76%

Food Name	Serving Size	Calories	Prot. gms	Carbs gms	Sod. mgs	Fiber gms	Fat gms	Sat. Fat gms	Chol. mgs	% Fat Cal.
....	1 tbsp	60	0.1	3.4	(mq)	(mq)	5.2	0.8	12	77%
(Best Foods)	1 tbsp	50	0.0	2.0	170	(mq)	5.0	1.0	5	85%
(Hellmann's)	1 tbsp	50	0.0	2.0	170	(mq)	5.0	1.0	5	85%
(Kraft)	1 tbsp	50	0.0	3.0	95	(mq)	5.0	1.0	5	79%
SPREADS. See CHEESE SPREAD; SPREAD, VEGETARIAN; and individual listings.										
SPRING ONION. See ONION, GREEN.										
SPRINKLES										
milk chocolate *(Snack Pack)*	3.88 oz	178	2.0	28.4	156	.3	6.3	1.7	1	32%
vanilla chocolate *(Snack Pack)*	3.88 oz	166	1.5	26.3	132	.1	6.1	1.7	0	33%
SQUAB/pigeon										
Raw										
breast meat only	1 oz	38	6.2	0.0	(mq)	0	1.3	0.3	26	32%
giblets	100 gm	154	19.8	1.2	70	0	7.2	2.0	350	44%
light meat w/o skin	1 lb	202	32.9	0.0	83	0	6.8	1.8	136	32%
meat and skin	1 oz	83	5.2	0.0	(mq)	0	6.7	2.4	(mq)	74%
meat and skin, approx 7 oz	1 squab	584	36.8	0.0	(mq)	0	47.4	16.8	(mq)	74%
meat only	1 oz	40	5.0	0.0	(mq)	0	2.1	0.6	(mq)	49%
SQUASH SEED. See PUMPKIN SEED.										
SQUASH, ACORN/table queen squash										
boiled, mashed	1/2 cup	41	0.8	10.7	4	>1.4 c	0.1	0.0	0	2%
boiled, mashed	4 oz	39	0.8	10.0	3	>1.3 c	0.1	<.1	0	2%
raw *(Frieda's)*	1 lb	249	8.6	63.5	45	(mq)	0.5	na	0	2%
raw *(Frieda's)*	1 oz	16	0.5	4.0	3	(mq)	<.1	tr	0	<5%
raw, approx 4 inch diam	1 squash	172	3.5	44.9	13	>6.0 c	0.4	0.1	0	2%
raw, cubes	1/2 cup	28	0.6	7.3	3	>1.0 c	0.1	<.1	0	3%
raw, trimmed	1 oz	11	0.2	3.0	1	>.4 c	<.1	tr	0	<7%
raw, untrimmed	1 lb	138	2.8	35.9	11	>4.8 c	0.3	0.1	0	2%
SQUASH, BANANA										
baked *(Frieda's)*	1 lb	286	8.2	69.9	45	(mq)	1.8	na	0	5%
baked *(Frieda's)*	1 oz	18	0.5	4.4	3	(mq)	0.1	na	0	4%
SQUASH, BUTTERNUT										
baked	4 oz	45	1.0	11.9	5	>1.4 c	0.1	<.1	0	2%
baked, cubes	1/2 cup	41	0.9	10.7	4	>1.3 c	0.1	0.0	0	2%
boiled, mashed	1/2 cup	47	1.5	12.1	2	>1.0 c	0.1	0.0	0	2%
raw, cubes	1/2 cup	32	0.7	8.2	3	>1.0 c	0.1	0.0	0	3%
raw, trimmed	1 oz	13	0.3	3.3	1	>.4 c	<.1	tr	0	<6%
raw, untrimmed	1 lb	172	3.8	44.6	15	>5.3 c	0.4	0.1	0	2%
SQUASH, CORN AND BUTTERNUT *(Earth's Best)*	4.5 oz	90	2.0	15.0	0	na	2.0	na	na	21%
SQUASH, CROOKNECK										
boiled, drained	4 oz	23	1.0	4.9	1	1.2	0.4	0.1	0	13%
boiled, drained, slices	1/2 cup	18	0.8	3.9	1	>.5 c	0.3	0.1	0	13%
canned, drained, no salt added	4 oz	15	0.7	3.4	6	1.1	0.1	<.1	0	5%
canned, yellow, cut *(Allens)*	1/2 cup	16	1.0	3.0	230	(mq)	<1.0	(tr)	0	<36%
frozen, boiled, drained	4 oz	28	1.5	6.3	7	1.4	0.2	<.1	0	6%
frozen, cooked *(Kohl's)*	4 oz	45	1.0	11.0	0	(mq)	<1.0	(tr)	0	<16%
frozen, yellow *(Seabrook)*	3.3 oz	18	1.0	4.0	1	>1.0 c	0.0	0.0	0	0%
frozen, yellow *(Southern)*	3.5 oz	21	1.5	4.1	20	(mq)	0.1	(tr)	0	4%
raw, ends trimmed	1 oz	5	0.3	1.1	1	.3	0.1	<.1	0	14%
raw, slices	1/2 cup	12	0.6	2.6	1	>.4 c	0.2	0.0	0	12%
raw, untrimmed	1 lb	84	4.2	18.2	7	4.9	1.1	0.2	0	10%
SQUASH, HUBBARD										
baked	4 oz	57	2.8	12.3	9	>2.0 c	0.7	0.1	0	9%
baked, cubes	1/2 cup	51	2.5	11.0	8	>1.8 c	0.6	0.1	0	9%
boiled, mashed	1/2 cup	35	1.8	7.6	6	3.4	0.4	0.1	0	9%

Food Name	Serving Size	Calories	Prot. gms	Carbs gms	Sod. mgs	Fiber gms	Fat gms	Sat. Fat gms	Chol. mgs	% Fat Cal.
boiled, mashed	4 oz	34	1.7	7.3	6	3.4	0.4	0.1	0	9%
raw, cubes	1/2 cup	23	1.2	5.1	4	>.8 c	0.3	0.1	0	10%
raw, trimmed	1 oz	11	0.6	2.5	2	>.4 c	0.1	<.1	0	7%
raw, untrimmed	1 lb	116	5.8	25.3	20	>4.1 c	1.5	0.3	0	10%
SQUASH, MARROW / vegetable marrow squash										
raw, trimmed	1 oz	4	0.2	1.0	na	>.1 c	<.1	tr	0	<16%
SQUASH, SCALLOP / cymling / pattypan squash										
boiled, drained	4 oz	18	1.2	3.7	1	>.5 c	0.2	<.1	0	8%
boiled, drained, mashed	1/2 cup	19	1.2	4.0	1	>.6 c	0.2	0.0	0	8%
boiled, drained, slices	1/2 cup	14	0.9	3.0	1	>.4 c	0.2	0.0	0	10%
raw, slices	1/2 cup	12	0.8	2.5	1	>.4 c	0.1	0.0	0	6%
raw, trimmed	1 oz	5	0.3	1.1	<1	>.2 c	0.1	<.1	0	14%
raw, untrimmed	1 lb	81	5.3	17.1	5	>2.5 c	0.9	0.2	0	8%
SQUASH, SPAGHETTI										
baked or boiled, drained	4 oz	33	0.7	7.3	20	>1.6 c	0.3	0.1	0	8%
baked or boiled, drained	1/2 cup	23	0.5	5.0	14	1.1	0.2	0.1	0	8%
raw, cubes	1/2 cup	16	0.3	3.5	9	>.7 c	0.3	0.1	0	15%
raw, trimmed	1 oz	9	0.2	2.0	5	>.4 c	0.2	<.1	0	17%
raw, untrimmed	1 lb	106	2.1	22.3	55	>4.5 c	1.8	0.4	0	14%
SQUASH, STRAIGHTNECK, raw, slices	1/2 cup	12	0.6	2.6	1	>.4 c	0.2	0.0	0	12%
SQUASH, SUMMER, all varieties										
boiled, drained	4 oz	23	1.0	4.9	1	1.6	0.4	0.1	0	13%
boiled, drained, slices	1/2 cup	18	0.8	3.9	1	1.3	0.3	0.1	0	13%
raw, slices	1/2 cup	13	0.8	2.8	1	.8	0.1	0.0	0	6%
raw, trimmed	1 oz	6	0.3	1.2	1	.3	0.1	<.1	0	13%
raw, untrimmed	1 lb	87	5.1	18.7	8	5.2	0.9	0.2	0	8%
SQUASH, WINTER, all varieties										
baked	4 oz	44	1.0	9.9	1	3.2	0.7	0.1	0	13%
baked, cubes	1/2 cup	40	0.9	8.9	1	2.9	0.6	0.1	0	12%
frozen, cooked (Birds Eye)	4 oz	45	1.0	11.0	0	2.0	0.0	na	0	0%
frozen, cooked (Seabrook)	4 oz	45	1.0	11.0	2	2.0	0.0	0.0	0	0%
raw, cubes	1/2 cup	21	0.8	5.1	2	1.0	0.1	0.0	0	4%
raw, trimmed	1 oz	11	0.4	2.5	1	5.0	0.1	<.1	0	7%
raw, untrimmed	1 lb	119	4.7	28.4	12	5.8	0.7	0.1	0	5%
SQUID, MIXED SPECIES / calamari										
fried	3 oz	149	15.2	6.6	260	>.1 c	6.4	1.6	221	40%
raw	1 lb	416	70.7	14.0	199	0	6.3	1.6	1059	14%
raw	3 oz	78	13.2	2.6	37	0	1.2	0.3	198	15%
raw	1 oz	26	4.4	0.9	12	0	0.4	0.1	66	15%
SQUIRREL										
raw	1 oz	34	5.9	0.0	29	0	0.9	0.1	23	26%
roasted	4 oz	154	27.4	0.0	107	0	4.1	0.5	108	25%
roasted, diced	1 cup	190	33.8	0.0	132	0	5.1	0.6	133	25%
STAR APPLE. See CAIMIT.										
STAR FRUIT / carambola										
cubed	1 cup	45	0.7	10.7	3	3.7	0.5	na	0	9%
trimmed	1 oz	9	0.2	2.2	1	.3	0.1	(tr)	0	9%
untrimmed	1 lb	142	2.3	33.7	7	5.0	1.5	na	0	9%
STEAK SEASONING 'Spice Blends' (Schilling)	1/4 tsp	1	0.1	0.1	273	na	(tr)	(tr)	0	0%
STIR-FRY ENTRÉE KIT										
(Tyson)	9 oz	230	22.0	15.0	480	na	9.0	na	80	35%
(Tyson) 'Yoshida Oriental Sauce'	1.6 oz	100	2.0	22.0	1260	na	1.0	na	0	9%
STIR-FRY SEASONING (Gilroy)	1 tsp	6	0.2	1.0	5	na	0.0	0.0	na	0%
STRAIGHTNECK SQUASH. See SQUASH, STRAIGHTNECK.										

Food Name	Serving Size	Calories	Prot. gms	Carbs gms	Sod. mgs	Fiber gms	Fat gms	Sat. Fat gms	Chol. mgs	% Fat Cal.
STRAWBERRY										
trimmed	1 pint	96	2.0	22.5	3	8.3	1.2	0.1	0	10%
trimmed	1 cup	45	0.9	10.5	1	3.9	0.6	0.0	0	11%
trimmed	1 oz	9	0.2	2.0	<1	.7	0.1	tr	0	9%
untrimmed	1 lb	130	2.6	30.0	5	11.1	1.6	0.1	0	10%
Canned, in heavy syrup	4 oz	104	0.6	26.7	5	(mq)	0.3	<.1	0	2%
Freeze-dried (Mountain House) prepared	1/4 cup	45	1.0	12.0	<1	(mq)	0.0	0.0	0	0%
Frozen										
in lite syrup, halves 'Quick Thaw Pouch' (Birds Eye)	5 oz	90	1.0	22.0	5	1.0	0.0	0.0	0	0%
in lite syrup, whole (Birds Eye)	4 oz	80	1.0	20.0	0	2.0	0.0	0.0	0	0%
sweetened, sliced	10-oz pkg	273	1.5	73.6	9	5.4	0.4	0.0	0	1%
sweetened, sliced	1 cup	245	1.4	66.1	8	4.8	0.3	0.0	0	1%
sweetened, sliced	4 oz	109	0.6	29.4	3	2.2	0.1	tr	0	1%
sweetened, sliced (Finast)	3.3 oz	125	1.0	30.0	5	(mq)	0.0	0.0	0	0%
sweetened, whole	10-oz pkg	222	1.5	59.6	3	5.4	0.4	0.0	0	2%
sweetened, whole	1 cup	199	1.3	53.5	3	4.8	0.4	0.0	0	2%
sweetened, whole	4 oz	88	0.6	23.8	1	2.1	0.2	tr	0	2%
unsweetened	20-oz pkg	198	2.4	51.8	11	11.9	0.6	0.0	0	2%
unsweetened	1 cup	52	0.6	13.6	3	3.1	0.2	0.0	0	3%
unsweetened	4 oz	40	0.5	10.4	2	4.8	0.1	tr	0	2%
STRAWBERRY-BANANA NECTAR (Kern's)	6 oz	110	0.0	28.0	0	na	0.0	na	na	0%
STRAWBERRY COLADA. See ALCOHOLIC BEVERAGES.										
STRAWBERRY DAIQUIRI. See ALCOHOLIC BEVERAGES.										
STRAWBERRY DRINK										
(Snapple) 'Strawberry Passion Awareness' real fruit	8 oz	120	0.0	31.0	25	na	0.0	na	na	0%
STRAWBERRY FLAVOR DRINK										
(Ensure) liquid nutrition	8 oz	250	8.8	34.3	200	na	8.8	na	5	32%
(Ensure) liquid nutrition 'Plus'	8 oz	355	13.0	47.3	250	na	12.6	na	5	32%
(Frostee)	8 oz	100	2.0	27.0	150	(tr)	7.0	(mq)	na	35%
(Sego) 'Lite'	10 oz	150	11.0	17.0	390	(tr)	4.0	(mq)	5	24%
(Sego) 'Very Strawberry'	10 oz	225	11.0	34.0	360	(tr)	5.0	(mq)	5	20%
(Squeezit) 'Silly Billy Strawberry'	6.75 oz	90	0.0	23.0	5	na	0.0	na	na	0%
(Tang)	8.45 oz	120	0.0	32.0	10	na	0.0	na	0	0%
(10-K)	8 oz	60	0.0	15.0	55	na	0.0	na	na	0%
STRAWBERRY FLAVOR DRINK MIX, PREPARED										
(Kool-Aid) presweetened	8 oz	80	0.0	20.0	0	(tr)	0.0	0.0	0	0%
(Nestlé) 'Quik' 2 1/2 heap tsp w/whole milk	8 oz	220	8.0	32.0	120	(tr)	8.0	(mq)	(mq)	31%
(Nestlé) 'Quik' 2 1/2 heap tsp w/2% milk	8 oz	200	8.0	32.0	120	(tr)	5.0	(mq)	(mq)	22%
(Nestlé) 'Quik' 2 1/2 heap tsp w/skim milk	8 oz	160	8.0	32.0	125	(tr)	0.0	0.0	na	0%
(Turbo Nutrition) weight gain protein powder,										
2 oz w/whole milk	8 oz	360	36.0	33.0	420	na	9.0	na	na	23%
(Wylers) 'Crystals'	8 oz	85	0.0	20.7	43	(tr)	0.3	na	0	3%
STRAWBERRY GUAVA JUICE (Knudsen & Sons)	8 oz	105	<1.0	26.0	na	na	0.0	na	na	0%
STRAWBERRY GUAVA NECTAR										
(Santa Cruz Natural) organic	8 oz	90	<1.0	24.0	na	na	<1.0	na	na	<8%
STRAWBERRY JUICE DRINK										
(Knudsen & Sons) float	8 oz	130	2.0	32.0	na	na	0.0	na	na	0%
(Tang) 'Fruit Box'	8.45 oz	120	0.0	32.0	10	(tr)	0.0	0.0	0	0%
(Wyler's) 'Fruit Slush'	4 oz	157	0.0	39.3	10	(tr)	0.0	0.0	0	0%
STRAWBERRY LEMONADE										
(Kern's)	6 oz	110	0.0	28.0	0	na	0.0	na	na	0%
(Knudsen & Sons)	8 oz	90	<1.0	21.0	na	na	0.0	na	na	0%
(Santa Cruz Natural) organic	8 oz	60	<1.0	20.0	na	na	<1.0	na	na	<10%
(Snapple)	8 oz	110	0.0	26.0	5	na	0.0	0.0	0	0%

Food Name	Serving Size	Calories	Prot. gms	Carbs gms	Sod. mgs	Fiber gms	Fat gms	Sat. Fat gms	Chol. mgs	% Fat Cal.
STRAWBERRY NECTAR										
(Knudsen & Sons)	8 oz	105	<1.0	29.0	na	na	0.0	na	na	0%
(Libby's)	6 oz	110	0.0	27.0	0	(mq)	0.0	0.0	0	0%
STRAWBERRY PUNCH DRINK										
(Arizona) 'Cowboy Cocktail'	8 oz	120	0.0	30.0	20	na	0.0	na	na	0%
STRAWBERRY PUNCH MIX										
(Kool-Aid) sugar-sweetened, prepared	8 oz	80	0.0	20.0	0	na	0.0	na	0	0%
(Kool-Aid) unsweetened, prepared w/sugar	8 oz	100	0.0	25.0	25	na	0.0	na	0	0%
(Kool-Aid) unsweetened, prepared w/o sugar	8 oz	2	0.0	0.0	25	na	0.0	na	0	0%
STRAWBERRY SYRUP										
(Knott's Berry Farm)	1 oz	120	0.0	30.0	0	na	0.0	na	na	0%
(Knudsen & Sons)	1 oz	75	<1.0	18.0	na	na	<1.0	na	na	<11%
(S&W) w/saccharin	1 tsp	4	0.0	1.0	25	na	0.0	0.0	0	0%
STRAWBERRY TOPPING										
(Kraft)	1 tbsp	50	0.0	14.0	5	na	0.0	0.0	0	0%
(Smucker's)	2 tbsp	120	0.0	30.0	0	na	0.0	0.0	0	0%
(Smucker's) fat-free 'Light'	2 tbsp	55	0.0	14.0	0	na	0.0	0.0	na	0%
STRING BEAN. See GREEN BEAN.										
STROGANOFF DINNER. See BEEF ENTRÉE.										
STRUDEL. See INDIVIDUAL LISTINGS.										
STUFFED PEPPER										
(Celentano) sweet red, frozen	13 oz	350	28.0	28.0	810	(mq)	20.0	(mq)	(mq)	45%
(Stouffer's) green, w/beef in tomato sauce, frozen	7.75 oz	200	9.0	22.0	650	na	8.0	na	na	37%
(Stouffer's) single serving	10 oz	220	10.0	28.0	1010	na	8.0	na	na	32%
STUFFING										
(Betty Crocker)										
chicken, dry	1/6 pkg	110	4.0	21.0	530	na	1.0	na	na	8%
traditional herb, dry	1/6 pkg	110	4.0	22.0	550	na	1.0	na	na	8%
traditional herb, prepared w/salted butter	1/2 cup	190	4.0	22.0	640	(mq)	9.0	(mq)	na	44%
(Brownberry)										
corn, dry	1 oz	103	3.7	20.6	350	1.5	1.6	na	0	13%
herb, dry	1 oz	100	3.6	20.7	297	1.6	1.3	na	0	11%
(Croutettes) dry	.7 oz	70	3.0	14.0	260	0	0.0	0.0	0	0%
(General Mills)										
chicken, dry	1/6 pkg	110	4.0	21.0	530	na	1.0	na	na	8%
chicken, prepared w/margarine	1/2 cup	180	4.0	21.0	620	na	9.0	na	na	45%
traditional herb, dry	1/6 pkg	110	4.0	22.0	550	na	<1.0	na	na	<8%
traditional herb, prepared w/margarine	1/2 cup	180	4.0	22.0	640	na	8.0	na	na	41%
(Golden Dipt)										
Cajun style, dry	1/4 cup	40	1.0	9.0	590	na	0.0	0.0	0	0%
cheddar and French, dry	1/2 cup	80	4.0	9.0	580	na	3.0	2.0	14	34%
garden herb, dry	1/4 cup	40	1.0	9.0	330	na	0.0	0.0	0	0%
(Golden Grain)										
chicken, dry	1 oz	106	3.9	20.0	637	1.2	1.2	0.3	<1	10%
cornbread, dry	1 oz	105	3.3	20.9	774	1.2	1.0	0.1	<1	9%
herb and butter, dry	1 oz	104	3.7	19.7	713	1.4	1.1	0.2	<1	10%
w/wild rice, dry	1 oz	108	3.6	20.9	611	1.3	1.1	0.2	<1	9%
(Pepperidge Farm)										
apple and raisin 'Distinctive Stuffing' dry	1 oz	110	3.0	21.0	410	(mq)	1.0	na	na	9%
classic chicken 'Distinctive Stuffing' dry	1 oz	110	4.0	20.0	410	(mq)	1.0	na	na	9%
cornbread, dry	1 oz	110	3.0	22.0	320	(mq)	1.0	na	na	8%
country style, dry	1 oz	100	4.0	21.0	400	(mq)	1.0	na	na	8%
cube, dry	1 oz	110	3.0	22.0	400	(mq)	1.0	na	na	8%
herb, country garden 'Distinctive Stuffing' dry	1 oz	120	4.0	18.0	300	(mq)	4.0	(mq)	na	29%

Food Name	Serving Size	Calories	Prot. gms	Carbs gms	Sod. mgs	Fiber gms	Fat gms	Sat. Fat gms	Chol. mgs	% Fat Cal.
herb, dry	1 oz	110	3.0	22.0	380	(mq)	1.0	na	na	8%
vegetable, harvest, w/almonds 'Distinctive' dry	1 oz	110	4.0	19.0	250	(mq)	3.0	(mq)	na	23%
wild rice and mushroom 'Distinctive Stuffing' dry	1 oz	130	4.0	17.0	310	(mq)	5.0	(mq)	na	35%
(Stove Top)										
Americana San Francisco, prepared w/salted butter	1/2 cup	170	4.0	20.0	650	(mq)	9.0	(mq)	20	46%
beef, prepared w/salted butter	1/2 cup	180	4.0	21.0	590	(mq)	9.0	(mq)	20	45%
chicken flavor, prepared w/salted butter	1/2 cup	180	4.0	20.0	570	(mq)	9.0	(mq)	20	46%
cornbread 'Flexible Serving' prepared w/salted butter	1/2 cup	170	4.0	20.0	580	(mq)	9.0	(mq)	15	46%
cornbread, prepared w/salted butter	1/2 cup	170	3.0	21.0	570	(mq)	9.0	(mq)	20	46%
cornbread, prepared w/salted margarine	1/2 cup	180	4.0	22.0	590	na	9.0	na	0	44%
homestyle herb 'Flexible Serving' prepared w/salted butter	1/2 cup	170	4.0	20.0	520	(mq)	9.0	(mq)	15	46%
long grain and wild rice, prepared w/salted butter	1/2 cup	180	4.0	22.0	560	(mq)	9.0	(mq)	20	44%
mushroom and onion, prepared w/salted butter	1/2 cup	180	4.0	20.0	490	(mq)	9.0	(mq)	20	46%
pork 'Flexible Serving' prepared w/salted butter	1/2 cup	170	4.0	20.0	630	(mq)	9.0	(mq)	15	46%
pork, prepared w/salted butter	1/2 cup	170	4.0	20.0	570	(mq)	9.0	(mq)	20	46%
savory herbs, prepared w/salted butter	1/2 cup	170	4.0	20.0	590	(mq)	9.0	(mq)	20	46%
turkey, prepared w/salted butter	1/2 cup	170	4.0	20.0	640	(mq)	9.0	(mq)	20	46%
turkey, prepared w/salted margarine	1/2 cup	180	4.0	20.0	630	na	9.0	na	0	46%
STUFFING, FROZEN										
chicken 'Stuffing Originals' *(Green Giant)*	1/2 cup	170	4.0	21.0	670	(mq)	7.0	(mq)	na	39%
cornbread 'Stuffing Originals' *(Green Giant)*	1/2 cup	170	3.0	25.0	660	(mq)	6.0	(mq)	na	33%
mushroom 'Stuffing Originals' *(Green Giant)*	1/2 cup	150	4.0	19.0	780	(mq)	7.0	(mq)	na	41%
wild rice 'Stuffing Originals' *(Green Giant)*	1/2 cup	160	3.0	21.0	540	(mq)	7.0	(mq)	na	40%
STUFFING MIX, MICROWAVE										
broccoli and cheese, prepared w/salted butter										
(Stove Top)	1/2 cup	170	4.0	20.0	580	(mq)	8.0	(mq)	15	43%
cornbread, homestyle, prepared w/salted butter										
(Stove Top)	1/2 cup	160	3.0	20.0	450	(mq)	7.0	(mq)	10	41%
mushroom and onion, prepared w/salted butter										
(Stove Top)	1/2 cup	170	4.0	21.0	510	(mq)	7.0	(mq)	10	39%
STURGEON, MIXED SPECIES										
baked	4 oz	153	23.5	0.0	(mq)	0	5.9	1.3	(mq)	36%
broiled	4 oz	153	23.5	0.0	(mq)	0	5.9	1.3	(mq)	36%
dry-heat cooked	3 oz	115	17.6	0.0	59	0	4.4	1.0	65	36%
microwaved	4 oz	153	23.5	0.0	(mq)	0	5.9	1.3	(mq)	36%
raw	1 lb	478	73.2	0.0	(mq)	0	18.3	4.2	(mq)	36%
raw	3 oz	89	13.7	0.0	46	0	3.4	0.8	51	36%
raw	1 oz	30	4.6	0.0	(mq)	0	1.1	0.3	(mq)	35%
smoked	4 oz	196	35.4	0.0	(mq)	0	5.0	1.2	(mq)	24%
SUCCOTASH										
boiled, drained	4 oz	130	5.7	27.6	19	>1.5 c	0.9	0.2	0	6%
boiled, drained	1/2 cup	110	4.9	23.4	16	>1.3 c	0.8	0.1	0	6%
raw	1 lb	451	22.8	88.9	19	11.8	4.6	0.9	0	9%
raw	1 oz	28	1.4	5.6	1	.7	0.3	0.1	0	9%
Canned										
(S&W) 'Country Style'	1/2 cup	80	4.0	16.0	250	(mq)	1.0	(tr)	0	10%
(Stokely)	1/2 cup	90	3.0	20.0	300	(mq)	0.0	0.0	0	0%
Frozen										
boiled, drained	4 oz	105	4.9	22.6	51	>1.2 c	1.0	0.2	0	8%
boiled, drained	1/2 cup	79	3.7	17.0	38	>.9 c	0.8	0.1	0	8%
unprepared	1/2 cup	73	3.4	15.6	35	4.9	0.7	0.1	0	8%
(Frosty Acres)	3.3 oz	100	4.0	19.0	47	>1.0 c	0.0	0.0	0	0%
(Seabrook)	3.3 oz	100	4.0	19.0	47	>1.0 c	0.0	0.0	0	0%

Food Name	Serving Size	Calories	Prot. gms	Carbs gms	Sod. mgs	Fiber gms	Fat gms	Sat. Fat gms	Chol. mgs	% Fat Cal.
SUCKER										
dry-heat cooked	3 oz	101	18.3	0.0	43	0	2.5	0.5	45	24%
raw	1 lb	419	76.0	0.0	181	0	10.5	2.1	187	24%
SUGAR, ALTERNATIVE										
(Equal) aspartame	1 pkg	4	0.0	<1.0	0	0	0.0	0.0	0	0%
(Featherweight) saccharin	1 tablet	0	0.0	0.0	8	0	0.0	0.0	0	0%
(Featherweight) saccharin, liquid	3 drops	0	0.0	0.0	0	0	0.0	0.0	0	0%
(Nutra Taste) saccharin	1 pkt	4	0.0	1.0	0	na	0.0	0.0	na	0%
(NutraSweet) aspartame 'Spoonful'	1 tsp	2	0.0	<1.0	0	na	0.0	0.0	na	0%
(S&W Nutradiet) saccharin, liquid	1/8 tsp	0	0.0	0.0	0	0	0.0	0.0	0	0%
(Sprinkle Sweet)	1 tsp	2	0.0	0.5	19	0	0.0	0.0	0	0%
(Sugar Twin) saccharin	1 pkt	4	0.0	<1.0	0	na	0.0	0.0	na	0%
(Sugar Twin) saccharin 'Plus'	1 pkt	3	0.0	<1.0	0	na	0.0	0.0	na	0%
(Sweet 'n Low)	1 pkt	4	0.0	1.0	0	0	0.0	0.0	0	0%
(Sweet One)	1 pkt	4	0.0	1.0	0	na	0.0	na	na	0%
(Sweet Plus)	1 pkt	4	0.0	1.0	0	na	0.0	0.0	na	0%
(Sweet•10)	1/8 tsp	0	0.0	0.0	2	0	0.0	0.0	0	0%
(Weight Watchers) 'Sweet'ner'	1 pkt	4	0.0	1.0	30	0	0.0	0.0	0	0%
SUGAR, BEET OR CANE. See also SUGAR, ALTERNATIVE; SUGAR, DEXTROSE; SUGAR, MAPLE; SUGAR, TURBINADO; SUGAR CANE BATON.										
BROWN										
dark, 'Old Fashioned' *(Domino)*	1 tsp	16	0.0	4.0	0	na	0.0	0.0	na	0%
golden, fresh from Hawaii *(C&H)*	1 tsp	16	0.0	4.0	0	na	0.0	na	na	0%
light, 'Brownulated' *(Domino)*	1 tsp	12	0.0	3.0	0	na	0.0	0.0	na	0%
light, golden, packed *(Domino)*	1 tsp	16	0.0	4.0	0	na	0.0	0.0	na	0%
packed	1 cup	827	0.0	214.1	86	0	0.0	na	0	0%
packed	1 oz	106	0.0	27.3	1	0	0.0	0.0	0	0%
unpacked	1 cup	545	0.0	141.1	57	0	0.0	na	0	0%
CONFECTIONER'S /powdered										
sifted	1 cup	385	0.0	99.5	1	0	0.0	0.0	0	0%
sifted	1 oz	109	0.0	28.2	<1	0	0.0	0.0	0	0%
sifted, 10-X *(Domino)*	1/2 cup	240	0.0	60.0	0	na	0.0	0.0	na	0%
unsifted	1 cup	462	0.0	119.4	1	0	0.0	0.0	0	0%
unsifted	1 tbsp	31	0.0	8.0	tr	0	0.0	0.0	0	0%
GRANULATED										
	1 cup	774	0.0	199.8	2	0	0.0	na	0	0%
	1 oz	109	0.0	28.2	<1	0	0.0	0.0	0	0%
	1 tsp	15	0.0	4.0	0	0	0.0	na	0	0%
cubes 'Dots' *(Domino)*	1 cube	8	0.0	2.0	0	na	0.0	0.0	na	0%
cubes, 1/2 inch	2 cubes	19	0.0	5.0	tr	0	0.0	0.0	0	0%
juice, organic *(Sucanat)*	1 tsp	12	0.0	3.0	0	na	0.0	0.0	0	0%
lumps, 1 1/8 x 3/4 x 5/16 inches	1 lump	19	0.0	5.0	tr	0	0.0	0.0	0	0%
packet, approx .2 oz	1 pkt	23	0.0	6.0	tr	0	0.0	0.0	0	0%
'Packets' *(Domino)*	1 pkt	16	0.0	4.0	0	na	0.0	0.0	na	0%
SUPERFINE, instant dissolving *(Domino)*	1 tsp	16	0.0	4.0	0	na	0.0	0.0	na	0%
SUGAR, DEXTROSE										
anhydrous	100 gm	366	0.0	99.5	0	0	0.0	0.0	0	0%
anhydrous	1 oz	104	0.0	28.2	tr	0	0.0	0.0	0	0%
crystallized	100 gm	335	0.0	91.0	0	0	0.0	0.0	0	0%
crystallized	1 oz	95	0.0	25.8	tr	0	0.0	0.0	0	0%
SUGAR, MAPLE										
	100 gm	354	0.1	90.9	11	0	0.2	na	0	1%
	1-oz piece	100	0.0	25.8	3	0	0.1	na	0	1%
SUGAR, TURBINADO *(Hain)*	1 tbsp	50	0.0	12.0	0	0	0.0	0.0	0	0%

Food Name	Serving Size	Calories	Prot. gms	Carbs gms	Sod. mgs	Fiber gms	Fat gms	Sat. Fat gms	Chol. mgs	% Fat Cal.
SUGAR APPLE/sweetsop										
raw, approx 2 7/8 inch diam	1 med	146	3.2	36.6	14	6.8	0.5	na	0	3%
raw, pulp	1 cup	235	5.2	59.1	23	11.0	0.7	na	0	2%
trimmed	1/2 cup	118	2.6	29.6	12	3.4	0.4	(tr)	0	3%
trimmed	1 oz	27	0.6	6.7	3	.8	0.1	(tr)	0	3%
untrimmed	1 lb	236	5.1	59.0	24	12.8	0.7	(tr)	0	2%
SUGAR CANE BATON (Frieda's)	1 oz	21	<.1	49.9	na	(tr)	0.1	(tr)	0	0%
SUGAR CANE JUICE	1 oz	21	0.1	5.1	na	tr	tr	0.0	0	0%
SUMMER SAUSAGE										
(Eckrich)	1-oz slice	80	4.0	1.0	320	0	7.0	(mq)	(mq)	76%
(Hillshire Farm)	2 oz	180	9.0	1.0	670	0	16.0	(mq)	(mq)	78%
(Hormel) 'Perma-Fresh'	2 slices	140	10.0	0.0	706	0	11.0	(mq)	(mq)	71%
(Hormel) 'Tangy Chub'	1 oz	90	5.0	0.0	317	0	7.0	(mq)	(mq)	76%
(Hormel) 'Thuringer'	1 oz	90	4.0	0.0	332	0	9.0	(mq)	(mq)	84%
BEEF										
(Hillshire Farm)	2 oz	190	9.0	1.0	(mq)	0	17.0	(mq)	(mq)	79%
(Hormel) 'Beefy'	1 oz	100	5.0	0.0	313	0	9.0	(mq)	(mq)	80%
(Lean & Lite)	1 oz	43	6.1	1.0	(mq)	0	2.3	(mq)	18	42%
(Light & Lean)	2 slices	100	6.0	0.0	(mq)	0	8.0	(mq)	(mq)	75%
(OHSE)	1 oz	75	5.0	2.0	340	0	5.0	(mq)	(mq)	62%
(Oscar Mayer)	.8-oz slice	69	3.5	0.2	331	0	6.1	2.7	19	79%
TURKEY (Louis Rich)	1-oz slice	55	4.7	0.4	326	0	3.9	1.2	21	63%
W/CHEESE (Hillshire Farm)	2 oz	200	9.0	1.0	(mq)	0	18.0	(mq)	(mq)	80%
SUNCHOKE. See ARTICHOKE, JERUSALEM.										
SUN-DRIED TOMATOES, in oil and herbs (Bella Sun Luci)	2/3 oz	60	2.0	6.0	20	2.0	3.0	0.0	0	46%
SUNFISH/calico bass/crappie/pumpkinseed										
dry-heat cooked	3 oz	97	21.1	0.0	88	0	0.8	0.2	73	8%
raw	1 lb	404	88.0	0.0	368	0	3.2	0.6	304	8%
raw	3 oz	76	10.5	0.0	68	0	0.6	0.1	57	8%
raw	1 oz	25	5.5	0.0	23	0	0.2	<.1	19	8%
SUNFLOWER BUTTER										
	1 oz	165	5.6	7.8	1	1.4	13.6	1.4	0	70%
	1 tbsp	93	3.2	4.4	1	.8	7.6	0.8	0	69%
gourmet (Roaster Fresh)	1 oz	160	6.0	5.0	1	na	13.6	1.6	na	74%
roasted (Maranatha Natural)	2 tbsp	170	4.0	8.0	5	na	14.0	na	0	72%
SUNFLOWER OIL										
hydrogenated	1/2 cup	964	0.0	0.0	0	0	109.0	14.2	0	100%
hydrogenated	1 oz	251	0.0	0.0	0	0	28.4	3.7	0	100%
linoleic	1/2 cup	964	0.0	0.0	0	0	109.0	11.3	0	100%
linoleic	1 oz	251	0.0	0.0	0	0	28.4	2.9	0	100%
(Hain)	1 tbsp	120	0.0	0.0	0	0	14.0	2.0	0	100%
(IGA)	1 tbsp	120	0.0	0.0	0	0	14.0	2.0	0	100%
(Kroger)	1 tbsp	122	0.0	0.0	0	0	13.6	1.7	0	100%
(Pathmark)	1 tbsp	130	0.0	0.0	0	0	14.0	2.0	0	100%
(Spectrum Naturals)	1 tbsp	120	0.0	0.0	0	(tr)	14.0	1.5	(tr)	100%
(Wesson)	1 tbsp	122	0.0	0.0	0	0	13.6	1.6	0	100%
SUNFLOWER SEED KERNELS										
Dried										
	1 cup	821	32.8	27.0	4	15.1	71.4	7.5	0	73%
	1 oz	162	6.5	5.3	1	3.0	14.1	1.5	0	73%
in shell	1 lb	1397	55.8	46.0	8	na	121.4	12.7	0	73%
(Arrowhead Mills)	1 oz	160	7.0	6.0	3	4.4	13.0	(mq)	0	69%
(Frito-Lay's)	1 oz	160	7.0	6.0	265	na	14.0	na	0	71%

Food Name	Serving Size	Calories	Prot. gms	Carbs gms	Sod. mgs	Fiber gms	Fat gms	Sat. Fat gms	Chol. mgs	% Fat Cal.
Dry-roasted										
. . . .	1 cup	745	24.8	30.8	4	11.5	63.7	6.7	0	72%
. . . .	1 oz	165	5.5	6.8	1	2.5	14.1	1.5	0	72%
salted	1 cup	745	24.8	30.8	998	8.7	63.7	6.7	0	72%
salted	1 oz	165	5.5	6.8	221	1.9	14.1	1.5	0	72%
(Fisher)	1 oz	170	6.0	6.0	200	na	15.0	2.0	0	74%
(Fisher) in shell	1 oz	170	6.0	6.0	110	na	15.0	1.0	0	74%
(Fisher) in shell, salted	1 oz	170	6.0	6.0	110	na	14.0	1.0	0	72%
(Flavor House)	1 oz	180	8.0	4.0	200	(mq)	15.0	(mq)	0	74%
(Pathmark)	1 oz	180	5.0	7.0	150	(mq)	14.0	(mq)	0	72%
(Planters)	1 oz	160	6.0	6.0	170	na	14.0	2.0	0	72%
Oil-roasted										
. . . .	1 cup	830	28.8	19.9	4	9.2	77.6	8.1	0	78%
. . . .	1 oz	175	6.1	4.2	1	1.9	16.3	1.7	0	78%
salted	1 cup	830	28.8	19.9	814	9.2	77.6	8.1	0	78%
salted	1 oz	175	6.1	4.2	171	1.9	16.3	1.7	0	78%
(Fisher)	1 oz	170	6.0	4.0	170	na	16.0	2.0	0	78%
(Planters)	1 oz	170	6.0	5.0	135	na	15.0	4.0	0	75%
Toasted										
. . . .	1 cup	829	23.1	27.6	4	>2.4 c	76.1	8.0	0	77%
. . . .	1 oz	176	4.9	5.9	1	>.5 c	16.1	1.7	0	77%
salted	1 cup	829	23.1	27.6	821	>2.4 c	76.1	8.0	0	77%
salted	1 oz	176	4.9	5.9	174	>.5 c	16.1	1.7	0	77%
(Fisher)	1 oz	170	6.0	6.0	0	na	14.0	1.0	0	72%
SUNFLOWER SEED FLOUR										
partially defatted	1 cup	261	38.5	28.7	2	4.2	1.3	0.1	0	4%
partially defatted	1 oz	92	13.6	10.2	1	1.5	0.5	<.1	0	5%
partially defatted	1 tbsp	16	2.4	1.8	0	.3	0.1	0.0	0	5%
SUNSHINE JUICE, organic (Santa Cruz Natural)	8 oz	100	1.0	23.0	na	na	1.0	na	na	9%
SURIMI										
. . . .	3 oz	84	12.9	5.8	122	0	0.8	0.2	25	9%
leg style 'Classic Seablends' 10% crab										
(Peter Pan Seafoods)	3.5 oz	85	9.8	na	890	na	0.4	na	31	8%
leg style 'Standard Seablends' (Peter Pan Seafoods)	3.5 oz	88	9.0	na	845	na	0.4	na	34	9%
salad style 'Classic Seablends Combo' 10% crab										
(Peter Pan Seafoods)	3.5 oz	85	9.8	na	890	na	0.4	na	31	8%
salad style 'Standard Seablends Combo'										
(Peter Pan Seafoods)	3.5 oz	88	9.0	na	845	na	0.4	na	34	9%
SURINAM CHERRY. See PITANGA.										
SWAMP CABBAGE. See CABBAGE, SKUNK.										
SWEDISH MEATBALL DINNER/ENTRÉE										
frozen dinner, 'Classics' (Armour)	11.25 oz	330	19.0	23.0	1140	na	18.0	na	80	49%
frozen entrée, w/parsley noodles, gravy										
'Lean Cuisine' (Stouffer's)	9.25 oz	420	24.0	32.0	740	na	21.0	na	na	46%
frozen entrée, w/pasta, gravy 'Lean Cuisine' (Stouffer's) . .	9 1/8 oz	290	23.0	31.0	550	na	8.0	3.0	55	25%
SWEDISH TURNIP										
boiled, drained	4 oz	39	1.2	8.8	20	>1.2 c	0.2	<.1	0	4%
boiled, drained, cubed	1/2 cup	29	0.9	6.6	15	>.9 c	0.2	<.1	0	6%
boiled, drained, mashed	1/2 cup	41	1.3	9.3	22	>1.3 c	0.2	<.1	0	4%
raw, cubed	1/2 cup	25	0.8	5.7	14	>.8 c	0.1	<.1	0	3%
raw, trimmed	1 oz	10	0.3	2.3	6	>.3 c	0.1	tr	0	8%
raw, untrimmed	1 lb	140	4.6	31.4	77	>4.2 c	0.8	0.1	0	5%
SWEET AND SOUR DINNER (LaChoy)	4.48 oz	89	1.1	21.7	838	2.0	0.2	0.0	0	2%

Food Name	Serving Size	Calories	Prot. gms	Carbs gms	Sod. mgs	Fiber gms	Fat gms	Sat. Fat gms	Chol. mgs	% Fat Cal.
SWEET POTATO. See also YAM.										
baked in skin, pulp only	4 oz	117	2.0	27.5	11	3.4	0.1	<.1	0	1%
baked in skin, pulp only, 5 inches long, 2 inches diam	1 potato	118	2.0	27.7	12	3.4	0.1	<.1	0	1%
baked in skin, pulp only, mashed	1/2 cup	103	1.7	24.3	10	3.0	0.1	0.0	0	1%
boiled, w/o skin	4 oz	119	1.9	27.5	15	>1.0 c	0.3	0.1	0	2%
boiled, w/o skin, mashed	1/2 cup	172	2.7	39.8	21	>1.4 c	0.5	0.1	0	3%
dehydrated flakes, dry	1 cup	455	5.0	108.0	217	>3.8 c	0.7	0.0	0	1%
dehydrated flakes, prepared w/water	1 lb	431	4.5	102.6	204	>3.6 c	0.5	0.0	0	1%
dehydrated flakes, prepared w/water	1 cup	242	2.5	57.6	115	>2.0 c	0.3	0.0	0	1%
raw, cubes	1 cup	140	2.2	32.3	17	4.0	0.4	0.1	0	3%
raw, 5 inches long, 2 inches diam	1 potato	136	2.2	31.6	17	3.9	0.4	0.1	0	3%
raw, trimmed	1 oz	30	0.5	6.9	4	.9	0.1	<.1	0	3%
raw, untrimmed	1 lb	343	5.4	79.3	44	9.8	1.0	0.2	0	3%
SWEET POTATO, CANNED										
Candied										
(Joan of Arc)	1/2 cup	240	1.0	60.0	15	(mq)	0.0	0.0	0	0%
(Princella)	1/2 cup	240	1.0	60.0	15	(mq)	0.0	0.0	0	0%
(Royal Prince)	1/2 cup	240	1.0	60.0	15	(mq)	0.0	0.0	0	0%
(S&W)	1/2 cup	180	1.0	44.0	355	(mq)	0.0	0.0	0	0%
In extra heavy syrup (S&W) 'Southern'	1/2 cup	139	1.0	31.0	27	(mq)	1.0	(tr)	0	7%
In heavy syrup										
(Joan of Arc)	1/2 cup	130	1.0	34.0	35	(mq)	0.0	0.0	0	0%
(Princella)	1/2 cup	130	1.0	34.0	35	(mq)	0.0	0.0	0	0%
(Royal Prince)	1/2 cup	130	1.0	34.0	35	(mq)	0.0	0.0	0	0%
In light syrup										
(Finast)	1/2 cup	110	2.0	25.0	45	(mq)	<1.0	(tr)	0	<8%
(Joan of Arc)	1/2 cup	110	1.0	28.0	25	(mq)	0.0	0.0	0	0%
(Princella)	1/2 cup	110	1.0	28.0	25	(mq)	0.0	0.0	0	0%
(Royal Prince)	1/2 cup	110	1.0	28.0	25	(mq)	0.0	0.0	0	0%
In pineapple-orange sauce										
(Joan of Arc)	1/2 cup	210	1.0	54.0	35	(mq)	0.0	0.0	0	0%
(Princella)	1/2 cup	210	1.0	54.0	35	(mq)	0.0	0.0	0	0%
(Royal Prince)	1/2 cup	210	1.0	54.0	35	(mq)	0.0	0.0	0	0%
In syrup										
(Allens) cut	1/2 cup	90	2.0	20.0	20	(mq)	<1.0	(tr)	0	<9%
(Allens) whole	1/2 cup	90	2.0	20.0	40	(mq)	<1.0	(tr)	0	<9%
(Joan of Arc)	1/2 cup	90	1.0	24.0	45	(mq)	0.0	0.0	0	0%
(Kohl's) cut	1/2 cup	110	1.0	31.0	30	(mq)	<1.0	(tr)	0	<7%
(Pathmark) 'No Frills'	1/2 cup	105	1.0	25.0	33	(mq)	0.0	0.0	0	0%
(Pathmark) 'Southern'	1 cup	230	2.0	55.0	100	(mq)	0.0	0.0	0	0%
(Princella)	1/2 cup	90	1.0	24.0	45	(mq)	0.0	0.0	0	0%
(Royal Prince)	1/2 cup	90	1.0	24.0	45	(mq)	0.0	0.0	0	0%
(Taylor's Brand) whole and cut	1 cup	240	3.0	58.0	56	(mq)	0.0	0.0	0	0%
In water (Allens) cut	1/2 cup	70	1.0	16.0	20	(mq)	<1.0	(tr)	0	<12%
SWEET POTATO, FROZEN										
unprepared, cubes	1/2 cup	84	1.5	19.5	5	>.7 c	0.2	0.0	0	2%
(Mrs. Paul's) candied	4 oz	170	1.0	42.0	40	(mq)	0.0	0.0	0	0%
(Mrs. Paul's) candied, w/apples 'Sweets 'n Apples'	4 oz	160	1.0	38.0	60	(mq)	0.0	0.0	0	0%
SWEET POTATO LEAF										
raw, approx 12 1/4 inches long	1 leaf	6	0.6	1.0	1	>.2 c	0.1	0.0	0	12%
raw, chopped	1 cup	12	1.4	2.2	3	>.4 c	0.1	0.0	0	6%
raw, trimmed	1 oz	10	1.1	1.8	3	>.3 c	0.1	<.1	0	7%
raw, untrimmed	1 lb	149	17.1	27.2	38	>5.1 c	1.3	0.3	0	6%
steamed	4 oz	39	2.6	8.3	15	2.1	0.3	0.1	0	6%

Food Name	Serving Size	Calories	Prot. gms	Carbs gms	Sod. mgs	Fiber gms	Fat gms	Sat. Fat gms	Chol. mgs	% Fat Cal.
steamed	1/2 cup	11	0.7	2.3	4	.6	0.1	.1	0	7%

SWEETBREAD. See BEEF, PANCREAS; BEEF, THYMUS; LAMB, PANCREAS; VEAL, PANCREAS; VEAL, THYMUS.

SWEETENERS. See SUGAR, ALTERNATIVE; SUGAR, BEET OR CANE; SUGAR, MAPLE; SUGAR, TURBINADO.

SWEETSOP. See SUGAR APPLE.

SWISS CHARD/chard

Food Name	Serving Size	Calories	Prot. gms	Carbs gms	Sod. mgs	Fiber gms	Fat gms	Sat. Fat gms	Chol. mgs	% Fat Cal.
boiled, drained	4 oz	23	2.1	4.7	203	>1.1 c	0.1	(tr)	0	3%
boiled, drained, chopped	1/2 cup	18	1.6	3.6	158	1.9	0.1	na	0	4%
raw, chopped	1/2 cup	3	0.3	0.7	38	.3	0.0	na	0	0%
raw, trimmed	1 oz	5	0.5	1.1	60	>.2 c	0.1	(tr)	0	12%
raw, untrimmed	1 lb	81	7.5	15.6	888	>3.3 c	0.8	(tr)	0	7%

SWISS STEAK DINNER

Food Name	Serving Size	Calories	Prot. gms	Carbs gms	Sod. mgs	Fiber gms	Fat gms	Sat. Fat gms	Chol. mgs	% Fat Cal.
frozen (Budget Gourmet)	11.2 oz	450	23.0	40.0	1110	(mq)	22.0	(mq)	70	44%
frozen (Swanson)	10 oz	350	26.0	37.0	700	(mq)	11.0	(mq)	(mq)	28%

SWISS STEAK SEASONING MIX

Food Name	Serving Size	Calories	Prot. gms	Carbs gms	Sod. mgs	Fiber gms	Fat gms	Sat. Fat gms	Chol. mgs	% Fat Cal.
'Bag'n Season' (Schilling)	1 pkg	81	1.9	17.0	2651	na	0.4	na	1	5%

SWORDFISH

Food Name	Serving Size	Calories	Prot. gms	Carbs gms	Sod. mgs	Fiber gms	Fat gms	Sat. Fat gms	Chol. mgs	% Fat Cal.
baked	4 oz	176	28.8	0.0	130	0	5.8	1.6	57	31%
broiled	4 oz	176	28.8	0.0	130	0	5.8	1.6	57	31%
dry-heat cooked	3 oz	132	21.6	0.0	98	0	4.4	1.2	43	31%
frozen, steaks, w/o seasoning mix (SeaPak)	6-oz pkg	210	34.0	0.0	155	0	7.0	(mq)	70	32%
microwaved	4 oz	176	28.8	0.0	130	0	5.8	1.6	57	31%
raw	1 lb	548	89.8	0.0	408	0	18.2	5.0	178	31%
raw	3 oz	103	16.8	0.0	77	0	3.4	0.9	33	31%
raw	1 oz	34	5.6	0.0	26	0	1.1	0.3	11	31%
raw (Peter Pan Seafoods)	3.5 oz	118	19.1	na	102	na	4.0	na	39	32%

T

Food Name	Serving Size	Calories	Prot. gms	Carbs gms	Sod. mgs	Fiber gms	Fat gms	Sat. Fat gms	Chol. mgs	% Fat Cal.

TABBOULEH MIX

Food Name	Serving Size	Calories	Prot. gms	Carbs gms	Sod. mgs	Fiber gms	Fat gms	Sat. Fat gms	Chol. mgs	% Fat Cal.
(Casbah) dry	1 oz	126	4.0	28.0	(mq)	(mq)	1.0	na	0	7%
(Fantastic Foods) prepared w/oil and tomatoes	1/2 cup	161	2.0	17.0	250	(mq)	10.0	(mq)	0	54%
(Fantastic Foods) prepared w/o oil	1/2 cup	85	3.0	17.0	265	na	0.5	na	na	5%
(Near East) prepared	1/2 cup	170	3.0	20.0	290	(mq)	9.0	(mq)	0	47%

TABLE QUEEN SQUASH. See SQUASH, ACORN.

TACO DIP. See DIP, TACO.

TACO KIT

Food Name	Serving Size	Calories	Prot. gms	Carbs gms	Sod. mgs	Fiber gms	Fat gms	Sat. Fat gms	Chol. mgs	% Fat Cal.
(Natural Touch) vegetarian	2 tbsp	90	10.0	6.0	(mq)	(mq)	2.0	(mq)	0	22%
(Old El Paso) prepared	1 taco	67	2.0	8.0	423	(mq)	3.0	(mq)	na	40%
(Tio Sancho) 'Dinner Kit' prepared	1 taco	64	1.1	8.1	1	>.5 c	3.1	(mq)	na	43%

TACO SEASONING MIX

Food Name	Serving Size	Calories	Prot. gms	Carbs gms	Sod. mgs	Fiber gms	Fat gms	Sat. Fat gms	Chol. mgs	% Fat Cal.
(Hain)	1/10 pkg	10	1.0	2.0	200	(mq)	0.0	0.0	0	0%
(Lawry's) 'Seasoning Blends'	1 pkg	118	3.4	23.6	1441	>1.0 c	1.1	na	0	8%
(Old El Paso)	1 pkg	100	1.0	21.0	3570	(mq)	1.0	na	na	9%
(Old El Paso)	1/12 pkg	8	<1.0	2.0	298	(mq)	<1.0	na	0	<43%
(Schilling)	1/4 pkg	31	1.0	6.0	675	(mq)	0.5	na	0	14%
(Tio Sancho)	1.51 oz	132	2.9	26.0	2623	>2.0 c	1.7	na	0	12%
(Tio Sancho) 'Dinner Kit' taco seasoning	1.25 oz	104	2.1	20.9	2500	>1.7 c	1.4	na	na	12%

TACO SHELL

Food Name	Serving Size	Calories	Prot. gms	Carbs gms	Sod. mgs	Fiber gms	Fat gms	Sat. Fat gms	Chol. mgs	% Fat Cal.
(Azteca) corn	1 shell	60	1.0	7.0	65	(mq)	3.0	(mq)	0	46%
(Azteca) flour	1 shell	200	3.0	18.0	130	(mq)	12.0	(mq)	na	56%
(Chi-Chi's)	1 shell	140	2.0	17.0	5	na	7.0	na	0	45%

Food Name	Serving Size	Calories	Prot. gms	Carbs gms	Sod. mgs	Fiber gms	Fat gms	Sat. Fat gms	Chol. mgs	% Fat Cal.
(Gebhardt)	1 shell	50	1.0	7.0	<1	<1.0	2.0	1.8	0	36%
(Lawry's)	1 shell	50	0.8	8.0	123	>.2 c	2.1	(mq)	0	35%
(Lawry's) 'Super'	1 shell	86	1.4	13.0	210	>.4 c	3.6	(mq)	0	36%
(Old El Paso)	1 shell	50	0.0	6.0	50	.5	3.0	na	0	53%
(Old El Paso) 'Mini'	3 shells	70	1.0	7.0	60	.5	4.0	na	0	53%
(Old El Paso) 'Super Size'	1 shell	100	1.0	11.0	95	1.5	6.0	(mq)	0	53%
(Ortega)	1 shell	50	0.0	8.0	5	(mq)	2.0	(mq)	0	36%
(Rosarita)	1 shell	50	1.0	7.0	<1	<1.0	2.0	1.8	0	36%
(Tio Sancho)	1 shell	64	1.1	8.1	1	>.5 c	3.1	(mq)	0	43%
(Tio Sancho) 'Super'	1 shell	94	1.6	11.3	2	>.7 c	4.7	(mq)	0	45%
TAFFY. See CANDY.										
TAHINI MIX										
(Arrowhead Mills) organic	1 oz	170	6.0	4.0	<1	2.6	17.0	(mq)	0	79%
(Casbah) dry	1 oz	25	2.0	2.0	(mq)	(mq)	5.0	(mq)	0	74%
(Erewhon) 'Sesame Tahini'	2 tbsp	200	6.0	3.0	65	na	18.0	na	na	82%
(Maranatha Natural) 'Sesame Tahini'	2 tbsp	210	8.0	3.0	20	na	19.0	na	0	80%
(Westbrae) raw, organic	2 tbsp	210	8.0	1.0	0	na	19.0	na	na	83%
(Westbrae) toasted, organic	2 tbsp	220	8.0	3.0	0	na	19.0	na	na	80%
TAMALE										
(Derby) beef	2 tamales	160	8.0	15.0	570	1.0	7.0	3.0	24	41%
(Gebhardt)	2 tamales	290	5.0	19.0	730	2.0	22.0	8.0	54	67%
(Gebhardt) jumbo	2 tamales	400	7.0	26.0	1025	3.0	30.0	11.4	75	67%
Canned										
(Derby) beef	6.561 oz	253	7.3	20.8	1034	4.0	17.4	8.2	23	58%
(Gebhardt)	5.75 oz	269	4.6	18.6	770	2.6	20.7	9.5	28	67%
(Gebhardt) beef	4 oz	230	4.0	15.0	620	(mq)	17.0	(mq)	(mq)	67%
(Gebhardt) jumbo	6.949 oz	332	5.6	24.0	930	3.2	25.2	11.6	34	66%
(Hormel)	7.5 oz	280	6.0	19.0	990	na	20.0	na	35	64%
(Hormel) beef	2 tamales	140	4.0	8.0	550	(mq)	10.0	(mq)	(mq)	65%
(Hormel) hot 'n spicy	7.5 oz	280	6.0	19.0	990	na	20.0	na	35	64%
(Libby's) beef, w/sauce	7.5 oz	408	8.9	26.4	1200	na	30.2	13.2	43	66%
(Old El Paso)	2 tamales	190	5.0	16.0	380	(mq)	12.0	(mq)	20	56%
(Van Camp's) w/sauce	1 cup	293	8.3	28.6	1132	>2.2 c	16.2	(mq)	(mq)	50%
(Wolf Brand)	7.75 oz	328	8.3	24.9	1181	>1.5 c	24.5	(mq)	(mq)	62%
Frozen										
(Amy's Kitchen) 'Mexican' organic	8 oz	170	6.0	36.0	190	5.0	3.0	na	0	14%
(Hormel) beef	1 tamale	140	6.0	13.0	555	(mq)	7.0	(mq)	(mq)	45%
(Patio) dinner	13 oz	470	12.0	58.0	1850	(mq)	21.0	(mq)	35	40%
TAMALITO (Dennison's) in chili gravy, canned	7.5 oz	310	6.0	37.0	1395	(mq)	16.0	(mq)	(mq)	46%
TAMARIND / Indian date										
pulp	1 cup	287	3.4	75.0	34	>6.1 c	0.7	0.3	0	2%
'Tamarindos' (Frieda's)	3.5 oz	239	2.8	62.5	51	(mq)	0.6	(mq)	0	2%
trimmed	1 oz	68	0.8	17.7	8	>1.4 c	0.2	0.1	0	2%
untrimmed	1 lb	369	4.3	96.4	43	>7.9 c	0.9	0.4	0	2%
TANGELO JUICE, fresh	100 gm	41	0.5	9.7	1	0	0.1	0.0	0	2%
TANGERINE										
peeled, seeded	1 oz	12	0.2	3.2	<1	>.1 c	0.1	tr	0	6%
sections, w/o membrane	1/2 cup	43	0.6	10.9	2	>.3 c	0.2	<.1	0	4%
untrimmed	1 lb	144	2.1	36.6	4	>1.1 c	0.6	0.1	0	3%
TANGERINE, CANNED										
in heavy syrup (S&W)	1/2 cup	76	0.0	20.0	10	(mq)	0.0	0.0	0	0%
in juice	4 oz	42	0.7	10.9	6	.9	<.1	tr	0	<2%
in light syrup	4 oz	69	0.5	18.4	7	.9	0.1	<.1	0	1%
in light syrup (A&P)	1/2 cup	80	<1.0	20.0	0	(mq)	<1.0	(tr)	0	<10%

Food Name	Serving Size	Calories	Prot. gms	Carbs gms	Sod. mgs	Fiber gms	Fat gms	Sat. Fat gms	Chol. mgs	% Fat Cal.
in light syrup (Dole)	1/2 cup	76	0.6	20.0	0	(mq)	0.1	(tr)	0	1%
in light syrup (Empress)	5.5 oz	100	0.0	25.0	10	(mq)	0.0	0.0	0	0%
in light syrup (Finast)	5.5 oz	100	0.0	25.0	na	(mq)	0.0	0.0	0	0%
'Natural Style' (S&W)	1/2 cup	60	0.0	15.0	10	(mq)	0.0	0.0	0	0%
sections, in water (Featherweight)	1/2 cup	35	0.0	8.0	10	(mq)	0.0	0.0	0	0%
unsweetened (S&W Nutradiet)	1/2 cup	28	0.0	7.0	10	(mq)	0.0	0.0	0	0%
TANGERINE JUICE										
canned, sweetened	1 cup	125	1.3	29.9	2	.5	0.5	0.0	0	4%
canned, sweetened	1 oz	16	0.2	3.7	0	.1	0.1	0.0	0	6%
chilled 'Pure & Light Mandarin Tangerine' (Dole)	6 oz	97	0.6	25.0	20	(mq)	0.1	(tr)	0	1%
fresh	1 cup	106	1.2	25.0	2	.5	0.5	0.1	0	4%
fresh	1 oz	13	0.2	3.1	0	.1	0.1	0.0	0	6%
frozen concentrate, sweetened, diluted w/3 vol water	1 cup	111	1.0	26.7	2	na	0.3	0.0	0	2%
frozen concentrate, sweetened, diluted w/3 vol water	1 oz	14	0.1	3.3	0	na	0.0	0.0	0	0%
frozen concentrate, sweetened, undiluted	6 oz	345	3.2	83.1	6	1.3	0.8	0.1	0	2%
frozen or chilled (Minute Maid)	6 oz	90	1.0	23.0	0	na	0.0	na	na	0%
TANGERINE ORANGE DRINK										
'Thirst Quencher Light' (Gatorade)	8 oz	25	0.0	7.0	80	na	0.0	na	na	0%
TAPIOCA, PEARL										
dry	1 cup	518	0.3	134.8	2	1.6	0.0	na	0	0%
dry	1 oz	97	<.1	25.1	tr	.3	tr	(tr)	0	0%
TARO										
cooked	4 oz	161	0.6	39.2	11	>1.0 c	0.1	<.1	0	1%
cooked, slices	1/2 cup	94	0.3	22.8	10	3.4	0.1	0.0	0	1%
raw, slices	1/2 cup	56	0.8	13.8	6	2.1	0.1	0.0	0	2%
raw, trimmed	1 oz	30	0.4	7.5	3	>.2 c	0.1	<.1	0	3%
raw, untrimmed	1 lb	419	5.9	103.2	43	>3.1 c	0.8	0.2	0	2%
TARO, TAHITIAN										
cooked	4 oz	50	4.7	7.8	61	>2.6 c	0.8	0.2	0	13%
cooked, slices	1/2 cup	30	2.8	4.7	37	>1.5 c	0.5	0.1	0	13%
raw, slices	1/2 cup	25	1.7	4.3	31	>1.1 c	0.6	0.1	0	18%
raw, trimmed	1 lb	181	12.7	31.3	227	>7.9 c	4.4	0.9	0	18%
raw, trimmed	1 oz	11	0.8	2.0	14	>.5 c	0.3	0.1	0	19%
TARO LEAF										
raw	1 cup	12	1.4	1.9	1	1.0	0.2	0.0	0	12%
raw, 11 x 6 1/2 inches	1 leaf	4	0.5	0.7	0	.4	0.1	0.0	0	16%
raw, trimmed	1 oz	12	1.4	1.9	1	>.6 c	0.2	<.1	0	12%
raw, untrimmed	1 lb	115	13.5	18.3	8	>5.5 c	2.0	0.4	0	12%
steamed	4 oz	27	3.1	4.6	2	>.6 c	0.5	0.1	0	13%
steamed	1/2 cup	18	2.0	3.0	1	>.4 c	0.3	0.1	0	12%
TARO SHOOTS										
cooked	4 oz	16	0.8	3.6	2	>.6 c	0.1	<.1	0	5%
cooked, slices	1/2 cup	10	0.5	2.2	1	>.4 c	0.1	0.0	0	8%
raw, 15 x 5 inches	1 shoot	9	0.8	1.9	1	>.5 c	0.1	0.0	0	8%
raw, slices	1/2 cup	5	0.4	1.0	0	>.3 c	0.0	0.0	0	0%
raw, trimmed	1 oz	3	0.3	0.7	<1	>.2 c	<.1	tr	0	<18%
raw, untrimmed	1 lb	45	3.7	9.3	4	>2.3 c	0.4	0.1	0	7%
TARPON, ATLANTIC										
raw	1 lb	422	94.8	0.0	(mq)	0	1.8	(mq)	(mq)	4%
raw	1 oz	26	5.0	0.0	(mq)	0	0.1	(mq)	(mq)	4%
TARRAGON										
ground	1 oz	84	6.5	14.2	18	2.1	2.1	(mq)	0	19%
ground	1 tbsp	14	1.1	2.4	3	.4	0.4	na	0	21%
ground	1 tsp	5	0.4	0.8	1	.1	0.1	na	0	16%

Food Name	Serving Size	Calories	Prot. gms	Carbs gms	Sod. mgs	Fiber gms	Fat gms	Sat. Fat gms	Chol. mgs	% Fat Cal.
ground *(Durkee)*	1 tsp	10	0.0	0.0	0	0	<0.1	na	na	<18%
ground *(Laurel Leaf)*	1 tsp	10	0.0	0.0	0	0	<0.1	na	na	<18%
ground *(Spice Islands)*	1 tsp	5	0.3	0.7	1	.1	0.1	na	0	18%
TEA										
Brewed										
prepared w/distilled water	6 oz	2	0.0	0.5	0	0	0.0	0.0	0	0%
prepared w/tap water	6 oz	2	0.0	0.5	5	0	0.0	0.0	0	0%
(Celestial Seasonings) caffeine-free	8 oz	4	tr	0.8	5	tr	tr	(tr)	0	0%
(Nestea)	6 oz	0	0.0	0.0	0	0	0.0	0.0	0	0%
Instant										
decaffeinated *(Lipton)*	6 oz	0	0.0	0.0	0	0	0.0	0.0	0	0%
lemon flavor *(Lipton)*	6 oz	3	0.1	0.6	1	0	0.0	0.0	0	0%
regular *(Lipton)*	6 oz	0	0.0	0.0	0	0	0.0	0.0	0	0%
TEA, FLAVORED										
(Bigelow)										
'Chinese Fortune'	5.25 oz	1	<.1	0.1	<1	0	tr	(tr)	0	0%
'Cinnamon Stick'	5.25 oz	1	<.1	0.1	<1	0	tr	(tr)	0	0%
'Constant Comment'	5.25 oz	1	<.1	0.1	<1	0	tr	(tr)	0	0%
'Darjeeling'	5.25 oz	1	<.1	0.1	<1	0	tr	(tr)	0	0%
'Earl Grey'	5.25 oz	1	<.1	0.1	1	0	tr	(tr)	0	0%
'English Teatime'	5.25 oz	1	<.1	0.1	tr	0	tr	(tr)	0	0%
'Lemon Lift'	5.25 oz	1	<.1	0.2	<1	0	tr	(tr)	0	0%
'Plantation Mint'	5.25 oz	1	<.1	0.1	1	0	tr	(tr)	0	0%
'Raspberry Royale'	5.25 oz	1	<.1	0.1	<1	0	tr	(tr)	0	0%
(Celestial Seasonings)										
'Amaretto Nights'	8 oz	3	tr	0.6	1	tr	tr	(tr)	0	0%
apple spice 'Fruit & Tea'	8 oz	3	<.1	0.2	1	tr	tr	(tr)	0	0%
'Bavarian Chocolate Orange'	8 oz	7	tr	1.6	5	tr	tr	(tr)	0	0%
'Cinnamon Vienna'	8 oz	2	tr	0.4	2	tr	tr	(tr)	0	0%
'Classic English Breakfast'	8 oz	3	tr	0.4	<1	tr	tr	(tr)	0	0%
'Darjeeling Gardens'	8 oz	3	tr	0.5	<1	tr	tr	(tr)	0	0%
'Extraordinary Earl Grey'	8 oz	3	tr	0.5	<1	tr	tr	(tr)	0	0%
'Irish Cream Mist'	8 oz	3	tr	0.6	1	tr	tr	(tr)	0	0%
lemon 'Fruit & Tea'	8 oz	3	tr	0.5	<1	tr	tr	(tr)	0	0%
mint, Swiss	8 oz	3	tr	0.4	<1	tr	tr	(tr)	0	0%
'Morning Thunder'	8 oz	3	tr	0.4	<1	tr	tr	(tr)	0	0%
orange spice 'Fruit & Tea'	8 oz	3	tr	0.4	<1	tr	tr	(tr)	0	0%
raspberry 'Fruit & Tea'	8 oz	2	tr	0.5	<1	tr	tr	(tr)	0	0%
(Nestea)										
apple spice	16 oz	180	2.0	44.0	50	na	0.0	0.0	0	0%
apple spice	6 oz	66	1.0	16.5	18	na	0.0	0.0	0	0%
lemon, natural	16 oz	180	2.0	44.0	50	na	0.0	0.0	0	0%
lemon, natural	6 oz	66	1.0	16.5	18	na	0.0	0.0	0	0%
lemon, natural, diet	16 oz	180	2.0	44.0	50	na	0.0	0.0	0	0%
lemon, natural, diet	6 oz	66	1.0	16.5	18	na	0.0	0.0	0	0%
peach	16 oz	180	2.0	44.0	50	na	0.0	0.0	0	0%
peach	6 oz	66	1.0	16.5	18	na	0.0	0.0	0	0%
raspberry	16 oz	180	2.0	44.0	50	na	0.0	0.0	0	0%
raspberry	6 oz	66	1.0	16.5	18	na	0.0	0.0	0	0%
tropical	16 oz	180	2.0	44.0	50	na	0.0	0.0	0	0%
tropical	6 oz	66	1.0	16.5	18	na	0.0	0.0	0	0%
(Tetley)										
'Apple Freeze'	8 oz	79	tr	20.0	<1	na	0.0	na	na	0%
'Classic'	8 oz	69	tr	17.0	<1	na	0.0	na	na	0%

Food Name	Serving Size	Calories	Prot. gms	Carbs gms	Sod. mgs	Fiber gms	Fat gms	Sat. Fat gms	Chol. mgs	% Fat Cal.
'Classic Lemon'	8 oz	108	0.1	27.0	<1	na	0.0	na	na	0%
'Diet Lemon Frost'	8 oz	10	0.1	2.3	<1	na	0.0	na	na	0%
'Diet Raspberry Blizzard'	8 oz	10	0.1	2.4	<1	na	0.0	na	na	0%
'Lemon Frost'	8 oz	89	tr	22.0	<1	na	0.0	na	na	0%
'Orange Glazier'	8 oz	79	tr	20.0	<1	na	0.0	na	na	0%
'Peach Chiller'	8 oz	79	tr	20.0	<1	na	0.0	na	na	0%
'Raspberry Blizzard'	8 oz	95	tr	24.0	<1	na	0.0	na	na	0%
(Wyler's) 'Fruit Tea Punch'	12 oz	118	0.0	29.6	1	0	0.0	0.0	0	0%
TEA, HERBAL										
(Bigelow)										
almond orange	5 oz	<1	<.1	<.1	<1	0	tr	(tr)	0	0%
'Apple Orchard'	5.25 oz	5	<.1	1.2	1	0	tr	(tr)	0	0%
apple spice	5 oz	<1	tr	<.1	1	0	tr	(tr)	0	0%
chamomile	5 oz	<1	<.1	tr	2	0	tr	(tr)	0	0%
chamomile mint	5 oz	<1	tr	tr	1	0	tr	(tr)	0	0%
cinnamon orange	5 oz	<1	<.1	0.1	<1	0	tr	(tr)	0	0%
cranberry apple	5 oz	1	0.1	0.3	1	0	tr	(tr)	0	0%
'Fruit & Almond'	5.25 oz	1	<.1	<.1	<1	0	tr	(tr)	0	0%
grains, roasted, w/carob	5 oz	3	<.1	0.6	1	0	tr	(tr)	0	0%
hibiscus and rose hips	5 oz	1	<.1	0.2	1	0	tr	(tr)	0	0%
'I Love Lemon'	5.25 oz	1	<.1	<.1	<1	0	tr	(tr)	0	0%
'Lemon & C'	5 oz	<1	tr	<.1	<1	0	tr	(tr)	0	0%
'Mint Blend'	5 oz	<1	<.1	0.2	3	0	tr	(tr)	0	0%
'Mint Medley'	5.25 oz	1	<.1	0.2	<1	0	tr	(tr)	0	0%
'Orange & C'	5 oz	<1	tr	<.1	<1	0	tr	(tr)	0	0%
'Orange & Spice'	5.25 oz	1	<.1	<.1	1	0	tr	(tr)	0	0%
peppermint	5 oz	<1	<.1	<.1	2	0	<.1	(tr)	0	<53%
red raspberry	5 oz	1	0.1	0.2	<1	0	tr	(tr)	0	0%
spearmint	5 oz	<1	<.1	<.1	1	0	tr	(tr)	0	0%
'Specially Strawberry'	5 oz	1	0.1	0.2	<1	0	tr	(tr)	0	0%
'Sweet Dreams'	5.25 oz	1	<.1	0.1	1	0	tr	(tr)	0	0%
'Take-A-Break'	5.25 oz	1	<.1	0.6	1	0	tr	(tr)	0	0%
(Celestial Seasonings)										
'Almond Sunset'	8 oz	3	tr	1.1	2	tr	tr	(tr)	0	0%
chamomile	8 oz	2	tr	0.5	5	tr	tr	(tr)	0	0%
'Cinnamon Apple Spice'	8 oz	3	tr	0.4	1	tr	tr	(tr)	0	0%
'Cinnamon Rose'	8 oz	2	tr	1.1	1	tr	tr	(tr)	0	0%
'Country Peach Spice'	8 oz	3	tr	0.7	3	tr	tr	(tr)	0	0%
'Cranberry Cone'	8 oz	3	tr	0.7	1	tr	tr	(tr)	0	0%
'Emperor's Choice'	8 oz	4	<.1	0.9	2	<.1	<.1	(tr)	0	<18%
'Ginseng Plus'	8 oz	3	tr	<.5	4	tr	tr	(tr)	0	0%
'Grandma's Tummy Mint'	8 oz	2	tr	<.3	7	tr	tr	(tr)	0	0%
'Lemon Mist'	8 oz	2	tr	<.5	3	tr	tr	(tr)	0	0%
'Lemon Zinger'	8 oz	4	<.1	0.7	1	tr	tr	(tr)	0	0%
'Mandarin Orange Spice'	8 oz	5	tr	1.1	2	tr	tr	(tr)	0	0%
'Mellow Mint'	8 oz	2	tr	0.4	4	tr	tr	(tr)	0	0%
'Mint Magic'	8 oz	1	tr	0.4	3	tr	tr	(tr)	0	0%
'Mo's 24'	8 oz	2	<.1	0.2	4	tr	tr	(tr)	0	0%
'Orange Zinger'	8 oz	5	tr	1.2	1	tr	tr	(tr)	0	0%
peppermint	8 oz	2	tr	1.1	8	tr	tr	(tr)	0	0%
'Raspberry Patch'	8 oz	4	tr	1.1	1	tr	tr	(tr)	0	0%
'Red Zinger'	8 oz	4	tr	1.1	2	<.1	tr	(tr)	0	0%
'Roastaroma'	8 oz	11	<.1	2.0	4	<.1	<.1	(tr)	0	<10%
'Sleepytime'	8 oz	5	tr	1.1	2	<.1	tr	(tr)	0	0%

Food Name	Serving Size	Calories	Prot. gms	Carbs gms	Sod. mgs	Fiber gms	Fat gms	Sat. Fat gms	Chol. mgs	% Fat Cal.
spearmint	8 oz	5	<.1	0.2	6	<.1	<.1	(tr)	0	<43%
'Strawberry Fields'	8 oz	4	tr	0.8	1	tr	tr	(tr)	0	0%
'Sunburst C'	8 oz	3	tr	1.1	6	<.1	tr	(tr)	0	0%
'Wild Forest Blackberry'	8 oz	2	tr	1.8	1	tr	tr	(tr)	0	0%
(Lipton)										
'Almond Pleasure'	8 oz	4	0.0	1.0	0	0	0.0	0.0	0	0%
chamomile	8 oz	4	0.0	1.0	0	0	0.0	0.0	0	0%
cinnamon apple	8 oz	2	0.0	<1.0	0	0	0.0	0.0	0	0%
'Citrus Sunset'	8 oz	4	0.0	1.0	0	0	0.0	0.0	0	0%
'Gentle/Tangy Orange'	8 oz	4	0.0	1.0	0	0	0.0	0.0	0	0%
'Lemon Soother'	8 oz	4	0.0	1.0	0	0	0.0	0.0	0	0%
'Toasty Spice'	8 oz	6	0.0	1.0	0	0	0.0	0.0	0	0%

TEA, ICED

CAN, BOTTLE, OR BOX

(Arizona)

Food Name	Serving Size	Calories	Prot. gms	Carbs gms	Sod. mgs	Fiber gms	Fat gms	Sat. Fat gms	Chol. mgs	% Fat Cal.
'Diet'	8 oz	4	0.0	0.0	15	na	0.0	na	na	0%
'Diet' with lemon	8 oz	4	0.0	0.0	15	na	0.0	na	na	0%
raspberry flavor, sun-brewed style	8 oz	95	0.0	25.0	20	na	0.0	na	na	0%
(Lipton) w/lemon, aseptic box	8.45 oz	96	1.6	24.0	20	0	0.3	(tr)	0	3%
(Nestea)										
	8 oz	90	0.0	22.0	35	na	0.0	na	na	0%
diet	8 oz	4	0.0	1.0	35	na	0.0	na	na	0%
(Shasta)	12 oz	124	0.0	34.0	28	0	0.0	0.0	0	0%
(Snapple)										
cranberry	8 oz	110	0.0	27.0	10	na	0.0	0.0	0	0%
'Diet'	8 oz	0	0.0	1.0	10	na	0.0	0.0	0	0%
lemon	8 oz	110	0.0	27.0	10	na	0.0	0.0	0	0%
mango	8 oz	110	0.0	27.0	5	na	0.0	0.0	0	0%
mint	8 oz	120	0.0	29.0	10	na	0.0	0.0	0	0%
old fashioned	8 oz	80	0.0	20.0	10	na	0.0	0.0	0	0%
orange	8 oz	110	0.0	27.0	10	na	0.0	0.0	0	0%
peach	8 oz	110	0.0	27.0	10	na	0.0	0.0	0	0%
peach 'Diet'	8 oz	0	0.0	1.0	10	na	0.0	0.0	0	0%
raspberry	8 oz	120	0.0	29.0	10	na	0.0	0.0	0	0%
raspberry 'Diet'	8 oz	0	0.0	1.0	10	na	0.0	0.0	0	0%
strawberry	8 oz	100	0.0	26.0	10	na	0.0	0.0	0	0%
w/lemon, 'Diet'	8 oz	4	<1.0	<1.0	15	na	<1.0	na	na	<53%
(Tetley)										
brewed	8 oz	74	0.0	19.0	20	na	0.0	na	na	0%
brewed, w/lemon	8 oz	74	0.0	19.0	20	na	0.0	na	na	0%
sweetened	8 oz	74	0.0	19.0	20	na	0.0	na	na	0%
(Veryfine)										
peach kiwi flavored, brewed, 'Chillers'	8 oz	80	0.0	18.0	5	0	0.0	0.0	0	0%
w/lemon	8 oz	80	<1.0	16.0	10	0	0.0	0.0	0	0%

PREPARED FROM MIX

(Crystal Light)

Food Name	Serving Size	Calories	Prot. gms	Carbs gms	Sod. mgs	Fiber gms	Fat gms	Sat. Fat gms	Chol. mgs	% Fat Cal.
w/NutraSweet	8 oz	4	0.0	0.0	0	na	0.0	na	0	0%
w/Nutrasweet, decaffeinated	8 oz	4	0.0	0.0	0	0	0.0	0.0	0	0%
(Lipton)										
lemon flavor	6 oz	55	0.0	14.3	1	0	0.0	0.0	0	0%
lemon flavor, decaffeinated	6 oz	55	0.0	14.2	<1	0	0.0	0.0	0	0%
lemon flavor, w/NutraSweet	8 oz	5	0.1	1.2	2	0	0.0	0.0	0	0%
'Sugar-free'	8 oz	1	0.0	0.3	6	0	0.0	0.0	0	0%
'Sugar-free' decaffeinated	8 oz	1	0.0	0.3	5	0	0.0	0.0	0	0%

Food Name	Serving Size	Calories	Prot. gms	Carbs gms	Sod. mgs	Fiber gms	Fat gms	Sat. Fat gms	Chol. mgs	% Fat Cal.
(Nestea)										
'Ice Teasers' all flavors	8 oz	6	0.0	1.0	0	0	0.0	0.0	0	0%
lemon flavor	8 oz	6	0.0	1.0	0	0	0.0	0.0	0	0%
lemon flavor, sugar-free	8 oz	4	0.0	1.0	0	0	0.0	0.0	0	0%
lemon flavor, sugar-free, decaffeinated	2 tsp	6	0.0	1.0	0	0	0.0	0.0	0	0%
'100%'	8 oz	2	0.0	0.0	0	na	0.0	na	na	0%
'100%' decaffeinated	8 oz	0	0.0	0.0	0	0	0.0	0.0	0	0%
sugar-free	8 oz	6	0.0	1.0	5	na	0.0	na	na	0%
w/sugar and lemon	8 oz	70	0.0	19.0	0	na	0.0	na	na	0%
(Pathmark)										
lemon flavor, low-calorie	8 oz	4	0.0	1.0	0	0	0.0	0.0	0	0%
lemon flavor, low-calorie, decaffeinated	8 oz	4	0.0	1.0	0	0	0.0	0.0	0	0%
lemon flavor, sugar-sweetened, decaffeinated	2 tbsp	80	0.0	20.0	0	0	0.0	0.0	0	0%
TEA FLAVORED DRINK *(10-K)*	8 oz	60	0.0	15.0	55	na	0.0	na	na	0%
TEASEED OIL										
	1 cup	1927	0.0	0.0	0	0	218.0	46.0	0	100%
	1 oz	251	0.0	0.0	0	0	28.4	6.0	0	100%
	1 tbsp	120	0.0	0.0	0	0	13.6	2.9	0	100%
TEFF FLOUR, whole-grain *(Arrowhead Mills)*	2 oz	200	7.0	41.0	6	7.7	1.0	na	0	5%
TEFF SEED *(Arrowhead Mills)*	1/2 cup	165	15.7	14.1	5	>2.5 c	6.4	0.9	0	33%
TEMPEH	1 oz	56	5.4	4.8	2	>.8 c	2.2	0.3	0	33%
TENDERGREEN. See MUSTARD SPINACH.										
TEQUILA. See ALCOHOLIC BEVERAGES.										
TEQUILA SUNRISE. See ALCOHOLIC BEVERAGES.										
TERIYAKI MARINADE										
(Lawry's)	2 tbsp	72	6.4	11.0	7100	.2	0.4	0.2	0	5%
(Lawry's) barbecue	1/4 cup	164	8.0	27.4	12330	.1	2.3	na	na	13%
TERRAPIN, diamond back, raw	100 gm	111	18.6	0.0	50	0	3.5	0.0	50	30%
THURINGER CERVELAT										
(Hillshire Farm)	2 oz	180	9.0	1.0	650	0	15.0	(mq)	(mq)	77%
(Hormel) 'Old Smokehouse'	1 oz	90	4.0	1.0	328	0	8.0	(mq)	(mq)	78%
(Hormel) 'Old Smokehouse Chub'	1 oz	100	5.0	0.0	332	0	9.0	(mq)	(mq)	80%
(Hormel) 'Old Smokehouse Sliced'	1 oz	100	5.0	0.0	321	0	9.0	(mq)	(mq)	80%
(Hormel) 'Viking Club Cervelat'	1 oz	90	5.0	0.0	325	0	8.0	(mq)	(mq)	78%
(JM) beef	1-oz slice	80	5.0	1.0	340	0	7.0	(mq)	(mq)	72%
(JM) 'Cervelat'	1-oz slice	70	4.0	1.0	260	0	6.0	(mq)	(mq)	73%
THYME										
ground	1 oz	78	2.6	18.1	16	5.3	2.1	0.8	0	19%
ground	1 tbsp	12	0.4	2.8	2	.8	0.3	0.1	0	17%
ground	1 tsp	4	0.1	0.9	1	.3	0.1	0.0	0	18%
ground *(Durkee)*	1 tsp	5	0.0	0.0	0	0	tr	na	na	tr
ground *(Laurel Leaf)*	1 tsp	5	0.0	0.0	0	0	tr	na	na	tr
ground *(Spice Islands)*	1 tsp	5	0.1	1.0	1	.4	0.1	(tr)	0	17%
TILEFISH										
broiled	4 oz	167	27.8	0.0	67	0	5.3	1.0	(mq)	30%
dry-heat cooked	4 oz	167	27.8	0.0	67	0	5.3	1.0	(mq)	30%
dry-heat cooked	3 oz	125	20.8	0.0	50	0	4.0	0.7	54	30%
microwaved	4 oz	167	27.8	0.0	67	0	5.3	1.0	(mq)	30%
raw	1 lb	433	79.4	0.0	239	0	10.5	2.0	(mq)	23%
raw	3 oz	82	14.9	0.0	45	0	2.0	0.4	43	23%
raw	1 oz	27	5.0	0.0	15	0	0.7	0.1	(mq)	24%
TOASTED SESAME OIL. See SESAME OIL.										
TOASTER BISCUIT. See BISCUIT, TOASTER.										
TOASTER MUFFIN/PASTRY. See MUFFIN/PASTRY, TOASTER.										

Food Name	Serving Size	Calories	Prot. gms	Carbs gms	Sod. mgs	Fiber gms	Fat gms	Sat. Fat gms	Chol. mgs	% Fat Cal.
TOFFEE. See CANDY.										
TOFU /soybean curd cake										
raw	1 oz	22	2.3	0.5	2	.3	1.4	0.2	0	53%
raw	1/2 cup	94	10.0	2.3	9	1.5	5.9	0.9	0	52%
Flavored										
Chinese 5-spice (Nasoya)	5 oz	150	15.0	2.0	15	(mq)	8.0	(mq)	0	51%
French, country herb (Nasoya)	5 oz	150	15.0	2.0	15	(mq)	8.0	(mq)	0	51%
pasteurized (Frieda's)	4.2 oz	86	9.6	2.9	8	(mq)	(mq)	0.8	0	0%
Freeze-dried/koyadofu	1 oz	136	13.6	4.1	2	>.1 c	8.6	1.2	0	52%
Fried	1 oz	77	4.9	3.0	5	>.1 c	5.7	0.8	0	62%
Grilled/yakidofu	1 oz	25	2.2	0.3	5	(mq)	1.7	(mq)	0	61%
Okara	1 oz	22	0.9	3.6	3	>1.2 c	0.5	0.1	0	20%
Salted and fermented/fuyu	1 oz	33	2.3	1.5	814	>.1 c	2.3	0.3	0	58%
Silken (Mori-Nu)	1/2 pkg	90	10.0	4.0	50	na	4.0	na	0	39%
TOFU PATTY, FROZEN										
garden (Natural Touch)	2.5-oz patty	90	10.0	3.0	260	(mq)	4.0	1.0	0	41%
okara (Natural Touch)	2.25-oz patty	160	11.0	7.0	420	(mq)	10.0	1.0	0	56%
TOFU SPREAD										
green chili 'Tofu Topper' canned (Natural Touch)	2 tbsp	50	2.0	2.0	(mq)	(mq)	4.0	(mq)	0	69%
herb and spice 'Tofu Topper' canned (Natural Touch)	2 tbsp	50	2.0	2.0	(mq)	(mq)	4.0	(mq)	0	69%
Mexican 'Tofu Topper' canned (Natural Touch)	2 tbsp	60	2.0	2.0	(mq)	(mq)	5.0	(mq)	0	74%
TOM COLLINS. See ALCOHOLIC BEVERAGES.										
TOMATILLO /ground husk tomato										
fresh (Frieda's)	3.5 oz	25	1.4	4.2	na	(mq)	0.5	na	0	17%
raw	1 med	11	0.3	2.0	0	na	0.4	na	0	28%
raw, chopped	1/2 cup	21	0.6	3.8	1	na	0.7	na	0	26%
TOMATO. See also TOMATO, SUN-DRIED.										
Green										
raw, 2 3/5 inch diam	1 tomato	30	1.5	6.3	16	1.8	0.3	0.0	0	8%
trimmed	1 oz	7	0.3	1.4	4	>.1 c	0.1	tr	0	12%
untrimmed	1 lb	99	5.0	21.1	55	>2.1 c	0.8	0.1	0	7%
Red										
boiled	1/2 cup	32	1.3	7.0	13	1.2	0.5	0.1	0	12%
boiled	4 oz	31	1.2	6.6	12	1.1	0.5	0.1	0	13%
raw, chopped	1/2 cup	19	0.8	4.2	8	1.2	0.3	<.1	0	12%
raw, 2 3/5 inch diam, 4.75 oz	1 tomato	26	1.0	5.7	11	1.6	0.4	0.1	0	12%
raw, trimmed	1 oz	6	0.2	1.3	3	.4	0.1	<.1	0	13%
raw, untrimmed	1 lb	88	3.5	19.2	36	5.4	1.4	0.2	0	12%
stewed	1 cup	80	2.0	13.2	460	1.7	2.7	0.5	0	29%
stewed	4 oz	90	2.2	14.8	516	1.9	3.0	0.6	0	28%
TOMATO, CANNED										
(A&P)										
sliced	1/2 cup	35	1.0	8.0	350	(mq)	<1.0	(tr)	0	<20%
whole	1/2 cup	25	1.0	6.0	220	(mq)	<1.0	(tr)	0	<24%
(Angela Mia)										
chopped, 'Premium Choice'	4 oz	24	1.7	4.1	254	1.2	0.4	0.0	0	13%
crushed	4 oz	25	2.5	5.1	463	2.0	0.2	0.0	0	6%
crushed, chunky	4 oz	26	2.0	5.1	378	2.0	0.3	0.0	0	9%
crushed, 'Premium Choice'	2.222 oz	29	1.7	5.6	25	.9	0.4	0.0	0	11%
(Contadina)										
crushed, in purée	1/2 cup	30	1.0	6.0	350	(mq)	<1.0	(tr)	0	<24%
Italian style	1/2 cup	35	1.0	8.0	250	(mq)	<1.0	(tr)	0	<20%
Italian style, pear	1/2 cup	25	1.0	5.0	220	(mq)	<1.0	(tr)	0	<27%
'Recipe Ready'	1/2 cup	25	1.0	5.0	570	na	0.2	0.1	0	7%

Food Name	Serving Size	Calories	Prot. gms	Carbs gms	Sod. mgs	Fiber gms	Fat gms	Sat. Fat gms	Chol. mgs	% Fat Cal.
stewed	1/2 cup	35	1.0	8.0	350	(mq)	<1.0	(tr)	0	<20%
stewed, Mexican style	1/2 cup	35	1.0	8.0	230	na	0.3	0.1	0	7%
whole, peeled	1/2 cup	25	1.0	5.0	260	(mq)	<1.0	(tr)	0	<27%
w/jalapeños	1/2 cup	35	1.0	8.0	250	(mq)	<1.0	(tr)	0	<20%
(Del Monte)										
stewed	1/2 cup	35	1.0	8.0	355	(mq)	0.0	0.0	0	0%
stewed, 'No Salt Added'	1/2 cup	35	1.0	8.0	45	(mq)	0.0	0.0	0	0%
wedges, w/liquid	1/2 cup	30	1.0	8.0	355	(mq)	0.0	0.0	0	0%
whole, peeled, w/liquid	1/2 cup	25	1.0	5.0	220	(mq)	0.0	0.0	0	0%
(Eden Foods) crushed, organic, no salt added	4 oz	35	2.0	6.0	0	na	0.0	0.0	0	0%
(Featherweight)	1/2 cup	20	1.0	4.0	<1	(mq)	0.0	0.0	0	0%
(Finast)										
sliced	1/2 cup	35	1.0	9.0	355	(mq)	0.0	0.0	0	0%
whole, peeled	1/2 cup	25	1.0	6.0	195	(mq)	0.0	0.0	0	0%
(Hunt's)										
choice cut	4 oz	19	1.1	4.0	278	.5	0.0	0.0	0	0%
crushed	4 oz	31	0.9	7.2	317	1.1	0.4	0.0	0	10%
crushed, 'Angela Mia'	4 oz	35	1.0	7.0	260	<1.0	<1.0	na	0	<22%
crushed, Italian flavored	4 oz	40	2.0	9.0	460	<1.0	<1.0	na	0	<17%
diced, in juice	4 oz	19	1.1	4.0	477	.5	0.1	0.0	0	4%
diced, in juice, 'No Salt Added'	4 oz	20	1.1	4.1	8	.5	0.1	0.0	0	4%
diced, in purée	4 oz	23	1.3	4.7	304	.6	0.2	0.0	0	7%
diced, w/green chilies	.3527 oz	2	0.1	0.2	33	.1	0.1	0.0	0	43%
pear shaped	4.868 oz	21	1.5	4.1	285	1.2	0.1	0.0	0	4%
pear shaped	4.832 oz	21	1.5	4.1	373	.6	0.1	0.0	0	4%
pear shaped	4.656 oz	20	1.4	3.9	360	.6	0.1	0.0	0	4%
pear shaped, Italian flavored	4 oz	20	1.0	5.0	320	<1.0	<1.0	na	0	<27%
peeled, choice cut	4 oz	20	1.0	5.0	460	1.0	<1.0	na	0	<27%
stewed	4 oz	33	1.2	6.7	357	.8	0.1	0.0	0	3%
stewed, 'Food Service'	4 oz	29	1.2	6.7	262	.8	0.1	0.0	0	3%
stewed, Italian flavored	4 oz	35	1.0	8.0	400	<1.0	<1.0	na	0	<20%
stewed, 'No Salt Added'	1/2 cup	35	1.0	8.0	20	(mq)	0.0	0.0	0	0%
whole	4 oz	20	1.0	5.0	415	(mq)	0.0	0.0	0	0%
whole, Italian flavored	4 oz	25	1.0	6.0	420	<1.0	<1.0	na	0	<24%
whole, 'No Salt Added'	4 oz	20	1.0	5.0	20	(mq)	0.0	0.0	0	0%
whole, peeled	5.608 oz	24	1.7	4.7	433	.7	0.3	0.0	0	10%
whole, peeled	5.22 oz	22	1.6	4.4	333	.6	0.1	0.0	0	4%
whole, peeled	5.009 oz	22	1.5	4.2	387	.6	0.1	0.0	0	4%
whole, peeled	4.832 oz	21	1.5	4.1	373	.6	0.1	0.0	0	4%
whole, peeled, 'No Salt Added'	4.832 oz	21	1.5	4.1	9	.6	0.1	0.0	0	4%
(Old El Paso) w/green chilies	1/4 cup	14	0.0	3.0	480	(mq)	0.0	0.0	0	0%
(Ortega) w/jalapeños	1 oz	8	0.0	1.0	120	(mq)	0.0	0.0	0	0%
(Pathmark)										
crushed	1/2 cup	40	1.0	9.0	210	(mq)	0.0	0.0	0	0%
crushed, 'No Frills'	1 cup	90	3.0	20.0	510	(mq)	0.0	0.0	0	0%
'No Frills'	1 cup	50	2.0	11.0	440	(mq)	0.0	0.0	0	0%
sliced	1/2 cup	35	1.0	9.0	360	(mq)	0.0	0.0	0	0%
whole, peeled, 'No Salt Added'	1/2 cup	25	1.0	6.0	20	(mq)	0.0	0.0	0	0%
whole, peeled, w/tomato juice	1/2 cup	25	1.0	6.0	220	(mq)	0.0	0.0	0	0%
(S&W)										
aspic, supreme	1/2 cup	60	1.0	16.0	860	(mq)	0.0	0.0	0	0%
cut, peeled 'Ready-Cut'	1/2 cup	25	1.0	6.0	220	(mq)	0.0	0.0	0	0%
diced, in rich purée	1/2 cup	35	1.0	8.0	290	(mq)	0.0	0.0	0	0%
Italian, sliced	1/2 cup	35	1.0	9.0	355	(mq)	0.0	0.0	0	0%

Food Name	Serving Size	Calories	Prot. gms	Carbs gms	Sod. mgs	Fiber gms	Fat gms	Sat. Fat gms	Chol. mgs	% Fat Cal.
Mexican style	1/2 cup	40	1.0	8.0	360	(mq)	0.0	0.0	0	0%
sliced	1/2 cup	35	1.0	9.0	355	(mq)	0.0	0.0	0	0%
stewed, '50% Salt Reduced'	1/2 cup	35	1.0	9.0	180	(mq)	0.0	0.0	0	0%
whole, peeled	1/2 cup	25	1.0	6.0	220	(mq)	0.0	0.0	0	0%
whole, peeled, Italian-style pear, w/basil	1/2 cup	25	1.0	5.0	200	(mq)	0.0	0.0	0	0%
(S&W Nutradiet) whole	1/2 cup	25	1.0	5.0	20	(mq)	0.0	0.0	0	0%
(Stokely)										
stewed	1/2 cup	35	1.0	8.0	220	(mq)	0.0	0.0	0	0%
whole	1/2 cup	25	1.0	5.0	190	(mq)	0.0	0.0	0	0%
TOMATO, PICKLED, kosher (Claussen)	1 oz	5	0.2	1.0	330	(mq)	0.0	na	00	0%
TOMATO-BEEF COCKTAIL (Beefamato)	6 oz	80	1.0	19.0	240	(mq)	0.0	0.0	na	0%
TOMATO-CHILE COCKTAIL (Snap-E-Tom)	6 oz	40	2.0	7.0	980	(mq)	0.0	0.0	0	0%
TOMATO-CLAM COCKTAIL (Clamato)	6 oz	96	1.0	23.0	815	(mq)	0.0	0.0	na	0%
TOMATO JUICE										
(A&P)	6 oz	30	1.0	7.0	550	(mq)	0.0	0.0	0	0%
(Biotta)	6 oz	28	1.3	5.8	277	(mq)	0.1	(tr)	0	3%
(Campbell's)	6 oz	40	1.0	8.0	540	(mq)	0.0	0.0	0	0%
(Featherweight)	6 oz	35	1.0	8.0	10	(mq)	0.0	0.0	0	0%
(Hunt's)	9.03 oz	33	2.1	6.5	608	.8	0.2	0.0	0	5%
(Hunt's)	7.16 oz	28	1.8	5.5	513	.7	0.2	0.0	0	6%
(Hunt's)	6 oz	30	1.0	7.0	640	(mq)	0.0	0.0	0	0%
(Hunt's)	5.467 oz	22	1.4	4.2	399	.5	0.1	0.0	0	4%
(Hunt's) 'No Salt Added'	6 oz	45	2.0	11.0	30	(mq)	0.0	0.0	0	0%
(Knudsen & Sons) organic	8 oz	50	<1.0	10.0	na	na	0.0	na	na	0%
(Libby's)	6 oz	35	2.0	7.0	500	na	0.0	na	na	0%
(Pathmark)	6 oz	30	1.0	6.0	510	(mq)	0.0	0.0	0	0%
(Pathmark) frozen, diluted	6 oz	35	1.0	8.0	450	(mq)	0.0	0.0	0	0%
(S&W) 'California'	6 oz	35	1.0	8.0	600	(mq)	0.0	0.0	0	0%
(S&W Nutradiet)	6 oz	35	1.0	8.0	20	(mq)	0.0	0.0	0	0%
(Stokely)	4 oz	20	1.0	4.0	330	(mq)	0.0	0.0	0	0%
(Welch's)	6 oz	35	1.0	7.0	550	0	0.0	0.0	0	0%
TOMATO PASTE										
(Contadina)	2 oz	50	2.0	11.0	40	na	<1.0	na	na	<15%
(Contadina) Italian style	2 oz	65	2.0	12.0	520	na	1.0	na	na	14%
(Hunt's)	1.164 oz	24	1.4	4.9	81	.7	0.2	0.0	0	7%
(Hunt's) 'Food Service'	1.164 oz	24	1.4	4.9	101	.7	0.2	0.0	0	7%
(Hunt's) Italian style	1.164 oz	25	1.5	4.7	255	.8	0.4	0.0	0	13%
(Hunt's) 'No Salt Added'	1.164 oz	24	1.4	4.9	11	.7	0.2	0.0	0	7%
(Hunt's) w/garlic	2 oz	50	2.0	11.0	440	2.0	<1.0	na	0	<15%
(Hunt's) w/garlic	1.164 oz	26	1.6	5.1	247	.8	0.3	0.0	0	9%
TOMATO POWDER										
ground	1 oz	86	3.7	21.2	38	>1.9 c	0.1	<.1	0	1%
ground	100 gm	302	12.9	74.7	134	>6.7 c	0.4	0.1	0	1%
TOMATO PURÉE										
(Angela Mia)	2.187 oz	16	0.9	2.9	21	.4	0.3	0.0	0	15%
(Contadina)	1/2 cup	40	2.0	8.0	35	na	<1.0	na	na	<18%
(Contadina) w/crushed tomatoes	1/2 cup	30	1.0	6.0	350	na	<1.0	na	na	<24%
(Hunt's)	2.187 oz	23	1.6	4.3	98	.7	0.3	0.0	0	10%
(Hunt's) 'Food Service'	2.222 oz	26	1.5	5.0	22	.8	0.4	0.0	0	12%
TOMATO SAUCE										
CANNED										
(A&P)	1/2 cup	45	2.0	9.0	600	(mq)	<1.0	(tr)	0	<17%
(Contadina)	1/2 cup	30	1.0	7.0	580	(mq)	<1.0	(tr)	0	<22%
(Del Monte)	1 cup	70	3.0	16.0	1330	(mq)	1.0	(tr)	0	11%

Food Name	Serving Size	Calories	Prot. gms	Carbs gms	Sod. mgs	Fiber gms	Fat gms	Sat. Fat gms	Chol. mgs	% Fat Cal.
(Finast)	1/2 cup	45	2.0	9.0	650	(mq)	0.0	0.0	0	0%
(Health Valley)	1 cup	70	2.4	13.0	460	.3	0.5	(tr)	0	7%
(Hunt's)	4 oz	30	1.0	7.0	730	(mq)	0.0	0.0	0	0%
(Hunt's)	2.187 oz	16	1.0	2.6	360	.1	0.2	0.0	0	11%
(Pathmark)	1/2 cup	40	2.0	9.0	620	(mq)	0.0	0.0	0	0%
(S&W)	1/2 cup	40	2.0	9.0	620	(mq)	0.0	0.0	0	0%
(Stokely)	1/2 cup	30	2.0	7.0	810	(mq)	0.0	0.0	0	0%
Casera (Hunt's)	2.187 oz	22	0.7	5.2	293	.8	0.1	0.0	0	4%
Chunky										
(Hunt's) chili	2.222 oz	21	1.0	4.1	320	1.4	0.4	0.0	0	15%
(Hunt's) 'Food Service'	2.187 oz	15	1.1	2.8	360	.5	0.2	0.0	0	10%
(Hunt's) Italian	2.222 oz	29	1.0	4.5	293	1.4	1.1	0.2	0	31%
(Hunt's) Mexican	2.222 oz	19	0.7	3.8	369	1.2	0.4	0.0	0	17%
(Hunt's) tomato	2.187 oz	13	0.7	2.9	405	1.1	0.1	0.0	0	6%
Garden vegetable (Contadina)	5 oz	80	2.0	9.0	580	na	3.0	<1.0	0	38%
Herb flavored (Hunt's)	4 oz	70	2.0	12.0	470	2.0	2.0	0.6	<1	24%
Hot, Maya (Hunt's)	1.058 oz	6	0.3	1.1	174	.2	0.2	0.0	0	24%
Italian style										
(Contadina)	1/2 cup	30	1.0	7.0	670	(mq)	<1.0	(tr)	0	<22%
(Contadina) sausage	5 oz	110	5.0	8.0	570	na	6.0	2.0	15	51%
(Hunt's)	4 oz	60	2.0	11.0	520	(mq)	2.0	(mq)	na	26%
(Hunt's)	2.222 oz	26	1.1	5.2	251	1.4	0.5	0.0	0	15%
(Rokeach)	3 oz	60	1.0	8.0	243	(mq)	2.0	(mq)	0	33%
Low sodium (Rokeach)	3 oz	50	1.0	8.0	124	(mq)	2.0	na	0	33%
Marinara										
(Buitoni)	1/2 cup	70	1.0	11.0	570	(mq)	3.0	<1.0	0	36%
(Contadina)	4 oz	80	2.0	8.0	460	na	4.0	<1.0	0	47%
(Pathmark) 'No Frills'	1/2 cup	80	1.0	12.0	620	(mq)	3.0	(mq)	0	34%
(Rokeach)	3 oz	60	1.0	9.0	257	(mq)	2.0	(mq)	0	31%
'Meatloaf Fixin's' (Hunt's)	2 oz	20	<1.0	5.0	580	<1.0	<1.0	na	0	<27%
No salt added										
(Del Monte)	1 cup	70	3.0	16.0	50	(mq)	1.0	(tr)	0	11%
(Finast)	8 oz	90	4.0	18.0	10	(mq)	0.0	0.0	0	0%
(Health Valley)	1 cup	70	2.4	13.0	43	.3	0.5	(tr)	0	7%
(Hunt's)	4 oz	35	1.0	8.0	25	(mq)	0.0	0.0	0	0%
(Hunt's)	2.187 oz	16	1.0	2.6	11	.1	0.2	0.0	0	11%
(Pathmark)	1/2 cup	45	2.0	9.0	25	(mq)	0.0	0.0	0	0%
Pesto (Contadina)	2.33 oz	350	7.0	5.0	440	na	34.0	5.0	10	86%
Plum (Contadina)	5 oz	80	2.0	8.0	420	na	4.0	<1.0	5	47%
'Special'										
(Hunt's)	4 oz	35	1.0	8.0	320	(mq)	0.0	0.0	0	0%
(Hunt's)	2.187 oz	21	0.8	3.8	144	.6	0.6	0.0	0	23%
'Thick and Zesty' (Contadina)	1/2 cup	40	2.0	8.0	650	(mq)	<1.0	(tr)	0	<18%
W/bits (Hunt's)	4 oz	30	1.0	7.0	620	2.0	<1.0	na	0	<22%
W/garlic										
(Hunt's)	4 oz	70	2.0	10.0	480	2.0	2.0	0.3	0	27%
(Hunt's)	2.258 oz	29	1.0	4.9	269	1.8	1.0	0.1	0	28%
W/green chilies (Old El Paso)	1/4 cup	14	<1.0	3.0	480	(mq)	<1.0	na	0	<36%
W/herbs (Hunt's)	2.187 oz	33	1.3	4.9	255	.8	1.3	0.3	0	32%
W/jalapeños (Old El Paso)	1/4 cup	11	1.0	2.0	150	(mq)	1.0	0.0	0	43%
W/mushrooms (Hunt's)	4 oz	25	1.0	6.0	710	2.0	<1.0	na	0	<24%
W/onions										
(Del Monte)	1 cup	100	3.0	23.0	1150	(mq)	1.0	na	0	8%
(Hunt's)	4 oz	40	1.0	9.0	650	2.0	<1.0	na	0	<18%

Food Name	Serving Size	Calories	Prot. gms	Carbs gms	Sod. mgs	Fiber gms	Fat gms	Sat. Fat gms	Chol. mgs	% Fat Cal.
REFRIGERATED										
(Contadina) 'Light'	.5 oz	50	2.0	9.0	570	na	0.0	na	0	0%
(Contadina) marinara 'Fresh'	7.5 oz	100	4.0	12.0	700	(mq)	4.0	(mq)	0	36%
(Contadina) plum w/basil 'Fresh'	7.5 oz	100	3.0	14.0	700	(mq)	4.0	(mq)	5	35%
TOMATOES, SUN-DRIED. See SUN-DRIED TOMATOES.										
TOMATOSEED OIL										
	1/2 cup	964	0.0	0.0	0	0	109.0	21.5	0	100%
	1 oz	251	0.0	0.0	0	0	28.4	5.6	0	100%
	1 tbsp	120	0.0	0.0	0	0	13.6	2.7	0	100%
TOM COLLINS. See ALCOHOLIC BEVERAGES.										
TONIC. See SOFT DRINKS AND MIXERS.										
TORSK. See CUSK.										
TORTELLINI PASTA, NONDAIRY										
regular (Tofutti) frozen	2 oz	210	12.0	32.0	158	(mq)	4.0	(mq)	0	17%
spinach (Tofutti) frozen	2 oz	210	12.0	32.0	158	(mq)	4.0	(mq)	0	17%
TORTELLINI PASTA, REFRIGERATED										
CHEESE (DiGiorno) approx 1 cup cooked	1/3 pkg	270	13.0	41.0	240	na	6.0	3.0	35	20%
CHICKEN AND HERB (DiGiorno) approx 1 cup cooked	1/3 pkg	240	14.0	37.0	230	na	5.0	2.0	40	18%
EGG										
w/cheese, 'Fresh' (Contadina)	4.5 oz	380	21.0	60.0	570	(mq)	6.0	(mq)	70	14%
w/cheese, 'Fresh' (Contadina)	3 oz	260	13.0	39.0	310	na	6.0	2.0	40	21%
w/chicken and prosciutto, 'Fresh' (Contadina)	4.5 oz	370	24.0	53.0	560	(mq)	7.0	(mq)	75	17%
w/meat, 'Fresh' (Contadina)	4.5 oz	380	22.0	60.0	580	(mq)	6.0	(mq)	75	14%
MOZZARELLA GARLIC (DiGiorno) approx 1 cup cooked	1/3 pkg	260	13.0	35.0	270	na	8.0	4.0	40	27%
SAUSAGE, Italian, 'Fresh' (Contadina)	3 oz	260	11.0	37.0	290	na	7.0	2.0	65	25%
SPINACH										
w/cheese, 'Fresh' (Contadina)	4.5 oz	380	21.0	60.0	590	(mq)	6.0	(mq)	70	14%
w/cheese, 'Fresh' (Contadina)	3 oz	260	13.0	38.0	360	na	6.0	2.0	45	21%
w/chicken and prosciutto, 'Fresh' (Contadina)	4.5 oz	340	24.0	53.0	580	(mq)	7.0	(mq)	75	17%
w/meat, 'Fresh' (Contadina)	4.5 oz	380	22.0	60.0	610	(mq)	6.0	(mq)	75	14%
W/CHICKEN AND PROSCIUTTO (Contadina)	3 oz	250	15.0	34.0	370	na	6.0	2.0	50	22%
W/MEAT										
(Contadina) 'Fresh'	3 oz	260	13.0	39.0	380	na	6.0	2.0	45	21%
(DiGiorno) approx 1 cup cooked	1/3 pkg	280	12.0	38.0	360	na	9.0	4.0	40	29%
TORTELLINI DISH/ENTRÉE, FROZEN										
(Birds Eye) in tomato sauce 'For One'	5.5 oz	210	11.0	31.0	500	0	5.0	(mq)	30	21%
(Budget Gourmet) 'Side Dish'	5.5 oz	180	7.0	25.0	400	(mq)	9.0	(mq)	15	39%
(Green Giant) marinara 'One Serving'	5.5 oz	260	8.0	37.0	660	(mq)	9.0	3.0	25	31%
(Green Giant) Provençal 'Microwave Garden Gourmet'	1 pkg	260	10.0	44.0	840	3.0	6.0	2.0	15	20%
(Le Menu) and meat sauce 'LightStyle'	8 oz	250	11.0	34.0	480	(mq)	8.0	1.0	15	29%
(Stouffer's) in Alfredo sauce	8 7/8 oz	580	26.0	35.0	830	na	37.0	na	na	58%
(Stouffer's) w/tomato sauce	9.25 oz	360	18.0	39.0	720	na	15.0	na	na	37%
(Top Shelf) in marinara sauce	10 oz	211	10.0	37.0	663	(mq)	3.0	(mq)	35	13%
(Top Shelf) w/shrimp and seafood	10 oz	278	16.0	36.0	1341	(mq)	8.0	(mq)	89	26%
(Weight Watchers)	9 oz	310	14.0	50.0	570	na	6.0	1.0	15	17%
TORTILLA, CORN										
(Azteca)	1 tortilla	45	1.0	9.0	10	0	0.0	0.0	0	0%
(Old El Paso)	1 tortilla	60	1.0	10.0	170	na	1.0	na	0	17%
TORTILLA, FLOUR										
(Azteca) 9 inch diam	1 tortilla	130	3.0	23.0	180	0	3.0	(mq)	0	21%
(Azteca) 7 inch diam	1 tortilla	80	2.0	14.0	110	0	2.0	(mq)	0	22%
(Mission) 'Light'	1 tortilla	70	2.0	16.0	280	4.0	1.0	<.5	0	11%
(Old El Paso)	1 tortilla	150	4.0	27.0	360	na	3.0	(mq)	0	18%

Food Name	Serving Size	Calories	Prot. gms	Carbs gms	Sod. mgs	Fiber gms	Fat gms	Sat. Fat gms	Chol. mgs	% Fat Cal.
Burrito style										
(Garcia's)	1 tortilla	220	5.0	37.0	220	2.0	5.0	1.5	0	21%
(Mission) 'Premium'	1 tortilla	230	6.0	40.0	395	na	6.0	na	0	23%
(Tyson)	1 tortilla	173	5.0	29.0	40	na	4.0	na	0	21%
(Tyson) large, heat-pressed	1 tortilla	182	5.0	33.0	90	na	4.0	na	0	19%
(Tyson) small, hand-stretched	1 tortilla	106	3.0	19.0	50	na	2.0	na	0	17%
Fajita style										
(Fry's) extra soft	1 tortilla	100	2.0	17.0	160	na	2.0	na	0	19%
(Garcia's)	1 tortilla	100	2.0	17.0	220	<1.0	2.5	0.5	0	23%
(Tyson)	1 tortilla	84	3.0	18.0	20	na	2.0	na	0	18%
Taco size										
(Mission) soft	1 tortilla	150	4.0	25.0	255	na	4.0	na	0	24%
(Tyson) soft	1 tortilla	121	4.0	20.0	30	na	3.0	na	0	22%
TORTILLA CHIPS. See also CORN CHIPS AND SNACKS.										
(Bachman)										
nacho	1 oz	140	2.0	18.0	210	(mq)	6.0	(mq)	0	40%
'No Salt'	1 oz	140	2.0	19.0	0	(mq)	6.0	(mq)	0	39%
(Barbara's Bakery)										
yellow corn, organic	1 oz	140	2.0	18.0	120	na	7.0	na	0	44%
yellow corn, organic, no salt added	1 oz	140	2.0	18.0	15	na	7.0	na	0	44%
(Bearitos)										
blue corn 'Organic'	1 oz	146	2.9	17.4	29	.6	7.0	(mq)	0	44%
blue corn 'Organic No Salt'	1 oz	137	2.6	17.1	3	1.0	6.5	(mq)	0	43%
yellow corn 'Organic'	1 oz	143	2.1	18.1	58	1.1	6.4	(mq)	0	42%
yellow corn 'Organic No Salt'	1 oz	148	2.2	17.2	2	1.4	7.2	(mq)	0	46%
(Bravos)										
nacho cheese flavored, jalapeño	1 oz	150	2.0	19.0	170	(mq)	7.0	(mq)	0	43%
nacho cheese flavored, round, crispy	1 oz	150	2.0	18.0	180	(mq)	8.0	(mq)	0	47%
nacho cheese flavored, strips	1 oz	140	2.0	18.0	220	(mq)	7.0	(mq)	0	44%
(Buenitos)										
'Tortilla Chips'	1 oz	150	2.0	18.0	80	3.6	8.0	(mq)	0	47%
'Tortilla Chips, No Salt Added'	1 oz	150	2.0	18.0	1	3.6	8.0	(mq)	0	47%
(Doritos)										
'Cool Ranch'	1 oz	140	2.0	18.0	170	1.5	7.0	na	0	44%
'Cool Ranch Light'	1 oz	120	2.0	21.0	240	(mq)	4.0	(mq)	0	28%
'Jumpin' Jack'	1 oz	140	2.0	18.0	220	1.5	7.0	na	0	44%
nacho cheese	1 oz	140	2.0	18.0	240	(mq)	7.0	(mq)	0	44%
nacho cheese 'Light'	1 oz	120	2.0	21.0	290	(mq)	4.0	(mq)	0	28%
salsa 'n cheese 'Thins'	1 oz	150	2.0	17.0	180	na	8.0	na	0	49%
'Salsa Rio'	1 oz	140	2.0	18.0	190	1.5	7.0	na	0	44%
taco	1 oz	140	2.0	18.0	250	1.5	7.0	na	0	44%
toasted corn	1 oz	140	2.0	19.0	80	1.5	7.0	na	0	43%
white corn, lightly salted 'Thins'	1 oz	140	2.0	19.0	135	na	7.0	na	0	43%
(Eagle) ranch	1 oz	140	2.0	17.0	190	(mq)	8.0	(mq)	1	49%
(Featherweight)										
'Low Salt'	1 oz	150	2.0	18.0	10	(mq)	8.0	(mq)	0	47%
nacho	1 oz	150	2.0	18.0	45	(mq)	8.0	(mq)	0	47%
(Guiltless Gourmet)										
white corn, baked, salted	1 oz	110	3.0	22.0	160	2.0	1.5	0.0	0	12%
yellow corn, baked, salted	1 oz	110	3.0	22.0	140	3.0	1.5	0.0	0	12%
yellow corn, baked, unsalted	1 oz	110	3.0	22.0	25	3.0	1.5	0.0	0	12%
(Hain)										
sesame	1 oz	140	2.0	19.0	190	(mq)	7.0	(mq)	0	43%
sesame, cheese	1 oz	160	2.0	20.0	270	(mq)	8.0	(mq)	5	45%

Food Name	Serving Size	Calories	Prot. gms	Carbs gms	Sod. mgs	Fiber gms	Fat gms	Sat. Fat gms	Chol. mgs	% Fat Cal.
sesame, 'No Salt Added'	1 oz	140	2.0	19.0	0	(mq)	7.0	(mq)	5	43%
taco	1 oz	160	2.0	15.0	320	(mq)	11.0	(mq)	5	59%
(Keebler)										
cinnamon crispaña, flour 'Chacho's'	1 oz	140	2.0	19.0	70	na	7.0	1.0	0	43%
original, restaurant style 'Chacho's'	1 oz	140	3.0	18.0	180	na	7.0	1.0	5	43%
(Kettle Ties)										
blue corn, lightly salted	1 oz	140	3.0	18.0	80	2.0	6.0	0.5	0	39%
blue corn, no salt	1 oz	140	3.0	18.0	2	2.0	6.0	0.5	0	39%
yellow corn, lightly salted	1 oz	140	2.0	19.0	80	2.0	7.0	0.5	0	43%
yellow corn, no salt	1 oz	140	2.0	19.0	3	2.0	7.0	0.5	0	43%
(La Famous)										
'No Salt Added'	1 oz	140	2.0	18.0	5	(mq)	7.0	(mq)	0	44%
plain	1 oz	140	2.0	18.0	180	(mq)	7.0	(mq)	0	44%
(Laura Scudder's)										
lightly salted 'Restaurant Style'	1 oz	140	2.0	18.0	90	(mq)	7.0	(mq)	0	44%
nacho, jalapeño 'Strips'	1 oz	150	2.0	19.0	170	(mq)	7.0	(mq)	0	43%
nacho, 'Triangles'	1 oz	140	2.0	18.0	220	(mq)	7.0	(mq)	0	44%
picante 'Restaurant Style Strips'	1 oz	150	2.0	19.0	190	(mq)	7.0	(mq)	0	43%
(Old El Paso)										
crispy	1 oz	150	2.0	17.0	105	.5	8.0	(mq)	0	49%
white, round 'NaChips' low sodium	1 oz	160	2.0	17.0	5	na	9.0	na	0	52%
(Planters)										
nacho cheese	1 oz	150	2.0	18.0	160	na	8.0	2.0	0	47%
traditional	1 oz	150	2.0	18.0	150	na	8.0	2.0	0	47%
(Slimchips) fat-free	.4 oz	44	<1.0	10.0	60	<.5	<.5	na	0	<9%
(Tio Sancho)										
'Microwave Snacks'	4 oz	567	8.5	74.4	590	>4.0 c	26.1	(mq)	na	42%
nacho	.5 oz	70	4.1	0.7	282	>.1 c	5.7	(mq)	na	73%
(Tostitos)										
nacho, sharp	1 oz	150	2.0	17.0	200	(mq)	8.0	(mq)	0	49%
white corn, baked 'Cool Ranch'	1 oz	130	2.0	21.0	170	na	3.0	na	0	23%
white corn, baked, no salt	1 oz	110	2.0	24.0	0	na	1.0	na	0	8%
white corn, baked 'Original'	1 oz	110	2.0	24.0	140	na	1.0	na	0	8%
(Wise) nacho cheese flavored, crispy, round	1 oz	150	2.0	18.0	180	na	8.0	na	na	47%
TORULA YEAST. See YEAST, TORULA.										
TOSTACO SHELL *(Old El Paso)*	1 shell	100	1.0	11.0	10	1.0	5.0	na	0	48%
TOSTADA SHELL										
(Lawry's)	1 shell	73	1.2	9.5	147	>.4 c	3.5	(mq)	0	42%
(Old El Paso)	1 shell	55	<1.0	6.0	65	.5	3.0	na	0	49%
(Ortega)	1 shell	50	0.0	8.0	5	(mq)	2.0	(mq)	0	36%
(Pancho Villa)	1 shell	55	<1.0	6.0	65	na	3.0	na	0	49%
(Rosarita)	1 shell	60	1.0	8.0	<1	<1.0	3.0	2.2	0	43%
(Tio Sancho)	1 shell	67	1.2	8.4	1	>.5 c	3.2	(mq)	0	43%
TOWEL GOURD. See GOURD, DISHCLOTH.										
TRAIL MIX										
(Harmony) 'Delux Super'	1/4 cup	150	3.0	23.0	35	3.0	7.0	2.5	0	38%
(Harmony) nut and berry mix	1/4 cup	160	5.0	21.0	0	3.0	8.0	1.0	0	41%
TREE FERN										
cooked	4 oz	45	0.3	12.5	6	.7	0.1	(tr)	0	2%
cooked, chopped	1/2 cup	28	0.2	7.8	4	2.6	0.1	na	0	3%
TRITICALE										
whole grain	1/2 cup	323	12.5	69.2	5	>2.5 c	2.0	0.4	0	5%
whole grain	1 oz	95	3.7	20.4	1	5.1	0.6	0.1	0	5%

Food Name	Serving Size	Calories	Prot. gms	Carbs gms	Sod. mgs	Fiber gms	Fat gms	Sat. Fat gms	Chol. mgs	% Fat Cal.
TRITICALE FLOUR										
whole grain	1/2 cup	220	8.6	47.5	1	9.5	1.2	0.2	0	5%
whole grain	1 oz	96	3.7	20.7	<1	4.1	0.5	0.1	0	4%
TROPICAL CITRUS DRINK										
chilled *(Five Alive)*	6 oz	90	0.0	21.0	20	na	0.0	na	na	0%
frozen, prepared *(Five Alive)*	6 oz	90	0.0	21.0	0	na	0.0	na	na	0%
TROPICAL FRUIT DRINK										
bottled 'Thirst Quencher' *(Gatorade)*	8 oz	50	0.0	14.0	110	na	0.0	na	na	0%
mix 'Thirst Quencher' prepared *(Gatorade)*	8 oz	60	0.0	15.0	110	na	0.0	na	na	0%
TROPICAL FRUIT JUICE										
bottled *(Juicy Juice)*	6 oz	110	1.0	26.0	10	na	0.0	na	na	0%
boxed *(Juicy Juice)*	8.45 oz	150	1.0	36.0	10	na	0.0	na	na	0%
TROPICAL LIME COOLER *(Knudsen & Sons)*	8 oz	130	<1.0	32.0	na	na	0.0	na	na	0%
TROPICAL NECTAR, can or bottle *(Kern's)*	6 oz	110	0.0	27.0	5	na	0.0	na	na	0%
TROPICAL ORANGE DRINK, 'Fruit Box' *(Tang)*	8.45 oz	150	0.0	37.0	10	na	0.0	na	0	0%
TROPICAL PASSION JUICE *(Knudsen & Sons)*	8 oz	80	<1.0	20.0	na	na	0.0	na	na	0%
TROPICAL PUNCH										
Can, bottle, or box										
(Knudsen & Sons)	8 oz	105	<1.0	33.0	na	na	0.0	na	na	0%
(Kool-Aid) 'Koolers'	8.45 oz	130	0.0	35.0	10	na	0.0	na	0	0%
(Minute Maid)	6 oz	90	0.0	22.0	20	na	0.0	na	na	0%
(Santa Cruz Natural) organic	8 oz	110	<1.0	26.0	na	na	<1.0	na	na	<8%
Mix										
(Kool-Aid) sugar-free, w/NutraSweet, prepared	8 oz	4	0.0	0.0	10	na	0.0	na	0	0%
(Kool-Aid) sugar-sweetened, prepared	8 oz	80	0.0	21.0	0	na	0.0	na	0	0%
(Kool-Aid) unsweetened, prepared w/sugar	8 oz	100	0.0	25.0	0	na	0.0	na	0	0%
(Kool-Aid) unsweetened, prepared w/o sugar	8 oz	2	0.0	0.0	0	na	0.0	na	0	0%
TROPICAL SALAD										
(Sun Fresh) chilled, packed in light syrup	3.5 oz	88	1.2	18.7	39	2.3	0.9	0.3	1	9%
TROUT, MIXED SPECIES										
dry-heat cooked	3 oz	161	22.6	0.0	57	0	7.2	1.3	63	42%
raw	1 lb	673	94.2	0.0	236	0	30.0	5.2	264	42%
raw	3 oz	126	17.6	0.0	44	0	5.6	1.0	49	42%
raw	1 oz	42	5.9	0.0	15	0	1.9	0.3	16	42%
raw, approx 2.8 oz	1 fillet	117	16.4	0.0	41	0	5.2	0.9	46	42%
TROUT, RAINBOW										
farmed, dry-heat cooked	3 oz	144	20.6	0.0	36	0	6.1	1.8	58	40%
farmed, raw	3 oz	117	17.7	0.0	30	0	4.6	1.3	50	37%
wild, dry-heat cooked	3 oz	127	19.5	0.0	48	0	4.9	1.4	59	36%
wild, raw	3 oz	101	17.4	0.0	26	0	2.9	0.6	50	27%
wild, raw, approx 2.8 oz	1 fillet	189	32.6	0.0	49	0	5.5	1.1	94	28%
TROUT, SEA, MIXED SPECIES										
raw	1 lb	472	76.0	0.0	263	0	16.4	4.6	376	33%
raw	3 oz	88	14.2	0.0	49	0	3.1	0.9	71	33%
raw	1 oz	29	4.7	0.0	16	0	1.0	0.3	24	32%
TUMERIC. See TURMERIC.										
TUNA, ALBACORE. See TUNA, CANNED; TUNA, FROZEN.										
TUNA, ALTERNATIVE, frozen 'Tuno' *(Worthington)*	2 oz	100	5.0	3.0	310	(mq)	7.0	1.0	0	66%
TUNA, BLUEFIN										
dry-heat cooked	4 oz	209	33.9	0.0	57	0	7.1	1.8	56	32%
dry-heat cooked	3 oz	156	25.4	0.0	43	0	5.3	1.4	42	32%
raw	1 lb	652	105.8	0.0	177	0	22.2	5.7	173	32%
raw	3 oz	122	19.8	0.0	33	0	4.2	1.1	32	32%
raw	1 oz	41	6.6	0.0	11	0	1.4	0.4	11	32%

Food Name	Serving Size	Calories	Prot. gms	Carbs gms	Sod. mgs	Fiber gms	Fat gms	Sat. Fat gms	Chol. mgs	% Fat Cal.
TUNA, CANNED										
LIGHT										
In canola oil, chunk *(Chicken of the Sea)*	2 oz	160	12.0	<1.0	250	na	12.0	1.0	na	68%
In oil										
drained	3 oz	168	24.8	0.0	301	0	7.0	1.3	15	39%
drained, approx 6 oz	1 can	339	49.8	0.0	605	0	14.0	2.6	31	39%
w/o salt, drained	3 oz	168	24.8	0.0	43	0	7.0	1.3	15	39%
w/o salt, drained, approx 6 oz	1 can	339	49.8	0.0	86	0	14.0	2.6	31	39%
In pure vegetable oil, chunk, w/liquid *(Chicken of the Sea)* . .	2 oz	160	12.0	<1.0	250	na	12.0	na	na	68%
In soybean oil										
chunk, drained	1 oz	56	8.3	0.0	100	0	2.3	0.4	5	38%
chunk, drained *(A&P)*	2 oz	150	13.0	<1.0	310	0	13.0	(mq)	(mq)	68%
chunk, drained *(Bumble Bee)*	2 oz	110	12.0	0.0	310	0	12.0	3.0	30	69%
chunk, drained *(Finast)*	2 oz	150	13.0	<1.0	310	0	13.0	(mq)	(mq)	68%
chunk, drained *(Star-Kist)*	2 oz	150	13.0	<1.0	310	0	13.0	1.0	25	68%
chunk 'Fancy' drained *(S&W)*	2 oz	140	13.0	0.0	450	0	10.0	(mq)	(mq)	63%
solid, drained *(Progresso)*	1/3 cup	150	13.0	<1.0	400	0	13.0	(mq)	(mq)	68%
solid, drained *(Star-Kist)*	2 oz	150	13.0	<1.0	310	0	13.0	1.0	25	68%
w/o salt, drained	1 oz	56	8.3	0.0	14	0	2.3	0.4	5	38%
In spring water, chunk, w/liquid *(Chicken of the Sea)*	2 oz	60	12.0	<1.0	250	na	1.0	na	na	15%
In water										
chunk, drained *(Bumble Bee)*	2 oz	50	12.0	0.0	310	0	1.0	0.5	30	16%
chunk, drained *(Finast)*	2 oz	60	13.0	<1.0	310	0	<1.0	(mq)	(mq)	<14%
chunk, drained *(Pathmark)*	2 oz	70	15.0	0.0	310	0	2.0	(mq)	(mq)	23%
chunk, drained *(Star-Kist)*	2 oz	60	13.0	<1.0	310	0	<1.0	0.2	25	<14%
chunk, diet, drained *(Star-Kist)*	2 oz	65	14.0	<1.0	35	0	<1.0	0.2	25	<13%
chunk 'Fancy' drained *(S&W)*	2 oz	60	13.0	0.0	500	0	1.0	(mq)	(mq)	15%
chunk 'No Salt Added' drained *(Weight Watchers)*	2 oz	60	14.0	<1.0	210	0	<1.0	0.2	25	<13%
chunk '00% Less Salt' drained *(Star-Kist)*	2 oz	65	14.0	<1.0	120	0	1.0	0.2	25	13%
drained	3 oz	111	25.1	0.0	303	0	0.4	0.1	15	4%
drained	1 oz	37	8.4	0.0	101	0	0.1	<.1	(mq)	3%
drained, approx 6.3 oz	1 can	216	48.8	0.0	587	0	0.8	0.3	30	4%
drained *(A&P)*	2 oz	60	13.0	<1.0	310	0	<1.0	(mq)	(mq)	<14%
drained *(Empress)*	2 oz	60	12.0	0.0	310	0	1.0	(mq)	(mq)	16%
solid, drained *(Star-Kist)*	2 oz	60	14.0	<1.0	310	0	<1.0	0.2	25	<13%
solid 'Prime Catch' drained *(Star-Kist)*	2 oz	60	14.0	<1.0	310	0	<1.0	0.2	25	<13%
w/o salt, drained	3 oz	111	25.1	0.0	43	0	0.4	0.1	15	4%
w/o salt, drained	1 oz	37	8.4	0.0	14	0	0.1	<.1	(mq)	3%
w/o salt, drained, approx 6.3 oz	1 can	216	48.8	0.0	83	0	0.8	0.3	30	4%
WHITE										
In oil										
drained	3 oz	158	22.5	0.0	337	0	6.9	1.4	26	41%
drained, approx 6.3 oz	1 can	331	47.2	0.0	705	0	14.4	2.9	55	41%
w/o salt, drained	3 oz	158	22.5	0.0	43	0	6.9	1.4	26	41%
w/o salt, drained, approx 6.3 oz	1 can	331	47.2	0.0	89	0	14.4	2.9	55	41%
In soybean oil										
chunk, drained	1 oz	53	7.5	0.0	112	0	2.3	(mq)	9	41%
chunk, drained *(A&P)*	2 oz	150	13.0	<1.0	310	0	10.0	(mq)	(mq)	62%
chunk, drained *(Bumble Bee)*	2 oz	110	12.0	0.0	310	0	12.0	3.0	30	69%
chunk, drained *(Star-Kist)*	2 oz	140	14.0	<1.0	310	0	10.0	1.0	25	60%
solid, albacore, drained *(Bumble Bee)*	2 oz	100	14.0	0.0	310	0	8.0	2.0	30	56%
solid, albacore, drained *(Finast)*	2 oz	145	14.0	<1.0	320	0	10.0	(mq)	(mq)	60%
solid, albacore, drained *(S&W)*	2 oz	160	13.0	0.0	450	0	12.0	(mq)	(mq)	68%
solid, albacore, drained *(Star-Kist)*	2 oz	140	14.0	<1.0	310	0	10.0	1.0	25	60%

Food Name	Serving Size	Calories	Prot. gms	Carbs gms	Sod. mgs	Fiber gms	Fat gms	Sat. Fat gms	Chol. mgs	% Fat Cal.
w/o salt, drained	1 oz	53	7.5	0.0	14	0	2.3	(mq)	0	41%
In spring water, solid, fancy albacore (Chicken of the Sea)	2 oz	60	14.0	<1.0	250	na	1.0	na	na	13%
In water										
chunk, diet, drained (Star-Kist)	2 oz	70	15.0	<1.0	30	0	1.0	0.2	25	12%
chunk, drained (A&P)	2 oz	100	12.0	<1.0	310	0	5.0	(mq)	(mq)	46%
chunk, drained (Bumble Bee)	2 oz	60	12.0	0.0	310	0	2.0	1.0	30	27%
chunk '60% Less Salt' drained (Star-Kist)	2 oz	70	15.0	<1.0	120	0	<1.0	0.2	25	<12%
drained	3 oz	116	22.7	0.0	333	0	2.1	0.6	36	17%
drained, approx 6.1 oz	1 can	234	45.9	0.0	674	0	4.2	1.1	72	17%
solid, albacore, drained (A&P)	2 oz	70	15.0	<1.0	310	0	<1.0	(mq)	(mq)	<12%
solid, albacore, drained (Bumble Bee)	2 oz	60	14.0	0.0	310	0	2.0	1.0	30	24%
solid, albacore, drained (Finast)	2 oz	70	15.0	<1.0	310	0	1.0	(mq)	(mq)	12%
solid, albacore, drained (Pathmark)	2 oz	70	15.0	0.0	310	0	2.0	(mq)	(mq)	23%
solid, albacore, drained (Star-Kist)	2 oz	70	15.0	<1.0	310	0	1.0	0.2	25	12%
solid, albacore, drained (Weight Watchers)	2 oz	70	15.0	<1.0	210	0	1.0	0.2	25	12%
w/o salt, drained	3 oz	116	22.7	0.0	43	0	2.1	0.6	36	17%
w/o salt, drained	1 oz	39	7.6	0.0	14	0	0.7	0.2	12	17%
w/o salt, drained, approx 6.1 oz	1 can	234	45.9	0.0	86	0	4.2	1.1	72	17%
TUNA, FROZEN										
(Peter Pan Seafoods) albacore, white, steaks, skinless, boneless, raw	3.5 oz	102	18.8	na	51	na	4.9	na	54	37%
(Peter Pan Seafoods) yellowfin, steaks, skinless, boneless, raw	3.5 oz	131	23.4	na	61	na	4.1	na	45	28%
(SeaPak) steak, w/o seasoning mix	6-oz pkg	180	40.0	0.0	65	0	2.0	(mq)	75	10%
TUNA, SKIPJACK / aku / arctic bonito / katsuo / oceanic bonito. See also BONITO.										
dry-heat cooked	3 oz	112	24.0	0.0	40	0	1.1	0.4	51	9%
raw	1 lb	468	99.8	0.0	167	0	4.6	1.5	213	9%
raw	3 oz	88	18.7	0.0	31	0	0.9	0.3	40	10%
raw	1 oz	29	6.2	0.0	10	0	0.3	0.1	13	10%
raw, approx 7 oz	1/2 fillet	204	43.6	0.0	73	0	2.0	0.7	93	9%
TUNA, YELLOWFIN / ahi										
dry-heat cooked	3 oz	118	25.5	0.0	40	0	1.0	0.3	na	8%
raw	1 lb	492	106.0	0.0	168	0	4.3	1.1	203	8%
raw	3 oz	92	19.9	0.0	31	0	0.8	0.2	38	8%
raw	1 oz	31	6.6	0.0	10	0	0.3	0.1	13	9%
TUNA ENTRÉE, FROZEN										
noodle casserole (Stouffer's)	10 oz	280	17.0	33.0	1090	na	15.0	na	na	40%
noodle casserole (Weight Watchers)	9 oz	230	15.0	27.0	550	na	7.0	2.0	20	27%
pie (Banquet)	7 oz	540	17.0	44.0	810	(mq)	33.0	(mq)	30	55%
TUNA ENTRÉE, MIX										
au gratin, dry mix (Tuna Helper)	1/5 pkg	180	6.0	27.0	800	(mq)	5.0	(mq)	na	25%
buttery rice, dry mix (Tuna Helper)	1/5 pkg	160	4.0	32.0	830	(mq)	2.0	(mq)	na	11%
cheesy noodle, dry mix (Tuna Helper)	1/5 pkg	160	5.0	27.0	810	(mq)	4.0	(mq)	na	22%
creamy broccoli, dry mix (Tuna Helper)	1/5 pkg	200	6.0	35.0	800	na	4.0	na	na	18%
fettuccine Alfredo, dry mix (Tuna Helper)	1/5 pkg	160	6.0	28.0	760	(mq)	3.0	(mq)	na	17%
mushroom, creamy, dry mix (Tuna Helper)	1/5 pkg	140	5.0	28.0	580	(mq)	1.0	na	na	6%
noodle, creamy, dry mix (Tuna Helper)	1/5 pkg	210	5.0	29.0	790	(mq)	8.0	(mq)	na	35%
pot pie, dry mix (Tuna Helper)	1/6 pkg	290	4.0	31.0	730	(mq)	17.0	(mq)	na	52%
salad, dry mix (Tuna Helper)	1/5 pkg	140	5.0	28.0	580	(mq)	1.0	na	na	6%
tetrazzini, dry mix (Tuna Helper)	1/5 pkg	160	6.0	26.0	620	(mq)	3.0	(mq)	na	17%
TUNA LUNCH KIT										
'Charlie's Lunch Kit' w/1 mayo packet (Star-Kist)	4.6 oz	290	24.0	16.0	780	na	15.0	na	na	46%
'Charlie's Lunch Kit' w/2 mayo packets (Star-Kist)	5 oz	370	24.0	16.0	845	na	15.0	na	na	46%

Food Name	Serving Size	Calories	Prot. gms	Carbs gms	Sod. mgs	Fiber gms	Fat gms	Sat. Fat gms	Chol. mgs	% Fat Cal.
TUNA MIX										
classic Italian 'Tuna Mix-ins' dry mix *(Bumble Bee)*	1 oz	25	0.0	5.0	5	na	0.0	na	0	0%
garden and herb 'Tuna Mix-ins' dry mix *(Bumble Bee)*	1 oz	25	0.0	5.0	5	na	0.0	na	0	0%
lemon herb 'Tuna Mix-ins' dry mix *(Bumble Bee)*	1 oz	25	0.0	6.0	5	na	0.0	na	0	0%
zesty tomato 'Tuna Mix-ins' dry mix *(Bumble Bee)*	1 oz	25	0.0	5.0	5	na	0.0	na	0	0%
TUNA SALAD										
(Longacre)	1 oz	58	2.0	3.0	130	na	4.0	(mq)	10	64%
(Longacre) 'Saladfest'	1 oz	52	3.0	2.0	180	na	4.0	(mq)	10	64%
TUNA SALAD SPREAD *(Libby's)* 'Spreadables'	1.9 oz	80	5.0	5.0	220	1.9	5.0	1.0	na	53%
TUNKA. See GOURD, WHITE.										
TURBOT, DOMESTIC										
raw	1 lb	845	65.2	0.0	363	0	62.8	11.0	209	68%
raw	1 oz	53	4.1	0.0	23	0	3.9	0.7	13	68%
raw, approx 7.2 oz	1/2 fillet	380	29.3	0.0	163	0	28.2	4.9	94	68%
TURBOT, EUROPEAN										
dry-heat cooked	3 oz	104	17.5	0.0	163	0	3.2	na	53	29%
raw	1 lb	432	72.8	0.0	678	0	13.4	(mq)	(mq)	29%
raw	3 oz	81	13.6	0.0	127	0	2.5	0.6	41	29%
raw	1 oz	27	4.6	0.0	43	0	0.8	(mq)	(mq)	28%
raw, approx 7.2 oz	1/2 fillet	194	32.7	0.0	306	0	6.0	1.5	98	29%
TURKEY, ALL CLASSES										
BACK MEAT W/SKIN										
raw	1 lb	896	81.6	0.0	304	0	59.2	16.0	336	62%
raw	1 oz	56	5.1	0.0	19	0	3.7	1.0	21	62%
roasted	4 oz	276	30.2	0.0	83	0	16.3	4.7	103	55%
BREAST MEAT W/SKIN										
raw	1 lb	720	99.2	0.0	272	0	32.0	8.0	288	42%
raw	1 oz	45	6.2	0.0	17	0	2.0	0.5	18	42%
roasted	4 oz	214	32.6	0.0	71	0	8.4	2.4	84	37%
DARK MEAT ONLY										
raw	1 lb	560	91.2	0.0	352	0	19.2	6.4	320	32%
raw	1 oz	35	5.7	0.0	22	0	1.2	0.4	20	32%
roasted	1 cup	262	40.0	0.0	111	0	10.1	3.4	119	36%
roasted	4 oz	212	32.4	0.0	90	0	8.2	2.7	96	36%
DARK MEAT W/SKIN										
raw	1 lb	720	86.4	0.0	320	0	40.0	11.2	320	51%
raw	1 oz	45	5.4	0.0	20	0	2.5	0.7	20	51%
roasted	4 oz	251	31.2	0.0	86	0	13.1	4.0	101	49%
LEG MEAT W/SKIN										
raw	1 lb	656	88.0	0.0	336	0	30.4	9.6	320	44%
raw	1 oz	41	5.5	0.0	21	0	1.9	0.6	20	44%
roasted	4 oz	236	31.6	0.0	87	0	11.1	3.5	96	44%
LIGHT MEAT ONLY										
raw	1 lb	528	107.2	0.0	288	0	6.4	1.6	272	12%
raw	1 oz	33	6.7	0.0	18	0	0.4	0.1	17	12%
roasted	4 oz	178	33.9	0.0	73	0	3.7	1.2	78	20%
roasted, diced	1 cup	220	41.9	0.0	90	0	4.5	1.4	97	20%
LIGHT MEAT W/SKIN										
raw	1 lb	72.0	97.6	0.0	272	0	33.6	9.6	288	44%
raw	1 oz	45	6.1	0.0	17	0	2.1	0.6	18	44%
roasted	4 oz	223	32.4	0.0	71	0	9.4	2.7	86	40%
NECK MEAT ONLY										
raw	1 lb	608	91.2	0.0	416	0	24.0	8.0	352	37%
raw	1 oz	38	5.7	0.0	26	0	1.5	0.5	22	37%

Food Name	Serving Size	Calories	Prot. gms	Carbs gms	Sod. mgs	Fiber gms	Fat gms	Sat. Fat gms	Chol. mgs	% Fat Cal.
simmered	4 oz	204	30.4	0.0	64	0	8.2	2.8	100	00%
SKIN ONLY
raw	1 lb	1760	57.6	0.0	160	0	168.0	43.2	576	87%
raw	1 oz	110	3.6	0.0	10	0	10.5	2.7	26	87%
roasted	1 oz	125	5.6	0.0	15	0	11.2	2.9	32	82%
WING MEAT W/SKIN
raw	1 lb	896	91.2	0.0	256	0	56.0	14.4	320	58%
raw	1 oz	56	5.7	0.0	16	0	3.5	0.9	20	58%
roasted	4 oz	260	31.0	0.0	69	0	14.1	3.8	92	51%
TURKEY, ALTERNATIVE
(Worthington) roll, smoked, frozen	4 slices	180	13.0	5.0	820	(mq)	12.0	(mq)	0	60%
(Worthington) sliced, smoked, frozen	4 slices	180	13.0	5.0	820	(mq)	12.0	(mq)	0	60%
(Worthington) 'Turkee Slices' canned	2 slices	130	9.0	3.0	430	(mq)	9.0	(mq)	0	63%
(Worthington) '209' canned, drained	2 slices	120	8.0	3.0	(mq)	(mq)	8.0	(mq)	0	62%
TURKEY, BONELESS. See also LUNCHEON MEAT.
BREAST
(Butterball) 'Slice 'n Serve'	1 oz	35	5.0	<1.0	230	0	1.0	(mq)	(mq)	27%
(Longacre) 'Gourmet'	1 oz	35	5.0	1.0	300	0	1.0	(mq)	15	27%
(Longacre) 'Gourmet Low Salt'	1 oz	30	6.0	1.0	150	0	<1.0	(mq)	10	<24%
(Longacre) 'Premium'	1 oz	30	4.0	1.0	250	0	1.0	(mq)	10	31%
(Longacre) 'Salt Watchers'	1 oz	32	7.0	0.0	10	0	<1.0	(mq)	15	<24%
(Mr. Turkey)	1 oz	31	5.8	0.3	233	0	0.7	(mq)	10	21%
Barbecue seasoned *(Butterball)* Slice 'n Serve	1 oz	40	5.0	1.0	210	0	2.0	(mq)	(mq)	43%
Browned
(Longacre) glazed 'Gourmet'	1 oz	35	5.0	1.0	240	0	1.0	(mq)	15	27%
(Longacre) glazed 'Premium'	1 oz	30	4.0	1.0	300	0	1.0	(mq)	10	31%
(Longacre) roasted 'Gourmet'	1 oz	35	5.0	1.0	260	0	1.0	(mq)	15	27%
(Longacre) roasted 'Premium'	1 oz	30	4.0	1.0	300	0	1.0	(mq)	10	31%
Golden
(Boar's Head)	1 oz	35	6.0	<1.0	200	0	1.0	(mq)	20	24%
(Boar's Head) skinless	1 oz	30	6.0	<1.0	(mq)	0	<1.0	(mq)	10	<24%
Hickory smoked *(Butterball)* 'Slice 'n Serve'	1 oz	35	5.0	1.0	250	0	1.0	(mq)	(mq)	27%
Honey roasted *(Louis Rich)*	1 oz	32	4.9	1.2	315	0	0.8	0.3	11	23%
Lean, lite
(Longacre) 'Deli'	1 oz	35	6.0	0.0	160	0	1.0	(mq)	15	27%
(Longacre) skinless 'Deli'	1 oz	35	6.0	0.0	160	0	<1.0	(mq)	15	<27%
(Longacre) smoked 'Deli'	1 oz	35	6.0	0.0	160	0	1.0	(mq)	15	27%
Skinless
(Longacre) 'Catering'	1 oz	35	6.0	<1.0	280	0	<1.0	(mq)	15	<24%
(Longacre) 'Gourmet'	1 oz	30	5.0	1.0	260	0	<1.0	(mq)	15	<27%
(Longacre) 'Premium'	1 oz	30	4.0	1.0	250	0	<1.0	(mq)	10	<31%
(Norbest) 'Blue Label'	1 oz	26	5.1	0.4	252	0	0.4	(mq)	(mq)	14%
(Norbest) 'Norfresh'	1 oz	27	5.2	0.5	269	0	0.3	(mq)	(mq)	11%
(Norbest) 'Norfresh Blue Label'	1 oz	24	4.4	0.7	253	0	0.3	(mq)	(mq)	12%
(Norbest) 'Norfresh Yellow Label'	1 oz	24	4.4	0.4	284	0	0.5	(mq)	(mq)	19%
(Norbest) 'Orange Label'	1 oz	26	5.1	0.5	239	0	0.2	(mq)	(mq)	7%
(Norbest) salt-free 'Blue Label'	1 oz	33	7.7	<.1	13	0	0.3	(mq)	(mq)	8%
(Norbest) 'Tan Label'	1 oz	24	4.3	0.5	354	0	0.5	(mq)	(mq)	19%
(Norbest) 'Yellow Label'	1 oz	26	4.3	0.8	272	0	0.5	(mq)	(mq)	18%
Smoked
(Healthy Deli) 'Gourmet'	1 oz	31	5.8	0.4	170	0	0.5	(mq)	11	15%
(Hormel) 'Perma-Fresh'	2 slices	60	10.0	0.0	540	0	2.0	(mq)	(mq)	31%
(Longacre)	1 oz	35	6.0	0.0	240	0	1.0	(mq)	15	27%
(Norbest) 'Gold Label'	1 oz	29	6.4	0.1	270	0	<.6	(mq)	(mq)	<17%

Food Name	Serving Size	Calories	Prot. gms	Carbs gms	Sod. mgs	Fiber gms	Fat gms	Sat. Fat gms	Chol. mgs	% Fat Cal.
(OHSE)	1 oz	30	5.0	1.0	340	0	1.0	(mq)	(mq)	27%
W/skin										
(Norbest) 'Blue Label'	1 oz	28	5.1	0.2	239	0	0.7	(mq)	(mq)	23%
(Norbest) 'Norfresh Orange Label'	1 oz	26	5.3	0.1	256	0	0.3	(mq)	(mq)	11%
(Norbest) 'Norfresh Yellow Label'	1 oz	25	4.8	0.1	244	0	0.5	(mq)	(mq)	19%
(Norbest) 'Orange Label'	1 oz	28	5.7	0.1	232	0	0.3	(mq)	(mq)	10%
(Norbest) prebrowned 'Orange Label'	1 oz	29	5.1	0.2	259	0	0.8	(mq)	(mq)	25%
(Norbest) salt-free 'Blue Label'	1 oz	35	7.5	0.2	13	0	0.5	(mq)	(mq)	13%
(Norbest) smoked 'Orange Label'	1 oz	30	5.3	0.9	284	0	0.5	(mq)	(mq)	15%
(Norbest) 'Yellow Label'	1 oz	26	5.1	0.1	271	0	0.4	(mq)	(mq)	15%
BREAST AND LIGHT MEAT										
(Longacre) browned and roasted	1 oz	40	5.0	1.0	240	0	2.0	(mq)	15	43%
(Longacre) 'Deli Chef'	1 oz	35	5.0	1.0	240	0	1.0	(mq)	15	27%
(Longacre) skinless 'Deli Chef'	1 oz	40	4.0	1.0	240	0	2.0	(mq)	15	47%
BREAST AND THIGH (Norbest) 'Blue Label'	1 oz	31	5.8	0.2	238	0	0.9	(mq)	(mq)	25%
DARK MEAT (Norbest) ham flavor, hickory smoked	1 oz	39	4.6	0.1	335	0	2.2	(mq)	(mq)	51%
OVEN COOKED (OHSE)	1 oz	30	5.0	1.0	190	0	1.0	(mq)	(mq)	27%
ROLL										
(Norbest) white meat 'Orange Label'	1 oz	29	4.1	0.5	299	0	0.9	(mq)	(mq)	31%
(Norbest) white and dark meat 'Orange Label'	1 oz	36	4.0	0.3	314	0	2.0	(mq)	(mq)	51%
SMOKED (Louis Rich)	1 oz	32	5.4	0.4	284	0	1.0	0.4	14	28%
W/PORK (Healthy Favorites) 'Breakfast Strips'	11 grams	18	1.8	0.4	145	0	1.0	0.3	9	51%
TURKEY, CANNED										
(Hormel) chunk	6.75 oz	230	37.0	0.0	1278	0	10.0	(mq)	(mq)	38%
(Hormel) chunk	2.5 oz	80	13.0	1.0	420	0	3.0	1.0	45	33%
(Swanson) white	2.5 oz	80	17.0	1.0	260	0	1.0	na	(mq)	11%
(Tyson) 'Wholesale Club Item'	3.5 oz	120	23.0	0.0	360	na	3.0	na	na	23%
TURKEY, FROZEN/REFRIGERATED										
BREAST										
Cooked										
(Land O'Lakes)	3 oz	100	20.0	0.0	55	0	1.0	<1.0	50	10%
(Longacre) 'Cook-N-Bag'	1 oz	38	8.0	<1.0	85	0	<1.0	(mq)	15	<20%
(Louis Rich)	1 oz	47	8.1	0.1	21	0	1.5	0.6	21	29%
(Louis Rich) barbecue	1 oz	33	5.3	0.9	315	0	1.0	0.3	12	27%
(Louis Rich) hen, w/o wings	1 oz	50	7.9	0.1	19	0	2.0	0.4	19	36%
(Louis Rich) hickory smoked	1 oz	33	5.4	0.8	346	0	1.0	0.3	13	27%
(Louis Rich) honey roasted	1 oz	33	5.3	1.1	318	0	0.8	0.3	12	22%
(Louis Rich) oven roasted	1 oz	31	5.3	0.4	296	0	0.9	0.2	13	26%
(Louis Rich) roast	1 oz	42	8.3	0.2	20	0	0.8	0.3	19	18%
(Louis Rich) slices	1 oz	39	8.4	0.1	24	0	0.5	0.1	17	12%
(Louis Rich) smoked	1 oz	33	5.7	0.2	268	0	1.0	0.4	11	28%
(Louis Rich) steaks	1 oz	39	8.4	0.1	24	0	0.5	0.1	17	12%
(Louis Rich) tenderloins	1 oz	39	8.5	0.2	24	0	0.5	0.2	18	12%
(Mr. Turkey) barbecue, quarter 'Chub'	1 oz	34	5.4	1.0	251	0	1.0	(mq)	11	26%
(Mr. Turkey) oven roasted, quarter 'Chub'	1 oz	34	5.8	0.4	266	0	1.0	(mq)	12	27%
(Mr. Turkey) smoked, quarter 'Chub'	1 oz	35	6.1	0.3	263	0	1.0	(mq)	10	26%
(Tyson) skinless, boneless 'Wholesale Club Item'	3.5 oz	160	30.0	0.0	65	na	3.0	na	70	18%
w/skin, roasted, broth pre-basted	4 oz	143	25.1	0.0	450	0	3.9	1.1	48	26%
Raw										
(Longacre) 'Cook-N-Bag'	1 oz	27	6.0	<1.0	120	0	<1.0	(mq)	10	<24%
(Longacre) 'Ready-to-Cook'	1 oz	39	8.0	0.0	150	0	<1.0	(mq)	(mq)	<22%
(Norbest) steaks, cubed	4 oz	135	27.8	<.1	81	0	2.0	(mq)	(mq)	14%
(Norbest) strips and tips 'Tasti-Lean'	4 oz	135	27.8	<.1	81	0	2.0	(mq)	(mq)	14%
(Norbest) tenderloin 'Tasti-Lean Tenders'	4 oz	135	27.8	<.1	81	0	2.0	(mq)	(mq)	14%

Food Name	Serving Size	Calories	Prot. gms	Carbs gms	Sod. mgs	Fiber gms	Fat gms	Sat. Fat gms	Chol. mgs	% Fat Cal.
(Norbest) w/gravy	4 oz	115	20.7	1.1	492	0	2.4	(mq)	(mq)	20%
CUTLET (Norbest) raw 'Tasti-Lean'	4 oz	135	27.8	<.1	81	0	2.0	(mq)	(mq)	14%
DARK MEAT (Butterball) w/o skin, roasted, approx 3.5 oz	2 slices	195	25.0	na	90	0	10.0	(mq)	130	47%
DRUMSTICK										
(Land O'Lakes)	3 oz	120	17.0	0.0	85	0	5.0	2.0	(mq)	40%
(Louis Rich) cooked	1 oz	56	7.9	0.1	22	0	2.6	0.9	27	42%
(Louis Rich) cooked 'Fresh Turkey Cuts'	1 oz	55	8.0	<1.0	25	na	3.0	na	30	43%
HINDQUARTER ROAST (Land O'Lakes)	3 oz	140	17.0	0.0	80	0	8.0	3.0	(mq)	51%
LIGHT AND DARK MEAT										
roasted, then seasoned	4 oz	176	24.2	3.5	771	na	6.6	(mq)	(mq)	35%
seasoned raw, then roasted	1 lb	544	79.8	29.0	3075	na	10.0	(mq)	(mq)	17%
seasoned raw, then roasted	1 oz	34	5.0	1.8	192	na	0.6	(mq)	(mq)	17%
(Butterball) w/skin, roasted, approx 3.5 oz	2 slices	195	27.0	na	115	0	10.0	(mq)	100	46%
LIGHT MEAT (Butterball) w/o skin, roasted, approx 3.5 oz	2 slices	160	30.0	na	130	0	4.0	(mq)	80	23%
THIGH										
w/skin, roasted, pre-basted w/broth	4 oz	178	21.3	0.0	496	0	9.7	3.0	70	51%
(Land O'Lakes)	3 oz	150	17.0	0.0	75	0	10.0	4.0	(mq)	57%
(Louis Rich) cooked	1 oz	64	7.5	0.1	20	0	3.7	1.0	27	52%
(Louis Rich) cooked 'Fresh Turkey Cuts'	1 oz	65	7.0	<1.0	20	na	4.0	na	30	53%
WHOLE										
(Louis Rich) w/o giblets, cooked	1 oz	52	7.7	0.1	23	0	2.3	0.7	22	40%
(Louis Rich) w/o giblets, cooked 'Fresh Whole Turkey'	1 oz	50	8.0	<1.0	25	na	2.0	na	25	33%
(Norbest) boneless, cooked	1 oz	42	6.2	0.3	105	0	1.5	(mq)	(mq)	34%
(Norbest) boneless, smoked, cooked	1 oz	42	6.4	0.3	218	0	1.6	(mq)	(mq)	35%
WING										
(Land O'Lakes)	3 oz	120	18.0	0.0	65	0	5.0	2.0	(mq)	39%
(Louis Rich) cooked	1 oz	54	7.2	0.1	20	0	2.7	0.8	31	45%
(Louis Rich) cooked 'Drumettes'	1 oz	51	7.8	0.1	20	0	2.2	0.7	29	39%
(Louis Rich) cooked 'Fresh Turkey Cuts'	1 oz	55	7.0	<1.0	20	na	3.0	na	30	46%
(Louis Rich) drumettes, cooked 'Fresh Turkey Cuts'	1 oz	50	8.0	<1.0	20	na	2.0	na	30	33%
(Louis Rich) portions, cooked	1 oz	54	6.9	0.1	17	0	2.9	0.7	29	48%
(Louis Rich) portions, cooked 'Fresh Turkey Cuts'	1 oz	55	7.0	<1.0	20	na	3.0	na	30	46%
W/GRAVY (Norbest) raw	4 oz	115	20.3	1.1	600	0	2.7	(mq)	(mq)	22%
YOUNG										
(Land O'Lakes)	3 oz	130	17.0	<1.0	55	0	7.0	2.0	65	47%
(Land O'Lakes) butter-basted	3 oz	140	17.0	<1.0	135	0	8.0	3.0	85	50%
(Land O'Lakes) self-basting, w/broth	3 oz	120	18.0	<1.0	145	0	5.0	2.0	77	37%
TURKEY, FRYER-ROASTER										
BACK MEAT ONLY										
raw	1 lb	544	94.4	0.0	288	0	16.0	4.8	336	28%
raw	1 oz	34	5.9	0.0	18	0	1.0	0.3	21	28%
roasted	4 oz	193	31.8	0.0	83	0	6.4	2.1	108	31%
BACK MEAT W/SKIN										
raw	1 lb	688	89.6	0.0	272	0	336.0	9.6	384	46%
raw	1 oz	43	5.6	0.0	17	0	2.1	0.6	24	46%
roasted	4 oz	231	29.7	0.0	79	0	11.6	3.4	122	47%
BREAST MEAT ONLY										
raw	1 lb	496	112.0	0.0	224	0	3.2	1.6	288	6%
raw	1 oz	31	7.0	0.0	14	0	0.2	0.1	18	6%
roasted	4 oz	153	34.1	0.0	59	0	0.8	0.3	94	5%
BREAST MEAT W/SKIN										
raw	1 lb	560	107.2	0.0	224	0	12.8	3.2	320	21%
raw	1 oz	35	6.7	0.0	14	0	0.8	0.2	20	21%
roasted	4 oz	174	33.0	0.0	60	0	3.6	1.0	102	20%

Food Name	Serving Size	Calories	Prot. gms	Carbs gms	Sod. mgs	Fiber gms	Fat gms	Sat. Fat gms	Chol. mgs	% Fat Cal.
DARK MEAT ONLY										
raw	1 lb	496	92.8	0.0	320	0	12.8	4.8	368	24%
raw	1 oz	31	5.8	0.0	20	0	0.8	0.3	23	24%
roasted	4 oz	184	32.7	0.0	90	0	4.9	1.6	127	25%
roasted, diced	1 cup	227	40.4	0.0	111	0	6.0	2.0	157	25%
DARK MEAT W/SKIN										
raw	1 lb	592	91.2	0.0	304	0	22.4	6.4	400	36%
raw	1 oz	37	5.7	0.0	19	0	1.4	0.4	25	36%
roasted	4 oz	206	31.4	0.0	86	0	8.0	2.4	133	36%
LEG MEAT ONLY										
raw	1 lb	496	92.8	0.0	320	0	11.2	3.2	384	21%
raw	1 oz	31	5.8	0.0	20	0	0.7	0.2	24	21%
roasted	4 oz	180	33.1	0.0	92	0	4.3	1.4	135	23%
LEG MEAT W/SKIN										
raw	1 lb	528	91.2	0.0	320	0	16.0	4.8	400	28%
raw	1 oz	33	5.7	0.0	20	0	1.0	0.3	25	28%
roasted	4 oz	193	32.3	0.0	91	0	6.1	1.9	79	30%
LIGHT MEAT ONLY										
raw	1 lb	496	110.4	0.0	240	0	1.6	<1.6	304	3%
raw	1 oz	31	6.9	0.0	15	0	0.1	<.1	19	3%
roasted	4 oz	159	34.2	0.0	64	0	1.3	0.4	98	8%
roasted, diced	1 cup	196	42.3	0.0	78	0	1.6	0.5	120	8%
LIGHT MEAT W/SKIN										
raw	1 lb	608	104.0	0.0	224	0	17.6	4.8	352	28%
raw	1 oz	38	6.5	0.0	14	0	1.1	0.3	22	28%
roasted	4 oz	186	32.6	0.0	65	0	5.2	1.4	108	26%
SKIN ONLY										
raw	1 lb	1280	75.2	0.0	160	0	107.2	27.2	624	70%
raw	1 oz	80	4.7	0.0	10	0	6.7	1.7	39	76%
WING MEAT ONLY										
raw	1 lb	480	102.4	0.0	288	0	4.8	1.6	368	10%
raw	1 oz	30	6.4	0.0	18	0	0.3	0.1	23	10%
roasted	4 oz	185	35.0	0.0	88	0	3.9	1.2	116	20%
WING MEAT W/SKIN										
raw	1 lb	720	94.4	0.0	256	0	35.2	9.6	448	46%
raw	1 oz	45	5.9	0.0	16	0	2.2	0.6	28	46%
roasted	4 oz	235	31.4	0.0	83	0	11.2	3.1	130	45%
TURKEY, GROUND										
Cooked										
	4 oz	260	27.7	0.0	94	0	15.6	4.3	78	56%
approx 2.9 oz	1 patty	193	22.4	0.0	88	0	10.8	2.8	84	52%
yield from 1 lb raw	11.6 oz	754	80.4	0.0	273	0	45.5	12.4	227	56%
(Hudson's)	1 oz	55	5.0	0.0	35	0	3.7	(mq)	(mq)	63%
(Longacre)	1 oz	60	5.0	0.0	20	0	4.0	(mq)	30	64%
(Louis Rich) 85% fat-free	1 oz	60	7.0	<1.0	30	na	3.0	na	30	46%
(Louis Rich) 90% fat-free	1 oz	50	7.0	<1.0	30	na	3.0	na	25	46%
(Louis Rich) 90% fat-free, natural flavorings	1 oz	50	7.0	<1.0	35	na	2.0	na	25	36%
(Mr. Turkey)	1 oz	54	4.5	0.0	27	0	4.0	(mq)	20	67%
Raw										
	1 lb	676	79.2	0.0	426	0	37.5	10.2	358	52%
	1 oz	40	4.9	0.0	27	0	2.1	0.6	21	49%
(Norbest)	1 oz	45	5.2	0.1	34	0	2.6	(mq)	(mq)	53%
(Louis Rich) w/natural flavoring	1 oz	50	7.5	0.0	33	0	2.2	0.7	24	40%

Food Name	Serving Size	Calories	Prot. gms	Carbs gms	Sod. mgs	Fiber gms	Fat gms	Sat. Fat gms	Chol. mgs	% Fat Cal.
TURKEY, YOUNG HEN										
BACK MEAT W/SKIN										
raw	1 lb	992	80.0	0.0	272	0	72.0	20.8	304	67%
raw	1 oz	62	5.0	0.0	17	0	4.5	1.3	19	67%
roasted	4 oz	288	29.9	0.0	78	0	17.7	5.1	96	57%
BREAST MEAT W/SKIN										
raw	1 lb	752	97.6	0.0	256	0	38.4	9.6	288	47%
raw	1 oz	47	6.1	0.0	16	0	2.4	0.6	18	47%
roasted	4 oz	220	32.7	0.0	66	0	8.9	2.6	82	38%
DARK MEAT ONLY										
raw	1 lb	592	91.2	0.0	336	0	22.4	8.0	288	36%
raw	1 oz	37	5.7	0.0	21	0	1.4	0.5	18	36%
roasted	4 oz	218	32.2	0.0	85	0	8.8	3.0	91	38%
roasted, diced	1 cup	269	39.8	0.0	105	0	10.9	3.7	112	38%
DARK MEAT W/SKIN										
raw	1 lb	784	84.8	0.0	304	0	46.4	12.8	288	55%
raw	1 oz	49	5.3	0.0	19	0	2.9	0.8	18	55%
roasted	4 oz	263	31.0	0.0	82	0	14.5	4.4	95	51%
LEG MEAT W/SKIN										
raw	1 lb	688	88.0	0.0	320	0	33.6	9.6	288	46%
raw	1 oz	43	5.5	0.0	20	0	2.1	0.6	18	46%
roasted	4 oz	242	31.4	0.0	83	0	11.9	3.7	93	46%
LIGHT MEAT ONLY										
raw	1 lb	528	107.2	0.0	272	0	8.0	3.2	256	14%
raw	1 oz	33	6.7	0.0	17	0	0.5	0.2	16	14%
roasted	4 oz	183	33.9	0.0	68	0	4.2	1.3	77	22%
roasted, diced	1 cup	225	41.8	0.0	84	0	5.2	1.7	95	22%
LIGHT MEAT W/SKIN										
raw	1 lb	752	97.6	0.0	256	0	36.8	9.6	288	46%
raw	1 oz	47	6.1	0.0	16	0	2.3	0.6	18	46%
roasted	4 oz	235	32.5	0.0	66	0	10.7	3.0	84	43%
SKIN ONLY										
roasted	1 oz	137	5.4	0.0	12	0	12.6	3.3	30	84%
WING MEAT W/SKIN										
raw	1 lb	960	91.2	0.0	224	0	62.4	16.0	288	61%
raw	1 oz	60	5.7	0.0	14	0	3.9	1.0	18	61%
roasted	4 oz	270	31.0	0.0	64	0	15.3	4.2	87	53%
TURKEY, YOUNG TOM										
BACK MEAT W/SKIN										
raw	1 lb	81.6	83.2	0.0	320	0	51.2	14.4	352	58%
raw	1 oz	51	5.2	0.0	20	0	3.2	0.9	22	58%
roasted	4 oz	270	30.4	0.0	87	0	15.5	4.5	107	53%
BREAST MEAT W/SKIN										
raw	1 lb	688	99.2	0.0	288	0	28.8	8.0	112	40%
raw	1 oz	43	6.2	0.0	18	0	1.8	0.5	7	40%
roasted	4 oz	214	32.4	0.0	76	0	8.4	2.4	85	37%
DARK MEAT ONLY										
raw	1 lb	560	91.2	0.0	368	0	19.2	6.4	336	32%
raw	1 oz	35	5.7	0.0	23	0	1.2	0.4	21	32%
roasted	4 oz	210	32.5	0.0	93	0	7.9	2.7	100	35%
roasted, diced	1 cup	259	40.1	0.0	115	0	9.8	3.3	123	36%
DARK MEAT W/SKIN										
raw	1 lb	688	86.4	0.0	336	0	35.2	11.2	352	48%
raw	1 oz	43	5.4	0.0	21	0	2.2	0.7	22	48%

Food Name	Serving Size	Calories	Prot. gms	Carbs gms	Sod. mgs	Fiber gms	Fat gms	Sat. Fat gms	Chol. mgs	% Fat Cal.
roasted	4 oz	245	31.3	0.0	91	0	12.3	3.7	103	47%
LEG MEAT W/SKIN										
raw	1 lb	640	88.0	0.0	352	0	28.8	8.0	352	42%
raw	1 oz	40	5.5	0.0	22	0	1.8	0.5	22	42%
roasted	4 oz	234	31.7	0.0	91	0	10.9	3.4	102	44%
LIGHT MEAT ONLY										
raw	1 lb	512	105.6	0.0	304	0	6.4	1.6	288	12%
raw	1 oz	32	6.6	0.0	19	0	0.4	0.1	18	12%
roasted	4 oz	175	33.9	0.0	77	0	3.3	1.1	78	18%
roasted, diced	1 cup	216	41.8	0.0	95	0	4.1	1.3	97	18%
LIGHT MEAT W/SKIN										
raw	1 lb	704	97.6	0.0	288	0	32.0	8.0	304	41%
raw	1 oz	44	6.1	0.0	18	0	2.0	0.5	19	43%
roasted	4 oz	217	32.3	0.0	76	0	8.7	2.4	85	38%
SKIN ONLY										
raw	1 lb	1664	60.8	0.0	176	0	157.0	42.0	432	85%
raw	1 oz	104	3.8	0.0	11	0	9.8	2.6	27	85%
roasted	1 oz	120	5.7	0.0	17	0	10.6	2.8	33	81%
WING MEAT W/SKIN										
raw	1 lb	848	92.8	0.0	272	0	51.2	12.8	320	55%
raw	1 oz	53	5.8	0.0	17	0	3.2	0.8	20	55%
roasted	4 oz	251	31.1	0.0	75	0	13.0	3.5	92	49%
TURKEY BREAST										
BARBECUED *(Louis Rich)* skinless	1 oz	30	6.0	<1.0	280	na	<1.0	na	10	<24%
HONEY ROASTED										
(Louis Rich) 95% fat-free	1-oz slice	35	5.0	1.0	315	na	1.0	na	10	27%
(Louis Rich) skinless	1 oz	30	6.0	<1.0	295	na	<1.0	na	10	<24%
OVEN ROASTED										
(Louis Rich) 'Carving Board'	22 grams	21	4.5	0.1	272	0	0.3	0.1	9	13%
(Louis Rich) 'Fresh Turkey Cuts'	1 oz	45	8.0	<1.0	20	na	2.0	na	20	33%
(Louis Rich) 96% fat-free 'Deli-Thin'	1 slice	10	2.0	<1.0	130	na	<1.0	na	5	<43%
(Louis Rich) 97% fat-free	1-oz slice	30	5.0	1.0	315	na	<1.0	na	10	<27%
(Louis Rich) 97% fat-free 'Deli-Thin'	1 slice	10	2.0	<1.0	125	na	<1.0	na	5	<43%
(Louis Rich) roast 'Fresh Turkey Cuts'	1 oz	40	8.0	<1.0	20	na	<1.0	na	20	<20%
(Louis Rich) skinless	1 oz	25	6.0	<1.0	275	na	<1.0	na	10	<24%
(Louis Rich) slices 'Fresh Turkey Cuts'	1 oz	40	8.0	<1.0	25	na	<1.0	na	15	<20%
(Louis Rich) steaks 'Fresh Turkey Cuts'	1 oz	40	8.0	<1.0	25	na	<1.0	na	20	<20%
(Louis Rich) tenderloins 'Fresh Turkey Cuts'	1 oz	40	8.0	<1.0	25	na	<1.0	na	20	<20%
SMOKED										
(Louis Rich) 'Carving Board'	10 grams	9	2.0	0.1	124	0	0.1	0.0	4	10%
(Louis Rich) 96% fat-free	1 oz	35	6.0	<1.0	270	na	1.0	na	10	24%
(Louis Rich) 97% fat-free 'Deli-Thin'	1 slice	10	2.0	<1.0	110	na	<1.0	na	5	<43%
(Louis Rich) 98% fat-free	1-oz slice	20	4.0	<1.0	210	na	<1.0	na	10	<31%
(Louis Rich) skinless	1 oz	30	6.0	<1.0	330	na	<1.0	na	10	<24%
TURKEY DINNER, FROZEN										
(Banquet)	10.5 oz	390	18.0	35.0	1110	(mq)	20.0	(mq)	40	46%
(Banquet) 'Extra Helping'	19 oz	750	29.0	68.0	1980	(mq)	42.0	(mq)	65	49%
(Morton)	10 oz	230	15.0	28.0	1300	(mq)	6.0	(mq)	45	24%
(Swanson)	11.5 oz	350	21.0	42.0	1090	(mq)	11.0	(mq)	(mq)	28%
(Swanson) 'Hungry Man'	17 oz	550	36.0	61.0	1810	(mq)	18.0	(mq)	(mq)	30%
BREAST										
(Budget Gourmet) Dijon	11.2 oz	340	20.0	37.0	860	(mq)	12.0	(mq)	65	32%
(Budget Gourmet) sliced	11.1 oz	290	16.0	36.0	1200	(mq)	9.0	(mq)	45	28%
(Healthy Choice) medallions, w/vegetables 'Classics'	12.5 oz	350	29.0	45.0	480	na	6.0	3.0	60	15%

Food Name	Serving Size	Calories	Prot. gms	Carbs gms	Sod. mgs	Fiber gms	Fat gms	Sat. Fat gms	Chol. mgs	% Fat Cal.
(Le Menu) sliced, w/mushroom gravy	10.5 oz	300	22.0	38.0	1020	(mq)	7.0	(mq)	(mq)	21%
(Swanson) w/pasta	11.25 oz	310	22.0	36.0	670	na	9.0	na	35	26%
DIVAN (Le Menu) 'LightStyle'	10 oz	260	25.0	23.0	420	(mq)	7.0	(mq)	60	25%
SLICED										
(Freezer Queen)	10 oz	280	16.0	36.0	1210	(mq)	8.0	(mq)	(mq)	26%
(Le Menu) 'LightStyle'	10 oz	210	21.0	21.0	540	(mq)	5.0	(mq)	30	21%
TETRAZZINI (Healthy Choice)	12.6 oz	340	23.0	49.0	490	na	6.0	3.0	40	16%
W/DRESSING AND GRAVY										
(Armour) 'Classics'	11.5 oz	320	19.0	34.0	1280	(mq)	12.0	(mq)	50	34%
(Banquet) w/dressing and gravy 'Healthy Balance'	11.25 oz	270	16.0	41.0	750	na	5.0	2.0	40	17%
TURKEY ENTRÉE										
(Dinty Moore) w/dressing and gravy 'American Classics' ..	10 oz	290	28.0	33.0	910	na	5.0	1.0	40	16%
(Hormel) and vegetables 'Health Selections' microwave cup	7.25 oz	220	15.0	35.0	420	na	2.0	1.0	20	8%
(Libby's) w/dressing and gravy 'Diner' microwave cup	7 oz	170	11.0	15.0	830	1.2	7.0	2.0	35	38%
(Mountain House) tetrazzini, freeze-dried, prepared	1 cup	200	13.0	20.0	(mq)	(mq)	8.0	(mq)	(mq)	35%
(Turkey by George) hickory barbecue	5 oz	190	28.0	8.0	840	na	5.0	na	65	24%
(Turkey by George) Italian Parmesan	5 oz	170	28.0	3.0	860	na	5.0	na	70	27%
(Turkey by George) lemon pepper	5 oz	160	28.0	4.0	830	na	4.0	1.0	60	22%
(Turkey by George) mustard tarragon	5 oz	180	29.0	3.0	830	na	6.0	na	80	30%
(Ultra Slim Fast) glazed, w/dressing	10.5 oz	340	28.0	49.0	570	na	5.0	na	50	13%
(Ultra Slim Fast) medallions, in herb sauce	12 oz	280	23.0	33.0	950	na	6.0	na	40	19%
TURKEY ENTRÉE, FROZEN										
À LA KING (Budget Gourmet) w/rice	10 oz	390	20.0	36.0	740	(mq)	18.0	(mq)	75	42%
BREAST										
(Healthy Choice) sliced, w/dressing and gravy 'Classics' ..	10 oz	270	27.0	30.0	530	na	4.0	2.0	50	14%
(Lean Cuisine) sliced, w/dressing	7 7/8 oz	200	16.0	23.0	590	na	5.0	1.0	25	22%
(Lean Cuisine) sliced, w/mushroom sauce and rice	8 oz	230	17.0	24.0	540	na	7.0	2.0	35	28%
(Stouffer's) roast, w/stuffing and gravy	7 7/8 oz	270	19.0	27.0	920	na	9.0	na	na	31%
(Tyson) 'Gourmet Selections'	11.5 oz	380	19.0	51.0	1350	(mq)	11.0	(mq)	(mq)	26%
(Weight Watchers) stuffed	8.5 oz	270	18.0	31.0	520	na	8.0	3.0	60	27%
CASSEROLE (Pillsbury) 'Microwave Classic'	1 pkg	430	20.0	31.0	880	(mq)	25.0	(mq)	(mq)	52%
CROQUETTES (Freezer Queen) breaded, w/gravy	7 oz	250	13.0	19.0	940	(mq)	13.0	(mq)	(mq)	48%
DIJON (Lean Cuisine)	9.5 oz	210	20.0	20.0	590	na	6.0	2.0	45	25%
GLAZED (Le Menu) 'LightStyle'	8.25 oz	260	18.0	34.0	720	(mq)	6.0	(mq)	35	21%
HOMESTYLE (Lean Cuisine) w/vegetables and pasta	9 3/8 oz	230	21.0	25.0	550	na	5.0	2.0	50	20%
MEDALLIONS (Smart Ones) roasted, w/mushroom sauce ...	8.5 oz	200	13.0	35.0	440	na	1.0	<1.0	25	5%
PIE										
(Banquet)	7 oz	510	16.0	39.0	860	(mq)	31.0	(mq)	40	56%
(Banquet) 'Supreme Microwave'	7 oz	430	15.0	30.0	740	(mq)	27.0	(mq)	35	57%
(Mrs. Paterson's) w/broccoli 'Aussie Pie'	5.5 oz	460	16.0	42.0	790	na	26.0	10.0	95	50%
(Stouffer's)	10 oz	410	16.0	3.0	750	na	24.0	na	na	74%
(Swanson) 'Hungry Man'	16 oz	650	24.0	57.0	1470	(mq)	36.0	(mq)	(mq)	50%
(Swanson) 'Pot Pie'	7 oz	380	11.0	36.0	720	(mq)	21.0	(mq)	(mq)	50%
(Tyson)	9 oz	370	13.0	39.0	981	na	18.0	na	34	44%
ROASTED (Healthy Choice) and mushrooms in gravy	8.5 oz	200	18.0	26.0	380	na	3.0	1.0	40	13%
SLICED										
(Banquet) w/gravy 'Cookin' Bags'	5 oz	100	7.0	5.0	(mq)	na	6.0	(mq)	(mq)	53%
(Banquet) w/gravy 'Family Entrees'	8 oz	150	12.0	8.0	(mq)	na	8.0	(mq)	(mq)	47%
(Freezer Queen) w/dressing and gravy 'Single Serve'	9 oz	230	17.0	32.0	1130	(mq)	5.0	(mq)	(mq)	19%
(Freezer Queen) w/gravy 'Cook-In-Pouch'	5 oz	70	7.0	6.0	880	na	2.0	(mq)	(mq)	26%
(Freezer Queen) w/gravy 'Family Suppers'	7 oz	110	9.0	8.0	1160	na	5.0	(mq)	(mq)	40%
(Right Course) in mild curry sauce, w/rice pilaf	8.75 oz	320	23.0	40.0	570	(mq)	8.0	2.0	50	22%
TETRAZZINI (Stouffer's)	10 oz	400	22.0	26.0	960	na	23.0	na	na	52%

Food Name	Serving Size	Calories	Prot. gms	Carbs gms	Sod. mgs	Fiber gms	Fat gms	Sat. Fat gms	Chol. mgs	% Fat Cal.
W/DRESSING										
(Freezer Queen) w/dressing and gravy 'Deluxe Family' . . .	7 oz	160	12.0	18.0	1130	(mq)	5.0	(mq)	(mq)	27%
(Tyson) 'Looney Tunes Elmer Fudd'	6.55 oz	260	10.0	40.0	510	na	7.0	na	18	24%
W/DRESSING AND POTATOES										
(Swanson) 'Homestyle Recipe'	9 oz	290	18.0	30.0	1010	(mq)	11.0	(mq)	(mq)	34%
W/GRAVY (Tyson) 'Gourmet Selections'	9.5 oz	320	19.0	34.0	900	na	12.0	na	35	34%
W/VEGETABLES (Healthy Choice) low fat 'Homestyle'	9.5 oz	230	24.0	28.0	470	na	3.0	1.0	35	12%
WHITE MEAT (Le Menu) w/stuffing and gravy	8 oz	200	19.0	19.0	610	(mq)	5.0	1.0	25	23%
TURKEY FAT										
. . . .	1 cup	1846	0.0	0.0	0	0	204.6	60.3	209	100%
. . . .	1 oz	255	0.0	0.0	0	0	28.3	8.3	29	100%
. . . .	1 tbsp	115	0.0	0.0	0	0	12.8	3.8	13	100%
TURKEY GIBLETS										
raw	1 oz	37	5.5	0.6	25	0	1.2	0.4	80	31%
raw: 1 gizzard, 1 heart, and 1 liver, approx 8.6 oz	1 pkt	315	47.2	5.1	212	0	10.2	3.1	688	31%
simmered	4 oz	189	30.1	2.4	67	0	5.8	1.7	474	29%
simmered, chopped or diced	1 cup	243	38.5	3.0	85	0	7.4	2.2	606	29%
simmered, w/giblet fat	1 cup	242	38.5	3.0	86	0	7.4	2.2	606	29%
TURKEY GIZZARD										
raw	1 oz	33	5.4	0.2	23	0	1.0	0.3	45	29%
raw, approx 4 oz	1 gizzard	132	21.6	0.7	90	0	4.2	1.2	179	30%
simmered	1 cup	236	42.7	0.9	78	0	5.6	1.6	336	22%
simmered	4 oz	185	33.4	0.7	61	0	4.4	1.3	263	23%
TURKEY HAM SALAD										
(Longacre)	1 oz	53	2.0	3.0	190	na	4.0	(mq)	10	64%
(Longacre) 'Saladfest'	1 oz	58	2.0	2.0	270	na	4.0	(mq)	10	69%
TURKEY HEART										
raw	1 oz	41	5.2	0.2	25	0	2.0	0.6	33	46%
raw, approx 1 oz	1 heart	41	5.2	0.2	25	0	2.0	0.6	33	46%
simmered	1 cup	257	38.8	3.0	80	0	8.9	2.5	328	32%
simmered	4 oz	201	30.3	2.3	62	0	6.9	2.0	256	32%
TURKEY LIVER										
raw	1 oz	39	5.7	1.2	27	0	1.1	0.4	132	26%
raw, approx 3.6 oz	1 liver	140	20.4	4.2	98	0	4.1	1.3	475	27%
simmered	1 cup	237	33.6	4.8	90	0	8.3	2.6	876	33%
simmered	4 oz	192	27.2	3.9	73	0	6.7	2.1	710	33%
TURKEY NUGGET										
(Louis Rich) 80% fat-free, breaded, cooked	3/4 oz	60	3.0	3.0	155	na	4.0	na	10	60%
TURKEY SALAD										
(Longacre)	1 oz	70	3.0	3.0	200	na	5.0	(mq)	10	65%
(Longacre) 'Saladfest'	1 oz	68	3.0	2.0	180	na	5.0	(mq)	15	69%
TURKEY SEASONING MIX										
(Schilling) roast 'Bag'n Season'	1 pkg	146	6.0	20.0	1935	na	5.0	na	na	30%
TURKEY SPREAD										
(Libby's) 'Spreadables'	1.9 oz	100	5.0	6.0	260	1.9	6.0	1.0	15	55%
(Underwood) chunky 'Light'	2 1/8 oz	75	11.0	2.0	330	na	2.0	<1.0	25	26%
TURKEY STICK										
(Louis Rich) cooked, breaded, 80% fat-free	.95 oz	80	4.0	5.0	195	na	5.0	na	10	56%
(Louis Rich) cooked, prepared	1 oz	81	4.1	4.8	197	(mq)	5.0	1.0	12	56%
(The Turkey Store) breast meat, cheese 'Gobble Stix'	1 stick	30	6.0	0.5	na	na	0.8	0.4	10	22%
(The Turkey Store) breast meat, smoked 'Gobble Stix'	1 stick	25	5.0	0.1	na	na	0.2	0.0	10	8%
TURMERIC										
ground	1 oz	100	2.2	18.4	11	>1.9 c	2.8	(mq)	0	23%
ground	1 tbsp	24	0.5	4.4	3	1.4	0.7	na	0	24%

Food Name	Serving Size	Calories	Prot. gms	Carbs gms	Sod. mgs	Fiber gms	Fat gms	Sat. Fat gms	Chol. mgs	% Fat Cal.
ground	1 tsp	8	0.2	1.4	1	.5	0.2	na	0	00%
ground (Durkee)	1 tsp	9	0.0	0.0	0	0	tr	na	na	tr
ground (Laurel Leaf)	1 tsp	9	0.0	0.0	0	0	tr	na	na	tr
ground (Spice Islands)	1 tsp	7	0.2	1.3	<1	>.1 c	0.2	na	0	23%
TURNIP										
boiled, drained	4 oz	20	0.8	5.6	57	2.3	0.1	tr	0	3%
boiled, drained, cubed	1/2 cup	14	0.6	3.8	39	1.6	0.1	0.0	0	5%
boiled, drained, mashed	1/2 cup	21	0.8	5.6	58	2.3	0.1	0.0	0	3%
raw, cubed	1/2 cup	18	0.6	4.1	44	1.2	0.1	0.0	0	5%
raw, trimmed	1 oz	8	0.3	1.8	19	.5	<.1	tr	0	<10%
raw, untrimmed	1 lb	100	3.3	22.9	248	6.6	0.4	<.1	0	3%
Canned										
(Allens) diced	1/2 cup	16	2.0	2.0	25	(mq)	<1.0	(tr)	0	<36%
(Stokely)	1/2 cup	20	2.0	3.0	350	(mq)	0.0	0.0	0	0%
Frozen										
boiled, drained	4 oz	26	1.7	4.9	41	>.8 c	0.3	<.1	0	9%
mashed	3 1/3 oz	15	1.0	2.8	23	1.7	0.2	0.0	0	11%
(Southern) diced	3.5 oz	17	1.0	2.9	50	(mq)	0.2	(tr)	0	10%
TURNIP GREENS										
boiled, drained	4 oz	23	1.3	4.9	33	3.5	0.3	0.1	0	10%
boiled, drained, chopped	1/2 cup	14	0.8	3.1	21	2.2	0.2	0.0	0	10%
raw, chopped	1/2 cup	8	0.4	1.6	11	.7	0.1	0.0	0	10%
raw, untrimmed	1 lb	85	4.8	18.2	126	7.6	1.0	0.2	0	9%
TURNIP GREENS, CANNED										
Chopped										
(Allens)	1/2 cup	21	2.0	3.0	15	(mq)	<1.0	(tr)	0	<31%
(Bush's Best)	1/2 cup	20	2.0	3.0	310	na	0.0	na	na	0%
W/diced turnips										
(Allens) chopped	1/2 cup	19	2.0	1.0	15	(mq)	<1.0	(tr)	0	<43%
(Bush's Best)	1/2 cup	25	1.0	4.0	370	2.0	0.0	na	na	0%
(Stokely)	1/2 cup	20	2.0	0.0	340	(mq)	0.0	0.0	0	0%
W/liquid	1/2 cup	16	1.6	2.8	324	1.5	0.4	0.1	0	17%
TURNIP GREENS, FROZEN										
boiled, drained	10 oz	66	7.4	11.0	33	>2.3 c	0.9	0.2	0	10%
boiled, drained	4 oz	34	3.8	5.6	17	>1.2 c	0.5	0.1	0	11%
boiled, drained	1/2 cup	25	2.8	4.1	12	>.8 c	0.3	0.1	0	9%
chopped	10 oz	62	7.0	10.4	34	6.8	0.9	0.2	0	10%
chopped	1/2 cup	18	2.0	3.0	10	2.0	0.3	0.1	0	12%
chopped (Frosty Acres)	3.3 oz	20	2.0	4.0	10	>1.0 c	0.0	0.0	0	0%
chopped (Seabrook)	3.3 oz	20	2.0	4.0	11	>1.0 c	0.0	0.0	0	0%
chopped (Southern)	3.5 oz	25	2.5	3.6	70	(mq)	0.3	(tr)	0	10%
w/turnips	10 oz	60	7.0	9.7	51	6.8	0.5	0.1	0	6%
w/turnips (Seabrook)	3.3 oz	20	3.0	3.0	na	(mq)	0.0	0.0	0	0%
w/turnips, boiled, drained	4 oz	19	2.4	3.3	17	>.6 c	0.2	<.1	0	7%
TURNIP-ROOTED PARSLEY. See PARSLEY ROOT.										
TURNOVER. See also PASTRY.										
apple, frozen (Pepperidge Farm)	1 turnover	300	3.0	34.0	210	(mq)	17.0	(mq)	na	51%
apple, refrigerated (Pillsbury)	1 turnover	170	2.0	23.0	320	(mq)	8.0	2.0	0	42%
blueberry, frozen (Pepperidge Farm)	1 turnover	310	3.0	32.0	230	(mq)	19.0	(mq)	na	55%
cherry, frozen (Pepperidge Farm)	1 turnover	310	3.0	32.0	280	(mq)	19.0	(mq)	na	55%
cherry, refrigerated (Pillsbury)	1 turnover	170	2.0	23.0	320	(mq)	8.0	2.0	0	42%
peach, frozen (Pepperidge Farm)	1 turnover	310	3.0	34.0	260	(mq)	18.0	(mq)	na	52%
raspberry, frozen (Pepperidge Farm)	1 turnover	310	4.0	36.0	260	(mq)	17.0	(mq)	na	49%

Food Name	Serving Size	Calories	Prot. gms	Carbs gms	Sod. mgs	Fiber gms	Fat gms	Sat. Fat gms	Chol. mgs	% Fat Cal.
TURTLE, GREEN										
canned	100 gm	106	23.4	0.0	68	0	0.7	0.0	50	6%
raw	100 gm	89	19.8	0.0	68	0	0.5	0.0	50	5%
TUSK. See CUSK.										

U

Food Name	Serving Size	Calories	Prot. gms	Carbs gms	Sod. mgs	Fiber gms	Fat gms	Sat. Fat gms	Chol. mgs	% Fat Cal.

UDON NOODLE. See NOODLE, JAPANESE.
ULTRA SLIM FAST. See DIET DRINK.
UMEBOSHI PLUM. See PLUM, JAPANESE.

V

Food Name	Serving Size	Calories	Prot. gms	Carbs gms	Sod. mgs	Fiber gms	Fat gms	Sat. Fat gms	Chol. mgs	% Fat Cal.
VANILLA BAKING CHIPS (Hershey's)	1/4 cup	240	3.0	25.0	65	na	14.0	na	na	53%
VANILLA EXTRACT, pure (Virginia Dare)	1 tsp	10	0.0	0.3	0	0	0.0	0.0	0	0%
VANILLA FLAVOR DRINK, CANNED										
(Ensure) liquid nutrition	8 oz	250	8.8	34.3	200	na	8.8	na	5	32%
(Ensure) liquid nutrition 'Plus'	8 oz	355	13.0	47.3	250	na	12.6	na	5	32%
(Ensure) liquid nutrition, w/fiber	8 oz	260	9.4	38.3	200	na	8.8	na	5	29%
(Sego) 'Lite'	10 oz	150	11.0	17.0	390	na	4.0	(mq)	5	24%
(Sego) 'Lite French Vanilla'	10 oz	150	11.0	17.0	390	na	4.0	(mq)	5	24%
(Sego) 'Very Vanilla'	10 oz	225	11.0	34.0	360	na	5.0	(mq)	5	20%
(Sustacal) liquid food, nutritionally complete	8 oz	240	14.5	33.0	220	na	5.5	na	na	21%
VEAL										
(NOTE: TRIMMED = Lean; separable fat removed. UNTRIMMED = Separable fat not removed.)										
BRAINS										
braised	3 oz	116	9.8	0.0	133	0	8.2	1.9	2635	65%
pan-fried	3 oz	181	12.3	0.0	150	0	14.2	3.4	1802	72%
raw	1 oz	33	2.9	0.0	36	na	2.3	0.5	445	64%
GROUND										
broiled	1 cup	200	28.3	0.0	96	0	8.8	3.5	119	41%
broiled	3 oz	146	20.7	0.0	71	na	6.4	2.6	88	41%
raw	1 cup	325	43.7	0.0	185	0	15.3	6.3	185	44%
raw	1 oz	40	5.4	0.0	23	na	1.9	0.8	23	44%
HEART										
braised	3 oz	158	24.7	0.1	49	0	5.7	1.5	150	34%
raw	1 oz	31	4.8	0.0	22	0	1.1	0.3	29	34%
simmered	4 oz	368	57.7	0.3	116	0	13.4	3.6	349	34%
KIDNEYS										
braised	3 oz	139	22.4	0.0	94	na	4.8	1.5	672	33%
raw	1 oz	28	4.4	0.2	50	na	0.9	0.3	102	31%
LEG										
Trimmed										
braised	3 oz	173	31.2	0.0	57	0	4.3	1.6	115	24%
pan-fried	3 oz	156	28.2	0.0	65	0	3.9	1.1	91	24%
raw	1 oz	30	6.0	0.0	18	0	0.5	0.2	22	16%
roasted	3 oz	127	23.9	0.0	58	0	2.9	1.0	88	21%

Food Name	Serving Size	Calories	Prot. gms	Carbs gms	Sod. mgs	Fiber gms	Fat gms	Sat. Fat gms	Chol. mgs	% Fat Cal.
Untrimmed										
braised	3 oz	179	30.7	0.0	57	0	5.4	2.2	114	28%
pan-fried	3 oz	179	27.0	0.0	65	0	7.1	2.7	89	37%
raw	1 oz	33	5.9	0.0	18	0	0.9	0.3	22	26%
roasted	3 oz	136	23.5	0.0	58	0	4.0	1.6	88	28%
LEG AND SHOULDER										
raw, trimmed	1 oz	31	5.7	0.0	23	0	0.7	0.2	24	22%
trimmed, braised	3 oz	160	29.7	0.0	79	0	3.7	1.1	123	22%
LIVER										
braised	3 oz	140	18.4	2.3	45	na	5.9	2.2	477	39%
pan-fried	3 oz	208	25.3	3.3	112	na	9.7	3.6	281	43%
raw	4 oz	152	20.3	5.2	70	na	5.0	1.9	350	31%
raw	1 oz	38	5.0	1.3	17	na	1.2	0.5	87	30%
LOIN										
Trimmed										
braised	3 oz	192	28.5	0.0	71	0	7.8	2.2	106	38%
raw	1 oz	32	5.7	0.0	25	0	0.9	0.3	22	26%
roasted	3 oz	149	22.4	0.0	82	0	5.9	2.2	90	37%
stewed	4 oz	256	38.1	0.0	95	0	10.4	2.9	142	38%
Untrimmed										
braised	3 oz	241	25.7	0.0	68	0	14.6	5.7	100	56%
raw	1 oz	46	5.3	0.0	24	0	2.6	1.1	22	53%
roasted	3 oz	184	21.1	0.0	79	0	10.5	4.5	88	53%
stewed	4 oz	322	34.2	0.0	91	0	19.5	7.6	134	56%
LUNGS										
braised	3 oz	88	15.9	0.0	48	0	2.2	0.8	224	24%
raw	1 oz	25	4.6	0.0	30	0	0.6	0.2	64	23%
PANCREAS										
braised	3 oz	218	24.7	0.0	58	0	12.4	7.2	na	53%
raw	1 oz	51	4.2	0.0	19	0	3.7	1.3	48	67%
RIB										
Trimmed										
braised	3 oz	185	29.3	0.0	84	0	6.6	2.2	122	34%
raw	1 lb	544	90.6	0.0	431	0	17.6	5.3	376	30%
raw	1 oz	34	5.6	0.0	27	0	1.1	0.3	23	31%
roasted	3 oz	150	21.9	0.0	82	0	6.3	1.8	98	39%
stewed	4 oz	247	39.1	0.0	112	0	8.9	2.9	163	34%
Untrimmed										
braised	3 oz	213	27.6	0.0	81	0	10.6	4.2	118	46%
raw	1 lb	735	85.6	0.0	404	0	40.9	16.8	372	52%
raw	1 oz	45	5.3	0.0	25	0	2.5	1.0	23	52%
roasted	3 oz	194	20.4	0.0	78	0	11.9	4.6	94	57%
stewed	4 oz	285	36.8	0.0	108	0	14.2	5.6	158	47%
SHOULDER, ARM										
Trimmed										
braised	3 oz	171	30.4	0.0	77	0	4.5	1.3	132	25%
braised, approx 5.6 oz	1 steak	321	57.1	0.0	143	0	8.5	2.4	248	25%
raw	1 oz	29	5.6	0.0	24	0	0.6	0.2	23	19%
roasted	3 oz	139	22.2	0.0	77	0	4.9	2.0	93	33%
roasted, approx 9.6 oz	1 steak	447	71.2	0.0	248	0	15.8	6.3	298	33%
Untrimmed										
braised	3 oz	201	28.6	0.0	74	0	8.7	3.4	126	41%
braised, approx 6.1 oz	1 steak	409	58.2	0.0	151	0	17.7	6.9	257	41%
raw	1 oz	37	5.4	0.0	23	0	1.5	0.6	23	39%

Food Name	Serving Size	Calories	Prot. gms	Carbs gms	Sod. mgs	Fiber gms	Fat gms	Sat. Fat gms	Chol. mgs	% Fat Cal.
roasted	3 oz	156	21.6	0.0	77	0	7.0	3.0	92	42%
SHOULDER, BLADE										
Trimmed										
braised	3 oz	168	27.8	0.0	86	0	5.5	1.5	134	31%
diced, braised	1 cup	277	45.7	0.0	141	0	9.1	2.5	221	31%
diced, roasted	1 cup	239	35.9	0.0	143	0	9.6	3.6	167	38%
diced, stewed	1 cup	277	45.7	0.0	141	0	9.1	2.5	221	31%
raw	1 lb	513	89.1	0.0	440	0	14.8	4.4	408	27%
raw	1 oz	32	5.5	0.0	27	0	0.9	0.3	25	27%
roasted	3 oz	145	21.8	0.0	87	0	5.8	2.2	101	37%
stewed	4 oz	224	37.0	0.0	115	0	7.3	2.1	179	31%
Untrimmed										
braised	3 oz	191	26.6	0.0	83	0	8.6	3.1	130	42%
diced, braised	1 cup	315	43.8	0.0	137	0	14.1	5.1	214	42%
diced, roasted	1 cup	260	35.2	0.0	140	0	12.1	4.8	164	44%
diced, stewed	1 cup	315	43.8	0.0	137	0	14.1	5.1	214	42%
raw	1 lb	585	87.2	0.0	431	0	23.6	8.8	408	38%
raw	1 oz	36	5.4	0.0	27	0	1.5	0.5	25	39%
roasted	3 oz	158	21.4	0.0	85	0	7.4	2.9	99	44%
stewed	4 oz	255	35.4	0.0	111	0	11.4	4.1	174	42%
SHOULDER, WHOLE										
Trimmed										
braised	3 oz	169	28.6	0.0	82	0	5.2	1.4	110	29%
diced, braised	1 cup	279	47.2	0.0	136	0	8.5	2.4	182	29%
diced, roasted	1 cup	238	36.1	0.0	136	0	9.3	3.5	160	37%
diced, stewed	1 cup	279	47.2	0.0	136	0	8.5	2.4	182	29%
raw	1 lb	508	89.8	0.0	417	0	13.6	4.1	390	25%
raw	1 oz	31	5.5	0.0	26	0	0.8	0.3	24	25%
roasted	3 oz	144	21.9	0.0	82	0	5.6	2.1	97	37%
stewed	4 oz	226	38.2	0.0	110	0	6.9	1.9	147	29%
Untrimmed										
braised	3 oz	194	27.2	0.0	81	0	8.6	3.2	107	42%
diced, braised	1 cup	319	44.9	0.0	133	0	14.2	5.3	176	42%
diced, roasted	1 cup	258	35.4	0.0	134	0	11.8	4.8	158	43%
diced, stewed	1 cup	319	44.9	0.0	133	0	14.2	5.3	176	42%
raw	1 lb	590	87.4	0.0	413	0	24.0	9.3	395	38%
raw	1 oz	36	5.4	0.0	25	0	1.5	0.6	24	39%
roasted	3 oz	156	21.5	0.0	82	0	7.2	2.9	96	43%
stewed	4 oz	259	36.4	0.0	108	0	11.5	4.3	143	42%
SIRLOIN										
Trimmed										
braised	3 oz	173	28.9	0.0	69	0	5.5	1.5	96	30%
diced, braised	1 cup	286	47.5	0.0	113	0	9.1	2.5	158	30%
diced, roasted	1 cup	235	36.8	0.0	119	0	8.7	3.4	146	35%
diced, stewed	1 cup	286	47.5	0.0	113	0	9.1	2.5	158	30%
raw	1 lb	499	91.6	0.0	363	0	11.7	3.5	358	22%
raw	1 oz	31	5.7	0.0	22	0	0.7	0.2	22	22%
roasted	3 oz	143	22.4	0.0	72	0	5.3	2.0	88	35%
stewed	4 oz	231	38.5	0.0	92	0	7.4	2.1	128	30%
Untrimmed										
braised	3 oz	214	26.6	0.0	67	0	11.2	4.4	92	49%
diced, braised	1 cup	353	43.8	0.0	111	0	18.4	7.3	151	49%
diced, roasted	1 cup	283	35.2	0.0	116	0	14.6	6.3	143	48%
diced, stewed	1 cup	353	43.8	0.0	111	0	18.4	7.3	151	49%

Food Name	Serving Size	Calories	Prot. gms	Carbs gms	Sod. mgs	Fiber gms	Fat gms	Sat. Fat gms	Chol. mgs	% Fat Cal.
raw	1 lb	689	86.5	0.0	345	0	35.4	15.2	354	48%
raw	1 oz	43	5.3	0.0	21	0	2.2	0.9	22	48%
roasted	3 oz	172	21.4	0.0	71	0	8.9	3.8	87	48%
stewed	4 oz	286	35.4	0.0	90	0	14.9	5.9	122	49%
SPLEEN										
braised	3 oz	110	20.5	0.0	49	0	2.5	0.8	380	22%
raw	1 oz	27	5.1	0.0	27	0	0.6	0.2	95	21%
THYMUS										
braised	3 oz	148	26.8	0.0	56	0	3.7	1.3	399	24%
raw	1 oz	28	5.0	0.0	23	0	0.7	0.2	75	24%
TONGUE										
braised	3 oz	172	22.0	0.0	54	0	8.6	3.7	202	47%
raw	1 oz	37	4.8	0.5	23	0	1.5	0.7	17	39%
TOP ROUND										
Trimmed										
braised	4 oz	230	41.6	0.0	76	0	5.8	2.2	159	24%
diced, braised	1 cup	284	51.4	0.0	94	0	7.1	2.7	189	24%
diced, roasted	1 cup	210	39.3	0.0	95	0	4.7	1.7	144	21%
diced, stewed	1 cup	284	51.4	0.0	94	0	7.1	2.7	189	24%
pan-fried in vegetable oil	4 oz	208	37.6	0.0	87	0	5.2	1.5	121	24%
roasted	4 oz	170	31.8	0.0	77	0	3.8	1.4	177	21%
stewed	4 oz	230	41.6	0.0	76	0	5.8	2.2	159	24%
Untrimmed										
diced, roasted	1 cup	224	38.8	0.0	95	0	6.5	2.6	144	27%
diced, stewed	1 cup	295	50.6	0.0	94	0	8.9	3.5	188	28%
pan-fried in vegetable oil	4 oz	239	36.0	0.0	86	0	9.5	3.6	119	37%
roasted	4 oz	181	31.4	0.0	77	0	5.3	2.1	117	28%
stewed	4 oz	239	41.0	0.0	76	0	7.2	2.9	152	28%
VEAL ENTRÉE, FROZEN										
MARSALA *(Le Menu)* 'LightStyle'	10 oz	230	22.0	28.0	700	(mq)	3.0	(mq)	75	12%
PARMIGIANA										
(Armour) 'Classics'	11.25 oz	400	18.0	34.0	1320	(mq)	22.0	(mq)	55	49%
(Le Menu)	11.5 oz	390	24.0	36.0	840	(mq)	17.0	(mq)	(mq)	39%
(Morton)	10 oz	260	10.0	35.0	1510	(mq)	8.0	(mq)	35	29%
(Swanson)	12.25 oz	430	20.0	42.0	1010	(mq)	20.0	(mq)	(mq)	42%
(Swanson) 'Homestyle Recipe'	10 oz	330	19.0	33.0	960	(mq)	13.0	(mq)	(mq)	36%
(Swanson) 'Hungry Man'	18.25 oz	590	32.0	57.0	1840	(mq)	26.0	(mq)	(mq)	40%
(Ultimate 200)	8.2 oz	150	22.0	5.0	550	na	4.0	1.0	50	25%
Breaded										
(Banquet) 'Cookin' Bags'	4 oz	230	10.0	20.0	(mq)	(mq)	11.0	(mq)	(mq)	45%
(Banquet) 'Family Entrées'	8 oz	370	18.0	33.0	(mq)	(mq)	18.0	(mq)	(mq)	44%
(Freezer Queen)	5 oz	220	11.0	17.0	560	(mq)	12.0	(mq)	(mq)	49%
(Freezer Queen) 'Cook-In-Pouch'	5 oz	220	11.0	17.0	560	(mq)	12.0	(mq)	(mq)	49%
(Freezer Queen) 'Deluxe Family Suppers'	7 oz	300	17.0	22.0	820	(mq)	15.0	(mq)	(mq)	46%
Platter *(Freezer Queen)*	10 oz	400	22.0	32.0	870	(mq)	20.0	(mq)	(mq)	46%
W/pasta Alfredo *(Stouffer's)* homestyle	9.25 oz	350	28.0	26.0	1060	na	15.0	na	na	39%
STEAK										
(Hormel)	4 oz	130	22.0	2.0	(mq)	na	4.0	(mq)	(mq)	27%
(Hormel) breaded	4 oz	240	17.0	13.0	(mq)	(mq)	13.0	(mq)	(mq)	49%
VEGETABLE. See individual listings.										
VEGETABLE DISH, CANNED. See also individual listings.										
Corn, beans, and carrots, w/pasta, in tomato sauce										
(Green Giant)	1/2 cup	80	2.0	17.0	330	3.0	2.0	0.0	0	19%

Food Name	Serving Size	Calories	Prot. gms	Carbs gms	Sod. mgs	Fiber gms	Fat gms	Sat. Fat gms	Chol. mgs	% Fat Cal.
Green beans, potatoes, and mushrooms, in sauce										
(Green Giant)	1/2 cup	50	1.0	9.0	430	2.0	2.0	<1.0	0	31%
Snap beans, potatoes, and mushrooms, in sauce										
(Green Giant)	1/2 cup	50	1.0	9.0	430	2.0	2.0	<1.0	0	31%
String beans, potatoes, and mushrooms, in sauce										
(Green Giant)	1/2 cup	50	1.0	9.0	430	2.0	2.0	<1.0	0	31%
VEGETABLE DISH, FROZEN. See also individual listings.										
Broccoli, cauliflower, carrots										
(Birds Eye) 'Butter Sauce'	3.3 oz	45	2.0	6.0	290	2.0	2.0	na	5	36%
(Birds Eye) 'Cheese Sauce'	4.5 oz	110	5.0	11.0	410	2.0	5.0	na	5	41%
(Birds Eye) 'Farm Fresh'	4 oz	35	2.0	7.0	40	3.0	0.0	na	0	0%
(Green Giant) 'Butter Sauce'	1/2 cup	30	2.0	4.0	240	3.0	1.0	<1.0	5	27%
(Green Giant) in cheese sauce	1/2 cup	60	3.0	9.0	490	2.0	2.0	<1.0	2	27%
(Green Giant) 'One Serving'	1 pkg	30	3.0	7.0	40	3.0	0.0	0.0	0	0%
(Stokely) 'Singles' w/baby carrots	3 oz	25	2.0	5.0	25	(mq)	1.0	(tr)	0	24%
(Stokely) w/baby carrots, in cheese sauce	4 oz	70	4.0	8.0	180	(mq)	3.0	(mq)	15	36%
Broccoli, cauliflower, peppers, w/red peppers 'Farm Fresh'										
(Birds Eye)	4 oz	30	3.0	5.0	25	3.0	0.0	na	0	0%
Broccoli, corn, peppers, w/red peppers 'Farm Fresh'										
(Birds Eye)	4 oz	60	3.0	14.0	15	3.0	1.0	na	0	12%
Broccoli, green beans, onions, peppers, w/pearl onions										
and red peppers (Birds Eye)	4 oz	35	2.0	7.0	15	3.0	0.0	na	0	0%
Broccoli, peppers, bamboo shoots, mushrooms, w/red										
peppers (Birds Eye)	4 oz	30	3.0	5.0	20	3.0	0.0	0.0	0	0%
Broccoli and carrots, w/rotini, in cheese sauce										
(Green Giant)	1 pkg	100	5.0	17.0	440	3.0	2.0	na	5	17%
Brussels sprouts, cauliflower, carrots (Birds Eye)	4 oz	40	3.0	8.0	30	4.0	0.0	0.0	0	0%
Cauliflower, broccoli, carrots, in cheese sauce										
(Freezer Queen)	5 oz	60	2.0	10.0	360	(mq)	1.0	(mq)	na	16%
Cauliflower, carrots, snow peas, w/baby carrots and snow										
pea pods (Birds Eye)	4 oz	40	2.0	8.0	35	3.0	0.0	0.0	0	0%
Cauliflower, zucchini, carrots, peppers, w/red peppers										
(Birds Eye)	4 oz	30	2.0	6.0	25	2.0	0.0	na	0	0%
Peas, carrots, water chestnuts, w/sugar snap peas and										
baby carrots (Birds Eye)	3.2 oz	50	2.0	11.0	20	4.0	0.0	na	0	0%
Zucchini, carrots, onions, mushrooms, w/pearl onions										
(Birds Eye)	4 oz	30	1.0	7.0	15	1.0	0.0	na	0	0%
VEGETABLE ENTRÉE										
Chinese style, w/chicken, frozen (Budget Gourmet)	10 oz	280	11.0	47.0	590	na	7.0	1.0	10	21%
Country style, w/beef tips (Ultra Slim Fast)	12 oz	230	21.0	26.0	960	na	5.0	na	45	19%
Italian style, w/chicken, frozen (Budget Gourmet)	10.25 oz	310	14.0	50.0	690	na	8.0	2.0	30	22%
Pot pie, frozen										
(Amy's Kitchen) organic	8 oz	347	9.0	45.0	260	3.0	16.0	na	na	40%
(Morton) w/beef	7 oz	430	11.0	27.0	740	(mq)	31.0	(mq)	30	65%
(Morton) w/chicken	7 oz	420	14.0	27.0	740	(mq)	28.0	(mq)	35	61%
(Morton) w/turkey	7 oz	420	14.0	27.0	740	(mq)	28.0	(mq)	40	61%
Stir-fry, frozen (Shanghai)	5.1 oz	75	6.0	11.0	510	na	1.0	na	0	12%
VEGETABLE FLAKES (French's) dehydrated	1 tbsp	12	0.0	3.0	20	(mq)	0.0	0.0	0	0%
VEGETABLE JUICE										
cocktail, canned	6 oz	35	1.1	8.3	664	1.5	0.2	0.0	0	5%
cocktail, canned	1/2 cup	23	0.8	5.5	442	1.0	0.1	0.0	0	3%
(Biotta) 'Breuss Juice'	6 oz	67	1.9	13.2	147	(mq)	0.1	(tr)	0	2%
(Biotta) 'Cocktail'	6 oz	50	1.7	10.1	497	(mq)	0.1	(tr)	0	2%
(Knudsen & Sons) 'Very Veggie'	8 oz	40	<1.0	8.0	na	na	0.0	na	na	0%

Food Name	Serving Size	Calories	Prot. gms	Carbs gms	Sod. mgs	Fiber gms	Fat gms	Sat. Fat gms	Chol. mgs	% Fat Cal.
(Knudsen & Sons) 'Very Veggie' low sodium	8 oz	40	2.0	8.0	32	na	0.0	na	na	0%
(Knudsen & Sons) 'Very Veggie' organic	8 oz	40	2.0	8.0	na	na	0.0	na	na	0%
(Knudsen & Sons) 'Very Veggie' spicy	8 oz	40	2.0	8.0	560	na	0.0	na	na	0%
(Smucker's) hearty	8 oz	58	0.6	13.0	714	(mq)	<.1	(tr)	0	<2%
(Smucker's) hot and spicy	8 oz	58	0.6	13.0	650	(mq)	<.1	(tr)	0	<2%
(V•8)	6 oz	35	1.0	8.0	560	(mq)	0.0	0.0	0	0%
(V•8) 'Light'n Tangy'	6 oz	40	1.0	8.0	240	na	0.0	0.0	0	0%
(V•8) 'No Salt Added'	6 oz	35	1.0	8.0	45	(mq)	0.0	0.0	0	0%
(V•8) 'Picante' mild	6 oz	35	1.0	8.0	520	na	0.0	0.0	0	0%
(V•8) spicy hot	6 oz	35	1.0	8.0	650	(mq)	0.0	0.0	0	0%
(Veryfine) '100%'	6 oz	32	1.6	6.0	600	(mq)	0.0	0.0	0	0%
VEGETABLE MARROW SQUASH. See SQUASH, MARROW.										
VEGETABLE OIL. See also individual listings.										
(Crisco)	1 tbsp	120	0.0	0.0	0	0	14.0	2.0	0	100%
(Finast)	1 tbsp	120	0.0	0.0	0	0	14.0	2.0	0	100%
(Hain) 'All Blend'	1 tbsp	120	0.0	0.0	0	0	14.0	2.0	0	100%
(Hain) w/garlic 'Garlic & Oil'	1 tbsp	120	0.0	0.0	0	0	14.0	3.0	0	100%
(Kroger)	1 tbsp	122	0.0	0.0	0	0	13.6	2.1	0	100%
(Pathmark)	1 tbsp	120	0.0	0.0	0	0	14.0	2.0	0	100%
(Pathmark) 'No Frills'	1 tbsp	130	0.0	0.0	0	0	14.0	2.0	0	100%
(Puritan)	1 tbsp	120	0.0	0.0	0	0	14.0	1.0	0	100%
(Wesson)	1 tbsp	120	0.0	0.0	0	0	14.0	2.0	0	100%
VEGETABLE OIL SPRAY. See COOKING SPRAY.										
VEGETABLE OIL SPREAD. See MARGARINE SPREAD.										
VEGETABLE OYSTER. See SALSIFY.										
VEGETABLE SPONGE. See GOURD, DISHCLOTH.										
VEGETABLE STICKS, breaded, frozen (Farm Rich)	4 oz	240	4.0	34.0	980	(mq)	10.0	(mq)	na	37%
VEGETABLES, MIXED, CANNED										
drained	4 oz	53	2.9	10.5	169	2.7	0.3	0.1	0	5%
drained	1/2 cup	39	2.1	7.6	122	>1.1 c	0.2	0.0	0	4%
w/liquid	4 oz	41	1.6	8.1	254	>1.3 c	0.3	0.1	0	7%
w/liquid	1/2 cup	40	2.0	7.0	355	(mq)	0.0	0.0	0	0%
(A&P) 'Eastern'	1/2 cup	45	2.0	8.0	330	(mq)	<1.0	(tr)	0	<18%
(A&P) 'No Salt Added'	1/2 cup	40	1.0	9.0	20	(mq)	<1.0	(tr)	0	<18%
(A&P) 'Western'	1/2 cup	40	1.0	9.0	380	(mq)	<1.0	(tr)	0	<18%
(Bush's Best) 'Mixed Greens'	1/2 cup	20	2.0	3.0	300	na	0.0	na	na	0%
(Featherweight)	1/2 cup	40	2.0	8.0	25	(mq)	0.0	0.0	0	0%
(Finast)	1/2 cup	40	1.0	8.0	390	(mq)	0.0	0.0	0	0%
(Finast) 'No Salt Added'	1/2 cup	40	2.0	8.0	25	(mq)	0.0	0.0	0	0%
(Freshlike) water packed, w/o salt	1/2 cup	35	2.0	8.0	25	na	0.0	na	na	0%
(Freshlike) water packed, w/o sugar or salt	1/2 cup	35	2.0	8.0	25	na	0.0	na	na	0%
(Green Giant) 'Garden Medley'	1/2 cup	35	1.0	9.0	350	1.0	0.0	0.0	0	0%
(Green Giant) 'Pantry Express'	1/2 cup	35	1.0	8.0	300	1.0	<1.0	0.0	0	<20%
(LaChoy) 'Chinese'	1/2 cup	12	1.0	2.0	30	1.1	0.1	(tr)	0	7%
(LaChoy) 'Chop Suey'	1/2 cup	9	0.7	2.0	330	1.0	0.1	(tr)	0	8%
(LaChoy) 'Fancy Mix'	1/2 cup	12	1.0	2.0	30	1.0	<1.0	(mq)	0	<43%
(P&Q) 'Chunky Eastern'	1/2 cup	40	2.0	8.0	330	(mq)	<1.0	(tr)	0	<18%
(P&Q) 'Chunky Western'	1/2 cup	40	1.0	9.0	380	(mq)	<1.0	(tr)	0	<18%
(Pathmark)	1/2 cup	35	2.0	8.0	320	(mq)	0.0	0.0	0	0%
(Pathmark) 'No Salt Added'	1/2 cup	35	2.0	7.0	25	(mq)	0.0	0.0	0	0%
(S&W) 'Old Fashioned Harvest'	1/2 cup	35	1.0	6.0	380	(mq)	0.0	0.0	0	0%
(Stokely)	1/2 cup	40	2.0	8.0	300	(mq)	0.0	0.0	0	0%
(Stokely) 'No Salt or Sugar Added'	1/2 cup	40	2.0	8.0	25	(mq)	0.0	0.0	0	0%
(Veg•All) 'Homestyle Large Cut'	1/2 cup	35	2.0	9.0	380	na	0.0	na	na	0%

Food Name	Serving Size	Calories	Prot. gms	Carbs gms	Sod. mgs	Fiber gms	Fat gms	Sat. Fat gms	Chol. mgs	% Fat Cal.
(Veg•All) 'Lite'	1/2 cup	35	2.0	8.0	25	na	0.0	na	na	0%
(Veg•All) 'Original'	1/2 cup	35	2.0	8.0	320	na	0.0	na	na	0%
VEGETABLES, MIXED, FROZEN										
boiled, drained	10-oz pkg	162	7.9	36.0	96	10.5	0.4	0.1	0	2%
boiled, drained	4 oz	67	3.2	14.8	40	4.3	0.2	<.1	0	2%
boiled, drained	1/2 cup	54	2.6	11.9	32	3.5	0.1	0.0	0	2%
(A&P)	3.3 oz	65	3.0	13.0	55	(mq)	<1.0	(tr)	0	<12%
(Birds Eye)	3.3 oz	60	3.0	13.0	40	2.0	0.0	0.0	0	0%
(Birds Eye) 'Portion Pack'	3 oz	50	2.0	12.0	35	2.0	0.0	0.0	0	0%
(Freshlike)	3.3 oz	70	3.0	13.0	45	na	0.0	na	na	0%
(Frosty Acres)	3.3 oz	65	3.0	13.0	50	>1.0 c	0.0	0.0	0	0%
(Green Giant)	1/2 cup	40	2.0	9.0	40	2.0	0.0	0.0	0	0%
(Green Giant) 'Harvest Fresh'	1/2 cup	40	2.0	9.0	125	2.0	0.0	0.0	0	0%
(Green Giant) 'Plain Polybag'	1/2 cup	40	2.0	9.0	40	2.0	0.0	0.0	0	0%
(Health Valley)	1/2 cup	68	3.0	14.0	39	1.9	0.0	0.0	0	0%
(Seabrook)	3.3 oz	65	3.0	13.0	50	>1.0 c	0.0	0.0	0	0%
(Southern)	3.5 oz	69	3.2	13.9	60	(mq)	0.0	0.0	0	0%
(Stokely) 'Singles'	3 oz	60	3.0	12.0	40	(mq)	1.0	(tr)	0	13%
(Veg•All)	3.3 oz	70	3.0	13.0	45	na	0.0	na	na	0%
CALIFORNIA STYLE										
(A&P) 'California Blend'	3.3 oz	25	2.0	5.0	25	(mq)	<1.0	(tr)	0	<24%
(Freshlike) 'California Blend'	3.3 oz	30	2.0	6.0	20	na	0.0	na	na	0%
(Green Giant) 'American Mixtures'	1/2 cup	25	2.0	6.0	40	2.0	0.0	0.0	0	0%
(Veg•All) 'California Blend'	3.3 oz	30	2.0	6.0	20	na	0.0	na	na	0%
CHINESE STYLE										
(Birds Eye) chow mein, w/Oriental sauce 'Custom Cuisine'	4.6 oz	80	3.0	14.0	570	1.0	2.0	(mq)	0	21%
(Birds Eye) chow mein, w/seasoned sauce	3.3 oz	90	2.0	12.0	370	1.0	4.0	(mq)	0	39%
(Birds Eye) 'Stir-Fry'	3.3 oz	35	2.0	8.0	540	2.0	0.0	0.0	0	0%
CHUCKWAGON STYLE										
(Freshlike) 'Chuckwagon Blend'	3.3 oz	70	2.0	16.0	5	na	1.0	na	na	11%
(Veg•All) 'Chuckwagon Blend'	3.3 oz	70	2.0	16.0	5	na	1.0	na	na	11%
COUNTRY STYLE										
(Birds Eye) 'International Rice Recipes'	3.3 oz	90	2.0	19.0	380	1.0	0.0	na	0	0%
(Freshlike) 'Country Blend'	3.3 oz	50	2.0	12.0	15	na	0.0	na	na	0%
(Green Giant) 'American Mixtures Heartland'	1/2 cup	25	1.0	6.0	35	2.0	0.0	0.0	0	0%
(Veg•All) 'Country Blend'	3.3 oz	50	2.0	12.0	15	na	0.0	na	na	0%
DUTCH STYLE (Frosty Acres)	3.2 oz	30	2.0	5.0	30	(mq)	0.0	0.0	0	0%
FOR BEEF										
(Birds Eye) Oriental style, w/sauce	4.6 oz	90	6.0	11.0	350	2.0	4.0	(mq)	0	35%
(Birds Eye) w/cream mushroom 'Custom Cuisine'	4.6 oz	60	3.0	9.0	450	2.0	2.0	na	5	27%
FOR CHICKEN										
(Birds Eye) w/tomato basil sauce	4.6 oz	110	5.0	17.0	360	1.0	3.0	na	0	24%
(Birds Eye) w/wild rice, in white wine sauce	4.6 oz	100	3.0	19.0	510	1.0	0.0	0.0	0	0%
FOR CHICKEN OR FISH (Birds Eye) w/Dijon mustard sauce	4.6 oz	70	4.0	9.0	310	1.0	3.0	na	5	34%
FOR CHICKEN OR SHRIMP (Birds Eye) w/delicate herb sauce	4.6 oz	90	3.0	8.0	460	2.0	5.0	na	0	51%
FOR SOUP										
(Freshlike)	3.3 oz	50	2.0	11.0	40	na	0.0	na	na	0%
(Veg•All)	3.3 oz	50	2.0	11.0	40	na	0.0	na	na	0%
FOR STEW										
(A&P)	4 oz	60	1.0	13.0	30	(mq)	<1.0	(tr)	0	<14%
(Freshlike) 5-ways	3.3 oz	50	1.0	12.0	40	na	0.0	na	na	0%
(Freshlike) 4-ways	3.3 oz	50	1.0	11.0	40	na	0.0	na	na	0%
(Frosty Acres)	3 oz	42	3.0	10.0	21	(mq)	0.0	0.0	0	0%
(Kohl's)	3.3 oz	50	1.0	10.0	30	(mq)	<1.0	(tr)	0	<17%

Food Name	Serving Size	Calories	Prot. gms	Carbs gms	Sod. mgs	Fiber gms	Fat gms	Sat. Fat gms	Chol. mgs	% Fat Cal.
(Ore-Ida)	3 oz	60	1.0	12.0	40	(mq)	<1.0	(tr)	0	<15%
(Veg•All) 5-ways	3.3 oz	50	1.0	12.0	40	na	0.0	na	na	0%
(Veg•All) 4-ways	3.3 oz	50	1.0	11.0	40	na	0.0	na	na	0%
FRENCH STYLE *(Birds Eye)* 'International Recipes'	3.3 oz	110	3.0	23.0	610	na	0.0	na	0	0%
IN BUTTER SAUCE										
(Finast)	3.3 oz	70	4.0	15.0	340	(mq)	4.0	(mq)	na	32%
(Green Giant)	1/2 cup	60	2.0	11.0	300	2.0	2.0	<1.0	5	26%
ITALIAN STYLE										
(A&P) blend	3.3 oz	40	2.0	8.0	35	(mq)	<1.0	(tr)	0	<18%
(Birds Eye) 'International Recipes'	3.3 oz	100	2.0	11.0	490	2.0	5.0	na	0	46%
(Freshlike) 'Italian Blend'	3.3 oz	30	2.0	7.0	20	na	0.0	na	na	0%
(Freshlike) 'Italian Blend' food service	3.3 oz	25	1.0	5.0	20	na	0.0	na	na	0%
(Veg•All) 'Italian Blend'	3.3 oz	30	2.0	7.0	20	na	0.0	na	na	0%
(Veg•All) 'Italian Blend' food service	3.3 oz	25	1.0	5.0	20	na	0.0	na	na	0%
JAPANESE STYLE										
(Birds Eye) 'International Recipes'	3.3 oz	90	2.0	10.0	420	2.0	5.0	(mq)	0	48%
(Birds Eye) 'Stir-Fry'	3.3 oz	30	2.0	7.0	510	2.0	0.0	0.0	0	0%
LE SUEUR STYLE *(Green Giant)* 'Valley Combinations'	1/2 cup	70	4.0	12.0	400	2.0	2.0	0.0	0	22%
MANHATTAN STYLE *(Green Giant)* 'American Mixtures'	1/2 cup	25	2.0	5.0	15	2.0	0.0	0.0	0	0%
MIDWESTERN STYLE										
(Freshlike) 'Midwestern Blend'	3.3 oz	40	2.0	8.0	30	na	0.0	na	na	0%
(Veg•All) 'Midwestern Blend'	3.3 oz	40	2.0	8.0	30	na	0.0	na	na	0%
NEW ENGLAND STYLE										
(Birds Eye) 'International Recipes'	3.3 oz	130	3.0	14.0	430	2.0	7.0	(mq)	0	48%
(Green Giant) 'American Mixtures'	1/2 cup	70	3.0	14.0	75	4.0	1.0	na	0	12%
ORIENTAL STYLE										
(A&P) blend	3.3 oz	25	2.0	5.0	15	(mq)	<1.0	(tr)	0	<24%
(Birds Eye) 'International Recipes'	3.3 oz	70	2.0	8.0	300	1.0	4.0	(mq)	0	47%
(Freshlike) 'Oriental Blend'	3.3 oz	25	3.0	5.0	10	na	0.0	na	na	0%
(Frosty Acres)	3.2 oz	25	2.0	5.0	15	(mq)	0.0	0.0	0	0%
(Veg•All) 'Oriental Blend'	3.3 oz	25	3.0	5.0	10	na	0.0	na	na	0%
SAN FRANCISCO STYLE										
(Birds Eye) 'International Recipes'	3.3 oz	100	2.0	11.0	400	1.0	5.0	na	0	46%
(Green Giant) 'American Mixtures'	1/2 cup	25	1.0	7.0	35	2.0	0.0	0.0	0	0%
SANTA FE STYLE *(Green Giant)* 'American Mixtures'	1/2 cup	70	2.0	16.0	0	2.0	1.0	na	0	11%
SCANDINAVIAN STYLE										
(Freshlike) 'Scandinavian Blend'	3.3 oz	45	2.0	9.0	30	na	0.0	na	na	0%
(Veg•All) 'Scandinavian Blend'	3.3 oz	45	2.0	9.0	30	na	0.0	na	na	0%
SEATTLE STYLE *(Green Giant)* 'American Mixtures'	1/2 cup	25	2.0	7.0	35	2.0	0.0	0.0	0	0%
SPANISH STYLE *(Birds Eye)* 'International Recipes'	3.3 oz	110	3.0	24.0	540	na	0.0	na	0	0%
WESTERN STYLE *(Green Giant)* 'American Mixtures'	1/2 cup	60	2.0	12.0	25	2.0	2.0	0.0	0	24%
WINTER VEGETABLES										
(A&P) blend	3.3 oz	24	2.0	6.0	190	(mq)	<1.0	(tr)	0	<22%
(Freshlike) 'Winter Blend'	3.3 oz	25	3.0	5.0	25	na	0.0	na	na	0%
(Veg•All) 'Winter Blend'	3.3 oz	25	3.0	5.0	25	na	0.0	na	na	0%
W/PASTA										
(Birds Eye) cheese tortellini, in tomato sauce 'For One'	5.5 oz	210	11.0	31.0	500	0	5.0	na	30	21%
(Birds Eye) in Stroganoff sauce 'Custom Cuisine'	4.6 oz	120	5.0	15.0	700	0	5.0	na	30	36%
(Birds Eye) in white cheese sauce 'Custom Cuisine'	4.6 oz	150	7.0	19.0	440	1.0	6.0	na	15	34%
(Birds Eye) primavera style, w/seasoned sauce	3.3 oz	120	5.0	14.0	340	2.0	5.0	(mq)	5	37%
(Stokely) rotini, in cheddar cheese sauce 'Singles'	4 oz	100	4.0	15.0	380	(mq)	3.0	(mq)	10	26%
(Stokely) shells, in Italian style sauce 'Singles'	4 oz	170	3.0	5.0	270	(mq)	15.0	(mq)	5	81%
W/TERIYAKI SAUCE *(Stokely)* 'Singles'	4 oz	100	3.0	24.0	580	(mq)	0.0	0.0	0	0%
W/WHITE AND WILD RICE, pilaf *(Stokely)* 'Singles'	4 oz	80	3.0	17.0	290	(mq)	0.0	0.0	5	0%

Food Name	Serving Size	Calories	Prot. gms	Carbs gms	Sod. mgs	Fiber gms	Fat gms	Sat. Fat gms	Chol. mgs	% Fat Cal.
VEGETABLES, MIXED, MICROWAVE										
(Green Giant) 'Microwave Shelf-Pack'	1/2 cup	35	1.0	8.0	300	1.0	<1.0	0.0	0	<20%
(Pantry Express) 'Microwave Shelf-Pack'	1/2 cup	35	1.0	8.0	300	1.0	<1.0	0.0	0	<20%
VEGETARIAN ENTRÉE. See also individual listings.										
(Amy's Kitchen) Salisbury steak, organic, frozen										
'Country Dinner'	11 oz	482	12.0	48.0	760	4.0	19.0	na	32	42%
(Ken & Robert's) patty, frozen 'Truly Amazing'	2.5-oz patty	110	5.0	19.0	390	na	2.0	0.0	0	16%
(LaChoy) chow mein, w/o meat, canned	3/4 cup	35	2.0	6.0	820	2.2	0.4	na	0	10%
(Natural Touch) patty, frozen 'Dinner Entree'	3 oz	230	20.0	6.0	300	(mq)	14.0	2.0	0	55%
(Tofutti) tortellini, meatless, frozen	2 oz	220	12.0	38.0	110	(mq)	2.0	(mq)	0	8%
(Worthington) roast, frozen 'Dinner Roast'	2 oz	120	7.0	5.0	440	(mq)	8.0	1.0	0	60%
VEGETARIAN ENTRÉE MIX. See also individual listings.										
(Tofu Classics) stroganoff, creamy, prepared w/tofu	1/2 cup	94	7.0	11.0	264	(mq)	3.0	(mq)	0	27%
(Tofu Classics) stroganoff, creamy, prepared w/tofu and										
salted butter	1/2 cup	127	7.0	11.0	310	(mq)	7.0	(mq)	(mq)	47%
VEGETARIAN FOODS. See BACON, ALTERNATIVE; BEEF, ALTERNATIVE; BEEF JERKY, ALTERNATIVE; BURGER, VEGETARIAN; BURGER MIX, VEGETARIAN; CHICKEN, ALTERNATIVE; CRAB, ALTERNATIVE; FISH FILLET, ALTERNATIVE; HAM, ALTERNATIVE; LUNCHEON MEAT, ALTERNATIVE; MEAT, ALTERNATIVE; MEAT LOAF MIX, ALTERNATIVE; SAUSAGE, ALTERNATIVE; SCALLOP, ALTERNATIVE; SPREAD, VEGETARIAN; TUNA, ALTERNATIVE; TURKEY, ALTERNATIVE; VEGETARIAN ENTRÉE; and individual listings.										
VENISON. See ANTELOPE; CARIBOU; DEER; ELK; MOOSE.										
VIENNA SAUSAGE, CANNED										
beef and pork	1 oz	79	2.9	0.6	270	0	7.1	2.6	15	82%
2 inches long, 7/8 inch diam	1 sausage	45	1.6	0.3	152	0	4.0	1.5	8	83%
(Armour) chicken, in beef stock 'Premium' lite	2 oz	150	6.0	1.0	400	na	13.0	na	na	81%
(Armour) hot and spicy	2.5 oz	190	6.0	3.0	860	na	17.0	na	na	81%
(Armour) in barbecue sauce	2.5 oz	190	6.0	4.0	760	na	17.0	na	na	79%
(Armour) in beef stock	2 oz	180	5.0	1.0	530	na	17.0	na	na	86%
(Armour) in beef stock, lite	2 oz	150	6.0	1.0	400	na	13.0	na	na	81%
(Armour) smoked	2 oz	180	5.0	1.0	530	na	17.0	na	na	86%
(Hormel)	1 oz	69	3.0	2.0	225	na	7.0	2.0	15	76%
(Hormel) chicken	1 oz	56	3.0	1.0	220	na	5.0	1.0	27	74%
(Hormel) w/o broth	4 links	200	7.0	1.0	479	0	18.0	(mq)	(mq)	84%
(Libby's) chicken, in beef broth	2 oz	130	7.0	3.0	560	na	10.0	na	na	69%
(Libby's) in barbecue sauce	2.5 oz	180	8.0	2.0	420	0	15.0	(mq)	(mq)	77%
(Libby's) in beef broth	2 oz	160	6.0	1.0	330	0	15.0	(mq)	(mq)	83%
VINE SPINACH / basella										
raw	1 lb	86	8.2	15.4	(mq)	>3.2 c	1.4	(mq)	0	12%
raw	3.5 oz	19	1.8	3.4	24	>.7 c	0.3	na	0	12%
VINEGAR										
APPLE CIDER										
	1 cup	34	0.0	14.2	2	0	0.0	0.0	0	0%
	1 tbsp	2	0.0	0.9	0	0	0.0	0.0	0	0%
(Great Impressions)	1 tbsp	7	0.0	0.9	<1	0	0.0	0.0	0	0%
(Hain)	1 tbsp	2	0.0	4.0	1	0	0.0	0.0	0	0%
(Heinz)	.51 oz	2	0.0	0.0	1	0	0.0	0.0	0	0%
(Heinz) gourmet 'Decanter'	.51 oz	4	0.0	0.0	0	na	0.0	na	na	0%
(Indian Summer)	1 cup	40	<1.0	14.0	5	0	<1.0	0.0	0	<13%
(Lucky Leaf)	1 oz	4	0.0	2.0	0	0	0.0	0.0	0	0%
(Musselman's)	1 oz	4	0.0	2.0	0	0	0.0	0.0	0	0%
(Spectrum Naturals) filtered	1 tbsp	7	0.0	2.0	55	(tr)	0.0	0.0	0	0%
(Spectrum Naturals) unfiltered	1 tbsp	7	0.0	2.0	55	(tr)	0.0	0.0	0	0%
(White House)	1 oz	4	0.0	2.0	5	0	0.0	0.0	0	0%
BROWN RICE										
(Spectrum Naturals) organic	1 tbsp	0	0.0	0.0	0	(tr)	0.0	0.0	0	0%

Food Name	Serving Size	Calories	Prot. gms	Carbs gms	Sod. mgs	Fiber gms	Fat gms	Sat. Fat gms	Chol. mgs	% Fat Cal.
(Spectrum Naturals) organic, seasoned .... 1 tbsp		10	0.0	2.0	240	(tr)	0.0	0.0	0	0%

WHITE

Food Name	Serving Size	Calories	Prot. gms	Carbs gms	Sod. mgs	Fiber gms	Fat gms	Sat. Fat gms	Chol. mgs	% Fat Cal.
.... 1 cup		29	0.0	12.0	2	0	0.0	0.0	0	0%
.... 1 tbsp		2	0.0	0.8	0	0	0.0	0.0	0	0%
(Heinz) .... 1 tbsp		2	0.0	0.0	1	0	0.0	0.0	0	0%
(Indian Summer) .... 1 cup		30	<1.0	12.0	5	0	<1.0	0.0	0	<15%
(Lucky Leaf) .... 1 oz		4	0.0	2.0	0	0	0.0	0.0	0	0%
(Musselman's) .... 1 oz		4	0.0	2.0	0	0	0.0	0.0	0	0%
(Spectrum Naturals) organic .... 1 tbsp		0	0.0	0.0	0	(tr)	0.0	0.0	0	0%

WINE

Food Name	Serving Size	Calories	Prot. gms	Carbs gms	Sod. mgs	Fiber gms	Fat gms	Sat. Fat gms	Chol. mgs	% Fat Cal.
(Great Impressions) basil .... 1 tbsp		7	0.0	0.6	<1	0	0.0	0.0	0	0%
(Great Impressions) paprika, hot ..... 1 tbsp		6	0.0	0.6	<1	0	0.0	0.0	0	0%
(Great Impressions) raspberry .... 1 tbsp		7	0.0	1.0	<1	0	0.0	0.0	0	0%
(Heinz) gourmet 'Decanter' .... .51 oz		4	0.0	0.0	0	na	0.0	na	na	0%
(Heinz) tarragon, gourmet 'Decanter' .. .51 oz		2	0.0	0.0	0	na	0.0	na	na	0%
(Lucky Leaf) red .... 1 oz		0	0.0	0.0	0	0	0.0	0.0	0	0%
(Musselman's) red .... 1 oz		0	0.0	0.0	0	0	0.0	0.0	0	0%
(Regina) all varieties .... 1 oz		4	0.0	0.0	0	0	0.0	0.0	0	0%
(Spectrum Naturals) garlic, organic ... 1 tbsp		0	0.0	0.0	0	(tr)	0.0	0.0	0	0%
(Spectrum Naturals) Italian herb, organic ... 1 tbsp		0	0.0	0.0	0	(tr)	0.0	0.0	0	0%
(Spectrum Naturals) raspberry, organic ... 1 tbsp		10	2.0	0.0	0	(tr)	0.0	0.0	0	0%
(Spectrum Naturals) red, organic ..... 1 tbsp		0	0.0	0.0	0	(tr)	0.0	0.0	0	0%
(Spectrum Naturals) white, organic ... 1 tbsp		0	0.0	0.0	0	(tr)	0.0	0.0	0	0%
VITA JUICE *(Knudsen & Sons)* .... 8 oz		90	1.0	21.0	na	na	0.0	na	na	0%

VODKA. See ALCOHOLIC BEVERAGES.

Food Name	Serving Size	Calories	Prot. gms	Carbs gms	Sod. mgs	Fiber gms	Fat gms	Sat. Fat gms	Chol. mgs	% Fat Cal.

WAFFLE, FROZEN

Food Name	Serving Size	Calories	Prot. gms	Carbs gms	Sod. mgs	Fiber gms	Fat gms	Sat. Fat gms	Chol. mgs	% Fat Cal.
(Aunt Jemima) 'Original' 2.5 oz ..... 1 waffle		173	4.3	27.8	591	1.5	5.6	1.4	6	28%
(Downyflake) .... 2 waffles		120	3.0	20.0	420	(mq)	3.0	1.0	0	23%
(Downyflake) 'Crisp & Healthy' ...... 1 waffle		80	2.0	16.0	180	1.0	1.0	0.0	0	11%
(Downyflake) 'Hot-N-Buttery' .... 2 waffles		180	4.0	27.0	620	(mq)	6.0	(mq)	na	30%
(Downyflake) 'Jumbo' .... 2 waffles		170	4.0	30.0	570	(mq)	4.0	1.0	0	21%
(Eggo) 'Homestyle' .... 1 waffle		120	3.0	16.0	250	(mq)	5.0	(mq)	10	37%
(Eggo) 'Nutri-Grain' .... 1 waffle		130	3.0	18.0	250	2.0	5.0	(mq)	0	35%
(Roman Meal) .... 2 waffles		280	5.0	33.0	680	3.0	14.0	(mq)	4	45%
APPLE *(Eggo)* 'Fruit Top' .... 3.1 oz		190	3.0	32.0	250	na	6.0	1.0	0	28%

APPLE CINNAMON

Food Name	Serving Size	Calories	Prot. gms	Carbs gms	Sod. mgs	Fiber gms	Fat gms	Sat. Fat gms	Chol. mgs	% Fat Cal.
(Aunt Jemima) 2.5 oz .... 1 waffle		176	4.5	28.8	616	2.0	5.6	1.3	6	28%
(Downyflake) 'Crisp & Healthy' ...... 1 waffle		80	2.0	16.0	180	1.0	1.0	0.0	0	11%
(Eggo) .... 1 waffle		130	3.0	18.0	250	(mq)	5.0	(mq)	na	35%
(Van's) .... 1 waffle		75	2.8	8.4	68	3.3	2.0	na	0	29%

BLUEBERRY

Food Name	Serving Size	Calories	Prot. gms	Carbs gms	Sod. mgs	Fiber gms	Fat gms	Sat. Fat gms	Chol. mgs	% Fat Cal.
(Aunt Jemima) 2.5 oz .... 1 waffle		175	4.2	29.2	684	1.3	5.2	1.3	5	26%
(Downyflake) .... 2 waffles		180	4.0	32.0	570	(mq)	4.0	(mq)	0	20%
(Eggo) .... 1 waffle		130	3.0	18.0	250	(mq)	5.0	(mq)	na	35%
(Eggo) 'Fruit Top' .... 3.1 oz		190	3.0	32.0	250	na	6.0	1.0	0	28%
(Krusteaz) 1.2 oz .... 1 waffle		110	3.0	19.0	210	2.0	3.0	0.6	3	24%

BUTTERMILK

Food Name	Serving Size	Calories	Prot. gms	Carbs gms	Sod. mgs	Fiber gms	Fat gms	Sat. Fat gms	Chol. mgs	% Fat Cal.
(Aunt Jemima) 2.5 oz .... 1 waffle		179	4.4	28.7	615	1.3	5.8	1.4	7	28%

Food Name	Serving Size	Calories	Prot. gms	Carbs gms	Sod. mgs	Fiber gms	Fat gms	Sat. Fat gms	Chol. mgs	% Fat Cal.
(Downyflake)	2 waffles	190	5.0	32.0	750	(mq)	5.0	(mq)	0	23%
(Downyflake) 'Jumbo'	2 waffles	170	4.0	30.0	630	na	4.0	1.0	na	21%
(Eggo)	1 waffle	120	3.0	16.0	250	(mq)	5.0	(mq)	10	37%
(Krusteaz) 1.2 oz	1 waffle	100	3.0	16.0	190	2.0	2.0	na	4	19%
GOLDEN (Krusteaz) 1.2 oz	1 waffle	100	2.0	16.0	190	2.0	2.0	na	3	20%
HONEY ALMOND (Van's)	1 waffle	75	2.8	8.4	68	3.3	2.0	na	0	29%
MULTIGRAIN										
(Downyflake)	2 waffles	250	6.0	28.0	500	3.5	4.0	(mq)	0	21%
(Van's)	1 waffle	75	2.8	8.4	68	3.3	2.0	na	0	29%
OAT BRAN										
(Aunt Jemima)	2.5 oz	154	5.9	29.4	676	3.0	2.8	(mq)	na	15%
(Downyflake)	2 waffles	260	6.0	30.0	650	3.0	13.0	(mq)	0	45%
(Eggo) 'Common Sense'	1 waffle	110	3.0	16.0	220	2.0	4.0	(mq)	0	32%
(Eggo) w/fruit and nut 'Common Sense'	1 waffle	120	3.0	17.0	220	2.0	5.0	(mq)	0	36%
(Van's) 'Belgian'	1 waffle	89	3.3	11.0	124	na	2.0	na	0	24%
ORIGINAL (Van's) 'Belgian'	1 waffle	86	2.6	14.0	54	na	2.0	na	0	21%
PEACH (Eggo) 'Fruit Top'	3.1 oz	190	3.0	30.0	240	na	6.0	1.0	0	29%
RAISIN BRAN (Eggo) 'Nutri-Grain'	1 waffle	130	3.0	18.0	250	2.0	5.0	(mq)	0	35%
RICE BRAN (Downyflake)	2 waffles	210	5.0	25.0	230	3.5	11.0	(mq)	0	45%
SEVEN GRAIN (Van's) 'Belgian'	1 waffle	88	3.3	9.9	81	na	2.0	na	0	25%
STRAWBERRY										
(Eggo)	1 waffle	130	3.0	18.0	250	(mq)	5.0	(mq)	na	35%
(Eggo) 'Fruit Top'	1 waffle	190	3.0	31.0	230	na	6.0	1.0	0	28%
WHOLE-GRAIN WHEAT (Aunt Jemima)	1 waffle	154	5.9	29.4	676	3.0	2.8	(mq)	na	15%
WAFFLE BREAKFAST, FROZEN										
(Swanson) Belgian, w/sausage 'Great Starts'	2.85 oz	280	7.0	21.0	420	(mq)	19.0	(mq)	(mq)	60%
(Swanson) Belgian, w/strawberries and sausage	3.5 oz	210	3.0	31.0	240	(mq)	8.0	(mq)	(mq)	35%
(Swanson) w/bacon 'Great Starts'	2.2 oz	230	7.0	19.0	710	(mq)	14.0	(mq)	(mq)	55%
WAFFLE MIX. See PANCAKE/WAFFLE MIX.										
WAKAME. See SEAWEED.										
WALNUT, BLACK										
Dried										
	1 oz	172	6.9	3.4	0	1.4	16.1	1.0	0	78%
chopped	1 cup	759	30.4	15.1	1	6.3	70.7	4.5	0	78%
finely ground	1 cup	486	19.5	9.7	1	4.0	45.3	2.9	0	78%
in shell	1 lb	661	26.5	13.2	2	5.4	61.6	3.9	0	78%
Raw (Planters)	1 oz	180	7.0	3.0	0	na	17.0	1.0	0	79%
Shelled (Fisher)	1 oz	170	7.0	3.0	0	na	16.0	1.0	0	78%
WALNUT, ENGLISH										
Dried										
	1 lb	1310	29.2	37.4	21	9.8	126.3	11.4	0	81%
halves	1 cup	642	14.3	18.3	10	4.8	61.9	5.6	0	81%
halves, approx 14	1 oz	182	4.1	5.2	3	1.4	17.6	1.6	0	81%
in shell	1 lb	1310	29.2	37.4	21	9.8	126.3	11.4	0	81%
pieces or chips	1 cup	770	17.2	22.0	12	5.8	74.2	6.7	0	81%
(Diamond)	1 oz	192	5.0	4.0	na	(mq)	19.0	(mq)	0	83%
(Fisher) chopped	1 oz	180	4.0	5.0	0	na	18.0	2.0	0	82%
(Fisher) ground	1 oz	180	4.0	5.0	0	na	18.0	2.0	0	82%
(Planters) halves	1 oz	190	4.0	3.0	0	(mq)	20.0	2.0	0	87%
(Planters) pieces	1 oz	190	4.0	3.0	0	(mq)	20.0	2.0	0	87%
(Planters) whole	1 oz	190	4.0	3.0	0	(mq)	20.0	2.0	0	87%
Raw (Fisher)	1 oz	180	4.0	5.0	0	na	18.0	2.0	0	82%
WALNUT, PERSIAN										
Dried, in shell	1 lb	1310	29.2	37.4	21	9.8	126.3	11.4	0	81%

Food Name	Serving Size	Calories	Prot. gms	Carbs gms	Sod. mgs	Fiber gms	Fat gms	Sat. Fat gms	Chol. mgs	% Fat Cal.
Dried, shelled										
halves	1 cup	642	14.3	18.3	10	4.8	61.9	5.6	0	81%
halves, approx 14	1 oz	182	4.1	5.2	3	1.4	17.6	1.6	0	81%
pieces or chips	1 cup	770	17.2	22.0	12	5.8	74.2	6.7	0	81%
(Diamond)	1 oz	192	5.0	4.0	na	(mq)	19.0	(mq)	0	83%
(Planters) halves	1 oz	190	4.0	3.0	0	(mq)	20.0	2.0	0	87%
(Planters) pieces	1 oz	190	4.0	3.0	0	(mq)	20.0	2.0	0	87%
(Planters) whole	1 oz	190	4.0	3.0	0	(mq)	20.0	2.0	0	87%
WALNUT OIL										
	1 cup	1927	0.0	0.0	0	0	218.0	19.8	0	100%
	1 tbsp	120	0.0	0.0	0	0	13.6	1.2	0	100%
(Hain)	1 tbsp	120	0.0	0.0	0	0	14.0	2.0	0	100%
(Spectrum Naturals)	1 tbsp	120	0.0	0.0	0	(tr)	14.0	1.0	(tr)	100%
WASABI	1/4 oz	24	0.8	4.9	2	na	<.1	0.0	0	<4%
WATER, BOTTLED										
(Perrier)	1 cup	0	0.0	0.0	2	0	0.0	0.0	0	0%
(Perrier)	6.5-oz bottle	0	0.0	0.0	2	0	0.0	0.0	0	0%
(Poland Spring)	1 cup	0	0.0	0.0	2	0	0.0	0.0	0	0%
distilled (Arrowhead)	1 liter	0	0.0	0.0	0	0	0.0	0.0	0	0%
drinking (Arrowhead)	1 liter	0	0.0	0.0	16	0	0.0	0.0	0	0%
fluoridated (Arrowhead)	1 liter	0	0.0	0.0	16	0	0.0	0.0	0	0%
mineral (Perrier)	1 liter	0	0.0	0.0	19	0	0.0	0.0	0	0%
sparkling, natural, unflavored (Clearly Canadian)	6 oz	0	0.0	0.0	3	na	0.0	0.0	na	0%
spring (Arrowhead)	1 liter	0	0.0	0.0	9	0	0.0	0.0	0	0%
spring, Arizona Tule (Arrowhead)	1 liter	0	0.0	0.0	7	0	0.0	0.0	0	0%
Vichy (Schweppes)	6 oz	0	0.0	0.0	76	0	0.0	0.0	0	0%
WATER, SPARKLING, FLAVORED. See also SOFT DRINKS AND MIXERS.										
BLACK CHERRY										
'Refresher' (Quest)	10 oz	2	0.0	0.0	40	na	0.0	na	na	0%
'Refresher' (Quest)	8 oz	2	0.0	0.0	35	na	0.0	na	na	0%
BLACKBERRY, 'Mountain Blackberry' (Clearly Canadian)	6 oz	70	0.0	16.0	10	na	0.0	0.0	na	0%
CHERRY, 'Wild Cherry' (Clearly Canadian)	6 oz	70	0.0	16.0	10	na	0.0	0.0	na	0%
CHERRY-BLACKBERRY, w/juice (Cascadia)	6 oz	2	0.0	0.0	0	na	0.0	na	na	0%
CRANBERRY, 'Coastal Cranberry' (Clearly Canadian)	6 oz	70	0.0	16.0	10	na	0.0	0.0	na	0%
GRAPEFRUIT, w/juice (Cascadia)	6 oz	2	0.0	0.0	0	na	0.0	na	na	0%
GUAVA-BERRY, w/juice (Cascadia)	6 oz	2	0.0	0.0	0	na	0.0	na	na	0%
LEMONAID, w/juice (Cascadia)	6 oz	2	0.0	0.0	0	na	0.0	na	na	0%
LEMON-LIME (H2OH!)	6 oz	0	0.0	0.0	0	na	0.0	na	na	0%
LOGANBERRY, 'Western Loganberry' (Clearly Canadian)	6 oz	70	0.0	16.0	10	na	0.0	0.0	na	0%
NATURAL BERRY (H2OH!)	6 oz	0	0.0	0.0	0	na	0.0	na	na	0%
PEACH, 'Orchard Peach' (Clearly Canadian)	6 oz	70	0.0	16.0	10	na	0.0	0.0	na	0%
PEACH-CITRUS										
'Refresher' (Quest)	10 oz	2	0.0	0.0	40	na	0.0	na	na	0%
'Refresher' (Quest)	8 oz	2	0.0	0.0	35	na	0.0	na	na	0%
RASPBERRY										
'Country Raspberry' (Clearly Canadian)	6 oz	70	0.0	16.0	10	na	0.0	0.0	na	0%
'Refresher' (Quest)	10 oz	2	0.0	0.0	40	na	0.0	na	na	0%
'Refresher' (Quest)	8 oz	2	0.0	0.0	35	na	0.0	na	na	0%
RED RASPBERRY										
'Refresher' (Quest)	10 oz	2	0.0	0.0	40	na	0.0	na	na	0%
'Refresher' (Quest)	8 oz	2	0.0	0.0	35	na	0.0	na	na	0%
STRAWBERRY-KIWI										
'Refresher' (Quest)	10 oz	2	0.0	0.0	40	na	0.0	na	na	0%
'Refresher' (Quest)	8 oz	2	0.0	0.0	35	na	0.0	na	na	0%

Food Name	Serving Size	Calories	Prot. gms	Carbs gms	Sod. mgs	Fiber gms	Fat gms	Sat. Fat gms	Chol. mgs	% Fat Cal.
TANGERINE-LIME										
'Refresher' (Quest)	10 oz	2	0.0	0.0	40	na	0.0	na	na	0%
'Refresher' (Quest)	8 oz	2	0.0	0.0	35	na	0.0	na	na	0%
WATER BUFFALO										
raw	1 lb	449	92.5	0.0	240	na	6.2	2.1	209	13%
raw	1 oz	28	5.7	0.0	15	na	0.4	0.1	13	14%
roasted	3 oz	111	22.8	0.0	48	na	1.5	0.5	52	13%
roasted, diced, approx 4.9 oz	1 cup	183	37.6	0.0	78	0	2.5	0.8	85	13%
WATER CHESTNUT, CHINESE/matai										
approx 1.7 oz	4 fruits	38	0.5	8.6	5	1.1	0.0	na	0	0%
slices	1/2 cup	66	0.9	14.8	9	1.9	0.1	na	0	1%
trimmed	1 oz	30	0.4	6.8	4	>.2 c	<.1	(tr)	0	<3%
untrimmed	1 lb	369	4.9	83.6	50	>2.8 c	0.4	na	0	1%
Canned										
sliced, w/liquid	1/2 cup	35	0.6	8.7	6	1.8	0.0	na	0	0%
w/liquid	4 oz	57	1.0	14.1	9	>.7 c	0.1	(tr)	0	2%
w/liquid	4 fruits	14	0.3	3.5	2	.7	0.0	na	0	0%
(LaChoy)	1.28 oz	18	0.3	4.5	3	(mq)	<.1	(tr)	0	<5%
(LaChoy) chopped	.6349 oz	9	0.2	2.2	2	.9	0.1	0.0	0	9%
(LaChoy) sliced	1/4 cup	18	<1.0	4.0	3	<1.0	<1.0	(mq)	0	<31%
(LaChoy) sliced	.776 oz	11	0.2	2.7	3	1.1	0.1	0.0	0	7%
(LaChoy) whole	4 fruits	14	<1.0	4.0	2	<1.0	<1.0	(mq)	0	<31%
(LaChoy) whole	.6702 oz	10	0.2	2.3	2	.9	0.1	0.0	0	8%
WATER CONVOLVULUS. See CABBAGE, SKUNK.										
WATERCRESS										
chopped	1/2 cup	2	0.4	0.2	7	.4	0.0	0.0	0	0%
fresh	1 sprig	0	0.1	0.0	1	.1	0.0	0.0	0	0%
trimmed	1 oz	3	0.7	0.4	12	.7	<.1	tr	0	<17%
untrimmed	1 lb	46	9.6	5.4	170	9.6	0.4	0.1	0	6%
WATERMELON										
diced	1 cup	51	1.0	11.5	3	.6	0.7	na	0	11%
diced	1/2 cup	25	0.5	5.7	2	.3	0.3	(tr)	0	10%
sliced, 1/16 of 10-inch-diam fruit	1 slice	154	3.0	34.6	10	1.9	2.1	na	0	11%
trimmed	1 oz	9	0.2	2.0	1	.1	0.1	(tr)	0	9%
untrimmed	1 lb	74	1.5	16.9	5	.9	1.0	na	0	11%
WATERMELON SEED, DRIED										
in hard coat	1 lb	935	47.5	25.7	166	>5.1 c	79.5	16.4	0	71%
kernels	1 cup	602	30.6	16.5	107	>3.3 c	51.2	10.6	0	71%
kernels	1 oz	158	8.1	4.3	28	>.9 c	13.4	2.8	0	71%
WAX BEAN, CANNED										
(Allens)	1/2 cup	15	1.0	3.0	260	(mq)	<1.0	(tr)	0	<36%
(Del Monte) golden, cut	1/2 cup	20	0.0	4.0	355	(mq)	0.0	0.0	0	0%
(Del Monte) golden, French style	1/2 cup	20	0.0	4.0	355	(mq)	0.0	0.0	0	0%
(Stokely)	1/2 cup	20	1.0	4.0	360	(mq)	0.0	0.0	0	0%
(Stokely) 'No Salt or Sugar'	1/2 cup	20	1.0	4.0	5	(mq)	0.0	0.0	0	0%
WAX BEAN, FROZEN										
(Frosty Acres)	3 oz	25	2.0	5.0	1	>1.0 c	0.0	0.0	0	0%
(Seabrook) cut	3 oz	25	2.0	5.0	1	>1.0 c	0.0	0.0	0	0%
WAX GOURD. See GOURD, WAX.										
WELSH ONION. See ONION, WELSH.										
WELSH RAREBIT										
(Snow's) canned	1/2 cup	170	9.0	10.0	460	na	11.0	(mq)	(mq)	57%
(Stouffer's) frozen	5 oz	270	13.0	9.0	460	na	20.0	na	na	67%

Food Name	Serving Size	Calories	Prot. gms	Carbs gms	Sod. mgs	Fiber gms	Fat gms	Sat. Fat gms	Chol. mgs	% Fat Cal.
WESTERN DINNER, FROZEN										
(Banquet)	11 oz	630	28.0	40.0	720	(mq)	41.0	(mq)	90	58%
(Morton)	10 oz	290	14.0	29.0	1450	(mq)	14.0	(mq)	35	42%
(Swanson)	11.5 oz	430	22.0	43.0	1060	(mq)	19.0	(mq)	(mq)	40%
WHALE, raw	100 gm	156	20.6	0.0	78	0	7.5	1.3	50	45%
WHEAT, SPROUTED										
	1/3 cup	71	2.7	15.3	6	.4	0.5	0.1	0	6%
	1 oz	56	2.1	12.1	5	(mq)	0.4	0.1	0	6%
WHEAT, WHOLE GRAIN										
DURUM										
	1 cup	650	26.3	136.6	3	(mq)	4.7	0.9	0	6%
	1/2 cup	325	13.1	68.3	2	>2.2 c	2.4	0.4	0	6%
	1 oz	96	3.9	20.2	<1	(mq)	0.7	0.1	0	6%
HARD RED										
spring	1 cup	631	29.6	130.6	4	24.2	3.7	0.6	0	5%
spring	1/2 cup	316	14.8	65.3	2	12.1	1.8	0.3	0	5%
spring	1 oz	93	4.4	19.3	<1	>.6 c	0.5	0.1	0	5%
spring or winter (Arrowhead Mills)	2 oz	190	8.0	41.0	1	8.3	1.0	na	0	4%
winter	1 cup	628	24.2	136.7	4	24.2	3.0	0.5	0	4%
winter	1/2 cup	314	12.1	68.3	2	12.1	1.5	0.3	0	4%
winter	1 oz	93	3.6	20.2	<1	>.6 c	0.4	0.1	0	4%
HARD WHITE										
	1 cup	656	21.7	145.7	na	(mq)	3.3	0.5	0	4%
	1/2 cup	328	10.9	72.9	2	>2.2 c	1.6	0.3	0	4%
	1 oz	97	3.2	21.5	na	(mq)	0.5	0.1	0	4%
SOFT RED										
for pastry (Arrowhead Mills)	2 oz	190	8.0	41.0	1	8.3	1.0	na	0	4%
winter	1 cup	556	17.4	124.7	4	>2.9 c	2.6	0.5	0	4%
winter	1/2 cup	278	8.7	62.4	2	>1.4 c	1.3	0.2	0	4%
winter	1 oz	94	2.9	21.0	<1	>.5 c	0.4	0.1	0	4%
SOFT WHITE										
	1 cup	571	18.0	126.6	na	(mq)	3.3	0.6	0	5%
	1/2 cup	286	9.0	63.3	2	>1.4 c	1.7	0.3	0	5%
	1 oz	96	3.0	21.4	na	(mq)	0.6	0.1	0	5%
WHEAT BRAN										
crude	1/2 cup	65	4.7	19.4	1	12.8	1.3	0.2	0	11%
crude	1 oz	61	4.4	18.3	<1	12.0	1.2	0.2	0	11%
crude	2 tbsp	15	1.1	4.5	0	3.0	0.3	0.0	0	11%
crude (Arrowhead Mills)	2 oz	50	10.0	30.0	3	24.4	2.0	(mq)	0	10%
toasted (Kretschmer)	1 oz	57	5.7	14.8	2	11.4	2.3	0.2	0	20%
unprocessed (Quaker)	2 tbsp	8	1.0	3.8	0	3.3	0.2	0.0	0	9%
WHEAT CAKE										
(Quaker) 'Grain Cakes'	1 cake	34	1.4	6.7	52	.8	0.3	0.1	0	8%
(Quaker) lightly salted	1 cake	35	1.0	7.0	50	na	0.0	na	0	0%
WHEAT FLAKES (Arrowhead Mills)	2 oz	210	8.0	42.0	1	6.7	1.0	na	0	4%
WHEAT FLOUR										
RYE										
(Pillsbury's Best) medium-colored	1 cup	400	12.0	83.0	0	9	2.0	0.0	0	5%
(Pillsbury's Best) w/wheat 'Bohemian Style'	1 cup	400	11.0	86.0	0	na	1.0	na	0	2%
WHITE										
(Drifted Snow)	1 cup	400	11.0	87.0	0	(mq)	1.0	(mq)	0	2%
(Softasilk)	1/4 cup	100	2.0	23.0	0	(mq)	0.0	0.0	0	0%
(Wondra)	1 cup	400	11.0	87.0	0	(mq)	1.0	(mq)	0	2%

Food Name	Serving Size	Calories	Prot. gms	Carbs gms	Sod. mgs	Fiber gms	Fat gms	Sat. Fat gms	Chol. mgs	% Fat Cal.
All-purpose										
enriched	1/2 cup	226	6.4	47.3	1	1.7	0.6	0.1	0	3%
enriched	1 oz	103	2.9	21.6	<1	.8	0.3	<.1	0	3%
enriched, calcium-fortified	1/2 cup	226	6.4	47.3	1	>.2 c	0.6	0.1	0	3%
(Ballard)	1 cup	400	11.0	87.0	0	(mq)	1.0	(mq)	0	2%
(Ceresota)	4 oz	390	12.5	82.5	0	(mq)	1.0	(mq)	0	2%
(Gold Medal)	1 cup	400	11.0	87.0	0	(mq)	1.0	(mq)	0	2%
(Heckers)	4 oz	390	12.5	82.5	0	(mq)	1.0	(mq)	0	2%
(Pillsbury's Best)	1 cup	400	11.0	87.0	0	(mq)	1.0	(mq)	0	2%
(Red Band)	1 cup	390	10.0	85.0	0	(mq)	1.0	(mq)	0	2%
(Robin Hood)	1 cup	400	13.0	85.0	0	(mq)	1.0	(mq)	0	2%
(White Deer)	1 cup	400	11.0	87.0	0	(mq)	1.0	(mq)	0	2%
All-purpose, unbleached										
enriched	1/2 cup	226	6.4	47.3	1	>.2 c	0.6	0.1	0	3%
(Arrowhead Mills)	2 oz	200	7.0	53.0	1	(mq)	1.0	(mq)	0	4%
(Gold Medal)	1 cup	400	11.0	87.0	0	(mq)	1.0	(mq)	0	2%
(Pillsbury's Best)	1 cup	400	12.0	86.0	0	(mq)	1.0	(mq)	0	2%
(Robin Hood)	1 cup	400	13.0	85.0	0	(mq)	1.0	(mq)	0	2%
Bread										
enriched	1/2 cup	249	8.3	50.0	1	1.7	1.1	0.2	0	4%
enriched	1 oz	102	3.4	20.6	<1	(mq)	0.5	0.1	0	5%
(Gold Medal) 'Better for Bread'	1 cup	400	14.0	83.0	0	(mq)	1.0	(mq)	0	2%
(Pillsbury's Best)	1 cup	400	14.0	83.0	0	(mq)	2.0	(mq)	0	4%
Cake										
enriched	1/2 cup	195	4.4	42.1	1	.9	0.5	0.1	0	2%
enriched	1 oz	103	2.3	22.1	<1	(mq)	0.2	<.1	0	2%
Self-rising										
enriched	1/2 cup	219	6.1	46.0	787	2.0	0.6	0.1	0	3%
enriched	1 oz	100	2.8	21.0	360	<.1	0.3	<.1	0	3%
(Aunt Jemima) enriched	1 oz	109	3.0	23.6	368	>.1 c	0.3	na	0	3%
(Ballard)	1 cup	380	9.0	84.0	1290	(mq)	1.0	(mq)	0	2%
(Gold Medal)	1 cup	380	10.0	83.0	1520	(mq)	1.0	(mq)	0	2%
(Pillsbury's Best)	1 cup	380	9.0	84.0	1290	2	1.0	(mq)	0	2%
(Pillsbury's Best) unbleached	1 cup	380	9.0	84.0	1290	2	1.0	0.0	0	2%
(Red Band)	1 cup	380	9.0	83.0	1520	(mq)	1.0	(mq)	0	2%
(Robin Hood)	1 cup	380	10.0	83.0	1520	(mq)	1.0	(mq)	0	2%
Shake and blend (Pillsbury's Best)	2 tbsp	50	1.0	11.0	0	na	0.0	0.0	0	0%
Tortilla mix										
enriched	1/3 cup	150	3.6	24.8	250	>.1 c	3.9	1.5	0	24%
enriched	1 oz	115	2.7	19.0	192	<.1	3.0	1.2	0	24%
WHOLE GRAIN										
	1/2 cup	203	8.2	43.5	3	7.3	1.1	0.2	0	5%
	1 oz	96	3.9	20.6	1	3.6	0.5	0.1	0	4%
(Arrowhead Mills) pastry	2 oz	180	6.0	41.0	1	6.8	1.0	(mq)	0	5%
(Arrowhead Mills) stone ground	2 oz	200	8.0	40.0	1	6.7	1.0	(mq)	0	5%
(Ceresota)	4 oz	400	15.0	80.0	0	(mq)	2.0	(mq)	0	5%
(Gold Medal)	1 cup	350	16.0	78.0	0	10.0	2.0	(mq)	0	5%
(Gold Medal) blend	1 cup	380	14.0	84.0	0	8.0	2.0	(mq)	0	4%
(Heckers)	4 oz	400	15.0	80.0	0	(mq)	2.0	(mq)	0	5%
(Krusteaz)	1 cup	450	17.0	90.0	5	15.0	2.0	<1.0	0	4%
(Pillsbury's Best)	1 cup	400	15.0	80.0	10	(mq)	2.0	(mq)	0	5%
WHEAT GERM										
crude	1/4 cup	104	6.7	15.0	3	3.8	2.8	0.5	0	23%
crude	1 oz	102	6.6	14.7	3	4.3	2.8	0.5	0	23%

Food Name	Serving Size	Calories	Prot. gms	Carbs gms	Sod. mgs	Fiber gms	Fat gms	Sat. Fat gms	Chol. mgs	% Fat Cal.
toasted	1 cup	431	32.9	56.1	4	14.6	12.1	2.1	0	23%
toasted	1 oz	108	8.3	14.1	1	3.7	3.0	0.5	0	23%
(Arrowhead Mills) raw	2 oz	210	15.0	26.0	1	6.5	6.0	(mq)	0	25%
(Kretschmer)	1 oz	103	9.3	12.3	2	3.3	3.4	0.5	0	26%
(Kretschmer) honey crunch	1 oz	105	7.6	15.2	2	3.0	2.8	0.4	0	22%
WHEAT GERM OIL										
	1 cup	1927	0.0	0.0	0	0	218.0	41.0	0	100%
	1 tbsp	120	0.0	0.0	0	0	13.6	2.6	0	100%
(Spectrum Naturals) unrefined	1 tbsp	120	0.0	0.0	0	(tr)	14.0	1.0	(tr)	100%
WHEAT GLUTEN (Arrowhead Mills) 'Vita 1' toasted	1 oz	100	15.0	9.0	1	.9	1.0	na	0	9%
WHEAT NUTS										
macadamia flavor, w/o salt	1 oz	176	3.2	7.9	13	1.5	16.0	2.4	0	76%
other flavors, w/o salt	1 oz	184	3.7	5.9	26	1.5	17.7	2.7	0	81%
unflavored, w/salt added	1 oz	177	3.9	6.7	143	1.5	16.4	2.5	0	78%
WHEAT PILAF MIX, dry mix (Casbah)	1 oz	100	3.0	20.0	(mq)	(mq)	0.0	0.0	0	0%
WHELK										
moist-heat cooked	3 oz	234	40.5	13.2	350	0	0.7	0.1	110	3%
raw	1 lb	623	108.1	35.2	934	0	1.8	0.1	294	3%
raw	3 oz	116	20.3	6.6	175	0	0.3	0.0	55	2%
raw	1 oz	39	6.8	2.2	54	0	0.1	<.1	18	2%
WHEY										
Acid										
dry	1 cup	193	6.7	41.9	552	0	0.3	0.2	2	1%
dry	1 oz	96	3.3	20.8	274	0	0.2	0.1	(tr)	2%
dry	1 tbsp	10	0.3	2.1	28	0	0.0	0.0	0	0%
fluid	1 quart	235	7.5	50.4	473	0	0.9	0.6	5	3%
fluid	1 cup	59	1.9	12.6	118	0	0.2	0.1	1	3%
fluid	1 oz	7	0.2	1.5	14	0	<.1	<.1	(tr)	<12%
Sweet										
dry	1 cup	512	18.8	108.0	1565	0	1.5	1.0	9	3%
dry	1 oz	100	3.7	21.1	306	0	0.3	0.2	2	3%
dry	1 tbsp	26	1.0	5.6	81	0	0.1	0.1	0	3%
fluid	1 quart	263	8.4	50.6	526	0	3.5	2.3	20	12%
fluid	1 cup	66	2.1	12.6	132	0	0.9	0.6	5	12%
fluid	1 oz	8	0.2	1.5	15	0	0.1	<.1	<1	12%
WHIPPED TOPPING. See CREAM TOPPING.										
WHISKEY. See ALCOHOLIC BEVERAGES.										
WHISKEY SOUR. See ALCOHOLIC BEVERAGES.										
WHITE BEAN										
boiled	4 oz	158	11.0	28.5	7	>2.8 c	0.4	0.1	0	2%
boiled	1/2 cup	125	8.8	22.6	5	5.7	0.3	0.1	0	2%
raw	1/2 cup	336	23.6	60.9	16	15.4	0.9	0.2	0	2%
raw	1 oz	94	6.6	17.1	5	>1.7 c	0.2	0.1	0	2%
small, boiled	4 oz	161	10.2	29.3	2	5.0	0.7	0.2	0	4%
small, boiled	1/2 cup	128	8.1	23.2	2	>2.2 c	0.6	0.2	0	4%
small, raw	1/2 cup	363	22.8	67.2	13	>2.9 c	1.3	0.3	0	3%
small, raw	1 oz	95	6.0	17.6	3	2.9	0.3	0.1	0	3%
WHITE BEAN, CANNED										
	1/2 cup	153	9.5	28.7	7	6.3	0.4	0.1	0	2%
w/liquid	4 oz	133	8.2	24.9	515	>.8 c	0.3	0.1	0	2%
WHITE-FLOWERED GOURD. See GOURD, BOTTLE.										
WHITE GOURD. See GOURD, WHITE.										
WHITEFISH										
dry-heat cooked	3 oz	146	20.8	0.0	55	0	6.4	1.0	65	41%

Food Name	Serving Size	Calories	Prot. gms	Carbs gms	Sod. mgs	Fiber gms	Fat gms	Sat. Fat gms	Chol. mgs	% Fat Cal.
dry-heat cooked, approx 7 oz	1 fillet	265	37.7	0.0	100	0	11.6	1.8	119	41%
raw	1 lb	610	86.6	0.0	232	0	26.6	4.1	272	41%
raw	3 oz	114	16.2	0.0	43	0	5.0	0.8	51	41%
raw	1 oz	38	5.4	0.0	14	0	1.7	0.3	17	42%
raw, approx 7 oz	1 fillet	265	37.8	0.0	101	0	11.6	1.8	119	41%
smoked	4 oz	122	26.5	0.0	1156	0	1.1	0.3	37	9%
smoked	3 oz	92	19.9	0.0	866	0	0.8	0.2	28	8%
smoked	1 oz	30	6.6	0.0	285	0	0.3	0.1	9	9%
WHITING, MIXED SPECIES/silver hake										
dry-heat cooked	4 oz	130	26.6	0.0	150	0	1.9	0.4	95	14%
dry-heat cooked	3 oz	98	20.0	0.0	112	0	1.4	0.3	7	14%
raw	1 lb	408	83.1	0.0	326	0	6.0	1.1	303	14%
raw	3 oz	77	15.6	0.0	61	0	1.1	0.2	57	14%
raw	1 oz	26	5.2	0.0	20	0	0.4	<.1	19	15%
WHITING, MIXED SPECIES										
(Booth) frozen	4 oz	100	19.0	0.0	90	0	1.0	(mq)	(mq)	11%
(Booth) 'Individually Wrapped' frozen	4 oz	80	19.0	0.0	85	0	1.0	(mq)	(mq)	11%
WILD BERRY DRINK										
(Hi-C)	6 oz	92	0.1	22.5	17	(tr)	0.1	(tr)	0	1%
(Hi-C) aseptic box or chilled	6 oz	90	0.0	22.0	20	na	0.0	na	na	0%
(Hi-C) boxed	8.45 oz	129	0.1	31.7	24	(tr)	0.1	(tr)	0	1%
(Hi-C) chilled	6 oz	90	0.0	22.0	20	na	0.0	na	na	0%
(Tropicana) 'Juice Sparkler'	8 oz	110	(tr)	27.0	15	(tr)	0.0	0.0	0	0%
WINE. See ALCOHOLIC BEVERAGES.										
WINE, COOKING. See also ALCOHOLIC BEVERAGES.										
Burgundy (Regina)	1/4 cup	2	<1.0	<1.0	365	0	<1.0	(tr)	0	<53%
Marsala (Holland House)	1 oz	9	0.0	2.3	186	0	0.0	0.0	0	0%
red (Holland House)	1 oz	6	0.0	1.5	186	0	0.0	0.0	0	0%
Sauternes (Regina)	1/4 cup	2	<1.0	<1.0	365	0	<1.0	(tr)	0	<53%
sherry (Holland House)	1 oz	5	0.0	1.2	186	0	0.0	0.0	0	0%
sherry (Regina)	1/4 cup	20	<1.0	5.0	70	0	<1.0	(tr)	0	<27%
vermouth (Holland House)	1 oz	2	0.0	<1.0	186	0	0.0	0.0	0	0%
white (Holland House)	1 oz	2	0.0	<1.0	186	0	0.0	0.0	0	0%
WINGED BEAN/goa bean										
boiled, drained	4 oz	43	6.0	3.6	5	>1.6 c	0.7	0.2	0	14%
immature seeds, boiled, drained	1/2 cup	12	1.6	1.0	1	>.4 c	0.2	0.1	0	15%
immature seeds, raw, approx .6 oz	1 pod	8	1.1	0.7	1	>.4 c	0.1	0.0	0	11%
immature seeds, slices, raw	1 cup	22	3.1	1.9	2	>1.1 c	0.4	0.1	0	15%
mature seeds, boiled, drained	1/2 cup	126	9.1	12.8	11	>2.1 c	5.0	0.7	0	34%
mature seeds, raw	1/2 cup	372	27.0	38.0	35	>6.2 c	14.9	2.1	0	34%
trimmed, raw	1 oz	14	2.0	1.2	1	>.7 c	0.2	0.1	0	12%
untrimmed, raw	1 lb	218	30.9	19.2	17	>11.4 c	3.9	1.1	0	15%
WINGED BEAN, DRIED										
boiled	4 oz	167	12.0	16.9	15	>2.8 c	6.6	0.9	0	34%
boiled	1/2 cup	126	9.1	12.8	11	>2.1 c	5.0	0.7	0	34%
raw	1/2 cup	372	27.0	38.0	35	14.1 c	14.9	2.1	0	34%
raw	1 oz	116	8.4	11.8	11	4.4	4.6	0.7	0	34%
WINGED BEAN LEAVES										
trimmed	1 lb	336	26.5	64.0	na	>11.3 c	5.0	1.2	0	11%
trimmed	1 oz	21	1.7	4.0	na	>.7 c	0.3	0.1	0	11%
WOLF FISH/ocean catfish										
dry-heat cooked	3 oz	105	19.1	0.0	93	0	2.6	0.4	50	23%
frozen (Booth)	4 oz	115	20.0	0.0	85	0	20.0	(mq)	(mq)	69%
raw	1 lb	437	79.4	0.0	386	0	10.8	1.7	209	23%

Food Name	Serving Size	Calories	Prot. gms	Carbs gms	Sod. mgs	Fiber gms	Fat gms	Sat. Fat gms	Chol. mgs	% Fat Cal.
raw	3 oz	82	11.0	0.0	72	0	2.0	0.3	39	23%
raw	1 oz	27	5.0	0.0	24	0	0.7	0.1	13	24%
raw, approx 5.4 oz	1/2 fillet	147	26.8	0.0	130	0	3.7	0.6	70	24%
WON TON SKIN										
....	1 oz	83	2.8	16.4	162	na	0.4	0.1	3	5%
....	1 wrapper	23	0.8	4.6	46	na	0.1	0.0	1	4%
(Nasoya)	1 wrapper	23	1.0	4.5	19	(mq)	0.0	0.0	0	0%
WON TON SOUP. See SOUP.										

Y

Food Name	Serving Size	Calories	Prot. gms	Carbs gms	Sod. mgs	Fiber gms	Fat gms	Sat. Fat gms	Chol. mgs	% Fat Cal.
YAKIDOFU. See TOFU.										
YAM										
boiled and drained, or baked	4 oz	132	1.7	31.2	9	(mq)	0.2	<.1	0	1%
boiled and drained, or baked, cubed	1/2 cup	79	1.0	18.8	5	2.7	0.1	0.0	0	1%
raw, cubed	1/2 cup	89	1.1	20.9	7	3.1	0.1	0.0	0	1%
raw, trimmed	1 oz	33	0.4	7.9	3	(mq)	<.1	<.1	0	<3%
raw, untrimmed	1 lb	460	6.0	108.8	37	(mq)	0.7	0.1	0	1%
Mountain/Hawaiian										
raw, approx 8.25 inches long	1 yam	281	5.6	68.5	55	>1.9 c	0.4	0.1	0	1%
raw, cubed	1/2 cup	46	0.9	11.1	9	>.3 c	0.1	0.0	0	2%
raw, trimmed	1 oz	19	0.4	4.6	4	>.1 c	<.1	0.0	tr	<4%
raw, untrimmed	1 lb	253	5.0	61.4	49	>1.7 c	0.4	0.1	0	1%
steamed	4 oz	93	2.0	22.7	14	>.6 c	0.1	<.1	0	1%
steamed, cubed	1/2 cup	59	1.2	14.4	9	>.4 c	0.1	<.1	0	1%
YAM, CANNED *(Bush's Best)*	1/2 cup	120	1.0	28.0	20	na	0.0	na	na	0%
YAM BEAN TUBER. See JICAMA.										
YARDLONG BEAN/asparagus bean										
boiled, drained	4 oz	53	2.9	10.4	5	>1.7 c	0.1	<.1	0	2%
boiled, drained, approx 13.25 inches long	1 pod	7	0.4	1.3	1	>.2 c	0.0	0.0	0	0%
boiled, drained, sliced	1 cup	49	2.6	9.6	4	1.6	0.1	0.0	0	2%
boiled, drained, sliced	1/2 cup	25	1.3	4.8	2	>.8 c	0.1	<.1	0	4%
mature, boiled	1/2 cup	101	7.1	18.1	4	>1.4 c	0.4	0.1	0	3%
mature, raw	1/2 cup	291	20.4	52.0	14	>4.0 c	1.1	0.3	0	3%
raw, approx 13.25 inches long	1 pod	6	0.3	1.0	0	>.1 c	0.1	0.0	0	15%
raw, sliced	1 cup	43	2.5	7.6	4	>.6 c	0.4	0.1	0	8%
raw, sliced	1/2 cup	22	1.3	3.8	2	(mq)	0.2	<.1	0	8%
raw, trimmed	1 oz	13	0.8	2.4	1	(mq)	0.1	<.1	0	7%
raw, untrimmed	1 lb	203	12.1	36.0	17	(mq)	1.7	0.5	0	7%
Dried										
boiled	4 oz	134	9.4	23.9	6	>1.8 c	0.5	0.1	0	3%
boiled	1/2 cup	102	7.1	18.1	4	>1.4 c	0.4	0.1	0	3%
raw	1/2 cup	292	20.4	52.0	14	>4.0 c	1.1	0.3	0	3%
raw	1 oz	98	6.9	17.6	5	>1.4 c	0.4	0.1	0	4%
YEAST, BAKER'S										
active dry	1 oz	79	10.3	10.9	15	0	0.5	0.0	0	5%
active dry	1 tbsp	35	4.6	4.6	6	3.3	0.6	0.1	0	13%
active dry	.25-oz pkg	21	2.7	2.7	4	1.9	0.3	0.0	0	11%
compressed	100 gm	105	8.4	18.1	30	9.3	1.9	0.2	0	14%
compressed	.6-oz cake	18	1.4	3.1	5	1.6	0.3	0.0	0	13%
compressed, fortified	1 oz	24	3.4	3.1	4	>.2 c	0.1	0.0	0	3%

Food Name	Serving Size	Calories	Prot. gms	Carbs gms	Sod. mgs	Fiber gms	Fat gms	Sat. Fat gms	Chol. mgs	% Fat Cal.
compressed, not fortified	1 oz	24	3.4	3.1	4	>.2 c	0.1	0.0	0	3%
YEAST, BREWER'S										
debittered	1 oz	79	10.9	10.8	34	>.5 c	0.3	0.0	0	3%
debittered	1 tbsp	23	3.1	3.1	10	>.1 c	0.1	0.0	0	4%
(Fleischmann's) 'Active Dry/RapidRise'	1/4 oz	20	3.0	3.0	10	(mq)	0.0	0.0	0	0%
(Red Star) 'Active Dry'	1/4 oz	15	2.0	2.0	5	(mq)	0.0	0.0	0	0%
YEAST, TORULA	1 oz	78	10.8	10.4	4	>.9 c	0.3	0.0	0	3%
YELLOW BEAN										
mature, boiled	1/2 cup	127	8.1	22.2	4	>1.0 c	1.0	0.3	0	7%
mature, raw	1/2 cup	338	21.6	59.5	12	>2.7 c	2.5	0.7	0	7%
Dried										
boiled	4 oz	163	10.4	28.7	6	>1.3 c	1.2	0.3	0	7%
boiled	1/2 cup	126	8.1	22.2	4	>1.0 c	1.0	0.2	0	7%
raw	1/2 cup	338	21.6	59.5	12	>2.7 c	2.6	0.7	0	7%
raw	1 oz	98	6.2	17.2	3	>.8 c	0.7	0.2	0	6%
YELLOW MOMBIN. See JOBO.										
YELLOWEYE BEAN *(B&M)* canned, baked style	8 oz	326	15.0	50.0	770	15.0	7.0	(mq)	4	20%
YELLOW-EYED PEAS. See BLACK-EYED PEAS.										
YELLOWTAIL, MIXED SPECIES										
dry-heat cooked	3 oz	159	25.2	0.0	43	0	5.7	na	60	34%
raw	1 lb	662	105.0	0.0	177	0	23.8	(mq)	(mq)	34%
raw	3 oz	124	19.7	0.0	33	0	4.4	1.1	47	33%
raw	1 oz	41	6.6	0.0	11	0	1.5	(mq)	(mq)	34%
YOGURT										
(Colombo) 'Fruit on the Bottom' all flavors	8 oz	230	7.0	36.0	140	(mq)	6.0	(mq)	(mq)	24%
(Colombo) 'Nonfat Fruit on the Bottom' all flavors	8 oz	190	8.0	38.0	140	(mq)	<1.0	na	5	<5%
(Colombo) 'Nonfat Lite Minipack' all flavors	4.4 oz	100	5.0	20.0	70	(mq)	0.0	0.0	(mq)	0%
(Crowley) 'Sundae Style' all flavors	8 oz	250	9.0	47.0	170	(mq)	2.0	(mq)	10	7%
(Crowley) 'Swiss Style' all flavors	8 oz	240	8.0	40.0	150	(mq)	2.0	(mq)	10	7%
(Dannon) 'Extra Smooth' all flavors	4.4 oz	130	5.0	24.0	80	(mq)	2.0	(mq)	10	13%
(Dannon) 'Hearty Nuts & Raisins' all flavors except vanilla	8 oz	260	11.0	48.0	120	(mq)	3.0	(mq)	10	10%
(Knudsen) 'Lowfat' all flavors except strawberry	8 oz	240	11.0	43.0	135	(mq)	4.0	2.0	15	14%
(Light n' Lively) 'Free' all flavors except strawberry	4.4 oz	50	4.0	8.0	60	(mq)	0.0	0.0	0	0%
(Ripple) '70' fat-free, all flavors	6 oz	70	5.0	13.0	85	(mq)	0.0	0.0	5	0%
(Yoplait) 'Fat-free' all flavors	6 oz	150	7.0	31.0	95	(mq)	0.0	0.0	5	0%
(Yoplait) 'Light' all flavors	6 oz	90	7.0	14.0	100	(mq)	0.0	0.0	5	0%
(Yoplait) 'Light' all flavors	4 oz	60	5.0	9.0	65	(mq)	0.0	0.0	5	0%
APPLE CRISP *(New Country)* 'Lowfat'	6 oz	150	5.0	30.0	85	(mq)	2.0	(mq)	(mq)	11%
BANANA										
(Dannon) 'Sprinkl'ins' lowfat	4.1 oz	140	5.0	24.0	80	na	2.0	na	5	13%
(Yoplait) 'Custard Style'	6 oz	180	7.0	30.0	105	na	3.0	na	na	15%
BANANA BERRY										
(Light n' Lively) lowfat, 1% milkfat, cultured	4.4 oz	130	5.0	24.0	75	na	1.0	1.0	10	7%
BERRIES *(Yoplait)* 'Breakfast' w/wheat, raisins, and walnuts	6 oz	200	8.0	39.0	125	na	2.0	na	na	9%
BLACK CHERRY										
(Alta•Dena) 'Blended European Style'	8 oz	190	8.0	38.0	140	na	<1.0	na	na	<5%
(Alta•Dena) 'Naja' fruit-on-the-bottom	8 oz	240	12.0	40.0	150	na	4.0	na	na	15%
(Breyers) 'Lowfat'	8 oz	260	9.0	49.0	120	(mq)	3.0	1.0	10	10%
(Knudsen) 'Cal 70'	6 oz	70	5.0	12.0	75	(mq)	0.0	0.0	5	0%
(Light n' Lively)	8 oz	230	9.0	44.0	125	(mq)	2.0	1.0	15	8%
(Light n' Lively) '100'	8 oz	100	8.0	17.0	100	(mq)	0.0	0.0	0	0%
(Mountain High) 'Honey Light' natural	8 oz	190	9.0	35.0	140	na	1.0	na	5	5%
(TCBY) 'Light'	8 oz	100	8.0	17.0	180	na	0.0	na	na	0%

Food Name	Serving Size	Calories	Prot. gms	Carbs gms	Sod. mgs	Fiber gms	Fat gms	Sat. Fat gms	Chol. mgs	% Fat Cal.
BLUEBERRY										
(Alta•Dena) 'Maya' fruit-on-the-bottom	8 oz	280	11.0	39.0	170	na	9.0	na	na	29%
(Breyers) 'Lowfat'	8 oz	250	9.0	48.0	120	(mq)	2.0	1.0	10	7%
(Dannon) 'Blended' fat-free	6 oz	160	7.0	33.0	105	na	0.0	0.0	5	0%
(Dannon) 'Light' nonfat	8 oz	100	9.0	19.0	135	na	0.0	0.0	<5	0%
(Knudsen) 'Cal 70'	6 oz	70	6.0	11.0	80	(mq)	0.0	0.0	5	0%
(Light n' Lively)	8 oz	240	8.0	46.0	130	(mq)	2.0	1.0	10	8%
(Light n' Lively)	4.4 oz	130	5.0	26.0	79	(mq)	1.0	1.0	5	7%
(Light n' Lively) 'Free' nonfat	4.4 oz	50	4.0	8.0	60	na	0.0	0.0	0	0%
(Light n' Lively) '100'	8 oz	90	8.0	15.0	110	(mq)	0.0	0.0	0	0%
(Mountain High) 'Honey Light' natural	8 oz	190	9.0	35.0	140	na	<1.0	na	5	<5%
(Mountain High) w/other natural flavors	8 oz	220	10.0	31.0	140	(mq)	6.0	(mq)	(mq)	25%
(New Country) 'Supreme'	6 oz	150	5.0	31.0	90	(mq)	2.0	(mq)	(mq)	11%
(TCBY)	8 oz	220	9.0	42.0	150	na	2.0	na	na	8%
(TCBY) 'Light' nonfat, w/aspartame	8 oz	100	8.0	17.0	210	na	0.0	0.0	na	0%
(Weight Watchers) 'Ultimate 90'	8 oz	90	10.0	13.0	120	na	0.0	na	5	0%
(Yogi) 'Sundae' cheesecake, w/gelatin	5.6 oz	50	6.0	14.0	75	na	<1.0	na	4	<10%
(Yoplait) 'Fruit-on-the-Bottom'	6 oz	170	7.0	35.0	105	na	0.0	na	5	0%
(Yoplait) 'Light' fat-free	6 oz	90	5.0	16.0	70	na	0.0	na	5	0%
(Yoplait) 'Original' 99% fat-free	6 oz	180	8.0	32.0	130	na	2.0	na	na	10%
(Yoplait) 'Parfait Style' blueberry and vanilla	6 oz	200	8.0	34.0	120	na	3.0	na	na	14%
BOYSENBERRY (Yoplait) 'Original' 99% fat-free	6 oz	180	8.0	32.0	130	na	2.0	na	na	10%
CAPPUCCINO (Dannon) 'Light' nonfat	8 oz	100	9.0	16.0	135	na	0.0	0.0	<5	0%
CHERRIES JUBILEE (Weight Watchers) 'Ultimate 90'	8 oz	90	10.0	13.0	120	na	0.0	na	5	0%
CHERRY										
(Dannon) 'Sprinkl'ins' lowfat	4.1 oz	140	5.0	24.0	80	na	2.0	na	5	13%
(Light n' Lively)	4.4 oz	140	5.0	27.0	70	(mq)	1.0	1.0	5	7%
(New Country) 'Supreme'	6 oz	150	5.0	32.0	90	(mq)	2.0	(mq)	(mq)	11%
(Yoplait) 'Breakfast Yogurt' w/almonds	6 oz	200	8.0	38.0	90	2.0	3.0	2.0	10	13%
(Yoplait) 'Custard Style'	6 oz	180	7.0	30.0	95	(mq)	4.0	(mq)	20	20%
(Yoplait) 'Light' fat-free	6 oz	90	5.0	16.0	70	na	0.0	na	5	0%
(Yoplait) 'Original' 99% fat-free	6 oz	180	8.0	32.0	130	na	2.0	na	na	10%
(Yoplait) 'Parfait Style' cherry and vanilla	6 oz	200	8.0	34.0	120	na	3.0	na	na	14%
CHERRY-VANILLA										
(Dannon) 'Light' nonfat	8 oz	100	9.0	18.0	135	na	0.0	0.0	<5	0%
(Dannon) 'Sprinkl'ins' lowfat	4.1 oz	140	5.0	24.0	95	na	2.0	na	5	13%
(Lite-Line) 'Swiss Style 1%'	8 oz	240	10.0	45.0	150	(mq)	2.0	(mq)	(mq)	8%
(TCBY)	8 oz	220	9.0	42.0	150	na	2.0	na	na	8%
(Yogi) w/gelatin 'Sundae'	5.6 oz	50	6.0	14.0	75	na	<1.0	na	4	<10%
(Yoplait) fat-free 'Light Custard Style'	6 oz	90	6.0	17.0	85	na	0.0	na	5	0%
COFFEE										
(Bison) 'Lowfat'	8 oz	210	11.0	33.0	160	0	4.0	(mq)	10	17%
(Dannon) 'Fresh Flavors'	8 oz	200	10.0	34.0	140	0	3.0	(mq)	10	13%
(Friendship) 'Lowfat'	8 oz	210	11.0	35.0	170	0	3.0	(mq)	14	13%
CRANBERRY-RASPBERRY (Weight Watchers) 'Ultimate 90' . .	8 oz	90	10.0	13.0	120	na	0.0	na	5	0%
FRUIT CRUNCH (New Country) 'Lowfat'	6 oz	150	5.0	30.0	90	(mq)	2.0	(mq)	(mq)	11%
GRAPE										
(Dannon) lowfat 'Sprinkl'ins'	4.1 oz	140	5.0	24.0	110	na	2.0	na	5	13%
(Light n' Lively)	4.4 oz	130	6.0	24.0	70	(mq)	1.0	1.0	10	7%
HAWAIIAN SALAD (New Country) 'Lowfat'	6 oz	150	5.0	31.0	90	(mq)	2.0	(mq)	(mq)	11%
LEMON										
(Alta•Dena) 'Naja' fruit-on-the-bottom	8 oz	240	12.0	40.0	150	na	4.0	na	na	15%
(Bison) 'Lowfat'	8 oz	210	11.0	33.0	160	na	4.0	(mq)	10	17%
(Dannon) 'Fresh Flavors'	8 oz	200	10.0	34.0	140	na	3.0	(mq)	10	13%

Food Name	Serving Size	Calories	Prot. gms	Carbs gms	Sod. mgs	Fiber gms	Fat gms	Sat. Fat gms	Chol. mgs	% Fat Cal.
(Knudsen) 'Cal 70'	6 oz	70	6.0	12.0	125	na	0.0	0.0	0	0%
(Light n' Lively) '100'	8 oz	100	9.0	16.0	150	na	0.0	0.0	5	0%
(Mountain High) 'Natural'	8 oz	220	10.0	31.0	140	na	6.0	na	na	25%
(New Country) 'Supreme'	6 oz	150	5.0	31.0	90	na	2.0	(mq)	(mq)	11%
(Weight Watchers) 'Ultimate 90'	1 cup	90	10.0	13.0	120	na	0.0	na	5	0%
(Yoplait) 'Original' 99% fat-free	6 oz	180	8.0	32.0	130	na	2.0	na	na	10%
LEMON CHIFFON										
(Dannon) 'Blended' fat-free	6 oz	150	8.0	30.0	110	na	0.0	na	5	0%
(Dannon) 'Light' non-fat	8 oz	100	9.0	15.0	135	na	0.0	0.0	<5	0%
(Yogi) 'Sundae' w/gelatin	5.6 oz	50	6.0	14.0	75	na	<1.0	na	4	<10%
MIXED BERRIES										
(Alta•Dena) 'Blended European Style'	8 oz	190	8.0	39.0	140	na	<1.0	na	na	<5%
(Breyers) 'Lowfat'	8 oz	250	9.0	48.0	120	(mq)	2.0	1.0	10	7%
(New Country) 'Lowfat'	6 oz	150	5.0	31.0	85	(mq)	2.0	(mq)	(mq)	11%
(Yoplait) 'Custard Style'	6 oz	180	7.0	30.0	95	(mq)	4.0	(mq)	20	20%
(Yoplait) 'Original' 99% fat-free	6 oz	180	8.0	32.0	130	na	2.0	na	na	10%
ORANGE										
(Dannon) 'Fruit-on-the-Bottom'	8 oz	230	9.0	44.0	130	na	3.0	na	10	11%
(New Country) 'Supreme'	6 oz	150	5.0	31.0	90	na	2.0	(mq)	(mq)	11%
ORANGE-PINEAPPLE (Yogi) 'Sundae' w/gelatin	5.6 oz	50	6.0	14.0	75	na	<1.0	na	4	<10%
PEACH										
(Alta•Dena) 'Naja' fruit-on-the-bottom	8 oz	240	12.0	40.0	150	na	4.0	na	na	15%
(Alta•Dena) nonfat, fruit-on-the-bottom	8 oz	190	12.0	36.0	128	na	<1.0	na	na	<5%
(Breyers) 'Lowfat'	8 oz	250	9.0	48.0	120	(mq)	2.0	1.0	10	7%
(Carnation) 'Smooth'n Creamy' fruit on the bottom	8 oz	250	8.0	47.0	130	na	3.0	na	na	11%
(Dannon) 'Fruit-on-the-Bottom'	8 oz	230	9.0	44.0	140	na	3.0	na	10	11%
(Dannon) 'Light' nonfat	8 oz	100	9.0	17.0	135	na	0.0	0.0	5	0%
(Knudsen) 'Cal 70'	6 oz	70	6.0	11.0	95	(mq)	0.0	0.0	0	0%
(Light n' Lively)	8 oz	240	9.0	46.0	120	(mq)	2.0	1.0	15	8%
(Light n' Lively)	4.4 oz	130	5.0	26.0	65	(mq)	1.0	1.0	10	7%
(Light n' Lively) '100'	8 oz	100	9.0	16.0	115	(mq)	0.0	0.0	5	0%
(Lite-Line) 'Swiss Style 1%'	8 oz	230	10.0	42.0	150	(mq)	2.0	(mq)	(mq)	8%
(Mountain High) 'Natural'	8 oz	220	10.0	31.0	140	na	6.0	na	na	25%
(New Country) 'Lowfat' 'n cream	6 oz	150	5.0	31.0	90	(mq)	2.0	(mq)	(mq)	11%
(TCBY)	8 oz	220	9.0	36.0	150	na	2.0	na	na	9%
(Weight Watchers) 'Ultimate 90'	8 oz	90	10.0	13.0	120	na	0.0	na	5	0%
(Yogi) 'Sundae' peachy peach, w/gelatin	5.6 oz	50	6.0	14.0	75	na	<1.0	na	4	<10%
(Yoplait) 'Crunch 'N Yogurt' nonfat, w/granola	7 oz	220	8.0	43.0	125	na	2.0	na	5	8%
(Yoplait) 'Fruit-on-the-Bottom'	6 oz	170	7.0	35.0	105	na	0.0	na	5	0%
(Yoplait) 'Light' fat-free	6 oz	90	5.0	16.0	70	na	0.0	na	5	0%
(Yoplait) 'Light Custard Style' fat-free	6 oz	90	6.0	17.0	85	na	0.0	na	5	0%
(Yoplait) 'Original' 99% fat-free	6 oz	180	8.0	32.0	130	na	2.0	na	na	10%
(Yoplait) 'Parfait Style' peach and vanilla	6 oz	200	8.0	34.0	120	na	3.0	na	na	14%
PIÑA COLADA										
(Yoplait)	6 oz	190	8.0	32.0	110	(mq)	3.0	(mq)	10	14%
(Yoplait) 'Original' 99% fat-free	6 oz	180	8.0	32.0	130	na	2.0	na	na	10%
PINEAPPLE										
(Breyers) 'Lowfat'	8 oz	250	9.0	50.0	120	(mq)	2.0	1.0	10	7%
(Knudsen) 'Cal 70'	6 oz	70	6.0	12.0	125	(mq)	0.0	0.0	0	0%
(Light n' Lively)	8 oz	230	9.0	47.0	120	(mq)	2.0	1.0	10	7%
(Light n' Lively)	4.4 oz	130	5.0	26.0	65	(mq)	1.0	1.0	5	7%
(Yoplait) 'Original' 99% fat-free	6 oz	180	8.0	32.0	130	na	2.0	na	na	10%
PLAIN										
(Alta•Dena) nonfat	8 oz	100	13.0	13.0	160	na	<1.0	na	na	<8%

Food Name	Serving Size	Calories	Prot. gms	Carbs gms	Sod. mgs	Fiber gms	Fat gms	Sat. Fat gms	Chol. mgs	% Fat Cal.
(Bison) 'Lowfat'	8 oz	150	12.0	17.0	180	0	4.0	(mq)	10	24%
(Bison) 'Nonfat'	8 oz	120	12.0	16.0	170	0	0.0	0.0	0	0%
(Breyers) 'Lowfat'	8 oz	140	12.0	16.0	170	0	3.0	2.0	20	19%
(Colombo)	8 oz	160	9.0	13.0	160	0	8.0	(mq)	(mq)	45%
(Colombo) 'Nonfat Lite'	8 oz	110	11.0	17.0	160	0	<1.0	na	5	<7%
(Crowley)	8 oz	160	10.0	14.0	150	0	8.0	(mq)	30	43%
(Crowley) 'Lowfat'	8 oz	140	12.0	17.0	180	0	2.0	(mq)	10	13%
(Crowley) 'Nonfat'	8 oz	120	13.0	17.0	180	0	<1.0	0.0	<1	<7%
(Dannon) 'Lowfat'	8 oz	140	10.0	16.0	160	0	4.0	(mq)	15	26%
(Dannon) 'Nonfat'	8 oz	110	11.0	16.0	160	0	0.0	0.0	5	0%
(Friendship) 'Lowfat 1.5%'	8 oz	150	12.0	17.0	190	0	3.0	(mq)	14	19%
(Knudsen)	8 oz	200	12.0	16.0	170	0	9.0	5.0	35	42%
(Knudsen) 'Lowfat'	8 oz	160	12.0	17.0	180	0	5.0	1.0	25	28%
(Lite-Line) 'Swiss Style 1.5%'	8 oz	140	12.0	18.0	150	0	2.0	(mq)	(mq)	13%
(Meadow Gold) lowfat, 2% milkfat	8 oz	160	12.0	16.0	160	0	5.0	(mq)	(mq)	29%
(Mountain High)	8 oz	200	12.0	16.0	140	0	9.0	(mq)	(mq)	42%
(Weight Watchers) 'Nonfat'	8 oz	90	10.0	13.0	135	0	<1.0	0.0	5	<9%
(Yoplait)	6 oz	130	10.0	15.0	140	0	3.0	(mq)	15	21%
(Yoplait) fat-free	8 oz	120	13.0	17.0	170	na	0.0	na	10	0%
(Yoplait) 'Nonfat'	8 oz	120	13.0	18.0	160	0	0.0	0.0	5	0%
(Yoplait) 'Original' 98% fat-free	6 oz	120	10.0	15.0	150	na	2.0	na	15	15%
RAINBOW PUNCH (Yoplait) 'Trix'	6 oz	190	9.0	31.0	120	na	3.0	na	na	14%
RASPBERRY										
(Alta•Dena) 'Blended European Style'	8 oz	180	8.0	37.0	140	na	<1.0	na	na	<5%
(Dannon) 'Blended' fat-free	6 oz	150	8.0	30.0	110	na	0.0	na	5	0%
(Dannon) 'Fruit-on-the-Bottom'	8 oz	240	9.0	45.0	140	na	3.0	na	10	11%
(Dannon) 'Light' nonfat	8 oz	100	9.0	18.0	135	na	0.0	0.0	5	0%
(Meadow Gold) 'Sundae Style' lowfat, natural	8 oz	250	10.0	42.0	160	na	4.0	na	na	15%
(Mountain High) 'Honey Light' natural	8 oz	190	9.0	35.0	140	na	<1.0	na	5	<5%
(TCBY)	8 oz	220	9.0	42.0	150	na	2.0	na	na	8%
(Weight Watchers) 'Ultimate 90'	8 oz	90	10.0	13.0	120	na	0.0	na	5	0%
(Yoplait) fat-free 'Light'	6 oz	90	5.0	16.0	70	na	0.0	na	5	0%
(Yoplait) 'Fruit-on-the-Bottom'	6 oz	170	7.0	35.0	105	na	0.0	na	5	0%
(Yoplait) 'Original' 99% fat-free	6 oz	180	8.0	32.0	130	na	2.0	na	na	10%
RED RASPBERRY										
(Alta•Dena) 'Naja' fruit-on-the-bottom	8 oz	240	12.0	40.0	150	na	4.0	na	na	15%
(Breyers) 'Lowfat'	8 oz	250	9.0	48.0	120	(mq)	2.0	1.0	10	7%
(Carnation) 'Smooth'n Creamy' fruit on the bottom	8 oz	250	8.0	47.0	130	na	3.0	na	na	11%
(Knudsen) 'Cal 70'	6 oz	70	6.0	11.0	80	(mq)	0.0	0.0	5	0%
(Light n' Lively)	8 oz	230	9.0	43.0	130	(mq)	2.0	1.0	10	8%
(Light n' Lively)	4.4 oz	130	5.0	24.0	70	(mq)	1.0	1.0	5	7%
(Light n' Lively) 'Free' nonfat	4.4 oz	50	4.0	8.0	60	(mq)	0.0	0.0	0	0%
(Light n' Lively) '100'	8 oz	90	8.0	15.0	105	(mq)	0.0	0.0	0	0%
(Meadow Gold) lowfat, 1.5% milkfat	8 oz	250	10.0	42.0	160	(mq)	4.0	(mq)	(mq)	15%
(New Country) 'Supreme'	6 oz	150	5.0	31.0	90	(mq)	2.0	(mq)	(mq)	11%
STRAWBERRY										
(Alta•Dena) 'Blended European Style'	8 oz	180	8.0	37.0	140	na	<1.0	na	na	<5%
(Alta•Dena) 'Maya' fruit-on-the-bottom	8 oz	280	11.0	39.0	170	na	9.0	na	na	29%
(Alta•Dena) 'Naja' fruit-on-the-bottom	8 oz	240	12.0	40.0	150	na	4.0	na	na	15%
(Breyers) 'Lowfat'	8 oz	250	9.0	48.0	120	(mq)	2.0	1.0	10	7%
(Carnation) 'Smooth'n Creamy' fruit on the bottom	8 oz	230	8.0	44.0	115	na	3.0	na	na	12%
(Colombo)	8 oz	210	8.0	29.0	140	(mq)	7.0	(mq)	(mq)	30%
(Crowley) 'Nonfat'	8 oz	190	12.0	35.0	190	(mq)	<1.0	na	<1	<5%
(Dannon) 'Blended' fat-free	6 oz	150	8.0	30.0	110	na	0.0	na	5	0%

Food Name	Serving Size	Calories	Prot. gms	Carbs gms	Sod. mgs	Fiber gms	Fat gms	Sat. Fat gms	Chol. mgs	% Fat Cal.
(Dannon) 'Fruit-on-the-Bottom'	8 oz	230	9.0	45.0	140	na	3.0	na	10	11%
(Dannon) 'Light' nonfat	8 oz	100	9.0	17.0	135	na	0.0	0.0	5	0%
(Dannon) 'Sprinkl'ins' lowfat	4.1 oz	140	5.0	24.0	95	na	2.0	na	5	13%
(Knudsen) 'Cal 70'	6 oz	70	6.0	11.0	85	(mq)	0.0	0.0	0	0%
(Knudsen) 'Lowfat'	8 oz	250	10.0	45.0	135	(mq)	4.0	2.0	15	14%
(Light n' Lively)	8 oz	240	9.0	45.0	130	(mq)	2.0	2.0	15	8%
(Light n' Lively)	4.4 oz	130	5.0	25.0	70	(mq)	1.0	1.0	10	7%
(Light n' Lively) 'Free'	4.4 oz	50	4.0	8.0	60	(mq)	0.0	0.0	0	0%
(Light n' Lively) '100'	8 oz	90	8.0	15.0	105	(mq)	0.0	0.0	5	0%
(Lite-Line) 'Lowfat 1%'	8 oz	240	10.0	46.0	150	(mq)	2.0	(mq)	(mq)	7%
(Mountain High) 'Honey Light' natural	8 oz	190	9.0	35.0	140	na	<1.0	na	5	<5%
(New Country) 'Supreme'	6 oz	150	5.0	30.0	90	(mq)	2.0	(mq)	(mq)	11%
(TCBY)	8 oz	220	9.0	43.0	150	na	2.0	na	na	8%
(Weight Watchers) 'Ultimate 90'	8 oz	90	10.0	13.0	120	na	0.0	na	5	0%
(Yoplait) 'Custard Style'	6 oz	180	7.0	30.0	105	na	3.0	na	na	15%
(Yoplait) 'Fruit-on-the-Bottom'	6 oz	170	7.0	35.0	105	na	0.0	na	5	0%
(Yoplait) 'Light' fat-free	6 oz	90	5.0	16.0	70	na	0.0	na	5	0%
(Yoplait) 'Light Custard Style' fat-free	6 oz	90	6.0	17.0	85	na	0.0	na	5	0%
(Yoplait) 'Original' 99% fat-free	6 oz	180	8.0	32.0	130	na	2.0	na	na	10%
(Yoplait) 'Parfait Style' strawberry and vanilla	6 oz	200	8.0	34.0	120	na	3.0	na	na	14%
STRAWBERRY CHEESECAKE (Yogi) 'Sundae' w/gelatin	5.6 oz	50	6.0	14.0	75	na	<1.0	na	4	<10%
STRAWBERRY FRUIT BASKET (Knudsen) 'Cal 70'	6 oz	70	6.0	11.0	75	(mq)	0.0	0.0	5	0%
STRAWBERRY FRUIT CUP										
(Dannon) 'Light' nonfat	8 oz	100	9.0	17.0	135	na	0.0	0.0	5	0%
(Light n' Lively)	8 oz	240	9.0	47.0	120	(mq)	2.0	1.0	15	7%
(Light n' Lively)	4.4 oz	130	5.0	26.0	65	(mq)	1.0	1.0	10	7%
(Light n' Lively) 'Free' nonfat	4.4 oz	50	4.0	8.0	55	(mq)	0.0	0.0	0	0%
(Light n' Lively) '100'	8 oz	90	8.0	15.0	100	(mq)	0.0	0.0	0	0%
(New Country) 'Lowfat'	6 oz	150	5.0	30.0	85	(mq)	2.0	(mq)	(mq)	11%
STRAWBERRY-ALMOND (Yoplait) 'Breakfast Yogurt'	6 oz	200	8.0	38.0	90	2.0	3.0	2.0	10	13%
STRAWBERRY-BANANA										
(Alta•Dena) nonfat, fruit-on-the-bottom	8 oz	180	12.0	35.0	128	na	<1.0	na	na	<5%
(Breyers) 'Lowfat'	8 oz	250	9.0	50.0	120	(mq)	2.0	1.0	10	7%
(Carnation) 'Smooth'n Creamy' fruit on the bottom	8 oz	240	9.0	42.0	125	na	4.0	na	na	15%
(Dannon) 'Fruit-on-the-Bottom'	8 oz	230	9.0	44.0	140	na	3.0	na	10	11%
(Dannon) 'Light' nonfat	8 oz	100	9.0	17.0	135	na	0.0	0.0	<5	0%
(Dannon) lowfat 'Sprinkl'ins'	4.1 oz	140	5.0	24.0	95	na	2.0	na	5	13%
(Knudsen) 'Cal 70'	6 oz	70	6.0	12.0	80	(mq)	0.0	0.0	0	0%
(Light n' Lively)	8 oz	260	9.0	52.0	120	(mq)	2.0	1.0	10	7%
(Light n' Lively)	4.4 oz	140	5.0	29.0	65	(mq)	1.0	1.0	5	6%
(Light n' Lively) 'Free' nonfat	4.4 oz	50	4.0	8.0	60	na	0.0	0.0	0	0%
(Mountain High) 'Honey Light' natural	8 oz	190	9.0	35.0	140	na	<1.0	na	5	<5%
(New Country)	6 oz	150	5.0	31.0	85	(mq)	2.0	(mq)	(mq)	11%
(TCBY)	8 oz	220	9.0	43.0	150	na	2.0	na	na	8%
(Weight Watchers) 'Ultimate 90'	8 oz	90	10.0	13.0	120	na	0.0	na	5	0%
(Yoplait) 'Breakfast' w/wheat and walnuts	6 oz	200	8.0	40.0	110	na	2.0	na	na	9%
(Yoplait) 'Fruit-on-the-Bottom'	6 oz	170	7.0	35.0	105	na	0.0	na	5	0%
(Yoplait) 'Light' fat-free	6 oz	90	5.0	16.0	70	na	0.0	na	5	0%
(Yoplait) 'Original' 99% fat-free	6 oz	180	8.0	32.0	130	na	2.0	na	na	10%
(Yoplait) 'Trix' bash	6 oz	190	9.0	31.0	120	na	3.0	na	na	14%
STRAWBERRY-RHUBARB (Yoplait)	6 oz	190	8.0	32.0	110	(mq)	3.0	(mq)	10	14%
TRIPLE CHERRY (Yoplait) 'Trix'	6 oz	190	9.0	31.0	120	na	3.0	na	na	14%
TROPICAL FRUIT										
(Dannon) 'Light' nonfat	8 oz	100	9.0	18.0	135	na	0.0	0.0	<5	0%

Food Name	Serving Size	Calories	Prot. gms	Carbs gms	Sod. mgs	Fiber gms	Fat gms	Sat. Fat gms	Chol. mgs	% Fat Cal.
(Ripple) '70'	6 oz	70	5.0	13.0	85	(mq)	0.0	0.0	5	0%
(Weight Watchers) 'Ultimate 90'	8 oz	90	10.0	13.0	120	na	0.0	na	5	0%
(Yoplait) 'Breakfast' w/wheat, raisins, and nuts	6 oz	200	8.0	41.0	110	na	3.0	na	na	12%
VANILLA										
(Bison) 'Lowfat'	8 oz	210	11.0	33.0	160	0	4.0	(mq)	10	17%
(Breyers) 'Lowfat' vanilla bean	8 oz	230	11.0	41.0	150	0	3.0	2.0	20	12%
(Colombo) French	8 oz	215	8.0	30.0	140	0	7.0	(mq)	(mq)	29%
(Colombo) 'Nonfat Lite'	8 oz	160	10.0	30.0	140	0	<1.0	na	5	<5%
(Crowley) 'Lowfat'	8 oz	200	12.0	33.0	170	0	2.0	(mq)	10	9%
(Dannon) 'Blended' French, fat-free	6 oz	150	7.0	31.0	100	na	0.0	0.0	5	0%
(Dannon) 'Fresh Flavors'	8 oz	200	10.0	34.0	140	0	3.0	(mq)	10	13%
(Dannon) 'Fresh Flavors'	4.4 oz	110	5.0	20.0	90	0	2.0	(mq)	5	15%
(Dannon) 'Hearty Nuts & Raisins' w/wheat	8 oz	270	9.0	48.0	120	(mq)	5.0	(mq)	10	17%
(Dannon) 'Light' nonfat	8 oz	100	9.0	16.0	135	na	0.0	0.0	<5	0%
(Friendship) 'Lowfat'	8 oz	210	11.0	35.0	170	0	3.0	(mq)	14	13%
(Knudsen) 'Cal 70'	6 oz	70	6.0	11.0	90	0	0.0	0.0	0	0%
(Knudsen) 'Lowfat'	8 oz	240	11.0	43.0	135	0	4.0	2.0	15	14%
(New Country) 'Lowfat' French	6 oz	150	5.0	31.0	90	0	2.0	(mq)	(mq)	11%
(Weight Watchers) 'Ultimate 90'	1 cup	90	10.0	13.0	120	na	0.0	na	5	0%
(Yoplait)	6 oz	180	9.0	29.0	120	0	3.0	(mq)	15	15%
(Yoplait) 'Crunch 'N Yogurt' w/granola, nonfat	7 oz	220	8.0	43.0	125	na	2.0	na	5	8%
(Yoplait) 'Custard Style'	6 oz	180	7.0	30.0	110	0	4.0	(mq)	20	20%
(Yoplait) 'Custard Style'	4 oz	130	5.0	20.0	70	0	3.0	(mq)	15	21%
(Yoplait) 'Fat-free'	6 oz	150	8.0	28.0	110	0	0.0	0.0	5	0%
(Yoplait) 'Light Custard Style' fat-free	6 oz	90	6.0	17.0	85	na	0.0	na	5	0%
(Yoplait) 'Nonfat'	8 oz	180	11.0	35.0	140	0	0.0	0.0	5	0%
WILD BERRY (Light n' Lively) lowfat, 1% milkfat, cultured	4.4 oz	140	5.0	28.0	70	na	1.0	1.0	5	6%
YOGURT, FROZEN										
(Alta•Dena) apricot mango, nonfat	4 oz	90	3.0	20.0	210	na	0.0	0.1	0	0%
(Baskin Robbins) See Part III.										
(Ben & Jerry's)										
apple pie	1/2 cup	170	4.0	32.0	90	0	3.0	2.0	10	16%
banana strawberry	1/2 cup	160	4.0	32.0	60	1.0	2.0	1.0	5	11%
blueberry	1/2 cup	160	4.0	32.0	60	1.0	2.0	1.0	5	11%
cherry garcia	1/2 cup	170	4.0	31.0	70	0	3.0	2.0	10	16%
chocolate fudge brownie	1/2 cup	190	6.0	35.0	130	2.0	4.0	2.0	10	19%
chocolate raspberry swirl	1/2 cup	200	5.0	40.0	72	1.0	2.5	1.5	5	11%
coffee almond fudge	1/2 cup	200	6.0	30.0	82	1.0	7.0	2.0	15	32%
English toffee crunch	1/2 cup	190	4.0	32.0	110	0	6.0	2.5	10	28%
(Bison) chocolate	3.5 oz	94	3.0	18.0	50	(tr)	2.0	(mq)	5	18%
(Breyers)										
black cherry	1/2 cup	120	3.0	24.0	50	(tr)	1.0	(mq)	10	8%
chocolate	1/2 cup	120	3.0	24.0	65	(tr)	1.0	(mq)	10	8%
peach	1/2 cup	110	3.0	22.0	50	(tr)	1.0	(mq)	10	8%
red raspberry	1/2 cup	120	3.0	23.0	50	(tr)	1.0	(mq)	10	8%
strawberry	1/2 cup	110	3.0	22.0	45	(tr)	1.0	(mq)	10	8%
strawberry-banana	1/2 cup	110	3.0	22.0	45	(tr)	1.0	(mq)	10	8%
vanilla	1/2 cup	120	3.0	23.0	55	0	1.0	(mq)	15	8%
(Colombo)										
banana split, lowfat, 'Sundae Style'	3 oz	100	2.0	20.0	50	na	1.0	na	5	9%
Bavarian chocolate chunk, 'Gourmet'	3 oz	120	3.0	18.0	40	(tr)	4.0	(mq)	10	30%
caramel fudge sundae, lowfat, 'Sundae Style'	3 oz	100	3.0	21.0	60	na	1.0	na	5	9%
caramel-pecan chunk, 'Gourmet'	3 oz	120	4.0	19.0	150	(tr)	3.0	(mq)	10	23%
chocolate peanut butter twist, 'Sundae Style'	3 oz	110	3.0	18.0	65	na	3.0	na	5	24%

Food Name	Serving Size	Calories	Prot. gms	Carbs gms	Sod. mgs	Fiber gms	Fat gms	Sat. Fat gms	Chol. mgs	% Fat Cal.
dream, 'Gourmet'	3 oz	90	3.0	16.0	45	0	2.0	(mq)	10	19%
Heath bar crunch, 'Gourmet'	3 oz	130	3.0	19.0	75	(tr)	5.0	(mq)	15	34%
mocha Swiss almond, 'Gourmet'	3 oz	120	3.0	17.0	45	(tr)	5.0	(mq)	10	36%
nonfat, lite	4 oz	95	4.0	21.0	70	na	0.0	na	0	0%
peanut butter cup, 'Gourmet'	3 oz	140	4.0	16.0	90	(tr)	7.0	(mq)	5	44%
plain, lowfat	4 oz	99	3.0	18.0	35	na	2.0	na	10	18%
plain, 'Nonfat Lite'	4 oz	95	4.0	21.0	70	na	0.0	na	0	0%
strawberry passion, 'Gourmet'	3 oz	100	1.0	18.0	40	(tr)	2.0	(mq)	5	19%
wild raspberry cheesecake, 'Gourmet'	3 oz	100	2.0	18.0	40	(tr)	2.0	(mq)	5	18%
(Crowley)										
cherry	3 oz	80	2.0	16.0	40	(tr)	1.0	(mq)	5	11%
chocolate	3 oz	80	2.0	15.0	40	(tr)	2.0	(mq)	10	21%
peach	3 oz	80	2.0	16.0	40	(tr)	1.0	(mq)	5	11%
raspberry	3 oz	80	2.0	16.0	40	(tr)	1.0	(mq)	5	11%
strawberry	3 oz	80	2.0	16.0	40	(tr)	1.0	(mq)	5	11%
vanilla	3 oz	80	2.0	15.0	40	0	2.0	(mq)	10	21%
(Dannon)										
cappuccino, nonfat, 'Light'	4 oz	80	4.0	19.0	70	na	0.0	na	0	0%
caramel pecan, 'Pure Indulgence'	4 oz	180	4.0	22.0	70	na	8.0	na	20	41%
cherry vanilla swirl, nonfat, 'Light'	4 oz	90	4.0	21.0	65	na	0.0	na	0	0%
chocolate, nonfat, 'Light'	4 oz	80	4.0	19.0	70	na	<1.0	na	0	<9%
chocolate, 'Pure Indulgence'	3 oz	130	5.0	24.0	75	na	3.0	na	10	19%
chocolate nut, chunky, 'Pure Indulgence'	4 oz	190	5.0	24.0	60	na	9.0	na	20	41%
chunky chocolate nut, 'Pure Indulgence'	4 oz	190	5.0	24.0	60	na	9.0	na	20	41%
cookies and cream, 'Pure Indulgence'	4 oz	180	4.0	18.0	95	na	7.0	na	20	42%
Heath bar crunch, 'Pure Indulgence'	4 oz	170	4.0	25.0	100	na	7.0	na	25	35%
peach, nonfat, 'Light'	4 oz	80	4.0	19.0	70	na	0.0	na	0	0%
red raspberry, nonfat, 'Light'	4 oz	90	3.0	21.0	65	(tr)	0.0	0.0	0	0%
strawberry, nonfat, 'Light'	4 oz	80	4.0	19.0	70	na	0.0	na	0	0%
vanilla, nonfat, 'Light'	4 oz	80	4.0	20.0	70	na	0.0	na	0	0%
vanilla, 'Pure Indulgence'	3 oz	130	5.0	25.0	50	na	3.0	na	10	18%
(Dreyer's)										
black cherry vanilla, nonfat, 'Inspirations'	4 oz	90	4.0	19.0	80	na	0.0	na	0	0%
blueberry, 'Inspirations'	3 oz	80	2.0	15.0	40	(tr)	1.0	(mq)	5	12%
cherry, 'Inspirations'	3 oz	80	2.0	15.0	40	(tr)	1.0	(mq)	5	12%
chocolate, 'Inspirations'	3 oz	80	2.0	15.0	40	(tr)	1.0	(mq)	5	12%
peach, 'Inspirations Perfectly Peach'	3 oz	80	2.0	15.0	40	(tr)	1.0	(mq)	5	12%
raspberry, 'Inspirations'	3 oz	80	2.0	15.0	40	(tr)	1.0	(mq)	5	12%
strawberry, 'Inspirations'	3 oz	80	2.0	15.0	40	(tr)	1.0	(mq)	5	12%
strawberry-banana, 'Inspirations'	3 oz	80	2.0	15.0	40	(tr)	1.0	(mq)	5	12%
vanilla chocolate swirl, nonfat, 'Inspirations'	4 oz	90	4.0	19.0	85	na	0.0	na	0	0%
vanilla-raspberry swirl, 'Inspirations'	3 oz	80	2.0	15.0	45	(tr)	1.0	(mq)	5	12%
(Elan) chocolate almond	1/2 cup	160	5.0	23.0	65	(tr)	7.0	(mq)	(mq)	36%
(Häagen-Dazs)										
chocolate	3 oz	130	6.0	21.0	40	(tr)	3.0	2.0	25	20%
peach	3 oz	120	4.0	20.0	30	(tr)	3.0	1.5	31	22%
praline pandemonium, 'Extrãas'	4 oz	240	7.0	33.0	115	na	9.0	4.0	45	34%
strawberry	3 oz	120	4.0	21.0	30	(tr)	3.0	1.6	29	21%
strawberry cheesecake craze, 'Extrãas'	4 oz	210	7.0	31.0	100	na	7.0	3.0	50	29%
vanilla almond crunch	3 oz	150	5.0	22.0	65	(tr)	5.0	1.5	33	29%
(Natural Nectar) chocolate, 'Fi-Bar Lite'	2.5 oz	190	4.0	29.0	140	na	6.0	na	5	29%
(Sealtest)										
black cherry, nonfat, 'Free'	1/2 cup	110	2.0	24.0	50	(tr)	0.0	0.0	0	0%
chocolate, nonfat, 'Free'	1/2 cup	110	3.0	24.0	55	(tr)	0.0	0.0	0	0%

Food Name	Serving Size	Calories	Prot. gms	Carbs gms	Sod. mgs	Fiber gms	Fat gms	Sat. Fat gms	Chol. mgs	% Fat Cal.
peach, nonfat, 'Free'	1/2 cup	100	2.0	23.0	35	(tr)	0.0	0.0	0	0%
red raspberry, nonfat, 'Free'	1/2 cup	100	2.0	23.0	40	(tr)	0.0	0.0	0	0%
strawberry, nonfat, 'Free'	1/2 cup	100	2.0	22.0	35	(tr)	0.0	0.0	0	0%
(TCBY) See Part III.										
YOGURT, FROZEN, SOFT-SERVE										
(Bresler's)										
'Gourmet' all flavors, 1 oz	1/2 cup	29	0.9	5.5	15	(tr)	0.5	na	2	15%
'Lite' all flavors, 1 oz	1/2 cup	27	1.1	6.0	11	(tr)	0.0	0.0	0	0%
(Crowley)										
banana, 'Peaks of Perfection,' 3.5 oz	1/2 cup	100	3.0	19.0	50	(tr)	2.0	(mq)	5	17%
chocolate, 'Peaks of Perfection,' 3.5 oz	1/2 cup	100	4.0	19.0	60	(tr)	2.0	(mq)	5	16%
lemon, 'Peaks of Perfection,' 3.5 oz	1/2 cup	100	3.0	19.0	50	(tr)	2.0	(mq)	5	17%
plain, 'Peaks of Perfection,' 3.5 oz	1/2 cup	90	2.0	20.0	40	0	1.0	(mq)	5	9%
raspberry, 'Peaks of Perfection,' 3.5 oz	1/2 cup	100	3.0	19.0	50	(tr)	2.0	(mq)	5	17%
strawberry, 'Peaks of Perfection,' 3.5 oz	1/2 cup	100	3.0	19.0	50	(tr)	2.0	(mq)	5	17%
vanilla, 'Peaks of Perfection,' 3.5 oz	1/2 cup	100	3.0	19.0	50	0	2.0	(mq)	5	17%
(Dannon)										
blueberry	1/2 cup	100	3.0	18.0	50	(tr)	2.0	(mq)	5	18%
butter pecan	1/2 cup	100	3.0	18.0	55	(tr)	2.0	(mq)	5	18%
cappuccino	1/2 cup	100	3.0	18.0	55	0	2.0	(mq)	5	18%
cheesecake	1/2 cup	100	4.0	18.0	55	0	2.0	(mq)	5	17%
chocolate	1/2 cup	120	5.0	23.0	65	(tr)	2.0	(mq)	5	14%
lemon meringue	1/2 cup	100	4.0	18.0	55	(tr)	2.0	(mq)	5	17%
peach	1/2 cup	100	4.0	18.0	55	(tr)	2.0	(mq)	5	17%
piña colada	1/2 cup	100	4.0	18.0	55	(tr)	2.0	(mq)	5	17%
raspberry	1/2 cup	100	3.0	18.0	50	(tr)	2.0	(mq)	5	18%
red raspberry, 'Nonfat'	1/2 cup	90	3.0	21.0	65	(tr)	0.0	0.0	0	0%
strawberry	1/2 cup	100	3.0	18.0	50	(tr)	2.0	(mq)	5	18%
strawberry-banana	1/2 cup	100	3.0	18.0	50	(tr)	2.0	(mq)	5	18%
(Häagen-Dazs)										
banana, nonfat	1 oz	25	1.0	5.0	15	na	0.0	0.0	0	0%
chocolate	1 oz	30	1.0	4.0	13	(tr)	1.0	na	3	31%
chocolate, nonfat	1 oz	30	1.0	6.0	20	(tr)	0.0	0.0	0	0%
coffee	1 oz	28	1.0	4.0	13	0	1.0	na	3	31%
raspberry	1 oz	30	1.0	5.0	15	na	1.0	na	3	27%
strawberry, nonfat	1 oz	25	1.0	5.0	10	na	0.0	0.0	0	0%
vanilla	1 oz	28	1.0	4.0	13	0	1.0	na	3	31%
YOGURT BAR, FROZEN										
(Dole)										
cherry 'Fruit & Yogurt'	1 bar	80	2.0	17.0	22	na	<1.0	na	na	<11%
raspberry 'Fruit & Yogurt'	1 bar	70	1.0	17.0	18	na	<1.0	na	na	<11%
strawberry 'Fruit & Yogurt'	1 bar	70	1.0	17.0	16	na	<1.0	na	na	<11%
(Häagen-Dazs)										
cherry chocolate fudge	1 bar	230	5.0	28.0	50	na	12.0	7.0	35	45%
peach	1 bar	100	2.0	18.0	20	na	1.0	1.0	15	10%
piña colada	1 bar	100	2.0	21.0	25	na	1.0	<1.0	15	9%
raspberry and vanilla	1 bar	100	3.0	19.0	20	na	1.0	1.0	15	9%
strawberry daiquiri	1 bar	100	2.0	20.0	20	na	1.0	<1.0	20	9%
tropical orange passion	1 bar	100	2.0	21.0	30	na	1.0	<1.0	20	9%
YOGURT DESSERT *(Sara Lee)* 'Free & Light'	1/10 pkg	120	2.0	26.0	90	na	1.0	na	0	7%
YOGURT FLAVORED DRINK										
(Dannon) all flavors	8 oz	190	6.0	32.0	110	(tr)	4.0	(mq)	10	19%
(Yogloo) fruit basket	10 oz	170	3.0	40.0	80	na	0.0	0.0	na	0%
(Yogloo) original	10 oz	170	3.0	40.0	80	na	0.0	0.0	na	0%

Food Name	Serving Size	Calories	Prot. gms	Carbs gms	Sod. mgs	Fiber gms	Fat gms	Sat. Fat gms	Chol. mgs	% Fat Cal.
(Yogloo) peach	10 oz	170	3.0	40.0	80	na	0.0	0.0	na	0%
(Yogloo) strawberry	10 oz	170	3.0	40.0	80	na	0.0	0.0	na	0%
YOKAN	1 oz	74	0.9	17.2	24	0	(tr)	0.0	0	0%

YUCA. See CASSAVA.

Z

Food Name	Serving Size	Calories	Prot. gms	Carbs gms	Sod. mgs	Fiber gms	Fat gms	Sat. Fat gms	Chol. mgs	% Fat Cal.
ZITI ENTRÉE, FROZEN										
(Budget Gourmet) 'Side Dish' in marinara sauce	6.25 oz	220	9.0	25.0	380	(mq)	9.0	(mq)	15	37%
ZUCCHINI. See also SQUASH, SUMMER.										
baby, raw	1 large	3	0.4	0.5	0	na	0.1	0.0	0	20%
baby, raw	1 med	2	0.3	0.3	0	na	0.0	0.0	0	0%
boiled, drained	4 oz	18	0.7	4.5	3	>.6 c	0.1	<.1	0	4%
raw	1 lb	62	5.0	12.5	11	2.2	0.6	0.1	0	7%
raw, trimmed	1 oz	4	0.3	0.8	1	.1	<.1	tr	0	<17%
w/skin, boiled, drained, mashed	1/2 cup	19	0.8	4.7	4	1.7	0.1	0.0	0	4%
w/skin, boiled, drained, sliced	1/2 cup	14	0.6	3.5	3	1.3	0.0	0.0	0	0%
w/skin, raw, sliced	1/2 cup	9	0.8	1.9	2	.8	0.1	0.0	0	8%
Canned										
in tomato juice	1/2 cup	33	1.2	7.8	424	>.6 c	0.1	<.1	0	2%
Italian style	1/2 cup	33	1.2	7.8	426	>.6 c	0.1	0.0	0	2%
(Del Monte) in tomato sauce	1/2 cup	30	1.0	8.0	485	(mq)	0.0	0.0	0	0%
(Progresso) Italian style	1/2 cup	50	1.0	8.0	540	2.0	2.0	<1.0	<1	33%
Frozen										
w/skin, unprepared	10-oz pkg	48	3.3	10.2	6	3.4	0.4	0.1	0	6%
(Seabrook)	3.3 oz	16	1.0	3.0	2	>1.0 c	0.0	0.0	0	0%
(Southern)	3.5 oz	18	1.2	3.6	20	(mq)	0.1	(tr)	0	5%
(Stilwell) 'Quick Krisp' breaded	3.3 oz	200	4.0	24.0	410	(mq)	10.0	(mq)	15	45%

PART TWO

VITAMIN AND MINERAL VALUES

Vitamin A • Thiamine • Riboflavin • Niacin •
Vitamin B_6 • Folic Acid • Vitamin B_{12} • Vitamin C •
Calcium • Iron • Magnesium • Potassium • Zinc

A

Food Name	Serving Size	A I.U.	Thi mg	Rib mg	Nia mg	B$_6$ mg	Fol mcg	B$_{12}$ mcg	C mg	Calc mg	Iron mg	Mag mg	Pot mg	Zn mg
ABALONE, MIXED SPECIES, raw .... 3 oz		4	.16	.09	1.27	.13	4.3	.62	1.7	26.35	2.71	40.8	212.5	.7
ACEROLA CHERRY / Barbados cherry														
trimmed .... 1 cup		752	.02	.06	.39	.01	na	0	1644.1	11.76	.2	17.64	143.08	na
trimmed .... 1 fruit		37	0	0	.02	0	na	0	80.5	.58	.01	.86	7.01	na
ACEROLA CHERRY JUICE / Barbados cherry juice														
.... 1 cup		1232	.05	.15	.97	.01	na	0	3872.0	24.2	1.21	29.04	234.74	na
.... 1 oz		154	.01	.02	.12	0	na	0	483.2	3.02	.15	3.62	29.29	na
ACORN														
dried .... 1 oz		0	.04	.04	.68	.2	32.6	0	0.0	15.34	.3	23.29	201.36	.19
raw, shelled .... 1 oz		11	.03	.03	.52	.15	24.7	0	0.0	11.64	.22	17.61	153.08	.14
ACORN FLOUR, full fat .... 1 oz		14	.04	.04	.68	.2	32.2	0	0.0	12.21	.34	31.24	202.21	.18
ACORN SQUASH. See SQUASH, ACORN.														
ADZUKI BEAN														
boiled, mature seeds .... 1/2 cup		7	.13	.07	.82	.11	139.3	0	0.0	32.2	2.3	59.8	611.8	2.04
raw, mature seeds .... 1/2 cup		17	.45	.22	2.58	.34	609.5	0	0.0	64.68	4.88	124.46	1228.92	4.94
yokan, mature seeds, 1/4-inch slice .... 1 slice		0	0	0	.01	0	1.2	0	0.0	3.78	.16	2.52	6.3	.01
ADZUKI BEAN, CANNED														
mature seeds, sweetened .... 1/2 cup		7	.15	.08	.93	.12	157.8	0	0.0	32.56	1.67	45.88	176.12	2.31
organic, no salt added (Eden Foods) ...... 1/2 cup		na	na	na	na	na	na	na	na	na	na	na	230	na
organic, w/liquid (Eden Foods) .... 1/2 cup		na	na	na	na	na	na	na	na	na	na	na	250	na
AGAR														
dried .... 100 gm		0	.01	.22	.2	.3	580.2	0	0.0	625.0	21.4	770.0	1125.0	5.8
raw .... 100 gm		0	.01	.02	.06	.03	84.8	0	0.0	54.0	1.86	67.0	226.0	.58
AHI. See TUNA, YELLOWFIN.														
AKU. See TUNA, SKIPJACK.														
ALBACORE. See TUNA, CANNED.														
ALCOHOL-FREE BEVERAGES														
BEER														
(Cutter) .... 12 oz		na	na	na	na	na	na	na	na	.26	na	na	3.39	na
(Kaliber) .... 12 oz		na	na	na	na	na	na	na	na	na	na	na	25	na
MIXED-DRINK MIXERS														
Banana Daiquiri, frozen, diluted w/water														
(Bacardi) .... 7 oz		na	na	na	na	na	na	na	2.0	na	na	na	90	na
Bloody Mary, bottled (Mr. & Mrs. T) .... 4.5 oz		na	na	na	na	na	na	na	na	5	1	na	130	na
Lime Daiquiri, shelf stable, w/water (Bacardi) .. 7 oz		na	na	na	na	na	na	na	2.0	na	na	na	30	na
Margarita														
bottled (Mr. & Mrs. T) .... 3 oz		na	na	na	na	na	na	na	na	na	na	na	25	na
frozen, diluted w/water (Bacardi) .... 7 oz		na	na	na	na	na	na	na	6.0	na	na	na	25	na
shelf stable, w/water (Bacardi) .... 7 oz		na	na	na	na	na	na	na	2.0	na	na	na	30	na
Peach Daiquiri, frozen, diluted w/water														
(Bacardi) .... 7 oz		na	na	na	na	na	na	na	9.0	na	na	na	50	na
Piña Colada														
bottled (Mr. & Mrs. T) .... 4 oz		na	na	na	na	na	na	na	na	na	na	na	30	na
frozen, diluted w/water (Bacardi) .... 7 oz		na	na	na	na	na	na	na	9.0	na	na	na	170	na
shelf stable, w/water (Bacardi) .... 7 oz		na	na	na	na	na	na	na	1.0	na	na	na	65	na
Rum Runner, shelf stable, w/water (Bacardi) ... 7 oz		na	na	na	na	na	na	na	6.0	na	na	na	85	na
Strawberry Colada, shelf stable, w/water														
(Bacardi) .... 7 oz		na	na	na	na	na	na	na	6.0	na	na	na	50	na
Strawberry Daiquiri														
frozen, diluted w/water (Bacardi) .... 7 oz		na	na	na	na	na	na	na	9.0	na	na	na	35	na
shelf stable, w/water (Bacardi) .... 7 oz		na	na	na	na	na	na	na	1.0	na	na	na	15	na
ALCOHOLIC BEVERAGES. See also ALCOHOL-FREE BEVERAGES.														
BEER, ALE, and MALT LIQUOR														
(Coors) .... 12 oz		na	na	na	na	na	na	na	na	.62	na	na	5.78	na

Food Name	Serving Size	A I.U.	Thi mg	Rib mg	Nia mg	B$_6$ mg	Fol mcg	B$_{12}$ mcg	C mg	Calc mg	Iron mg	Mag mg	Pot mg	Zn mg
(Coors) 'Dry'	12 oz	na	na	na	na	na	na	na	na	.71	na	na	5.37	na
(Coors) 'Dry' 3.2%	12 oz	na	na	na	na	na	na	na	na	.85	na	na	5.02	na
(Coors) 'Extra Gold'	12 oz	na	na	na	na	na	na	na	na	.56	na	na	6.49	na
(Coors) 'Extra Gold' 3.2%	12 oz	na	na	na	na	na	na	na	na	.7	na	na	5.9	na
(Coors) 'Light'	12 oz	na	na	na	na	na	na	na	na	.74	na	na	5.02	na
(Coors) 'Light' 3.2%	12 oz	na	na	na	na	na	na	na	na	.74	na	na	4.87	na
(Coors) 3.2%	12 oz	na	na	na	na	na	na	na	na	.64	na	na	5.13	na
(Keystone)	12 oz	na	na	na	na	na	na	na	na	.74	na	na	4.63	na
(Keystone) 'Dry'	12 oz	na	na	na	na	na	na	na	na	.67	na	na	4.96	na
(Keystone) 'Light'	12 oz	na	na	na	na	na	na	na	na	.74	na	na	4.63	na
(Keystone) 'Light' 3.2%	12 oz	na	na	na	na	na	na	na	na	.77	na	na	4.66	na
(Keystone) 3.2%	12 oz	na	na	na	na	na	na	na	na	.77	na	na	4.66	na
(Killian's)	12 oz	na	na	na	na	na	na	na	na	.59	na	na	6.64	na
(Killian's) 3.2%	12 oz	na	na	na	na	na	na	na	na	.59	na	na	5.6	na
(Zima)	12 oz	na	na	na	na	na	na	na	na	.32	na	na	4.36	na
LIQUOR AND LIQUEUR														
Coffee Liqueur														
53 proof	1 oz	0	0	0	.05	0	0.0	0	0.0	.35	.02	1.04	10.44	.01
63 proof	1 oz	0	0	0	.05	0	0.0	0	0.0	.35	.02	1.04	10.44	.01
Creme de Menthe, 72 proof	1 oz	0	0	0	0	0	0.0	0	0.0	0	.02	0	0	.01
Gin														
80 proof, distilled	1 oz	0	0	0	0	0	0.0	0	0.0	0	.01	0	.56	.01
86 proof, distilled	1 oz	0	0	0	0	0	0.0	0	0.0	0	.01	0	.56	.01
90 proof, distilled	1 oz	0	0	0	0	0	0.0	0	0.0	0	.01	0	.56	.01
94 proof, distilled	1 oz	0	0	0	0	0	0.0	0	0.0	0	.01	0	.56	.01
100 proof, distilled	1 oz	0	0	0	0	0	0.0	0	0.0	0	.01	0	.56	.01
Rum														
80 proof, distilled	1 oz	0	0	0	0	0	0.0	0	0.0	0	.03	0	.56	.02
86 proof, distilled	1 oz	0	0	0	0	0	0.0	0	0.0	0	.01	0	.56	.01
90 proof, distilled	1 oz	0	0	0	0	0	0.0	0	0.0	0	.01	0	.56	.01
94 proof, distilled	1 oz	0	0	0	0	0	0.0	0	0.0	0	.01	0	.56	.01
100 proof, distilled	1 oz	0	0	0	0	0	0.0	0	0.0	0	.01	0	.56	.01
Vodka														
80 proof, distilled	1 oz	0	0	0	0	0	0.0	0	0.0	0	0	0	.28	0
86 proof, distilled	1 oz	0	0	0	0	0	0.0	0	0.0	0	.01	0	.56	.01
90 proof, distilled	1 oz	0	0	0	0	0	0.0	0	0.0	0	.01	0	.56	.01
94 proof, distilled	1 oz	0	0	0	0	0	0.0	0	0.0	0	.01	0	.56	.01
100 proof, distilled	1 oz	0	0	0	0	0	0.0	0	0.0	0	.01	0	.56	.01
Whiskey														
80 proof, distilled	1 oz	0	0	0	0	0	0.0	0	0.0	0	.01	0	.56	.01
86 proof, distilled	1 oz	0	0	0	0	0	0.0	0	0.0	0	.01	0	.56	.01
90 proof, distilled	1 oz	0	0	0	0	0	0.0	0	0.0	0	.01	0	.56	.01
94 proof, distilled	1 oz	0	0	0	0	0	0.0	0	0.0	0	.01	0	.56	.01
100 proof, distilled	1 oz	0	0	0	0	0	0.0	0	0.0	0	.01	0	.56	.01
MIXED DRINKS. See also ALCOHOL-FREE BEVERAGES, MIXED-DRINK MIXERS.														
Banana Daiquiri, frozen, prepared w/1/2 can rum, diluted as directed (Bacardi)	7 oz	na	na	na	na	na	na	na	2.0	na	na	na	90	na
Bloody Mary, prepared from recipe	5 oz	508	.05	.03	.64	.11	19.7	0	20.4	10.36	.55	11.84	216.08	.13
Bourbon and Soda, prepared from recipe	4 oz	0	0	0	.02	0	0.0	0	0.0	3.48	.02	1.16	2.32	.09
Daiquiri, prepared from recipe	1 oz	1	0	0	.01	0	0.6	0	0.5	.91	.05	.6	6.34	.02
Gin and Tonic, prepared from recipe	1 oz	0	0	0	0	0	0.2	0	0.1	.6	.01	.3	1.5	.02
Lime Daiquiri, mix, shelf stable, prepared w/1/2 can rum (Bacardi)	7 oz	na	na	na	na	na	na	na	2.0	na	na	na	30	na
Manhattan, prepared from recipe	1 oz	0	0	0	.03	0	0.0	0	0.0	.57	.03	.57	7.41	.01
Margarita														
frozen, prepared w/1/2 can rum, diluted as directed (Bacardi)	7 oz	na	na	na	na	na	na	na	6.0	na	na	na	25	na

Food Name	Serving Size	A I.U.	Thi mg	Rib mg	Nia mg	B₆ mg	Fol mcg	B₁₂ mcg	C mg	Calc mg	Iron mg	Mag mg	Pot mg	Zn mg
shelf stable, prepared w/1/2 can rum														
(Bacardi)	7 oz	na	na	na	na	na	na	na	2.0	na	na	na	30	na
Martini, prepared from recipe	1 oz	0	0	0	0	0	0.1	0	0.0	.56	.03	.56	5.08	.01
Peach Daiquiri, frozen, prepared w/1/2 can														
rum, diluted as directed (Bacardi)	7 oz	na	na	na	na	na	na	na	9.0	na	na	na	50	na
Piña Colada														
frozen, prepared w/1/2 can rum, diluted as														
directed (Bacardi)	7 oz	na	na	na	na	na	na	na	9.0	na	na	na	170	na
mix, shelf stable, prepared w/1/2 can rum														
(Bacardi)	7 oz	na	na	na	na	na	na	na	1.0	na	na	na	65	na
prepared from recipe	1 oz	1	.01	0	.04	.01	3.2	0	1.5	2.51	.07	2.51	22.29	.04
Rum Runner, shelf stable, prepared w/1/2 can														
rum (Bacardi)	7 oz	na	na	na	na	na	na	na	6.0	na	na	na	85	na
Screwdriver, prepared from recipe	1 oz	19	.02	0	.05	.01	10.7	0	9.5	2.13	.02	2.43	46.51	.01
Strawberry Colada, mix, shelf stable, prepared														
w/1/2 can rum (Bacardi)	7 oz	na	na	na	na	na	na	na	6.0	na	na	na	50	na
Strawberry Daiquiri														
frozen, prepared w/1/2 can rum, diluted as														
directed (Bacardi)	7 oz	na	na	na	na	na	na	na	9.0	na	na	na	35	na
mix, shelf stable, prepared w/1/2 can rum														
(Bacardi)	7 oz	na	na	na	na	na	na	na	1.0	na	na	na	15	na
Tequila Sunrise, prepared from recipe	1 oz	30	.01	0	.06	.02	3.3	0	6.0	1.87	.00	2.18	32.45	.02
Tom Collins, prepared from recipe	1 oz	0	0	0	0	0	0.2	0	0.5	1.18	0	.3	2.37	.02
Whiskey Sour, prepared from recipe	1 oz	2	.06	0	.04	.01	1.6	0	3.8	1.79	.02	1.2	15.85	.01
ALFALFA SEEDS, sprouted, raw	1 tbsp	5	0	0	.01	0	1.1	0	0.3	.96	.03	.81	2.37	.03
ALLSPICE														
ground	1 tbsp	32	.01	0	.17	na	na	0	2.4	39.63	.42	8.08	62.64	.06
ground	1 tsp	10	0	0	.05	na	na	0	0.7	12.55	.13	2.56	19.84	.02
ground (Durkee)	1 tsp	.19	.04	.02	0	na	na	na	.01	0	0	na	0	na
ground (Laurel Leaf)	1 tsp	.19	.04	.02	0	na	na	na	.01	0	0	na	0	na
ALMOND														
whole kernels	1 cup	0	.3	1.11	4.77	.16	83.4	0	0.9	377.72	5.2	420.32	1039.44	4.15
whole kernels, approx 24	1 oz	0	.06	.22	.95	.03	16.7	0	0.2	75.54	1.04	84.06	207.89	.83
Blanched														
whole kernels	1 cup	0	.23	.98	4.59	.15	55.7	0	0.9	358.15	5.26	414.7	1087.5	4.58
whole kernels	1 oz	0	.05	.19	.9	.03	10.9	0	0.2	70.15	1.03	81.22	213.0	.9
Honey roasted														
whole kernels	1 cup	0	.16	1.37	4.06	.12	46.1	0	1.0	378.72	4.08	345.6	806.4	3.74
whole kernels	1 oz	0	.03	.27	.8	.02	9.1	0	0.2	74.56	.8	68.04	158.76	.74
Toasted, unblanched	1 oz	0	.04	.17	.8	.02	18.2	0	0.2	80.37	1.4	86.62	219.53	1.4
ALMOND BUTTER														
Plain, roasted (Maranatha Natural)	2 tbsp	na	na	na	na	na	na	na	na	na	na	na	280	na
ALMOND OIL	1 tbsp	0	0	0	0	0	0.0	0	0.0	0	0	0	0	0
ALMOND PASTE														
	1 oz	0	.06	.21	.82	.03	15.8	0	0.1	65.32	.9	73.56	183.75	.73
firmly packed	1 cup	0	.47	1.67	6.56	.22	126.2	0	1.1	522.1	7.17	587.93	1468.69	5.86
ALMOND POWDER														
full-fat	1 oz	0	.06	.34	.67	.03	16.8	0	0.1	61.91	.8	87.47	201.36	.06
full-fat, not packed	1 cup	0	.13	.77	1.53	.07	38.5	0	0.3	141.7	1.82	200.2	460.85	.14
partially defatted	1 oz	0	.04	.18	.86	.03	10.5	0	0.2	67.31	.99	77.82	204.2	.86
partially defatted, not packed	1 cup	0	.1	.42	1.97	.06	23.9	0	0.4	154.05	2.26	178.1	467.35	1.97
AMARANTH														
boiled, drained	1/2 cup	1828	.01	.09	.37	.12	37.5	0	27.1	137.94	1.49	36.3	423.06	.58
raw	1 cup	817	.01	.04	.18	.05	23.9	0	12.1	60.2	.65	15.4	171.08	.25
ANCHOVY, CANNED														
in olive oil, drained, yield from 2-oz can	1.6 oz	32	.04	.16	8.96	.09	5.6	.4	0.0	104.4	2.08	31.05	244.8	1.1

ANGLER FISH. See MONKFISH.

Food Name	Serving Size	A I.U.	Thi mg	Rib mg	Nia mg	B₆ mg	Fol mcg	B₁₂ mcg	C mg	Calc mg	Iron mg	Mag mg	Pot mg	Zn mg
ANISE SEED														
whole	1 tbsp	21	.02	.02	.21	.02	0.7	0	1.4	43.26	2.48	11.39	96.55	.36
whole	1 tsp	7	.01	.01	.06	.01	0.2	0	0.4	13.56	.78	3.57	30.26	.11
ANTELOPE														
raw	1 oz	0	.09	.16	na	na	na	na	0.0	.84	.89	7.56	98.84	.36
roasted	3 oz	0	.22	.62	na	na	na	na	0.0	3.4	3.57	23.8	316.2	1.43
APPLE														
boiled, unpeeled slices	1/2 cup	38	.01	.01	.08	.04	0.5	0	0.2	4.3	.16	2.58	75.68	.03
microwaved, unpeeled slices	1/2 cup	34	.01	.01	.05	.04	0.5	0	0.3	4.25	.14	2.55	79.05	.03
raw, peeled slices	1 cup	48	.02	.01	.1	.05	0.4	0	4.4	4.4	.08	3.3	124.3	.04
raw, peeled whole fruit, approx 3 per lb	1 med	56	.02	.01	.12	.06	0.5	0	5.1	5.12	.09	3.84	144.64	.05
raw, unpeeled slices	1 cup	58	.02	.02	.08	.05	3.1	0	6.3	7.7	.2	5.5	126.5	.04
raw, unpeeled whole fruit, approx 3 per lb	1 med	73	.02	.02	.11	.07	3.9	0	7.9	9.66	.25	6.9	158.7	.06
APPLE, DEHYDRATED/SULFURED														
stewed, low moisture	1/2 cup	18	.01	.03	.14	.05	0.1	0	0.6	3.88	.42	4.85	131.92	.06
uncooked, low moisture	1/2 cup	24	.01	.04	.2	.08	0.3	0	0.7	5.7	.6	6.6	192.0	.09
APPLE, DRIED														
sulfured, stewed	1/2 cup	22	.01	.02	.17	.06	0.0	0	1.3	3.84	.42	5.12	134.4	.06
sulfured, uncooked	1 cup	0	0	.14	.8	.11	0.0	0	3.4	12.04	1.2	13.76	387.0	.17
APPLE, FROZEN														
unsweetened, heated, sliced	1/2 cup	21	.01	.01	.04	.03	0.6	0	0.4	5.15	.2	3.09	78.28	.05
APPLE BUTTER														
	1 cup	0	.03	.02	.21	.1	0.0	0	5.1	14.1	.37	8.46	256.62	.17
	1 tbsp	0	0	0	.01	.01	0.0	0	0.3	.9	.02	.54	16.38	.01
APPLE CIDER (S. Martinelli) 'Sparkling'	6 oz	na	na	na	na	na	na	na	112.0	6	1.0	na	230	na
APPLE CIDER MIX (Swiss Miss)	.776 oz	na	na	na	na	na	na	na	107.8	.27	.3	na	na	na
APPLE DRINK														
(Hi-C) 'Jamin' Apple Drink,' aseptic box	6 oz	na	na	na	na	na	na	na	60.0	na	na	na	25	na
(10-K)	8 oz	na	na	na	na	na	na	na	na	5	0	na	30	na
APPLE JUICE														
Can, bottle, or box														
(J. Hungerford)	9.03 oz	na	na	na	na	na	na	na	100.0	.5	1.3	na	na	na
(J. Hungerford) 50% juice	9.03 oz	na	na	na	na	na	na	na	100.0	.6	1.7	na	na	na
(J. Hungerford) 100% juice	9.03 oz	na	na	na	na	na	na	na	100.0	1.5	3.4	na	na	na
(Minute Maid) aseptic box	6 oz	na	na	na	na	na	na	na	1.0	na	na	na	230	na
(Minute Maid) 'Juices to Go'	6 oz	na	na	na	na	na	na	na	1.0	na	na	na	230	na
(Ocean Spray)	6 oz	na	na	4	na	na	na	na	na	na	4	na	160	na
(S. Martinelli)	6 oz	na	na	na	na	na	na	na	112.0	6	1.0	na	230	na
(S. Martinelli) 'Sparkling'	6 oz	na	na	na	na	na	na	na	112.0	6	1.0	na	230	na
Chilled or frozen														
(Minute Maid) diluted as directed	6 oz	na	na	na	na	na	na	na	1.0	na	na	na	230	na
APPLE PUNCH														
(Minute Maid) chilled	6 oz	na	na	na	na	na	na	na	1.0	na	na	na	30	na
(Minute Maid) frozen concentrate	6 oz	na	na	na	na	na	na	na	1.0	na	na	na	30	na
APPLE STRAWBERRY NECTAR														
(Kern's) can or bottle	6 oz	na	na	na	na	na	na	na	na	na	na	na	120	na
APRICOT														
candied	100 gm	2700	.03	.04	.6	na	na	na	10.0	17.0	.5	na	281.0	na
raw, halves	1 cup	4049	.05	.06	.93	.08	13.3	0	15.5	21.7	.84	12.4	458.8	.4
APRICOT, CANNED														
In heavy syrup, peeled, halves	1 cup	3173	.05	.06	.97	.14	4.4	0	8.0	23.22	.77	18.06	361.2	.28
APRICOT, DEHYDRATED/SULFURED														
stewed, low-moisture	1/2 cup	5465	.02	.08	2.02	.2	1.9	0	8.8	29.76	3.08	31.0	902.72	.48
uncooked, low-moisture	1/2 cup	7601	.03	.09	2.15	.31	2.6	0	5.7	36.6	3.79	37.8	1110.0	.6
APRICOT, DRIED														
sulfured, stewed, halves	1/2 cup	2954	.01	.04	1.18	.14	0.0	0	2.0	20.0	2.09	21.25	611.25	.33
sulfured, uncooked, halves	1 cup	9412	.01	.2	3.9	.2	13.4	0	3.1	58.5	6.11	61.1	1791.4	.96

Food Name	Serving Size	A I.U.	Thi mg	Rib mg	Nia mg	B₆ mg	Fol mcg	B₁₂ mcg	C mg	Calc mg	Iron mg	Mag mg	Pot mg	Zn mg
(Mariani) California, sun dried, premium	1/4 cup	na	na	na	na	na	na	na	na	na	na	na	765	na
(Mariani) Mediterranean, sun dried, premium	1/4 cup	na	na	na	na	na	na	na	na	na	na	na	765	na
APRICOT, FROZEN, sweetened, unthawed	1 cup	4066	.05	.1	1.94	.15	4.1	0	21.8	24.2	2.18	21.78	554.18	.24
APRICOT NECTAR														
(Kern's)	6 oz	na	na	na	na	na	na	na	na	na	na	na	200	na
(Libby's)	6 oz	na	na	na	na	na	na	na	na	na	na	na	180	na
ARCTIC BONITO. See TUNA, SKIPJACK.														
ARROWHEAD														
boiled, drained	1 med	0	.02	.01	.14	.02	1.1	0	0.0	.84	.15	5.88	105.72	.03
raw	1 large	0	.04	.02	.41	.07	3.5	0	0.3	2.5	.64	12.75	230.5	.07
raw	1 med	0	.02	.01	.2	.03	1.7	0	0.1	1.2	.31	6.12	110.64	.03
ARROWROOT FLOUR	1/3 cup	0	0	0	0	0	3.0	0	0.0	17.2	.14	1.29	4.73	.03
ARTICHOKE HEARTS														
frozen, 'Deluxe' *(Birds Eye)*	3 oz	na	na	na	na	na	na	na	na	na	na	na	210	na
ARTICHOKES, FRENCH														
boiled, drained	1 med	212	.08	.08	1.2	.13	61.2	0	12.0	54.0	1.55	72.0	424.8	.59
boiled, drained, hearts	1/2 cup	149	.05	.06	.84	.09	42.8	0	8.4	37.8	1.08	50.4	297.36	.41
frozen, boiled, drained	3 oz	131	.05	.13	.73	.07	95.0	0	4.0	16.8	.45	24.8	211.2	.29
raw	1 large	300	.12	.11	1.69	.19	110.2	0	19.0	71.28	2.07	97.2	599.4	.79
raw	1 med	237	.09	.08	1.34	.15	87.0	0	15.0	56.32	1.64	76.8	473.6	.63
ARTICHOKES, GLOBE														
boiled, drained	1 med	212	.08	.08	1.2	.13	61.2	0	12.0	54.0	1.55	72.0	424.8	.59
boiled, drained, hearts	1/2 cup	149	.05	.06	.84	.09	42.8	0	8.4	37.8	1.08	50.4	297.36	.41
fresh *(Dole)*	1 large	0	na	na	na	na	na	na	7.0	na	na	na	241	na
frozen, boiled, drained	3 oz	131	.05	.13	.73	.07	95.0	0	4.0	16.8	.45	24.8	211.2	.29
frozen, unprepared	9 oz	393	.15	.36	2.19	.21	320.3	0	13.5	48.45	1.28	68.85	632.4	.82
raw	1 large	300	.12	.11	1.69	.19	110.2	0	19.0	71.28	2.07	97.2	599.4	.79
raw	1 med	237	.09	.08	1.34	.15	87.0	0	15.0	56.32	1.64	76.8	473.6	.63
ARTICHOKES, JERUSALEM, raw, slices	1/2 cup	15	.15	.05	.98	.06	10.1	0	3.0	10.5	2.55	12.75	321.75	.09
ARUGULA/rocket/roquette/ruculo/rugula														
raw	1 leaf	47	0	0	.01	0	1.9	0	0.3	3.2	.03	.94	7.38	.01
raw	1/2 cup	237	0	.01	.03	.01	9.7	0	1.5	16.0	.15	4.7	36.9	.05
ASPARAGUS														
boiled, drained	1/2 cup	485	.11	.11	.97	.11	131.4	0	9.7	18.0	.66	9.0	144.0	.38
fresh *(Dole)*	5 spears	604	na	na	na	na	na	na	9.0	na	na	na	264	na
ASPARAGUS, FROZEN														
boiled, drained	10-oz pkg	2397	.19	.3	3.04	.06	394.7	0	71.5	67.39	1.88	38.09	638.74	1.64
cuts *(Birds Eye)*	3.3 oz	na	na	na	na	na	na	na	na	na	na	na	240	na
spears *(Birds Eye)*	3.3 oz	na	na	na	na	na	na	na	na	na	na	na	260	na
unprepared	10-oz pkg	2692	.34	.37	3.41	.32	541.6	0	90.3	71.0	2.07	39.76	718.52	1.68
AUBERGINE. See EGGPLANT.														
AU JUS. See GRAVY.														
AVOCADO														
California, puréed	1/2 cup	704	.12	.14	2.20	.32	75.4	0	9.0	13.0	1.36	47	729	.49
Florida, puréed	1/2 cup	704	.12	.14	2.20	.32	61.3	0	9.0	13.0	.61	39	561	.49
AWA/milkfish														
dry-heat cooked	3 oz	93	.01	.06	7.02	.41	15.3	2.78	0.0	55.25	.35	32.3	317.9	.89

B

Food Name	Serving Size	A I.U.	Thi mg	Rib mg	Nia mg	B₆ mg	Fol mcg	B₁₂ mcg	C mg	Calc mg	Iron mg	Mag mg	Pot mg	Zn mg

BABASSU OIL. See PALM KERNEL OIL.

Food Name	Serving Size	A I.U.	Thi mg	Rib mg	Nia mg	B$_6$ mg	Fol mcg	B$_{12}$ mcg	C mg	Calc mg	Iron mg	Mag mg	Pot mg	Zn mg
BABY FOOD														
CEREAL														
Barley														
dry	1 tbsp	180	.01	.06	.06	.03	4.2	.09	0.9	30.72	.6	3.84	49.92	.36
dry	.5 oz	2	.39	.38	5.11	.05	4.1	0	0.3	112.89	10.62	16.33	56.09	.44
prepared w/whole milk	3.5 oz	105	.48	.58	5.98	.1	8.9	.3	na	230.0	12.34	30.0	192.0	.83
Cereal w/egg yolks														
junior	7.5 oz	307	.02	.1	.1	.04	7.0	.13	1.5	51.12	1.09	6.39	74.55	.62
junior	1 oz	41	0	.01	.01	.01	0.9	.02	0.2	6.8	.14	.85	9.92	.08
strained	1 oz	40	0	.01	.01	.01	0.9	.02	0.2	6.8	.13	.85	11.06	.08
w/bacon, junior	4.5 oz	120	.06	.1	.34	.03	5.3	.12	1.2	35.84	.6	6.4	44.8	.35
w/bacon, junior	1 oz	27	.01	.02	.08	.01	1.2	.03	0.3	7.94	.13	1.42	9.92	.08
w/bacon, strained	7.5 oz	143	.04	.11	.34	.06	9.4	.17	2.6	53.25	1.07	10.65	78.81	.61
w/bacon, strained	1 oz	19	.01	.01	.05	.01	1.3	.02	0.3	7.09	.14	1.42	10.49	.08
Cereal w/eggs														
strained	4.5 oz	206	.01	.06	.07	.03	12.0	.1	1.0	34.56	.69	3.84	56.32	.42
strained	1 oz	46	0	.01	.02	.01	2.7	.02	0.2	7.65	.15	.85	12.47	.09
Grits and egg yolks														
strained	4.5 oz	156	.04	.09	.38	.03	3.7	.05	0.6	35.84	.64	6.4	71.68	.29
strained	1 oz	35	.01	.02	.08	.01	0.8	.01	0.1	7.94	.14	1.42	15.88	.06
High-protein														
instant, dry	1 tbsp	0	.06	.06	.82	.01	4.6	0	0.1	17.38	1.77	5.47	32.47	.11
instant, dry	.5 oz	2	.38	.38	4.84	.07	27.0	0	0.3	102.81	10.45	32.38	192.13	.63
instant, 1 oz cereal prepared w/whole milk	1 serving	30	.13	.16	1.61	.03	10.0	.09	na	61.8	3.44	13.61	98.94	.3
instant, w/apple and orange, dry	1 tbsp	1	.09	.1	.57	.01	4.6	.01	0.1	18.02	2.1	3.82	31.92	.06
instant, w/apple and orange, dry	.5 oz	8	.54	.61	3.38	.05	27.0	.04	0.4	106.64	12.43	22.58	188.86	.38
instant, w/apple and orange, 1 oz cereal prepared w/whole milk	1 serving	na	.19	.24	1.13	.03	7.8	.1	na	63.22	4.09	10.49	98.09	.22
Mixed														
dry	1 tbsp	0	.06	.07	.83	0	1.0	0	0.1	17.59	1.52	2.4	10.49	.06
dry	.5 oz	3	.35	.39	4.93	.03	6.1	0	0.3	104.09	8.97	14.2	62.05	.34
1 oz cereal prepared w/whole milk	1 serving	30	.12	.16	1.64	.02	3.2	.09	na	62.37	2.96	7.65	56.42	.2
w/applesauce and bananas, junior	7.75 oz	42	.63	.78	8.89	.31	8.1	0	20.0	8.8	12.34	15.4	70.4	.48
w/applesauce and bananas, junior	1 oz	5	.08	.1	1.15	.04	1.1	0	2.6	1.13	1.59	1.98	9.07	.06
w/applesauce and bananas, '2nd Foods' (Gerber)	7 tbsp	na	.2	.24	3.17	.16	na	na	13.9	5	3.0	na	51	na
w/applesauce and bananas, strained	4.75 oz	24	.38	.47	5.35	.18	4.9	0	34.4	8.1	8.94	10.8	55.35	.26
w/applesauce and bananas, strained	1 oz	5	.08	.1	1.12	.04	1.0	0	7.2	1.7	1.88	2.27	11.62	.05
w/applesauce and bananas, '3rd Foods' (Gerber)	7 tbsp	na	.13	.16	2.12	.11	na	na	9.3	5	2.6	na	58	na
w/bananas, dry	1 tbsp	3	.09	.09	.49	.01	0.4	.01	0.1	16.7	1.62	2.16	16.03	.03
w/bananas, dry	.5 oz	18	.54	.51	2.92	.06	2.4	.03	0.5	98.83	9.6	12.78	94.86	.2
w/bananas, 1 oz cereal prepared w/whole milk	1 serving	na	.19	.2	.98	.03	2.0	.1	na	60.67	3.16	7.37	67.19	.16
w/honey, dry	1 tbsp	1	.06	.07	.9	0	1.1	0	0.0	28.39	1.64	2.47	6.46	.06
w/honey, dry	.5 oz	3	.36	.39	5.35	.03	6.3	0	0.0	167.99	9.7	14.63	38.2	.35
w/honey, 1 oz cereal prepared w/whole milk	1 serving	na	.13	.17	1.77	.02	3.2	.09	na	83.35	3.2	7.94	48.48	.2
Oatmeal														
instant, dry	1 tbsp	0	.07	.06	.86	0	0.9	0	0.1	17.59	1.77	3.48	11.28	.09
instant, dry	.5 oz	2	.41	.37	5.11	.02	5.0	0	0.5	104.09	10.45	20.59	66.74	.52
prepared w/whole milk	1 oz	30	.14	.16	1.7	.02	2.8	.09	na	62.37	3.44	9.92	57.83	.26
w/applesauce and bananas, '2nd Foods' (Gerber)	7 tbsp	na	.2	.24	3.17	.16	na	na	13.9	6	6.0	na	65	na
w/applesauce and bananas, '3rd Foods' (Gerber)	7 tbsp	na	.13	.16	2.12	.11	na	na	9.3	6	2.6	na	64	na
w/applesauce and bananas, junior	7.75 oz	62	.53	1.06	7.37	.53	7.7	0	42.0	13.2	12.12	24.2	105.6	.73
w/applesauce and bananas, junior	1 oz	8	.07	.14	.95	.07	1.0	0	5.4	1.7	1.56	3.12	13.61	.09

Food Name	Serving Size	A I.U.	Thi mg	Rib mg	Nia mg	B$_6$ mg	Fol mcg	B$_{12}$ mcg	C mg	Calc mg	Iron mg	Mag mg	Pot mg	Zn mg
w/applesauce and bananas, strained	4.75 oz	41	.57	.49	6.81	.27	4.7	0	29.4	12.15	7.63	14.85	63.45	.47
w/applesauce and bananas, strained	1 oz	9	.12	.1	1.43	.06	1.0	0	6.2	2.55	1.6	3.12	13.32	.1
w/bananas, dry	1 tbsp	2	.09	.09	.48	.01	0.5	.01	0.1	15.62	1.63	2.83	17.54	.05
w/bananas, dry	.5 oz	10	.51	.53	2.86	.06	2.7	.03	0.7	92.44	9.67	16.76	103.8	.27
w/bananas, prepared w/whole milk	1 oz	28	.18	.21	.96	.03	2.1	.09	0.5	58.4	3.18	8.51	70.02	.18
w/bananas, prepared w/whole milk	3.5 oz	99	.62	.74	3.38	.1	7.3	.33	1.6	206.0	11.23	30.0	247.0	.63
w/honey, dry	1 tbsp	1	.07	.07	.87	0	0.9	0	0.0	27.7	1.61	3.5	6.22	.09
w/honey, dry	.5 oz	3	.39	.4	5.15	.02	5.0	0	0.0	163.87	9.55	20.73	36.78	.53
w/honey, prepared w/whole milk	1 oz	na	.14	.17	1.71	.02	2.8	.09	na	81.93	3.14	9.92	48.19	.26
Rice														
dry	1 tbsp	0	.06	.05	.75	.01	0.6	0	0.1	20.4	1.77	4.94	9.24	.05
dry	.5 oz	2	.38	.32	4.44	.07	3.5	0	0.3	120.7	10.49	29.25	54.67	.28
dry, prepared w/whole milk	1 oz	30	.13	.14	1.48	.03	2.3	.09	na	67.76	3.46	12.76	53.87	.18
w/applesauce and bananas, '2nd Foods'														
(Gerber)	7 tbsp	na	.2	.24	3.17	.16	na	na	13.9	16	6.0	na	48	na
w/applesauce and bananas, strained	4.75 oz	28	.35	.57	5.42	0	3.4	na	42.7	22.95	9.09	4.05	37.8	.11
w/applesauce and bananas, strained	1 oz	6	.07	.12	1.14	0	0.7	na	9.0	4.82	1.91	.85	7.94	.02
w/bananas, dry	1 tbsp	1	.1	.09	.56	.02	0.3	.01	0.1	16.58	1.61	3.38	18.46	.04
w/bananas, dry	.5 oz	4	.56	.54	3.31	.1	1.7	.03	0.3	98.12	9.5	20.02	109.2	.21
w/bananas, prepared w/whole milk	1 oz	na	.19	.22	1.11	.04	1.8	.09	na	60.39	3.13	9.64	71.73	.16
w/honey, dry	1 tbsp	1	.06	.07	.88	.01	0.6	0	0.0	28.03	1.57	5.04	1.99	.05
w/honey, dry	.5 oz	4	.38	.41	5.2	.07	3.5	0	0.0	165.86	9.31	29.82	11.79	.29
w/honey, prepared w/whole milk	1 oz	na	.13	.17	1.72	.03	2.4	.09	na	82.5	3.06	12.76	39.97	.18
w/mixed fruit, junior	7.75 oz	33	.55	1.31	6.01	.54	5.9	.09	44.4	44.0	10.36	11.0	72.6	.4
w/mixed fruit, junior	1 oz	4	.07	.17	.77	.07	0.8	.01	5.7	5.67	1.34	1.42	9.36	.05
w/mixed fruit, '3rd Foods' (Gerber)	7 tbsp	na	.13	.16	2.12	.11	na	na	9.3	16	2.6	na	50	na
DESSERTS AND SNACKS														
Apple betty														
junior	7.75 oz	35	.02	.11	.1	.03	0.9	.09	59.6	35.2	.44	4.4	116.6	.06
junior	1 oz	5	0	.01	.01	0	0.1	.01	7.7	4.54	.06	.57	15.03	.01
strained	4.75 oz	23	.02	.05	.06	.02	0.5	.05	46.9	25.65	.24	2.7	67.5	.01
strained	1 oz	5	0	.01	.01	0	0.1	.01	9.8	5.39	.05	.57	14.17	0
Banana yogurt, '2nd Foods' (Gerber)	7 tbsp	2	.01	.04	na	.9	na	na	13.9	32	.1	na	114	na
Banana-apple dessert, '2nd Foods'														
(Gerber)	7 tbsp	2	.02	.02	.11	.07	na	na	13.9	3	.1	na	69	na
Banana-vanilla dessert, 'Tropical Foods'														
(Gerber)	7 tbsp	3	.02	.05	.18	.1	na	na	13.9	15	.2	na	90	na
Cereal snack														
apple-banana finger snacks, 'Graduates'														
(Gerber)	3.2 oz	250	.18	.2	2.25	.1	na	na	10.0	388	43.5	na	286	na
apple-cinnamon finger snacks, 'Graduates'														
(Gerber)	3.2 oz	250	.18	.2	2.25	.1	na	na	10.0	368	43.5	na	271	na
Cherry vanilla dessert														
junior	7.75 oz	440	.02	.02	.08	.03	0.7	na	2.4	11.0	.37	4.4	72.6	.07
junior	1 oz	57	0	0	.01	0	0.1	na	0.3	1.42	.05	.57	9.36	.01
strained	4.75 oz	270	.01	.01	.05	.01	0.4	na	1.5	6.75	.26	2.7	45.9	.05
strained	1 oz	57	0	0	.01	0	0.1	na	0.3	1.42	.05	.57	9.64	.01
Cookies and crackers														
animal-shaped, baked, chunky (Gerber)	3.5 oz	4	.5	.47	3.4	.22	na	na	7.0	42	2.1	na	231	na
arrowroot		0	.14	.12	1.63	.01	2.8	.02	1.6	9.07	.85	6.24	44.23	.15
baked, chunky, 'Biter Biscuit' (Gerber)	1 biscuit	11	.17	.41	2.77	.12	na	na	na	94	3.3	na	304	na
cinnamon animal crackers, baked, 'Graduates'														
(Gerber)	3.5 oz	15	.44	.32	3.8	.1	na	na	5.3	31.5	4.4	na	160	na
pretzel	1 oz	2	.13	.1	1.01	.02	5.7	0	1.1	7.09	1.07	7.94	38.84	.22
teething biscuit	1 biscuit	13	.03	.06	.48	.01	2.2	.01	1.0	28.93	.39	3.85	35.53	.1
teething biscuit	1 oz	33	.07	.15	1.23	.03	5.7	.02	2.6	74.56	1.01	9.92	91.57	.26

Food Name	Serving Size	A I.U.	Thi mg	Rib mg	Nia mg	B₆ mg	Fol mcg	B₁₂ mcg	C mg	Calc mg	Iron mg	Mag mg	Pot mg	Zn mg
Cottage cheese w/pineapple														
junior	7.75 oz	35	.03	.11	.1	.02	11.2	.15	52.4	68.2	.29	8.8	92.4	.38
junior	1 oz	5	0	.01	.01	0	1.5	.02	6.8	8.79	.04	1.13	11.91	.05
strained	4.75 oz	39	.02	.07	.05	.02	6.1	.11	31.5	35.1	.15	5.4	58.05	.21
strained	1 oz	8	.01	.02	.01	0	1.3	.02	6.6	7.37	.03	1.13	12.19	.04
Custard/pudding														
caramel pudding, junior	7.75 oz	70	.01	.15	.08	.04	1.9	.02	4.7	117.15	.34	10.65	123.54	.56
caramel pudding, junior	1 oz	9	0	.02	.01	.01	0.3	0	0.6	15.59	.05	1.42	16.44	.07
caramel pudding, strained	4.75 oz	49	.01	.11	.05	.03	1.2	.01	3.0	59.4	.23	6.75	70.2	.37
caramel pudding, strained	1 oz	10	0	.02	.01	.01	0.3	0	0.6	12.47	.05	1.42	14.74	.08
cherry vanilla pudding, '2nd Foods' (Gerber)	7 tbsp	2	.01	.02	.04	.01	na	na	0.2	5	.1	na	43	na
chocolate custard, junior	7.75 oz	101	.03	.24	.24	.03	10.6	.02	2.4	134.2	.88	22.0	195.8	.73
chocolate custard, junior	1 oz	13	0	.03	.03	0	1.4	0	0.3	17.29	.11	2.84	25.23	.09
chocolate custard, strained	4.75 oz	59	.02	.13	.13	.02	5.8	.01	1.9	78.08	.49	12.8	110.08	.41
chocolate custard, strained	1 oz	13	0	.03	.03	0	1.3	0	0.4	17.29	.11	2.84	24.38	.09
orange pudding, strained	4.75 oz	155	.05	.08	.16	.04	10.5	.01	12.3	43.2	.14	6.75	116.1	.23
orange pudding, strained	1 oz	33	.01	.02	.03	.01	2.2	0	2.6	9.07	.03	1.42	24.38	.05
pineapple pudding, junior	7.75 oz	81	.09	.11	.27	.09	12.3	.13	58.7	74.8	.42	19.8	198.0	.42
pineapple pudding, junior	1 oz	10	.01	.01	.03	.01	1.6	.02	7.6	9.64	.05	2.55	25.51	.05
pineapple pudding, strained	4.75 oz	51	.05	.06	.14	.05	6.7	.08	34.8	39.68	.23	11.52	103.68	.26
pineapple pudding, strained	1 oz	11	.01	.01	.03	.01	1.5	.02	7.7	8.79	.05	2.55	22.96	.06
vanilla custard, junior	7.75 oz	79	.03	.17	.09	.04	13.6	.02	1.8	123.2	.57	11.0	136.4	.61
vanilla custard, junior	1 oz	10	0	.02	.01	.01	1.8	0	0.2	15.88	.07	1.42	17.58	.08
vanilla custard, '2nd Foods' (Gerber)	7 tbsp	13	.01	.05	.05	.02	na	na	0.8	53	.2	na	64	na
vanilla custard, strained	4.75 oz	82	.02	.1	.05	.03	7.7	.01	1.0	70.4	.31	6.4	84.48	.36
vanilla custard, strained	1 oz	18	0	.02	.01	.01	1.7	0	0.2	15.59	.07	1.42	18.71	.08
vanilla custard, '3rd Foods' (Gerber)	7 tbsp	13	.01	.05	.05	.02	na	na	0.9	53	.2	na	67	na
Dutch apple dessert														
junior	7.75 oz	110	.03	.03	.11	.03	1.5	0	47.1	8.8	.44	4.4	81.4	.05
junior	1 oz	14	0	0	.01	0	0.2	0	6.1	1.13	.06	.57	10.49	.01
'2nd Foods' (Gerber)	7 tbsp	3	.01	.01	.03	.01	na	na	13.9	3	.1	na	36	na
strained	4.75 oz	66	.01	.02	.06	.01	0.9	0	28.9	6.75	.27	2.7	44.55	.01
strained	1 oz	14	0	0	.01	0	0.2	0	6.1	1.42	.06	.57	9.36	0
'3rd Foods' (Gerber)	7 tbsp	3	.01	.02	.04	.01	na	na	9.3	3	.1	na	40	na
Fruit dessert														
'2nd Foods' (Gerber)	7 tbsp	11	.02	.01	.38	.03	na	na	13.9	7	.2	na	99	na
'3rd Foods' (Gerber)	7 tbsp	40	.02	.01	.15	.04	na	na	0.6	9	.2	na	79	na
w/o ascorbic acid, junior	7.75 oz	526	.05	.03	.32	.07	7.7	0	6.6	19.8	.46	11.0	209.0	.11
w/o ascorbic acid, junior	1 oz	68	.01	0	.04	.01	1.0	0	0.9	2.55	.06	1.42	26.93	.01
w/o ascorbic acid, strained	4.75 oz	339	.02	.01	.19	.05	4.5	0	3.4	12.15	.3	6.75	126.9	.05
w/o ascorbic acid, strained	1 oz	71	0	0	.04	.01	0.9	0	0.7	2.55	.06	1.42	26.65	.01
Guava dessert, w/tapioca, 'Tropical Foods' (Gerber)	7 tbsp	4	.01	.01	.28	.02	na	na	13.9	4	.1	na	70	na
Hawaiian dessert														
'2nd Foods' (Gerber)	7 tbsp	1	.04	.03	.14	.04	na	na	13.9	41	.1	na	82	na
'3rd Foods' (Gerber)	7 tbsp	na	.04	.05	.08	.04	na	na	9.3	40	.1	na	76	na
Mango dessert, w/tapioca 'Tropical Foods' (Gerber)	7 tbsp	97	.02	.01	.25	.07	na	na	13.9	6	.1	na	64	na
Mango-banana dessert, w/passion fruit 'Tropical Foods' (Gerber)	7 tbsp	25	.01	.01	.27	.07	na	na	13.9	3	.1	na	87	na
Mixed fruit yogurt, '2nd Foods' (Gerber)	7 tbsp	12	.02	.04	.28	.04	na	na	13.9	30	.1	na	131	na
Papaya dessert, w/tapioca, 'Tropical Foods' (Gerber)	7 tbsp	9	.01	.01	.11	0	na	na	13.9	7	.1	na	64	na
Papaya-pineapple dessert, 'Tropical Foods' (Gerber)	7 tbsp	13	.02	.03	.12	.02	na	na	13.9	10	.3	na	96	na
Peach cobbler														
junior	7.75 oz	312	.02	.03	.57	.02	2.4	0	45.1	8.8	.22	4.4	123.2	.07

Food Name	Serving Size	A I.U.	Thi mg	Rib mg	Nia mg	B$_6$ mg	Fol mcg	B$_{12}$ mcg	C mg	Calc mg	Iron mg	Mag mg	Pot mg	Zn mg
junior	1 oz	40	0	0	.07	0	0.3	0	5.8	1.13	.03	.57	15.88	.01
'2nd Foods' (Gerber)	7 tbsp	14	.01	.01	.34	.01	na	na	13.9	4	.1	na	67	na
strained	4.75 oz	192	.01	.02	.35	.01	1.5	0	27.7	5.4	.14	2.7	72.9	.41
strained	1 oz	40	0	0	.07	0	0.3	0	5.8	1.13	.03	.57	15.31	.09
'3rd Foods' (Gerber)	7 tbsp	13	.02	.01	.34	.01	na	na	9.3	4	.1	na	85	na
Peach melba														
junior	7.75 oz	431	.02	.07	.6	.01	4.2	0	57.2	24.2	.66	4.4	204.6	.62
junior	1 oz	56	0	.01	.08	0	0.5	0	7.4	3.12	.09	.57	26.37	.08
strained	4.75 oz	248	.01	.05	.46	.01	2.6	0	42.4	13.5	.45	2.7	112.05	.38
strained	1 oz	52	0	.01	.1	0	0.5	0	8.9	2.84	.09	.57	23.53	.08
Peach yogurt, '2nd Foods' (Gerber)	7 tbsp	20	.01	.04	.37	.02	na	na	13.9	25	.2	na	121	na
Peach-mango dessert, 'Tropical Foods' (Gerber)	7 tbsp	42	.01	.01	.25	.02	na	na	13.9	4	.1	na	57	na
Pear yogurt														
pineapple-banana dessert, 'Tropical Foods' (Gerber)	7 tbsp	3	.03	.05	.15	.09	na	na	13.9	8	.3	na	80	na
Pineapple-orange dessert														
strained	4.75 oz	73	.02	.03	.06	.04	3.3	.06	18.3	14.08	.23	5.12	60.16	.22
strained	1 oz	16	0	.01	.01	.01	0.7	.01	4.1	3.12	.05	1.13	13.32	.05
Tropical fruit dessert														
junior	7.75 oz	44	.02	.07	.18	.07	7.3	0	41.4	22.0	.57	11.0	127.6	.1
junior	1 oz	6	0	.01	.02	.01	0.9	0	5.3	2.84	.07	1.42	16.44	.01
medley, 'Tropical Foods' (Gerber)	7 tbsp	20	.02	.01	.12	.05	na	na	13.9	5	.1	na	39	na
DINNERS AND MAIN DISHES														
Apples and chicken dinner, 'Simple Recipe' '2nd Foods' (Gerber)	7 tbsp	1	.02	.08	.59	.06	na	na	0.1	23	.4	na	na	na
Apples and ham dinner, 'Simple Recipe' '2nd Foods' (Gerber)	7 tbsp	0	.07	.06	.68	.08	na	na	0.1	4	.3	na	na	na
Apples and turkey dinner 'Simple Recipe,' '2nd Foods' (Gerber)	7 tbsp	1	.02	.09	.66	.07	na	na	0.1	5	.5	na	na	na
Beans and rice dinner 'Tropical Foods' (Gerber)	7 tbsp	na	.03	.02	.18	.06	na	na	na	14	.8	na	118	na
Beef and egg noodle dinner '3rd Foods' (Gerber)	7 tbsp	236	.02	.03	.71	.05	na	na	1.4	11	.4	na	94	na
Beef and rice dinner														
toddler	6.25 oz	889	.03	.12	2.38	.25	10.6	.9	6.9	19.47	1.22	14.16	212.4	1.62
toddler	1 oz	142	0	.02	.38	.04	1.7	.14	1.1	3.12	.2	2.27	34.02	.26
Beef lasagna dinner														
toddler	6.25 oz	2059	.13	.16	2.39	.13	10.6	.9	3.4	31.86	1.54	19.47	215.94	1.24
toddler	1 oz	330	.02	.03	.38	.02	1.7	.14	0.5	5.1	.25	3.12	34.59	.2
Beef noodle dinner														
junior	7.5 oz	1397	.06	.08	1.24	.07	11.7	.21	3.0	17.04	.92	14.91	97.98	.85
junior	1 oz	186	.01	.01	.16	.01	1.6	.03	0.4	2.27	.12	1.98	13.04	.11
strained	4.5 oz	1053	.04	.05	.93	.06	6.5	.12	1.5	11.52	.52	8.96	60.16	.48
strained	1 oz	233	.01	.01	.2	.01	1.5	.03	0.3	2.55	.12	1.98	13.32	.11
Beef stew														
toddler	6.25 oz	2919	.02	.12	2.32	.13	10.6	.9	5.3	15.93	1.27	19.47	251.34	1.54
toddler	1 oz	467	0	.02	.37	.02	1.7	.14	0.9	2.55	.2	3.12	40.26	.25
Beef vegetable dinner														
high-meat, junior	4.5 oz	1014	.05	.1	1.82	.11	8.3	.74	2.4	15.36	1.01	10.24	190.72	1.79
high-meat, junior	1 oz	225	.01	.02	.4	.02	1.8	.16	0.5	3.4	.22	2.27	42.24	.4
high-meat, strained	4.5 oz	1004	.04	.08	1.7	.11	7.3	.65	2.4	15.36	.93	10.24	179.2	1.66
high-meat, strained	1 oz	222	.01	.02	.38	.02	1.6	.14	0.5	3.4	.21	2.27	39.69	.37
Broccoli-chicken dinner, 'Simple Recipe' '2nd Foods' (Gerber)	7 tbsp	58	.02	.09	.68	.09	na	na	17.1	39	.7	na	175	na

Food Name	Serving Size	A I.U.	Thi mg	Rib mg	Nia mg	B$_6$ mg	Fol mcg	B$_{12}$ mcg	C mg	Calc mg	Iron mg	Mag mg	Pot mg	Zn mg
Carrots and beef dinner, 'Simple Recipe'														
'2nd Foods' (Gerber)	7 tbsp	1198	.03	.06	.86	.12	na	na	0.8	23	.5	na	209	na
Chicken noodle dinner														
junior	7.5 oz	1906	.06	.07	1.1	.06	11.3	.28	2.6	36.21	.83	19.17	74.55	.63
junior	1 oz	254	.01	.01	.15	.01	1.5	.04	0.3	4.82	.11	2.55	9.92	.08
'2nd Foods' (Gerber)	7 tbsp	81	.03	.04	.72	.05	na	na	1.3	25	.3	na	79	na
strained	4.5 oz	1158	.04	.07	.6	.04	6.9	.17	1.3	28.16	.58	11.52	49.92	.38
strained	1 oz	257	.01	.02	.13	.01	1.5	.04	0.3	6.24	.13	2.55	11.06	.09
'3rd Foods' (Gerber)	7 tbsp	111	.02	.03	.8	.06	na	na	0.0	14	.3	na	84	na
Chicken rice dinner														
'Tropical Foods' (Gerber)	7 tbsp	na	.02	.03	.62	.07	na	na	0.1	16	.3	na	59	na
Chicken stew dinner														
toddler	6 oz	1717	.05	.13	1.96	.08	1.7	.24	3.2	61.2	1.12	17.0	156.4	.7
toddler	1 oz	286	.01	.02	.33	.01	0.3	.04	0.5	10.21	.19	2.84	26.08	.12
w/noodles, 'Graduates'	3.2 oz	141	.04	.08	1.04	.11	na	na	0.1	14	.5	na	108	na
Chicken vegetable dinner														
high-meat, junior	4.5 oz	1071	.04	.09	1.26	.05	1.4	.2	1.4	55.04	.95	8.96	79.36	1.28
high-meat, junior	1 oz	237	.01	.02	.28	.01	0.3	.05	0.3	12.19	.21	1.98	17.58	.28
high-meat, strained	4.5 oz	737	.03	.09	1.31	.08	1.4	.18	0.9	66.56	1.27	8.96	75.52	1.22
high-meat, strained	1 oz	163	.01	.02	.29	.02	0.3	.04	0.2	14.74	.28	1.98	16.73	.27
Green bean dinner, w/turkey, 'Simple Recipe,'														
'2nd Foods' (Gerber)	7 tbsp	44	.03	.11	1.14	.08	na	na	2.2	31	.7	na	188	na
Ham vegetable dinner														
high-meat, junior	4.5 oz	333	.14	.11	1.48	.12	8.3	.36	2.4	12.8	.76	11.52	207.36	1.38
high-meat, junior	1 oz	74	.03	.02	.33	.03	1.8	.08	0.5	2.84	.17	2.55	45.93	.31
high-meat, strained	4.5 oz	214	.13	.11	1.8	.14	8.1	.35	2.3	14.08	.76	11.52	198.4	1.28
high-meat, strained	1 oz	47	.03	.02	.4	.03	1.8	.08	0.5	3.12	.17	2.55	43.94	.28
Lamb noodle dinner														
junior	7.5 oz	1668	.08	.14	1.43	.11	9.2	.4	4.1	38.34	.77	17.04	164.01	.56
junior	1 oz	222	.01	.02	.19	.01	1.2	.05	0.5	5.1	.1	2.27	21.83	.07
Macaroni dinner														
tomato beef, '2nd Foods' (Gerber)	7 tbsp	97	.04	.04	.65	.08	na	na	1.2	18	.5	na	123	na
tomato beef, '3rd Foods' (Gerber)	7 tbsp	122	.01	.03	.67	.06	na	na	1.3	7	.4	na	117	na
w/bacon, junior	7.5 oz	2471	.1	.18	1.34	.04	3.4	.06	4.5	151.23	.81	17.04	178.92	.75
w/bacon, junior	1 oz	329	.01	.02	.18	.01	0.5	.01	0.6	20.13	.11	2.27	23.81	.1
w/cheese, junior	7.5 oz	28	.12	.14	1.16	.03	3.2	.06	2.8	108.63	.64	14.91	93.72	.68
w/cheese, junior	1 oz	4	.02	.02	.15	0	0.4	.01	0.4	14.46	.09	1.98	12.47	.09
w/cheese, strained	4.5 oz	35	.07	.09	.56	.02	1.8	.04	1.7	69.12	.4	10.24	58.88	.44
w/cheese, strained	1 oz	8	.02	.02	.13	0	0.4	.01	0.4	15.31	.09	2.27	13.04	.1
w/cheese, '2nd Foods' (Gerber)	7 tbsp	10	.03	.04	.53	.03	na	na	1.0	55	.2	na	54	na
Macaroni main dish														
alphabets w/beef and tomato sauce, chunky (Gerber)	7 tbsp	15	.06	.07	1.09	.06	na	na	2.5	9	.6	na	139	na
w/beef, in sauce, 'Graduates' (Gerber)	3.2 oz	15	.07	.09	151	.11	na	na	0.3	15	.7	na	207	na
w/ham, junior	7.5 oz	1120	.12	.21	1.73	.03	4.3	.06	4.7	159.75	.81	14.91	225.78	.76
w/ham, junior	1 oz	149	.02	.03	.23	0	0.6	.01	0.6	21.26	.11	1.98	30.05	.1
w/tomato and beef, junior	7.5 oz	1472	.1	.12	1.6	.1	13.9	.51	3.2	29.82	.77	14.91	153.36	.77
w/tomato and beef, junior	1 oz	196	.01	.02	.21	.01	1.8	.07	0.4	3.97	.1	1.98	20.41	.1
w/tomato and beef, strained	4.5 oz	680	.09	.08	1.05	.06	25.7	.29	1.9	20.48	.63	11.52	122.88	.4
w/tomato and beef, strained	1 oz	151	.02	.02	.23	.01	5.7	.07	0.4	4.54	.14	2.55	27.22	.09
Mixed vegetable dinner														
junior	7.5 oz	5206	.03	.05	.88	.16	14.3	0	7.0	36.21	.66	21.3	238.56	.51
junior	1 oz	693	0	.01	.12	.02	1.9	0	0.9	4.82	.09	2.84	31.75	.07
strained	4.5 oz	3492	.02	.04	.64	.1	10.2	0	3.6	28.16	.42	14.08	154.88	.21
strained	1 oz	773	0	.01	.14	.02	2.3	0	0.8	6.24	.09	3.12	34.3	.05
Noodle main dish														
w/beef, chunky, 'Homestyle' (Gerber)	7 tbsp	116	.04	.07	.83	.05	na	na	1.5	29	.5	na	99	na

Food Name	Serving Size	A I.U.	Thi mg	Rib mg	Nia mg	B₆ mg	Fol mcg	B₁₂ mcg	C mg	Calc mg	Iron mg	Mag mg	Pot mg	Zn mg
w/chicken, carrots, and peas, chunky														
(Gerber) .... 7 tbsp	7 tbsp	188	.03	.04	1.16	.06	na	na	2.9	12	.4	na	96	na
Ravioli														
beef, w/tomato sauce, 'Graduates' (Gerber)	3.2 oz	119	.39	.12	1.38	.4	na	na	0.1	38	.7	na	na	na
cheese, w/tomato sauce, 'Graduates'														
(Gerber)	3.2 oz	124	.12	.14	1.65	.09	na	na	0.1	54	.8	na	na	na
Rice main dish														
saucy, w/chicken, chunky (Gerber) .... 7 tbsp	7 tbsp	136	.03	.04	.87	.07	na	na	2.7	18	.3	na	90	na
w/beef and tomato sauce, chunky (Gerber) .. 7 tbsp	7 tbsp	104	.03	.05	.8	.08	na	na	3.7	13	.5	na	157	na
Spaghetti														
w/mini meatballs and sauce, 'Graduates'														
(Gerber)	3.2 oz	13	.07	.07	1.19	.07	na	na	0.1	17	.6	na	186	na
w/tomato and meat, junior	7.5 oz	1476	.14	.15	2.34	.13	15.1	.02	4.7	38.34	1.17	17.04	230.04	.89
w/tomato and meat, junior	1 oz	196	.02	.02	.31	.02	2.0	0	0.6	5.1	.16	2.27	30.62	.12
w/tomato and meat, toddler	6.25 oz	784	.11	.18	2.76	.15	10.6	.41	7.3	38.94	1.59	26.55	288.51	.85
w/tomato and meat, toddler	1 oz	126	.02	.03	.44	.02	1.7	.07	1.2	6.24	.26	4.25	46.21	.14
w/tomato sauce and beef, chunky (Gerber) .. 7 tbsp	7 tbsp	24	.08	.11	1.64	.09	na	na	5.2	28	.7	na	248	na
w/tomato sauce and beef, '3rd Foods'														
(Gerber) .... 7 tbsp	7 tbsp	110	.05	.05	1.0	.06	na	na	0.5	15	.5	na	128	na
Split pea and ham dinner														
junior	7.5 oz	1284	.1	.1	1.02	.09	27.7	.11	4.1	48.99	1.07	na	289.68	1.37
junior	1 oz	171	.01	.01	.14	.01	3.7	.01	0.5	6.52	.14	na	38.56	.18
Turkey rice dinner														
junior	7.5 oz	2256	.02	.06	.59	.06	6.6	.21	2.6	48.99	.62	17.04	72.42	.52
junior	1 oz	300	0	.01	.08	.01	0.9	.03	0.3	6.52	.08	2.27	9.64	.07
'2nd Foods' (Gerber)	7 tbsp	154	.02	.03	.73	.07	na	na	1.1	8	.03	na	91	na
strained	4.5 oz	782	.01	.03	.39	.04	4.1	.13	1.5	26.88	.33	10.24	52.48	.32
strained	1 oz	173	0	.01	.09	.01	0.9	.03	0.3	5.95	.07	2.27	11.62	.07
'3rd Foods' (Gerber)	7 tbsp	270	.01	.04	.76	.06	na	na	1.7	11	.3	na	112	na
Turkey stew main dish, w/rice, 'Graduates'														
(Gerber)	3.2 oz	1405	.02	.04	1.14	.07	na	na	0.0	9	.3	na	114	na
Turkey vegetable dinner														
high-meat, junior	4.5 oz	810	.01	.09	1.03	.05	12.7	.58	1.7	90.88	1.0	10.24	136.96	1.16
high-meat, junior	1 oz	179	0	.02	.23	.01	2.8	.13	0.4	20.13	.22	2.27	30.33	.26
high-meat, strained	4.5 oz	420	.01	.09	1.29	.05	12.3	.56	1.9	79.36	.88	10.24	153.6	1.28
high-meat, strained	1 oz	93	0	.02	.28	.01	2.7	.12	0.4	17.58	.2	2.27	34.02	.28
Veal vegetable dinner														
high-meat, junior	4.5 oz	544	.03	.1	1.97	.09	7.7	.59	2.2	14.08	1.14	11.52	200.96	1.41
high-meat, junior	1 oz	120	.01	.02	.44	.02	1.7	.13	0.5	3.12	.25	2.55	44.51	.31
high-meat, strained	4.5 oz	349	.03	.09	2.06	.11	7.7	.58	2.4	11.52	.77	10.24	195.84	1.28
high-meat, strained	1 oz	77	.01	.02	.46	.02	1.7	.13	0.5	2.55	.17	2.27	43.38	.28
Vegetable bacon dinner														
junior	7.5 oz	3357	.11	.06	1.16	.14	19.2	.21	2.3	23.43	.87	17.04	183.18	.56
junior	1 oz	447	.01	.01	.15	.02	2.6	.03	0.3	3.12	.12	2.27	24.38	.08
strained	4.5 oz	3409	.04	.04	.68	.1	11.8	.13	1.7	17.92	.46	8.96	113.92	.32
'3rd Foods' (Gerber)	7 tbsp	364	.03	.03	.45	.06	na	na	0.1	16	.3	na	92	na
Vegetable beef dinner														
junior	7.5 oz	3012	.07	.07	1.4	.14	10.4	.55	3.2	21.3	1.0	12.78	223.65	.88
junior	1 oz	401	.01	.01	.19	.02	1.4	.07	0.4	2.84	.13	1.7	29.77	.12
'2nd Foods' (Gerber)	7 tbsp	198	.02	.03	.57	.05	na	na	0.9	8	.3	na	98	na
strained	4.5 oz	755	.01	.01	.15	.02	2.6	.03	0.4	3.97	.1	1.98	25.23	.07
strained	1 oz	337	.01	.01	.14	.02	1.3	.07	0.3	3.4	.11	1.42	28.63	.09
'3rd Foods' (Gerber)	7 tbsp	344	.02	.03	.62	.08	na	na	0.1	13	.4	na	144	na
Vegetable chicken dinner														
junior	7.5 oz	2545	.03	.04	.71	.08	8.1	.21	3.0	29.82	.64	19.17	55.38	.66
junior	1 oz	339	0	.01	.09	.01	1.1	.03	0.4	3.97	.09	2.55	7.37	.09
'2nd Foods' (Gerber)	7 tbsp	137	.02	.02	.59	.06	na	na	0.7	18	.3	na	78	na

Food Name	Serving Size	A I.U.	Thi mg	Rib mg	Nia mg	B$_6$ mg	Fol mcg	B$_{12}$ mcg	C mg	Calc mg	Iron mg	Mag mg	Pot mg	Zn mg
strained	4.5 oz	1416	.02	.02	.24	.03	4.1	.13	1.4	17.00	.25	10.24	38.4	.33
strained	1 oz	314	0	.01	.05	.01	0.9	.03	0.3	3.97	.08	2.27	8.51	.07
'3rd Foods' (Gerber)	7 tbsp	177	.01	.02	.59	.05	na	na	na	17	.2	na	86	na
Vegetable dumpling dinner														
w/beef, junior	7.5 oz	1406	.08	.08	1.04	.1	15.8	.19	1.7	29.82	1.0	14.91	100.11	.7
w/beef, junior	1 oz	187	.01	.01	.14	.01	2.1	.03	0.2	3.97	.13	1.98	13.32	.09
w/beef, strained	4.5 oz	532	.06	.05	.73	.06	9.2	.12	1.0	17.92	.5	7.68	58.88	.51
w/beef, strained	1 oz	118	.01	.01	.16	.01	2.0	.03	0.2	3.97	.11	1.7	13.04	.11
Vegetable ham dinner														
junior	7.5 oz	1310	.08	.05	.75	.07	11.3	.11	2.8	17.04	.47	10.65	195.96	.47
junior	1 oz	174	.01	.01	.1	.01	1.5	.01	0.4	2.27	.06	1.42	26.08	.06
'2nd Foods' (Gerber)	7 tbsp	123	.04	.03	.51	.05	na	na	0.8	7	.2	na	77	na
strained	4.5 oz	873	.04	.04	.52	.04	6.3	.05	2.1	10.24	.38	6.4	108.8	.25
strained	1 oz	193	.01	.01	.11	.01	1.4	.01	0.5	2.27	.09	1.42	24.1	.05
'3rd Foods' (Gerber)	7 tbsp	296	.02	.02	.58	.06	na	na	1.4	9	.2	na	102	na
toddler	6.25 oz	628	.08	.1	1.24	.15	8.9	.25	6.6	40.71	1.24	30.09	270.81	.83
toddler	1 oz	101	.01	.02	.2	.02	1.4	.04	1.1	6.52	.2	4.82	43.38	.13
Vegetable lamb dinner														
junior	7.5 oz	3159	.04	.07	1.18	.09	7.7	.34	3.6	27.69	.72	14.91	202.35	.47
junior	1 oz	420	.01	.01	.16	.01	1.0	.05	0.5	3.69	.1	1.98	26.93	.06
strained	4.5 oz	2554	.02	.04	.68	.06	4.6	.2	1.5	15.36	.45	8.96	120.32	.28
strained	1 oz	566	.01	.01	.15	.01	1.0	.05	0.3	3.4	.1	1.98	26.65	.06
Vegetable liver dinner														
junior	7.5 oz	8369	.05	.48	2.46	.21	68.2	3.86	3.8	21.3	3.86	25.56	189.57	.81
junior	1 oz	1114	.01	.06	.33	.03	9.1	.51	0.5	2.84	.51	3.4	25.23	.11
strained	4.5 oz	3981	.02	.34	1.54	.1	36.7	2.32	2.3	8.96	2.83	15.36	120.32	.49
strained	1 oz	882	.01	.08	.34	.02	8.1	.51	0.5	1.98	.63	3.4	26.65	.11
Vegetable main dish														
w/beef, chunky (Gerber)	7 tbsp	219	.03	.05	.86	.09	na	na	3.3	12	.5	na	162	na
w/chicken, chunky (Gerber)	7 tbsp	304	.02	.04	.96	.07	na	na	2.9	22	.4	na	127	na
w/ham, chunky (Gerber)	7 tbsp	177	.06	.04	.78	.06	na	na	2.3	12	.4	na	111	na
w/turkey, chunky (Gerber)	7 tbsp	166	.02	.05	.83	.05	na	na	1.6	22	.4	na	105	na
Vegetable noodle dinner														
w/chicken, junior	7.5 oz	2239	.09	.08	1.44	.05	7.2	.19	1.7	55.38	1.04	23.43	125.67	.68
w/chicken, junior	1 oz	298	.01	.01	.19	.01	1.0	.03	0.2	7.37	.14	3.12	16.73	.09
w/chicken, strained	4.5 oz	1814	.04	.06	.52	.03	4.1	.1	0.9	35.84	.45	12.8	70.4	.32
w/chicken, strained	1 oz	402	.01	.01	.12	.01	0.9	.02	0.2	7.94	.1	2.84	15.59	.07
w/turkey, junior	7.5 oz	2117	.05	.09	.64	.04	6.0	.26	1.7	68.16	.55	19.17	155.49	.64
w/turkey, junior	1 oz	282	.01	.01	.08	.01	0.8	.03	0.2	9.07	.07	2.55	20.7	.09
w/turkey, strained	4.5 oz	1268	.02	.06	.32	.02	3.1	.13	1.0	40.96	.24	10.24	80.64	.35
w/turkey, strained	1 oz	281	.01	.01	.07	0	0.7	.03	0.2	9.07	.05	2.27	17.86	.08
Vegetable stew														
w/beef, 'Graduates' (Gerber)	3.2 oz	170	.03	.07	1.23	.09	na	na	0.6	18	.6	na	176	na
Vegetable turkey dinner														
junior	7.5 oz	1908	.03	.04	.53	.05	6.2	.19	2.3	27.69	.68	19.17	53.25	.54
junior	1 oz	254	0	0	.07	.01	0.8	.03	0.3	3.69	.09	2.55	7.09	.07
'2nd Foods' (Gerber)	7 tbsp	107	.02	.04	.64	.05	na	na	1.0	18	.3	na	74	na
'3rd Foods' (Gerber)	7 tbsp	134	.02	.02	.55	.04	na	na	1.6	10	.2	na	78	na
strained	4.5 oz	1068	.01	.02	.39	.04	3.3	.12	1.4	20.48	.35	10.24	56.32	.29
strained	1 oz	236	0	0	.09	.01	0.7	.03	0.3	4.54	.08	2.27	12.47	.06
toddler	6.25 oz	3715	.04	.16	1.04	.11	5.3	.78	6.0	81.42	1.06	28.32	200.82	.57
toddler	1 oz	595	.01	.03	.17	.02	0.9	.12	1.0	13.04	.17	4.54	47.06	.09
EGG YOLK														
'2nd Foods' (Gerber)	7 tbsp	158	.06	022	.03	.16	na	na	1.4	71	2.0	na	70	na
strained	3.3 oz	1176	.07	.25	.02	.15	86.6	1.45	1.3	71.44	2.59	6.58	72.38	1.8
strained	1 oz	355	.02	.08	.01	.05	26.1	.44	0.4	21.55	.78	1.98	21.83	.54

Food Name	Serving Size	A I.U.	Thi mg	Rib mg	Nia mg	B$_6$ mg	Fol mcg	B$_{12}$ mcg	C mg	Calc mg	Iron mg	Mag mg	Pot mg	Zn mg
FRUIT														
Apple and blueberry														
junior	7.75 oz	92	.04	.09	.23	.09	7.7	0	30.6	11.0	.88	6.6	143.0	.08
junior	1 oz	12	.01	.01	.03	.01	1.0	0	3.9	1.42	.11	.85	18.43	.01
'2nd Foods' (Gerber)	7 tbsp	1	.03	.02	.11	.03	na	na	13.9	4	.1	na	77	na
strained	4.75 oz	27	.02	.05	.16	.05	4.7	0	37.5	5.4	.27	4.05	93.15	.05
strained	1 oz	6	0	.01	.03	.01	1.0	0	7.9	1.13	.06	.85	19.56	.01
'3rd Foods' (Gerber)	7 tbsp	na	.02	.04	.11	.04	na	na	9.3	4	.1	na	91	na
Apple and raspberry														
w/sugar, junior	7.75 oz	66	.03	.06	.23	.07	7.3	0	63.6	11.0	.48	8.8	158.4	.07
w/sugar, junior	1 oz	9	0	.01	.03	.01	0.9	0	8.2	1.42	.06	1.13	20.41	.01
w/sugar, strained	4.75 oz	30	.02	.04	.14	.05	4.6	0	36.2	6.75	.3	5.4	108.0	.04
w/sugar, strained	1 oz	6	0	.01	.03	.01	1.0	0	7.6	1.42	.06	1.13	22.68	.01
Applesauce														
'1st Foods' (Gerber)	7 tbsp	4	.02	.03	.08	.05	na	na	22.2	4	.1	na	102	na
junior	7.5 oz	19	.03	.06	.13	.06	3.6	0	80.5	10.65	.47	6.39	164.01	.09
junior	1 oz	3	0	.01	.02	.01	0.5	0	10.7	1.42	.06	.85	21.83	.01
'2nd Foods' (Gerber)	7 tbsp	4	.02	.03	.08	.04	na	na	13.9	4	.1	na	77	na
strained	4.5 oz	22	.02	.04	.08	.04	2.4	0	49.0	5.12	.28	3.84	90.88	.03
strained	1 oz	5	0	.01	.02	.01	0.5	0	10.9	1.13	.06	.85	20.13	.01
'3rd Foods' (Gerber)	7 tbsp	na	.02	.03	.08	.04	na	na	9.3	4	.1	na	93	na
w/apricot, junior	7.75 oz	746	.03	.07	.32	.07	3.1	0	39.4	13.2	.57	8.8	239.8	.07
w/apricot, junior	1 oz	96	0	.01	.04	.01	0.4	0	5.1	1.7	.07	1.13	30.9	.01
w/apricot, '2nd Foods' (Gerber)	7 tbsp	63	.02	.03	.16	.04	na	na	13.9	6	.2	na	119	na
w/apricot, strained	4.75 oz	522	.02	.04	.19	.04	1.8	0	25.5	8.1	.34	5.4	162.0	.06
w/apricot, strained	1 oz	110	0	.01	.04	.01	0.4	0	5.4	1.7	.07	1.13	34.02	.01
w/cherry, junior	7.75 oz	90	.03	.1	.22	.09	0.9	0	51.0	19.8	.9	8.8	213.4	.06
w/cherry, junior	1 oz	12	0	.01	.03	.01	0.1	0	6.6	2.55	.12	1.13	27.5	.01
w/cherry, strained	4.75 oz	53	.02	.06	.13	.05	0.5	0	45.2	13.5	.53	5.4	129.6	.04
w/cherry, strained	1 oz	11	0	.01	.03	.01	0.1	0	9.5	2.84	.11	1.13	27.22	.01
w/pineapple, junior	7.5 oz	45	.05	.06	.17	.08	4.3	0	57.1	8.52	.21	8.52	161.88	.06
w/pineapple, junior	1 oz	6	.01	.01	.02	.01	0.6	0	7.6	1.13	.03	1.13	21.55	.01
w/pineapple, strained	4.5 oz	26	.03	.03	.1	.05	2.4	0	36.0	5.12	.13	3.84	99.84	.02
w/pineapple, strained	1 oz	6	.01	.01	.02	.01	0.5	0	8.0	1.13	.03	.85	22.11	0
Apricot														
w/tapioca, junior	7.75 oz	1591	.02	.03	.43	.06	3.5	0	39.4	17.6	.59	8.8	275.0	.09
w/tapioca, junior	1 oz	205	0	0	.06	.01	0.5	0	5.1	2.27	.08	1.13	35.44	.01
w/tapioca, '2nd Foods' (Gerber)	7 tbsp	149	.01	.01	.23	.04	na	na	13.9	7	.2	na	108	na
w/tapioca, strained	4.75 oz	979	.01	.02	.26	.04	2.0	0	29.2	12.15	.41	5.4	163.35	.06
w/tapioca, strained	1 oz	206	0	0	.06	.01	0.4	0	6.1	2.55	.09	1.13	34.3	.01
w/tapioca, '3rd Foods' (Gerber)	7 tbsp	89	.01	.01	.23	.04	na	na	9.3	8	.2	na	134	na
Banana														
'1st Foods' (Gerber)	7 tbsp	9	.03	.07	.61	.39	na	na	22.2	4	.2	na	312	na
w/pineapple and tapioca, '2nd Foods' (Gerber)	7 tbsp	5	.02	.03	.17	.14	na	na	13.9	4	.1	na	98	na
w/pineapple and tapioca,'3rd Foods' (Gerber)	7 tbsp	4	.02	.02	.16	.12	na	na	9.3	5	.1	na	110	na
w/tapioca, junior	7.75 oz	97	.03	.04	.48	.31	14.1	0	56.5	17.6	.66	26.4	237.6	.15
w/tapioca, junior	1 oz	12	0	.01	.06	.04	1.8	0	7.3	2.27	.09	3.4	30.62	.02
w/tapioca, '2nd Foods' (Gerber)	7 tbsp	3	.02	.04	.23	.15	na	na	13.9	4	.1	na	149	na
w/tapioca, '3rd Foods' (Gerber)	7 tbsp	4	.01	.04	.23	.17	na	na	9.3	4	.1	na	142	na
w/tapioca, strained	4.75 oz	58	.02	.04	.25	.16	7.4	0	22.6	6.75	.27	13.5	118.8	.08
w/tapioca, strained	1 oz	12	0	.01	.05	.03	1.6	0	4.7	1.42	.06	2.84	24.95	.02
Banana and pineapple														
w/tapioca, junior	4.75 oz	54	.02	.03	.25	.12	7.4	0	28.6	9.45	.18	8.1	105.3	.04
w/tapioca, junior	1 oz	11	0	.01	.05	.03	1.6	0	6.0	1.98	.04	1.7	22.11	.01
w/tapioca, strained	7.75 oz	90	.04	.04	.37	.18	11.9	0	42.2	15.4	.51	13.2	149.6	.09

Food Name	Serving Size	A I.U.	Thi mg	Rib mg	Nia mg	B6 mg	Fol mcg	B12 mcg	C mg	Calc mg	Iron mg	Mag mg	Pot mg	Zn mg
w/tapioca, strained	1 oz	12	.01	.01	.05	.02	1.5	0	5.4	1.98	.07	1.7	19.28	.01
Guava														
w/tapioca, strained	4.5 oz	383	.02	.09	.5	.05	2.6	0	96.5	8.96	.26	2.56	93.44	.1
w/tapioca, strained	1 oz	85	0	.02	.11	.01	0.6	0	21.4	1.98	.06	.57	20.7	.02
Guava and papaya														
w/tapioca, strained	4.5 oz	236	.01	.03	.34	.02	2.6	0	103.6	8.96	.26	6.4	94.72	.08
w/tapioca, strained	1 oz	52	0	.01	.07	0	0.6	0	22.9	1.98	.06	1.42	20.98	.02
Mango														
w/tapioca, strained	4.75 oz	898	.03	.04	.34	.16	2.7	0	167.9	5.4	.14	5.4	79.65	.08
w/tapioca, strained	1 oz	189	.01	.01	.07	.03	0.6	0	35.3	1.13	.03	1.13	16.73	.02
Papaya and applesauce														
w/tapioca, strained	4.5 oz	97	.01	.04	.14	.03	2.6	0	144.8	8.96	.56	6.4	101.12	.04
w/tapioca, strained	1 oz	22	0	.01	.03	.01	0.6	0	32.1	1.98	.12	1.42	22.4	.01
Peach														
'1st Foods' (Gerber)	7 tbsp	66	.02	.04	.78	.02	na	na	22.2	4	.1	na	157	na
'2nd Foods' (Gerber)	7 tbsp	30	.01	.03	.77	.02	na	na	13.9	4	.1	na	148	na
'3rd Foods' (Gerber)	7 tbsp	29	.02	.03	.75	.02	na	na	9.3	4	.1	na	164	na
w/sugar, junior	7.75 oz	392	.03	.07	1.42	.04	8.6	0	41.6	11.0	.59	11.0	341.0	.13
w/sugar, junior	1 oz	50	0	.01	.18	.01	1.1	0	5.4	1.42	.08	1.42	43.94	.02
w/sugar, strained	4.75 oz	217	.01	.04	.82	.02	5.3	0	42.4	8.1	.32	8.1	218.7	.11
w/sugar, strained	1 oz	46	0	.01	.17	0	1.1	0	8.9	1.7	.07	1.7	45.93	.02
Pear														
'1st Foods' (Gerber)	7 tbsp	3	.03	.03	.23	.02	na	na	22.2	10	.1	na	121	na
junior	7.5 oz	72	.03	.06	.4	.02	8.1	0	46.9	17.04	.53	19.17	244.95	.17
junior	1 oz	10	0	.01	.05	0	1.1	0	6.2	2.27	.07	2.55	32.6	.02
'2nd Foods' (Gerber)	7 tbsp	2	.02	.03	.2	.01	na	na	13.9	10	.1	na	103	na
strained	4.5 oz	42	.02	.04	.24	.01	4.6	0	31.4	10.24	.31	10.24	166.4	.1
strained	1 oz	9	0	.01	.05	0	1.0	0	7.0	2.27	.07	2.27	36.85	.02
'3rd Foods' (Gerber)	7 tbsp	3	.01	.03	.21	.01	na	na	9.3	9	.1	na	121	na
Pear and pineapple														
junior	7.5 oz	68	.05	.05	.39	.03	6.2	0	35.8	21.3	.45	14.91	251.34	.27
junior	1 oz	9	.01	.01	.05	0	0.8	0	4.8	2.84	.06	1.98	33.45	.04
'2nd Foods' (Gerber)	7 tbsp	3	.02	.03	.19	.02	na	na	13.9	9	.1	na	102	na
strained	4.5 oz	37	.03	.04	.26	.02	3.6	0	35.2	12.8	.32	8.96	148.48	.08
strained	1 oz	8	.01	.01	.06	0	0.8	0	7.8	2.84	.07	1.98	32.89	.02
'3rd Foods' (Gerber)	7 tbsp	4	.03	.02	.2	.02	na	na	9.3	10	.1	na	116	na
Plum														
w/tapioca, '2nd Foods' (Gerber)	7 tbsp	18	.01	.03	.23	.03	na	na	1.4	7	.1	na	81	na
w/tapioca, '3rd Foods' (Gerber)	7 tbsp	5	.01	.04	.2	.04	na	na	0.9	7	.1	na	102	na
w/tapioca, w/o ascorbic acid, junior	7.75 oz	207	.01	.07	.45	.06	2.0	0	1.8	13.2	.48	8.8	182.6	.18
w/tapioca, w/o ascorbic acid, junior	1 oz	27	0	.01	.06	.01	0.3	0	0.2	1.7	.06	1.13	23.53	.02
w/tapioca, w/o ascorbic acid, strained	4.75 oz	128	.01	.04	.29	.03	1.2	0	1.5	8.1	.27	5.4	114.75	.11
w/tapioca, w/o ascorbic acid, strained	1 oz	27	0	.01	.06	.01	0.3	0	0.3	1.7	.06	1.13	24.1	.02
Prune														
'1st Foods' (Gerber)	7 tbsp	6	.02	.21	.72	.11	na	na	na	21	.4	na	306	na
w/tapioca, '2nd Foods' (Gerber)	7 tbsp	30	.02	.09	.45	.09	na	na	2.9	14	.2	na	167	na
w/tapioca, w/o ascorbic acid, junior	7.75 oz	895	.05	.18	1.16	.19	0.4	0	1.8	33.0	.73	22.0	356.4	.22
w/tapioca, w/o ascorbic acid, junior	1 oz	115	.01	.02	.15	.02	0.1	0	0.2	4.25	.09	2.84	45.93	.03
w/tapioca, w/o ascorbic acid, strained	4.75 oz	612	.03	.1	.71	.11	0.3	0	1.1	20.25	.47	13.5	238.95	.12
w/tapioca, w/o ascorbic acid, strained	1 oz	128	.01	.02	.15	.02	0.1	0	0.2	4.25	.1	2.84	50.18	.03
INFANT FORMULA														
Mix														
liquid, iron-fortified, prepared, 'Follow-Up' (Carnation)	5 oz	250	80	96	1280	66	16.0	.32	8.0	135	1.9	8.4	135	.63
liquid, iron-fortified, prepared, 'Good Start' (Carnation)	5 oz	300	60	135	750	75	9.0	.22	8.0	64	1.5	6.7	98	.75
liquid, low-iron, prepared (Enfamil)	5 oz	310	78	150	1250	63	15.6	.23	8.1	78	.5	7.8	108	.78

Food Name	Serving Size	A I.U.	Thi mg	Rib mg	Nia mg	B_6 mg	Fol mcg	B_{12} mcg	C mg	Calc mg	Iron mg	Mag mg	Pot mg	Zn mg
liquid, low-iron, prepared (Gerber)	5 oz	300	60	90	1350	60	15.0	.45	9.0	94	.5	8.0	115	.75
liquid, low-iron, prepared (Similac)	5 oz	300	100	150	1050	60	15.0	.25	9.0	73	.22	6	105	.75
liquid, soy, iron-fortified, milk-free (Nursoy)	5 oz	300	100	150	750	62.5	7.5	.3	8.3	90	1.8	10	105	.8
liquid, soy, iron-fortified, milk-free, prepared (Gerber)	5 oz	300	60	90	1350	60	15.0	.45	9.0	94	1.8	8.0	115	.75
liquid, soy, iron-fortified, milk-free, prepared (ProSobee)	5 oz	310	78	94	1250	63	15.6	.31	8.1	94	1.88	10.9	122	.78
liquid, soy, w/iron, milk-free, prepared (Isomil)	5 oz	300	60	90	1350	60	15.0	.45	9.0	105	1.8	7.5	108	.75
liquid, w/iron, prepared (Enfamil)	5 oz	310	78	150	1250	63	15.6	.23	8.1	78	1.88	7.8	108	.78
liquid, w/iron, prepared (Gerber)	5 oz	300	100	150	1050	60	15.0	.25	9.0	75	1.8	6.0	108	.75
liquid, w/iron, prepared (Similac)	5 oz	300	100	150	1050	60	15.0	.25	9.0	73	1.8	6	105	.75
powder, iron-fortified, prepared, 'Follow-Up' (Carnation)	5 oz	250	80	96	1280	66	16.0	.32	8.0	135	1.9	8.4	135	.63
powder, iron-fortified, prepared, 'Good Start' (Carnation)	5 oz	300	60	135	750	75	9.0	.22	8.0	64	1.5	6.7	98	.75
powder, low-iron, prepared (Enfamil)	5 oz	310	78	150	1250	63	15.6	.23	8.1	78	.5	7.8	108	.78
powder, low-iron, prepared (Gerber)	5 oz	300	60	90	1350	60	15.0	.45	9.0	94	.5	8.0	115	.75
powder, low-iron, prepared (Similac)	5 oz	300	100	150	1050	60	15.0	.25	9.0	73	.22	6	105	.75
powder, soy, iron-fortified, milk-free, prepared (Gerber)	5 oz	300	60	90	1350	60	15.0	.45	9.0	94	1.8	8.0	115	.75
powder, soy, iron-fortified, milk-free, prepared (ProSobee)	5 oz	310	78	94	1250	63	15.6	.31	8.1	94	1.88	10.9	122	.78
powder, soy, w/iron, milk-free, prepared (Isomil)	5 oz	300	60	90	1350	60	15.0	.45	9.0	105	1.8	7.5	108	.75
powder, w/iron, prepared (Enfamil)	5 oz	310	78	150	1250	63	15.6	.23	8.1	78	1.88	7.8	108	.78
powder, w/iron, prepared (Gerber)	5 oz	300	100	150	1050	60	15.0	.25	9.0	75	1.8	na	108	.75
powder, w/iron, prepared (Similac)	5 oz	300	100	150	1050	60	15.0	.25	9.0	73	1.8	6	105	.75
Ready to use														
iron-fortified, 'Follow-Up' (Carnation)	5 oz	250	80	00	1280	66	16.0	.32	8.0	135	1.9	8.4	135	.63
iron-fortified, 'Good Start' (Carnation)	5 oz	300	60	135	750	75	9.0	.22	8.0	64	1.5	6.7	98	.75
low-iron (Enfamil)	5 oz	310	78	150	1250	63	15.6	.23	8.1	78	.5	7.8	108	.78
low-iron (Gerber)	5 oz	300	60	90	1350	60	15.0	.45	9.0	94	.5	8.0	115	.75
low-iron (Similac)	5 oz	300	100	150	1050	60	15.0	.25	9.0	73	.22	6	105	.75
soy, iron-fortified, milk-free (Gerber)	5 oz	300	60	90	1350	60	15.0	.45	9.0	94	1.8	8.0	115	.75
soy, iron-fortified, milk-free (ProSobee)	5 oz	310	78	94	1250	63	15.6	.31	8.1	94	1.88	10.9	122	.78
soy, w/iron, milk-free (Isomil)	5 oz	300	60	90	1350	60	15.0	.45	9.0	105	1.8	7.5	108	.75
w/iron (Enfamil)	5 oz	310	78	150	1250	63	15.6	.23	8.1	78	1.88	7.8	108	.78
w/iron (Gerber)	5 oz	300	100	150	1050	60	15.0	.25	9.0	75	1.8	6.0	108	.75
w/iron (Similac)	5 oz	300	100	150	1050	60	15.0	.25	9.0	73	1.8	6	105	.75
JUICE														
Apple														
	4.2 oz	23	.01	.02	.11	.04	0.1	0	75.3	5.2	.74	3.9	118.3	.04
	1 oz	6	0	0	.03	.01	0.0	0	18.0	1.24	.18	.93	28.21	.01
'Graduates' (Gerber)	3.2 oz	na	na	.02	.09	.03	na	na	21.5	86	.3	na	89	na
strained, '1st Foods' (Gerber)	3.2 oz	na	.01	.01	.09	.03	na	na	33.5	3	.1	na	89	na
w/yogurt, 2nd Foods' (Gerber)	3.2 oz	1	.03	.07	.11	.02	na	na	33.9	73	.2	na	143	na
Apple-banana														
'Graduates' (Gerber)	3.2 oz	2	.01	.03	.16	.08	na	na	21.5	86	.2	na	123	na
'2nd Foods' (Gerber)	3.2 oz	2	.01	.02	.14	.06	na	na	33.5	7	.3	na	123	na
Apple-carrot, '3rd Foods' (Gerber)	3.2 oz	194	.01	.03	.08	.05	na	na	34.1	14	.3	na	81	na
Apple-cherry														
	4.2 oz	7	.01	.02	.12	.04	0.4	0	75.8	6.5	.86	3.9	127.4	.04
	1 oz	2	0	0	.03	.01	0.1	0	18.1	1.55	.2	.93	30.38	.01
'Graduates' (Gerber)	6 oz	1	.01	.03	.11	.03	na	na	21.5	86	.2	na	115	na
'2nd Foods' (Gerber)	3.2 oz	1	.01	.02	.1	.03	na	na	33.5	8	.3	na	115	na
Apple-cranberry 'Stages 2' (Beech-Nut)	4 oz	na	na	na	na	na	na	na	na	na	na	na	120	na

Food Name	Serving Size	A I.U.	Thi mg	Rib mg	Nia mg	B$_6$ mg	Fol mcg	B$_{12}$ mcg	C mg	Calc mg	Iron mg	Mag mg	Pot mg	Zn mg
Apple-grape														
....	4.2 oz	8	.01	.03	.14	.04	0.4	0	69.7	7.8	.51	3.9	117.0	.05
....	1 oz	2	0	.01	.03	.01	0.1	0	16.6	1.86	.12	.93	27.9	.01
'Graduates' (Gerber)	3.2 oz	na	.01	.02	.1	.05	na	na	21.5	86	.2	na	97	na
'2nd Foods' (Gerber)	3.2 oz	2	.01	.02	.11	.03	na	na	33.5	8	.2	na	97	na
'Stages 2' (Beech-Nut)	4 oz	na	na	na	na	na	na	na	na	na	na	na	105	na
Apple-peach														
....	4.2 oz	82	.01	.01	.28	.03	1.7	0	76.1	3.9	.73	3.9	126.1	.03
....	1 oz	20	0	0	.07	.01	0.4	0	18.1	.93	.17	.93	30.07	.01
'2nd Foods' (Gerber)	3.2 oz	6	.01	.01	.2	.03	na	na	33.5	7	.3	na	117	na
Apple-plum														
....	4.2 oz	56	.03	.02	.25	.04	0.3	0	75.7	6.5	.81	3.9	131.3	.04
....	1 oz	13	.01	.01	.06	.01	0.1	0	18.0	1.55	.19	.93	31.31	.01
'2nd Foods' (Gerber)	3.2 oz	2	.01	.02	.17	.03	na	na	33.5	8	.2	na	110	na
Apple-prune														
....	4.2 oz	21	.01	0	.39	.05	0.1	0	87.8	11.7	1.24	9.1	192.4	.06
....	1 oz	5	0	0	.09	.01	0.0	0	20.9	2.79	.29	2.17	45.88	.01
'2nd Foods' (Gerber)	3.2 oz	1	.01	.08	.22	15.32	na	na	33.5	10	.4	na	139	na
Apple-sweet potato, '3rd Foods' (Gerber) ...	3.2 oz	172	.01	.03	.1	.07	na	na	34.1	15	.3	na	137	na
Banana														
w/yogurt, '2nd Foods' (Gerber)	3.2 oz	3	.03	.08	.24	.09	na	na	33.9	71	.1	na	173	na
Grape														
red, '1st Foods' (Gerber)	3.2 oz	na	.02	.01	.13	.06	na	na	33.5	12	.2	na	52	na
white, '1st Foods' (Gerber)	3.2 oz	na	.01	.01	.09	.06	na	na	33.5	13	.1	na	41	na
Guava, w/mixed fruit, 'Tropical Foods'														
(Gerber)	3.2 oz	1	.02	.03	.28	.04	na	na	33.5	16	.2	na	121	na
Mango, w/mixed fruit 'Tropical Foods'														
(Gerber)	3.2 oz	7	.02	.03	.29	.07	na	na	33.5	13	.3	na	102	na
Mixed fruit														
....	4.2 oz	55	.03	.02	.16	.06	8.7	0	82.7	10.4	.44	6.5	131.3	.04
....	1 oz	13	.01	0	.04	.01	2.1	0	19.7	2.48	.11	1.55	31.31	.01
'2nd Foods' (Gerber)	3.2 oz	4	.03	.01	.13	.04	na	na	33.5	10	.2	na	120	na
w/yogurt, '2nd Foods' (Gerber)	3.2 oz	2	.04	.08	.15	.03	na	na	33.9	71	.2	na	152	na
Orange														
....	4.2 oz	72	.06	.04	.31	.07	34.3	0	81.3	15.6	.22	11.7	239.2	.07
....	1 oz	17	.01	.01	.07	.02	8.2	0	19.4	3.72	.05	2.79	57.04	.02
'2nd Foods' (Gerber)	3.2 oz	35	.07	.03	.24	.05	na	na	33.5	11	.1	na	168	na
Orange-apple														
....	4.2 oz	95	.05	.04	.24	.05	15.9	0	100.0	13.0	.26	6.5	179.4	.03
....	1 oz	23	.01	.01	.06	.01	3.8	0	23.8	3.1	.06	1.55	42.78	.01
w/banana	4.2 oz	35	.06	.04	.34	.08	12.6	0	41.7	6.5	.46	7.8	174.2	.03
w/banana	1 oz	8	.01	.01	.08	.02	3.0	0	10.0	1.55	.11	1.86	41.54	.01
Orange-apricot														
....	4.2 oz	281	.08	.04	.35	.07	25.9	0	111.7	7.8	.49	9.1	258.7	.05
....	1 oz	67	.02	.01	.08	.02	6.2	0	26.6	1.86	.12	2.17	61.69	.01
Orange-banana														
....	4.2 oz	60	.07	.05	.23	.07	31.7	0	44.2	22.1	.14	18.2	260.0	.11
....	1 oz	14	.02	.01	.06	.02	7.6	0	10.5	5.27	.03	4.34	62.0	.03
Orange-carrot, '3rd Foods' (Gerber)	3.2 oz	188	.06	.05	.21	.05	na	na	34.1	16	.2	na	174	na
Orange-pineapple														
....	4.2 oz	40	.07	.03	.25	.08	24.2	0	69.4	10.4	.55	11.7	183.3	.05
....	1 oz	10	.02	.01	.06	.02	5.8	0	16.6	2.48	.13	2.79	43.71	.01
Papaya, w/mixed fruit, 'Tropical Foods'														
(Gerber)	3.2 oz	8	.02	.05	.6	.06	na	na	33.5	14	.2	na	106	na
Pear, strained, '1st Foods' (Gerber)	3.2 oz	na	.01	.02	.15	.02	na	na	33.5	3	.1	na	89	na
Pear-peach														
w/yogurt, '2nd Foods' (Gerber)	3.2 oz	17	.03	.08	.39	.02	na	na	33.9	71	.1	na	171	na

Food Name	Serving Size	A I.U.	Thi mg	Rib mg	Nia mg	B$_6$ mg	Fol mcg	B$_{12}$ mcg	C mg	Calc mg	Iron mg	Mag mg	Pot mg	Zn mg
Pineapple-carrot, '3rd Foods' (Gerber)	3.2 oz	170	.06	.04	.19	.07	na	na	34.1	16	.3	na	115	na
Prune-orange														
	4.2 oz	170	.06	.16	.51	.08	17.0	0	82.9	15.6	1.13	10.4	235.3	.05
	1 oz	41	.01	.04	.12	.02	4.1	0	19.8	3.72	.27	2.48	56.11	.01
MEAT														
Beef														
junior	3.5 oz	102	.01	.16	3.25	.12	5.6	1.46	1.9	7.92	1.63	8.91	188.1	1.98
junior	1 oz	29	0	.05	.93	.03	1.6	.42	0.5	2.27	.47	2.55	53.87	.57
'2nd Foods' (Gerber)	7 tbsp	7	.01	.12	3.04	.12	na	na	1.9	6	1.5	na	212	na
strained	3.5 oz	183	.01	.14	2.82	.14	5.4	1.41	2.1	6.93	1.46	16.83	217.8	2.43
strained	1 oz	52	0	.04	.81	.04	1.6	.4	0.6	1.98	.42	4.82	62.37	.7
'3rd Foods' (Gerber)	7 tbsp	7	.02	.13	3.06	.12	na	na	2.2	6	1.7	na	216	na
w/beef heart, strained	3.5 oz	125	.02	.35	3.85	.12	5.0	6.75	2.1	3.96	1.97	11.88	198.0	1.82
w/beef heart, strained	1 oz	36	.01	.1	1.1	.03	1.4	1.93	0.6	1.13	.56	3.4	56.7	.52
Chicken														
junior	3.5 oz	184	.01	.16	3.39	.19	11.0	.4	1.5	54.45	.98	10.89	120.78	1.0
junior	1 oz	53	0	.05	.97	.05	3.2	.11	0.4	15.59	.28	3.12	34.59	.29
'2nd Foods' (Gerber)	7 tbsp	2	.02	.11	4.07	.21	na	na	2.0	60	1.0	na	175	na
strained	3.5 oz	134	.01	.15	3.22	.2	10.3	.4	1.7	63.36	1.39	12.87	139.59	1.2
strained	1 oz	38	0	.04	.92	.06	3.0	.11	0.5	18.14	.4	3.69	39.97	.34
'3rd Foods' (Gerber)	7 tbsp	1	.02	.07	3.98	.17	na	na	1.9	30	.9	na	168	na
Chicken sticks														
finger snacks, 'Graduates' (Gerber)	10 sticks	2	.02	.14	2.72	.1	na	na	2.3	58	1.1	na	128	na
junior	1 stick	318	0	.02	.2	.01	1.1	.04	0.2	7.3	.16	1.4	10.6	.1
Ham														
junior	3.5 oz	32	.14	.19	2.81	.2	2.1	.1	2.1	4.95	1.0	10.89	207.9	1.68
junior	1 oz	9	.04	.05	.81	.06	0.6	.03	0.6	1.42	.29	3.12	59.53	.48
'2nd Foods' (Gerber)	7 tbsp	3	.1	.14	2.76	.17	na	na	2.1	5	.9	na	232	na
strained	3.5 oz	38	.14	.15	2.61	.25	2.0	.1	2.1	5.94	1.02	12.87	201.96	2.22
strained	1 oz	11	.04	.04	.75	.07	0.6	.03	0.6	1.7	.29	3.69	57.83	.64
'3rd Foods' (Gerber)	7 tbsp	3	.1	.15	3.04	.18	na	na	2.0	5	1.0	na	237	na
Lamb														
junior	3.5 oz	27	.02	.19	3.16	.18	2.0	2.25	1.7	6.93	1.64	9.9	208.89	2.57
junior	1 oz	8	.01	.05	.91	.05	0.6	.64	0.5	1.98	.47	2.84	59.82	.74
strained	3.5 oz	85	.02	.2	2.9	.15	2.3	2.17	1.2	6.93	1.48	12.87	202.95	2.73
strained	1 oz	24	.01	.06	.83	.04	0.7	.62	0.3	1.98	.42	3.69	58.12	.78
Liver														
strained	3.5 oz	37754	.05	1.8	8.24	.34	334.0	2.14	19.1	3.96	5.24	12.87	224.73	2.95
strained	1 oz	10811	.01	.51	2.36	.1	95.7	.61	5.5	1.13	1.5	3.69	64.35	.84
Meat sticks														
finger snacks, 'Graduates' (Gerber)	10 sticks	4	.07	.14	1.8	.09	na	na	1.5	27	1.5	na	125	na
junior	1 stick	7	.01	.02	.15	.01	0.9	.03	0.2	3.4	.14	1.1	11.4	.19
Pork														
strained	3.5 oz	38	.14	.2	2.25	.2	1.9	.98	1.8	4.95	.99	9.9	220.77	2.25
strained	1 oz	11	.04	.06	.64	.06	0.5	.28	0.5	1.42	.28	2.84	63.22	.64
Turkey														
junior	3.5 oz	562	.02	.25	3.45	.16	12.0	1.06	2.4	27.72	1.34	11.88	178.2	1.78
junior	1 oz	161	0	.07	.99	.05	3.4	.3	0.7	7.94	.38	3.4	51.03	.51
'2nd Foods' (Gerber)	7 tbsp	1	.02	.12	3.61	.13	na	na	2.9	4	1.2	na	209	na
strained	3.5 oz	554	.02	.21	3.63	.18	11.2	.99	2.2	22.77	1.19	13.86	228.69	1.81
strained	1 oz	159	.01	.06	1.04	.05	3.2	.28	0.6	6.52	.34	3.97	65.49	.52
'3rd Foods' (Gerber)	7 tbsp	1	.02	.13	3.22	.19	na	na	2.1	4	.8	na	203	na
Turkey sticks														
finger snacks, 'Graduates' (Gerber)	10 sticks	3	.02	.15	2.02	.08	na	na	1.9	27	1.2	na	122	na
junior	1 stick	23	0	.02	.18	.01	1.1	.1	0.2	7.2	.12	1.6	9.1	.18

Food Name	Serving Size	A I.U.	Thi mg	Rib mg	Nia mg	B$_6$ mg	Fol mcg	B$_{12}$ mcg	C mg	Calc mg	Iron mg	Mag mg	Pot mg	Zn mg
Veal														
junior	3.5 oz	50	.02	.18	3.77	.12	6.6	1.29	2.1	5.94	1.24	10.89	233.64	2.49
junior	1 oz	14	.01	.05	1.08	.03	1.9	.37	0.6	1.7	.35	3.12	66.91	.71
'2nd Foods' (Gerber)	7 tbsp	5	.02	.15	3.7	.13	na	na	2.8	4	.9	na	224	na
strained	3.5 oz	46	.02	.16	3.52	.15	5.8	1.29	2.3	6.93	1.26	11.88	213.84	1.98
strained	1 oz	13	0	.05	1.01	.04	1.7	.37	0.7	1.98	.36	3.4	61.24	.57
'3rd Foods' (Gerber)	7 tbsp	4	.02	.15	3.84	.12	na	na	2.3	5	1.0	na	224	na
SOUP														
Chicken														
strained	4.5 oz	1772	.02	.04	.38	.05	6.7	.15	1.3	47.36	.35	6.4	84.48	.28
strained	1 oz	392	0	.01	.08	.01	1.5	.03	0.3	10.49	.08	1.42	18.71	.06
Cream of broccoli, '3rd Foods' (Gerber)	3.2 oz	3	.01	.03	.17	.02	na	na	0.2	50	.2	na	38	na
Cream of chicken														
strained	4.5 oz	929	.01	.06	.48	.06	7.9	.08	1.7	44.8	.38	7.68	99.84	.33
strained	1 oz	206	0	.01	.11	.01	1.8	.02	0.4	9.92	.09	1.7	22.11	.07
Cream of potato, '3rd Foods' (Gerber)	3.2 oz	1	.02	.05	.53	.05	na	na	0.5	50	.3	na	122	na
Cream of tomato, '3rd Foods' (Gerber)	3.2 oz	13	.03	.08	.57	.09	na	na	0.4	50	.4	na	296	na
Cream of vegetable, '3rd Foods' (Gerber)	3.2 oz	27	.02	.05	.2	.03	na	na	0.1	50	.2	na	78	na
VEGETABLES														
Beet														
'2nd Foods' (Gerber)	7 tbsp	2	.02	.04	.12	.03	na	na	0.5	14	.3	na	219	na
strained	4.5 oz	42	.01	.06	.17	.03	39.4	0	3.1	17.92	.41	17.92	232.96	.15
strained	1 oz	9	0	.01	.04	.01	8.7	0	0.7	3.97	.09	3.97	51.6	.03
Broccoli, carrot, and cheese, '3rd Foods' (Gerber)	7 tbsp	264	.02	.03	.29	.05	na	na	4.5	29	.2	na	98	na
Carrot														
buttered, junior	7.5 oz	20959	.04	.12	1.1	na	18.3	na	16.2	74.55	.66	na	308.85	na
buttered, junior	1 oz	2790	.01	.02	.15	na	2.4	na	2.2	9.92	.09	na	41.11	na
buttered, strained	4.5 oz	13860	.02	.07	.76	na	12.0	na	11.7	44.8	.36	na	291.84	na
buttered, strained	1 oz	3070	0	.02	.17	na	2.7	na	2.6	9.92	.08	na	64.64	na
diced, 'Graduates' (Gerber)	3.2 oz	8571	.02	.03	.25	.02	na	na	0.7	19.2	.2	na	129	na
'1st Foods' (Gerber)	7 tbsp	1590	.03	.04	.58	.1	na	na	0.7	26	.2	na	234	na
junior	7.5 oz	25155	.05	.09	1.06	.17	36.9	0	11.7	48.99	.83	23.43	430.26	.37
junior	1 oz	3348	.01	.01	.14	.02	4.9	0	1.6	6.52	.11	3.12	57.27	.05
'2nd Foods' (Gerber)	7 tbsp	1569	.02	.03	.42	.09	na	na	0.6	22	.2	na	191	na
strained	4.5 oz	14670	.03	.05	.59	.09	19.1	0	7.3	28.16	.47	11.52	250.88	.19
strained	1 oz	3249	.01	.01	.13	.02	4.2	0	1.6	6.24	.1	2.55	55.57	.04
'3rd Foods' (Gerber)	7 tbsp	1508	.02	.03	.44	.09	na	na	0.2	23	.2	na	176	na
Corn, creamed														
junior	7.5 oz	164	.03	.1	1.07	.09	27.1	.04	4.7	38.34	.58	17.04	172.53	.49
junior	1 oz	22	0	.01	.14	.01	3.6	.01	0.6	5.1	.08	2.27	22.96	.07
'2nd Foods' (Gerber)	7 tbsp	4	.02	.04	.53	.04	na	na	0.3	19	.1	na	101	na
strained	4.5 oz	96	.02	.06	.66	.05	14.5	.03	2.7	25.6	.36	10.24	115.2	.24
strained	1 oz	21	0	.01	.15	.01	3.2	.01	0.6	5.67	.08	2.27	25.51	.05
Garden vegetable														
'2nd Foods' (Gerber)	7 tbsp	561	.06	.06	.77	.09	na	na	2.5	31	.7	na	169	na
strained	4.5 oz	7766	.08	.09	1.0	.13	51.5	0	7.3	35.84	1.06	26.88	215.04	.33
strained	1 oz	1720	.02	.02	.22	.03	11.4	0	1.6	7.94	.24	5.95	47.63	.07
Green bean														
buttered, junior	7.25 oz	787	.00	.20	.66	na	56.2	na	17.7	142.14	2.37	na	352.26	na
buttered, junior	1 oz	108	0	.03	.09	na	7.7	na	2.4	19.56	.33	na	48.48	na
buttered, strained	4.5 oz	584	.02	.14	.44	na	36.5	na	10.6	81.92	1.64	na	204.8	na
buttered, strained	1 oz	129	.01	.03	.1	na	8.1	na	2.4	18.14	.36	na	45.36	na
creamed, junior	7.5 oz	320	.05	.12	.5	.03	84.6	.11	5.8	68.16	.55	14.91	138.45	.34
creamed, junior	1 oz	43	.01	.02	.07	0	11.3	.01	0.8	9.07	.07	1.98	18.43	.05
creamed, '3rd Foods' (Gerber)	7 tbsp	8	.02	.05	.32	.04	na	na	0.5	35	.3	na	114	na
diced, 'Graduates' (Gerber)	3.2 oz	153	.02	.05	.23	.03	na	na	0.9	23.3	.4	na	75	na

Food Name	Serving Size	A I.U.	Thi mg	Rib mg	Nia mg	B$_6$ mg	Fol mcg	B$_{12}$ mcg	C mg	Calc mg	Iron mg	Mag mg	Pot mg	Zn mg
'1st Foods' (Gerber)	7 tbsp	41	.04	.08	.31	.05	na	na	1.2	40	.6	na	182	na
junior	7.25 oz	892	.04	.21	.66	.07	67.4	0	17.3	133.9	2.22	45.32	263.68	.4
junior	1 oz	123	.01	.03	.09	.01	9.3	0	2.4	18.43	.31	6.24	36.29	.05
'2nd Foods' (Gerber)	7 tbsp	37	.04	.06	.43	.06	na	na	2.0	36	.5	na	155	na
strained	4.5 oz	573	.03	.11	.44	.05	44.3	0	6.7	49.92	.96	30.72	202.24	.26
strained	1 oz	127	.01	.02	.1	.01	9.8	0	1.5	11.06	.21	6.8	44.79	.06
Mixed														
junior	7.5 oz	8935	.06	.07	1.42	.17	8.7	0	5.3	23.43	.87	23.43	362.1	.58
junior	1 oz	1189	.01	.01	.19	.02	1.2	0	0.7	3.12	.12	3.12	48.19	.08
'2nd Foods' (Gerber)	7 tbsp	612	.03	.02	.31	.07	na	na	0.1	15	.3	na	120	na
strained	4.5 oz	5108	.03	.03	.42	.07	5.0	0	2.2	16.64	.41	12.8	162.56	.19
strained	1 oz	1131	.01	.01	.09	.02	1.1	0	0.5	3.69	.09	2.84	36.0	.04
'3rd Foods' (Gerber)	7 tbsp	526	.03	.03	.6	.1	na	na	0.4	15	.4	na	144	na
Peas														
buttered, junior	7.25 oz	845	.15	.16	2.84	na	74.6	na	26.2	92.7	2.14	na	241.02	na
buttered, junior	1 oz	116	.02	.02	.39	na	10.3	na	3.6	12.76	.29	na	33.17	na
buttered, strained	4.5 oz	422	.1	.09	1.75	na	44.4	na	15.4	49.92	1.41	na	124.16	na
buttered, strained	1 oz	94	.02	.02	.39	na	9.8	na	3.4	11.06	.31	na	27.5	na
creamed, strained	4.5 oz	110	.11	.07	1.04	.06	29.1	.1	2.1	16.64	.72	20.48	112.64	.5
creamed, strained	1 oz	24	.02	.02	.23	.01	6.4	.02	0.5	3.69	.16	4.54	24.95	.11
diced, 'Graduates' (Gerber)	3.2 oz	234	.1	.07	1.08	.05	na	na	5.8	17.5	1.1	na	88	na
'1st Foods' (Gerber)	7 tbsp	37	.08	.07	.93	.06	na	na	0.8	21	1.0	na	87	na
'2nd Foods' (Gerber)	7 tbsp	33	.07	.05	.98	.07	na	na	3.2	21	.9	na	102	na
strained	4.5 oz	723	.1	.08	1.3	.09	33.2	0	8.8	25.6	1.23	19.2	143.36	.45
strained	1 oz	160	.02	.02	.29	.02	7.3	0	2.0	5.67	.27	4.25	31.75	.1
'3rd Foods' (Gerber)	7 tbsp	35	.03	.05	1.3	.08	na	na	2.0	20	1.0	na	91	na
Potato, diced, 'Graduates' (Gerber)	3.2 oz	na	.03	.02	.61	.1	na	na	4.0	3.3	.3	na	158	na
Spinach, creamed														
junior	7.5 oz	7830	.05	.18	.55	.12	146.5	.15	7.7	240.69	2.98	134.19	470.73	.75
junior	1 oz	1042	.01	.02	.07	.02	19.5	.02	1.0	32.04	.4	17.86	62.65	.1
'2nd Foods' (Gerber)	7 tbsp	300	.03	.11	.32	.08	na	na	5.7	88	.7	na	202	na
strained	4.5 oz	5338	.02	.13	.28	.1	77.8	.08	11.1	113.92	.79	70.4	244.48	.4
strained	1 oz	1182	0	.03	.06	.02	17.2	.02	2.5	25.23	.18	15.59	54.15	.09
Squash														
buttered, junior	7.5 oz	3259	.02	.14	.67	na	4.9	na	16.2	66.03	.89	na	287.55	na
buttered, junior	1 oz	434	0	.02	.09	na	3.3	na	2.2	8.79	.12	na	38.27	na
buttered, strained	4.5 oz	2122	.01	.09	.46	na	15.1	na	9.7	42.24	.52	na	162.56	na
buttered, strained	1 oz	470	0	.02	.1	na	3.4	na	2.2	9.36	.12	na	36.0	na
'1st Foods' (Gerber)	7 tbsp	127	.03	.04	.5	.07	na	na	3.1	26	.2	na	192	na
junior	7.5 oz	4290	.02	.14	.81	.15	32.8	0	16.6	51.12	.75	25.56	394.05	.17
junior	1 oz	571	0	.02	.11	.02	4.4	0	2.2	6.8	.1	3.4	52.45	.02
'2nd Foods' (Gerber)	7 tbsp	142	.02	.04	.4	.07	na	na	4.2	28	.2	na	166	na
strained	4.5 oz	2589	.01	.07	.45	.08	19.7	0	9.9	30.72	.38	15.36	229.12	.18
strained	1 oz	574	0	.02	.1	.02	4.4	0	2.2	6.8	.09	3.4	50.75	.04
'3rd Foods' (Gerber)	7 tbsp	169	.02	.04	.38	.07	na	na	3.6	28	.2	na	167	na
Sweet potato														
buttered, junior	7.75 oz	13295	.04	.1	.65	na	29.5	na	20.5	61.6	.88	na	475.2	na
buttered, junior	1 oz	1713	0	.01	.08	na	3.8	na	2.6	7.94	.11	na	61.24	na
buttered, strained	4.75 oz	9199	.02	.05	.37	na	17.7	na	12.3	28.35	.61	na	280.8	na
buttered, strained	1 oz	1932	.01	.01	.08	na	3.7	na	2.6	5.95	.13	na	58.97	na
'1st Foods' (Gerber)	7 tbsp	854	.03	.03	.4	.1	na	na	0.7	14	.3	na	254	na
junior	7.75 oz	14599	.06	.07	.84	.25	22.7	0	21.1	35.2	.86	26.4	534.6	.24
junior	1 oz	1881	.01	.01	.11	.03	2.9	0	2.7	4.54	.11	3.4	68.89	.03
'2nd Foods' (Gerber)	7 tbsp	645	.03	.04	.38	.12	na	na	1.8	14	.3	na	236	na
strained	4.75 oz	8691	.04	.04	.48	.13	13.2	0	13.4	21.6	.5	17.55	355.05	.28
strained	1 oz	1825	.01	.01	.1	.03	2.8	0	2.8	4.54	.1	3.69	74.56	.06
'3rd Foods' (Gerber)	7 tbsp	698	.02	.04	.36	.13	na	na	1.3	14	.3	na	255	na

Food Name	Serving Size	A I.U.	Thi mg	Rib mg	Nia mg	B₆ mg	Fol mcg	B₁₂ mcg	C mg	Calc mg	Iron mg	Mag mg	Pot mg	Zn mg
BACON														
cured, breakfast strips, cooked	3 slices	0	.25	.13	2.58	.12	1.4	.6	14.8	4.76	.67	8.84	158.44	1.25
cured, broiled	4.5 oz	0	.88	.36	9.3	.34	6.4	2.22	42.5	15.24	2.04	30.48	617.22	4.14
cured, broiled	3 med slices	0	.13	.05	1.39	.05	1.0	.33	6.4	2.28	.31	4.56	92.34	.62
cured, canned	100 gm	0	.23	.1	1.5	na	na	na	0.0	15.0	.6	na	130.0	na
cured, pan-fried	4.5 oz	0	.88	.36	9.3	.34	6.4	2.22	42.5	15.24	2.04	30.48	617.22	4.14
cured, pan-fried	3 med slices	0	.13	.05	1.39	.05	1.0	.33	6.4	2.28	.31	4.56	92.34	.62
cured, roasted	4.5 oz	0	.88	.36	9.3	.34	6.4	2.22	42.5	15.24	2.04	30.48	617.22	4.14
cured, roasted	3 med slices	0	.13	.05	1.39	.05	1.0	.33	6.4	2.28	.31	4.56	92.34	.62
cured, strips, cooked	6 oz	0	1.25	.63	12.91	.58	6.8	3.01	73.8	23.8	3.35	44.2	792.2	6.26
cured, 12 slices per lb, raw	1 slice	0	.14	.04	1.05	.05	0.8	.35	8.3	2.66	.23	3.42	58.14	.44
cured, strips, 15 slices per 12 oz, raw	3 slices	0	.32	.12	2.48	.14	2.0	.67	18.5	5.44	.64	8.16	138.72	1.13
BACON, ALTERNATIVE														
VEGETARIAN														
	1 cup	127	6.34	.69	10.89	.69	59.8	0	0.0	33.12	3.47	27.36	244.8	.6
	1 oz	7	.35	.04	.6	.04	3.3	0	0.0	1.84	.19	1.52	13.6	.03
BACON, CANADIAN-STYLE														
cured, grilled	2 slices	0	.38	.09	3.22	.21	1.9	.36	10.0	4.65	.38	9.76	181.35	.79
cured, grilled, yield from 6 oz raw	4.9 oz	0	1.15	.27	9.61	.63	5.6	1.08	30.0	13.9	1.14	29.19	542.1	2.36
cured, packed 6 slices per 6 oz, unheated	2 slices	0	.43	.1	3.53	.22	2.3	.38	12.4	4.54	.39	9.64	195.05	.79
cured, unheated	6 oz	0	1.28	.29	10.59	.66	6.8	1.14	37.2	13.6	1.16	28.9	584.8	2.36
BACON BITS (Hormel)	1 oz	na	na	na	na	na	na	na	na	na	na	na	336	na
BACON PIECES (Hormel)	1 oz	na	na	na	na	na	na	na	na	na	na	na	228	na
BAGEL														
EGG	1 oz	31	.15	.07	.98	.02	6.2	.05	0.2	3.69	1.13	7.09	19.28	.22
ONION														
enriched, 3.5 inch diam	1 bagel	0	.38	.22	3.24	.04	15.6	0	0.0	12.78	2.53	20.59	71.71	.62
enriched, w/calcium proprianate, 3.5 inch diam	1 bagel	0	.38	.22	3.24	.04	15.6	0	0.0	52.54	2.53	20.59	71.71	.62
enriched, w/calcium proprianate, toasted	1 oz	0	.13	.09	1.25	.01	4.8	0	0.0	22.68	1.08	8.79	30.9	.27
unenriched, 3.5 inch diam	1 bagel	0	.12	.04	1.25	.04	15.6	0	0.0	12.78	.97	20.59	71.71	.62
unenriched, w/calcium proprianate, 3.5 inch diam	1 bagel	0	.12	.04	1.25	.04	15.6	0	0.0	52.54	.97	20.59	71.71	.62
PLAIN														
enriched, 3.5 inch diam	1 bagel	0	.38	.22	3.24	.04	15.6	0	0.0	12.78	2.53	20.59	71.71	.62
enriched, w/calcium proprianate, 3.5 inch diam	1 bagel	0	.38	.22	3.24	.04	15.6	0	0.0	52.54	2.53	20.59	71.71	.62
unenriched, 3.5 inch diam	1 bagel	0	.12	.04	1.25	.04	15.6	0	0.0	12.78	.97	20.59	71.71	.62
unenriched, w/calcium proprianate, 3.5 inch diam	1 bagel	0	.12	.04	1.25	.04	15.6	0	0.0	52.54	.97	20.59	71.71	.62
POPPY SEED														
enriched, 3.5 inch diam	1 bagel	0	.38	.22	3.24	.04	15.6	0	0.0	12.78	2.53	20.59	71.71	.62
enriched, w/calcium proprianate, 3.5 inch diam	1 bagel	0	.38	.22	3.24	.04	15.6	0	0.0	52.54	2.53	20.59	71.71	.62
enriched, w/calcium proprianate, toasted	1 oz	0	.13	.09	1.25	.01	4.8	0	0.0	22.68	1.08	8.79	30.9	.27
unenriched, 3.5 inch diam	1 bagel	0	.12	.04	1.25	.04	15.6	0	0.0	12.78	.97	20.59	71.71	.62
unenriched, w/calcium proprianate, 3.5 inch diam	1 bagel	0	.12	.04	1.25	.04	15.6	0	0.0	52.54	.97	20.59	71.71	.62
SESAME														
enriched, 3.5 inch diam	1 bagel	0	.38	.22	3.24	.04	15.6	0	0.0	12.78	2.53	20.59	71.71	.62
enriched, w/calcium proprianate, 3.5 inch diam	1 bagel	0	.38	.22	3.24	.04	15.6	0	0.0	52.54	2.53	20.59	71.71	.62
enriched, w/calcium proprianate, toasted	1 oz	0	.13	.09	1.25	.01	4.8	0	0.0	22.68	1.08	8.79	30.9	.27
unenriched, 3.5 inch diam	1 bagel	0	.12	.04	1.25	.04	15.6	0	0.0	12.78	.97	20.59	71.71	.62
unenriched, w/calcium proprianate, 3.5 inch diam	1 bagel	0	.12	.04	1.25	.04	15.6	0	0.0	52.54	.97	20.59	71.71	.62

Food Name	Serving Size	A I.U.	Thi mg	Rib mg	Nia mg	B$_6$ mg	Fol mcg	B$_{12}$ mcg	C mg	Calc mg	Iron mg	Mag mg	Pot mg	Zn mg
BAKED BEANS, CANNED. See also BEANS, CANNED.														
(Open Range)	4.656 oz	na	na	na	na	na	na	na	6.9	8.46	12.62	na	na	na
(Van Camp's)	1 cup	0	.12	.14	1.2	na	na	na	0.0	100	3.6	na	na	na
Boston, w/ham 'Homestyle' (Hunt's)	9.03 oz	na	na	na	na	na	na	na	16.3	19.49	23.13	na	na	na
brown sugar (Van Camp's)	1 cup	0	.09	.14	.86	na	na	na	0.0	121	2.7	na	535	na
'Deluxe' (Van Camp's)	1 cup	0	.3	.1	.8	na	na	na	0.0	60	3.6	na	690	na
vegetarian	1/2 cup	217	.19	.08	.54	.17	30.4	0	3.9	63.5	.37	40.64	375.92	1.78
w/beef	1/2 cup	283	.07	.06	1.25	.12	57.7	0	2.4	59.85	2.13	33.25	425.6	1.6
w/franks	1/2 cup	197	.07	.07	1.15	.06	38.4	0	2.9	61.44	2.21	35.84	300.8	2.39
w/franks, 'Beanee Weenee' (Van Camp's)	1 cup	294	.13	.17	2.0	na	na	na	na	95	4.27	na	565	na
w/pork	1/2 cup	224	.07	.05	.56	.08	45.7	0	2.5	66.78	2.14	42.84	389.34	1.84
w/pork (Van Camp's)	1 cup	164	.12	.12	.99	na	na	na	2.4	100	4.29	na	563	na
w/pork and sweet sauce	1/2 cup	144	.06	.08	.44	.11	47.1	0	3.8	76.86	2.09	42.84	335.16	1.89
w/pork and tomato sauce	1/2 cup	156	.07	.06	.63	.09	28.4	0	3.9	70.56	4.13	44.1	378.0	7.38
BAKING POWDER														
	1 tbsp	0	0	0	0	na	na	na	0.0	663.6	0	na	15.75	na
	1 tsp	0	0	0	0	na	na	na	0.0	183.28	0	na	4.35	na
commercial	3 1/2 oz	0	0	0	0	na	na	na	0.0	0	0	na	0	na
cream of tartar, w/tartaric acid	1 tbsp	0	0	0	0	na	na	na	0.0	0	0	na	361.0	na
double-acting, sodium aluminum sulfate	1 tsp	0	0	0	0	0	0.0	0	0.0	270.3	.51	1.24	.92	0
double-acting, straight phosphate	1 tsp	0	0	0	0	0	0.0	0	0.0	338.74	.52	1.79	.23	0
low-sodium	1 tsp	0	0	0	0	0	0.0	0	0.0	216.6	.41	1.45	505.0	.04
low-sodium, commercial	1 tbsp	0	0	0	0	na	na	na	0.0	650.16	0	na	1477.98	na
low-sodium, commercial	1 tsp	0	0	0	0	na	na	na	0.0	207.09	0	na	470.76	na
low-sodium, non-commercial	1 tsp	0	0	0	0	na	na	na	0.0	144.48	0	na	621.87	na
w/monohydrate	1 tbsp	0	0	0	0	na	na	na	0.0	212.52	0	na	16.5	na
w/monohydrate	1 tsp	0	0	0	0	na	na	na	0.0	57.96	0	na	4.5	na
w/straight phosphate	1 tbsp	0	0	0	0	na	na	na	0.0	784.88	0	na	21.25	na
w/straight phosphate	1 tsp	0	0	0	0	na	na	na	0.0	238.6	0	na	6.46	na
BALSAM PEAR / bitter melon														
Leafy tips														
boiled, drained	1/2 cup	503	.04	.08	.29	.22	25.4	0	16.1	12.18	.3	27.26	174.58	.09
raw	1/2 cup	416	.04	.09	.27	.19	30.7	0	21.1	20.16	.49	20.4	145.92	.07
Pods														
boiled, drained, 1/2-inch pieces	1/2 cup	70	.03	.03	.17	.03	31.7	0	20.5	5.58	.24	9.92	197.78	.48
raw	1 pear	471	.05	.05	.5	.05	89.3	0	104.2	23.56	.53	21.08	367.04	.99
raw, 1/2-Inch pieces	1 cup	353	.04	.04	.37	.04	67.0	0	78.1	17.67	.4	15.81	275.28	.74
BAMBOO SHOOTS														
boiled, drained, 1/2-inch slices	1 cup	0	.02	.06	.36	.12	2.8	0	0.0	14.4	.29	3.6	639.6	.56
canned (LaChoy)	2 tbsp	na	na	na	na	na	na	na	0.0	.01	.07	na	na	na
canned, drained solids, 1/8-inch slices	1 cup	10	.03	.03	.18	.18	4.2	0	1.4	10.48	.42	5.24	104.8	.85
raw, 1/2-inch slices	1 cup	30	.23	.11	.91	.36	10.7	0	6.0	19.63	.76	4.53	804.83	1.66
BANANA														
fresh (Dole)	1 fruit	70	na	na	na	na	na	na	11.0	na	na	na	380	na
raw, w/o skin and seeds	1 fruit	92	.05	.11	.62	.66	21.8	0	10.4	6.84	.35	33.06	451.44	.18
BANANA, RED, raw	100 gm	400	.05	.04	.6	na	na	na	10.0	10.0	.8	na	370.0	na
BANANA BERRY DRINK														
'Stompin' Banana Berry Drink' (Hi-C)	6 oz	na	na	na	na	na	na	na	60.0	na	na	na	30	na
BANANA CHIPS														
	1 oz	24	.02	0	.2	.07	4.0	0	1.8	5.1	.35	21.55	151.96	.21
premium (Mariani)	1 oz	na	na	na	na	na	na	na	na	na	na	na	415	na
BANANA NECTAR (Libby's)	6 oz	na	na	na	na	na	na	na	na	na	na	na	110	na
BANANA PINEAPPLE NECTAR (Kern's)	6 oz	na	na	na	na	na	na	na	na	na	na	na	160	na
BARBADOS CHERRY. See ACEROLA CHERRY.														
BARBADOS CHERRY JUICE. See ACEROLA CHERRY JUICE.														
BARBECUE SAUCE														
(Healthy Choice) original	1.1 oz	na	na	na	na	na	na	na	2.4	1.1	1.77	na	na	na

Food Name	Serving Size	A I.U.	Thi mg	Rib mg	Nia mg	B$_6$ mg	Fol mcg	B$_{12}$ mcg	C mg	Calc mg	Iron mg	Mag mg	Pot mg	Zn mg
(Heinz) 'Select'	1 oz	na	na	na	na	na	na	na	na	na	na	na	115	na
(Heinz) 'Thick and Rich' old fashioned	1 oz	na	na	na	na	na	na	na	na	na	na	na	95	na
(Heinz) 'Thick and Rich' original	1 oz	na	na	na	na	na	na	na	na	na	na	na	90	na
(Hunt's) 'Bold' original	1.2 oz	na	na	na	na	na	na	na	2.9	1.05	.15	na	na	na
(Hunt's) 'Light' original	1.1 oz	na	na	na	na	na	na	na	0.9	.63	1.09	na	na	na
(Hunt's) original	1.2 oz	na	na	na	na	na	na	na	2.4	1.19	1.25	na	na	na
(Open Range) original	1.2 oz	na	na	na	na	na	na	na	2.0	1.68	1.43	na	na	na
CAJUN STYLE (Heinz) 'Thick and Rich'	1 oz	na	na	na	na	na	na	na	na	na	na	na	100	na
CHUNKY (Heinz) 'Thick and Rich'	1 oz	na	na	na	na	na	na	na	na	na	na	na	100	na
COUNTRY STYLE (Hunt's)	1.2 oz	na	na	na	na	na	na	na	1.6	.75	.71	na	na	na
HAWAIIAN STYLE (Heinz) 'Thick and Rich'	1 oz	na	na	na	na	na	na	na	na	na	na	na	65	na
HICKORY														
(Healthy Choice)	1.1 oz	na	na	na	na	na	na	na	3.9	.63	.68	na	na	na
(Heinz) 'Select'	1 oz	na	na	na	na	na	na	na	na	na	na	na	105	na
(Hunt's) bold	1.2 oz	na	na	na	na	na	na	na	4.5	1.34	1.58	na	na	na
(Hunt's) 'Light'	1.1 oz	na	na	na	na	na	na	na	1.0	.75	.91	na	na	na
(Open Range)	1.2 oz	na	na	na	na	na	na	na	3.7	1.77	1.52	na	na	na
HICKORY SMOKE (Heinz) 'Thick and Rich'	1 oz	na	na	na	na	na	na	na	na	na	na	na	90	na
HOMESTYLE (Hunt's)	1.2 oz	na	na	na	na	na	na	na	1.2	.51	.64	na	na	na
HONEY MUSTARD (Hunt's)	1.2 oz	na	na	na	na	na	na	na	3.3	1.26	1.45	na	na	na
HOT														
(Healthy Choice) and spicy	1.1 oz	na	na	na	na	na	na	na	2.4	1.1	1.77	na	na	na
(Hunt's) and spicy	1.2 oz	na	na	na	na	na	na	na	3.3	1.26	1.45	na	na	na
KANSAS CITY STYLE (Hunt's)	1.2 oz	na	na	na	na	na	na	na	2.1	.68	.74	na	na	na
MESQUITE SMOKE (Heinz) 'Thick and Rich'	1 oz	na	na	na	na	na	na	na	na	na	na	na	90	na
MUSHROOM (Heinz) 'Thick and Rich'	1 oz	na	na	na	na	na	na	na	na	na	na	na	100	na
NEW ORLEANS STYLE (Hunt's)	1.2 oz	na	na	na	na	na	na	na	1.0	.64	.7	na	na	na
ONION (Heinz) 'Thick and Rich'	1 oz	na	na	na	na	na	na	na	na	na	na	na	95	na
TEXAS STYLE (Heinz) hot 'Thick and Rich'	1 oz	na	na	na	na	na	na	na	na	na	na	na	85	na
BARLEY														
	1 cup	40	1.19	.52	8.47	.59	35.0	0	0.0	60.72	6.62	244.72	831.68	5.1
pearled, cooked	1 cup	11	.13	.1	3.24	.18	25.1	0	0.0	17.27	2.09	34.54	146.01	1.29
pearled, raw	1 cup	44	.38	.23	9.21	.52	46.0	0	0.0	58.0	5.0	158.0	560.0	4.26
pearled, raw, medium 'Scotch Brand' 1.7 oz (Quaker)	1/4 cup	11	.11	.06	2.22	.13	32.0	0	0.0	11	1.24	34	130	0
pearled, raw, quick 'Scotch Brand' (Quaker)	1/3 cup	11	.11	.06	1.2	.13	32.0	0	0.0	11	1.24	34	130	0
BARRACUDA, PACIFIC, raw	100 gm	50	.04	.1	13.3	na	na	na	0.0	16.0	1.6	na	293.0	na
BASELLA. See VINE SPINACH.														
BASIL														
dried, crumbled	1 tbsp	422	.01	.01	.31	na	na	0	2.8	95.1	1.89	18.99	154.48	.26
dried, ground (Durkee)	1 tsp	2.94	.03	.06	0	na	na	na	.01	0	.01	na	0	na
dried, ground (Laurel Leaf)	1 tsp	2.94	.03	.06	0	na	na	na	.01	0	.01	na	0	na
fresh	2 tbsp	205	0	0	.05	.01	3.4	0	1.0	8.16	.17	4.29	24.49	.05
fresh	5 leaves	97	0	0	.02	0	1.6	0	0.5	3.85	.08	2.03	11.55	.02
BASS, FRESHWATER, MIXED SPECIES														
dry-heat cooked	3 oz	98	.07	.08	1.29	.12	14.5	1.96	1.8	87.55	1.62	32.3	387.6	.71
raw	3 oz	85	.06	.06	1.06	.1	12.8	1.7	1.7	68.0	1.27	25.5	302.6	.55
BASS, SEA, MIXED SPECIES														
dry heat cooked	3 oz	181	.11	.13	1.61	.39	4.9	.26	0.0	11.05	.31	45.05	278.8	.44
raw	3 oz	156	.09	.1	1.36	.34	4.3	.26	0.0	8.5	.25	34.85	217.6	.34
BASS, STRIPED														
dry-heat cooked	3 oz	88	.1	.03	2.17	.29	8.5	3.75	0.0	16.15	.92	43.35	278.8	.43
raw	3 oz	77	.09	.03	1.78	.26	7.7	3.25	0.0	12.75	.71	34.0	217.6	.34
BAY LEAF														
dried, crumbled	1 tbsp	111	0	.01	.04	na	na	0	0.8	15.02	.77	2.16	9.53	.07
dried, crumbled	1 tsp	37	0	0	.01	na	na	0	0.3	5.01	.26	.72	3.18	.02

Food Name	Serving Size	A I.U.	Thi mg	Rib mg	Nia mg	B_6 mg	Fol mcg	B_{12} mcg	C mg	Calc mg	Iron mg	Mag mg	Pot mg	Zn mg
dried, crumbled (Durkee)	1 tsp	.22	0	.02	0	na	na	na	0	0	0	na	0	na
dried, crumbled (Laurel Leaf)	1 tsp	.22	0	.02	0	na	na	na	0	0	0	na	0	na

BEAN. See individual listings.

BEAN ENTRÉE, MICROWAVE

Food Name	Serving Size	A I.U.	Thi mg	Rib mg	Nia mg	B_6 mg	Fol mcg	B_{12} mcg	C mg	Calc mg	Iron mg	Mag mg	Pot mg	Zn mg
w/wieners, microwave cup (Kid's Kitchen)	7.5 oz	na	na	na	na	na	na	na	na	na	na	na	731	na

BEAN SPROUTS, CANNED (LaChoy)

Food Name	Serving Size	A I.U.	Thi mg	Rib mg	Nia mg	B_6 mg	Fol mcg	B_{12} mcg	C mg	Calc mg	Iron mg	Mag mg	Pot mg	Zn mg
BEAN SPROUTS, CANNED (LaChoy)	2.928 oz	na	na	na	na	na	na	na	23.7	.97	1.39	na	na	na

BEANS, BAKED. See BAKED BEANS, CANNED.

BEANS, CANNED. See also BAKED BEANS, CANNED; BEAN SPROUTS, CANNED; and individual listings.

Food Name	Serving Size	A I.U.	Thi mg	Rib mg	Nia mg	B_6 mg	Fol mcg	B_{12} mcg	C mg	Calc mg	Iron mg	Mag mg	Pot mg	Zn mg
barbecue (Open Range)	4.75 oz	na	na	na	na	na	na	na	18.7	9.1	15.65	na	na	na
'Beans 'N' Fixins' (Big John's)	4.7 oz	na	na	na	na	na	na	na	4.7	7.17	14.83	na	na	na
'Mix and Serve' (Hunt's)	4.75 oz	na	na	na	na	na	na	na	3.8	7.35	10.78	na	na	na
'Pork and Beans' (Hunt's)	4.5 oz	na	na	na	na	na	na	na	2.6	4.53	4.64	na	na	na
'Pork and Beans' (Open Range)	4.6 oz	na	na	na	na	na	na	na	6.9	7.25	11.76	na	na	na
ranch (Open Ranch)	4.7 oz	na	na	na	na	na	na	na	3.0	na	10.66	na	na	na
spiced (Gebhardt)	4.5 oz	na	na	na	na	na	na	na	2.8	4.89	4.72	na	na	na
'Vegetarian Style' (Van Camp's)	1 cup	179	.13	.12	1.0	na	na	na	2.4	100	3.6	na	602	na
w/beef, 'Homestyle' (Hunt's)	9 oz	na	na	na	na	na	na	na	13.2	11.72	15.36	na	na	na
w/franks, 'Homestyle' (Hunt's)	9 oz	na	na	na	na	na	na	na	12.5	22.11	20.05	na	na	na
w/sausage, 'Homestyle' (Hunt's)	9 oz	na	na	na	na	na	na	na	9.9	12.32	20.65	na	na	na

BEAR

Food Name	Serving Size	A I.U.	Thi mg	Rib mg	Nia mg	B_6 mg	Fol mcg	B_{12} mcg	C mg	Calc mg	Iron mg	Mag mg	Pot mg	Zn mg
raw	1 lb	0	.73	3.08	14.52	na	na	na	0.0	13.61	30.16	na	na	na
raw	1 oz	0	.04	.19	.9	na	na	na	0.0	.84	1.86	na	na	na
simmered	3 oz	0	.09	.7	2.85	na	na	na	0.0	4.25	9.12	na	na	na

BEAVER

Food Name	Serving Size	A I.U.	Thi mg	Rib mg	Nia mg	B_6 mg	Fol mcg	B_{12} mcg	C mg	Calc mg	Iron mg	Mag mg	Pot mg	Zn mg
raw	1 lb	0	.27	1.0	8.62	na	na	na	9.1	68.04	31.3	113.4	1578.53	na
raw	1 oz	0	.02	.06	.53	na	na	na	0.6	4.2	1.93	7.0	97.44	na
roasted	3 oz	0	.04	.26	1.87	.37	9.4	7.06	2.6	18.7	8.5	24.65	342.55	na

BEECHNUT, DRIED, shelled

Food Name	Serving Size	A I.U.	Thi mg	Rib mg	Nia mg	B_6 mg	Fol mcg	B_{12} mcg	C mg	Calc mg	Iron mg	Mag mg	Pot mg	Zn mg
BEECHNUT, DRIED, shelled	1 oz	0	.09	.11	.25	.19	32.0	0	4.4	.28	.7	0	288.83	.1

BEEF

(NOTE: TRIMMED = Lean; separable fat removed after cooking. UNTRIMMED = Separable fat not removed.)

BRAIN

Food Name	Serving Size	A I.U.	Thi mg	Rib mg	Nia mg	B_6 mg	Fol mcg	B_{12} mcg	C mg	Calc mg	Iron mg	Mag mg	Pot mg	Zn mg
pan-fried	3 oz	0	.11	.22	3.21	.33	5.1	12.92	2.8	7.65	1.89	12.75	300.9	1.15
raw	4 oz	0	.17	.31	5.17	.29	4.5	12.32	18.8	9.04	2.42	14.69	362.73	1.38

BRISKET, FLAT HALF

Trimmed

Food Name	Serving Size	A I.U.	Thi mg	Rib mg	Nia mg	B_6 mg	Fol mcg	B_{12} mcg	C mg	Calc mg	Iron mg	Mag mg	Pot mg	Zn mg
all grades, 0-inch fat, braised	3 oz	0	.06	.19	3.28	.26	6.8	2.24	0.0	4.25	2.41	21.25	253.3	5.41
all grades, 1/4-inch fat, braised	3 oz	0	.06	.19	3.28	.26	6.8	2.24	0.0	4.25	2.41	21.25	253.3	5.41
all grades, 1/2-inch fat, braised	3 oz	0	.06	.19	3.28	.26	6.8	2.24	0.0	4.25	2.41	21.25	253.3	5.41

Untrimmed

Food Name	Serving Size	A I.U.	Thi mg	Rib mg	Nia mg	B_6 mg	Fol mcg	B_{12} mcg	C mg	Calc mg	Iron mg	Mag mg	Pot mg	Zn mg
all grades, 1/4-inch fat, braised	3 oz	0	.05	.15	2.67	.22	5.1	1.97	0.0	6.8	1.95	16.15	206.55	4.1
all grades, 1/4-inch fat, raw	4 oz	0	.1	.17	4.02	.42	6.8	2.44	0.0	6.78	1.81	20.34	307.36	3.23
all grades, 1/2-inch fat, braised	3 oz	0	.05	.15	2.63	.21	5.1	1.95	0.0	6.8	1.91	16.15	203.15	4.01
all grades, 1/2-inch fat, raw	1 lb	0	.38	.67	15.79	1.63	27.2	9.71	0.0	27.22	7.08	81.65	1202.04	12.7
all grades, 1/2-inch fat, raw	1 oz	0	.02	.04	.99	.1	1.7	.61	0.0	1.7	.44	5.1	75.13	.79

BRISKET, POINT HALF

Trimmed

Food Name	Serving Size	A I.U.	Thi mg	Rib mg	Nia mg	B_6 mg	Fol mcg	B_{12} mcg	C mg	Calc mg	Iron mg	Mag mg	Pot mg	Zn mg
all grades, 0-inch fat, braised	3 oz	0	.06	.2	3.03	.24	6.8	2.19	0.0	5.1	2.37	18.7	232.05	6.28
all grades, 1/4-inch fat, braised	3 oz	0	.06	.2	3.03	.24	6.8	2.19	0.0	5.1	2.37	18.7	232.05	6.28
all grades, 1/2-inch fat, braised	3 oz	0	.06	.19	3.03	.24	6.8	2.19	0.0	5.1	2.37	18.7	232.05	6.28

Untrimmed

Food Name	Serving Size	A I.U.	Thi mg	Rib mg	Nia mg	B_6 mg	Fol mcg	B_{12} mcg	C mg	Calc mg	Iron mg	Mag mg	Pot mg	Zn mg
all grades, 0-inch fat, braised	3 oz	0	.05	.16	2.58	.2	6.0	1.98	0.0	6.8	1.99	15.3	198.05	4.96
all grades, 1/4-inch fat, braised	3 oz	0	.05	.15	2.45	.2	5.1	1.91	0.0	7.65	1.87	14.45	187.85	4.55
all grades, 1/4-inch fat, raw	1 lb	0	.32	.59	12.88	1.5	27.2	9.57	0.0	31.75	6.99	72.58	1047.82	16.83
all grades, 1/4-inch fat, raw	1 oz	0	.02	.04	.81	.09	1.7	.6	0.0	1.98	.44	4.54	65.49	1.05
all grades, 1/2-inch fat, braised	3 oz	0	.05	.15	2.43	.2	5.1	1.9	0.0	7.65	1.85	13.6	186.15	4.51
all grades, 1/2-inch fat, raw	1 lb	0	.32	.59	12.61	1.45	27.2	9.43	0.0	31.75	6.85	68.04	1016.06	16.33
all grades, 1/2-inch fat, raw	1 oz	0	.02	.04	.79	.09	1.7	.59	0.0	1.98	.43	4.25	63.5	1.02

Food Name	Serving Size	A I.U.	Thi mg	Rib mg	Nia mg	B$_6$ mg	Fol mcg	B$_{12}$ mcg	C mg	Calc mg	Iron mg	Mag mg	Pot mg	Zn mg
BRISKET, WHOLE														
Trimmed														
all grades, 0-inch fat, braised	3 oz	0	.06	.19	3.15	.25	6.8	2.21	0.0	5.1	2.39	19.55	242.25	5.86
all grades, 1/4-inch fat, braised	3 oz	0	.06	.19	3.15	.25	6.8	2.21	0.0	5.1	2.39	19.55	242.25	5.86
all grades, 1/2-inch fat, braised	3 oz	0	.06	.19	3.19	.26	6.8	2.17	0.0	5.1	2.35	19.55	243.95	5.85
Untrimmed														
all grades, 0-inch fat, braised	3 oz	0	.06	.17	2.86	.23	6.0	2.08	0.0	5.95	2.15	17.85	220.15	5.07
all grades, 1/4-inch fat, braised	3 oz	0	.05	.15	2.55	.2	5.1	1.94	0.0	6.8	1.9	15.3	196.35	4.33
all grades, 1/4-inch fat, raw	1 lb	0	.36	.64	14.42	1.59	27.2	9.66	0.0	31.75	7.12	77.11	1134.0	15.01
all grades, 1/4-inch fat, raw	1 oz	0	.02	.04	.9	.1	1.7	.6	0.0	1.98	.45	4.82	70.88	.94
all grades, 1/2-inch fat, braised	3 oz	0	.05	.15	2.55	.21	5.1	1.9	0.0	7.65	1.86	15.3	194.65	4.26
all grades, 1/2-inch fat, raw	1 lb	0	.35	.63	14.17	1.54	27.2	9.43	0.0	31.75	7.12	77.11	1097.71	14.61
all grades, 1/2-inch fat, raw	1 oz	0	.02	.04	.89	.1	1.7	.59	0.0	1.98	.45	4.82	68.61	.91
CHUCK, ARM POT ROAST														
Trimmed														
all grades, 0-inch fat, braised	3 oz	0	.07	.25	3.16	.28	9.4	2.89	0.0	7.65	3.22	20.4	245.65	7.36
all grades, 1/4-inch fat, braised	3 oz	0	.07	.25	3.16	.28	9.4	2.89	0.0	7.65	3.22	20.4	245.65	7.36
all grades, 1/2-inch fat, braised	3 oz	0	.07	.25	3.16	.28	9.4	2.89	0.0	7.65	3.22	20.4	245.65	7.36
choice, 0-inch fat, braised	3 oz	0	.07	.25	3.16	.28	9.4	2.89	0.0	7.65	3.22	20.4	245.65	7.36
choice, 1/4-inch fat, braised	3 oz	0	.07	.25	3.16	.28	9.4	2.89	0.0	7.65	3.22	20.4	245.65	7.36
choice, 1/2-inch fat, braised	3 oz	0	.07	.25	3.16	.28	9.4	2.89	0.0	7.65	3.22	20.4	245.65	7.36
prime, 1/2-inch fat, braised	3 oz	0	.07	.25	3.16	.28	9.4	2.89	0.0	7.65	3.22	20.4	245.65	7.36
prime, 1/2-inch fat, raw	1 lb	0	.58	.93	16.91	2.0	36.3	15.79	0.0	27.22	11.2	108.86	1687.39	22.0
prime, 1/2-inch fat, raw	1 oz	0	.04	.06	1.06	.12	2.3	.99	0.0	1.7	.7	6.8	105.46	1.37
select, 0-inch fat, braised	3 oz	0	.07	.25	3.16	.28	9.4	2.89	0.0	7.65	3.22	20.4	245.65	7.36
select, 1/4-inch fat, braised	3 oz	0	.07	.25	3.16	.28	9.4	2.89	0.0	7.65	3.22	20.4	245.65	7.36
select, 1/2-inch fat, braised	3 oz	0	.07	.25	3.16	.28	9.4	2.89	0.0	7.65	3.22	20.4	245.65	7.36
Untrimmed														
all grades, 0-inch fat, braised	3 oz	0	.06	.22	2.88	.26	8.5	2.66	0.0	8.5	2.87	17.85	223.55	6.43
all grades, 1/4-inch fat, braised	3 oz	0	.06	.2	2.7	.24	7.7	2.51	0.0	8.5	2.64	16.15	209.1	5.81
all grades, 1/4-inch fat, raw	1 lb	0	.5	.82	14.7	1.72	31.8	13.88	0.0	31.75	9.57	90.72	1397.09	18.33
all grades, 1/4-inch fat, raw	1 oz	0	.03	.05	.92	.11	2.0	.87	0.0	1.98	.6	5.67	87.32	1.15
all grades, 1/2-inch fat, braised	3 oz	0	.06	.2	2.67	.24	7.7	2.49	0.0	8.5	2.61	16.15	207.4	5.73
all grades, 1/2-inch fat, raw	1 lb	0	.49	.79	14.55	1.72	31.8	13.74	0.0	31.75	9.43	86.18	1374.41	18.05
all grades, 1/2-inch fat, raw	1 oz	0	.03	.05	.91	.11	2.0	.86	0.0	1.98	.59	5.39	85.9	1.13
choice, 0-inch fat, braised	3 oz	0	.06	.22	2.86	.26	8.5	2.65	0.0	8.5	2.85	17.85	222.7	6.38
choice, 1/4-inch fat, braised	3 oz	0	.06	.2	2.66	.24	7.7	2.48	0.0	8.5	2.59	16.15	206.55	5.69
choice, 1/4-inch fat, raw	1 lb	0	.5	.82	14.61	1.72	31.8	13.79	0.0	31.75	9.48	86.18	1383.48	18.14
choice, 1/4-inch fat, raw	1 oz	0	.03	.05	.91	.11	2.0	.86	0.0	1.98	.59	5.39	86.47	1.13
choice, 1/2-inch fat, braised	3 oz	0	.06	.2	2.66	.24	7.7	2.48	0.0	8.5	2.59	16.15	206.55	5.69
choice, 1/2-inch fat, raw	1 lb	0	.49	.79	14.47	1.68	31.8	13.65	0.0	31.75	9.39	86.18	1360.8	17.92
choice, 1/2-inch fat, raw	1 oz	0	.03	.05	.9	.1	2.0	.85	0.0	1.98	.59	5.39	85.05	1.12
prime, 1/2-inch fat, braised	3 oz	0	.06	.19	2.59	.23	7.7	2.42	0.0	8.5	2.5	16.15	201.45	5.46
prime, 1/2-inch fat, raw	1 lb	0	.47	.77	14.09	1.63	31.8	13.34	0.0	31.75	9.12	81.65	1310.9	17.28
prime, 1/2-inch fat, raw	1 oz	0	.03	.05	.88	.1	2.0	.83	0.0	1.98	.57	5.1	81.93	1.08
select, 0-inch fat, braised	3 oz	0	.06	.22	2.92	.26	8.5	2.69	0.0	8.5	2.92	18.7	226.95	6.56
select, 1/4-inch fat, braised	3 oz	0	.06	.2	2.74	.25	7.7	2.54	0.0	8.5	2.69	17.0	212.5	5.94
select, 1/4-inch fat, raw	1 lb	0	.5	.82	14.83	1.77	31.8	13.97	0.0	31.75	9.66	90.72	1410.7	18.51
select, 1/4-inch fat, raw	1 oz	0	.03	.05	.93	.11	2.0	.87	0.0	1.98	.6	5.67	88.17	1.16
select, 1/2-inch fat, braised	3 oz	0	.00	.2	2.7	.24	7.7	2.51	0.0	8.5	2.63	17.0	209.1	5.81
select, 1/2-inch fat, raw	1 lb	0	.5	.81	14.84	1.72	31.8	14.02	0.0	31.75	9.00	90.72	1410.7	18.55
select, 1/2-inch fat, raw	1 oz	0	.03	.05	.93	.11	2.0	.88	0.0	1.98	.6	5.67	88.17	1.16
CHUCK, BLADE ROAST														
Trimmed														
all grades, 0-inch fat, braised	3 oz	0	.07	.24	2.27	.25	5.1	2.1	0.0	11.05	3.13	19.55	223.55	8.73
all grades, 1/4-inch fat, braised	3 oz	0	.07	.24	2.27	.25	5.1	2.1	0.0	11.05	3.13	19.55	223.55	8.73
all grades, 1/2-inch fat, braised	3 oz	0	.07	.24	2.27	.25	5.1	2.1	0.0	11.05	3.13	19.55	223.55	8.73

Food Name	Serving Size	A I.U.	Thi mg	Rib mg	Nia mg	B6 mg	Fol mcg	B12 mcg	C mg	Calc mg	Iron mg	Mag mg	Pot mg	Zn mg
choice, 0-inch fat, braised	3 oz	0	.07	.24	2.27	.25	5.1	2.1	0.0	11.05	3.13	19.55	223.55	8.73
choice, 1/4-inch fat, braised	3 oz	0	.07	.24	2.27	.25	5.1	2.1	0.0	11.05	3.13	19.55	223.55	8.73
choice, 1/2-inch fat, braised	3 oz	0	.07	.24	2.27	.25	5.1	2.1	0.0	11.05	3.13	19.55	223.55	8.73
prime, 1/2-inch fat, braised	3 oz	0	.07	.24	2.27	.25	5.1	2.1	0.0	11.05	3.13	19.55	223.55	8.73
prime, 1/2-inch fat, raw	1 lb	0	.49	.86	10.7	1.81	27.2	17.46	0.0	45.36	10.61	90.72	1446.98	26.81
prime, 1/2-inch fat, raw	1 oz	0	.03	.05	.67	.11	1.7	1.09	0.0	2.84	.66	5.67	90.44	1.68
select, 0-inch fat, braised	3 oz	0	.07	.24	2.27	.25	5.1	2.1	0.0	11.05	3.13	19.55	223.55	8.73
select, 1/4-inch fat, braised	3 oz	0	.07	.24	2.27	.25	5.1	2.1	0.0	11.05	3.13	19.55	223.55	8.73
select, 1/2-inch fat, braised	3 oz	0	.07	.24	2.27	.25	5.1	2.1	0.0	11.05	3.13	19.55	223.55	8.73
Untrimmed														
all grades, 0-inch fat, braised	3 oz	0	.06	.21	2.08	.22	4.3	1.96	0.0	11.05	2.7	17.0	200.6	7.29
all grades, 1/4-inch fat, braised	3 oz	0	.06	.2	2.06	.22	4.3	1.94	0.0	11.05	2.63	16.15	196.35	7.07
all grades, 1/4-inch fat, raw	1 lb	0	.41	.77	9.84	1.59	22.7	15.29	0.0	45.36	9.16	77.11	1215.65	22.36
all grades, 1/4-inch fat, raw	1 oz	0	.03	.05	.62	.1	1.4	.96	0.0	2.84	.57	4.82	75.98	1.4
all grades, 1/2-inch fat, braised	3 oz	0	.06	.2	2.01	.21	4.3	1.9	0.0	11.05	2.52	15.3	189.55	6.66
all grades, 1/2-inch fat, raw	1 lb	0	.42	.73	9.69	1.59	22.7	14.92	0.0	45.36	8.89	72.58	1174.82	21.59
all grades, 1/2-inch fat, raw	1 oz	0	.03	.05	.61	.1	1.4	.93	0.0	2.84	.56	4.54	73.43	1.35
choice, 0-inch fat, braised	3 oz	0	.06	.21	2.07	.22	4.3	1.95	0.0	11.05	2.69	17.0	198.9	7.23
choice, 1/4-inch fat, braised	3 oz	0	.06	.2	2.04	.21	4.3	1.93	0.0	11.05	2.59	16.15	193.8	6.92
choice, 1/4-inch fat, raw	1 lb	0	.41	.73	9.75	1.59	22.7	15.06	0.0	45.36	9.03	72.58	1192.97	21.91
choice, 1/4-inch fat, raw	1 oz	0	.03	.05	.61	.1	1.4	.94	0.0	2.84	.56	4.54	74.56	1.37
choice, 1/2-inch fat, braised	3 oz	0	.06	.19	2.0	.21	4.3	1.9	0.0	11.05	2.51	15.3	189.55	6.62
choice, 1/2-inch fat, raw	1 lb	0	.41	.73	9.66	1.54	22.7	14.83	0.0	45.36	8.85	72.58	1165.75	21.41
choice, 1/2-inch fat, raw	1 oz	0	.03	.05	.6	.1	1.4	.93	0.0	2.84	.55	4.54	72.86	1.34
prime, 1/2-inch fat, braised	3 oz	0	.06	.2	2.01	.21	4.3	1.9	0.0	11.05	2.52	15.3	189.55	6.67
prime, 1/2-inch fat, raw	1 lb	0	.41	.72	9.57	1.54	22.7	14.61	0.0	45.36	8.71	72.58	1143.07	20.96
prime, 1/2-inch fat, raw	1 oz	0	.03	.04	.6	.1	1.4	.91	0.0	2.84	.54	4.54	71.44	1.31
select, 0-inch fat, braised	3 oz	0	.06	.21	2.11	.22	4.3	1.98	0.0	11.05	2.75	17.0	203.15	7.45
select, 1/4-inch fat, braised	3 oz	0	.06	.21	2.07	.22	4.3	1.95	0.0	11.05	2.69	17.0	198.0	7.20
select, 1/4-inch fat, raw	1 lb	0	.45	.77	0.00	1.03	22.7	15.51	0.0	45.36	9.3	77.11	1238.33	22.82
select, 1/4-inch fat, raw	1 oz	0	.03	.05	.62	.1	1.4	.97	0.0	2.84	.58	4.82	77.4	1.43
select, 1/2-inch fat, braised	3 oz	0	.06	.2	2.02	.21	4.3	1.91	0.0	11.05	2.55	15.3	191.25	6.77
select, 1/2-inch fat, raw	1 lb	0	.43	.75	9.82	1.59	22.7	15.2	0.0	45.36	9.12	77.11	1206.58	22.23
select, 1/2-inch fat, raw	1 oz	0	.03	.05	.61	.1	1.4	.95	0.0	2.84	.57	4.82	75.41	1.39
FLANK														
Trimmed														
choice, 0-inch fat, braised	3 oz	0	.12	.16	3.91	.31	7.7	2.9	0.0	5.1	2.95	20.4	298.35	5.14
choice, 0-inch fat, broiled	3 oz	0	.09	.16	4.28	.29	6.8	2.76	0.0	5.95	2.18	20.4	351.9	4.08
Untrimmed														
choice, 0-inch fat, braised	3 oz	0	.12	.15	3.76	.3	7.7	2.81	0.0	5.1	2.83	19.55	286.45	4.9
choice, 0-inch fat, broiled	3 oz	0	.09	.15	4.17	.29	6.8	2.71	0.0	5.95	2.13	19.55	341.7	3.96
choice, 0-inch fat, raw	1 oz	0	.03	.04	1.29	.12	2.0	.84	0.0	1.42	.56	5.67	99.23	.98
choice, 0-inch fat, raw	4 oz	0	.12	.17	5.14	.47	7.9	3.36	0.0	5.65	2.23	22.6	395.5	3.92
HEART														
raw	4 oz	0	.21	1.15	10.69	.49	2.3	15.44	7.1	2.26	5.21	25.99	300.58	2.69
simmered	3 oz	0	.12	1.31	3.46	.18	1.7	12.16	1.3	5.1	6.38	21.25	198.05	2.66
KIDNEY														
raw	4 oz	994	.43	2.88	8.98	.58	90.4	30.53	10.1	6.78	8.32	19.21	290.41	2.09
simmered	3 oz	1055	.16	3.45	5.12	.44	83.3	43.6	0.7	14.45	6.21	15.3	152.15	3.59
LIVER														
braised	3 oz	30327	.17	3.49	9.11	.77	184.5	60.35	19.6	5.95	5.75	17.0	199.75	5.16
pan-fried	3 oz	30689	.18	3.52	12.27	1.22	187.0	95.03	19.6	9.35	5.34	19.55	309.4	4.63
raw	4 oz	39941	.29	3.14	14.44	1.06	280.2	78.18	24.9	6.78	7.71	21.47	364.99	4.43
LUNG														
braised	3 oz	33	.03	.12	2.12	.02	6.8	2.2	27.8	9.35	4.59	8.5	147.05	1.39
raw	4 oz	52	.05	.26	4.52	.05	12.4	4.31	43.5	11.3	8.98	15.82	384.2	1.82

Food Name	Serving Size	A I.U.	Thi mg	Rib mg	Nia mg	B₆ mg	Fol mcg	B₁₂ mcg	C mg	Calc mg	Iron mg	Mag mg	Pot mg	Zn mg
PANCREAS														
braised	3 oz	0	.15	.41	3.37	.15	2.6	14.11	17.3	13.6	2.22	17.85	209.1	3.91
raw	4 oz	0	.16	.5	5.03	.23	3.4	15.82	15.5	10.17	2.51	20.34	311.88	2.92
PORTERHOUSE														
Trimmed														
choice, 1/4-inch fat, broiled	3 oz	0	.09	.21	3.94	.34	6.8	1.93	0.0	5.95	2.55	24.65	345.95	4.59
choice, 1/2-inch fat, broiled	3 oz	0	.09	.21	3.94	.34	6.8	1.93	0.0	5.95	2.55	24.65	345.95	4.59
Untrimmed														
choice, 1/4-inch fat, broiled	3 oz	0	.09	.19	3.44	.3	6.0	1.83	0.0	6.8	2.24	21.25	299.2	3.94
choice, 1/4-inch fat, raw	1 lb	0	.45	.77	15.56	1.63	27.2	12.02	0.0	27.22	7.98	86.18	1338.12	13.93
choice, 1/4-inch fat, raw	1 oz	0	.03	.05	.97	.1	1.7	.75	0.0	1.7	.5	5.39	83.63	.87
choice, 1/2-inch fat, broiled	3 oz	0	.08	.19	3.48	.3	6.0	1.84	0.0	6.8	2.26	21.25	302.6	3.99
choice, 1/2-inch fat, raw	1 lb	0	.44	.74	15.26	1.63	27.2	11.84	0.0	27.22	7.85	81.65	1306.37	13.65
choice, 1/2-inch fat, raw	1 oz	0	.03	.05	.95	.1	1.7	.74	0.0	1.7	.49	5.1	81.65	.85
RIB, LARGE END														
Trimmed														
all grades, ribs 6-9, 0-inch fat, roasted	3 oz	0	.08	.19	3.78	.22	7.7	2.22	0.0	6.8	2.4	21.25	303.45	6.34
all grades, ribs 6-9, 1/4-inch fat, broiled	3 oz	0	.07	.16	2.7	.22	6.0	2.81	0.0	7.65	2.18	19.55	316.2	5.34
all grades, ribs 6-9, 1/4-inch fat, roasted	3 oz	0	.08	.19	3.78	.22	7.7	2.22	0.0	6.8	2.4	21.25	303.45	6.34
all grades, ribs 6-9, 1/2-inch fat, broiled	3 oz	0	.07	.17	2.61	.27	6.0	2.77	0.0	6.8	2.11	20.4	313.65	5.31
all grades, ribs 6-9, 1/2-inch fat, roasted	3 oz	0	.07	.19	3.78	.22	7.7	2.22	0.0	6.8	2.4	21.25	303.45	6.34
choice, ribs 6-9, 0-inch fat, roasted	3 oz	0	.08	.19	3.78	.22	7.7	2.22	0.0	6.8	2.4	21.25	303.45	6.34
choice, ribs 6-9, 1/4-inch fat, broiled	3 oz	0	.07	.16	2.7	.22	6.0	2.81	0.0	7.65	2.18	19.55	316.2	5.34
choice, ribs 6-9, 1/4-inch fat, roasted	3 oz	0	.08	.19	3.78	.22	7.7	2.22	0.0	6.8	2.4	21.25	303.45	6.34
choice, ribs 6-9, 1/2-inch fat, broiled	3 oz	0	.07	.17	2.61	.27	6.0	2.77	0.0	6.8	2.11	20.4	313.65	5.31
choice, ribs 6-9, 1/2-inch fat, roasted	3 oz	0	.07	.19	3.78	.22	7.7	2.22	0.0	6.8	2.4	21.25	303.45	6.34
prime, ribs 6-9, 1/4-inch fat, broiled	3 oz	0	.08	.17	2.61	.27	6.0	2.77	0.0	6.8	2.11	20.4	313.65	5.31
prime, ribs 6-9, 1/4-inch fat, roasted	3 oz	0	.08	.19	3.78	.22	7.7	2.22	0.0	6.8	2.4	21.25	303.45	6.34
prime, ribs 6-9, 1/2-inch fat, broiled	3 oz	0	.07	.17	2.61	.27	6.0	2.77	0.0	6.8	2.11	20.4	31.45	5.31
prime, ribs 6-9, 1/2-inch fat, roasted	3 oz	0	.07	.19	3.78	.22	7.7	2.22	0.0	6.8	2.4	21.25	303.45	6.34
select, ribs 6-9, 0-inch fat, roasted	3 oz	0	.08	.19	3.78	.22	7.7	2.22	0.0	6.8	2.4	21.25	303.45	6.34
select, ribs 6-9, 1/4-inch fat, broiled	3 oz	0	.07	.16	2.7	.22	6.0	2.81	0.0	7.65	2.18	19.55	316.2	5.34
select, ribs 6-9, 1/4-inch fat, roasted	3 oz	0	.08	.19	3.78	.22	7.7	2.22	0.0	6.8	2.4	21.25	303.45	6.34
select, ribs 6-9, 1/2-inch fat, broiled	3 oz	0	.07	.17	2.61	.27	6.0	2.77	0.0	6.8	2.11	20.4	313.65	5.31
select, ribs 6-9, 1/2-inch fat, roasted	3 oz	0	.07	.19	3.78	.22	7.7	2.22	0.0	6.8	2.4	21.25	303.45	6.34
Untrimmed														
all grades, ribs 6-9, 0-inch fat, roasted	3 oz	0	.06	.16	3.15	.2	6.0	2.0	0.0	8.5	2.01	17.0	250.75	5.0
all grades, ribs 6-9, 1/4-inch fat, broiled	3 oz	0	.06	.14	2.33	.2	5.1	2.43	0.0	8.5	1.84	15.3	257.55	4.22
all grades, ribs 6-9, 1/4-inch fat, raw	1 lb	0	.36	.59	11.7	1.32	22.7	12.16	0.0	36.29	7.67	68.04	1161.22	16.74
all grades, ribs 6-9, 1/4-inch fat, raw	1 oz	0	.02	.04	.73	.08	1.4	.76	0.0	2.27	.48	4.25	72.58	1.05
all grades, ribs 6-9, 1/4-inch fat, roasted	3 oz	0	.06	.15	3.07	.2	6.0	1.97	0.0	8.5	1.96	16.15	244.8	4.84
all grades, ribs 6-9, 1/2-inch fat, broiled	3 oz	0	.06	.14	2.19	.22	5.1	2.32	0.0	8.5	1.72	15.3	244.8	3.98
all grades, ribs 6-9, 1/2-inch fat, raw	1 lb	0	.34	.58	11.35	1.27	22.7	11.79	0.0	36.29	7.35	68.04	1102.25	15.92
all grades, ribs 6-9, 1/2-inch fat, raw	1 oz	0	.02	.04	.71	.08	1.4	.74	0.0	2.27	.46	4.25	68.89	1.0
all grades, ribs 6-9, 1/2-inch fat, roasted	3 oz	0	.06	.16	3.08	.19	6.0	1.98	0.0	8.5	1.97	16.15	245.65	4.87
choice, ribs 6-9, 0-inch fat, roasted	3 oz	0	.06	.16	3.09	.2	6.0	1.98	0.0	8.5	1.98	17.0	246.5	4.9
choice, ribs 6-9, 1/4-inch fat, broiled	3 oz	0	.06	.14	2.3	.2	5.1	2.4	0.0	8.5	1.81	15.3	253.3	4.14
choice, ribs 6-9, 1/4-inch fat, raw	1 lb	0	.36	.59	11.48	1.27	22.7	11.93	0.0	36.29	7.48	68.04	1120.39	16.19
choice, ribs 6-9, 1/4-inch fat, raw	1 oz	0	.02	.04	.72	.08	1.4	.75	0.0	2.27	.47	4.25	70.02	1.01
choice, ribs 6-9, 1/4-inch fat, roasted	3 oz	0	.06	.15	3.02	.19	6.0	1.95	0.0	8.5	1.93	16.15	240.55	4.74
choice, ribs 6-9, 1/2-inch fat, broiled	3 oz	0	.06	.14	2.19	.22	5.1	2.31	0.0	8.5	1.71	15.3	243.95	3.95
choice, ribs 6-9, 1/2-inch fat, raw	1 lb	0	.34	.58	11.3	1.27	22.7	11.7	0.0	36.29	7.3	68.04	1093.18	15.79
choice, ribs 6-9, 1/2-inch fat, raw	1 oz	0	.02	.04	.71	.08	1.4	.73	0.0	2.27	.46	4.25	68.32	.99
choice, ribs 6-9, 1/2-inch fat, roasted	3 oz	0	.06	.16	3.07	.19	6.0	1.98	0.0	8.5	1.96	16.15	244.8	4.86
prime, ribs 6-9, 1/4-inch fat, broiled	3 oz	0	.06	.14	2.21	.22	5.1	2.34	0.0	8.5	1.73	15.3	247.35	4.04
prime, ribs 6-9, 1/4-inch fat, raw	1 lb	0	.36	.59	11.34	1.27	22.7	11.75	0.0	36.29	7.35	68.04	1097.71	15.88
prime, ribs 6-9, 1/4-inch fat, raw	1 oz	0	.02	.04	.71	.08	1.4	.73	0.0	2.27	.46	4.25	68.61	.99

Food Name	Serving Size	A I.U.	Thi mg	Rib mg	Nia mg	B_6 mg	Fol mcg	B_{12} mcg	C mg	Calc mg	Iron mg	Mag mg	Pot mg	Zn mg
prime, ribs 6-9, 1/4-inch fat, roasted	3 oz	0	.06	.15	3.04	.19	6.0	1.96	0.0	8.5	1.95	16.15	243.1	4.79
prime, ribs 6-9, 1/2-inch fat, broiled	3 oz	0	.06	.14	2.17	.22	5.1	2.3	0.0	8.5	1.69	15.3	241.4	3.91
prime, ribs 6-9, 1/2-inch fat, raw	1 lb	0	.34	.58	11.23	1.27	22.7	11.66	0.0	36.29	7.26	63.5	1084.1	15.65
prime, ribs 6-9, 1/2-inch fat, raw	1 oz	0	.02	.04	.7	.08	1.4	.73	0.0	2.27	.45	3.97	67.76	.98
prime, ribs 6-9, 1/2-inch fat, roasted	3 oz	0	.06	.15	3.01	.19	6.0	1.95	0.0	8.5	1.93	16.15	239.7	4.73
select, ribs 6-9, 0-inch fat, roasted	3 oz	0	.06	.16	3.19	.2	6.8	2.01	0.0	7.65	2.04	17.0	255.0	5.11
select, ribs 6-9, 1/4-inch fat, broiled	3 oz	0	.06	.14	2.36	.2	5.1	2.46	0.0	8.5	1.86	16.15	261.8	4.3
select, ribs 6-9, 1/4-inch fat, raw	1 lb	0	.36	.59	11.84	1.32	22.7	12.34	0.0	36.29	7.8	72.58	1183.9	17.1
select, ribs 6-9, 1/4-inch fat, raw	1 oz	0	.02	.04	.74	.08	1.4	.77	0.0	2.27	.49	4.54	73.99	1.07
select, ribs 6-9, 1/4-inch fat, roasted	3 oz	0	.06	.16	3.15	.2	6.0	2.0	0.0	8.5	2.01	17.0	250.75	5.0
select, ribs 6-9, 1/2-inch fat, broiled	3 oz	0	.06	.14	2.22	.23	5.1	2.35	0.0	8.5	1.74	16.15	249.9	4.08
select, ribs 6-9, 1/2-inch fat, raw	1 lb	0	.34	.59	11.56	1.27	22.7	11.98	0.0	36.29	7.53	68.04	1138.54	16.37
select, ribs 6-9, 1/2-inch fat, raw	1 oz	0	.02	.04	.72	.08	1.4	.75	0.0	2.27	.47	4.25	71.16	1.02
select, ribs 6-9, 1/2-inch fat, roasted	3 oz	0	.06	.16	3.09	.19	6.0	1.98	0.0	8.5	1.98	16.15	246.5	4.9
RIB, SHORTRIB														
Trimmed, choice, braised	3 oz	0	.06	.17	2.73	.24	6.0	2.94	0.0	9.35	2.86	18.7	266.05	6.63
Untrimmed														
choice, braised	3 oz	0	.04	.13	2.08	.19	4.3	2.23	0.0	10.2	1.96	12.75	190.4	4.15
choice, raw	1 lb	0	.32	.54	11.59	1.36	22.7	11.61	0.0	40.82	7.03	63.5	1052.35	14.33
choice, raw	1 oz	0	.02	.03	.72	.09	1.4	.73	0.0	2.55	.44	3.97	65.77	.9
RIB, SMALL END														
Trimmed														
all grades, ribs 10-12, 0-inch fat, broiled	3 oz	0	.09	.19	4.08	.34	6.8	2.82	0.0	11.05	2.18	22.95	334.9	5.94
all grades, ribs 10-12, 1/4-inch fat, roasted	3 oz	0	.06	.16	3.18	.24	6.8	2.83	0.0	10.2	2.47	21.25	338.3	5.28
all grades, ribs 10-12, 1/2-inch fat, broiled	3 oz	0	.09	.18	4.08	.34	6.8	2.82	0.0	11.05	2.18	22.95	334.9	5.94
all grades, ribs 10-12, 1/2-inch fat, roasted	3 oz	0	.07	.17	3.09	.31	6.8	2.86	0.0	11.05	1.95	21.25	343.4	5.26
all grades, ribs 10-12, 1/4-inch fat, broiled	3 oz	0	.09	.19	4.08	.34	6.8	2.82	0.0	11.05	2.18	22.95	334.9	5.94
choice, ribs 10-12, 0-inch fat, broiled	3 oz	0	.09	.19	4.08	.34	6.8	2.82	0.0	11.05	2.18	22.95	334.9	5.94
choice, ribs 10-12, 1/4-inch fat, broiled	3 oz	0	.09	.19	4.08	.34	6.8	2.82	0.0	11.05	2.18	22.95	334.0	5.94
choice, ribs 10-12, 1/4-inch fat, roasted	3 oz	0	.06	.16	3.18	.24	0.8	2.83	0.0	10.2	2.47	21.25	338.3	5.28
choice, ribs 10-12, 1/2-inch fat, broiled	3 oz	0	.09	.18	4.08	.34	6.8	2.82	0.0	11.05	2.18	22.95	334.9	5.94
choice, ribs 10-12, 1/2-inch fat, roasted	3 oz	0	.07	.17	3.09	.31	6.8	2.86	0.0	11.05	1.95	21.25	343.4	5.26
prime, ribs 10-12, 1/4-inch fat, broiled	3 oz	0	.09	.19	4.08	.34	6.8	2.82	0.0	11.05	2.18	22.95	334.9	5.94
prime, ribs 10-12, 1/4-inch fat, roasted	3 oz	0	.07	.16	3.09	.31	6.8	2.86	0.0	11.05	1.95	21.25	343.4	5.26
prime, ribs 10-12, 1/2-inch fat, broiled	3 oz	0	.09	.18	4.08	.34	6.8	2.82	0.0	11.05	2.18	22.95	334.9	5.94
prime, ribs 10-12, 1/2-inch fat, roasted	3 oz	0	.07	.17	3.09	.31	6.8	2.86	0.0	11.05	1.95	21.25	343.4	5.26
select, ribs 10-12, 0-inch fat, broiled	3 oz	0	.09	.19	4.08	.34	6.8	2.82	0.0	11.05	2.18	22.95	334.9	5.94
select, ribs 10-12, 1/4-inch fat, broiled	3 oz	0	.09	.19	4.08	.34	6.8	2.82	0.0	11.05	2.18	22.95	334.9	5.94
select, ribs 10-12, 1/4-inch fat, roasted	3 oz	0	.06	.16	3.18	.24	6.8	2.83	0.0	10.2	2.47	21.25	338.3	5.28
select, ribs 10-12, 1/2-inch fat, broiled	3 oz	0	.09	.18	4.08	.34	6.8	2.82	0.0	11.05	2.18	22.95	334.9	5.94
select, ribs 10-12, 1/2-inch fat, roasted	3 oz	0	.07	.17	3.09	.31	6.8	2.86	0.0	11.05	1.95	21.25	343.4	5.26
Untrimmed														
all grades, ribs 10-12, 0-inch fat, broiled	3 oz	0	.08	.16	3.59	.3	6.0	2.56	0.0	11.05	1.95	19.55	292.4	5.08
all grades, ribs 10-12, 1/4-inch fat, broiled	3 oz	0	.08	.15	3.39	.28	6.0	2.46	0.0	11.05	1.86	18.7	276.25	4.75
all grades, ribs 10-12, 1/4-inch fat, raw	1 lb	0	.36	.59	14.02	1.59	22.7	13.52	0.0	45.36	8.07	77.11	1301.83	16.51
all grades, ribs 10-12, 1/4-inch fat, raw	1 oz	0	.02	.04	.88	.1	1.4	.84	0.0	2.84	.5	4.82	81.36	1.03
all grades, ribs 10-12, 1/4-inch fat, roasted	3 oz	0	.05	.14	2.66	.2	5.1	2.42	0.0	11.05	2.03	17.0	272.0	4.14
all grades, ribs 10-12, 1/2-inch fat, broiled	3 oz	0	.07	.16	3.45	.29	6.0	2.49	0.0	11.05	1.89	18.7	281.35	4.84
all grades, ribs 10-12, 1/2-inch fat, raw	1 lb	0	.36	.57	13.97	1.59	22.7	13.47	0.0	45.36	8.03	77.11	1292.76	16.42
all grades, ribs 10-12, 1/2-inch fat, raw	1 oz	0	.02	.04	.87	.1	1.4	.84	0.0	2.84	.5	4.82	80.8	1.03
all grades, ribs 10-12, 1/2-inch fat, roasted	3 oz	0	.06	.14	2.59	.26	6.0	2.45	0.0	11.05	1.66	17.0	276.25	4.13
choice, ribs 10-12, 0-inch fat, broiled	3 oz	0	.08	.16	3.55	.3	6.0	2.55	0.0	11.05	1.94	19.55	290.7	5.04
choice, ribs 10-12, 1/4-inch fat, broiled	3 oz	0	.08	.15	3.37	.28	6.0	2.45	0.0	11.05	1.85	18.7	273.7	4.71
choice, ribs 10-12, 1/4-inch fat, raw	1 lb	0	.36	.54	13.83	1.54	22.7	13.34	0.0	45.36	7.94	72.58	1274.62	16.15
choice, ribs 10-12, 1/4-inch fat, raw	1 oz	0	.02	.03	.86	.1	1.4	.83	0.0	2.84	.5	4.54	79.66	1.01
choice, ribs 10-12, 1/4-inch fat, roasted	3 oz	0	.05	.14	2.63	.2	5.1	2.4	0.0	11.05	2.0	16.15	266.9	4.05
choice, ribs 10-12, 1/2-inch fat, broiled	3 oz	0	.07	.16	3.43	.29	6.0	2.48	0.0	11.05	1.88	18.7	280.5	4.83

Food Name	Serving Size	A I.U.	Thi mg	Rib mg	Nia mg	B₆ mg	Fol mcg	B₁₂ mcg	C mg	Calc mg	Iron mg	Mag mg	Pot mg	Zn mg
choice, ribs 10-12, 1/2-inch fat, raw	1 lb	0	.35	.56	13.89	1.59	22.7	13.38	0.0	16.26	7.98	77.11	1283.69	16.28
choice, ribs 10-12, 1/2-inch fat, raw	1 oz	0	.02	.04	.87	.1	1.4	.84	0.0	2.84	.5	4.82	80.23	1.02
choice, ribs 10-12, 1/2-inch fat, roasted	3 oz	0	.05	.14	2.58	.26	6.0	2.44	0.0	11.05	1.66	17.0	274.55	4.11
prime, ribs 10-12, 1/4-inch fat, broiled	3 oz	0	.08	.16	3.42	.29	6.0	2.47	0.0	11.05	1.88	18.7	278.8	4.8
prime, ribs 10-12, 1/4-inch fat, raw	1 lb	0	.36	.54	13.83	1.54	22.7	13.34	0.0	45.36	7.94	72.58	1274.62	16.15
prime, ribs 10-12, 1/4-inch fat, raw	1 oz	0	.02	.03	.86	.1	1.4	.83	0.0	2.84	.5	4.54	79.66	1.01
prime, ribs 10-12, 1/4-inch fat, roasted	3 oz	0	.05	.14	2.56	.26	5.1	2.41	0.0	11.05	1.64	16.15	270.3	4.04
prime, ribs 10-12, 1/2-inch fat, broiled	3 oz	0	.07	.16	3.39	.29	6.0	2.47	0.0	11.05	1.86	18.7	277.1	4.76
prime, ribs 10-12, 1/2-inch fat, raw	1 lb	0	.35	.56	13.66	1.54	22.7	13.2	0.0	45.36	7.85	72.58	1251.94	15.92
prime, ribs 10-12, 1/2-inch fat, raw	1 oz	0	.02	.03	.85	.1	1.4	.82	0.0	2.84	.49	4.54	78.25	1.0
prime, ribs 10-12, 1/2-inch fat, roasted	3 oz	0	.05	.14	2.54	.26	6.0	2.41	0.0	11.05	1.63	16.15	268.6	4.0
select, ribs 10-12, 0-inch fat, broiled	3 oz	0	.08	.16	3.59	.3	6.0	2.56	0.0	11.05	1.95	19.55	292.4	5.08
select, ribs 10-12, 1/4-inch fat, broiled	3 oz	0	.08	.16	3.42	.29	6.0	2.47	0.0	11.05	1.88	18.7	278.8	4.8
select, ribs 10-12, 1/4-inch fat, raw	1 lb	0	.36	.59	14.11	1.59	22.7	13.61	0.0	45.36	8.12	77.11	1315.44	16.65
select, ribs 10-12, 1/4-inch fat, raw	1 oz	0	.02	.04	.88	.1	1.4	.85	0.0	2.84	.51	4.82	82.22	1.04
select, ribs 10-12, 1/4-inch fat, roasted	3 oz	0	.05	.14	2.68	.2	5.1	2.44	0.0	11.05	2.05	17.0	274.55	4.17
select, ribs 10-12, 1/2-inch fat, broiled	3 oz	0	.08	.16	3.49	.29	6.0	2.52	0.0	11.05	1.9	19.55	285.6	4.92
select, ribs 10-12, 1/2-inch fat, raw	1 lb	0	.36	.58	14.22	1.59	22.7	13.7	0.0	45.36	8.21	77.11	1329.05	16.83
select, ribs 10-12, 1/2-inch fat, raw	1 oz	0	.02	.04	.89	.1	1.4	.86	0.0	2.84	.51	4.82	83.07	1.05
select, ribs 10-12, 1/2-inch fat, roasted	3 oz	0	.06	.14	2.64	.26	6.0	2.49	0.0	11.05	1.68	17.0	282.2	4.22

RIB, WHOLE

Trimmed

Food Name	Serving Size	A I.U.	Thi mg	Rib mg	Nia mg	B₆ mg	Fol mcg	B₁₂ mcg	C mg	Calc mg	Iron mg	Mag mg	Pot mg	Zn mg
all grades, ribs 6-12, 1/4-inch fat, broiled	3 oz	0	.08	.17	3.26	.27	6.0	2.82	0.0	9.35	2.18	21.25	323.85	5.58
all grades, ribs 6-12, 1/4-inch fat, roasted	3 oz	0	.07	.18	3.54	.23	6.8	2.47	0.0	8.5	2.43	21.25	317.9	5.91
all grades, ribs 6-12, 1/2-inch fat, broiled	3 oz	0	.08	.18	3.21	.3	6.8	2.79	0.0	8.5	2.14	21.25	322.15	5.57
all grades, ribs 6-12, 1/2-inch fat, roasted	3 oz	0	.07	.18	3.5	.26	6.8	2.48	0.0	8.5	2.22	21.25	319.6	5.9
choice, ribs 6-12, 1/4-inch fat, broiled	3 oz	0	.08	.17	3.26	.27	6.0	2.82	0.0	9.35	2.18	21.25	323.85	5.58
choice, ribs 6-12, 1/4-inch fat, roasted	3 oz	0	.07	.18	3.54	.23	6.8	2.47	0.0	8.5	2.43	21.25	317.9	5.91
choice, ribs 6-12, 1/2-inch fat, broiled	3 oz	0	.08	.18	3.21	.3	6.8	2.79	0.0	8.5	2.14	21.25	322.15	5.57
choice, ribs 6-12, 1/2-inch fat, roasted	3 oz	0	.07	.18	3.5	.26	6.8	2.48	0.0	8.5	2.22	21.25	319.6	5.9
prime, ribs 6-12, 1/4-inch fat, broiled	3 oz	0	.08	.18	3.21	.3	6.0	2.79	0.0	8.5	2.14	21.25	322.15	5.57
prime, ribs 6-12, 1/4-inch fat, roasted	3 oz	0	.07	.18	3.49	.26	7.7	2.48	0.0	8.5	2.22	21.25	319.6	5.9
prime, ribs 6-12, 1/2-inch fat, broiled	3 oz	0	.08	.18	3.21	.3	6.8	2.79	0.0	8.5	2.14	21.25	322.15	5.57
prime, ribs 6-12, 1/2-inch fat, roasted	3 oz	0	.07	.18	3.5	.26	6.8	2.48	0.0	8.5	2.22	21.25	319.6	5.9
select, ribs 6-12, 1/4-inch fat, broiled	3 oz	0	.08	.17	3.26	.27	6.0	2.82	0.0	9.35	2.18	21.25	323.85	5.58
select, ribs 6-12, 1/4-inch fat, roasted	3 oz	0	.07	.18	3.54	.23	6.8	2.47	0.0	8.5	2.43	21.25	317.9	5.91
select, ribs 6-12, 1/2-inch fat, broiled	3 oz	0	.08	.18	3.21	.3	6.8	2.79	0.0	8.5	2.14	21.25	322.15	5.57
select, ribs 6-12, 1/2-inch fat, roasted	3 oz	0	.07	.18	3.5	.26	6.8	2.48	0.0	8.5	2.22	21.25	319.6	5.9

Untrimmed

Food Name	Serving Size	A I.U.	Thi mg	Rib mg	Nia mg	B₆ mg	Fol mcg	B₁₂ mcg	C mg	Calc mg	Iron mg	Mag mg	Pot mg	Zn mg
all grades, ribs 6-12, 1/4-inch fat, broiled	3 oz	0	.07	.14	2.76	.23	5.1	2.44	0.0	10.2	1.84	17.0	265.2	4.44
all grades, ribs 6-12, 1/4-inch fat, raw	1 lb	0	.36	.59	12.61	1.41	22.7	12.7	0.0	40.82	7.8	72.58	1215.65	16.65
all grades, ribs 6-12, 1/4-inch fat, raw	1 oz	0	.02	.04	.79	.09	1.4	.79	0.0	2.55	.49	4.54	75.98	1.04
all grades, ribs 6-12, 1/4-inch fat, roasted	3 oz	0	.06	.14	2.9	.2	6.0	2.16	0.0	9.35	1.99	17.0	255.85	4.55
all grades, ribs 6-12, 1/2-inch fat, broiled	3 oz	0	.06	.15	2.65	.25	5.1	2.37	0.0	9.35	1.77	17.0	256.7	4.28
all grades, ribs 6-12, 1/2-inch fat, raw	1 lb	0	.35	.58	12.38	1.41	22.7	12.43	0.0	40.82	7.62	72.58	1179.36	16.15
all grades, ribs 6-12, 1/2-inch fat, raw	1 oz	0	.02	.04	.77	.09	1.4	.78	0.0	2.55	.48	4.54	73.71	1.01
all grades, ribs 6-12, 1/2-inch fat, roasted	3 oz	0	.06	.15	2.8	.21	6.0	2.13	0.0	9.35	1.79	16.15	249.9	4.39
choice, ribs 6-12, 1/4-inch fat, broiled	3 oz	0	.07	.14	2.73	.23	5.1	2.41	0.0	10.2	1.83	16.15	261.8	4.36
choice, ribs 6-12, 1/4-inch fat, raw	1 lb	0	.36	.59	12.38	1.41	22.7	12.47	0.0	40.82	7.67	68.04	1183.9	16.19
choice, ribs 6-12, 1/4-inch fat, raw	1 oz	0	.02	.04	.77	.09	1.4	.78	0.0	2.55	.48	4.25	73.99	1.01
choice, ribs 6-12, 1/4-inch fat, roasted	3 oz	0	.06	.14	2.86	.2	6.0	2.14	0.0	9.35	1.90	16.15	251.6	4.45
choice, ribs 6-12, 1/2-inch fat, broiled	3 oz	0	.06	.15	2.64	.25	5.1	2.36	0.0	9.35	1.76	17.0	255.85	4.25
choice, ribs 6-12, 1/2-inch fat, raw	1 lb	0	.34	.58	12.32	1.41	22.7	12.38	0.0	40.82	7.58	68.04	1170.29	16.01
choice, ribs 6-12, 1/2-inch fat, raw	1 oz	0	.02	.04	.77	.09	1.4	.77	0.0	2.55	.47	4.25	73.14	1.0
choice, ribs 6-12, 1/2-inch fat, roasted	3 oz	0	.06	.15	2.79	.21	6.0	2.13	0.0	9.35	1.79	16.15	249.05	4.38
prime, ribs 6-12, 1/4-inch fat, broiled	3 oz	0	.07	.14	2.68	.25	5.1	2.4	0.0	9.35	1.79	17.0	260.1	4.34
prime, ribs 6-12, 1/4-inch fat, raw	1 lb	0	.36	.59	12.25	1.36	22.7	12.34	0.0	40.82	7.58	68.04	1165.75	15.97

Food Name	Serving Size	A I.U.	Thi mg	Rib mg	Nia mg	B_6 mg	Fol mcg	B_{12} mcg	C mg	Calc mg	Iron mg	Mag mg	Pot mg	Zn mg
prime, ribs 6-12, 1/4-inch fat, raw	1 oz	0	.02	.04	.77	.09	1.4	.77	0.0	2.55	.47	4.25	72.86	1.0
prime, ribs 6-12, 1/4-inch fat, roasted	3 oz	0	.06	.14	2.84	.22	6.0	2.15	0.0	9.35	1.82	16.15	254.15	4.48
prime, ribs 6-12, 1/2-inch fat, broiled	3 oz	0	.06	.14	2.6	.25	5.1	2.34	0.0	10.2	1.74	16.15	251.6	4.17
prime, ribs 6-12, 1/2-inch fat, raw	1 lb	0	.34	.57	12.16	1.36	22.7	12.25	0.0	40.82	7.48	68.04	1147.61	15.74
prime, ribs 6-12, 1/2-inch fat, raw	1 oz	0	.02	.04	.76	.09	1.4	.77	0.0	2.55	.47	4.25	71.73	.98
prime, ribs 6-12, 1/2-inch fat, roasted	3 oz	0	.06	.14	2.75	.21	6.0	2.1	0.0	9.35	1.77	15.3	244.8	4.28
select, ribs 6-12, 1/4-inch fat, broiled	3 oz	0	.07	.14	2.8	.23	5.1	2.47	0.0	9.35	1.87	17.0	268.6	4.51
select, ribs 6-12, 1/4-inch fat, raw	1 lb	0	.36	.59	12.75	1.41	22.7	12.84	0.0	40.82	7.94	72.58	1238.33	16.92
select, ribs 6-12, 1/4-inch fat, raw	1 oz	0	.02	.04	.8	.09	1.4	.8	0.0	2.55	.5	4.54	77.4	1.06
select, ribs 6-12, 1/4-inch fat, roasted	3 oz	0	.06	.15	2.95	.2	6.0	2.18	0.0	9.35	2.02	17.0	260.1	4.66
select, ribs 6-12, 1/2-inch fat, broiled	3 oz	0	.07	.15	2.69	.25	5.1	2.41	0.0	9.35	1.8	17.0	261.8	4.37
select, ribs 6-12, 1/2-inch fat, raw	1 lb	0	.35	.59	12.59	1.41	22.7	12.66	0.0	40.82	7.8	72.58	1211.11	16.56
select, ribs 6-12, 1/2-inch fat, raw	1 oz	0	.02	.04	.79	.09	1.4	.79	0.0	2.55	.49	4.54	75.69	1.03
select, ribs 6-12, 1/2-inch fat, roasted	3 oz	0	.06	.15	2.85	.21	6.0	2.16	0.0	9.35	1.83	16.15	255.0	4.51
RIB EYE, SMALL END														
Trimmed														
choice, ribs 10-12, 0-inch fat, broiled	3 oz	0	.09	.19	4.08	.34	6.8	2.82	0.0	11.05	2.18	22.95	334.9	5.94
Untrimmed														
choice, ribs 10-12, 0-inch fat, broiled	3 oz	0	.08	.16	3.59	.3	6.0	2.56	0.0	11.05	1.95	19.55	292.4	5.08
choice, ribs 10-12, 0-inch fat, raw	1 lb	0	.36	.59	14.65	1.63	22.7	14.11	0.0	45.36	8.48	81.65	1383.48	17.46
choice, ribs 10-12, 0-inch fat, raw	1 oz	0	.02	.04	.92	.1	1.4	.88	0.0	2.84	.53	5.1	86.47	1.09
ROUND, BOTTOM														
Trimmed														
all grades, 0-inch fat, braised	3 oz	0	.06	.22	3.47	.31	9.4	2.1	0.0	4.25	2.94	21.25	261.8	4.66
all grades, 0-inch fat, roasted	3 oz	0	.07	.2	3.46	.31	10.2	2.3	0.0	4.25	2.66	23.8	332.35	3.93
all grades, 1/4-inch fat, braised	3 oz	0	.06	.22	3.47	.31	9.4	2.1	0.0	4.25	2.94	21.25	261.8	4.66
all grades, 1/4-inch fat, roasted	3 oz	0	.07	.2	3.46	.31	10.2	2.3	0.0	4.25	2.66	23.8	332.35	3.93
all grades, 1/2-inch fat, braised	3 oz	0	.06	.22	3.47	.31	9.4	2.1	0.0	4.25	2.94	21.25	261.8	4.66
choice, 0-inch fat, braised	3 oz	0	.06	.22	3.47	.31	9.4	2.1	0.0	4.25	2.94	21.25	261.8	4.66
choice, 0-inch fat, roasted	3 oz	0	.07	.2	3.46	.01	10.2	2.3	0.0	4.25	2.66	23.8	332.35	3.93
choice, 1/4-inch fat, braised	3 oz	0	.06	.22	3.47	.31	9.4	2.1	0.0	4.25	2.94	21.25	261.8	4.66
choice, 1/4-inch fat, roasted	3 oz	0	.07	.2	3.46	.31	10.2	2.3	0.0	4.25	2.66	23.8	332.35	3.93
choice, 1/2-inch fat, braised	3 oz	0	.06	.22	3.47	.31	9.4	2.1	0.0	4.25	2.94	21.25	261.8	4.66
prime, 1/2-inch fat, braised	3 oz	0	.06	.22	3.47	.31	9.4	2.1	0.0	4.25	2.94	21.25	261.8	4.66
prime, 1/2-inch fat, raw	1 lb	0	.53	.89	18.72	2.59	45.4	13.29	0.0	18.14	10.8	113.4	1682.86	15.92
prime, 1/2-inch fat, raw	1 oz	0	.03	.06	1.17	.16	2.8	.83	0.0	1.13	.67	7.09	105.18	1.0
select, 0-inch fat, braised	3 oz	0	.06	.22	3.47	.31	9.4	2.1	0.0	4.25	2.94	21.25	261.8	4.66
select, 0-inch fat, roasted	3 oz	0	.07	.2	3.46	.31	10.2	2.3	0.0	4.25	2.66	23.8	332.35	3.93
select, 1/4-inch fat, braised	3 oz	0	.06	.22	3.47	.31	9.4	2.1	0.0	4.25	2.94	21.25	261.8	4.66
select, 1/4-inch fat, roasted	3 oz	0	.07	.2	3.46	.31	10.2	2.3	0.0	4.25	2.66	23.8	332.35	3.93
select, 1/2-inch fat, braised	3 oz	0	.06	.22	3.47	.31	9.4	2.1	0.0	4.25	2.94	21.25	261.8	4.66
Untrimmed														
all grades, 0-inch fat, braised	3 oz	0	.06	.22	3.43	.31	9.4	2.08	0.0	4.25	2.9	21.25	258.4	4.59
all grades, 0-inch fat, roasted	3 oz	0	.07	.2	3.44	.31	10.2	2.29	0.0	4.25	2.64	23.8	329.8	3.9
all grades, 1/4-inch fat, braised	3 oz	0	.06	.2	3.17	.28	8.5	2.0	0.0	5.1	2.65	18.7	239.7	4.17
all grades, 1/4-inch fat, raw	1 lb	0	.5	.82	17.24	2.36	40.8	12.47	0.0	22.68	9.89	99.79	1515.02	14.56
all grades, 1/4-inch fat, raw	1 oz	0	.03	.05	1.08	.15	2.6	.78	0.0	1.42	.62	6.24	94.69	.91
all grades, 1/4-inch fat, roasted	3 oz	0	.07	.2	3.2	.3	9.4	2.18	0.0	5.1	2.45	21.25	304.3	3.6
all grades, 1/2-inch fat, braised	3 oz	0	.06	.21	3.29	.29	9.4	2.04	0.0	5.1	2.76	19.55	248.2	4.36
all grades, 1/2-inch fat, raw	1 lb	0	.48	.8	16.94	2.31	40.8	12.29	0.0	22.68	9.71	99.79	1483.27	14.29
all grades, 1/2-inch fat, raw	1 oz	0	.03	.05	1.06	.14	2.6	.77	0.0	1.42	.61	6.24	92.7	.89
choice, 0-inch fat, braised	3 oz	0	.06	.21	3.41	.3	9.4	2.07	0.0	4.25	2.88	20.4	256.7	4.56
choice, 0-inch fat, roasted	3 oz	0	.07	.2	3.42	.31	10.2	2.28	0.0	4.25	2.63	23.8	327.25	3.87
choice, 1/4-inch fat, braised	3 oz	0	.06	.2	3.17	.28	8.5	2.0	0.0	5.1	2.65	18.7	239.7	4.17
choice, 1/4-inch fat, raw	1 lb	0	.5	.82	17.15	2.36	40.8	12.43	0.0	22.68	9.84	99.79	1501.42	14.42
choice, 1/4-inch fat, raw	1 oz	0	.03	.05	1.07	.15	2.6	.78	0.0	1.42	.62	6.24	93.84	.9
choice, 1/4-inch fat, roasted	3 oz	0	.07	.19	3.19	.29	9.4	2.18	0.0	5.1	2.43	21.25	301.75	3.57

Food Name	Serving Size	A I.U.	Thi mg	Rib mg	Nia mg	B_6 mg	Fol mcg	B_{12} mcg	C mg	Calc mg	Iron mg	Mag mg	Pot mg	Zn mg
choice, 1/2-inch fat, braised	3 oz	0	.06	.21	3.29	.29	9.4	2.04	0.0	5.1	2.70	19.55	248.2	4.36
choice, 1/2-inch fat, raw	1 lb	0	.48	.8	16.91	2.31	40.8	12.29	0.0	22.68	9.71	95.26	1478.74	14.24
choice, 1/2-inch fat, raw	1 oz	0	.03	.05	1.06	.14	2.6	.77	0.0	1.42	.61	5.95	92.42	.89
prime, 1/2-inch fat, braised	3 oz	0	.06	.2	3.23	.29	8.5	2.01	0.0	5.1	2.71	19.55	243.95	4.27
prime, 1/2-inch fat, raw	1 lb	0	.49	.82	17.16	2.36	40.8	12.43	0.0	22.68	9.84	99.79	1510.49	14.47
prime, 1/2-inch fat, raw	1 oz	0	.03	.05	1.07	.15	2.6	.78	0.0	1.42	.62	6.24	94.41	.9
select, 0-inch fat, braised	3 oz	0	.06	.22	3.43	.31	9.4	2.08	0.0	4.25	2.9	21.25	258.4	4.59
select, 0-inch fat, roasted	3 oz	0	.07	.2	3.44	.31	10.2	2.29	0.0	4.25	2.64	23.8	329.8	3.9
select, 1/4-inch fat, braised	3 oz	0	.06	.2	3.19	.28	8.5	2.01	0.0	5.1	2.68	19.55	240.55	4.21
select, 1/4-inch fat, raw	1 lb	0	.5	.82	17.37	2.4	40.8	12.56	0.0	22.68	9.98	104.33	1528.63	14.65
select, 1/4-inch fat, raw	1 oz	0	.03	.05	1.09	.15	2.6	.79	0.0	1.42	.62	6.52	95.54	.92
select, 1/4-inch fat, roasted	3 oz	0	.07	.2	3.23	.3	9.4	2.19	0.0	5.1	2.47	22.1	306.85	3.62
select, 1/2-inch fat, braised	3 oz	0	.06	.21	3.29	.29	9.4	2.04	0.0	5.1	2.77	20.4	249.05	4.37
select, 1/2-inch fat, raw	1 lb	0	.48	.81	17.07	2.36	40.8	12.38	0.0	22.68	9.8	99.79	1496.88	14.42
select, 1/2-inch fat, raw	1 oz	0	.03	.05	1.07	.15	2.6	.77	0.0	1.42	.61	6.24	93.56	.9
ROUND, EYE OF														
Trimmed														
all grades, 0-inch fat, roasted	3 oz	0	.08	.14	3.19	.32	6.0	1.84	0.0	4.25	1.66	22.95	335.75	4.03
all grades, 1/4-inch fat, roasted	3 oz	0	.08	.14	3.19	.32	6.0	1.84	0.0	4.25	1.66	22.95	335.75	4.03
all grades, 1/2-inch fat, roasted	3 oz	0	.07	.15	3.19	.32	6.0	1.84	0.0	4.25	1.66	22.95	335.75	4.03
choice, 0-inch fat, roasted	3 oz	0	.08	.14	3.19	.32	6.0	1.84	0.0	4.25	1.66	22.95	335.75	4.03
choice, 1/4-inch fat, roasted	3 oz	0	.08	.14	3.19	.32	6.0	1.84	0.0	4.25	1.66	22.95	335.75	4.03
choice, 1/2-inch fat, roasted	3 oz	0	.07	.15	3.19	.32	6.0	1.84	0.0	4.25	1.66	22.95	335.75	4.03
prime, 1/2-inch fat, roasted	3 oz	0	.07	.14	2.99	.3	6.0	1.79	0.0	5.1	1.57	21.25	311.1	3.72
prime, 1/2-inch fat, raw	1 lb	0	.44	.62	16.81	2.04	31.8	14.52	0.0	18.14	6.62	104.33	1737.29	13.25
prime, 1/2-inch fat, raw	1 oz	0	.03	.04	1.05	.13	2.0	.91	0.0	1.13	.41	6.52	108.58	.83
prime, 1/2-inch fat, roasted	3 oz	0	.07	.15	3.19	.32	6.0	1.84	0.0	4.25	1.66	22.95	335.75	4.03
select, 0-inch fat, roasted	3 oz	0	.08	.14	3.19	.32	6.0	1.84	0.0	4.25	1.66	22.95	335.75	4.03
select, 1/2-inch fat, roasted	3 oz	0	.08	.14	3.19	.32	6.0	1.84	0.0	4.25	1.66	22.95	335.75	4.03
select, 1/2-inch fat, roasted	3 oz	0	.07	.15	3.19	.32	6.0	1.84	0.0	4.25	1.66	22.95	335.75	4.03
Untrimmed														
all grades, 0-inch fat, roasted	3 oz	0	.08	.14	3.17	.32	6.0	1.84	0.0	4.25	1.65	22.95	333.2	4.0
all grades, 1/4-inch fat, raw	1 lb	0	.41	.59	15.24	1.86	27.2	13.34	0.0	22.68	6.12	90.72	1519.56	11.93
all grades, 1/4-inch fat, raw	1 oz	0	.03	.04	.95	.12	1.7	.83	0.0	1.42	.38	5.67	94.97	.75
choice, 0-inch fat, braised	3 oz	0	.06	.21	3.24	.24	7.7	2.3	0.0	3.4	2.82	22.1	283.9	3.88
all grades, 1/4-inch fat, roasted	3 oz	0	.07	.14	2.97	.3	6.0	1.78	0.0	5.1	1.56	20.4	307.7	3.69
all grades, 1/2-inch fat, raw	1 lb	0	.4	.58	15.51	1.91	27.2	13.52	0.0	22.68	6.21	95.26	1560.38	12.16
all grades, 1/2-inch fat, raw	1 oz	0	.03	.04	.97	.12	1.7	.84	0.0	1.42	.39	5.95	97.52	.76
all grades, 1/2-inch fat, roasted	3 oz	0	.07	.14	2.96	.3	6.0	1.78	0.0	5.1	1.56	21.25	307.7	3.68
choice, 0-inch fat, roasted	3 oz	0	.08	.14	3.17	.32	6.0	1.84	0.0	4.25	1.65	22.95	333.2	4.0
choice, 1/4-inch fat, raw	1 lb	0	.41	.59	15.24	1.86	27.2	13.34	0.0	22.68	6.12	90.72	1519.56	11.93
choice, 1/4-inch fat, raw	1 oz	0	.03	.04	.95	.12	1.7	.83	0.0	1.42	.38	5.67	94.97	.75
choice, 1/4-inch fat, roasted	3 oz	0	.07	.14	2.95	.3	5.1	1.78	0.0	5.1	1.56	20.4	305.15	3.66
choice, 1/2-inch fat, raw	1 lb	0	.4	.58	15.48	1.86	27.2	13.52	0.0	22.68	6.21	95.26	1555.85	12.11
choice, 1/2-inch fat, raw	1 oz	0	.03	.04	.97	.12	1.7	.84	0.0	1.42	.39	5.95	97.24	.76
choice, 1/2-inch fat, roasted	3 oz	0	.07	.14	2.96	.3	6.0	1.78	0.0	5.1	1.56	21.25	307.7	3.68
prime, 1/2-inch fat, raw	1 lb	0	.4	.58	15.4	1.86	27.2	13.43	0.0	22.68	6.17	95.26	1542.24	12.07
prime, 1/2-inch fat, raw	1 oz	0	.02	.04	.96	.12	1.7	.84	0.0	1.42	.39	5.95	96.39	.75
select, 0-inch fat, roasted	3 oz	0	.08	.14	3.17	.32	6.0	1.84	0.0	4.25	1.65	22.95	333.2	4.0
select, 1/4-inch fat, raw	1 lb	0	.41	.59	15.08	1.86	27.2	13.43	0.0	22.68	6.17	90.72	1537.7	12.02
select, 1/4-inch fat, raw	1 oz	0	.03	.04	.96	.12	1.7	.84	0.0	1.42	.39	5.67	96.11	.75
select, 1/4-inch fat, roasted	1 oz	0	.07	.14	2.98	.3	6.0	1.79	0.0	5.1	1.57	21.25	310.25	3.71
select, 1/2-inch fat, raw	1 lb	0	.4	.58	15.63	1.91	27.2	13.61	0.0	22.68	6.26	95.26	1573.99	12.25
select, 1/2-inch fat, raw	1 oz	0	.03	.04	.98	.12	1.7	.85	0.0	1.42	.39	5.95	98.37	.77
select, 1/2-inch fat, roasted	3 oz	0	.07	.14	2.97	.3	6.0	1.78	0.0	5.1	1.56	21.25	308.55	3.69

Food Name	Serving Size	A I.U.	Thi mg	Rib mg	Nia mg	B₆ mg	Fol mcg	B₁₂ mcg	C mg	Calc mg	Iron mg	Mag mg	Pot mg	Zn mg
ROUND, FULL CUT														
Trimmed														
choice, 1/4-inch fat, broiled	3 oz	0	.09	.19	3.62	.34	8.5	2.69	0.0	4.25	2.3	23.8	358.7	3.94
select, 1/4-inch fat, broiled	3 oz	0	.09	.19	3.63	.35	8.5	2.69	0.0	4.25	2.3	23.8	359.55	3.96
select, 1/2-inch fat, broiled	3 oz	0	.09	.19	3.54	.43	8.5	2.53	0.0	4.25	2.29	23.8	352.75	3.98
Untrimmed														
choice, 1/4-inch fat, broiled	3 oz	0	.08	.18	3.39	.32	7.7	2.56	0.0	5.1	2.15	21.25	333.2	3.67
choice, 1/4-inch fat, raw	1 lb	0	.45	.77	16.83	2.13	36.3	12.7	0.0	18.14	8.94	99.79	1533.17	14.52
choice, 1/4-inch fat, raw	1 oz	0	.03	.05	1.05	.13	2.3	.79	0.0	1.13	.56	6.24	95.82	.91
choice, 1/2-inch fat, broiled	3 oz	0	.08	.18	3.18	.37	7.7	2.34	0.0	5.95	2.06	20.4	311.1	3.51
choice, 1/2-inch fat, raw	1 lb	0	.44	.75	15.97	2.04	36.3	12.2	0.0	22.68	8.53	90.72	1433.38	13.74
choice, 1/2-inch fat, raw	1 oz	0	.03	.05	1.0	.13	2.3	.76	0.0	1.42	.53	5.67	89.59	.86
select, 1/4-inch fat, broiled	3 oz	0	.08	.18	3.4	.32	7.7	2.57	0.0	5.1	2.16	22.1	333.2	3.68
select, 1/4-inch fat, raw	1 lb	0	.45	.77	16.83	2.13	36.3	12.7	0.0	18.14	8.98	99.79	1533.17	14.56
select, 1/4-inch fat, raw	1 oz	0	.03	.05	1.05	.13	2.3	.79	0.0	1.13	.56	6.24	95.82	.91
select, 1/2-inch fat, raw	1 lb	0	.44	.75	16.08	2.04	36.3	12.29	0.0	22.68	8.57	95.26	1446.98	13.88
select, 1/2-inch fat, raw	1 oz	0	.03	.05	1.01	.13	2.3	.77	0.0	1.42	.54	5.95	90.44	.87
ROUND, TIP														
Trimmed														
all grades, 0-inch fat, roasted	3 oz	0	.09	.23	3.18	.34	6.8	2.46	0.0	4.25	2.5	22.95	328.1	6.01
all grades, 1/4-inch fat, roasted	3 oz	0	.09	.23	3.18	.34	6.8	2.46	0.0	4.25	2.5	22.95	328.1	6.01
all grades, 1/2-inch fat, roasted	3 oz	0	.08	.23	3.18	.34	6.8	2.46	0.0	4.25	2.5	22.95	328.1	6.01
choice, 0-inch fat, roasted	3 oz	0	.09	.23	3.18	.34	6.8	2.46	0.0	4.25	2.5	22.95	328.1	6.01
choice, 1/4-inch fat, roasted	3 oz	0	.09	.23	3.18	.34	6.8	2.46	0.0	4.25	2.5	22.95	328.1	6.01
choice, 1/2-inch fat, roasted	3 oz	0	.08	.23	3.18	.34	6.8	2.46	0.0	4.25	2.5	22.95	328.1	6.01
prime, 1/4-inch fat, roasted	3 oz	0	.09	.23	3.18	.34	6.8	2.46	0.0	4.25	2.5	22.95	328.1	6.01
prime, 1/2-inch fat, roasted	3 oz	0	.08	.23	3.18	.34	6.8	2.46	0.0	4.25	2.5	22.95	328.1	6.01
select, 0-inch fat, roasted	3 oz	0	.09	.23	3.18	.34	6.8	2.46	0.0	4.25	2.5	22.95	328.1	6.01
select, 1/4-inch fat, roasted	3 oz	0	.09	.23	3.18	.34	6.8	2.46	0.0	4.25	2.5	22.95	328.1	6.01
select, 1/2-inch fat, roasted	3 oz	0	.08	.20	3.18	.34	6.8	2.46	0.0	4.25	2.5	22.95	328.1	6.01
Untrimmed														
all grades, 0-inch fat, roasted	3 oz	0	.09	.22	3.12	.33	6.8	2.42	0.0	4.25	2.45	22.1	321.3	5.86
all grades, 1/4-inch fat, raw	1 lb	0	.5	.82	14.11	1.81	31.8	13.47	0.0	22.68	8.94	95.26	1460.59	19.6
all grades, 1/4-inch fat, raw	1 oz	0	.03	.05	.88	.11	2.0	.84	0.0	1.42	.56	5.95	91.29	1.22
all grades, 1/4-inch fat, roasted	3 oz	0	.08	.21	2.99	.31	6.0	2.35	0.0	5.1	2.34	21.25	305.15	5.53
all grades, 1/2-inch fat, raw	1 lb	0	.48	.81	14.11	1.81	31.8	13.47	0.0	22.68	8.94	95.26	1460.59	19.55
all grades, 1/2-inch fat, raw	1 oz	0	.03	.05	.88	.11	2.0	.84	0.0	1.42	.56	5.95	91.29	1.22
all grades, 1/2-inch fat, roasted	3 oz	0	.08	.21	2.95	.31	6.0	2.33	0.0	5.1	2.3	21.25	300.05	5.41
choice, 0-inch fat, roasted	3 oz	0	.09	.22	3.1	.33	6.8	2.41	0.0	4.25	2.43	22.1	318.75	5.81
choice, 1/4-inch fat, raw	1 lb	0	.5	.82	14.02	1.81	31.8	13.43	0.0	22.68	8.89	95.26	1446.98	19.41
choice, 1/4-inch fat, raw	1 oz	0	.03	.05	.88	.11	2.0	.84	0.0	1.42	.56	5.95	90.44	1.21
choice, 1/4-inch fat, roasted	3 oz	0	.08	.21	2.96	.31	6.0	2.33	0.0	5.1	2.3	20.4	300.9	5.43
choice, 1/2-inch fat, raw	1 lb	0	.48	.81	14.08	1.81	31.8	13.47	0.0	22.68	8.94	95.26	1456.06	19.5
choice, 1/2-inch fat, raw	1 oz	0	.03	.05	.88	.11	2.0	.84	0.0	1.42	.56	5.95	91.0	1.22
choice, 1/2-inch fat, roasted	3 oz	0	.08	.21	2.94	.31	6.0	2.32	0.0	5.95	2.3	21.25	299.2	5.4
prime, 1/4-inch fat, raw	1 lb	0	.5	.82	14.2	1.81	31.8	13.56	0.0	22.68	9.03	95.26	1474.2	19.78
prime, 1/4-inch fat, raw	1 oz	0	.03	.05	.89	.11	2.0	.85	0.0	1.42	.56	5.95	92.14	1.24
prime, 1/4-inch fat, roasted	3 oz	0	.08	.2	2.94	.31	6.0	2.31	0.0	5.1	2.3	20.4	298.35	5.38
prime, 1/2-inch fat, raw	1 lb	0	.48	.8	14.01	1.81	31.8	13.38	0.0	22.68	8.89	90.72	1442.45	19.37
prime, 1/2-inch fat, raw	1 oz	0	.03	.05	.88	.11	2.0	.84	0.0	1.42	.56	5.67	90.15	1.21
prime, 1/2-inch fat, roasted	3 oz	0	.07	.2	2.9	.31	6.0	2.3	0.0	5.95	2.25	20.4	294.1	5.28
select, 0-inch fat, roasted	3 oz	0	.09	.22	3.12	.33	6.8	2.42	0.0	4.25	2.45	22.1	321.3	5.86
select, 1/4-inch fat, raw	1 lb	0	0	.01	.14	.02	0.3	.14	0.0	.23	.09	.95	14.88	.2
select, 1/4-inch fat, raw	1 oz	0	.03	.05	.89	.12	2.0	.85	0.0	1.42	.57	5.95	92.99	1.25
select, 1/4-inch fat, roasted	3 oz	0	.08	.21	3.01	.32	6.8	2.36	0.0	5.1	2.35	21.25	307.7	5.58
select, 1/2-inch fat, raw	1 lb	0	.49	.82	14.25	1.86	31.8	13.61	0.0	22.68	9.03	95.26	1478.74	19.82
select, 1/2-inch fat, raw	1 oz	0	.03	.05	.89	.12	2.0	.85	0.0	1.42	.56	5.95	92.42	1.24

Food Name	Serving Size	A I.U.	Thi mg	Rib mg	Nia mg	B_6 mg	Fol mcg	B_{12} mcg	C mg	Calc mg	Iron mg	Mag mg	Pot mg	Zn mg
select, 1/2-inch fat, roasted	3 oz	0	.08	.21	2.96	.31	6.0	2.34	0.0	5.1	2.31	21.05	301.75	5.45
ROUND, TOP														
Trimmed														
all grades, 0-inch fat, braised	3 oz	0	.06	.21	3.24	.24	7.7	2.3	0.0	3.4	2.82	22.1	283.9	3.88
all grades, 1/4-inch fat, braised	3 oz	0	.06	.21	3.24	.24	7.7	2.3	0.0	3.4	2.82	22.1	283.9	3.88
all grades, 1/4-inch fat, broiled	3 oz	0	.1	.23	5.13	.48	10.2	2.11	0.0	5.1	2.45	26.35	375.7	4.73
all grades, 1/2-inch fat, broiled	3 oz	0	.1	.23	5.13	.48	10.2	2.11	0.0	5.1	2.45	26.35	375.7	4.73
choice, 1/4-inch fat, braised	3 oz	0	.06	.21	3.24	.24	7.7	2.3	0.0	3.4	2.82	22.1	283.9	3.88
choice, 1/4-inch fat, broiled	3 oz	0	.1	.23	5.13	.48	10.2	2.11	0.0	5.1	2.45	26.35	375.7	4.73
choice, 1/4-inch fat, pan-fried	3 oz	0	.09	.24	4.66	.52	11.1	2.92	0.0	4.25	2.68	29.75	436.05	3.93
choice, 1/2-inch fat, broiled	3 oz	0	.1	.23	5.13	.48	10.2	2.11	0.0	5.1	2.45	26.35	375.7	4.73
choice, 1/2-inch fat, pan-fried	3 oz	0	.1	.24	4.66	.52	11.1	2.92	0.0	4.25	2.68	29.75	436.05	3.93
prime, 1/4-inch fat, broiled	3 oz	0	.1	.23	5.13	.48	10.2	2.11	0.0	5.1	2.45	26.35	375.7	4.73
prime, 1/2-inch fat, broiled	3 oz	0	.1	.23	5.13	.48	10.2	2.11	0.0	5.1	2.45	26.35	375.7	4.73
select, 0-inch fat, braised	3 oz	0	.06	.21	3.24	.24	7.7	2.3	0.0	3.4	2.82	22.1	283.9	3.88
select, 1/4-inch fat, braised	3 oz	0	.06	.21	3.24	.24	7.7	2.3	0.0	3.4	2.82	22.1	283.9	3.88
select, 1/4-inch fat, broiled	3 oz	0	.1	.23	5.13	.48	10.2	2.11	0.0	5.1	2.45	26.35	375.7	4.73
select, 1/2-inch fat, broiled	3 oz	0	.1	.23	5.13	.48	10.2	2.11	0.0	5.1	2.45	26.35	375.7	4.73
Untrimmed														
all grades, 0-inch fat, braised	3 oz	0	.06	.21	3.2	.24	7.7	2.28	0.0	3.4	2.78	21.25	280.5	3.83
all grades, 1/4-inch fat, braised	3 oz	0	.06	.2	3.07	.23	7.7	2.21	0.0	4.25	2.65	20.4	267.75	3.64
all grades, 1/4-inch fat, broiled	3 oz	0	.09	.22	4.85	.45	9.4	2.06	0.0	5.95	2.34	24.65	356.15	4.48
all grades, 1/4-inch fat, raw	1 lb	0	.41	.82	18.6	2.18	36.3	12.34	0.0	18.14	8.94	104.33	1605.74	12.25
all grades, 1/4-inch fat, raw	1 oz	0	.03	.05	1.16	.14	2.3	.77	0.0	1.13	.56	6.52	100.36	.77
all grades, 1/2-inch fat, broiled	3 oz	0	.1	.22	4.98	.46	10.2	2.07	0.0	5.1	2.39	25.5	364.65	4.59
all grades, 1/2-inch fat, raw	1 lb	0	.43	.81	18.84	2.22	40.8	12.43	0.0	18.14	9.07	104.33	1637.5	12.43
all grades, 1/2-inch fat, raw	1 oz	0	.03	.05	1.18	.14	2.6	.78	0.0	1.13	.57	6.52	102.34	.78
choice, 0-inch fat, braised	3 oz	0	.06	.21	3.2	.24	7.7	2.28	0.0	3.4	2.78	21.25	280.5	3.83
choice, 1/4-inch fat, broiled	3 oz	0	.09	.22	4.85	.45	9.4	2.06	0.0	5.95	2.34	24.65	356.15	4.48
choice, 1/4-inch fat, pan-fried	3 oz	0	.09	.22	4.29	.48	10.2	2.75	0.0	5.1	2.48	27.2	399.5	3.63
choice, 1/4-inch fat, raw	1 lb	0	.41	.82	18.6	2.18	36.3	12.34	0.0	18.14	8.94	104.33	1605.74	12.25
choice, 1/4-inch fat, raw	1 oz	0	.03	.05	1.16	.14	2.3	.77	0.0	1.13	.56	6.52	100.36	.77
choice, 1/2-inch fat, braised	3 oz	0	.06	.2	3.04	.23	7.7	2.2	0.0	4.25	2.63	20.4	265.2	3.6
choice, 1/2-inch fat, broiled	3 oz	0	.1	.22	4.98	.47	10.2	2.07	0.0	5.1	2.39	25.5	364.65	4.59
choice, 1/2-inch fat, pan-fried	3 oz	0	.09	.21	4.2	.47	9.4	2.7	0.0	5.1	2.43	26.35	390.15	3.55
choice, 1/2-inch fat, raw	1 lb	0	.43	.81	18.84	2.22	40.8	12.43	0.0	18.14	9.07	104.33	1637.5	12.43
choice, 1/2-inch fat, raw	1 oz	0	.03	.05	1.18	.14	2.6	.78	0.0	1.13	.57	6.52	102.34	.78
prime, 1/4-inch fat, broiled	3 oz	0	.1	.22	5.01	.47	10.2	2.08	0.0	5.1	2.41	25.5	367.2	4.62
prime, 1/4-inch fat, raw	1 lb	0	.45	.82	19.14	2.22	40.8	12.56	0.0	13.61	9.16	108.86	1664.71	12.61
prime, 1/4-inch fat, raw	1 oz	0	.03	.05	1.2	.14	2.6	.79	0.0	.85	.57	6.8	104.04	.79
prime, 1/2-inch fat, broiled	3 oz	0	.1	.22	4.96	.46	9.4	2.07	0.0	5.1	2.38	25.5	362.95	4.57
prime, 1/2-inch fat, raw	1 lb	0	.44	.82	18.9	2.22	40.8	12.43	0.0	18.14	9.07	104.33	1642.03	12.47
prime, 1/2-inch fat, raw	1 oz	0	.03	.05	1.18	.14	2.6	.78	0.0	1.13	.57	6.52	102.63	.78
select, 0-inch fat, braised	3 oz	0	.06	.21	3.2	.24	7.7	2.28	0.0	3.4	2.78	21.25	280.5	3.83
select, 1/4-inch fat, braised	3 oz	0	.06	.2	3.09	.23	7.7	2.22	0.0	4.25	2.67	20.4	269.45	3.66
select, 1/4-inch fat, broiled	3 oz	0	.09	.22	4.85	.45	9.4	2.06	0.0	5.95	2.34	24.65	356.15	4.48
select, 1/4-inch fat, raw	1 lb	0	.45	.82	18.73	2.18	40.8	12.38	0.0	18.14	8.98	104.33	1623.89	12.34
select, 1/4-inch fat, raw	1 oz	0	.03	.05	1.17	.14	2.6	.77	0.0	1.13	.56	6.52	101.49	.77
select, 1/2-inch fat, broiled	3 oz	0	.1	.22	4.96	.46	9.4	2.07	0.0	5.1	2.38	25.5	362.95	4.57
select, 1/2-inch fat, raw	1 lb	0	.43	.81	10.07	2.22	40.8	12.43	0.0	18.14	9.07	104.33	1637.5	12.43
select, 1/2-inch fat, raw	1 oz	0	.03	.05	1.18	.14	2.6	.78	0.0	1.13	.57	6.52	102.34	.78
SIRLOIN, TOP														
Trimmed														
all grades, 0-inch fat, broiled	3 oz	0	.11	.25	3.64	.38	8.5	2.42	0.0	9.35	2.86	27.2	342.55	5.54
all grades, 1/4-inch fat, broiled	3 oz	0	.11	.25	3.64	.38	8.5	2.42	0.0	9.35	2.86	27.2	342.55	5.54
all grades, 1/2-inch fat, broiled	3 oz	0	.11	.25	3.64	.38	8.5	2.42	0.0	9.35	2.86	27.2	342.55	5.54
choice, 0-inch fat, broiled	3 oz	0	.11	.25	3.64	.38	8.5	2.42	0.0	9.35	2.86	27.2	342.55	5.54

Food Name	Serving Size	A I.U.	Thi mg	Rib mg	Nia mg	B6 mg	Fol mcg	B12 mcg	C mg	Calc mg	Iron mg	Mag mg	Pot mg	Zn mg
choice, 1/4-inch fat, broiled	3 oz	0	.11	.25	3.64	.38	8.5	2.42	0.0	9.35	2.86	27.2	342.55	5.54
choice, 1/4-inch fat, pan-fried	3 oz	0	.12	.28	3.65	.43	8.5	3.14	0.0	9.35	3.31	28.05	395.25	5.44
choice, 1/2-inch fat, broiled	3 oz	0	.11	.25	3.64	.38	8.5	2.42	0.0	9.35	2.86	27.2	342.55	5.54
choice, 1/2-inch fat, pan-fried	3 oz	0	.12	.28	3.66	.43	8.5	3.14	0.0	9.35	3.31	28.05	395.25	5.44
prime, 1/2-inch fat, broiled	3 oz	0	.11	.25	3.64	.38	8.5	2.42	0.0	9.35	2.86	27.2	342.55	5.54
prime, 1/2-inch fat, raw	1 lb	0	.6	1.05	16.16	2.0	36.3	14.38	0.0	31.75	12.2	108.86	1637.5	18.78
prime, 1/2-inch fat, raw	1 oz	0	.04	.07	1.01	.12	2.3	.9	0.0	1.98	.76	6.8	102.34	1.17
select, 0-inch fat, broiled	3 oz	0	.11	.25	3.64	.38	8.5	2.42	0.0	9.35	2.86	27.2	342.55	5.54
select, 1/4-inch fat, broiled	3 oz	0	.11	.25	3.64	.38	8.5	2.42	0.0	9.35	2.86	27.2	342.55	5.54
select, 1/2-inch fat, broiled	3 oz	0	.11	.25	3.64	.38	8.5	2.42	0.0	9.35	2.86	27.2	342.55	5.54
Untrimmed														
all grades, 0-inch fat, broiled	3 oz	0	.1	.24	3.52	.37	8.5	2.37	0.0	9.35	2.75	26.35	330.65	5.32
all grades, 1/4-inch fat, broiled	3 oz	0	.09	.23	3.34	.35	7.7	2.29	0.0	9.35	2.6	24.65	311.1	4.97
all grades, 1/4-inch fat, raw	1 lb	0	.54	.95	14.61	1.81	31.8	13.15	0.0	31.75	10.8	95.26	1424.3	16.51
all grades, 1/4-inch fat, raw	1 oz	0	.03	.06	.91	.11	2.0	.82	0.0	1.98	.67	5.95	89.02	1.03
all grades, 1/2-inch fat, broiled	3 oz	0	.1	.22	3.29	.34	7.7	2.26	0.0	9.35	2.56	23.8	306.0	4.89
all grades, 1/2-inch fat, raw	1 lb	0	.5	.88	13.92	1.72	31.8	12.56	0.0	36.29	10.16	90.72	1329.05	15.51
all grades, 1/2-inch fat, raw	1 oz	0	.03	.05	.87	.11	2.0	.79	0.0	2.27	.64	5.67	83.07	.97
choice, 0-inch fat, broiled	3 oz	0	.1	.24	3.5	.37	8.5	2.36	0.0	9.35	2.74	25.5	328.1	5.28
choice, 1/4-inch fat, broiled	3 oz	0	.09	.23	3.31	.35	7.7	2.28	0.0	9.35	2.58	23.8	308.55	4.93
choice, 1/4-inch fat, pan-fried	3 oz	0	.1	.24	3.19	.37	7.7	2.79	0.0	10.2	2.83	23.8	336.6	4.59
choice, 1/4-inch fat, raw	1 lb	0	.54	.91	14.52	1.77	31.8	13.06	0.0	36.29	10.7	90.72	1410.7	16.37
choice, 1/4-inch fat, raw	1 oz	0	.03	.06	.91	.11	2.0	.82	0.0	2.27	.67	5.67	88.17	1.02
choice, 1/2-inch fat, broiled	3 oz	0	.09	.22	3.28	.34	7.7	2.26	0.0	9.35	2.55	23.8	305.15	4.87
choice, 1/2-inch fat, pan-fried	3 oz	0	.1	.23	3.12	.36	7.7	2.73	0.0	9.35	2.76	22.95	327.25	4.46
choice, 1/2-inch fat, raw	1 lb	0	.5	.88	13.87	1.72	31.8	12.56	0.0	36.29	10.16	86.18	1324.51	15.42
choice, 1/2-inch fat, raw	1 oz	0	.03	.05	.87	.11	2.0	.79	0.0	2.27	.64	5.39	82.78	.96
prime, 1/2-inch fat, broiled	3 oz	0	.09	.22	3.21	.33	7.7	2.23	0.0	9.35	2.49	22.95	296.65	4.73
prime, 1/2-inch fat, raw	1 lb	0	.49	.86	13.61	1.68	27.2	12.34	0.0	36.29	9.89	86.18	1299.22	15.00
prime, 1/2-inch fat, raw	1 oz	0	.00	.05	.85	.1	1.7	.77	0.0	2.27	.62	5.39	80.51	.94
select, 0-inch fat, broiled	3 oz	0	.1	.25	3.57	.37	8.5	2.39	0.0	9.35	2.79	26.35	334.05	5.4
select, 1/4-inch fat, broiled	3 oz	0	.09	.23	3.36	.35	7.7	2.3	0.0	9.35	2.62	24.65	313.65	5.02
select, 1/4-inch fat, raw	1 lb	0	.54	.95	14.7	1.81	31.8	13.2	0.0	31.75	10.89	95.26	1437.91	16.65
select, 1/4-inch fat, raw	1 oz	0	.03	.06	.92	.11	2.0	.82	0.0	1.98	.68	5.95	89.87	1.04
select, 1/2-inch fat, broiled	3 oz	0	.09	.22	3.28	.34	7.7	2.26	0.0	9.35	2.55	23.8	305.15	4.87
select, 1/2-inch fat, raw	1 lb	0	.51	.89	14.1	1.72	31.8	12.75	0.0	36.29	10.34	90.72	1356.26	15.79
select, 1/2-inch fat, raw	1 oz	0	.03	.06	.88	.11	2.0	.8	0.0	2.27	.65	5.67	84.77	.99
SHANK CROSSCUTS														
Trimmed														
choice, 1/4-inch fat, simmered	3 oz	0	.12	.18	5.01	.31	8.5	3.22	0.0	27.2	3.28	25.5	379.95	8.92
choice, 1/2-inch fat, simmered	3 oz	0	.12	.18	5.01	.31	8.5	3.22	0.0	27.2	3.28	25.5	379.95	8.92
Untrimmed														
choice, 1/4-inch fat, raw	1 oz	0	.03	.06	1.52	.12	2.3	.9	0.0	5.39	.62	3.69	101.49	1.82
choice, 1/4-inch fat, raw	3 oz	0	.09	.17	4.55	.37	6.8	2.69	0.0	16.15	1.85	11.05	304.3	5.45
choice, 1/4-inch fat, simmered	3 oz	0	.1	.17	4.53	.29	7.7	2.98	0.0	25.5	2.98	22.95	343.4	7.91
choice, 1/2-inch fat, raw	1 lb	0	.46	.95	24.89	2.04	36.3	14.61	0.0	90.72	10.12	58.97	1673.78	29.89
choice, 1/2-inch fat, raw	1 oz	0	.03	.06	1.56	.13	2.3	.91	0.0	5.67	.63	3.69	104.61	1.87
choice, 1/2-inch fat, simmered	3 oz	0	.11	.17	4.68	.29	7.7	3.05	0.0	25.5	3.07	23.8	354.45	8.22
SPLEEN														
braised	3 oz	0	.04	.26	4.73	.03	3.4	4.27	42.8	10.2	33.46	16.15	241.4	2.37
calf, raw	100 gm	20	.53	.37	8.2	na	na	na	2.0	5.0	10.6	na	193.0	na
raw	4 oz	0	.06	.42	9.49	.08	4.5	6.42	51.4	10.17	50.34	24.86	484.77	2.38
T-BONE														
Trimmed														
choice, 1/4-inch fat, broiled	3 oz	0	.09	.21	3.94	.33	6.8	1.93	0.0	5.95	2.55	24.65	345.95	4.59
choice, 1/2-inch fat, broiled	3 oz	0	.09	.21	3.94	.33	6.8	1.93	0.0	5.95	2.55	24.65	345.95	4.59

Food Name	Serving Size	A I.U.	Thi mg	Rib mg	Nia mg	B6 mg	Fol mcg	B12 mcg	C mg	Calc mg	Iron mg	Mag mg	Pot mg	Zn mg
Untrimmed														
choice, 1/4-inch fat, broiled	3 oz	0	.09	.19	3.47	.29	6.0	1.83	0.0	6.8	2.25	21.25	301.75	3.98
choice, 1/4-inch fat, raw	1 lb	0	.45	.77	15.56	1.63	27.2	12.02	0.0	27.22	7.98	86.18	1338.12	13.93
choice, 1/4-inch fat, raw	1 oz	0	.03	.05	.97	.1	1.7	.75	0.0	1.7	.5	5.39	83.63	.87
choice, 1/2-inch fat, broiled	3 oz	0	.08	.18	3.32	.28	6.0	1.8	0.0	7.65	2.16	20.4	288.15	3.79
choice, 1/2-inch fat, raw	1 lb	0	.42	.71	14.76	1.59	27.2	11.57	0.0	31.75	7.58	77.11	1247.4	13.11
choice, 1/2-inch fat, raw	1 oz	0	.03	.04	.92	.1	1.7	.72	0.0	1.98	.47	4.82	77.96	.82
TENDERLOIN														
Trimmed														
all grades, 0-inch fat, broiled	3 oz	0	.11	.26	3.33	.37	6.0	2.18	0.0	5.95	3.04	25.5	356.15	4.75
all grades, 1/4-inch fat, broiled	3 oz	0	.11	.26	3.33	.37	6.0	2.18	0.0	5.95	3.04	25.5	356.15	4.75
all grades, 1/4-inch fat, roasted	3 oz	0	.09	.26	2.9	.25	7.7	2.3	0.0	5.95	3.14	22.95	332.35	4.07
all grades, 1/2-inch fat, broiled	3 oz	0	.11	.25	3.33	.37	6.0	2.18	0.0	5.95	3.04	25.5	356.15	4.75
all grades, 1/2-inch fat, roasted	3 oz	0	.09	.27	2.88	.32	6.8	2.35	0.0	5.95	3.11	22.95	334.05	4.39
choice, 0-inch fat, broiled	3 oz	0	.11	.26	3.33	.37	6.0	2.18	0.0	5.95	3.04	25.5	356.15	4.75
choice, 1/4-inch fat, broiled	3 oz	0	.11	.26	3.33	.37	6.0	2.18	0.0	5.95	3.04	25.5	356.15	4.75
choice, 1/4-inch fat, roasted	3 oz	0	.15	.28	3.87	.48	7.7	3.29	0.0	6.8	3.14	27.2	415.65	4.07
choice, 1/2-inch fat, broiled	3 oz	0	.11	.25	3.33	.37	6.0	2.18	0.0	5.95	3.04	25.5	356.15	4.75
choice, 1/2-inch fat, roasted	3 oz	0	.09	.27	2.88	.32	6.8	2.35	0.0	5.95	3.11	22.95	334.05	4.39
prime, 1/4-inch fat, broiled	3 oz	0	.11	.26	3.33	.37	6.0	2.18	0.0	5.95	3.04	25.5	356.15	4.75
prime, 1/4-inch fat, roasted	3 oz	0	.09	.27	2.88	.32	6.8	2.35	0.0	5.95	3.11	22.95	334.05	4.39
prime, 1/2-inch fat, broiled	3 oz	0	.11	.25	3.33	.37	6.0	2.18	0.0	5.95	3.04	25.5	356.15	4.75
prime, 1/2-inch fat, roasted	3 oz	0	.09	.27	2.88	.32	6.8	2.35	0.0	5.95	3.11	22.95	334.05	4.39
select, 0-inch fat, broiled	3 oz	0	.11	.26	3.33	.37	6.0	2.18	0.0	5.95	3.04	25.5	356.15	4.75
select, 1/4-inch fat, broiled	3 oz	0	.11	.26	3.33	.37	6.0	2.18	0.0	5.95	3.04	25.5	356.15	4.75
select, 1/4-inch fat, roasted	3 oz	0	.09	.26	2.9	.25	7.7	2.3	0.0	5.95	3.14	22.95	332.35	4.07
select, 1/2-inch fat, broiled	3 oz	0	.11	.25	3.33	.37	6.0	2.18	0.0	5.95	3.04	25.5	356.15	4.75
select, 1/2-inch fat, roasted	3 oz	0	.09	.27	2.88	.32	6.8	2.35	0.0	5.95	3.11	22.95	334.05	4.39
Untrimmed														
all grades, 0-inch fat, broiled	3 oz	0	.1	.25	3.21	.36	6.0	2.13	0.0	5.95	2.92	24.65	340.85	4.54
all grades, 1/4-inch fat, broiled	3 oz	0	.09	.22	2.99	.33	5.1	2.05	0.0	6.8	2.68	22.1	312.8	4.15
all grades, 1/4-inch fat, raw	1 lb	0	.5	.91	13.29	1.68	27.2	11.57	0.0	31.75	10.39	86.18	1338.12	13.47
all grades, 1/4-inch fat, raw	1 oz	0	.03	.06	.83	.1	1.7	.72	0.0	1.98	.65	5.39	83.63	.84
all grades, 1/4-inch fat, roasted	3 oz	0	.07	.22	2.52	.21	6.0	2.08	0.0	7.65	2.6	18.7	277.1	3.37
all grades, 1/2-inch fat, broiled	3 oz	0	.1	.23	3.07	.34	0.9	2.08	0.0	6.8	2.76	22.95	323.0	4.28
all grades, 1/2-inch fat, raw	1 lb	0	.54	.97	13.86	1.72	27.2	12.02	0.0	31.75	10.93	95.26	1424.3	14.2
all grades, 1/2-inch fat, roasted	3 oz	0	.08	.24	2.6	.29	6.0	2.18	0.0	6.8	2.71	19.55	291.55	3.81
choice, 0-inch fat, broiled	3 oz	0	.1	.24	3.2	.36	6.0	2.13	0.0	5.95	2.89	23.8	338.3	4.51
choice, 1/4-inch fat, broiled	3 oz	0	.09	.22	2.98	.33	5.1	2.04	0.0	6.8	2.66	22.1	310.25	4.11
choice, 1/4-inch fat, raw	1 lb	0	.5	.91	13.29	1.68	27.2	11.57	0.0	31.75	10.39	86.18	1338.12	13.47
choice, 1/4-inch fat, raw	1 oz	0	.03	.06	.83	.1	1.7	.72	0.0	1.98	.65	5.39	83.63	.84
choice, 1/4-inch fat, roasted	3 oz	0	.13	.23	3.26	.4	6.8	2.83	0.0	7.65	2.6	22.1	340.0	3.37
choice, 1/2-inch fat, broiled	3 oz	0	.1	.23	3.06	.34	6.0	2.07	0.0	6.8	2.75	22.95	322.15	4.27
choice, 1/2-inch fat, raw	1 lb	0	.54	.97	13.82	1.72	27.2	11.98	0.0	31.75	10.89	90.72	1415.23	14.11
choice, 1/2-inch fat, roasted	3 oz	0	.08	.23	2.59	.29	6.0	2.17	0.0	6.8	2.69	19.55	289.85	3.8
prime, 1/4-inch fat, broiled	3 oz	0	.09	.22	2.95	.32	5.1	2.03	0.0	6.8	2.63	21.25	307.7	4.07
prime, 1/4-inch fat, raw	1 lb	0	.5	.95	13.38	1.68	27.2	11.66	0.0	31.75	10.48	86.18	1351.73	13.61
prime, 1/4-inch fat, raw	1 oz	0	.03	.06	.84	.1	1.7	.73	0.0	1.98	.65	5.39	84.48	.85
prime, 1/4 inch fat, roasted	3 oz	0	.08	.23	2.52	.28	6.0	2.13	0.0	7.65	2.6	18.7	280.5	3.66
prime, 1/4-inch fat, broiled	3 oz	0	.09	.22	2.95	.32	6.0	2.03	0.0	6.8	2.63	22.1	307.7	4.07
prime, 1/2-inch fat, raw	1 lb	0	.51	.93	13.33	1.68	27.2	11.61	0.0	31.75	10.39	86.18	1342.66	13.47
prime, 1/2-inch fat, roasted	3 oz	0	.07	.22	2.5	.27	6.0	2.12	0.0	7.65	2.58	18.7	277.1	3.61
select, 0-inch fat, broiled	3 oz	0	.1	.25	3.21	.36	6.0	2.13	0.0	5.95	2.92	24.65	340.85	4.54
select, 1/4-inch fat, broiled	3 oz	0	.1	.23	3.03	.33	5.1	2.07	0.0	6.8	2.72	22.1	317.9	4.22
select, 1/4-inch fat, raw	1 lb	0	.5	.91	13.29	1.68	27.2	11.57	0.0	31.75	10.39	86.18	1338.12	13.47
select, 1/4-inch fat, raw	1 oz	0	.03	.06	.83	.1	1.7	.72	0.0	1.98	.65	5.39	83.63	.84
select, 1/4-inch fat, roasted	3 oz	0	.07	.22	2.52	.21	6.0	2.08	0.0	7.65	2.6	18.7	277.1	3.37

Food Name	Serving Size	A I.U.	Thi mg	Rib mg	Nia mg	B₆ mg	Fol mcg	B₁₂ mcg	C mg	Calc mg	Iron mg	Mag mg	Pot mg	Zn mg
select, 1/2-inch fat, broiled	3 oz	0	.1	.23	3.09	.34	6.0	2.09	0.0	6.8	2.79	23.8	325.55	4.33
select, 1/2-inch fat, raw	1 lb	0	.54	.98	13.96	1.77	27.2	12.07	0.0	31.75	11.02	95.26	1437.91	14.29
select, 1/2-inch fat, roasted	3 oz	0	.08	.24	2.62	.29	6.0	2.18	0.0	6.8	2.74	19.55	294.1	3.85
THYMUS														
braised	3 oz	0	.07	.19	1.56	.07	0.9	1.28	25.7	8.5	1.27	8.5	368.05	1.87
raw	4 oz	0	.12	.39	3.9	.18	2.3	2.41	38.4	7.91	2.37	15.82	406.8	2.33
TONGUE														
potted or deviled	100 gm	0	.04	.11	1.3	.14	4.0	5.02	0.0	20.0	2.7	13.0	164.0	3.79
raw	4 oz	0	.14	.38	4.79	.35	7.9	4.28	3.5	6.78	3.33	18.08	355.95	3.24
simmered	3 oz	0	.03	.3	1.83	.14	4.3	5.01	0.4	5.95	2.88	14.45	153.0	4.08
smoked	100 gm	0	.04	.21	3.0	na	na	na	0.0	8.0	1.6	na	197.0	na
whole, canned or pickled	100 gm	0	.12	.29	5.0	.14	4.0	5.21	0.0	8.0	3.2	16.0	197.0	4.54
TOP LOIN														
Trimmed														
all grades, 0-inch fat, broiled	3 oz	0	.08	.17	4.54	.36	6.8	1.7	0.0	6.8	2.1	22.95	336.6	4.44
all grades, 1/4-inch fat, broiled	3 oz	0	.08	.17	4.54	.36	6.8	1.7	0.0	6.8	2.1	22.95	336.6	4.44
all grades, 1/2-inch fat, broiled	3 oz	0	.08	.17	4.54	.36	6.8	1.7	0.0	6.8	2.1	22.95	336.6	4.44
choice, 0-inch fat, broiled	3 oz	0	.08	.17	4.54	.36	6.8	1.7	0.0	6.8	2.1	22.95	336.6	4.44
choice, 1/4-inch fat, broiled	3 oz	0	.08	.17	4.54	.36	6.8	1.7	0.0	6.8	2.1	22.95	336.6	4.44
choice, 1/2-inch fat, broiled	3 oz	0	.08	.17	4.54	.36	6.8	1.7	0.0	6.8	2.1	22.95	336.6	4.44
prime, 1/4-inch fat, broiled	3 oz	0	.08	.17	4.54	.36	6.8	1.7	0.0	6.8	2.1	22.95	336.6	4.44
prime, 1/2-inch fat, broiled	3 oz	0	.08	.17	4.54	.36	6.8	1.7	0.0	6.8	2.1	22.95	336.6	4.44
select, 0-inch fat, broiled	3 oz	0	.08	.17	4.54	.36	6.8	1.7	0.0	6.8	2.1	22.95	336.6	4.44
select, 1/4-inch fat, broiled	3 oz	0	.08	.17	4.54	.36	6.8	1.7	0.0	6.8	2.1	22.95	336.6	4.44
select, 1/2-inch fat, broiled	3 oz	0	.08	.17	4.54	.36	6.8	1.7	0.0	6.8	2.1	22.95	336.6	4.44
Untrimmed														
all grades, 0-inch fat, broiled	3 oz	0	.08	.16	4.45	.35	6.8	1.69	0.0	6.8	2.07	22.1	329.8	4.34
all grades, 1/4-inch fat, broiled	3 oz	0	.07	.15	3.99	.31	6.0	1.65	0.0	7.65	1.9	19.55	296.65	3.88
all grades, 1/4-inch fat, raw	1 lb	0	.41	.64	17.6	1.77	27.2	12.47	0.0	27.22	7.17	81.65	1338.12	14.21
all grades, 1/2-inch fat, broiled	3 oz	0	.07	.15	4.02	.31	6.0	1.65	0.0	7.65	1.9	20.4	298.35	3.91
all grades, 1/2-inch fat, raw	1 lb	0	.38	.59	16.7	1.68	27.2	12.02	0.0	31.75	6.89	81.65	1256.47	13.47
choice, 0-inch fat, broiled	3 oz	0	.08	.16	4.41	.35	6.8	1.68	0.0	6.8	2.05	22.1	327.25	4.31
choice, 1/4-inch fat, broiled	3 oz	0	.07	.15	3.96	.31	6.0	1.64	0.0	7.65	1.89	19.55	294.1	3.85
choice, 1/4-inch fat, raw	1 lb	0	.41	.59	17.33	1.72	27.2	12.34	0.0	27.22	7.08	81.65	1315.44	14.02
choice, 1/2-inch fat, broiled	3 oz	0	.07	.15	4.0	.31	6.0	1.65	0.0	7.65	1.9	20.4	297.5	3.89
choice, 1/2-inch fat, raw	1 lb	0	.37	.59	16.62	1.68	27.2	11.98	0.0	31.75	6.85	77.11	1251.94	13.38
prime, 1/4-inch fat, broiled	3 oz	0	.07	.15	3.96	.31	6.0	1.64	0.0	7.65	1.89	19.55	294.1	3.85
prime, 1/4-inch fat, raw	1 lb	0	.36	.59	16.87	1.72	27.2	12.11	0.0	27.22	6.94	77.11	1274.62	13.65
prime, 1/2-inch fat, broiled	3 oz	0	.07	.15	3.84	.31	6.0	1.63	0.0	7.65	1.84	19.55	285.6	3.73
prime, 1/2-inch fat, raw	1 lb	0	.37	.59	16.41	1.68	27.2	11.84	0.0	31.75	6.8	77.11	1229.26	13.2
select, 0-inch fat, broiled	3 oz	0	.08	.16	4.45	.35	6.8	1.69	0.0	6.8	2.07	22.1	329.8	4.34
select, 1/4-inch fat, broiled	3 oz	0	.07	.15	4.05	.32	6.0	1.65	0.0	7.65	1.92	20.4	300.9	3.95
select, 1/4-inch fat, raw	1 lb	0	.41	.64	17.74	1.77	27.2	12.52	0.0	27.22	7.21	86.18	1351.73	14.33
select, 1/2-inch fat, broiled	3 oz	0	.07	.15	4.07	.32	6.0	1.65	0.0	7.65	1.92	20.4	301.75	3.96
select, 1/2-inch fat, raw	1 lb	0	.38	.6	16.99	1.72	27.2	12.16	0.0	27.22	6.99	81.65	1283.69	13.7
TRIPE														
pickled	100 gm	0	0	.15	1.6	.14	4.0	5.02	0.0	127.0	1.6	13.0	19.0	3.79
raw	4 oz	0	.01	.19	.07	.05	2.3	1.74	3.8	10.17	2.2	9.04	305.1	2.79
BEEF, CORNED														
brisket, cured, cooked	3 oz	0	.02	.14	2.58	.2	5.1	1.39	13.6	6.8	1.58	10.2	123.25	3.89
brisket, cured, raw	1 lb	0	.2	.71	16.6	1.32	22.7	8.07	122.5	31.75	7.67	63.5	1347.19	12.93
brisket, cured, raw	1 oz	0	.01	.04	1.04	.08	1.4	.5	7.7	1.98	.48	3.97	84.2	.81
canned, cured	1 oz	0	.01	.04	.69	.04	2.6	.46	0.4	3.4	.59	3.97	38.56	1.01
BEEF, CORNED, HASH														
canned (Mary Kitchen)	1 oz	na	na	na	na	na	na	na	na	na	na	na	70	na
canned, w/potato	1 cup	0	.02	.2	4.62	na	na	na	0.0	28.6	4.4	na	440.0	na

Food Name	Serving Size	A I.U.	Thi mg	Rib mg	Nia mg	B_6 mg	Fol mcg	B_{12} mcg	C mg	Calc mg	Iron mg	Mag mg	Pot mg	Zn mg
BEEF, DRIED														
chipped, cooked, creamed	1 cup	882	.15	.47	1.47	na	na	na	1.5	257.25	1.96	na	374.85	na
cured	1 oz	0	.02	.06	1.55	.1	3.1	.75	4.2	1.7	1.28	9.07	125.87	1.49
BEEF, GROUND														
Extra lean														
baked, medium-cooked	3 oz	0	.03	.2	3.54	.19	7.7	1.47	0.0	5.95	1.94	14.45	190.4	4.54
baked, well-done	3 oz	0	.04	.26	4.6	.25	9.4	1.58	0.0	7.65	2.52	18.7	247.35	5.9
broiled, medium-cooked	3 oz	0	.05	.23	4.22	.23	7.7	1.84	0.0	5.95	2.0	17.85	266.05	4.63
broiled, well-done	3 oz	0	.06	.27	4.97	.27	9.4	2.18	0.0	7.65	2.35	21.25	313.65	5.47
pan-fried, medium-cooked	3 oz	0	.05	.22	4.0	.23	7.7	1.7	0.0	5.95	2.01	17.85	265.2	4.61
pan-fried, well-done	3 oz	0	.06	.26	4.62	.26	8.5	1.97	0.0	6.8	2.32	20.4	306.0	5.33
raw	1 oz	0	.02	.07	1.28	.07	2.3	.58	0.0	1.98	.55	5.67	80.51	1.17
raw	4 oz	0	.07	.28	5.12	.29	9.0	2.33	0.0	7.91	2.2	22.6	320.92	4.68
Lean														
baked, medium-cooked	3 oz	0	.04	.16	3.64	.17	7.7	1.5	0.0	7.65	1.78	14.45	190.4	4.33
baked, well-done	3 oz	0	.06	.2	4.64	.22	10.2	1.92	0.0	10.2	2.26	17.85	243.1	5.53
broiled, medium-cooked	3 oz	0	.04	.18	4.39	.22	7.7	2.0	0.0	9.35	1.79	17.85	255.85	4.56
broiled, well-done	3 oz	0	.05	.2	5.07	.26	9.4	2.31	0.0	10.2	2.08	20.4	296.65	5.27
pan-fried, medium-cooked	3 oz	0	.04	.19	4.07	.24	7.7	1.93	0.0	8.5	1.85	17.0	254.15	4.42
pan-fried, well-done	3 oz	0	.05	.2	4.63	.27	8.5	2.19	0.0	9.35	2.11	19.55	289.0	5.02
raw	1 oz	0	.01	.06	1.28	.07	2.3	.66	0.0	2.27	.5	5.1	73.99	1.09
raw	4 oz	0	.06	.24	5.1	.28	9.0	2.64	0.0	9.04	2.0	20.34	294.93	4.36
Regular														
baked, medium-cooked	3 oz	0	.03	.14	4.04	.2	7.7	1.99	0.0	8.5	2.05	12.75	187.85	4.16
baked, well-done	3 oz	0	.03	.17	5.01	.25	9.4	2.47	0.0	10.2	2.54	16.15	232.9	5.16
broiled, frozen patty, medium-cooked	3 oz	0	.04	.17	4.48	.22	7.7	2.1	0.0	9.35	1.78	17.0	249.9	4.59
broiled, medium-cooked	3 oz	0	.03	.16	4.9	.23	7.7	2.49	0.0	9.35	2.07	17.0	248.2	4.4
broiled, well-done	3 oz	0	.03	.18	5.5	.26	8.5	2.79	0.0	10.2	2.33	18.7	277.95	4.94
pan-fried, medium-cooked	3 oz	0	.03	.17	4.96	.2	7.7	2.3	0.0	9.35	2.08	17.0	255.0	4.31
pan-fried well-done	3 oz	0	.03	.18	5.49	.23	8.5	2.55	0.0	11.05	2.3	18.7	282.2	4.78
raw	1 oz	0	.01	.04	1.27	.07	2.0	.75	0.0	2.27	.49	4.54	64.64	1.01
raw	4 oz	0	.04	.17	5.06	.27	7.9	2.99	0.0	9.04	1.95	18.08	257.64	4.01
raw, frozen patty	3 oz	0	.04	.16	3.83	.21	6.0	2.04	0.0	6.8	1.51	14.45	210.8	3.23
BEEF DINNER, FROZEN. See also BEEF ENTRÉE, FROZEN.														
'Extra Helping' (Banquet)	16 oz	na	na	na	na	na	na	na	na	na	na	na	720	na
Salisbury steak 'Classics' (Armour)	11.25 oz	na	na	na	na	na	na	na	na	na	na	na	530	na
Salisbury steak 'Classics Lite' (Armour)	11.5 oz	na	na	na	na	na	na	na	na	na	na	na	660	na
Salisbury steak, parmigiana 'Classics' (Armour)	11.5 oz	na	na	na	na	na	na	na	na	na	na	na	540	na
BEEF ENTRÉE, CANNED														
chow mein, 'Bi-Pack' (LaChoy)	8.748 oz	na	na	na	na	na	na	na	10.8	3.43	11.58	na	na	na
Oriental, w/noodles, 'Bi-Pack' (LaChoy)	9 oz	na	na	na	na	na	na	na	33.8	2.29	15.76	na	na	na
pepper Oriental, 'Bi-Pack' (LaChoy)	8.783 oz	na	na	na	na	na	na	na	11.6	2.36	12.17	na	na	na
stew (Dinty Moore)	8 oz	na	na	na	na	na	na	na	na	na	na	na	527	na
stew (Wolf Brand)	1 cup	8090	.02	.3	3.49	.17	13.0	2	na	34	1.89	26	417	2
BEEF ENTRÉE, FROZEN. See also BEEF DINNER, FROZEN.														
creamed, chipped (Stouffer's)	5.5 oz	na	na	na	na	na	na	na	na	na	na	na	310	na
homestyle, w/noodles, gravy, and vegetable (Stouffer's)	8 3/8 oz	na	na	na	na	na	na	na	na	na	na	na	400	na
pepper, Oriental (Chun King)	13 oz	na	na	na	na	na	na	na	na	na	na	na	370	na
pie (Stouffer's)	10 oz	na	na	na	na	na	na	na	na	na	na	na	300	na
Salisbury steak (Dining Lite)	9 oz	na	na	na	na	na	na	na	na	na	na	na	650	na
Salisbury steak, homestyle, w/gravy, macaroni and cheese (Stouffer's)	9 5/8 oz	na	na	na	na	na	na	na	na	na	na	na	310	na
steak and mushroom hand-held pie, 'Aussie Pie' (Mrs. Paterson's)	5.5 oz	na	na	na	na	na	na	na	na	na	na	na	351	na
BEEF POT PIE. See BEEF ENTRÉE, FROZEN.														

Food Name	Serving Size	A I.U.	Thi mg	Rib mg	Nia mg	B$_6$ mg	Fol mcg	B$_{12}$ mcg	C mg	Calc mg	Iron mg	Mag mg	Pot mg	Zn mg
BEEF STEW. See BEEF ENTRÉE, CANNED.														
BEEF SUET, raw	1 oz	0	0	0	.07	.01	0.3	.08	0.0	.57	.05	.28	4.54	.06
BEEF TALLOW														
	1 cup	0	0	0	0	0	0.0	0	0.0	0	0	0	.02	0
	1 tbsp	0	0	0	0	0	0.0	0	0.0	0	0	0	0	0
BEEFALO														
raw	1 lb	0	.18	.41	21.05	na	68.0	10.98	31.8	81.65	10.52	na	1977.7	22.04
raw	1 oz	0	.01	.03	1.3	na	4.2	.68	2.0	5.04	.65	na	122.08	1.36
roasted	3 oz	0	.03	.09	4.16	na	15.3	2.17	7.7	20.4	2.59	na	390.15	5.44
BEER. See ALCOHOLIC BEVERAGES.														
BEER, NONALCOHOLIC. See ALCOHOL-FREE BEVERAGES.														
BEERWURST														
beef, 4 inch diam	1/8-inch slice	0	.02	.03	.78	.04	0.7	.45	3.7	2.07	.35	2.76	40.02	.56
beef, 2.75 inch diam	1/16-inch slice	0	0	.01	.2	.01	0.2	.12	1.0	.54	.09	.72	10.44	.15
pork, 4 inch diam	1/8-inch slice	0	.13	.04	.75	.08	0.7	.2	6.7	1.84	.17	2.99	58.19	.4
pork, 2.75 inch diam	1/16-inch slice	0	.03	.01	.2	.02	0.2	.05	1.7	.48	.05	.78	15.18	.1
pork, cured, 4 inch diam	1/8-inch slice	0	.13	.04	.75	.08	0.7	.2	6.7	1.84	.17	2.99	58.19	.4
pork, cured, 2.75 inch diam	1/16-inch slice	0	.03	.01	.2	.02	0.2	.05	1.7	.48	.05	.78	15.18	.1
BEET														
boiled, drained, sliced	1/2 cup	30	.02	.03	.28	.06	68.0	0	3.1	13.6	.67	19.55	259.25	.3
raw, sliced	1/2 cup	26	.02	.03	.23	.05	74.1	0	3.3	10.88	.54	15.64	221.0	.24
BEET, CANNED														
Harvard, sliced, w/liquid	1/2 cup	14	.01	.06	.1	.07	35.7	0	3.0	13.53	.44	23.37	201.72	.28
pickled *(Freshlike)*	1/2 cup	na	na	na	na	na	na	na	na	na	na	na	210	na
pickled, sliced, w/liquid	1/2 cup	13	.01	.05	.29	.06	30.2	0	2.6	12.54	.47	17.1	168.72	.3
regular pack, w/liquid	1/2 cup	14	.01	.05	.19	.07	35.7	0	4.8	17.22	.82	19.68	174.66	.28
sliced, drained	1/2 cup	9	.01	.03	.13	.05	25.7	0	3.5	12.75	1.55	14.45	125.8	.18
sliced, water packed, w/o salt *(Freshlike)*	1/2 cup	na	na	na	na	na	na	na	na	na	na	na	210	na
sliced, water packed, w/o sugar or salt *(Freshlike)*	1/2 cup	na	na	na	na	na	na	na	na	na	na	na	210	na
small, sliced *(Freshlike)*	1/2 cup	na	na	na	na	na	na	na	na	na	na	na	210	na
small, whole *(Freshlike)*	1/2 cup	na	na	na	na	na	na	na	na	na	na	na	210	na
special dietary pack, w/liquid	1/2 cup	14	.01	.05	.19	.07	35.7	0	4.8	17.22	.82	19.68	174.66	.28
BEET GREENS														
boiled, drained, 1-inch pieces	1/2 cup	3672	.08	.21	.36	.1	10.3	0	17.9	82.08	1.37	48.96	654.48	.36
raw, approx 2 oz	1 leaf	1952	.03	.07	.13	.03	4.7	0	9.6	38.08	1.06	23.04	175.04	.12
raw, 1-inch pieces	1/2 cup	1159	.02	.04	.08	.02	2.8	0	5.7	22.61	.63	13.68	103.93	.07
BELLYFISH. See MONKFISH.														
BERLINER														
beef and pork	1 oz	0	.11	.06	.88	.06	1.4	.76	2.0	3.4	.33	4.25	80.23	.7
beef and pork, 2.5 inch diam	1/4-inch slice	0	.09	.05	.72	.05	1.2	.61	1.6	2.76	.26	3.45	65.09	.57
BERRY DRINK														
berry citrus drink, frozen, prepared *(Five Alive)*	6 oz	na	na	na	na	na	na	na	6.0	na	na	na	90	na
berry punch, aseptic box or chilled *(Minute Maid)*	6 oz	na	na	na	na	na	na	na	1.0	na	na	na	20	na
berry punch, frozen concentrate *(Minute Maid)*	6 oz	na	na	na	na	na	na	na	1.0	na	na	na	20	na
'Bopin' Berry' *(Hi-C)*	6 oz	na	na	na	na	na	na	na	60.0	na	na	na	20	na
Mountain Berry Punch *(Kool-Aid)* 'Koolers'	8.45 oz	na	na	na	na	na	na	na	na	na	na	na	40	na
BERRY DRINK MIX														
berry blend, sugar-free w/NutraSweet, prepared *(Crystal Light)*	8 oz	na	na	na	na	na	na	na	na	na	na	na	45	na

BEVERAGES. See ALCOHOL-FREE BEVERAGES; ALCOHOLIC BEVERAGES; COFFEE; MILK; SOFT DRINKS AND MIXERS; SPORTS DRINK; TEA; WATER; and individual listings.

BIBB LETTUCE. See LETTUCE.

Food Name	Serving Size	A IU	Thi mg	Rib mg	Nia mg	B6 mg	Fol mcg	B12 mcg	C mg	Calc mg	Iron mg	Mag mg	Pot mg	Zn mg
BISCUIT, REFRIGERATED														
(Ballard) buttermilk, extra lights, 'Ovenready'	1 biscuit	na	na	na	na	na	na	na	na	na	na	na	105	na
(Ballard) extra lights, 'Ovenready'	1 biscuit	na	na	na	na	na	na	na	na	na	na	na	105	na
(Big Country) 'Butter Tastin'	1 biscuit	na	na	na	na	na	na	na	na	na	na	na	90	na
(Big Country) buttermilk	1 biscuit	na	na	na	na	na	na	na	na	na	na	na	90	na
(Big Country) Southern style	1 biscuit	na	na	na	na	na	na	na	na	na	na	na	90	na
(1869 Brand) baking powder	1 biscuit	na	na	na	na	na	na	na	na	na	na	na	30	na
(1869 Brand) 'Butter Tastin'	1 biscuit	na	na	na	na	na	na	na	na	na	na	na	25	na
(1869 Brand) buttermilk	1 biscuit	na	na	na	na	na	na	na	na	na	na	na	30	na
(Good 'N Buttery) fluffy	1 biscuit	na	na	na	na	na	na	na	na	na	na	na	75	na
(Grands Inch) 'Butter Tastin'	1 biscuit	na	na	na	na	na	na	na	na	na	na	na	65	na
(Grands Inch) cinnamon raisin	1 biscuit	na	na	na	na	na	na	na	na	na	na	na	95	na
(Grands Inch) flaky	1 biscuit	na	na	na	na	na	na	na	na	na	na	na	35	na
(Hungry Jack) buttermilk, 'Extra Rich'	1 biscuit	na	na	na	na	na	na	na	na	na	na	na	100	na
(Hungry Jack) buttermilk, flaky	1 biscuit	na	na	na	na	na	na	na	na	na	na	na	15	na
(Hungry Jack) buttermilk, fluffy	1 biscuit	na	na	na	na	na	na	na	na	na	na	na	15	na
(Hungry Jack) flaky	1 biscuit	na	na	na	na	na	na	na	na	na	na	na	15	na
(Hungry Jack) flaky, 'Butter Tastin"	1 biscuit	na	na	na	na	na	na	na	na	na	na	na	15	na
(Hungry Jack) honey, flaky, 'Honey Tastin"	1 biscuit	na	na	na	na	na	na	na	na	na	na	na	15	na
(Hungry Jack) Southern style, flaky	1 biscuit	na	na	na	na	na	na	na	na	na	na	na	15	na
(Pillsbury) 'Big Premium Heat 'n Eat'	2 biscuits	na	na	na	na	na	na	na	na	na	na	na	75	na
(Pillsbury) butter	1 biscuit	na	na	na	na	na	na	na	na	na	na	na	105	na
(Pillsbury) buttermilk	1 biscuit	na	na	na	na	na	na	na	na	na	na	na	105	na
(Pillsbury) buttermilk, 'Heat 'n Eat'	2 biscuits	na	na	na	na	na	na	na	na	na	na	na	55	na
(Pillsbury) buttermilk, 'Tender Layer'	1 biscuit	na	na	na	na	na	na	na	na	na	na	na	100	na
(Pillsbury) 'Country'	1 biscuit	na	na	na	na	na	na	na	na	na	na	na	105	na
BISON. See BUFFALO, AMERICAN.														
BLACK BEAN														
boiled	1/2 cup	5	.21	.05	.43	.06	128.0	0	0.0	23.22	1.81	60.2	305.3	.96
raw	1/2 cup	16	.87	.19	1.9	.28	431.0	0	0.0	119.31	4.87	165.87	1438.51	3.54
BLACK BEAN, CANNED														
(Eden Foods) organic, very low sodium, no salt added	1/2 cup	na	na	na	na	na	na	na	na	na	na	na	260	na
BLACK PUDDING. See BLOOD SAUSAGE.														
BLACK TURTLE BEAN														
boiled	1/2 cup	6	.21	.05	.48	.07	78.7	0	0.0	50.6	2.62	45.08	398.36	.7
canned	1/2 cup	5	.17	.14	.74	.07	73.0	0	3.2	42.0	2.28	42.0	369.6	.65
raw	1/2 cup	16	.83	.18	1.8	.26	408.8	0	0.0	147.2	8.0	147.2	1380.0	2.02
BLACKBERRY, raw	1/2 cup	119	.02	.03	.29	.04	24.5	0	15.1	23.04	.41	14.4	141.12	.19
BLACKBERRY, CANNED														
in heavy syrup, w/liquid	1/2 cup	280	.03	.05	.37	.05	33.9	0	3.6	26.88	.83	21.76	126.72	.23
BLACKBERRY, FROZEN														
unsweetened	18-oz pkg	581	.15	.23	6.16	.31	173.4	0	15.8	147.9	4.08	112.2	714.0	1.28
unsweetened	1 cup	172	.04	.07	1.82	.09	51.3	0	4.7	43.79	1.21	33.22	211.4	.38
BLOOD PUDDING. See BLOOD SAUSAGE.														
BLOOD SAUSAGE / black pudding / blood pudding	1 oz	0	.02	.04	.34	.01	1.4	.28	0.0	1.7	1.81	2.27	10.77	.37
approx 5 inches x 4 5/8 inches	1/16-inch slice	0	.02	.03	.3	.01	1.3	.25	0.0	1.5	1.6	2.0	9.5	.33
BLOODY MARY. See ALCOHOLIC BEVERAGES.														
BLOODY MARY MIX. See ALCOHOL-FREE BEVERAGES.														
BLUEBERRY														
trimmed	1 pint	402	.19	.2	1.44	.14	25.7	0	52.3	24.12	.68	20.1	357.78	.44
trimmed	1 cup	145	.07	.07	.52	.05	9.3	0	18.9	8.7	.25	7.25	129.05	.16
BLUEBERRY, CANNED														
in heavy syrup, w/liquid	1/2 cup	82	.04	.07	.14	.05	2.1	0	1.4	6.4	.42	5.12	51.2	.09
BLUEBERRY, FROZEN														
sweetened	10-oz pkg	125	.06	.15	.72	.17	19.0	0	2.8	17.04	1.11	5.68	170.4	.17

Food Name	Serving Size	A I.U.	Thi mg	Rib mg	Nia mg	B_6 mg	Fol mcg	B_{12} mcg	C mg	Calc mg	Iron mg	Mag mg	Pot mg	Zn mg
unsweetened	20-oz pkg	459	.18	.21	2.95	.33	38.0	0	14.2	45.36	1.02	28.35	306.18	.4
unsweetened	1 cup	126	.05	.06	.81	.09	10.4	0	3.9	12.4	.28	7.75	83.7	.11
BLUEFISH														
dry-heat cooked	3 oz	390	.06	.08	6.16	.39	1.7	5.29	0.0	7.65	.53	35.7	405.45	.88
raw	3 oz	338	.05	.07	5.06	.34	1.4	4.58	0.0	5.95	.41	28.05	316.2	.69
BOAR, WILD														
raw	1 lb	0	1.77	.5	18.14	na	na	na	0.0	54.43	na	na	na	na
raw	1 oz	0	.11	.03	1.12	na	na	na	0.0	3.36	na	na	na	na
roasted	3 oz	0	.26	.12	3.58	na	na	na	0.0	13.6	na	na	na	na
BOCKWURST														
	1 oz	7	.12	.05	1.17	.07	1.7	.23	0.0	4.54	.18	5.1	76.55	.44
7 links per lb	1 link	15	.27	.11	2.68	.15	3.9	.53	0.0	10.4	.42	11.7	175.5	1.01
BOK CHOY														
boiled, drained, shredded	1/2 cup	2183	.03	.05	.36	.14	34.5	0	22.1	79.05	.88	9.35	315.35	.14
raw, shredded	1 cup	2100	.03	.05	.35	.14	46.0	0	31.5	73.5	.56	13.3	176.4	.13
shredded *(Dole)*	1/2 cup	1050	na	na	na	na	na	na	16.0	na	na	na	88	na
BORAGE														
boiled, drained	3.5 oz	4385	.06	.16	.94	.09	10.0	0	32.5	102.0	3.64	57.0	491.0	.22
raw, 1-inch pieces	1/2 cup	1848	.03	.07	.4	.04	5.8	0	15.4	40.92	1.45	22.88	206.8	.09
BORECOLE. See KALE.														
BOUILLON. See SOUP.														
BOYSENBERRY, CANNED, in heavy syrup	1/2 cup	51	.03	.04	.29	.05	44.0	0	7.9	23.04	.55	14.08	115.2	.24
BOYSENBERRY, FROZEN														
unsweetened, unthawed	10-oz pkg	190	.15	.11	2.18	.16	179.8	0	8.8	76.68	2.41	45.44	394.76	.62
unsweetened, unthawed	1 cup	88	.07	.05	1.01	.07	83.6	0	4.1	35.64	1.12	21.12	183.48	.29
BRAMBLE. See RASPBERRY.														
BRAZIL NUT/butternut/cream nut/paranut														
shelled, unblanched, approx 6-8 kernels	1 oz	0	.28	.03	.46	.07	1.1	0	0.2	49.98	.97	63.9	170.4	1.3
shelled, unblanched, approx 32 kernels	1 cup	0	1.4	.17	2.27	.35	5.6	0	1.0	246.4	4.76	315.0	840.0	6.43
BREAD. See also BAGEL; BISCUIT; BUN; CROISSANT; ENGLISH MUFFIN; ROLL; MUFFIN/PASTRY, TOASTER.														
BRAN, 'Gold'N Bran' *(Earth Grains)*	1 oz	na	na	na	na	na	na	na	na	na	na	na	55	na
BROWN														
Boston, w/white corn meal, 3.25 inch diam	1/2-inch slice	0	.06	.04	.68	na	na	na	0.0	40.5	.94	na	131.4	na
Boston, w/yellow corn meal, 3.25 inch diam	1/2-inch slice	32	.06	.04	.68	na	na	na	0.0	40.5	.94	na	131.4	na
canned, Boston	1 oz	25	0	.03	.32	.02	2.0	0	0.0	19.85	.6	17.86	90.15	.14
BUTTERMILK														
(Grant's Farm)	1-oz slice	na	na	na	na	na	na	na	na	na	na	na	50	na
CRISP, hard crispbread or toast	4 oz	260	.09	.25	1.24	na	na	na	0.0	22.6	1.47	na	181.93	na
EGG	1 oz	22	.12	.12	1.37	.02	19.9	.03	0.0	26.37	.86	5.39	32.6	.22
FRENCH														
enriched	1 oz	0	.15	.09	1.35	.01	8.8	0	0.0	21.26	.72	7.65	32.04	.25
enriched, 5 inches x 2.5 inches	1 slice	0	.14	.09	1.16	na	na	na	0.0	15.05	.98	na	31.5	na
unenriched, 5 inches x 2.5 inches	1 slice	0	.03	.03	.28	na	na	na	0.0	15.05	.25	na	31.5	na
GRAIN														
honey grain *(Grant's Farm)*	1-oz slice	na	na	na	na	na	na	na	na	na	na	na	45	na
honey grain, 'Family Recipe' *(Colonial)*	1-oz slice	na	na	na	na	na	na	na	na	na	na	na	55	na
honey grain, 'Family Recipe' *(Kilpatrick's)*	1-oz slice	na	na	na	na	na	na	na	na	na	na	na	40	na
honey grain, 'Family Recipe' *(Rainbo)*	1-oz slice	na	na	na	na	na	na	na	na	na	na	na	55	na
mixed grain, toasted	1 oz	0	.1	.09	1.21	.09	10.5	.02	0.1	28.07	1.07	16.44	62.94	.39
mixed grain, whole grain	1 oz	0	.12	.1	1.24	.09	13.6	.02	0.1	25.8	.98	15.03	57.83	.36
multi-grain *(Hearty Grains)*	1 slice	na	na	na	na	na	na	na	na	na	na	na	180	na
7-grain *(Grant's Farm)*	1-oz slice	na	na	na	na	na	na	na	na	na	na	na	60	na
7-grain, 'Light' *(Grant's Farm)*	.75-oz slice	na	na	na	na	na	na	na	na	na	na	na	20	na
12-grain *(Earth Grains)*	1 oz	na	na	na	na	na	na	na	na	na	na	na	50	na
HIGH-CALCIUM														
dark	1 oz	1	.11	.11	1.13	.04	6.2	0	0.0	242.68	1.1	21.26	62.94	.47
light	1 oz	1	.13	.09	1.17	.01	6.0	.01	0.0	204.69	1.01	10.77	53.87	.31

Food Name	Serving Size	A I.U.	Thi mg	Rib mg	Nia mg	B$_6$ mg	Fol mcg	B$_{12}$ mcg	C mg	Calc mg	Iron mg	Mag mg	Pot mg	Zn mg
HONEY OAT NUT *(Earth Grains)*	1 oz	na	na	na	na	na	na	na	na	na	na	na	40	na
HONEY WHEAT BRAN *(Grant's Farm)*	1-oz slice	na	na	na	na	na	na	na	na	na	na	na	70	na
HONEY WHEATBERRY *(Earth Grains)*	1 oz	na	na	na	na	na	na	na	na	na	na	na	50	na
INDIAN FRY, Navajo, 5-inch diam	1 slice	0	.39	.27	3.27	.02	11.7	0	0.0	209.7	3.24	14.4	66.6	.45
OAT														
split top, 'Family Recipe' *(Colonial)*	1-oz slice	na	na	na	na	na	na	na	na	na	na	na	40	na
split top, 'Family Recipe' *(Kilpatrick's)*	1-oz slice	na	na	na	na	na	na	na	na	na	na	na	40	na
split top, 'Family Recipe' *(Rainbo)*	1-oz slice	na	na	na	na	na	na	na	na	na	na	na	40	na
OAT BRAN														
(Grant's Farm)	1-oz slice	na	na	na	na	na	na	na	na	na	na	na	50	na
honey *(Earth Grains)*	1 oz	na	na	na	na	na	na	na	na	na	na	na	50	na
OATMEAL														
country twists *(Hearty Grains)*	1 slice	na	na	na	na	na	na	na	na	na	na	na	150	na
toasted almond *(Grant's Farm)*	1-oz slice	na	na	na	na	na	na	na	na	na	na	na	50	na
PITA														
white, enriched	1 oz	0	.17	.09	1.31	.01	6.8	0	0.0	24.38	.74	7.37	34.02	.24
white, enriched	1 pita	0	.36	.2	2.78	.02	14.4	0	0.0	51.6	1.57	15.6	72.0	.5
white, unenriched	1 oz	0	.08	.03	.61	.01	6.8	0	0.0	24.38	.4	7.37	34.02	.24
white, unenriched	1 pita	0	.16	.06	1.29	.02	14.4	0	0.0	51.6	.84	15.6	72.0	.5
whole-wheat	1 oz	0	.1	.02	.81	.07	9.9	0	0.0	4.25	.82	19.56	48.19	.43
whole-wheat	1 pita	0	.22	.05	1.82	.15	22.4	0	0.0	9.6	1.85	44.16	108.8	.97
PROTEIN, includes gluten	1 oz	1	.1	.11	1.22	.02	9.9	0	0.0	35.15	1.18	14.46	89.3	.3
PUMPERNICKEL														
	1 oz	0	.09	.09	.88	.04	9.6	0	0.0	19.28	.81	15.31	58.97	.42
toasted	1 oz	0	.08	.09	.87	.04	7.4	0	0.0	20.98	.89	17.01	64.64	.46
toasted	1 slice	0	.08	.09	.89	.04	7.5	0	0.0	21.46	.91	17.4	66.12	.47
RAISIN, unenriched	1 oz	1	.05	.05	.46	.02	7.4	0	0.1	20.41	.56	7.94	69.74	.22
RYE														
honey cracked *(Grant's Farm)*	1-oz slice	na	na	na	na	na	na	na	na	na	na	na	55	na
very thin, light *(Earth Grains)*	1 oz	na	na	na	na	na	na	na	na	na	na	na	45	na
SOURDOUGH, 'Light' *(Earth Grains)*	.75 oz	na	na	na	na	na	na	na	na	na	na	na	20	na
WHEAT														
	1 oz	0	.12	.08	1.17	.03	11.6	0	0.0	29.77	.94	13.04	56.98	.29
cracked	1 oz	0	.1	.07	1.04	.09	11.1	.01	0.0	12.19	.8	14.74	50.18	.35
cracked *(Earth Grains)*	1 oz	na	na	na	na	na	na	na	na	na	na	na	50	na
cracked wheat and honey twists														
(Hearty Grains)	1 serving	na	na	na	na	na	na	na	na	na	na	na	150	na
'Family Recipe' *(Colonial)*	1-oz slice	na	na	na	na	na	na	na	na	na	na	na	45	na
'Family Recipe' *(Kilpatrick's)*	1-oz slice	na	na	na	na	na	na	na	na	na	na	na	45	na
'Family Recipe' *(Rainbo)*	1-oz slice	na	na	na	na	na	na	na	na	na	na	na	55	na
'Light' *(Grant's Farm)*	.75-oz slice	na	na	na	na	na	na	na	na	na	na	na	115	na
'Light 35' *(Earth Grains)*	1 oz	na	na	na	na	na	na	na	na	na	na	na	25	na
loaf *(Pipin' Hot)*	1-inch slice	na	na	na	na	na	na	na	na	na	na	na	15	na
stone ground *(Grant's Farm)*	1-oz slice	na	na	na	na	na	na	na	na	na	na	na	60	na
stone ground, 'Family Recipe' *(Kilpatrick's)*	1-oz slice	na	na	na	na	na	na	na	na	na	na	na	45	na
stone ground, 'Family Recipe' *(Rainbo)*	1-oz slice	na	na	na	na	na	na	na	na	na	na	na	45	na
very thin *(Earth Grains)*	1 oz	na	na	na	na	na	na	na	na	na	na	na	30	na
WHEAT GERM	1 oz	0	.1	.11	1.28	.03	15.6	.02	0.1	25.23	.98	9.92	72.01	.38
WHEATBERRY *(Grant's Farm)*	1-oz slice	na	na	na	na	na	na	na	na	na	na	na	190	na
WHITE														
	1 oz	0	.13	.1	1.13	.02	9.6	.01	0.0	30.62	.86	6.8	33.74	.18
'Light' *(Grant's Farm)*	.75-oz slice	na	na	na	na	na	na	na	na	na	na	na	20	na
'Light 35' *(Earth Grains)*	1 oz	na	na	na	na	na	na	na	na	na	na	na	15	na
special recipe, 'Iron Kids' *(Rainbo)*	1 slice	na	na	na	na	na	na	na	na	na	na	na	30	na
very thin *(Earth Grains)*	1 oz	na	na	na	na	na	na	na	na	na	na	na	40	na
white loaf *(Pipin' Hot)*	1-inch slice	na	na	na	na	na	na	na	na	na	na	na	20	na

Food Name	Serving Size	A I.U.	Thi mg	Rib mg	Nia mg	B$_6$ mg	Fol mcg	B$_{12}$ mcg	C mg	Calc mg	Iron mg	Mag mg	Pot mg	Zn mg
WHOLE WHEAT														
.... 1 oz	1 oz	0	.1	.06	1.09	.05	14.2	0	0.0	20.41	.94	24.38	71.44	.55
100% whole wheat (Earth Grains) .... 1 oz	1 oz	na	na	na	na	na	na	na	na	na	na	na	60	na
BREAD, QUICK, MIX														
CORNBREAD														
(Ballard) mix only, dry .... 1/16 pkg	1/16 pkg	na	na	na	na	na	na	na	na	na	na	na	45	na
(Ballard) prepared w/1 cup milk, 1 egg .... 1/16 pan	1/16 pan	na	na	na	na	na	na	na	na	na	na	na	100	na
BREAD CRUMBS														
plain .... 1 cup	1 cup	1	.83	.47	7.4	.11	27.0	.02	0.0	245.16	6.61	49.68	238.68	1.32
plain .... 1 oz	1 oz	0	.22	.12	1.94	.03	7.1	.01	0.0	64.35	1.74	13.04	62.65	.35
seasoned .... 1 cup	1 cup	17	.19	.2	3.28	.16	24.0	.04	0.5	118.8	3.82	45.6	324.0	1.09
seasoned .... 1 oz	1 oz	4	.05	.05	.77	.04	5.7	.01	0.1	28.07	.9	10.77	76.55	.26
seasoned (Contadina) .... 1 cup	1 cup	109	.5	.5	6.5	na	na	na	1.4	106	4.98	40.6	164	1.1
seasoned (Contadina) .... 1 tbsp	1 tbsp	9	.04	.04	.55	na	na	na	0.1	8.85	.42	3.39	13.7	.14
BREAD DOUGH														
cornbread twists, refrigerated (Pillsbury) ... 1 twist	1 twist	na	na	na	na	na	na	na	na	na	na	na	15	na
BREADFRUIT														
raw .... 1 cup	1 cup	88	.24	.07	1.98	na	na	0	63.8	37.4	1.19	55.0	1078.0	.26
raw .... 1/4 small	1/4 small	38	.11	.03	.86	na	na	0	27.8	16.32	.52	24.0	470.4	.12
BREADFRUIT SEEDS														
boiled .... 1 oz	1 oz	68	.08	.05	1.51	.08	13.9	0	1.7	17.32	.17	14.2	248.5	.24
raw .... 1 oz	1 oz	73	.14	.09	.12	.09	15.0	0	1.9	10.22	1.04	15.34	267.24	.26
roasted .... 1 oz	1 oz	84	.12	.07	2.1	.12	16.8	0	2.2	24.42	.26	17.61	307.29	.29
BREADNUT TREE SEEDS/Jamaican breadnut														
dried .... 1 oz	1 oz	61	.01	.04	.6	.19	32.1	0	13.2	26.7	1.31	32.66	571.12	.54
raw .... 1 oz	1 oz	70	.02	.02	.25	.11	18.9	0	7.8	27.83	.59	19.31	335.97	.32
BREADSTICK														
soft, refrigerated (Pillsbury) .... 1 stick	1 stick	na	na	na	na	na	na	na	na	na	na	na	25	na
BREAKFAST BAR. See SNACK BAR.														
BREAKFAST DRINK MIX, INSTANT														
CHOCOLATE FLAVOR														
(Carnation) 'Diet Instant Breakfast' dry mix .. 1 pouch	1 pouch	1750	.3	.1	5	.4	100.0	.6	27.0	60	4.5	80	240	3
(Carnation) 'Diet Instant Breakfast' dry mix .. 1 pouch	1 pouch	1750	.3	.17	5	.4	100.0	.6	27.0	100	4.5	80	380	3
(Carnation) 'Instant Breakfast' dry mix ..... 1 pouch	1 pouch	1750	.3	.1	5	.4	100.0	.6	27.0	80	4.5	80	260	3
COFFEE FLAVOR (Carnation) 'Instant Breakfast'														
dry mix .... 1 pouch	1 pouch	1750	.3	.17	5	.4	100.0	.6	27.0	150	4.5	80	340	3
VANILLA FLAVOR														
(Carnation) 'Diet Instant Breakfast' dry mix .. 1 pouch	1 pouch	1750	.3	.17	5	.4	100.0	.6	27.0	150	4.5	80	290	3
(Carnation) 'Instant Breakfast' dry mix ..... 1 pouch	1 pouch	1750	.3	.17	5	.4	100.0	.6	27.0	150	4.5	80	300	3
BREAKFAST STRIPS. See also BACON; BACON, ALTERNATIVE.														
beef, cured, cooked .... 6 oz	6 oz	0	.15	.44	11.0	.53	13.6	5.86	61.2	15.3	5.34	45.9	700.4	10.83
beef, cured, cooked .... 3 slices	3 slices	0	.03	.09	2.2	.11	2.7	1.17	12.2	3.06	1.07	9.18	140.08	2.17
beef, cured, raw .... 3 slices	3 slices	0	.04	.08	2.02	.12	3.4	1.12	16.3	2.72	.84	7.48	104.04	1.63
beef, cured, unheated .... 3 slices	3 slices	0	.04	.08	2.02	.12	3.4	1.12	16.3	2.72	.84	7.48	104.04	1.63
BROAD BEAN														
immature, boiled, drained .... 100 gm	100 gm	270	.13	.09	1.2	.03	57.8	0	19.8	18.0	1.5	31.0	193.0	.47
immature, raw .... 1 cup	1 cup	382	.19	.12	1.64	.04	105.0	0	36.0	23.98	2.07	41.42	272.5	.63
mature, boiled .... 1/2 cup	1/2 cup	13	.08	.08	.6	.06	88.5	0	0.3	30.6	1.27	36.55	227.8	.86
mature, raw .... 1/2 cup	1/2 cup	40	.42	.25	2.12	.27	317.2	0	1.1	77.25	5.03	144.0	796.5	2.36
BROCCOLI														
boiled, drained, chopped .... 1/2 cup	1/2 cup	1083	.04	.09	.45	.11	39.0	0	58.2	35.88	.66	18.72	227.76	.3
florets, raw, chopped .... 1/2 cup	1/2 cup	1320	.03	.05	.28	.07	31.2	0	41.0	21.12	.39	11.0	143.0	.18
fresh (Dole) .... 1 med spear	1 med spear	721	na	na	na	na	na	na	139.0	na	na	na	572	na
leaves, raw, chopped .... 1/2 cup	1/2 cup	7040	.03	.05	.28	.07	31.2	0	41.0	21.12	.39	11.0	143.0	.18
raw, chopped .... 1/2 cup	1/2 cup	678	.03	.05	.28	.07	31.2	0	41.0	21.12	.39	11.0	143.0	.18
BROCCOLI, FROZEN														
chopped (Birds Eye) .... 3.3 oz	3.3 oz	na	na	na	na	na	na	na	na	na	na	na	190	na

Food Name	Serving Size	A I.U.	Thi mg	Rib mg	Nia mg	B6 mg	Fol mcg	B12 mcg	C mg	Calc mg	Iron mg	Mag mg	Pot mg	Zn mg
chopped, boiled, drained	1/2 cup	1741	.05	.07	.42	.12	51.9	0	36.9	46.92	.56	10.4	106.6	.28
chopped, unprepared	10-oz pkg	5867	.15	.27	1.33	.37	190.3	0	160.2	155.04	2.3	51.12	602.08	1.36
cuts (Birds Eye)	3.2 oz	na	na	na	na	na	na	na	na	na	na	na	200	na
florets, 'Deluxe' (Birds Eye)	3.3 oz	na	na	na	na	na	na	na	na	na	na	na	220	na
spears (Birds Eye)	3.3 oz	na	na	na	na	na	na	na	na	na	na	na	220	na
spears, baby, 'Deluxe' (Birds Eye)	3.3 oz	na	na	na	na	na	na	na	na	na	na	na	250	na
spears, boiled, drained	10-oz pkg	4730	.14	.2	1.15	.33	75.0	0	100.3	127.5	1.52	50.0	450.0	.75
spears, boiled, drained	1/2 cup	1741	.05	.07	.42	.12	27.6	0	36.9	46.92	.56	18.4	165.6	.28
spears, unprepared	10-oz pkg	4058	.2	.32	1.31	.5	267.8	0	194.0	116.44	2.04	45.44	710.0	.97
spears and florets, 'Deluxe' (Birds Eye)	3.3 oz	na	na	na	na	na	na	na	na	na	na	na	220	na

BROTH. See SOUP.

BROWN BREAD. See BREAD.

BRUSSELS SPROUTS

boiled, drained	1/2 cup	561	.08	.06	.47	.14	46.8	0	48.4	28.08	.94	15.6	247.26	.26
boiled, drained	1 sprout	151	.02	.02	.13	.04	12.6	0	13.0	7.56	.25	4.2	66.57	.07
fresh (Dole)	1/2 cup	389	na	na	na	na	na	na	37.0	na	na	na	171	na
raw	1/2 cup	389	.06	.04	.33	.1	26.9	0	37.4	18.48	.62	10.12	171.16	.18
raw	1 sprout	168	.03	.02	.14	.04	11.6	0	16.2	7.98	.27	4.37	73.91	.08

BRUSSELS SPROUTS, FROZEN

boiled, drained	1/2 cup	459	.08	.09	.42	.23	78.9	0	35.7	18.72	.58	18.72	253.5	.28
(Birds Eye)	3.3 oz	na	na	na	na	na	na	na	na	na	na	na	330	na

BUCKWHEAT, whole-grain	1/2 cup	0	.09	.36	5.97	.18	25.5	0	0.0	15.3	1.87	196.35	391.0	2.04
BUCKWHEAT FLOUR, whole-groat	1/2 cup	0	.25	.11	3.69	.35	32.4	0	0.0	24.6	2.44	150.6	346.2	1.87

BUCKWHEAT GROATS/kasha

roasted, cooked	1/2 cup	0	.04	.04	.93	.08	13.9	0	0.0	6.93	.79	50.49	87.12	.6
roasted, dry	1/2 cup	0	.18	.22	4.21	.29	34.4	0	0.0	13.94	2.03	181.22	262.4	1.98

BUFFALO, AMERICAN/bison

raw	1 lb	0	na	na	na	na	na	na	0.0	27.22	11.79	113.4	1555.85	12.7
raw	1 oz	0	na	na	na	na	na	na	0.0	1.68	.73	7.0	96.04	.78

BULGUR

cooked	1/2 cup	0	.05	.03	.91	.08	16.4	0	0.0	9.1	.87	29.12	61.88	.52
dry	1/2 cup	0	.16	.08	3.58	.24	18.9	0	0.0	24.5	1.72	114.8	287.0	1.35

BULLOCK'S HEART. See CUSTARD APPLE.

BUN. See also BISCUIT; CROISSANT; ENGLISH MUFFIN; ROLL.

brown and serve, partially baked	2.5-inch roll	0	.02	.02	.21	na	na	na	0.0	13.26	.18	na	26.0	na
brown and serve, partially baked, unbrowned	2.5-inch roll	0	.01	.02	.19	na	na	na	0.0	12.22	.18	na	23.66	na
enriched, browned	2.5-inch roll	0	.1	.08	.86	na	na	na	0.0	13.26	.78	na	26.0	na
enriched, unbrowned	2.5-inch roll	0	.1	.08	.84	na	na	na	0.0	13.16	.76	na	25.48	na
hard, enriched, ready to cook	3.75-inch roll	0	.2	.12	1.65	na	na	na	0.0	23.5	1.4	na	48.5	na
hard, enriched, ready to cook	2.5-inch roll	0	.1	.06	.83	na	na	na	0.0	11.75	.7	na	24.25	na
hard, unenriched, ready to cook	3.75-inch roll	0	.02	.05	.4	na	na	na	0.0	23.5	.4	na	48.5	na
hard, unenriched, ready to cook	2.5-inch roll	0	.01	.02	.2	na	na	na	0.0	11.75	.2	na	24.25	na

BUN, FRANKFURTER

plain	1 bun	0	.21	.13	1.69	.02	11.6	.01	0.0	59.77	1.36	8.6	60.63	.27
reduced calorie	1 bun	2	.17	.08	2.12	.02	12.9	.11	0.2	25.37	1.29	12.04	33.54	.39
reduced calorie	1 oz	1	.11	.05	1.4	.02	8.5	.07	0.1	16.73	.85	7.94	22.11	.26

BUN, HAMBURGER

mixed grain	1 bun	0	.2	.13	1.92	.04	12.0	0	0.0	40.85	1.7	20.64	64.5	.46
mixed grain	1 oz	0	.13	.09	1.27	.03	7.9	0	0.0	26.93	1.12	13.61	42.53	.3
plain	1 bun	0	.21	.13	1.69	.02	11.6	.01	0.0	59.77	1.36	8.6	60.63	.27
plain	1 oz	0	.14	.09	1.12	.01	7.7	.01	0.0	39.41	.9	5.67	39.97	.18
reduced calorie	1 bun	2	.17	.08	2.12	.02	12.9	.11	0.2	25.37	1.29	12.04	33.54	.39
reduced calorie	1 oz	1	.11	.05	1.4	.02	8.5	.07	0.1	16.73	.85	7.94	22.11	.26

BUN, SWEET

apple honey, multi pak, 1.5 oz (Break Cake)	1 bun	na	na	na	na	na	na	na	na	na	na	na	35	na

Food Name	Serving Size	A I.U.	Thi mg	Rib mg	Nia mg	B₆ mg	Fol mcg	B₁₂ mcg	C mg	Calc mg	Iron mg	Mag mg	Pot mg	Zn mg
honey *(Break Cake)* 3 oz	1 bun	na	na	na	na	na	na	na	na	na	na	na	80	na
honey, multi pak *(Break Cake)*	1 bun	na	na	na	na	na	na	na	na	na	na	na	75	na
BURBOT														
dry-heat cooked	3 oz	14	.36	.15	1.68	.29	0.9	.78	0.0	54.4	.98	34.85	440.3	.82
raw	3 oz	13	.32	.12	1.38	.26	0.9	.68	0.0	42.5	.77	27.2	343.4	.65
BURDOCK ROOT / gobo														
boiled, drained	1 root	0	.06	.1	.53	.46	32.4	0	4.3	81.34	1.28	64.74	597.6	.63
boiled, drained	1 cup	0	.05	.07	.4	.35	24.4	0	3.3	61.25	.96	48.75	450.0	.48
raw	1 root	0	.02	.05	.47	.37	35.6	0	4.7	63.96	1.25	59.28	480.48	.51
raw, 1-inch pieces	1 cup	0	.01	.04	.35	.28	26.9	0	3.5	48.38	.94	44.84	363.44	.39
BURGER, VEGETARIAN														
frozen, organic *(Amy's Kitchen)*	2.5 oz	na	na	na	na	na	na	na	na	na	na	na	232	na
BURRITO, FROZEN														
(Amy's Kitchen) bean and rice	6 oz	na	na	na	na	na	na	na	na	na	na	na	351	na
BURRITO DINNER MIX														
(Amy's Kitchen) beans, rice, and cheese, organic	6 oz	na	na	na	na	na	na	na	na	na	na	na	337	na
BURRITO DINNER, FROZEN														
beef steak fajita, 'Supreme' 5-oz pkg *(Ruiz)*	1 burrito	na	na	na	na	na	na	na	na	na	na	na	70	na
chicken fajita, 'Supreme' 5-oz pkg *(Ruiz)*	1 burrito	na	na	na	na	na	na	na	na	na	na	na	300	na
BUSH NUT. See MACADAMIA NUT.														
BUTTER, CLARIFIED. See GHEE.														
BUTTER, REGULAR														
lightly salted *(Land O'Lakes)*	1 tbsp	na	na	na	na	na	na	na	na	na	na	na	0	na
unsalted	4-oz stick	3468	.01	.04	.05	0	3.2	.14	0.0	26.65	.18	2.47	29.48	.06
unsalted	1 pat	153	0	0	0	0	0.1	.01	0.0	1.17	.01	.11	1.3	0
BUTTER, WHIPPED														
lightly salted *(Land O'Lakes)*	1 tbsp	na	na	na	na	na	na	na	na	na	na	na	0	na
unsalted *(Land O'Lakes)*	1 tbsp	na	na	na	na	na	na	na	na	na	na	na	0	na
BUTTER FLAVORED OIL *(Wesson)*	1 tbsp	na	na	na	na	na	na	na	0.0	0	0	na	na	na
BUTTER OIL														
anhydrous	1 cup	7688	0	.01	.01	0	0.4	.02	0.0	7.99	0	.9	10.05	.02
anhydrous	1 tbsp	480	0	0	0	0	0.0	0	0.0	.5	0	.06	.63	0
BUTTERBEAN. See LIMA BEAN.														
BUTTERBUR / Fuki														
raw	1 cup	47	.02	.02	.19	.09	9.8	0	29.6	96.82	.09	13.16	615.7	.15
BUTTERBUR, CANNED														
chopped	1 cup	0	.01	.01	.17	.04	3.2	0	14.8	42.16	.78	2.48	14.88	.07
stalks	3 stalks	0	0	0	.06	.01	1.2	0	5.4	15.3	.28	.9	5.4	.03
BUTTERFISH														
dry-heat cooked	3 oz	93	.12	.16	4.9	.29	14.5	1.56	0.0	23.8	.54	27.2	408.85	.84
raw	3 oz	85	.1	.13	3.83	.26	12.8	1.61	0.0	18.7	.43	21.25	318.75	.65
BUTTERHEAD LETTUCE . See LETTUCE.														
BUTTERMILK														
blend, cultured, dry *(Saco Foods)*	3.5 tbsp	na	na	.36	na	na	na	na	na	176	na	na	na	na
BUTTERNUT. See BRAZIL NUT.														
BUTTERNUT SQUASH. See SQUASH, BUTTERNUT.														
BUTTERSCOTCH TOPPING	2 tbsp	37	0	.04	.02	.01	0.8	.04	0.1	21.73	.08	2.87	34.44	.08

C

Food Name	Serving Size	A I.U.	Thi mg	Rib mg	Nia mg	B₆ mg	Fol mcg	B₁₂ mcg	C mg	Calc mg	Iron mg	Mag mg	Pot mg	Zn mg
CABBAGE														
boiled, drained	1 head	1000	.72	.69	3.56	1.43	252.4	0	253.7	391.22	2.15	100.96	1224.14	1.14
boiled, drained, shredded	1/2 cup	99	.04	.04	.21	.08	15.0	0	15.1	23.25	.13	6.0	72.75	.07

Food Name	Serving Size	A I.U.	Thi mg	Rib mg	Nia mg	B₆ mg	Fol mcg	B₁₂ mcg	C mg	Calc mg	Iron mg	Mag mg	Pot mg	Zn mg
raw, approx 2.5 lbs	1 head	1208	.45	.36	2.72	.87	390.4	0	292.4	426.76	5.36	136.2	2233.68	1.63
raw, medium size (Dole)	1/12 head	69	na	na	na	na	na	na	41.0	na	na	na	187	na
raw, shredded	1/2 cup	47	.02	.01	.11	.03	15.1	0	11.3	16.45	.21	5.25	86.1	.06
CABBAGE, DANISH														
fresh	1 head	1144	.45	.27	2.72	.86	514.8	0	463.1	426.76	5.08	136.2	2233.68	1.63
fresh, shredded	1/2 cup	44	.02	.01	.11	.03	19.9	0	17.9	16.45	.2	5.25	86.1	.06
CABBAGE, NAPPA / Chinese cabbage														
boiled, drained	1 leaf	135	.01	.01	.07	.02	7.5	0	2.2	4.48	.04	1.4	31.5	.03
boiled, drained, shredded	1/2 cup	2183	.03	.05	.36	.14	34.5	0	22.1	79.05	.88	9.35	315.35	.14
raw, shredded	1/2 cup	1050	.01	.02	.18	.07	23.0	0	15.8	36.75	.28	6.65	88.2	.07
CABBAGE, RED														
boiled, drained, shredded	1/2 cup	20	.03	.02	.15	.11	9.5	0	25.8	27.75	.26	8.25	105.0	.11
raw, shredded	1/2 cup	14	.02	.01	.11	.07	7.3	0	20.0	17.85	.17	5.25	72.1	.07
CABBAGE, SAVOY														
boiled, drained, shredded	1/2 cup	649	.04	.01	.02	.11	33.8	0	12.4	21.9	.28	17.52	134.32	.17
raw, shredded	1/2 cup	350	.02	.01	.11	.07	28.1	0	10.9	12.25	.14	9.8	80.5	.09
CABBAGE, SKUNK / swamp cabbage / water convolvulus														
boiled, drained, chopped	1/2 cup	2548	.02	.04	.25	.04	17.1	0	7.8	26.46	.65	14.7	139.16	.08
raw	1 shoot	819	0	.01	.12	.01	7.4	0	7.2	10.01	.22	9.23	40.56	.02
CABBAGE TURNIP. See KOHLRABI.														
CAESAR SALAD, Saco Easy Caesar Kit	.75 oz	na	na	na	na	na	na	na	na	na	na	na	227	na
CAKE MIX														
Cheesecake														
lemon 'No Bake' dry mix (Jell-O)	1 pkg	na	na	na	na	na	na	na	na	na	na	na	135	na
New York style 'No Bake' dry mix (Jell-O)	1 pkg	na	na	na	na	na	na	na	na	na	na	na	150	na
'No Bake' dry mix (Jell-O)	1 pkg	na	na	na	na	na	na	na	na	na	na	na	125	na
CALAMARI. See SQUID, MIXED SPECIES.														
CALICO BASS. See SUNFISH.														
CALIFORNIA SHEEPSHEAD. See SHEEPSHEAD.														
CANADIAN BACON. See BACON, CANADIAN-STYLE.														
CANDY														
ALMOND, 'Golden Almond Solitaires' chocolate														
covered (Hershey's)	3 oz	43	.05	.43	.92	.04	17.9	.4	0.2	305.15	1.19	100.3	428.4	1.56
AMARETTO CHOCOLATE, 'Buffalo Ball' confection														
(Great Cakes)	1 ball	na	na	na	na	na	na	na	na	na	na	na	80	na
BAR														
'Almond Joy' 1.76 oz (Hershey's)	1 bar	7	.02	.08	.23	.03	4.0	.06	0.1	39.5	.6	33.0	185.5	.4
'Almond Joy' snack size (Hershey's)	1 bar	3	.01	.03	.09	.01	1.6	.02	0.0	15.8	.24	13.2	74.2	.16
'Alpine White' white chocolate w/almonds														
(Nestlé)	1 bar	29	.03	.15	.03	.03	4.6	.3	0.1	80.85	.2	13.3	146.3	.4
'Alpine White' white chocolate w/almonds,														
2.2 oz (Nestlé)	1 bar	52	.05	.26	.05	.05	8.1	.53	0.3	143.22	.35	23.56	259.16	.7
'A-Ok' fruit juice sweetened														
(Natures Warehouse)	1 oz	na	na	na	na	na	na	na	na	na	na	na	109.7	na
'Baby Ruth' chocolate w/peanuts (Nestlé)	1 bar	0	.06	.05	2.1	.06	30.6	.01	0.0	23.4	.49	42.6	129.0	.41
'Bar None' 1.5 oz (Bar None)	1 bar	57	.03	.12	.68	.03	12.0	.18	0.0	62.35	.52	30.96	168.13	.53
'Brazil Nut Crunch' (Yogafection)	1 oz	na	na	na	na	na	na	na	na	na	na	na	140	na
'Butterfinger' 2.16 oz (Nestlé)	1 bar	40	.09	.03	2.01	.04	18.9	.09	1.7	14.64	.64	27.45	129.32	.45
'Butterfinger' snack size (Nestlé)	1 bar	14	.03	.01	.69	.01	6.5	.03	0.6	5.04	.22	9.45	44.52	.15
'Caramello' 5 oz (Cadbury)	1 bar	466	.07	.57	1.63	.07	9.9	.89	0.7	281.16	1.56	59.64	482.8	1.35
'Caramello' 1.6 oz (Cadbury)	1 bar	148	.02	.18	.52	.02	3.2	.28	0.2	89.1	.5	18.9	153.0	.43
'Cashew Nut Crunch' (Yogafection)	1 oz	na	na	na	na	na	na	na	na	na	na	na	140	na
'Chunky' 1.4 oz (Nestlé)	1 bar	25	.03	.16	.76	.05	8.8	.15	0.1	57.2	.5	29.2	213.6	.74
'Chunky' 1.25 oz (Nestlé)	1 bar	22	.03	.14	.67	.04	7.7	.13	0.1	50.05	.44	25.55	186.9	.64
'Crunch' milk chocolate w/crisp rice,														
snack size (Nestlé)	1 bar	6	.01	.03	.05	.01	0.9	.04	0.0	16.9	.07	4.6	34.4	.11

Food Name	Serving Size	A I.U.	Thi mg	Rib mg	Nia mg	B$_6$ mg	Fol mcg	B$_{12}$ mcg	C mg	Calc mg	Iron mg	Mag mg	Pot mg	Zn mg
'5th Avenue' 4.2 oz (Hershey's)	1 pkg	36	.02	.26	3.89	.11	65.5	.21	0.0	83.3	1.19	74.97	390.32	1.29
'5th Avenue' 2.1 oz (Hershey's)	1 bar	18	.01	.13	1.96	.06	33.0	.11	0.0	42.0	.6	37.8	196.8	.65
'Golden Almond' chocolate w/almonds, 3 oz (Hershey's)	1 bar	125	.05	.45	.9	.04	20.4	.37	0.2	278.8	1.27	94.35	400.35	1.44
'Golden III' 3.2 oz	1 bar	82	.06	.25	.15	.1	10.9	.41	0.8	274.82	.55	60.97	413.14	1.0
'Kit Kat' chocolate covered wafer, 3.375 oz (Hershey's)	1 bar	104	.06	.25	.39	.05	0.0	.66	1.7	172.8	.81	42.24	295.68	.96
'Kit Kat' chocolate covered wafer, 1.625 oz (Hershey's)	1 bar	50	.03	.12	.19	.02	0.0	.32	0.8	82.8	.39	20.24	141.68	.46
'Krackel' chocolate w/rice crisps, 2.6 oz (Hershey's)	1 bar	36	.04	.22	.33	.02	5.9	.43	0.3	132.46	.6	40.7	253.08	.9
'Krackel' chocolate w/rice crisps, 1.65 oz (Hershey's)	1 bar	23	.02	.14	.21	.02	3.8	.27	0.2	84.13	.38	25.85	160.74	.57
'Mars Almond, 1.76 oz (M&M/Mars)	1 bar	81	.02	.16	.47	.03	7.0	.15	0.5	84.0	.55	36.0	162.5	.56
'Milky Way' milk chocolate, 2.1 oz (M&M/Mars)	1 bar	105	.02	.13	.21	.03	5.4	.31	0.5	78.0	.46	20.4	144.6	.43
'Milky Way' milk chocolate, snack size (M&M/Mars)	1 bar	32	.01	.04	.06	.01	1.6	.09	0.2	23.4	.14	6.12	43.38	.13
'Mounds' chocolate covered coconut, 1.9 oz (Hershey's)	1 pkg	5	.01	.03	.02	.02	1.6	0	0.1	12.42	2.04	36.72	113.4	.56
'Mounds' chocolate covered coconut, snack size (Hershey's)	1 bar	2	0	.01	.01	.01	0.6	0	0.0	4.6	.75	13.6	42.0	.21
'Mr. GoodBar' milk chocolate w/peanuts, 2.8 oz (Hershey's)	1 bar	32	.04	.21	3.72	.1	56.9	.36	0.0	87.69	.95	75.05	355.5	1.42
'Mr. GoodBar' milk chocolate w/peanuts, 1.75 oz (Hershey's)	1 bar	20	.02	.14	2.35	.06	36.0	.23	0.0	55.5	.6	47.5	225.0	.9
'My O My' fruit juice sweetened (Natures Warehouse)	1 oz	na	na	na	na	na	na	na	na	na	na	na	103.5	na
'No How' peanut butter, fruit juice sweetened (Natures Warehouse)	1 oz	na	na	na	na	na	na	na	na	na	na	na	129.5	na
'Non Stop' fruit juice sweetened (Natures Warehouse)	1 oz	na	na	na	na	na	na	na	na	na	na	na	92.9	na
'Nut Wit' carob, caramel, and peanuts (Natures Warehouse)	1 oz	na	na	na	na	na	na	na	na	na	na	na	109.7	na
'Oh Henry!' chocolate covered caramel w/peanuts, 2 oz (Nestlé)	1 bar	27	.01	.09	1.6	.04	18.8	.19	0.1	62.13	.32	35.23	184.68	.7
'100 Grand' 1.5 oz (Nestlé)	1 bar	33	.02	.1	.1	.02	2.2	.16	0.0	49.88	.29	14.19	106.64	.26
'Protein Blast' high-energy, chocolate (Weider)	1 bar	na	na	na	na	na	na	na	na	na	na	na	300	na
'Skor' toffee, 1.4 oz (Hershey's)	1 bar	112	.01	.14	.04	.01	2.4	.11	0.1	44.8	.16	13.6	95.2	.3
'Snickers' 2.16 oz (M&M/Mars)	1 bar	72	.03	.11	1.82	.11	24.4	.25	0.2	70.15	.48	36.6	198.86	.7
'Snickers' snack size (M&M/Mars)	1 bar	18	.01	.03	.45	.03	6.0	.06	0.1	17.25	.12	9.0	48.9	.17
'Special Dark' sweet chocolate bar, 2.8 oz (Hershey's)	1 bar	16	.02	.19	.53	.04	3.2	0	0.0	15.01	1.66	90.85	268.6	1.18
'Special Dark' sweet chocolate bar, 1.45 oz (Hershey's)	1 bar	8	.01	.1	.27	.02	1.6	0	0.0	7.79	.86	47.15	139.4	.62
'Symphony' milk chocolate, 2.4 oz (Hershey's)	1 bar	48	.06	.26	.22	.03	4.8	.27	0.3	159.8	.68	37.4	261.8	.77
'Symphony' milk chocolate, 1.4 oz (Hershey's)	1 bar	28	.04	.15	.13	.02	2.8	.16	0.2	94.0	.4	22.0	154.0	.45
'3 Musketeers' 2.13 oz (M&M/Mars)	1 bar	63	.02	.08	.14	.01	0.0	.13	0.2	50.4	.44	17.4	79.8	.33
'3 Musketeers' snack size (M&M/Mars)	1 bar	19	.01	.03	.04	0	0.0	.04	0.1	15.12	.13	5.22	23.94	.1
'Twix' caramel, 2.0 oz (M&M/Mars)	1 pkg	67	.03	.11	.21	.02	4.0	.22	0.1	67.26	.38	16.53	117.42	.39
'Twix' peanut butter, 1.77 oz (M&M/Mars) ...	1 pkg	29	.05	.09	1.73	.05	11.0	.11	0.5	58.5	1.06	38.5	158.0	.73
'Whatchamacallit' 1.8 oz (Hershey's)	1 bar	36	.31	.14	1.06	.03	5.1	.2	0.2	62.22	.46	29.07	177.48	.57
CARAMEL, 'Nip' (Pearson)	1 oz	na	na	na	na	na	na	na	na	na	na	na	70	na
CHERRY, 'Nibs' (Y&S)	1 oz	6	.01	.01	.03	0	0	0	0.0	18.43	.17	1.7	18.14	.05
CHOCOLATE														
'Choc'Oh's' (Saco Foods)	1.5 oz	6	0	.01	.05	na	na	na	0.0	6.85	.21	na	20.0	na

Food Name	Serving Size	A I.U.	Thi mg	Rib mg	Nia mg	B_6 mg	Fol mcg	B_{12} mcg	C mg	Calc mg	Iron mg	Mag mg	Pot mg	Zn mg
chunks *(Saco Foods)*	3.5 oz	0	.02	.08	.53	na	na	na	0.0	27.46	2.4	na	292.21	na
'M&M's' plain *(M&M/Mars)*	10 pieces	7	0	.02	.04	0	0.6	.03	0.0	11.83	.11	4.69	27.37	.09
'M&M's' plain, 1.69 oz *(M&M/Mars)*	1 pkg	49	.03	.12	.26	.03	3.8	.2	0.0	81.12	.73	32.16	187.68	.61
COFFEE, 'Nip' *(Pearson)*	1 oz	na	na	na	na	na	na	na	na	na	na	na	50	na
FONDANT, candy corn	1 cup	0	0	0	0	na	na	na	0.0	28.0	2.2	na	10.0	na
FRUIT														
'Skittles' *(M&M/Mars)* candy coated, bite size, 2.3 oz	1 pkg	0	0	0	0	0	0.0	0	0.0	1.95	.07	.65	14.95	.01
'Twizzlers' *(Y&S)*														
strawberry sticks, 5 oz	1 pkg	0	.03	.06	.14	.01	0.0	0	0.0	49.7	.71	8.52	90.88	.23
strawberry sticks, 2.5 oz	1 pkg	0	.01	.03	.07	.01	0.0	0	0.0	24.85	.35	4.26	45.44	.11
FUDGE, chews, 2.07 oz	1 pkg	0	0	0	0	0	0.0	0	31.2	2.36	.08	.59	1.18	0
LICORICE, 'Nip' *(Pearson)*	1 oz	na	na	na	na	na	na	na	na	na	na	na	50	na
MINT														
'After Eight' dark chocolate *(Rowntree)*	1 mint	na	na	na	na	na	na	na	na	na	na	na	15	na
'Nip' chocolate *(Pearson)*	1 oz	na	na	na	na	na	na	na	na	na	na	na	60	na
'Mint'Oh's' *(Saco Foods)*	1.5 oz	6	0	.01	.05	na	na	na	0.0	6.85	.21	na	20.0	na
'Peppermint Pattie' large patties *(York)*	1 piece	2	.01	.04	.37	0	1.7	.01	0.0	7.31	.65	27.09	50.31	.33
'Peppermint Pattie' small patties *(York)*	1 piece	1	0	.01	.09	0	0.4	0	0.0	1.87	.16	6.93	12.87	.08
PEANUT														
'Goobers' chocolate covered *(Nestlé)*	10 pieces	0	.01	.02	.52	.02	0.8	.03	0.0	12.7	.13	11.9	50.2	.22
'M&M's' candy coated chocolate peanuts *(M&M/Mars)*	10 pieces	7	.01	.04	.64	.04	11.2	.07	0.0	26.6	.3	16.4	78.0	.3
PEANUT BUTTER														
'Reese's Peanut Butter Cups' *(Hershey's)*	1.8 oz	40	.02	.11	2.02	.04	14.3	.23	0.0	39.78	.56	43.35	204.0	.71
'Reese's Peanut Butter Cups' miniatures *(Hershey's)*	6 cups	33	.02	.09	1.67	.04	11.8	.19	0.0	32.76	.46	35.7	168.0	.59
'Reese's Pieces' candy coated *(Hershey's)*	10 pieces	2	0	.02	.46	.01	4.5	.03	0.0	10.64	.12	6.48	35.2	.09
'Reese's Pieces' candy coated, 1.95 oz *(Hershey's)*	1 pkg	11	.03	.13	3.13	.07	30.8	.18	0.3	73.15	.83	44.55	242.0	.61
PECAN, 'Demet's Turtles' milk chocolate, pecans, caramel *(Demet's)*	1 piece	28	.03	.04	.06	.01	1.7	.07	0.1	26.86	.23	8.91	52.36	.24
RAISIN														
'Raisinets' chocolate covered *(Nestlé)*	10 pieces	4	.01	.02	.04	.01	0.5	.02	0.0	10.8	.12	4.5	51.4	.08
'Raisinets' chocolate covered *(Nestlé)*	1.58 oz	17	.04	.1	.18	.05	2.3	.09	0.1	48.6	.54	20.25	231.3	.36
CANNELLONI ENTRÉE, frozen														
cheese *(Dining Lite)*	9 oz	na	na	na	na	na	na	na	na	na	na	na	520	na
CANOLA OIL														
	1 tbsp	0	0	0	0	0	0.0	0	0.0	0	0	0	0	0
(Kroger)	1 tbsp	na	na	na	na	na	na	na	0.0	0	0	na	na	na
(Wesson) 'Food Service'	1 tbsp	na	na	na	na	na	na	na	0.0	0	0	na	na	na
CANTALOUPE / muskmelon														
approx 5 inch diam	1/2 fruit	8608	.1	.06	1.53	.31	45.4	0	112.7	29.37	.56	29.37	825.03	.43
untrimmed *(Dole)*	1/4 fruit	6382	na	na	na	na	na	na	63.0	na	na	na	120	na
CAPE GOOSEBERRY / ground cherry / poha														
raw	1/2 cup	504	.08	.03	1.96	na	na	0	7.7	6.3	.7	na	na	na
CAPPUCCINO. See COFFEE, FLAVORED.														
CARAMBOLA. See STAR FRUIT.														
CARAWAY SEED														
whole	1 tbsp	24	.03	.03	.24	na	na	0	1.4	46.16	1.09	17.29	90.52	.37
whole	1 tsp	8	.01	.01	.08	na	na	0	0.4	14.47	.34	5.42	28.37	.12
whole *(Durkee)*	1 tsp	.14	.15	.15	0	na	na	na	na	0	0	na	0	na
whole *(Laurel Leaf)*	1 tsp	.14	.15	.15	0	na	na	na	na	0	0	na	0	na
CARDAMOM														
ground	1 tbsp	0	.01	.01	.06	na	na	0	na	22.22	.81	13.26	64.89	.43
ground	1 tsp	0	0	0	.02	na	na	0	na	7.66	.28	4.57	22.38	.15
ground *(Durkee)*	1 tsp	na	.07	.09	0	na	na	na	na	0	0	na	0	na

Food Name	Serving Size	A I.U.	Thi mg	Rib mg	Nia mg	B₆ mg	Fol mcg	B₁₂ mcg	C mg	Calc mg	Iron mg	Mag mg	Pot mg	Zn mg
ground *(Laurel Leaf)*	1 tsp	na	.07	.09	0	na	na	na	na	0	0	na	0	na
CARDONI. See CARDOON.														
CARDOON/cardoni														
raw, shredded	1 cup	214	.04	.05	.53	.08	50.4	0	3.6	124.6	1.25	74.76	712.0	.3
raw, shredded	1/2 cup	107	.02	.03	.27	.04	25.2	0	1.8	62.3	.62	37.38	356.0	.15
CARIBOU														
raw	1 lb	0	1.45	3.27	24.95	1.68	18.1	28.62	0.0	77.11	21.27	117.94	1338.12	18.14
raw	1 oz	0	.09	.2	1.54	.1	1.1	1.77	0.0	4.76	1.31	7.28	82.6	1.12
roasted	3 oz	0	.21	.77	4.92	.27	4.3	5.64	2.6	18.7	5.24	22.95	263.5	4.47
CARISSA/natal plum														
raw, sliced	1 cup	60	.06	.09	.3	na	na	0	57.0	16.5	1.96	24.0	390.0	na
raw, w/o skin and seeds, approx .8 oz	1 fruit	8	.01	.01	.04	na	na	0	7.6	2.2	.26	3.2	52.0	na
CAROB FLAVOR DRINK, mix, powder	3 tsp	0	0	0	.09	.01	0.0	0	0.0	3.84	.55	.6	12.48	.01
CAROB FLOUR														
	1 cup	14	.05	.47	1.95	.38	29.9	0	0.2	358.44	3.03	55.62	851.81	.95
	1 tbsp	1	0	.04	.15	.03	2.3	0	0.0	27.84	.24	4.32	66.16	.07
CARP														
dry-heat cooked	3 oz	27	.12	.06	1.78	.19	14.7	1.25	1.4	44.2	1.35	32.3	362.95	1.61
dry-heat cooked, approx 7.7 oz raw wt	1 fillet	54	.24	.12	3.57	.37	29.4	2.5	2.7	88.4	2.7	64.6	725.9	3.23
raw	3 oz	25	.1	.05	1.39	.16	12.8	1.3	1.4	34.85	1.05	24.65	283.05	1.26
raw, approx 7.7 oz	1 fillet	63	.25	.12	3.58	.41	32.7	3.34	3.5	89.38	2.7	63.22	725.94	3.23
CARROT														
baby, raw	1 large	296	0	.01	.13	.01	5.0	0	1.3	3.45	.12	1.8	41.85	.02
baby, raw	1 med	197	0	0	.09	.01	3.3	0	0.8	2.3	.08	1.2	27.9	.02
boiled, drained	1 med	11295	.02	.03	.23	.11	6.4	0	1.1	14.26	.29	5.98	104.42	.14
boiled, drained, sliced	1/2 cup	19152	.03	.04	.39	.19	10.8	0	1.8	24.18	.48	10.14	177.06	.23
raw	1 med	20253	.07	.04	.67	.11	10.1	0	6.7	19.44	.36	10.8	232.56	.14
raw *(Dole)*	1 med	16065	na	na	na	na	na	na	6.0	na	na	na	311	na
raw, shredded	1/2 cup	15471	.05	.03	.51	.08	7.7	0	5.1	14.85	.28	8.25	177.65	.11
CARROT, CANNED														
Crinkle sliced														
(Freshlike)	1/2 cup	na	na	na	na	na	na	na	na	na	na	na	200	na
(Veg•All)	1/2 cup	na	na	na	na	na	na	na	na	na	na	na	200	na
Sliced														
regular pack, drained	1/2 cup	10055	.01	.02	.4	.08	6.7	0	2.0	18.25	.47	5.84	130.67	.19
regular pack, w/liquid	1/2 cup	16197	.02	.03	.52	.14	10.0	0	3.4	30.75	.75	11.07	212.79	.36
special dietary pack, drained	1/2 cup	10055	.01	.02	.4	.08	6.7	0	2.0	18.25	.47	5.84	130.67	.19
special dietary pack, w/liquid	1/2 cup	16197	.02	.03	.52	.14	10.0	0	3.4	30.75	.75	11.07	212.79	.36
water-packed, w/o salt *(Freshlike)*	1/2 cup	na	na	na	na	na	na	na	na	na	na	na	200	na
water-packed, w/o sugar or salt *(Freshlike)*	1/2 cup	na	na	na	na	na	na	na	na	na	na	na	200	na
CARROT, FROZEN														
baby, whole 'Deluxe' *(Bird's Eye)*	3.3 oz	na	na	na	na	na	na	na	na	na	na	na	200	na
Parisienne 'Deluxe' *(Deluxe)*	2.6 oz	na	na	na	na	na	na	na	na	na	na	na	160	na
sliced *(Birds Eye)*	3.2 oz	na	na	na	na	na	na	na	na	na	na	na	200	na
sliced, boiled, drained	1/2 cup	12922	.02	.03	.32	.09	7.9	0	2.0	20.44	.34	7.3	115.34	.18
sliced, unprepared	1/2 cup	13620	.02	.03	.4	.12	6.1	0	2.8	20.48	.39	7.04	115.84	.16
w/sweet peas, pearl onions 'Deluxe' *(Birds Eye)*	3.3 oz	na	na	na	na	na	na	na	na	na	na	na	180	na
CARROT JUICE														
canned	6 oz	47382	.17	.1	.71	.4	7.0	0	15.6	44.16	.85	25.76	537.28	.33
canned	1/2 cup	31674	.11	.07	.47	.27	4.7	0	10.5	29.52	.57	17.22	359.16	.22
CASABA MELON														
cubed	1 cup	51	.1	.03	.68	na	na	0	27.2	8.5	.68	13.6	357.0	na
1/10 of 7.75-inch melon	2-inch slice	49	.1	.03	.66	na	na	0	26.2	8.2	.66	13.12	344.4	na
CASHEW/heart nut														
Dry roasted														
salted	1 oz	0	.06	.06	.4	.07	19.7	0	0.0	12.78	1.7	73.84	160.46	1.59

Food Name	Serving Size	A I.U.	Thi mg	Rib mg	Nia mg	B₆ mg	Fol mcg	B₁₂ mcg	C mg	Calc mg	Iron mg	Mag mg	Pot mg	Zn mg
salted, wholes and halves	1 cup	0	.27	.27	1.92	.35	94.8	0	0.0	61.65	8.22	356.2	774.05	7.67
unsalted	1 oz	0	.06	.06	.4	.07	19.7	0	0.0	12.78	1.7	73.84	160.46	1.59
Honey roasted (Frito-Lays)	1 oz	na	na	na	na	na	na	na	na	na	na	na	115	na
Oil roasted														
salted	1 oz	0	.12	.05	.51	.07	19.2	0	0.0	11.64	1.16	72.42	150.52	1.35
salted, wholes and halves	1 cup	0	.55	.23	2.34	.33	88.0	0	0.0	53.3	5.33	331.5	689.0	6.18
unsalted	1 oz	0	.12	.05	.51	.07	19.2	0	0.0	11.64	1.16	72.42	150.52	1.35
unsalted, halves	1 cup	0	.55	.23	2.34	.33	88.0	0	0.0	53.3	5.33	331.5	689.0	6.18
CASHEW BUTTER														
peanut date (Maranatha Natural)	2 tbsp	na	na	na	na	na	na	na	na	na	na	na	240	na
plain	1 oz	0	.09	.05	.45	.07	19.4	0	0.0	12.21	1.43	73.27	155.06	1.47
plain	1 tbsp	0	.05	.03	.26	.04	10.9	0	0.0	6.88	.8	41.28	87.36	.83
roasted (Maranatha Natural)	2 tbsp	na	na	na	na	na	na	na	na	na	na	na	250	na
CASSAVA / manioc														
raw	100 gm	10	.23	.1	1.4	.3	22.1	0	48.2	91.0	3.6	66.0	764.0	.25
CATFISH, CHANNEL														
Farmed														
dry-heat cooked	3 oz	43	.36	.06	2.14	.14	6.0	2.38	0.7	7.65	.7	22.1	272.85	.89
raw	3 oz	43	.31	.06	1.96	.16	8.5	2.1	0.5	7.65	.43	19.55	254.15	.63
Wild														
dry-heat cooked	3 oz	43	.19	.06	2.03	.09	8.5	2.47	0.7	9.35	.3	23.8	356.15	.52
raw	3 oz	43	.18	.06	1.62	.1	8.5	1.9	0.6	11.9	.26	19.55	304.3	.43
CATFISH, OCEAN. See WOLF FISH.														
CATSUP / ketchup														
	1 tbsp	152	.01	.01	.21	.03	2.3	0	2.3	2.85	.11	3.3	72.15	.03
	.2-oz pkt	61	.01	0	.08	.01	0.9	0	0.9	1.14	.04	1.32	28.86	.01
(Healthy Choice)	.5 oz	na	na	na	na	na	na	na	2.1	.28	.56	na	na	na
(Heinz)	1 tbsp	na	na	na	na	na	na	na	na	na	na	na	50	na
(Hunt's)	1 tbsp	na	na	na	na	na	na	na	2.3	.31	.57	na	na	na
(Snider's)	1 tbsp	na	na	na	na	na	na	na	4.1	0	0	na	na	na
'Food Service' (Hunt's)	1 tbsp	na	na	na	na	na	na	na	3.8	0	0	na	na	na
fruit-sweetened (Westbrae)	1 tbsp	na	na	na	na	na	na	na	na	na	na	na	50	na
fruit-sweetened, no salt (Westbrae)	1 tbsp	na	na	na	na	na	na	na	na	na	na	na	85	na
hot (Heinz)	1 tbsp	na	na	na	na	na	na	na	na	na	na	na	60	na
'Lite' (Heinz)	1 tbsp	na	na	na	na	na	na	na	na	na	na	na	65	na
low-sodium	1 tbsp	152	.01	.01	.21	.03	2.3	0	2.3	2.85	.11	3.3	72.15	.03
low-sodium	.2-oz pkt	61	.01	0	.08	.01	0.9	0	0.9	1.14	.04	1.32	28.86	.01
portion pack (Hunt's)	.3175 oz	na	na	na	na	na	na	na	2.7	0	0	na	na	na
CAULIFLOWER														
boiled, drained, approx 1.9 oz	3 flowerets	9	.02	.03	.22	.09	23.8	0	23.9	8.64	.18	4.86	76.68	.1
boiled, drained, 1-inch pieces	1/2 cup	11	.03	.03	.25	.11	27.3	0	27.5	9.92	.2	5.58	88.04	.11
fresh, medium size (Dole)	1/6 head	17	na	na	na	na	na	na	53.0	na	na	na	250	na
green, fresh (Dole)	1/5 head	na	na	na	na	na	na	na	na	na	na	na	280	na
raw, approx 5 oz	3 flowerets	11	.03	.04	.29	.12	31.9	0	26.0	12.32	.25	8.4	169.68	.16
raw, 1-inch pieces	1/2 cup	10	.03	.03	.26	.11	28.5	0	23.2	11.0	.22	7.5	151.5	.14
Frozen														
(Birds Eye)	3.3 oz	na	na	na	na	na	na	na	na	na	na	na	190	na
boiled, drained, 1-inch pieces	1/2 cup	20	.03	.05	.28	.08	36.9	0	28.2	15.3	.37	8.1	125.1	.12
unprepared, 1-inch pieces	1/2 cup	20	.03	.05	.28	.08	42.2	0	32.2	14.52	.36	7.92	127.38	.11
CAVIAR														
black, granular	1 oz	523	.05	.17	.03	.09	14.0	5.6	0.0	77.0	3.33	84.0	50.68	.27
black, granular	1 tbsp	299	.03	.1	.02	.05	8.0	3.2	0.0	44.0	1.9	48.0	28.96	.15
red, granular	1 oz	523	.05	.17	.03	.09	14.0	5.6	0.0	77.0	3.33	na	50.68	.27
red, granular	1 tbsp	299	.03	.1	.02	.05	8.0	3.2	0.0	44.0	1.9	na	28.96	.15
CAYENNE PEPPER														
	1 tbsp	2205	.02	.05	.46	na	na	0	4.1	7.86	.41	8.04	106.74	.13
	1 tsp	749	.01	.02	.16	na	na	0	1.4	2.67	.14	2.73	36.25	.04

Food Name	Serving Size	A I.U.	Thi mg	Rib mg	Nia mg	B₆ mg	Fol mcg	B₁₂ mcg	C mg	Calc mg	Iron mg	Mag mg	Pot mg	Zn mg
CECI. See GARBANZO BEAN.														
CELERIAC / celery root														
boiled, drained	100 gm	0	.03	.04	.43	.1	3.4	0	3.6	26.0	.43	12.0	173.0	.2
raw	1/2 cup	0	.04	.05	.55	.13	5.9	0	6.2	33.54	.55	15.6	234.0	.26
CELERY														
boiled, drained, diced	1/2 cup	99	.03	.04	.24	.06	16.5	0	4.6	31.5	.31	9.0	213.0	.11
fresh, medium size (Dole)	2 stalks	156	na	na	na	na	na	na	9.0	na	na	na	355	na
raw, diced	1/2 cup	80	.03	.03	.19	.05	16.8	0	4.2	24.0	.24	6.6	172.2	.08
CELERY SEED														
whole	1 tbsp	3	na	na	na	na	na	0	1.1	114.83	2.92	28.6	91.0	.45
whole	1 tsp	1	na	na	na	na	na	0	0.3	35.33	.9	8.8	28.0	.14
whole (Durkee)	1 tsp	.02	.16	.2	0	na	na	na	.01	0	.02	na	0	na
whole (Laurel Leaf)	1 tsp	.02	.16	.2	0	na	na	na	.01	0	.02	na	0	na
CELTUCE, raw, approx .4 oz	1 leaf	280	0	.01	.04	0	3.7	0	1.6	3.12	.04	2.24	26.4	.02
CEREAL, HOT														
(NOTE: All of the following hot cereals are dry unless otherwise noted.)														
BARLEY (Erewhon) organic plus	1 oz	na	na	na	na	na	na	na	na	na	na	na	85	na
CORN GRITS. See GRITS.														
FARINA (Malt•O•Meal) 'Maple Brown Sugar'														
30% formulation	1 oz	na	na	na	na	na	na	na	na	na	na	na	20	na
GRAIN, MIXED														
(Malt•O•Meal) wheat and barley,														
chocolate flavor	1 tbsp	0	.13	.09	1.81	.01	2.5	0	0.0	1.44	2.95	1.34	9.68	.05
(Malt•O•Meal) wheat and barley, plain	1 tbsp	0	.13	.09	1.81	.01	2.5	0	0.0	1.44	2.95	1.34	9.68	.05
OAT BRAN														
(Erewhon) toasted wheat germ	1 oz	na	na	na	na	na	na	na	na	na	na	na	210	na
(Malt•O•Meal) 'Plus 40% Oat Bran'	1.3 oz	na	na	na	na	na	na	na	na	na	na	na	110	na
(Quaker)	1 oz	26	.27	.08	.28	.04	14.0	na	0.0	22	1.84	69	169	1.19
OATMEAL AND OATS														
(Erewhon) instant, apple and cinnamon	1.25 oz	na	na	na	na	na	na	na	na	na	na	na	140	na
(Erewhon) instant, apple and raisin	1.3 oz	na	na	na	na	na	na	na	na	na	na	na	150	na
(Erewhon) instant, maple spice	1.2 oz	na	na	na	na	na	na	na	na	na	na	na	115	na
(Erewhon) instant, oat bran	1.25 oz	na	na	na	na	na	na	na	na	na	na	na	130	na
(Erewhon) instant, raisins, dates, and														
walnuts	1.2 oz	na	na	na	na	na	na	na	na	na	na	na	160	na
(Maypo)	1 cup	4974	1.5	1.69	19.93	1.97	25.4	5.92	60.2	265.08	17.86	108.1	449.32	3.15
(Quaker) 'Extra'	1 pkt	5115	1.5	1.7	21.57	2.0	400.0	6.0	60.0	222	18.0	na	104	15.0
(Quaker) 'Extra' apples and spice	1 pkt	5001	1.5	1.7	20.0	2.0	400.0	6.0	60.0	220	18.0	na	116	15.0
(Quaker) 'Extra' raisins and cinnamon	1 pkt	5001	1.5	1.7	20.0	2.0	400.0	6.0	60.0	278	18.0	na	139	15.0
(Quaker) instant	1 pkt	1237	.44	.21	3.64	.47	122.0	na	0.0	170	8.35	39	103	.88
(Quaker) instant, apple and cinnamon	1 pkt	1233	.37	.21	3.69	.43	113.0	0	0.2	168	5.89	39	108	.66
(Quaker) instant, cinnamon and spice	1 pkt	1309	.39	.23	3.72	.46	120.0	na	0.0	178	8.08	40	117	.84
(Quaker) instant, maple and brown sugar	1 pkt	1380	.4	.23	3.77	.44	116.0	na	0.0	170	8.35	42	116	.85
(Quaker) instant, peaches and cream	1 pkt	1245	.33	.22	3.65	.41	121.0	na	0.0	146	5.71	35	140	.67
(Quaker) instant, raisins and spice	1 pkt	1298	.36	.23	3.68	.44	103.0	.08	0.0	165	6.23	39	152	.91
(Quaker) instant, raisins, dates, and walnuts	1 pkt	988	.3	.2	3.14	.37	95.0	na	0.0	134	5.33	39	127	.77
(Quaker) instant, strawberries and cream	1 pkt	1186	.31	.21	3.25	.37	118.0	na	0.0	157	5.48	35	140	.67
(Quaker) 'Old Fashioned'	1 oz	26	.14	.03	.22	.03	7.0	na	0.0	15	1.08	38	109	.87
(Quaker) 'Quick'	1 oz	26	.14	.03	.22	.03	7.0	na	0.0	15	1.08	38	109	.87
(Ralston)	1 cup	0	.64	.57	6.16	.34	70.8	.33	0.0	41.3	4.96	179.36	462.56	4.25
(Roman Meal)	1 cup	42	.62	.44	6.53	.76	70.0	0	0.0	55.0	2.81	150.0	513.0	3.91
RICE														
(Cream of Rice)	1 tbsp	0	.02	.01	.31	.02	3.0	0	0.0	2.45	.13	2.35	14.59	.11
(Lundberg Family) 'Hot 'n Creamy' cooked	1 oz	na	na	na	na	na	na	na	na	na	na	na	140	na
RICE, BROWN (Erewhon) cream of brown rice	1 oz	na	na	na	na	na	na	na	na	na	na	na	140	na
WHEAT														
(Cream of Wheat)	1 tbsp	0	.05	.02	.45	.01	3.6	0	0.0	14.95	3.03	2.86	12.72	.09

Food Name	Serving Size	A I.U.	Thi mg	Rib mg	Nia mg	B6 mg	Fol mcg	B12 mcg	C mg	Calc mg	Iron mg	Mag mg	Pot mg	Zn mg
(Cream of Wheat) instant	1 oz	na	na	na	na	na	na	na	na	na	na	na	35	na
(Cream of Wheat) instant	1 tbsp	0	.06	.02	.48	.01	3.9	0	0.0	16.21	3.29	3.91	13.22	.11
(Cream of Wheat) 'Mix'n Eat' instant	1 oz	na	na	na	na	na	na	na	na	na	na	na	30	na
(Cream of Wheat) 'Mix'n Eat' instant, apple and cinnamon	1 oz	na	na	na	na	na	na	na	na	na	na	na	45	na
(Cream of Wheat) 'Mix'n Eat' instant, apple, banana, and maple	1 pkt	1250	.39	.25	4.99	.5	99.8	0	0.0	40.0	8.11	9.2	54.87	.23
(Cream of Wheat) 'Mix'n Eat' instant, brown sugar and cinnamon	1 oz	na	na	na	na	na	na	na	na	na	na	na	65	na
(Cream of Wheat) 'Mix'n Eat' instant, maple and brown sugar	1 oz	na	na	na	na	na	na	na	na	na	na	na	40	na
(Cream of Wheat) 'Quick'	1 tbsp	0	.05	.02	.45	.01	3.6	0	0.0	14.95	3.03	3.5	13.78	.1
(General Mills) 'Wheat Hearts'	1 oz	na	na	na	na	na	na	na	na	na	na	na	105	na
(Maltex)	1 cup	0	.79	.3	7.04	.23	86.1	0	0.0	54.36	5.29	167.61	786.71	5.5
(Quaker)	1/3 cup	26	.09	.03	1.3	.04	13.0	na	0.0	10	.96	31	125	.73

CEREAL, READY-TO-SERVE

(NOTE: All of the following ready-to-serve cereals are in their dry form.)

Food Name	Serving Size	A I.U.	Thi mg	Rib mg	Nia mg	B6 mg	Fol mcg	B12 mcg	C mg	Calc mg	Iron mg	Mag mg	Pot mg	Zn mg
'All Bran' extra fiber (Kellogg's)	1 oz	750	.38	.43	5	.5	na	2	15.0	28	4.5	113	330	3.75
'All Bran' wheat bran (Kellogg's)	1 oz	1252	.37	.43	5.0	.51	100.3	0	15.1	23.0	4.52	105.93	350.46	3.75
'Almond Raisin' low fat (Golden Temple)	1 oz	41	.13	.07	.83	na	na	na	na	14.0	1.0	na	94	na
'Alpha Bits' oat and other grains (Post)	1 oz	1252	.37	.43	5.0	.51	100.3	1.51	0.0	8.24	2.7	16.76	110.19	1.51
'Apple Almond Müesli' (Ralston)	1.45 oz	na	na	na	na	na	na	na	na	na	na	na	170	na
'Apple & Cinnamon Toasted Oat' (Malt•O•Meal)	1 oz	na	na	na	na	na	na	na	na	na	na	na	6	na
'Apple Cinnamon Cheerios' (General Mills)	1 oz	na	na	na	na	na	na	na	na	na	na	na	70	na
'Apple Cinnamon Corn Flakes' (Wonder)	1 oz	na	na	na	na	na	na	na	na	na	na	na	25	na
'Apple Cinnamon' low fat (Golden Temple)	1 oz	44	.13	.07	.88	na	na	na	na	17.0	1.0	na	85	na
'Apple Cinnamon Squares' (Kellogg's)	1 oz	0	.38	.43	5	.5	na	2	tr	11	8.1	25	85	1.5
'Apple Jacks' corn and other grains (Kellogg's)	1 oz	1252	.37	.43	5.0	.51	100.3	0	15.1	3.12	4.52	6.25	23.0	3.75
'Apple Raisin Crisp' (Kellogg's)	1 oz	750	.38	.43	5	.5	na	2	tr	10	1.8	7	115	1.5
'Banana O's' (Erewhon)	1 oz	na	na	na	na	na	na	na	na	na	na	na	150	na
'Banana Walnut Müesli' (Ralston)	1.45 oz	na	na	na	na	na	na	na	na	na	na	na	170	na
'Basic 4' (General Mills)	3/4 cup	na	na	na	na	na	na	na	na	na	na	na	300	na
'Berry Berry Kix' (General Mills)	1 oz	na	na	na	na	na	na	na	na	na	na	na	35	na
'Blueberry Squares' (Kellogg's)	1 oz	0	.38	.43	5	.5	na	2	tr	10	8.1	26	85	1.5
'Body Buddies Natural Fruit' (General Mills)	1 oz	na	na	na	na	na	na	na	na	na	na	na	40	na
'Booberry' (General Mills)	1 oz	na	na	na	na	na	na	na	na	na	na	na	45	na
'Bran Buds' wheat bran (Kellogg's)	1 oz	1252	.37	.43	5.0	.51	100.3	0	15.1	19.03	4.52	90.31	474.85	3.75
'Bran Chex' wheat bran and corn (Kellogg's)	1 oz	62	.37	.15	5.0	.51	100.3	1.51	15.1	17.04	4.52	72.99	228.34	1.24
'Bran Flakes' (Kellogg's)	1 oz	750	.38	.43	5	.5	na	2	tr	15	18	50	160	3.75
'Bran Flakes' (Malt•O•Meal)	1 oz	na	na	na	na	na	na	na	na	na	na	na	210	na
'Buñuelitos' (General Mills)	1 oz	na	na	na	na	na	na	na	na	na	na	na	25	na
'C.W. Post Hearty Granola Cereal' (Post)	1 oz	na	na	na	na	na	na	na	na	na	na	na	55	na
'C.W. Post' oats and other grains (Post)	1 oz	1252	.37	.43	5.0	.51	100.3	1.51	0.0	13.63	4.52	19.6	57.94	.48
'C.W. Post' oats and other grains, raisins (Post)	1 oz	1252	.37	.43	5.0	.51	100.3	1.51	0.0	13.92	4.52	20.45	71.85	.45
'Captain Crunch' corn and other grains (Quaker)	1 oz	11	.61	.55	6.63	.77	182.6	1.8	0.0	4.83	7.55	11.64	36.64	3.08
'Captain Crunch Crunchberries' corn and oat (Quaker)	1 oz	36	.48	.55	6.6	.75	103.7	2.03	0.0	8.8	7.33	11.08	39.76	2.89
'Captain Crunch Peanut Butter' corn (Quaker)	1 oz	44	.49	.57	7.28	.85	197.7	1.87	0.0	5.68	7.39	15.05	46.01	3.07
'Cashew Almond Granola' (Golden Temple)	1 oz	2	.17	.04	.24	na	na	na	na	15.0	1.0	na	112	na
'Cheerios' oat and wheat (General Mills)	1 oz	1252	.37	.43	5.0	.51	6.3	1.51	15.1	48.56	4.52	39.19	101.39	.79
'Cinnamon & Raisin' 100% natural (Nature Valley)	1 oz	na	na	na	na	na	na	na	na	na	na	na	80	na

Food Name	Serving Size	A I.U.	Thi mg	Rib mg	Nia mg	B$_6$ mg	Fol mcg	B$_{12}$ mcg	C mg	Calc mg	Iron mg	Mag mg	Pot mg	Zn mg
'Cinnamon & Spice Crunch' psyllium and chia seed (Golden Temple)	1 oz	29	.15	.08	.55	na	na	na	na	30.0	1.0	na	89	na
'Cinnamon Apple Raisin Granola' (Golden Temple)	1 oz	2	.16	.04	.22	na	na	na	na	16.0	1.0	na	112	na
'Cinnamon Mini Buns' (Kellogg's)	1 oz	750	.38	.43	5	.5	na	na	15.0	4	4.5	12	40	3.75
'Cinnamon Toast Crunch' (General Mills)	1 oz	na	na	na	na	na	na	na	na	na	na	na	45	na
'Cinnamon Toast Crunch' breakfast pack (General Mills)	1 oz	na	na	na	na	na	na	na	na	na	na	na	50	na
'Clusters' (General Mills)	1 oz	na	na	na	na	na	na	na	na	na	na	na	105	na
'Cocoa Krispies' rice (Kellogg's)	1 oz	1252	.37	.43	5.0	.51	100.3	.01	15.1	5.11	1.79	9.37	42.03	1.51
'Cocoa Pebbles' rice (Post)	1 oz	1252	.37	.43	5.0	.51	100.3	1.51	0.0	4.83	1.79	11.64	46.86	1.51
'Cocoa Puffs' (General Mills)	1 oz	na	na	na	na	na	na	na	na	na	na	na	55	na
'Coconut Almond Granola' (Golden Temple)	1 oz	2	.14	.04	.22	na	na	na	na	14.0	1.0	na	97	na
'Common Sense Oat Bran' (Kellogg's)	1 oz	750	.38	.43	5	.5	na	2	tr	14	8.1	45	125	3.75
'Common Sense Oat Bran' raisins (Kellogg's)	3/4 cup	750	.38	.43	5	.5	na	2	tr	14	8.1	45	125	3.75
'Cookie-Crisp' chocolate chip and vanilla (Ralston)	1 oz	1252	.37	.43	5.0	.51	3.1	1.51	15.1	5.4	4.52	7.95	27.83	.27
'Corn Bran' corn bran and other grains (Ralston)	1 oz	60	.3	.55	8.57	.68	183.2	1.1	0.0	32.66	9.66	14.48	55.38	3.16
'Corn Chex' (Ralston)	1 oz	143	.37	.07	5.0	.51	100.3	1.51	15.1	3.12	1.79	3.98	23.0	.1
'Corn Flakes' (Kellogg's)	1 oz	1252	.37	.43	5.0	.51	100.3	0	15.1	.85	1.79	3.41	26.13	.08
'Corn Flakes' (Malt•O•Meal)	1 oz	na	na	na	na	na	na	na	na	na	na	na	25	na
'Corn Flakes' (Ralston)	1 oz	108	.14	.03	1.19	.02	2.0	0	0.0	1.99	.71	3.12	24.99	.07
'Corn Flakes' sugar frosted (Kellogg's)	1 oz	1252	.37	.43	5.0	.51	100.3	0	15.1	1.14	1.79	2.27	18.18	.04
'Corn Flakes' sugar frosted (Ralston)	1 oz	1252	.37	.43	5.0	.51	2.0	1.51	15.1	3.12	.71	1.99	17.89	.61
'Corn Pops' (Kellogg's)	1 oz	750	.38	.43	5	.5	na	na	15.0	2	1.8	2	20	1.5
'Count Chocula' (General Mills)	1 oz	na	na	na	na	na	na	na	na	na	na	na	55	na
'Country Corn Flakes' (General Mills)	1 oz	na	na	na	na	na	na	na	na	na	na	na	30	na
'Cracklin' Bran' wheat bran and other grains (Kellogg's)	1 oz	1252	.37	.43	5.0	.51	100.3	0	15.1	18.74	1.79	55.1	167.84	1.51
'Cracklin' Oat Bran' (Kellogg's)	1 oz	750	.38	.43	5	.5	na	na	15.0	15	1.8	45	160	1.5
'Cranberry Walnut Müesli' (Ralston)	1.45 oz	na	na	na	na	na	na	na	na	na	na	na	170	na
'Crisp N' Crackling Rice' (Malt•O•Meal)	1 oz	na	na	na	na	na	na	na	na	na	na	na	40	na
'Crispix' (Kellogg's)	1 oz	750	.38	.43	5	.5	na	na	15.0	3	1.8	7	30	1.5
'Crispy Wheats 'N Raisins' wheat (General Mills)	1 oz	1252	.37	.43	5.0	.51	9.7	1.51	0.0	46.86	4.52	22.72	114.74	.34
'Crunch Graham Oat Rings' (Wonder)	1 oz	na	na	na	na	na	na	na	na	na	na	na	50	na
'Date Almond Müesli' (Ralston)	1.45 oz	na	na	na	na	na	na	na	na	na	na	na	200	na
'Double Chex' (Ralston)	1 oz	na	na	na	na	na	na	na	na	na	na	na	25	na
'Double Dip Crunch' (Kellogg's)	1 oz	750	.38	.43	5	.5	na	na	15.0	5	1.8	5	45	1.5
'Fiber One' aspartame (General Mills)	1 oz	na	na	na	na	na	na	na	na	na	na	na	220	na
'Fiberwise' (Kellogg's)	1 oz	750	.38	.43	5	.5	na	na	15.0	19	4.5	32	160	1.5
'40% Bran Flakes' wheat bran (Kellogg's)	1 oz	1252	.37	.43	5.0	.51	100.3	1.51	0.0	13.92	18.03	51.69	180.34	3.75
'40% Bran Flakes' wheat bran (Post)	1 oz	1252	.37	.43	5.0	.51	100.3	1.51	0.0	12.5	4.52	61.34	151.37	1.51
'40% Bran Flakes' wheat bran (Ralston)	1 oz	1252	.37	.43	5.0	.51	100.3	1.51	15.1	13.06	4.52	68.16	165.86	1.18
'Frankenberry' (General Mills)	1 oz	na	na	na	na	na	na	na	na	na	na	na	45	na
'Froot Loops' corn and other grains (Kellogg's)	1 oz	1252	.37	.43	5.0	.51	100.3	0	15.1	2.84	4.52	7.1	26.13	3.75
'Frosted Chex Juniors' (Ralston)	1 oz	na	na	na	na	na	na	na	na	na	na	na	15	na
'Frosted Flakes' (Kellogg's)	1 oz	750	.38	.43	5	.5	na	na	15.0	2	1.8	7	25	.28
'Frosted Krispies' (Kellogg's)	1 oz	750	.38	.43	5	.5	na	na	15.0	2	1.8	7	25	.28
'Frosted Mini Wheats' (Kellogg's)	1 oz	0	.38	.43	5	.5	na	2	tr	10	1.8	29	80	1.5
'Frosted Mini Wheats' bite size (Kellogg's)	1 oz	0	.38	.43	5	.5	na	2	tr	9	1.8	27	100	1.5
'Frosted Mini Wheats' brown sugar and cinnamon (Kellogg's)	1 oz	1252	.37	.43	5.0	.51	100.3	0	15.1	9.37	1.79	23.29	96.84	1.51
'Frosted Rice Krispies' rice (Kellogg's)	1 oz	1252	.37	.43	5.0	.51	100.3	0	15.1	1.14	1.79	5.11	21.02	.31
'Fruit & Fibre' oat, dates, raisins, and walnuts (Post)	1.25 oz	na	na	na	na	na	na	na	na	na	na	na	200	na

Food Name	Serving Size	A I.U.	Thi mg	Rib mg	Nia mg	B6 mg	Fol mcg	B12 mcg	C mg	Calc mg	Iron mg	Mag mg	Pot mg	Zn mg
'Fruit & Fibre' oat, peaches, raisins, and almonds (Post)	1.25 oz	na	na	na	na	na	na	na	na	na	na	na	210	na
'Fruit & Fibre' oat, tropical fruit (Post)	1.25 oz	na	na	na	na	na	na	na	na	na	na	na	210	na
'Fruit & Frosted O's' mixed grain (Malt•O•Meal)	1 oz	na	na	na	na	na	na	na	na	na	na	na	30	na
'Fruit & Nut' 100% natural (Nature Valley)	1 oz	na	na	na	na	na	na	na	na	na	na	na	90	na
'Fruit 'N Nut Granola' (Golden Temple)	1 oz	2	.17	.04	.24	na	na	na	na	16.0	1.0	na	116	na
'Fruit 'n Wheat' (Erewhon)	1 oz	na	na	na	na	na	na	na	na	na	na	na	160	na
'Fruitful Bran' fruit (Kellogg's)	1 oz	750	.38	.43	5	.5	na	2	tr	19	4.5	.56	230	1.08
'Fruity Marshmallow Krispies' (Kellogg's)	1 1/4 cups	750	.38	.43	5	.5	na	na	15.0	2	1.8	7	20	.32
'Fruity Pebbles' rice (Post)	1 oz	1252	.37	.43	5.0	.51	100.3	1.51	0.0	3.41	1.79	8.24	21.58	1.51
'Golden Crisp' (Post)	1 oz	na	na	na	na	na	na	na	na	na	na	na	50	na
'Golden Grahams' corn and wheat (General Mills)	1 oz	1252	.37	.43	5.0	.51	4.3	1.51	15.1	17.32	4.52	11.64	62.76	.25
'Golden Granola' (Golden Temple)	1 oz	2	.17	.04	.26	na	na	na	na	19.0	1.0	na	96	na
'Granola' toasted oat mix (Nature Valley)	1 oz	19	.1	.05	.21	.02	21.3	0	0.0	17.89	.95	28.97	97.7	.55
'Grape-Nuts' wheat and barley (Post)	1 oz	1252	.37	.43	5.0	.51	100.3	1.51	0.0	2.7	1.23	19.03	94.86	.62
'Grape-Nuts Flakes' wheat and barley (Post)	1 oz	1252	.37	.43	5.0	.51	100.3	1.51	0.0	11.36	8.12	31.24	98.83	.57
'Hawaiian Granola' (Golden Temple)	1 oz	2	.16	.04	.24	na	na	na	na	14.0	1.0	na	117	na
'Hazelnut Boysenberry' organic oats (Golden Temple)	1 oz	2	.17	.04	.21	na	na	na	na	14.0	1.0	na	88	na
'Heartland Natural' oat and wheat germ	1 oz	16	.09	.04	.4	.05	15.9	0	0.3	18.46	1.07	36.35	95.14	.75
'Heartland Natural' oat and wheat germ, coconut	1 oz	15	.09	.04	.48	.04	15.3	0	0.3	17.89	1.46	37.2	103.94	.74
'Heartland Natural' oat and wheat germ, raisins	1 oz	16	.08	.04	.4	.05	11.4	0	0.3	17.04	1.04	36.35	107.07	.73
'High Protein Granola' (Golden Temple)	1 oz	2	.17	.04	.25	na	na	na	na	24.0	1.0	na	119	na
'Honey Almond Granola' (Golden Temple)	1 oz	2	.16	.04	.19	na	na	na	na	14.0	1.0	na	85	na
'Honey & Nut Toasted Oat' (Malt•O•Meal)	1 oz	na	na	na	na	na	na	na	na	na	na	na	90	na
'Honey Blueberry Apple Granola' (Golden Temple)	1 oz	2	.16	.03	.2	na	na	na	na	12.0	1.0	na	82	na
'Honey Bunches of Oats' almonds (Post)	1 oz	na	na	na	na	na	na	na	na	na	na	na	60	na
'Honey Bunches of Oats' honey roasted (Post)	1 oz	na	na	na	na	na	na	na	na	na	na	na	50	na
'Honey Nut Cheerios' oat and wheat (General Mills)	1 oz	1252	.37	.43	5.0	.51	18.5	1.51	15.1	19.88	4.52	33.23	99.12	.74
'Honey Nut Cheerios' oat and wheat, breakfast pack (General Mills)	4/5 oz	na	na	na	na	na	na	na	na	na	na	na	75	na
'Honey Nut Crispy Rice' (Wonder)	1 oz	na	na	na	na	na	na	na	na	na	na	na	35	na
'HoneyComb' corn and oats (Post)	1 oz	1252	.37	.43	5.0	.51	100.3	1.51	0.0	4.83	2.7	9.66	90.88	1.51
'Just Right' fiber nuggets (Kellogg's)	1 oz	5000	1.5	1.7	20	2	na	6	tr	9	18	18	70	15
'Just Right' raisins, dates, and nuts (Kellogg's)	3/4 cup	5000	1.5	1.7	20	2	na	6	tr	16	18	26	120	15
'Kaboom' (General Mills)	1 oz	na	na	na	na	na	na	na	na	na	na	na	60	na
'Kamut Flakes' (Erewhon)	1 oz	na	na	na	na	na	na	na	na	na	na	na	90	na
'Kenmei Rice Bran' (Kellogg's)	1 oz	750	.38	.43	5	.5	na	2	tr	54	.5	35	75	1.5
'King Vitaman' corn and other grains	1 oz	3229	1.25	1.43	17.46	1.6	386.8	5.58	44.9	2.27	17.23	9.66	34.93	.22
'Kix' corn and other grains (General Mills)	1 oz	1252	.37	.43	5.0	.51	100.3	1.51	15.1	35.5	8.12	12.21	44.59	.25
'Life' oat and other grains (Quaker Oat)	1 oz	19	.62	.64	7.51	.05	23.9	0	na	99.4	7.5	9.09	126.95	.94
'Life' oat and other grains, cinnamon (Quaker Oat)	1 oz	19	.62	.64	7.51	.05	23.9	0	na	99.4	7.5	9.09	126.95	.94
'Lite Müesli' (Golden Temple)	1 oz	72	.17	.11	1.16	na	na	na	na	13.0	1.0	na	115	na
'Lite 'N Crunchy Granola' (Golden Temple)	1 oz	9	.18	.05	.35	na	na	na	na	18.0	1.0	na	116	na
'Lucky Charms' oat and other grains (General Mills)	1 oz	1252	.37	.43	5.0	.51	5.7	1.51	15.1	32.09	4.52	23.86	58.79	.5
'Lucky Charms' oat and other grains, breakfast pack (General Mills)	7/8 oz	na	na	na	na	na	na	na	na	na	na	na	55	na

Food Name	Serving Size	A I.U.	Thi mg	Rib mg	Nia mg	B_6 mg	Fol mcg	B_{12} mcg	C mg	Calc mg	Iron mg	Mag mg	Pot mg	Zn mg
'Maple Almond Granola' (Golden Temple)	1 oz	2	.16	.04	.19	na	na	na	na	15.0	1.0	na	8	na
'Maple Frosted Corn' mini puffs (Glenny's)	1 oz	na	na	na	na	na	na	na	na	na	na	na	40	na
'Most' wheat bran and wheat	1 oz	5009	1.51	1.7	20.02	2.02	400.7	6.02	60.2	43.17	18.03	56.23	185.45	1.51
'Müeslix Crispy Blend' (Kellogg's)	2/3 cup	750	.38	.43	5	.5	na	2	tr	35	4.5	36	160	3.75
'Müeslix Golden Crunch' (Kellogg's)	1/2 cup	750	.38	.43	5	.5	na	1	tr	19	4.5	34	115	3
'Multi Grain Cheerios' (General Mills)	1 oz	na	na	na	na	na	na	na	na	na	na	na	90	na
'Multi-Bran Chex' (Ralston)	1 oz	na	na	na	na	na	na	na	na	na	na	na	125	na
'Natural Blueberry Granola' (Golden Temple)	1 oz	2	.17	.04	.23	na	na	na	na	14.0	1.0	na	108	na
'Natural Blueberry Granola' coconut-free (Golden Temple)	1 oz	2	.18	.04	.24	na	na	na	na	14.0	1.0	na	108	na
'Natural Bran Flakes' (Post)	1 oz	na	na	na	na	na	na	na	na	na	na	na	200	na
'Natural Delite Granola' (Golden Temple)	1 oz	2	.16	.04	.23	na	na	na	na	16.0	1.0	na	99	na
'Natural Foods Apple Cinnamon' low fat (Golden Temple)	1 oz	2	.15	.04	.21	na	na	na	na	17.0	1.0	na	103	na
'Natural Foods Raisin Almond' low fat (Golden Temple)	1 oz	2	.15	.04	.21	na	na	na	na	14.0	1.0	na	111	na
'Natural Foods Strawberry/Raspberry' low fat (Golden Temple)	1 oz	2	.16	.04	.21	na	na	na	na	13.0	1.0	na	104	na
'Natural Raisin Bran' (Post)	1.4 oz	na	na	na	na	na	na	na	na	na	na	na	260	na
'Nut & Honey Crunch' (Kellogg's)	1 oz	750	.38	.43	5	.5	na	na	15.0	4	1.8	6	40	.1
'Nut & Honey Crunch O's' (Kellogg's)	1 oz	750	.38	.43	5	.5	na	na	15.0	19	1.8	14	70	1.5
'Nutri-Grain' barley (Kellogg's)	1 oz	1252	.37	.43	5.0	.51	100.3	1.51	15.1	7.67	1.0	22.44	74.69	3.75
'Nutri-Grain' corn (Kellogg's)	1 oz	1252	.37	.43	5.0	.51	100.3	1.51	15.1	.85	.6	18.18	66.17	3.75
'Nutri-Grain' rye (Kellogg's)	1 oz	1252	.37	.43	5.0	.51	100.3	1.51	15.1	5.96	.8	21.58	50.84	3.75
'Nutri-Grain' wheat (Kellogg's)	1 oz	1252	.37	.43	5.0	.51	100.3	1.51	15.1	7.95	.8	22.15	77.25	3.75
'Nutri-Grain Almond Raisin' (Kellogg's)	2/3 cup	0	.38	.43	5	.5	na	2	tr	16	.8	11	130	3.75
'Nutri-Grain Raisin Bran' (Kellogg's)	1 cup	0	.38	.43	5	.5	na	2	tr	200	1.9	52	250	3.75
'Oat Bran Almond' (Golden Temple)	1 oz	2	.19	.05	.22	na	na	na	na	18.0	1.0	na	126	na
'Oat Bran Apple' (Golden Temple)	1 oz	2	.2	.04	.25	na	na	na	na	15.0	1.0	na	120	na
'Oat Bran Granola' berries (Golden Temple)	1 oz	0	.10	.04	.24	na	na	na	na	15.0	1.0	na	119	na
'Oat Bran Granola' raisins and almonds (Golden Temple)	1 oz	2	.18	.04	.24	na	na	na	na	16.0	1.0	na	125	na
'Oat Bran Müesli' dates and almonds (Golden Temple)	1 oz	98	.19	.15	1.65	na	na	na	na	14.0	1.0	na	105	na
'Oat Bran Müesli' raisins and hazelnuts (Golden Temple)	1 oz	104	.2	.14	1.62	na	na	na	na	16.0	5.0	na	160	na
'Oat Bran Oregonberry' (Golden Temple)	1 oz	2	.2	.04	.24	na	na	na	na	15.0	1.0	na	123	na
'Oat Flakes' (Post)	1 oz	na	na	na	na	na	na	na	na	na	na	na	135	na
'Oat Mini Puffs' (Glenny's)	1 oz	na	na	na	na	na	na	na	na	na	na	na	40	na
'Oat Mini Puffs' w/o salt, w/o sugar (Glenny's)	1 oz	na	na	na	na	na	na	na	na	na	na	na	10	na
'Oatbake Honey Bran' (Kellogg's)	1 oz	750	.38	.43	5	.5	na	na	15.0	15	4.5	28	100	3.75
'Oatbake Raisin Nut' (Kellogg's)	1 oz	750	.38	.43	5	.5	na	na	15.0	14	4.5	26	110	3.75
'Oatmeal Crisp' (General Mills)	1 oz	na	na	na	na	na	na	na	na	na	na	na	75	na
'Oatmeal Raisin Crisp' (General Mills)	1/2 cup	na	na	na	na	na	na	na	na	na	na	na	120	na
'100% Bran' wheat bran and barley (Nabisco)	1 oz	0	.68	.77	9.0	.91	20.2	2.7	27.0	19.88	3.49	134.33	354.43	2.47
'100% Natural Almond' (Golden Temple)	1 oz	6	.11	.04	.32	na	na	na	na	24.0	1.0	na	106	na
'100% Natural Apple/Cinnamon' (Golden Temple)	1 oz	6	.11	.04	.33	na	na	na	na	25.0	1.0	na	103	na
'100% Natural' mixed grain (Quaker)	1 oz	0	.08	.07	.4	.05	12.0	.26	0.0	43	.79	31	134	.63
'100% Natural Oat Bran' (Golden Temple)	1 oz	0	.33	.06	.27	na	na	na	na	17.0	2.0	na	161	na
'100% Natural' oats and wheat (Quaker)	1 oz	16	.09	.15	.65	.05	8.5	.04	0.0	49.42	.84	34.08	140.3	.64
'100% Natural' oats and wheat, apple and cinnamon (Quaker)	1 oz	16	.09	.16	.51	.03	4.5	.08	0.3	42.88	.79	19.6	140.3	.55
'100% Natural' oats and wheat, raisins and dates (Quaker)	1 oz	16	.08	.17	.54	.04	11.6	.04	0.0	41.18	.81	32.09	138.88	.55

Food Name	Serving Size	A I.U.	Thi mg	Rib mg	Nia mg	B$_6$ mg	Fol mcg	B$_{12}$ mcg	C mg	Calc mg	Iron mg	Mag mg	Pot mg	Zn mg
'100% Natural Raisin/Almond' *(Golden Temple)*	1 oz	6	.11	.04	.33	na	na	na	na	22.0	1.0	na	115	na
'Orange Almond Granola' *(Golden Temple)*	1 oz	2	.16	.04	.2	na	na	na	na	13.0	1.0	na	88	na
'Peach Pecan Müesli' *(Ralston)*	1.45 oz	na	na	na	na	na	na	na	na	na	na	na	170	na
'Post Toasties Corn Flakes' *(Post)*	1 oz	na	na	na	na	na	na	na	na	na	na	na	35	na
'Product 19' corn and other grains *(Kellogg's)*	1 oz	5009	1.51	1.7	20.02	2.02	400.7	6.02	60.2	3.41	18.03	10.51	44.3	.43
'Puffed Rice' *(Malt•O•Meal)*	.5 oz	na	na	na	na	na	na	na	na	na	na	na	20	na
'Puffed Wheat' *(Malt•O•Meal)*	.5 oz	na	na	na	na	na	na	na	na	na	na	na	55	na
'Raisin Apricot-Date Granola' *(Golden Temple)*	1 oz	5	.16	.04	.23	na	na	na	na	12.0	1.0	na	93	na
'Raisin Bran' *(Erewhon)*	1 oz	na	na	na	na	na	na	na	na	na	na	na	60	na
'Raisin Bran' wheat *(Kellogg's)*	1.3 oz	1250	.37	.44	5.02	.52	100.0	1.51	0.0	12.92	16.75	47.6	191.88	3.76
'Raisin Bran' wheat *(Post)*	1 oz	1252	.37	.43	5.0	.51	100.3	1.51	0.0	13.35	4.52	48.28	174.94	1.51
'Raisin Bran' wheat *(Ralston)*	1 1/3 oz	1250	.38	.42	4.99	.49	100.2	1.51	1.1	18.14	18.45	57.08	193.91	1.13
'Raisin Bran Flakes' *(Malt•O•Meal)*	1.4 oz	na	na	na	na	na	na	na	na	na	na	na	230	na
'Raisin Grape-Nuts' *(Post)*	1 oz	na	na	na	na	na	na	na	na	na	na	na	110	na
'Raisin Squares' *(Kellogg's)*	1 oz	0	.38	.43	5	.5	na	2	tr	10	8.1	26	110	1.5
'Raspberry Almond Müesli' *(Ralston)*	1.45 oz	na	na	na	na	na	na	na	na	na	na	na	170	na
'Rice Chex' *(Ralston)*	1 oz	17	.37	.01	5.0	.51	100.3	1.51	15.1	3.98	1.79	7.1	32.94	.39
'Rice Krispies' *(Kellogg's)*	1 oz	1252	.37	.43	5.0	.51	100.3	0	15.1	3.98	1.79	10.22	29.54	.48
'Rice Mini Puffs' *(Glenny's)*	1 oz	na	na	na	na	na	na	na	na	na	na	na	40	na
'Shredded Wheat' *(Nabisco)*	1 biscuit	na	na	na	na	na	na	na	na	na	na	na	95	na
'Shredded Wheat 'n Bran' *(Nabisco)*	1 oz	na	na	na	na	na	na	na	na	na	na	na	140	na
'Shredded Wheat With Oat Bran' *(Nabisco)*	1 oz	na	na	na	na	na	na	na	na	na	na	na	130	na
'6-Grain Crisp' fruit and flaxseed *(Golden Temple)*	1 oz	106	.21	.15	1.55	na	na	na	na	16.0	5.0	na	127	na
'Smacks' *(Kellogg's)*	1 oz	750	.38	.43	5	.5	na	na	15.0	3	1.8	14	40	.31
'Smacks' wheat *(Kellogg's)*	1 oz	1252	.37	.43	5.0	.51	100.3	0	15.1	3.12	1.79	13.63	42.03	.28
'S'Mores Grahams' *(General Mills)*	1 oz	na	na	na	na	na	na	na	na	na	na	na	45	na
'Smurf-Magic Berries' *(Post)*	1 oz	na	na	na	na	na	na	na	na	na	na	na	25	na
'Special K' rice and wheat *(Kellogg's)*	1 oz	1252	.37	.43	5.0	.51	100.3	.01	15.1	8.24	4.52	15.62	49.13	3.75
'Spoon Size Shredded Wheat' *(Nabisco)*	1 oz	na	na	na	na	na	na	na	na	na	na	na	120	na
'Sprinkle Spangles' corn puffs, sprinkles *(General Mills)*	1 oz	na	na	na	na	na	na	na	na	na	na	na	35	na
'Strawberry Squares' *(Kellogg's)*	1 oz	0	.38	.43	5	.5	na	2	tr	11	8.1	28	90	1.5
'Sugar Corn Pops' *(Kellogg's)*	1 oz	1252	.37	.43	5.0	.51	100.3	0	15.1	1.14	1.79	1.99	17.32	1.51
'Sugar Frosted Flakes' *(Malt•O•Meal)*	1 oz	na	na	na	na	na	na	na	na	na	na	na	20	na
'Super Nutty Granola' *(Golden Temple)*	1 oz	2	.17	.04	.22	na	na	na	na	16.0	1.0	na	89	na
'Super O's' *(Erewhon)*	1 oz	na	na	na	na	na	na	na	na	na	na	na	55	na
'Super Sugar Crisp' wheat *(Post)*	1 oz	1252	.37	.43	5.0	.51	100.3	1.51	0.0	5.96	1.79	17.04	105.65	1.51
'Sweet Home Farm Almond' *(Golden Temple)*	1 oz	6	.11	.04	.32	na	na	na	na	24.0	1.0	na	106	na
'Sweet Home Farm Crunchy Müesli' low fat *(Golden Temple)*	1 oz	130	.18	.17	2.0	na	na	na	na	15.0	4.0	na	92	na
'Sweet Home Farm Granola' low fat *(Golden Temple)*	1 oz	0	6.0	2.0	2.0	na	na	na	na	2.0	4.0	na	105	na
'Sweet Home Farm Raisin' *(Golden Temple)*	1 oz	6	.1	.04	.03	na	na	na	na	22.0	0	na	117	na
'Sweetened Puffed Wheat' *(Malt•O•Meal)*	1 oz	na	na	na	na	na	na	na	na	na	na	na	50	na
'Swiss Style Müesli' *(Golden Temple)*	1 oz	19	.15	.06	.53	na	na	na	na	16.0	1.0	na	118	na
'Tasteeos' oat and other grains	1 oz	1252	.37	.43	5.0	.51	11.1	1.51	15.1	13.06	4.52	30.96	84.06	.81
'Team' rice and other grains *(Nabisco)*	1 oz	1252	.37	.43	5.0	.51	4.5	1.51	15.1	4.26	1.74	12.5	48.0	.39
'35% Fruit Müesli' *(Golden Temple)*	1 oz	21	.14	.06	.51	na	na	na	na	13.0	1.0	na	122	na
'Toasted Oat' 100% natural *(Nature Valley)*	1 oz	na	na	na	na	na	na	na	na	na	na	na	75	na
'Toasted Oats' *(Malt•O•Meal)*	1 oz	na	na	na	na	na	na	na	na	na	na	na	90	na
'Toasties' corn *(Post)*	1 oz	1252	.37	.43	5.0	.51	100.3	1.51	na	1.14	.75	4.26	32.94	.08
'Total Corn Flakes' *(General Mills)*	1 oz	na	na	na	na	na	na	na	na	na	na	na	35	na
'Total Raisin Bran' *(General Mills)*	1.5 oz	na	na	na	na	na	na	na	na	na	na	na	230	na

Food Name	Serving Size	A I.U.	Thi mg	Rib mg	Nia mg	B₆ mg	Fol mcg	B₁₂ mcg	C mg	Calc mg	Iron mg	Mag mg	Pot mg	Zn mg
'Total' wheat *(General Mills)*	1 oz	5009	1.51	1.7	20.02	2.02	400.7	6.02	60.2	242.54	18.03	31.81	105.93	.67
'Triples' *(General Mills)*	1 oz	na	na	na	na	na	na	na	na	na	na	na	35	na
'Triples' breakfast pack *(General Mills)*	1 oz	na	na	na	na	na	na	na	na	na	na	na	30	na
'Trix' corn and other grains *(General Mills)*	1 oz	1252	.37	.43	5.0	.51	2.6	1.51	15.1	5.68	4.52	6.25	26.7	.13
'Uncle Sam' *(US Mills)*	1 oz	na	na	na	na	na	na	na	na	na	na	na	135	na
'Urkel-O's' *(Ralston)*	1 oz	na	na	na	na	na	na	na	na	na	na	na	40	na
'Waffelos' wheat and other grains	1 oz	1252	.37	.43	5.0	.51	3.1	1.51	15.1	7.95	4.52	5.96	24.99	.23
'Wheat Chex' *(Ralston)*	1 oz	0	.37	.1	5.0	.51	100.3	1.51	15.1	11.08	4.52	36.07	107.07	.76
'Wheat Flakes' *(Erewhon)*	1 oz	na	na	na	na	na	na	na	na	na	na	na	35	na
'Wheat 'n Raisin Chex' *(Ralston)*	1 1/3 oz	1	.38	.42	4.99	.49	100.2	1.51	1.1	17.01	5.41	37.04	158.76	.83
'Wheaties' *(General Mills)*	1 oz	1252	.37	.43	5.0	.51	100.3	1.51	15.1	42.88	4.52	30.96	106.22	.63
'Wheaties Honey Gold' *(General Mills)*	1 oz	na	na	na	na	na	na	na	na	na	na	na	60	na
'Whole-Grain Shredded Wheat' *(Kellogg's)*	1 oz	0	.38	.43	5	.5	na	2	tr	11	1.8	38	120	1.5
'Whole-Grain Wheat Chex' *(Ralston)*	1 oz	na	na	na	na	na	na	na	na	na	na	na	115	na

CEREAL SNACK. See GRANOLA AND CEREAL BAR.

CHARD. See SWISS CHARD.

CHAYOTE

Food Name	Serving Size	A I.U.	Thi mg	Rib mg	Nia mg	B₆ mg	Fol mcg	B₁₂ mcg	C mg	Calc mg	Iron mg	Mag mg	Pot mg	Zn mg
boiled, drained, 1-inch pieces	1/2 cup	38	.02	.03	.34	.09	14.5	0	6.4	10.4	.18	9.6	138.4	.25
raw, approx 7.2 oz	1 med	114	.06	.08	1.02	.27	56.0	0	22.3	38.57	.81	28.42	304.5	.71

CHEESE. See also CHEESE, ALTERNATIVE; CHEESE FOOD; CHEESE SPREAD.

AMERICAN

Food Name	Serving Size	A I.U.	Thi mg	Rib mg	Nia mg	B₆ mg	Fol mcg	B₁₂ mcg	C mg	Calc mg	Iron mg	Mag mg	Pot mg	Zn mg
(Hoffman's)	1 oz	na	na	na	na	na	na	na	na	146	na	na	na	na
(Land O'Lakes)	1 oz	na	na	na	na	na	na	na	na	na	na	na	30	na
(Land O'Lakes) sharp	1 oz	na	na	na	na	na	na	na	na	na	na	na	25	na

BLUE

Food Name	Serving Size	A I.U.	Thi mg	Rib mg	Nia mg	B₆ mg	Fol mcg	B₁₂ mcg	C mg	Calc mg	Iron mg	Mag mg	Pot mg	Zn mg
crumbled, not packed	1 cup	973	.04	.52	1.37	.22	49.1	1.64	0.0	712.26	.42	30.96	346.0	3.59
(Kraft)	1 oz	na	na	na	na	na	na	na	na	na	na	na	25	na

BRICK

Food Name	Serving Size	A I.U.	Thi mg	Rib mg	Nia mg	B₆ mg	Fol mcg	B₁₂ mcg	C mg	Calc mg	Iron mg	Mag mg	Pot mg	Zn mg
(Kraft)	1 oz	na	na	na	na	na	na	na	na	na	na	na	20	na
(Land O'Lakes)	1 oz	na	na	na	na	na	na	na	na	na	na	na	40	na
CAMEMBERT, domestic	1 oz	258	.01	.14	.18	.06	17.4	.36	0.0	108.53	.09	5.59	52.25	.67
CARAWAY	1 oz	295	.01	.13	.05	.02	5.1	.08	0.0	188.52	.18	6.19	26.04	.82

CHEDDAR

Food Name	Serving Size	A I.U.	Thi mg	Rib mg	Nia mg	B₆ mg	Fol mcg	B₁₂ mcg	C mg	Calc mg	Iron mg	Mag mg	Pot mg	Zn mg
American domestic	1 oz	297	.01	.11	.02	.02	5.1	.23	0.0	201.96	.19	7.78	27.55	.87
American domestic, shredded, not packed	1 cup	1197	.03	.42	.09	.08	20.6	.93	0.0	815.07	.77	31.39	111.19	3.51
(Hoffman's) super sharp processed	1 oz	na	na	na	na	na	na	na	na	146	na	na	na	na
CHESHIRE	1 oz	276	.01	.08	.02	.02	5.1	.23	0.0	180.04	.06	5.85	26.6	.78

COTTAGE CHEESE

Creamed

Food Name	Serving Size	A I.U.	Thi mg	Rib mg	Nia mg	B₆ mg	Fol mcg	B₁₂ mcg	C mg	Calc mg	Iron mg	Mag mg	Pot mg	Zn mg
large curd	4 oz	184	.02	.18	.14	.08	13.8	.7	0.0	67.8	.16	5.94	95.26	.42
large curd, not packed	1 cup	342	.04	.34	.26	.14	25.6	1.31	0.0	126.0	.29	11.05	177.03	.78
small curd	4 oz	184	.02	.18	.14	.08	13.8	.7	0.0	67.8	.16	5.94	95.26	.42
small curd, not packed	1 cup	342	.04	.34	.26	.14	25.6	1.31	0.0	126.0	.29	11.05	177.03	.78
(Breakstone's) lowfat 2%	4 oz	na	na	na	na	na	na	na	na	na	na	na	90	na
(Knudsen) 4% fat, large curd	4 oz	na	na	na	na	na	na	na	na	na	na	na	70	na
(Knudsen) 4% fat, small curd	4 oz	na	na	na	na	na	na	na	na	na	na	na	60	na

Lowfat

Food Name	Serving Size	A I.U.	Thi mg	Rib mg	Nia mg	B₆ mg	Fol mcg	B₁₂ mcg	C mg	Calc mg	Iron mg	Mag mg	Pot mg	Zn mg
1%, not packed	1 cup	84	.05	.37	.29	.15	28.0	1.43	0.0	137.63	.32	12.07	193.23	.86
2%, not packed	1 cup	158	.05	.42	.33	.17	29.6	1.61	0.0	154.81	.36	13.56	217.41	.95
(Knudsen) 2%	4 oz	na	na	na	na	na	na	na	na	na	na	na	80	na
(Knudsen) 2%, w/fruit cocktail	4 oz	na	na	na	na	na	na	na	na	na	na	na	190	na
(Knudsen) 2%, w/Mandarin orange	4 oz	na	na	na	na	na	na	na	na	na	na	na	100	na
(Knudsen) 2%, w/peach	6 oz	na	na	na	na	na	na	na	na	na	na	na	105	na
(Knudsen) 2%, w/pear	4 oz	na	na	na	na	na	na	na	na	na	na	na	105	na
(Knudsen) 2%, w/pineapple	6 oz	na	na	na	na	na	na	na	na	na	na	na	110	na
(Knudsen) 2%, w/spiced apple	6 oz	na	na	na	na	na	na	na	na	na	na	na	120	na
(Knudsen) 2%, w/strawberry	6 oz	na	na	na	na	na	na	na	na	na	na	na	100	na

Food Name	Serving Size	A I.U.	Thi mg	Rib mg	Nia mg	B₆ mg	Fol mcg	B₁₂ mcg	C mg	Calc mg	Iron mg	Mag mg	Pot mg	Zn mg
(Light n' Lively) 1%	4 oz	na	na	na	na	na	na	na	na	na	na	na	130	na
(Light n' Lively) 1%, garden salad	4 oz	na	na	na	na	na	na	na	na	na	na	na	140	na
(Sealtest) 2%	4 oz	na	na	na	na	na	na	na	na	na	na	na	250	na
Nonfat *(Knudsen)*	4 oz	na	na	na	na	na	na	na	na	na	na	na	60	na
Uncreamed														
dry, large curd	4 oz	34	.03	.16	.18	.09	16.7	.93	0.0	35.82	.26	4.45	36.61	.53
dry, large curd, not packed	1 cup	44	.04	.21	.22	.12	21.5	1.2	0.0	45.96	.33	5.71	46.98	.68
dry, small curd	4 oz	34	.03	.16	.18	.09	16.7	.93	0.0	35.82	.26	4.45	36.61	.53
dry, small curd, not packed	1 cup	44	.04	.21	.22	.12	21.5	1.2	0.0	45.96	.33	5.71	46.98	.68
CREAM CHEESE														
natural	1 oz	400	0	.06	.03	.01	3.7	.12	0.0	22.37	.34	1.8	33.43	.15
(Philadelphia Brand)	1 oz	na	na	na	na	na	na	na	na	na	na	na	25	na
(Philadelphia Brand) pasteurized process														
'Light'	1 oz	na	na	na	na	na	na	na	na	na	na	na	60	na
(Philadelphia Brand) w/chives	1 oz	na	na	na	na	na	na	na	na	na	na	na	30	na
(Philadelphia Brand) w/pimento	1 oz	na	na	na	na	na	na	na	na	na	na	na	30	na
Soft														
(Philadelphia Brand)	1 oz	na	na	na	na	na	na	na	na	na	na	na	55	na
(Philadelphia Brand) w/chives and onion	1 oz	na	na	na	na	na	na	na	na	na	na	na	45	na
(Philadelphia Brand) w/herb and garlic	1 oz	na	na	na	na	na	na	na	na	na	na	na	70	na
(Philadelphia Brand) w/olives and pimento	1 oz	na	na	na	na	na	na	na	na	na	na	na	40	na
(Philadelphia Brand) w/pineapple	1 oz	na	na	na	na	na	na	na	na	na	na	na	40	na
(Philadelphia Brand) w/smoked salmon	1 oz	na	na	na	na	na	na	na	na	na	na	na	40	na
(Philadelphia Brand) w/strawberries	1 oz	na	na	na	na	na	na	na	na	na	na	na	65	na
Whipped														
(Philadelphia Brand)	1 oz	na	na	na	na	na	na	na	na	na	na	na	30	na
(Philadelphia Brand) w/chives	1 oz	na	na	na	na	na	na	na	na	na	na	na	40	na
(Philadelphia Brand) w/onions	1 oz	na	na	na	na	na	na	na	na	na	na	na	45	na
(Philadelphia Brand) w/smoked salmon	1 oz	na	na	na	na	na	na	na	na	na	na	na	45	na
EDAM *(May-Bud)*	1 oz	na	na	na	na	na	na	na	na	207	na	na	na	na
FARMER *(May-Bud)*	1 oz	na	na	na	na	na	na	na	na	150	na	na	na	na
FRENCH ONION *(Alouette)*	1 oz	na	na	na	na	na	na	na	na	na	na	na	35	na
GOAT														
hard type	1 oz	156	.04	.34	.68	.02	1.1	.03	0.0	253.73	.53	15.31	13.61	.45
semisoft type	1 oz	162	.02	.19	.33	.02	0.6	.06	0.0	84.48	.46	8.22	44.79	.19
soft type	1 oz	130	.02	.11	.12	.07	3.4	.05	0.0	39.69	.54	4.54	7.37	.26
GOUDA *(May-Bud)*	1 oz	na	na	na	na	na	na	na	na	198	na	na	na	na
GRUYERE	1 oz	341	.02	.08	.03	.02	2.9	.45	0.0	283.08	.05	10.05	22.68	1.09
MONTEREY	1 oz	266	0	.11	.03	.02	5.1	.23	0.0	208.99	.2	7.56	22.6	.84
MONTEREY JACK *(May-Bud)*	1 oz	na	na	na	na	na	na	na	na	212	na	na	na	na
NEUFCHATEL *(Philadelphia Brand)* 'Light'	1 oz	na	na	na	na	na	na	na	na	na	na	na	30	na
PARMESAN														
natural, piece	1 oz	169	.01	.09	.08	.03	1.9	.34	0.0	331.38	.23	12.24	25.82	.77
natural, shredded	1 oz	179	.01	.1	.08	.03	2.2	.39	0.0	350.84	.24	14.22	27.16	.89
natural, shredded	1 tbsp	32	0	.02	.01	.01	0.4	.07	0.0	62.65	.04	2.54	4.85	.16
Grated														
natural	1 oz	196	.01	.11	.09	.03	2.2	.39	0.0	385.2	.27	14.22	29.99	.89
natural	1 tbsp	35	0	.02	.02	.01	0.4	.07	0.0	68.79	.05	2.54	5.36	.16
ROQUEFORT	1 oz	293	.01	.16	.21	.03	13.7	.18	0.0	185.3	.16	8.27	25.4	.58
SMOKED *(Hoffman's)* sharp, processed	1 oz	na	na	na	na	na	na	na	na	136	na	na	na	na
SWISS														
domestic	1 oz	237	.01	.1	.03	.02	1.8	.47	0.0	269.05	.05	10.05	31.0	1.09
domestic	1-inch cube	127	0	.05	.01	.01	1.0	.25	0.0	144.14	.03	5.39	16.61	.58
Processed														
(Borden) fat-free, low cholesterol	1 oz	na	na	na	na	na	na	na	na	na	na	na	70	na
(Hoffman's) smoky, w/cheddar	1 oz	na	na	na	na	na	na	na	na	170	na	na	na	na
TILSIT, whole milk	1 oz	293	.02	.1	.06	.02	5.6	.59	0.0	196.0	.06	3.64	18.06	.98

Food Name	Serving Size	A I.U.	Thi mg	Rib mg	Nia mg	B₆ mg	Fol mcg	B₁₂ mcg	C mg	Calc mg	Iron mg	Mag mg	Pot mg	Zn mg
CHEESE, ALTERNATIVE														
American style (Delicia)	1 oz	na	na	na	na	na	na	na	na	233	na	na	na	na
American style, hickory smoked (Delicia)	1 oz	na	na	na	na	na	na	na	na	237	na	na	na	na
American style, w/hot pepper (Delicia)	1 oz	na	na	na	na	na	na	na	na	215	na	na	na	na
mild cheddar style 'TofuRella' (Sharon's Finest)	1 oz	na	na	na	na	na	na	na	na	140	na	na	na	na
mild cheddar style 'TofuRella' slices (Sharon's Finest)	3/4 oz	na	na	na	na	na	na	na	na	150	na	na	na	na
CHEESE FLAVORED SNACKS														
(Chee•tos)														
cheddar valley	1 oz	na	na	na	na	na	na	na	na	na	na	na	45	na
crunchy	1 oz	na	na	na	na	na	na	na	na	na	na	na	40	na
curls	1 oz	na	na	na	na	na	na	na	na	na	na	na	40	na
flamin' hot	1 oz	na	na	na	na	na	na	na	na	na	na	na	50	na
light	1 oz	na	na	na	na	na	na	na	na	na	na	na	75	na
paws	1 oz	na	na	na	na	na	na	na	na	na	na	na	45	na
puffed balls	1 oz	na	na	na	na	na	na	na	na	na	na	na	50	na
puffs	1 oz	na	na	na	na	na	na	na	na	na	na	na	50	na
CHEESE FOOD														
AMERICAN														
colored (Hoffman's)	1 oz	na	na	na	na	na	na	na	na	146	na	na	na	na
w/Swiss cheese (Land O'Lakes)	1 oz	na	na	na	na	na	na	na	na	na	na	na	25	na
BACON, 'Chees'N Bacon' (Hoffman's)	1 oz	na	na	na	na	na	na	na	na	132	na	na	na	na
CARAWAY, 'Swisson Rye' (Hoffman's)	1 oz	na	na	na	na	na	na	na	na	151	na	na	na	na
JALAPEÑO (Hoffman's)	1 oz	na	na	na	na	na	na	na	na	150	na	na	na	na
ONION, 'Chees'N Onion' (Hoffman's)	1 oz	na	na	na	na	na	na	na	na	148	na	na	na	na
SALAMI, 'Chees'N Salami' (Hoffman's)	1 oz	na	na	na	na	na	na	na	na	140	na	na	na	na
CHEESE SPREAD														
AMERICAN, 'Easy Cheese American' (Nabisco)	1 oz	na	na	na	na	na	na	na	na	na	na	na	70	na
CHEDDAR														
'Easy Cheese Cheddar' (Nabisco)	1 oz	na	na	na	na	na	na	na	na	na	na	na	70	na
'Easy Cheese Cheddar 'n Bacon' (Nabisco)	1 oz	na	na	na	na	na	na	na	na	na	na	na	75	na
'Easy Cheese Sharp Cheddar' (Nabisco)	1 oz	na	na	na	na	na	na	na	na	na	na	na	75	na
FRENCH ONION (Alouette)	1 oz	na	na	na	na	na	na	na	na	na	na	na	35	na
GARLIC, and spices (Alouette)	1 oz	na	na	na	na	na	na	na	na	na	na	na	30	na
MEXICAN, 'Easy Cheese Nacho' (Nabisco)	1 oz	na	na	na	na	na	na	na	na	na	na	na	75	na
SALMON (Alouette)	1 oz	na	na	na	na	na	na	na	na	na	na	na	45	na
SPINACH, creamy (Alouette)	1 oz	na	na	na	na	na	na	na	na	na	na	na	40	na
CHEESE STRAW														
made w/lard, 5 x 3/8 x 3/8 inches	10 straws	234	.14	.19	1.26	na	na	na	0.0	155.4	1.32	na	37.8	na
made w/vegetable shortening, 5 x 3/8 x 3/8 inches	10 straws	234	.14	.19	1.26	na	na	na	0.0	155.4	1.32	na	37.8	na
CHEESECAKE FILLING														
'No-Bake' lite (Royal)	1/8 pie	na	na	na	na	na	na	na	na	na	na	na	190	na
'No-Bake' real (Royal)	1/8 pie	na	na	na	na	na	na	na	na	na	na	na	115	na
CHERIMOYA. See CUSTARD APPLE.														
CHERRY														
SOUR, RED														
trimmed, w/pits	1 cup	1321	.03	.04	.41	.05	7.7	0	10.3	16.48	.33	9.27	178.19	.1
trimmed, w/o pits	1 cup	1989	.05	.06	.62	.07	11.6	0	15.5	24.8	.5	13.95	268.15	.15
SWEET														
trimmed, w/pits	1 cup	310	.07	.09	.58	.05	6.1	0	10.2	21.75	.57	15.95	324.8	.09
trimmed, w/pits, approx 2.6 oz	10 med	146	.03	.04	.27	.02	2.9	0	4.8	10.2	.27	7.48	152.32	.04
untrimmed (Dole)	1 cup	64	na	na	na	na	na	na	11.0	na	na	na	270	na
CHERRY, CANNED														
SOUR, RED														
in extra heavy syrup	1/2 cup	905	.02	.05	.21	.06	9.6	0	2.5	13.0	1.64	6.5	118.3	.08

Food Name	Serving Size	A I.U.	Thi mg	Rib mg	Nia mg	B6 mg	Fol mcg	B12 mcg	C mg	Calc mg	Iron mg	Mag mg	Pot mg	Zn mg
in heavy syrup	1/2 cup	914	.02	.05	.22	.06	9.7	0	2.6	12.8	1.66	7.68	119.04	.08
in light syrup	1/2 cup	915	.02	.05	.21	.06	9.7	0	2.5	12.6	1.66	7.56	119.7	.09
in water	1/2 cup	920	.02	.05	.22	.05	9.8	0	2.6	13.42	1.67	7.32	119.56	.09
SWEET														
Pitted														
in extra heavy syrup	1/2 cup	196	.03	.05	.5	.04	5.5	0	4.7	11.7	.46	10.4	184.6	.13
in heavy syrup	1/2 cup	199	.03	.05	.51	.04	5.4	0	4.6	11.61	.45	11.61	187.05	.13
in juice	1/2 cup	156	.02	.03	.51	.04	5.3	0	3.1	17.5	.73	15.0	163.75	.12
in light syrup	1/2 cup	198	.03	.05	.51	.04	5.3	0	4.7	11.34	.45	11.34	186.48	.13
in water	1/2 cup	198	.03	.05	.51	.04	5.2	0	2.7	13.64	.45	11.16	162.44	.1
CHERRY, FROZEN														
SWEET														
sweetened	10-oz pkg	537	.08	.13	.5	.1	11.9	0	2.8	34.08	.99	28.4	565.16	.11
sweetened	1 cup	490	.07	.12	.46	.09	10.9	0	2.6	31.08	.91	25.9	515.41	.1
CHERRY DRINK														
(Hi-C) aseptic box	6 oz	na	na	na	na	na	na	na	60.0	na	na	na	25	na
(Hi-C) chilled	6 oz	na	na	na	na	na	na	na	60.0	na	na	na	25	na
(Kool-Aid) 'Koolers'	8.45 oz	na	na	na	na	na	na	na	na	na	na	na	40	na
CHERRY DRINK MIX														
(Kool-Aid) sugar-sweetened, prepared	8 oz	na	na	na	na	na	na	na	na	na	na	na	0	na
(Kool-Aid) unsweetened, prepared w/sugar	8 oz	na	na	na	na	na	na	na	na	na	na	na	0	na
(Kool-Aid) unsweetened, prepared w/o sugar	8 oz	na	na	na	na	na	na	na	na	na	na	na	0	na
(Kool-Aid) w/NutraSweet, prepared	8 oz	na	na	na	na	na	na	na	na	na	na	na	0	na
CHERRY JUICE DRINK (Tang) 'Fruit Box'	8.45 oz	na	na	na	na	na	na	na	na	na	na	na	30	na
CHERVIL														
dried	1 tbsp	na	na	na	na	.02	na	0	na	25.57	.61	2.47	90.06	.17
dried	1 tsp	na	na	na	na	.01	na	0	na	8.08	.19	.78	28.44	.05
CHESTNUT, CHINESE														
boiled or steamed	1 oz	39	.03	.03	.16	.08	13.2	0	7.0	3.41	.28	16.47	86.9	.17
dried	1 oz	93	.07	.08	.37	.19	31.2	0	16.6	8.24	.65	38.91	206.18	.4
raw	1 oz	57	.05	.05	.23	.12	19.2	0	10.2	5.11	.4	23.86	126.95	.25
roasted	1 oz	1	.04	.03	.43	.12	20.5	0	10.9	5.4	.43	25.56	135.47	.26
CHESTNUT, EUROPEAN/Italian chestnut/sweet chestnut														
dried, shelled, peeled	1 oz	0	.1	.02	.24	.19	31.2	0	4.3	18.18	.68	21.02	281.44	.1
dried, shelled, unpeeled	1 oz	0	.08	.1	.24	.19	31.0	0	4.3	19.03	.68	21.02	280.02	.1
raw, shelled, peeled	1 oz	7	.04	0	.31	.1	16.5	0	11.4	5.4	.27	8.52	137.46	.14
raw, shelled, unpeeled	1 cup	41	.35	.24	1.71	.55	89.9	0	62.4	39.15	1.46	46.4	751.1	.75
raw, shelled, unpeeled	1 oz	8	.07	.05	.33	.11	17.6	0	12.2	7.67	.29	9.09	147.11	.15
roasted, in shell	1 cup	34	.35	.25	1.92	.71	100.1	0	37.2	41.47	1.3	47.19	846.56	.82
roasted, in shell	1 oz	7	.07	.05	.38	.14	19.9	0	7.4	8.24	.26	9.37	168.13	.16
CHESTNUT, ITALIAN. See CHESTNUT, EUROPEAN.														
CHESTNUT, JAPANESE														
boiled or steamed	1 oz	4	.04	.02	.15	.03	4.8	0	2.7	3.12	.15	5.11	33.8	.11
dried, shelled	1 oz	24	.23	.11	.99	.19	30.9	0	17.4	20.45	.96	32.66	218.11	.73
dried, shelled	1 cup	133	1.24	.59	5.43	1.02	168.5	0	95.0	111.6	5.24	178.25	1190.4	3.98
raw, shelled	1 oz	11	.1	.05	.43	.08	13.2	0	7.5	8.8	.41	13.92	93.44	.31
roasted	1 oz	21	.13	na	.2	.12	16.7	0	8.0	9.94	.6	18.18	121.27	.41
CHESTNUT, SWEET. See CHESTNUT, EUROPEAN.														
CHESTNUT FLOUR	100 gm	0	.23	.37	1.0	na	na	na	0.0	50.0	3.2	na	847.0	na
CHIA SEEDS, dried	1 oz	10	.25	.05	1.65	.2	32.5	0	4.5	150.24	2.84	21.87	292.8	1.51
CHICK PEA. See GARBANZO BEAN.														
CHICKEN. For fresh chicken see CHICKEN, BROILER-FRYER; CHICKEN, CAPON; CHICKEN, ROASTER; CHICKEN, STEWING.														
CHICKEN, BROILER-FRYER														
BACK MEAT ONLY														
raw	1 lb	31	.02	.05	2.07	.1	2.8	.11	1.0	5.27	.32	6.82	63.24	.57
BREAST MEAT AND SKIN														
raw	1 lb	72	.05	.07	8.62	.46	3.5	.3	0.9	9.57	.64	21.75	191.4	.7

Food Name	Serving Size	A I.U.	Thi mg	Rib mg	Nia mg	B_6 mg	Fol mcg	B_{12} mcg	C mg	Calc mg	Iron mg	Mag mg	Pot mg	Zn mg
BREAST MEAT ONLY														
raw	1 lb	15	.05	.07	7.95	.39	2.8	.27	0.9	7.81	.51	19.88	181.05	.57
DARK MEAT AND SKIN														
raw	1 lb	272	.1	.23	8.34	.4	11.2	.46	3.4	17.6	1.57	30.4	284.8	2.53
DARK MEAT ONLY														
fried, chopped or diced	1 cup	111	.13	.35	9.9	.52	12.6	.46	0.0	25.2	2.09	35.0	354.2	4.07
raw	1 lb	78	.08	.2	6.81	.36	10.9	.39	3.4	13.08	1.12	25.07	241.98	2.18
roasted	1 cup	101	.1	.32	9.17	.5	11.2	.45	0.0	21.0	1.86	32.2	336.0	3.92
stewed	1 cup	97	.08	.28	6.63	.29	9.8	.31	0.0	19.6	1.9	28.0	253.4	3.72
DRUMSTICK MEAT AND SKIN														
raw	1 lb	42	.03	.08	2.4	.13	4.0	.15	1.2	4.84	.45	9.24	90.64	.88
DRUMSTICK MEAT ONLY														
raw	1 lb	21	.03	.07	2.14	.13	3.7	.14	1.2	4.07	.38	8.51	83.62	.82
LEG MEAT AND SKIN														
raw	1 lb	124	.07	.17	5.49	.29	11.1	.32	2.5	10.1	1.02	21.21	199.98	1.79
LEG MEAT ONLY														
raw	1 lb	48	.06	.15	4.73	.26	7.8	.28	2.5	8.58	.8	17.94	178.62	1.61
LIGHT MEAT AND SKIN														
raw	1 lb	115	.07	.1	10.33	.56	4.6	.39	1.0	12.76	.92	26.68	236.64	1.08
LIGHT MEAT ONLY														
fried	8 oz	42	.1	.18	18.71	.88	5.6	.5	0.0	22.4	1.6	40.6	368.2	1.78
raw	1 lb	25	.06	.08	9.33	.48	3.5	.33	1.1	10.56	.64	23.76	210.32	.85
roasted, chopped or diced	1 cup	41	.09	.16	17.39	.84	5.6	.48	0.0	21.0	1.48	37.8	345.8	1.72
NECK MEAT AND SKIN														
raw	1 lb	32	.01	.03	.54	.03	0.8	.04	0.2	2.7	.29	1.95	20.55	.28
NECK MEAT ONLY														
raw	1 lb	9	0	.01	.25	.02	0.5	.02	0.2	1.62	.12	1.02	10.5	.16
THIGH MEAT AND SKIN														
raw	1 lb	83	.04	.09	3.09	.15	4.0	.17	1.3	5.7	.56	11.4	109.44	.01
THIGH MEAT ONLY														
raw	1 lb	27	.03	.08	2.59	.14	4.1	.14	1.3	4.1	.43	9.84	94.71	.78
WING MEAT AND SKIN														
raw	1 lb	43	.01	.03	1.72	.1	1.2	.09	0.2	3.48	.28	5.22	45.24	.39
WING MEAT ONLY														
raw	1 lb	10	.01	.02	1.25	.09	0.7	.06	0.2	2.21	.15	3.74	32.98	.28
CHICKEN, CAPON														
GIBLETS														
raw	1 lb	2622	.02	.2	1.26	.08	70.9	2.33	3.3	1.8	1.13	3.24	40.68	.61
simmered	1 cup	19236	.14	1.54	5.97	.55	600.3	1.65	13.1	18.85	9.86	29.0	221.85	6.77
MEAT AND SKIN														
raw	1 lb	383	.19	.38	21.6	1.07	17.8	1.01	5.1	32.67	3.24	62.37	644.49	3.47
CHICKEN, ROASTER														
GIBLETS, simmered	1 cup	11797	.11	1.17	5.85	.43	439.4	12.25	9.4	17.4	8.83	29.0	232.0	6.71
MEAT AND SKIN														
raw	1 lb	384	.17	.34	19.26	.94	17.6	.91	4.4	29.3	2.96	55.67	574.28	3.14
CHICKEN, STEWING														
DARK MEAT ONLY														
raw	1 lb	142	.17	.29	5.68	.36	10.5	.39	4.8	10.5	1.28	24.15	254.1	2.18
stewed	1 cup	203	.18	.49	6.38	.34	11.2	.35	0.0	16.8	2.3	30.8	285.6	4.37
GIBLETS														
raw	1 lb	2939	.03	.31	2.39	.15	98.0	3.03	3.2	2.8	1.66	5.04	63.28	.84
simmered	1 cup	13827	.13	1.52	7.21	.59	532.2	13.75	8.0	18.85	9.34	29.0	223.3	6.21
LIGHT MEAT ONLY														
raw	1 lb	62	.12	.11	8.82	.51	3.6	.36	1.6	9.79	.82	23.14	232.29	.53
stewed	1 cup	102	.13	.27	11.95	.55	5.6	.38	0.0	19.6	1.67	32.2	278.6	1.16
MEAT AND SKIN														
raw	1 lb	402	.31	.45	16.97	.89	16.3	.87	6.5	27.1	2.82	54.2	552.84	3.22

Food Name	Serving Size	A I.U.	Thi mg	Rib mg	Nia mg	B_6 mg	Fol mcg	B_{12} mcg	C mg	Calc mg	Iron mg	Mag mg	Pot mg	Zn mg
CHICKEN DINNER/ENTRÉE, CANNED														
(LaChoy)														
chow mein 'Bi-Pack'	8.642 oz	na	na	na	na	na	na	na	11.4	3.38	5.3	na	na	na
Oriental w/noodles 'Bi-Pack'	9 oz	na	na	na	na	na	na	na	41.7	2.04	7.74	na	na	na
sweet and sour 'Bi-Pack'	8.959 oz	na	na	na	na	na	na	na	21.6	3.08	10.74	na	na	na
teriyaki 'Bi-Pack'	8.642 oz	na	na	na	na	na	na	na	11.4	3.06	10.06	na	na	na
CHICKEN DINNER/ENTRÉE, FROZEN														
(Armour)														
à la king 'Classics Lite'	11.25 oz	na	na	na	na	na	na	na	na	na	na	na	370	na
and noodles 'Classics'	11 oz	na	na	na	na	na	na	na	na	na	na	na	540	na
Burgundy 'Classics Lite'	10 oz	na	na	na	na	na	na	na	na	na	na	na	510	na
fettuccini 'Classics'	11 oz	na	na	na	na	na	na	na	na	na	na	na	400	na
glazed, 'Classics'	10.75 oz	na	na	na	na	na	na	na	na	na	na	na	400	na
mesquite 'Classics'	9.5 oz	na	na	na	na	na	na	na	na	na	na	na	810	na
Oriental 'Classics Lite'	10 oz	na	na	na	na	na	na	na	na	na	na	na	510	na
parmigiana 'Classics'	11.5 oz	na	na	na	na	na	na	na	na	na	na	na	540	na
sweet and sour 'Classics Lite'	11 oz	na	na	na	na	na	na	na	na	na	na	na	490	na
w/wine and mushroom sauce 'Classics'	10.75 oz	na	na	na	na	na	na	na	na	na	na	na	550	na
(Banquet)														
nuggets, w/barbecue sauce 'Extra Helping'	10 oz	na	na	na	na	na	na	na	na	na	na	na	710	na
nuggets, w/sweet and sour sauce 'Extra Helping'	10 oz	na	na	na	na	na	na	na	na	na	na	na	710	na
(Chun King)														
chow mein	13 oz	na	na	na	na	na	na	na	na	na	na	na	260	na
Imperial	13 oz	na	na	na	na	na	na	na	na	na	na	na	260	na
walnut, crunchy	13 oz	na	na	na	na	na	na	na	na	na	na	na	200	na
(Dining Lite)														
à la king	9 oz	na	na	na	na	na	na	na	na	na	na	na	220	na
and noodles	9 oz	na	na	na	na	na	na	na	na	na	na	na	300	na
chow mein	9 oz	na	na	na	na	na	na	na	na	na	na	na	180	na
(Mrs. Paterson's) 'Aussie Pie'	5.5 oz	na	na	na	na	na	na	na	na	na	na	na	329	na
(Stouffer's)														
à la king, w/rice	9.5 oz	na	na	na	na	na	na	na	na	na	na	na	260	na
and noodles, homestyle	10 oz	na	na	na	na	na	na	na	na	na	na	na	400	na
breast, baked, in gravy, w/potato, homestyle	8 7/8 oz	na	na	na	na	na	na	na	na	na	na	na	520	na
breast, fried, and whipped potatoes, homestyle	7 1/8 oz	na	na	na	na	na	na	na	na	na	na	na	440	na
breast, grilled, in barbecue sauce, homestyle	7 5/8 oz	na	na	na	na	na	na	na	na	na	na	na	700	na
chow mein, w/rice	10.75 oz	na	na	na	na	na	na	na	na	na	na	na	340	na
creamed	6.5 oz	na	na	na	na	na	na	na	na	na	na	na	230	na
Divan	8 oz	na	na	na	na	na	na	na	na	na	na	na	490	na
escalloped, and noodles	10 oz	na	na	na	na	na	na	na	na	na	na	na	300	na
fettuccini, w/vegetable medley, homestyle	9.5 oz	na	na	na	na	na	na	na	na	na	na	na	640	na
parmigiana and pasta Alfredo, homestyle	9 7/8 oz	na	na	na	na	na	na	na	na	na	na	na	800	na
pie	10 oz	na	na	na	na	na	na	na	na	na	na	na	320	na
tenders, breaded, w/potatoes, homestyle	8 3/8 oz	na	na	na	na	na	na	na	na	na	na	na	600	na
CHICKEN DINNER/ENTRÉE, PACKAGED														
(Chicken By George)														
Cajun	5 oz	na	na	na	na	na	na	na	na	na	na	na	698	na
lemon herb	5 oz	na	na	na	na	na	na	na	na	na	na	na	816	na
mesquite barbecue	5 oz	na	na	na	na	na	na	na	na	na	na	na	747	na
teriyaki	5 oz	na	na	na	na	na	na	na	na	na	na	na	749	na
(LaChoy) sweet and sour, w/noodles	9.383 oz	na	na	na	na	na	na	na	11.7	2.93	1.92	na	na	na
(Top Shelf)														
breast, glazed	10 oz	na	na	na	na	na	na	na	na	na	na	na	804	na

Food Name	Serving Size	A I.U.	Thi mg	Rib mg	Nia mg	B$_6$ mg	Fol mcg	B$_{12}$ mcg	C mg	Calc mg	Iron mg	Mag mg	Pot mg	Zn mg
breast, w/Spanish rice	10 oz	na	na	na	na	na	na	na	na	na	na	na	584	na
CHICKEN FAT														
	1 cup	0	0	0	0	0	0.0	0	0.0	0	0	0	0	0
	1 tbsp	0	0	0	0	0	0.0	0	0.0	0	0	0	0	0
CHICKEN GIBLETS														
fried	1 cup	17297	.14	2.21	15.93	.88	549.6	19.3	12.6	26.1	14.96	36.25	478.5	9.09
simmered	1 cup	10775	.13	1.38	5.95	.49	545.2	14.7	11.6	17.4	9.34	29.0	229.1	6.63
CHICKEN GIZZARD, all classes, simmered	1 cup	273	.04	.35	5.76	.17	76.9	2.81	2.3	14.5	6.02	29.0	259.55	6.35
CHICKEN HEART, all classes, simmered	1 cup	41	.1	1.07	4.06	.46	116.0	10.57	2.6	27.55	13.09	29.0	191.4	10.58
CHICKEN LIVER, all classes, simmered	1 cup	22925	.21	2.45	6.23	.81	1078.0	27.15	22.1	19.6	11.86	29.4	196.0	6.08
CHICKEN STEW (Dinty Moore) canned	7.5 oz	na	na	na	na	na	na	na	na	na	na	na	512	na
CHICORY, WITLOOF														
raw	1/2 cup	13	.03	.01	.07	.02	16.7	0	1.3	8.55	.11	4.5	94.95	.07
raw, approx 2.1 oz	1 head	15	.03	.01	.08	.02	19.6	0	1.5	10.07	.13	5.3	111.83	.08
CHICORY GREENS, trimmed, chopped	1/2 cup	3600	.05	.09	.45	.09	98.6	0	21.6	90.0	.81	27.0	378.0	.38
CHICORY ROOT														
raw, approx 2.6 oz	1 root	4	.02	.02	.24	.14	13.7	0	3.0	24.6	.48	13.2	174.0	.2
raw, 1-inch pieces	1/2 cup	3	.02	.01	.18	.11	10.3	0	2.3	18.45	.36	9.9	130.5	.15
CHILI, CANNED														
vegetarian, plain (Gebhardt)	4.339 oz	na	na	na	na	na	na	na	10.8	3.6	6.82	na	na	na
vegetarian, plain (Open Range)	4.409 oz	na	na	na	na	na	na	na	9.7	3.15	1.46	na	na	na
vegetarian, w/beans (Gebhardt)	4.444 oz	na	na	na	na	na	na	na	8.0	5.07	5.45	na	na	na
vegetarian, w/beans (Just Rite)	4.55 oz	na	na	na	na	na	na	na	2.9	5.05	3.36	na	na	na
vegetarian, w/beans (Open Range)	4.5 oz	na	na	na	na	na	na	na	7.3	5.57	6.7	na	na	na
vegetarian, w/beans, 'Longhorn' (Gebhardt)	4.55 oz	na	na	na	na	na	na	na	4.8	4.16	3.21	na	na	na
w/beans	1/2 cup	431	.06	.13	.46	.17	29.1	0	2.2	60.16	4.39	57.6	467.2	2.56
w/beans (Van Camp's)	1 cup	3428	.09	.22	2.39	na	na	na	na	63	4.83	na	537	na
w/beans (Wolf Brand)	8 oz	3940	.09	.82	2.68	.25	32.0	0	na	59	2.54	57	633	2
w/beans, extra spicy (Wolf Brand)	7.75 oz	3690	.08	.77	2.51	.23	30.0	0	na	55	2.38	53	603	2
w/o beans (Van Camp's)	1 cup	4938	.06	.20	3.22	na	na	na	na	46	3.48	na	370	na
w/o beans (Wolf Brand)	8 oz	4770	.11	1.27	3.86	.1	25.0	1	na	64	3.86	30	717	2
w/o beans 'Chili-Mac' (Wolf Brand)	7.75 oz	2450	.08	.53	3.51	.13	40.0	2	na	28	1.87	28	337	2
w/o beans, extra spicy (Wolf Brand)	7.5 oz	4470	.1	1.19	3.62	.09	23.0	1	na	60	3.62	28	672	2
CHILI, FROZEN, con carne, w/beans (Stouffer's)	8.75 oz	na	na	na	na	na	na	na	na	na	na	na	700	na
CHILI, MIX, 'Homestyle Chili Fixins' (Hunt's)	4.656 oz	na	na	na	na	na	na	na	12.2	3.6	.07	na	na	na
CHILI BEAN, CANNED . See also KIDNEY BEAN, CANNED; PINTO BEAN.														
(Gebhardt)	4.586 oz	na	na	na	na	na	na	na	2.7	6.41	12.84	na	na	na
(Hunt's)	4.48 oz	na	na	na	na	na	na	na	2.4	4.08	2.81	na	na	na
Mexican style (Van Camp's)	1 cup	1595	.12	.14	.89	na	na	na	1.2	80	4.42	na	640	na
CHILI POWDER														
(Durkee)	1 tsp	35	.4	1.12	.01	na	na	na	.04	0	.01	na	0	na
(Laurel Leaf)	1 tsp	35	.4	1.12	.01	na	na	na	.04	0	.01	na	0	na
CHILI SAUCE. See SAUCE.														
CHINESE CABBAGE. See CABBAGE, NAPA.														
CHINESE GOOSEBERRY. See KIWI FRUIT.														
CHINESE NOODLE. See NOODLE, CHINESE.														
CHINESE WATERMELON														
boiled, drained, cubes	1/2 cup	0	.03	0	.33	.03	3.2	0	9.1	15.66	.33	8.7	4.35	.51
raw, cubes	1 cup	0	.05	.15	.53	.05	6.9	0	17.2	25.08	.53	13.2	7.92	.81
CHIVES														
freeze-dried	1 tbsp	137	0	0	.01	0	0.2	0	1.3	1.63	.04	1.28	5.92	.01
freeze-dried	1/4 cup	546	.01	.01	.05	.02	0.9	0	5.3	6.5	.16	5.12	23.68	.04
raw, chopped	1 tbsp	131	0	0	.02	0	3.2	0	1.7	2.76	.05	1.26	8.88	.02
raw, chopped	1 tsp	44	0	0	.01	0	1.1	0	0.6	.92	.02	.42	2.96	.01
CHOCOLATE, BAKING														
Bar														
semi-sweet (Baker's)	1 oz	na	na	na	na	na	na	na	na	na	na	na	115	na

Food Name	Serving Size	A I.U.	Thi mg	Rib mg	Nia mg	B₆ mg	Fol mcg	B₁₂ mcg	C mg	Calc mg	Iron mg	Mag mg	Pot mg	Zn mg
semi-sweet (Nestlé)	1 oz	na	na	na	na	na	na	na	na	na	na	na	110	na
sweet 'German' (Baker's)	1 oz	na	na	na	na	na	na	na	na	na	na	na	80	na
unsweetened (Baker's)	1 oz	na	na	na	na	na	na	na	na	na	na	na	250	na
unsweetened (Nestlé)	1 oz	na	na	na	na	na	na	na	na	na	na	na	220	na
white 'Premier' (Nestlé)	1 oz	na	na	na	na	na	na	na	na	na	na	na	95	na
Chips														
milk chocolate (Baker's)	1 oz	na	na	na	na	na	na	na	na	na	na	na	95	na
milk chocolate 'Big Chips' (Baker's)	1/4 cup	na	na	na	na	na	na	na	na	na	na	na	150	na
semi-sweet (Baker's)	1/4 cup	na	na	na	na	na	na	na	na	na	na	na	220	na
semi-sweet 'Big Chips' (Baker's)	1/4 cup	na	na	na	na	na	na	na	na	na	na	na	150	na
semi-sweet, real chocolate (Baker's)	1/4 cup	na	na	na	na	na	na	na	na	na	na	na	135	na
Grated, bitter	1 cup	79	.07	.32	1.98	na	na	na	0.0	102.96	8.84	na	1095.6	na
Powder, cocoa 'Premium' (Saco Foods)	1 tbsp	1	.01	.03	.1	na	na	na	na	10.86	.8	na	46.5	na
Premelted, unsweetened 'Choco Bake'														
(Nestlé)	1 oz	na	na	na	na	na	na	na	na	na	na	na	129	na
Squares														
unsweetened, grated	1 cup	129	.11	.22	1.47	.13	9.2	0	0.0	97.68	8.34	409.2	1099.56	5.29
unsweetened, 1 oz	1 square	28	.02	.05	.32	.03	2.0	0	0.0	20.98	1.79	87.88	236.16	1.14
CHOCOLATE FLAVOR DRINK														
Mix/powder														
'Chocolate Milk Maker' (Swiss Miss)	.6702 oz	na	na	na	na	na	na	na	0.0	.45	3.65	na	na	na
dairy, reduced calorie, w/aspartame	.75-oz pkt	245	.02	.41	.27	.02	9.0	.51	0.3	187.44	1.64	44.73	477.12	.77
CHOCOLATE MILK														
whole	1 cup	303	.09	.41	.31	.1	11.8	.83	2.3	280.25	.6	32.57	417.25	1.02
2% fat	1 cup	500	.09	.41	.32	.1	12.0	.85	2.3	284.0	.6	33.0	422.0	1.02
1% fat	1 cup	500	.1	.42	.32	.1	12.0	.86	2.3	286.75	.6	33.33	425.5	1.02
CHOCOLATE SYRUP														
fudge-type	1 cup	306	.1	.75	.68	.12	13.6	1.02	1.7	340.0	4.08	163.2	731.0	2.72
fudge type	1 oz	56	.02	.08	.15	na	na	na	0.0	47.62	.49	na	106.5	na
fudge-type	1 tbsp	19	.01	.05	.04	.01	0.8	.06	0.1	21.0	.25	10.08	45.15	.17
unsweetened, 1 oz	1 pkt	5	.01	.04	.6	.02	1.7	0	0.0	15.31	1.18	75.13	330.56	1.04
w/added nutrients	1 cup	13035	.01	2.48	100.76	.06	12.0	0	2.7	42.0	40.65	195.0	1443.0	2.19
w/added nutrients	1 tbsp	817	0	.16	6.31	0	0.8	0	0.2	2.63	2.55	12.22	90.43	.14
w/o added nutrients	1 cup	90	.03	.15	.97	.02	12.0	0	0.6	42.0	6.33	195.0	672.0	2.19
w/o added nutrients	1 oz	11	0	.02	.12	0	1.5	0	0.1	5.25	.79	24.38	84.0	.27
CHORIZO														
	1 oz	0	.18	.09	1.45	.15	0.6	.57	0.0	2.27	.45	5.1	112.83	.97
4 inches	1 link	0	.38	.18	3.08	.32	1.2	1.2	0.0	4.8	.95	10.8	238.8	2.05
CHOW MEIN, chicken, w/o noodles, can	1 cup	150	.05	.1	1.0	na	na	na	12.5	45.0	1.25	na	417.5	na
CHRYSANTHEMUM GARLAND														
boiled, drained, 1-inch pieces	1/2 cup	2525	.01	.08	.36	.06	25.1	0	12.0	34.5	1.87	9.0	284.5	.1
raw, 1-inch pieces	1 cup	3669	.01	.06	.22	.03	19.1	0	9.3	14.0	.78	4.25	142.75	.05
raw, 8.75 inches long	1 stem	2055	0	.03	.12	.02	10.7	0	5.2	7.84	.44	2.38	79.94	.03
CHUB/cisco														
smoked	1 oz	264	.01	.04	.65	.08	0.6	1.19	0.0	7.28	.14	4.76	82.04	.08
CINNAMON														
ground	1 tbsp	18	.01	.01	.09	na	na	0	1.9	83.54	2.59	3.78	33.99	.13
ground	1 tsp	6	0	0	.03	na	na	0	0.7	28.25	.88	1.28	11.5	.05
ground (Durkee)	1 tsp	.14	.07	.11	0	na	na	na	.02	0	0	na	0	na
ground (Laurel Leaf)	1 tsp	.14	.07	.11	0	na	na	na	.02	0	0	na	0	na
CISCO. See CHUB.														
CITRON, candied	1 oz	0	0	0	0	na	na	na	0.0	23.24	.22	na	33.6	na
CITRUS DRINK (Five Alive) chilled	6 oz	na	na	na	na	na	na	na	30.0	na	na	na	130	na
CITRUS DRINK MIX														
(Crystal Light) blend, sugar-free,														
w/NutraSweet	8 oz	na	na	na	na	na	na	na	na	na	na	na	45	na
(Five Alive) frozen, diluted	6 oz	na	na	na	na	na	na	na	27.0	na	na	na	130	na

Food Name	Serving Size	A I.U.	Thi mg	Rib mg	Nia mg	B₆ mg	Fol mcg	B₁₂ mcg	C mg	Calc mg	Iron mg	Mag mg	Pot mg	Zn mg
CITRUS FRUIT JUICE DRINK														
frozen concentrate	12-oz can	618	.22	.16	2.67	.36	29.6	0	403.1	105.75	16.67	84.6	1662.39	.51
frozen concentrate, diluted	1 cup	104	.03	.03	.45	.06	5.0	0	67.2	22.32	2.78	14.88	277.76	.12
CITRUS PUNCH														
(Minute Maid) can or bottle 'Juices To Go' ..	6 oz	na	na	na	na	na	na	na	9.0	na	na	na	70	na
(Minute Maid) chilled	6 oz	na	na	na	na	na	na	na	9.0	na	na	na	70	na
CLAM, CANNED														
mixed species, drained	1 cup	912	.24	.68	5.37	.18	46.1	158.22	35.4	147.2	44.74	28.8	1004.8	4.37
mixed species, drained	3 oz	485	.13	.36	2.85	.09	24.5	84.05	18.8	78.2	23.77	15.3	533.8	2.32
mixed species, liquid only	1 cup	72	.02	.05	.43	.02	4.8	12.0	2.4	31.2	.72	26.4	357.6	.24
mixed species, liquid only	3 oz	26	.01	.02	.15	.01	1.7	4.25	0.9	11.05	.26	9.35	126.65	.09
CLAM, MIXED SPECIES														
breaded and fried	20 small	568	.19	.46	3.88	.11	34.2	75.71	18.8	118.44	26.15	26.32	612.88	2.74
breaded and fried	3 oz	257	.09	.21	1.75	.05	15.5	34.23	8.5	53.55	11.82	11.9	277.1	1.24
moist-heat cooked	20 small	513	.14	.38	3.02	.1	25.9	89.0	19.9	82.8	25.16	16.2	565.2	2.46
moist-heat cooked	3 oz	485	.13	.36	2.85	.09	24.5	84.05	18.8	78.2	23.77	15.3	533.8	2.32
raw	20 small	540	.14	.38	3.18	.11	28.8	89.0	23.4	82.8	25.16	na	565.2	2.47
raw	9 large	540	.14	.38	3.18	.11	28.8	89.0	23.4	82.8	25.16	16.2	565.2	2.47
raw	3 oz	255	.07	.18	1.5	.05	13.6	42.03	11.1	39.1	11.88	7.65	266.9	1.16
CLAM TOMATO JUICE, canned	5.5 oz	357	.07	.05	.32	.14	26.4	50.8	6.8	19.92	1.0	36.52	149.4	1.79
CLEARMALT. See ALCOHOLIC BEVERAGES.														
CLOVES														
ground	1 tbsp	35	.01	.02	.1	na	na	0	5.3	42.61	.57	17.42	72.71	.07
ground	1 tsp	11	0	.01	.03	na	na	0	1.7	13.56	.18	5.54	23.14	.02
ground (Durkee)	1 tsp	.23	.05	na	0	na	na	na	.04	0	0	na	0	na
ground (Laurel Leaf)	1 tsp	.23	.05	na	0	na	na	na	.04	0	0	na	0	na
COCOA BUTTER OIL														
....	1 cup	0	0	0	0	0	0.0	0	0.0	0	0	0	0	0
....	1 tbsp	0	0	0	0	0	0.0	0	0.0	0	0	0	0	0
COCOA MIX														
chocolate almond mocha (Swiss Miss)	1.235 oz	na	na	na	na	na	na	na	0.0	3.88	3.41	na	na	na
chocolate Bavarian mint (Swiss Miss)	1.235 oz	na	na	na	na	na	na	na	0.0	4.3	4.78	na	na	na
chocolate English toffee (Swiss Miss)	1.235 oz	na	na	na	na	na	na	na	0.0	3.98	3.45	na	na	na
chocolate praline and creme (Swiss Miss) ..	1.235 oz	na	na	na	na	na	na	na	0.0	3.98	3.45	na	na	na
chocolate raspberry truffle (Swiss Miss)	1.235 oz	na	na	na	na	na	na	na	0.0	4.21	3.92	na	na	na
dark chocolate truffle (Swiss Miss)	1.235 oz	na	na	na	na	na	na	na	0.0	4.3	3.43	na	na	na
diet 'Hot Cocoa Mix' (Swiss Miss)	.26 oz	na	na	na	na	na	na	na	0.0	3.24	.38	na	na	na
fat-free 'Hot Cocoa Mix' (Swiss Miss)	.5 oz	na	na	na	na	na	na	na	0.0	11.54	5.6	na	na	na
lite 'Hot Cocoa Mix' (Swiss Miss)	.7407 oz	na	na	na	na	na	na	na	0.0	4.63	2.48	na	na	na
marshmallow lovers 'Hot Cocoa Mix'														
(Swiss Miss)	1.199 oz	na	na	na	na	na	na	na	0.0	3.97	2.12	na	na	na
milk chocolate 'Hot Cocoa Mix' (Swiss Miss)	1.199 oz	na	na	na	na	na	na	na	0.0	4.02	2.14	na	na	na
milk chocolate 'Hot Cocoa Mix' (Swiss Miss)	1 oz	na	na	na	na	na	na	na	0.0	3.31	1.76	na	na	na
milk chocolate w/mini marshmallows 'Hot														
Cocoa Mix' (Swiss Miss)	1.199 oz	na	na	na	na	na	na	na	0.0	4.38	2.27	na	na	
milk chocolate w/mini marshmallows 'Hot														
Cocoa Mix' (Swiss Miss)	1 oz	na	na	na	na	na	na	na	0.0	3.61	1.87	na	na	na
rich, sugar-free 'Hot Cocoa Mix' (Swiss Miss)	.5 oz	na	na	na	na	na	na	na	0.0	4.34	.47	na	na	na
rich chocolate 'Hot Cocoa Mix' (Swiss Miss)	1 oz	na	na	na	na	na	na	na	0.0	1.91	.44	na	na	na
sugar-free 'Hot Cocoa Mix' (Swiss Miss)	.7055 oz	na	na	na	na	na	na	na	0.0	10.65	5.59	na	na	na
sugar-free 'Hot Cocoa Mix' (Swiss Miss)	.5 oz	na	na	na	na	na	na	na	0.0	7.85	4.12	na	na	na
sugar-free, w/mini marshmallows 'Hot Cocoa														
Mix' (Swiss Miss)	.7055 oz	na	na	na	na	na	na	na	0.0	3.69	.55	na	na	na
sugar-free, w/mini marshmallows 'Hot Cocoa														
Mix' (Swiss Miss)	.5 oz	na	na	na	na	na	na	na	0.0	2.8	.42	na	na	na
vending 'Hot Cocoa Mix' (Swiss Miss)	1.34 oz	na	na	na	na	na	na	na	0.0	4.4	2.35	na	na	na

Food Name	Serving Size	A I.U.	Thi mg	Rib mg	Nia mg	B₆ mg	Fol mcg	B₁₂ mcg	C mg	Calc mg	Iron mg	Mag mg	Pot mg	Zn mg
white chocolate 'Hot Cocoa Mix'														
(Swiss Miss)	1 oz	na	na	na	na	na	na	na	0.0	3.36	.2	na	na	na
w/added nutrients	1-oz pkt	500	.15	.17	2.0	.04	0.0	.41	6.0	100.15	1.8	22.15	404.04	.22
w/added nutrients, prepared	1 pkt	502	.15	.17	2.0	na	0.0	.42	6.1	104.5	1.82	22.99	405.46	.27
w/aspartame	.53-oz pkt	240	.04	.21	.16	.05	2.3	.29	0.0	218.88	.75	32.64	405.12	.56
w/aspartame, w/added calcium and														
potassium	.53-oz pkt	240	.04	.21	.16	.05	2.2	.29	0.0	216.0	.74	31.2	405.3	.52
w/aspartame, w/added sodium and														
vitamin A	.53-oz pkt	5	.04	.21	.16	.05	2.2	.29	0.0	86.4	.74	31.2	405.3	.52
w/o added nutrients	1-oz pkt	4	.03	.16	.17	.03	0.0	.37	0.5	92.58	.34	23.57	202.21	.41
w/o added nutrients, prepared	3-4 heaping tsp	4	.03	.16	.17	.03	0.0	.37	0.4	96.82	.35	24.72	201.88	.45
COCOA POWDER. See also CHOCOLATE, BAKING.														
(Hershey's) unsweetened, European style	1 cup	17	.02	.22	2.92	.1	27.5	0	0.0	129.0	29.76	473.0	4411.8	6.28
(Hershey's) unsweetened, European style	1 tbsp	1	0	.01	.17	.01	1.6	0	0.0	7.5	1.73	27.5	256.5	.36
COCONUT														
meat, raw, 2 x 2 x 1/2 inch	1 piece	0	.03	.01	.24	.02	11.9	0	1.5	6.3	1.09	14.4	160.2	.5
meat, raw, shredded	1 cup	0	.05	.02	.43	.04	21.1	0	2.6	11.2	1.94	25.6	284.8	.88
COCONUT, DRIED														
creamed	1 oz	0	.02	.03	.17	.09	2.6	0	0.4	7.38	.95	26.13	156.48	.58
sweetened, flaked, canned	4 oz	0	.03	.02	.35	.27	8.1	0	0.0	15.96	2.1	55.86	369.36	1.81
sweetened, flaked, canned	1 cup	0	.02	.02	.23	.18	5.5	0	0.0	10.78	1.42	37.73	249.48	1.22
sweetened, flaked, packaged	7-oz pkg	0	.06	.04	.6	.52	15.5	0	0.0	27.86	3.58	95.52	628.84	3.48
sweetened, flaked, packaged	1 cup	0	.02	.01	.22	.19	5.8	0	0.0	10.36	1.33	35.52	233.84	1.3
sweetened, shredded	7-oz pkg	0	.06	.04	.94	.54	16.1	0	1.4	29.85	3.82	99.5	670.63	3.62
sweetened, shredded	1 cup	0	.03	.02	.44	.25	7.5	0	0.7	13.95	1.79	46.5	313.41	1.69
sweetened, shredded, toasted	1 oz	0	.02	.03	.17	.09	2.6	0	0.4	7.67	.96	26.13	157.34	.58
sweetened, shredded, toasted 'Angel Flake'														
(Baker's)	1/3 cup	na	na	na	na	na	na	na	na	na	na	na	130	na
COCONUT CREAM														
Canned														
liquid expressed from grated meat	1 cup	0	.07	.12	.11	.09	42.3	0	5.3	2.96	1.51	50.32	298.96	1.78
liquid expressed from grated meat	1 tbsp	0	0	.01	.01	.01	2.7	0	0.3	.19	.1	3.23	19.19	.11
Raw														
liquid expressed from grated meat	1 cup	0	.07	0	2.14	.11	55.2	0	6.7	26.4	5.47	67.2	780.0	2.3
liquid expressed from grated meat	1 tbsp	0	0	0	.13	.01	3.5	0	0.4	1.65	.34	4.2	48.75	.14
COCONUT MILK														
canned	1 cup	0	.05	0	1.44	.06	30.5	0	2.3	40.68	7.46	103.96	497.2	1.27
canned	1 tbsp	0	0	0	.1	0	2.0	0	0.2	2.7	.5	6.9	33.0	.08
frozen	1 cup	0	.06	0	1.61	.07	34.1	0	2.6	9.6	1.94	76.8	556.8	1.42
frozen	1 tbsp	0	0	0	.1	0	2.1	0	0.2	.6	.12	4.8	34.8	.09
raw	1 cup	0	.06	0	1.82	.08	38.6	0	6.7	38.4	3.94	88.8	631.2	1.61
raw	1 tbsp	0	0	0	.11	0	2.4	0	0.4	2.4	.25	5.55	39.45	.1
COCONUT PINEAPPLE NECTAR														
can or bottle (Kern's)	6 oz	na	na	na	na	na	na	na	na	na	na	na	120	na
COCONUT VEGETABLE OIL														
	1 cup	0	0	0	0	0	0.0	0	0.0	0	.09	0	0	0
	1 tbsp	0	0	0	0	0	0.0	0	0.0	0	.01	0	0	0
COCONUT WATER														
	1 cup	0	.07	.14	.19	.08	6.0	0	5.8	57.6	.7	60.0	600.0	.24
	1 tbsp	0	0	.01	.01	0	0.4	0	0.4	3.6	.04	3.75	37.5	.01
COD, ATLANTIC														
dried and salted	3 oz	120	.23	.2	6.38	.73	21.0	8.5	3.0	136.0	2.13	113.05	1239.3	1.35
dry-heat cooked	3 oz	39	.07	.07	2.14	.24	6.9	.89	0.9	11.9	.42	35.7	207.4	.49
raw	3 oz	34	.06	.06	1.75	.21	6.0	.77	0.9	13.6	.32	27.2	351.05	.38
COD, PACIFIC														
dry-heat cooked	3 oz	27	.02	.04	2.11	.39	6.8	.88	2.6	7.65	.28	26.35	439.45	.43
raw	3 oz	24	.02	.04	1.73	.34	5.6	.77	2.5	5.95	.22	20.4	342.55	.34

Food Name	Serving Size	A I.U.	Thi mg	Rib mg	Nia mg	B₆ mg	Fol mcg	B₁₂ mcg	C mg	Calc mg	Iron mg	Mag mg	Pot mg	Zn mg
COD LIVER OIL														
regular	1 cup	0	na	0	0	0	0.0	0	0.0	0	0	0	0	0
regular	1 tbsp	0	na	0	0	0	0.0	0	0.0	0	0	0	0	0
COFFEE, brewed	6 oz	0	0	0	.39	0	0.2	0	0.0	3.54	.09	10.62	122.13	.02
COFFEE, ALTERNATIVE														
cereal grain beverage, powder, dry	1 tsp	0	.01	0	.39	.02	0.6	0	0.0	1.2	.11	5.61	42.32	.01
cereal grain beverage, powder, 'Instant,' prepared (Postum)	6 oz	na	na	na	na	na	na	na	na	na	na	na	95	na
cereal grain beverage, prepared w/ water	1 tsp	0	.01	0	.39	.02	0.5	0	0.0	5.4	.11	7.2	43.2	.05
cereal grain beverage, prepared w/whole milk	6 oz	229	.07	.3	.54	.08	9.1	.65	1.7	220.15	.2	29.6	318.2	.7
COFFEE, DECAFFEINATED														
instant, powder	1 round tsp	0	0	.02	.51	0	0.0	0	0.0	2.52	.07	5.6	63.02	0
instant, powder, prepared	6 oz	0	0	.03	.5	0	0.0	0	0.0	5.37	.07	7.16	62.65	.05
COFFEE, FLAVORED														
'Cafe Amaretto International' prepared (General Foods)	6 oz	na	na	na	na	na	na	na	na	na	na	na	260	na
'Cafe Français International' prepared (General Foods)	6 oz	na	na	na	na	na	na	na	na	na	na	na	220	na
'Cafe Français International' sugar-free, prepared (General Foods)	6 oz	na	na	na	na	na	na	na	na	na	na	na	280	na
'Cafe Irish Creme International' prepared (General Foods)	6 oz	na	na	na	na	na	na	na	na	na	na	na	260	na
'Cafe Vienna International' prepared (General Foods)	6 oz	na	na	na	na	na	na	na	na	na	na	na	110	na
'Cafe Vienna International' sugar-free, prepared (General Foods)	6 oz	na	na	na	na	na	na	na	na	na	na	na	105	na
'Double Dutch Chocolate International' prepared (General Foods)	6 oz	na	na	na	na	na	na	na	na	na	na	na	120	na
'Dutch Chocolate Mint International' prepared (General Foods)	6 oz	na	na	na	na	na	na	na	na	na	na	na	110	na
'Orange Cappuccino International' prepared (General Foods)	6 oz	na	na	na	na	na	na	na	na	na	na	na	140	na
'Orange Cappuccino International sugar-free, prepared (General Foods)	6 oz	na	na	na	na	na	na	na	na	na	na	na	125	na
COFFEE, INSTANT														
regular, powder	1 round tsp	0	0	0	.51	0	0.0	0	0.0	2.54	.08	5.89	63.63	.01
regular, prepared	6 oz	0	0	0	.51	0	0.0	0	0.0	5.37	.09	7.16	64.44	.05
'Suisse Mocha International' prepared (General Foods)	6 oz	na	na	na	na	na	na	na	na	na	na	na	170	na
'Suisse Mocha International' sugar-free, prepared (General Foods)	6 oz	na	na	na	na	na	na	na	na	na	na	na	130	na
w/chicory, powder	1 round tsp	0	0	.01	.39	0	0.0	0	0.0	1.85	.09	3.83	61.11	.01
w/chicory, prepared	6 oz	0	0	.01	.39	0	0.0	0	0.0	5.37	.09	5.37	60.86	.05
w/sugar, cappuccino flavor, powder	2 round tsp	0	.02	.01	.32	0	0.0	0	0.0	3.69	.14	7.38	118.0	.04
w/sugar, cappucino flavor, prepared	6 oz	0	.02	.01	.32	0	0.0	0	0.0	7.68	.15	9.6	119.04	.08
w/sugar, French flavor, powder	2 round tsp	0	0	0	.67	0	0.0	0	0.0	4.14	.08	5.29	136.16	.01
w/sugar, French flavor, prepared	6 oz	0	0	0	.67	0	0.0	0	0.0	7.56	.02	1.89	136.08	.04
w/sugar, mocha flavor, powder	2 round tsp	0	0	0	.26	0	0.0	0	0.0	3.68	.23	7.82	118.79	.11
w/sugar, mocha flavor, prepared	6 oz	0	0	0	.26	0	0.0	0	0.0	7.52	.24	9.4	118.44	.15
COFFEE LIQUEUR. See ALCOHOLIC BEVERAGES.														
COLE. See KALE.														
COLEWART. See KALE.														
COLESLAW														
fresh	1/2 cup	381	.04	.04	.16	.08	15.9	0	19.6	27.0	.35	6.0	108.6	.12
fresh	1 tbsp	51	.01	0	.02	.01	2.1	0	2.6	3.6	.05	.8	14.48	.02

Food Name	Serving Size	A I.U.	Thi mg	Rib mg	Nia mg	B$_6$ mg	Fol mcg	B$_{12}$ mcg	C mg	Calc mg	Iron mg	Mag mg	Pot mg	Zn mg
COLLARDS														
boiled, drained, chopped	1/2 cup	1745	.01	.03	.19	.03	3.8	0	7.7	14.72	.1	4.48	83.84	.07
raw, chopped	1/2 cup	599	.01	.01	.07	.01	2.2	0	4.2	5.22	.03	1.62	30.42	.02
Frozen														
chopped, boiled, drained	1/2 cup	5084	.04	.1	.54	.1	64.7	0	22.4	178.5	.95	25.5	213.35	.23
chopped, unprepared	10-oz pkg	16225	.14	.31	1.82	.33	207.6	0	113.6	570.84	3.04	82.36	718.52	.74
CONCORD PUNCH, 'Juices To Go'														
(Minute Maid)	6 oz	na	na	na	na	na	na	na	1.0	na	na	na	40	na
CONDIMENTS. See individual listings.														
COOKIE														
ALMOND														
(Health Valley) date 'Fruit Jumbos'	1 cookie	na	na	na	na	na	na	na	na	na	na	na	100	na
(Mother's) shortbread	2 cookies	na	na	na	na	na	na	na	na	na	na	na	35	na
ANIMAL CRACKERS														
(Grandma's) candied, 5 cookies	1 oz	na	na	na	na	na	na	na	na	na	na	na	25	na
(Mother's) circus animal	4 cookies	na	na	na	na	na	na	na	na	na	na	na	25	na
(Nabisco) 'Barnum's Animals' 5 1/2 pieces ...	.5 oz	na	na	na	na	na	na	na	na	na	na	na	15	na
APPLE														
(Bakery Wagon) cinnamon	1 cookie	na	na	na	na	na	na	na	na	na	na	na	20	na
(Bakery Wagon) filled oatmeal	1 cookie	na	na	na	na	na	na	na	na	na	na	na	55	na
(Bakery Wagon) walnut raisin	1 cookie	na	na	na	na	na	na	na	na	na	na	na	55	na
(Break Cake) sandwich	1 cookie	na	na	na	na	na	na	na	na	na	na	na	30	na
(Frookie) cinnamon oat bran	1 cookie	na	na	na	na	na	na	na	na	na	na	na	40	na
(Frookie) 'Fruitins'	1 cookie	na	na	na	na	na	na	na	na	na	na	na	25	na
(Frookie) spice, fat-free	1 cookie	na	na	na	na	na	na	na	na	na	na	na	20	na
(Great Cakes)	4.5 oz	na	na	na	na	na	na	na	na	na	na	na	380	na
(Health Valley) 'Fruit Centers' fat-free	1 cookie	na	na	na	na	na	na	na	na	na	na	na	60	na
(Health Valley) raisin 'Fruit Chunks'	3 cookies	na	na	na	na	na	na	na	na	na	na	na	110	na
(Nabisco) 'Newtons' .75 oz	1 cookie	na	na	na	na	na	na	na	na	na	na	na	25	na
(Nabisco) 'Newtons' fat-free, .75 oz	1 cookie	na	na	na	na	na	na	na	na	na	na	na	20	na
ARROWROOT (Nabisco) 'National Arrowroot														
Biscuit' 6 pieces	1 oz	na	na	na	na	na	na	na	na	na	na	na	25	na
BANANA														
(Break Cake) creme	1 cookie	na	na	na	na	na	na	na	na	na	na	na	50	na
(Frookie) fat-free	1 cookie	na	na	na	na	na	na	na	na	na	na	na	30	na
(Natures Warehouse) wheat-free, fat-free ...	1 oz	na	na	na	na	na	na	na	na	na	na	na	184	na
BLUEBERRY (Great Cakes)	4.5 oz	na	na	na	na	na	na	na	na	na	na	na	380	na
BROWNIE (Break Cake) creme	1 cookie	na	na	na	na	na	na	na	na	na	na	na	85	na
BUTTER (Mother's) flavored	5 cookies	na	na	na	na	na	na	na	na	na	na	na	30	na
CARAMEL (Natures Warehouse) crisp, wheat-free,														
fat-free	1 oz	na	na	na	na	na	na	na	na	na	na	na	184	na
CHERRY														
(Great Cakes) carob	4.5 oz	na	na	na	na	na	na	na	na	na	na	na	380	na
(Natures Warehouse) wheat-free, fat-free ...	1 oz	na	na	na	na	na	na	na	na	na	na	na	184	na
CHIPS AND CREME														
(Break Cake)	1 cookie	na	na	na	na	na	na	na	na	na	na	na	45	na
(Frookie) and vanilla sandwich 'Frookwich' ..	1 cookie	na	na	na	na	na	na	na	na	na	na	na	20	na
CHOCOLATE														
(Frookie) 'Animal Frackers	6 cookies	na	na	na	na	na	na	na	na	na	na	na	55	na
(Frookie) 'Funky Monkeys'	8 cookies	na	na	na	na	na	na	na	na	na	na	na	30	na
(Grandma's) 'Chocolate Cookie Bits'														
8 cookies	1 oz	na	na	na	na	na	na	na	na	na	na	na	55	na
(Nabisco) 'Chocolate Snap' 4 pieces	.5 oz	na	na	na	na	na	na	na	na	na	na	na	30	na
(Nabisco) 'Pure Chocolate Middles'	.5 oz cookie	na	na	na	na	na	na	na	na	na	na	na	20	na
CHOCOLATE CHIP														
(Almost Home)	.5 oz	na	na	na	na	na	na	na	na	na	na	na	20	na
(Break Cake) approx 1 oz	5 cookies	na	na	na	na	na	na	na	na	na	na	na	35	na

Food Name	Serving Size	A I.U.	Thi mg	Rib mg	Nia mg	B6 mg	Fol mcg	B12 mcg	C mg	Calc mg	Iron mg	Mag mg	Pot mg	Zn mg
(Chips Ahoy!)	.5 oz	na	na	na	na	na	na	na	na	na	na	na	15	na
(Chips Ahoy!) 'Mini'	.5 oz	na	na	na	na	na	na	na	na	na	na	na	20	na
(Chips Ahoy!) pecan 'Selections'	.5 oz	na	na	na	na	na	na	na	na	na	na	na	na	na
(Chips Ahoy!) 'Sprinkled'	.5 oz	na	na	na	na	na	na	na	na	na	na	na	15	na
(Chips Ahoy!) 'Striped'	.5 oz	na	na	na	na	na	na	na	na	na	na	na	25	na
(Chips Ahoy!) walnut 'Selections'	.5 oz	na	na	na	na	na	na	na	na	na	na	na	30	na
(Frookie)	1 cookie	na	na	na	na	na	na	na	na	na	na	na	40	na
(Frookie) Mandarin	1 cookie	na	na	na	na	na	na	na	na	na	na	na	40	na
(Frookie) mint	1 cookie	na	na	na	na	na	na	na	na	na	na	na	40	na
(Grandma's) 'Big Cookies' 2.75 oz	2 cookies	na	na	na	na	na	na	na	na	na	na	na	160	na
(Grandma's) 'Rich'N Chewy' 3 cookies	1 oz	na	na	na	na	na	na	na	na	na	na	na	40	na
(Mother's)	1 cookie	na	na	na	na	na	na	na	na	na	na	na	30	na
(Mother's) angel	2 cookies	na	na	na	na	na	na	na	na	na	na	na	40	na
(Nabisco) 'Chocolate Chip Snaps' 3 piece	.5 oz	na	na	na	na	na	na	na	na	na	na	na	0	na
CHOCOLATE CHUNK (Chips Ahoy!) 'Selections'	.5 oz	na	na	na	na	na	na	na	na	na	na	na	25	na
CHOCOLATE GRAHAM (Nabisco) 'Chocolate Grahams'	.5 oz	na	na	na	na	na	na	na	na	na	na	na	125	na
CHOCOLATE SANDWICH														
(Frookie) 'Frookwich'	1 cookie	na	na	na	na	na	na	na	na	na	na	na	20	na
(Oreo) 'Big Stuf'	.25 oz	na	na	na	na	na	na	na	na	na	na	na	80	na
(Oreo) 'Halloween Treats' 1 oz	2 cookies	na	na	na	na	na	na	na	na	na	na	na	40	na
(Oreo) 2 1/2 cookies	1 oz	na	na	na	na	na	na	na	na	na	na	na	50	na
CINNAMON														
(Frookie) 'Animal Frackers'	6 cookies	na	na	na	na	na	na	na	na	na	na	na	55	na
(Mother's) dinosaur, mini	7 cookies	na	na	na	na	na	na	na	na	na	na	na	15	na
(Mother's) dinosaur grahams	1 cookie	na	na	na	na	na	na	na	na	na	na	na	30	na
COCONUT														
(Break Cake) macaroons	2 cookies	na	na	na	na	na	na	na	na	na	na	na	160	na
(Mother's) cocadas	4 cookies	na	na	na	na	na	na	na	na	na	na	na	30	na
(Mother's) macaroons	1 cookie	na	na	na	na	na	na	na	na	na	na	na	35	na
CRANBERRY (Frookie) orange, fat-free	1 cookie	na	na	na	na	na	na	na	na	na	na	na	20	na
DATE														
(Bakery Wagon) filled oatmeal	1 cookie	na	na	na	na	na	na	na	na	na	na	na	55	na
(Break Cake) creme	1 cookie	na	na	na	na	na	na	na	na	na	na	na	45	na
DEVIL'S FOOD (Break Cake) creme	1 cookie	na	na	na	na	na	na	na	na	na	na	na	60	na
DUPLEX SANDWICH (Mother's)	2 cookies	na	na	na	na	na	na	na	na	na	na	na	40	na
ENGLISH TEA (Mother's) sandwich	1 cookie	na	na	na	na	na	na	na	na	na	na	na	35	na
FIG														
(Frookie) 'Fruitins'	1 cookie	na	na	na	na	na	na	na	na	na	na	na	25	na
(Frookie) 'Fruitins' fat-free	2 cookies	na	na	na	na	na	na	na	na	na	na	na	80	na
(Mother's) bar	2 cookies	na	na	na	na	na	na	na	na	na	na	na	95	na
(Mother's) whole wheat	2 cookies	na	na	na	na	na	na	na	na	na	na	na	120	na
(Nabisco) 'Newtons'	.5 oz	na	na	na	na	na	na	na	na	na	na	na	40	na
(Nabisco) 'Newtons Cookie Variety'	1 oz	na	na	na	na	na	na	na	na	na	na	na	50	na
(Nabisco) 'Newtons' fat-free, one piece	.75 oz	na	na	na	na	na	na	na	na	na	na	na	50	na
(Natures Warehouse) bar, apple cinnamon, wheat-free	1 oz	na	na	na	na	na	na	na	na	na	na	na	109	na
(Natures Warehouse) bar, raspberry, wheat-free	1 oz	na	na	na	na	na	na	na	na	na	na	na	109	na
(Natures Warehouse) bar, wheat-free	1 oz	na	na	na	na	na	na	na	na	na	na	na	109	na
(Natures Warehouse) bar, whole wheat	1 oz	na	na	na	na	na	na	na	na	na	na	na	109	na
FORTUNE (LaChoy)	1 oz	na	na	na	na	na	na	na	0.0	.37	.94	na	na	na
FRUIT (Health Valley) Hawaiian, fat-free	3 cookies	na	na	na	na	na	na	na	na	na	na	na	110	na
FUDGE														
(Almost Home) chocolate chip	.5 oz	na	na	na	na	na	na	na	na	na	na	na	20	na
(Chips Ahoy!) mini bites 'Little Fudgies'	1 oz	na	na	na	na	na	na	na	na	na	na	na	70	na
(Grandma's) 'Big Cookies' 2.75 oz	2 cookies	na	na	na	na	na	na	na	na	na	na	na	160	na

Food Name	Serving Size	A I.U.	Thi mg	Rib mg	Nia mg	B₆ mg	Fol mcg	B₁₂ mcg	C mg	Calc mg	Iron mg	Mag mg	Pot mg	Zn mg
(Mother's) double fudge sandwich	2 cookies	na	na	na	na	na	na	na	na	na	na	na	60	na
(Mother's) wafer 'Flaky Flix'	2 cookies	na	na	na	na	na	na	na	na	na	na	na	90	na
(Nabisco) caramel, peanut 'Heyday Bars' 1 piece	.75 oz	na	na	na	na	na	na	na	na	na	na	na	70	na
GINGER (Frookie) spice	1 cookie	na	na	na	na	na	na	na	na	na	na	na	40	na
GINGERSNAPS (Break Cake) approx 1 oz	5 cookies	na	na	na	na	na	na	na	na	na	na	na	40	na
GRAHAM														
(Mother's) dinosaur, mini	7 cookies	na	na	na	na	na	na	na	na	na	na	na	20	na
(Mother's) dinosaur, original	1 cookie	na	na	na	na	na	na	na	na	na	na	na	25	na
(Nabisco) 'Bugs Bunny' 5 pieces	.5 oz	na	na	na	na	na	na	na	na	na	na	na	15	na
'HERMIT' (Break Cake)	1 cookie	na	na	na	na	na	na	na	na	na	na	na	100	na
HONEY (Bakery Wagon) fruit bar	1 cookie	na	na	na	na	na	na	na	na	na	na	na	55	na
LEMON (Frookie) sandwich 'Frookwich'	1 cookie	na	na	na	na	na	na	na	na	na	na	na	20	na
MARSHMALLOW														
(Nabisco) fudge cake 'Puffs'	.75 oz	na	na	na	na	na	na	na	na	na	na	na	45	na
(Nabisco) fudge cake 'Twirls'	1 oz	na	na	na	na	na	na	na	na	na	na	na	50	na
(Nabisco) 'Pinwheels'	1 cookie	na	na	na	na	na	na	na	na	na	na	na	45	na
MINT (Nabisco) sandwich 'Mystic Mint'	.5 oz	na	na	na	na	na	na	na	na	na	na	na	30	na
MOLASSES														
(Bakery Wagon) iced	1 cookie	na	na	na	na	na	na	na	na	na	na	na	40	na
(Grandma's) 'Old Time Big Cookies'	2 cookies	na	na	na	na	na	na	na	na	na	na	na	190	na
OAT BRAN (Frookie) muffin	1 cookie	na	na	na	na	na	na	na	na	na	na	na	40	na
OATMEAL														
(Almost Home) raisin	.5 oz	na	na	na	na	na	na	na	na	na	na	na	50	na
(Bakery Wagon) soft	1 cookie	na	na	na	na	na	na	na	na	na	na	na	65	na
(Break Cake) approx 1 oz	5 cookies	na	na	na	na	na	na	na	na	na	na	na	35	na
(Chips Ahoy!) chocolate chip 'Selections'	.5 oz	na	na	na	na	na	na	na	na	na	na	na	30	na
(Frookie) raisin	1 cookie	na	na	na	na	na	na	na	na	na	na	na	40	na
(Frookie) raisin, fat-free	1 cookie	na	na	na	na	na	na	na	na	na	na	na	20	na
(Frookie) 7-grain oatmeal	1 cookie	na	na	na	na	na	na	na	na	na	na	na	40	na
(Glenny's) wheat-free 'Noah 'N Friends Animal'	.5 oz	na	na	na	na	na	na	na	na	na	na	na	50	na
(Grandma's) apple spice 'Big Cookies' 2.75 oz	2 cookies	na	na	na	na	na	na	na	na	na	na	na	180	na
(Mother's)	1 cookie	na	na	na	na	na	na	na	na	na	na	na	25	na
(Mother's) chocolate chip	1 cookie	na	na	na	na	na	na	na	na	na	na	na	40	na
(Mother's) iced	1 cookie	na	na	na	na	na	na	na	na	na	na	na	25	na
(Mother's) walnut chocolate chip	1 cookie	na	na	na	na	na	na	na	na	na	na	na	40	na
PEACH (Great Cakes)	4.5 oz	na	na	na	na	na	na	na	na	na	na	na	380	na
PEANUT BUTTER														
(Bakery Wagon) oatmeal	1 cookie	na	na	na	na	na	na	na	na	na	na	na	75	na
(Break Cake)	1 cookie	na	na	na	na	na	na	na	na	na	na	na	45	na
(Break Cake) wafer	1 wafer	na	na	na	na	na	na	na	na	na	na	na	60	na
(Frookie) sandwich 'Frookwich'	1 cookie	na	na	na	na	na	na	na	na	na	na	na	20	na
(Glenny's) 'Noah 'N Friends Animal Cookies'	.5 oz	na	na	na	na	na	na	na	na	na	na	na	60	na
(Grandma's) 'Big Cookies' 2.75 oz	2 cookies	na	na	na	na	na	na	na	na	na	na	na	160	na
(Grandma's) cookie bits, 8 cookies	1 oz	na	na	na	na	na	na	na	na	na	na	na	55	na
(Great Cakes) and jelly	4.5 oz	na	na	na	na	na	na	na	na	na	na	na	380	na
(Mother's) sandwich 'Gaucho'	1 cookie	na	na	na	na	na	na	na	na	na	na	na	40	na
(Nabisco) 'Ideal Bars'	.5 oz cookie	na	na	na	na	na	na	na	na	na	na	na	50	na
(Nabisco) 'Nutter Butter Peanut Sandwich'	.5 oz	na	na	na	na	na	na	na	na	na	na	na	30	na
PEANUT CREME (Nabisco) 'Nutter Butter Patties'	.5 oz	na	na	na	na	na	na	na	na	na	na	na	45	na
RAISIN														
(Break Cake) creme	1 cookie	na	na	na	na	na	na	na	na	na	na	na	30	na
(Grandma's) soft 'Big Cookies' approx 2.75 oz	2 cookies	na	na	na	na	na	na	na	na	na	na	na	135	na

Food Name	Serving Size	A I.U.	Thi mg	Rib mg	Nia mg	B₆ mg	Fol mcg	B₁₂ mcg	C mg	Calc mg	Iron mg	Mag mg	Pot mg	Zn mg
(Mother's) iced	1 cookie	na	na	na	na	na	na	na	na	na	na	na	35	na
RASPBERRY														
(Bakery Wagon) filled	1 cookie	na	na	na	na	na	na	na	na	na	na	na	50	na
(Frookie) 'Fruitins' fat-free	2 cookies	na	na	na	na	na	na	na	na	na	na	na	80	na
(Great Cakes)	4.5 oz	na	na	na	na	na	na	na	na	na	na	na	380	na
(Natures Warehouse) wheat-free, fat-free	1 oz	na	na	na	na	na	na	na	na	na	na	na	184	na
SHORTBREAD														
(Break Cake) approx 1 oz	5 cookies	na	na	na	na	na	na	na	na	na	na	na	25	na
(Lorna Doone) .5 oz	3 cookies	na	na	na	na	na	na	na	na	na	na	na	15	na
(Mother's) striped	2 cookies	na	na	na	na	na	na	na	na	na	na	na	40	na
SUGAR														
(Almost Home) 'Old Fashioned'	.5 oz	na	na	na	na	na	na	na	na	na	na	na	15	na
(Mother's)	1 cookie	na	na	na	na	na	na	na	na	na	na	na	15	na
TAFFY (Mother's) sandwich	1 cookie	na	na	na	na	na	na	na	na	na	na	na	25	na
TEA BISCUIT (Nabisco) 'Social Tea Biscuit' 3 pieces	.5 oz	na	na	na	na	na	na	na	na	na	na	na	15	na
TOFFEE (Chips Ahoy!) chunk, Heath 'Selections'	1 cookie	na	na	na	na	na	na	na	na	na	na	na	20	na
VANILLA														
(Frookie) sandwich 'Frookwich'	1 cookie	na	na	na	na	na	na	na	na	na	na	na	20	na
(Glenny's) 'Noah 'N Friends Animal Cookies'	.5 oz	na	na	na	na	na	na	na	na	na	na	na	45	na
(Grandma's) cookie bits, artificially flavored	1 oz	na	na	na	na	na	na	na	na	na	na	na	40	na
(Nabisco) creme sandwich 'Cookie Break'	1 cookie	na	na	na	na	na	na	na	na	na	na	na	5	na
WAFER														
(Break Cake) chocolate, sugar	4 wafers	na	na	na	na	na	na	na	na	na	na	na	55	na
(Break Cake) 'Striper Wafer'	1 wafer	na	na	na	na	na	na	na	na	na	na	na	75	na
(Break Cake) vanilla, sugar	4 wafers	na	na	na	na	na	na	na	na	na	na	na	30	na
(Mother's) checkerboard	5 wafers	na	na	na	na	na	na	na	na	na	na	na	25	na
(Mother's) vanilla, 'Flaky Flix'	2 cookies	na	na	na	na	na	na	na	na	na	na	na	75	na
(Nabisco) 'Brown Edge Wafers' 2 1/2 wafers	.5 oz	na	na	na	na	na	na	na	na	na	na	na	15	na
(Nabisco) 'Famous Chocolate Wafers' 2 1/2 wafers	.5 oz	na	na	na	na	na	na	na	na	na	na	na	35	na
(Nabisco) striped wafer 'Cookies 'N Fudge'	1 wafer	na	na	na	na	na	na	na	na	na	na	na	70	na
(Weider) 'Victory Explosive Workout'	6 wafers	na	na	na	na	na	450	na	na	na	na	8	100	na
WALNUT (Mother's) fudge	1 cookie	na	na	na	na	na	na	na	na	na	na	na	35	na
COOKIE DOUGH, PREPARED														
chocolate chip	1 oz	17	.05	.05	.56	.01	2.6	.02	0.0	7.09	.64	6.8	51.03	.14
chocolate chip	1 cookie	9	.03	.03	.32	.01	1.4	.01	0.0	4.0	.36	3.84	28.8	.08
chocolate chip, baked	1 oz	17	.05	.05	.56	0	2.0	.02	0.0	7.94	.71	7.65	56.7	.16
chocolate chip, baked	1 cookie	7	.02	.02	.24	0	0.8	.01	0.0	3.36	.3	3.24	24.0	.07
oatmeal	1 oz	20	.07	.04	.53	.02	2.6	.01	0.0	8.79	.61	7.94	41.67	.18
oatmeal	1 cookie	11	.04	.02	.3	.01	1.4	.01	0.0	4.96	.34	4.48	23.52	.1
oatmeal, baked	1 oz	20	.06	.04	.53	.02	2.0	.01	0.0	9.92	.67	9.07	46.21	.2
oatmeal, baked	1 cookie	8	.02	.02	.22	.01	0.8	0	0.0	4.2	.29	3.84	19.56	.09
sugar	1 oz	10	.06	.03	.68	.01	2.3	.02	0.0	22.96	.47	1.98	41.67	.07
sugar	1 cookie	6	.03	.02	.39	0	1.3	.01	0.0	12.96	.26	1.12	23.52	.04
sugar, baked	1 oz	10	.05	.03	.68	.01	1.7	.02	0.0	25.51	.52	2.27	46.21	.08
COOKING SPRAY (Wesson) no-stick	.25 gm	na	na	na	na	na	na	na	0.0	0	0	na	na	na
CORIANDER / Chinese parsley														
raw	1 tbsp	na	.02	.03	.19	na	na	0	10.3	22.52	.77	12.54	80.75	na
raw	1 tsp	na	.01	.01	.06	na	na	0	3.4	7.51	.26	4.18	26.92	na
raw, approx .8 oz	9 plants	553	.01	.02	.15	.02	2.1	0	2.1	19.6	.39	5.2	108.4	.09
CORIANDER SEED / Chinese parsley seed														
whole	1 tbsp	0	.01	.01	.11	na	0.0	0	na	35.43	.82	16.51	63.35	.23
whole	1 tsp	0	0	.01	.04	na	0.0	0	na	12.76	.29	5.94	22.81	.08
whole (Durkee)	1 tsp	na	.08	.07	0	na	na	na	na	0	0	na	0	na
whole (Laurel Leaf)	1 tsp	na	.08	.07	0	na	na	na	na	0	0	na	0	na

Food Name	Serving Size	A I.U.	Thi mg	Rib mg	Nia mg	B6 mg	Fol mcg	B12 mcg	C mg	Calc mg	Iron mg	Mag mg	Pot mg	Zn mg
CORN														
cooked	1/2 cup	40	.04	.02	.39	.04	4.2	0	0.0	.7	.18	25.2	21.7	.44
dry	1 cup	179	.24	.09	2.55	.22	26.3	0	0.0	4.2	.98	124.95	308.7	1.88
dry	2 oz	97	.13	.05	1.39	.12	14.3	0	0.0	2.28	.53	67.83	167.58	1.02
sweet, white, boiled, drained, cut	1/2 cup	0	.18	.06	1.32	.05	38.1	0	5.1	1.64	.5	26.24	204.18	.39
sweet, white, kernels, boiled, drained	1 ear	0	.17	.06	1.24	.05	35.7	0	4.8	1.54	.47	24.64	191.73	.37
sweet, white, kernels from cob, raw	1 ear	0	.18	.05	1.53	.05	41.2	0	6.1	1.8	.47	33.3	243.0	.41
sweet, white, raw, cut	1/2 cup	0	.15	.05	1.31	.04	35.3	0	5.2	1.54	.4	28.49	207.9	.35
sweet, yellow, boiled, drained, cut	1/2 cup	178	.18	.06	1.32	.05	38.1	0	5.1	1.64	.5	26.24	204.18	.39
sweet, yellow, kernels, boiled, drained	1 ear	167	.17	.06	1.24	.05	35.7	0	4.8	1.54	.47	24.64	191.73	.37
sweet, yellow, kernels from cob, raw	1 ear	253	.18	.05	1.53	.05	41.2	0	6.1	1.8	.47	33.3	243.0	.41
sweet, yellow, raw, cut	1/2 cup	216	.15	.05	1.31	.04	35.3	0	5.2	1.54	.4	28.49	207.9	.35
white	1/2 cup	0	.32	.17	3.01	.52	na	0	0.0	5.81	2.25	105.41	238.21	1.83
yellow	1/2 cup	389	.32	.17	3.01	.52	15.8	0	0.0	5.81	2.25	105.41	238.21	1.83
CORN, CANNED														
'Crisp 'N Sweet' vacuum packed *(Freshlike)*	1/2 cup	na	na	na	na	na	na	na	na	na	na	na	160	na
golden, cream style *(Freshlike)*	1/2 cup	na	na	na	na	na	na	na	na	na	na	na	150	na
golden, cream style *(Veg•All)*	1/2 cup	na	na	na	na	na	na	na	na	na	na	na	150	na
golden, cream style, no salt added *(Freshlike)*	1/2 cup	na	na	na	na	na	na	na	na	na	na	na	150	na
golden, whole kernel *(Veg•All)*	1/2 cup	na	na	na	na	na	na	na	na	na	na	na	150	na
golden, whole kernel, vacuum packed *(Freshlike)*	1/2 cup	na	na	na	na	na	na	na	na	na	na	na	170	na
golden, whole kernel, water packed, w/o salt *(Freshlike)*	1/2 cup	na	na	na	na	na	na	na	na	na	na	na	150	na
golden, whole kernel, water packed, w/o sugar and salt *(Freshlike)*	1/2 cup	na	na	na	na	na	na	na	na	na	na	na	150	na
sweet, white, brine pack, drained solids	1/2 cup	0	.03	.06	.98	.04	39.9	0	7.0	4.1	.71	16.4	159.9	.32
sweet, white, brine pack, regular, w/liquid	1/2 cup	0	.03	.08	1.2	.05	48.8	0	8.6	5.12	.45	20.48	195.84	.46
sweet, white, brine pack, dietary, w/liquid	1/2 cup	0	.03	.08	1.2	.05	48.8	0	8.6	5.12	.45	20.48	195.84	.46
sweet, white, cream style, regular pack	1/2 cup	0	.03	.07	1.23	.08	57.3	0	5.9	3.84	.49	21.76	171.52	.68
sweet, white, cream style, special dietary pack	1/2 cup	0	.03	.07	1.23	.08	57.3	0	5.9	3.84	.49	21.76	171.52	.68
sweet, white, vacuum pack, regular pack	1/2 cup	0	.04	.08	1.23	.06	51.8	0	8.5	5.25	.44	24.15	195.3	.48
sweet, white, vacuum pack, special dietary pack	1/2 cup	0	.04	.08	1.23	.06	51.8	0	8.5	5.25	.44	24.15	195.3	.48
sweet, yellow, brine pack, drained solids	1/2 cup	128	.03	.06	.98	.04	39.9	0	7.0	4.1	.71	16.4	159.9	.32
sweet, yellow, brine pack, regular, w/liquid	1/2 cup	154	.03	.08	1.2	.05	48.8	0	8.6	5.12	.45	20.48	195.84	.46
sweet, yellow, brine pack, dietary, w/liquid	1/2 cup	154	.03	.08	1.2	.05	48.8	0	8.6	5.12	.45	20.48	195.84	.46
sweet, yellow, cream style, regular pack	1/2 cup	124	.03	.07	1.23	.08	57.3	0	5.9	3.84	.49	21.76	171.52	.68
sweet, yellow, cream style, special dietary pack	1/2 cup	124	.03	.07	1.23	.08	57.3	0	5.9	3.84	.49	21.76	171.52	.68
sweet, yellow, vacuum pack, regular pack	1/2 cup	253	.04	.08	1.23	.06	51.8	0	8.5	5.25	.44	24.15	195.3	.48
sweet, yellow, vacuum pack, special dietary pack	1/2 cup	253	.04	.08	1.23	.06	51.8	0	8.5	5.25	.44	24.15	195.3	.48
CORN, FROZEN														
kernel, cut, petite 'Deluxe' *(Birds Eye)*	2.6 oz	na	na	na	na	na	na	na	na	na	na	na	160	na
kernel 'Tender Sweet Deluxe' *(Birds Eye)*	3.3 oz	na	na	na	na	na	na	na	na	na	na	na	200	na
on the cob *(Birds Eye)*	1 ear	na	na	na	na	na	na	na	na	na	na	na	380	na
on the cob, baby 'Deluxe' *(Birds Eye)*	2.6 oz	na	na	na	na	na	na	na	na	na	na	na	380	na
on the cob 'Big Ears' *(Birds Eye)*	1 ear	na	na	na	na	na	na	na	na	na	na	na	490	na
on the cob 'Little Ears' *(Birds Eye)*	2 ears	na	na	na	na	na	na	na	na	na	na	na	400	na
sweet *(Birds Eye)*	3.3 oz	na	na	na	na	na	na	na	na	na	na	na	200	na
sweet, tender 'Deluxe' *(Birds Eye)*	3.3 oz	na	na	na	na	na	na	na	na	na	na	na	200	na
sweet, white, kernels, boiled, drained	1 ear	0	.11	.04	.96	.14	19.2	0	3.0	1.89	.38	18.27	158.13	.4
sweet, white, kernels, boiled, drained	1/2 cup	0	.14	.06	1.24	.18	25.0	0	3.9	2.46	.5	23.78	205.82	.52

Food Name	Serving Size	A I.U.	Thi mg	Rib mg	Nia mg	B$_6$ mg	Fol mcg	B$_{12}$ mcg	C mg	Calc mg	Iron mg	Mag mg	Pot mg	Zn mg
sweet, white, kernels, unprepared	1/2 cup	0	.07	.06	1.42	.15	29.3	0	5.3	3.28	.34	14.76	172.2	.3
sweet, yellow, kernels, boiled, drained	1 ear	133	.11	.04	.96	.14	19.2	0	3.0	1.89	.38	18.27	158.13	.4
sweet, yellow, kernels, boiled, drained	1/2 cup	173	.14	.06	1.24	.18	25.0	0	3.9	2.46	.5	23.78	205.82	.52
sweet, yellow, kernels, unprepared	1/2 cup	107	.07	.06	1.42	.15	29.3	0	5.3	3.28	.34	14.76	172.2	.3
CORN AND PEPPERS, CANNED														
red and green peppers, solid and liquid	1/2 cup	264	.03	.09	1.08	.11	38.7	0	10.0	5.7	.9	28.5	174.42	.42
vacuum packed (Freshlike)	1/2 cup	na	na	na	na	na	na	na	na	na	na	na	170	na
CORN BRAN, crude	1 cup	54	.01	.08	2.08	.12	3.0	0	0.0	31.92	2.12	48.64	33.44	1.19
CORN CAKE														
apple cinnamon flavor (Roman Meal)	1 cake	na	na	na	na	na	na	na	na	na	na	na	25	na
cheddar flavor (Roman Meal)	1 cake	na	na	na	na	na	na	na	na	na	na	na	23	na
plain	1 cake	22	.02	0	.46	.01	1.7	0	0.0	1.71	.13	10.26	14.13	.18
popcorn	1 cake	7	.01	.02	.6	.02	1.8	0	0.0	.9	.19	15.9	32.7	.4
very low sodium	1 cake	0	0	0	0	0	0.0	0	0.0	.45	.01	.18	1.98	.02
CORN CHIPS AND SNACKS. See also TORTILLA CHIPS.														
barbecue 'Rowdy Rustlers' 34 chips (Fritos)	1 oz	na	na	na	na	na	na	na	na	na	na	na	45	na
bare bean 'Garden Vegetable Chips' (Harry's)	1 oz	12	na	na	na	na	na	na	0.2	21	.45	na	na	na
bare bean 'Offbeat Originals' (Peddlers)	1 oz	12	na	na	na	na	na	na	0.2	21	.45	na	na	na
beet garlic 'Garden Vegetable Chips' (Harry's)	1 oz	12	na	na	na	na	na	na	0.3	27	.48	na	na	na
beet garlic 'Offbeat Originals' (Peddlers)	1 oz	12	na	na	na	na	na	na	0.3	27	.18	na	na	na
bell pepper 'Garden Vegetable Chips' (Harry's)	1 oz	26	na	na	na	na	na	na	2.5	27	.4	na	na	na
bell pepper 'Offbeat Originals' (Peddlers)	1 oz	26	na	na	na	na	na	na	2.5	27	.4	na	na	na
blue garlic 'Garden Vegetable Chips' (Harry's)	1 oz	12	na	na	na	na	na	na	0.2	24	.54	na	na	na
blue garlic 'Offbeat Originals' (Peddlers)	1 oz	12	na	na	na	na	na	na	0.2	24	.54	na	na	na
carrot caraway 'Garden Vegetable Chips' (Harry's)	1 oz	221	na	na	na	na	na	na	1.7	26	.4	na	na	na
carrot caraway 'Offbeat Originals' (Peddlers)	1 oz	221	na	na	na	na	na	na	1.7	26	.4	na	na	na
chili cheese, 34 chips (Fritos)	1 oz	na	na	na	na	na	na	na	na	na	na	na	55	na
cones, nacho-flavor	1 oz	89	.06	.03	.4	.03	1.4	0	0.0	10.21	.36	7.09	34.87	.14
cones, plain	1 oz	90	.09	.07	.4	.01	0.9	0	0.0	.85	.72	3.12	22.96	.06
cool ranch (Doritos)	1 oz	na	na	na	na	na	na	na	na	na	na	na	65	na
'Crisp 'N Thin' 18 chips (Fritos)	1 oz	na	na	na	na	na	na	na	na	na	na	na	40	na
curls, ranch flavored (Weight Watchers)	.5 oz	na	na	na	na	na	na	na	na	na	na	na	170	na
'Dip Size Fritos' 13 pieces (Fritos)	1 oz	na	na	na	na	na	na	na	na	na	na	na	40	na
'Fritos' 34 pieces (Fritos)	1 oz	na	na	na	na	na	na	na	na	na	na	na	45	na
mild bean 'Garden Vegetable Chips' (Harry's)	1 oz	12	na	na	na	na	na	na	0.2	21	.45	na	na	na
mild bean 'Offbeat Originals' (Peddlers)	1 oz	12	na	na	na	na	na	na	0.2	21	.45	na	na	na
nacho cheese flavor (Doritos)	1 oz	na	na	na	na	na	na	na	na	na	na	na	65	na
nacho cheese 'Non-Stop' 34 chips (Fritos)	1 oz	na	na	na	na	na	na	na	na	na	na	na	55	na
onion-flavor	1 oz	34	.06	.09	.9	.04	4.5	0	0.5	8.22	1.05	7.94	40.54	.09
plain	1 oz	27	.01	.04	.34	.07	5.7	0	0.0	36.0	.37	21.55	40.26	.36
puffs, cheese-flavor	1 oz	75	.07	.1	.92	.04	34.0	.04	0.1	16.44	.67	5.1	47.06	.11
puffs, cheese-flavor, enriched	1 oz	69	.07	.01	1.46	.04	5.4	0	0.0	5.39	.4	32.32	44.51	.57
toasted corn, crunchy, barbecue (Cornuts)	2 oz	192	.2	.08	.85	.11	0.0	0	0.2	9.64	.96	61.8	162.16	1.07
toasted corn, crunchy, barbecue (Cornuts)	1 oz	96	.1	.04	.43	.05	0.0	0	0.1	4.82	.48	30.9	81.08	.53
toasted corn, crunchy, nacho (Cornuts)	2 oz	22	.21	.04	.69	.12	8.5	0	8.8	19.85	.95	61.8	176.34	1.02
toasted corn, crunchy, nacho (Cornuts)	1 oz	11	.1	.02	.34	.06	4.3	0	4.4	9.92	.48	30.9	88.17	.51
toasted corn, crunchy, original (Cornuts)	2 oz	0	.02	.07	.96	.13	0.0	0	0.0	5.1	.95	64.07	157.63	1.01
toasted corn, crunchy, original (Cornuts)	1 oz	0	.01	.04	.48	.06	0.0	0	0.0	2.55	.47	32.04	78.81	.5
veggie 'Garden Vegetable Chips' (Harry's)	1 oz	456	na	na	na	na	na	na	1.0	40	.65	na	na	na
veggie 'Offbeat Originals' (Peddlers)	1 oz	456	na	na	na	na	na	na	1.0	40	.65	na	na	na
wild bean 'Garden Vegetable Chips' (Harry's)	1 oz	12	na	na	na	na	na	na	0.5	24	.48	na	na	na

Food Name	Serving Size	A I.U.	Thi mg	Rib mg	Nia mg	B_6 mg	Fol mcg	B_{12} mcg	C mg	Calc mg	Iron mg	Mag mg	Pot mg	Zn mg
wild bean 'Offbeat Originals' (Peddlers)	1 oz	12	na	na	na	na	na	na	0.5	24	.40	na	na	na
'Wild 'N Mild' 32 chips (Fritos)	1 oz	na	na	na	na	na	na	na	na	na	na	na	55	na
CORN FLOUR														
masa, enriched, white	1 cup	0	1.63	.86	11.22	.42	27.4	0	0.0	160.74	8.22	125.4	339.72	2.03
masa, enriched, yellow	1 cup	535	1.63	.86	11.22	.42	27.4	0	0.0	160.74	8.22	125.4	339.72	2.03
'Masa Harina De Maiz' approx 1/3 cup														
(Quaker)	1.3 oz	0	.38	.29	3.49	.19	17.0	0	0.0	60	1.8	41	115	1
'Masa Trigo' approx 1/3 cup (Quaker)	1.3 oz	0	.39	.24	3.12	.01	29.0	0	0.0	66	1.8	8	36	0
whole-grain, white	1/2 cup	0	.14	.05	1.1	na	14.5	0	0.0	4.06	1.38	53.94	182.7	1.0
whole-grain, yellow	1/2 cup	272	.14	.05	1.1	.21	14.5	0	0.0	4.06	1.38	53.94	182.7	1.0
CORN GRITS. See GRITS.														
CORN OIL														
(Kroger)	1 tbsp	na	na	na	na	na	na	na	0.0	0	0	na	na	na
(Wesson)	1 tbsp	na	na	na	na	na	na	na	0.0	0	0	na	na	na
CORN OIL SPREAD														
(Fleischmann's) 60% oil 'Light'	1 tbsp	na	na	na	na	na	na	na	na	na	na	na	10	na
(Fleischmann's) 40% oil 'Extra Light'	1 tbsp	na	na	na	na	na	na	na	na	na	na	na	5	na
CORN SALAD, raw	1/2 cup	1986	.02	.02	.12	.08	3.8	0	10.7	10.64	.61	3.64	128.52	.17
CORN SOUFFLÉ, FROZEN, 1 pkg (Stouffer's) ...	6 oz	na	na	na	na	na	na	na	na	na	na	na	200	na
CORN SYRUP														
dark	1 cup	0	.04	.03	.07	.03	0.0	0	0.0	59.04	1.21	26.24	144.32	.13
dark	1 tbsp	0	0	0	0	0	0.0	0	0.0	3.6	.07	1.6	8.8	.01
high-fructose	1 cup	0	0	.06	0	0	0.0	0	0.0	0	.09	0	0	.06
high-fructose	1 tbsp	0	0	0	0	0	0.0	0	0.0	0	.01	0	0	0
light	1 cup	0	.04	.03	.07	.03	0.0	0	0.0	9.84	.16	6.56	13.12	.07
light	1 tbsp	0	0	0	0	0	0.0	0	0.0	.6	.01	.4	.8	0
table blends, refiner, and sugar	1 cup	0	.02	.15	.06	.03	9.5	0	0.0	72.68	2.34	28.44	199.08	.09
table blends, refiner, and sugar	1 tbsp	0	0	.01	0	0	0.6	0	0.0	4.6	.15	1.8	12.6	.01
CORNMEAL														
degermed, enriched, white	1 cup	0	.99	.56	6.95	.35	66.2	0	0.0	6.9	5.7	55.2	223.56	.99
degermed, enriched, yellow	1 cup	570	.99	.56	6.95	.35	66.2	0	0.0	6.9	5.7	55.2	223.56	.99
degermed, unenriched, white	1 cup	0	.19	.07	1.38	.35	66.2	0	0.0	6.9	1.52	55.2	223.56	.99
degermed, unenriched, yellow	1 cup	570	.19	.07	1.38	.35	66.2	0	0.0	6.9	1.52	55.2	223.56	.99
white, bolted (Aunt Jemima)	1 oz	0	.22	.14	1.6	.14	19.0	0	0.0	60	1.08	21	68	0
white, dry (Albers)	1 oz	200	.13	.08	1.2	.04	0.0	0	0.0	1	.8	7.7	39	0
white, enriched (Aunt Jemima)	1 oz	0	.12	.07	1.0	.1	15.0	0	0.0	1	.81	12	51	0
white, whole-grain	1 cup	0	.47	.25	4.43	.37	na	0	0.0	7.32	4.21	154.94	350.14	2.22
yellow, dry (Albers)	1 oz	200	.13	.08	1.2	.04	0.0	0	0.0	1	.8	7.7	39	0
yellow, enriched (Aunt Jemima)	1 oz	115	.12	.07	1.0	.1	15.0	0	0.0	1	.81	12	51	0
yellow, whole-grain	1 cup	572	.47	.25	4.43	.37	31.0	0	0.0	7.32	4.21	154.94	350.14	2.22
CORNMEAL, SELF-RISING														
white (Aunt Jemima)	1 oz	0	.12	.07	1.0	.11	9.0	0	0.0	109	.81	14	45	0
white, bolted, enriched (Aunt Jemima)	1 oz	0	.12	.07	1.0	.15	16.0	0	0.0	109	.81	24	78	1
white, bolted, plain, enriched	1 cup	0	.81	.49	6.46	.66	69.5	0	0.0	440.42	7.03	104.92	311.1	2.44
white, bolted, wheat flour added, enriched ..	1 cup	0	1.21	.74	8.84	.65	112.2	0	0.0	508.3	8.41	91.8	351.9	2.36
white, buttermilk (Aunt Jemima)	3 tbsp	0	.22	.14	1.6	.12	10.0	0	0.0	60	1.08	25	87	1
white, degermed, enriched	1 cup	0	.94	.53	6.3	.54	42.8	0	0.0	483.0	6.53	67.62	234.6	1.38
yellow (Aunt Jemima)	3 tbsp	0	.23	.14	1.6	na	na	na	0.0	60	1.08	na	30	na
yellow, bolted, plain, enriched ,,,,,,,,,	1 cup	572	.81	.49	6.46	.66	69.5	0	0.0	440.42	7.03	104.92	311.1	2.44
yellow, bolted, wheat flour added, enriched ..	1 cup	488	1.21	.74	8.84	.65	112.2	0	0.0	508.3	8.41	91.8	351.9	2.36
yellow, degermed, enriched	1 cup	570	.94	.53	6.3	.54	42.8	0	0.0	483.0	6.53	67.62	234.6	1.38
CORNED BEEF. See BEEF, CORNED.														
CORNSTARCH	1 cup	0	0	0	0	0	0.0	0	0.0	2.56	.6	3.84	3.84	.08
COTTAGE CHEESE. See CHEESE.														
COTTONSEED FLOUR														
lowfat	1 oz	123	.59	.11	1.15	.22	64.7	0	0.7	134.62	3.57	203.34	500.12	3.3
partially defatted	1 cup	408	1.98	.38	3.82	.72	215.5	0	2.3	449.32	11.9	677.74	1665.68	10.99

Food Name	Serving Size	A I.U.	Thi mg	Rib mg	Nia mg	B$_6$ mg	Fol mcg	B$_{12}$ mcg	C mg	Calc mg	Iron mg	Mag mg	Pot mg	Zn mg
partially defatted	1 tbsp	22	.11	.02	.2	.04	11.5	0	0.1	23.9	.63	36.05	88.6	.58
COTTONSEED KERNELS														
roasted	1 cup	659	1.12	.38	4.47	1.17	347.6	0	13.4	149.0	8.05	655.6	2011.5	8.94
roasted	1 tbsp	44	.08	.03	.3	.08	23.3	0	0.9	10.0	.54	44.0	135.0	.6
COTTONSEED MEAL, partially defatted	1 oz	130	.63	.12	1.22	.23	68.6	0	0.7	143.14	3.79	215.84	530.8	3.5
COTTONSEED OIL														
	1 cup	0	0	na	0	0	0.0	0	0.0	0	0	0	0	0
	1 tbsp	0	0	na	0	0	0.0	0	0.0	0	0	0	0	0
(Wesson)	1 tbsp	na	na	na	na	na	na	na	0.0	0	0	na	na	na
COUSCOUS														
cooked	1/2 cup	40	.37	.2	3.96	.23	58.5	0	1.2	98.1	3.05	144.9	583.2	2.83
dry	1/2 cup	0	.15	.07	3.21	.1	18.4	0	0.0	22.08	.99	40.48	152.72	.76
COWPEA. See BLACK-EYED PEAS.														
CRAB														
ALASKA KING														
moist-heat cooked	3 oz	25	.05	.05	1.14	.15	43.4	9.77	6.5	50.15	.65	53.55	222.7	6.48
raw	3 oz	20	.04	.04	.94	.13	37.4	7.65	6.0	39.1	.5	41.65	173.4	5.06
BLUE														
canned	1 cup	7	.11	.11	1.85	.2	57.4	.62	3.7	136.35	1.13	52.65	504.9	5.43
canned	3 oz	4	.07	.07	1.16	.13	36.1	.39	2.3	85.85	.71	33.15	317.9	3.42
moist-heat cooked	1 cup	8	.14	.07	4.46	.24	68.6	9.85	4.5	140.4	1.23	44.55	437.4	5.7
moist-heat cooked	3 oz	5	.09	.04	2.81	.15	43.2	6.21	2.8	88.4	.77	28.05	275.4	3.59
raw	3 oz	4	.07	.03	2.3	.13	37.4	7.65	2.6	75.65	.63	28.9	279.65	3.01
DUNGENESS														
moist-heat cooked	3 oz	88	.05	.17	3.08	.15	35.7	8.82	3.1	50.15	.37	49.3	346.8	4.65
raw	3 oz	77	.04	.14	2.67	.13	37.4	7.65	3.0	39.1	.31	38.25	300.9	3.63
IMPERIAL	1 cup	684	.13	.26	2.42	na	na	na	11.0	132.0	1.98	na	288.2	na
QUEEN														
moist-heat cooked	100 gm	173	.1	.24	2.88	.17	42.0	10.38	7.2	33.0	2.88	63.0	200.0	0.59
moist-heat cooked	3 oz	147	.08	.21	2.45	.15	35.7	8.82	6.1	28.05	2.45	53.55	170.0	3.05
raw	3 oz	128	.07	.17	2.13	.13	37.4	7.65	6.0	22.1	2.13	41.65	147.05	2.38
CRAB, ALTERNATIVE, Alaskan king, made from														
surimi	3 oz	56	.03	.02	.15	.03	1.4	1.36	0.0	11.05	.33	36.55	76.5	.28
CRAB, DEVILED	1 cup	1601	.19	.26	3.6	na	na	na	14.4	112.8	2.88	na	398.4	na
CRAB CAKE														
	100 gm	71	.26	.15	4.12	.42	19.0	14.45	2.4	381.0	1.27	75.0	548.0	6.44
	1 cake	43	.16	.09	2.47	.25	11.4	8.67	1.4	228.6	.76	45.0	328.8	3.86
blue crab	1 cake	151	.05	.05	1.74	.1	24.9	3.56	1.7	63.0	.65	19.8	194.4	2.45
CRABAPPLE														
raw	100 gm	40	.03	.02	.1	na	na	0	8.0	18.0	.36	7.0	194.0	na
raw, slices, w/skin	1 cup	44	.03	.02	.11	na	na	0	8.8	19.8	.4	7.7	213.4	na
CRACKER														
butter, country flavor (McCrakens)	1 oz	na	na	na	na	na	na	na	na	na	na	na	65	na
cheese 'Better Cheddars' (Nabisco)	.5 oz	na	na	na	na	na	na	na	na	na	na	na	15	na
cheese 'Better Cheddars' low salt (Nabisco)	.5 oz	na	na	na	na	na	na	na	na	na	na	na	15	na
cheese, cheddar, approx 13-16 crackers (Frito-Lay's)	.5 oz	na	na	na	na	na	na	na	na	na	na	na	20	na
cheese, cheddar, baked, cracker chips 'Zings' (Nabisco)	.5 oz	na	na	na	na	na	na	na	na	na	na	na	50	na
cheese, cheddar, tangy (McCrakens)	1 oz	na	na	na	na	na	na	na	na	na	na	na	65	na
cheese 'Cheddar Wedges' 31 pieces (Nabisco)	.5 oz	na	na	na	na	na	na	na	na	na	na	na	15	na
cheese 'Cheese Nips' 13 pieces (Nabisco)	.5 oz	na	na	na	na	na	na	na	na	na	na	na	25	na
cheese 'Cheese Peanut Butter Sandwich' 4 pieces (Nabisco)	1 oz	na	na	na	na	na	na	na	na	na	na	na	20	na
cheese 'Cheese Ritz Bits Mini Ritz' 22 pieces (Ritz)	.5 oz	na	na	na	na	na	na	na	na	na	na	na	15	na

Food Name	Serving Size	A I.U.	Thi mg	Rib mg	Nia mg	B6 mg	Fol mcg	B12 mcg	C mg	Calc mg	Iron mg	Mag mg	Pot mg	Zn mg
cheese, sandwich-type w/peanut butter filling	.5 oz	45	.06	.05	.92	.21	3.5	0	0.0	11.2	.41	8.22	34.73	.15
cheese 'Tid-Bits' 15 pieces (Nabisco)	.5 oz	na	na	na	na	na	na	na	na	na	na	na	20	na
cheese flavor, organic, fat-free (Health Valley)	.5 oz	na	na	na	na	na	na	na	na	na	na	na	75	na
cheese-filled, 6 crackers (Frito-Lay's)	1.5 oz	na	na	na	na	na	na	na	na	na	na	na	170	na
chicken flavor 'Chicken in a Biskit' 7 pieces (Nabisco)	.5 oz	na	na	na	na	na	na	na	na	na	na	na	15	na
5-spice wafer (Westbrae)	4.5 wafers	na	na	na	na	na	na	na	na	na	na	na	20	na
herb, organic, fat-free (Health Valley)	.5 oz	na	na	na	na	na	na	na	na	na	na	na	75	na
matzo, egg	.5 oz	6	.09	.09	.72	.01	4.1	.07	0.0	5.67	.38	3.26	21.26	.1
matzo, egg, 1 oz	1 matzo	12	.18	.18	1.44	.02	8.2	.14	0.0	11.34	.77	6.52	42.53	.21
matzo, egg and onion	.5 oz	8	.08	.06	.69	.02	1.4	.03	0.0	5.1	.62	4.25	11.77	.1
matzo, egg and onion, 1 oz	1 matzo	17	.16	.12	1.39	.03	2.8	.06	0.1	10.21	1.24	8.51	23.53	.21
matzo, plain	.5 oz	0	.05	.04	.55	.02	2.0	0	0.0	1.84	.45	3.54	15.88	.1
matzo, plain, 1 oz	1 matzo	0	.11	.08	1.1	.03	4.0	0	0.0	3.69	.9	7.09	31.75	.19
matzo, whole-wheat	.5 oz	0	.05	.04	.77	.02	5.0	0	0.0	3.26	.66	18.99	44.79	.37
matzo, whole-wheat, 1 oz	1 matzo	0	.1	.08	1.53	.05	9.9	0	0.0	6.52	1.32	37.99	89.59	.74
melba toast, plain	.5 oz	0	.06	.04	.58	.01	3.7	0	0.0	13.18	.52	8.36	28.63	.28
melba toast, plain, w/o salt	.5 oz	0	.06	.04	.58	.01	3.7	0	0.0	13.18	.52	8.36	28.63	.28
melba toast, rye	.5 oz	0	.07	.04	.67	.01	3.1	0	0.0	11.06	.52	5.53	27.36	.19
melba toast, wheat	.5 oz	0	.06	.04	.72	.01	3.4	0	0.0	6.1	.64	7.94	20.98	.21
milk	.5 oz	5	.08	.06	.63	.01	2.3	.01	0.0	24.38	.51	3.12	16.16	.09
oat 'Oat Thins' approx .5 oz (Nabisco)	8 crackers	na	na	na	na	na	na	na	na	na	na	na	30	na
onion, minced, approx .5 oz (American Classic)	4 crackers	na	na	na	na	na	na	na	na	na	na	na	20	na
onion, organic, fat-free (Health Valley)	.5 oz	na	na	na	na	na	na	na	na	na	na	na	75	na
onion garlic wafer (Westbrae)	4.5 crackers	na	na	na	na	na	na	na	na	na	na	na	20	na
oyster	.5 oz	0	.08	.07	.74	.01	4.4	0	0.0	16.87	.77	3.83	18.14	.11
oyster (Premium)	20 crackers	na	na	na	na	na	na	na	na	na	na	na	15	na
oyster, low salt	.5 oz	0	.08	.07	.74	.01	4.4	0	0.0	16.87	.77	3.83	102.63	.11
oyster, unsalted tops	.5 oz	0	.08	.07	.74	.01	4.4	0	0.0	16.87	.77	3.83	18.14	.11
peanut butter 'Toast Sandwich' 4 pieces (Nabisco)	1 oz	na	na	na	na	na	na	na	na	na	na	na	55	na
peanut butter bar (Frito-Lay's)	1.75 oz	na	na	na	na	na	na	na	na	na	na	na	100	na
peanut butter-filled, 6 crackers (Frito-Lay's)	1.5 oz	na	na	na	na	na	na	na	na	na	na	na	120	na
poppy, toasted, approx .5 oz (American Classic)	4 crackers	na	na	na	na	na	na	na	na	na	na	na	30	na
'Royal Lunch Milk Crackers' .5 oz (Nabisco)	1 cracker	na	na	na	na	na	na	na	na	na	na	na	15	na
rusk toast	.5 oz	7	.06	.06	.66	.01	9.1	.01	0.0	3.83	.39	5.1	34.73	.16
rye	.5 oz	0	.03	.02	.15	.03	3.1	0	0.0	4.39	.34	11.06	45.22	.34
rye 'RyKrisp' (Ralston)	.5 oz	na	na	na	na	na	na	na	na	na	na	na	70	na
rye, sandwich-type w/cheese filling	.5 oz	3	.09	.07	.51	.03	2.3	.01	0.0	31.47	.35	5.24	48.48	.1
rye, seasoned 'Rykrisp' (Ralston)	.5 oz	na	na	na	na	na	na	na	na	na	na	na	65	na
rye, sesame 'Rykrisp' 2 triple pieces (Ralston)	.5 oz	na	na	na	na	na	na	na	na	na	na	na	65	na
rye wafers, plain	.5 oz	3	.06	.04	.22	.04	6.4	0	0.0	5.67	.84	17.15	70.17	.4
rye wafers, seasoned	.5 oz	3	.04	.00	.25	.03	7.4	0	0.0	6.24	.43	15.03	64.35	.36
salt sticks, Vienna bread type, 6.5 inches long	1 stick	0	.02	.03	.28				0.0	15.75	.28	na	32.9	na
saltine 'Bits, Mini Saltine Crackers' .5 oz (Premium)	16 crackers	na	na	na	na	na	na	na	na	na	na	na	15	na
saltine, crumbs, not packed	1 cup	0	.32	.25	3.08	na	na	na	0.0	14.7	3.36	na	84.0	na
saltine 'Fat-Free' .5 oz (Premium)	4 crackers	na	na	na	na	na	na	na	na	na	na	na	25	na
saltine, low salt	.5 oz	0	.08	.07	.74	.01	4.4	0	0.0	16.87	.77	3.83	102.63	.11

Food Name	Serving Size	A I.U.	Thi mg	Rib mg	Nia mg	B₆ mg	Fol mcg	B₁₂ mcg	C mg	Calc mg	Iron mg	Mag mg	Pot mg	Zn mg
saltine 'Low Salt' approx .5 oz														
(Premium)	5 crackers	na	na	na	na	na	na	na	na	na	na	na	105	na
saltine, 1 7/8-inch square	10 crackers	0	.13	.1	1.25	na	na	na	0.0	5.96	1.36	na	34.08	na
saltine, original, .5 oz (Premium)	5 crackers	na	na	na	na	na	na	na	na	na	na	na	25	na
saltine, unsalted tops	.5 oz	0	.08	.07	.74	.01	4.4	0	0.0	16.87	.77	3.83	18.14	.11
saltine 'Unsalted Tops' approx .5 oz														
(Premium)	5 crackers	na	na	na	na	na	na	na	na	na	na	na	20	na
sandwich, peanut-cheese, 6 sandwiches	1 pkt	17	.49	.13	2.6	na	na	na	0.0	23.52	1.51	na	94.92	na
sandwich, peanut-cheese, 4 sandwiches	1 pkt	11	.33	.09	1.74	na	na	na	0.0	15.68	1.01	na	63.28	na
sandwich, w/cheese filling	.5 oz	4	.06	.1	.53	.01	2.0	.01	0.0	36.43	.34	5.1	60.81	.09
sandwich, w/peanut butter filling	.5 oz	0	.06	.05	.83	.01	4.8	0	0.0	13.75	.43	7.51	31.61	.15
sesame wafer (Westbrae)	4.5 wafers	na	na	na	na	na	na	na	na	na	na	na	30	na
seven-grain vegetable, organic, fat-free														
(Health Valley)	.5 oz	na	na	na	na	na	na	na	na	na	na	na	75	na
seven-grain vegetable, organic, no salt added														
(Health Valley)	.5 oz	na	na	na	na	na	na	na	na	na	na	na	75	na
'Sociables' approx .5 oz (Nabisco)	6 crackers	na	na	na	na	na	na	na	na	na	na	na	20	na
soda, low salt	.5 oz	0	.08	.07	.74	.01	4.4	0	0.0	16.87	.77	3.83	102.63	.11
soda, unsalted tops	.5 oz	0	.08	.07	.74	.01	4.4	0	0.0	16.87	.77	3.83	18.14	.11
soup, low salt	.5 oz	0	.08	.07	.74	.01	4.4	0	0.0	16.87	.77	3.83	102.63	.11
soup, unsalted tops	.5 oz	0	.08	.07	.74	.01	4.4	0	0.0	16.87	.77	3.83	18.14	.11
sour cream and chive flavor (McCrakens)	1 oz	na	na	na	na	na	na	na	na	na	na	na	65	na
tamari wafer (Westbrae)	4.5 crackers	na	na	na	na	na	na	na	na	na	na	na	15	na
'Vegetable Thins' (Nabisco)	7 crackers	na	na	na	na	na	na	na	na	na	na	na	35	na
wafer, no salt (Westbrae)	4.5 wafers	na	na	na	na	na	na	na	na	na	na	na	20	na
wheat, low salt	.5 oz	0	.07	.05	.7	.02	2.6	0	0.0	6.95	.62	8.79	28.78	.23
wheat, regular	.5 oz	0	.07	.05	.7	.02	2.6	0	0.0	6.95	.62	8.79	25.94	.23
wheat, sandwich, w/cheese filling	.5 oz	10	.05	.06	.45	.04	2.7	.01	0.2	28.92	.37	7.65	43.38	.12
wheat, sandwich, w/peanut butter filling	.5 oz	0	.06	.04	.83	.02	5.2	0	0.0	24.1	.38	5.39	42.1	.10
wheat, toasted (McCrakens)	1 oz	na	na	na	na	na	na	na	na	na	na	na	65	na
wheat 'Wheat Krisp' (Ralston)	.5 oz	na	na	na	na	na	na	na	na	na	na	na	90	na
wheat 'Wheat Thins' (Nabisco)	8 crackers	na	na	na	na	na	na	na	na	na	na	na	30	na
whole-wheat	.5 oz	0	.03	.01	.64	.03	4.0	0	0.0	7.09	.44	14.03	42.1	.3
whole wheat, approx .5 oz (Ritz)	5 crackers	na	na	na	na	na	na	na	na	na	na	na	15	na
whole wheat, low salt	.5 oz	0	.03	.01	.64	.03	4.0	0	0.0	7.09	.44	14.03	42.1	.3
whole wheat, organic, fat-free (Health Valley)	.5 oz	na	na	na	na	na	na	na	na	na	na	na	75	na
zesty Italian, approx 13-16 crackers														
(Frito-Lay's)	.5 oz	na	na	na	na	na	na	na	na	na	na	na	20	na
zwieback	1 oz	16	.06	.07	.37	.02	5.7	0	1.5	5.67	.17	3.97	86.47	.15
CRACKER CRUMBS AND MEAL														
meal	1 cup	0	.8	.54	6.56	.04	25.3	0	0.0	26.45	5.34	27.6	132.25	.79
meal	1 oz	0	.2	.13	1.62	.01	6.2	0	0.0	6.52	1.32	6.8	32.6	.2
CRANBERRY														
raw (Ocean Spray) approx 2 oz	1/2 cup	na	na	na	na	na	na	na	10.0	na	na	na	42	na
raw, chopped	1 cup	51	.03	.02	.11	.07	1.9	0	14.9	7.7	.22	5.5	78.1	.14
raw, whole	1 cup	44	.03	.02	.09	.06	1.6	0	12.8	6.65	.19	4.75	67.45	.12
CRANBERRY APPLE COCKTAIL														
(Minute Maid) 'Juices To Go'	6 oz	na	na	na	na	na	na	na	1.0	na	na	na	25	na
CRANBERRY APPLE DRINK														
	6 oz	6	.01	.04	.11	.04	0.4	0	58.9	12.88	.11	3.68	49.68	.07
(Ocean Spray) 'Cran•Apple'	6 oz	na	na	na	na	na	na	na	100.0	na	na	na	20	na
(Ocean Spray) 'Cran•Apple Low Calorie'	6 oz	na	na	4	na	na	na	na	100.0	na	na	4	65	na
CRANBERRY APRICOT DRINK														
	6 oz	852	.01	.02	.22	.04	1.1	0	0.0	16.56	.28	5.52	112.24	.07
'Cranicot' (Ocean Spray)	6 oz	45	na	na	na	na	na	na	na	na	na	na	85	na
CRANBERRY BEAN/borlotti/Roman bean/rose coco														
boiled	1 cup	0	.37	.12	.91	.14	366.0	0	0.0	88.5	3.7	88.5	684.99	2.02

Food Name	Serving Size	A I.U.	Thi mg	Rib mg	Nia mg	B_6 mg	Fol mcg	B_{12} mcg	C mg	Calc mg	Iron mg	Mag mg	Pot mg	Zn mg
raw	1 cup	4	1.46	.42	2.84	.6	1178.6	0	0.0	247.65	9.75	304.2	2507.4	7.09
CRANBERRY BEAN, CANNED	1 cup	0	.1	.1	1.31	.14	201.2	0	2.1	88.4	4.03	83.2	676.0	2.18
CRANBERRY COCKTAIL JUICE														
(J. Hungerford)	9.03 oz	na	na	na	na	na	na	na	100.0	.1	.3	na	na	na
(J. Hungerford) 50% juice	9.03 oz	na	na	na	na	na	na	na	100.0	.5	1.4	na	na	na
(J. Hungerford) 100% juice	9.03 oz	na	na	na	na	na	na	na	100.0	1.52	4.0	na	na	na
CRANBERRY DRINK														
(Ocean Spray) 'Cran•Blueberry'	6 oz	na	na	4	na	na	na	na	100.0	na	1	na	25	na
(Ocean Spray) 'Cran•Raspberry'	6 oz	na	na	na	na	na	na	na	100.0	na	na	na	25	na
(Ocean Spray) 'Cran•Raspberry Low Calorie'	6 oz	na	na	2	na	na	na	na	100.0	na	2	na	80	na
(Ocean Spray) 'Cran•Strawberry'	6 oz	na	na	na	na	na	na	na	100.0	na	na	na	20	na
CRANBERRY GRAPE DRINK														
(Ocean Spray) 'Cran•Grape'	6 oz	na	na	4	na	na	na	na	100.0	na	2	na	10	na
CRANBERRY JUICE														
(Ocean Spray) 'Cran•tastic'	6 oz	na	na	4	na	na	na	na	100.0	na	na	na	30	na
CRANBERRY JUICE COCKTAIL														
	1 cup	10	.02	.02	.09	.05	0.5	0	89.6	7.59	.38	5.06	45.54	.18
	6 oz	8	.02	.02	.07	.04	0.4	0	67.3	5.7	.28	3.8	34.2	.13
(Ocean Spray) 'Low Calorie'	6 oz	na	na	2	na	na	na	na	100.0	na	2	na	25	na
CRANBERRY JUICE DRINK														
citrus 'Refreshers' (Ocean Spray)	6 oz	na	na	na	na	na	na	na	100.0	na	na	na	40	na
CRANBERRY SAUCE														
canned, sweetened	1 cup	55	.04	.06	.28	.04	na	0	5.5	11.08	.61	8.31	72.02	.14
jellied (Ocean Spray)	2 oz	na	na	na	na	na	na	na	na	na	na	na	10	na
whole berry (Ocean Spray)	2 oz	na	na	na	na	na	na	na	na	na	na	na	15	na
CRANBERRY STRAWBERRY SAUCE, crushed,														
for chicken 'Cran•Fruit' (Ocean Spray)	2 oz	na	na	na	na	na	na	na	na	na	na	na	25	na
CRAPPIE. See SUNFISH.														
CRAYFISH, MIXED SPECIES														
farmed, moist-heat cooked	100 gm	50	.05	.08	1.67	.13	11.0	3.1	0.5	51.0	1.11	33.0	238.0	1.48
farmed, moist-heat cooked	3 oz	43	.04	.07	1.42	.11	9.4	2.63	0.4	43.35	.94	28.05	202.3	1.26
farmed, raw	3 oz	43	.04	.03	1.59	.06	25.5	1.78	0.4	21.25	.47	25.5	221.85	.86
farmed, raw	8 crayfish	14	.01	.01	.5	.02	8.1	.57	0.1	6.75	.15	8.1	70.47	.27
wild, moist-heat cooked	100 gm	50	.05	.09	2.28	.08	44.0	2.15	0.9	60.0	.83	33.0	296.0	1.76
wild, moist-heat cooked	3 oz	43	.04	.07	1.94	.06	37.4	1.83	0.8	51.0	.71	28.05	251.6	1.5
wild, raw	3 oz	44	.06	.03	1.88	.09	31.5	1.7	1.0	22.95	.71	22.95	256.7	1.1
wild, raw	8 crayfish	14	.02	.01	.6	.03	10.0	.54	0.3	7.29	.23	7.29	81.54	.35
CREAM														
half and half	1 cup	1050	.08	.36	.19	.09	6.1	.8	2.1	253.86	.17	24.61	313.63	1.23
half and half	1 tbsp	65	.01	.02	.01	.01	0.4	.05	0.1	15.74	.01	1.53	19.44	.08
heavy whipping	1 cup	3499	.05	.26	.09	.06	8.8	.43	1.4	153.75	.07	16.73	179.45	.55
heavy, whipping	1 tbsp	221	0	.02	.01	0	0.6	.03	0.1	9.69	0	1.05	11.31	.03
light whipping	1 cup	2694	.06	.3	.1	.07	8.8	.47	1.5	165.87	.07	17.28	231.35	.6
light whipping	1 tbsp	169	0	.02	.01	0	0.6	.03	0.1	10.41	0	1.08	14.52	.04
light, coffee or table	1 cup	1728	.08	.36	.14	.08	5.5	.53	1.8	230.88	.1	20.76	292.08	.65
light, coffee or table	1 tbsp	108	0	.02	.01	0	0.3	.03	0.1	14.43	.01	1.3	18.25	.04
medium, 25% fat	1 cup	2251	.07	.33	.12	.07	5.5	.52	1.7	215.58	.1	20.03	273.66	.62
medium, 25% fat	1 tbsp	141	0	.02	.01	0	0.3	.03	0.1	13.53	.01	1.26	17.18	.04
CREAM CHEESE. See CHEESE.														
CREAM NUT. See BRAZIL NUT.														
CREAM OF TARTAR	1 tsp	0	0	0	0	0	0.0	0	0.0	.24	.11	.06	495.0	.01
CREAM SODA. See SOFT DRINKS AND MIXERS.														
CREAM TOPPING														
creamy white 'Dolci Frutta Crema Bianca'														
(Saco Foods)	1 box	6	.65	.33	.17	na	na	na	0.1	244.05	.21	na	337.93	na
dark chocolate 'Dolci Frutta Con Cioccolatta'														
(Saco Foods)	1 box	48	.21	.11	.37	na	na	na	0.2	54.82	1.65	na	159.97	na

Food Name	Serving Size	A I.U.	Thi mg	Rib mg	Nia mg	B₆ mg	Fol mcg	B₁₂ mcg	C mg	Calc mg	Iron mg	Mag mg	Pot mg	Zn mg
pressurized can, whipped	1 cup	548	.02	.04	.04	.02	1.6	.18	0.0	60.6	.03	6.47	88.38	.22
pressurized can, whipped	1 tbsp	27	0	0	0	0	0.1	.01	0.0	3.03	0	.32	4.42	.01
CREAM TOPPING, NONDAIRY														
frozen, chocolate 'Cool Whip' (Birds Eye) ...	1 tbsp	na	na	na	na	na	na	na	na	na	na	na	0	na
frozen 'Cool Whip' (Birds Eye)	1 tbsp	na	na	na	na	na	na	na	na	na	na	na	0	na
frozen 'Cool Whip Lite' (Birds Eye)	1 tbsp	na	na	na	na	na	na	na	na	na	na	na	0	na
frozen, extra creamy 'Cool Whip Dairy Recipe'														
(Birds Eye)	1 tbsp	na	na	na	na	na	na	na	na	na	na	na	0	na
frozen, semisolid	1 cup	646	0	0	0	0	0.0	0	0.0	4.72	.09	1.34	13.65	.02
frozen, semisolid	1 tbsp	34	0	0	0	0	0.0	0	0.0	.25	0	.07	.73	0
mix, prepared (D-Zerta)	1 tbsp	na	na	na	na	na	na	na	na	na	na	na	10	na
reduced calorie (D-Zerta)	1 tbsp	na	na	na	na	na	na	na	na	na	na	na	10	na
CREAMER, NONDAIRY														
Liquid														
w/hydrogenated vegetable oil and soy														
protein	1/2 cup	107	0	0	0	0	0.0	0	0.0	11.16	.04	.4	228.6	.02
w/hydrogenated vegetable oil and soy														
protein	1/2 oz	13	0	0	0	0	0.0	0	0.0	1.4	0	.05	28.58	0
w/lauric acid oil and sodium caseinate	1/2 cup	107	0	0	0	0	0.0	0	0.0	11.16	.04	.4	228.6	.02
w/lauric acid oil and sodium caseinate	1/2 oz	13	0	0	0	0	0.0	0	0.0	1.4	0	.05	28.58	0
(Westbrae)	1 tbsp	na	na	na	na	na	na	na	na	na	na	na	20	na
Powder (Coffee-Mate) 'Lite'	1 tsp	na	na	na	na	na	na	na	na	na	na	na	15	na
CREME DE MENTHE. See ALCOHOLIC BEVERAGES.														
CRESS, GARDEN														
boiled, drained	1/2 cup	5236	.04	.11	.54	.11	25.2	0	15.6	41.48	.54	17.68	240.04	.1
raw	1/2 cup	2325	.02	.07	.25	.06	20.1	0	17.3	20.25	.33	9.5	151.5	.06
CROAKER, ATLANTIC														
raw	3 oz	51	.06	.08	3.57	.26	12.8	2.13	0.0	12.75	.31	34.0	293.25	.36
raw, approx 2.8 oz	1 fillet	47	.06	.08	3.32	.24	11.9	1.98	0.0	11.85	.29	31.6	272.55	.33
CROOKNECK SQUASH. See SQUASH, CROOKNECK.														
CROUTONS														
plain	1 cup	0	.19	.08	1.63	.01	6.6	0	0.0	22.8	1.22	9.3	37.2	.27
plain	.5 oz	0	.09	.04	.77	0	3.1	0	0.0	10.77	.58	4.39	17.58	.13
seasoned	1 cup	8	.2	.17	1.86	.03	16.0	.03	0.0	38.4	1.13	16.8	72.4	.38
seasoned	.5 oz	3	.07	.06	.66	.01	5.7	.01	0.0	13.61	.4	5.95	25.66	.13
CUCUMBER														
raw, approx 10.9 oz	1 med	647	.07	.07	.67	.13	39.1	0	16.0	42.14	.78	33.11	433.44	.6
raw, slices	1/2 cup	112	.01	.01	.11	.02	6.8	0	2.8	7.28	.14	5.72	74.88	.1
CUMIN SEED														
whole	1 tbsp	76	.04	.02	.27	na	na	0	0.5	55.84	3.98	21.93	107.25	.29
whole	1 tsp	27	.01	.01	.1	na	na	0	0.2	19.54	1.39	7.68	37.54	.1
whole (Durkee)	1 tsp	.56	.32	.17	0	na	na	na	.01	0	.02	na	0	na
whole (Laurel Leaf)	1 tsp	.56	.32	.17	0	na	na	na	.01	0	.02	na	0	na
CUPU ASSU OIL	1 tbsp	0	0	0	0	0	0.0	0	0.0	0	na	0	0	0
CURRANT, BLACK /European currant														
raw	1 cup	258	.06	.06	.34	.07	na	0	202.7	61.6	1.72	26.88	360.64	.3
CURRANT, RED														
raw	1 cup	134	.04	.06	.11	.08	na	0	45.9	36.96	1.12	14.56	308.0	.26
CURRANT, WHITE														
raw	1 cup	134	.04	.06	.11	.08	na	0	45.9	36.96	1.12	na	308.0	.26
CURRANT, ZANTE														
dried	1 cup	105	.23	.2	2.33	.43	14.7	0	6.8	123.84	4.69	59.04	1284.48	.95
CURRY POWDER														
ground	1 tbsp	62	.02	.02	.22	na	na	0	0.7	30.11	1.86	16.0	97.21	.26
ground	1 tsp	20	.01	.01	.07	na	na	0	0.2	9.56	.59	5.08	30.86	.08
CUSK / torsk / tusk														
dry-heat cooked	3 oz	59	.04	.14	2.78	.38	1.7	1.02	0.0	11.05	.9	34.0	427.55	.42

Food Name	Serving Size	A I.U.	Thi mg	Rib mg	Nia mg	B₆ mg	Fol mcg	B₁₂ mcg	C mg	Calc mg	Iron mg	Mag mg	Pot mg	Zn mg
raw	3 oz	51	.04	.11	2.28	.33	1.7	.89	0.0	8.5	.71	26.35	333.2	.00
raw, approx 4.3 oz	1 fillet	73	.05	.16	3.28	.47	2.4	1.27	0.0	12.2	1.01	37.82	478.24	.46
CUSTARD. See PUDDING MIX.														
CUSTARD APPLE/ bullock's heart/cherimoya														
raw	100 gm	33	.08	.1	.5	.22	na	0	19.2	30.0	.71	18.0	382.0	na
CUTTLEFISH, MIXED SPECIES														
moist-heat cooked	100 gm	675	.02	1.73	2.19	.27	24.0	5.4	8.5	180.0	10.84	60.0	637.0	3.46
moist-heat cooked	3 oz	574	.01	1.47	1.86	.23	20.4	4.59	7.2	153.0	9.21	51.0	541.45	2.94
CYMLING. See SQUASH, SCALLOP.														

D

Food Name	Serving Size	A I.U.	Thi mg	Rib mg	Nia mg	B₆ mg	Fol mcg	B₁₂ mcg	C mg	Calc mg	Iron mg	Mag mg	Pot mg	Zn mg
DAIQUIRI. See ALCOHOLIC BEVERAGES.														
DANDELION GREENS														
boiled, drained, chopped	1 cup	12285	.14	.18	.54	.17	13.1	0	18.9	147.0	1.89	25.2	243.6	.29
DANISH CABBAGE. See CABBAGE, DANISH.														
DATES														
(Amport Foods) chopped	1.5 oz	na	na	na	na	na	na	na	na	na	na	na	323	na
(Amport Foods) whole	1.5 oz	na	na	na	na	na	na	na	na	na	na	na	323	na
DEER														
raw	1 lb	0	1.0	2.18	28.89	na	na	na	0.0	22.68	15.42	104.33	1442.45	9.48
raw	1 oz	0	.06	.13	1.78	na	na	na	0.0	1.4	.95	6.44	89.04	.59
roasted	3 oz	0	.15	.51	5.7	na	na	na	0.0	5.95	3.8	20.4	284.75	2.34
DILL SEED														
whole	1 tbsp	4	.03	.02	.19	na	na	0	na	100.03	1.08	16.89	78.28	.34
whole	1 tsp	1	.01	.01	.06	na	na	0	na	31.83	.34	5.37	24.91	.11
whole (Durkee)	1 tsp	.02	.19	.12	0	na	na	na	na	0	.01	na	0	na
whole (Laurel Leaf)	1 tsp	.02	.19	.12	0	na	na	na	na	0	.01	na	0	na
DILL WEED														
dried	1 tbsp	na	.01	.01	.09	.05	na	0	na	55.31	1.51	13.98	102.53	.1
dried	1 tsp	na	0	0	.03	.01	na	0	na	17.84	.49	4.51	33.08	.03
fresh, sprigs	1 cup	687	.01	.03	.14	.02	13.4	0	7.6	18.51	.59	4.89	65.68	.08
DIP														
BACON AND HORSERADISH (Breakstone's)	2 tbsp	na	na	na	na	na	na	na	na	na	na	na	40	na
BACON AND ONION (Breakstone's) 'Gourmet'	2 tbsp	na	na	na	na	na	na	na	na	na	na	na	40	na
CHEDDAR CHEESE (Frito-Lay's)	1 oz	na	na	na	na	na	na	na	na	na	na	na	35	na
CLAM														
(Breakstone's)	2 tbsp	na	na	na	na	na	na	na	na	na	na	na	40	na
(Breakstone's) 'Gourmet Chesapeake'	2 tbsp	na	na	na	na	na	na	na	na	na	na	na	40	na
CUCUMBER AND ONION (Breakstone's)	2 tbsp	na	na	na	na	na	na	na	na	na	na	na	40	na
FRENCH ONION (Breakstone's)	2 tbsp	na	na	na	na	na	na	na	na	na	na	na	40	na
JALAPEÑO														
(Breakstone's) cheddar 'Gourmet'	2 tbsp	na	na	na	na	na	na	na	na	na	na	na	40	na
(Frito-Lay's)	1 oz	na	na	na	na	na	na	na	na	na	na	na	105	na
MUSHROOM AND HERB														
(Breakstone's) 'Gourmet'	2 tbsp	na	na	na	na	na	na	na	na	na	na	na	40	na
ONION (Breakstone's) toasted 'Gourmet'	2 tbsp	na	na	na	na	na	na	na	na	na	na	na	40	na
PICANTE SAUCE (Frito-Lay's)	1 oz	na	na	na	na	na	na	na	na	na	na	na	80	na
DISHCLOTH GOURD. See GOURD, DISHCLOTH.														
DOCK														
boiled, drained	100 gm	3474	.03	.09	.41	.1	7.8	0	26.3	38.0	2.08	89.0	321.0	.17
raw, chopped	1/2 cup	2680	.03	.07	.34	.08	8.8	0	32.2	29.48	1.61	69.01	261.3	.13
DOLPHIN FISH. See MAHI MAHI.														

Food Name	Serving Size	A I.U.	Thi mg	Rib mg	Nia mg	B_6 mg	Fol mcg	B_{12} mcg	C mg	Calc mg	Iron mg	Mag mg	Pot mg	Zn mg
DONUT														
(Break Cake)														
chocolate, 1 oz	1 donut	na	na	na	na	na	na	na	na	na	na	na	40	na
chocolate, gem, .5 oz	1 donut	na	na	na	na	na	na	na	na	na	na	na	20	na
chocolate, gem, .5 oz	6 donuts	na	na	na	na	na	na	na	na	na	na	na	125	na
cinnamon, 1 oz	1 donut	na	na	na	na	na	na	na	na	na	na	na	35	na
cinnamon, gem, .5 oz	1 donut	na	na	na	na	na	na	na	na	na	na	na	15	na
powdered, 1 oz	1 donut	na	na	na	na	na	na	na	na	na	na	na	35	na
powdered, gem, .5 oz	1 donut	na	na	na	na	na	na	na	na	na	na	na	20	na
powdered, gem, .5 oz	6 donuts	na	na	na	na	na	na	na	na	na	na	na	110	na
DRINKS. See ALCOHOL-FREE BEVERAGES; ALCOHOLIC BEVERAGES; COFFEE; MILK; SOFT DRINKS AND MIXERS; SPORTS DRINK; TEA; WATER; and individual listings.														
DRINK MIX. See individual drink mix flavors.														
DRUM, FRESHWATER														
dry-heat cooked	3 oz	167	.07	.18	2.43	.29	14.5	1.96	0.9	65.45	.98	32.3	300.05	.72
raw	3 oz	145	.06	.14	2.0	.26	12.8	1.7	0.9	51.0	.77	25.5	233.75	.56
DUCK FAT														
	1 cup	0	0	0	0	0	0.0	0	0.0	0	0	0	0	0
	1 tbsp	0	0	0	0	0	0.0	0	0.0	0	0	0	0	0
DULSE, raw	100 gm	0	0	0	0	na	na	na	0.0	296.0	0	na	8060.0	na

E

Food Name	Serving Size	A I.U.	Thi mg	Rib mg	Nia mg	B_6 mg	Fol mcg	B_{12} mcg	C mg	Calc mg	Iron mg	Mag mg	Pot mg	Zn mg
EEL, MIXED SPECIES, dry-heat cooked	3 oz	3219	.16	.04	3.81	.07	14.7	2.45	1.5	22.1	.54	22.1	296.65	1.77
EGG, ALTERNATIVE														
Frozen														
(Fleischmann's) 'Egg Beaters' cheese omelet	1/2 cup	na	na	na	na	na	na	na	na	na	na	na	135	na
(Fleischmann's) 'Egg Beaters' vegetable omelet	1/2 cup	na	na	na	na	na	na	na	na	na	na	na	180	na
Refrigerated														
(Fleischmann's) 'Egg Beaters'	1/4 cup	na	na	na	na	na	na	na	na	na	na	na	75	na
EGG, CHICKEN. See also EGG WHITE, CHICKEN; EGG YOLK, CHICKEN.														
Cooked														
hard-boiled, chopped	1 cup	762	.09	.7	.09	.16	59.8	1.51	0.0	68.0	1.62	13.6	171.36	1.43
poached	1 large	316	.02	.22	.03	.06	17.5	.4	0.0	24.5	.72	5.0	60.0	.55
scrambled	1 cup	1500	.11	.96	.17	.26	66.0	1.69	0.4	156.2	2.64	26.4	303.6	2.2
scrambled	1 large	409	.03	.26	.05	.07	18.0	.46	0.1	42.6	.72	7.2	82.8	.6
Dried														
	1 tbsp	98	.02	.06	.01	.02	9.2	.5	0.0	10.58	.39	2.32	24.49	.27
sifted	1 cup	1658	.26	1.0	.21	.34	156.2	8.5	0.0	179.78	6.7	39.38	416.25	4.62
stabilized, glucose reduced	1 tbsp	103	.02	.06	.01	.02	9.7	.53	0.0	11.12	.41	2.44	25.74	.29
stabilized, glucose reduced, sifted	1 cup	1743	.28	1.05	.22	.36	164.2	8.94	0.0	188.95	7.04	41.4	437.58	4.85
EGG, DUCK, raw	1 large	930	.11	.28	.14	.18	56.0	3.78	0.0	44.59	2.69	11.55	155.61	.99
EGG, GOOSE, raw	1 large	1843	.21	.55	.27	.34	108.9	7.34	0.0	86.69	5.24	22.46	302.4	1.92
EGG, QUAIL, raw	1 large	27	.01	.07	.01	.01	6.0	.14	0.0	5.76	.33	1.13	11.92	.13
EGG, TURKEY, raw	1 large	438	.09	.37	.02	.1	56.2	1.34	0.0	78.21	3.24	10.62	112.26	1.25
EGG NOODLE. See NOODLE, EGG.														
EGG ROLL														
Frozen *(Chun King)*														
chicken	3.6 oz	na	na	na	na	na	na	na	na	na	na	na	120	na
meat and shrimp	3.6 oz	na	na	na	na	na	na	na	na	na	na	na	130	na
pork 'Restaurant Style'	3 oz	na	na	na	na	na	na	na	na	na	na	na	250	na
shrimp	3.6 oz	na	na	na	na	na	na	na	na	na	na	na	80	na

Food Name	Serving Size	A I.U.	Thi mg	Rib mg	Nia mg	B$_6$ mg	Fol mcg	B$_{12}$ mcg	C mg	Calc mg	Iron mg	Mag mg	Pot mg	Zn mg
EGG WHITE, CHICKEN														
Raw														
fresh or frozen	1 cup	0	.01	1.1	.22	.01	7.3	.49	0.0	14.58	.07	26.73	347.49	.02
fresh or frozen	1 large	0	0	.15	.03	0	1.0	.07	0.0	2.0	.01	3.67	47.76	0
EGG YOLK, CHICKEN														
Dried														
sifted	1 cup	2293	.29	.54	.09	.39	142.5	4.74	0.0	189.01	6.95	18.97	112.43	4.12
sifted	1 tbsp	137	.02	.03	.01	.02	8.5	.28	0.0	11.28	.42	1.13	6.71	.25
Raw														
fresh	1 cup	4726	.41	1.55	.04	.95	354.8	7.56	0.0	332.91	8.58	21.87	228.42	7.56
fresh	1 large	323	.03	.11	0	.07	24.2	.52	0.0	22.74	.59	1.49	15.6	.52
frozen, salted	100 gm	1475	.13	.55	.03	.3	110.0	2.35	0.0	109.0	2.75	8.0	91.0	2.38
frozen, sugared	100 gm	1475	.13	.55	.03	.3	110.0	2.35	0.0	105.0	2.74	8.0	90.0	2.38
EGGNOG MIX														
dry, 2 heaping tsp	1 oz	10	0	0	.04	0	0.6	.02	0.0	.85	.26	0	1.42	.02
1 oz powder, prepared w/whole milk	1 cup	307	.09	.39	.25	.1	12.2	.87	2.2	291.04	.38	32.64	369.92	.92
EGGPLANT/aubergine														
boiled, drained, 1-inch cubes	1 cup	61	.07	.02	.58	.08	13.8	0	1.3	5.76	.34	12.48	238.08	.14
raw, 1-inch pieces	1/2 cup	34	.02	.01	.25	.03	7.8	0	0.7	2.87	.11	5.74	88.97	.06
raw, peeled, approx 1 lb	1 eggplant	385	.24	.16	2.74	.38	87.0	0	7.8	32.06	1.24	64.12	993.86	.64
ELDERBERRY, fresh	1 cup	870	.1	.09	.73	.33	na	0	52.2	55.1	2.32	na	406.0	na
ELK														
raw	1 lb	0	na	na	na	na	na	na	0.0	18.14	12.52	104.33	1415.23	10.89
raw	1 oz	0	na	na	na	na	na	na	0.0	1.12	.77	6.44	87.36	.67
roasted	3 oz	0	na	na	na	na	na	na	0.0	4.25	3.09	20.4	278.8	2.69
ENCHILADA ENTRÉE, FROZEN														
BLACK BEAN-VEGETABLE (*Amy's Kitchen*)	4.75 oz	na	na	na	na	na	na	na	na	na	na	na	167	na
CHEESE														
(*Amy's Kitchen*) organic	4.75 oz	na	na	na	na	na	na	na	na	na	na	na	108	na
(*Stouffer's*)	9.75 oz	na	na	na	na	na	na	na	na	na	na	na	400	na
CHICKEN														
(*Stouffer's*)	10 oz	na	na	na	na	na	na	na	na	na	na	na	420	na
ENDIVE														
approx 1.3 lb	1 head	10517	.41	.38	2.05	.1	728.5	0	33.4	266.76	4.26	76.95	1610.82	4.05
chopped	1/2 cup	513	.02	.02	.1	.01	35.5	0	1.6	13.0	.21	3.75	78.5	.2
ENGLISH MUFFIN														
(*Earth Grains*)														
oat bran, 12-oz pkg	1 muffin	na	na	na	na	na	na	na	na	na	na	na	85	na
plain, 12.5-oz pkg	1 muffin	na	na	na	na	na	na	na	na	na	na	na	60	na
plain, 12-oz pkg	1 muffin	na	na	na	na	na	na	na	na	na	na	na	60	na
raisin, 14-oz pkg	1 muffin	na	na	na	na	na	na	na	na	na	na	na	130	na
raisin, 'Sun Maid' 15-oz pkg	1 muffin	na	na	na	na	na	na	na	na	na	na	na	160	na
sourdough, 12.5-oz pkg	1 muffin	na	na	na	na	na	na	na	na	na	na	na	60	na
sourdough, 12-oz pkg	1 muffin	na	na	na	na	na	na	na	na	na	na	na	60	na
whole wheat, 15-oz pkg	1 muffin	na	na	na	na	na	na	na	na	na	na	na	150	na
whole wheat, 14-oz pkg	1 muffin	na	na	na	na	na	na	na	na	na	na	na	140	na
ENTRÉES. See individual entrées.														
EPPAW, raw	1/2 cup	0	.06	.06	.15	.09	12.2	0	6.5	55.0	.58	16.0	170.0	.58

F

Food Name	Serving Size	A I.U.	Thi mg	Rib mg	Nia mg	B$_6$ mg	Fol mcg	B$_{12}$ mcg	C mg	Calc mg	Iron mg	Mag mg	Pot mg	Zn mg

FARINA. See CEREAL, HOT.
FATHEAD. See SHEEPSHEAD.

Food Name	Serving Size	A I.U.	Thi mg	Rib mg	Nia mg	B₆ mg	Fol mcg	B₁₂ mcg	C mg	Calc mg	Iron mg	Mag mg	Pot mg	Zn mg
FAVA BEAN/horse bean/jack bean														
mature seeds, boiled	1/2 cup	13	.08	.08	.6	.06	88.5	0	0.3	30.6	1.27	36.55	227.8	.86
mature seeds, raw	1/2 cup	40	.42	.25	2.12	.27	317.2	0	1.1	77.25	5.03	144.0	796.5	2.36
Canned, mature seeds	1/2 cup	13	.03	.06	1.23	.06	41.9	0	2.3	33.28	1.28	40.96	309.76	.79
FEIJAO														
raw	1 fruit	0	0	.02	.14	.02	19.0	0	10.2	8.5	.04	4.5	77.5	.02
raw, purée	1 cup	0	.02	.08	.7	.12	92.3	0	49.3	41.31	.19	21.87	376.65	.1
FENNEL/finocchio														
raw, bulb	1 bulb	314	.02	.07	1.5	.11	63.2	0	28.1	114.66	1.7	39.78	968.76	.47
raw, leaves	100 gm	3500	.06	.1	.5	na	na	na	31.0	100.0	2.7	na	397.0	na
raw, sliced	1 cup	117	.01	.03	.56	.04	23.5	0	10.4	42.63	.63	14.79	360.18	.17
FENNEL SEED														
whole	1 tbsp	8	.02	.02	.35	na	na	0	na	69.39	1.08	22.33	98.24	.21
whole	1 tsp	3	.01	.01	.12	na	na	0	na	23.93	.37	7.7	33.88	.07
whole (Durkee)	1 tsp	.05	.16	.14	0	na	na	na	na	0	0	na	0	na
whole (Laurel Leaf)	1 tsp	.05	.16	.14	0	na	na	na	na	0	0	na	0	na
FENUGREEK SEED														
whole	1 tbsp	na	.04	.04	.18	na	6.3	0	0.3	19.5	3.72	21.16	85.45	.28
whole	1 tsp	na	.01	.01	.06	na	2.1	0	0.1	6.5	1.24	7.05	28.48	.09
FETTUCCINE ENTRÉE, FROZEN														
Alfredo, 10-oz pkg (Stouffer's)	5 oz	na	na	na	na	na	na	na	na	na	na	na	100	na
FIG														
candied	100 gm	80	.1	.1	.7	na	na	na	0.0	126.0	3.0	na	640.0	na
raw, w/o stem	1 large	91	.04	.03	.26	.07	na	0	1.3	22.4	.24	10.88	148.48	.1
raw, w/o stem	1 med	71	.03	.02	.2	.06	na	0	1.0	17.5	.19	8.5	116.0	.08
Canned														
in extra heavy syrup, solid and liquid	1 cup	94	.06	.09	1.09	na	na	0	2.6	67.86	.73	26.1	253.17	.29
In extra heavy syrup, w/1.75 tbsp liquid	3 fruits	31	.02	.03	.36	na	na	0	0.9	22.1	.24	8.5	82.45	.09
in heavy syrup, solid and liquid	1 cup	96	.06	.1	1.11	na	na	0	2.6	69.93	.73	25.9	256.41	.28
in heavy syrup, w/1.75 tbsp liquid	3 fruits	01	.02	.03	.36	na	na	0	0.9	22.95	.24	8.5	84.15	.09
in light syrup, solid and liquid	1 cup	93	.06	.1	1.1	na	na	0	2.5	68.04	.73	25.2	257.04	.28
in light syrup, w/1.75 tbsp liquid	3 fruits	31	.02	.03	.37	na	na	0	0.9	22.95	.25	8.5	86.7	.09
in water, solid and liquid	1 cup	94	.06	.09	1.1	na	na	0	2.5	69.44	.72	24.8	255.44	.3
in water, w/1.75 tbsp liquid	3 fruits	30	.02	.03	.36	na	na	0	0.8	22.4	.23	8.0	82.4	.1
Dried														
stewed	1/2 cup	207	.01	.14	.83	.17	1.3	0	5.7	79.3	1.22	32.5	391.3	.27
uncooked	1 cup	265	.14	.18	1.38	.45	14.9	0	1.6	286.56	4.44	117.41	1416.88	1.01
uncooked, trimmed	10 fruits	249	.13	.16	1.3	.42	14.0	0	1.5	269.28	4.17	110.33	1331.44	.95
FILBERT BUTTER														
roasted (Maranatha Natural)	2 tbsp	na	na	na	na	na	na	na	na	na	na	na	180	na
FISH. See individual listings.														
FISH CAKE														
fried	1 cake	0	.02	.04	.96	na	na	na	0.0	6.6	.24	na	208.8	na
fried, bite size	5 cakes	0	.02	.04	.96	na	na	na	0.0	6.6	.24	na	208.8	na
FISH FILLET, FROZEN														
breaded, 8 fillets (Healthy Choice)	2.5 oz	na	na	na	na	na	na	na	na	na	na	na	165	na
breaded, 4 fillets (Healthy Choice)	3 oz	na	na	na	na	na	na	na	na	na	na	na	195	na
breaded, 2 fillets (Healthy Choice)	3.5 oz	na	na	na	na	na	na	na	na	na	na	na	230	na
FISH LOAF, cooked	1 loaf	0	.85	7.53	26.73	na	na	na	0.0	133.65	4.86	na	4228.2	na
FISH OIL														
herring	1 cup	0	0	0	0	0	0.0	0	0.0	0	0	0	0	0
herring	1 tbsp	0	0	0	0	0	0.0	0	0.0	0	0	0	0	0
menhaden	1 cup	0	0	0	0	0	0.0	0	0.0	0	0	0	0	0
menhaden	1 tbsp	0	0	0	0	0	0.0	0	0.0	0	0	0	0	0
menhaden, fully hydrogenated	1 cup	0	0	0	0	0	0.0	0	0.0	0	0	0	0	0
menhaden, fully hydrogenated	1 tbsp	0	0	0	0	0	0.0	0	0.0	0	0	0	0	0
salmon	1 cup	0	0	0	0	0	0.0	0	0.0	0	0	0	0	0

Food Name	Serving Size	A I.U.	Thi mg	Rib mg	Nia mg	B_6 mg	Fol mcg	B_{12} mcg	C mg	Calc mg	Iron mg	Mag mg	Pot mg	Zn mg
salmon	1 tbsp	0	0	0	0	0	0.0	0	0.0	0	0	0	0	0
sardine	1 cup	0	0	0	0	0	0.0	0	0.0	0	0	0	0	0
sardine	1 tbsp	0	0	0	0	0	0.0	0	0.0	0	0	0	0	0
FLAN. See PUDDING MIX.														
FLATFISH. See FLOUNDER; HALIBUT; SOLE.														
FLOUNDER														
dry-heat cooked	3 oz	32	.07	.1	1.85	.2	7.8	2.13	0.0	15.3	.29	49.3	292.4	.54
raw	3 oz	28	.08	.06	2.46	.18	6.8	1.29	1.4	15.3	.31	26.35	306.85	.38
FLOUR. See individual listings.														
FONDANT. See CANDY.														
FORMULA, INFANT. See BABY FOOD.														
FRANKFURTER														
chicken, 1 oz	1 frank	37	.02	.03	.88	.09	1.1	.07	0.0	26.93	.57	2.84	23.81	.29
raw, beef and pork, 2 oz	1 frank	0	.11	.07	1.5	.07	2.3	.74	14.8	6.27	.66	5.7	95.19	1.05
raw, w/nonfat dry milk and cereal, 2 oz	1 frank	0	.09	.11	1.54	na	na	na	0.0	11.4	1.08	na	125.4	na
turkey, 1 oz	1 frank	0	.01	.05	1.17	.07	2.3	.08	0.0	30.05	.52	3.97	50.75	.88
FRENCH ARTICHOKE. See ARTICHOKES, FRENCH.														
FRENCH BEAN														
boiled	4 oz	3	.11	.05	.47	.09	64.2	0	1.0	54.18	.93	48.16	318.2	.55
dried, boiled	1/2 cup													
raw	1/2 cup	7	.49	.2	1.92	.37	366.6	0	4.2	171.12	3.13	172.96	1210.72	1.75
FROG'S LEGS , raw	100 gm	0	.14	.25	1.2	na	na	na	0.0	18.0	1.5	na	285.0	na
FROGFISH. See MONKFISH.														
FRUIT. See individual listings.														
FRUIT, MIXED														
Frozen														
(Birds Eye) in syrup 'Quick Thaw pouch'	5 oz	na	na	na	na	na	na	na	na	na	na	na	160	na
FRUIT BAR, FROZEN. See ICE BARS AND DESSERTS; SHERBET; SORBET.														
FRUIT COCKTAIL, CANNED														
in extra heavy syrup, solid and liquid	1/2 cup	261	.02	.02	.48	.06	3.4	0	2.5	7.8	.36	6.5	111.8	.1
in extra light syrup, solid and liquid	1/2 cup	287	.04	.01	.62	.06	3.3	0	3.7	9.84	.37	7.38	127.92	.1
in heavy syrup, solid and liquid	1/2 cup	262	.02	.02	.48	.06	3.3	0	2.4	7.68	.37	6.4	112.64	.1
in juice, solid and liquid	1/2 cup	378	.01	.02	.5	.06	3.1	0	3.4	9.92	.26	8.68	117.8	.11
in light syrup, solid and liquid	1/2 cup	262	.02	.02	.48	.06	3.4	0	2.4	7.56	.37	6.3	112.14	.11
in water, solid and liquid	1/2 cup	305	.02	.01	.44	.06	3.3	0	2.6	6.1	.31	8.54	114.68	.11
FRUIT DRINK														
(Hi-C) 'Double Fruit Cooler'	6 oz	na	na	na	na	na	na	na	60.0	na	na	na	20	na
(Hi-C) 'Double Fruit Cooler' aseptic box	6 oz	na	na	na	na	na	na	na	60.0	na	na	na	20	na
(Hi-C) 'Ecto Cooler'	6 oz	na	na	na	na	na	na	na	60.0	na	na	na	105	na
(Hi-C) 'Ecto Cooler' aseptic box	6 oz	na	na	na	na	na	na	na	60.0	na	na	na	105	na
(Hi-C) 'Hula Cooler'	6 oz	na	na	na	na	na	na	na	60.0	na	na	na	35	na
FRUIT JUICE														
(Juicy Juice) bottled	6 oz	na	na	na	na	na	na	na	na	na	na	na	130	na
(Juicy Juice) boxed	8.45 oz	na	na	na	na	na	na	na	na	na	na	na	180	na
FRUIT JUICE DRINK														
mixed 'Fruit Box' *(Tang)*	8.45 oz	na	na	na	na	na	na	na	na	na	na	na	30	na
FRUIT JUICE PUNCH DRINK														
frozen, concentrate, prepared w/water	1 cup	15	0	.16	.15	.03	0.0	0	13.9	17.36	.57	9.92	190.96	.55
frozen, concentrate, prepared w/water	1 oz	2	0	.02	.02	0	0.0	0	1.7	2.17	.07	1.24	23.87	.07
FRUIT PUNCH														
(Bright & Early) frozen 'Bright & Early Fruit Punch' prepared	6 oz	na	na	na	na	na	na	na	60.0	na	na	na	0	na
(Juicy Juice) can, bottle, or box	6 oz	na	na	na	na	na	na	na	na	na	na	na	130	na
(Minute Maid) aseptic box, canned, or chilled	6 oz	na	na	na	na	na	na	na	1.0	na	na	na	25	na
(Minute Maid) frozen, concentrate, prepared	6 oz	na	na	na	na	na	na	na	1.0	na	na	na	25	na

Food Name	Serving Size	A I.U.	Thi mg	Rib mg	Nia mg	B₆ mg	Fol mcg	B₁₂ mcg	C mg	Calc mg	Iron mg	Mag mg	Pot mg	Zn mg
FRUIT PUNCH DRINK														
(All Sport) thirst quencher, caffeine-free	8 oz	na	na	na	na	na	na	na	na	na	na	na	55	na
(J. Hungerford) 20% juice	9.03 oz	na	na	na	na	na	na	na	0.0	.41	.02	na	na	na
(J. Hungerford) 50% juice	9.03 oz	na	na	na	na	na	na	na	100.0	1.0	1.7	na	na	na
(J. Hungerford) 100% juice	9.03 oz	na	na	na	na	na	na	na	100.0	1.6	3.1	na	na	na
(PowerAde) thirst quencher, high energy ...	8 oz	na	na	na	na	na	na	na	na	na	na	na	30	na
(10-K)	8 oz	na	na	na	na	na	na	na	na	5	0	na	30	na
FRUIT PUNCH DRINK MIX														
frozen concentrate, prepared	12 oz	163	.14	.19	.31	.09	13.8	0	650.4	33.44	1.25	25.08	183.92	.29
frozen, prepared w/water	1 cup	27	.02	.03	.05	.01	2.2	0	108.4	9.88	.22	4.94	32.11	.1
frozen, prepared w/water	1 oz	3	0	0	.01	0	0.3	0	13.6	1.24	.03	.62	4.02	.01
powder, w/added sodium, dry	2 rounded tbsp	1	0	.01	0	0	0.2	0	31.0	36.07	.13	.25	1.27	.03
powder, w/o added sodium, dry	2 rounded tbsp	1	0	.01	0	0	0.2	0	31.0	36.07	.13	.25	1.27	.03
sugar-free, prepared (Crystal Light)	8 oz	na	na	na	na	na	na	na	na	na	na	na	45	na
sugar-free, w/NutraSweet, prepared (Crystal Light)	8 oz	na	na	na	na	na	na	na	na	na	na	na	45	na

FRUIT SALAD, CANNED. See FRUIT COCKTAIL, CANNED.
FUKI. See BUTTERBUR.

G

Food Name	Serving Size	A I.U.	Thi mg	Rib mg	Nia mg	B₆ mg	Fol mcg	B₁₂ mcg	C mg	Calc mg	Iron mg	Mag mg	Pot mg	Zn mg
GARBANZO BEAN / ceci / chick pea														
boiled	1/2 cup	22	.1	.05	.43	.11	141.0	0	1.1	40.18	2.37	39.36	238.62	1.25
raw	1/2 cup	67	.48	.21	1.54	.53	556.6	0	4.0	105.0	6.24	115.0	875.0	3.43
Canned														
(Eden Foods) organic, very low sodium, no salt added	1/2 cup	na	na	na	na	na	na	na	na	na	na	na	220	na
(Eden Foods) organic, w/liquid	1/2 cup	na	na	na	na	na	na	na	na	na	na	na	150	na
GARLIC POWDER														
dry	1 tbsp	0	.04	.01	.06	na	na	0	na	6.68	.23	4.9	92.5	.22
dry	1 tsp	0	.01	0	.02	na	na	0	na	2.23	.08	1.63	30.84	.07
dry (Durkee)	1 tsp	na	.53	.06	0	na	na	na	na	0	0	na	0	na
dry (Laurel Leaf)	1 tsp	na	.53	.06	0	na	na	na	na	0	0	na	0	na
GARLIC SEASONING														
(Gilroy) crushed	1 tsp	na	na	na	na	na	na	na	na	na	na	na	26	na
(Gilroy) minced	1 tsp	na	na	na	na	na	na	na	na	na	na	na	27	na
GATORADE. See individual flavors.														
GELATIN DESSERT														
PREPARED FROM MIX														
(D-Zerta)														
all flavors	1/2 cup	na	na	na	na	na	na	na	na	na	na	na	50	na
all flavors, low calorie, w/aspartame	1/2 cup	na	na	na	na	na	na	na	na	na	na	na	50	na
(Jell-O)														
berry blue	1/2 cup	na	na	na	na	na	na	na	na	na	na	na	0	na
black raspberry	1/2 cup	na	na	na	na	na	na	na	na	na	na	na	0	na
cherry	1/2 cup	na	na	na	na	na	na	na	na	na	na	na	0	na
cherry, sugar-free	1/2 cup	na	na	na	na	na	na	na	na	na	na	na	0	na
concord grape	1/2 cup	na	na	na	na	na	na	na	na	na	na	na	0	na
lemon	1/2 cup	na	na	na	na	na	na	na	na	na	na	na	0	na
lemon, sugar-free	1/2 cup	na	na	na	na	na	na	na	na	na	na	na	0	na
lime	1/2 cup	na	na	na	na	na	na	na	na	na	na	na	0	na
lime, sugar-free	1/2 cup	na	na	na	na	na	na	na	na	na	na	na	0	na
orange, sugar-free	1/2 cup	na	na	na	na	na	na	na	na	na	na	na	0	na

Food Name	Serving Size	A I.U.	Thi mg	Rib mg	Nia mg	B₆ mg	Fol mcg	B₁₂ mcg	C mg	Calc mg	Iron mg	Mag mg	Pot mg	Zn mg
orange-pineapple	1/2 cup	na	na	na	na	na	na	na	na	na	na	na	0	na
raspberry, sugar-free	1/2 cup	na	na	na	na	na	na	na	na	na	na	na	0	na
strawberry, sugar-free	1/2 cup	na	na	na	na	na	na	na	na	na	na	na	0	na
strawberry banana, sugar-free	1/2 cup	na	na	na	na	na	na	na	na	na	na	na	0	na
watermelon	1/2 cup	na	na	na	na	na	na	na	na	na	na	na	0	na
wild strawberry	1/2 cup	na	na	na	na	na	na	na	na	na	na	na	0	na
(Royal)														
apple	1/2 cup	na	na	na	na	na	na	na	na	na	na	na	0	na
blackberry	1/2 cup	na	na	na	na	na	na	na	na	na	na	na	0	na
cherry	1/2 cup	na	na	na	na	na	na	na	na	na	na	na	0	na
cherry, sugar-free	1/2 cup	na	na	na	na	na	na	na	na	na	na	na	0	na
concord grape	1/2 cup	na	na	na	na	na	na	na	na	na	na	na	0	na
fruit punch	1/2 cup	na	na	na	na	na	na	na	na	na	na	na	0	na
lemon	1/2 cup	na	na	na	na	na	na	na	na	na	na	na	0	na
lemon-lime	1/2 cup	na	na	na	na	na	na	na	na	na	na	na	0	na
lime	1/2 cup	na	na	na	na	na	na	na	na	na	na	na	0	na
lime, sugar-free	1/2 cup	na	na	na	na	na	na	na	na	na	na	na	0	na
mixed berry	1/2 cup	na	na	na	na	na	na	na	na	na	na	na	0	na
orange	1/2 cup	na	na	na	na	na	na	na	na	na	na	na	0	na
orange, sugar-free	1/2 cup	na	na	na	na	na	na	na	na	na	na	na	0	na
peach	1/2 cup	na	na	na	na	na	na	na	na	na	na	na	0	na
pineapple	1/2 cup	na	na	na	na	na	na	na	na	na	na	na	0	na
raspberry	1/2 cup	na	na	na	na	na	na	na	na	na	na	na	0	na
raspberry, sugar-free	1/2 cup	na	na	na	na	na	na	na	na	na	na	na	0	na
strawberry	1/2 cup	na	na	na	na	na	na	na	na	na	na	na	0	na
strawberry, sugar-free	1/2 cup	na	na	na	na	na	na	na	na	na	na	na	0	na
strawberry banana	1/2 cup	na	na	na	na	na	na	na	na	na	na	na	0	na
strawberry banana, sugar-free	1/2 cup	na	na	na	na	na	na	na	na	na	na	na	0	na
strawberry orange	1/2 cup	na	na	na	na	na	na	na	na	na	na	na	0	na
tropical fruit	1/2 cup	na	na	na	na	na	na	na	na	na	na	na	0	na
GERMAN SAUSAGE. See individual listings.														
GIN. See ALCOHOLIC BEVERAGES.														
GINGER														
ground	1 tbsp	8	0	.01	.28	na	na	0	na	6.26	.62	9.94	72.49	.25
ground	1 tsp	3	0	0	.09	na	na	0	na	2.09	.21	3.31	24.16	.08
ground *(Durkee)*	1 tsp	.05	.02	.04	0	na	na	na	na	0	0	na	0	na
ground *(Laurel Leaf)*	1 tsp	.05	.02	.04	0	na	na	na	na	0	0	na	0	na
GINGER ROOT														
candied, crystallized	1 lb	454	.91	1.82	31.78	na	na	na	181.6	1044.2	95.34	na	11985.6	na
candied, crystallized	1 oz	28	.06	.11	1.96	na	na	na	11.2	64.4	5.88	na	739.2	na
raw, slices, 1-inch diam	1/4 cup	0	.01	.01	.17	.04	2.7	0	1.2	4.32	.12	10.32	99.6	.08
raw, slices, 1-inch diam	5 slices	0	0	0	.08	.02	1.2	0	0.6	1.98	.06	4.73	45.65	.04
GINKGO NUT														
canned	1 cup	522	.21	.08	5.62	.31	50.7	0	14.1	6.2	.45	24.8	279.0	.33
canned, approx 9 large, 14 medium, or 22 small kernels	1 oz	96	.04	.02	1.03	.06	9.3	0	2.6	1.14	.08	4.54	51.12	.06
dried	1 oz	310	.12	.05	3.33	.18	30.0	0	8.3	5.68	.45	15.05	283.43	.19
raw	1 oz	158	.06	.03	1.7	.09	15.4	0	4.3	.57	.28	7.67	144.84	.1
GLOBE ARTICHOKE. See ARTICHOKES, GLOBE.														
GOA BEAN. See WINGED BEAN.														
GOAT														
raw	1 lb	0	.5	2.22	17.01	na	22.7	5.13	0.0	58.97	12.84	na	1746.36	18.14
raw	1 oz	0	.03	.14	1.05	na	1.4	.32	0.0	3.64	.79	na	107.8	1.12
GOBO. See BURDOCK ROOT.														
GOOSE FAT	1 tbsp	0	0	0	0	0	0.0	0	0.0	0	0	0	0	0
GOOSE GIBLETS, raw	100 gm	4530	.16	1.36	4.9	na	na	na	0.0	14.0	4.5	na	172.0	na

Food Name	Serving Size	A I.U.	Thi mg	Rib mg	Nia mg	B₆ mg	Fol mcg	B₁₂ mcg	C mg	Calc mg	Iron mg	Mag mg	Pot mg	Zn mg
GOOSE GIZZARD, raw	100 gm	0	.02	.2	4.5	na	na	na	0.0	10.0	2.9	na	240.0	na
GOOSE LIVER, raw	1 lb	3410	.06	.1	.72	.08	81.2	5.94	0.5	4.73	3.36	2.64	25.3	.34
GOOSEBERRY, whole	1 cup	435	.06	.05	.45	.12	na	0	41.6	37.5	.47	15.0	297.0	.18
GOOSEFISH. See MONKFISH.														
GOURD, DISHCLOTH / loofah gourd / rag gourd / sponge gourd / towel gourd / vegetable sponge														
boiled, drained, 1-inch slices	1/2 cup	231	.04	.04	.23	.09	10.7	0	5.1	8.01	.32	17.8	403.17	.15
raw, approx 8.6 oz	1 med	730	.09	.11	.71	.08	11.9	0	21.4	35.6	.64	24.92	247.42	.12
raw, 1-inch slices	1 cup	390	.05	.06	.38	.04	6.4	0	11.4	19.0	.34	13.3	132.05	.07
GOURD, SPONGE. See GOURD, DISHCLOTH.														
GOURD, RAG. See GOURD, DISHCLOTH.														
GOURD, WAX														
boiled, drained, cubes	1/2 cup	0	.03	0	.33	.03	3.2	0	9.1	15.66	.33	8.7	4.35	.51
raw, cubes	1 cup	0	.05	.15	.53	.05	6.9	0	17.2	25.08	.53	13.2	7.92	.81
GOURD, WHITE / tunka														
boiled, drained, cubes	1/2 cup	0	.03	0	.33	.03	3.2	0	9.1	15.66	.33	8.7	4.35	.51
raw, cubes	1 cup	0	.05	.15	.53	.05	6.9	0	17.2	25.08	.53	13.2	7.92	.81
GRANOLA. See CEREAL, READY-TO-SERVE.														
GRANOLA AND CEREAL BAR. See also GRANOLA SNACKS.														
(Bear Valley)														
carob-cocoa, food bar 'Pemmican' 3.75 oz	1 bar	na	na	na	na	na	na	na	na	na	na	na	720	na
coconut almond, food bar														
'Meal Pack' 3.75 oz	1 bar	na	na	na	na	na	na	na	na	na	na	na	650	na
sesame lemon, food bar 'Meal Pack' 3.75 oz	1 bar	na	na	na	na	na	na	na	na	na	na	na	650	na
fruit 'n nut, food bar 'Pemmican' 3.75 oz	1 bar	na	na	na	na	na	na	na	na	na	na	na	720	na
(Golden Temple)														
cashew almond 'Wha Guru Chew Bar'	1 bar	0	.14	.06	.51	na	na	na	na	22.0	1.0	na	104	na
peanut cashew 'Wha Guru Chew Bar'	1 bar	0	.15	.03	1.42	na	na	na	na	28.0	1.0	na	113	na
sesame almond 'Wha Guru Chew Bar'	1 bar	0	.17	.07	.65	na	na	na	na	56.0	1.0	na	107	na
(Natural Nectar)														
apple-oatmeal spice, 'Fi-Bar A.M.'	1 bar	na	na	na	na	na	na	na	na	na	na	na	190	na
banana nut, 'Fi-Bar A.M.'	1 bar	na	na	na	na	na	na	na	na	na	na	na	190	na
cocoa almond, 'Fi-Bar Chewy & Nutty'	1 bar	na	na	na	na	na	na	na	na	na	na	na	100	na
cocoa almond crunch,														
'Canadian Chewy & Nutty'	1 bar	na	na	na	na	na	na	na	na	na	na	na	100	na
cocoa peanut, 'Fi-Bar Chewy & Nutty'	1 bar	na	na	na	na	na	na	na	na	na	na	na	100	na
cocoa peanut butter crunch, 'Chewy & Nutty'	1 bar	na	na	na	na	na	na	na	na	na	na	na	85	na
coconut	1 bar	na	na	na	na	na	na	na	na	na	na	na	100	na
cranberry, w/wild berries 'Original Fruit Bar'	1 bar	na	na	na	na	na	na	na	na	na	na	na	125	na
peanut butter	1 bar	na	na	na	na	na	na	na	na	na	na	na	100	na
raisin nut bran, 'Fi-Bar A.M.'	1 bar	na	na	na	na	na	na	na	na	na	na	na	130	na
raspberry 'Canadian'	1 bar	na	na	na	na	na	na	na	na	na	na	na	130	na
raspberry 'Original Fruit Bar'	1 bar	na	na	na	na	na	na	na	na	na	na	na	130	na
strawberry 'Canadian'	1 bar	na	na	na	na	na	na	na	na	na	na	na	130	na
strawberry 'Original Fruit Bar'	1 bar	na	na	na	na	na	na	na	na	na	na	na	125	na
strawberry-oatmeal w/almonds, 'Fi-Bar A.M.'	1 bar	na	na	na	na	na	na	na	na	na	na	na	190	na
vanilla almond, 'Fi-Bar Chewy & Nutty'	1 bar	na	na	na	na	na	na	na	na	na	na	na	100	na
vanilla almond crunch,														
'Canadian Chewy & Nutty'	1 bar	na	na	na	na	na	na	na	na	na	na	na	100	na
vanilla peanut, 'Fi-Bar Chewy & Nutty'	1 bar	na	na	na	na	na	na	na	na	na	na	na	100	na
wild cranberry 'Canadian'	1 bar	na	na	na	na	na	na	na	na	na	na	na	130	na
GRANOLA SNACKS. See also GRANOLA AND CEREAL BAR.														
(Nature Valley) apple-cinnamon 'Granola Bites'	1 pkg	na	na	na	na	na	na	na	na	na	na	na	75	na
GRAPE														
AMERICAN (Concord, Delaware, Niagara)														
Slipskin														
trimmed	10 fruits	24	.02	.01	.07	.03	0.9	0	1.0	3.36	.07	1.2	45.84	.01
untrimmed	1 cup	92	.08	.05	.28	.1	3.6	0	3.7	12.88	.27	4.6	175.72	.04

Food Name	Serving Size	A III	Thi mg	Rib mg	Nia mg	B6 mg	Fol mcg	B12 mcg	C mg	Calc mg	Iron mg	Mag mg	Pot mg	Zn mg
EUROPEAN (Muskat, Tokay, Thompson)														
Adherent skin														
trimmed	10 fruits	37	.05	.03	.15	.06	2.0	0	5.4	5.5	.13	3.0	92.5	.02
untrimmed	1 cup	117	.15	.09	.48	.18	6.2	0	17.3	17.6	.42	9.6	296.0	.08
GRAPE, CANNED														
THOMPSON, seedless, in water	1 cup	162	.08	.06	.32	.16	6.4	0	2.5	24.5	2.4	14.7	262.15	.12
GRAPE DRINK														
Can, bottle, or box														
(All Sport) thirst quencher, caffeine-free	8 oz	na	na	na	na	na	na	na	na	na	na	na	55	na
(Bright & Early) frozen, diluted	6 oz	na	na	na	na	na	na	na	60.0	na	na	na	0	na
(J. Hungerford)	9.03 oz	0	na	na	na	na	na	na	0.7	0	0	na	na	na
(Kool-Aid) 'Koolers'	8.45 oz	na	na	na	na	na	na	na	na	na	na	na	30	na
(10-K) 'Clear'	8 oz	na	na	na	na	na	na	na	na	5	0	na	30	na
Prepared from mix														
(Kool-Aid) sugar-sweetened	8 oz	na	na	na	na	na	na	na	na	na	na	na	0	na
(Kool-Aid) unsweetened, prepared w/sugar	8 oz	na	na	na	na	na	na	na	na	na	na	na	0	na
(Kool-Aid) unsweetened, prepared w/o sugar	8 oz	na	na	na	na	na	na	na	na	na	na	na	0	na
(Kool-Aid) w/NutraSweet	8 oz	na	na	na	na	na	na	na	na	na	na	na	0	na
GRAPE JUICE														
Can, bottle, or box														
(J. Hungerford)	9.03 oz	na	na	na	na	na	na	na	100.0	.4	.7	na	na	na
(J. Hungerford) 100% juice	9.03 oz	na	na	na	na	na	na	na	100.0	1.3	2.9	na	na	na
(J. Hungerford) 50% juice	9.03 oz	na	na	na	na	na	na	na	100.0	.5	.8	na	na	na
(J. Hungerford) 20% juice	9.03 oz	na	na	na	na	na	na	na	0.7	0	0	na	na	na
(Juicy Juice) bottled	6 oz	na	na	na	na	na	na	na	na	na	na	na	122	na
(Juicy Juice) boxed	8.45 oz	na	na	na	na	na	na	na	na	na	na	na	180	na
Frozen, diluted as directed														
(Minute Maid)	6 oz	na	na	na	na	na	na	na	5.0	na	na	na	125	na
GRAPE JUICE DRINK (Tang) 'Fruit Box'	8.45 oz	na	na	na	na	na	na	na	na	na	na	na	40	na
GRAPE PUNCH														
(Minute Maid) chilled	6 oz	na	na	na	na	na	na	na	1.0	na	na	na	40	na
(Minute Maid) frozen concentrate	6 oz	na	na	na	na	na	na	na	1.0	na	na	na	40	na
GRAPEFRUIT														
PINK AND RED														
Arizona/California														
fresh, 3.75 inch diam	1/2 fruit	319	.04	.02	.23	.05	15.0	0	46.9	13.53	.1	11.07	180.81	.09
sections w/juice	1 cup	596	.08	.05	.44	.1	28.1	0	87.6	25.3	.18	20.7	338.1	.16
Florida														
fresh (Ocean Spray)	1/2 med	na	na	na	na	na	na	na	70.0	na	na	na	166	na
fresh, 3.75 inch diam	1/2 fruit	319	.05	.02	.25	.05	11.6	0	45.5	18.45	.15	9.84	156.21	.09
sections w/juice	1 cup	596	.09	.05	.46	.1	21.6	0	85.1	34.5	.28	18.4	292.1	.16
WHITE														
California														
fresh, 3.75 inch diam	1/2 fruit	12	.04	.02	.32	.05	13.9	0	39.3	14.16	.09	10.62	168.74	.08
sections w/juice	1 cup	23	.09	.05	.62	.1	27.1	0	76.6	27.6	.18	20.7	328.9	.16
Florida														
fresh (Ocean Spray)	1/2 med	na	na	na	na	na	na	na	70.0	na	na	na	159	na
fresh, 3.75 inch diam	1/2 fruit	12	.05	.02	.24	.05	11.1	0	43.7	17.7	.06	10.62	177.0	.08
sections w/juice	1 cup	23	.09	.05	.46	.1	21.6	0	85.1	34.5	.11	20.7	345.0	.16
GRAPEFRUIT JUICE														
Can, bottle, or box														
(J. Hungerford) 100% juice	9.03 oz	na	na	na	na	na	na	na	100.0	1.4	2.2	na	na	na
(J. Hungerford) 50% juice	9.03 oz	na	na	na	na	na	na	na	100.0	.9	.9	na	na	na
(Libby's)	6 oz	na	na	na	na	na	na	na	na	na	na	na	280	na
(Minute Maid)	6 oz	na	na	na	na	na	na	na	60.0	na	na	na	240	na

Food Name	Serving Size	A I.U.	Thi mg	Rib mg	Nia mg	B$_6$ mg	Fol mcg	B$_{12}$ mcg	C mg	Calc mg	Iron mg	Mag mg	Pot mg	Zn mg
(Minute Maid) 'Juices to Go'	6 oz	na	na	na	na	na	na	na	60.0	na	na	na	240	na
(Ocean Spray) 100%	6 oz	na	na	na	na	na	na	na	100.0	na	na	na	150	na
(Ocean Spray) 'Ruby Red'	6 oz	na	na	na	na	na	na	na	100.0	na	2	na	55	na
Fresh														
pink	1 cup	1087	.1	.05	.49	.11	25.2	0	93.9	22.23	.49	29.64	400.14	.12
white	1 cup	25	.1	.05	.49	.11	25.2	0	93.9	22.23	.49	29.64	400.14	.12
GRAPEFRUIT JUICE COCKTAIL														
(Minute Maid) 'Juices To Go'	6 oz	na	na	na	na	na	na	na	30.0	na	na	na	115	na
(Ocean Spray)	6 oz	na	na	na	na	na	na	na	100.0	na	na	na	90	na
GRAPESEED OIL														
	1 cup	0	0	0	0	0	0.0	0	0.0	0	0	0	0	0
	1 tbsp	0	0	0	0	0	0.0	0	0.0	0	0	0	0	0
GRAVY. See also SAUCE.														
AU JUS														
Canned or in jars *(Heinz)* 'HomeStyle'	1/4 cup	na	na	na	na	na	na	na	na	na	na	na	20	na
BROWN														
Canned or in jars														
(Heinz) 'HomeStyle'	1/4 cup	na	na	na	na	na	na	na	na	na	na	na	10	na
(Heinz) 'HomeStyle' w/onions	1/4 cup	na	na	na	na	na	na	na	na	na	na	na	25	na
CHICKEN														
Canned or in jars														
(Heinz) 'HomeStyle'	1/4 cup	na	na	na	na	na	na	na	na	na	na	na	40	na
(Heinz) 'Homestyle'														
w/mushrooms and onions	1/4 cup	na	na	na	na	na	na	na	na	na	na	na	na	na
MUSHROOM														
Canned or in jars *(Heinz)* 'HomeStyle'	1/4 cup	na	na	na	na	na	na	na	na	na	na	na	25	na
PORK, Canned or in jars *(Heinz)* 'HomeStyle'	1/4 cup	na	na	na	na	na	na	na	na	na	na	na	10	na
TURKEY, Canned or in jars *(Heinz)* 'HomeStyle'	1/4 cup	na	na	na	na	na	na	na	na	na	na	na	30	na
GREAT NORTHERN BEAN														
boiled, mature seeds	1/2 cup	1	.14	.05	.6	.1	89.9	0	1.1	59.84	1.87	44.0	344.08	.77
raw	1/2 cup	3	.59	.22	1.78	.41	438.6	0	4.8	159.25	4.98	171.99	1262.17	2.1
Canned														
(Eden Foods) organically grown, w/liquid	1/2 cup	na	na	na	na	na	na	na	na	na	na	na	310	na
GREEN BEAN, CANNED														
Cut														
(Freshlike)	1/2 cup	na	na	na	na	na	na	na	na	na	na	na	120	na
(Freshlike) no sugar or salt, in water	1/2 cup	na	na	na	na	na	na	na	na	na	na	na	120	na
(Freshlike) wax, water packed, w/o salt	1/2 cup	na	na	na	na	na	na	na	na	na	na	na	115	na
(Freshlike) wax, water packed, w/o sugar														
or salt	1/2 cup	na	na	na	na	na	na	na	na	na	na	na	115	na
(Veg•All)	1/2 cup	na	Thi	Rib	na	na	na	na	na	na	na	na	120	na
French style														
(Freshlike)	1/2 cup	na	na	na	na	na	na	na	na	na	na	na	120	na
(Freshlike) in water, w/o salt	1/2 cup	na	na	na	na	na	na	na	na	na	na	na	120	na
(Veg•All)	1/2 cup	na	na	na	na	na	na	na	na	na	na	na	120	na
Whole *(Freshlike)*	1/2 cup	na	na	na	na	na	na	na	na	na	na	na	120	na
GREEN BEAN, FROZEN														
Cut														
(Birds Eye)	3 oz	na	na	na	na	na	na	na	na	na	na	na	130	na
(Freshlike)	3 oz	na	na	na	na	na	na	na	na	na	na	na	125	na
French style														
(Birds Eye)	3 oz	na	na	na	na	na	na	na	na	na	na	na	140	na
(Freshlike)	3 oz	na	na	na	na	na	na	na	na	na	na	na	150	na
(Veg•All)	3 oz	na	na	na	na	na	na	na	na	na	na	na	120	na
Italian														
(Birds Eye)	3 oz	na	na	na	na	na	na	na	na	na	na	na	180	na
(Freshlike)	3 oz	na	na	na	na	na	na	na	na	na	na	na	220	na

Food Name	Serving Size	A I.U.	Thi mg	Rib mg	Nia mg	B$_6$ mg	Fol mcg	B$_{12}$ mcg	C mg	Calc mg	Iron mg	Mag mg	Pot mg	Zn mg
Whole														
(Birds Eye) 'Deluxe'	3 oz	na	na	na	na	na	na	na	na	na	na	na	150	na
(Bird's Eye) petite 'Deluxe'	2.6 oz	na	na	na	na	na	na	na	na	na	na	na	135	na
(Freshlike)	3 oz	na	na	na	na	na	na	na	na	na	na	na	150	na
GRITS														
Dry														
white, enriched	1 cup	0	1.0	.59	7.74	.23	7.8	0	na	3.12	6.1	42.12	213.72	.64
white, enriched	1 tbsp	0	.06	.04	.48	.01	0.5	0	na	.19	.38	2.62	13.29	.04
white, enriched 'Regular/Quick'														
(Aunt Jemima)	3 tbsp	0	.12	.07	1.0	.03	3.0	0	0.0	1	.81	6	39	0
white, unenriched	1 cup	0	.2	.06	1.87	.23	7.8	0	na	3.12	1.56	42.12	213.72	.64
white, unenriched	1 tbsp	0	.01	0	.12	.01	0.5	0	na	.19	.1	2.62	13.29	.04
yellow, enriched	1 cup	686	1.0	.59	7.74	.23	7.8	0	na	3.12	6.1	42.12	213.72	.64
yellow, enriched	1 tbsp	43	.06	.04	.48	.01	0.5	0	na	.19	.38	2.62	13.29	.04
yellow, unenriched	1 cup	686	.2	.06	1.87	.23	7.8	0	na	3.12	1.56	42.12	213.72	.64
yellow, unenriched	1 tbsp	43	.01	0	.12	.01	0.5	0	na	.19	.1	2.62	13.29	.04
Prepared														
white, enriched, cooked w/water	1 cup	0	.24	.15	1.96	.06	2.4	0	na	0	1.55	9.68	53.24	.17
white, unenriched, cooked w/water	1 cup	0	.05	.02	.48	.06	2.4	0	na	0	.48	9.68	53.24	.17
yellow, enriched, cooked w/water	1 cup	145	.24	.15	1.96	.06	2.4	0	na	0	1.55	9.68	53.24	.17
yellow, unenriched, cooked w/water	1 cup	145	.05	.02	.48	.06	2.4	0	na	0	.48	9.68	53.24	.17
GRITS, CANNED														
white	1 cup	0	0	.01	.05	.01	1.6	0	0.0	16.0	.99	25.6	14.4	1.68
yellow	1 cup	176	0	.01	.05	.01	1.6	0	0.0	16.0	.99	25.6	14.4	1.68
GRITS, INSTANT														
white, hominy product, dry, one packet														
(Quaker)	.8 oz	0	.12	.07	1.0	.05	2.0	0	0.0	7	8.1	5	28	0
w/imitation bacon bits, dry, one packet														
(Quaker)	1 oz	0	.12	.07	1.0	.05	2.0	0	0.0	7	8.1	9	62	0
w/imitation ham bits, dry, one packet														
(Quaker)	1 oz	0	.12	.07	1.0	.06	1.0	0	0.0	7	8.1	9	56	0
w/real cheddar cheese flavor, dry, one packet														
(Quaker)	1 oz	400	.12	.07	1.0	.07	10.0	0	0.0	14	8.1	10	40	0
GRITS, QUICK-COOKING														
Dry														
white, enriched	1 cup	0	1.0	.59	7.74	.23	7.8	0	na	3.12	6.1	na	213.72	.64
white, enriched	1 tbsp	0	.06	.04	.48	.01	0.5	0	na	.19	.38	na	13.29	.04
white, unenriched	1 cup	0	.2	.06	1.87	.23	7.8	0	na	3.12	1.56	42.12	213.72	.64
white, unenriched	1 tbsp	0	.01	0	.12	.01	0.5	0	na	.19	.1	2.62	13.29	.04
yellow, enriched	1 cup	686	1.0	.59	7.74	.23	7.8	0	na	3.12	6.1	42.12	213.72	.64
yellow, enriched	1 tbsp	43	.06	.04	.48	.01	0.5	0	na	.19	.38	2.62	13.29	.04
yellow, enriched 'Quick' (Quaker)	3 tbsp	0	.12	.07	1.0	.05	3.0	0	0.0	1	.81	6	30	0
yellow, unenriched	1 cup	686	.2	.06	1.87	.23	7.8	0	na	3.12	1.56	42.12	213.72	.64
yellow, unenriched	1 tbsp	43	.01	0	.12	.01	0.5	0	na	.19	.1	2.62	13.29	.04
Prepared														
white, enriched, cooked w/water	1 cup	0	.24	.15	1.96	.06	2.4	0	na	0	1.55	9.68	53.24	.17
white, unenriched, cooked w/water	1 cup	0	.05	.02	.48	.06	2.4	0	na	0	.48	9.68	53.24	.17
yellow, enriched, cooked w/water	1 cup	145	.24	.15	1.96	.06	2.4	0	na	0	1.55	9.68	53.24	.17
yellow, unenriched, cooked w/water	1 cup	145	.05	.02	.48	.06	2.4	0	na	0	.48	9.68	53.24	.17
GROUND CHERRY. See CAPE GOOSEBERRY.														
GROUND HUSK TOMATO. See TOMATILLO.														
GROUPER, MIXED SPECIES														
dry-heat cooked	3 oz	140	.07	.01	.32	.3	8.7	.59	0.0	17.85	.97	31.45	403.75	.43
raw	3 oz	122	.06	0	.27	.26	7.5	.51	0.0	22.95	.76	26.35	410.55	.41
GUANABANA NECTAR (Libby's)	6 oz	na	na	na	na	na	na	na	na	na	na	na	75	na
GUAVA														
trimmed	1 cup	1307	.08	.08	1.98	.24	na	0	302.8	33.0	.51	16.5	468.6	.38

Food Name	Serving Size	A I.U.	Thi mg	Rib mg	Nia mg	B$_6$ mg	Fol mcg	B$_{12}$ mcg	C mg	Calc mg	Iron mg	Mag mg	Pot mg	Zn mg
trimmed	1 fruit	713	.04	.04	1.08	.13	na	0	165.2	18.0	.28	9.0	255.6	.21
GUAVA, STRAWBERRY														
trimmed	1 cup	220	.07	.07	1.46	na	na	0	90.3	51.24	.54	41.48	712.48	na
trimmed	1 fruit	5	0	0	.04	na	na	0	2.2	1.26	.01	1.02	17.52	na
GUAVA FRUIT DRINK														
Hawaiian 'Mauna La'i' (Ocean Spray)	6 oz	na	na	na	na	na	na	na	100.0	na	na	na	30	na
GUAVA NECTAR														
(Kern's)	6 oz	na	na	na	na	na	na	na	na	na	na	na	60	na
(Libby's)	6 oz	na	na	na	na	na	na	na	na	na	na	na	70	na
GUAVA PASSION DRINK														
Hawaiian 'Mauna La'i' (Ocean Spray)	6 oz	45	na	na	na	na	na	na	100.0	na	na	na	60	na
GUINEA HEN														
giblets, raw	100 gm	4530	.16	1.36	4.9	na	na	na	0.0	14.0	4.5	na	172.0	na
meat and skin, raw	1 lb	330	.21	.37	27.52	1.36	18.0	1.22	4.7	39.49	3.02	78.98	692.87	4.06

GUMBO. See OKRA.

H

Food Name	Serving Size	A I.U.	Thi mg	Rib mg	Nia mg	B$_6$ mg	Fol mcg	B$_{12}$ mcg	C mg	Calc mg	Iron mg	Mag mg	Pot mg	Zn mg
HADDOCK														
dry-heat cooked	3 oz	54	.03	.04	3.94	.29	11.3	1.18	0.0	35.7	1.15	42.5	339.15	.41
raw	3 oz	47	.03	.03	3.23	.26	9.8	1.02	0.0	28.05	.89	33.15	264.35	.31
smoked	3 oz	62	.04	.04	4.31	.34	13.0	1.36	0.0	41.65	1.19	45.9	352.75	.43
HALIBUT														
ATLANTIC														
dry-heat cooked	3 oz	152	.06	.08	6.05	.34	11.7	1.16	0.0	51.0	.91	90.95	489.6	.45
raw	3 oz	132	.05	.06	4.97	.29	10.2	1.01	0.0	39.95	.71	70.55	382.5	.36
GREENLAND														
dry-heat cooked	3 oz	51	.06	.09	1.63	.41	0.9	.82	0.0	3.4	.72	28.05	292.4	.43
raw	3 oz	47	.05	.07	1.27	.36	0.9	.85	0.0	2.55	.56	22.1	227.8	.34
PACIFIC														
dry-heat cooked	3 oz	152	.06	.08	6.05	.34	11.7	1.16	0.0	51.0	.91	90.95	489.6	.45
raw	3 oz	132	.05	.06	4.97	.29	10.2	1.01	0.0	39.95	.71	70.55	382.5	.36
HAM. See HAM, CANNED; HAM, CURED; HAM, FRESH; HAM PATTY.														
HAM, CANNED														
chopped	1 oz	0	.15	.05	.91	.09	0.3	.2	0.5	1.98	.27	3.69	80.51	.52
cured, extra lean, approx 4% fat, baked	3 oz	0	.88	.21	4.16	.38	4.3	.6	23.4	5.1	.78	17.85	295.8	1.9
cured, extra lean, approx 4% fat, unheated	1 oz	0	.24	.07	1.5	.13	1.7	.23	7.6	1.7	.27	4.82	103.19	.55
cured, extra lean and regular, baked	3 oz	0	.82	.21	4.28	.34	4.3	.71	19.5	5.95	.91	17.0	298.35	1.97
cured, extra lean and regular, unheated	1 oz	0	.25	.07	1.3	.13	1.7	.23	7.1	1.7	.26	4.54	94.69	.52
cured, regular, approx 13% fat, baked	3 oz	0	.7	.22	4.51	.26	4.3	.9	11.9	6.8	1.16	14.45	303.45	2.13
cured, regular, approx 13% fat, unheated	1 oz	0	.27	.07	.91	.14	1.4	.22	6.2	1.7	.24	3.97	89.59	.47
HAM, CURED														
(NOTE: TRIMMED = Lean, separable fat removed. UNTRIMMED = Separable fat not removed.)														
BONELESS														
center slice, country-style, trimmed, unheated	1 oz	0	.16	.07	1.1	.12	1.4	.25	0.0	2.84	.31	7.09	144.59	.8
center slice, untrimmed, unheated	1 oz	0	.24	.06	1.36	.13	1.1	.23	0.0	1.98	.21	4.54	95.54	.53
extra lean, approx 5% fat, baked	3 oz	0	.64	.17	3.42	.34	2.6	.55	17.9	6.8	1.26	11.9	243.95	2.45
extra lean and regular, baked	3 oz	0	.63	.24	4.53	.3	2.6	.58	18.7	6.8	1.19	16.15	307.7	2.24
extra lean and regular, unheated, 4 x 6 1/4 inch slice	1 slice	0	.25	.07	1.44	.11	0.9	.23	7.7	1.98	.26	5.1	84.2	.58
regular, approx 11% fat, baked	3 oz	0	.62	.28	5.23	.26	2.6	.6	19.3	6.8	1.14	18.7	347.65	2.1
WHOLE														
trimmed, fully cooked, baked	3 oz	0	.58	.22	4.27	.4	3.4	.6	na	5.95	.8	18.7	268.6	2.18

Food Name	Serving Size	A I.U.	Thi mg	Rib mg	Nia mg	B$_6$ mg	Fol mcg	B$_{12}$ mcg	C mg	Calc mg	Iron mg	Mag mg	Pot mg	Zn mg
trimmed, fully cooked, unheated	1 oz	0	.26	.06	1.49	.15	1.1	.25	na	1.98	.23	5.1	105.18	.58
untrimmed, fully cooked, baked	3 oz	0	.51	.19	3.79	.32	2.6	.54	na	5.95	.74	16.15	243.1	1.97
untrimmed, fully cooked, unheated	1 oz	0	.22	.05	1.27	.12	1.1	.21	na	1.98	.2	4.25	87.88	.5

HAM, FRESH. See also PORK.
(NOTE: TRIMMED = Lean; separable fat removed. UNTRIMMED = Separable fat not removed.)

LEG, RUMP HALF
  Trimmed

Food Name	Serving Size	A I.U.	Thi mg	Rib mg	Nia mg	B$_6$ mg	Fol mcg	B$_{12}$ mcg	C mg	Calc mg	Iron mg	Mag mg	Pot mg	Zn mg
raw	1 lb	27	4.87	1.29	22.04	2.1	13.6	3.22	5.9	27.22	3.95	113.4	1705.54	8.89
raw	1 oz	2	.3	.08	1.38	.13	0.9	.2	0.4	1.7	.25	7.09	106.6	.56
roasted	3 oz	8	.68	.3	4.18	.29	2.6	.64	0.2	5.95	.97	24.65	332.35	2.56
roasted, diced	1 cup	12	1.08	.48	6.64	.46	4.1	1.01	0.3	9.45	1.54	39.15	527.85	4.06

  Untrimmed

Food Name	Serving Size	A I.U.	Thi mg	Rib mg	Nia mg	B$_6$ mg	Fol mcg	B$_{12}$ mcg	C mg	Calc mg	Iron mg	Mag mg	Pot mg	Zn mg
raw	1 lb	32	4.22	1.15	19.71	1.78	13.6	2.9	5.0	22.68	3.49	95.26	1510.49	7.94
raw	1 oz	2	.26	.07	1.23	.11	0.9	.18	0.3	1.42	.22	5.95	94.41	.5
roasted	3 oz	8	.64	.28	3.96	.27	2.6	.61	0.2	10.2	.89	22.95	317.9	2.4
roasted, diced	1 cup	12	1.01	.44	6.28	.43	4.1	.97	0.3	16.2	1.42	36.45	504.9	3.81

LEG, SHANK HALF
  Trimmed

Food Name	Serving Size	A I.U.	Thi mg	Rib mg	Nia mg	B$_6$ mg	Fol mcg	B$_{12}$ mcg	C mg	Calc mg	Iron mg	Mag mg	Pot mg	Zn mg
raw	1 lb	27	4.04	1.26	20.89	2.31	22.7	3.13	4.1	31.75	4.26	113.4	1542.24	10.48
raw	1 oz	2	.25	.08	1.31	.14	1.4	.2	0.3	1.98	.27	7.09	96.39	.65
roasted	3 oz	7	.54	.29	4.15	.39	5.1	.6	0.3	5.95	.94	21.25	306.0	2.93
roasted, diced	1 cup	11	.85	.46	6.59	.62	8.1	.96	0.5	9.45	1.5	33.75	486.0	4.66

  Untrimmed

Food Name	Serving Size	A I.U.	Thi mg	Rib mg	Nia mg	B$_6$ mg	Fol mcg	B$_{12}$ mcg	C mg	Calc mg	Iron mg	Mag mg	Pot mg	Zn mg
raw	1 lb	32	3.29	1.06	17.73	1.78	18.1	2.72	3.2	27.22	3.54	86.18	1292.76	8.66
raw	1 oz	2	.21	.07	1.11	.11	1.1	.17	0.2	1.7	.22	5.39	80.8	.54
roasted	3 oz	8	.49	.26	3.79	.34	4.3	.56	0.3	12.75	.83	18.7	287.3	2.6
roasted, diced	1 cup	12	.78	.41	6.02	.54	6.8	.89	0.4	20.25	1.32	29.7	456.3	4.13

LEG, WHOLE
  Trimmed

Food Name	Serving Size	A I.U.	Thi mg	Rib mg	Nia mg	B$_6$ mg	Fol mcg	B$_{12}$ mcg	C mg	Calc mg	Iron mg	Mag mg	Pot mg	Zn mg
raw	1 lb	27	3.97	1.03	24.21	2.27	40.8	3.22	4.1	27.22	4.58	113.4	1673.78	10.3
raw	1 oz	2	.25	.06	1.51	.14	2.6	.2	0.3	1.7	.29	7.09	104.61	.64
roasted	3 oz	8	.59	.3	4.19	.38	10.2	.61	0.3	5.95	.95	21.25	317.05	2.77
roasted	1 cup	12	.93	.47	6.66	.61	16.2	.97	0.5	9.45	1.51	33.75	503.55	4.4

  Untrimmed

Food Name	Serving Size	A I.U.	Thi mg	Rib mg	Nia mg	B$_6$ mg	Fol mcg	B$_{12}$ mcg	C mg	Calc mg	Iron mg	Mag mg	Pot mg	Zn mg
raw	1 lb	32	3.34	.91	20.75	1.82	31.8	2.86	3.2	22.68	3.86	90.72	1428.84	8.75
raw	1 oz	2	.21	.06	1.3	.11	2.0	.18	0.2	1.42	.24	5.67	89.3	.55
roasted	3 oz	9	.54	.27	3.89	.34	8.5	.58	0.3	11.9	.86	18.7	299.2	2.52
roasted, diced	1 cup	14	.86	.42	6.17	.54	13.5	.92	0.4	18.9	1.36	29.7	475.2	4.0

HAM, MINCED

Food Name	Serving Size	A I.U.	Thi mg	Rib mg	Nia mg	B$_6$ mg	Fol mcg	B$_{12}$ mcg	C mg	Calc mg	Iron mg	Mag mg	Pot mg	Zn mg
HAM, MINCED	1 oz	0	.2	.05	1.18	.07	0.3	.27	8.4	2.84	.22	4.54	88.17	.54

HAM ENTRÉE, FROZEN

Food Name	Serving Size	A I.U.	Thi mg	Rib mg	Nia mg	B$_6$ mg	Fol mcg	B$_{12}$ mcg	C mg	Calc mg	Iron mg	Mag mg	Pot mg	Zn mg
and asparagus bake (Stouffer's)	9.5 oz	na	na	na	na	na	na	na	na	na	na	na	360	na

HAM PATTY

Food Name	Serving Size	A I.U.	Thi mg	Rib mg	Nia mg	B$_6$ mg	Fol mcg	B$_{12}$ mcg	C mg	Calc mg	Iron mg	Mag mg	Pot mg	Zn mg
cured, boneless steak, extra lean, unheated	2-oz slice	0	.45	.11	2.88	.21	2.3	.45	18.3	2.27	.57	10.77	184.28	1.15
cured, unheated	1 oz	0	.13	.04	.85	.05	0.9	.31	0.0	2.27	.3	2.84	67.76	.45

HAM SPREAD

Food Name	Serving Size	A I.U.	Thi mg	Rib mg	Nia mg	B$_6$ mg	Fol mcg	B$_{12}$ mcg	C mg	Calc mg	Iron mg	Mag mg	Pot mg	Zn mg
deviled	1 cup	0	.32	.23	3.6	na	na	na	0.0	18.0	1.4	na	499.5	na
deviled	4.5-oz can	0	.18	.13	2.05	na	na	na	0.0	10.24	.79	na	284.16	na
ham and cheese	1 oz	86	.09	.06	.61	.04	0.9	.21	2.0	61.52	.22	5.1	45.93	.64
ham and cheese	1 tbsp	46	.05	.03	.32	.02	0.5	.11	1.1	32.55	.11	2.7	24.3	.34
ham salad	1 oz	0	.12	.03	.59	.04	0.3	.22	1.7	2.27	.17	2.84	42.53	.31
ham salad	1 tbsp	0	.07	.02	.31	.02	0.2	.11	0.9	1.2	.09	1.5	22.5	.17

HAMBURGER. See BEEF, GROUND.
HAMBURGER BUN. See BUN, HAMBURGER.
HAWAIIAN YAM. See YAM, MOUNTAIN.
HAWS/hawthorn tree fruit

Food Name	Serving Size	A I.U.	Thi mg	Rib mg	Nia mg	B$_6$ mg	Fol mcg	B$_{12}$ mcg	C mg	Calc mg	Iron mg	Mag mg	Pot mg	Zn mg
scarlet, flesh and skin, raw	100 gm	0	0	0	0	na	na	na	0.0	0	0	na	0	na

Food Name	Serving Size	A I.U.	Thi mg	Rib mg	Nia mg	B$_6$ mg	Fol mcg	B$_{12}$ mcg	C mg	Calc mg	Iron mg	Mag mg	Pot mg	Zn mg
HAZELNUT OIL														
....	1 cup	0	0	0	0	0	0.0	0	0.0	0	0	0	0	0
....	1 tbsp	0	0	0	0	0	0.0	0	0.0	0	0	0	0	0
HEART NUT. See CASHEW.														
HERRING														
ATLANTIC														
dry-heat cooked	3 oz	87	.1	.25	3.51	.3	9.8	11.17	0.6	62.9	1.2	34.85	356.15	1.08
raw	3 oz	80	.08	.2	2.73	.26	8.5	11.62	0.6	48.45	.94	27.2	277.95	.84
PACIFIC														
dry-heat cooked	3 oz	99	.06	.22	2.4	.44	5.1	8.18	0.0	90.1	1.22	34.85	460.7	.58
raw	3 oz	90	.05	.17	1.87	.38	4.3	8.5	0.0	70.55	.95	27.2	359.55	.45
HICKORY NUT, shelled	1 oz	37	.25	.04	.26	.05	11.4	0	0.6	17.32	.6	49.13	123.82	1.22
HOMINY GRITS. See GRITS.														
HONEY														
extracted	1 cup	0	.02	.14	1.02	na	na	na	3.4	16.95	1.69	na	172.89	na
extracted	1 tbsp	0	0	.01	.06	na	na	na	0.2	1.05	.11	na	10.71	na
strained	1 cup	0	.02	.14	1.02	na	na	na	3.4	16.95	1.69	na	172.89	na
strained	1 tbsp	0	0	.01	.06	na	na	na	0.2	1.05	.11	na	10.71	na
HONEY ROLL SAUSAGE														
....	1 oz	0	.02	.05	1.18	.08	1.1	.67	4.8	2.55	.62	4.54	82.5	.92
4 inch diam	1/8-inch slice	0	.02	.04	.96	.06	0.9	.54	3.9	2.07	.51	3.68	66.93	.75
HONEYDEW MELON														
raw, cubed	1 cup	68	.13	.03	1.02	.1	na	0	42.2	10.2	.12	11.9	460.7	na
raw, wedge	7 x 2 inches	52	.1	.02	.77	.08	na	0	32.0	7.74	.09	9.03	349.59	na
HORSE														
roasted	3 oz	0	.09	.1	4.11	.28	na	2.69	1.7	6.8	4.28	21.25	322.15	3.25
raw	1 lb	0	.59	.45	20.87	1.72	na	13.61	4.5	27.22	17.33	108.86	1632.96	13.15
raw	1 oz	0	.04	.03	1.29	.11	na	.84	0.3	1.68	1.07	6.72	100.8	.81
HORSE BEAN. See FAVA BEAN.														
HORSERADISH														
Prepared														
....	1 tbsp	0	0	0	0	na	na	na	0.0	9.15	.14	na	43.5	na
....	1 tsp	0	0	0	0	na	na	na	0.0	3.05	.05	na	14.5	na
Raw	1 lb	0	.23	0	0	na	na	na	268.5	463.99	4.64	na	1869.21	na
HORSERADISH TREE														
Leafy tips														
boiled, drained, chopped	1 cup	2945	.09	.21	.84	.39	9.5	0	13.0	63.42	.97	63.42	144.48	.21
raw, chopped	1 cup	1588	.05	.14	.47	.25	8.4	0	10.9	38.85	.84	30.87	70.77	.13
Pods														
boiled, drained, sliced	1 cup	83	.05	.08	.7	.13	35.9	0	114.5	23.6	.53	49.56	539.26	.5
raw, sliced	1 cup	74	.05	.07	.62	.12	44.3	0	141.0	30.0	.36	45.0	461.0	.45
raw, whole, approx 15 1/3 inches long	1 pod	8	.01	.01	.07	.01	4.9	0	15.5	3.3	.04	4.95	50.71	.05
HOT CHOCOLATE. See COCOA MIX.														
HOT DOG. See FRANKFURTER.														
HOT DOG BUN. See BUN, FRANKFURTER.														
HUBBARD SQUASH. See SQUASH, HUBBARD.														
HYACINTH BEAN														
immature, boiled, drained	1/2 cup	62	.02	.04	.21	.01	20.5	0	2.2	18.04	.33	18.48	115.28	.17
immature, raw	1/2 cup	44	.03	.04	.21	.01	24.6	0	5.2	20.0	.3	16.0	100.8	.15
mature, boiled	1/2 cup	0	.26	.04	.4	.04	3.7	0	0.0	38.8	4.44	79.54	326.89	2.76
mature, raw	1/2 cup	0	1.19	.14	1.69	.16	23.6	0	0.0	136.5	5.35	297.15	1296.75	9.77

I

Food Name	Serving Size	A I.U.	Thi mg	Rib mg	Nia mg	B₆ mg	Fol mcg	B₁₂ mcg	C mg	Calc mg	Iron mg	Mag mg	Pot mg	Zn mg
ICE BARS AND DESSERTS. See also SHERBET; SORBET.														
BAR														
Fruit														
and juice, 3 oz	1 bar	27	.01	.02	.15	.02	5.5	0	8.7	4.6	.17	3.68	48.76	.05
and water, aspartame-sweetened	1 bar	1	0	0	.08	0	0.0	0	0.0	1.02	.07	1.02	13.26	.02
DESSERT														
lime	4 oz	0	0	0	.01	0	0.0	0	1.0	1.92	.15	.96	2.88	.02
pineapple-coconut	4 oz	0	.01	0	.03	.02	1.0	0	12.7	0	3.39	4.8	16.32	.11
ICE CREAM. See also ICE CREAM BAR; ICE MILK.														
BORDEAUX CHERRY														
(Healthy Choice) 'Dairy Dessert'	4 oz	na	na	na	na	na	na	na	na	na	na	na	150	na
BUTTER ALMOND (Breyers)	4 oz	na	na	na	na	na	na	na	na	na	na	na	150	na
BUTTER CRUNCH (Sealtest)	4 oz	na	na	na	na	na	na	na	na	na	na	na	120	na
BUTTER PECAN														
(Breyers)	4 oz	na	na	na	na	na	na	na	na	na	na	na	170	na
(Frusen Glädjé)	4 oz	na	na	na	na	na	na	na	na	na	na	na	220	na
(Sealtest)	4 oz	na	na	na	na	na	na	na	na	na	na	na	140	na
BUTTER PECAN CRUNCH														
(Healthy Choice) 'Dairy Dessert'	4 oz	na	na	na	na	na	na	na	na	na	na	na	150	na
CHERRY (Breyers) vanilla	4 oz	na	na	na	na	na	na	na	na	na	na	na	160	na
CHOCOLATE														
(Breyers)	4 oz	na	na	na	na	na	na	na	na	na	na	na	150	na
(Frusen Glädjé)	4 oz	na	na	na	na	na	na	na	na	na	na	na	230	na
(Healthy Choice) 'Dairy Dessert'	4 oz	na	na	na	na	na	na	na	na	na	na	na	190	na
(Sealtest)	4 oz	na	na	na	na	na	na	na	na	na	na	na	170	na
CHOCOLATE CHIP														
(Healthy Choice) 'Dairy Dessert'	4 oz	na	na	na	na	na	na	na	na	na	na	na	160	na
(Sealtest)	4 oz	na	na	na	na	na	na	na	na	na	na	na	140	na
CHOCOLATE CHOCOLATE CHIP														
(Frusen Glädjé)	4 oz	na	na	na	na	na	na	na	na	na	na	na	270	na
CHOCOLATE TRIPLE STRIPES (Sealtest)	4 oz	na	na	na	na	na	na	na	na	na	na	na	160	na
COFFEE														
(Breyers)	4 oz	na	na	na	na	na	na	na	na	na	na	na	150	na
(Sealtest)	4 oz	na	na	na	na	na	na	na	na	na	na	na	170	na
COFFEE TOFFEE														
(Healthy Choice) 'Dairy Dessert'	4 oz	na	na	na	na	na	na	na	na	na	na	na	160	na
COOKIES 'N' CREAM														
(Breyers)	4 oz	na	na	na	na	na	na	na	na	na	na	na	170	na
(Healthy Choice) 'Dairy Dessert'	4 oz	na	na	na	na	na	na	na	na	na	na	na	180	na
FUDGE BROWNIE														
(Healthy Choice) 'Dairy Dessert'	4 oz	na	na	na	na	na	na	na	na	na	na	na	190	na
FUDGE ROYALE (Sealtest)	4 oz	na	na	na	na	na	na	na	na	na	na	na	150	na
FUDGE SWIRL, DOUBLE														
(Healthy Choice) 'Dairy Dessert'	4 oz	na	na	na	na	na	na	na	na	na	na	na	210	na
HEAVENLY HASH (Sealtest)	4 oz	na	na	na	na	na	na	na	na	na	na	na	150	na
MAPLE WALNUT (Sealtest)	4 oz	na	na	na	na	na	na	na	na	na	na	na	130	na
MINT CHOCOLATE (Breyers)	4 oz	na	na	na	na	na	na	na	na	na	na	na	170	na
MINT CHOCOLATE CHIP														
(Healthy Choice) 'Dairy Dessert'	4 oz	na	na	na	na	na	na	na	na	na	na	na	170	na
NEAPOLITAN														
(Healthy Choice) 'Dairy Dessert'	4 oz	na	na	na	na	na	na	na	na	na	na	na	160	na
PEACH (Breyers) natural	4 oz	na	na	na	na	na	na	na	na	na	na	na	135	na

Food Name	Serving Size	A I.U.	Thi mg	Rib mg	Nia mg	B_6 mg	Fol mcg	B_{12} mcg	C mg	Calc mg	Iron mg	Mag mg	Pot mg	Zn mg
PRALINE *(Healthy Choice)* and caramel 'Dairy Dessert' .... 4 oz		na	na	na	na	na	na	na	na	na	na	na	160	na
RASPBERRY SWIRL														
(Healthy Choice) 'Dairy Dessert' .... 4 oz		na	na	na	na	na	na	na	na	na	na	na	160	na
ROCKY ROAD														
(Healthy Choice) 'Dairy Dessert' .... 4 oz		na	na	na	na	na	na	na	na	na	na	na	190	na
STRAWBERRY														
(Breyers) .... 4 oz		na	na	na	na	na	na	na	na	na	na	na	125	na
(Frusen Glädjé) .... 4 oz		na	na	na	na	na	na	na	na	na	na	na	200	na
(Healthy Choice) 'Dairy Dessert' .... 4 oz		na	na	na	na	na	na	na	na	na	na	na	140	na
(Sealtest) .... 4 oz		na	na	na	na	na	na	na	na	na	na	na	130	na
SUNDAE														
(Sealtest) chocolate-marshmallow .... 4 oz		na	na	na	na	na	na	na	na	na	na	na	160	na
(Sealtest) peanut fudge .... 4 oz		na	na	na	na	na	na	na	na	na	na	na	140	na
SWISS CHOCOLATE CANDY ALMOND														
(Frusen Glädjé) .... 4 oz		na	na	na	na	na	na	na	na	na	na	na	280	na
VANILLA														
(Breyers) .... 4 oz		na	na	na	na	na	na	na	na	na	na	na	140	na
(Frusen Glädjé) .... 4 oz		na	na	na	na	na	na	na	na	na	na	na	200	na
(Healthy Choice) 'Dairy Dessert' .... 4 oz		na	na	na	na	na	na	na	na	na	na	na	180	na
(Sealtest) .... 4 oz		na	na	na	na	na	na	na	na	na	na	na	150	na
VANILLA, FRENCH *(Sealtest)* .... 4 oz		na	na	na	na	na	na	na	na	na	na	na	140	na
VANILLA FUDGE TWIRL *(Breyers)* .... 4 oz		na	na	na	na	na	na	na	na	na	na	na	170	na
VANILLA SWISS ALMOND *(Frusen Glädjé)* ..... 4 oz		na	na	na	na	na	na	na	na	na	na	na	240	na
VANILLA-CHOCOLATE *(Breyers)* .... 4 oz		na	na	na	na	na	na	na	na	na	na	na	145	na
VANILLA-CHOCOLATE-STRAWBERRY														
(Breyers) .... 4 oz		na	na	na	na	na	na	na	na	na	na	na	140	na
(Sealtest) .... 4 oz		na	na	na	na	na	na	na	na	na	na	na	140	na
(Sealtest) 'Cubic Scoops' .... 4 oz		na	na	na	na	na	na	na	na	na	na	na	140	na
ICE CREAM BAR														
CHOCOLATE FUDGE														
(Baker's) sundae, crunchy 'Fudgetastic' 4 oz	1 bar	na	na	na	na	na	na	na	na	na	na	na	170	na
(Baker's) sundae 'Fudgetastic' 4 oz	1 bar	na	na	na	na	na	na	na	na	na	na	na	170	na
ICE CREAM CONE														
Cup-style, wafer *(Bozo)* cake	1 cone	0	0	0	na	na	na	na	0.0	1	0	na	na	na
ICE MILK														
CARAMEL NUT *(Light n' Lively)* .... 4 oz		na	na	na	na	na	na	na	na	na	na	na	150	na
CHOCOLATE *(Breyers)* 'Light' .... 4 oz		na	na	na	na	na	na	na	na	na	na	na	180	na
CHOCOLATE CHIP *(Light n' Lively)* .... 4 oz		na	na	na	na	na	na	na	na	na	na	na	150	na
CHOCOLATE FUDGE TWIRL *(Breyers)* 'Light' .... 4 oz		na	na	na	na	na	na	na	na	na	na	na	200	na
COFFEE *(Light n' Lively)* .... 4 oz		na	na	na	na	na	na	na	na	na	na	na	115	na
COOKIES N' CREAM *(Light n' Lively)* .... 4 oz		na	na	na	na	na	na	na	na	na	na	na	160	na
HEAVENLY HASH														
(Breyers) 'Light' .... 4 oz		na	na	na	na	na	na	na	na	na	na	na	170	na
(Light n' Lively) .... 4 oz		na	na	na	na	na	na	na	na	na	na	na	140	na
PRALINE ALMOND *(Breyers)* 'Light' .... 4 oz		na	na	na	na	na	na	na	na	na	na	na	160	na
STRAWBERRY *(Breyers)* 'Light' .... 4 oz		na	na	na	na	na	na	na	na	na	na	na	150	na
TOFFEE FUDGE PARFAIT *(Breyers)* 'Light' ..... 4 oz		na	na	na	na	na	na	na	na	na	na	na	170	na
VANILLA														
(Breyers) 'Light' .... 4 oz		na	na	na	na	na	na	na	na	na	na	na	160	na
(Light n' Lively) .... 4 oz		na	na	na	na	na	na	na	na	na	na	na	150	na
(Light n' Lively) w/chocolate covered almonds .... 4 oz		na	na	na	na	na	na	na	na	na	na	na	140	na
VANILLA-CHOCOLATE-STRAWBERRY														
(Breyers) 'Light' .... 4 oz		na	na	na	na	na	na	na	na	na	na	na	160	na
(Light n' Lively) .... 4 oz		na	na	na	na	na	na	na	na	na	na	na	130	na

Food Name	Serving Size	A I.U.	Thi mg	Rib mg	Nia mg	B₆ mg	Fol mcg	B₁₂ mcg	C mg	Calc mg	Iron mg	Mag mg	Pot mg	Zn mg
VANILLA-RASPBERRY														
(Breyers) parfait 'Light'	4 oz	na	na	na	na	na	na	na	na	na	na	na	150	na
(Light n' Lively) swirl	4 oz	na	na	na	na	na	na	na	na	na	na	na	130	na

ICED TEA. See TEA, ICED.
INDIAN DATE. See TAMARIND.
INDIAN FRY BREAD. See BREAD.
INFANT FORMULA. See BABY FOOD.
IRISH MOSS. See SEAWEED.
ITALIAN STONE PINE NUT. See PINE NUT.

J

Food Name	Serving Size	A I.U.	Thi mg	Rib mg	Nia mg	B₆ mg	Fol mcg	B₁₂ mcg	C mg	Calc mg	Iron mg	Mag mg	Pot mg	Zn mg
JACK BEAN. See FAVA BEAN.														
JALAPEÑO. See PEPPER, JALAPEÑO.														
JAMAICAN BREADNUT. See BREADNUT TREE SEEDS.														
JAMBOLAN. See JAVA PLUM.														
JAPANESE MEDLAR. See LOQUAT.														
JAVA PLUM / jambolan														
raw	1 cup	4	.01	.02	.35	.05	na	0	19.3	25.65	.26	20.25	106.65	na
raw	3 fruits	0	0	0	.02	0	na	0	1.3	1.71	.02	1.35	7.11	na
JERUSALEM ARTICHOKE. See ARTICHOKES, JERUSALEM.														
JUICE. See individual listings.														
JUJUBE, CHINESE														
dried	100 gm	na	.21	.36	.5	na	na	0	13.0	79.0	1.8	37.0	531.0	.19
raw	100 gm	40	.02	.04	.9	.08	na	0	69.0	21.0	.48	10.0	250.0	.05
JUNKET MIX														
CHOCOLATE														
mix only, dry	1 tbsp	0	0	.01	.03	0	0.5	0	0.0	14.94	.23	7.29	38.7	.14
prepared w/2% milk	1/2 cup	252	.05	.21	.15	.06	6.8	.45	1.2	171.36	.41	27.2	247.52	.69
prepared w/whole milk	1/2 cup	155	.05	.21	.14	.06	6.8	.44	1.1	168.64	.41	27.2	243.44	.68
STRAWBERRY OR RASPBERRY														
mix only, dry	1.5-oz pkg	0	0	0	0	na	na	na	0.0	73.1	0	na	0	na
mix only, dry	1 tbsp	0	0	0	0	na	na	na	0.0	17.0	0	na	0	na
prepared w/whole milk	1 cup	375	.08	.4	.25	na	na	na	2.5	302.5	0	na	320.0	na
VANILLA														
mix only, dry	1.5-oz pkg	0	0	.01	0	0	0.0	0	0.0	50.31	.03	.43	1.29	.02
mix only, dry	1 tbsp	0	0	0	0	0	0.0	0	0.0	12.64	.01	.11	.32	0
prepared w/2% milk	1/2 cup	251	.05	.2	.11	.05	6.7	.44	1.2	160.93	.07	17.29	188.86	.48
prepared w/whole milk	1/2 cup	154	.05	.2	.1	.05	6.7	.44	1.2	158.27	.07	15.96	186.2	.47

K

Food Name	Serving Size	A I.U.	Thi mg	Rib mg	Nia mg	B₆ mg	Fol mcg	B₁₂ mcg	C mg	Calc mg	Iron mg	Mag mg	Pot mg	Zn mg
KALE/borecole/cole/colewort														
boiled, drained, chopped	1 cup	9620	.07	.09	.65	.18	17.3	0	53.3	93.6	1.17	23.4	296.4	.31
chopped (Dole)	1/2 cup	3026	na	na	na	na	na	na	41.0	na	na	na	152	na
raw, chopped	1 cup	5963	.07	.09	.67	.18	19.6	0	80.4	90.45	1.14	22.78	299.49	.29
Frozen														
boiled, drained, chopped	1 cup	8260	.06	.15	.87	.11	18.6	0	32.8	179.4	1.22	23.4	417.3	.23
unprepared 10-oz pkg	3.3 oz	5878	.05	.11	.66	.08	15.7	0	36.9	127.84	.87	16.92	313.02	.17
KALE, SCOTCH														
boiled, drained, chopped	1 cup	2592	.05	.05	1.03	.18	17.3	0	68.6	171.6	2.51	74.1	356.2	.31

Food Name	Serving Size	A I.U.	Thi mg	Rib mg	Nia mg	B$_6$ mg	Fol mcg	B$_{12}$ mcg	C mg	Calc mg	Iron mg	Mag mg	Pot mg	Zn mg
raw, chopped	1 cup	2077	.05	.04	.87	.15	18.8	0	87.1	137.35	2.01	58.96	301.5	.25
KANPYO/dried gourd strips	1/2 cup	0	0	.01	.78	.14	16.5	0	0.1	75.6	1.38	33.75	427.14	1.58
KASHA. See BUCKWHEAT GROATS.														
KATSUO. See TUNA, SKIPJACK.														
KELP. See SEAWEED.														
KETCHUP. See CATSUP.														
KIDNEY BEAN														
California red, mature														
boiled	1/2 cup	3	.11	.05	.48	.09	64.9	0	1.1	58.08	2.62	42.24	368.72	.76
raw	1/2 cup	7	.49	.2	1.9	.37	362.6	0	4.1	179.4	8.6	147.2	1370.8	2.35
Red, mature														
boiled	1/2 cup	0	.14	.05	.51	.11	114.1	0	1.1	24.64	2.59	39.6	354.64	.94
raw	1/2 cup	7	.56	.2	1.94	.37	362.6	0	4.1	76.36	6.15	126.96	1250.28	2.57
Royal red, mature														
boiled	1/2 cup	3	.08	.06	.49	.09	64.9	0	1.1	38.72	2.44	36.96	332.64	.79
raw	1/2 cup	7	.36	.22	1.94	.36	361.9	0	4.1	120.52	8.0	126.96	1238.32	2.45
Sprouted, mature, raw	1 cup	4	.68	.46	5.37	.16	108.4	0	71.2	31.28	1.49	38.64	344.08	.74
KIDNEY BEAN, CANNED														
Dark red (Van Camp's)	1 cup	0	.16	.1	1.0	na	na	na	0.0	52	3.31	na	549	na
Light red (Van Camp's)	1 cup	0	.17	.11	.94	na	na	na	0.0	55	2.96	na	494	na
Red														
(Eden Foods) organic, very low sodium, no salt added	1/2 cup	na	na	na	na	na	na	na	na	na	na	na	420	na
(Van Camp's)	1 cup	0	.17	.11	.94	na	na	na	0.0	55	2.96	na	494	na
(Van Camp's) 'New Orleans Style'	1 cup	0	.16	.1	1.2	na	na	na	0.0	60	3.1	na	586	na
KIWI FRUIT/Chinese gooseberry														
fresh, raw, w/o skin	1 large	159	.02	.05	.46	na	na	0	89.2	23.66	.37	27.3	302.12	na
fresh, raw, w/o skin	1 med	133	.02	.04	.38	na	na	0	74.5	19.76	.31	22.8	252.32	na
untrimmed (Dole)	2 fruits	136	na	na	na	na	na	na	143.0	na	na	na	450	na
KNACKWURST														
	4-inch link	0	.23	.1	1.86	.12	1.4	.8	18.4	7.48	.62	7.48	135.32	1.13
	1 oz	0	.1	.04	.78	.05	0.6	.33	7.7	3.12	.26	3.12	56.42	.47
KOHLRABI/cabbage turnip														
boiled, drained, sliced	1/2 cup	29	.03	.02	.32	.13	9.9	0	44.3	20.5	.33	15.58	278.8	.25
raw, sliced	1/2 cup	25	.03	.01	.28	.11	11.3	0	43.4	16.8	.28	13.3	245.0	.02
KOLBASSY. See KIELBASA.														
KOOL-AID. See individual flavors.														
KUMQUAT, raw, trimmed	1 fruit	57	.02	.02	.1	na	na	0	7.1	8.36	.07	2.47	37.05	.02

L

Food Name	Serving Size	A I.U.	Thi mg	Rib mg	Nia mg	B$_6$ mg	Fol mcg	B$_{12}$ mcg	C mg	Calc mg	Iron mg	Mag mg	Pot mg	Zn mg
LAMB, DOMESTIC														
(NOTE: All USDA choice grade. TRIMMED = Lean; separable fat removed. UNTRIMMED = Separable fat not removed.)														
BRAINS														
braised	3 oz	0	.09	.2	2.1	.09	4.3	7.86	10.2	10.2	1.43	11.9	174.25	1.16
braised, yield from 1 lb raw	12.25 oz	0	.38	.83	8.57	.38	17.4	32.1	41.6	41.64	5.83	48.58	711.35	4.72
pan-fried	3 oz	0	.14	.31	3.87	.2	6.0	20.48	19.6	17.85	1.73	18.7	304.3	1.7
raw	4 oz	0	.15	.34	4.42	.33	3.4	12.81	18.1	10.21	1.98	13.61	335.66	1.33
COMPOSITE CUTS/LEG AND SHOULDER														
Trimmed														
braised, cubes	3 oz	0	.06	.2	5.06	.1	17.9	2.32	0.0	12.75	2.38	23.8	221.0	5.59
broiled, cubes	3 oz	0	.09	.26	5.62	.12	19.6	2.58	0.0	11.05	1.99	26.35	284.75	4.9
broiled, ground	3 oz	0	.09	.21	5.69	.12	16.2	2.22	na	18.7	1.52	20.4	288.15	3.97
raw, cubes	1 lb	0	.59	1.09	26.99	.73	104.3	12.38	0.0	40.82	8.03	117.94	1288.22	18.82

Food Name	Serving Size	A I.U.	Thi mg	Rib mg	Nia mg	B₆ mg	Fol mcg	B₁₂ mcg	C mg	Calc mg	Iron mg	Mag mg	Pot mg	Zn mg
raw, cubes	1 oz	0	.04	.07	1.67	.04	6.4	.76	0.0	2.52	.5	7.28	79.52	1.16
raw, ground	1 lb	0	.5	.95	27.03	.59	81.7	10.48	na	72.58	7.03	95.26	1006.99	15.47
raw, ground	1 oz	0	.03	.06	1.67	.04	5.0	.65	na	4.48	.43	5.88	62.16	.95
HEART														
braised	3 oz	0	.14	1.01	3.71	.26	1.7	9.52	6.0	11.9	4.69	20.4	159.8	3.13
raw	4 oz	0	.42	1.12	6.96	.44	2.3	11.62	5.7	6.8	5.22	19.28	358.34	2.12
KIDNEYS														
braised	3 oz	387	.3	1.76	5.09	.1	68.9	67.07	10.2	15.3	10.54	17.0	151.3	3.23
raw	4 oz	358	.7	2.54	8.52	.25	31.8	59.43	12.5	14.74	7.23	19.28	314.12	2.54
LEG/FORESHANK														
Trimmed														
braised	3 oz	0	.03	.16	4.31	.09	16.2	1.92	0.0	17.0	1.93	19.55	226.95	7.36
raw	1 lb	0	.45	.91	24.09	.77	99.8	11.11	0.0	40.82	8.12	113.4	1075.03	26.99
raw	1 oz	0	.03	.06	1.49	.05	6.2	.69	0.0	2.52	.5	7.0	66.36	1.67
Untrimmed														
braised	3 oz	0	.04	.16	4.64	.09	14.5	1.94	0.0	17.0	1.82	18.7	218.45	6.54
raw	1 lb	0	.45	.86	24.81	.68	86.2	10.61	0.0	49.9	7.58	99.79	970.7	23.68
raw	1 oz	0	.03	.05	1.53	.04	5.3	.66	0.0	3.08	.47	6.16	59.92	1.46
LEG/SHANK														
Trimmed														
raw	1 lb	0	.64	1.13	28.08	.77	104.3	11.98	0.0	27.22	8.26	122.47	1315.44	17.65
raw	1 oz	0	.04	.07	1.73	.05	6.4	.74	0.0	1.68	.51	7.56	81.2	1.09
roasted	3 oz	0	.09	.24	5.43	.14	20.4	2.3	0.0	6.8	1.75	22.1	290.7	4.27
Untrimmed														
raw	1 lb	0	.59	1.04	28.21	.68	90.7	11.39	0.0	36.29	7.76	108.86	1183.9	15.88
raw	1 oz	0	.04	.06	1.74	.04	5.6	.7	0.0	2.24	.48	6.72	73.08	.98
roasted	3 oz	0	.09	.23	5.57	.14	18.7	2.27	0.0	8.5	1.68	21.25	277.1	3.96
LEG/SIRLOIN														
Trimmed														
raw	1 lb	0	.64	1.13	28.71	.77	108.9	12.52	0.0	31.75	8.3	122.47	1288.22	17.1
raw	1 oz	0	.04	.07	1.77	.05	6.7	.77	0.0	1.96	.51	7.56	79.52	1.06
roasted	3 oz	0	.1	.26	5.33	.14	17.9	2.19	0.0	6.8	1.87	21.25	283.05	4.12
Untrimmed														
raw	1 lb	0	.54	1.04	28.76	.64	81.7	11.25	0.0	45.36	7.3	99.79	1047.82	13.97
raw	1 oz	0	.03	.06	1.78	.04	5.0	.69	0.0	2.8	.45	6.16	64.68	.86
roasted	3 oz	0	.09	.24	5.63	.12	14.5	2.15	0.0	9.35	1.7	18.7	255.85	3.51
LEG/WHOLE														
Trimmed														
raw	1 lb	0	.64	1.13	28.26	.77	104.3	12.25	0.0	27.22	8.26	122.47	1310.9	17.42
raw	1 oz	0	.04	.07	1.74	.05	6.4	.76	0.0	1.68	.51	7.56	80.92	1.08
roasted	3 oz	0	.09	.25	5.39	.14	19.6	2.24	0.0	6.8	1.8	22.1	287.3	4.2
Untrimmed														
raw	1 lb	0	.59	1.04	28.4	.68	86.2	11.34	0.0	40.82	7.53	104.33	1129.46	15.06
raw	1 oz	0	.04	.06	1.75	.04	5.3	.7	0.0	2.52	.46	6.44	69.72	.93
roasted	3 oz	0	.09	.23	5.6	.13	17.0	2.2	0.0	9.35	1.68	20.4	266.05	3.74
LIVER														
braised	3 oz	21203	.2	3.43	10.33	.42	62.1	65.03	3.4	6.8	7.04	18.7	187.85	6.71
pan-fried	3 oz	22098	.3	3.9	14.18	.81	340.0	72.84	11.1	7.65	8.67	19.55	299.2	4.79
raw	4 oz	27910	.39	4.12	18.27	1.02	260.8	102.12	4.5	7.94	8.36	21.55	354.94	5.28
LOIN														
Trimmed														
broiled	3 oz	0	.09	.24	5.82	.14	20.4	2.14	0.0	16.15	1.7	23.8	319.6	3.51
raw	1 oz	0	.04	.06	1.82	.05	6.7	.62	0.0	3.36	.53	7.56	77.28	.89
roasted	3 oz	0	.09	.23	5.81	.14	21.3	1.84	0.0	14.45	2.07	22.95	226.95	3.45

Food Name	Serving Size	A I.U.	Thi mg	Rib mg	Nia mg	B$_6$ mg	Fol mcg	B$_{12}$ mcg	C mg	Calc mg	Iron mg	Mag mg	Pot mg	Zn mg
Untrimmed														
broiled	3 oz	0	.09	.21	6.04	.11	15.3	2.1	0.0	17.0	1.54	20.4	277.95	2.96
roasted	3 oz	0	.09	.2	6.04	.09	16.2	1.88	0.0	15.3	1.8	19.55	209.1	2.9
LUNGS														
braised	3 oz	90	.03	.12	2.06	.05	6.8	2.14	23.8	10.2	3.88	9.35	107.95	1.64
raw	4 oz	101	.05	.27	4.68	.12	13.6	4.46	35.2	11.34	7.26	15.88	269.89	2.04
PANCREAS														
braised	3 oz	0	.02	.18	2.18	.04	11.1	4.71	17.0	10.2	1.8	16.15	247.35	2.28
raw	4 oz	0	.03	.28	4.2	.08	14.7	6.8	20.4	9.07	2.61	23.81	476.28	2.19
RIB														
Trimmed														
broiled	3 oz	0	.09	.21	5.57	.13	17.9	2.24	0.0	13.6	1.88	24.65	266.05	4.48
raw	1 lb	0	.54	.91	26.72	.73	95.3	10.8	0.0	54.43	7.58	113.4	1202.04	17.24
raw	1 oz	0	.03	.06	1.65	.04	5.9	.67	0.0	3.36	.47	7.0	74.2	1.06
roasted	3 oz	0	.08	.2	5.24	.13	18.7	1.84	0.0	17.85	1.5	19.55	267.75	3.8
Untrimmed														
broiled	3 oz	0	.08	.19	5.95	.09	11.9	2.16	0.0	16.15	1.6	19.55	229.5	3.4
raw	1 lb	0	.45	.86	27.62	.5	63.5	9.48	0.0	68.04	6.31	81.65	861.84	12.29
raw	1 oz	0	.03	.05	1.71	.03	3.9	.59	0.0	4.2	.39	5.04	53.2	.76
roasted	3 oz	0	.08	.18	5.74	.09	12.8	1.9	0.0	18.7	1.36	17.0	230.35	2.97
SHOULDER/ARM														
Trimmed														
braised	3 oz	0	.06	.23	5.38	.11	18.7	2.25	0.0	22.1	2.3	24.65	287.3	6.21
broiled	3 oz	0	.09	.25	5.79	.12	19.6	2.55	0.0	14.45	1.96	25.5	289.0	4.87
raw	1 oz	0	.03	.06	1.68	.04	6.7	.75	0.0	3.36	.49	7.0	80.36	1.16
roasted	3 oz	0	.09	.23	5.39	.12	21.3	2.22	0.0	13.6	1.9	22.1	235.45	4.46
Untrimmed														
braised	3 oz	0	.06	.21	5.66	.09	15.3	2.19	0.0	21.25	2.03	22.1	260.1	5.17
broiled	3 oz	0	.09	.23	5.97	.1	15.3	2.43	0.0	15.3	1.78	22.1	262.65	4.16
raw	1 oz	0	.03	.06	1.71	.04	5.3	.68	0.0	3.92	.44	5.88	66.64	.96
roasted	3 oz	0	.08	.21	5.66	.1	17.0	2.17	0.0	15.3	1.73	19.55	220.15	3.81
SHOULDER/BLADE														
Trimmed														
braised	1 oz	0	.02	.06	1.58	.03	5.9	.82	0.0	7.84	.73	7.28	71.12	2.26
broiled	3 oz	0	.09	.22	5.16	.14	17.9	2.39	0.0	20.4	1.54	22.1	312.8	5.51
raw	3 oz	0	.1	.19	4.41	.14	19.6	2.41	0.0	13.6	1.38	20.4	227.8	4.34
roasted	3 oz	0	.08	.21	4.65	.13	21.3	2.33	0.0	17.85	1.76	21.25	219.3	5.51
Untrimmed														
braised	3 oz	0	.05	.18	5.13	.09	15.3	2.41	0.0	22.95	2.0	20.4	206.55	5.83
broiled	3 oz	0	.08	.21	5.42	.13	15.3	2.32	0.0	20.4	1.46	20.4	285.6	4.78
raw	1 lb	0	.5	.91	24.63	.64	86.2	11.75	0.0	77.11	6.71	95.26	1038.74	19.41
raw	1 oz	0	.03	.06	1.52	.04	5.3	.73	0.0	4.76	.41	5.88	64.12	1.2
roasted	3 oz	0	.08	.2	5.02	.09	17.9	2.27	0.0	17.85	1.63	18.7	209.1	4.74
SPLEEN														
braised	3 oz	0	.04	.27	4.99	.07	3.4	4.5	22.1	11.05	32.87	17.85	210.8	3.35
raw	4 oz	0	.05	.39	8.95	.12	4.5	6.06	26.1	10.21	47.5	23.81	405.97	3.22
TONGUE														
braised	3 oz	0	.07	.36	3.14	.14	2.6	5.35	6.0	8.5	2.24	13.6	134.3	2.54
raw	4 oz	0	.17	.43	5.27	.2	4.5	8.16	6.8	10.21	3.01	23.81	291.44	2.63
LAMB, NEW ZEALAND, FROZEN														
LEG/FORESHANK														
Trimmed														
braised	3 oz	0	.06	.31	4.79	.08	0.9	2.08	0.0	8.5	1.89	13.6	106.25	4.76
raw	1 lb	0	.68	1.81	28.26	.59	4.5	12.38	0.0	31.75	7.12	77.11	680.4	18.14
raw	1 oz	0	.04	.11	1.74	.04	0.3	.76	0.0	1.96	.44	4.76	42.0	1.12
Untrimmed														
braised	3 oz	0	.06	.28	5.16	.07	0.9	2.07	0.0	11.9	1.76	12.75	100.3	4.08

Food Name	Serving Size	A I.U.	Thi mg	Rib mg	Nia mg	B$_6$ mg	Fol mcg	B$_{12}$ mcg	C mg	Calc mg	Iron mg	Mag mg	Pot mg	Zn mg
raw	1 lb	0	.59	1.63	28.58	.5	4.5	11.48	0.0	45.36	6.76	68.04	594.22	15.29
raw	1 oz	0	.04	.1	1.76	.03	0.3	.71	0.0	2.8	.42	4.2	36.68	.94
LEG/WHOLE														
Trimmed														
raw	1 lb	0	.68	1.91	31.39	.68	0.0	11.79	0.0	18.14	7.62	90.72	811.94	13.83
raw	1 oz	0	.04	.12	1.94	.04	0.0	.73	0.0	1.12	.47	5.6	50.12	.85
roasted	3 oz	0	.1	.43	6.38	.12	0.0	2.24	0.0	5.95	1.9	17.85	155.55	3.43
Untrimmed														
raw	1 lb	0	.64	1.72	31.07	.59	4.5	11.11	0.0	36.29	7.17	77.11	707.62	12.02
raw	1 oz	0	.04	.11	1.92	.04	0.3	.69	0.0	2.24	.44	4.76	43.68	.74
roasted	3 oz	0	.1	.38	6.45	.11	0.9	2.21	0.0	8.5	1.78	17.0	141.95	3.04
LOIN														
Trimmed														
raw	1 oz	0	.04	.1	1.95	.04	0.0	.64	0.0	4.2	.5	5.32	43.96	.66
roasted	3 oz	0	.11	.37	6.71	.12	0.0	2.19	0.0	17.85	1.99	18.7	160.65	2.8
Untrimmed														
broiled	3 oz	0	.1	.31	6.74	.09	0.9	2.15	0.0	19.55	1.74	16.15	135.15	2.25
raw	1 oz	0	.04	.08	1.91	.03	0.3	.59	0.0	4.76	.43	4.2	33.88	.52
RIB														
Trimmed														
raw	1 lb	0	.68	1.41	27.9	.54	0.0	11.25	0.0	49.9	7.12	77.11	707.62	13.06
raw	1 oz	0	.04	.09	1.72	.03	0.0	.69	0.0	3.08	.44	4.76	43.68	.81
roasted	3 oz	0	.09	.28	5.21	.09	0.0	1.94	0.0	11.9	1.61	13.6	124.1	2.92
Untrimmed														
raw	1 lb	0	.5	1.13	28.67	.36	4.5	9.84	0.0	72.58	6.31	58.97	512.57	9.25
raw	1 oz	0	.03	.07	1.77	.02	0.3	.61	0.0	4.48	.39	3.64	31.64	.57
roasted	3 oz	0	.08	.23	5.81	.07	0.9	1.98	0.0	16.15	1.45	11.9	105.4	2.21
SHOULDER/WHOLE														
Trimmed														
braised	3 oz	0	.07	.31	4.97	.07	0.0	3.15	0.0	22.95	1.99	17.0	141.1	4.76
raw	1 lb	0	.64	1.63	23.22	.45	0.0	16.15	0.0	68.04	6.49	81.65	739.37	15.97
raw	1 oz	0	.04	.1	1.45	.03	0.0	1.01	0.0	4.26	.41	5.11	46.29	1.0
Untrimmed														
braised	3 oz	0	.07	.27	5.41	.06	0.9	2.89	0.0	22.95	1.79	15.3	124.95	3.85
raw	1 lb	0	.54	1.36	24.99	.36	4.5	13.93	0.0	77.11	6.12	68.04	603.29	12.7
LAMB'S-QUARTER														
boiled, drained, chopped	1 cup	17460	.18	.47	1.62	.31	24.5	0	66.6	464.4	1.26	41.4	518.4	.54
raw	100 gm	11600	.16	.44	1.2	.27	29.6	0	80.0	309.0	1.2	34.0	452.0	.44
LARD														
pork, fresh	1 cup	0	0	0	0	0	0.0	0	0.0	0	0	0	0	.23
pork, fresh	1 tbsp	0	0	0	0	0	0.0	0	0.0	0	0	0	0	.01
pork leaf, fresh	1 oz	0	.03	.02	.35	.01	0.0	.07	0.0	.28	.03	.28	8.79	.05
LASAGNA ENTRÉE, FROZEN														
(Stouffer's) 96-oz tray	9.75 oz	na	na	na	na	na	na	na	na	na	na	na	490	na
(Stouffer's) 21-oz pkg	10.5 oz	na	na	na	na	na	na	na	na	na	na	na	570	na
(Stouffer's) 10-oz pkg	10 oz	na	na	na	na	na	na	na	na	na	na	na	570	na
TOFU														
(Amy's Kitchen) vegetable, organic	9.5 oz	na	na	na	na	na	na	na	na	na	na	na	461	na
VEGETABLE														
(Amy's Kitchen) organic	9.5 oz	na	na	na	na	na	na	na	na	na	na	na	530	na
(Stouffer's)	10.5 oz	na	na	na	na	na	na	na	na	na	na	na	450	na
(Stouffer's) 96-oz tray	9.5 oz	na	na	na	na	na	na	na	na	na	na	na	350	na
LASAGNA ENTRÉE, PACKAGED														
(Top Shelf) Italian	10 oz	na	na	na	na	na	na	na	na	na	na	na	728	na

LASAGNA NOODLE. See PASTA.

LAVER. See SEAWEED.

Food Name	Serving Size	A I.U.	Thi mg	Rib mg	Nia mg	B$_6$ mg	Fol mcg	B$_{12}$ mcg	C mg	Calc mg	Iron mg	Mag mg	Pot mg	Zn mg
LEEK, boiled, drained, chopped	1/4 cup	12	.01	.01	.05	.03	6.3	0	1.1	7.8	.29	3.64	22.62	.02
LEEK, FREEZE-DRIED														
bulb-lower leaf portion	1/4 cup	2	.01	0	.03	.01	2.9	0	0.9	2.88	.06	1.29	19.2	.01
bulb-lower leaf portion	1 tbsp	1	0	0	.01	0	0.7	0	0.2	.72	.02	.32	4.8	0
LEMON														
w/peel, approx 3.9 oz	1 med	32	.05	.04	.22	.12	na	0	83.2	65.88	.76	12.96	156.6	.11
w/o peel, approx 3.9 oz	1 med	17	.02	.01	.06	.05	6.2	0	30.7	15.08	.35	4.64	80.04	.03
w/o peel, approx 5.6 oz	1 large	24	.03	.02	.08	.07	8.9	0	44.5	21.84	.5	6.72	115.92	.05
w/o peel, trimmed	1-oz wedge	8	.01	.01	.05	.03	na	0	20.8	16.47	.19	3.24	39.15	.03
LEMON DRINK. See also LEMONADE.														
(Gatorade) 'Thirst Quencher'	8 oz	na	na	na	na	na	na	na	na	na	na	na	30	na
LEMON JUICE														
. . . .	1 cup	49	.07	.02	.24	.12	31.5	0	112.2	17.08	.07	14.64	302.56	.12
. . . .	1 tbsp	3	0	0	.02	.01	2.0	0	7.0	1.06	0	.91	18.85	.01
Frozen *(Minute Maid)* concentrate	6 oz	na	na	na	na	na	na	na	9.0	na	na	na	30	na
LEMON PEEL														
candied	1 oz	0	0	0	0	na	na	na	0.0	0	0	na	0	na
raw	1 tbsp	3	0	0	.02	.01	na	0	7.7	8.04	.05	.9	9.6	na
raw	1 tsp	1	0	0	.01	0	na	0	2.6	2.68	.02	.3	3.2	na
LEMONADE														
Can, bottle, or box														
(J. Hungerford) pink, 20% plus juice	9.03 oz	na	na	na	na	na	na	na	3.3	2.58	.12	na	na	na
(Minute Maid)	6 oz	na	na	na	na	na	na	na	9.0	na	na	na	25	na
(Minute Maid) country style	6 oz	na	na	na	na	na	na	na	9.0	na	na	na	25	na
(Minute Maid) cranberry	6 oz	na	na	na	na	na	na	na	6.0	na	na	na	20	na
(Minute Maid) pink	6 oz	na	na	na	na	na	na	na	9.0	na	na	na	25	na
(Minute Maid) raspberry	6 oz	na	na	na	na	na	na	na	6.0	na	na	na	20	na
(10-K) pink	8 oz	na	na	na	na	na	na	na	na	5	0	na	30	na
LEMONADE DRINK MIX														
Prepared from dry mix														
(Country Time)	8 oz	na	na	na	na	na	na	na	na	na	na	na	10	na
(Country Time) pink	8 oz	na	na	na	na	na	na	na	na	na	na	<a	10	na
(Country Time) pink, 'Sugar Free'	8 oz	na	na	na	na	na	na	na	na	na	na	na	40	na
(Country Time) pink, sugar sweetened	8 oz	na	na	na	na	na	na	na	na	na	na	na	10	na
(Country Time) pink, sugar-free, w/NutraSweet	8 oz	na	na	na	na	na	na	na	na	na	na	na	40	na
(Country Time) 'Sugar-free'	8 oz	na	na	na	na	na	na	na	na	na	na	na	40	na
(Crystal Light) 'Sugar-free'	8 oz	na	na	na	na	na	na	na	na	na	na	na	60	na
(Crystal Light) sugar-free, w/NutraSweet	8 oz	na	na	na	na	na	na	na	na	na	na	na	60	na
(Kool-Aid) pink, unsweetened, prepared w/sugar	8 oz	na	na	na	na	na	na	na	na	na	na	na	0	na
(Kool-Aid) pink, unsweetened, prepared w/o sugar	8 oz	na	na	na	na	na	na	na	na	na	na	na	0	na
(Kool-Aid) sugar free, w/NutraSweet	8 oz	na	na	na	na	na	na	na	na	na	na	na	0	na
(Kool-Aid) sugar sweetened	8 oz	na	na	na	na	na	na	na	na	na	na	na	0	na
Prepared from frozen concentrate														
(Minute Maid)	6 oz	na	na	na	na	na	na	na	9.0	na	na	na	25	na
(Minute Maid) country style	6 oz	na	na	na	na	na	na	na	9.0	na	na	na	25	na
(Minute Maid) cranberry	6 oz	na	na	na	na	na	na	na	6.0	na	na	na	20	na
(Minute Maid) pink	6 oz	na	na	na	na	na	na	na	9.0	na	na	na	25	na
(Minute Maid) raspberry	6 oz	na	na	na	na	na	na	na	6.0	na	na	na	20	na
LEMON-LIME DRINK														
Can, bottle, or box														
(All-Sports) thirst quencher, caffeine-free . . .	8 oz	na	na	na	na	na	na	na	na	na	na	na	55	na
(PowerAde) thirst quencher, high energy . . .	8 oz	na	na	na	na	na	na	na	na	na	na	na	30	na
(10-K)	8 oz	na	na	na	na	na	na	na	na	5	0	na	30	na

Food Name	Serving Size	A I.U.	Thi mg	Rib mg	Nia mg	B6 mg	Fol mcg	B12 mcg	C mg	Calc mg	Iron mg	Mag mg	Pot mg	Zn mg
Prepared from dry mix														
(Crystal Light) w/NutraSweet	8 oz	na	na	na	na	na	na	na	na	na	na	na	5	na
(Kool-Aid) unsweetened, prepared w/sugar . .	8 oz	na	na	na	na	na	na	na	na	na	na	na	0	na
(Kool-Aid) unsweetened, prepared w/o sugar	8 oz	na	na	na	na	na	na	na	na	na	na	na	0	na
LETTUCE														
BIBB, BOSTON, OR BUTTERHEAD														
raw, approx 7.75 oz, 5 inch diam	1 head	1581	.1	.1	.49	.08	119.5	0	13.0	52.16	.49	21.19	418.91	.28
COS, raw, shredded	1/2 cup	728	.03	.03	.14	.01	38.0	0	6.7	10.08	.31	1.68	81.2	.07
ICEBERG, raw, 6 inch diam	1 head	1779	.25	.16	1.01	.22	301.8	0	21.0	102.41	2.69	48.51	851.62	1.19
LEAF, shredded (Dole)	1.5 cups	1596	na	na	na	na	na	na	15.0	na	na	na	220	na
LOOSELEAF, raw, shredded	1/2 cup	532	.01	.02	.11	.02	13.9	0	5.0	19.04	.39	3.08	73.92	.08
ROMAINE, raw, shredded	1/2 cup	728	.03	.03	.14	.01	38.0	0	6.7	10.08	.31	1.68	81.2	.07
LIMA BEAN/butterbean														
MATURE, DRY														
Baby														
boiled, thin-seeded	1/2 cup	0	.15	.05	.6	.07	136.4	0	0.0	26.39	2.18	48.23	364.91	.94
raw, thin-seeded	1/2 cup	5	.58	.22	1.73	.33	404.2	0	0.0	81.81	6.25	189.88	1417.03	2.63
Large, boiled	1/2 cup	0	.15	.05	.4	.15	78.1	0	0.0	15.98	2.25	40.42	477.52	.89
LIMA BEAN, CANNED														
(Freshlike)	1/2 cup	na	na	na	na	na	na	na	na	na	na	na	270	na
(Freshlike) water packed, w/o salt	1/2 cup	na	na	na	na	na	na	na	na	na	na	na	270	na
(Veg•All)	1/2 cup	na	na	na	na	na	na	na	na	na	na	na	270	na
LIMA BEAN, FROZEN														
BABY														
boiled, drained, immature seeds	10-oz pkg	519	.22	.17	2.39	.36	48.2	0	18.0	87.08	6.1	174.16	1278.21	1.71
boiled, drained, immature seeds	1/2 cup	150	.06	.05	.69	.1	14.0	0	5.2	25.2	1.76	50.4	369.9	.5
unprepared, immature seeds	10-oz pkg	537	.32	.21	2.91	.45	78.4	0	23.6	99.4	6.28	142.0	1283.68	1.79
unprepared, immature seeds	1/2 cup	155	.09	.06	.84	.13	22.6	0	6.8	28.7	1.81	41.0	370.64	.52
(Birds Eye)	3.3 oz	na	na	na	na	na	na	na	na	na	na	na	470	na
(Freshlike)	3.3 oz	na	na	na	na	na	na	na	na	na	na	na	470	na
FORDHOOK														
boiled, drained, immature seeds	10-oz pkg	591	.23	.19	3.32	.38	65.9	0	39.8	68.42	4.23	105.74	1268.88	1.37
boiled, drained, immature seeds	1/2 cup	162	.06	.05	.91	.1	18.0	0	10.9	18.7	1.16	28.9	346.8	.37
unprepared, immature seeds	1/2 cup	178	.07	.05	.95	.11	25.5	0	15.4	19.2	1.21	30.4	382.4	.39
(Birds Eye)	3.3 oz	na	na	na	na	na	na	na	na	na	na	na	480	na
LIME, raw, 2 inch diam	1 med	7	.02	.01	.13	.03	5.5	0	19.5	22.11	.4	4.02	68.34	.07
LIME JUICE														
fresh	1 cup	25	.05	.02	.25	.11	20.2	0	72.1	22.14	.07	14.76	268.14	.15
fresh	1 tbsp	2	0	0	.02	.01	1.3	0	4.5	1.39	0	.92	16.79	.01
Canned or bottled														
unsweetened	1 cup	39	.08	.01	.4	.07	19.4	0	15.7	29.52	.57	17.22	184.5	.15
unsweetened	1 tbsp	2	.01	0	.03	0	1.2	0	1.0	1.85	.04	1.08	11.55	.01
LIMEADE														
(Minute Maid) frozen concentrate, diluted ...	6 oz	na	na	na	na	na	na	na	5.0	na	na	na	15	na
LING														
dry-heat cooked	3 oz	98	.11	.2	2.38	.3	6.8	.55	0.0	37.4	.71	68.85	413.1	.85
raw	3 oz	85	.09	.16	1.95	.26	6.0	.48	0.0	28.9	.55	53.55	322.15	.66
LINGCOD														
dry-heat cooked	3 oz	49	.03	.12	1.97	.29	8.5	3.53	0.0	15.3	.35	28.05	476.0	.49
raw	3 oz	43	.03	.1	1.61	.26	7.7	3.06	0.0	11.9	.27	22.1	371.45	.38
LINGUINE ENTRÉE														
Refrigerated														
(Contadina) egg, angel hair 'Fresh'	3 oz	75	.3	.26	2.0	.03	17.8	.22	0.0	20	2.7	45.6	150	.94
(DiGiorno) herb, approx 1 1/3 cups cooked . .	3 oz	na	na	na	na	na	na	na	na	na	na	na	170	na
LINGUINE NOODLE. See PASTA.														
LIQUEUR. See ALCOHOLIC BEVERAGES.														
LIQUOR. See ALCOHOLIC BEVERAGES.														

Food Name	Serving Size	A I.U.	Thi mg	Rib mg	Nia mg	B$_6$ mg	Fol mcg	B$_{12}$ mcg	C mg	Calc mg	Iron mg	Mag mg	Pot mg	Zn mg
LITCHI/lychee														
Dried	100 gm	0	.01	.57	3.1	na	na	0	183.0	33.0	1.7	42.0	1110.0	.28
LIVER. See individual animal listings.														
LOBSTER, NORTHERN														
moist-heat cooked	1 cup	126	.01	.1	1.55	.11	16.1	4.51	0.0	88.45	.57	50.75	510.4	4.23
moist-heat cooked	3 oz	74	.01	.06	.91	.07	9.4	2.64	0.0	51.85	.33	29.75	299.2	2.48
raw	3 oz	60	.01	.04	1.24	.05	7.7	.79	0.0	40.8	.26	22.95	233.75	2.57
LOBSTER, SPINY, MIXED SPECIES														
moist-heat cooked	3 oz	17	.01	.05	4.16	.15	0.9	3.43	1.8	53.55	1.2	43.35	176.8	6.18
raw	3 oz	14	.01	.04	3.61	.13	0.5	2.98	1.7	41.65	1.04	34.0	153.0	4.82
LOBSTER PASTE, canned	1 tsp	4	0	.02	.13	na	na	na	0.0	8.05	.22	na	8.54	na
LOGANBERRY, frozen	1 cup	51	.07	.05	1.23	.1	37.8	0	22.5	38.22	.94	30.87	213.15	.5
LONGAN, DRIED	100 gm	0	.04	.5	1.0	.1	na	0	28.0	45.0	5.4	46.0	658.0	.22
LOOFAH GOURD. See GOURD, DISHCLOTH.														
LOQUAT/Japanese medlar														
trimmed, .6 oz	1 med	151	0	0	.02	na	na	0	0.1	1.58	.03	1.29	26.33	0
LOTTE. See MONKFISH.														
LOTUS ROOT														
boiled, drained, 2.5 inch diam	10 slices	0	.11	.01	.27	.19	7.0	0	24.4	23.14	.8	19.58	323.07	.29
raw, 2.5 inch diam	10 slices	0	.13	.18	.32	.21	10.3	0	35.6	36.45	.94	18.63	450.36	.32
raw, 9.5 inches long	1 root	0	.18	.25	.46	.3	14.6	0	50.6	51.75	1.33	26.45	639.4	.45
LOTUS SEED														
dried	1 cup	16	.2	.05	.51	.2	33.2	0	0.0	52.16	1.13	67.2	437.76	.34
dried, approx 42 medium seeds	1 oz	14	.18	.04	.45	.18	29.5	0	0.0	46.29	1.0	59.64	388.51	.3
raw	1 oz	4	.05	.01	.12	.05	7.9	0	0.0	12.5	.27	15.9	104.23	.08
LOX. See SALMON, CHINOOK.														
LUNCHEON MEAT, CANNED. See also POTTED MEAT SPREAD; SANDWICH SPREAD.														
(Spam)	1 oz	na	na	na	na	na	na	na	na	na	na	na	116	na
(Spam) less salt	2 oz	na	na	na	na	na	na	na	na	na	na	na	320	na
(Spam) lite	2 oz	na	na	na	na	na	na	na	na	na	na	na	350	na
LUPIN, mature seeds														
boiled	1/2 cup	6	.11	.04	.41	.01	49.2	0	0.9	42.33	1.0	44.82	203.35	1.15
raw	1/2 cup	21	.58	.2	1.97	.32	319.5	0	4.3	158.4	3.92	178.2	911.7	4.28
LYCHEE. See LITCHI.														

M

Food Name	Serving Size	A I.U.	Thi mg	Rib mg	Nia mg	B$_6$ mg	Fol mcg	B$_{12}$ mcg	C mg	Calc mg	Iron mg	Mag mg	Pot mg	Zn mg
MACADAMIA NUT/bushnut														
shelled	1 cup	0	.47	.15	2.87	.26	21.0	0	0.0	93.8	3.23	155.44	493.12	2.29
shelled	1 oz	0	.1	.03	.61	.06	4.5	0	0.0	19.88	.68	32.94	104.51	.49
shelled, oil roasted, kernels, 10-12	1 oz	3	.06	.03	.57	.06	4.5	0	0.0	12.78	.51	33.23	93.44	.31
shelled, oil roasted, whole or halves	1 cup	12	.29	.15	2.71	.27	21.3	0	0.0	60.3	2.41	156.78	440.86	1.47
MACADAMIA NUT BUTTER, roasted														
(Maranatha Natural)	2 tbsp	na	na	na	na	na	na	na	na	na	na	na	115	na
MACARONI. See PASTA.														
MACARONI ENTRÉE, FROZEN														
W/BEEF														
W/tomatoes (Stouffer's) 11.5-oz pkg	11.5-oz pkg	na	na	na	na	na	na	na	na	na	na	na	300	na
W/CHEESE														
(Stouffer's) 76-oz pkg	9.5 oz	na	na	na	na	na	na	na	na	na	na	na	260	na
(Stouffer's) 20-oz pkg	5 oz	na	na	na	na	na	na	na	na	na	na	na	120	na
(Stouffer's) 12-oz pkg	6 oz	na	na	na	na	na	na	na	na	na	na	na	140	na
Organic (Amy's Kitchen)	9 oz	na	na	na	na	na	na	na	na	na	na	na	334	na

Food Name	Serving Size	A I.U.	Thi mg	Rib mg	Nia mg	B6 mg	Fol mcg	B12 mcg	C mg	Calc mg	Iron mg	Mag mg	Pot mg	Zn mg
MACARONI ENTRÉE, MICROWAVE														
W/CHEESE														
(Kid's Kitchen) microwave cup	7.5 oz	na	na	na	na	na	na	na	na	na	na	na	209	na
MACE														
ground	1 tbsp	42	.02	.02	.07	na	na	0	na	13.37	.74	8.66	24.53	.12
ground	1 tsp	14	.01	.01	.02	na	na	0	na	4.29	.24	2.78	7.87	.04
ground (Durkee)	1 tsp	.23	.11	.16	0	na	na	na	na	0	0	na	0	na
ground (Laurel Leaf)	1 tsp	.23	.11	.16	0	na	na	na	na	0	0	na	0	na
MACKEREL														
ATLANTIC														
dry-heat cooked	3 oz	153	.14	.35	5.82	.39	1.3	16.15	0.3	12.75	1.33	82.45	340.85	.8
raw	3 oz	140	.15	.27	7.72	.34	1.1	7.4	0.3	10.2	1.39	64.6	266.9	.54
JACK, mixed species														
canned, drained	1 cup	825	.08	.4	11.74	.4	9.5	13.19	1.7	457.9	3.88	70.3	368.6	1.94
dry-heat cooked	3 oz	40	.11	.46	9.07	.32	1.7	3.6	1.8	24.65	1.27	30.6	442.85	.73
raw	3 oz	37	.09	.36	7.07	.28	1.7	3.74	1.7	19.55	.99	23.8	345.1	.57
KING														
dry-heat cooked	3 oz	713	.1	.49	8.89	.43	7.7	15.3	1.4	34.0	1.94	34.85	474.3	.61
raw	3 oz	618	.09	.4	7.3	.38	6.5	13.26	1.4	26.35	1.51	27.2	369.75	.48
PACIFIC, mixed species														
dry-heat cooked	3 oz	40	.11	.46	9.07	.32	1.7	3.6	1.8	24.65	1.27	30.6	442.85	.73
raw	3 oz	37	.09	.36	7.07	.28	1.7	3.74	1.7	19.55	.99	23.8	345.1	.57
SPANISH														
dry-heat cooked	3 oz	93	.11	.18	4.25	.39	1.0	5.95	1.4	11.05	.63	32.3	470.9	.53
raw	3 oz	85	.11	.14	1.95	.34	0.9	2.04	1.4	9.35	.37	28.05	379.1	.42
MAHI MAHI / dolphin fish														
dry-heat cooked	3 oz	177	.02	.07	6.31	.39	5.1	.59	0.0	16.15	1.23	32.3	453.05	.5
raw	3 oz	153	.02	.06	5.18	.34	4.3	.51	0.0	12.75	.96	25.5	353.6	.39
MALT, DRY	1 oz	0	.14	.09	2.52	na	na	na	0.0	13.44	1.12	na	64.4	na
MALT EXTRACT, DRIED	1 oz	0	.1	.13	2.74	na	na	na	0.0	13.44	2.44	na	64.4	na
MALT LIQUOR. See ALCOHOLIC BEVERAGES.														
MALT SYRUP														
....	1 cup	0	.04	1.51	31.18	1.92	46.1	0	0.0	234.24	3.69	276.48	1228.8	.54
....	1 tbsp	0	0	.09	1.95	.12	2.9	0	0.0	14.64	.23	17.28	76.8	.03
MALTED MILK DRINK MIX. See also BREAKFAST DRINK MIX, INSTANT.														
CHOCOLATE FLAVOR, w/added nutrients	4-5 heap tsp	2751	.64	.86	10.7	.92	19.6	.04	31.5	93.03	3.65	20.16	250.53	.22
NATURAL FLAVOR														
w/added nutrients	4-5 heap tsp	2222	.62	.75	10.2	.76	9.7	.16	27.2	78.96	3.49	13.86	203.49	.15
w/o added nutrients	3/4 oz	61	.11	.19	1.1	.09	9.7	.16	0.6	62.58	.15	19.53	159.18	.21
MAMMY APPLE														
raw	3 1/2 oz	230	.02	.04	.4	na	na	0	14.0	11.0	.7	na	47.0	na
raw, trimmed, approx 3.1 lb	1 med	1946	.17	.34	3.38	na	na	0	118.4	93.06	5.92	na	397.62	na
MANGO														
raw, sliced	1 cup	6425	.1	.09	.96	.22	na	0	45.7	16.5	.21	14.85	257.4	.07
raw, trimmed, approx 10.6 oz	1 med	8061	.12	.12	1.21	.28	na	0	57.3	20.7	.27	18.63	322.92	.08
MANGO DRINK														
(Kern's) nectar, canned or bottled	6 oz	na	na	na	na	na	na	na	na	na	na	na	60	na
(Libby's) nectar, canned or bottled	6 oz	na	na	na	na	na	na	na	na	na	na	na	30	na
MAPLE SYRUP. See also PANCAKE SYRUP.														
....	1 cup	0	.02	.03	.09	.01	0.0	0	0.0	211.05	3.78	44.1	642.6	13.1
....	1 tbsp	0	0	0	.01	0	0.0	0	0.0	13.4	.24	2.8	40.8	.83
MARGARINE														
hydrogenated and regular corn oil	1 stick	3750	.01	.04	.03	.01	1.3	.11	0.2	33.91	0	2.95	48.08	0
hydrogenated and regular corn oil	1 tsp	155	0	0	0	0	0.1	0	0.0	1.41	0	.12	1.99	0
hydrogenated and regular soybean oil	1 stick	3750	.01	.04	.03	.01	1.3	.11	0.2	33.91	0	2.95	48.08	na
hydrogenated and regular soybean oil	1 tsp	155	0	0	0	0	0.1	0	0.0	1.41	0	.12	1.99	na
hydrogenated safflower and soybean oil ...	1 stick	3750	.01	.04	.03	.01	1.3	.11	0.2	33.91	0	2.95	48.08	0

Food Name	Serving Size	A I.U.	Thi mg	Rib mg	Nia mg	B$_6$ mg	Fol mcg	B$_{12}$ mcg	C mg	Calc mg	Iron mg	Mag mg	Pot mg	Zn mg
hydrogenated safflower and soybean oil	1 tsp	155	0	0	0	0	0.1	0	0.0	1.41	0	.12	1.99	0
hydrogenated soybean and cottonseed oil	1 stick	3750	.01	.04	.03	.01	1.3	.11	0.2	33.91	0	2.95	48.08	0
hydrogenated soybean and cottonseed oil	1 tsp	155	0	0	0	0	0.1	0	0.0	1.41	0	.12	1.99	0
(Blue Bonnet) stick	1 tbsp	na	na	na	na	na	na	na	na	na	na	na	5	na
(Fleischmann's)														
reduced calorie, 'Diet'	1 tbsp	na	na	na	na	na	na	na	na	na	na	na	70	na
stick	1 tbsp	na	na	na	na	na	na	na	na	na	na	na	5	na
unsalted, stick	1 tbsp	na	na	na	na	na	na	na	na	na	na	na	0	na
MARGARINE, ALTERNATIVE														
hydrogenated and regular corn oil	1 cup	7672	.01	.05	.03	.01	1.7	.13	0.2	41.3	0	3.6	58.7	0
hydrogenated and regular corn oil	1 tsp	159	0	0	0	0	0.0	0	0.0	.85	0	.07	1.21	0
hydrogenated soybean and cottonseed oil	1 cup	7672	.01	.05	.03	.01	1.7	.13	0.2	41.3	0	3.6	58.7	0
hydrogenated soybean and cottonseed oil	1 tsp	159	0	0	0	0	0.0	0	0.0	.85	0	.07	1.21	0
hydrogenated soybean oil	1 cup	7672	.01	.05	.03	.01	1.7	.13	0.2	41.3	0	3.6	58.7	0
hydrogenated soybean oil	1 tsp	159	0	0	0	0	0.0	0	0.0	.85	0	.07	1.21	0
MARGARINE, SOFT														
(Blue Bonnet)	1 tbsp	na	na	na	na	na	na	na	na	na	na	na	5	na
(Fleischmann's)														
lightly salted	1 tbsp	na	na	na	na	na	na	na	na	na	na	na	5	na
unsalted	1 tbsp	na	na	na	na	na	na	na	na	na	na	na	0	na
MARGARINE, WHIPPED														
(Blue Bonnet) stick	1 tbsp	na	na	na	na	na	na	na	na	na	na	na	0	na
(Fleischmann's)														
lightly salted	1 tbsp	na	na	na	na	na	na	na	na	na	na	na	0	na
unsalted	1 tbsp	na	na	na	na	na	na	na	na	na	na	na	0	na
MARGARINE SPREAD														
hydrogenated soybean and cottonseed oil, tub	1 cup	7573	.02	.06	.04	.01	1.9	.15	0.3	47.86	0	4.17	68.24	0
hydrogenated soybean and cottonseed oil, tub	1 tsp	159	0	0	0	0	0.0	0	0.0	1.0	0	.09	1.43	0
hydrogenated soybean and hydrogenated and regular palm oils	1 tsp	159	0	0	0	0	0.0	0	0.0	1.0	0	.09	1.43	0
hydrogenated soybean and hydrogenated and regular palm oils, tub	1 cup	7573	.02	.06	.04	.01	1.9	.15	0.3	47.86	0	4.17	68.24	0
hydrogenated soybean and palm oil, stick	1 cup	7573	.02	.06	.04	.01	1.9	.15	0.3	47.86	0	4.17	68.24	0
hydrogenated soybean and palm oil, stick	1 tsp	159	0	0	0	0	0.0	0	0.0	1.0	0	.09	1.43	0
60% corn oil margarine, 40% butter	1 stick	3624	.01	.04	.04	.01	2.3	.07	0.1	31.64	.07	2.26	40.68	.02
60% corn oil margarine, 40% butter	1 tsp	160	0	0	0	0	0.1	0	0.0	1.4	0	.1	1.8	0
(Blue Bonnet)														
48% vegetable oil	1 tbsp	na	na	na	na	na	na	na	na	na	na	na	5	na
whipped, 60% vegetable oil	1 tbsp	na	na	na	na	na	na	na	na	na	na	na	5	na
(Blue Bonnet) 'Better Blend'														
soft	1 tbsp	na	na	na	na	na	na	na	na	na	na	na	10	na
unsalted	1 tbsp	na	na	na	na	na	na	na	na	na	na	na	0	na
MARGARITA. See ALCOHOLIC BEVERAGES.														
MARINADE. See individual listings.														
MARJORAM														
dried	1 tbsp	137	0	.01	.07	na	na	0	0.9	33.83	1.41	5.88	25.87	.06
dried	1 tsp	48	0	0	.02	na	na	0	0.3	11.94	.5	2.08	9.13	.02
dried (Durkee)	1 tsp	.29	.01	.01	0	na	na	na	0	0	0	na	0	na
dried (Laurel Leaf)	1 tsp	.29	.01	.01	0	na	na	na	0	0	0	na	0	na
MARMALADE PLUM. See SAPOTE.														
MARSHMALLOW														
(Kraft) 'Jet Puffed'	1 piece	na	na	na	na	na	na	na	na	na	na	na	0	na
(Kraft) miniature	10 pieces	na	na	na	na	na	na	na	na	na	na	na	0	na
MARTINI. See ALCOHOLIC BEVERAGES.														
MASA HARINA. See CORN FLOUR.														

Food Name	Serving Size	A I.U.	Thi mg	Rib mg	Nia mg	B6 mg	Fol mcg	B12 mcg	C mg	Calc mg	Iron mg	Mag mg	Pot mg	Zn mg
MATAI. See WATER CHESTNUT, CHINESE.														
MATZO. See CRACKER.														
MAYONNAISE														
(Westbrae)	1 tbsp	na	na	na	na	na	na	na	na	na	na	na	75	na
CANOLA (Westbrae)	1 tbsp	na	na	na	na	na	na	na	na	na	na	na	7	na
MEAT. See individual listings.														
MEAT, ALTERNATIVE. See individual listings.														
MEAT EXTENDER														
soybean	1 cup	28	.62	.78	19.38	1.18	174.2	5.28	0.0	179.52	10.55	190.08	1673.76	1.94
soybean	1 oz	9	.2	.25	6.17	.37	55.4	1.68	0.0	57.12	3.36	60.48	532.56	.62
MEAT LOAF ENTRÉE, FROZEN														
(Armour) 'Classics'	11.25 oz	na	na	na	na	na	na	na	na	na	na	na	590	na
(Stouffer's) homestyle, in gravy, w/whipped														
potatoes	9 7/8 oz	na	na	na	na	na	na	na	na	na	na	na	490	na
MEAT LOAF MIX														
(Hunt's) 'Meatloaf Fixins'	2.222 oz	na	na	na	na	na	na	na	4.2	1.09	2.41	na	na	na
MEAT STICKS														
smoked	1 oz	428	.04	.12	1.29	.06	0.0	.28	1.9	19.28	.96	5.95	72.86	.69
smoked	1 stick	299	.03	.09	.9	.04	0.0	.2	1.4	13.46	.67	4.16	50.89	.48
MEATBALL ENTRÉE														
Canned, stew (Dinty Moore)	8 oz	na	na	na	na	na	na	na	na	na	na	na	525	na
Microwave (Dinty Moore) microwave cup	7.5 oz	na	na	na	na	na	na	na	na	na	na	na	525	na
MELBA TOAST. See CRACKER.														
MELON. See individual listings.														
MELON, BITTER. See BALSAM PEAR.														
MELON BALLS, FROZEN														
cantaloupe and honeydew	1 cup	3069	.29	.04	1.11	.18	44.5	0	10.7	17.3	.5	24.22	484.4	.29
MENUDO MIX (Gebhardt) spice	.0141 oz	na	na	na	na	na	na	na	0.6	.08	.17	na	na	na
MEXICAN FOODS. See individual listings.														
MEXICAN STYLE DINNER, FROZEN. See individual listings.														
MILK, COW'S, CANNED														
CONDENSED, SWEETENED														
	1 cup	1004	.28	1.27	.64	.16	34.3	1.36	8.0	867.51	.58	78.49	1136.48	2.88
(Carnation)	1/3 cup	302	.09	.32	.2	.08	10.4	.83	1.4	260	.07	22.8	370	.84
EVAPORATED														
	1/2 cup	306	.06	.4	.24	.06	10.0	.21	2.4	328.61	.24	30.48	381.91	.97
(Carnation)	1/2 cup	200	.06	.4	.24	.06	10.0	.2	0.6	329	.24	30	380	.97
Low-fat (Carnation)	1/2 cup	500	.04	.39	.2	.06	10.0	.27	0.8	320	.29	36	400	1.01
Skim														
	1/2 cup	502	.06	.4	.22	.07	11.0	.31	1.6	370.56	.37	34.56	424.32	1.15
(Carnation) 'Lite'	1/2 cup	500	.06	.39	.22	.07	11.0	.3	1.6	369	.37	34	420	1.15
MILK, COW'S, DRY														
SKIM														
(Saco Foods)	5 tbsp	na	na	na	na	na	na	na	na	na	na	na	390	na
(Sanalac) reconstituted	9.03 oz	na	na	na	na	na	na	na	2.5	28.5	.3	na	na	na
MILK, COW'S, FLUID														
WHOLE (Carnation)	1 cup	307	.09	.4	.2	.1	12.0	.87	3.3	291	.12	33	370	.93
Low-sodium	1 cup	317	.05	.26	.1	.08	12.2	.88	2.3	245.95	.12	12.2	616.83	.93
3.7% fat	1 cup	337	.09	.39	.2	.1	12.2	.87	3.6	290.36	.12	32.7	368.44	.93
3.3% fat	1 cup	307	.09	.4	.2	.1	12.2	.87	2.3	291.34	.12	32.79	369.66	.93
2% FAT	1 cup	500	.1	.4	.21	.1	12.4	.89	2.3	296.7	.12	33.35	376.74	.95
Protein-fortified	1 cup	499	.11	.48	.25	.13	14.8	1.05	2.8	352.03	.15	39.56	446.98	1.11
1% FAT														
Protein-fortified	1 cup	499	.11	.47	.25	.12	14.5	1.05	2.8	349.32	.15	39.26	443.54	1.11
W/non-fat milk solids added	1 cup	500	.1	.42	.22	.11	13.0	.94	2.5	312.87	.12	35.16	397.15	.98

Food Name	Serving Size	A I.U.	Thi mg	Rib mg	Nia mg	B₆ mg	Fol mcg	B₁₂ mcg	C mg	Calc mg	Iron mg	Mag mg	Pot mg	Zn mg
SKIM														
Protein-fortified														
W/non-fat milk solids added	1 cup	500	.1	.43	.22	.11	13.2	.95	2.5	316.3	.12	35.55	418.22	1.0
W/vitamin A added	1 cup	500	.09	.34	.22	.1	12.7	.93	2.4	302.33	.1	27.83	405.72	.98
MILK, GOAT'S														
evaporated *(Meyenberg)* canned, undiluted	4 oz	270	.07	.37	.64	.08	0.1	.04	na	244	.35	36	120	.94
fluid, whole	1 cup	451	.12	.34	.68	.11	1.5	.16	3.2	325.74	.12	34.09	498.74	.73
MILK, HUMAN														
fluid, whole	1 cup	593	.03	.09	.44	.03	12.8	.11	12.3	79.21	.07	8.36	125.95	.42
fluid, whole	1 oz	74	0	.01	.05	0	1.6	.01	1.5	9.92	.01	1.05	15.77	.05
MILK, INDIA BUFFALO, fluid, whole	1 cup	434	.13	.33	.22	.06	13.7	.89	5.5	412.36	.29	75.93	433.59	.54
MILK, REINDEER	1 cup	372	.07	.42	.25	na	na	na	2.5	629.92	.25	na	394.32	na
MILK, SHEEP'S, fluid, whole	1 cup	360	.16	.87	1.02	.15	17.2	1.74	10.2	473.83	.25	44.98	334.42	1.32
MILKFISH. See AWA.														
MILKSHAKE														
chocolate, thick	10.6 oz	258	.14	.67	.37	.07	14.7	.95	0.0	396.0	.93	48.0	672.0	1.44
vanilla, thick	11 oz	357	.09	.61	.46	.13	20.7	1.63	0.0	457.29	.31	36.81	571.85	1.22
MILLET														
pearl, cooked	1/2 cup	0	.13	.1	1.6	.13	22.8	0	0.0	3.6	.76	52.8	74.4	1.09
pearl, raw	1/2 cup	0	.42	.29	4.72	.38	85.0	0	0.0	8.0	3.01	114.0	·195.0	1.68
MISO														
	1/2 cup	120	.13	.35	1.19	.3	45.5	0	0.0	91.08	3.78	57.96	226.32	4.58
soybean and rice/kome, organic														
(Eden Foods)	1 tbsp	na	na	na	na	na	na	na	na	na	na	na	55	na
MOLASSES														
	1 cup	0	.13	.01	3.05	2.2	0.0	0	0.0	672.4	15.48	793.76	4801.92	.95
	1 tbsp	0	.01	0	.19	.13	0.0	0	0.0	41.0	.94	48.4	292.8	.06
Barbados	1 cup	0	.2	.66	.66	na	na	na	0.0	803.6	14.1	na	3007.76	na
Barbados	1 oz	0	.02	.08	.08	na	na	na	0.0	100.45	1.76	na	375.97	na
1st extraction/light	1 cup	0	.20	.2	.66	na	na	na	0.0	541.2	14.1	na	3007.76	na
1st extraction/light	1 oz	0	.03	.02	.08	na	na	na	0.0	67.65	1.76	na	375.97	na
2nd extraction/medium	1 cup	0	.3	.39	3.94	na	na	na	0.0	951.2	19.68	na	3486.64	na
2nd extraction/medium	1 oz	0	.04	.05	.49	na	na	na	0.0	118.9	2.46	na	435.83	na
3rd extraction/blackstrap	1 cup	0	.11	.17	3.54	2.3	3.3	0	0.0	2820.8	57.4	705.2	8173.76	3.28
3rd extraction/blackstrap	1 tbsp	0	.01	.01	.22	.14	0.2	0	0.0	172.0	3.5	43.0	498.4	.2
(Br'er Rabbit) dark	1 oz	na	na	na	na	na	na	na	na	na	na	na	750	na
(Br'er Rabbit) light	1 oz	na	na	na	na	na	na	na	na	na	na	na	670	na
(LaChoy) bead	.7055 oz	na	na	na	na	na	na	na	0.0	19.21	25.95	na	na	na
MONKFISH/angler fish/bellyfish/frogfish/goosefish/lotte/sea devil														
dry-heat cooked	3 oz	39	.02	.06	2.17	.24	6.8	.88	0.9	8.5	.35	22.95	436.05	.45
raw	3 oz	34	.02	.05	1.78	.2	6.0	.77	0.9	6.8	.27	17.85	340.0	.35
MOOSE														
raw	1 lb	0	.27	1.22	22.68	na	na	na	18.1	22.68	14.56	104.33	1437.91	12.7
raw	1 oz	0	.02	.08	1.4	na	na	na	1.1	1.4	.9	6.44	88.76	.78
roasted	3 oz	0	.04	.29	4.47	na	na	na	4.3	5.1	3.59	20.4	283.9	3.13
MOTH BEAN														
boiled	1/2 cup	9	.11	.02	.59	.08	126.1	0	0.9	2.64	2.76	91.52	267.52	.52
raw	1/2 cup	31	.55	.09	2.74	.36	635.9	0	3.9	147.0	10.63	373.38	1167.18	1.88
MOUNTAIN YAM. See YAM.														
MOUSSE MIX														
(Jell-O) 'Rich & Luscious' chocolate, dry mix	1 pkg	na	na	na	na	na	na	na	na	na	na	na	170	na
(Jell-O) 'Rich & Luscious' chocolate, prepared	1/2 cup	na	na	na	na	na	na	na	na	na	na	na	260	na
(Jell-O) 'Rich & Luscious' chocolate fudge, dry mix	1 pkg	na	na	na	na	na	na	na	na	na	na	na	230	na

Food Name	Serving Size	A I.U.	Thi mg	Rib mg	Nia mg	B6 mg	Fol mcg	B12 mcg	C mg	Calc mg	Iron mg	Mag mg	Pot mg	Zn mg
(Jell-O) 'Rich & Luscious' chocolate fudge, prepared	1/2 cup	na	na	na	na	na	na	na	na	na	na	na	320	na
MUFFIN. See also ENGLISH MUFFIN.														
BANANA NUT *(Break Cake)* .5-oz muffin	1 muffin	na	na	na	na	na	na	na	na	na	na	na	25	na
BLUEBERRY *(Break Cake)*	1 muffin	na	na	na	na	na	na	na	na	na	na	na	15	na
MUFFIN / PASTRY, TOASTER														
APPLE														
(Pastry Poppers) fruit juice sweetened, low-sodium, 2 oz each	1 pastry	na	na	na	na	na	na	na	na	49	na	na	.28	na
(Toastettes) 'Frosted Tarts' 1.5 oz each	1 pastry	na	na	na	na	na	na	na	na	na	na	na	45	na
(Toastettes) 'Tarts' 1.5 oz each	1 pastry	na	na	na	na	na	na	na	na	na	na	na	45	na
BANANA NUT														
(Pastry Poppers) fruit juice sweetened, low-sodium, 2 oz each	1 pastry	na	na	na	na	na	na	na	na	54	na	na	.28	na
BLUEBERRY														
(Toastettes) 'Frosted Tarts' 1.5 oz each	1 pastry	na	na	na	na	na	na	na	na	na	na	na	50	na
(Toastettes) 'Tarts' 1.5 oz each	1 pastry	na	na	na	na	na	na	na	na	na	na	na	50	na
BROWN SUGAR-CINNAMON														
(Toastettes) 'Frosted Tarts' 1.5 oz each	1 pastry	na	na	na	na	na	na	na	na	na	na	na	65	na
CHERRY														
(Toastettes) 'Frosted Tarts' 1.5 oz each	1 pastry	na	na	na	na	na	na	na	na	na	na	na	50	na
(Toastettes) 'Tarts' 1.5 oz each	1 pastry	na	na	na	na	na	na	na	na	na	na	na	50	na
FRUIT PUNCH														
(Toastettes) 'Frosted Tarts' 1.5 oz each	1 pastry	na	na	na	na	na	na	na	na	na	na	na	50	na
FUDGE														
(Toastettes) 'Frosted Tarts' 1.5 oz each	1 pastry	na	na	na	na	na	na	na	na	na	na	na	80	na
PEACH-APRICOT														
(Pastry Poppers) fruit juice sweetened, low-sodium, 2 oz each	1 pastry	na	na	na	na	na	na	na	na	54	na	na	.28	na
RASPBERRY														
(Pastry Poppers) fruit juice sweetened, low-sodium, 2 oz each	1 pastry	na	na	na	na	na	na	na	na	54	na	na	.28	na
STRAWBERRY														
(Pastry Poppers) fruit juice sweetened, low-sodium, 2 oz each	1 pastry	na	na	na	na	na	na	na	na	54	na	na	.28	na
(Toastettes) 'Frosted Tarts' 1.5 oz each	1 pastry	na	na	na	na	na	na	na	na	na	na	na	50	na
(Toastettes) 'Tarts' 1.5 oz each	1 pastry	na	na	na	na	na	na	na	na	na	na	na	50	na
MULBERRY, raw	1 cup	35	.04	.14	.87	na	na	0	51.0	54.6	2.59	25.2	271.6	na
MULLET, STRIPED														
dry-heat cooked	3 oz	120	.09	.09	5.35	.42	8.3	.21	1.0	26.35	1.2	28.05	389.3	.75
raw	3 oz	104	.08	.07	4.42	.36	7.2	.19	1.0	34.85	.87	24.65	303.45	.44
MUNG BEAN														
boiled	1/2 cup	24	.17	.06	.58	.07	160.4	0	1.0	27.27	1.41	48.48	268.66	.85
raw	1/2 cup	119	.65	.24	2.34	.4	649.9	0	5.0	137.28	7.01	196.56	1295.84	2.79
sprouted, boiled, drained	1/2 cup	9	.03	.06	.51	.03	18.2	0	7.1	7.44	.4	8.68	62.62	.29
sprouted, raw	1/2 cup	11	.04	.06	.39	.05	31.6	0	6.9	6.76	.47	10.92	77.48	.21
sprouted, stir-fried	1/2 cup	19	.09	.11	.74	.08	43.2	0	9.9	8.06	1.18	20.46	135.78	.56
MUNG BEAN, CANNED, sprouted, drained	1/2 cup	14	.02	.04	.14	.02	6.0	0	0.2	8.68	.27	5.58	16.74	.17
MUNG BEAN LONG RICE, dehydrated	1/2 cup	0	.11	0	.14	.03	1.4	0	0.0	17.5	1.52	2.1	7.0	.29
MUNGO BEAN														
boiled	1/2 cup	28	.14	.07	1.35	.05	85.0	0	0.9	47.7	1.58	56.7	207.9	.75
raw	1/2 cup	119	.37	.29	1.87	.29	653.3	0	5.0	203.84	7.11	270.4	1066.0	3.2
MUSHROOM, ENOKI														
raw	1 large	0	0	.01	.18	0	1.5	0	0.6	.05	.04	.8	19.05	.03
raw	1 med	0	0	0	.11	0	0.9	0	0.4	.03	.03	.48	11.43	.02
MUSHROOM, SHIITAKE, cooked, pieces	1 cup	0	.05	.25	2.17	.23	30.3	0	0.4	4.35	.64	20.3	169.65	1.93

Food Name	Serving Size	A I.U.	Thi mg	Rib mg	Nia mg	B₆ mg	Fol mcg	B₁₂ mcg	C mg	Calc mg	Iron mg	Mag mg	Pot mg	Zn mg
MUSHROOM, WHITE														
boiled, drained, pieces	1/2 cup	0	.06	.23	3.48	.07	14.2	0	3.1	4.68	1.36	9.36	277.68	.68
raw, pieces	1/2 cup	0	.04	.16	1.44	.03	7.4	0	1.2	1.75	.43	3.5	129.5	.26
Canned, pieces, drained	1/2 cup	0	.07	.02	1.24	.05	9.6	0	0.0	8.58	.62	11.7	100.62	.56
Frozen														
(Birds Eye) whole, 'Deluxe'	2.6 oz	na	na	na	na	na	na	na	na	na	na	na	280	na
(Freshlike)	3.5 oz	na	na	na	na	na	na	na	na	na	na	na	410	na
MUSKMELON. See CANTALOUPE.														
MUSKRAT														
raw	1 lb	0	.41	2.36	28.12	na	na	na	22.7	113.4	na	99.79	1251.94	na
raw	1 oz	0	.03	.15	1.74	na	na	na	1.4	7.0	na	6.16	77.28	na
roasted	3 oz	0	.07	.6	6.11	.4	9.4	7.06	6.0	30.6	6.04	22.1	272.0	1.93
MUSSEL, BLUE														
moist-heat cooked	3 oz	258	.26	.36	2.55	.09	64.3	20.4	11.6	28.05	5.71	31.45	227.8	2.27
raw	1 cup	240	.24	.31	2.4	.07	63.0	18.0	12.0	39.0	5.93	51.0	480.0	2.4
raw	3 oz	136	.14	.18	1.36	.04	35.7	10.2	6.8	22.1	3.36	28.9	272.0	1.36
MUSTARD, PREPARED														
(Grey Poupon) 'Parisian'	1 tsp	na	na	na	na	na	na	na	na	na	na	na	5	na
(Westbrae) 'Mt. Fuji'	1 tbsp	na	na	na	na	na	na	na	na	na	na	na	40	na
DIJON														
(Grey Poupon) 'Country style'	1 tsp	na	na	na	na	na	na	na	na	na	na	na	10	na
(Westbrae)	1 tbsp	na	na	na	na	na	na	na	na	na	na	na	40	na
SPICY (Heinz) 'Brown'	1 tbsp	na	na	na	na	na	na	na	na	na	na	na	20	na
STONE GROUND (Westbrae)	1 tbsp	na	na	na	na	na	na	na	na	na	na	na	40	na
YELLOW														
(Heinz) 'Mild'	1 tbsp	na	na	na	na	na	na	na	na	na	na	na	20	na
(Westbrae)	1 tbsp	na	na	na	na	na	na	na	na	na	na	na	40	na
MUSTARD GREENS														
boiled, drained, chopped	1/2 cup	2122	.03	.04	.3	.07	51.4	0	17.7	51.8	.49	10.5	141.4	.08
raw, chopped	1/2 cup	1484	.02	.03	.22	.05	52.5	0	19.0	28.84	.41	8.96	99.12	.06
Frozen														
boiled, drained	10-oz pkg	9476	.08	.11	.55	.23	147.3	0	29.3	214.12	2.37	27.56	294.68	.42
boiled, drained, chopped	1/2 cup	3353	.03	.04	.19	.08	52.1	0	10.4	75.75	.84	9.75	104.25	.15
chopped	1/2 cup	3763	.04	.04	.23	.1	101.0	0	18.5	84.68	.94	10.95	124.1	.17
unprepared	10-oz pkg	14640	.14	.17	.89	.37	392.8	0	71.9	329.44	3.66	42.6	482.8	.65
MUSTARD OIL														
	1 cup	0	0	0	0	0	0.0	0	0.0	0	0	0	0	0
	1 tbsp	0	0	0	0	0	0.0	0	0.0	0	0	0	0	0
MUSTARD POWDER														
ground (Durkee)	1 tsp	.07	.71	.49	.01	na	na	na	.02	0	.01	na	0	na
ground (Laurel Leaf)	1 tsp	.07	.71	.49	.01	na	na	na	.02	0	.01	na	0	na
MUSTARD SEED, YELLOW														
whole	1 tbsp	7	.06	.04	.88	na	na	0	na	58.37	1.12	33.42	76.43	.64
whole	1 tsp	2	.02	.01	.26	na	na	0	na	17.2	.33	9.85	22.52	.19
MUSTARD SPINACH / tendergreen														
boiled, drained, chopped	1/2 cup	7380	.04	.06	.39	.09	65.5	0	58.5	142.2	.72	6.3	256.5	.1
raw, chopped	1/2 cup	7425	.05	.07	.51	.11	119.2	0	97.5	157.5	1.13	8.25	336.75	.13
MUTTON TALLOW														
	1 cup	0	0	0	0	0	0.0	0	0.0	0	0	0	0	0
	1 tbsp	0	0	0	0	0	0.0	0	0.0	0	0	0	0	0

MUTTONFISH. See OCEAN POUT.

N

Food Name	Serving Size	A I.U.	Thi mg	Rib mg	Nia mg	B$_6$ mg	Fol mcg	B$_{12}$ mcg	C mg	Calc mg	Iron mg	Mag mg	Pot mg	Zn mg
NACHO CHIPS. See CORN CHIPS AND SNACKS.														
NATAL PLUM. See CARISSA.														
NATTO. See SOYBEAN, FERMENTED.														
NAVY BEAN														
boiled	1/2 cup	2	.18	.06	.48	.15	127.3	0	0.8	63.7	2.26	53.69	334.88	.96
raw	1/2 cup	4	.67	.24	2.15	.45	384.5	0	3.1	161.2	6.7	179.92	1185.6	2.64
NAVY BEAN, CANNED														
(Eden Foods) organic, very low sodium	1/2 cup	na	na	na	na	na	na	na	na	na	na	na	280	na
(Hunt's) w/ham 'Homestyle'	9.03 oz	na	na	na	na	na	na	na	8.5	16.11	22.61	na	na	na
NAVY BEAN, SPROUTED														
raw	1/2 cup	2	.2	.11	.63	.1	68.6	0	9.8	7.8	1.0	52.52	159.64	.46
NECTAR. See individual flavors.														
NECTARINE														
sliced	1 cup	1016	.02	.06	1.37	.03	5.1	0	7.5	6.9	.21	11.04	292.56	.12
trimmed, approx 2.5 inch diam	1 med	1001	.02	.06	1.35	.03	5.0	0	7.3	6.8	.2	10.88	288.32	.12
NEW ZEALAND SPINACH. See SPINACH, NEW ZEALAND.														
NOODLE. See NOODLE, CHINESE; NOODLE, EGG; NOODLE, JAPANESE; PASTA.														
NOODLE, CHINESE														
chow mein	1 cup	38	.26	.19	2.68	.05	9.9	0	0.0	9.0	2.13	23.4	54.0	.63
chow mein	1.5 oz	37	.25	.18	2.56	.05	9.5	0	0.0	8.6	2.03	22.36	51.6	.6
NOODLE, EGG														
(NOTE: All of the following egg noodles are dry unless otherwise noted.)														
DUMPLING (Creamette) w/pasteurized eggs	2 oz	na	na	na	na	na	na	na	na	na	na	na	110	na
ENRICHED														
	2 oz	35	.6	.27	4.58	.07	16.5	.23	0.0	17.67	2.59	34.2	133.38	.91
cooked	1 cup	32	.3	.13	2.38	.06	11.2	.14	0.0	19.2	2.54	30.4	44.8	.99
FINE (Herb's)	2 oz	na	na	na	na	na	na	na	na	na	na	na	135	na
SPINACH														
enriched	1 cup	120	.41	.18	2.5	.16	33.4	.15	0.0	21.28	1.6	31.16	134.9	.7
enriched	2 oz	180	.62	.27	3.75	.23	50.2	.23	0.0	31.92	2.39	46.74	202.35	1.04
enriched, cooked	1 cup	165	.39	.2	2.36	.18	33.6	.22	0.0	30.4	1.74	38.4	59.2	1.01
UNENRICHED														
	2 oz	0	.09	.01	.84	.05	1.7	0	0.0	5.7	.68	6.84	19.95	.28
cooked	1 cup	32	.05	.03	.64	.06	11.2	.14	0.0	19.2	.96	30.4	44.8	.99
WIDE														
(Creamette) w/pasteurized eggs 'Fancy'	2 oz	na	na	na	na	na	na	na	na	na	na	na	110	na
NOODLE, JAPANESE														
SOBA / BUCKWHEAT														
cooked	1 cup	0	.11	.03	.58	.05	8.0	0	0.0	4.56	.55	10.26	39.9	.14
dry	2 oz	0	.27	.07	1.83	.14	34.2	0	0.0	19.95	1.54	54.15	143.64	.97
SOMEN / WHEAT														
cooked	1 cup	0	.04	.06	.17	.02	3.5	0	0.0	14.08	.92	3.52	51.04	.39
dry	2 oz	0	.06	.01	.5	.03	8.0	0	0.0	13.11	.75	15.96	93.48	.26
NOODLE ENTRÉE / DISH														
(LaChoy)														
and beef	9.03 oz	na	na	na	na	na	na	na	8.1	3.28	4.4	na	na	na
and chicken	8.995 oz	na	na	na	na	na	na	na	5.1	3.13	8.07	na	na	na
and vegetables	9.383 oz	na	na	na	na	na	na	na	3.8	3.16	3.34	na	na	na
chow mein	2 tbsp	na	na	na	na	na	na	na	0.0	.68	2.52	na	na	na
crispy, wide	2 tbsp	na	na	na	na	na	na	na	0.0	.58	2.99	na	na	na
rice	2 tbsp	na	na	na	na	na	na	na	0.0	.48	1.73	na	na	na
NOODLE ENTRÉE / DISH, CANNED														
(Van Camp's) w/franks 'Noodle Weenee'	1 cup	672	.12	.2	2.11	na	na	na	na	47	5.98	na	289	na

Food Name	Serving Size	A I.U.	Thi mg	Rib mg	Nia mg	B₆ mg	Fol mcg	B₁₂ mcg	C mg	Calc mg	Iron mg	Mag mg	Pot mg	Zn mg
NOODLE ENTRÉE/DISH, FROZEN														
(Stouffer's) Romanoff	6 oz	na	na	na	na	na	na	na	na	na	na	na	90	na
NUTMEG														
ground	1 tbsp	7	.02	0	.09	na	na	0	na	12.91	.21	12.83	24.47	.15
ground	1 tsp	2	.01	0	.03	na	na	0	na	4.06	.07	4.03	7.69	.05
ground (Durkee)	1 tsp	.05	.17	.12	0	na	na	na	na	0	0	na	0	na
ground (Laurel Leaf)	1 tsp	.05	.17	.12	0	na	na	na	na	0	0	na	0	na
NUTMEG BUTTER OIL														
	1 cup	0	0	0	0	0	0.0	0	0.0	0	0	0	0	0
	1 tbsp	0	0	0	0	0	0.0	0	0.0	0	0	0	0	0
NUTS, MIXED														
Dry roasted														
w/peanuts	1 cup	21	.27	.27	6.44	.41	69.1	0	0.6	95.9	5.07	308.25	817.89	5.21
w/peanuts	1 oz	4	.06	.06	1.33	.08	14.3	0	0.1	19.88	1.05	63.9	169.55	1.08
w/peanuts, salted	1 cup	21	.27	.27	6.44	.41	69.1	0	0.6	95.9	5.07	308.25	817.89	5.21
w/peanuts, salted	1 oz	4	.06	.06	1.33	.08	14.3	0	0.1	19.88	1.05	63.9	169.55	1.08
Oil roasted														
salted	1 cup	29	.73	.7	2.83	.26	81.2	0	0.7	152.64	3.7	361.44	783.36	6.71
salted	1 oz	6	.14	.14	.56	.05	16.0	0	0.1	30.1	.73	71.28	154.5	1.32
w/peanuts	1 cup	27	.71	.32	7.19	.34	117.9	0	0.7	153.36	4.56	333.7	825.02	7.21
w/peanuts	1 oz	5	.14	.06	1.44	.07	23.6	0	0.1	30.67	.91	66.74	165.0	1.44
w/peanuts, salted	1 cup	27	.71	.32	7.19	.34	117.9	0	0.7	153.36	4.56	333.7	825.02	7.21
w/peanuts, salted	1 oz	5	.14	.06	1.44	.07	23.6	0	0.1	30.67	.91	66.74	165.0	1.44

O

Food Name	Serving Size	A I.U.	Thi mg	Rib mg	Nia mg	B₆ mg	Fol mcg	B₁₂ mcg	C mg	Calc mg	Iron mg	Mag mg	Pot mg	Zn mg
OAT. See CEREAL, HOT.														
OAT BRAN. See CEREAL, HOT.														
OAT VEGETABLE OIL														
	1 cup	0	0	0	0	0	0.0	0	0.0	0	0	0	0	0
	1 tbsp	0	0	0	0	0	0.0	0	0.0	0	0	0	0	0
OATMEAL. See CEREAL, HOT.														
OCEAN CATFISH. See WOLF FISH.														
OCEAN PERCH, ATLANTIC/red perch/redfish/rosefish/sea perch														
dry-heat cooked	3 oz	39	.11	.11	2.07	.23	8.8	.98	0.7	116.45	1.0	33.15	297.5	.52
OCEAN POUT/muttonfish														
dry-heat cooked	3 oz	39	.08	.06	2.17	.24	6.8	.88	0.0	11.05	.31	14.45	436.05	1.12
OCEANIC BONITO. See TUNA, SKIPJACK.														
OCTOPUS														
moist-heat cooked	3 oz	230	.05	.06	3.21	.55	20.4	30.6	6.8	90.1	8.11	51.0	535.5	2.86
OHELOBERRY														
raw	1 cup	1162	.02	.05	.38	na	na	0	8.4	9.8	.13	8.4	53.2	na
raw, approx .4 oz	10 fruits	91	0	0	.03	na	na	0	0.7	.77	.01	.66	4.18	na
OIL. See individual listings.														
OKRA/gumbo														
boiled, drained, approx 3 inches long	8 pods	489	.11	.05	.74	.16	38.9	0	13.9	53.55	.38	48.45	273.7	.47
boiled, drained, sliced	1/2 cup	460	.11	.04	.7	.15	36.6	0	13.0	50.4	.36	45.6	257.6	.44
raw, approx 3 inches long	8 pods	627	.19	.06	.95	.2	83.4	0	20.1	76.95	.76	54.15	287.85	.57
raw, sliced	1/2 cup	330	.1	.03	.5	.11	43.9	0	10.6	40.5	.4	28.5	151.5	.3
OKRA, FROZEN														
boiled, drained	10 oz	1311	.25	.31	2.0	.12	371.3	0	31.1	244.8	1.71	130.05	596.7	1.58
boiled, drained, sliced	1/2 cup	473	.09	.11	.72	.04	134.0	0	11.2	88.32	.62	46.92	215.28	.57
cut (Freshlike)	3.3 oz	na	na	na	na	na	na	na	na	na	na	na	180	na
whole (Freshlike)	3.3 oz	na	na	na	na	na	na	na	na	na	na	na	220	na

Food Name	Serving Size	A I.U.	Thi mg	Rib mg	Nia mg	B6 mg	Fol mcg	B12 mcg	C mg	Calc mg	Iron mg	Mag mg	Pot mg	Zn mg
OLIVE														
black, jumbo, canned	1 olive	29	0	0	0	0	0.0	0	0.1	7.8	.28	.33	.75	.02
black, large, canned	1 olive	18	0	0	0	0	0.0	0	0.0	3.87	.15	.18	.35	.01
black, small, canned	1 olive	13	0	0	0	0	0.0	0	0.0	2.82	.11	.13	.26	.01
black, super colossal, canned	1 olive	53	0	0	0	0	0.0	0	0.2	14.29	.5	.61	1.37	.03
ONION														
Mature														
chopped, boiled, drained	1/2 cup	0	.04	.02	.17	.14	15.8	0	5.5	23.1	.25	11.55	174.3	.22
chopped, boiled, drained	1 tbsp	0	.01	0	.02	.02	2.3	0	0.8	3.3	.04	1.65	24.9	.03
raw (Dole)	1 med	0	na	na	na	na	na	na	11.0	na	na	na	208	na
raw, chopped	1/2 cup	0	.03	.02	.12	.09	15.2	0	5.1	16.0	.18	8.0	125.6	.15
ONION, CANNED														
w/liquid, chopped	1/2 cup	0	.04	.01	.07	.15	10.9	0	4.8	50.4	.15	6.72	124.32	.32
ONION, DRIED														
flakes	1/4 cup	0	.07	.01	.14	.22	23.2	0	10.5	35.98	.22	12.88	227.08	.26
flakes	1 tbsp	0	.03	0	.05	.08	8.3	0	3.8	12.85	.08	4.6	81.1	.09
ONION, FROZEN														
Chopped														
boiled, drained	1/2 cup	36	.02	.03	.15	.07	14.1	0	2.7	16.8	.32	6.3	113.4	.07
boiled, drained	1 tbsp	5	0	0	.02	.01	2.0	0	0.4	2.4	.05	.9	16.2	.01
unprepared	10 oz	99	.09	.08	.43	.21	49.1	0	9.4	48.28	.94	19.88	352.16	.2
Diiced (Freshlike)	3.3 oz	na	na	na	na	na	na	na	na	na	na	na	35	na
Whole														
(Birds Eye) small	4 oz	na	na	na	na	na	na	na	na	na	na	na	160	na
(Freshlike)	3.3 oz	na	na	na	na	na	na	na	na	na	na	na	135	na
ONION, GREEN														
trimmed, w/top, chopped	1/2 cup	193	.03	.04	.26	.03	32.0	na	9.4	36.0	.74	10.0	138.0	.19
trimmed, w/top, chopped	1 tbsp	23	0	0	.03	0	3.8	na	1.1	4.32	.09	1.2	16.56	.02
ONION, SPRING. See ONION, GREEN.														
ONION POWDER														
ground	1 tbsp	0	.03	0	.04	na	na	0	1.0	23.59	.17	7.9	61.32	.15
ground	1 tsp	0	.01	0	.01	na	na	0	0.3	7.62	.05	2.55	19.81	.05
ground (Durkee)	1 tsp	na	.19	.03	0	na	na	na	.01	0	0	na	0	na
ground (Laurel Leaf)	1 tsp	na	.19	.03	0	na	na	na	.01	0	0	na	0	na
ONION RINGS, FROZEN														
breaded, partially fried in vegetable oil, prepared in oven	2 rings	45	.06	.03	.72	.02	2.6	0	0.3	6.2	.34	3.8	25.8	.08
breaded, partially fried in vegetable oil, unprepared	16 oz	790	.45	.36	3.15	.6	87.6	0	20.9	208.84	4.22	63.56	862.6	1.63
OPOSSUM, roasted	3 oz	0	.09	.31	na	na	na	na	0.0	na	na	na	na	na
ORANGE														
All commercial varieties														
approx 2 5/8 inch diam	1 med	269	.11	.05	.37	.08	39.7	0	69.7	52.4	.13	13.1	237.11	.09
sections, w/o membrane	1 cup	369	.16	.07	.51	.11	54.5	0	95.8	72.0	.18	18.0	325.8	.13
California Navel														
approx 2 7/8 inch diam	1 med	256	.12	.06	.41	.1	47.2	0	80.2	56.0	.17	14.0	249.2	.08
sections, w/o membrane	1 cup	302	.14	.07	.48	.11	55.6	0	94.6	66.0	.2	16.5	293.7	.1
California Valencia														
approx 2 5/8 inch diam	1 med	278	.11	.05	.33	.08	46.7	0	58.7	48.4	.11	12.1	216.59	.07
sections, w/o membrane	1 cup	414	.16	.07	.49	.11	69.5	0	87.3	72.0	.16	18.0	322.2	.11
Florida														
approx 2 5/8 inch diam	1 med	302	.15	.06	.6	.08	26.1	0	68.0	64.93	.14	15.1	255.19	.12
sections, w/o membrane	1 cup	370	.19	.07	.74	.09	32.0	0	83.3	79.55	.17	18.5	312.65	.15
ORANGE APRICOT JUICE DRINK	1 oz	181	.01	0	.06	.01	1.8	0	6.2	1.56	.03	1.25	24.96	.02

Food Name	Serving Size	A I.U.	Thi mg	Rib mg	Nia mg	B$_6$ mg	Fol mcg	B$_{12}$ mcg	C mg	Calc mg	Iron mg	Mag mg	Pot mg	Zn mg
ORANGE CRANBERRY JUICE DRINK														
(Ocean Spray) 'Refreshers'	6 oz	na	na	na	na	na	na	na	100.0	na	na	na	55	na
ORANGE DRINK														
Can, bottle, or box														
(J. Hungerford) 20% plus juice	9.03 oz	na	na	na	na	na	na	na	2.2	.52	0	na	na	na
Frozen, w/juice and pulp, diluted	6 oz	11	.2	1.96	.48	.13	60.7	0	103.6	219.96	.15	20.68	253.8	.09
Mix														
(Kool-Aid) sugar-sweetened, prepared	8 oz	na	na	na	na	na	na	na	na	na	na	na	0	na
(Kool-Aid) unsweetened, prepared w/sugar . .	8 oz	na	na	na	na	na	na	na	na	na	na	na	0	na
(Kool-Aid) unsweetened, prepared w/o sugar	8 oz	na	na	na	na	na	na	na	na	na	na	na	0	na
ORANGE FLAVOR DRINK														
Mix														
(Tang) crystals, prepared	6 oz	na	na	na	na	na	na	na	na	na	na	na	45	na
(Tang) crystals 'Sugar-free' prepared	6 oz	na	na	na	na	na	na	na	na	na	na	na	50	na
ORANGE GRAPEFRUIT JUICE														
canned	8 oz	294	.14	.07	.83	.06	35.3	0	71.9	19.76	1.14	24.7	390.26	.17
canned	1 oz	37	.02	.01	.1	.01	4.4	0	9.0	2.47	.14	3.09	48.82	.02
ORANGE JUICE														
fresh-squeezed	8 oz	496	.22	.07	.99	.1	75.1	0	124.0	27.28	.5	27.28	496.0	.12
Can, bottle, or box														
(J. Hungerford)	9.03 oz	na	na	na	na	na	na	na	100.0	.8	0	na	na	na
(Minute Maid) blend 'Juices to Go'	6 oz	na	na	na	na	na	na	na	48.0	na	na	na	310	na
(Ocean Spray)	6 oz	na	na	na	na	na	na	na	100.0	na	na	na	290	na
Chilled														
(Minute Maid) calcium fortified	6 oz	na	na	na	na	na	na	na	72.0	na	na	na	350	na
(Minute Maid) country style	6 oz	na	na	na	na	na	na	na	72.0	na	na	na	350	na
(Minute Maid) country style, premium choice	6 oz	na	na	na	na	na	na	na	60.0	na	na	na	370	na
(Minute Maid) premium choice	6 oz	na	na	na	na	na	na	na	60.0	na	na	na	370	na
(Minute Maid) regular	6 oz	na	na	na	na	na	na	na	72.0	na	na	na	350	na
Frozen														
(Minute Maid) calcium fortified	6 oz	na	na	na	na	na	na	na	72.0	na	na	na	350	na
(Minute Maid) country style	6 oz	na	na	na	na	na	na	na	72.0	na	na	na	350	na
(Minute Maid) reduced acid	6 oz	na	na	na	na	na	na	na	72.0	na	na	na	350	na
(Minute Maid) regular	6 oz	na	na	na	na	na	na	na	72.0	na	na	na	350	na
ORANGE JUICE COCKTAIL (Ocean Spray) . . .	6 oz	30	na	na	na	na	na	na	100.0	na	na	na	100	na
ORANGE JUICE DRINK (Tang) 'Fruit Box'	8.45 oz	na	na	na	na	na	na	na	na	na	na	na	230	na
ORANGE PEEL, candied	1 oz	0	0	0	0	na	na	na	0.0	0	0	na	0	na
ORANGE ROUGHY / slimehead														
dry-heat cooked	3 oz	69	.1	.16	3.11	.29	6.8	1.96	0.0	32.3	.2	32.3	327.25	.82
OREGANO														
ground	1 tbsp	311	.02	na	.28	na	na	0	na	70.93	1.98	12.15	75.09	.2
ground	1 tsp	104	.01	na	.09	na	na	0	na	23.64	.66	4.05	25.03	.07
ground (Durkee)	1 tsp	1.55	.08	na	0	na	na	na	na	0	.01	na	0	na
ground (Laurel Leaf)	1 tsp	1.55	.08	na	0	na	na	na	na	0	.01	na	0	na
OYSTER, CANNED														
Eastern	1 cup	744	.37	.41	3.09	.24	22.1	47.45	12.4	111.6	16.62	133.92	567.92	225.56
Eastern	3 oz	255	.13	.14	1.06	.08	7.6	16.26	4.3	38.25	5.69	45.9	194.65	77.31
OYSTER, EASTERN														
Farmed														
dry-heat cooked	3 oz	54	.11	.05	1.52	.06	20.4	20.66	5.1	na	6.6	28.05	129.2	38.38
dry-heat cooked	6 med	37	.08	.03	1.06	.04	14.2	14.34	3.5	na	4.58	19.47	89.68	26.64
raw, approx 3 oz	6 med	21	.09	.05	1.06	.05	15.1	13.61	4.0	na	4.86	27.72	104.16	31.85
Wild														
dry-heat cooked	3 oz	0	.07	.07	1.42	.08	15.3	23.63	3.5	na	3.68	39.1	142.8	62.56
dry-heat cooked	6 med	0	.05	.05	.99	.06	10.6	16.4	2.4	na	2.55	27.14	99.12	43.42
moist-heat cooked	3 oz	153	.16	.15	2.11	.1	11.9	29.77	5.1	76.5	10.19	80.75	238.85	154.37

Food Name	Serving Size	A I.U.	Thi mg	Rib mg	Nia mg	B$_6$ mg	Fol mcg	B$_{12}$ mcg	C mg	Calc mg	Iron mg	Mag mg	Pot mg	Zn mg
moist-heat cooked, approx 1.5 oz	6 med	76	.08	.08	1.04	.05	5.9	14.71	2.5	37.8	5.04	39.9	118.02	76.28
raw	1 cup	248	.25	.24	3.42	.15	24.8	48.26	9.2	111.6	16.52	116.56	386.88	225.21
raw, approx 3 oz	6 med	84	.08	.08	1.16	.05	8.4	16.35	3.1	37.8	5.59	39.48	131.04	76.28
OYSTER, PACIFIC														
moist-heat cooked	3 oz	413	.11	.38	3.08	.08	12.8	24.48	10.9	13.6	7.82	37.4	256.7	28.25
moist-heat cooked	1 med	122	.03	.11	.9	.02	3.8	7.2	3.2	4.0	2.3	11.0	75.5	8.31
raw	3 oz	230	.06	.2	1.71	.04	8.5	13.6	6.8	6.8	4.34	18.7	142.8	14.13
raw, approx 1.75 oz	1 med	135	.03	.12	1.0	.02	5.0	8.0	4.0	4.0	2.56	11.0	84.0	8.31

OYSTER PLANT. See SALSIFY.
OYSTER STEW. See SOUP.

P

Food Name	Serving Size	A I.U.	Thi mg	Rib mg	Nia mg	B$_6$ mg	Fol mcg	B$_{12}$ mcg	C mg	Calc mg	Iron mg	Mag mg	Pot mg	Zn mg
PALM KERNEL OIL/babassu oil	1 cup	0	0	0	0	0	0.0	0	0.0	0	.02	0	0	na
PALM OIL	1 tbsp	0	0	0	0	0	0.0	0	0.0	0	0	0	0	na
PANCAKE SYRUP. See also MAPLE SYRUP.														
15% maple	1 cup	0	.03	.03	.07	.03	0.0	0	0.0	40.95	2.58	12.6	107.1	2.02
15% maple	1 tbsp	0	0	0	0	0	0.0	0	0.0	2.6	.16	.8	6.8	.13
2% maple	1 cup	646	0	.07	.11	.06	104.0	0	27.7	63.0	1.54	12.6	242.55	.19
2% maple	1 tbsp	41	0	0	.01	0	6.6	0	1.8	4.0	.1	.8	15.4	.01
reduced calorie	100 gm	0	.01	.01	.02	0	0.0	0	0.0	1.0	.02	0	3.0	.02
(Aunt Jemima)														
'Lite'	1 oz	na	na	na	na	na	na	na	na	na	2	na	5	na
'Original' rich maple taste	1 oz	na	na	na	na	na	na	na	na	na	na	na	1	na
(Br'er Rabbit)														
dark	1 oz	na	na	na	na	na	na	na	na	na	na	na	135	na
light	1 oz	na	na	na	na	na	na	na	na	na	na	na	85	na
PAPAYA														
raw, approx 3 1/2 inch diam	1 med	863	.08	.1	1.03	.06	115.5	0	187.9	72.96	.3	30.4	781.28	.21
raw, cubed	1 cup	398	.04	.04	.47	.03	53.2	0	86.5	33.6	.14	14.0	359.8	.1
PAPAYA NECTAR														
canned	1 cup	278	.02	.01	.38	.02	5.3	0	7.5	25.0	.85	7.5	77.5	.38
canned	1 oz	35	0	0	.05	0	0.7	0	0.9	3.12	.11	.94	9.67	.05
(Kern's)	6 oz	na	na	na	na	na	na	na	na	na	na	na	90	na
(Libby's)	6 oz	na	na	na	na	na	na	na	na	na	na	na	0	na
PAPRIKA														
ground	1 tbsp	4182	.04	.12	1.06	na	na	0	4.9	12.21	1.63	12.74	161.77	.28
ground	1 tsp	1273	.01	.04	.32	na	na	0	1.5	3.72	.5	3.88	49.23	.09
ground *(Durkee)*	1 tsp	2.56	.26	.6	.01	na	na	na	.03	0	.01	na	0	na
ground *(Laurel Leaf)*	1 tsp	2.56	.26	.6	.01	na	na	na	.03	0	.01	na	0	na
PARANUT. See BRAZIL NUT.														
PARFAIT														
chocolate *(Pearson)*	1 oz	na	na	na	na	na	na	na	na	na	na	na	70	na
chocolate vanilla, fat-free *(Swiss Miss)*	4 oz	na	na	na	na	na	na	na	0.0	4.15	1.39	na	na	na
peanut butter *(Pearson)*	1 oz	na	na	na	na	na	na	na	na	na	na	na	70	na
vanilla chocolate *(Swiss Miss)*	4 oz	na	na	na	na	na	na	na	0.0	8.8	2.27	na	na	na
PARSLEY														
dried	1 tbsp	303	0	.02	.1	.01	na	0	1.6	19.08	1.27	3.24	49.46	.06
dried	1 tsp	70	0	0	.02	0	na	0	0.4	4.4	.29	.75	11.41	.01
dried flakes *(Durkee)*	1 tsp	.02	0	.01	0	na	na	na	0	0	0	na	0	na
dried flakes *(Laurel Leaf)*	1 tsp	.02	0	.01	0	na	na	na	0	0	0	na	0	na
freeze-dried	1/4 cup	885	.01	.03	.15	.02	21.5	0	2.1	2.46	.75	5.21	88.2	.09
freeze-dried	1 tbsp	253	0	.01	.04	.01	6.1	0	0.6	.7	.22	1.49	25.2	.02

Food Name	Serving Size	A I.U.	Thi mg	Rib mg	Nia mg	B6 mg	Fol mcg	B12 mcg	C mg	Calc mg	Iron mg	Mag mg	Pot mg	Zn mg
raw	10 sprigs	520	.01	.01	.13	.01	15.2	0	13.3	13.8	.62	5.0	55.4	.11
raw, chopped	1/2 cup	1560	.03	.03	.39	.03	45.6	0	39.9	41.4	1.86	15.0	166.2	.32
PARSNIP														
boiled, drained, 9 inches long	1 parsnip	0	.13	.08	1.16	.15	93.1	0	20.8	59.2	.93	46.4	587.2	.42
boiled, drained, slices	1/2 cup	0	.06	.04	.56	.07	45.4	0	10.1	28.86	.45	22.62	286.26	.2
raw, slices	1/2 cup	0	.06	.03	.47	.06	44.8	0	11.4	24.12	.4	19.43	251.25	.4
PASSION FRUIT/granadilla														
purple, trimmed, approx 1.2 oz	1 med	126	0	.02	.27	na	na	0	5.4	2.16	.29	5.22	62.64	na
PASSION FRUIT BEVERAGES														
COCKTAIL														
fresh, purple	1 cup	1771	0	.32	3.61	na	na	0	73.6	9.88	.59	41.99	686.66	na
fresh, purple	1 oz	222	0	.04	.45	na	na	0	9.2	1.24	.07	5.25	85.9	na
fresh, yellow	1 cup	5953	0	.25	5.53	na	na	0	45.0	9.88	.89	41.99	686.66	na
JUICE, fresh, yellow	1 oz	745	0	.03	.69	na	na	0	5.6	1.24	.11	5.25	85.9	na
PASTA/macaroni. See also NOODLE, CHINESE; NOODLE, EGG; NOODLE, JAPANESE; TORTELLINI PASTA.														
(NOTE: 2 ounces uncooked pasta = approximately 1 cup cooked.)														
AGNOLOTTI, refrigerated, 'Fresh' (Contadina)	3 oz	75	.3	.26	2.0	.03	11.6	.1	0.9	158	1.8	40.0	150	.75
ANGEL HAIR														
Dry														
corn (Westbrae)	2 oz	na	na	na	na	na	na	na	na	na	na	na	140	na
wheat (DiGiorno)	3 oz	na	na	na	na	na	na	na	na	na	na	na	160	na
Refrigerated, fresh														
'Fresh' (Contadina)	3 oz	75	.3	.26	2.0	.03	17.8	.22	0.0	20	2.7	45.6	150	.94
ELBOW														
Dry, corn (Westbrae)	2 oz	na	na	na	na	na	na	na	na	na	na	na	140	na
FETUCCINE														
Dry														
spinach (DiGiorno)	3 oz	na	na	na	na	na	na	na	na	na	na	na	310	na
wheat (DiGiorno)	3 oz	na	na	na	na	na	na	na	na	na	na	na	160	na
wheat, bell pepper/basil, organic (Herb'b)	2 oz	na	na	na	na	na	na	na	na	na	na	na	115	na
Refrigerated, fresh														
spinach 'Fresh' (Contadina)	3 oz	75	.38	.34	2.0	.1	18.5	.23	0.6	60	3.6	71.5	350	1.09
LASAGNA														
Dry, 100% semolina (Creamette)	2 oz	na	na	na	na	na	na	na	na	na	na	na	80	na
LINGUINE														
Dry, wheat (Creamette)	2 oz	na	na	na	na	na	na	na	na	na	na	na	80	na
Refrigerated, fresh (DiGiorno)	3 oz	na	na	na	na	na	na	na	na	na	na	na	160	na
RIBBON														
Dry														
wheat, mixed vegetable, organic (Herb's)	2 oz	na	na	na	na	na	na	na	na	na	na	na	115	na
wheat, paella, w/saffron, organic (Eden Foods)	2 oz	na	na	na	na	na	na	na	na	na	na	na	5	na
wheat, parsley garlic, organic (Eden Foods)	2 oz	na	na	na	na	na	na	na	na	na	na	na	5	na
RIGATONI														
Refrigerated, fresh, 'Fresh' (Contadina)	2.3 oz	75	.3	.26	2.0	.03	14.5	.19	0.0	20	1.8	33.4	115	7.11
ROTELLE														
Dry														
quinoa 'Supergrain Wheat Free' (Ancient Harvest)	2 oz	na	na	na	na	na	na	na	na	na	na	na	57	1.8
wheat (Ronzoni)	2 oz	na	na	na	na	na	na	na	na	na	na	na	2.0	na
ROTINI														
Dry, quinoa 'Supergrain' (Ancient Harvest)	2 oz	na	na	na	na	na	na	na	na	na	na	na	90	1.1
SHELL														
Dry														
corn (Westbrae)	2 oz	na	na	na	na	na	na	na	na	na	na	na	140	na

Food Name	Serving Size	A I.U.	Thi mg	Rib mg	Nia mg	B$_6$ mg	Fol mcg	B$_{12}$ mcg	C mg	Calc mg	Iron mg	Mag mg	Pot mg	Zn mg
wheat, vegetable, no eggs, organic														
(Eden Foods)	2 oz	na	na	na	na	na	na	na	na	na	na	na	5	na
SPAGHETTI														
Dry														
corn (Westbrae)	2 oz	na	na	na	na	na	na	na	na	na	na	na	140	na
protein-fortified	2 oz	na	.68	.27	4.36	.1	11.4	0	0.0	22.23	2.37	37.05	114.57	1.02
spinach	2 oz	263	.21	.11	2.59	.18	27.4	0	0.0	33.06	1.21	99.18	214.32	1.57
thin (Creamette)	2 oz	na	na	na	na	na	na	na	na	na	na	na	80	na
unenriched	2 oz	0	.05	.03	.97	.06	10.3	0	0.0	10.26	.74	27.36	92.34	.69
wheat (DiGiorno)	3 oz	na	na	na	na	na	na	na	na	na	na	na	160	na
whole-wheat	2 oz	0	.28	.08	2.92	.13	32.5	0	0.0	22.8	2.07	81.51	122.55	1.35
SPIRAL														
Dry														
wheat, sesame rice, organic (Eden Foods)	2 oz	na	na	na	na	na	na	na	na	na	na	na	260	na
wheat, vegetable, no eggs, organic														
(Eden Foods)	2 oz	na	na	na	na	na	na	na	na	na	na	na	5	na
VERMICELLI														
Dry, extra thin (Creamette)	2 oz	na	na	na	na	na	na	na	na	na	na	na	80	na

PASTA ENTRÉE, CANNED. See NOODLE ENTRÉE/DISH, CANNED; RAVIOLI ENTRÉE; SPAGHETTI ENTRÉE, CANNED.

PASTA ENTRÉE, FROZEN. See also NOODLE ENTRÉE/DISH, FROZEN; RAVIOLI ENTRÉE; SPAGHETTI ENTRÉE, FROZEN; TORTELLINI PASTA DISH/ENTRÉE, FROZEN.

Food Name	Serving Size	A I.U.	Thi mg	Rib mg	Nia mg	B$_6$ mg	Fol mcg	B$_{12}$ mcg	C mg	Calc mg	Iron mg	Mag mg	Pot mg	Zn mg
shells, cheese, w/tomato sauce (Stouffer's)	9.25 oz	na	na	na	na	na	na	na	na	na	na	na	480	na

PASTRY. See also BUN, SWEET; MUFFIN; PIE; ROLL, SWEET.

Food Name	Serving Size	A I.U.	Thi mg	Rib mg	Nia mg	B$_6$ mg	Fol mcg	B$_{12}$ mcg	C mg	Calc mg	Iron mg	Mag mg	Pot mg	Zn mg
(Charlette Russe) w/lady fingers, whipped														
cream filling	1 serving	844	.13	.17	.8	na	na	na	0.3	52.44	1.14	na	72.96	na
PATÉ, CANNED														
chicken liver	1 oz	205	.01	.4	2.13	.07	91.0	2.29	2.8	2.84	2.61	3.69	26.93	.61
chicken liver	1 tbsp	94	.01	.18	.98	.03	41.7	1.05	1.3	1.3	1.19	1.69	12.35	.28
foie gras, goose liver, smoked	1 oz	945	.02	.08	.71	.02	17.0	2.66	0.6	19.85	1.56	3.69	39.12	.26
foie gras, goose liver, smoked	1 tbsp	433	.01	.04	.33	.01	7.8	1.22	0.3	9.1	.72	1.69	17.94	.12

PATTYPAN SQUASH. See SQUASH, SCALLOP.

Food Name	Serving Size	A I.U.	Thi mg	Rib mg	Nia mg	B$_6$ mg	Fol mcg	B$_{12}$ mcg	C mg	Calc mg	Iron mg	Mag mg	Pot mg	Zn mg
PEACH														
raw, approx 4 oz	1 med	465	.01	.04	.86	.02	3.0	0	5.7	4.35	.1	6.09	171.39	.12
raw, slices	1 cup	910	.03	.07	1.68	.03	5.8	0	11.2	8.5	.19	11.9	334.9	.24
PEACH, FROZEN														
slices, sweetened	10-oz pkg	807	.04	.1	1.85	.05	9.1	0	267.5	8.52	1.05	14.2	369.2	.14
PEACH DRINK														
(Ocean Spray) citrus 'Refreshers'	6 oz	15	na	na	na	na	na	na	100.0	na	na	na	55	na
PEACH NECTAR														
w/added ascorbic acid	1 cup	642	.01	.03	.72	.02	3.5	0	66.7	12.45	.47	9.96	99.6	.2
w/added ascorbic acid	1 oz	80	0	0	.09	0	0.4	0	8.3	1.56	.06	1.24	12.44	.02
w/o added ascorbic acid	1 cup	642	.01	.03	.72	.02	3.5	0	13.2	12.45	.47	9.96	99.6	.2
w/o added ascorbic acid	1 oz	80	0	0	.09	0	0.4	0	1.7	1.56	.06	1.24	12.44	.02
(Kern's)	6 oz	na	na	na	na	na	na	na	na	na	na	na	120	na
(Libby's)	6 oz	na	na	na	na	na	na	na	na	na	na	na	110	na
PEANUT, SPANISH														
OIL-ROASTED, unsalted	1 oz	0	.09	.02	4.18	.07	35.3	0	0.0	28.0	.64	47.04	217.28	.56
RAW	1 oz	0	.19	.04	4.46	.1	67.2	0	0.0	29.68	1.09	52.64	208.32	.59
PEANUT, VALENCIA														
oil-roasted	1 cup	0	.13	.22	20.65	.35	180.7	0	0.0	77.76	2.38	230.4	881.28	4.44
raw	1 oz	0	.18	.08	3.61	.1	68.7	0	0.0	17.36	.59	51.52	92.96	.94
PEANUT, VIRGINIA														
oil-roasted, unsalted	1 cup	0	.39	.16	21.02	.36	179.3	0	0.0	122.98	2.39	268.84	932.36	9.47
oil-roasted, unsalted	1 oz	0	.08	.03	4.12	.07	35.1	0	0.0	24.08	.47	52.64	182.56	1.85
raw	1 cup	0	.95	.19	18.07	.51	348.5	0	0.0	129.94	3.72	249.66	1007.4	6.47
raw	1 oz	0	.18	.04	3.47	.1	66.8	0	0.0	24.92	.71	47.88	193.2	1.24

Food Name	Serving Size	A I.U.	Thi mg	Rib mg	Nia mg	B₆ mg	Fol mcg	B₁₂ mcg	C mg	Calc mg	Iron mg	Mag mg	Pot mg	Zn mg
PEANUT BUTTER														
CHUNKY														
(Jif) 'Simply Jif'	2 tbsp	na	na	na	na	na	na	na	na	na	na	na	244	na
(Maranatha Natural) crunchy	2 tbsp	na	na	na	na	na	na	na	na	na	na	na	350	na
SMOOTH														
(Jif) 'Simply Jif'	2 tbsp	na	na	na	na	na	na	na	na	na	na	na	244	na
PEANUT FLOUR														
defatted	1 cup	0	.42	.29	16.2	.3	148.9	0	0.0	84.0	1.26	222.0	774.0	3.06
defatted	1 oz	0	.2	.13	7.56	.14	69.5	0	0.0	39.2	.59	103.6	361.2	1.43
low-fat	1 cup	0	.27	.1	6.9	.18	80.0	0	0.0	78.0	2.84	28.8	814.8	3.59
low-fat	1 oz	0	.13	.05	3.22	.09	37.3	0	0.0	36.4	1.33	13.44	380.24	1.68
PEANUT OIL *(Wesson)*	1 tbsp	na	na	na	na	na	na	na	0.0	0	0	na	na	na
PEAR														
Asian, raw	1 fruit	0	.02	.03	.6	.06	22.0	0	10.5	11.0	0	22.0	332.75	.06
Asian, raw	1 fruit	0	.01	.01	.27	.03	9.8	0	4.6	4.88	0	9.76	147.62	.02
raw, slices	1 cup	33	.03	.07	.16	.03	12.0	0	6.6	18.15	.41	9.9	206.25	.2
PEAR, CANNED														
in extra heavy syrup, solid and liquid, halves	1 cup	0	.03	.06	.62	.04	3.1	0	2.9	13.05	.57	10.44	167.04	.21
in extra light syrup, solid and liquid, halves	1 cup	0	.02	.05	.99	.03	3.0	0	4.9	17.29	.49	12.35	111.15	.17
in heavy syrup, solid and liquid, halves	1 cup	0	.03	.06	.62	.04	3.1	0	2.8	12.75	.56	10.2	165.75	.2
in juice, solid and liquid, halves	1 cup	15	.03	.03	.5	.03	3.0	0	4.0	22.32	.72	17.36	238.08	.22
in light syrup, solid and liquid, halves	1 cup	0	.03	.04	.39	.04	3.0	0	1.8	12.55	.7	10.04	165.66	.2
in water, solid and liquid, halves	1 cup	0	.02	.02	.13	.03	2.9	0	2.4	9.76	.51	9.76	129.32	.22
PEAR, DRIED														
Sulfured														
stewed, w/added sugar, halves	1/2 cup	56	.01	.03	.47	.05	0.0	0	5.3	21.0	1.36	21.0	343.0	.25
stewed, w/o added sugar, halves	1/2 cup	54	.01	.03	.45	.04	0.0	0	5.1	20.48	1.31	20.48	330.24	.24
uncooked	10 halves	5	.01	.25	2.4	.13	0.0	0	12.3	59.5	3.67	57.75	932.75	.68
PEAR NECTAR														
(Kern's)	6 oz	na	na	na	na	na	na	na	na	na	na	na	90	na
(Libby's)	6 oz	na	na	na	na	na	na	na	na	na	na	na	65	na
PEAS, GREEN														
(NOTE: All peas are shelled unless otherwise noted.)														
boiled, drained	1/2 cup	478	.21	.12	1.62	.17	50.6	0	11.4	21.6	1.23	31.2	216.8	.95
boiled, drained, in pod	1/2 cup	105	.1	.06	.43	.12	23.3	0	38.3	33.6	1.58	20.8	192.0	.3
raw	1/2 cup	461	.19	.1	1.5	.12	46.8	0	28.8	18.0	1.06	23.76	175.68	.89
CANNED														
dietary pack, drained solids	1/2 cup	653	.1	.07	.62	.05	37.7	0	8.2	17.0	.81	14.45	147.05	.6
dietary pack, solids and liquid	1/2 cup	470	.14	.09	1.04	.08	35.3	0	13.5	22.32	1.38	21.08	107.88	.87
regular pack, drained solids	1/2 cup	653	.1	.07	.62	.05	37.7	0	8.2	17.0	.81	14.45	147.05	.6
regular pack, solids and liquid	1/2 cup	470	.14	.09	1.04	.08	35.3	0	13.5	22.32	1.38	21.08	107.88	.87
Sweet														
wrinkled, dietary pack, drained, low sodium	1 lb	0	.54	.23	4.99	na	na	na	45.4	40.86	4.99	na	435.84	na
wrinkled, dietary pack, drained, low sodium	1 oz	0	.03	.01	.31	na	na	na	2.8	2.52	.31	na	26.88	na
wrinkled, regular pack, drained	1 lb	0	.54	.23	4.99	na	na	na	45.4	40.86	4.99	na	435.84	na
wrinkled, regular pack, drained	1 oz	0	.03	.01	.31	na	na	na	2.8	2.52	.31	na	26.88	na
FROZEN														
boiled, drained	1/2 cup	534	.23	.08	1.18	.09	46.9	0	7.9	19.2	1.26	23.2	134.4	.75
unprepared	1/2 cup	523	.19	.07	1.23	.09	38.2	0	13.0	15.84	1.1	18.0	107.28	.58
(Birds Eye)	3.3 oz	na	na	na	na	na	na	na	na	na	na	na	160	na
Tiny *(Birds Eye)* tender, 'Deluxe'	3.3 oz	na	na	na	na	na	na	na	na	na	na	na	135	na
PEAS, PIGEON														
immature seeds, boiled, drained	1/2 cup	100	.27	.13	1.66	.04	77.0	0	21.6	31.57	1.21	na	na	.63
immature seeds, raw	10 seeds	6	.02	.01	.09	0	6.9	0	1.6	1.68	.06	2.72	22.08	.04
red gram, mature seeds, boiled	1/2 cup	3	.12	.05	.66	.04	93.1	0	0.0	36.12	.93	38.64	322.56	.76
red gram, mature seeds, raw	1/2 cup	29	.66	.19	3.02	.29	465.1	0	0.0	132.6	5.33	186.66	1419.84	2.82
PEAS, SNAP *(Birds Eye)* 'Deluxe'	2.6 oz	na	na	na	na	na	na	na	na	na	na	na	95	na

Food Name	Serving Size	A I.U.	Thi mg	Rib mg	Nia mg	B6 mg	Fol mcg	B12 mcg	C mg	Calc mg	Iron mg	Mag mg	Pot mg	Zn mg
PEAS AND CARROTS, CANNED														
regular pack, solid and liquid	1/2 cup	7386	.09	.07	.74	.11	23.4	0	8.5	29.44	.96	17.92	128.0	.74
special dietary pack, solid and liquid	1/2 cup	7386	.09	.07	.74	.11	23.4	0	8.5	29.44	.96	17.92	128.0	.74
(Freshlike)	1/2 cup	na	na	na	na	na	na	na	na	na	na	na	170	na
(Freshlike) water pack, w/o salt	1/2 cup	na	na	na	na	na	na	na	na	na	na	na	170	na
(Freshlike) water pack, w/o sugar, salt	1/2 cup	na	na	na	na	na	na	na	na	na	na	na	170	na
(Veg•All)	1/2 cup	na	na	na	na	na	na	na	na	na	na	na	170	na
PEAS AND CARROTS, FROZEN														
boiled, drained	10-oz pkg	21576	.63	.18	3.21	.24	72.3	0	22.5	63.94	2.61	44.48	439.24	1.25
boiled, drained	1/2 cup	6209	.18	.05	.92	.07	20.8	0	6.5	18.4	.75	12.8	126.4	.36
unprepared	10-oz pkg	26971	.54	.23	4.01	.29	101.4	0	31.8	76.68	3.1	51.12	550.96	1.48
unprepared	1/2 cup	6648	.13	.06	.99	.07	25.0	0	7.8	18.9	.76	12.6	135.8	.36
(Freshlike)	3.3 oz	na	na	na	na	na	na	na	na	na	na	na	180	na
PEAS AND ONIONS, CANNED														
solid and liquid	1/2 cup	97	.06	.04	.77	.12	16.0	0	1.8	10.2	.52	9.6	57.6	.35
(Freshlike) sweet peas, tiny onions	1/2 cup	na	na	na	na	na	na	na	na	na	na	na	130	na
PEAS AND ONIONS, FROZEN														
boiled, drained	1/2 cup	312	.14	.06	.94	.08	17.9	0	6.2	12.6	.85	11.7	105.3	.26
unprepared	10-oz pkg	1545	.84	.32	4.88	.41	126.4	0	39.8	65.32	4.37	59.64	576.52	1.36
unprepared	1/2 cup	375	.2	.08	1.19	.1	30.7	0	9.7	15.87	1.06	14.49	140.07	.33
(Freshlike)	3.3 oz	na	na	na	na	na	na	na	na	na	na	na	140	na
PECAN, SHELLED														
dried, 31 large or 20 medium halves	1 oz	36	.24	.04	.25	.05	11.1	0	0.6	10.22	.6	36.35	111.33	1.55
dry-roasted	1 oz	38	.09	.03	.26	.06	11.6	0	0.6	9.94	.62	37.77	105.08	1.61
oil-roasted	1 cup	142	.34	.11	.98	.21	43.3	0	2.2	37.4	2.32	141.9	394.9	6.05
oil-roasted, 15 halves	1 oz	37	.09	.03	.25	.05	11.2	0	0.6	9.66	.6	36.64	101.96	1.56
PECAN FLOUR	1 oz	34	.23	.03	.24	.05	10.4	0	0.5	9.09	.56	34.08	94.86	1.46
PECTIN, unsweetened, dry mix	.5 oz	0	0	.01	0	0	0.1	0	0.0	.84	.33	.12	.84	.06
PEPPER, BELL. See PEPPER, SWEET.														
PEPPER, CHILI														
green, raw, approx 1.6 oz	1 med	347	.04	.04	.43	.13	10.5	0	109.1	8.1	.54	11.25	153.0	.14
green, raw, chopped	1/2 cup	578	.07	.07	.71	.21	17.6	0	181.9	13.5	.9	18.75	255.0	.23
red, raw, approx 1.6 oz	1 med	4838	.04	.04	.43	.13	10.5	0	109.1	8.1	.54	11.25	153.0	.14
red, raw, chopped	1/2 cup	8063	.07	.07	.71	.21	17.6	0	181.9	13.5	.9	18.75	255.0	.23
Canned														
green, diced (Rosarita)	1.058 oz	na	na	na	na	na	na	na	10.7	2.32	.78	na	na	na
green, whole (Rosarita)	1.235 oz	na	na	na	na	na	na	na	11.2	1.66	.75	na	na	na
hot, green, pods, w/o seeds, solid and liquid, chopped	1/2 cup	415	.01	.03	.54	.1	6.8	0	46.2	4.76	.34	9.52	127.16	.12
PEPPER, GREEN. See PEPPER, SWEET.														
PEPPER, GROUND														
black	1 tbsp	12	.01	.02	.07	na	na	0	na	27.94	1.85	12.39	80.58	.09
black	1 tsp	4	0	.01	.02	na	na	0	na	9.17	.61	4.06	26.44	.03
black (Durkee)	1 tsp	.08	.03	.09	0	na	na	na	na	0	.01	na	0	na
black (Laurel Leaf)	1 tsp	.08	.03	.09	0	na	na	na	na	0	.01	na	0	na
cayenne/red	1 tbsp	2205	.02	.05	.46	na	na	0	4.1	7.86	.41	8.04	106.74	.13
cayenne/red	1 tsp	749	.01	.02	.16	na	na	0	1.4	2.67	.14	2.73	36.25	.04
cayenne/red (Durkee)	1 tsp	10.17	.17	.3	0	na	na	na	.01	0	0	na	0	na
cayenne/red (Laurel Leaf)	1 tsp	10.17	.17	.3	0	na	na	na	.01	0	0	na	0	na
white	1 tbsp	0	0	.01	.02	na	na	0	na	18.84	1.02	6.42	5.15	.08
white	1 tsp	0	0	0	.01	na	na	0	na	6.37	.34	2.17	1.74	.03
white (Durkee)	1 tsp	na	.01	.07	0	na	na	na	na	0	0	na	0	na
white (Laurel Leaf)	1 tsp	na	.01	.07	0	na	na	na	na	0	0	na	0	na
PEPPER, JALAPEÑO														
diced (Rosarita)	1.058 oz	na	na	na	na	na	na	na	1.4	.97	1.05	na	na	na
nacho sliced (Rosarita)	1.058 oz	na	na	na	na	na	na	na	7.7	4.01	.83	na	na	na
whole (Rosarita)	1.34 oz	na	na	na	na	na	na	na	9.8	5.08	1.06	na	na	na

Food Name	Serving Size	A I.U.	Thi mg	Rib mg	Nia mg	B₆ mg	Fol mcg	B₁₂ mcg	C mg	Calc mg	Iron mg	Mag mg	Pot mg	Zn mg
whole, w/escabeche *(Rosarita)*	1.164 oz	na	na	na	na	na	na	na	14.6	1.8	.75	na	na	na
PEPPER, SWEET/bell pepper/green pepper/red pepper/yellow pepper														
boiled, drained, approx 2.6 oz	1 med	432	.04	.02	.35	.17	11.7	0	54.3	6.57	.34	7.3	121.18	.09
boiled, drained, chopped	1/2 cup	403	.04	.02	.32	.16	10.9	0	50.6	6.12	.31	6.8	112.88	.08
raw *(Dole)*	1 med	415	na	na	na	na	na	na	117.0	na	na	na	281	na
raw, approx 3.2 oz	1 med	468	.05	.02	.38	.18	16.3	0	66.1	6.66	.34	7.4	130.98	.09
raw, chopped	1/2 cup	316	.03	.02	.25	.12	11.0	0	44.7	4.5	.23	5.0	88.5	.06
red, boiled, drained, approx 2.6 oz	1 med	2745	.04	.02	.35	.17	11.7	0	124.8	6.57	.34	7.3	121.18	.09
red, boiled, drained, chopped	1/2 cup	2557	.04	.02	.32	.16	10.9	0	116.3	6.12	.31	6.8	112.88	.08
red, raw, approx 3.2 oz	1 med	4218	.05	.02	.38	.18	16.3	0	140.6	6.66	.34	7.4	130.98	.09
red, raw, chopped	1/2 cup	2850	.03	.02	.25	.12	11.0	0	95.0	4.5	.23	5.0	88.5	.06
yellow, raw, approx 3.2 oz	1 med	443	.05	.05	1.66	.31	48.4	0	341.3	20.46	.86	22.32	394.32	.32
Canned														
solid and liquid, halves	1/2 cup	109	.02	.02	.39	.12	11.4	0	32.6	28.7	.56	7.7	102.2	.13
red, solid and liquid, halves	1/2 cup	364	.02	na	na	na	na	na	32.6	28.7	.56	7.7	102.2	.13
Freeze-dried														
	1/4 cup	100	.02	.02	.12	.04	3.7	0	30.4	2.14	.17	3.01	50.72	.04
red	1/4 cup	1236	.02	.02	.12	.04	3.7	0	30.4	2.14	.17	3.01	50.72	.04
Frozen														
chopped, unprepared	10-oz pkg	1042	.2	.11	3.89	.39	40.0	0	166.7	25.56	1.76	22.72	258.44	.17
chopped, unprepared	1 oz	103	.02	.01	.38	.04	4.0	0	16.4	2.52	.17	2.24	25.48	.02
red, chopped, unprepared	10-oz pkg	13524	.2	.11	3.89	.39	40.0	0	166.7	25.56	1.76	22.72	258.44	.17
red, chopped, unprepared	1 oz	1333	.02	.01	.38	.04	4.0	0	16.4	2.52	.17	2.24	25.48	.02
PEPPER STEAK DINNER														
(Armour) frozen, beef 'Classics Lite'	11.25 oz	na	na	na	na	na	na	na	na	na	na	na	320	na
(LaChoy)	3.81 oz	na	na	na	na	na	na	na	4.9	2.07	2.4	na	na	na
PEPPER STEAK ENTRÉE														
(Stouffer's) frozen, green, w/rice	10.5 oz	na	na	na	na	na	na	na	na	na	na	na	410	na
PERCH														
mixed species, dry-heat cooked	3 oz	27	.07	.1	1.01	.12	4.9	1.87	1.4	86.7	.99	32.3	292.4	1.22
mixed species, raw	3 oz	24	.06	.09	1.29	.1	4.3	1.61	1.4	68.0	.77	25.5	228.65	.94
PERSIMMON														
Japanese, raw, 2.5 inch diam	1 med	3641	.05	.03	.17	na	12.6	0	12.6	13.44	.25	15.12	270.48	.18
native, raw, trimmed, approx 1.1 oz	1 med	na	na	na	na	na	na	0	16.5	6.75	.63	na	77.5	na
PE-TSAI. See CABBAGE, NAPA.														
PHYLLO DOUGH, 1 sheet	1 oz	0	.15	.1	1.15	.01	5.1	0	0.0	3.12	.91	4.25	20.98	.14
PICKLES														
BREAD AND BUTTER														
fresh	2 slices	21	0	0	0	na	na	na	1.4	4.8	.27	na	30.0	na
slices	1 cup	238	0	.05	0	na	na	na	15.3	54.4	3.06	na	340.0	na
PIE														
CHERRY, Fresh *(McMillin's)*	4 oz	na	na	na	na	na	na	na	na	na	na	na	70	na
CHOCOLATE, Fresh *(McMillin's)* chocolate pudding	4 oz	na	na	na	na	na	na	na	na	na	na	na	95	na
COCONUT, Fresh *(McMillin's)* coconut pudding	4 oz	na	na	na	na	na	na	na	na	na	na	na	60	na
LEMON, Fresh *(McMillin's)*	4 oz	na	na	na	na	na	na	na	na	na	na	na	50	na
STRAWBERRY, Fresh *(McMillin's)*	4 oz	na	na	na	na	na	na	na	na	na	na	na	70	na
PIE, SNACK														
APPLE *(Break Cake)* 'Fried Pie' 4.5 oz	2 pies	na	na	na	na	na	na	na	na	na	na	na	95	na
CHERRY *(Break Cake)* 'Fried Pie' 4.5 oz	2 pies	na	na	na	na	na	na	na	na	na	na	na	95	na
LEMON *(Break Cake)* 'Fried Pie' 4.5 oz	2 pies	na	na	na	na	na	na	na	na	na	na	na	95	na
PIE MIX														
BANANA CREAM														
(Jell-O) 'No Bake' dry	1 pkg	na	na	na	na	na	na	na	na	na	na	na	15	na
(Jell-O) 'No Bake' prepared	1/8 pie	na	na	na	na	na	na	na	na	na	na	na	95	na
BOSTON CREAM														
(Jell-O) mousse 'No Bake' dry	1 pkg	na	na	na	na	na	na	na	na	na	na	na	160	na

Food Name	Serving Size	A I.U.	Thi mg	Rib mg	Nia mg	B₆ mg	Fol mcg	B₁₂ mcg	C mg	Calc mg	Iron mg	Mag mg	Pot mg	Zn mg
(Jell-O) mousse 'No Bake' prepared	1/8 pie	na	na	na	na	na	na	na	na	na	na	na	240	na
COCONUT CREAM														
(Jell-O) 'No Bake' dry	1 pkg	na	na	na	na	na	na	na	na	na	na	na	40	na
(Jell-O) 'No Bake' prepared	1/8 pie	na	na	na	na	na	na	na	na	na	na	na	115	na
KEY LIME *(Royal)* dry	1 serving	na	na	na	na	na	na	na	na	na	na	na	40	na
LEMON *(Royal)* dry	1 serving	na	na	na	na	na	na	na	na	na	na	na	40	na
PUMPKIN														
(Jell-O) 'No Bake' dry	1 pkg	na	na	na	na	na	na	na	na	na	na	na	25	na
(Jell-O) 'No Bake' prepared	1/8 pie	na	na	na	na	na	na	na	na	na	na	na	140	na
PIGEON. See SQUAB.														
PIGNOLIA. See PINE NUT.														
PIG'S FEET														
pickled, cured	1 lb	0	.03	.19	1.66	1.72	18.1	2.81	na	145.15	2.81	18.14	1065.96	5.62
pickled, cured	1 oz	0	0	.01	.1	.11	1.1	.18	na	9.07	.18	1.13	66.62	.35
raw	1 oz	0	.01	.03	.31	.03	0.6	.08	0.0	16.73	.14	1.98	77.68	.37
simmered	5 oz	0	.01	.09	.74	.13	1.4	.26	0.0	63.9	.67	7.1	207.32	1.53
PIG'S HEART														
braised	1 cup	32	.8	2.47	8.77	.57	5.8	5.5	2.9	10.15	8.45	34.8	298.7	4.48
raw	1 oz	7	.17	.34	1.92	.11	1.1	1.07	1.5	1.42	1.33	5.39	83.35	.79
PIG'S JOWL, raw	1 oz	3	.11	.07	1.29	.03	0.3	.23	na	1.13	.12	.85	41.96	.24
PIG'S TAIL														
raw	1 oz	0	.06	.03	.58	.1	1.4	.25	0.0	5.1	.28	2.27	98.94	.65
simmered	3 oz	0	.06	.06	.95	.23	3.4	.47	0.0	11.9	.67	5.95	133.45	1.39
PIG'S TONGUE														
braised	3 oz	0	.27	.43	4.54	.2	3.4	2.03	1.4	16.15	4.24	17.0	201.45	3.85
raw	1 oz	0	.14	.14	1.5	.07	1.1	.81	1.3	4.54	.95	5.1	68.89	.85
PIKE, NORTHERN														
dry-heat cooked	3 oz	69	.06	.07	2.38	.11	14.7	1.95	3.2	62.05	.6	34.0	281.35	.73
raw	3 oz	60	.05	.05	1.95	.1	12.8	1.7	3.2	48.45	.47	26.35	220.15	.57
PIKE, WALLEYE														
dry-heat cooked	3 oz	69	.27	.17	2.38	.12	14.5	1.96	0.0	119.85	1.42	32.3	424.15	.67
raw	3 oz	60	.23	.14	1.95	.1	12.8	1.7	0.0	93.5	1.1	25.5	330.65	.53
PILI NUT, CANARY TREE														
dried	1 cup	49	1.1	.11	.62	.14	71.6	0	0.7	174.0	4.24	362.4	608.4	3.56
dried, 15 kernels	1 oz	12	.26	.03	.15	.03	17.0	0	0.2	41.18	1.0	85.77	143.99	.84
PIÑA COLADA. See ALCOHOLIC BEVERAGES.														
PINE NUT /Colorado pinyon pine nut / Italian stone pine nut / pignolia / pinocchio / piñon														
whole	1 oz	8	.23	.05	1.01	.03	16.3	0	0.5	7.38	2.61	66.17	170.12	1.21
whole	1 tbsp	3	.08	.02	.36	.01	5.7	0	0.2	2.6	.92	23.3	59.9	.43
whole	10 kernels	0	.01	0	.04	0	0.6	0	0.0	.08	.03	2.34	6.28	.04
PINEAPPLE														
candied, approx 1/2 cup	4-oz container	113	.52	.14	2.03	na	na	na	94.9	88.14	2.03	na	1066.72	na
raw, diced pieces	1 cup	36	.14	.06	.65	.13	16.4	0	23.9	10.85	.57	21.7	175.15	.12
raw, 3 1/2 inch diam	1 slice	19	.08	.03	.35	.07	8.9	0	12.9	5.88	.31	11.76	94.92	.07
untrimmed *(Dole)*	2 slices	46	na	na	na	na	na	na	16.0	na	na	na	165	na
PINEAPPLE, CANNED														
in extra heavy syrup, w/1.25 tbsp liquid	1 slice	8	.05	.01	.16	.04	2.7	0	4.2	8.12	.22	8.7	59.16	.06
in heavy syrup, chunks or crushed, w/liquid	1 cup	36	.23	.06	.73	.19	11.7	0	18.9	35.7	.97	40.8	265.2	.31
in heavy syrup, w/1.25 tbsp liquid	1 slice	8	.05	.01	.17	.04	2.7	0	4.3	8.12	.22	9.28	60.32	.07
in juice, chunks or tidbits, w/liquid	1 cup	95	.24	.05	.71	.19	12.0	0	23.8	35.0	.7	35.0	305.0	.25
in juice, w/1.25 tbsp liquid	1 slice	22	.06	.01	.16	.04	2.8	0	5.5	8.12	.16	8.12	70.76	.06
in light syrup, w/liquid	1 cup	38	.23	.06	.74	.19	11.8	0	18.9	35.28	.98	40.32	264.6	.3
in light syrup, w/1.75 tbsp liquid	1 slice	9	.05	.01	.17	.04	2.7	0	4.4	8.12	.23	9.28	60.9	.07
in water, tidbits, w/liquid	1 cup	37	.23	.06	.73	.18	11.8	0	18.9	36.9	.98	44.28	312.42	.3
in water, w/1.25 tbsp liquid	1 slice	9	.05	.02	.17	.04	2.8	0	4.5	8.7	.23	10.44	73.66	.07
PINEAPPLE, FROZEN														
sweetened, chunks	1/2 cup	37	.12	.04	.37	.09	12.9	0	9.8	10.98	.49	12.2	122.0	.13

Food Name	Serving Size	A I.U.	Thi mg	Rib mg	Nia mg	B₆ mg	Fol mcg	B₁₂ mcg	C mg	Calc mg	Iron mg	Mag mg	Pot mg	Zn mg
PINEAPPLE DRINK, frozen 'Bright & Early														
Pineapple' prepared *(Bright & Early)* ..... 6 oz		na	na	na	na	na	na	na	60.0	na	na	na	75	na
PINEAPPLE GRAPEFRUIT JUICE														
canned .... 1 cup		88	.08	.04	.67	.1	26.3	0	115.0	17.5	.78	15.0	152.5	.15
canned .... 1 oz		11	.01	.01	.08	.01	3.3	0	14.4	2.19	.1	1.88	19.09	.02
PINEAPPLE JUICE														
Can, bottle, or box														
(Minute Maid) .... 6 oz		na	na	na	na	na	na	na	21.0	na	na	na	250	na
50% juice *(J. Hungerford)* ...... 9.03 oz		na	na	na	na	na	na	na	100.0	1.3	1.7	na	na	na
100% juice *(J. Hungerford)* ...... 9.03 oz		na	na	na	na	na	na	na	100.0	2.0	3.5	na	na	na
regular *(J. Hungerford)* ...... 9.03 oz		na	na	na	na	na	na	na	100.0	1.1	1.5	na	na	na
unsweetened, w/added ascorbic acid ..... 1 cup		13	.14	.05	.64	.24	57.8	0	96.3	42.5	.65	32.5	335.0	.28
unsweetened, w/added ascorbic acid ..... 1 oz		2	.02	.01	.08	.03	7.2	0	12.1	5.32	.08	4.07	41.94	.03
unsweetened, w/o added ascorbic acid .... 1 cup		13	.14	.05	.64	.24	57.8	0	26.8	42.5	.65	32.5	335.0	.28
unsweetened, w/o added ascorbic acid .... 1 oz		2	.02	.01	.08	.03	7.2	0	3.4	5.32	.08	4.07	41.94	.03
Frozen or chilled														
(Minute Maid) .... 6 oz		na	na	na	na	na	na	na	21.0	na	na	na	250	na
unsweetened concentrate, diluted .... 1 cup		25	.18	.05	.5	.19	26.5	0	30.0	27.5	.75	22.5	340.0	.28
unsweetened concentrate, diluted .... 1 oz		3	.02	.01	.06	.02	3.3	0	3.7	3.43	.09	2.81	42.43	.03
unsweetened concentrate, undiluted ..... 6 oz		108	.5	.13	1.94	.55	79.5	0	90.7	84.24	1.94	75.6	1019.52	.86
PINEAPPLE NECTAR *(Libby's)* .... 6 oz		na	na	na	na	na	na	na	na	na	na	na	65	na
PINEAPPLE ORANGE JUICE, frozen or chilled														
(Minute Maid) .... 6 oz		na	na	na	na	na	na	na	27.0	na	na	na	260	na
PINEAPPLE TOPPING														
.... 1 cup		71	.1	.03	.31	.07	10.2	0	199.2	74.8	1.63	6.8	1077.8	1.63
.... 2 tbsp		9	.01	0	.04	.01	1.3	0	24.6	9.24	.2	.84	133.14	.2
PINK BEAN														
mature seeds, boiled .... 1/2 cup		0	.22	.05	.48	.15	141.4	0	0.0	43.68	1.93	54.6	426.72	.81
mature seeds, raw .... 1/2 cup		0	.81	.2	1.99	.55	486.4	0	0.0	136.5	7.11	191.1	1537.2	2.68
PINOCCHIO. See PINE NUT.														
PIÑON. See PINE NUT.														
PINTO BEAN														
mature seeds, boiled .... 1/2 cup		2	.16	.08	.34	.13	146.2	0	1.8	40.8	2.22	46.75	397.8	.92
mature seeds, raw .... 1/2 cup		5	.53	.23	1.39	.43	486.1	0	7.0	116.16	5.64	152.64	1274.88	2.44
Canned														
(Gebhardt) .... 4 oz		na	na	na	na	na	na	na	0.0	5.25	7.47	na	na	na
mature seeds .... 1/2 cup		1	.12	.08	.35	.09	72.2	0	0.8	44.4	1.93	32.4	361.2	.83
organic, very low sodium, no salt added														
(Eden Foods) .... 1/2 cup		na	na	na	na	na	na	na	na	na	na	na	330	na
organic, w/liquid *(Eden Foods)* .... 1/2 cup		na	na	na	na	na	na	na	na	na	na	na	300	na
Frozen														
immature seeds, boiled, drained, 10-oz pkg	1/3 pkg	0	.26	.1	.59	.18	31.5	0	0.7	48.88	2.55	50.76	607.24	.65
immature seeds, unprepared, 10-oz pkg ...	1/3 pkg	0	.32	.11	.66	.2	47.4	0	0.9	54.52	2.82	56.4	710.64	.72
PISTACHIO BUTTER, roasted														
(Maranatha Natural) .... 2 tbsp		na	na	na	na	na	na	na	na	na	na	na	210	na
PISTACHIO NUT														
Shelled														
dried .... 1 cup		298	1.05	.22	1.38	.32	74.2	0	9.2	172.8	8.68	202.24	1399.04	1.72
dried, approx 47 kernels .... 1 oz		66	.23	.05	.31	.07	16.5	0	2.0	38.34	1.93	44.87	310.41	.38
dry-roasted .... 1 cup		305	.54	.31	1.8	.33	75.7	0	9.3	89.6	4.06	166.4	1241.6	1.74
dry-roasted .... 1 oz		68	.12	.07	.4	.07	16.8	0	2.1	19.88	.9	36.92	275.48	.39
PITANGA / Surinam cherry														
raw .... 1 cup		2595	.05	.07	.52	na	na	0	45.5	15.57	.35	20.76	178.19	na
raw, trimmed, approx .3 oz .... 1 med		105	0	0	.02	na	na	0	1.8	.63	.01	.84	7.21	na
PIZZA, FRENCH BREAD, FROZEN														
Canadian style bacon, 1 pkg *(Stouffer's)* ... 5.5 oz		na	na	na	na	na	na	na	na	na	na	na	300	na

Food Name	Serving Size	A I.U.	Thi mg	Rib mg	Nia mg	B$_6$ mg	Fol mcg	B$_{12}$ mcg	C mg	Calc mg	Iron mg	Mag mg	Pot mg	Zn mg
cheese *(Healthy Choice)*	5.6 oz	na	na	na	na	na	na	na	na	na	na	na	310	na
cheese, microwave *(Oven Lovin')*	1 serving	na	na	na	na	na	na	na	na	na	na	na	210	na
cheese, 1 pkg *(Stouffer's)*	5 1/8 oz	na	na	na	na	na	na	na	na	na	na	na	300	na
combination, microwave *(Oven Lovin')*	1 serving	na	na	na	na	na	na	na	na	na	na	na	290	na
deluxe *(Healthy Choice)*	6.25 oz	na	na	na	na	na	na	na	na	na	na	na	350	na
deluxe, 1 pkg *(Stouffer's)*	6 1/8 oz	na	na	na	na	na	na	na	na	na	na	na	350	na
double cheese, 1 pkg *(Stouffer's)*	5 7/8 oz	na	na	na	na	na	na	na	na	na	na	na	320	na
hamburger, 1 pkg *(Stouffer's)*	6 oz	na	na	na	na	na	na	na	na	na	na	na	340	na
Italian turkey sausage *(Healthy Choice)*	6.45 oz	na	na	na	na	na	na	na	na	na	na	na	350	na
pepperoni, microwave *(Oven Lovin')*	1 serving	na	na	na	na	na	na	na	na	na	na	na	280	na
pepperoni *(Healthy Choice)*	6.25 oz	na	na	na	na	na	na	na	na	na	na	na	370	na
pepperoni, 1 pkg *(Stouffer's)*	5 3/4 oz	na	na	na	na	na	na	na	na	na	na	na	300	na
pepperoni and mushroom *(Stouffer's)*	6 oz	na	na	na	na	na	na	na	na	na	na	na	340	na
sausage *(Stouffer's)*	6 oz	na	na	na	na	na	na	na	na	na	na	na	340	na
sausage, microwave *(Oven Lovin')*	1 serving	na	na	na	na	na	na	na	na	na	na	na	270	na
sausage and pepperoni *(Stouffer's)*	6.25 oz	na	na	na	na	na	na	na	na	na	na	na	360	na
vegetable deluxe *(Stouffer's)*	6.5 oz	na	na	na	na	na	na	na	na	na	na	na	230	na
PIZZA, FROZEN														
(Banquet)														
pepperoni 'Pizza Pie'	6-oz pie	na	na	na	na	na	na	na	na	na	na	na	250	na
sausage 'Pizza Pie'	6-oz pie	na	na	na	na	na	na	na	na	na	na	na	230	na
sausage and pepperoni 'Pizza Pie'	6-oz pie	na	na	na	na	na	na	na	na	na	na	na	250	na
(Celeste)														
cheese	1/4 pie	na	na	na	na	na	na	na	na	na	na	na	268	na
cheese 'Pizza for One'	1 pie	na	na	na	na	na	na	na	na	na	na	na	342	na
deluxe	1/4 pie	na	na	na	na	na	na	na	na	na	na	na	352	na
deluxe 'Pizza for One'	1 pie	na	na	na	na	na	na	na	na	na	na	na	498	na
four cheese, original 'Pizza for One'	1 pie	na	na	na	na	na	na	na	na	na	na	na	410	na
four cheese, zesty 'Pizza for One'	1 pie	na	na	na	na	na	na	na	na	na	na	na	440	na
pepperoni	1/4 pie	na	na	na	na	na	na	na	na	na	na	na	284	na
pepperoni 'Pizza for One'	1 pie	na	na	na	na	na	na	na	na	na	na	na	416	na
sausage	1/4 pie	na	na	na	na	na	na	na	na	na	na	na	311	na
sausage 'Pizza for One'	1 pie	na	na	na	na	na	na	na	na	na	na	na	456	na
suprema	1/4 pie	na	na	na	na	na	na	na	na	na	na	na	342	na
suprema 'Pizza for One'	1 pie	na	na	na	na	na	na	na	na	na	na	na	528	na
vegetable 'Pizza for One'	1 pie	na	na	na	na	na	na	na	na	na	na	na	170	na
(Jeno's)														
combination 'Crisp 'N Tasty'	1/2 pizza	na	na	na	na	na	na	na	na	na	na	na	170	na
pepperoni 'Crisp 'N Tasty'	1/2 pizza	na	na	na	na	na	na	na	na	na	na	na	150	na
pepperoni 'Pizza Pocket'	1 serving	na	na	na	na	na	na	na	na	na	na	na	220	na
sausage 'Crisp'N Tasty'	1/2 pizza	na	na	na	na	na	na	na	na	na	na	na	170	na
sausage 'Pizza Pocket'	1 serving	na	na	na	na	na	na	na	na	na	na	na	190	na
sausage and pepperoni 'Pizza Pocket'	1 serving	na	na	na	na	na	na	na	na	na	na	na	200	na
supreme 'Pizza Pocket'	1 serving	na	na	na	na	na	na	na	na	na	na	na	300	na
(Oven Lovin')														
cheese, microwave	1/2 pie	na	na	na	na	na	na	na	na	na	na	na	140	na
combination, microwave	1/2 pie	na	na	na	na	na	na	na	na	na	na	na	190	na
pepperoni, microwave	1/2 pie	na	na	na	na	na	na	na	na	na	na	na	190	na
sausage, microwave	1/2 pie	na	na	na	na	na	na	na	na	na	na	na	180	na
supreme, microwave	1/2 pie	na	na	na	na	na	na	na	na	na	na	na	290	na
(Pappalo's)														
pepperoni, 9 inch, traditional crust	1/2 pie	na	na	na	na	na	na	na	na	na	na	na	400	na
pepperoni, 12 inch, traditional crust	1/4 pie	na	na	na	na	na	na	na	na	na	na	na	330	na
pepperoni, pan pizza	1/6 pie	na	na	na	na	na	na	na	na	na	na	na	300	na
sausage, 9 inch, traditional crust	1/2 pie	na	na	na	na	na	na	na	na	na	na	na	370	na
sausage, 12 inch, traditional crust	1/4 pie	na	na	na	na	na	na	na	na	na	na	na	290	na
sausage, pan pizza	1/5 pie	na	na	na	na	na	na	na	na	na	na	na	260	na

Food Name	Serving Size	A I.U.	Thi mg	Rib mg	Nia mg	B$_6$ mg	Fol mcg	B$_{12}$ mcg	C mg	Calc mg	Iron mg	Mag mg	Pot mg	Zn mg
sausage and pepperoni, 9 inch, traditional crust	1/2 pie	na	na	na	na	na	na	na	na	na	na	na	340	na
sausage and pepperoni, 12 inch, traditional crust	1/4 pie	na	na	na	na	na	na	na	na	na	na	na	320	na
sausage and pepperoni, pan pizza	1/5 pie	na	na	na	na	na	na	na	na	na	na	na	280	na
supreme, 9 inch, traditional crust	1/2 pie	na	na	na	na	na	na	na	na	na	na	na	370	na
supreme, 12 inch, traditional crust	1/4 pie	na	na	na	na	na	na	na	na	na	na	na	400	na
supreme, pan pizza	1/5 pie	na	na	na	na	na	na	na	na	na	na	na	370	na
three cheese, 9 inch, traditional crust	1/2 pie	na	na	na	na	na	na	na	na	na	na	na	300	na
three cheese, 12 inch, traditional crust	1/4 pie	na	na	na	na	na	na	na	na	na	na	na	260	na
three cheese, pan pizza	1/5 pie	na	na	na	na	na	na	na	na	na	na	na	250	na
(Tombstone)														
cheese, microwave, 7 inch	7.7 oz	na	na	na	na	na	na	na	na	na	na	na	510	na
cheese, original, 9 inch	5.6 oz	na	na	na	na	na	na	na	na	na	na	na	260	na
cheese and hamburger, original, 9 inch	6.3 oz	na	na	na	na	na	na	na	na	na	na	na	330	na
cheese and pepperoni, microwave, 7 inch	7.5 oz	na	na	na	na	na	na	na	na	na	na	na	480	na
cheese and pepperoni, original, 9 inch	6.3 oz	na	na	na	na	na	na	na	na	na	na	na	330	na
cheese and sausage, original, 9 inch	6.3 oz	na	na	na	na	na	na	na	na	na	na	na	350	na
chicken, 'Light' 8 inch	4.5 oz	na	na	na	na	na	na	na	na	na	na	na	290	na
deluxe, original, 9 inch	7.0 oz	na	na	na	na	na	na	na	na	na	na	na	400	na
four meat, 'Special Order' 9 inch	3.9 oz	na	na	na	na	na	na	na	na	na	na	na	230	na
Italian sausage, microwave, 7 inch	8.0 oz	na	na	na	na	na	na	na	na	na	na	na	540	na
pepperoni, 'Light' 8 inch	4.0 oz	na	na	na	na	na	na	na	na	na	na	na	330	na
pepperoni, 'Special Order' 9 inch	3.7 oz	na	na	na	na	na	na	na	na	na	na	na	210	na
pepperoni and sausage, original, 9 inch	6.6 oz	na	na	na	na	na	na	na	na	na	na	na	370	na
sausage and pepperoni, microwave, 7 inch	8 oz	na	na	na	na	na	na	na	na	na	na	na	550	na
sausage and pepperoni, 'Double Top' w/double cheese, 12 inch	4.8 oz	na	na	na	na	na	na	na	na	na	na	na	250	na
supreme, 'Light' 8 inch	4.6 oz	na	na	na	na	na	na	na	na	na	na	na	370	na
supreme, microwave, 7 inch	8.5 oz	na	na	na	na	na	na	na	na	na	na	na	610	na
supreme, 'Special Order' 9 inch	4.0 oz	na	na	na	na	na	na	na	na	na	na	na	230	na
taco, microwave, 7 inch	8.4 oz	na	na	na	na	na	na	na	na	na	na	na	570	na
three sausage, 'Special Order' 9 inch	3.8 oz	na	na	na	na	na	na	na	na	na	na	na	220	na
vegetable, 'Light' 8 inch	4.4 oz	na	na	na	na	na	na	na	na	na	na	na	320	na
(Totino's)														
Canadian bacon 'Party Pizza'	1/2 pie	na	na	na	na	na	na	na	na	na	na	na	240	na
cheese 'Pan Pizza'	1/6 pie	na	na	na	na	na	na	na	na	na	na	na	180	na
cheese 'Party Pizza'	1/2 pie	na	na	na	na	na	na	na	na	na	na	na	240	na
cheese 'Party Pizza Family Size'	1/3 pie	na	na	na	na	na	na	na	na	na	na	na	260	na
combination 'Party Pizza'	1/2 pie	na	na	na	na	na	na	na	na	na	na	na	300	na
combination 'Party Pizza Family Size'	1/3 pie	na	na	na	na	na	na	na	na	na	na	na	320	na
hamburger 'Party Pizza'	1/2 pie	na	na	na	na	na	na	na	na	na	na	na	270	na
pepperoni 'Pan Pizza'	1/6 pie	na	na	na	na	na	na	na	na	na	na	na	220	na
pepperoni 'Party Pizza'	1/2 pie	na	na	na	na	na	na	na	na	na	na	na	240	na
pepperoni 'Party Pizza Family Size'	1/3 pie	na	na	na	na	na	na	na	na	na	na	na	260	na
sausage 'Pan Pizza'	1/6 pie	na	na	na	na	na	na	na	na	na	na	na	210	na
sausage 'Party Pizza'	1/2 pie	na	na	na	na	na	na	na	na	na	na	na	270	na
sausage 'Party Pizza Family Size'	1/3 pie	na	na	na	na	na	na	na	na	na	na	na	300	na
sausage and pepperoni 'Pan Pizza'	1/6 pie	na	na	na	na	na	na	na	na	na	na	na	220	na

PIZZA ENTRÉE, FROZEN

Food Name	Serving Size	A I.U.	Thi mg	Rib mg	Nia mg	B$_6$ mg	Fol mcg	B$_{12}$ mcg	C mg	Calc mg	Iron mg	Mag mg	Pot mg	Zn mg
supreme, hand held 'Aussie Pie' *(Mrs. Paterson's)*	5.5 oz	na	na	na	na	na	na	na	na	na	na	na	294	na

PIZZA MIX

Food Name	Serving Size	A I.U.	Thi mg	Rib mg	Nia mg	B$_6$ mg	Fol mcg	B$_{12}$ mcg	C mg	Calc mg	Iron mg	Mag mg	Pot mg	Zn mg
cheese, kit *(Contadina)*	4.94 oz	na	na	na	na	na	na	na	na	na	na	na	250	na
pepperoni, kit *(Contadina)*	4.94 oz	na	na	na	na	na	na	na	na	na	na	na	270	na

PIZZA ROLL, FROZEN

Food Name	Serving Size	A I.U.	Thi mg	Rib mg	Nia mg	B$_6$ mg	Fol mcg	B$_{12}$ mcg	C mg	Calc mg	Iron mg	Mag mg	Pot mg	Zn mg
cheese, approx 6 rolls *(Jeno's)*	3 oz	na	na	na	na	na	na	na	na	na	na	na	140	na

Food Name	Serving Size	A I.U.	Thi mg	Rib mg	Nia mg	B₆ mg	Fol mcg	B₁₂ mcg	C mg	Calc mg	Iron mg	Mag mg	Pot mg	Zn mg
combination (Jeno's)	3 oz	na	na	na	na	na	na	na	na	na	na	na	200	na
hamburger, approx 6 rolls (Jeno's)	3 oz	na	na	na	na	na	na	na	na	na	na	na	200	na
pepperoni, approx 6 rolls (Jeno's)	3 oz	na	na	na	na	na	na	na	na	na	na	na	200	na
sausage (Jeno's)	3 oz	na	na	na	na	na	na	na	na	na	na	na	200	na
PLANTAIN														
cooked, sliced	1 cup	1400	.07	.08	1.16	.37	40.0	0	16.8	3.08	.89	49.28	716.1	.2
raw, sliced	1 cup	1668	.08	.08	1.02	.44	32.6	0	27.2	4.44	.89	54.76	738.52	.21
raw, trimmed, approx 9.7 oz	1 med	2017	.09	.1	1.23	.54	39.4	0	32.9	5.37	1.07	66.23	893.21	.25
PLUM														
raw, 2 1/8 inch diam	1 med	213	.03	.06	.33	.05	1.5	0	6.3	2.64	.07	4.62	113.52	.07
raw, sliced	1 cup	533	.07	.16	.83	.13	3.6	0	15.7	6.6	.16	11.55	283.8	.16
PLUM, PURPLE, CANNED														
in extra heavy syrup, w/liquid	1 cup	663	.04	.1	.74	.07	6.5	0	1.0	23.49	2.14	13.05	232.29	.18
in extra heavy syrup, w/2.75 tbsp liquid	3 plums	338	.02	.05	.38	.04	3.3	0	0.5	11.97	1.09	6.65	118.37	.09
in heavy syrup, w/liquid	1 cup	668	.04	.1	.75	.07	6.5	0	1.0	23.22	2.17	12.9	234.78	.18
in heavy syrup, w/2.75 tbsp liquid	3 plums	344	.02	.05	.39	.04	3.3	0	0.5	11.97	1.12	6.65	121.03	.09
POHA. See CAPE GOOSEBERRY.														
POI, fresh	1/2 cup	24	.16	.05	1.32	.33	25.7	0	4.8	19.2	1.06	28.8	219.6	.26
POKEBERRY SHOOTS														
boiled, drained	1/2 cup	7134	.06	.21	.9	.09	7.1	0	67.2	43.46	.98	11.48	150.88	.16
raw	1/2 cup	6960	.06	.26	.96	.12	12.6	0	108.8	42.4	1.36	14.4	193.6	.19
POLLACK, ATLANTIC, raw	3 oz	30	.04	.16	2.78	.24	2.6	2.71	0.0	51.0	.39	56.95	302.6	.4
POLLACK, WALLEYE														
dry-heat cooked	3 oz	65	.06	.06	1.4	.06	3.1	3.57	0.0	5.1	.24	62.05	328.95	.51
raw	3 oz	56	.06	.05	1.1	.05	2.6	2.63	0.0	4.25	.2	48.45	277.1	.37
POMEGRANATE/Chinese apple														
raw, approx 3 3/8 inch diam	1 med	0	.05	.05	.46	.16	na	0	9.4	4.62	.46	4.62	398.86	na
POMELO/pumelo														
raw, approx 5 1/2 inches diam, 2.4 lbs	1 med	0	.21	.16	1.34	.22	na	0	371.5	24.36	.67	36.54	1315.44	.49
POMPANO, FLORIDA														
dry-heat cooked	3 oz	102	.58	.13	3.23	.2	14.7	1.02	0.0	36.55	.57	26.35	540.6	.59
POPCORN														
(NOTE: All popcorn is popped unless otherwise noted.)														
(Orville Redenbacher)														
caramel 'Ready-to-Eat'	1 oz	na	na	na	na	na	na	na	0.0	1.44	.24	na	na	na
white cheddar cheese 'Ready-to-Eat'	1.058 oz	na	na	na	na	na	na	na	0.0	2.73	.83	na	na	na
POPCORN, MICROWAVE														
(NOTE: All microwave popcorn is popped unless otherwise noted.)														
(Orville Redenbacher)														
red herb and garlic flavor, 2 tbsp unpopped	1.27 oz	na	na	na	na	na	na	na	0.0	.95	3.75	na	na	na
zesty butter flavor 'Reddenbutter' 2 tbsp unpopped	1.27 oz	na	na	na	na	na	na	na	0.0	.75	4.16	na	na	na
POPCORN OIL														
(Wesson) buttery flavor popping oil	1 tbsp	na	na	na	na	na	na	na	0.0	0	0	na	na	na
(Wesson) popping and topping oil 'Food Service'	1 tbsp	na	na	na	na	na	na	na	0.0	0	0	na	na	na
POPPY SEED														
whole	1 tbsp	0	.07	.02	.09	.04	na	0	na	127.46	.83	29.17	61.56	.9
whole	1 tsp	0	.02	0	.03	.01	na	0	na	40.56	.26	9.28	19.59	.29
whole (Durkee)	1 tsp	na	.54	.14	0	na	na	na	na	0	.01	na	0	na
whole (Laurel Leaf)	1 tsp	na	.54	.14	0	na	na	na	na	0	.01	na	0	na
POPPY SEED OIL														
	1 cup	0	0	0	0	0	0.0	0	0.0	0	0	0	0	0
	1 tbsp	0	0	0	0	0	0.0	0	0.0	0	0	0	0	0

Food Name	Serving Size	A I.U.	Thi mg	Rib mg	Nia mg	B$_6$ mg	Fol mcg	B$_{12}$ mcg	C mg	Calc mg	Iron mg	Mag mg	Pot mg	Zn mg
PORK. See also HAM, CANNED; HAM, CURED; HAM, FRESH; HAM PATTY.														
(NOTE: TRIMMED = Lean; separable fat removed. UNTRIMMED = Separable fat not removed.)														
BACKFAT														
wholesale cuts, raw	1 lb	68	.38	.23	4.47	.18	4.5	.82	0.5	9.07	.82	9.07	294.84	1.68
wholesale cuts, raw	1 oz	4	.02	.01	.28	.01	0.3	.05	0.0	.57	.05	.57	18.43	.1
BACKRIB														
Untrimmed														
raw	1 lb	45	2.65	1.17	20.73	1.79	18.1	3.72	0.9	145.15	4.13	72.58	1056.89	10.48
raw	1 oz	3	.17	.07	1.3	.11	1.1	.23	0.1	9.07	.26	4.54	66.06	.65
roasted	3 oz	8	.36	.17	3.02	.26	2.6	.54	0.3	38.25	1.17	17.85	267.75	2.86
BELLY														
wholesale cuts, raw	1 lb	45	1.8	1.1	21.08	.59	4.5	3.81	1.4	22.68	2.36	18.14	839.16	4.63
wholesale cuts, raw	1 oz	3	.11	.07	1.32	.04	0.3	.24	0.1	1.42	.15	1.13	52.45	.29
BOSTON BUTT														
Trimmed														
cured, medium fat, chopped, roasted	1 cup	0	.9	.35	7.0	na	na	na	0.0	16.8	2.0	na	435.96	na
cured, medium fat, roasted	9.8 oz	0	1.79	.7	13.95	na	na	na	0.0	33.48	3.99	na	868.81	na
BRAINS														
braised	3 oz	0	.07	.19	2.83	.12	3.4	1.21	11.9	7.65	1.55	10.2	165.75	1.26
raw	1 oz	0	.04	.08	1.21	.05	1.7	.62	3.8	2.84	.45	3.97	73.14	.36
CENTER LOIN														
Trimmed														
braised	3 oz	6	.7	.19	4.13	.34	2.6	.43	0.9	19.55	.96	17.0	311.95	1.92
broiled	3 oz	7	.98	.26	4.71	.4	5.1	.63	0.3	26.35	.72	22.95	318.75	2.02
pan-fried	3 oz	7	1.06	.28	5.1	.44	5.1	.65	1.0	19.55	.83	27.2	381.65	2.07
roasted	3 oz	6	.78	.23	4.64	.32	3.4	.49	0.9	21.25	.88	18.7	307.7	1.78
Untrimmed														
braised	3 oz	7	.65	.18	3.92	.32	2.6	.43	0.8	22.1	.89	16.15	300.05	1.84
broiled	3 oz	8	.91	.24	4.45	.36	5.1	.62	0.3	28.05	.68	21.25	304.3	1.92
pan-fried	3 oz	7	.97	.26	4.76	.4	5.1	.62	0.9	22.95	.77	24.65	361.25	1.96
roasted	3 oz	6	.73	.22	4.43	.3	3.4	.48	0.8	22.95	.84	17.0	299.2	1.72
CENTER RIB														
Trimmed														
braised	3 oz	5	.53	.21	4.44	.29	1.7	.46	0.3	18.7	.82	16.15	344.25	1.78
broiled	3 oz	5	.95	.28	5.24	.4	2.6	.65	0.3	26.35	.7	23.8	357.0	2.02
pan-fried	3 oz	5	.74	.28	5.03	.33	2.6	.64	0.3	17.0	.65	22.95	386.75	1.77
raw	1 lb	27	4.41	1.16	26.38	2.16	13.6	2.95	1.4	95.26	3.45	104.33	1909.66	7.44
roasted	3 oz	5	.64	.27	5.46	.29	2.6	.58	0.3	22.1	.83	18.7	371.45	1.81
Untrimmed														
braised	3 oz	6	.5	.2	4.2	.27	1.7	.45	0.3	21.25	.77	15.3	328.95	1.71
broiled	3 oz	6	.88	.26	4.91	.37	2.6	.62	0.3	28.05	.65	22.1	340.85	1.92
pan-fried	3 oz	6	.68	.26	4.7	.31	2.6	.6	0.3	20.4	.61	21.25	365.5	1.69
roasted	3 oz	5	.62	.26	5.2	.28	2.6	.56	0.3	23.8	.8	17.85	357.85	1.75
CHITTERLINGS														
raw	1 oz	0	0	.02	.02	0	0.6	.23	1.3	5.67	.54	1.7	32.89	.59
simmered	3 oz	0	0	.07	.09	.01	2.6	.88	0.0	22.95	3.15	8.5	6.8	4.3
COMPOSITE CUTS														
Trimmed														
loin and shoulder, cooked	3 oz	6	.74	.29	4.46	.37	5.1	.64	0.3	18.7	.91	22.1	320.45	2.44
loin and shoulder, raw	1 lb	32	4.45	1.23	21.89	2.31	22.7	2.99	2.7	77.11	3.99	104.33	1741.82	9.03
loin and shoulder, raw	1 oz	2	.28	.08	1.37	.14	1.4	.19	0.2	4.82	.25	6.52	108.86	.56
roasted	3 oz	6	.72	.29	4.4	.37	5.1	.64	0.3	17.85	.94	22.1	318.75	2.52
Untrimmed														
loin and shoulder, cooked	3 oz	7	.72	.28	4.22	.34	5.1	.63	0.3	20.4	.84	20.4	307.7	2.23
loin and shoulder, raw	1 lb	32	4.05	1.15	20.38	2.07	22.7	2.86	2.7	86.18	3.72	95.26	1596.67	8.48
loin and shoulder, raw	1 oz	2	.25	.07	1.27	.13	1.4	.18	0.2	5.39	.23	5.95	99.79	.53
raw	1 lb	32	3.63	1.1	20.02	1.88	27.2	3.04	2.7	68.04	4.04	90.72	1469.66	9.57

Food Name	Serving Size	A I.U.	Thi mg	Rib mg	Nia mg	B$_6$ mg	Fol mcg	B$_{12}$ mcg	C mg	Calc mg	Iron mg	Mag mg	Pot mg	Zn mg
raw	1 oz	2	.23	.07	1.25	.12	1.7	.19	0.2	4.25	.25	5.67	91.85	.6
KIDNEYS														
braised	1 cup	364	.55	2.22	8.1	.64	57.4	10.91	14.8	18.2	7.41	25.2	200.2	5.81
braised	3 oz	221	.34	1.35	4.92	.39	34.9	6.62	9.0	11.05	4.5	15.3	121.55	3.53
raw	1 oz	56	.1	.48	2.33	.12	11.9	2.41	3.8	2.55	1.39	4.82	64.92	.78
LIVER														
braised	3 oz	15297	.22	1.87	7.17	.48	138.6	15.87	20.1	8.5	15.23	11.9	127.5	5.71
fried	3 oz	19717	.29	3.71	18.95	na	na	na	18.7	12.75	24.74	na	335.75	na
raw	1 oz	6138	.08	.85	4.34	.2	60.1	7.37	7.2	2.55	6.61	5.1	77.4	1.63
LOIN														
Trimmed														
blade, braised	3 oz	6	.45	.23	3.34	.3	2.6	.6	0.7	20.4	1.15	15.3	277.1	3.32
blade, broiled	3 oz	6	.63	.3	3.87	.38	3.4	.8	0.7	19.55	.93	22.1	317.9	3.37
blade, pan-fried	3 oz	6	.62	.3	3.77	.35	3.4	.82	0.7	18.7	.91	22.1	310.25	3.29
blade, raw	1 lb	32	3.67	1.27	19.61	2.22	18.1	3.81	3.6	104.33	4.63	95.26	1542.24	13.38
blade, roasted	3 oz	7	.49	.29	3.96	.37	4.3	.68	0.3	24.65	1.1	20.4	296.65	3.24
country-style ribs, braised	3 oz	6	.46	.24	3.48	.31	2.6	.63	0.7	21.25	1.17	15.3	293.25	3.39
country-style ribs, raw	1 lb	32	3.67	1.27	19.61	2.22	18.1	3.81	3.6	104.33	4.63	95.26	1542.24	13.38
country-style ribs, raw	1 oz	2	.23	.08	1.23	.14	1.1	.24	0.2	6.52	.29	5.95	96.39	.84
country-style ribs, roasted	3 oz	7	.49	.29	3.96	.37	4.3	.68	0.3	24.65	1.1	20.4	296.65	3.24
whole, braised	3 oz	6	.56	.23	3.9	.33	3.4	.47	0.5	15.3	.96	17.0	328.95	2.11
whole, broiled	3 oz	6	.78	.29	4.46	.42	5.1	.61	0.6	14.45	.77	24.65	372.3	2.11
whole, roasted	3 oz	7	.86	.28	5.01	.47	6.0	.62	0.5	15.3	.93	23.8	361.25	2.15
Untrimmed														
blade, braised	3 oz	7	.4	.2	3.05	.25	1.7	.55	0.5	26.35	.94	12.75	258.4	2.78
blade, broiled	3 oz	7	.55	.25	3.49	.32	3.4	.71	0.6	24.65	.79	18.7	292.4	2.86
blade, pan-fried	3 oz	7	.53	.25	3.35	.29	3.4	.71	0.5	25.5	.75	17.85	282.2	2.71
blade, raw	1 lb	36	2.97	1.05	16.56	1.68	13.6	.41	2.7	131.54	3.76	72.58	1274.62	10.66
blade, roasted	3 oz	8	.45	.25	3.6	.32	3.4	.62	0.2	28.9	.94	17.0	277.1	2.81
country-style ribs, braised	3 oz	7	.43	.22	3.27	.28	2.6	.59	0.6	24.65	1.04	14.45	278.8	3.03
country-style ribs, raw	1 lb	36	3.2	1.12	17.6	1.86	18.1	3.4	3.2	122.47	4.04	81.65	1369.87	11.61
country-style ribs, raw	1 oz	2	.2	.07	1.1	.12	1.1	.21	0.2	7.65	.25	5.1	85.62	.73
country-style ribs, roasted	3 oz	8	.76	.29	3.67	.38	4.3	.67	0.3	21.25	.9	19.55	292.4	2.01
whole, broiled	3 oz	6	.75	.27	4.28	.39	4.3	.6	0.5	16.15	.74	23.8	359.55	2.03
whole, raw	1 lb	32	4.09	1.12	20.77	2.14	22.7	2.4	2.7	81.65	3.58	95.26	1614.82	7.89
whole, roasted	3 oz	8	.84	.27	4.74	.44	5.1	.6	0.5	16.15	.84	22.1	346.8	1.97
LUNGS														
braised	3 oz	0	.07	.27	1.16	.07	1.7	1.73	6.7	6.8	13.95	10.2	128.35	2.08
raw	1 oz	0	.02	.12	.95	.03	0.9	.78	3.5	1.98	5.36	3.97	85.9	.58
PANCREAS														
braised	3 oz	0	.08	.56	2.73	.37	4.3	14.51	4.8	13.6	2.29	19.55	142.8	3.65
raw	1 oz	0	.03	.13	.98	.13	0.9	4.65	4.3	3.12	.6	4.82	55.85	.74
SHOULDER														
Trimmed														
arm picnic, braised	3 oz	7	.51	.31	5.05	.35	4.3	.6	0.3	6.8	1.66	18.7	344.25	4.22
arm picnic, raw	1 lb	23	3.96	1.39	20.99	2.22	18.1	3.31	4.1	27.22	5.4	95.26	1546.78	12.97
arm picnic, raw	1 oz	1	.25	.09	1.31	.14	1.1	.21	0.3	1.7	.34	5.95	96.67	.81
arm picnic, roasted	3 oz	6	.49	.3	3.67	.35	4.3	.66	0.3	7.65	1.21	17.0	298.35	3.46
Boston blade, braised	3 oz	8	.61	.34	3.64	.25	1.7	.83	0.3	24.65	1.74	17.0	350.2	4.73
Boston blade, broiled	3 oz	7	.64	.37	3.65	.26	4.3	.96	0.3	28.05	1.33	20.4	291.55	4.27
Boston blade, roasted	3 oz	8	.95	.34	4.22	.37	6.8	.99	0.9	22.95	1.33	22.1	362.95	3.6
whole, raw	1 lb	27	4.01	1.42	19.39	1.88	22.7	3.81	3.6	63.5	5.53	95.26	1546.78	14.24
whole, raw	1 oz	2	.25	.09	1.21	.12	1.4	.24	0.2	3.97	.35	5.95	96.67	.89
whole, roasted	3 oz	6	.53	.31	3.62	.27	4.3	.73	0.5	15.3	1.27	17.0	294.1	3.54
whole, roasted, diced	1 cup	9	.85	.5	5.75	.43	6.8	1.16	0.8	24.3	2.03	27.0	467.1	5.62
Untrimmed														
arm picnic, roasted	3 oz	7	.44	.26	3.33	.3	3.4	.6	0.2	16.15	1.0	14.45	276.25	2.93

Food Name	Serving Size	A I.U.	Thi mg	Rib mg	Nia mg	B$_6$ mg	Fol mcg	B$_{12}$ mcg	C mg	Calc mg	Iron mg	Mag mg	Pot mg	Zn mg
Boston blade, braised	3 oz	9	0	.31	3.45	.23	1.7	.77	0.3	27.2	1.56	15.3	330.65	4.27
Boston blade, broiled	3 oz	8	.59	.34	3.46	.24	3.4	.9	0.3	30.6	1.19	17.85	277.1	3.83
Boston blade, raw	1 lb	32	3.66	1.32	16.71	1.4	27.2	3.86	3.2	113.4	5.08	81.65	1419.77	13.74
Boston blade, roasted	3 oz	6	.54	.3	3.45	.2	4.3	.75	0.6	23.8	1.23	15.3	282.2	3.37
whole, diced, roasted	1 cup	11	.78	.44	5.39	.39	6.8	1.08	0.7	32.4	1.78	24.3	444.15	5.01
whole, raw	1 lb	32	3.48	1.25	17.39	1.58	22.7	3.36	3.2	68.04	4.76	81.65	1369.87	12.25
whole, raw	1 oz	2	.22	.08	1.09	.1	1.4	.21	0.2	4.25	.3	5.1	85.62	.77
whole, roasted	3 oz	7	.49	.28	3.39	.24	4.3	.68	0.4	20.4	1.12	15.3	279.65	3.15
SIRLOIN														
Trimmed														
boneless, braised	3 oz	6	.59	.24	3.36	.38	2.6	.48	0.8	11.05	.94	18.7	302.6	2.01
boneless, broiled	3 oz	7	.88	.34	4.05	.46	5.1	.71	0.3	15.3	1.05	22.95	320.45	2.26
boneless, raw	1 lb	32	4.93	1.32	19.99	2.86	22.7	3.13	4.1	58.97	3.95	117.94	1678.32	8.39
boneless, roasted	3 oz	6	.76	.32	4.36	.4	4.3	.65	0.9	14.45	1.01	22.95	344.25	2.15
braised	3 oz	6	.59	.24	3.36	.38	2.6	.48	0.8	11.05	1.08	17.0	285.6	2.21
broiled	3 oz	6	.87	.32	4.05	.51	4.3	.67	0.9	11.05	.91	26.35	340.85	2.33
raw, approx 3.1 oz	1 chop	7	1.02	.27	4.14	.59	4.7	.65	0.9	12.22	.82	24.44	347.8	1.74
roasted	3 oz	6	.68	.28	4.72	.36	5.1	.66	0.3	17.0	.95	21.25	311.1	2.18
Untrimmed														
boneless, braised	3 oz	6	.58	.23	3.32	.37	2.6	.48	0.7	11.05	.93	17.85	299.2	1.99
boneless, broiled	3 oz	7	.86	.33	3.99	.45	5.1	.71	0.3	15.3	1.03	22.95	316.2	2.23
boneless, raw	1 lb	32	4.8	1.3	19.6	2.77	22.7	3.08	4.1	58.97	3.86	113.4	1637.5	8.21
boneless, roasted	3 oz	6	.75	.32	4.32	.4	4.3	.64	0.9	13.6	.99	22.1	341.7	2.13
braised	3 oz	6	.56	.22	3.23	.35	2.6	.48	0.7	15.3	.99	16.15	276.25	2.08
broiled	3 oz	7	.81	.29	3.84	.46	4.3	.64	0.8	14.45	.84	24.65	325.55	2.18
roasted	3 oz	7	.64	.27	4.46	.33	5.1	.65	0.3	19.55	.88	20.4	297.5	2.07
SPARERIBS														
Untrimmed														
braised	3 oz	9	.35	.32	4.65	.3	3.4	.92	na	39.95	1.57	20.4	272.0	3.91
raw	1 lb	50	2.01	1.24	22.04	1.91	18.1	3.95	na	140.62	4.49	99.79	1174.82	12.25
raw	1 oz	3	.18	.08	1.38	.12	1.1	.25	na	8.79	.28	6.24	73.43	.77
SPLEEN														
braised	3 oz	0	.12	.22	5.05	.05	3.4	2.35	9.9	11.05	18.9	12.75	192.95	3.01
raw	1 oz	0	.04	.09	1.66	.02	1.1	.92	8.1	2.84	6.33	3.69	112.27	.72
STOMACH, raw	1 oz	0	.02	.03	1.26	.01	0.6	.28	na	2.84	.62	2.55	56.98	.57
TENDERLOIN														
Trimmed														
broiled	3 oz	6	.84	.33	4.36	.45	5.1	.85	0.9	4.25	1.22	30.6	383.35	2.51
raw	1 lb	27	4.42	1.27	20.09	2.36	22.7	3.67	4.1	22.68	5.58	117.94	1660.18	9.21
raw	1 oz	2	.28	.08	1.26	.15	1.4	.23	0.3	1.42	.35	7.37	103.76	.58
roasted	3 oz	6	.8	.33	4.0	.36	5.1	.47	0.3	5.1	1.25	23.8	371.45	2.24
Untrimmed														
broiled	3 oz	6	.82	.32	4.3	.44	5.1	.83	0.9	4.25	1.18	29.75	377.4	2.46
raw	1 lb	27	4.31	1.25	19.72	2.29	22.7	3.58	4.1	22.68	5.44	113.4	1628.42	9.03
raw	1 oz	2	.27	.08	1.23	.14	1.4	.22	0.3	1.42	.34	7.09	101.78	.56
roasted	3 oz	6	.79	.33	3.96	.35	5.1	.47	0.3	5.1	1.23	22.95	368.05	2.21
TOP LOIN														
Trimmed														
braised	3 oz	5	.49	.23	3.99	.29	4.3	.39	0.3	19.55	.86	17.0	357.85	1.85
broiled	3 oz	5	.76	.27	4.45	.34	7.7	.6	0.3	26.35	.7	23.8	357.0	2.02
pan-fried	3 oz	5	.71	.32	4.79	.36	6.8	.57	0.3	18.7	.72	25.5	425.0	1.95
roast, boneless, raw	1 lb	27	3.88	1.22	22.84	2.13	31.8	2.4	1.4	95.26	3.45	104.33	1909.66	7.44
roast, boneless, raw	1 oz	2	.24	.08	1.43	.13	2.0	.15	0.1	5.95	.22	6.52	119.35	.46
roasted	3 oz	7	.54	.27	4.55	.34	7.7	.47	0.3	4.25	.9	21.25	300.9	1.96
Untrimmed														
braised	3 oz	6	.47	.22	3.86	.28	3.4	.39	0.3	17.85	.82	16.15	345.95	1.79

Food Name	Serving Size	A I.U.	Thi mg	Rib mg	Nia mg	B6 mg	Fol mcg	B12 mcg	C mg	Calc mg	Iron mg	Mag mg	Pot mg	Zn mg
broiled	3 oz	5	.73	.26	4.29	.32	6.8	.59	0.3	24.65	.67	22.95	344.25	1.95
pan-fried	3 oz	6	.68	.3	4.57	.34	6.8	.55	0.3	17.85	.69	23.8	407.15	1.87
roast, boneless, raw	1 lb	27	3.6	1.14	21.36	1.94	27.2	2.31	1.4	86.18	3.22	95.26	1769.04	6.99
roast, boneless, raw	1 oz	2	.22	.07	1.34	.12	1.7	.14	0.1	5.39	.2	5.95	110.57	.44
roasted	3 oz	7	.52	.25	4.36	.32	6.8	.47	0.3	4.25	.68	19.55	290.7	1.88
PORK, CURED														
boneless, blade roll, untrimmed, roasted	3 oz	0	.39	.24	2.02	.18	2.6	.89	2.7	5.95	.76	11.05	164.9	2.08
boneless, blade roll, untrimmed, unheated	1 oz	0	.15	.06	.77	.07	0.9	.37	0.1	1.98	.23	3.69	83.63	.67
PORK, GROUND														
cooked	3 oz	7	.6	.19	3.58	.33	5.1	.46	0.6	18.7	1.1	20.4	307.7	2.73
raw	1 oz	2	.21	.07	1.23	.11	1.4	.2	0.2	3.97	.25	5.39	81.36	.62
PORK, SALT, cured, raw	1 oz	0	.06	.02	.46	.02	0.3	.08	0.0	1.7	.12	1.98	18.71	.26
PORK DINNER, FROZEN														
chow mein 'Bi-Pack' (LaChoy)	8.642 oz	na	na	na	na	na	na	na	4.1	3.23	7.9	na	na	na
PORK ENTRÉE														
Frozen, sweet and sour (Chun King)	13 oz	na	na	na	na	na	na	na	na	na	na	na	330	na
PORK FAT														
separable fat from ham and arm picnic, roasted	3 oz	0	.24	.08	1.89	.03	1.7	.36	0.0	6.8	.52	7.65	139.4	1.11
separable fat from ham and arm picnic, roasted	1 oz	0	.08	.03	.63	.01	0.6	.12	0.0	2.27	.17	2.55	46.49	.37
separable fat from ham and arm picnic, unheated	1 oz	0	.07	.02	.52	.01	0.3	.09	0.0	1.42	.11	1.7	29.77	.23
PORK RIND SNACK														
(Baken-ets)	1 oz	na	na	na	na	na	na	na	na	na	na	na	55	na
(Baken-ets) hot 'n spicy	1 oz	na	na	na	na	na	na	na	na	na	na	na	55	na
POT ROAST DINNER / ENTRÉE, FROZEN														
homestyle, w/browned potatoes (Stouffer's)	8 7/8 oz	na	na	na	na	na	na	na	na	na	na	na	800	na
POTATO														
Baked, pulp	1/2 cup	0	.06	.01	.85	.18	5.6	0	7.8	3.05	.21	15.25	238.51	.18
Boiled														
in skin, pulp only	1/2 cup	0	.08	.02	1.12	.23	7.8	0	10.1	3.9	.24	17.16	295.62	.23
in skin, pulp only, approx 2.5 inch diam	1 potato	0	.14	.03	1.96	.41	13.6	0	17.7	6.8	.42	29.92	515.44	.41
pulp only	1/2 cup	0	.08	.01	1.02	.21	6.9	0	5.8	6.24	.24	15.6	255.84	.21
pulp only, approx 2.5 inch diam	1 potato	0	.13	.03	1.77	.36	12.0	0	10.0	10.8	.42	27.0	442.8	.36
Microwaved, in skin, pulp only	1/2 cup	0	.1	.02	1.27	.25	9.7	0	11.8	3.9	.32	19.5	320.58	.26
Raw, pulp only, diced	1/2 cup	0	.07	.03	1.11	.2	9.6	0	14.8	5.25	.57	15.75	407.25	.29
POTATO CHIPS AND SNACKS														
(Funyuns) rings, onion flavor, approx 11 rings	1 oz	na	na	na	na	na	na	na	na	na	na	na	40	na
(Lay's)														
barbecue flavor, approx 15-20 chips	1 oz	na	na	na	na	na	na	na	na	na	na	na	350	na
barbecue flavor 'Kansas City Style' approx 15-20 chips	1 oz	na	na	na	na	na	na	na	na	na	na	na	400	na
Cajun flavor 'Crunch Tators Amazin Cajun'	1 oz	na	na	na	na	na	na	na	na	na	na	na	370	na
cheddar cheese flavor, approx 15-20 chips	1 oz	na	na	na	na	na	na	na	na	na	na	na	410	na
'Flamin' Hot' approx 15-20 chips	1 oz	na	na	na	na	na	na	na	na	na	na	na	380	na
jalapeño flavor 'Crunch Tators Hoppin' Jalapeño'	1 oz	na	na	na	na	na	na	na	na	na	na	na	400	na
mesquite flavor 'Crunch Tators Mighty Mesquite'	1 oz	na	na	na	na	na	na	na	na	na	na	na	390	na
original flavor, approx 15-20 chips	1 oz	na	na	na	na	na	na	na	na	na	na	na	380	na
original flavor 'Crunch Tators' approx 16 chips	1 oz	na	na	na	na	na	na	na	na	na	na	na	400	na
salt and vinegar flavor, approx 15-20 chips	1 oz	na	na	na	na	na	na	na	na	na	na	na	360	na
sour cream and onion flavor, approx 15-20 chips	1 oz	na	na	na	na	na	na	na	na	na	na	na	410	na
tangy ranch flavor, approx 15-20 chips	1 oz	na	na	na	na	na	na	na	na	na	na	na	340	na

Food Name	Serving Size	A I.U.	Thi mg	Rib mg	Nia mg	B$_6$ mg	Fol mcg	B$_{12}$ mcg	C mg	Calc mg	Iron mg	Mag mg	Pot mg	Zn mg
'Unsalted'	1 oz	na	na	na	na	na	na	na	na	na	na	na	410	na
(Munchos) plain, approx 16 chips	1 oz	na	na	na	na	na	na	na	na	na	na	na	180	na
(Nabisco) baked, cheddar cheese flavor, cracker														
chips 'Zings'	.5 oz	na	na	na	na	na	na	na	na	na	na	na	50	na
(Poore Brothers)														
barbecue flavor	1 oz	na	na	na	na	na	na	na	na	na	na	na	350	na
Cajun flavor	1 oz	na	na	na	na	na	na	na	na	na	na	na	360	na
dill pickle flavor	1 oz	na	na	na	na	na	na	na	na	na	na	na	360	na
grilled steak and onion flavor	1 oz	na	na	na	na	na	na	na	na	na	na	na	330	na
jalapeño flavor	1 oz	na	na	na	na	na	na	na	na	na	na	na	360	na
Parmesan and garlic flavor	1 oz	na	na	na	na	na	na	na	na	na	na	na	360	na
regular flavor	1 oz	na	na	na	na	na	na	na	na	na	na	na	370	na
salt and vinegar flavor	1 oz	na	na	na	na	na	na	na	na	na	na	na	340	na
unsalted	1 oz	na	na	na	na	na	na	na	na	na	na	na	390	na
(Ruffles)														
'Light Choice' 1/3 less fat	1 oz	na	na	na	na	na	na	na	na	na	na	na	490	na
mesquite barbecue flavor 'Mesquite Grille'	1 oz	na	na	na	na	na	na	na	na	na	na	na	370	na
ranch flavor	1 oz	na	na	na	na	na	na	na	na	na	na	na	360	na
regular flavor	1 oz	na	na	na	na	na	na	na	na	na	na	na	400	na
sour cream and onion flavor	1 oz	na	na	na	na	na	na	na	na	na	na	na	370	na
(Schlotzsky's) barbecue, deli style	1 oz	na	na	na	na	na	na	na	na	na	na	na	444	na
(Sun Chips)														
multi-grain snacks, French onion flavor	1 oz	na	na	na	na	na	na	na	na	na	na	na	60	na
multi-grain snacks, harvest cheddar flavor	1 oz	na	na	na	na	na	na	na	na	na	na	na	65	na
multi-grain snacks, original flavor	1 oz	na	na	na	na	na	na	na	na	na	na	na	45	na
(Westbrae)														
no salt	1 oz	na	na	na	na	na	na	na	na	na	na	na	320	na
'Ripple'	1 oz	na	na	na	na	na	na	na	na	na	na	na	320	na
salted	1 oz	na	na	na	na	na	na	na	na	na	na	na	320	na
POTATO DISH, FROZEN														
au gratin, side dish (Stouffer's)	5.75 oz	na	na	na	na	na	na	na	na	na	na	na	260	na
scalloped, side dish (Stouffer's)	5.75 oz	na	na	na	na	na	na	na	na	na	na	na	375	na
POTATO FLOUR	1/2 cup	0	.38	.13	3.06	.01	45.5	0	17.1	29.7	15.48	79.2	1429.2	1.47
POTATO STICKS. See POTATO CHIPS AND SNACKS.														
POTTED MEAT SPREAD. See also LUNCHEON MEAT, CANNED; SANDWICH SPREAD.														
beef	1 cup	0	.07	.5	2.7	na	na	na	0.0	22.5	2.7	na	517.5	na
chicken	1 cup	0	.07	.5	2.7	na	na	na	0.0	22.5	2.7	na	517.5	na
turkey	1 cup	0	.07	.5	2.7	na	na	na	0.0	22.5	2.7	na	517.5	na
POULTRY SEASONING														
dry	1 tbsp	97	.01	.01	.11	na	na	0	0.4	36.85	1.31	8.29	25.31	.12
dry	1 tsp	39	0	0	.04	na	na	0	0.2	14.94	.53	3.36	10.26	.05
PRETZELS														
BAVARIAN (Rold Gold) 1 oz	3 pretzels	na	na	na	na	na	na	na	na	na	na	na	50	na
CHEDDAR (Combos)	10 nuggets	20	.03	.17	.95	.01	2.4	.04	0.0	57.3	.91	6.6	39.0	.22
DUTCH STYLE														
	7.5-oz pkg	0	.04	.06	1.49	na	na	na	0.0	46.86	3.19	na	276.9	na
	1 pretzel	0	0	0	.11	na	na	na	0.0	3.52	.24	na	20.8	na
(Mister Salty) 1 oz	2 pretzels	na	na	na	na	na	na	na	na	na	na	na	20	na
HARD														
plain, made w/unenriched flour, salted	10 twists	0	.1	.12	2.3	.4	27.0	0	18.7	14.4	.98	40.2	765.0	.65
plain, made w/unenriched flour, unsalted	10 twists	0	.11	.06	1.15	.07	49.8	0	0.0	21.6	1.0	21.0	87.6	.51
plain, salted	10 twists	0	.28	.37	3.15	.07	49.8	0	0.0	21.6	2.59	21.0	87.6	.51
plain, unsalted	10 twists	0	.11	.06	1.15	.07	49.8	0	0.0	21.6	1.0	21.0	87.6	.51
whole wheat	2 oz	0	.25	.16	3.71	.16	30.6	0	0.6	15.88	1.53	17.01	243.81	.35
MINIS (Mister Salty) 1 oz	22 pretzels	na	na	na	na	na	na	na	na	na	na	na	45	na
RODS (Rold Gold)	1 oz	na	na	na	na	na	na	na	na	na	na	na	50	na

Food Name	Serving Size	A I.U.	Thi mg	Rib mg	Nia mg	B$_6$ mg	Fol mcg	B$_{12}$ mcg	C mg	Calc mg	Iron mg	Mag mg	Pot mg	Zn mg
STICKS														
(Mister Salty) fat-free	1 oz	na	na	na	na	na	na	na	na	na	na	na	30	na
(Mister Salty) very thin, 1 oz	92 sticks	na	na	na	na	na	na	na	na	na	na	na	40	na
(Rold Gold)	1 oz	na	na	na	na	na	na	na	na	na	na	na	50	na
TWISTS														
(Mister Salty) .5 oz	5 twists	na	na	na	na	na	na	na	na	na	na	na	35	na
(Mister Salty) fat-free, 1 oz	9 twists	na	na	na	na	na	na	na	na	na	na	na	30	na
(Rold Gold) thin, 1 oz	10 twists	na	na	na	na	na	na	na	na	na	na	na	55	na
(Rold Gold) tiny, 1 oz	15 twists	na	na	na	na	na	na	na	na	na	na	na	50	na
PRICKLY PEAR, raw, trimmed, approx 4.8 oz	1 fruit	53	.01	.06	.47	na	na	0	14.4	57.68	.31	87.55	226.6	na
PRUNE														
Canned														
in heavy syrup, w/liquid	1 cup	1865	.08	.29	2.03	.48	0.2	0	6.6	39.78	.96	35.1	528.84	.44
in heavy syrup, w/2 tbsp liquid	5 fruits	685	.03	.1	.74	.17	0.1	0	2.4	14.62	.35	12.9	194.36	.16
PRUNE, DRIED														
pitted	1 cup	3199	.13	.26	3.16	.43	6.0	0	5.3	82.11	3.99	72.45	1199.45	.85
pitted, approx 3 oz	10 fruits	1669	.07	.14	1.65	.22	3.1	0	2.8	42.84	2.08	37.8	625.8	.45
(Mariani) pitted, premium	1/4 cup	na	na	na	na	na	na	na	na	na	na	na	420	na
PRUNE JUICE (J. Hungerford) 100% juice	9.03 oz	na	na	na	na	na	na	na	100.0	3.1	16.4	na	na	na
PRUNE WHIP														
cold	1 cup	598	.03	.18	.65	na	na	na	2.6	28.6	1.69	na	377.0	na
hot	1 cup	414	.02	.13	.45	na	na	na	1.8	19.8	1.17	na	261.0	na
PUDDING, READY-TO-SERVE														
BANANA (Snack Pack)	4 oz	na	na	na	na	na	na	na	0.0	5.24	.06	na	na	na
BUTTERSCOTCH														
(Snack Pack)	4 oz	na	na	na	na	na	na	na	0.0	5.43	1.13	na	na	na
(Swiss Miss)	4 oz	na	na	na	na	na	na	na	0.0	6.19	0	na	na	na
CHOCOLATE														
(Jell-O) 'Light Pudding Snacks'	4 oz	na	na	na	na	na	na	na	na	na	na	na	200	na
(Jell-O) 'Pudding Snacks'	5.5 oz	na	na	na	na	na	na	na	na	na	na	na	350	na
(Jell-O) 'Pudding Snacks'	4 oz	na	na	na	na	na	na	na	na	na	na	na	270	na
(Snack Pack)	4 oz	na	na	na	na	na	na	na	0.0	5.23	.06	na	na	na
(Snack Pack) fat-free	4 oz	na	na	na	na	na	na	na	0.0	5.34	1.83	na	na	na
(Swiss Miss)	4 oz	na	na	na	na	na	na	na	0.0	8.29	4.03	na	na	na
(Swiss Miss) fat-free	4 oz	na	na	na	na	na	na	na	0.0	2.71	.63	na	na	na
CHOCOLATE FUDGE														
(Jell-O) 'Light Pudding Snacks'	4 oz	na	na	na	na	na	na	na	na	na	na	na	210	na
(Jell-O) 'Pudding Snacks'	4 oz	na	na	na	na	na	na	na	na	na	na	na	260	na
(Snack Pack)	4 oz	na	na	na	na	na	na	na	0.0	5.71	.06	na	na	na
(Swiss Miss)	4 oz	na	na	na	na	na	na	na	0.0	7.91	1.2	na	na	na
(Swiss Miss) fat-free	4 oz	na	na	na	na	na	na	na	0.0	2.71	.63	na	na	na
CHOCOLATE FUDGE-MILK CHOCOLATE SWIRL														
(Jell-O)	4 oz	na	na	na	na	na	na	na	na	na	na	na	260	na
CHOCOLATE-CARAMEL SWIRL														
(Jell-O) 'Pudding Snacks'	4 oz	na	na	na	na	na	na	na	na	na	na	na	230	na
(Snack Pack)	4 oz	na	na	na	na	na	na	na	0.0	6.04	3.34	na	na	na
(Swiss Miss)	4 oz	na	na	na	na	na	na	na	0.0	6.04	3.34	na	na	na
CHOCOLATE-MARSHMALLOW (Snack Pack)	4 oz	na	na	na	na	na	na	na	0.0	5.17	.06	na	na	na
CHOCOLATE-PEANUT BUTTER SWIRL														
(Snack Pack)	4 oz	na	na	na	na	na	na	na	0.0	6.91	3.09	na	na	na
CHOCOLATE-VANILLA SWIRL														
(Jell-O) combo 'Light Pudding Snacks'	4 oz	na	na	na	na	na	na	na	na	na	na	na	160	na
(Jell-O) 'Pudding Snacks'	5.5 oz	na	na	na	na	na	na	na	na	na	na	na	320	na
(Jell-O) 'Pudding Snacks'	4 oz	na	na	na	na	na	na	na	na	na	na	na	230	na
CHOCOLATE-VANILLA-CHOCOLATE SWIRL														
(Swiss Miss)	4 oz	na	na	na	na	na	na	na	0.0	6.79	1.32	na	na	na
LEMON (Snack Pack)	4 oz	na	na	na	na	na	na	na	0.0	3.21	.06	na	na	na

Food Name	Serving Size	A I.U.	Thi mg	Rib mg	Nia mg	B$_6$ mg	Fol mcg	B$_{12}$ mcg	C mg	Calc mg	Iron mg	Mag mg	Pot mg	Zn mg
MILK CHOCOLATE														
(Jell-O) 'Pudding Snacks'	4 oz	na	na	na	na	na	na	na	na	na	na	na	250	na
(Snack Pack)	4 oz	na	na	na	na	na	na	na	0.0	6.57	3.15	na	na	na
(Swiss Miss)	4 oz	na	na	na	na	na	na	na	0.0	6.57	3.15	na	na	na
S'MORES SWIRL (Snack Pack)	4 oz	na	na	na	na	na	na	na	0.0	5.08	.76	na	na	na
TAPIOCA														
(Jell-O) 'Pudding Snacks'	4 oz	na	na	na	na	na	na	na	na	na	na	na	150	na
(Snack Pack)	4 oz	na	na	na	na	na	na	na	0.0	6.47	1.13	na	na	na
(Snack Pack) fat-free	4 oz	na	na	na	na	na	na	na	0.0	5.69	.13	na	na	na
(Swiss Miss)	4 oz	na	na	na	na	na	na	na	0.0	8.46	.57	na	na	na
(Swiss Miss) fat-free	4 oz	na	na	na	na	na	na	na	0.0	4.48	.32	na	na	na
VANILLA														
(Jell-O) 'Light Pudding Snacks'	4 oz	na	na	na	na	na	na	na	na	na	na	na	120	na
(Jell-O) 'Pudding Snacks'	5.5 oz	na	na	na	na	na	na	na	na	na	na	na	200	na
(Jell-O) 'Pudding Snacks'	4 oz	na	na	na	na	na	na	na	na	na	na	na	150	na
(Snack Pack)	4 oz	na	na	na	na	na	na	na	0.0	5.24	.06	na	na	na
(Snack Pack) fat-free	4 oz	na	na	na	na	na	na	na	0.0	5.23	2.46	na	na	na
(Swiss Miss)	4 oz	na	na	na	na	na	na	na	0.0	8.29	.38	na	na	na
(Swiss Miss) fat-free	4 oz	na	na	na	na	na	na	na	0.0	4.25	.25	na	na	na
(Swiss Miss) sundae	4 oz	na	na	na	na	na	na	na	0.0	6.36	2.46	na	na	na
PUDDING MIX. See also PUDDING/PIE FILLING MIX.														
BANANA (Jell-O) 'Instant Sugar-free' prepared w/2% milk	1/2 cup	na	na	na	na	na	na	na	na	na	na	na	190	na
BANANA CREAM (Jell-O) 'Microwave' prepared	1/2 cup	na	na	na	na	na	na	na	na	na	na	na	190	na
BUTTER PECAN (Jell-O) 'Instant' prepared	1/2 cup	na	na	na	na	na	na	na	na	na	na	na	190	na
BUTTERSCOTCH														
(D-Zerta) low calorie, prepared w/skim milk	1/2 cup	na	na	na	na	na	na	na	na	na	na	na	240	na
(Jell-O) 'Instant' prepared	1/2 cup	na	na	na	na	na	na	na	na	na	na	na	190	na
(Jell-O) 'Instant Sugar-free' prepared w/2% milk	1/2 cup	na	na	na	na	na	na	na	na	na	na	na	190	na
(Jell-O) 'Microwave' prepared	1/2 cup	na	na	na	na	na	na	na	na	na	na	na	190	na
(Jell-O) prepared	1/2 cup	na	na	na	na	na	na	na	na	na	na	na	190	na
CHOCOLATE														
(D-Zerta) low calorie, prepared w/skim milk	1/2 cup	na	na	na	na	na	na	na	na	na	na	na	320	na
(Jell-O) 'Instant' prepared	1/2 cup	na	na	na	na	na	na	na	na	na	na	na	280	na
(Jell-O) 'Instant Sugar-free' prepared w/2% milk	1/2 cup	na	na	na	na	na	na	na	na	na	na	na	260	na
(Jell-O) 'Microwave' prepared	1/2 cup	na	na	na	na	na	na	na	na	na	na	na	310	na
(Jell-O) prepared	1/2 cup	na	na	na	na	na	na	na	na	na	na	na	310	na
CHOCOLATE FUDGE														
(Jell-O) 'Instant' prepared	1/2 cup	na	na	na	na	na	na	na	na	na	na	na	320	na
(Jell-O) 'Instant Sugar-free' prepared w/2% milk	1/2 cup	na	na	na	na	na	na	na	na	na	na	na	340	na
(Jell-O) prepared	1/2 cup	na	na	na	na	na	na	na	na	na	na	na	340	na
EGG (Jell-O) custard 'Americana' prepared	1/2 cup	na	na	na	na	na	na	na	na	na	na	na	280	na
FLAN (Jell-O) prepared	1/2 cup	na	na	na	na	na	na	na	na	na	na	na	190	na
FRENCH VANILLA														
(Jell-O) 'Instant' prepared	1/2 cup	na	na	na	na	na	na	na	na	na	na	na	190	na
(Jell-O) prepared	1/2 cup	na	na	na	na	na	na	na	na	na	na	na	190	na
KEY LIME (Royal) prepared	1/2 cup													
LEMON (Jell-O) 'Instant' prepared	1/2 cup	na	na	na	na	na	na	na	na	na	na	na	190	na
MILK CHOCOLATE														
(Jell-O) 'Instant' prepared	1/2 cup	na	na	na	na	na	na	na	na	na	na	na	280	na
(Jell-O) 'Microwave' prepared	1/2 cup	na	na	na	na	na	na	na	na	na	na	na	270	na
(Jell-O) prepared	1/2 cup	na	na	na	na	na	na	na	na	na	na	na	250	na
PISTACHIO														
(Jell-O) 'Instant' prepared	1/2 cup	na	na	na	na	na	na	na	na	na	na	na	190	na

Food Name	Serving Size	A I.U.	Thi mg	Rib mg	Nia mg	B_6 mg	Fol mcg	B_{12} mcg	C mg	Calc mg	Iron mg	Mag mg	Pot mg	Zn mg
(Jell-O) 'Instant Sugar-free' prepared w/2% milk	1/2 cup	na	na	na	na	na	na	na	na	na	na	na	200	na
RICE (Jell-O) 'Americana' prepared	1/2 cup	na	na	na	na	na	na	na	na	na	na	na	190	na
VANILLA														
(D-Zerta) low calorie, prepared w/skim milk	1/2 cup	na	na	na	na	na	na	na	na	na	na	na	200	na
(Jell-O) 'Instant' prepared	1/2 cup	na	na	na	na	na	na	na	na	na	na	na	190	na
(Jell-O) 'Instant Sugar-free' prepared w/2% milk	1/2 cup	na	na	na	na	na	na	na	na	na	na	na	190	na
(Jell-O) 'Microwave' prepared	1/2 cup	na	na	na	na	na	na	na	na	na	na	na	190	na
(Jell-O) prepared	1/2 cup	na	na	na	na	na	na	na	na	na	na	na	190	na
(Jell-O) tapioca 'Americana' prepared	1/2 cup	na	na	na	na	na	na	na	na	na	na	na	190	na
PUDDING/PIE FILLING MIX. See also PUDDING MIX.														
BANANA (Jell-O) instant, sugar-free, prepared w/2% milk	1/2 cup	na	na	na	na	na	na	na	na	na	na	na	190	na
BANANA CREAM														
(Jell-O) instant, prepared	1/2 cup	na	na	na	na	na	na	na	na	na	na	na	190	na
(Jell-O) microwave, prepared	1/2 cup	na	na	na	na	na	na	na	na	na	na	na	190	na
(Jell-O) prepared, w/o crust	1/6 pie	na	na	na	na	na	na	na	na	na	na	na	125	na
(Royal) dry	1 serving	na	na	na	na	na	na	na	na	na	na	na	0	na
(Royal) instant, dry	1 serving	na	na	na	na	na	na	na	na	na	na	na	25	na
BUTTER PECAN (Jell-O) instant, prepared	1/2 cup	na	na	na	na	na	na	na	na	na	na	na	390	na
BUTTERSCOTCH														
(D-Zerta) reduced calorie, prepared	1/2 cup	na	na	na	na	na	na	na	na	na	na	na	240	na
(Jell-O) instant, prepared	1/2 cup	na	na	na	na	na	na	na	na	na	na	na	190	na
(Jell-O) instant, sugar-free, prepared w/2% milk	1/2 cup	na	na	na	na	na	na	na	na	na	na	na	190	na
(Jell-O) microwave, prepared	1/2 cup	na	na	na	na	na	na	na	na	na	na	na	190	na
(Jell-O) prepared	1/2 cup	na	na	na	na	na	na	na	na	na	na	na	190	na
(Nabisco) 'My•T•Fine' prepared	1/2 cup	na	na	na	na	na	na	na	na	na	na	na	0	na
(Royal) instant, dry	1 serving	na	na	na	na	na	na	na	na	na	na	na	25	na
(Royal) prepared	1/2 cup	na	na	na	na	na	na	na	na	na	na	na	5	na
CHERRY-VANILLA (Royal) instant, dry	1 serving	na	na	na	na	na	na	na	na	na	na	na	35	na
CHOCOLATE														
(D-Zerta) reduced calorie, prepared	1/2 cup	na	na	na	na	na	na	na	na	na	na	na	320	na
(Jell-O) instant, prepared	1/2 cup	na	na	na	na	na	na	na	na	na	na	na	280	na
(Jell-O) instant, sugar-free, prepared w/2% milk	1/2 cup	na	na	na	na	na	na	na	na	na	na	na	260	na
(Jell-O) microwave, prepared	1/2 cup	na	na	na	na	na	na	na	na	na	na	na	310	na
(Jell-O) prepared	1/2 cup	na	na	na	na	na	na	na	na	na	na	na	310	na
(Jell-O) sugar-free, prepared w/2% milk	1/2 cup	na	na	na	na	na	na	na	na	na	na	na	310	na
(Nabisco) 'My•T•Fine' prepared	1/2 cup	na	na	na	na	na	na	na	na	na	na	na	15	na
(Royal) dark and sweet, instant, dry	1 serving	na	na	na	na	na	na	na	na	na	na	na	40	na
(Royal) dark and sweet, prepared	1/2 cup	na	na	na	na	na	na	na	na	na	na	na	30	na
(Royal) instant, dry	1 serving	na	na	na	na	na	na	na	na	na	na	na	75	na
(Royal) instant, sugar-free, prepared	1/2 cup	na	na	na	na	na	na	na	na	na	na	na	130	na
(Royal) prepared	1/2 cup	na	na	na	na	na	na	na	na	na	na	na	40	na
CHOCOLATE FUDGE														
(Jell-O) instant, prepared	1/2 cup	na	na	na	na	na	na	na	na	na	na	na	320	na
(Jell-O) instant, sugar-free, prepared w/2% milk	1/2 cup	na	na	na	na	na	na	na	na	na	na	na	340	na
(Jell-O) prepared	1/2 cup	na	na	na	na	na	na	na	na	na	na	na	340	na
(Nabisco) 'My•T•Fine' prepared	1/2 cup	na	na	na	na	na	na	na	na	na	na	na	15	na
CHOCOLATE-ALMOND														
(Nabisco) 'My•T•Fine' prepared	1/2 cup	na	na	na	na	na	na	na	na	na	na	na	20	na
CHOCOLATE-CHOCOLATE CHIP (Royal) instant, dry	1 serving	na	na	na	na	na	na	na	na	na	na	na	45	na

Food Name	Serving Size	A I.U.	Thi mg	Rib mg	Nia mg	B6 mg	Fol mcg	B12 mcg	C mg	Calc mg	Iron mg	Mag mg	Pot mg	Zn mg
CHOCOLATE-PEANUT BUTTER CHIP (Royal)														
instant, dry	1 serving	na	na	na	na	na	na	na	na	na	na	na	45	na
COCONUT CREAM														
(Jell-O) instant, prepared	1/2 cup	na	na	na	na	na	na	na	na	na	na	na	200	na
(Jell-O) prepared, w/o crust	1/6 pie	na	na	na	na	na	na	na	na	na	na	na	140	na
FLAN														
(Jell-O) prepared	1/2 cup	na	na	na	na	na	na	na	na	na	na	na	190	na
(Royal) caramel custard, prepared	1/2 cup	na	na	na	na	na	na	na	na	na	na	na	25	na
FRENCH VANILLA														
(Jell-O) instant, prepared	1/2 cup	na	na	na	na	na	na	na	na	na	na	na	190	na
(Jell-O) prepared	1/2 cup	na	na	na	na	na	na	na	na	na	na	na	190	na
LEMON														
(Jell-O) instant, prepared	1/2 cup	na	na	na	na	na	na	na	na	na	na	na	190	na
(Jell-O) prepared, w/o crust	1/6 pie	na	na	na	na	na	na	na	na	na	na	na	25	na
(Nabisco) 'My•T•Fine' dry	1 serving	na	na	na	na	na	na	na	na	na	na	na	15	na
(Royal) instant, dry	1 serving	na	na	na	na	na	na	na	na	na	na	na	0	na
MILK CHOCOLATE														
(Jell-O) instant, prepared	1/2 cup	na	na	na	na	na	na	na	na	na	na	na	280	na
(Jell-O) microwave, prepared	1/2 cup	na	na	na	na	na	na	na	na	na	na	na	270	na
(Jell-O) prepared	1/2 cup	na	na	na	na	na	na	na	na	na	na	na	250	na
PISTACHIO														
(Jell-O) instant, prepared	1/2 cup	na	na	na	na	na	na	na	na	na	na	na	190	na
(Jell-O) instant, sugar-free, prepared w/2% milk	1/2 cup	na	na	na	na	na	na	na	na	na	na	na	200	na
(Royal) instant, dry	1 serving	na	na	na	na	na	na	na	na	na	na	na	35	na
STRAWBERRY (Royal) instant, dry	1 serving	na	na	na	na	na	na	na	na	na	na	na	25	na
TAPIOCA (Nabisco) 'My•T•Fine' dry	1 serving	na	na	na	na	na	na	na	na	na	na	na	5	na
VANILLA														
(D-Zerta) reduced calorie, w/Aspartame, prepared	1/2 cup	na	na	na	na	na	na	na	na	na	na	na	200	na
(Jell-O) instant, prepared	1/2 cup	na	na	na	na	na	na	na	na	na	na	na	190	na
(Jell-O) instant, sugar-free, prepared w/2% milk	1/2 cup	na	na	na	na	na	na	na	na	na	na	na	190	na
(Jell-O) microwave, prepared	1/2 cup	na	na	na	na	na	na	na	na	na	na	na	190	na
(Jell-O) prepared	1/2 cup	na	na	na	na	na	na	na	na	na	na	na	190	na
(Jell-O) sugar-free, w/Aspartame, prepared w/2% milk	1/2 cup	na	na	na	na	na	na	na	na	na	na	na	190	na
(Nabisco) 'My•T•Fine' prepared	1/2 cup	na	na	na	na	na	na	na	na	na	na	na	0	na
(Royal) instant, dry	1 serving	na	na	na	na	na	na	na	na	na	na	na	5	na
VANILLA-CHOCOLATE CHIP (Royal) instant, dry	1 serving	na	na	na	na	na	na	na	na	na	na	na	30	na
PUFF PASTRY, FROZEN														
shell, ready to bake	1 shell	0	.19	.13	1.96	.01	6.1	0	0.0	4.7	1.2	7.52	28.67	.25
shell, ready to bake	1 oz	0	.11	.08	1.18	.01	3.7	0	0.0	2.84	.73	4.54	17.29	.15
PUMELO. See POMELO.														
PUMPKIN														
boiled, drained, mashed	1/2 cup	1320	.04	.1	.5	.05	10.4	0	5.7	18.3	.7	10.98	280.6	.28
raw, 1-inch cubes	1/2 cup	928	.03	.06	.35	.04	9.4	0	5.2	12.18	.46	6.96	197.2	.19
PUMPKIN, CANNED	1/2 cup	26908	.03	.07	.45	.07	15.0	0	5.1	31.72	1.7	28.06	251.32	.21
PUMPKIN FLOWER														
boiled, drained	1/2 cup	1162	.01	.02	.21	na	27.3	0	3.4	24.79	.59	16.75	71.02	na
raw	1 cup	643	.01	.02	.23	na	19.4	0	9.2	12.87	.23	7.92	57.09	na
PUMPKIN LEAF														
boiled, drained	1/2 cup	866	.02	.05	.3	.07	8.7	0	0.4	15.05	1.12	13.3	153.3	.07
raw	1/2 cup	388	.02	.03	.18	.04	7.2	0	2.2	7.8	.44	7.6	87.2	.04

Food Name	Serving Size	A I.U.	Thi mg	Rib mg	Nia mg	B$_6$ mg	Fol mcg	B$_{12}$ mcg	C mg	Calc mg	Iron mg	Mag mg	Pot mg	Zn mg
PUMPKIN PIE SPICE														
dried	1 tbsp	15	.01	.01	.13	na	na	0	1.3	38.19	1.1	7.62	37.13	.13
dried	1 tsp	4	0	0	.04	na	na	0	0.4	11.59	.34	2.31	11.27	.04
PUMPKIN SEED														
w/squash seeds, roasted	1 cup	40	.02	.03	.18	.02	5.8	0	0.2	35.2	2.12	167.68	588.16	6.59
w/squash seeds, roasted	1 oz	18	.01	.01	.08	.01	2.6	0	0.1	15.62	.94	74.41	261.0	2.93
PUMPKIN SEED, SHELLED														
w/squash seed kernels, dried	1 cup	524	.29	.44	2.41	.31	79.4	0	2.6	59.34	20.66	738.3	1113.66	10.29
w/squash seed kernels, dried, approx 142 kernels	1 oz	108	.06	.09	.5	.06	16.3	0	0.5	12.21	4.25	151.94	229.19	2.12
w/squash seed kernels, roasted	1 cup	863	.48	.72	3.95	.2	130.3	0	4.1	97.61	33.91	1212.18	1829.62	16.89
PUNCH. See also FRUIT PUNCH; and individual listings.														
(J. Hungerford)	9.03 oz	na	na	na	na	na	na	na	100.0	.1	.2	na	na	na
PURPLESAURUS REX DRINK MIX														
(Kool-Aid) sugar-free, w/NutraSweet, prepared	8 oz	na	na	na	na	na	na	na	na	na	na	na	0	na
(Kool-Aid) sugar-sweetened, prepared	8 oz	na	na	na	na	na	na	na	na	na	na	na	0	na
(Kool-Aid) unsweetened, prepared w/sugar	8 oz	na	na	na	na	na	na	na	na	na	na	na	0	na
(Kool-Aid) unsweetened, prepared w/o sugar	8 oz	na	na	na	na	na	na	na	na	na	na	na	0	na
PURSLANE / pussley														
boiled, drained	1/2 cup	1074	.02	.05	.27	.04	4.9	0	6.1	45.24	.45	38.86	283.04	.1
raw	1 cup	568	.02	.05	.21	.03	4.9	0	9.0	27.95	.86	29.24	212.42	.07

Q

Food Name	Serving Size	A I.U.	Thi mg	Rib mg	Nia mg	B$_6$ mg	Fol mcg	B$_{12}$ mcg	C mg	Calc mg	Iron mg	Mag mg	Pot mg	Zn mg
QUAIL GIBLETS, raw	3.5 oz	4530	.16	1.36	4.9	na	na	na	0.0	8.0	4.5	na	172.0	na
QUINCE, raw, trimmed	1 med	37	.02	.03	.18	.04	na	0	13.8	10.12	.64	7.36	181.24	na
QUINOA, WHOLE GRAIN														
dry	1/2 cup	0	.17	.34	2.49	.19	41.7	0	0.0	51.0	7.86	178.5	629.0	2.81
dry (Ancient Harvest)	1/4 cup	na	na	na	na	na	na	na	na	na	na	na	250	na
dry (Eden Foods)	2 oz	na	na	na	na	na	na	na	na	na	na	na	270	na
QUINOA FLOUR, WHOLE GRAIN														
non-gluten (Ancient Harvest)	1/4 cup	na	na	na	na	na	na	na	na	na	na	na	420	na

R

Food Name	Serving Size	A I.U.	Thi mg	Rib mg	Nia mg	B$_6$ mg	Fol mcg	B$_{12}$ mcg	C mg	Calc mg	Iron mg	Mag mg	Pot mg	Zn mg
RABBIT														
Domesticated														
raw	1 lb	0	.45	.68	32.98	2.27	36.3	32.48	0.0	58.97	7.12	86.18	1496.88	7.12
raw	1 oz	0	.03	.04	2.04	.14	2.2	2.0	0.0	3.64	.44	5.32	92.4	.44
roasted	3 oz	0	.08	.18	7.17	.4	9.4	7.06	0.0	16.15	1.93	17.85	325.55	1.93
stewed	3 oz	0	.05	.14	6.09	.29	7.7	5.53	0.0	17.0	2.01	17.0	255.0	2.01
Wild														
raw	1 lb	0	.14	.27	29.48	na	na	na	0.0	54.43	14.52	131.54	1714.61	na
raw	1 oz	0	.01	.02	1.82	na	na	na	0.0	3.36	.9	8.12	105.84	na
stewed	3 oz	0	.02	.06	5.44	na	na	na	0.0	15.3	4.12	26.35	291.55	na
RACCOON, roasted	3 oz	0	.5	.44	na	na	na	na	0.0	na	na	na	na	na
RADICCHIO														
raw	1 med	2	0	0	.02	0	4.8	0	0.6	1.52	.05	1.04	24.16	.05
raw, shredded	1/2 cup	5	0	.01	.05	.01	12.0	0	1.6	3.8	.11	2.6	60.4	.12

Food Name	Serving Size	A I.U.	Thi mg	Rib mg	Nia mg	B_6 mg	Fol mcg	B_{12} mcg	C mg	Calc mg	Iron mg	Mag mg	Pot mg	Zn mg
RADISH														
fresh *(Dole)*	7 med	na	na	na	na	na	na	na	19.0	na	na	na	200	na
raw, sliced	1/2 cup	5	0	.03	.17	.04	15.7	0	13.2	12.18	.17	5.22	134.56	.17
raw, 1 inch long, 3/4 inch diam	10 radishes	4	0	.02	.14	.03	12.2	0	10.3	9.45	.13	4.05	104.4	.14
RADISH, WHITE ICICLE														
raw	1 med	0	.01	0	.05	.01	2.4	0	4.9	4.59	.14	1.53	47.6	.02
raw, sliced	1/2 cup	0	.02	.01	.15	.04	7.0	0	14.5	13.5	.4	4.5	140.0	.07
RADISH SEED, sprouted, raw	1/2 cup	74	.02	.02	.54	.05	18.0	0	5.5	9.69	.16	8.36	16.34	.11
RAG GOURD. See GOURD, DISHCLOTH.														
RAINBOW PUNCH *(Kool-Aid)* 'Koolers'	8.45 oz	na	na	na	na	na	na	na	na	na	na	na	40	na
RAINBOW PUNCH MIX														
(Kool-Aid) sugar-sweetened	8 oz	na	na	na	na	na	na	na	na	na	na	na	0	na
(Kool-Aid) unsweetened, prepared w/sugar	8 oz	na	na	na	na	na	na	na	na	na	na	na	0	na
(Kool-Aid) unsweetened, prepared w/o sugar	8 oz	na	na	na	na	na	na	na	na	na	na	na	0	na
RAINBOW SMELT. See SMELT, RAINBOW.														
RAISIN														
Dark														
seedless	1 cup packed	13	.26	.15	1.35	.41	5.4	0	5.4	80.85	3.43	54.45	1239.15	.45
seedless	1 cup	12	.23	.13	1.19	.36	4.8	0	4.8	71.05	3.02	47.85	1088.95	.39
w/seeds	1 cup packed	0	.18	.3	1.84	.31	5.4	0	8.9	46.2	4.27	49.5	1361.25	.3
w/seeds	1 cup	0	.16	.26	1.62	.27	4.8	0	7.8	40.6	3.76	43.5	1196.25	.26
Golden														
seedless	1 cup packed	73	.01	.32	1.88	.53	5.4	0	5.3	87.45	2.95	57.75	1230.9	.53
seedless	1 cup	64	.01	.28	1.66	.47	4.8	0	4.6	76.85	2.6	50.75	1081.7	.46
RASPBERRY/*bramble*														
trimmed	1 pint	406	.09	.28	2.81	.18	81.1	0	78.0	68.64	1.78	56.16	474.24	1.44
trimmed	1 cup	160	.04	.11	1.11	.07	32.0	0	30.8	27.06	.7	22.14	186.96	.57
Canned														
red, in heavy syrup, solid and liquid	1/2 cup	42	.03	.04	.57	.05	13.4	0	11.1	14.08	.54	15.36	120.32	.2
Frozen														
red, in light syrup *(Birds Eye)* 'Quick Thaw Pouch'	5 oz	na	na	na	na	na	na	na	na	na	na	na	140	na
red, sweetened, unthawed	10 oz	170	.05	.13	.65	.1	73.8	0	46.9	42.6	1.85	36.92	323.76	.51
red, sweetened, unthawed	1 cup	150	.05	.11	.58	.09	65.0	0	41.3	37.5	1.62	32.5	285.0	.45
RASPBERRY PUNCH MIX														
(Kool-Aid) sugar-sweetened, prepared	8 oz	na	na	na	na	na	na	na	na	na	na	na	0	na
(Kool-Aid) unsweetened, prepared w/sugar	8 oz	na	na	na	na	na	na	na	na	na	na	na	0	na
(Kool-Aid) unsweetened, prepared w/o sugar	8 oz	na	na	na	na	na	na	na	na	na	na	na	0	na
RAVIOLI ENTRÉE														
FROZEN														
Cheese *(Amy's Kitchen)* organic	1 cup	na	na	na	na	na	na	na	na	na	na	na	152	na
MICROWAVE														
(Kid's Kitchen) mini microwave cup	7.5 oz	na	na	na	na	na	na	na	na	na	na	na	342	na
REFRIGERATED														
(Contadina) w/beef 'Fresh'	3 oz	75	.23	.26	3.0	.11	14.7	.87	0.5	40	2.7	39.8	200	2.21
(Contadina) w/cheese 'Fresh'	3 oz	75	.3	.26	1.96	.03	11.5	.26	0.3	200	1.44	31.9	160	.82
(DiGiorno) w/Italian herb cheese, cooked	1 cup	na	na	na	na	na	na	na	na	na	na	na	170	na
(DiGiorno) w/Italian sausage, cooked	1 cup	na	na	na	na	na	na	na	na	na	na	na	160	na
RED BEAN, CANNED														
(Van Camp's)	1 cup	0	.1	.1	.61	na	na	na	0.0	84	2.7	na	546	na
Small *(Hunt's)*	4.48 oz	na	na	na	na	na	na	na	0.8	3.15	3.53	na	na	na
RED CABBAGE. See CABBAGE, RED.														
RED PERCH. See OCEAN PERCH, ATLANTIC.														
REDFISH. See OCEAN PERCH, ATLANTIC.														
REDHEAD. See SHEEPSHEAD.														
REFRIED BEANS, CANNED														
	1/2 cup	0	.06	.07	.61	.13	105.2	0	7.6	57.96	2.23	49.14	495.18	1.73

Food Name	Serving Size	A I.U.	Thi mg	Rib mg	Nia mg	B6 mg	Fol mcg	B12 mcg	C mg	Calc mg	Iron mg	Mag mg	Pot mg	Zn mg
(Rosarita)	4.5 oz	na	na	na	na	na	na	na	0.0	4.29	11.12	na	na	na
NO-FAT (Rosarita)	4.5 oz	na	na	na	na	na	na	na	0.0	4.32	10.69	na	na	na
SPICY (Rosarita)	4.5 oz	na	na	na	na	na	na	na	0.0	4.57	10.83	na	na	na
VEGETARIAN (Rosarita)	4.5 oz	na	na	na	na	na	na	na	0.0	4.08	12.62	na	na	na
W/BACON (Rosarita)	4.5 oz	na	na	na	na	na	na	na	2.3	4.16	11.62	na	na	na
W/GREEN CHILIES (Rosarita)	4.5 oz	na	na	na	na	na	na	na	2.4	4.05	10.83	na	na	na
W/JALAPEÑO (Gebhardt)	4.5 oz	na	na	na	na	na	na	na	0.0	4.39	4.92	na		
W/NACHO CHEESE (Rosarita)	4.5 oz	na	na	na	na	na	na	na	0.0	4.53	10.41	na	22	na
W/ONION (Rosarita)	4.5 oz	na	na	na	na	na	na	na	2.0	4.56	10.91	na	na	na
REFRIED BEANS, DRIED (Rosarita)	1/3 cup	na	na	na	na	na	na	na	0.0	6.09	13.81	na	na	na
RELISH. See also specific listings.														
CHOWCHOW														
sour, w/cauliflower, onion, mustard	1 cup	240	0	.05	0	na	na	na	16.8	76.8	6.24	na	480.0	na
sweet, w/cauliflower, onion, mustard	1 cup	221	0	.05	0	na	na	na	14.7	56.35	3.67	na	490.0	na
CRANBERRY-ORANGE, canned	1/2 cup	97	.04	.03	.14	na	na	0	24.8	15.18	.28	5.52	52.44	na
HAMBURGER														
pickle	1/2 cup	326	.02	.05	.75	.02	1.2	0	2.8	4.88	1.39	8.54	92.72	.13
pickle	1 tbsp	40	0	.01	.09	0	0.2	0	0.3	.6	.17	1.05	11.4	.02
HOT DOG														
pickle	1/2 cup	204	.05	.05	.61	.02	1.2	0	1.2	6.1	1.52	23.18	95.16	.26
pickle	1 tbsp	25	.01	.01	.08	0	0.2	0	0.2	.75	.19	2.85	11.7	.03
PICKLE														
sweet	1/2 cup	189	0	.04	.28	.02	1.2	0	1.2	3.66	1.06	6.1	30.5	.17
sweet	1 tbsp	23	0	0	.03	0	0.2	0	0.2	.45	.13	.75	3.75	.02
SWEET														
chopped	1 cup	245	0	.05	0	na	na	na	14.7	49.0	1.96	na	490.0	na
chopped	1 tbsp	15	0	0	0	na	na	na	0.9	3.0	.12	na	30.0	na
finely cut	1 cup	245	0	.05	0	na	na	na	14.7	49.0	1.96	na	490.0	na
finely cut	1 tbsp	15	0	0	0	na	na	na	0.9	3.0	.12	na	30.0	na
RENNIN, enzyme tablet, unsweetened	1 tablet	0	0	0	0	0	0.0	0	0.0	33.6	.06	.16	2.63	.06
RHUBARB														
frozen, sweetened, cooked	1/2 cup	83	.02	.03	.24	.02	6.4	0	4.0	174.0	.25	14.4	115.2	.1
raw, diced	1/2 cup	61	.01	.02	.18	.01	4.3	0	4.9	52.46	.13	7.32	175.68	.06
RICE, BROWN														
(Lundberg Family) cooked	1 cup	na	na	na	na	na	na	na	na	23	na	na	na	na
LONG GRAIN														
cooked	1/2 cup	0	.09	.02	1.5	.14	3.9	0	0.0	9.8	.41	42.14	42.14	.62
dry	1/2 cup	0	.37	.09	4.68	.47	18.4	0	0.0	21.16	1.35	131.56	205.16	1.86
MEDIUM GRAIN														
cooked	1/2 cup	0	.1	.01	1.3	.15	3.9	0	0.0	9.8	.52	43.12	77.42	.61
dry	1/2 cup	0	.39	.04	4.09	.48	19.0	0	0.0	31.35	1.71	135.85	254.6	1.92
RICE, GLUTINOUS														
cooked	1/2 cup	0	.02	.02	.35	.03	1.2	0	0.0	2.4	.17	6.0	12.0	.49
dry	1/2 cup	0	.15	.01	1.37	.05	1.8	0	0.0	.92	1.34	7.36	23.92	.37
RICE, WHITE														
LONG GRAIN														
cooked	1/2 cup	0	.92	.17	.74	.13	41.1	0	0.0	45.82	4.27	185.65	447.14	2.46
raw, enriched	1/2 cup	0	.53	.05	3.86	.15	7.4	0	0.0	25.76	3.97	23.0	105.8	1.0
Parboiled														
cooked	1/2 cup	na	.02	.02	1.23	.02	3.5	0	0.0	16.72	.18	10.56	32.56	.27
enriched, cooked	1/2 cup	0	.22	.02	1.23	.02	3.5	0	0.0	16.72	.99	10.56	32.56	.27
unenriched, dry	1/2 cup	na	.09	.06	3.34	.32	15.6	0	0.0	55.2	1.38	28.52	110.4	.88
Precooked or instant														
dry	1/2 cup	0	.3	.03	2.63	.02	2.9	0	0.0	8.64	2.01	5.76	8.64	.46
enriched, cooked	1/2 cup	0	.06	.04	.72	.01	3.3	0	0.0	6.56	.52	4.1	3.28	.2
MEDIUM GRAIN														
cooked	1/2 cup	0	.55	.07	3.38	.33	15.8	0	0.0	55.8	3.31	28.83	111.6	.89

Food Name	Serving Size	A I.U.	Thi mg	Rib mg	Nia mg	B$_6$ mg	Fol mcg	B$_{12}$ mcg	C mg	Calc mg	Iron mg	Mag mg	Pot mg	Zn mg
enriched, dry	1/2 cup	0	.57	.05	4.99	.14	8.8	0	0.0	8.82	4.27	34.3	84.28	1.14
unenriched, cooked	1/2 cup	0	.02	.02	.41	.05	2.0	0	0.0	3.06	.2	13.26	29.58	.43
unenriched, dry	1/2 cup	na	.07	.05	1.57	.14	8.8	0	0.0	8.82	.78	34.3	84.28	1.14
SHORT GRAIN														
cooked	1/2 cup	0	.53	.04	3.83	.16	5.6	0	0.0	2.79	3.93	21.39	70.68	1.02
dry	1/2 cup	0	.17	.02	1.83	.05	2.0	0	0.0	3.0	1.49	13.0	29.0	.42
unenriched, cooked	1/2 cup	na	.02	.02	.41	.06	2.0	0	0.0	1.02	.2	8.16	26.52	.41
unenriched, dry	1/2 cup	na	.07	.05	1.6	.17	6.0	0	0.0	3.0	.8	23.0	76.0	1.1
RICE, WILD														
cooked	1/2 cup	0	.04	.07	1.06	.11	21.3	0	0.0	2.46	.49	26.24	82.82	1.1
dry	1/2 cup	15	.09	.21	5.39	.31	76.0	0	0.0	16.8	1.57	141.6	341.6	4.77
RICE BRAN, crude	1/3 cup	0	.77	.08	9.52	1.14	17.6	0	0.0	15.96	5.19	218.68	415.8	1.69
RICE BRAN OIL														
	1 cup	0	0	0	0	0	0.0	0	0.0	0	.15	0	0	0
	1 tbsp	0	0	0	0	0	0.0	0	0.0	0	.01	0	0	0
RICE CAKE														
(Lundberg Family) sodium-free, all flavors	1 cake	na	na	na	na	na	na	na	na	na	na	na	46	na
(Lundberg Family) very low sodium, all flavors	1 cake	na	na	na	na	na	na	na	na	na	na	na	46	na
BROWN RICE														
buckwheat	1 cake	0	.01	.01	.73	.01	1.9	0	0.0	.99	.1	13.59	26.91	.23
buckwheat, unsalted	1 cake	4	.01	.01	.7	.01	1.9	0	0.0	.99	.13	11.79	26.1	.27
corn	1 cake	0	.01	.01	.58	.01	1.7	0	0.0	.81	.11	10.26	24.75	.2
multi-grain	1 cake	0	.01	.02	.59	.01	1.8	0	0.0	1.89	.18	12.33	26.46	.23
multi-grain, unsalted	1 cake	0	.01	.01	.73	.01	1.9	0	0.0	.99	.1	13.59	26.91	.23
plain	1 cake	4	.01	.01	.7	.01	1.9	0	0.0	.99	.13	11.79	26.1	.27
rye	1 cake	0	.01	.01	.63	.01	0.5	0	0.0	1.89	.16	12.96	27.99	.27
sesame seed	1 cake	0	0	.01	.65	.01	1.6	0	0.3	1.08	.14	12.24	26.1	.27
sesame seed, unsalted	1 cake	0	.01	.02	.59	.01	1.8	0	0.0	1.89	.18	12.33	26.46	.23
unsalted	1 cake	0	.04	.06	.47	.01	7.5	0	0.0	3.24	.39	3.15	13.14	.08
SESAME (Westbrae) 'Double Sesame'	.28 oz	na	na	na	na	na	na	na	na	na	na	na	30	na
SESAME-GARLIC (Westbrae)	.28 oz	na	na	na	na	na	na	na	na	na	na	na	25	na
TERIYAKI (Westbrae)	.28 oz	na	na	na	na	na	na	na	na	na	na	na	20	na
RICE DISH														
CANNED														
Fried (LaChoy)	4.903 oz	na	na	na	na	na	na	na	0.0	1.71	4.63	na	na	na
Spanish (Van Camp's)	1 cup	1228	.06	.1	1.24	na	na	na	1.2	40	2.92	na	260	na
FROZEN														
Fried														
w/chicken (Chun King)	8 oz	na	na	na	na	na	na	na	na	na	na	na	190	na
w/pork (Chun King)	8 oz	na	na	na	na	na	na	na	na	na	na	na	180	na
RICE DISH MIX														
FRIED														
W/almonds														
(Rice-A-Roni) '1/2 less salt' dry mix	1/5 pkg	na	na	na	na	na	na	na	na	na	na	na	75	na
(Rice-A-Roni) '1/2 less salt' prepared	1/2 cup	na	na	na	na	na	na	na	na	na	na	na	75	na
RICE FLOUR														
brown	1/2 cup	0	.35	.06	5.01	.58	12.6	0	0.0	8.69	1.56	88.48	228.31	1.94
white	1/2 cup	0	.11	.02	2.05	.34	3.2	0	0.0	7.9	.28	27.65	60.04	.63
RIGATONI. See PASTA.														
RIGATONI ENTRÉE														
(Stouffer's) w/meat sauce, homestyle, frozen	12 oz	na	na	na	na	na	na	na	na	na	na	na	560	na
ROCKET. See ARUGULA.														
ROCKFISH, PACIFIC, MIXED SPECIES														
baked, broiled, or microwaved	3 oz	186	.04	.07	3.33	.23	8.8	1.02	0.0	10.2	.45	28.9	442.0	.45
raw	3 oz	162	.03	.06	2.74	.2	7.7	.85	0.0	7.65	.35	22.1	344.25	.35

Food Name	Serving Size	A I.U.	Thi mg	Rib mg	Nia mg	B6 mg	Fol mcg	B12 mcg	C mg	Calc mg	Iron mg	Mag mg	Pot mg	Zn mg
ROE, MIXED SPECIES														
dry-heat cooked	3 oz	258	.24	.81	1.86	.16	78.2	9.81	13.9	23.8	.65	22.1	240.55	1.09
dry-heat cooked	1 oz	86	.08	.27	.62	.05	26.1	3.27	4.7	7.94	.22	7.37	80.23	.36
raw	3 oz	224	.2	.63	1.53	.14	68.0	8.5	13.6	18.7	.51	17.0	187.85	.85
raw	1 oz	74	.07	.21	.5	.04	22.4	2.8	4.5	6.16	.17	5.6	61.88	.28
ROLL. See also BREAD; BUN ; CROISSANT ; ENGLISH MUFFIN.														
DINNER														
egg	1-oz roll	21	.15	.15	.93	.02	15.0	.07	0.0	16.73	1.0	7.09	29.77	.26
oat bran	1-oz roll	2	.13	.08	1.4	.01	8.8	0	0.0	24.1	1.17	8.51	30.9	.24
rye	1-oz roll	1	.11	.08	1.11	.02	6.2	0	0.0	8.51	.77	15.31	51.03	.29
wheat	1-oz roll	0	.12	.08	1.15	.02	4.3	0	0.0	49.9	1.01	11.91	37.71	.29
whole wheat	1-oz roll	0	.07	.04	1.04	.06	8.5	0	0.0	30.05	.69	24.1	77.11	.57
FRENCH STYLE	1 oz	1	.15	.09	1.23	.01	9.4	0	0.0	25.8	.77	5.67	32.32	.21
HARD	1 oz	0	.14	.1	1.2	.02	4.3	0	0.0	26.93	.93	7.65	30.62	.27
KAISER	1 oz	0	.14	.1	1.2	.02	4.3	0	0.0	26.93	.93	7.65	30.62	.27
ROLL, SWEET. See also BUN, SWEET.														
APPLE														
(Break Cake) 4.5 oz	2 rolls	na	na	na	na	na	na	na	na	na	na	na	180	na
(Break Cake) multi-pak, 1.4 oz	1 roll	na	na	na	na	na	na	na	na	na	na	na	55	na
CHEESE	1 oz	58	.04	.04	.24	.02	8.8	.05	0.1	33.45	.22	5.39	37.42	.18
CHERRY														
(Break Cake) 4.5 oz	2 rolls	na	na	na	na	na	na	na	na	na	na	na	150	na
(Break Cake) multi-pak, 1.4 oz	1 roll	na	na	na	na	na	na	na	na	na	na	na	50	na
CINNAMON														
(Break Cake) 4.5 oz	2 rolls	na	na	na	na	na	na	na	na	na	na	na	150	na
(Break Cake) multi-pak, 1.3 oz	1 roll	na	na	na	na	na	na	na	na	na	na	na	45	na
PECAN (Break Cake) multi-pak, 1.3 oz	1 roll	na	na	na	na	na	na	na	na	na	na	na	45	na
ROLL DOUGH, FROZEN														
unraised, enriched, 2 x 2 3/8 inches	1 roll	0	.11	.08	.9	na	na	na	0.0	9.24	.73	na	22.96	na
unraised, unenriched, 2 x 2 3/8 inches	1 roll	0	.02	.03	.27	na	na	na	0.0	9.24	.25	na	22.96	na
ROMAN BEAN. See CRANBERRY BEAN.														
ROOT BEER. See SOFT DRINKS AND MIXERS.														
ROQUETTE. See ARUGULA.														
ROSE APPLE, raw	100 gm	339	.02	.03	.8	na	na	0	22.3	29.0	.07	5.0	123.0	.06
ROSEFISH. See OCEAN PERCH, ATLANTIC.														
ROSELLE, raw, trimmed	1 cup	164	.01	.02	.18	na	na	0	6.8	122.55	.84	29.07	118.56	na
ROSEMARY														
dried	1 tbsp	103	.02	na	.03	na	na	0	2.0	42.24	.97	7.26	31.52	.11
dried	1 tsp	38	.01	na	.01	na	na	0	0.7	15.36	.35	2.64	11.46	.04
dried (Durkee)	1 tsp	.45	.07	na	0	na	na	na	.01	0	0	na	0	na
dried (Laurel Leaf)	1 tsp	.45	.07	na	0	na	na	na	.01	0	0	na	0	na
ROTINI. See PASTA.														
RUCULO. See ARUGULA.														
RUGULA. See ARUGULA.														
RUM. See ALCOHOLIC BEVERAGES.														
RUTABAGA														
boiled, drained, cubed	1/2 cup	477	.07	.03	.61	.09	12.8	0	16.0	40.8	.45	19.55	277.1	.3
boiled, drained, mashed	1/2 cup	673	.1	.05	.86	.12	18.0	0	22.6	57.6	.64	27.6	391.2	.42
raw, cubed	1/2 cup	406	.06	.03	.49	.07	14.7	0	17.5	32.9	.36	16.1	235.9	.24
RYE, flakes	1/2 cup	0	.27	.21	3.59	.25	50.4	0	0.0	27.72	2.24	101.64	221.76	3.13
RYE FLOUR														
dark	1/2 cup	0	.2	.16	2.73	.28	38.4	0	0.0	35.84	4.13	158.72	467.2	3.6
light	1/2 cup	0	.17	.05	.41	.12	11.2	0	0.0	10.71	.92	35.7	118.83	.89
medium	1/2 cup	0	.15	.06	.88	.14	9.7	0	0.0	12.24	1.08	38.25	173.4	1.01

S

Food Name	Serving Size	A I.U.	Thi mg	Rib mg	Nia mg	B$_6$ mg	Fol mcg	B$_{12}$ mcg	C mg	Calc mg	Iron mg	Mag mg	Pot mg	Zn mg
SABLEFISH/skil														
cooked	3 oz	287	.1	.1	4.36	.29	14.5	1.22	0.0	38.25	1.39	60.35	390.15	.35
raw	3 oz	264	.09	.08	3.4	.26	12.8	1.27	0.0	29.75	1.09	46.75	304.3	.27
raw, approx 6.8 oz	1/2 fillet	598	.19	.17	7.72	.58	29.0	2.9	0.0	67.55	2.47	106.15	690.94	.62
smoked	3 oz	347	.11	.1	4.51	.33	16.8	1.7	0.0	42.5	1.44	62.9	400.35	.37
SAFFLOWER OIL														
over 70% oleic	1 cup	0	0	0	0	0	0.0	0	0.0	0	0	0	0	0
over 70% oleic	1 tbsp	0	0	0	0	0	0.0	0	0.0	0	0	0	0	0
SAFFLOWER SEED, dried, kernels	1 oz	14	.33	.12	.65	.33	45.6	0	0.0	22.15	1.39	100.25	195.11	1.43
SAFFLOWER SEED MEAL, partially defatted	1 oz	14	.33	.12	.64	.33	45.2	0	0.0	21.87	1.38	99.4	19.31	1.42
SAFFRON														
dried	1 tbsp	na	na	na	na	na	na	0	na	2.33	.23	na	36.2	na
dried	1 tsp	na	na	na	na	na	na	0	na	.78	.08	na	12.07	na
SAGE														
ground	1 tbsp	118	.02	.01	.11	na	na	0	0.7	33.04	.56	8.56	21.4	.09
ground	1 tsp	41	.01	0	.04	na	na	0	0.2	11.56	.2	3.0	7.49	.03
ground (Durkee)	1 tsp	.29	.04	.02	0	na	na	na	0	0	0	na	0	na
ground (Laurel Leaf)	1 tsp	.29	.04	.02	0	na	na	na	0	0	0	na	0	na
SALAD DRESSING														
BACON (Kraft) creamy 'Reduced Calorie'	1 tbsp	na	na	na	na	na	na	na	na	na	na	na	10	na
BACON AND TOMATO														
(Kraft)	1 tbsp	na	na	na	na	na	na	na	na	na	na	na	15	na
(Kraft) 'Reduced Calorie'	1 tbsp	na	na	na	na	na	na	na	na	na	na	na	20	na
BLUE CHEESE														
	1 cup	515	.02	.25	.25	.09	19.8	.67	4.9	198.45	.49	0	90.65	0
	1 tbsp	32	0	.02	.02	.01	1.2	.04	0.3	12.39	.03	0	5.66	0
(Kraft) chunky	1 tbsp	na	na	na	na	na	na	na	na	na	na	na	5	na
(Kraft) chunky 'Reduced Calorie'	1 tbsp	na	na	na	na	na	na	na	na	na	na	na	5	na
BUTTERMILK														
(Kraft) creamy	1 tbsp	na	na	na	na	na	na	na	na	na	na	na	10	na
(Kraft) creamy 'Reduced Calorie'	1 tbsp	na	na	na	na	na	na	na	na	na	na	na	15	na
CAESAR (Kraft) golden	1 tbsp	na	na	na	na	na	na	na	na	na	na	na	5	na
CALIFORNIA FRENCH (Catalina) nonfat 'Free'	1 tbsp	na	na	na	na	na	na	na	na	na	na	na	20	na
CUCUMBER														
(Kraft) creamy	1 tbsp	na	na	na	na	na	na	na	na	na	na	na	10	na
(Kraft) creamy 'Reduced Calorie'	1 tbsp	na	na	na	na	na	na	na	na	na	na	na	10	na
FRENCH														
(Catalina)	1 tbsp	na	na	na	na	na	na	na	na	na	na	na	20	na
(Kraft)	1 tbsp	na	na	na	na	na	na	na	na	na	na	na	5	na
(Kraft) 'Miracle'	1 tbsp	na	na	na	na	na	na	na	na	na	na	na	15	na
(Kraft) nonfat 'Free'	1 tbsp	na	na	na	na	na	na	na	na	na	na	na	15	na
(Kraft) 'Reduced Calorie'	1 tbsp	na	na	na	na	na	na	na	na	na	na	na	5	na
GARLIC (Kraft) creamy	1 tbsp	na	na	na	na	na	na	na	na	na	na	na	10	na
ITALIAN														
(Kraft) house	1 tbsp	na	na	na	na	na	na	na	na	na	na	na	10	na
(Kraft) house 'Reduced Calorie'	1 tbsp	na	na	na	na	na	na	na	na	na	na	na	10	na
(Kraft) nonfat 'Free'	1 tbsp	na	na	na	na	na	na	na	na	na	na	na	5	na
(Kraft) oil-free 'Reduced Calorie'	1 tbsp	na	na	na	na	na	na	na	na	na	na	na	5	na
(Kraft) 'Presto'	1 tbsp	na	na	na	na	na	na	na	na	na	na	na	5	na
(Kraft) zesty	1 tbsp	na	na	na	na	na	na	na	na	na	na	na	5	na
(Kraft) zesty 'Reduced Calorie'	1 tbsp	na	na	na	na	na	na	na	na	na	na	na	5	na
ITALIAN, CREAMY														
(Kraft) 'Reduced Calorie'	1 tbsp	na	na	na	na	na	na	na	na	na	na	na	10	na
(Kraft) w/real sour cream	1 tbsp	na	na	na	na	na	na	na	na	na	na	na	10	na

Food Name	Serving Size	A I.U.	Thi mg	Rib mg	Nia mg	B₆ mg	Fol mcg	B₁₂ mcg	C mg	Calc mg	Iron mg	Mag mg	Pot mg	Zn mg
OIL AND VINEGAR														
W/olive oil *(Kraft)*	1 tbsp	na	na	na	na	na	na	na	na	na	na	na	0	na
W/red wine vinegar *(Kraft)*	1 tbsp	na	na	na	na	na	na	na	na	na	na	na	10	na
RANCH *(Kraft)* nonfat 'Free'	1 tbsp	na	na	na	na	na	na	na	na	na	na	na	20	na
RUSSIAN														
(Kraft) creamy	1 tbsp	na	na	na	na	na	na	na	na	na	na	na	25	na
(Kraft) 'Reduced Calorie'	1 tbsp	na	na	na	na	na	na	na	na	na	na	na	15	na
(Kraft) w/pure honey, low-calorie	1 tbsp	na	na	na	na	na	na	na	na	na	na	na	20	na
THOUSAND ISLAND														
(Kraft)	1 tbsp	na	na	na	na	na	na	na	na	na	na	na	15	na
(Kraft) and bacon	1 tbsp	na	na	na	na	na	na	na	na	na	na	na	20	na
(Kraft) nonfat 'Free'	1 tbsp	na	na	na	na	na	na	na	na	na	na	na	20	na
(Kraft) 'Reduced Calorie'	1 tbsp	na	na	na	na	na	na	na	na	na	na	na	5	na
SALISBURY STEAK DINNER. See BEEF DINNER, FROZEN.														
SALISBURY STEAK ENTRÉE. See BEEF ENTRÉE, FROZEN.														
SALMON, ATLANTIC														
Farmed														
dry-heat cooked	3 oz	43	.29	.11	6.84	.55	28.9	2.38	3.2	na	.29	25.5	326.4	.37
raw	3 oz	43	.29	.1	6.38	.54	22.1	2.38	3.3	na	.31	23.8	307.7	.34
Wild														
dry-heat cooked	3 oz	37	.23	.41	8.57	.8	24.7	2.59	0.0	12.75	.88	31.45	533.8	.7
raw	3 oz	34	.19	.32	6.68	.7	21.3	2.7	0.0	10.2	.68	24.65	416.5	.54
SALMON, CANNED														
CHUM *(Bumble Bee)* w/liquid	3.5 oz	na	na	na	na	na	na	na	na	na	na	na	340	na
PINK														
skinless, boneless, w/liquid *(Bumble Bee)*	3.5 oz	na	na	na	na	na	na	na	na	na	na	na	300	na
solids, w/bone and liquid	3 oz	47	.02	.16	5.56	.26	13.1	3.74	0.0	181.05	.71	28.9	277.1	.78
w/liquid *(Bumble Bee)*	3.5 oz	na	na	na	na	na	na	na	na	na	na	na	320	na
SOCKEYE														
skinless, boneless, w/liquid *(Bumble Bee)*	3.5 oz	na	na	na	na	na	na	na	na	na	na	na	310	na
solids, w/bone, drained	3 oz	150	.01	.16	4.66	.26	8.3	.26	0.0	203.15	.9	24.65	320.45	.87
solids, w/bone, drained, w/o salt	3 oz	150	.01	.16	4.66	.26	8.3	.26	0.0	203.15	.9	24.65	320.45	.87
w/liquid *(Bumble Bee)*	3.5 oz	na	na	na	na	na	na	na	na	na	na	na	370	na
SALMON, CHINOOK / king / lox / smoked														
dry-heat cooked	3 oz	422	.04	.13	8.54	.39	29.8	2.44	3.5	23.8	.77	103.7	429.25	.48
raw	3 oz	387	.03	.1	6.66	.34	25.5	2.54	3.4	18.7	.6	80.75	334.9	.37
smoked	3 oz	75	.02	.09	4.01	.24	1.6	2.77	0.0	9.35	.72	15.3	148.75	.26
smoked, lox	3 oz	75	.02	.09	4.01	.24	1.6	2.77	0.0	9.35	.72	15.3	148.75	.26
SALMON, CHUM / dog / keta														
dry-heat cooked	3 oz	97	.08	.19	7.25	.39	4.3	2.94	0.0	11.9	.6	23.8	467.5	.51
raw	3 oz	84	.07	.15	5.95	.34	3.4	2.55	0.0	9.35	.47	18.7	364.65	.4
raw, approx 7 oz	1/2 fillet	196	.16	.36	13.86	.79	7.9	5.94	0.0	21.78	1.09	43.56	849.42	.93
raw, solids, w/bone, drained, w/o salt	3 oz	52	.02	.14	5.95	.32	17.0	3.74	0.0	211.65	.6	25.5	255.0	.85
SALMON, COHO / silver														
Farmed														
dry-heat cooked	3 oz	167	.09	.1	6.28	.48	11.9	2.69	1.3	10.2	.33	28.9	391.0	.4
raw	3 oz	160	.08	.09	5.79	.56	11.1	2.27	0.9	10.2	.29	26.35	382.5	.37
Wild														
dry-heat cooked	3 oz	111	.06	.12	6.76	.48	11.1	4.25	1.2	na	.52	28.05	368.9	.48
moist-heat cooked	3 oz	92	.1	.14	6.61	.47	7.7	3.81	0.9	39.1	.6	29.75	386.75	.44
raw	3 oz	85	.1	.12	6.15	.47	7.7	3.54	0.9	30.6	.48	26.35	359.55	.35
raw, approx 7 oz	1/2 fillet	198	.22	.28	14.32	1.09	17.8	8.26	2.0	71.28	1.11	61.38	837.54	.81
SALMON, DOG. See SALMON, CHUM.														
SALMON, HUMPBACK. See SALMON, PINK.														
SALMON, KETA. See SALMON, CHUM.														

Food Name	Serving Size	A I.U.	Thi mg	Rib mg	Nia mg	B$_6$ mg	Fol mcg	B$_{12}$ mcg	C mg	Calc mg	Iron mg	Mag mg	Pot mg	Zn mg
SALMON, KING. See SALMON, CHINOOK.														
SALMON, PINK / humpback														
dry-heat cooked	3 oz	116	.17	.06	7.25	.2	4.3	2.94	0.0	14.45	.84	28.05	351.9	.6
raw	3 oz	100	.14	.05	5.95	.17	3.4	2.55	0.0	11.05	.65	22.1	274.55	.47
SALMON, RED. See SALMON, SOCKEYE.														
SALMON, REDEYE. See SALMON, SOCKEYE.														
SALMON, SILVER. See SALMON, COHO.														
SALMON, SMOKED. See SALMON, CHINOOK.														
SALMON, SOCKEYE / red / redeye														
dry-heat cooked	3 oz	178	.18	.15	5.67	.19	4.3	4.93	0.0	5.95	.47	26.35	318.75	.43
raw	3 oz	163	.17	.13	4.91	.16	3.4	4.25	0.0	5.1	.4	20.4	332.35	.46
raw, approx 7 oz	1/2 fillet	380	.4	.3	11.44	.38	7.9	9.9	0.0	11.88	.93	47.52	774.18	1.07
SALSA. See also SAUCE.														
GREEN CHILI														
(Ortega) hot	1 oz	na	na	na	na	na	na	na	na	na	na	na	65	na
(Ortega) medium	1 oz	na	na	na	na	na	na	na	na	na	na	na	55	na
(Ortega) mild	1 oz	na	na	na	na	na	na	na	na	na	na	na	70	na
(Rosarita) mild	1.093 oz	na	na	na	na	na	na	na	2.9	.94	.9	na	na	na
MEDIUM *(Rosarita)* 'Traditional'	1.093 oz	na	na	na	na	na	na	na	3.8	1.08	.7	na	na	na
MILD														
(Hunt's) 'Homestyle'	1.093 oz	na	na	na	na	na	na	na	7.9	1.02	.34	na	na	na
(Rosarita) 'Casa Mamita'	1.129 oz	na	na	na	na	na	na	na	1.2	2.86	.55	na	na	na
(Rosarita) roasted	1.093 oz	na	na	na	na	na	na	na	2.5	1.17	.8	na	na	na
(Rosarita) 'Traditional'	1.093 oz	na	na	na	na	na	na	na	2.8	1.26	.72	na	na	na
PICANTE														
(LàCasita) mild, chunky	2 oz	na	na	na	na	na	na	na	na	na	na	na	148	na
(Rosarita)	1.093 oz	na	na	na	na	na	na	na	0.6	.89	.75	na	na	na
TACO														
(Ortega) hot	1 oz	na	na	na	na	na	na	na	na	na	na	na	40	na
(Ortega) mild	1 oz	na	na	na	na	na	na	na	na	na	na	na	35	na
TOMATILLO *(Rosarita)* medium	1.093 oz	na	na	na	na	na	na	na	0.5	.5	.15	na	na	na
SALSIFY / oyster plant / vegetable oyster														
boiled, drained, sliced	1/2 cup	0	.04	.12	.27	.15	10.3	0	3.1	31.96	.37	12.24	192.44	.2
raw, sliced	1/2 cup	0	.05	.15	.34	.19	17.6	0	5.4	40.2	.47	15.41	254.6	.25
SALT														
plain	1 cup	0	0	0	0	na	na	na	0.0	130.5	.29	na	23.2	na
plain	1 tbsp	0	0	0	0	0	0.0	0	0.0	4.32	.06	.18	1.44	.02
plain	1 tsp	0	0	0	0	0	0.0	0	0.0	1.44	.02	.06	.48	.01
SANDWICH														
CANADIAN BACON														
(Quick Meal) muffin, w/egg and cheese	4.5 oz	na	na	na	na	na	na	na	na	na	na	na	270	na
PIZZA														
(Amy's Kitchen) frozen, pocket, cheese														
calzone, organic	4.5 oz	na	na	na	na	na	na	na	na	na	na	na	292	na
PORK *(Quick Meal)* barbecue	4.3 oz	na	na	na	na	na	na	na	na	na	na	na	326	na
SAUSAGE														
(Quick Meal) biscuit	3.7 oz	na	na	na	na	na	na	na	na	na	na	na	254	na
(Quick Meal) biscuit, w/cheese	4.3 oz	na	na	na	na	na	na	na	na	na	na	na	326	na
(Quick Meal) biscuit, w/egg	4.5 oz	na	na	na	na	na	na	na	na	na	na	na	294	na
(Quick Meal) muffin, w/egg and cheese	5.1 oz	na	na	na	na	na	na	na	na	na	na	na	56	na
VEGETABLE														
(Ken & Robert's) pocket, barbecue style, 'Truly Amazing'	5 oz	na	na	na	na	na	na	na	na	na	na	na	360	na
(Ken & Robert's) pocket, broccoli cheddar, 'Truly Amazing'	5 oz	na	na	na	na	na	na	na	na	na	na	na	238	na

Food Name	Serving Size	A I.U.	Thi mg	Rib mg	Nia mg	B₆ mg	Fol mcg	B₁₂ mcg	C mg	Calc mg	Iron mg	Mag mg	Pot mg	Zn mg
(Ken & Robert's) pocket, Greek style, 'Truly Amazing'	5 oz	na	na	na	na	na	na	na	na	na	na	na	230	na
(Ken & Robert's) pocket, Indian style, 'Truly Amazing'	5 oz	na	na	na	na	na	na	na	na	na	na	na	218	na
(Ken & Robert's) pocket, Oriental style, 'Truly Amazing'	5 oz	na	na	na	na	na	na	na	na	na	na	na	217	na
(Ken & Robert's) pocket, pizza style, 'Truly Amazing'	5 oz	na	na	na	na	na	na	na	na	na	na	na	313	na
(Ken & Robert's) pocket, Tex Mex style, 'Truly Amazing'	5 oz	na	na	na	na	na	na	na	na	na	na	na	256	na
SANDWICH SPREAD. See also LUNCHEON MEAT, CANNED; POTTED MEAT SPREAD.														
pork and beef	1 oz	25	.05	.04	.49	.03	0.6	.32	0.0	3.4	.22	2.27	31.19	.29
pork and beef	1 tbsp	13	.03	.02	.26	.02	0.3	.17	0.0	1.8	.12	1.2	16.5	.15
SAPODILLA														
approx 7.5 oz	1 med	102	0	.03	.34	.06	na	0	25.0	35.7	1.36	na	328.1	na
pulp	1 cup	145	0	.05	.48	.09	na	0	35.4	50.61	1.93	na	465.13	na
SAPOTE/marmalade plum														
trimmed, approx 11.2 oz	1 med	923	.02	.05	4.05	na	na	0	45.0	87.75	2.25	67.5	774.0	na
SARDINE														
ATLANTIC														
in soybean oil, drained	3.75-oz can	206	.07	.21	4.83	.15	10.9	8.22	0.0	351.44	2.69	35.88	365.24	1.21
in soybean oil, drained, approx .8 oz	2 med	54	.02	.05	1.26	.04	2.8	2.15	0.0	91.68	.7	9.36	95.28	.31
PACIFIC														
in tomato sauce, drained	13 oz	1351	.16	.86	15.54	.46	89.9	33.3	3.7	888.0	8.51	125.8	1261.7	5.18
in tomato sauce, drained, approx 1.3 oz	1 med	139	.02	.09	1.6	.05	9.2	3.42	0.4	91.2	.87	12.92	129.58	.53
SAUCE. See also BARBECUE SAUCE; CRANBERRY SAUCE; SALSA; TOMATO SAUCE.														
ALFREDO SAUCE														
(Contadina)	4 oz	100	.02	.17	.08	.03	3.5	.19	0.6	200	.18	15.5	105	.24
(DiGiorno) refrigerated	2 oz	na	na	na	na	na	na	na	na	na	na	na	55	na
BOLOGNESE SAUCE *(Contadina)*	5 oz	500	.06	.17	2.28	.23	11.6	1.13	0.9	38.7	2.16	34.8	410	2.71
BROWN GRAVY SAUCE *(LaChoy)*	3.139 oz	na	na	na	na	na	na	na	0.0	.56	.49	na	na	na
CARBONARA SAUCE *(DiGiorno)* refrigerated	2 oz	na	na	na	na	na	na	na	na	na	na	na	80	na
CHEDDAR CHEESE SAUCE														
(J. Hungerford) 'Stadium'	2.011 oz	na	na	na	na	na	na	na	1.0	6.0	1.0	na	na	na
CHILI SAUCE														
(Heinz)	1 oz	na	na	na	na	na	na	na	na	na	na	na	115	na
(Hunt's)	1.199 oz	na	na	na	na	na	na	na	1.8	.5	.63	na	na	na
(Wolf Brand) hot dog	1.25 oz	410	.06	.1	.35	.05	9.0	0	na	16	.57	15	102	0
CRANBERRY-ORANGE SAUCE														
(Ocean Spray) crushed, for chicken 'Cran•Fruit'	2 oz	na	na	na	na	na	na	na	na	na	na	na	15	na
CRANBERRY-RASPBERRY SAUCE														
(Ocean Spray) crushed, for chicken 'Cran•Fruit'	2 oz	na	na	na	na	na	na	na	na	na	na	na	20	na
FOUR CHEESE SAUCE														
(Contadina)	4 oz	100	.03	.26	.06	.03	4.0	.22	0.3	150	.09	10.9	115	.25
(DiGiorno) refrigerated	2 oz	na	na	na	na	na	na	na	na	na	na	na	70	na
GUAVA SAUCE, cooked	1/2 cup	337	.03	.02	.5	na	na	0	174.2	8.33	.21	8.33	267.75	.2
HORSERADISH SAUCE *(Heinz)*	1 tbsp	na	na	na	na	na	na	na	na	na	na	na	25	na
MARINARA SAUCE														
(Angela Mia)	4.409 oz	na	na	na	na	na	na	na	12.9	2.24	13.67	na	na	na
(DiGiorno) refrigerated	5 oz	na	na	na	na	na	na	na	na	na	na	na	590	na
(Westbrae)	4 oz	na	na	na	na	na	na	na	na	na	na	na	390	na
(Westbrae) w/mushrooms	4 oz	na	na	na	na	na	na	na	na	na	na	na	440	na
NACHO CHEESE SAUCE														
(J. Hungerford)	2.011 oz	na	na	na	na	na	na	na	1.0	10.0	1.0	na	na	na
(J. Hungerford) 'Stadium'	2.011 oz	na	na	na	na	na	na	na	1.0	6.0	1.0	na	na	na

Food Name	Serving Size	A I.U.	Thi mg	Rib mg	Nia mg	B$_6$ mg	Fol mcg	B$_{12}$ mcg	C mg	Calc mg	Iron mg	Mag mg	Pot mg	Zn mg
PASTA SAUCE / spaghetti sauce														
(Angela Mia)	4.409 oz	na	na	na	na	na	na	na	3.7	1.58	6.37	na	na	na
Garlic and herb														
(Hunt's) 'Classic'	4.409 oz	na	na	na	na	na	na	na	8.7	3.14	12.71	na	na	na
(Hunt's) 'Light'	4.409 oz	na	na	na	na	na	na	na	6.7	3.31	10.83	na	na	na
(Hunt's) 'Olde Country'	4.409 oz	na	na	na	na	na	na	na	11.9	2.86	1.32	na	na	na
Italian (Hunt's) vegetable 'Olde Country'	4.409 oz	na	na	na	na	na	na	na	11.5	2.66	1.66	na	na	na
Meat														
(Hunt's)	4.444 oz	na	na	na	na	na	na	na	22.2	2.63	8.89	na	na	na
(Hunt's) 'Homestyle'	4.409 oz	na	na	na	na	na	na	na	12.3	3.48	6.18	na	na	na
(Hunt's) 'Light'	4.409 oz	na	na	na	na	na	na	na	19.4	3.32	9.44	na	na	na
(Hunt's) 'Olde Country'	4.409 oz	na	na	na	na	na	na	na	17.6	3.1	.83	na	na	na
Meat flavor (Contadina) 'Original Recipe'	1/2 cup	841	.09	.1	1.74	.2	1.4	na	10.6	38	1.81	37	490	.43
Mushroom														
(Contadina) 'Original Recipe'	1/2 cup	858	.09	.11	1.74	.21	2.1	na	10.9	38	1.78	38	500	.46
(Hunt's)	4.444 oz	na	na	na	na	na	na	na	22.2	2.63	8.89	na	na	na
(Hunt's) 'Homestyle'	4.409 oz	na	na	na	na	na	na	na	12.3	3.48	6.18	na	na	na
(Hunt's) 'Light'	4.409 oz	na	na	na	na	na	na	na	6.7	3.31	10.83	na	na	na
(Hunt's) 'Olde Country'	4.409 oz	na	na	na	na	na	na	na	16.7	2.99	.56	na	na	na
Mushroom and tomato														
(DiGiorno) w/plum tomatoes, refrigerated	5 oz	na	na	na	na	na	na	na	na	na	na	na	520	na
No salt added (Eden Foods) organic	4 oz	na	na	na	na	na	na	na	na	na	na	na	610	na
Parmesan (Hunt's) 'Classic'	4.409 oz	na	na	na	na	na	na	na	5.3	3.86	6.67	na	na	na
Primavera														
(Westbrae)	4 oz	na	na	na	na	na	na	na	na	na	na	na	410	na
(Westbrae) no salt	4 oz	na	na	na	na	na	na	na	na	na	na	na	390	na
Tomato and basil (Hunt's) 'Classic'	4.409 oz	na	na	na	na	na	na	na	15.0	3.09	19.86	na	na	na
Traditional														
(Contadina) 'Original Recipe'	1/2 cup	851	.08	.1	1.61	.21	1.5	na	10.8	38	1.74	38	400	.44
(Hunt's) 'Homestyle'	4.409 oz	na	na	na	na	na	na	na	12.3	3.48	6.18	na	na	na
(Hunt's) 'Light'	4.409 oz	na	na	na	na	na	na	na	6.7	3.31	10.83	na	na	na
(Hunt's) 'Olde Country'	4.409 oz	na	na	na	na	na	na	na	16.7	2.99	.56	na	na	na
PESTO SAUCE (DiGiorno) refrigerated	2.3 oz	na	na	na	na	na	na	na	na	na	na	na	55	na
PICANTE SAUCE														
Hot (Rosarita) zesty jalapeño	1.093 oz	na	na	na	na	na	na	na	2.7	.8	.73	na	na	na
Medium (Rosarita) zesty jalapeño	1.093 oz	na	na	na	na	na	na	na	2.4	.69	.83	na	na	na
Mild														
(Hunt's) 'Homestyle'	1.093 oz	na	na	na	na	na	na	na	2.9	.47	.41	na	na	na
(Rosarita) zesty jalapeño	1.093 oz	na	na	na	na	na	na	na	2.4	.71	.71	na	na	na
PIZZA SAUCE														
(Angela Mia)	2.222 oz	na	na	na	na	na	na	na	23.1	1.29	1.58	na	na	na
(Angela Mia) super heavy 'Premium Choice'	2.258 oz	na	na	na	na	na	na	na	22.5	2.63	4.2	na	na	na
(Contadina) original 'Quick & Easy'	1/4 cup	669	.04	.02	.58	na	na	na	14.0	13	.72	8	220	na
(Contadina) 'Pizza Squeeze'	1/4 cup	669	.04	.02	.58	na	na	na	14.0	13	.72	8	220	na
(Contadina) w/Italian cheese	1/4 cup	664	.04	.02	.58	na	na	na	14.0	21	.71	8	280	na
(Contadina) w/pepperoni	1/4 cup	659	.04	.02	.06	na	na	na	13.0	13	.73	8	260	na
(Hunt's)	2.363 oz	na	na	na	na	na	na	na	2.8	2.06	.04	na	na	na
(Hunt's)	2.222 oz	na	na	na	na	na	na	na	8.2	1.56	7.26	na	na	na
RIGOLLETO SAUCE (DiGiorno) refrigerated	5 oz	na	na	na	na	na	na	na	na	na	na	na	480	na
SANDWICH SAUCE														
(Manwich) bold	2.222 oz	na	na	na	na	na	na	na	8.0	2.83	1.26	na	na	na
(Manwich) Mexican	2.258 oz	na	na	na	na	na	na	na	6.9	1.71	2.3	na	na	na
(Manwich) thick and chunky	2.293 oz	na	na	na	na	na	na	na	7.1	1.89	.51	na	na	na
SEAFOOD COCKTAIL SAUCE (Heinz)	1/4 cup	na	na	na	na	na	na	na	na	na	na	na	170	na
SPAGHETTI SAUCE. See PASTA SAUCE.														
STEAK SAUCE														
(Heinz) '57'	1 tbsp	na	na	na	na	na	na	na	na	na	na	na	50	na

Food Name	Serving Size	A I.U.	Thi mg	Rib mg	Nia mg	B₆ mg	Fol mcg	B₁₂ mcg	C mg	Calc mg	Iron mg	Mag mg	Pot mg	Zn mg
(Heinz) hickory smoke '57'	1 tbsp	na	na	na	na	na	na	na	na	na	na	na	50	na
(Heinz) traditional	1 tbsp	na	na	na	na	na	na	na	na	na	na	na	60	na
(Hunt's)	1 tbsp	na	na	na	na	na	na	na	1.9	.63	.01	na	na	na
STIR-FRY SAUCE														
(LaChoy) Mandarin	4.48 oz	na	na	na	na	na	na	na	5.9	1.21	4.44	na	na	na
(LaChoy) sweet and sour	4.797 oz	na	na	na	na	na	na	na	14.7	1.35	.76	na	na	na
(LaChoy) Szechwan	4.55 oz	na	na	na	na	na	na	na	5.6	1.17	5.57	na	na	na
SWEET AND SOUR SAUCE (Contadina)	1/2 cup	100	.02	.02	.38	.34	2.8	na	6.0	20.1	.36	8.0	120	.07
TACO SAUCE														
(Rosarita)	.1764 oz	na	na	na	na	na	na	na	0.2	.12	.25	na	na	na
Hot (Ortega)	1 oz	na	na	na	na	na	na	na	na	na	na	na	40	na
Mild (Ortega)	1 oz	na	na	na	na	na	na	na	na	na	na	na	35	na
TARTAR SAUCE (Heinz)	2 tbsp	na	na	na	na	na	na	na	na	na	na	na	15	na
TERIYAKI SAUCE (LaChoy) stir-fry sauce	4.621 oz	na	na	na	na	na	na	na	7.4	1.31	16.19	na	na	na
WORCESTERSHIRE SAUCE														
(Lea & Perrins)	1 tsp	na	na	na	na	na	na	na	na	na	na	na	22	na
(Lea & Perrins) white wine	1 tsp	na	na	na	na	na	na	na	na	na	na	na	17	na
SAUCE MIX														
HOLLANDAISE SAUCE														
(McCormick/Schilling) dry mix	1/4 pkg	na	na	na	na	na	na	na	na	na	na	na	20	na
SANDWICH SAUCE (Manwich) dry mix	.2469 oz	na	na	na	na	na	na	na	0.0	.8	.79	na	na	na
SAUERKRAUT, CANNED														
(Eden Foods) organic	1/2 cup	na	na	na	na	na	na	na	na	na	na	na	160	na
SAUERKRAUT JUICE, canned	1 cup	121	.07	.1	.48	na	na	na	43.6	89.54	2.66	na	338.8	na
SAUSAGE. See also individual listings.														
ITALIAN STYLE														
cooked	3 oz	0	.52	.19	3.46	.27	4.2	1.08	1.7	19.92	1.25	14.94	252.32	1.98
cooked	2.4 oz	0	.42	.16	2.79	.22	3.4	.87	1.3	16.08	1.0	12.06	203.68	1.59
raw	4 oz	0	.64	.19	3.67	.34	9.0	1.03	2.3	20.34	1.33	15.82	285.89	2.01
raw	3.2 oz	0	.52	.15	2.96	.27	7.3	.83	1.8	16.38	1.07	12.74	230.23	1.62
POLISH STYLE														
	1 oz	0	.14	.04	.98	.05	0.6	.28	0.3	3.4	.41	3.97	67.19	.55
10-inch sausage	1 link	0	1.14	.34	7.82	.43	4.5	2.22	2.3	27.24	3.27	31.78	537.99	4.38
PORK														
4-inch links, cooked	1 link	0	.1	.03	.59	.04	0.3	.22	0.3	4.16	.16	2.21	46.93	.33
4-inch links, raw	1 link	0	.15	.05	.79	.07	1.1	.32	0.6	5.04	.25	3.08	57.12	.45
patties, 1/4 inch x 3 7/8 inch diam, cooked	1 patty	0	.2	.07	1.22	.09	0.5	.47	0.5	8.64	.34	4.59	97.47	.68
patties, 1/4 inch x 3 7/8 inch diam, raw	1 patty	0	.31	.09	1.62	.14	2.3	.64	1.1	10.26	.52	6.27	116.28	.91
PORK AND BEEF														
fresh, 1/4 inch x 3 7/8 inch diam patties, cooked	1 patty	0	.1	.04	.91	.01	0.5	.12	0.0	2.7	.31	3.24	51.03	.5
fresh, 2 inch x 3/4 inch diam links, cooked	1 link	0	.05	.02	.44	.01	0.3	.06	0.0	1.3	.15	1.56	24.57	.24
smoked, 4 inch x 1 1/8 inch diam links	1 link	0	.18	.12	2.19	.12	1.4	1.03	12.9	6.8	.99	8.16	128.52	1.43
smoked, 2 inch x 3/4 inch diam links	1 link	0	.04	.03	.52	.03	0.3	.24	3.0	1.6	.23	1.92	30.24	.34
smoked, w/flour and nonfat dry milk added, 4 inch x 1 1/8 inch diam links	1 link	0	.16	.12	1.84	.09	1.4	.9	2.0	12.24	1.05	8.84	105.4	1.36
smoked, w/flour and nonfat dry milk added, 2 inch x 3/4 inch diam links	1 link	0	.04	.03	.43	.02	0.3	.21	0.5	2.88	.25	2.08	24.8	.32
smoked, w/nonfat dry milk added, 4 inch x 1 1/8 inch diam links	1 link	0	.13	.15	1.93	.12	1.4	1.07	14.3	27.88	1.0	10.88	194.48	1.33
smoked, w/nonfat dry milk added, 2 inch x 3/4 inch diam links	1 link	0	.03	.03	.46	.03	0.3	.25	3.4	6.56	.24	2.56	45.76	.31
SAVORY														
ground	1 tbsp	226	.02	na	.18	na	na	0	na	93.79	1.67	16.57	46.24	.19
ground	1 tsp	72	.01	na	.06	na	na	0	na	29.84	.53	5.27	14.71	.06
ground (Durkee)	1 tsp	1	.07	na	0	na	na	na	na	0	.01	na	0	na
ground (Laurel Leaf)	1 tsp	1	.07	na	0	na	na	na	na	0	.01	na	0	na

Food Name	Serving Size	A I.U.	Thi mg	Rib mg	Nia mg	B₆ mg	Fol mcg	B₁₂ mcg	C mg	Calc mg	Iron mg	Mag mg	Pot mg	Zn mg
SAVOY CABBAGE. See CABBAGE, SAVOY.														
SCALLOP, ALTERNATIVE														
mixed species, made from surimi	3 oz	56	.01	.01	.26	.03	1.4	1.36	0.0	6.8	.26	36.55	87.55	.28
SCALLOP, MIXED SPECIES														
raw	3 oz	43	.01	.06	.98	.13	13.6	1.3	2.6	20.4	.25	47.6	273.7	.81
SCALLOP SQUASH. See SQUASH, SCALLOP.														
SCRAPPLE	1 oz	0	.05	.03	.5	na	na	na	0.0	1.4	.34	na	75.32	na
SCREWDRIVER. See ALCOHOLIC BEVERAGES.														
SCUP / sea bream														
dry-heat cooked	3 oz	88	.11	.1	4.24	.29	14.5	1.38	0.0	43.35	.58	24.65	312.8	.53
raw	3 oz	77	.09	.09	3.49	.26	12.8	1.19	0.0	34.0	.45	19.55	243.95	.41
SEA BASS. See BASS, SEA, MIXED SPECIES.														
SEA BREAM. See SCUP.														
SEA DEVIL. See MONKFISH.														
SEA PERCH. See OCEAN PERCH, ATLANTIC.														
SEA TROUT. See TROUT, SEA, MIXED SPECIES.														
SEAFOOD ENTRÉE, CANNED. See individual listings.														
SEAFOOD ENTRÉE, FROZEN. See individual listings.														
SEAFOOD SALAD. See individual listings.														
SEAWEED														
Raw														
kelp	100 gm	116	.05	.15	.47	0	180.0	0	na	168.0	2.85	121.0	89.0	1.23
laver	100 gm	5202	.1	.45	1.47	.16	146.3	0	39.0	70.0	1.8	2.0	356.0	1.05
SEMOLINA														
enriched	1/2 cup	0	.15	.05	1.8	.09	5.9	0	0.0	9.24	1.34	19.32	64.68	1.01
unenriched	1/2 cup	0	.02	.01	.34	.08	2.5	0	0.0	8.4	.17	10.08	29.4	.41
SESAME BUTTER. See also TAHINI MIX.														
made from raw and stone ground kernels ..	1 oz	19	.36	.14	1.68	.04	27.8	0	0.0	119.28	.71	27.26	117.58	1.32
made from raw and stone ground kernels ..	1 tbsp	10	.19	.08	.89	.02	14.7	0	0.0	63.0	.38	14.4	62.1	.7
made from roasted kernels	1 oz	19	.35	.13	1.55	.04	27.8	0	0.0	120.98	2.54	26.98	117.58	1.31
made from roasted kernels	1 tbsp	10	.18	.07	.82	.02	14.7	0	0.0	63.9	1.34	14.25	62.1	.69
made from unroasted kernels	1 oz	19	.45	.03	1.6	.04	27.8	0	0.0	40.04	1.8	100.25	130.36	2.97
made from unroasted kernels	1 tbsp	9	.22	.02	.79	.02	13.7	0	0.0	19.74	.89	49.42	64.26	1.46
organic 'Natural' (Westbrae)	2 tbsp	na	na	na	na	na	na	na	na	na	na	na	150	na
paste	1 oz	14	.07	.06	1.9	.23	28.3	0	0.0	272.64	5.45	102.81	165.29	2.07
paste	1 tbsp	8	.04	.03	1.07	.13	16.0	0	0.0	153.6	3.07	57.92	93.12	1.17
SESAME FLOUR														
high-fat	1 oz	20	.76	.08	3.8	.04	8.8	0	0.0	45.16	4.31	102.52	120.13	3.03
low-fat	1 oz	18	.71	.08	3.56	.04	8.2	0	0.0	42.32	4.04	95.99	112.75	2.84
partially defatted	1 oz	20	.72	.08	3.58	.04	8.2	0	0.0	42.6	4.06	102.81	120.7	3.04
SESAME MEAL, partially defatted	1 oz	19	.73	.08	3.64	.04	8.4	0	0.0	43.45	4.13	98.26	115.3	2.91
SESAME SEED / sim sim														
Decorticated														
dried	1 tbsp	5	.06	.01	.37	.01	0.0	0	0.0	10.49	.62	27.73	32.53	.82
dried	1 tsp	2	.02	0	.13	0	0.0	0	0.0	3.54	.21	9.36	10.98	.28
Kernels														
dried	1 cup	99	1.08	.13	7.02	.22	144.0	0	0.0	196.5	11.7	520.5	610.5	15.38
dried	1 tbsp	5	.06	.01	.37	.01	7.7	0	0.0	10.48	.62	27.76	32.56	.82
dried, toasted	1 oz	19	.34	.13	1.54	.04	27.2	0	0.0	37.2	2.21	98.26	115.3	2.91
Whole														
dried	1 cup	13	1.14	.36	6.5	1.14	139.3	0	0.0	1404.0	20.95	505.44	673.92	11.16
dried	1 tbsp	1	.07	.02	.41	.07	8.7	0	0.0	87.75	1.31	31.59	42.12	.7
dried (Durkee)	1 tsp	.05	.58	.09	0	na	na	na	na	0	0	na	0	na
dried (Laurel Leaf)	1 tsp	.05	.58	.09	0	na	na	na	na	0	0	na	0	na
roasted	1 oz	3	.23	.07	1.3	.23	27.9	0	0.0	280.88	4.19	101.1	134.9	2.03

Food Name	Serving Size	A I.U.	Thi mg	Rib mg	Nia mg	B$_6$ mg	Fol mcg	B$_{12}$ mcg	C mg	Calc mg	Iron mg	Mag mg	Pot mg	Zn mg
SHAD, AMERICAN														
dry-heat cooked	3 oz	102	.16	.26	9.15	.39	14.5	.12	0.0	51.0	1.05	32.3	418.2	.4
raw	3 oz	94	.13	.2	7.14	.34	12.8	.13	0.0	39.95	.82	25.5	326.4	.31
SHALLOT														
freeze-dried	1/4 cup	2020	.01	0	.04	.06	4.2	0	1.4	6.59	.22	3.74	59.4	.07
freeze-dried	1 tbsp	505	0	0	.01	.02	1.1	0	0.4	1.65	.05	.94	14.85	.02
raw	100 gm	12484	.06	.02	.2	.34	34.2	0	8.0	37.0	1.2	21.0	334.0	.4
raw	1 tbsp	1248	.01	0	.02	.03	3.4	0	0.8	3.7	.12	2.1	33.4	.04
SHARK														
Mixed species														
batter-dipped, fried	3 oz	153	.06	.08	2.37	.26	4.4	1.03	0.0	42.5	.94	36.55	131.75	.41
raw	3 oz	198	.04	.05	2.5	.34	2.7	1.26	0.0	28.9	.71	41.65	136.0	.37
SHEANUT OIL	1 tbsp	0	0	0	0	0	0.0	0	0.0	0	0	0	0	0
SHEEPSHEAD / California sheepshead / fathead / redhead														
baked	3 oz	98	.01	.04	1.53	.3	14.7	1.95	0.0	31.45	.57	29.75	435.2	.54
raw	3 oz	85	.01	.03	1.27	.26	12.8	1.7	0.0	17.85	.39	27.2	343.4	.33
SHELLIE BEAN, CANNED, w/liquid	1/2 cup	278	.04	.07	.25	.06	22.0	0	3.8	35.38	1.21	18.3	132.98	.33
SHERBET. See also ICE BARS AND DESSERTS; SORBET.														
orange	1/2 cup	73	.02	.07	.09	.03	3.8	.12	4.1	51.84	.13	7.68	92.16	.46
vanilla-orange 'Cubic Scoops' *(Sealtest)*	4 oz	na	na	na	na	na	na	na	na	na	na	na	100	na
vanilla-red raspberry 'Cubic Scoops' *(Sealtest)*	4 oz	na	na	na	na	na	na	na	na	na	na	na	100	na
SHERBET BAR, orange	2.75-oz bar	50	.02	.04	.06	.02	2.6	.09	2.8	35.64	.09	5.28	63.36	.32
SHORTENING														
COMMERCIAL														
hydrogenated soybean oil and cottonseed oil	1 cup	0	0	0	0	0	0.0	0	0.0	0	0	0	0	0
hydrogenated soybean oil and cottonseed oil	1 tbsp	0	0	0	0	0	0.0	0	0.0	0	0	0	0	0
lard and vegetable oil	1 cup	0	0	0	0	0	0.0	0	0.0	0	0	0	0	0
lard and vegetable oil	1 tbsp	0	0	0	0	0	0.0	0	0.0	0	0	0	0	0
(Wesson) 'Crystal'	1 tbsp	na	na	na	na	na	na	na	0.0	0	0	na	na	na
(Wesson) 'Lo-Melt'	1 tbsp	na	na	na	na	na	na	na	0.0	0	0	na	na	na
(Wesson) 'Super'	1 tbsp	na	na	na	na	na	na	na	0.0	0	0	na	na	na
(Wesson) 'Wesgold'	1 tbsp	na	na	na	na	na	na	na	0.0	0	0	na	na	na
(Wesson) 'Wespour'	1 tbsp	na	na	na	na	na	na	na	0.0	0	0	na	na	na
For baking														
hydrogenated soybean, palm, and cottonseed oils	1 cup	0	0	0	0	0	0.0	0	0.0	0	0	0	0	0
hydrogenated soybean, palm, and cottonseed oils	1 tbsp	0	0	0	0	0	0.0	0	0.0	0	0	0	0	0
For bread														
hydrogenated soybean oil and cottonseed oil	1 cup	0	0	0	0	0	0.0	0	0.0	0	0	0	0	0
hydrogenaged soybean oil and cottonseed oil	1 tbsp	0	0	0	0	0	0.0	0	0.0	0	0	0	0	0
For cakes and frostings														
hydrogenated soybean and cottonseed oils	1 cup	0	0	0	0	0	0.0	0	0.0	0	0	0	0	0
hydrogenated soybean and cottonseed oils	1 tbsp	0	0	0	0	0	0.0	0	0.0	0	0	0	0	0
hydrogenated soybean oil	1 cup	0	0	0	0	0	0.0	0	0.0	0	0	0	0	0
hydrogenated soybean oil	1 tbsp	0	0	0	0	0	0.0	0	0.0	0	0	0	0	0
For confectionery														
fractionated palm oil	1 cup	0	0	0	0	0	0.0	0	0.0	0	0	0	0	0
fractionated palm oil	1 tbsp	0	0	0	0	0	0.0	0	0.0	0	0	0	0	0
hydrogenated coconut and/or palm kernel oil	1 cup	0	0	0	0	0	0.0	0	0.0	0	0	0	0	0
hydrogenated coconut and/or palm kernel oil	1 tbsp	0	0	0	0	0	0.0	0	0.0	0	0	0	0	0

Food Name	Serving Size	A I.U.	Thi mg	Rib mg	Nia mg	B₆ mg	Fol mcg	B₁₂ mcg	C mg	Calc mg	Iron mg	Mag mg	Pot mg	Zn mg
Heavy duty, for frying														
beef tallow and cottonseed oil	1 cup	0	0	0	0	0	0.0	0	0.0	0	0	0	0	0
beef tallow and cottonseed oil	1 tbsp	0	0	0	0	0	0.0	0	0.0	0	0	0	0	0
hydrogenated palm oil	1 cup	0	0	0	0	0	0.0	0	0.0	0	0	0	0	0
hydrogenated palm oil	1 tbsp	0	0	0	0	0	0.0	0	0.0	0	0	0	0	0
hydrogenated soybean and cottonseed oils	1 cup	0	0	0	0	0	0.0	0	0.0	0	0	0	0	0
hydrogenated soybean and cottonseed oils	1 tbsp	0	0	0	0	0	0.0	0	0.0	0	0	0	0	0
hydrogenated soybean oil, 30% linoleic	1 cup	0	0	0	0	0	0.0	0	0.0	0	0	0	0	0
hydrogenated soybean oil, 30% linoleic	1 tbsp	0	0	0	0	0	0.0	0	0.0	0	0	0	0	0
hydrogenated soybean oil, under 1% linoleic	1 cup	0	0	0	0	0	0.0	0	0.0	0	0	0	0	0
hydrogenated soybean oil, under 1% linoleic	1 tbsp	0	0	0	0	0	0.0	0	0.0	0	0	0	0	0
Multi-purpose														
hydrogenated soybean and palm oils	1 cup	0	0	0	0	0	0.0	0	0.0	0	0	0	0	0
hydrogenated soybean and palm oils	1 tbsp	0	0	0	0	0	0.0	0	0.0	0	0	0	0	0
HOUSEHOLD														
hydrogenated soybean and cottonseed oils	1 cup	0	0	0	0	0	0.0	0	0.0	0	0	0	0	0
hydrogenated soybean and cottonseed oils	1 tbsp	0	0	0	0	0	0.0	0	0.0	0	0	0	0	0
hydrogenated soybean oil and palm oil	1 cup	0	0	0	0	0	0.0	0	0.0	0	0	0	0	0
hydrogenated soybean oil and palm oil	1 tbsp	0	0	0	0	0	0.0	0	0.0	0	0	0	0	0
lard and vegetable oil	1 cup	0	0	0	0	0	0.0	0	0.0	0	0	0	0	0
lard and vegetable oil	1 tbsp	0	0	0	0	0	0.0	0	0.0	0	0	0	0	0
SHRIMP, ALTERNATIVE, made from surimi	3 oz	56	.02	.03	.14	.03	1.4	1.36	0.0	16.15	.51	36.55	75.65	.28
SHRIMP, MIXED SPECIES														
breaded, fried	3 oz	161	.11	.12	2.61	.08	6.9	1.59	1.3	56.95	1.07	34.0	191.25	1.17
breaded, fried, .8-oz size	4 shrimp	57	.04	.04	.92	.03	2.4	.56	0.5	20.1	.38	12.0	67.5	.41
moist-heat cooked	3 oz	186	.03	.03	2.2	.11	3.0	1.26	1.9	33.15	2.63	28.9	154.7	1.33
moist-heat cooked, .8-oz size	4 shrimp	48	.01	.01	.57	.03	0.8	.33	0.5	8.58	.68	7.48	40.04	.34
raw	3 oz	153	.02	.03	2.17	.09	2.6	.99	1.7	44.2	2.05	31.45	157.25	.94
raw, .8-oz size	4 shrimp	50	.01	.01	.71	.03	0.8	.33	0.6	14.56	67	10.36	51.8	.31
Canned														
drained	1 cup	77	.03	.05	3.53	.14	2.3	1.43	2.9	75.52	3.51	52.48	268.8	1.61
drained	3 oz	51	.02	.03	2.34	.09	1.5	.95	2.0	50.15	2.33	34.85	178.5	1.07
SHRIMP CHOW MEIN, canned														
(LaChoy) 'Bi-Pack'	8.536 oz	na	na	na	na	na	na	na	22.6	3.12	4.04	na	na	na
SHRIMP ENTRÉE, FROZEN														
CREOLE (Armour) 'Classics Lite'	11.25 oz	na	na	na	na	na	na	na	na	na	na	na	420	na
SHRIMP PASTE, canned	1 tsp	4	0	.02	.13	na	na	na	0.0	8.05	.22	na	8.54	na
SILVER HAKE. See WHITING, MIXED SPECIES.														
SIM SIM. See SESAME SEED.														
SISYMBRIUM SEED														
whole, dried	1 cup	47	.14	.31	12.45	.58	70.5	0	22.7	1208.42	.08	232.36	1576.2	.22
whole, dried	1 oz	18	.05	.12	4.78	.22	27.1	0	8.7	463.77	.03	89.18	604.92	.09
SKIL. See SABLEFISH.														
SKUNK CABBAGE. See CABBAGE, SKUNK.														
SLIMEHEAD. See ORANGE ROUGHY.														
SMELT, RAINBOW														
dry-heat cooked	3 oz	49	.01	.12	1.5	.14	3.9	3.37	0.0	65.45	.98	32.3	316.2	1.8
raw	3 oz	43	.01	.1	1.23	.13	3.4	2.92	0.0	51.0	.77	25.5	246.5	1.4
SNACK BAR														
(Bear Valley)														
carob-cocoa, food bar 'Pemmican'	3.75 oz	na	na	na	na	na	na	na	na	na	na	na	720	na
coconut almond, food bar 'Meal Pack'	3.75 oz	na	na	na	na	na	na	na	na	na	na	na	650	na
fruit 'n nut, food bar 'Pemmican'	3.75 oz	na	na	na	na	na	na	na	na	na	na	na	720	na
sesame lemon, food bar 'Meal Pack'	3.75 oz	na	na	na	na	na	na	na	na	na	na	na	650	na
(Carnation)														
chocolate chip, breakfast bar	1 bar	1750	.3	.03	5	.4	100.0	0	27.0	20	4.5	60	100	3
chocolate crunch, breakfast bar	1 bar	1750	.3	.03	5	.4	100.0	.6	27.0	20	4.5	60	130	3

Food Name	Serving Size	A I.U.	Thi mg	Rib mg	Nia mg	B$_6$ mg	Fol mcg	B$_{12}$ mcg	C mg	Calc mg	Iron mg	Mag mg	Pot mg	Zn mg
peanut butter chocolate chip, breakfast bar	1 bar	1750	.3	.03	5	.4	100.0	.6	27.0	20	4.5	60	110	3
peanut butter crunch, breakfast bar	1 bar	1750	.3	.03	5	.4	100.0	.6	27.0	20	4.5	60	110	3
(Earth Grains)														
banana apple walnut 'Bagel Power Bar'	1 bar	na	na	na	na	na	na	na	na	na	na	na	na	na
(Weider)														
'Sportsfood Enerquench Bar'	1 bar	na	na	na	na	na	na	na	na	na	na	na	150	na
'Sportsfood Protein Bar'	1 bar	na	na	na	na	na	na	na	na	na	na	na	200	na
SNACK MIX														
(Doo Dads) original recipe, 1 oz	1/2 cup	43	.1	.07	1.52	.06	11.3	0	0.0	20.98	.71	17.01	78.53	.64
(Ralston) 'Chex Traditional' 2/3 cup	1 oz	41	.44	.14	4.77	.44	0.0	3.52	13.5	9.92	7.0	17.86	76.26	.59
SNAPPER, RED, MIXED SPECIES														
dry-heat cooked	3 oz	98	.05	0	.29	.39	4.9	2.98	1.4	34.0	.2	31.45	443.7	.37
raw	3 oz	85	.04	0	.24	.34	4.3	2.55	1.4	27.2	.15	27.2	354.45	.31
SODA. See SOFT DRINKS AND MIXERS.														
SOFT DRINKS AND MIXERS. See also WATER, SPARKLING, FLAVORED.														
(A&W)														
cream soda	1 oz	na	na	na	na	na	na	na	na	.87	.02	na	1.54	na
cream soda, 'Diet'	1 oz	na	na	na	na	na	na	na	na	1.3	<.02	na	.8	na
root beer	1 oz	na	na	na	na	na	na	na	na	1.02	<.02	na	1.24	na
root beer, 'Diet'	1 oz	na	na	na	na	na	na	na	na	1.27	<.02	na	3.31	na
(Squirt)														
citrus	1 oz	na	na	na	na	na	na	na	na	1.14	<.02	na	.12	na
citrus, 'Diet'	1 oz	na	na	na	na	na	na	na	na	1.44	<.02	na	1.09	na
SOLE														
dry-heat cooked	3 oz	32	.07	.1	1.85	.2	7.8	2.13	0.0	15.3	.29	49.3	292.4	.54
raw	3 oz	28	.08	.06	2.46	.18	6.8	1.29	1.4	15.3	.31	26.35	306.85	.38
SORBET. See also ICE BARS AND DESSERTS; SHERBET.														
(Frusen Glädjé) raspberry	1/2 cup	na	na	na	na	na	na	na	na	na	na	na	20	na
SORGHUM, broomcorn, whole grain	100 gm	0	.73	.38	2.3	na	na	na	0.0	20.0	6.8	na	430.0	na
SORGHUM SYRUP	1/2 cup	0	.23	.14	2.81	na	na	0	0.0	26.88	4.22	na	336.0	na
SOUP, CANNED, CONDENSED														
(NOTE: Unless otherwise specified, PREPARED = prepared as directed w/water.)														
ASPARAGUS, CREAM OF														
prepared w/whole milk	8 oz	600	.1	.28	.88	.06	29.8	.5	4.0	173.6	.87	19.84	359.6	.93
unprepared	10.75 oz	1083	.13	.19	1.89	.03	58.0	.12	6.7	70.15	1.95	9.15	420.9	2.13
BEAN														
W/frankfurters														
prepared	1 cup	870	.11	.07	1.02	.13	30.0	.08	1.0	87.5	2.35	47.5	477.5	1.18
unprepared	11.25 oz	2112	.27	.16	2.49	.32	72.8	.18	2.4	212.45	5.71	115.33	1159.37	2.87
W/pork														
prepared	1 cup	888	.09	.03	.57	.04	31.9	.05	1.5	80.96	2.05	45.54	402.27	1.03
unprepared	11.5 oz	2155	.21	.08	1.38	.1	77.4	.12	3.7	196.48	4.97	110.52	976.26	2.51
BEEF MUSHROOM														
prepared	1 cup	0	.04	.06	.95	.05	9.8	.2	4.6	4.88	.88	9.76	153.72	1.46
unprepared	10.75 oz	0	.06	.18	2.74	.12	21.4	.49	0.0	12.2	2.13	21.35	384.3	3.36
BEEF NOODLE														
prepared	1 cup	630	.07	.06	1.07	.04	4.4	.2	0.2	14.64	1.1	4.88	100.04	1.54
unprepared	10.75 oz	1531	.17	.14	2.59	.09	10.7	.49	0.9	36.6	2.68	15.25	240.95	3.74
BLACK BEAN														
prepared	1 cup	506	.08	.05	.53	.09	24.7	.02	0.7	44.46	2.15	41.99	274.17	1.41
unprepared	11 oz	1230	.19	.13	1.3	.23	60.0	.06	1.8	108.0	5.22	102.0	666.0	3.43
CELERY, CREAM OF														
prepared	1 cup	307	.03	.05	.33	.01	2.4	.24	0.2	39.04	.63	7.32	122.0	.15
prepared w/whole milk	1 cup	461	.07	.25	.44	.06	8.4	.5	1.5	186.0	.69	22.32	310.0	.2
unprepared	10.75 oz	744	.07	.12	.81	.03	5.8	.12	0.6	97.6	1.52	15.25	298.9	.37
CHEESE														
prepared	1 cup	1087	.02	.14	.4	.02	4.9	0	0.0	140.79	.74	4.94	153.14	.64

Food Name	Serving Size	A I.U.	Thi mg	Rib mg	Nia mg	B$_6$ mg	Fol mcg	B$_{12}$ mcg	C mg	Calc mg	Iron mg	Mag mg	Pot mg	Zn mg
prepared w/whole milk	1 cup	1242	.06	.33	.5	.08	10.0	.43	1.3	288.65	.8	20.08	341.36	.69
unprepared	11 oz	2643	.04	.33	.97	.06	9.4	0	0.0	346.32	1.81	9.36	374.4	1.56
CHICKEN														
W/dumplings														
prepared	1 cup	518	.02	.07	1.75	.04	2.4	.17	0.0	14.46	.63	4.82	115.68	.37
unprepared	10.5 oz	1261	.04	.18	4.26	.09	6.0	.39	0.0	35.76	1.52	8.94	283.1	.89
W/rice														
prepared	1 cup	660	.02	.02	1.13	.02	1.0	.14	0.2	16.87	.75	0	101.22	.26
unprepared	10.5 oz	1606	.04	.06	2.74	.06	2.7	.39	0.3	41.72	1.82	0	244.36	.64
CHICKEN, CREAM OF														
prepared	1 cup	561	.03	.06	.82	.02	1.7	.1	0.2	34.16	.61	2.44	87.84	.63
unprepared	10.75 oz	1360	.07	.15	1.99	.04	4.0	.21	0.3	82.35	1.46	6.1	213.5	1.52
CHICKEN BROTH														
prepared	1 cup	0	.01	.07	3.35	.02	4.9	.24	0.0	9.76	.51	2.44	209.84	.25
unprepared	10.75 oz	0	.02	.14	6.8	.06	12.2	.61	0.0	18.3	1.25	6.1	518.5	.61
CHICKEN GUMBO														
prepared	1 cup	137	.02	.05	.66	.06	4.9	.02	4.9	24.4	.9	4.88	75.64	.38
unprepared	10.75 oz	329	.61	.91	1.62	.15	15.3	.06	12.2	57.95	2.17	9.15	183.0	.91
CHICKEN MUSHROOM														
prepared	1 cup	1135	.02	.11	1.63	.05	0.2	.05	0.0	29.28	.88	9.76	153.72	.98
unprepared	10.75 oz	2760	.06	.27	3.96	.12	6.1	.15	0.0	70.15	2.13	21.35	384.3	2.44
CHICKEN NOODLE														
prepared	1 cup	711	.05	.06	1.39	.03	2.2	.14	0.2	16.87	.77	4.82	55.43	.4
unprepared	10.5 oz	1585	.15	.16	3.66	.06	5.4	.39	0.0	32.78	1.85	11.92	134.1	.69
CHICKEN VEGETABLE														
prepared	1 cup	2656	.04	.06	1.23	.05	4.8	.12	1.0	16.87	.87	7.23	154.24	.37
unprepared	10.5 oz	6461	.11	.14	2.99	.12	11.9	.3	2.4	41.72	2.12	14.9	375.48	.89
CHILI BEEF														
prepared	1 cup	1510	.06	.08	1.07	.16	17.5	.33	4.0	42.5	2.13	30.0	525.0	1.4
unprepared	11.25 oz	3665	.14	.19	2.59	.38	44.7	.77	9.9	105.27	5.17	73.37	1276.0	3.39
CLAM CHOWDER														
Manhattan style														
prepared	1 cup	964	.03	.04	.82	.1	9.8	4.05	3.9	26.84	1.63	12.2	187.88	.98
unprepared	10.75 oz	2339	.07	.1	1.98	.24	24.4	9.85	9.8	57.95	3.96	24.4	457.5	2.26
New England style														
prepared	8 oz	7	.02	.04	.96	.08	3.7	8.0	2.0	43.92	1.49	7.32	146.4	.75
prepared w/whole milk	8 oz	164	.07	.24	1.03	.13	9.7	10.24	3.5	186.0	1.49	22.32	300.08	.8
CONSOMMÉ, Beef	10.5 oz	0	.05	.07	1.73	.06	7.2	0	2.1	20.86	1.28	0	372.5	.89
GREEN PEA														
prepared	1 cup	203	.11	.07	1.24	.05	1.8	0	1.8	27.5	1.95	40.0	190.0	1.71
prepared w/whole milk	1 cup	356	.15	.27	1.34	.1	7.9	.43	2.8	172.72	2.01	55.88	375.92	1.76
unprepared	11.25 oz	488	.26	.17	3.01	.13	4.5	0	4.2	66.99	4.72	95.7	462.55	4.15
MINESTRONE														
prepared	1 cup	2338	.05	.04	.94	.1	16.2	0	1.2	33.74	.92	7.23	313.3	.74
unprepared	10.5 oz	5686	.13	.11	2.29	.24	39.0	0	2.7	83.44	2.24	17.88	759.9	1.79
MUSHROOM														
W/beef stock														
prepared	1 cup	1254	.03	.1	1.21	.04	9.3	0	1.0	9.76	.83	9.76	158.6	1.38
unprepared	10.75 oz	3050	.09	.23	2.93	.09	22.3	0	2.4	24.4	2.04	21.35	384.3	3.36
MUSHROOM, CREAM OF														
prepared	1 cup	0	.05	.09	.72	.01	4.9	.05	1.0	46.36	.51	4.88	100.04	.59
prepared w/whole milk	1 cup	154	.08	.28	.91	.06	9.9	.5	2.2	178.56	.6	19.84	270.32	.64
unprepared	10.75 oz	0	.07	.2	1.97	.03	9.2	.3	2.7	79.3	1.28	12.2	204.35	1.44
MUSHROOM BARLEY														
prepared	1 cup	198	.02	.09	.88	.17	4.9	0	0.0	12.2	.51	9.76	92.72	.49
unprepared	10.75 oz	482	.06	.21	2.13	.43	15.3	0	0.0	30.5	1.22	21.35	231.8	1.22

Food Name	Serving Size	A I.U.	Thi mg	Rib mg	Nia mg	B_6 mg	Fol mcg	B_12 mcg	C mg	Calc mg	Iron mg	Mag mg	Pot mg	Zn mg
ONION														
prepared	1 cup	0	.03	.02	.6	.05	15.2	0	1.2	26.51	.67	2.41	67.48	.61
unprepared	10.5 oz	0	.08	.06	1.46	.12	37.0	0	3.0	65.56	1.64	5.96	166.88	1.49
unprepared	8 oz	0	.07	.05	1.21	.1	30.5	0	2.5	54.12	1.35	4.92	137.76	1.23
ONION, CREAM OF														
prepared	1 cup	295	.05	.08	.5	.02	6.8	.05	1.2	34.16	.63	4.88	119.56	.15
prepared w/whole milk	1 cup	451	.1	.27	.61	.07	12.4	.5	2.5	178.56	.69	22.32	310.0	.62
unprepared	10.75 oz	720	.12	.18	1.22	.06	17.4	.12	3.1	82.35	1.52	15.25	298.9	.37
OYSTER STEW														
prepared	1 cup	70	.02	.04	.23	.01	2.4	2.19	3.1	21.69	.99	4.82	48.2	10.29
prepared w/whole milk	1 cup	225	.07	.23	.34	.06	9.8	2.62	4.4	166.6	1.05	19.6	235.2	10.34
unprepared	10.5 oz	173	.05	.09	.57	.03	6.0	5.33	7.8	53.64	2.38	11.92	119.2	25.03
PEPPER POT														
prepared	1 cup	865	.05	.05	1.22	.06	9.6	.17	1.5	24.1	.89	4.82	151.83	1.22
unprepared	10.5 oz	2104	.13	.12	2.98	.15	23.8	.42	3.3	56.62	2.18	11.92	369.52	2.98
POTATO, CREAM OF														
prepared	1 cup	288	.03	.04	.54	.04	2.9	.05	0.0	19.52	.49	2.44	136.64	.63
prepared w/whole milk	1 cup	444	.08	.24	.64	.09	9.2	.5	1.2	166.16	.55	17.36	322.4	.67
unprepared	10.75 oz	702	.09	.09	1.31	.09	7.3	.12	0.0	48.8	1.16	3.05	332.45	1.52
SCOTCH BROTH														
prepared	1 cup	2179	.02	.05	1.16	.07	9.6	.27	1.0	14.46	.84	4.82	159.06	1.59
unprepared	10.5 oz	5301	.04	.11	2.83	.18	23.8	.66	2.1	35.76	2.03	8.94	387.4	3.87
SHRIMP, CREAM OF														
prepared	1 cup	159	.02	.03	.43	.05	3.7	.59	0.0	17.08	.54	9.76	58.56	.75
prepared w/whole milk	1 cup	312	.06	.23	.53	.45	9.9	1.04	1.2	163.68	.6	22.32	248.0	.8
unprepared	10.75 oz	384	.05	.07	1.04	.09	9.2	1.43	0.0	42.7	1.28	21.35	143.35	1.83
SPLIT PEA														
W/ham														
prepared	1 cup	445	.15	.08	1.47	.07	2.5	.25	1.5	22.77	2.28	48.07	399.74	1.32
unprepared	11.5 oz	1079	.36	.18	3.58	.16	6.2	.65	3.6	52.16	5.54	117.36	968.22	3.21
STOCKPOT														
prepared	1 cup	3979	.04	.05	1.22	.09	9.9	0	2.0	22.23	.86	4.94	237.12	1.16
unprepared	11 oz	9672	.11	.12	2.96	.22	25.0	0	5.0	53.04	2.12	9.36	577.2	2.81
TOMATO														
prepared	1 cup	688	.09	.05	1.42	.11	14.6	0	66.4	12.2	1.76	7.32	263.52	.24
prepared w/whole milk	1 cup	848	.13	.25	1.52	.16	20.8	.45	67.7	158.72	1.81	22.32	448.88	.29
unprepared	10.75 oz	1693	.21	.12	3.45	.27	35.7	0	161.7	33.55	4.27	18.3	640.5	.59
TOMATO BEEF W/NOODLES														
prepared	1 cup	534	.08	.09	1.87	.09	7.3	.2	0.0	17.08	1.12	7.32	219.6	.75
unprepared	10.75 oz	1296	.2	.22	4.54	.21	18.3	.46	0.0	42.7	2.71	18.3	536.8	1.83
TOMATO BISQUE														
prepared w/whole milk	1 cup	879	.11	.27	1.25	.14	21.3	.43	7.0	185.74	.88	25.1	604.91	.63
unprepared	11 oz	1753	.16	.17	2.79	.22	37.4	0	14.4	96.72	2.0	21.84	1014.0	1.43
TOMATO RICE														
prepared	1 cup	756	.06	.05	1.05	.08	13.6	0	14.8	22.23	.79	4.94	330.98	.51
unprepared	11 oz	1835	.15	.12	2.56	.19	34.3	0	35.9	56.16	1.93	12.48	801.84	1.25
TURKEY NOODLE														
prepared	1 cup	293	.07	.06	1.4	.04	2.2	.15	0.2	12.2	.95	4.88	75.64	.58
unprepared	10.75 oz	711	.18	.16	3.39	.09	5.5	.4	0.3	27.45	2.29	12.2	183.0	1.42
TURKEY VEGETABLE														
prepared	1 cup	2444	.03	.04	1.0	.05	4.8	.17	0.0	16.87	.77	4.82	175.93	.61
unprepared	10.5 oz	5948	.07	.1	2.44	.12	11.9	.42	0.0	41.72	1.85	8.94	426.14	1.49
VEGETABLE														
Vegetarian														
prepared	1 cup	3005	.05	.05	.92	.06	10.6	0	1.5	21.69	1.08	7.23	209.67	.46
unprepared	10.5 oz	7310	.13	.11	2.23	.13	25.6	0	3.6	50.66	2.62	17.88	509.58	1.12

Food Name	Serving Size	A I.U.	Thi mg	Rib mg	Nia mg	B₆ mg	Fol mcg	B₁₂ mcg	C mg	Calc mg	Iron mg	Mag mg	Pot mg	Zn mg
W/beef broth														
prepared	1 cup	2089	.05	.05	.97	.06	9.6	0	2.4	16.87	.96	7.23	192.8	.8
unprepared	10.5 oz	5087	.13	.11	2.35	.14	25.3	0	5.7	41.72	2.35	14.9	467.86	1.93
VEGETABLE BEEF														
prepared	1 cup	1891	.04	.05	1.03	.08	10.5	.32	2.4	17.08	1.12	4.88	173.24	1.54
unprepared	10.75 oz	4599	.09	.12	2.51	.18	25.6	.76	5.8	39.65	2.71	15.25	420.9	3.75
SOUP, CANNED, READY-TO-SERVE														
BEEF														
Bouillon	8 oz	0	0	.05	1.87	.02	4.8	.17	0.0	14.4	.41	4.8	129.6	0
Broth (College Inn)	7 oz	na	na	na	na	na	na	na	na	na	na	na	25	na
Hearty (Healthy Choice) 'Hearty Beef'	7.5 oz	na	na	na	na	na	na	na	na	na	na	na	280	na
W/tomato juice	1 oz	39	0	.01	.05	.01	1.3	.02	0.3	3.35	.18	.91	29.28	.01
CHICKEN														
Broth														
(College Inn)	7 oz	na	na	na	na	na	na	na	na	na	na	na	25	na
(College Inn) lower salt	7 oz	na	na	na	na	na	na	na	na	na	na	na	25	na
W/rice (Healthy Choice)	7.5 oz	na	na	na	na	na	na	na	na	na	na	na	140	na
CHICKEN NOODLE														
(Healthy Choice) 'Old Fashioned Chicken Noodle'	7.5 oz	na	na	na	na	na	na	na	na	na	na	na	130	na
CHICKEN RICE, Chunky	8 oz	5858	.02	.1	4.1	.05	3.8	.31	3.8	33.6	1.87	9.6	108.0	.96
CRAB	8 oz	505	.2	.07	1.34	.12	14.6	.2	0.0	65.88	1.22	14.64	326.96	1.46
GAZPACHO	8 oz	200	.05	.02	.93	.15	9.8	0	3.2	24.4	.98	7.32	224.48	.24
MINESTRONE														
(Health Valley) 'Real Italian Fat-Free'	7.5 oz	na	na	na	na	na	na	na	na	na	na	na	470	na
TURKEY	8 oz	7156	.04	.11	3.59	.31	11.1	2.12	6.4	49.56	1.91	23.6	361.08	2.12
VEGETABLE BEEF														
(Healthy Choice) 'Vegetable Beef'	7.5 oz	na	na	na	na	na	na	na	na	na	na	na	360	na
SOUP MIX														
(NOTE: Unless otherwise specified, PREPARED = prepared as directed w/water.)														
ASPARAGUS, prepared	8 oz	240	.03	.04	.43	.01	6.5	.03	0.7	19.45	.54	2.56	117.01	.6
ASPARAGUS, CREAM OF, prepared	8 oz	271	.05	.05	.5	.01	7.5	.03	0.8	22.57	.5	2.51	132.92	.68
BEAN W/BACON, prepared	1 cup	53	.05	.26	.4	.03	8.0	.03	1.1	55.63	1.32	29.14	325.83	.69
BEEF														
Broth														
cubed	1 cube	2	.01	.01	.12	.01	1.2	.04	0.0	2.16	.08	1.8	14.51	.01
cubed, prepared	6 oz	2	.01	.01	.12	0	1.8	0	0.0	1.81	.09	1.81	14.48	.01
powder, prepared	8 oz	5	0	.02	.36	0	0.0	0	0.0	9.76	.02	7.32	36.6	.07
BEEF NOODLE, prepared	8 oz	8	.12	.06	.69	.04	1.5	0	0.5	5.02	.33	10.04	80.32	.1
BOUILLON														
Beef flavor														
powder	1 pkt	3	0	.01	.27	.01	1.9	.06	0.0	3.6	.06	3.06	26.76	0
powder, prepared	8 oz	4	.01	.02	.36	.02	2.6	.08	0.0	4.8	.08	4.08	35.68	0
CAULIFLOWER, prepared	8 oz	5	.08	.08	.51	.03	2.6	.18	2.6	10.24	.51	2.56	105.0	.26
CELERY, prepared	8 oz	269	.03	.05	.3	0	2.0	.05	0.3	35.56	.51	5.08	109.22	.13
CHICKEN														
prepared	8 oz	407	.1	.2	2.61	.05	5.2	.26	0.5	75.72	.26	5.22	214.1	1.57
Broth														
cubed	1 cube	12	.01	.02	.19	0	1.5	.01	0.1	9.12	.09	2.69	17.95	.01
cubed, prepared	6 oz	13	.01	.02	.19	0	1.8	.02	0.0	9.1	.09	1.82	18.2	.01
CHICKEN NOODLE, prepared	1 cup	63	.07	.06	.88	.01	1.5	0	0.3	32.8	.5	7.57	30.28	.2
CHICKEN RICE, prepared	8 oz	0	0	0	.36	.03	0.5	.08	0.0	7.58	0	0	10.11	.13
CHICKEN VEGETABLE, prepared	8 oz	15	.07	.05	.69	.09	2.5	.1	1.3	15.04	.58	22.56	67.69	.21
CONSOMMÉ, w/gelatin, prepared	1 cup	7	0	.02	.57	.02	4.0	.12	0.0	7.47	.12	7.47	57.27	0
OXTAIL, prepared	8 oz	10	.03	.03	.76	.03	5.1	.25	0.0	10.12	.25	10.12	83.52	0
TOMATO VEGETABLE, prepared	8 oz	190	.06	.05	.79	.05	10.1	0	6.1	7.59	.63	20.24	103.73	.17

Food Name	Serving Size	A I.U.	Thi mg	Rib mg	Nia mg	B₆ mg	Fol mcg	B₁₂ mcg	C mg	Calc mg	Iron mg	Mag mg	Pot mg	Zn mg
VEGETABLE BEEF, prepared	8 oz	238	.03	.04	.46	.05	7.6	.25	1.3	12.66	.86	22.78	75.93	.27
SOUR CREAM														
....	1 cup	1817	.08	.34	.15	.04	24.8	.69	2.0	267.72	.14	25.83	331.2	.62
....	1 tbsp	95	0	.02	.01	0	1.3	.04	0.1	13.97	.01	1.35	17.28	.03
(Knudsen) 'Hampshire'	1 oz	na	na	na	na	na	na	na	na	na	na	na	40	na
HALF AND HALF														
(Breakstone's) 'Light Choice'	1 tbsp	na	na	na	na	na	na	na	na	na	na	na	30	na
Cultured	1 tbsp	68	.01	.02	.01	0	1.6	.05	0.1	15.66	.01	1.52	19.33	.08
LIGHT / LOW-FAT														
(Knudsen)	1 oz	na	na	na	na	na	na	na	na	na	na	na	60	na
(Land O'Lakes) 'Light'	2 tbsp	na	na	na	na	na	na	na	na	na	na	na	80	na
SOUR CREAM, ALTERNATIVE, NONDAIRY														
Cultured														
....	1 cup	0	0	0	0	0	0.0	0	0.0	5.75	.9	14.67	369.15	2.71
....	1 oz	0	0	0	0	0	0.0	0	0.0	.7	.11	1.79	44.94	.33
SOY BEVERAGE														
(Edensoy) 'Extra' original	8.45 oz	na	na	na	na	na	na	na	na	na	na	na	450	na
(Edensoy) original	8.45 oz	na	na	na	na	na	na	na	na	na	na	na	450	na
VANILLA FLAVOR														
(Edensoy) 'Extra'	8.45 oz	na	na	na	na	na	na	na	na	na	na	na	280	na
SOY FLOUR														
defatted, stirred	1/2 cup	20	.35	.13	1.31	.29	152.7	0	0.0	120.5	4.62	145.0	1192.0	1.23
full-fat, roasted, stirred	1/2 cup	46	.17	.4	1.38	.15	95.5	0	0.0	78.96	2.44	154.98	857.22	1.5
full-fat, stirred	1/2 cup	50	.24	.49	1.81	.19	144.9	0	0.0	86.52	2.68	180.18	1056.3	1.65
low-fat, stirred	1/2 cup	18	.17	.13	.95	.23	180.4	0	0.0	82.72	2.64	100.76	1130.8	.52
SOY MEAL, defatted, raw	1/2 cup	24	.42	.15	1.58	.35	184.6	0	0.0	148.84	8.36	186.66	1518.9	3.09
SOY MILK. See SOY BEVERAGE.														
SOY PROTEIN CONCENTRATE														
acid wash extracted	1 oz	0	.09	.04	.2	.04	95.2	0	0.0	101.64	3.02	39.2	126.0	1.23
alcohol extracted	1 oz	0	.09	.04	.2	.04	95.2	0	0.0	101.64	3.02	88.2	616.56	1.23
SOY PROTEIN ISOLATE														
....	1 oz	0	.05	.03	.4	.03	49.3	0	0.0	49.84	4.06	10.92	22.68	1.13
potassium type	1 oz	0	.05	.03	.4	.03	49.3	0	0.0	49.84	4.06	10.92	445.2	1.13
SOYBEAN														
Green														
boiled, drained	1/2 cup	140	.23	.14	1.13	.05	99.9	0	15.3	130.5	2.25	54.0	485.1	.82
raw	1/2 cup	230	.56	.22	2.11	.08	211.2	0	37.1	252.16	4.54	83.2	793.6	1.27
Kernels, roasted/toasted														
whole	1 cup	216	.11	.16	1.9	.32	243.5	0	2.4	149.04	4.81	186.84	1587.6	3.91
whole	1 oz	57	.03	.04	.5	.08	64.0	0	0.6	39.19	1.26	49.13	417.48	1.03
Mature														
boiled	1/2 cup	8	.13	.25	.34	.2	46.3	0	1.5	87.72	4.42	73.96	442.9	.99
dry-roasted	1/2 cup	20	.37	.65	.91	.19	176.0	0	4.0	232.2	3.4	196.08	1173.04	4.1
raw	1/2 cup	22	.81	.81	1.51	.35	348.8	0	5.6	257.61	14.6	260.4	1671.21	4.55
roasted	1/2 cup	172	.09	.12	1.21	.18	181.5	0	1.9	118.68	3.35	124.7	1264.2	2.7
Mature, sprouted														
boiled, drained	1 cup	100	.2	.19	.88	na	na	na	5.0	53.75	.88	na	195.0	na
raw	1/2 cup	4	.12	.04	.4	.06	60.2	0	5.4	23.45	.73	25.2	169.4	.41
steamed	1/2 cup	5	.1	.02	.51	.05	37.6	0	3.9	27.73	.62	28.2	166.85	.49
stir-fried	3.5 oz	17	.42	.19	1.1	.17	127.0	0	12.0	82.0	.4	96.0	567.0	2.1
SOYBEAN, FERMENTED. See also MISO.														
natto	1/2 cup	0	.14	.17	0	.11	7.0	0	11.4	190.96	7.57	101.2	641.52	2.67
SOYBEAN CURD CAKE. See TOFU.														
SOYBEAN OIL														
....	1 cup	0	0	0	0	0	0.0	0	0.0	.09	.04	.07	0	0
hydrogenated	1 cup	0	0	0	0	0	0.0	0	0.0	0	0	0	0	0

Food Name	Serving Size	A I.U.	Thi mg	Rib mg	Nia mg	B_6 mg	Fol mcg	B_{12} mcg	C mg	Calc mg	Iron mg	Mag mg	Pot mg	Zn mg
hydrogenated	1 tbsp	0	0	0	0	0	0.0	0	0.0	0	0	0	0	0
SPAGHETTI. See PASTA.														
SPAGHETTI ENTRÉE, CANNED														
W/frankfurters *(Van Camp's)*														
'Spaghettee Weenee'	1 cup	644	.11	.2	2.17	na	na	na	na	44	6.31	na	253	na
SPAGHETTI ENTRÉE, FROZEN														
Parmesan, w/Italian-style green beans														
(Stouffer's)	10.25 oz	na	na	na	na	na	na	na	na	na	na	na	650	na
W/meat sauce *(Stouffer's)*	12 7/8 oz	na	na	na	na	na	na	na	na	na	na	na	800	na
W/meatballs														
(Stouffer's) 19.5-oz pkg	1/2 pkg	na	na	na	na	na	na	na	na	na	na	na	550	na
(Stouffer's) 12 5/8-oz pkg	1 pkg	na	na	na	na	na	na	na	na	na	na	na	690	na
SPAGHETTI ENTRÉE, MICROWAVE														
Rings *(Kid's Kitchen)* microwave cup	7.5 oz	na	na	na	na	na	na	na	na	na	na	na	343	na
W/meatballs *(Kid's Kitchen)* microwave cup ...	7.5 oz	na	na	na	na	na	na	na	na	na	na	na	475	na
SPAGHETTI ENTRÉE, PACKAGED														
W/meat sauce *(Top Shelf)*	10 oz	na	na	na	na	na	na	na	na	na	na	na	879	na
SPAGHETTI SQUASH. See SQUASH, SPAGHETTI.														
SPAM. See LUNCHEON MEAT, CANNED.														
SPINACH														
boiled, drained	1/2 cup	7371	.09	.21	.44	.22	131.2	0	8.8	122.4	3.21	78.3	419.4	.68
raw	10-oz pkg	19071	.22	.54	2.06	.55	552.1	0	79.8	281.16	7.7	224.36	1584.72	1.51
raw *(Dole)*	3 oz	4751	na	na	na	na	na	na	21.0	na	na	na	379	na
raw, chopped	1/2 cup	1880	.02	.05	.2	.05	54.4	0	7.9	27.72	.76	22.12	156.24	.15
SPINACH, CANNED														
drained solids	1/2 cup	9390	.02	.15	.42	.11	104.7	0	15.3	135.89	2.46	81.32	370.22	.49
(Freshlike) cut	1/2 cup	na	na	na	na	na	na	na	na	na	na	na	330	na
(Freshlike) cut, water-packed, w/o salt	1/2 cup	na	na	na	na	na	na	na	na	na	na	na	330	na
(Freshlike) cut, water packed, w/o sugar														
or salt	1/2 cup	na	na	na	na	na	na	na	na	na	na	na	330	na
SPINACH, FROZEN														
Chopped														
boiled, drained	10-oz pkg	17125	.13	.37	.92	.32	236.5	0	27.1	321.2	3.34	151.8	655.6	1.54
boiled, drained	1/2 cup	7395	.06	.16	.4	.14	102.1	0	11.7	138.7	1.44	65.55	283.1	.67
unprepared	10-oz pkg	22033	.24	.43	1.24	.4	339.7	0	69.0	315.24	5.82	164.72	917.32	1.25
unprepared	1 cup	12102	.13	.24	.68	.22	186.6	0	37.9	173.16	3.2	90.48	503.88	.69
(Birds Eye)	3.3 oz	na	na	na	na	na	na	na	na	na	na	na	290	na
Leaf														
boiled, drained	10-oz pkg	17125	.13	.37	.92	.32	236.5	0	27.1	321.2	3.34	151.8	655.6	1.54
unprepared	10-oz pkg	22033	.24	.43	1.24	.4	339.7	0	69.0	315.24	5.82	164.72	917.32	1.25
unprepared	1 cup	12102	.13	.24	.68	.22	186.6	0	37.9	173.16	3.2	90.48	503.88	.69
(Birds Eye) whole leaf	3.3 oz	na	na	na	na	na	na	na	na	na	na	na	300	na
SPINACH, NEW ZEALAND														
boiled, drained, chopped	1/2 cup	3260	.03	.1	.35	.21	7.5	0	14.4	43.2	.59	28.8	91.8	.28
raw, chopped	1/2 cup	1232	.01	.04	.14	.09	4.1	0	8.4	16.24	.22	10.92	36.4	.11
SPINACH ENTRÉE, FROZEN														
creamed *(Stouffer's)*	4.5 oz	na	na	na	na	na	na	na	na	na	na	na	400	na
soufflé *(Stouffer's)*	6 oz	na	na	na	na	na	na	na	na	na	na	na	345	na
SPIRULINA														
dried	100 gm	570	2.38	3.67	12.82	.36	94.0	0	10.1	120.0	28.5	195.0	1363.0	2.0
raw	100 gm	56	.22	.34	1.2	.03	9.2	0	0.9	12.0	2.79	19.0	127.0	.2
SPLIT PEAS														
boiled, mature seeds	1/2 cup	7	.19	.05	.87	.05	63.6	0	0.4	13.72	1.26	35.28	354.76	.98
raw, mature seeds	1/2 cup	146	.71	.21	2.83	.17	268.3	0	1.8	53.9	4.34	112.7	961.38	2.95
SPONGE GOURD. See GOURD, DISHCLOTH.														

Food Name	Serving Size	A III	Thi mg	Rib mg	Nia mg	B₆ mg	Fol mcg	B₁₂ mcg	C mg	Calc mg	Iron mg	Mag mg	Pot mg	Zn mg
SPORTS DRINK														
CHOCOLATE														
(Weider) 'Dynamic Muscle Builder'	11 oz	na	na	na	na	na	na	na	na	na	na	na	460	na
(Weider) 'Dynamic Weight Gainer'	11 oz	na	na	na	na	na	na	na	na	na	na	na	640	na
(Weider) high-energy 'Protein Blast'	11.5 oz	na	na	na	na	na	na	na	na	na	na	na	640	na
(Weider) 'Sports Line Power Shake' Dutch chocolate	11 oz	na	na	na	na	na	na	na	na	na	na	na	470	na
ORANGE														
(All Sport) caffeine-free	8 oz	na	na	na	na	na	na	na	na	na	na	na	55	na
(PowerAde)	8 oz	na	na	na	na	na	na	na	na	na	na	na	30	na
(10-K)	8 oz	na	na	na	na	na	na	na	5	0	na	30	na
SPORTS DRINK MIX														
(Tiger's Milk)														
'Protein Booster' Dutch chocolate, dry	3 heap tbsp	na	na	na	na	na	na	na	na	na	na	na	340	na
(Weider)														
'Big' chocolate malt, sugar-free, dry	4 scoops	na	na	na	na	na	na	na	na	na	na	na	860	na
'Carbo Energizer' orange, dry	4 scoops	1750	.53	.6	7	.7	140.0	2.1	60.0	52	9	42	na	5.3
'Dynamic Body Shaper' Dutch chocolate, dry	2 scoops	na	na	na	na	na	na	na	na	na	na	na	100	na
'Dynamic Muscle Builder' natural chocolate, dry	2 scoops	na	na	na	na	na	na	na	na	na	na	na	100	na
'Dynamic Weight Gainer' peanut butter, dry	4 scoops	na	na	na	na	na	na	na	na	na	na	na	850	na
'90 Plus' vanilla, sugar-free, dry	2 scoops	500	na	.17	2	.2	40.0	.6	6.0	350	0	20	30	0
'N2itro-Fire' protein blend, dry	2 tbsp	1750	450	765	5	.5	100.0	1.8	18.0	550	3.6	100	340	3.75
'Victory Explosive Workout' citrus, dry	4 tbsp	na	1.5	2.0	25	5	50.0	6	100.0	100	na	40	110	1.5
SPOT, dry-heat cooked	3 oz	98	.16	.23	7.25	.39	5.1	2.94	0.0	15.3	.35	45.9	540.6	.55
SPREADS. See CHEESE SPREAD; and individual listings.														
SPRING ONION. See ONION, GREEN.														
SPRINKLES														
milk chocolate *(Snack Pack)*	3.88 oz	na	na	na	na	na	na	na	1.2	6.53	6.8	na	na	na
vanilla chocolate *(Snack Pack)*	3.88 oz	na	na	na	na	na	na	na	1.1	4.98	.43	na	na	na
SQUAB / pigeon														
Raw														
giblets	100 gm	4530	.16	1.36	4.9	na	na	na	0.0	14.0	4.5	na	172.0	na
light meat w/o skin	1 lb	86	.36	.37	11.06	.8	6.0	.71	7.7	15.1	3.49	42.28	392.6	4.08
SQUASH SEED. See PUMPKIN SEED.														
SQUASH, ACORN / table queen squash														
boiled, mashed	1/2 cup	315	.12	.01	.65	.14	13.8	0	7.9	31.72	.68	31.72	320.86	.13
raw, approx 4 inch diam	1 squash	1465	.6	.04	3.02	.66	72.0	0	47.4	142.23	3.02	137.92	1495.57	.56
SQUASH, BUTTERNUT														
baked, cubes	1/2 cup	7141	.07	.02	.99	.13	19.6	0	15.4	41.82	.61	29.58	289.68	.13
boiled, mashed	1/2 cup	4007	.06	.05	.56	.08	19.7	0	4.2	22.8	.7	10.8	159.6	.14
raw, cubes	1/2 cup	5460	.07	.01	.84	.11	18.7	0	14.7	33.6	.49	23.8	246.4	.11
SQUASH, CROOKNECK														
boiled, drained, slices	1/2 cup	258	.04	.04	.46	.08	18.1	0	5.0	24.3	.32	21.6	172.8	.35
raw, slices	1/2 cup	220	.03	.03	.3	.07	14.9	0	5.5	13.65	.31	13.65	137.8	.19
SQUASH, HUBBARD														
baked, cubes	1/2 cup	6156	.08	.05	.57	.18	16.5	na	9.7	17.34	.48	22.44	365.16	.15
boiled, mashed	1/2 cup	4726	.05	.03	.39	.12	11.5	0	7.7	11.8	.33	15.34	252.52	.12
raw, cubes	1/2 cup	3132	.04	.02	.29	.09	9.5	0	6.4	8.12	.23	11.02	185.6	.08
SQUASH, SCALLOP / cymling / pattypan squash														
boiled, drained, mashed	1/2 cup	102	.06	.03	.56	.1	24.8	0	13.0	18.0	.4	22.8	168.0	.29
boiled, drained, slices	1/2 cup	77	.05	.02	.42	.08	18.6	0	9.7	13.5	.3	17.1	126.0	.22
raw, slices	1/2 cup	72	.05	.02	.39	.07	19.6	0	11.7	12.35	.26	14.95	118.3	.19
SQUASH, SPAGHETTI														
baked or boiled, drained	1/2 cup	86	.03	.02	.63	.08	6.2	0	2.7	16.38	.27	8.58	91.26	.16
raw, cubes	1/2 cup	25	.02	.01	.48	.05	6.0	0	1.1	11.5	.15	6.0	54.0	.1
SQUASH, STRAIGHTNECK, raw, slices	1/2 cup	220	.03	.03	.3	.07	14.9	0	5.5	13.65	.31	13.65	137.8	.19

Food Name	Serving Size	A I.U.	Thi mg	Rib mg	Nia mg	B$_6$ mg	Fol mcg	B$_{12}$ mcg	C mg	Calc mg	Iron mg	Mag mg	Pot mg	Zn mg
SQUASH, SUMMER, all varieties														
boiled, drained, slices	1/2 cup	258	.04	.04	.46	.06	18.1	0	5.0	24.3	.32	21.6	172.8	.35
raw, slices	1/2 cup	127	.04	.02	.36	.07	16.6	0	9.6	13.0	.3	14.95	126.75	.17
SQUASH, WINTER, all varieties														
baked, cubes	1/2 cup	3628	.09	.02	.72	.07	28.6	0	9.8	14.28	.34	8.16	445.74	.27
frozen, cooked (Birds Eye)	4 oz	na	na	na	na	na	na	na	na	na	na	na	260	na
raw, cubes	1/2 cup	2355	.06	.02	.46	.05	12.6	0	7.1	17.98	.34	12.18	203.0	.08
SQUID, MIXED SPECIES / calamari														
fried	3 oz	30	.05	.39	2.21	.05	4.5	1.04	3.6	33.15	.86	32.3	237.15	1.48
raw	3 oz	28	.02	.35	1.85	.05	4.2	1.1	4.0	27.2	.58	28.05	209.1	1.3
SQUIRREL, raw	1 oz	0	.02	.06	1.12	na	na	na	0.0	.56	1.32	6.72	85.12	na
STAR FRUIT / carambola														
cubed	1 cup	675	.04	.04	.56	na	na	0	29.0	5.48	.36	na	223.31	.15
STIR-FRY SEASONING (Gilroy)	1 tsp	na	na	na	na	na	na	na	na	na	na	na	24	na
STRAIGHTNECK SQUASH. See SQUASH, STRAIGHTNECK.														
STRAWBERRY														
trimmed	1 pint	86	.06	.21	.74	.19	56.6	0	181.4	44.8	1.22	32.0	531.2	.42
trimmed	1 cup	40	.03	.1	.34	.09	26.4	0	84.5	20.86	.57	14.9	247.34	.19
Frozen														
in lite syrup, halves 'Quick Thaw Pouch'														
(Birds Eye)	5 oz	na	na	na	na	na	na	na	na	na	na	na	190	na
in lite syrup, whole (Birds Eye)	4 oz	na	na	na	na	na	na	na	na	na	na	na	140	na
sweetened, sliced	10-oz pkg	68	.05	.14	1.14	.09	42.3	0	117.6	31.24	1.68	19.88	278.32	.17
sweetened, sliced	1 cup	61	.04	.13	1.02	.08	38.0	0	105.6	28.05	1.5	17.85	249.9	.15
sweetened, whole	10-oz pkg	77	.04	.22	.83	.08	10.8	0	112.2	31.24	1.33	17.04	278.32	.14
sweetened, whole	1 cup	69	.04	.2	.75	.07	9.7	0	100.7	28.05	1.2	15.3	249.9	.13
unsweetened	20-oz pkg	255	.12	.21	2.62	.16	95.3	0	233.6	90.72	4.25	62.37	839.16	.74
unsweetened	1 cup	67	.03	.06	.69	.04	25.0	0	61.4	23.84	1.12	16.39	220.52	.19
STRAWBERRY-BANANA NECTAR (Kern's)	6 oz	na	na	na	na	na	na	na	na	na	na	na	110	na
STRAWBERRY COLADA. See ALCOHOLIC BEVERAGES.														
STRAWBERRY DAIQUIRI. See ALCOHOLIC BEVERAGES.														
STRAWBERRY FLAVOR DRINK (10-K)	8 oz	na	na	na	na	na	na	na	na	5	0	na	30	na
STRAWBERRY JUICE DRINK														
(Tang) 'Fruit Box'	8.45 oz	na	na	na	na	na	na	na	na	na	na	na	30	na
STRAWBERRY NECTAR (Libby's)	6 oz	na	na	na	na	na	na	na	na	na	na	na	60	na
STRAWBERRY PUNCH MIX														
(Kool-Aid) sugar-sweetened, prepared	8 oz	na	na	na	na	na	na	na	na	na	na	na	0	na
(Kool-Aid) unsweetened, prepared w/sugar	8 oz	na	na	na	na	na	na	na	na	na	na	na	0	na
(Kool-Aid) unsweetened, prepared w/o sugar	8 oz	na	na	na	na	na	na	na	na	na	na	na	0	na
STRING BEAN. See GREEN BEAN.														
STUFFED PEPPER														
(Stouffer's) single serving	10 oz	na	na	na	na	na	na	na	na	na	na	na	400	na
(Stouffer's) green, w/beef in tomato sauce, frozen	7.75 oz	na	na	na	na	na	na	na	na	na	na	na	380	na
STURGEON, MIXED SPECIES														
dry-heat cooked	3 oz	687	.07	.08	8.59	.2	14.7	2.13	0.0	14.45	.77	38.25	309.4	.46
raw	3 oz	595	.06	.06	7.06	.17	12.8	1.87	0.0	11.05	.6	29.75	241.4	.36
SUCCOTASH														
boiled, drained	1/2 cup	282	.16	.09	1.27	.11	31.5	0	7.9	16.32	1.46	50.88	393.6	.6
Frozen														
boiled, drained	1/2 cup	196	.06	.06	1.11	.08	28.2	0	5.0	12.75	.76	19.55	225.25	.38
unprepared	1/2 cup	200	.07	.06	1.07	.08	32.5	0	6.6	12.48	.73	18.72	230.1	.37
SUCKER, dry-heat cooked	3 oz	167	.01	.07	1.24	.2	14.5	1.96	0.0	76.5	1.42	32.3	413.95	.82
SUGAR, ALTERNATIVE (Sweet One)	1 pkt	na	na	na	na	na	na	na	na	na	na	na	11	na
SUGAR, BEET OR CANE. See also SUGAR, ALTERNATIVE; SUGAR, DEXTROSE; SUGAR, MAPLE.														
BROWN														
packed	1 cup	0	.02	.02	.18	.06	2.2	0	0.0	187.0	4.2	63.8	761.2	.4

Food Name	Serving Size	A I.U.	Thi mg	Rib mg	Nia mg	B₆ mg	Fol mcg	B₁₂ mcg	C mg	Calc mg	Iron mg	Mag mg	Pot mg	Zn mg
unpacked	1 cup	0	.01	.01	.12	.04	1.5	0	0.0	123.25	2.77	42.05	501.7	.26
GRANULATED														
	1 cup	0	0	.04	0	0	0.0	0	0.0	2.0	.12	0	4.0	.06
	1 tsp	0	0	0	0	0	0.0	0	0.0	.04	0	0	.08	0
SUGAR, DEXTROSE														
anhydrous	100 gm	0	0	0	0	na	na	na	0.0	0	0	na	0	na
crystallized	100 gm	0	0	0	0	na	na	na	0.0	0	0	na	0	na
SUGAR, MAPLE														
	100 gm	24	.01	.01	.04	0	0.0	0	0.0	90.0	1.61	19.0	274.0	6.06
	1-oz piece	7	0	0	.01	0	0.0	0	0.0	25.51	.46	5.39	77.68	1.72
SUGAR APPLE / sweetsop														
raw, approx 2 7/8 inch diam	1 med	9	.17	.18	1.37	.31	na	0	56.3	37.2	.93	32.55	382.85	na
raw, pulp	1 cup	15	.28	.28	2.21	.5	na	0	90.8	60.0	1.5	52.5	617.5	na
SUNFISH / calico bass / crappie / pumpkinseed														
dry-heat cooked	3 oz	49	.08	.07	1.24	.12	14.5	1.96	0.9	87.55	1.31	32.3	381.65	1.69
raw	3 oz	43	.07	.06	1.02	.1	12.8	1.7	0.9	68.0	1.02	25.5	297.5	1.32
SUNFLOWER BUTTER														
roasted (Maranatha Natural)	2 tbsp	na	na	na	na	na	na	na	na	na	na	na	180	na
SUNFLOWER OIL														
(Kroger)	1 tbsp	na	na	na	na	na	na	na	0.0	0	0	na	na	na
(Wesson)	1 tbsp	na	na	na	na	na	na	na	0.0	0	0	na	na	na
SUNFLOWER SEED FLOUR														
partially defatted	1 cup	39	2.55	.21	5.85	.6	177.8	0	1.0	91.2	5.3	276.8	53.6	3.96
partially defatted	1 tbsp	2	.16	.01	.37	.04	11.1	0	0.1	5.7	.33	17.3	3.35	.25
SURIMI	3 oz	56	.02	.02	.19	.03	1.4	1.36	0.0	7.65	.22	36.55	95.2	.28
SURINAM CHERRY. See PITANGA.														
SWAMP CABBAGE. See CABBAGE, SKUNK.														
SWEDISH MEATBALL DINNER/ENTRÉE														
frozen dinner, 'Classics' (Armour)	11.25 oz	na	na	na	na	na	na	na	na	na	na	na	460	na
frozen entrée, w/parsley noodles, gravy 'Lean Cuisine' (Stouffer's)	9.25 oz	na	na	na	na	na	na	na	na	na	na	na	350	na
SWEET POTATO. See also YAM.														
baked in skin, pulp only, mashed	1/2 cup	21822	.07	.13	.6	.24	22.6	0	24.6	28.0	.45	20.0	348.0	.29
boiled, w/o skin, mashed	1/2 cup	27969	.09	.23	1.05	.4	18.2	0	28.0	34.44	.92	16.4	301.76	.44
dehydrated flakes, dry	1 cup	56400	.07	.16	1.56	na	na	na	54.0	72.0	2.64	na	674.4	na
dehydrated flakes, prepared w/water	1 lb	54480	.09	.14	1.36	na	na	na	49.9	68.1	2.72	na	635.6	na
dehydrated flakes, prepared w/water	1 cup	30600	.05	.08	.77	na	na	na	28.1	38.25	1.53	na	357.0	na
raw, cubes	1 cup	26684	.09	.2	.9	.34	18.4	0	30.2	29.26	.78	13.3	271.32	.37
raw, 5 inches long, 2 inches diam	1 potato	26082	.09	.19	.88	.33	17.9	0	29.5	28.6	.77	13.0	265.2	.36
SWEET POTATO, FROZEN														
unprepared, cubes	1/2 cup	16400	.06	.04	.53	.16	18.7	0	11.7	32.56	.47	19.36	321.2	.27
SWEET POTATO LEAF														
raw, approx 12 1/4 inches long	1 leaf	164	.02	.06	.18	.03	12.8	0	1.8	5.92	.16	9.76	82.88	.05
raw, chopped	1 cup	360	.05	.12	.4	.07	28.0	0	3.9	12.95	.35	21.35	181.3	.1
SWEETBREAD. See BEEF, PANCREAS; BEEF, THYMUS; LAMB, PANCREAS; VEAL, PANCREAS; VEAL, THYMUS.														
SWEETENERS. See SUGAR, ALTERNATIVE; SUGAR, BEET OR CANE; SUGAR, MAPLE.														
SWEETSOP. See SUGAR APPLE.														
SWISS CHARD / chard														
boiled, drained, chopped	1/2 cup	2762	.03	.08	.32	.07	7.6	0	15.8	51.04	1.99	75.68	483.12	.29
raw, chopped	1/2 cup	594	.01	.02	.07	.02	2.5	0	5.4	9.18	.32	14.58	68.22	.06
SWORDFISH														
dry-heat cooked	3 oz	116	.04	.1	10.02	.32	2.0	1.72	0.9	5.1	.88	28.9	313.65	1.25
raw	3 oz	101	.03	.08	8.23	.28	1.7	1.49	0.9	3.4	.69	22.95	244.8	.98

T

Food Name	Serving Size	A I.U.	Thi mg	Rib mg	Nia mg	B₆ mg	Fol mcg	B₁₂ mcg	C mg	Calc mg	Iron mg	Mag mg	Pot mg	Zn mg
TABLE QUEEN SQUASH. See SQUASH, ACORN.														
TAHINI MIX														
(Maranatha Natural) 'Sesame Tahini'	2 tbsp	na	na	na	na	na	na	na	na	na	na	na	180	na
TAMALE														
Canned														
(Derby) beef	6.561 oz	na	na	na	na	na	na	na	11.0	2.95	3.62	na	na	na
(Gebhardt)	5.75 oz	na	na	na	na	na	na	na	3.4	2.65	4.43	na	na	na
(Gebhardt) jumbo	6.949 oz	na	na	na	na	na	na	na	3.5	3.55	4.04	na	na	na
(Van Camp's) w/sauce	1 cup	1906	.05	.16	2.08	na	na	na	na	36	2.71	na	236	na
(Wolf Brand)	7.75 oz	2150	.08	.49	1.94	.26	23.0	0	na	68	2.19	43	279	2
TAMARIND / Indian date														
pulp	1 cup	36	.51	.18	2.33	.08	na	0	4.2	88.8	3.36	110.4	753.6	na
TANGELO JUICE, fresh	100 gm	420	.06	.02	.1	na	na	na	27.0	18.0	.2	na	178.0	na
TANGERINE JUICE														
canned, sweetened	1 cup	1046	.15	.05	.25	.08	11.5	0	54.8	44.82	.5	19.92	443.22	.07
canned, sweetened	1 oz	131	.02	.01	.03	.01	1.4	0	6.8	5.6	.06	2.49	55.36	.01
fresh	1 cup	1037	.15	.05	.25	.1	11.4	0	76.6	44.46	.49	19.76	439.66	.07
fresh	1 oz	130	.02	.01	.03	.01	1.4	0	9.6	5.56	.06	2.47	55.0	.01
frozen concentrate, sweetened, diluted w/3 vol water	1 cup	1381	.13	.05	.22	.1	11.1	0	58.3	19.28	.24	19.28	272.33	.07
frozen concentrate, sweetened, diluted w/3 vol water	1 oz	172	.02	.01	.03	.01	1.4	0	7.3	2.41	.03	2.41	34.01	.01
frozen concentrate, sweetened, undiluted	6 oz	4310	.39	.14	.7	.31	34.7	0	182.1	57.78	.73	59.92	849.58	.19
frozen or chilled (Minute Maid)	6 oz	na	na	na	na	na	na	na	48.0	na	na	na	260	na
TAPIOCA, PEARL, dry	1 cup	0	.01	0	0	.01	6.1	0	0.0	30.4	2.4	1.52	16.72	.18
TARO														
cooked, slices	1/2 cup	0	.07	.02	.34	.22	12.7	0	3.3	11.88	.48	19.8	319.44	.18
raw, slices	1/2 cup	0	.05	.01	.31	.15	11.5	0	2.3	22.36	.29	17.16	307.32	.12
TARO, TAHITIAN, raw, slices	1/2 cup	1268	.04	.15	.62	.07	5.6	0	59.5	79.98	.81	29.14	375.72	.06
TARO LEAF														
raw	1 cup	1351	.06	.13	.42	.04	35.2	0	14.6	29.96	.63	12.6	181.44	.11
raw, 11 x 6 1/2 inches	1 leaf	483	.02	.05	.15	.01	12.6	0	5.2	10.7	.23	4.5	64.8	.04
steamed	1/2 cup	3136	.1	.28	.94	.05	35.7	0	26.3	63.64	.87	14.8	340.4	.16
TARO SHOOTS														
cooked, slices	1/2 cup	36	.03	.04	.57	.08	1.8	0	13.2	9.8	.29	5.6	240.8	.38
raw, 15 x 5 inches	1 shoot	42	.03	.04	.66	.09	2.7	0	17.4	9.96	.5	6.64	275.56	.42
raw, slices	1/2 cup	22	.02	.02	.34	.05	1.4	0	9.0	5.16	.26	3.44	142.76	.22
TARRAGON														
ground	1 tbsp	202	.01	.06	.43	na	na	0	na	54.68	1.55	16.64	144.94	.19
ground	1 tsp	67	0	.02	.14	na	na	0	na	18.23	.52	5.55	48.31	.06
ground (Durkee)	1 tsp	3.06	.18	.98	.01	na	na	na	na	0	.03	na	0	na
ground (Laurel Leaf)	1 tsp	3.06	.18	.98	.01	na	na	na	na	0	.03	na	0	na
TEA														
Brewed														
prepared w/distilled water	6 oz	0	0	.02	0	0	9.3	0	0.0	0	.02	1.78	37.38	.02
prepared w/tap water	6 oz	0	0	.02	0	0	9.3	0	0.0	0	.04	5.34	65.86	.04
(Nestea)	6 oz	na	na	na	na	na	na	na	na	na	na	na	60	na
TEA, ICED														
PREPARED FROM MIX														
(Crystal Light)														
w/NutraSweet	8 oz	na	na	na	na	na	na	na	na	na	na	na	15	na
w/Nutrasweet, decaffeinated	8 oz	na	na	na	na	na	na	na	na	na	na	na	15	na

Food Name	Serving Size	A IU	Thi mg	Rib mg	Nia mg	B$_6$ mg	Fol mcg	B$_{12}$ mcg	C mg	Calc mg	Iron mg	Mag mg	Pot mg	Zn mg
(Nestea)														
lemon flavor, sugar-free	8 oz	na	na	na	na	na	na	na	na	na	na	na	30	na
sugar free	8 oz	na	na	na	na	na	na	na	na	na	na	na	40	na
w/sugar and lemon	8 oz	na	na	na	na	na	na	na	na	na	na	na	40	na
TEASEED OIL														
	1 cup	0	0	0	0	0	0.0	0	0.0	0	0	0	0	0
	1 tbsp	0	0	0	0	0	0.0	0	0.0	0	0	0	0	0
TEQUILA SUNRISE. See ALCOHOLIC BEVERAGES.														
TERRAPIN, diamond back, raw	100 gm	170	.01	.04	1.5	na	na	na	1.0	50.0	3.2	na	286.0	na
THYME														
ground	1 tbsp	163	.02	.02	.21	na	na	0	na	81.25	5.31	9.48	35.01	.27
ground	1 tsp	53	.01	.01	.07	na	na	0	na	26.45	1.73	3.09	11.4	.09
ground *(Durkee)*	1 tsp	.74	.1	.08	0	na	na	na	na	0	.03	na	0	na
ground *(Laurel Leaf)*	1 tsp	.74	.1	.08	0	na	na	na	na	0	.03	na	0	na
TILEFISH														
dry-heat cooked	3 oz	59	.12	.16	2.98	.26	14.7	2.13	0.0	22.1	.26	28.05	435.2	.45
raw	3 oz	51	.1	.14	2.47	.22	12.8	1.87	0.0	22.1	.21	23.8	368.05	.31
TOASTER MUFFIN/PASTRY. See MUFFIN/PASTRY, TOASTER.														
TOM COLLINS. See ALCOHOLIC BEVERAGES.														
TOMATILLO /ground husk tomato														
raw	1 med	39	.01	.01	.63	.02	2.4	0	4.0	2.38	.21	6.8	91.12	.07
raw, chopped	1/2 cup	75	.03	.02	1.22	.04	4.6	0	7.7	4.62	.41	13.2	176.88	.15
TOMATO														
Green, raw, 2 3/5 inch diam	1 tomato	790	.07	.05	.62	.1	10.8	0	28.8	15.99	.63	12.3	250.92	.09
Red														
raw, chopped	1 cup	1121	.11	.09	1.13	.14	27.0	0	34.4	9.0	.81	19.8	399.6	.16
raw, 2 3/5 inch diam, 4.75 oz	1 tomato	766	.07	.06	.77	.1	18.5	0	23.5	6.15	.55	13.53	273.06	.11
stewed	1 cup	673	.11	.08	1.12	.09	11.1	0	18.4	26.26	1.07	15.15	249.47	.18
TOMATO, CANNED														
(Angela Mia)														
chopped, 'Premium Choice'	4 oz	na	na	na	na	na	na	na	23.8	1.07	2.83	na	na	na
crushed	4 oz	na	na	na	na	na	na	na	1.5	1.74	.07	na	na	na
crushed, chunky	4 oz	na	na	na	na	na	na	na	2.7	2.83	.07	na	na	na
crushed, 'Premium Choice'	2.222 oz	na	na	na	na	na	na	na	19.2	1.3	.76	na	na	na
(Contadina)														
crushed, in purée	1/2 cup	500	.03	.05	1.05	na	na	na	6.0	46	1.16	13	350	na
Italian style	1/2 cup	682	.06	.04	.8	na	na	na	16.0	43	.73	14	300	na
Italian style, pear	1/2 cup	703	.05	.04	.8	na	na	na	19.0	57	.72	18	280	na
'Recipe Ready'	1/2 cup	590	.07	.05	.7	na	na	na	10.0	40	.7	na	240	na
stewed	1/2 cup	682	.06	.04	.8	na	na	na	16.0	44	.74	15	350	na
stewed, Mexican style	1/2 cup	650	.1	.1	.8	na	na	na	12.0	46.8	.8	na	270	na
whole, peeled	1/2 cup	703	.05	.04	.8	na	na	na	19.0	57	.72	18	330	na
(Eden Foods)														
crushed, organic, no salt added	4 oz	na	na	na	na	na	na	na	na	na	na	na	350	na
(Hunt's)														
choice cut	4 oz	na	na	na	na	na	na	na	29.4	2.7	.4	na	na	na
crushed	4 oz	na	na	na	na	na	na	na	18.7	1.28	3.79	na	na	na
diced, in juice	4 oz	na	na	na	na	na	na	na	29.7	0	.37	na	na	na
diced, in juice, 'No Salt Added'	4 oz	na	na	na	na	na	na	na	29.7	0	.37	na	na	na
diced, in purée	4 oz	na	na	na	na	na	na	na	31.4	0	.7	na	na	na
diced, w/green chilies	.3527 oz	na	na	na	na	na	na	na	1.3	.76	.03	na	na	na
pear shaped	4.868 oz	na	na	na	na	na	na	na	29.1	3.2	.4	na	na	na
pear shaped	4.832 oz	na	na	na	na	na	na	na	28.9	3.2	.4	na	na	na
pear shaped	4.656 oz	na	na	na	na	na	na	na	27.8	3.1	.4	na	na	na
stewed	4 oz	na	na	na	na	na	na	na	14.0	3.5	2.6	na	na	na
stewed, 'Food Service'	4 oz	na	na	na	na	na	na	na	14.0	3.48	2.58	na	na	na

Food Name	Serving Size	A I.U.	Thi mg	Rib mg	Nia mg	B₆ mg	Fol mcg	B₁₂ mcg	C mg	Calc mg	Iron mg	Mag mg	Pot mg	Zn mg
whole, peeled	5.608 oz	na	na	na	na	na	na	na	33.5	3.7	.4	na	na	na
whole, peeled	5.22 oz	na	na	na	na	na	na	na	31.1	3.4	.4	na	na	na
whole, peeled	5.009 oz	na	na	na	na	na	na	na	29.9	3.3	.4	na	na	na
whole, peeled	4.832 oz	na	na	na	na	na	na	na	28.9	3.2	.4	na	na	na
whole, peeled, 'No Salt Added'	4.832 oz	na	na	na	na	na	na	na	28.9	3.2	.4	na	na	na
TOMATO JUICE														
(Hunt's)	9.03 oz	na	na	na	na	na	na	na	39.9	1.5	1.5	na	na	na
(Hunt's)	7.16 oz	na	na	na	na	na	na	na	25.2	1.3	1.2	na	na	na
(Hunt's)	5.467 oz	na	na	na	na	na	na	na	19.6	1.0	1.0	na	na	na
(Libby's)	6 oz	na	na	na	na	na	na	na	na	na	na	na	460	na
TOMATO PASTE														
(Contadina)	2 oz	1399	.09	.11	1.82	na	na	na	24.0	20	1.7	29	550	na
(Contadina) Italian style	2 oz	1290	.09	.12	1.6	na	na	na	22.0	38	1.65	42	460	na
(Hunt's)	1.164 oz	na	na	na	na	na	na	na	10.8	1.0	2.34	na	na	na
(Hunt's) 'Food Service'	1.164 oz	na	na	na	na	na	na	na	10.8	1.0	2.34	na	na	na
(Hunt's) Italian style	1.164 oz	na	na	na	na	na	na	na	13.2	1.35	3.04	na	na	na
(Hunt's) 'No Salt Added'	1.164 oz	na	na	na	na	na	na	na	10.8	1.0	2.34	na	na	na
(Hunt's) w/garlic	1.164 oz	na	na	na	na	na	na	na	6.7	1.46	1.83	na	na	na
TOMATO POWDER, ground	100 gm	17247	.91	.76	9.13	.46	119.9	0	116.7	166.0	4.56	178.0	1927.0	1.71
TOMATO PURÉE														
(Angela Mia)	2.187 oz	na	na	na	na	na	na	na	12.8	.7	0	na	na	na
(Contadina)	1/2 cup	1464	.08	.05	1.28	na	na	na	30.0	12	1.56	na	520	na
(Contadina) w/crushed tomatoes	1/2 cup	500	.03	.05	1.05	na	na	na	6.0	46	1.16	13	350	na
(Hunt's)	2.187 oz	na	na	na	na	na	na	na	16.0	1.0	.2	na	na	na
(Hunt's) 'Food Service'	2.222 oz	na	na	na	na	na	na	na	17.8	1.2	.5	na	na	na
TOMATO SAUCE														
CANNED														
(Contadina)	1/2 cup	1614	.08	.07	.85	na	na	na	25.0	23	.73	30	400	na
(Hunt's)	2.187 oz	na	na	na	na	na	na	na	10.9	.9	.2	na	na	na
Casera (Hunt's)	2.187 oz	na	na	na	na	na	na	na	12.5	.8	3.86	na	na	na
Chunky														
(Hunt's) chili	2.222 oz	na	na	na	na	na	na	na	4.5	4.35	1.15	na	na	na
(Hunt's) 'Food Service'	2.187 oz	na	na	na	na	na	na	na	11.4	na	.3	na	na	na
(Hunt's) Italian	2.222 oz	na	na	na	na	na	na	na	2.0	4.15	2.47	na	na	na
(Hunt's) Mexican	2.222 oz	na	na	na	na	na	na	na	5.2	4.0	2.36	na	na	na
(Hunt's) tomato	2.187 oz	na	na	na	na	na	na	na	16.1	.62	.62	na	na	na
Garden vegetable (Contadina)	5 oz	1815	.06	.14	1.85	.22	14.4	na	2.4	49.5	1.56	41.8	520	.48
Hot, Maya (Hunt's)	1.058 oz	na	na	na	na	na	na	na	0.6	.47	.02	na	na	na
Italian style														
(Contadina)	1/2 cup	975	.05	.04	1.23	na	na	na	25.0	29	.72	34	420	na
(Contadina) sausage	5 oz	1250	.12	.13	2.77	.29	12.1	.28	6.0	46.9	1.72	38	560	.93
(Hunt's)	2.222 oz	na	na	na	na	na	na	na	7.6	1.47	3.58	na	na	na
Marinara (Contadina)	4 oz	1000	.06	.07	1.43	.15	15.4	na	6.0	39	1.06	25.6	380	.3
No salt added (Hunt's)	2.187 oz	na	na	na	na	na	na	na	10.9	.9	.2	na	na	na
Pesto (Contadina)	2.33 oz	549	.06	.26	.4	.05	11.5	.13	0.9	200	.72	29.0	125	.63
Plum (Contadina)	5 oz	1000	.06	.09	1.41	.19	42.7	.01	4.8	41.5	1.08	34.6	400	.29
'Special' (Hunt's)	2.187 oz	na	na	na	na	na	na	na	8.6	.82	.27	na	na	na
'Thick and Zesty' (Contadina)	1/2 cup	1454	.08	.05	1.26	na	na	na	30.0	29	1.55	17	460	na
W/garlic (Hunt's)	2.258 oz	na	na	na	na	na	na	na	11.8	1.74	5.05	na	na	na
W/herbs (Hunt's)	2.187 oz		na	na	na	na	na	na	3.8	1.5	3.5	na	na	na
TOMATOSEED OIL	1 tbsp	0	0	0	0	0	0.0	0	0.0	0	0	0	0	0
TOM COLLINS. See ALCOHOLIC BEVERAGES.														
TORSK. See CUSK.														
TORTELLINI PASTA, REFRIGERATED														
CHEESE (DiGiorno) approx 1 cup cooked	1/3 pkg	na	na	na	na	na	na	na	na	na	na	na	135	na
CHICKEN AND HERB														
(DiGiorno) approx 1 cup cooked	1/3 pkg	na	na	na	na	na	na	na	na	na	na	na	150	na

Food Name	Serving Size	A IU	Thi mg	Rib mg	Nia mg	B₆ mg	Fol mcg	B₁₂ mcg	C mg	Calc mg	Iron mg	Mag mg	Pot mg	Zn mg
EGG, w/cheese, 'Fresh' (Contadina)	3 oz	75	.3	.26	2.0	.02	9.7	.11	0.1	150	1.8	34.9	125	.67
MOZZARELLA GARLIC														
(DiGiorno) approx 1 cup cooked	1/3 pkg	na	na	na	na	na	na	na	na	na	na	na	120	na
SAUSAGE, Italian, 'Fresh' (Contadina)	3 oz	75	.38	.17	2.0	.08	12.4	.39	0.9	40.0	1.44	32.8	160	1.01
SPINACH, w/cheese, 'Fresh' (Contadina)	3 oz	75	.3	.26	2.0	.05	10.0	.11	0.6	150	2.7	48.6	230	.76
W/CHICKEN AND PROSCIUTTO (Contadina)	3 oz	30	.3	.26	3.81	.09	8.8	.12	0.0	78	2.66	36.1	140	.85
W/MEAT														
(Contadina) 'Fresh'	3 oz	100	.45	.26	2.0	.09	9.8	.37	0.2	60	1.8	41.1	180	1.39
(DiGiorno) approx 1 cup cooked	1/3 pkg	na	na	na	na	na	na	na	na	na	na	na	140	na
TORTELLINI PASTA DISH/ENTRÉE, FROZEN														
(Stouffer's) in Alfredo sauce	8 7/8 oz	na	na	na	na	na	na	na	na	na	na	na	270	na
(Stouffer's) w/tomato sauce	9.25 oz	na	na	na	na	na	na	na	na	na	na	na	420	na
TORTILLA, FLOUR														
Fajita style (Fry's) extra soft	1 tortilla	na	na	na	na	na	na	na	na	na	na	na	190	na
TORTILLA CHIPS. See also CORN CHIPS AND SNACKS.														
(Doritos)														
'Cool Ranch'	1 oz	na	na	na	na	na	na	na	na	na	na	na	70	na
'Jumpin' Jack'	1 oz	na	na	na	na	na	na	na	na	na	na	na	60	na
nacho cheese	1 oz	na	na	na	na	na	na	na	na	na	na	na	60	na
'Salsa Rio'	1 oz	na	na	na	na	na	na	na	na	na	na	na	80	na
taco	1 oz	na	na	na	na	na	na	na	na	na	na	na	70	na
toasted corn	1 oz	na	na	na	na	na	na	na	na	na	na	na	55	na
TOWEL GOURD. See GOURD, DISHCLOTH.														
TREE FERN, cooked, chopped	1/2 cup	142	0	.21	2.49	.13	10.7	0	21.3	5.68	.11	3.55	3.55	.22
TRITICALE, whole grain	1/2 cup	0	.4	.13	1.37	.13	70.1	0	0.0	35.52	2.47	124.8	318.72	3.31
TRITICALE FLOUR														
whole grain	1/2 cup	0	.25	.09	1.86	.26	48.1	0	0.0	22.75	1.68	99.45	302.9	1.73
TROPICAL CITRUS DRINK														
chilled (Five Alive)	6 oz	na	na	na	na	na	na	na	21.0	na	na	na	130	na
frozen, prepared (Five Alive)	6 oz	na	na	na	na	na	na	na	21.0	na	na	na	130	na
TROPICAL NECTAR, can or bottle (Kern's)	6 oz	na	na	na	na	na	na	na	na	na	na	na	90	na
TROPICAL ORANGE DRINK, 'Fruit Box' (Tang)	8.45 oz	na	na	na	na	na	na	na	na	na	na	na	35	na
TROPICAL PUNCH														
Can, bottle, or box														
(Kool-Aid) 'Koolers'	8.45 oz	na	na	na	na	na	na	na	na	na	na	na	35	na
(Minute Maid)	6 oz	na	na	na	na	na	na	na	4.0	na	na	na	35	na
Mix														
(Kool-Aid) sugar-free, w/NutraSweet, prepared	8 oz	na	na	na	na	na	na	na	na	na	na	na	10	na
(Kool-Aid) sugar-sweetened, prepared	8 oz	na	na	na	na	na	na	na	na	na	na	na	0	na
(Kool-Aid) unsweetened, prepared w/sugar	8 oz	na	na	na	na	na	na	na	na	na	na	na	0	na
(Kool-Aid) unsweetened, prepared w/o sugar	8 oz	na	na	na	na	na	na	na	na	na	na	na	0	na
TROUT, MIXED SPECIES														
dry-heat cooked	3 oz	54	.36	.36	4.9	.2	12.8	6.37	0.4	46.75	1.63	23.8	393.55	.72
raw	3 oz	49	.3	.28	3.83	.17	11.1	6.62	0.4	36.55	1.27	18.7	306.85	.56
raw, approx 2.8 oz	1 fillet	46	.28	.26	3.56	.16	10.3	6.15	0.4	33.97	1.18	17.38	285.19	.52
TROUT, RAINBOW														
farmed, dry-heat cooked	3 oz	244	.2	.07	7.47	.34	20.4	4.22	2.8	na	.28	27.2	374.85	.42
farmed, raw	3 oz	236	.17	.06	6.99	.53	9.4	3.2	2.5	na	.23	27.2	383.35	.35
wild, dry-heat cooked	3 oz	43	.13	.08	4.9	.29	16.2	5.35	1.7	73.1	.32	26.35	380.8	.43
wild, raw	3 oz	53	.1	.09	4.58	.35	10.2	3.78	2.0	56.95	.6	26.35	408.85	.92
wild, raw, approx 2.8 oz	1 fillet	99	.2	.17	8.56	.65	19.1	7.08	3.8	106.53	1.11	49.29	764.79	1.72
TROUT, SEA, MIXED SPECIES, raw	3 oz	85	.05	.14	2.04	.34	4.3	2.55	0.0	14.45	.23	26.35	289.85	.38
TUMERIC. See TURMERIC.														
TUNA, ALBACORE. See TUNA, CANNED.														

Food Name	Serving Size	A I.U.	Thi mg	Rib mg	Nia mg	B$_6$ mg	Fol mcg	B$_{12}$ mcg	C mg	Calc mg	Iron mg	Mag mg	Pot mg	Zn mg
TUNA, BLUEFIN														
dry-heat cooked	3 oz	2142	.24	.26	8.96	.45	1.9	9.25	0.0	8.5	1.11	54.4	274.55	.65
raw	3 oz	1856	.2	.21	7.36	.39	1.6	8.01	0.0	6.8	.87	42.5	214.2	.51
TUNA, CANNED														
LIGHT														
In oil														
drained	3 oz	66	.03	.1	10.54	.09	4.5	1.87	0.0	11.05	1.18	26.35	175.95	.77
drained, approx 6 oz	1 can	133	.06	.21	21.2	.19	9.1	3.76	0.0	22.23	2.38	53.01	353.97	1.54
w/o salt, drained	3 oz	66	.03	.1	10.54	.09	4.5	1.87	0.0	11.05	1.18	26.35	175.95	.77
w/o salt, drained, approx 6 oz	1 can	133	.06	.21	21.2	.19	9.1	3.76	0.0	22.23	2.38	53.01	353.97	1.54
In soybean oil														
chunk, drained (Bumble Bee)	2 oz	na	na	na	na	na	na	na	na	na	na	na	120	na
In water														
chunk, drained (Bumble Bee)	2 oz	na	na	na	na	na	na	na	na	na	na	na	120	na
drained	3 oz	66	.03	.1	10.54	.32	4.0	1.87	0.0	10.2	2.72	24.65	266.9	.37
drained, approx 6.3 oz	1 can	129	.07	.2	20.46	.62	7.8	3.63	0.0	19.8	5.28	47.85	518.1	.73
w/o salt, drained	3 oz	66	.03	.1	10.54	.32	4.0	1.87	0.0	10.2	2.72	24.65	266.9	.37
w/o salt, drained, approx 6.3 oz	1 can	129	.07	.2	20.46	.62	7.8	3.63	0.0	19.8	5.28	47.85	518.1	.73
WHITE														
In oil														
drained	3 oz	68	.01	.07	9.94	.37	3.9	1.87	0.0	3.4	.55	28.9	283.05	.4
drained, approx 6.3 oz	1 can	142	.03	.14	20.82	.77	8.2	3.92	0.0	7.12	1.16	60.52	592.74	.84
w/o salt, drained	3 oz	68	.01	.07	9.94	.37	3.9	1.87	0.0	3.4	.55	28.9	283.05	.4
w/o salt, drained, approx 6.3 oz	1 can	142	.03	.14	20.82	.77	8.2	3.92	0.0	7.12	1.16	60.52	592.74	.84
In soybean oil														
chunk, drained (Bumble Bee)	2 oz	na	na	na	na	na	na	na	na	na	na	na	120	na
In water														
drained	3 oz	68	0	.04	4.93	.37	3.5	1.87	0.0	3.4	.51	28.9	240.55	.4
drained, approx 6.1 oz	1 can	138	.01	.08	9.97	.74	7.1	3.78	0.0	6.88	1.03	58.48	486.76	.81
w/o salt, drained	3 oz	68	0	.04	4.93	.37	3.5	1.87	0.0	3.4	.51	28.9	240.55	.4
w/o salt, drained, approx 6.1 oz	1 can	138	.01	.08	9.97	.74	7.1	3.78	0.0	6.88	1.03	58.48	486.76	.81
TUNA, SKIPJACK / aku / arctic bonito / katsuo / oceanic bonito														
dry-heat cooked	3 oz	51	.03	.1	15.94	.83	8.5	1.86	0.9	31.45	1.36	37.4	443.7	.89
raw	3 oz	44	.03	.09	13.09	.72	7.7	1.61	0.9	24.65	1.06	28.9	345.95	.7
raw, approx 7 oz	1/2 fillet	103	.07	.2	30.49	1.68	17.8	3.76	2.0	57.42	2.48	67.32	805.86	1.62
TUNA, YELLOWFIN / ahi														
dry-heat cooked	3 oz	58	.43	.05	10.15	.88	1.7	.51	0.9	17.85	.8	54.4	483.65	.57
raw	3 oz	50	.37	.04	8.33	.77	1.6	.44	0.9	13.6	.62	42.5	377.4	.44
TUNA ENTRÉE, FROZEN														
noodle casserole (Stouffer's)	10 oz	na	na	na	na	na	na	na	na	na	na	na	380	na
TUNKA. See GOURD, WHITE.														
TURBOT, EUROPEAN														
dry-heat cooked	3 oz	34	.06	.08	2.28	.21	7.7	2.16	1.4	19.55	.39	55.25	259.25	.24
raw	3 oz	30	.06	.07	1.87	.18	6.8	1.87	1.4	15.3	.31	43.35	202.3	.19
raw, approx 7.2 oz	1/2 fillet	71	.13	.16	4.49	.43	16.3	4.49	3.5	36.72	.73	104.04	485.52	.45
TURKEY, ALL CLASSES														
DARK MEAT ONLY														
roasted	1 cup	0	.09	.35	5.11	.5	12.6	.52	0.0	44.8	3.26	33.6	406.0	6.24
LIGHT MEAT ONLY														
roasted, diced	1 cup	0	.09	.18	9.57	.76	8.4	.52	0.0	26.6	1.89	39.2	427.0	2.86
TURKEY, FRYER-ROASTER														
DARK MEAT ONLY														
roasted, diced	1 cup	0	.07	.35	4.86	.53	14.0	.55	0.0	36.4	3.37	33.6	344.4	5.78
LIGHT MEAT ONLY														
roasted, diced	1 cup	0	.06	.19	9.71	.8	8.4	.55	0.0	21.0	2.2	39.2	387.8	2.91
TURKEY, GROUND														
Cooked, approx 2.9 oz	1 patty	0	.04	.14	3.95	.32	5.7	.27	0.0	20.5	1.58	19.68	221.4	2.35

Food Name	Serving Size	A I.U.	Thi mg	Rib mg	Nia mg	B$_6$ mg	Fol mcg	B$_{12}$ mcg	C mg	Calc mg	Iron mg	Mag mg	Pot mg	Zn mg
Raw	1 lb	23	.25	.6	15.84	1.59	31.8	1.54	0.0	58.97	5.67	86.18	1056.89	8.75
TURKEY, YOUNG HEN														
DARK MEAT ONLY														
roasted, diced	1 cup	0	.08	.33	5.26	.48	12.6	.5	0.0	42.0	3.26	35.0	408.8	6.15
LIGHT MEAT ONLY														
roasted, diced	1 cup	0	.08	.18	9.96	.73	8.4	.5	0.0	29.4	1.83	39.2	425.6	2.74
TURKEY, YOUNG TOM														
DARK MEAT ONLY														
roasted, diced	1 cup	0	.1	.37	4.99	.52	14.0	.53	0.0	49.0	3.26	32.2	410.2	6.38
LIGHT MEAT ONLY														
roasted, diced	1 cup	0	.09	.18	9.21	.77	8.4	.53	0.0	25.2	1.9	39.2	431.2	2.94
TURKEY DINNER, FROZEN														
W/DRESSING AND GRAVY (Armour) 'Classics'	11.5 oz	na	na	na	na	na	na	na	na	na	na	na	520	na
TURKEY ENTRÉE, FROZEN														
BREAST														
(Stouffer's) roast, w/stuffing and gravy	7 7/8 oz	na	na	na	na	na	na	na	na	na	na	na	310	na
PIE														
(Mrs. Paterson's) w/broccoli 'Aussie Pie'	5.5 oz	na	na	na	na	na	na	na	na	na	na	na	279	na
(Stouffer's)	10 oz	na	na	na	na	na	na	na	na	na	na	na	290	na
TETRAZZINI (Stouffer's)	10 oz	na	na	na	na	na	na	na	na	na	na	na	300	na
TURKEY FAT														
	1 cup	0	0	0	0	0	0.0	0	0.0	0	0	0	0	0
	1 tbsp	0	0	0	0	0	0.0	0	0.0	0	0	0	0	0
TURKEY GIBLETS														
raw: 1 gizzard, 1 heart, and 1 liver, approx 8.6 oz	1 pkt	18703	.19	2.79	15.44	1.05	834.5	69.27	9.3	19.52	16.69	46.36	771.04	5.83
simmered, w/giblet fat	1 cup	8752	.07	1.31	6.53	.48	500.3	34.84	2.5	18.85	9.73	24.65	290.0	5.34
TURKEY GIZZARD														
raw, approx 4 oz	1 gizzard	245	.06	.26	3.88	.16	58.8	2.4	3.6	10.17	4.29	19.21	387.59	2.27
simmered	1 cup	268	.05	.47	4.45	.17	75.4	2.76	2.3	21.75	7.89	27.55	305.95	6.03
TURKEY HEART														
raw, approx 1 oz	1 heart	9	.06	.32	1.19	.1	20.9	2.11	0.9	2.61	1.39	6.38	80.33	1.02
simmered	1 cup	41	.1	1.28	4.72	.46	114.6	10.37	2.5	18.85	9.99	31.9	265.35	7.64
TURKEY LIVER														
raw, approx 3.6 oz	1 liver	18403	.06	2.21	10.35	.78	752.8	64.6	4.6	7.14	10.99	21.42	302.94	2.53
simmered	1 cup	17613	.07	1.99	8.32	.73	932.4	66.5	2.7	15.4	10.92	21.0	271.6	4.33
TURMERIC														
ground	1 tbsp	0	.01	.02	.35	na	0.0	0	1.8	12.41	2.82	13.15	171.7	.3
ground	1 tsp	0	0	.01	.11	na	0.0	0	0.6	4.01	.91	4.25	55.55	.1
ground (Durkee)	1 tsp	na	.04	.09	0	na	na	na	.02	0	.02	na	0	na
ground (Laurel Leaf)	1 tsp	na	.04	.09	0	na	na	na	.02	0	.02	na	0	na
TURNIP														
boiled, drained, cubed	1/2 cup	0	.02	.02	.23	.05	7.2	0	9.1	17.16	.17	6.24	105.3	.16
boiled, drained, mashed	1/2 cup	0	.03	.03	.34	.08	10.6	0	13.3	25.3	.25	9.2	155.25	.23
raw, cubed	1/2 cup	0	.03	.02	.26	.06	9.4	0	13.7	19.5	.19	7.15	124.15	.18
TURNIP, Frozen, mashed	3 1/3 oz	24	.03	.02	.38	.05	7.2	0	4.1	21.62	.66	9.4	128.78	.13
TURNIP GREENS														
boiled, drained, chopped	1/2 cup	3959	.03	.05	.3	.13	85.3	0	19.7	98.64	.58	15.84	146.16	.1
raw, chopped	1/2 cup	2128	.02	.03	.17	.07	54.4	0	16.8	53.2	.31	8.68	82.88	.05
TURNIP GREENS, CANNED														
w/liquid	1/2 cup	4196	.01	.07	.42	.04	48.2	0	18.1	138.06	1.77	23.4	164.97	.27
TURNIP GREENS, FROZEN														
boiled, drained	10 oz	17545	.12	.16	1.03	.15	86.7	0	48.0	334.4	4.27	57.2	492.8	.9
boiled, drained	1/2 cup	6540	.04	.06	.38	.05	32.3	0	17.9	124.64	1.59	21.32	183.68	.34
chopped	10 oz	17563	.12	.26	1.09	.28	209.0	0	76.1	335.12	4.29	76.68	522.56	.48
chopped	1/2 cup	5071	.04	.07	.31	.08	60.4	0	22.0	96.76	1.24	22.14	150.88	.14
w/turnips	10 oz	17347	.12	.25	1.1	.21	115.3	0	73.3	323.76	4.63	51.12	232.88	.45

Food Name	Serving Size	A I.U.	Thi mg	Rib mg	Nia mg	B$_6$ mg	Fol mcg	B$_{12}$ mcg	C mg	Calc mg	Iron mg	Mag mg	Pot mg	Zn mg
TURTLE, GREEN														
canned	100 gm	100	.12	.15	1.1	.14	4.0	5.02	0.0	118.0	1.4	13.0	230.0	3.79
raw	100 gm	100	.12	.15	1.1	.14	4.0	5.02	0.0	118.0	1.4	13.0	230.0	3.79
TUSK. See CUSK.														

V

Food Name	Serving Size	A I.U.	Thi mg	Rib mg	Nia mg	B$_6$ mg	Fol mcg	B$_{12}$ mcg	C mg	Calc mg	Iron mg	Mag mg	Pot mg	Zn mg
VEAL														
(NOTE: TRIMMED = Lean; separable fat removed. UNTRIMMED = Separable fat not removed.)														
BRAINS														
braised	3 oz	0	.07	.17	2.07	.14	2.6	8.2	11.1	13.6	1.42	13.6	181.9	1.37
pan-fried	3 oz	0	.13	.31	4.78	.28	5.1	18.11	12.8	8.5	.91	15.3	401.2	1.55
raw	1 oz	0	.04	.07	1.2	.08	0.8	3.42	3.9	2.8	.6	3.92	88.2	.31
GROUND														
broiled	3 oz	na	.06	.23	6.83	.33	9.4	1.08	na	14.45	.84	20.4	286.45	3.29
raw	1 oz	na	.02	.08	2.1	.11	3.6	.38	na	4.2	.23	6.72	88.2	.86
HEART														
braised	3 oz	0	.3	.79	4.15	.18	1.7	12.29	8.5	6.8	3.67	15.3	169.15	1.9
raw	1 oz	0	.15	.28	1.79	.12	0.6	3.85	2.2	1.4	1.19	5.04	73.08	.41
KIDNEYS														
braised	3 oz	569	.16	1.69	3.94	.15	17.9	31.37	6.8	24.65	2.58	20.4	135.15	3.61
raw	1 oz	86	.09	.53	1.96	.1	5.9	7.9	1.4	3.08	.94	4.48	76.16	.55
LEG														
Trimmed														
braised	3 oz	0	.05	.31	9.11	.31	15.3	1.01	0.0	7.65	1.12	25.5	328.95	3.43
pan-fried	3 oz	0	.06	.31	10.74	.43	13.6	1.28	0.0	5.95	.74	27.2	375.7	2.87
raw	1 oz	0	.02	.08	2.68	.13	3.9	.29	0.0	1.4	.22	7.56	104.16	.66
roasted	3 oz	0	.05	.28	8.57	.26	13.6	1.0	0.0	5.1	.77	23.8	334.05	2.62
Untrimmed														
braised	3 oz	0	.05	.3	8.98	.31	15.3	.99	0.0	6.8	1.12	24.65	325.55	3.37
pan-fried	3 oz	0	.06	.3	10.24	.42	12.8	1.23	0.0	5.1	.75	26.35	361.25	2.75
raw	1 oz	0	.02	.08	2.64	.13	3.9	.29	0.0	1.4	.22	7.28	102.76	.64
roasted	3 oz	0	.05	.27	8.44	.26	13.6	.99	0.0	5.1	.77	23.8	330.65	2.58
LEG AND SHOULDER														
raw, trimmed	1 oz	0	.03	.08	2.07	.13	3.6	.42	0.0	4.76	.25	7.0	92.68	.97
trimmed, braised	3 oz	0	.06	.34	7.06	.32	13.6	1.42	0.0	24.65	1.22	23.8	290.7	5.11
LIVER														
braised	3 oz	22851	.11	1.65	7.21	.42	645.2	31.03	26.4	5.95	2.23	16.15	174.25	8.09
pan-fried	3 oz	15978	.21	2.86	14.38	.73	272.0	54.36	18.7	10.2	4.45	22.1	372.3	6.69
raw	4 oz	16720	.22	2.0	13.32	.84	728.0	53.07	25.0	10.21	5.43	20.41	331.13	4.57
raw	1 oz	4128	.05	.49	3.29	.21	179.8	13.1	6.2	2.52	1.34	5.04	81.76	1.13
LOIN														
Trimmed														
braised	3 oz	0	.04	.29	8.54	.24	12.8	1.12	0.0	27.2	.94	22.95	252.45	3.48
raw	1 oz	0	.02	.07	2.54	.16	3.9	.33	0.0	4.76	.21	7.0	90.72	.7
roasted	3 oz	0	.05	.26	8.04	.31	13.6	1.11	0.0	17.85	.72	22.1	289.0	2.75
Untrimmed														
braised	3 oz	0	.03	.26	7.68	.22	11.9	1.03	0.0	23.8	.93	20.4	238.0	3.09
raw	1 oz	0	.02	.07	2.37	.15	3.6	.31	0.0	4.48	.2	6.44	85.12	.65
roasted	3 oz	0	.04	.24	7.53	.29	12.8	1.05	0.0	16.15	.74	21.25	276.25	2.58
LUNGS														
braised	3 oz	0	.03	.11	1.95	.05	6.8	2.02	28.9	5.95	3.07	6.8	120.7	1.02
raw	1 oz	0	.01	.06	1.13	.03	3.1	1.07	10.9	1.96	1.46	3.36	76.72	.32
PANCREAS														

Food Name	Serving Size	A I.U.	Thi mg	Rib mg	Nia mg	B_6 mg	Fol mcg	B_{12} mcg	C mg	Calc mg	Iron mg	Mag mg	Pot mg	Zn mg
braised	3 oz	0	.16	.43	3.52	.16	2.6	14.73	5.1	15.3	2.02	20.4	236.3	4.42
raw	1 oz	0	.04	.12	1.19	.05	0.8	3.75	4.5	5.32	.59	5.04	77.84	.73
RIB														
Trimmed														
braised	3 oz	0	.05	.26	6.72	.29	13.6	1.3	0.0	20.4	1.23	22.1	270.3	5.08
raw	1 lb	0	.32	1.09	31.98	2.0	59.0	6.17	0.0	63.5	3.99	104.33	1388.02	15.74
raw	1 oz	0	.02	.07	1.97	.12	3.6	.38	0.0	3.92	.25	6.44	85.68	.97
roasted	3 oz	0	.05	.25	6.38	.23	11.9	1.34	0.0	10.2	.82	20.4	264.35	3.82
Untrimmed														
braised	3 oz	0	.04	.25	6.38	.27	13.6	1.23	0.0	18.7	1.2	21.25	260.1	4.73
raw	1 lb	0	.32	1.04	30.3	1.91	54.4	5.85	0.0	58.97	3.9	99.79	1315.44	14.7
raw	1 oz	0	.02	.06	1.87	.12	3.4	.36	0.0	3.64	.24	6.16	81.2	.91
roasted	3 oz	0	.04	.23	5.93	.21	11.1	1.24	0.0	9.35	.82	18.7	250.75	3.48
SHOULDER, ARM														
Trimmed														
braised	3 oz	0	.05	.28	9.1	.26	16.2	1.55	0.0	25.5	1.2	25.5	294.95	5.3
raw	1 oz	0	.02	.08	2.21	.13	4.5	.4	0.0	6.16	.29	7.28	94.92	.94
roasted	3 oz	0	.06	.28	7.0	.26	14.5	1.33	0.0	22.95	.99	22.95	302.6	3.67
Untrimmed														
braised	3 oz	0	.05	.26	8.57	.25	15.3	1.46	0.0	23.8	1.17	24.65	283.05	4.94
raw	1 oz	0	.02	.08	2.14	.12	4.2	.38	0.0	5.88	.28	7.0	91.56	.9
roasted	3 oz	0	.05	.27	6.82	.25	14.5	1.3	0.0	22.1	.98	22.1	295.8	3.55
SHOULDER, BLADE														
Trimmed														
braised	3 oz	0	.05	.31	4.83	.21	12.8	1.71	0.0	34.0	1.25	23.8	259.25	6.28
raw	1 lb	0	.41	1.41	25.17	1.68	45.4	8.44	0.0	104.33	3.99	104.33	1338.12	20.05
raw	1 oz	0	.03	.09	1.55	.1	2.8	.52	0.0	6.44	.25	6.44	82.6	1.24
roasted	3 oz	0	.06	.31	4.95	.2	9.4	1.75	0.0	23.8	.85	20.4	263.5	4.86
Untrimmed														
braised	3 oz	0	.05	.3	4.68	.2	12.8	1.64	0.0	32.3	1.22	22.1	252.45	5.95
raw	1 lb	0	.41	1.36	24.72	1.68	45.4	8.26	0.0	104.33	3.95	104.33	1310.9	19.55
raw	1 oz	0	.03	.08	1.53	.1	2.8	.51	0.0	6.44	.24	6.44	80.92	1.21
roasted	3 oz	0	.06	.3	4.87	.2	9.4	1.71	0.0	23.8	.85	20.4	260.1	4.74
SHOULDER, WHOLE														
Trimmed														
braised	3 oz	0	.05	.3	5.68	.22	13.6	1.65	0.0	31.45	1.23	23.8	271.15	5.95
raw	1 lb	0	.41	1.32	27.9	1.81	49.9	7.62	0.0	99.79	4.08	108.86	1410.7	18.42
raw	1 oz	0	.03	.08	1.72	.11	3.1	.47	0.0	6.16	.25	6.72	87.08	1.14
roasted	3 oz	0	.06	.29	5.47	.22	11.1	1.58	0.0	22.95	.88	21.25	277.95	4.46
Untrimmed														
braised	3 oz	0	.05	.29	5.46	.21	12.8	1.56	0.0	29.75	1.21	22.95	262.65	5.6
raw	1 lb	0	.41	1.32	28.08	1.77	54.4	7.58	0.0	99.79	4.13	104.33	1369.87	17.83
raw	1 oz	0	.03	.08	1.73	.11	3.4	.47	0.0	6.16	.25	6.44	84.56	1.1
roasted	3 oz	0	.06	.29	5.38	.22	10.2	1.55	0.0	22.95	.88	21.25	273.7	4.35
SIRLOIN														
Trimmed														
braised	3 oz	0	.05	.32	5.99	.32	13.6	1.35	0.0	16.15	1.05	24.65	288.15	4.04
raw	1 lb	0	.36	1.41	40.69	2.36	63.5	6.08	0.0	49.9	3.63	117.94	1578.53	12.38
raw	1 oz	0	.02	.09	2.51	.15	3.9	.38	0.0	3.08	.22	7.28	97.44	.76
roasted	3 oz	0	.05	.31	7.93	.29	13.6	1.27	0.0	11.9	.77	22.95	310.25	3.01
Untrimmed														
braised	3 oz	0	.04	.3	5.59	.3	12.8	1.26	0.0	14.45	1.02	22.95	272.85	3.67
raw	1 lb	0	.36	1.36	38.28	2.22	59.0	5.76	0.0	49.9	3.54	108.86	1492.34	11.57
raw	1 oz	0	.02	.08	2.36	.14	3.6	.36	0.0	3.08	.22	6.72	92.12	.71
roasted	3 oz	0	.05	.3	7.54	.27	12.8	1.21	0.0	11.05	.78	22.1	298.35	2.85
SPLEEN														
braised	3 oz	0	.04	.24	4.54	.06	3.4	4.1	34.0	5.95	6.26	11.9	182.75	1.62

Food Name	Serving Size	A I.U.	Thi mg	Rib mg	Nia mg	B₆ mg	Fol mcg	B₁₂ mcg	C mg	Calc mg	Iron mg	Mag mg	Pot mg	Zn mg
raw	1 oz	0	.01	.1	2.21	.03	1.1	1.5	11.5	1.68	2.61	4.76	101.36	.45
THYMUS														
braised	3 oz	0	.05	.14	1.73	.08	0.9	1.85	62.9	2.55	1.71	14.45	290.7	2.63
raw	1 oz	0	.02	.05	.72	.03	0.8	.88	15.7	.56	.53	4.48	121.24	.87
TONGUE														
braised	3 oz	0	.06	.3	1.25	.13	7.7	4.51	5.1	7.65	1.78	15.3	137.7	3.83
raw	1 oz	0	.05	.11	.62	.05	1.4	1.71	1.4	1.96	.76	4.76	75.88	.74
VEAL ENTRÉE, FROZEN														
PARMIGIANA														
(Armour) 'Classics'	11.25 oz	na	na	na	na	na	na	na	na	na	na	na	520	na
W/pasta Alfredo (Stouffer's) homestyle	9.25 oz	na	na	na	na	na	na	na	na	na	na	na	560	na
VEGETABLE. See individual listings.														
VEGETABLE ENTRÉE														
Pot pie, frozen (Amy's Kitchen) organic	8 oz	na	na	na	na	na	na	na	na	na	na	na	295	na
VEGETABLE JUICE														
cocktail, canned	6 oz	2129	.08	.05	1.32	.25	38.4	0	50.4	20.02	.76	20.02	351.26	.36
cocktail, canned	1/2 cup	1416	.05	.03	.88	.17	25.5	0	33.5	13.31	.51	13.31	233.53	.24
VEGETABLE OIL. See also individual listings.														
(Kroger)	1 tbsp	na	na	na	na	na	na	na	0.0	0	0	na	na	na
VEGETABLE OIL SPREAD. See MARGARINE SPREAD.														
VEGETABLE OYSTER. See SALSIFY.														
VEGETABLE SPONGE. See GOURD, DISHCLOTH.														
VEGETABLES, MIXED, CANNED														
drained	1/2 cup	9551	.04	.04	.47	.06	19.4	0	4.1	22.14	.86	13.12	238.62	.34
(Freshlike) water packed, w/o salt	1/2 cup	na	na	na	na	na	na	na	na	na	na	na	200	na
(Freshlike) water packed, w/o sugar or salt	1/2 cup	na	na	na	na	na	na	na	na	na	na	na	200	na
(Veg•All) 'Homestyle Large Cut'	1/2 cup	na	na	na	na	na	na	na	na	na	na	na	260	na
(Veg•All) 'Original'	1/2 cup	na	na	na	na	na	na	na	na	na	na	na	200	na
VEGETABLES, MIXED, FROZEN														
boiled, drained	10 oz pkg	11702	.2	.33	2.34	.2	52.3	0	8.8	68.75	2.25	60.5	464.75	1.35
boiled, drained	1/2 cup	3892	.06	.11	.77	.07	17.3	0	2.9	22.75	.75	20.02	153.79	.45
(Birds Eye)	3.3 oz	na	na	na	na	na	na	na	na	na	na	na	190	na
(Freshlike)	3.3 oz	na	na	na	na	na	na	na	na	na	na	na	200	na
CALIFORNIA STYLE														
(Freshlike) 'California Blend'	3.3 oz	na	na	na	na	na	na	na	na	na	na	na	200	na
CHUCKWAGON STYLE														
(Freshlike) 'Chuckwagon Blend'	3.3 oz	na	na	na	na	na	na	na	na	na	na	na	170	na
COUNTRY STYLE														
(Freshlike) 'Country Blend'	3.3 oz	na	na	na	na	na	na	na	na	na	na	na	170	na
FOR SOUP														
(Freshlike)	3.3 oz	na	na	na	na	na	na	na	na	na	na	na	190	na
FOR STEW														
(Freshlike) 5-ways	3.3 oz	na	na	na	na	na	na	na	na	na	na	na	190	na
(Freshlike) 4-ways	3.3 oz	na	na	na	na	na	na	na	na	na	na	na	190	na
ITALIAN STYLE														
(Freshlike) 'Italian Blend'	3.3 oz	na	na	na	na	na	na	na	na	na	na	na	170	na
(Freshlike) 'Italian Blend' food service	3.3 oz	na	na	na	na	na	na	na	na	na	na	na	140	na
MIDWESTERN STYLE														
(Freshlike) 'Midwestern Blend'	3.3 oz	na	na	na	na	na	na	na	na	na	na	na	210	na
ORIENTAL STYLE														
(Freshlike) 'Oriental Blend'	3.3 oz	na	na	na	na	na	na	na	na	na	na	na	200	na
SCANDINAVIAN STYLE														
(Freshlike) 'Scandinavian Blend'	3.3 oz	na	na	na	na	na	na	na	na	na	na	na	160	na
WINTER VEGETABLES														
(Freshlike) 'Winter Blend'	3.3 oz	na	na	na	na	na	na	na	na	na	na	na	200	na
VEGETARIAN ENTRÉE. See also individual listings.														
(Amy's Kitchen) Salisbury steak, organic, frozen														

Food Name	Serving Size	A I.U.	Thi mg	Rib mg	Nia mg	B₆ mg	Fol mcg	B₁₂ mcg	C mg	Calc mg	Iron mg	Mag mg	Pot mg	Zn mg
'Country Dinner'	11 oz	na	na	na	na	na	na	na	na	na	na	na	440	na

VEGETARIAN FOODS. See BACON, ALTERNATIVE; BURGER, VEGETARIAN; CRAB, ALTERNATIVE; SAUSAGE, ALTERNATIVE; SCALLOP, ALTERNATIVE; and individual listings.

VENISON. See ANTELOPE; CARIBOU; DEER; ELK; MOOSE.

VIENNA SAUSAGE, CANNED

Food Name	Serving Size	A I.U.	Thi mg	Rib mg	Nia mg	B₆ mg	Fol mcg	B₁₂ mcg	C mg	Calc mg	Iron mg	Mag mg	Pot mg	Zn mg
2 inches long, 7/8 inch diam	1 sausage	0	.01	.02	.26	.02	0.6	.16	0.0	1.6	.14	1.12	16.16	.26

VINE SPINACH / basella

raw	3.5 oz	8000	.05	.15	.5	.24	140.1	0	102.0	109.0	1.2	65.0	510.0	.43

VINEGAR

APPLE CIDER

....	1 cup	0	0	0	0	0	0.0	0	0.0	14.4	1.44	52.8	240.0	0
....	1 tbsp	0	0	0	0	0	0.0	0	0.0	.9	.09	3.3	15.0	0

WHITE

....	1 cup	0	0	0	0	.34	9.6	12.05	0.0	0	0	31.2	36.0	9.1
....	1 tbsp	0	0	0	0	.02	0.6	.75	0.0	0	0	1.95	2.25	.57

VODKA. See ALCOHOLIC BEVERAGES.

W

Food Name	Serving Size	A I.U.	Thi mg	Rib mg	Nia mg	B₆ mg	Fol mcg	B₁₂ mcg	C mg	Calc mg	Iron mg	Mag mg	Pot mg	Zn mg
WALNUT, BLACK														
Dried, chopped	1 cup	370	.27	.14	.86	.69	81.9	0	4.0	72.5	3.84	252.5	655.0	4.28
WALNUT, ENGLISH														
Dried														
halves, approx 14	1 oz	35	.11	.04	.3	.16	18.7	0	0.9	26.7	.69	48.0	142.57	.78
pieces or chips	1 cup	149	.46	.18	1.25	.67	79.2	0	3.8	112.8	2.93	202.8	602.4	3.28
WALNUT OIL														
....	1 cup	0	0	0	0	0	0.0	0	0.0	0	0	0	0	0
....	1 tbsp	0	0	0	0	0	0.0	0	0.0	0	0	0	0	0
WATER, BOTTLED														
(Perrier)	1 cup	0	0	0	0	0	0.0	0	0.0	33.18	0	0	0	0
(Perrier)	6.5-oz bottle	0	0	0	0	0	0.0	0	0.0	26.88	0	0	0	0
(Poland Spring)	1 cup	0	0	0	0	0	0.0	0	0.0	2.37	.02	2.37	0	0
sparkling, natural, unflavored (Clearly Canadian)	6 oz	na	na	na	na	na	na	na	na	15	na	7.8	.7	na
WATER, SPARKLING, FLAVORED. See also SOFT DRINKS AND MIXERS.														
BLACKBERRY, 'Mountain Blackberry'														
(Clearly Canadian)	6 oz	na	na	na	na	na	na	na	na	15	na	7.8	.7	na
CHERRY, 'Wild Cherry' (Clearly Canadian) ...	6 oz	na	na	na	na	na	na	na	na	15	na	7.8	.7	na
CRANBERRY, 'Coastal Cranberry' (Clearly Canadian)	6 oz	na	na	na	na	na	na	na	na	15	na	7.8	.7	na
LOGANBERRY, 'Western Loganberry' (Clearly Canadian)	6 oz	na	na	na	na	na	na	na	na	15	na	7.8	.7	na
PEACH, 'Orchard Peach' (Clearly Canadian)	6 oz	na	na	na	na	na	na	na	na	15	na	7.8	.7	na
RASPBERRY 'Country Raspberry' (Clearly Canadian)	6 oz	na	na	na	na	na	na	na	na	15	na	7.8	.7	na
WATER BUFFALO														
raw	1 lb	0	.18	.91	27.08	2.4	36.3	7.53	0.0	54.43	7.3	145.15	1347.19	8.75
raw	1 oz	0	.01	.06	1.67	.15	2.2	.46	0.0	3.36	.45	8.96	83.16	.54
roasted	3 oz	0	.03	.21	5.35	.39	7.7	1.49	0.0	12.75	1.8	28.05	266.05	2.16
WATER CHESTNUT, CHINESE / matai														
approx 1.7 oz	4 fruits	0	.05	.07	.36	.12	5.8	0	1.4	3.96	.02	7.92	210.24	.18
slices	1/2 cup	0	.09	.12	.62	.2	10.0	0	2.5	6.82	.04	13.64	362.08	.31

Food Name	Serving Size	A I.U.	Thi mg	Rib mg	Nia mg	B$_6$ mg	Fol mcg	B$_{12}$ mcg	C mg	Calc mg	Iron mg	Mag mg	Pot mg	Zn mg
Canned														
sliced, w/liquid	1/2 cup	3	.01	.02	.25	.11	4.1	0	0.9	2.8	.61	3.5	82.6	.27
w/liquid	4 fruits	1	0	.01	.1	.04	1.6	0	0.4	1.12	.24	1.4	33.04	.11
(LaChoy) chopped	.6349 oz	na	na	na	na	na	na	na	0.0	.06	.27	na	na	na
(LaChoy) sliced	.776 oz	na	na	na	na	na	na	na	0.0	.07	.33	na	na	na
(LaChoy) whole	.6702 oz	na	na	na	na	na	na	na	0.0	.06	.28	na	na	na
WATER CONVOLVULUS. See CABBAGE, SKUNK.														
WATERCRESS														
chopped	1/2 cup	799	.02	.02	.03	.02	1.6	0	7.3	20.4	.03	3.57	56.1	.02
fresh	1 sprig	118	0	0	0	0	0.2	0	1.1	3.0	0	.53	8.25	0
WATERMELON														
diced	1 cup	586	.13	.03	.32	.23	3.5	0	15.4	12.8	.27	17.6	185.6	.11
sliced, 1/16 of 10-inch-diam fruit	1 slice	1764	.39	.1	.96	.69	10.6	0	46.3	38.56	.82	53.02	559.12	.34
WATERMELON SEED, DRIED														
kernels	1 cup	0	.21	.16	3.83	.1	62.5	0	0.0	58.32	7.86	556.2	699.84	11.06
kernels	1 oz	0	.05	.04	1.01	.03	16.4	0	0.0	15.34	2.07	146.26	184.03	2.91
WAX GOURD. See GOURD, WAX.														
WELSH RAREBIT (Stouffer's) frozen	5 oz	na	na	na	na	na	na	na	na	na	na	na	140	na
WHALE, raw	100 gm	1860	.09	.08	8.2	.14	4.0	5.02	6.0	12.0	1.0	13.0	22.0	3.79
WHEAT, SPROUTED	1/3 cup	0	.08	.06	1.11	.1	13.7	0	0.9	10.08	.77	29.52	60.84	.59
WHEAT, WHOLE GRAIN														
DURUM	1/2 cup	0	.4	.12	6.47	.4	41.6	0	0.0	32.64	3.38	138.24	413.76	3.99
HARD RED														
spring	1/2 cup	0	.48	.11	5.48	.32	41.3	0	0.0	24.0	3.46	119.04	326.4	2.67
winter	1/2 cup	0	.37	.11	5.25	.29	36.5	0	0.0	27.84	3.06	120.96	348.48	2.54
HARD WHITE	1/2 cup	0	.37	.1	4.21	.35	36.1	0	0.0	30.72	4.38	89.28	414.72	3.2
SOFT RED, winter	1/2 cup	0	.33	.08	4.03	.23	34.4	0	0.0	22.68	2.7	105.84	333.48	2.21
SOFT WHITE	1/2 cup	0	.34	.09	4.0	.32	34.1	0	0.0	28.56	4.51	75.6	365.4	2.91
WHEAT BRAN														
crude	1/2 cup	0	.16	.17	4.07	.39	23.7	0	0.0	21.9	3.17	183.3	354.6	2.18
crude	2 tbsp	0	.04	.04	.95	.09	5.5	0	0.0	5.11	.74	42.77	82.74	.51
WHEAT FLOUR														
WHITE														
All-purpose														
enriched	1/2 cup	0	.49	.31	3.66	.03	16.1	0	0.0	9.3	2.88	13.64	66.34	.43
enriched, calcium-fortified	1/2 cup	na	.49	.31	3.66	.03	16.1	0	0.0	156.24	2.88	13.64	66.34	.43
All-purpose, unbleached, enriched	1/2 cup	0	.49	.31	3.66	.03	16.1	0	0.0	9.3	2.88	13.64	66.34	.43
Bread, enriched	1/2 cup	0	.56	.35	5.21	.03	20.0	0	0.0	10.35	3.04	17.25	69.0	.59
Cake, enriched	1/2 cup	0	.48	.23	3.67	.02	10.3	0	0.0	7.56	3.95	8.64	56.7	.33
Self-rising														
enriched	1/2 cup	0	.42	.26	3.62	.03	26.0	0	0.0	209.56	2.9	11.78	76.88	.38
(Aunt Jemima) enriched	1 oz	0	.18	.11	1.5	.01	12.0	0	0.0	60	1.25	6	32	0
Tortilla mix, enriched	1/3 cup	0	.27	.18	2.15	.01	8.7	0	0.0	75.85	2.61	7.77	37.0	.24
WHOLE GRAIN	1/2 cup	0	.27	.13	3.82	.2	26.4	0	0.0	20.4	2.33	82.8	243.0	1.76
WHEAT GERM, crude	1/4 cup	0	.55	.14	1.98	.38	81.5	0	0.0	11.31	1.82	69.31	258.68	3.56
WHEAT GERM OIL														
	1 cup	0	0	0	0	0	0.0	0	0.0	0	0	0	0	0
	1 tbsp	0	0	0	0	0	0.0	0	0.0	0	0	0	0	0
WHEAT NUTS														
macadamia flavor, w/o salt	1 oz	0	.06	.06	.28	.07	26.7	0	0.0	5.68	.57	16.47	74.12	.83
other flavors, w/o salt	1 oz	0	.11	.09	.43	.1	35.4	0	0.0	6.25	.74	16.76	90.88	.84
unflavored, w/salt added	1 oz	0	.09	.09	.43	.11	40.4	0	0.0	7.38	.68	16.47	90.31	.83
WHELK														
moist-heat cooked	3 oz	138	.04	.18	1.7	.55	9.7	15.42	5.8	96.05	8.55	146.2	589.9	2.77
raw	3 oz	72	.02	.09	.89	.29	5.4	7.71	3.4	48.45	4.28	73.1	294.95	1.39

Food Name	Serving Size	A I.U.	Thi mg	Rib mg	Nia mg	B₆ mg	Fol mcg	B₁₂ mcg	C mg	Calc mg	Iron mg	Mag mg	Pot mg	Zn mg
WHEY														
Acid														
dry	1 cup	33	.35	1.17	.66	.35	18.9	1.43	0.5	1171.01	.71	113.4	1304.44	3.6
dry	1 tbsp	2	.02	.06	.03	.02	1.0	.07	0.0	59.58	.04	5.77	66.37	.18
fluid	1 quart	69	.41	1.38	.78	.41	21.7	1.76	0.6	1010.57	.79	95.84	1408.1	4.23
fluid	1 cup	17	.1	.34	.19	.1	5.4	.44	0.2	252.64	.2	23.96	352.03	1.06
Sweet														
dry	1 cup	64	.75	3.2	1.82	.85	16.8	3.44	2.2	1154.34	1.28	255.34	3015.56	2.86
dry	1 tbsp	3	.04	.17	.09	.04	0.9	.18	0.1	59.71	.07	13.21	155.98	.15
fluid	1 quart	157	.35	1.55	.73	.31	7.9	2.73	1.0	460.51	.59	81.28	1584.24	1.28
fluid	1 cup	39	.09	.39	.18	.08	2.0	.68	0.3	115.13	.15	20.32	396.06	.32
WHISKEY. See ALCOHOLIC BEVERAGES.														
WHISKEY SOUR. See ALCOHOLIC BEVERAGES.														
WHITE BEAN														
boiled	1/2 cup	0	.11	.04	.13	.08	72.6	0	0.0	81.0	3.33	56.7	504.9	1.24
raw	1/2 cup	0	.44	.15	.48	.32	391.7	0	0.0	242.4	10.54	191.9	1812.95	3.71
small, boiled	1/2 cup	0	.21	.05	.24	.11	123.2	0	0.0	65.7	2.56	61.2	416.7	.98
small, raw	1/2 cup	0	.8	.22	1.45	.47	417.0	0	0.0	186.84	8.35	197.64	1665.36	3.03
WHITE BEAN, CANNED	1/2 cup	0	.13	.05	.15	.1	85.7	0	0.0	95.63	3.92	66.81	594.74	1.47
WHITE GOURD. See GOURD, WHITE.														
WHITEFISH														
dry-heat cooked	3 oz	111	.15	.13	3.27	.29	14.5	.82	0.0	28.05	.4	35.7	345.1	1.08
dry-heat cooked, approx 7 oz	1 fillet	202	.26	.24	5.92	.53	26.2	1.48	0.0	50.82	.72	64.68	625.24	1.96
raw	3 oz	102	.12	.1	2.55	.26	12.8	.85	0.0	22.1	.31	28.05	269.45	.84
raw, approx 7 oz	1 fillet	238	.28	.24	5.94	.59	29.7	1.98	0.0	51.48	.73	65.34	627.66	1.96
smoked	3 oz	162	.03	.09	2.04	.33	6.2	2.77	0.0	15.3	.43	19.55	359.55	.42
smoked	1 oz	53	.01	.03	.67	.11	2.0	.91	0.0	5.04	.14	6.44	118.44	.14
WHITING, MIXED SPECIES / silver hake														
dry-heat cooked	3 oz	97	.06	.05	1.42	.15	12.8	2.21	0.0	52.7	.36	22.95	368.9	.45
raw	3 oz	84	.05	.04	1.1	.13	11.1	1.95	0.0	40.8	.29	17.85	211.65	.75
WINGED BEAN / goa bean														
immature seeds, boiled, drained	1/2 cup	27	.03	.02	.2	.03	10.9	0	3.0	18.91	.34	9.3	84.94	.09
immature seeds, raw, approx .6 oz	1 pod	20	.02	.02	.14	.02	10.5	0	2.9	13.44	.24	5.44	35.68	.06
immature seeds, slices, raw	1 cup	56	.06	.04	.4	.05	28.9	0	8.1	36.96	.66	14.96	98.12	.17
mature seeds, boiled, drained	1/2 cup	0	.25	.11	.71	.04	8.9	0	0.0	122.12	3.72	46.44	240.8	1.24
mature seeds, raw	1/2 cup	0	.94	.41	2.81	.16	40.6	0	0.0	400.4	12.23	162.89	889.07	4.08
WOLF FISH / ocean catfish														
dry-heat cooked	3 oz	368	.18	.08	2.21	.39	5.1	2.0	0.0	6.8	.1	32.3	327.25	.85
raw	3 oz	319	.15	.07	1.81	.34	4.3	1.73	0.0	5.1	.08	25.5	255.0	.66
raw, approx 5.4 oz	1/2 fillet	574	.28	.12	3.26	.61	7.7	3.11	0.0	9.18	.14	45.9	459.0	1.19
WON TON SKIN														
	1 oz	4	.15	.11	1.54	.01	4.8	.01	0.0	13.32	.95	5.67	23.25	.2
	1 wrapper	1	.04	.03	.43	0	1.4	0	0.0	3.76	.27	1.6	6.56	.06

Y

Food Name	Serving Size	A I.U.	Thi mg	Rib mg	Nia mg	B₆ mg	Fol mcg	B₁₂ mcg	C mg	Calc mg	Iron mg	Mag mg	Pot mg	Zn mg
YAM														
boiled, drained, or baked, cubed	1/2 cup	0	.06	.02	.38	.16	10.9	0	8.2	9.52	.35	12.24	455.6	.14
raw, cubed	1/2 cup	0	.08	.02	.41	.22	17.3	0	12.8	12.75	.41	15.75	612.0	.18
Mountain/Hawaiian														
raw, approx 8.25 inches long	1 yam	0	.43	.08	2.02	.75	58.8	0	10.9	109.2	1.85	50.4	1755.6	1.13
raw, cubed	1/2 cup	0	.07	.01	.33	.12	9.5	0	1.8	17.68	.3	8.16	284.24	.18
YARDLONG BEAN / asparagus bean														
boiled, drained, approx 13.25 inches long	1 pod	63	.01	.01	.09	0	6.2	0	2.3	6.16	.14	5.88	40.6	.05

Food Name	Serving Size	A I.U.	Thi mg	Rib mg	Nia mg	B6 mg	Fol mcg	B12 mcg	C mg	Calc mg	Iron mg	Mag mg	Pot mg	Zn mg
boiled, drained, sliced	1 cup	468	.09	.1	.66	.02	46.3	0	16.9	45.76	1.02	43.68	301.6	.37
mature, boiled	1/2 cup	14	.18	.06	.47	.08	125.3	0	0.3	36.12	2.27	84.28	270.9	.93
mature, raw	1/2 cup	44	.75	.2	1.81	.31	552.6	0	1.3	115.92	7.23	283.92	971.88	2.94
raw, approx 13.25 inches long	1 pod	104	.01	.01	.05	0	7.4	0	2.3	6.0	.06	5.28	28.8	.04
raw, sliced	1 cup	787	.1	.1	.37	.02	56.1	0	17.1	45.5	.43	40.04	218.4	.34
YEAST, BAKERS														
active dry	1 oz	0	.65	1.51	10.28	.04	1.1	1.41	0.0	12.32	4.51	3.64	559.44	1.06
active dry	1 tbsp	0	.28	.66	4.77	.19	280.8	0	0.0	7.68	1.99	11.76	240.0	.77
active dry	.25-oz pkg	0	.17	.38	2.78	.11	163.8	0	0.0	4.48	1.16	6.86	140.0	.45
compressed	100 gm	0	1.88	1.13	12.3	.43	785.0	.01	0.1	19.0	3.25	40.0	601.0	9.97
compressed	.6-oz cake	0	.32	.19	2.09	.07	133.5	0	0.0	3.23	.55	6.8	102.17	1.69
compressed, fortified	1 oz	0	3.86	.46	40.32	.04	1.1	1.41	0.0	3.64	1.37	3.64	170.8	1.06
compressed, not fortified	1 oz	0	.2	.46	3.14	.04	1.1	1.41	0.0	3.64	1.37	3.64	170.8	1.06
YEAST, BREWERS														
debittered	1 oz	0	4.37	1.2	10.61	.04	1.1	1.41	0.0	58.8	4.84	3.64	530.32	1.06
debittered	1 tbsp	0	1.25	.34	3.03	.01	0.3	.4	0.0	16.8	1.38	1.04	151.52	.3
YEAST, TORULA	1 oz	0	3.92	1.42	12.43	.04	1.1	1.41	0.0	118.72	5.4	3.64	572.88	1.06
YELLOW BEAN														
mature, boiled	1/2 cup	2	.16	.09	.62	.11	71.2	0	1.6	54.56	2.18	65.12	286.0	.93
mature, raw	1/2 cup	6	.68	.32	2.38	.43	380.9	0	0.0	162.68	6.87	217.56	1021.16	2.77
YELLOWTAIL, mixed species														
dry-heat cooked	3 oz	88	.15	.04	7.41	.16	3.4	1.06	2.5	24.65	.54	32.3	457.3	.57
raw	3 oz	81	.12	.03	5.78	.14	3.2	1.1	2.4	19.55	.42	25.5	357.0	.44
YOGURT														
BLACK CHERRY														
(Breyers) 'Lowfat'	8 oz	na	na	na	na	na	na	na	na	na	na	na	430	na
(Knudsen) 'Cal 70'	6 oz	na	na	na	na	na	na	na	na	na	na	na	250	na
(Light n' Lively)	8 oz	na	na	na	na	na	na	na	na	na	na	na	390	na
(Light n' Lively) '100'	8 oz	na	na	na	na	na	na	na	na	na	na	na	340	na
BLUEBERRY														
(Breyers) 'Lowfat'	8 oz	na	na	na	na	na	na	na	na	na	na	na	320	na
(Dannon) 'Light' nonfat	8 oz	na	na	na	na	na	na	na	na	na	na	na	370	na
(Knudsen) 'Cal 70'	6 oz	na	na	na	na	na	na	na	na	na	na	na	250	na
(Light n' Lively)	8 oz	na	na	na	na	na	na	na	na	na	na	na	390	na
(Light n' Lively)	4.4 oz	na	na	na	na	na	na	na	na	na	na	na	210	na
(Light n' Lively) 'Free' nonfat	4.4 oz	na	na	na	na	na	na	na	na	na	na	na	190	na
(Light n' Lively) '100'	8 oz	na	na	na	na	na	na	na	na	na	na	na	340	na
CAPPUCCINO (Dannon) 'Light' nonfat	8 oz	na	na	na	na	na	na	na	na	na	na	na	350	na
CHERRY (Light n' Lively)	4.4 oz	na	na	na	na	na	na	na	na	na	na	na	200	na
CHERRY-VANILLA (Dannon) 'Light' nonfat	8 oz	na	na	na	na	na	na	na	na	na	na	na	400	na
GRAPE (Light n' Lively)	4.4 oz	na	na	na	na	na	na	na	na	na	na	na	220	na
LEMON														
(Knudsen) 'Cal 70'	6 oz	na	na	na	na	na	na	na	na	na	na	na	260	na
(Light n' Lively) '100'	8 oz	na	na	na	na	na	na	na	na	na	na	na	110	na
LEMON CHIFFON (Dannon) 'Light' non-fat	8 oz	na	na	na	na	na	na	na	na	na	na	na	350	na
MIXED BERRIES (Breyers) 'Lowfat'	8 oz	na	na	na	na	na	na	na	na	na	na	na	410	na
PEACH														
(Breyers) 'Lowfat'	8 oz	na	na	na	na	na	na	na	na	na	na	na	380	na
(Carnation) 'Smooth'n Creamy' fruit on the bottom	8 oz	1750	.3	.17	5	.4	100.0	.6	27.0	150	4.5	80	300	3
(Dannon) 'Light' nonfat	8 oz	na	na	na	na	na	na	na	na	na	na	na	380	na
(Knudsen) 'Cal 70'	6 oz	na	na	na	na	na	na	na	na	na	na	na	260	na
(Light n' Lively)	8 oz	na	na	na	na	na	na	na	na	na	na	na	380	na
(Light n' Lively)	4.4 oz	na	na	na	na	na	na	na	na	na	na	na	210	na
(Light n' Lively) '100'	8 oz	na	na	na	na	na	na	na	na	na	na	na	230	na
PINEAPPLE														
(Breyers) 'Lowfat'	8 oz	na	na	na	na	na	na	na	na	na	na	na	380	na

Food Name	Serving Size	A I.U.	Thi mg	Rib mg	Nia mg	B$_6$ mg	Fol mcg	B$_{12}$ mcg	C mg	Calc mg	Iron mg	Mag mg	Pot mg	Zn mg
(Knudsen) 'Cal 70'	6 oz	na	na	na	na	na	na	na	na	na	na	na	260	na
(Light n' Lively)	8 oz	na	na	na	na	na	na	na	na	na	na	na	440	na
(Light n' Lively)	4.4 oz	na	na	na	na	na	na	na	na	na	na	na	240	na
PLAIN (Breyers) 'Lowfat'	8 oz	na	na	na	na	na	na	na	na	na	na	na	500	na
RASPBERRY (Dannon) 'Light' nonfat	8 oz	na	na	na	na	na	na	na	na	na	na	na	380	na
RED RASPBERRY														
(Breyers) 'Lowfat'	8 oz	na	na	na	na	na	na	na	na	na	na	na	420	na
(Knudsen) 'Cal 70'	6 oz	na	na	na	na	na	na	na	na	na	na	na	270	na
(Light n' Lively)	8 oz	na	na	na	na	na	na	na	na	na	na	na	390	na
(Light n' Lively)	4.4 oz	na	na	na	na	na	na	na	na	na	na	na	210	na
(Light n' Lively) 'Free' nonfat	4.4 oz	na	na	na	na	na	na	na	na	na	na	na	190	na
(Light n' Lively) '100'	8 oz	na	na	na	na	na	na	na	na	na	na	na	350	na
STRAWBERRY														
(Breyers) 'Lowfat'	8 oz	na	na	na	na	na	na	na	na	na	na	na	390	na
(Dannon) 'Light' nonfat	8 oz	na	na	na	na	na	na	na	na	na	na	na	380	na
(Knudsen) 'Cal 70'	6 oz	na	na	na	na	na	na	na	na	na	na	na	270	na
(Light n' Lively)	8 oz	na	na	na	na	na	na	na	na	na	na	na	390	na
(Light n' Lively)	4.4 oz	na	na	na	na	na	na	na	na	na	na	na	220	na
(Light n' Lively) 'Free'	4.4 oz	na	na	na	na	na	na	na	na	na	na	na	200	na
(Light n' Lively) '100'	8 oz	na	na	na	na	na	na	na	na	na	na	na	360	na
STRAWBERRY FRUIT CUP														
(Dannon) 'Light' nonfat	8 oz	na	na	na	na	na	na	na	na	na	na	na	380	na
(Light n' Lively)	8 oz	na	na	na	na	na	na	na	na	na	na	na	390	na
(Light n' Lively)	4.4 oz	na	na	na	na	na	na	na	na	na	na	na	210	na
(Light n' Lively) 'Free' nonfat	4.4 oz	na	na	na	na	na	na	na	na	na	na	na	190	na
(Light n' Lively) '100'	8 oz	na	na	na	na	na	na	na	na	na	na	na	340	na
STRAWBERRY-BANANA														
(Breyers) 'Lowfat'	8 oz	na	na	na	na	na	na	na	na	na	na	na	390	na
(Dannon) 'Light' nonfat	8 oz	na	na	na	na	na	na	na	na	na	na	na	380	na
(Light n' Lively)	8 oz	na	na	na	na	na	na	na	na	na	na	na	390	na
(Light n' Lively)	4.4 oz	na	na	na	na	na	na	na	na	na	na	na	190	na
(Light n' Lively) 'Free' nonfat	4.4 oz	na	na	na	na	na	na	na	na	na	na	na	190	na
TROPICAL FRUIT (Dannon) 'Light' nonfat	8 oz	na	na	na	na	na	na	na	na	na	na	na	380	na
VANILLA														
(Breyers) 'Lowfat' vanilla bean	8 oz	na	na	na	na	na	na	na	na	na	na	na	450	na
(Dannon) 'Light' nonfat	8 oz	na	na	na	na	na	na	na	na	na	na	na	350	na

Z

Food Name	Serving Size	A I.U.	Thi mg	Rib mg	Nia mg	B$_6$ mg	Fol mcg	B$_{12}$ mcg	C mg	Calc mg	Iron mg	Mag mg	Pot mg	Zn mg
ZUCCHINI. See also SQUASH, SUMMER.														
baby, raw	1 large	78	.01	.01	.11	.02	3.2	0	5.5	3.36	.13	5.28	73.44	.13
baby, raw	1 med	54	0	0	.08	.02	2.2	0	3.8	2.31	.09	3.63	50.49	.09
w/skin, boiled, drained, mashed	1/2 cup	288	.05	.05	.51	.09	20.2	0	5.5	15.6	.42	26.4	303.6	.22
w/skin, boiled, drained, sliced	1/2 cup	216	.04	.04	.39	.07	15.1	0	4.1	11.7	.32	19.8	227.7	.16
w/skin, raw, sliced	1/2 cup	221	.05	.02	.26	.06	14.4	0	5.9	9.75	.27	14.3	161.2	.13
Canned, Italian style	1/2 cup	614	.05	.05	.6	.17	34.4	0	2.6	19.38	.78	15.96	312.36	.3
Frozen, w/skin, unprepared	10-oz pkg	1375	.14	.12	1.23	.14	28.1	0	15.1	51.12	1.45	36.92	619.12	.6

PART THREE

FAST FOOD VALUES

Calories • Protein • Carbohydrates • Sodium •
Fiber • Fat • Saturated Fat • Cholesterol •
Percentage of Calories From Fat

Food Name	Serving Size	Calories	Prot. gms	Carbs gms	Sod. mgs	Fiber gms	Fat gms	Sat. Fat gms	Chol. mgs	% Fat Cal.
ARBY'S										
AU JUS SAUCE	1 serving	7	1.0	1.0	750	na	0.0	0.0	0	0%
BARBECUE SANDWICH, 'Arby Q'	1 serving	389	17.6	48.2	1268	na	15.2	5.5	29	35%
BEEF SANDWICH										
'Beef'n Cheddar'	1 serving	508	24.6	43.2	1166	(mq)	26.5	7.7	52	47%
'Philly Beef 'n Swiss'	1 serving	467	24.1	38.2	1144	na	25.3	9.7	53	49%
BISCUIT, plain	1 serving	280	6.0	34.0	730	na	14.9	3.3	0	48%
BREAKFAST										
bacon platter	1 meal	593	21.8	51.0	880	na	33.0	9.2	458	50%
'Egg Platter'	1 meal	460	15.0	44.9	591	na	24.0	7.2	346	47%
'French Toastix' 3.5 oz	1 serving	420	8.0	43.0	440	na	25.0	4.6	20	54%
'Ham Platter'	1 meal	518	24.4	45.3	1177	na	26.2	7.9	374	46%
'Sausage Platter'	1 meal	640	21.0	45.9	861	na	41.0	13.3	406	58%
BREAKFAST SANDWICH										
'Bacon/Egg Croissant'	1 serving	430	17.4	28.8	720	na	30.0	15.4	245	63%
biscuit, w/bacon	1 serving	318	6.8	35.5	904	na	17.9	4.3	8	51%
'Ham Biscuit'	1 serving	323	13.0	34.3	1169	na	16.6	3.9	21	46%
'Ham/Cheese Croissant'	1 serving	345	16.0	29.3	939	na	20.7	12.1	90	54%
'Sausage Biscuit'	1 serving	460	12.0	35.0	1000	na	31.9	9.4	60	62%
'Sausage/Egg Croissant'	1 serving	519	17.5	29.3	632	na	39.2	18.6	271	68%
BROCCOLI SOUP, cream of	1 serving	166	7.7	18.0	1050	na	7.2	3.8	24	39%
CATSUP	1 serving	16	0.3	4.2	143	na	0.0	0.0	0	0%
CHEESE SOUP, Wisconsin cheese	1 serving	281	9.0	19.7	1084	na	18.0	9.0	32	58%
CHEESEBURGER, 'Bac'n Cheddar Deluxe'	1 serving	512	21.2	38.9	1094	na	31.5	8.7	38	55%
CHEESECAKE	1 serving	306	5.2	21.3	220	na	22.8	7.4	95	67%
CHICKEN NOODLE SOUP, 'Old Fashioned'	1 serving	99	6.0	14.8	929	na	1.8	0.5	25	16%
CHICKEN SANDWICH										
breast, fillet	1 serving	445	22.2	52.1	950	(mq)	22.5	3.0	45	46%
cordon bleu	1 serving	518	30.0	52.1	1463	na	27.1	5.3	92	47%
grilled, barbecue	1 serving	386	23.4	46.7	1002	na	13.1	3.6	43	31%
grilled, 'Deluxe'	1 serving	430	23.6	41.8	901	na	19.9	3.5	44	42%
roast, 'Club'	1 serving	503	30.5	36.6	1143	(mq)	27.0	6.9	46	48%
roast, 'Deluxe Light'	1 serving	276	24.0	33.0	777	na	7.0	1.7	33	23%
CHOWDER, Boston clam	1 serving	193	8.3	17.5	1032	na	10.0	4.5	26	47%
COFFEE	8 oz	3	0.0	0.0	3	na	0.0	0.0	0	0%
COOKIE, chocolate chip	1 serving	130	2.0	17.0	95	na	4.0	2.0	0	28%
CROISSANT, plain	1 serving	260	6.0	28.0	300	na	15.6	10.4	49	54%
CROISSANT SANDWICH, 'Mushroom/Cheese'	1 serving	493	13.0	34.0	935	na	37.7	15.2	116	69%
CROUTONS	1 serving	59	1.6	8.5	155	na	2.2	0.3	1	34%
DANISH, cinnamon nut	1 serving	360	6.0	60.0	105	na	11.0	1.0	0	28%
DESSERT										
'Butterfinger Polar Swirl'	1 serving	457	12.1	61.6	318	na	18.1	8.4	28	36%
'Heath Polar Swirl'	1 serving	543	10.6	76.3	346	na	21.8	5.2	39	36%
'Oreo Polar Swirl'	1 serving	482	10.5	65.8	521	na	19.7	10.4	35	37%
'Peanut Butter Cup Polar Swirl'	1 serving	517	14.0	61.4	385	na	24.0	8.1	34	42%
'Snickers Polar Swirl'	1 serving	511	12.2	73.3	351	na	18.8	6.7	33	33%
FISH SANDWICH, fillet	1 serving	526	23.0	50.0	872	na	27.0	7.0	44	46%
FRENCH DIP SANDWICH										
regular	1 serving	368	22.0	35.0	1018	na	15.4	5.6	43	38%
w/Swiss cheese	1 serving	429	28.7	35.5	1438	na	19.0	8.8	67	40%
FRENCH FRIES										
cheddar	1 serving	399	6.2	46.2	443	na	21.9	9.0	9	49%
curly	1 serving	337	4.2	43.2	167	na	17.7	7.4	0	47%
regular, small order, 2.5 oz	1 serving	246	2.1	29.8	114	(mq)	13.2	3.0	0	48%

Food Name	Serving Size	Calories	Prot. gms	Carbs gms	Sod. mgs	Fiber gms	Fat gms	Sat. Fat gms	Chol. mgs	% Fat Cal.
HAM AND CHEESE SANDWICH	1 serving	355	24.6	34.5	1400	(mq)	14.2	5.1	55	36%
HORSERADISH SAUCE, 'Horsey Sauce'	1 serving	55	0.1	2.6	105	na	5.0	2.0	0	82%
HOT CHOCOLATE	8 oz	110	2.0	23.0	120	na	1.2	0.7	0	10%
ICED TEA	16 oz	6	0.0	1.0	12	na	0.0	0.0	0	0%
MAYONNAISE	1 serving	90	0.0	0.0	75	na	10.0	1.0	0	100%
MILK, 2%	8 oz	121	8.0	12.0	122	na	4.4	3.0	18	33%
MILKSHAKE										
chocolate	1 serving	451	10.2	76.5	341	na	11.6	2.8	36	23%
jamocha	1 serving	368	9.3	59.1	262	na	10.5	2.5	35	26%
vanilla	1 serving	330	10.5	46.2	281	na	11.5	3.9	32	31%
MUFFIN, blueberry	1 muffin	240	4.0	40.0	200	na	7.0	1.0	22	26%
MUSTARD	1 serving	11	0.6	0.5	160	na	0.6	0.0	0	49%
ORANGE JUICE	6 oz	82	1.0	20.0	2	na	0.0	0.0	0	0%
POTATO, BAKED										
broccoli and cheddar	1 serving	417	10.5	55.0	361	na	17.9	6.9	22	39%
'Deluxe'	1 serving	621	17.2	58.9	605	na	36.4	18.1	58	53%
mushroom and cheese	1 serving	515	15.0	57.5	923	na	26.7	5.8	47	47%
plain	1 serving	240	5.8	50.2	58	na	1.9	0.0	0	7%
w/sour cream and butter	1 serving	463	7.7	52.7	203	na	25.2	12.1	40	49%
POTATO CAKES	3 oz	204	1.8	19.8	397	(mq)	12.0	2.2	0	53%
POTATO SOUP, w/bacon	1 serving	184	6.5	20.0	1068	na	8.8	4.3	20	43%
ROAST BEEF SANDWICH										
'Junior'	1 serving	233	11.5	22.8	519	na	10.8	4.1	22	42%
'Light Deluxe'	1 serving	294	18.0	33.0	826	na	10.0	3.5	42	31%
regular, 5.5 oz	1 serving	383	22.0	35.4	936	(mq)	18.2	7.0	43	43%
super	1 serving	552	23.7	54.1	1174	(mq)	28.3	7.6	43	46%
SALAD										
chef's	1 serving	205	18.5	13.0	796	na	9.5	3.9	126	42%
garden	1 serving	117	7.0	11.4	134	na	5.2	2.7	12	40%
roast chicken	1 serving	204	24.0	12.2	508	na	7.2	3.3	43	32%
side order	1 serving	25	2.0	4.0	30	na	0.3	0.0	0	11%
SALAD DRESSING										
blue cheese	1 serving	295	2.3	2.5	489	na	31.2	5.8	50	95%
buttermilk ranch	1 serving	349	0.3	1.9	471	na	38.5	5.6	6	99%
honey French	1 serving	322	0.2	21.8	486	na	26.9	3.9	0	75%
light Italian	1 serving	23	0.0	3.5	1110	na	1.1	0.1	0	43%
Thousand Island	1 serving	298	0.5	9.8	493	na	29.2	4.3	24	88%
SAUCE, Arby's	1 serving	15	0.1	3.3	113	na	0.2	0.0	0	12%
SOFT DRINK										
Coca-Cola Classic	12 oz	141	0.0	38.1	15	na	0.0	0.0	0	0%
Diet Coke	12 oz	1	0.0	0.0	30	na	0.0	0.0	0	0%
Diet 7Up	12 oz	4	0.3	0.0	22	na	0.0	0.0	0	0%
Nehi Orange	12 oz	190	0.0	47.4	21	na	0.0	0.0	0	0%
Pepsi Cola	12 oz	159	0.0	40.0	10	na	0.0	0.0	0	0%
R.C. Cola	12 oz	173	0.0	43.2	1	na	0.0	0.0	0	0%
R.C. Diet Rite	12 oz	1	0.0	0.2	10	na	0.0	0.0	0	0%
R.C. Root Beer	12 oz	173	0.0	42.9	16	na	0.0	0.0	0	0%
7Up	12 oz	144	0.0	38.0	34	na	0.0	0.0	0	0%
Upper Ten	12 oz	169	0.0	42.3	40	na	0.0	0.0	0	0%
SUBMARINE SANDWICH										
Italian	1 serving	671	34.1	47.4	2062	na	38.8	12.8	69	52%
roast beef	1 serving	623	37.7	46.8	1847	na	32.0	11.5	73	46%
tuna	1 serving	663	74.0	50.2	1342	na	37.0	8.2	43	50%
turkey	1 serving	486	32.8	46.5	2033	na	19.0	5.3	51	35%

Food Name	Serving Size	Calories	Prot. gms	Carbs gms	Sod. mgs	Fiber gms	Fat gms	Sat. Fat gms	Chol. mgs	% Fat Cal.
SUGAR SUBSTITUTE	1 serving	4	0.0	0.0	5	na	0.0	0.0	0	0%
SYRUP, maple, 1.5 oz	1 serving	120	0.0	29.0	52	na	0.1	0.0	0	1%
TURKEY SANDWICH, 'Light Roast Turkey Deluxe' 6.8 oz	1 serving	260	20.0	33.0	1262	na	6.0	1.6	33	21%
TURNOVER										
apple	1 serving	303	4.4	27.5	178	na	18.3	6.9	0	54%
blueberry	1 serving	320	3.0	32.0	240	na	19.0	6.3	0	53%
cherry	1 serving	280	4.6	25.4	200	na	17.8	5.3	0	57%
VEGETABLE SOUP, mixed vegetable, 'Lumberjack'	1 serving	89	2.3	12.6	1075	na	3.6	1.7	4	36%
ARTHUR TREACHER'S										
CHICKEN PATTIES, 4.8 oz	2 patties	369	27.1	16.5	495	(mq)	21.6	3.5	65	53%
CHICKEN SANDWICH, 5.5 oz	1 serving	413	16.2	44.0	708	(mq)	19.2	2.8	32	42%
COD FILLET, tail shape, 'Bake'n Broil' 5 oz	1 serving	245	19.6	9.7	144	(mq)	14.2	(mq)	(mq)	52%
COLESLAW, 3 oz	1 serving	123	1.0	11.1	266	(mq)	8.2	1.1	7	60%
DESSERT, 'Lemon Luv' 3 oz	1 serving	276	2.6	35.1	314	(mq)	13.9	2.2	<1	45%
FISH, 5.2 oz	2 pieces	355	19.2	25.4	450	(mq)	19.8	2.8	56	50%
FISH SANDWICH, 5.5 oz	1 serving	440	16.4	39.4	836	(mq)	24.0	4.2	42	49%
FRENCH FRIES, 'Chips' 4 oz	1 serving	276	4.0	34.9	39	(mq)	13.2	2.3	5	43%
HUSHPUPPY, 'Krunch Pup' 2 oz	1 piece	203	5.4	12.0	446	(mq)	14.8	3.7	25	66%
SHRIMP, 4.1 oz	7 pieces	381	13.1	27.2	538	(mq)	24.4	3.3	93	58%
AU BON PAIN										
BAGEL										
cinnamon	1 bagel	395	14.0	86.0	605	4.0	2.0	<1.0	0	5%
onion	1 bagel	390	16.0	81.0	665	4.0	2.0	<1.0	0	5%
plain	1 bagel	380	15.0	79.0	665	3.0	2.0	<1.0	0	5%
sesame	1 bagel	425	17.0	81.0	665	4.0	5.0	1.0	0	11%
BEEF BARLEY SOUP										
bowl	1 serving	112	9.0	15.0	901	na	3.0	na	18	24%
cup	1 serving	75	6.0	10.0	600	na	2.0	na	12	24%
BREAD										
baguette	1 loaf	810	27.0	166.0	1830	na	2.0	<1.0	0	2%
cheese	1 loaf	1670	70.0	269.0	4140	na	29.0	9.0	75	16%
four grain	1 loaf	1420	57.0	262.0	3050	na	11.0	<1.0	1	7%
onion herb	1 loaf	1430	52.0	263.0	2390	na	13.0	<1.0	0	8%
pita pocket	2 slices	80	2.7	18.0	na	na	<1.0	na	na	0%
Ponsienne	1 loaf	1490	49.0	166.0	3380	na	4.0	<1.0	0	2%
sandwich, multigrain	2 slices	391	16.0	77.0	2040	na	3.0	1.0	1	7%
sandwich, rye	2 slices	374	14.0	73.0	2170	na	4.0	1.0	na	10%
BROCCOLI SOUP, CREAM OF										
bowl	1 serving	302	8.0	18.0	219	na	26.0	12.0	54	77%
cup	1 serving	201	5.0	12.0	146	na	17.0	8.0	36	76%
CHEESE										
boursin, sandwich filling	1 serving	290	6.0	2.0	390	na	29.0	18.0	90	90%
brie, sandwich filling	1 serving	300	18.0	3.0	510	na	24.0	15.0	85	72%
cheddar, sandwich filling	1 serving	110	7.0	1.0	150	na	9.0	5.0	30	74%
provolone, sandwich filling	1 serving	155	9.9	<1.0	180	na	12.6	7.4	36	73%
Swiss, sandwich filling	1 serving	330	25.0	3.0	230	na	24.0	15.0	80	65%
CHICKEN NOODLE SOUP										
bowl	1 serving	119	12.0	14.0	743	na	1.7	<1.0	26	13%
cup	1 serving	79	8.0	9.0	495	na	1.0	<1.0	17	11%
CHICKEN POT PIE	1 serving	440	17.5	46.0	1109	na	21.0	7.0	45	43%
CHICKEN SANDWICH										
cracked pepper, on French roll	1 sandwich	440	33.0	66.0	1390	na	3.0	na	50	6%

Food Name	Serving Size	Calories	Prot. gms	Carbs gms	Sod. mgs	Fiber gms	Fat gms	Sat. Fat gms	Chol. mgs	% Fat Cal.
cracked pepper, on hearth roll	1 sandwich	490	39.0	70.0	1280	na	5.0	na	50	9%
cracked pepper, on soft roll	1 sandwich	430	31.0	51.0	1090	na	10.0	na	50	21%
grilled, on French roll	1 sandwich	450	33.0	66.0	1320	na	5.0	na	60	10%
grilled, on hearth roll	1 sandwich	500	39.0	70.0	1210	na	7.0	na	60	13%
grilled, on soft roll	1 sandwich	440	31.0	51.0	1020	na	12.0	na	60	25%
tarragon, on French roll	1 sandwich	590	34.0	68.0	1014	na	16.0	na	70	24%
tarragon, on hearth roll	1 sandwich	640	40.0	72.0	904	na	18.0	na	70	25%
tarragon, on soft roll	1 sandwich	580	32.0	53.0	714	na	23.0	na	70	36%
CHILI, VEGETARIAN										
bowl	1 serving	208	9.0	37.0	763	na	4.0	<1.0	0	17%
cup	1 serving	139	6.0	24.0	508	na	3.0	<1.0	0	19%
CHOWDER, clam										
bowl	1 serving	433	17.0	36.0	1029	na	27.0	15.0	90	56%
cup	1 serving	289	11.0	24.0	687	na	18.0	9.0	60	56%
COOKIE										
chocolate chip, 'Gourmet'	1 cookie	280	2.0	37.0	70	na	15.0	9.0	25	48%
chocolate chunk pecan, 'Gourmet'	1 cookie	290	3.0	37.0	200	na	17.0	6.0	10	53%
oatmeal raisin, 'Gourmet'	1 cookie	250	4.0	41.0	230	na	9.0	na	10	32%
peanut butter, 'Gourmet'	1 cookie	290	7.0	33.0	250	na	15.0	6.0	10	47%
shortbread, 'Gourmet'	1 cookie	425	5.0	46.0	385	na	26.0	16.0	68	55%
white chocolate chunk pecan, 'Gourmet'	1 cookie	300	3.0	37.0	200	na	17.0	6.0	10	51%
CROISSANT										
almond	1 croissant	420	8.0	41.0	250	na	25.0	12.0	95	54%
apple	1 croissant	250	4.0	38.0	150	na	10.0	6.0	25	36%
blueberry cheese	1 croissant	380	7.0	44.0	280	na	20.0	12.0	60	47%
chocolate	1 croissant	400	5.0	46.0	220	na	24.0	14.0	35	54%
cinnamon raisin	1 croissant	390	7.0	60.0	240	na	13.0	8.0	35	30%
coconut pecan	1 croissant	440	7.0	51.0	290	na	23.0	12.0	45	47%
hazelnut chocolate	1 croissant	480	6.0	56.0	220	na	28.0	14.0	35	53%
hot, filled w/ham and cheese	1 serving	370	10.0	38.0	280	na	20.0	12.0	55	49%
hot, filled w/spinach and cheese	1 serving	290	9.0	29.0	310	na	16.0	10.0	45	50%
hot, filled w/turkey and cheddar	1 serving	410	16.0	38.0	680	na	22.0	13.0	70	48%
hot, filled w/turkey and havarti	1 serving	410	17.0	38.0	630	na	21.0	13.0	70	46%
plain	1 croissant	220	5.0	29.0	240	na	10.0	6.0	25	41%
raspberry cheese	1 croissant	400	7.0	49.0	280	na	20.0	12.0	60	45%
strawberry cheese	1 croissant	400	7.0	49.0	280	na	20.0	12.0	60	45%
sweet cheese	1 croissant	420	8.0	45.0	310	na	23.0	14.0	70	49%
DANISH PASTRY										
cheese	1 Danish	390	8.0	43.0	530	2.0	22.0	12.0	78	51%
cherry	1 Danish	335	7.0	42.0	480	2.0	16.0	8.0	50	43%
cherry dumpling	1 Danish	360	5.0	59.0	255	1.0	13.0	2.0	0	33%
raspberry	1 Danish	335	6.0	43.0	480	2.0	16.0	8.0	50	43%
HAM SANDWICH										
country ham, on French roll	1 sandwich	470	27.0	68.0	1680	na	8.0	na	115	15%
country ham, on hearth roll	1 sandwich	520	33.0	72.0	1570	na	10.0	na	115	17%
country ham, on soft roll	1 sandwich	460	25.0	53.0	1380	na	15.0	na	115	29%
MINESTRONE SOUP, cup	1 serving	105	5.0	20.0	265	na	2.0	na	1	17%
MUFFIN										
blueberry, gourmet	1 muffin	390	8.0	66.0	410	na	4.0	na	40	9%
bran, gourmet	1 muffin	390	7.0	73.0	940	na	11.0	na	20	25%
carrot, gourmet	1 muffin	450	7.0	58.0	610	na	22.0	5.0	15	44%
corn, gourmet	1 muffin	460	8.0	71.0	510	na	17.0	3.0	25	33%
cranberry walnut, gourmet	1 muffin	350	7.0	53.0	730	na	13.0	na	15	33%
oat bran apple, gourmet	1 muffin	400	7.0	71.0	590	na	2.0	na	0	5%

Food Name	Serving Size	Calories	Prot. gms	Carbs gms	Sod. mgs	Fiber gms	Fat gms	Sat. Fat gms	Chol. mgs	% Fat Cal.
pumpkin, gourmet	1 muffin	410	6.0	63.0	500	na	16.0	2.0	20	35%
whole grain, gourmet	1 muffin	440	10.0	68.0	310	na	16.0	2.0	30	33%
ROAST BEEF SANDWICH										
on French roll	1 sandwich	500	34.0	66.0	1020	na	9.0	na	60	16%
on hearth roll	1 sandwich	550	40.0	70.0	910	na	11.0	na	60	18%
on soft roll	1 sandwich	490	32.0	51.0	720	na	16.0	na	60	29%
ROLL										
Alpine, fresh	1 roll	220	8.0	43.0	810	na	3.0	na	0	12%
country seed, fresh	1 roll	220	9.0	37.0	460	na	4.0	na	0	16%
hearth, fresh	1 roll	250	10.0	42.0	510	na	2.0	na	0	7%
'Petit Pain' fresh	1 roll	220	7.0	44.0	490	na	<1.0	na	0	0%
pumpernickel, fresh	1 roll	210	8.0	42.0	1005	na	2.0	na	0	9%
rye, fresh	1 roll	230	8.0	44.0	na	na	2.0	na	0	8%
sandwich, braided	1 roll	387	10.0	64.0	1540	na	11.0	3.0	34	26%
sandwich, croissant	1 roll	300	7.0	38.0	240	na	14.0	8.0	35	42%
sandwich, French	1 roll	320	10.0	65.0	710	na	<1.0	na	0	0%
sandwich, hearth	1 roll	370	16.0	69.0	600	na	3.0	na	0	7%
sandwich, soft	1 roll	310	8.0	50.0	410	na	8.0	na	0	23%
3 seed raisin, fresh	1 roll	250	8.0	46.0	480	na	4.0	na	0	14%
vegetable, fresh	1 roll	230	6.0	40.0	410	na	5.0	na	0	20%
SALAD										
garden, chicken tarragon	1 serving	310	24.0	11.0	332	na	15.0	na	70	44%
garden, cracked pepper chicken	1 serving	100	14.0	9.0	360	na	2.0	na	25	18%
garden, grilled chicken	1 serving	110	14.0	9.0	330	na	2.0	na	30	16%
garden, large	1 serving	40	3.0	8.0	20	na	<1.0	<1.0	0	0%
garden, shrimp	1 serving	102	11.0	8.0	193	na	2.0	na	105	18%
garden, small	1 serving	20	5.0	5.0	10	na	<1.0	na	0	0%
garden, tuna	1 serving	350	21.0	11.0	480	na	25.0	4.0	40	64%
Italian, low-calorie	1 serving	68	0.0	3.0	360	na	6.0	na	5	79%
SPLIT PEA SOUP										
bowl	1 serving	264	18.0	45.0	453	na	2.0	na	1	7%
cup	1 serving	176	12.0	30.0	303	na	1.0	na	1	5%
TOMATO SOUP, Florentine										
bowl	1 serving	92	4.0	15.0	221	na	1.7	<1.0	0	17%
cup	1 serving	61	3.0	10.0	147	na	1.0	<1.0	0	15%
TURKEY SANDWICH										
smoked turkey, on French roll	1 sandwich	420	32.0	65.0	1660	na	2.0	na	35	4%
smoked turkey, on hearth roll	1 sandwich	470	38.0	69.0	1550	na	4.0	na	35	8%
smoked turkey, on soft roll	1 sandwich	410	30.0	50.0	1360	na	9.0	na	35	20%
VEGETARIAN SOUP, garden										
bowl	1 serving	44	1.7	9.0	92	na	<1.0	<1.0	0	0%
cup	1 serving	29	1.0	6.0	61	na	<1.0	<1.0	0	0%
BASKIN ROBBINS										
ICE CREAM										
'Almond Buttercrunch' light	1 serving	130	3.0	16.0	na	na	6.0	na	12	42%
'Caramel Banana' fat-free	1 serving	100	2.0	23.0	na	na	0.0	na	1	0%
'Chocolate'	1 scoop	270	5.0	32.0	160	na	14.0	na	37	47%
'Chocolate Caramel Nut' light	1/2 cup	130	3.0	19.0	0	na	5.0	3.0	8	35%
'Chocolate Chip'	1 scoop	260	4.0	27.0	110	na	15.0	na	40	52%
'Chocolate Chip' sugar-free	1 serving	100	3.0	20.0	na	na	2.0	na	4	18%
'Chocolate Raspberry Truffle'	1 scoop	310	4.0	35.0	115	na	17.0	na	45	49%
'Chocolate Wonder' fat-free	1 serving	120	3.0	26.0	na	na	0.0	na	1	0%
'Chunky Banana' sugar-free	1/2 cup	100	3.0	20.0	50	na	1.0	na	3	9%

Food Name	Serving Size	Calories	Prot. gms	Carbs gms	Sod. mgs	Fiber gms	Fat gms	Sat. Fat gms	Chol. mgs	% Fat Cal.
'Double Raspberry' light	1 serving	120	2.0	19.0	na	na	4.0	na	9	30%
'Expresso and Cream' light	1/2 cup	120	3.0	15.0	0	na	5.0	3.0	12	38%
'French Vanilla'	1 scoop	280	4.0	25.0	90	na	18.0	na	90	58%
'Jamocha Almond Fudge'	1 scoop	270	5.0	30.0	115	na	14.0	na	32	47%
'Just Chocolate Vanilla' fat-free	1/2 cup	100	4.0	21.0	60	na	0.0	na	0	0%
'Just Peachy' fat-free	1/2 cup	100	3.0	22.0	60	na	0.0	na	0	0%
'Praline Dream' light	1/2 cup	130	3.0	17.0	85	na	6.0	na	11	42%
'Pralines 'N Cream'	1 scoop	280	4.0	35.0	180	na	14.0	na	36	45%
'Rocky Road'	1 scoop	300	5.0	39.0	135	na	14.0	na	32	42%
'Strawberry Royal,' light	1/2 cup	110	2.0	19.0	120	na	3.0	na	9	25%
'Strawberry' sugar-free	1 serving	80	2.0	17.0	70	na	1.0	na	3	11%
'Vanilla'	1 scoop	240	4.0	24.0	115	na	14.0	na	52	53%
'Very Berry Strawberry'	1 scoop	220	3.0	30.0	95	na	10.0	na	30	41%
'World Class Chocolate'	1 scoop	280	5.0	35.0	145	na	14.0	na	36	45%
ICE CREAM BAR										
chocolate, caramel ribbon, 'Sundae Bars' light	1 bar	150	3.0	24.0	75	na	5.0	na	11	30%
ICE CREAM CONE										
sugar	1 cone	60	1.0	11.0	45	na	1.0	na	0	15%
waffle	1 cone	140	3.0	28.0	5	na	2.0	na	0	13%
SHERBET/SORBET										
daiquiri ice	1 scoop	140	0.0	35.0	15	na	0.0	0.0	0	0%
fruit whip sorbet	1 serving	80	0.0	24.0	20	na	0.0	0.0	0	0%
rainbow sherbet	1 scoop	160	1.0	34.0	85	na	2.0	na	6	11%
red raspberry sorbet	1 scoop	140	0.0	34.0	25	na	0.0	0.0	0	0%
strawberry soft-serve sorbet	1 serving	100	0.0	20.0	20	na	0.0	na	0	0%
YOGURT, FROZEN										
cafe mocha, 'Trulyfree'	1 serving	70	4.0	16.0	14	na	0.0	0.0	0	0%
chocolate, low-fat, large	9 oz	315	9.0	54.0	90	na	9.0	na	9	26%
chocolate, low-fat, medium	7 oz	246	7.0	42.0	70	na	7.0	na	7	26%
chocolate, low-fat, small	5 oz	175	5.0	30.0	50	na	5.0	na	5	26%
coconut, nonfat, large	9 oz	180	9.0	45.0	90	na	0.0	na	0	0%
coconut, nonfat, medium	7 oz	140	7.0	35.0	70	na	0.0	na	0	0%
coconut, nonfat, small	5 oz	100	5.0	25.0	50	na	0.0	na	0	0%
raspberry, nonfat, large	9 oz	225	9.0	45.0	90	na	0.0	na	0	0%
raspberry, nonfat, medium	7 oz	164	7.0	35.0	70	na	0.0	na	0	0%
raspberry, nonfat, small	5 oz	125	5.0	25.0	50	na	0.0	na	0	0%
strawberry, low-fat, large	9 oz	270	9.0	54.0	90	na	9.0	na	9	30%
strawberry, low-fat, medium	7 oz	211	7.0	42.0	70	na	7.0	na	7	30%
strawberry, low-fat, small	5 oz	150	5.0	30.0	50	na	5.0	na	5	30%
strawberry, nonfat, large	9 oz	225	9.0	45.0	90	na	0.0	na	0	0%
strawberry, nonfat, medium	7 oz	176	7.0	35.0	70	na	0.0	na	0	0%
strawberry, nonfat, small	5 oz	125	5.0	25.0	50	na	0.0	na	0	0%
vanilla, low-fat, large	9 oz	270	9.0	54.0	90	na	9.0	na	9	30%
vanilla, low-fat, medium	7 oz	211	7.0	42.0	70	na	7.0	na	7	30%
vanilla, low-fat, small	5 oz	150	5.0	30.0	50	na	5.0	na	5	30%
BIG BOY RESTAURANT										
BEANS, green	1 serving	28	2.0	6.0	1	na	0.0	0.0	0	0%
CABBAGE SOUP										
bowl	1 serving	43	2.0	9.0	727	na	1.0	na	1	21%
cup	1 serving	37	2.0	8.0	623	na	0.0	0.0	1	0%
CARROTS	1 serving	35	1.0	8.0	38	na	0.0	0.0	0	0%
CHICKEN DINNER										
breast, salad w/o dressing, oat bran bread	1 serving	349	38.0	20.0	342	na	13.0	na	65	34%

Food Name	Serving Size	Calories	Prot. gms	Carbs gms	Sod. mgs	Fiber gms	Fat gms	Sat. Fat gms	Chol. mgs	% Fat Cal.
breast, w/mozzarella, salad w/o dressing, bread	1 serving	370	42.0	24.0	353	na	12.0	na	76	29%
Cajun, salad w/o dressing, oat bran bread	1 serving	349	38.0	20.0	612	na	13.0	na	65	34%
chicken and vegetable stir-fry	1 serving	562	43.0	68.0	750	na	14.0	na	68	22%
CHICKEN SANDWICH, pita, w/mozzarella, 'Heart Smart'	1 serving	404	42.0	26.0	421	na	13.0	na	76	29%
CORN	1 serving	90	3.0	21.0	1	na	1.0	na	0	10%
DESSERT, 'No-no' frozen dessert	1 serving	75	2.0	17.0	36	na	0.0	0.0	0	0%
FISH DINNER										
cod, baked, Dijon, salad w/o dressing, oat bran bread	1 serving	427	44.0	21.0	567	na	18.0	na	68	38%
cod, baked, salad w/o dressing, oat bran bread	1 serving	364	43.0	20.0	371	na	12.0	na	68	30%
cod, broiled, Dijon, salad w/o dressing, oat bran bread	1 serving	427	44.0	21.0	567	na	18.0	na	68	38%
cod, broiled, salad w/o dressing, oat bran bread	1 serving	364	43.0	20.0	371	na	12.0	na	68	30%
cod, Cajun, salad w/o dressing, oat bran bread	1 serving	364	43.0	20.0	461	na	12.0	na	68	30%
MIXED VEGETABLES	1 serving	27	2.0	5.0	42	na	0.0	0.0	0	0%
PEAS	1 serving	77	6.0	13.0	131	na	0.0	0.0	0	0%
POTATO, BAKED	1 serving	163	5.0	37.0	7	na	0.0	0.0	0	0%
RICE	1 serving	114	3.0	25.0	633	na	0.0	0.0	0	0%
ROLL	1 roll	139	3.0	30.0	187	na	0.0	0.0	2	0%
SALAD										
chicken breast, Dijon	1 serving	391	42.0	31.0	415	na	11.0	na	65	25%
dinner, w/o dressing	1 serving	19	1.0	4.0	11	na	0.0	na	0	0%
SALAD DRESSING, buttermilk	1 serving	36	0.0	4.0	151	na	2.0	na	10	50%
SPAGHETTI DINNER										
marinara, salad w/o dressing, oat bran bread	1 serving	450	15.0	87.0	761	na	6.0	na	8	12%
TURKEY SANDWICH, pita, 'Heart Smart'	1 serving	224	22.0	24.0	833	na	5.0	na	75	20%
VEGETABLE STIR-FRY	1 serving	408	9.0	74.0	703	na	10.0	na	0	22%
YOGURT, FROZEN										
regular	1 serving	72	2.0	16.0	31	na	0.0	0.0	0	0%
shake	1 serving	184	8.0	36.0	127	na	0.0	na	2	0%
BOJANGLES										
BISCUIT	1 serving	239	4.0	30.0	588	na	11.0	na	1	41%
CHICKEN										
breast, skin-free, 'Southern'	4 oz	271	28.0	11.0	869	na	13.0	na	104	43%
leg, skin-free, 'Southern'	1.8 oz	128	7.0	5.0	312	na	12.0	na	54	84%
thigh, skin-free, 'Southern'	3.2 oz	264	19.0	10.0	592	na	17.0	na	88	58%
CHICKEN SANDWICH, fillet, grilled, w/o mayonnaise	1 serving	329	27.0	37.0	418	na	7.0	na	59	19%
COLESLAW	1 serving	105	1.0	19.0	406	na	4.0	na	0	34%
PINTO BEANS, Cajun	1 serving	124	6.0	25.0	463	na	0.0	na	0	0%
RICE, 'Dirty'	1 serving	167	5.0	21.0	397	na	7.0	na	12	38%
BONANZA RESTAURANTS										
HALIBUT, fillet	6 oz	139	26.0	3.0	128	na	2.0	na	60	13%
RIB EYE STEAK	5.5 oz	196	28.0	1.0	563	na	8.0	na	50	37%
BOSTON ROTISSERIE CHICKEN										
BAKED BEANS, barbecue	7.10 oz	290	11.0	47.0	653	8.0	7.3	2.5	7	23%
BROWNIE	3.36 oz	452	6.0	47.0	188	3.0	26.8	7.8	81	53%
CHICKEN										
1/2 chicken, w/skin	10.05 oz	642	76.0	na	964	na	38.5	13.5	307	54%
1/4 chicken, dark meat, w/skin	4.67 oz	330	34.0	2.0	443	na	21.6	6.8	151	59%
1/4 chicken, dark meat, w/o skin	3.65 oz	218	28.0	na	342	na	11.9	3.4	121	49%
1/4 chicken, white meat, w/skin	5.39 oz	332	42.0	2.0	524	na	17.7	5.2	150	48%
1/4 chicken, white meat, w/o skin and wing	3.68 oz	164	32.0	na	356	na	4.0	1.5	89	22%

Food Name	Serving Size	Calories	Prot. gms	Carbs gms	Sod. mgs	Fiber gms	Fat gms	Sat. Fat gms	Chol. mgs	% Fat Cal.
CHICKEN ENTRÉE										
1/4 chicken, white meat, corn bread, corn, new potatoes	1 entrée	726	na	na	1203	na	20.7	5.3	118	26%
1/4 chicken, white meat, corn bread, cranberry, new potatoes	1 entrée	917	na	na	1016	na	20.7	4.6	118	20%
1/4 chicken, white meat, corn bread, vegetables, corn	1 entrée	633	na	na	1073	na	17.5	4.6	118	25%
1/4 chicken, white meat, corn bread, vegetables, fruit	1 entrée	502	na	na	899	na	12.4	3.6	118	22%
CHICKEN POT PIE	15.01 oz	703	35.0	65.0	1895	4.0	34.2	8.9	109	44%
CHICKEN SALAD, chunky	5.57 oz	460	27.0	2.0	781	na	38.2	5.1	145	75%
CHICKEN SANDWICH										
breast, 9.13 oz	1 sandwich	422	42.0	50.0	885	3.0	4.0	1.0	99	9%
breast, w/fruit salad	1 sandwich	471	na	na	892	na	4.0	1.0	99	8%
chunky chicken salad, 12.11 oz	1 sandwich	763	39.0	49.0	1362	3.0	43.1	6.7	170	51%
CHICKEN SOUP	6.8 oz	87	12.0	4.0	500	na	2.6	0.6	31	27%
CHICKEN SOUP ENTRÉE										
w/corn bread, steamed vegetables, new potatoes	1 entrée	505	na	na	1176	na	14.0	3.4	61	25%
CHOCOLATE CHIP COOKIE	2.79 oz	369	4.0	51.0	238	2.0	16.4	5.6	27	40%
COLESLAW	6.49 oz	289	2.0	33.0	632	2.0	16.9	2.6	13	53%
CORN, buttered	5.14 oz	181	5.0	31.0	187	5.0	5.7	1.1	1	28%
CORNBREAD	2.4 oz	253	4.0	43.0	505	1.0	7.7	2.1	30	27%
CRANBERRY RELISH	7.95 oz	371	2.0	82.0	1	5.0	5.5	0.3	1	13%
CUCUMBER SALAD	4.79 oz	79	1.0	4.0	182	1.0	6.5	1.0	1	74%
FRUIT SALAD	4.4 oz	49	1.0	11.0	7	1.0	1.0	1.0	1	18%
MACARONI AND CHEESE	6.76 oz	290	12.0	35.0	896	2.0	11.0	5.4	19	34%
OATMEAL RAISIN COOKIE	2.79 oz	341	5.0	51.0	270	3.0	13.3	3.0	28	35%
PASTA SALAD										
Mediterranean	4.54 oz	160	4.0	16.0	617	3.0	9.0	2.3	12	51%
tortellini	5.62 oz	430	14.0	38.0	660	2.0	24.9	5.0	55	52%
POTATOES										
mashed, homemade, w/gravy	6.69 oz	205	3.0	27.0	514	2.0	9.7	5.6	25	43%
new	4.61 oz	129	2.0	22.0	156	3.0	3.5	0.7	1	24%
RICE PILAF	5.13 oz	188	4.0	32.0	684	1.0	4.9	1.0	1	23%
SPINACH, creamed	6.37 oz	298	9.0	12.0	791	3.0	24.2	15.2	71	73%
SQUASH, butternut	6.79 oz	247	2.0	37.0	978	4.0	10.9	6.7	28	40%
STUFFING	6.14 oz	282	6.0	40.0	1052	3.0	11.3	2.1	1	36%
VEGETABLES, steamed	3.69 oz	32	2.0	6.0	13	2.0	0.2	1.0	1	6%
ZUCCHINI, marinara	6.68 oz	80	2.0	10.0	503	3.0	3.9	0.6	1	44%
BRAUM'S										
YOGURT, FROZEN										
diet, sugar-free w/NutraSweet	1 serving	90	3.0	13.0	na	na	3.0	na	na	30%
fat-free	1 serving	90	4.0	20.0	55	na	0.0	na	na	0%
regular	1 serving	180	3.0	16.0	35	na	3.0	na	na	15%
BRESLER'S										
ICE CREAM, 'Royal Lites' all flavors	1 serving	132	5.0	9.0	70	na	5.0	na	16	34%
SHERBET, all flavors	1 serving	160	1.0	34.0	na	na	2.0	na	6	11%
YOGURT, FROZEN										
gourmet, all flavors	1 serving	116	4.0	22.0	na	na	2.0	na	7	16%
lite, all flavors	1 serving	108	4.0	24.0	na	na	0.0	0.0	0	0%
BURGER CHEF										
APPLE TURNOVER	1 serving	237	2.0	38.0	na	na	9.0	na	na	34%
BREAKFAST										
scrambled eggs and bacon platter	1 serving	567	21.0	50.0	1108	na	31.0	na	na	49%

Food Name	Serving Size	Calories	Prot. gms	Carbs gms	Sod. mgs	Fiber gms	Fat gms	Sat. Fat gms	Chol. mgs	% Fat Cal.
scrambled eggs and sausage platter	1 serving	668	26.0	50.0	1411	na	40.0	na	479	54%
w/bacon, 'Sunrise'	1 serving	392	19.0	30.0	978	na	21.0	na	384	48%
w/sausage, 'Sunrise'	1 serving	526	26.0	30.0	1412	na	33.0	na	419	56%
BREAKFAST SANDWICH, sausage biscuit	1 serving	418	16.0	33.0	1313	na	25.0	na	45	54%
CHEESEBURGER										
double	1 serving	402	23.0	28.0	835	na	22.0	na	74	49%
regular	1 serving	278	14.0	28.0	641	na	12.0	na	37	39%
CLUB SANDWICH, chicken	1 serving	521	36.0	33.0	na	na	25.0	na	na	43%
FISH SANDWICH, 'Fisherman's Fillet'	1 serving	534	26.0	41.0	na	na	32.0	na	na	54%
FRENCH FRIES										
large order	1 serving	285	4.0	36.0	456	na	14.0	na	na	44%
regular order	1 serving	204	3.0	26.0	327	na	10.0	na	na	44%
HAMBURGER										
'Big Chef'	1 serving	556	22.0	37.0	840	na	36.0	na	78	58%
mushroom	1 serving	520	28.0	34.0	744	na	29.0	na	92	50%
regular	1 serving	235	11.0	27.0	480	na	9.0	na	27	34%
'Super Chef'	1 serving	604	27.0	35.0	1088	na	39.0	na	99	58%
'Top Chef'	1 serving	541	30.0	29.0	1007	na	33.0	na	100	55%
HAMBURGER MEAL, 'Funmeal'	1 serving	514	14.0	85.0	513	na	19.0	na	27	33%
MILKSHAKE										
chocolate	1 serving	403	10.0	72.0	378	na	9.0	na	36	20%
vanilla	1 serving	380	13.0	60.0	325	na	10.0	na	40	24%
POTATOES, HASH BROWN	1 serving	235	3.0	26.0	349	na	14.0	na	na	54%
SALAD	1 serving	11	1.0	3.0	8	na	0.0	0.0	na	0%
BURGER KING										
APPLE PIE	1 serving	311	3.0	44.0	412	(mq)	14.0	4.0	4	41%
BACON BITS	1 pkt	10	1.0	0.0	na	na	1.0	na	5	56%
BAGEL										
plain	1 bagel	272	10.0	44.0	438	(mq)	6.0	1.0	29	20%
w/cream cheese	1 bagel	370	12.0	45.0	523	(mq)	16.0	6.0	58	39%
BARBECUE SAUCE										
	1 oz	36	0.0	9.0	397	na	0.0	0.0	0	0%
'Bull's-Eye'	.5 oz	22	0.0	5.0	47	na	0.0	0.0	0	0%
BISCUIT, plain	1 serving	332	5.0	42.0	754	(mq)	17.0	3.0	2	46%
BREAKFAST										
French toast sticks	1 serving	440	4.0	60.0	490	(mq)	27.0	7.0	0	55%
scrambled egg platter, regular	1 serving	549	17.0	44.0	893	(mq)	34.0	9.0	365	56%
scrambled egg platter, w/bacon	1 serving	610	21.0	44.0	1043	(mq)	39.0	11.0	373	58%
scrambled egg platter, w/sausage	1 serving	768	26.0	47.0	1271	(mq)	53.0	15.0	412	62%
BREAKFAST SANDWICH										
bagel, w/bacon, egg, and cheese	1 serving	453	21.0	46.0	872	(mq)	20.0	7.0	252	40%
bagel, w/egg and cheese	1 serving	407	19.0	46.0	759	(mq)	16.0	5.0	247	35%
bagel, w/ham, egg, and cheese	1 serving	438	25.0	46.0	1114	(mq)	17.0	6.0	266	35%
bagel, w/sausage, egg, and cheese	1 serving	626	27.0	49.0	1137	(mq)	36.0	12.0	293	52%
biscuit, w/bacon	1 serving	378	8.0	42.0	867	(mq)	20.0	5.0	8	48%
biscuit, w/bacon and egg	1 serving	467	14.0	43.0	1033	(mq)	27.0	7.0	213	52%
biscuit, w/sausage	1 serving	478	11.0	44.0	1007	(mq)	29.0	8.0	33	55%
biscuit, w/sausage and egg	1 serving	568	17.0	45.0	1172	(mq)	36.0	10.0	238	57%
'Breakfast Buddy'	1 serving	255	11.0	15.0	492	na	16.0	6.0	127	56%
'Croissan'wich' w/bacon, egg, and cheese	1 serving	353	16.0	19.0	780	(mq)	23.0	8.0	230	59%
'Croissan'wich' w/egg and cheese	1 serving	315	13.0	19.0	607	(mq)	20.0	7.0	222	57%
'Croissan'wich' w/ham, egg, and cheese	1 serving	351	19.0	20.0	1373	(mq)	22.0	7.0	236	56%
'Croissan'wich' w/sausage, egg, and cheese	1 serving	534	21.0	22.0	985	(mq)	40.0	14.0	258	67%

Food Name	Serving Size	Calories	Prot. gms	Carbs gms	Sod. mgs	Fiber gms	Fat gms	Sat. Fat gms	Chol. mgs	% Fat Cal.
CHEESE										
American	.9 oz	92	5.0	1.0	312	0	7.0	5.0	25	68%
Swiss	.9 oz	82	6.0	1.0	352	0	6.0	4.0	20	66%
CHEESEBURGER										
bacon, double	1 serving	515	32.0	26.0	748	(mq)	31.0	14.0	105	54%
bacon, double, 'Deluxe'	1 serving	592	33.0	28.0	804	(mq)	39.0	16.0	111	59%
barbecue bacon, double	1 serving	536	32.0	31.0	795	(mq)	31.0	14.0	105	52%
'Deluxe'	1 serving	390	18.0	29.0	652	(mq)	23.0	8.0	56	53%
double	1 serving	483	30.0	29.0	851	(mq)	27.0	13.0	100	50%
'Mushroom Swiss' double	1 serving	473	31.0	27.0	746	(mq)	27.0	12.0	95	51%
regular	1 serving	318	17.0	28.0	651	(mq)	15.0	7.0	48	42%
'Whopper' double, w/cheese	1 serving	935	51.0	47.0	1245	(mq)	61.0	24.0	194	59%
'Whopper Jr.'	1 serving	380	16.0	29.0	660	na	22.0	7.0	50	52%
'Whopper' w/cheese	1 serving	706	32.0	47.0	1177	(mq)	44.0	16.0	115	56%
CHICKEN, 'Chicken Tenders'	6 pieces	236	16.0	14.0	541	(mq)	13.0	3.0	46	50%
CHICKEN SANDWICH										
'B.K. Broiler'	1 serving	379	24.0	31.0	764	(mq)	18.0	3.0	53	43%
regular	1 serving	685	26.0	56.0	1417	(mq)	40.0	8.0	82	53%
CREAM CHEESE	1 oz	98	2.0	1.0	86	0	10.0	5.0	28	92%
CROISSANT	1 serving	180	4.0	18.0	285	(mq)	10.0	2.0	4	50%
CROUTONS	.25 oz	31	1.0	5.0	90	na	1.0	na	na	29%
DANISH										
apple cinnamon	1 serving	390	6.0	62.0	305	(mq)	13.0	3.0	19	30%
cheese	1 serving	406	6.0	60.0	454	(mq)	16.0	5.0	7	35%
cinnamon raisin	1 serving	449	7.0	63.0	286	(mq)	18.0	4.0	15	36%
FISH SANDWICH, fillet, 'Ocean Catch'	1 serving	495	20.0	49.0	879	(mq)	25.0	4.0	57	45%
FRENCH FRIES, med order	1 serving	372	5.0	43.0	238	(mq)	20.0	5.0	0	48%
HAMBURGER										
'Burger Buddies'	1 serving	349	18.0	31.0	717	(mq)	17.0	7.0	52	44%
'Deluxe'	1 serving	344	15.0	28.0	496	(mq)	19.0	6.0	43	50%
regular	1 serving	272	15.0	28.0	505	(mq)	11.0	4.0	37	36%
'Whopper'	1 serving	614	27.0	45.0	865	(mq)	36.0	12.0	90	53%
'Whopper' double	1 serving	844	46.0	45.0	933	(mq)	53.0	19.0	169	57%
'Whopper Jr.'	1 serving	330	14.0	28.0	500	na	19.0	5.0	40	52%
HONEY SAUCE	1 oz	91	0.0	23.0	12	na	0.0	0.0	0	0%
LETTUCE	.75 oz	3	0.0	0.0	2	na	0.0	0.0	0	0%
MAYONNAISE	1 oz	194	0.0	2.0	142	0	21.0	4.0	16	97%
MILKSHAKE										
chocolate	1 serving	326	9.0	49.0	198	na	10.0	6.0	31	28%
chocolate, syrup added	1 serving	409	10.0	68.0	248	na	11.0	6.0	33	24%
strawberry, syrup added	1 serving	394	9.0	66.0	230	na	10.0	6.0	33	23%
vanilla	1 serving	334	9.0	51.0	213	(tr)	10.0	6.0	33	27%
MUFFIN										
blueberry, mini	1 serving	292	4.0	37.0	244	(mq)	14.0	3.0	72	43%
lemon poppyseed, mini	1 serving	318	5.0	33.0	253	(mq)	18.0	3.0	72	51%
MUSTARD	1 pkt	2	0.0	0.0	34	na	0.0	0.0	0	0%
ONION	.25 oz	5	0.0	1.0	0	(mq)	0.0	0.0	0	0%
ONION RINGS	1 serving	339	5.0	38.0	628	(mq)	19.0	5.0	0	50%
PICKLE	.5 oz	1	0.0	0.0	119	(mq)	0.0	0.0	0	0%
POTATOES, HASH BROWN, 'Tater Tenders'	1 serving	213	2.0	25.0	318	(mq)	12.0	3.0	0	51%
RANCH SAUCE	1 oz	171	0.0	2.0	208	na	18.0	3.0	0	95%
SALAD										
chef's, w/o dressing	1 serving	178	17.0	7.0	568	(mq)	9.0	4.0	103	46%
chunky chicken, w/o dressing	1 serving	142	20.0	8.0	443	(mq)	4.0	1.0	49	25%

Food Name	Serving Size	Calories	Prot. gms	Carbs gms	Sod. mgs	Fiber gms	Fat gms	Sat. Fat gms	Chol. mgs	% Fat Cal.
garden, w/o dressing	1 serving	95	6.0	8.0	125	(mq)	5.0	3.0	15	47%
side salad, w/o dressing	1 serving	25	1.0	5.0	27	(mq)	0.0	0.0	0	0%
SALAD DRESSING										
blue cheese, 'Newman's Own'	1 pkt	300	3.0	2.0	512	0	32.0	7.0	58	96%
French, 'Newman's Own'	1 pkt	290	0.0	23.0	400	na	22.0	3.0	0	68%
Italian, reduced calorie, 'Newman's Own'	1 pkt	170	0.0	3.0	762	na	18.0	3.0	0	95%
olive oil and vinegar, 'Newman's Own'	1 pkt	310	0.0	2.0	214	0	33.0	5.0	0	96%
ranch, 'Newman's Own'	1 pkt	350	1.0	4.0	316	na	37.0	7.0	20	95%
Thousand Island, 'Newman's Own'	1 pkt	290	1.0	15.0	403	na	26.0	5.0	36	81%
SANDWICH SAUCE										
'B.K. Broiler'	.5 oz	90	0.0	0.0	95	na	10.0	1.0	7	100%
'Burger King A.M. Express'	1 oz	84	0.0	21.0	18	na	0.0	0.0	0	0%
SWEET AND SOUR SAUCE	1 oz	45	0.0	11.0	52	na	0.0	0.0	0	0%
TARTAR SAUCE	1 oz	134	0.0	2.0	202	na	14.0	2.0	20	94%
TOMATO	1 oz	6	0.0	1.0	3	(mq)	0.0	0.0	0	0%
CAPTAIN D'S										
BEANS										
green, seasoned	1 serving	46	2.0	5.0	752	na	2.0	na	4	39%
white	1 serving	126	8.0	22.0	99	na	1.0	na	2	7%
BREADSTICKS	1 stick	91	3.0	17.0	210	na	1.0	na	0	10%
CHICKEN ENTRÉE, w/rice, green beans, breadstick, salad	1 serving	414	30.0	55.0	2615	na	8.0	na	71	17%
COCKTAIL SAUCE	2 tbsp	34	0.0	8.0	252	na	0.0	0.0	0	0%
CRACKER	4 crackers	50	1.0	8.0	147	na	1.0	na	3	18%
FISH DINNER										
baked, w/rice, green beans, breadstick, coleslaw	1 serving	659	36.0	62.0	1767	na	30.0	na	54	41%
orange roughy, w/rice, green beans, breadstick, salad	1 serving	537	35.0	56.0	2156	na	19.0	na	39	32%
RICE	1 serving	124	0.0	28.0	9	na	0.0	na	0	0%
SALAD, dinner, w/o dressing	1 serving	27	1.0	3.0	67	na	1.0	na	1	33%
SALAD DRESSING, Italian, low-calorie	2 tbsp	9	0.0	2.0	568	na	0.0	0.0	0	0%
SHRIMP ENTRÉE, w/rice, green beans, breadstick, salad	1 serving	457	56.0	34.0	2194	na	10.0	na	191	20%
SWEET AND SOUR SAUCE	2 tbsp	52	0.0	13.0	5	na	0.0	0.0	0	0%
CARL'S JR.										
BREAKFAST										
bacon, 2 strips, .4 oz	1 serving	50	3.0	0.0	200	0	4.0	3.0	8	72%
eggs, scrambled, 2.4 oz	1 serving	120	9.0	2.0	105	0	9.0	4.0	245	68%
French toast dips, w/o syrup	1 serving	480	8.0	54.0	576	(mq)	25.0	10.0	54	47%
hotcakes, w/margarine, w/o syrup	1 serving	360	7.0	59.0	1190	(mq)	12.0	3.0	15	30%
sausage, 1 patty, .5 oz	1 serving	190	7.0	1.0	275	0	17.0	4.0	25	81%
'Sunrise' w/bacon, 4.5 oz	1 serving	370	17.0	32.0	750	(mq)	19.0	8.0	120	46%
'Sunrise' w/sausage, 6.1 oz	1 serving	500	22.0	31.0	990	(mq)	32.0	12.0	165	58%
BROCCOLI SOUP, cream of	6.6 oz	140	7.0	14.0	845	(mq)	6.0	4.0	22	39%
BROWNIE, fudge, 4.5 oz	1 serving	597	8.0	88.0	295	(mq)	27.0	7.0	tr	41%
CAKE										
chocolate, 3 oz	1 serving	300	3.0	49.0	262	na	11.0	3.0	25	33%
fudge moussecake	4 oz	400	5.0	42.0	85	na	23.0	11.0	110	52%
CHEESE										
American, .6 oz	1 slice	60	4.0	1.0	290	na	5.0	3.0	15	75%
Swiss, .6 oz	1 slice	60	4.0	1.0	220	na	4.0	3.0	15	60%
CHEESEBURGER										
'Double Western Bacon' 11.6 oz	1 serving	1030	56.0	58.0	1810	na	63.0	32.0	145	55%
'Western Bacon' approx 8 oz	1 serving	730	34.0	59.0	1490	na	39.0	20.0	90	48%
CHEESECAKE	3.5 oz	310	7.0	32.0	200	na	17.0	8.0	60	49%

Food Name	Serving Size	Calories	Prot. gms	Carbs gms	Sod. mgs	Fiber gms	Fat gms	Sat. Fat gms	Chol. mgs	% Fat Cal.
CHICKEN NOODLE SOUP, 'Old Fashioned'	6.6 oz	80	4.0	11.0	605	(mq)	1.0	tr	14	11%
CHICKEN SANDWICH										
'Charbroiler BBQ' 'Lite Menu'	1 serving	310	25.0	34.0	680	na	6.0	2.0	30	17%
'Charbroiler Chicken Club' 8.8 oz	1 serving	570	35.0	42.0	1160	na	29.0	8.0	60	46%
'Santa Fe' 7.9 oz	1 serving	530	30.0	36.0	1230	na	29.0	7.0	85	49%
'Teriyaki' 'Lite Menu'	1 serving	330	28.0	42.0	830	na	6.0	2.0	55	16%
CHICKEN STRIPS	6 strips	260	19.0	11.0	600	na	19.0	5.0	25	66%
CHOWDER, Boston clam	6.6 oz	140	6.0	12.0	861	(mq)	8.0	3.0	22	51%
CINNAMON ROLL, 4 oz	1 serving	460	7.0	70.0	230	na	18.0	1.0	0	35%
COOKIE, chocolate chip, 2.5 oz	1 serving	330	4.0	41.0	170	na	17.0	7.0	5	46%
DANISH										
all varieties, except cheese	1 serving	520	7.0	75.0	230	na	16.0	4.0	0	28%
cheese	4 oz	520	7.0	75.0	230	na	22.0	4.0	0	38%
ENGLISH MUFFIN, w/margarine, 2 oz	1 muffin	180	4.0	28.0	275	(mq)	6.0	2.0	0	30%
FISH SANDWICH										
'Carl's Catch'	1 serving	560	17.0	54.0	1220	na	30.0	4.0	5	48%
fillet, 7.9 oz	1 serving	550	22.0	58.0	945	(mq)	26.0	11.0	90	43%
FRENCH FRIES										
'CrissCut' regular, approx 3.2 oz	1 serving	330	4.0	27.0	890	na	22.0	3.0	tr	60%
regular	1 serving	420	4.0	54.0	200	na	20.0	5.0	0	43%
HAMBURGER										
'Carl's Original' 6.8 oz	1 serving	460	25.0	46.0	810	na	20.0	9.0	50	39%
'Famous Star' 8.6 oz	1 serving	610	26.0	42.0	890	na	38.0	13.0	50	56%
'Happy Star' 3 oz	1 serving	220	12.0	26.0	445	(mq)	8.0	4.0	45	33%
'Old Time Star ' 5.9 oz	1 serving	400	24.0	38.0	760	(mq)	17.0	7.0	80	38%
regular, 4.3 oz	1 serving	320	17.0	33.0	590	na	14.0	5.0	35	39%
'Super Star' 11.25 oz	1 serving	820	43.0	41.0	1210	na	53.0	24.0	105	58%
ICED TEA, regular size	20 oz	2	0.0	0.0	0	na	0.0	0.0	0	0%
MILK, 1% lowfat	10 oz	150	14.0	19.0	200	na	3.0	2.0	13	18%
MILKSHAKE, regular	11.6 oz	350	11.0	61.0	230	na	7.0	4.0	15	18%
MUFFIN										
blueberry, 4.2 oz	1 muffin	340	5.0	61.0	300	na	9.0	1.0	45	24%
bran, 4.7 oz	1 muffin	310	6.0	52.0	370	na	7.0	0.0	60	20%
ONION RINGS										
5.3-oz order	1 serving	520	9.0	63.0	960	na	26.0	6.0	0	45%
3.2-oz order	1 serving	310	4.0	38.0	260	(mq)	15.0	7.0	10	44%
ORANGE JUICE, small, 8.7 oz	1 serving	90	2.0	21.0	2	na	1.0	0.0	0	10%
POTATO, BAKED, 'Fiesta' 15.2 oz	1 serving	550	25.0	60.0	1230	(mq)	23.0	9.0	40	38%
ROAST BEEF SANDWICH										
'California Roast Beef 'n Swiss'	1 serving	360	31.0	43.0	1070	(mq)	8.0	4.0	130	20%
'Club'	1 serving	620	30.0	48.0	1950	na	34.0	11.0	45	49%
'Deluxe' 9.3 oz	1 serving	540	28.0	46.0	1340	na	26.0	10.0	40	43%
SALAD										
salad-to-go, chef's, 10.7 oz	1 serving	180	19.0	11.0	581	(mq)	7.0	3.0	63	35%
salad-to-go, chicken, 'Lite Menu'	1 serving	200	24.0	8.0	300	na	8.0	4.0	70	36%
salad-to-go, chicken, 12 oz	1 serving	200	24.0	8.0	300	na	8.0	4.0	70	36%
salad-to-go, garden, 4.8 oz	1 serving	50	3.0	4.0	75	na	3.0	2.0	5	54%
salad-to-go, garden, 'Lite Menu'	1 serving	50	3.0	4.0	75	na	3.0	2.0	5	54%
salad-to-go, taco, 14.3 oz	1 serving	356	29.0	18.0	690	(mq)	19.0	6.0	99	48%
SALAD DRESSING										
1000 Island	1 oz	110	0.0	4.0	200	na	11.0	3.0	5	90%
blue cheese	1 oz	150	1.0	0.0	250	na	15.0	3.0	20	90%
French, reduced calorie	1 oz	40	0.0	5.0	292	na	2.0	0.0	0	45%
house	1 oz	110	1.0	2.0	170	(tr)	11.0	3.0	10	90%

Food Name	Serving Size	Calories	Prot. gms	Carbs gms	Sod. mgs	Fiber gms	Fat gms	Sat. Fat gms	Chol. mgs	% Fat Cal.
Italian	1 oz	120	0.0	1.0	210	(tr)	13.0	2.0	0	98%
Italian, reduced calorie	1 oz	40	0.0	5.0	290	na	2.0	0.0	0	45%
SALSA	1 oz	8	0.0	2.0	210	na	0.0	0.0	0	0%
STEAK SANDWICH, country-fried, 7.2 oz	1 serving	610	25.0	54.0	1290	(mq)	33.0	12.0	45	49%
TURKEY SANDWICH, 'Club' 9.3 oz	1 serving	530	30.0	50.0	2890	na	23.0	6.0	60	39%
VEGETABLE SOUP, 'Lumber Jack Mix'	6.6 oz	70	2.0	10.0	807	(mq)	3.0	tr	3	39%
ZUCCHINI										
fried, 4.3 oz	1 serving	300	5.0	33.0	480	(mq)	16.0	7.0	10	48%
fried, 6 oz	1 serving	390	7.0	38.0	1040	na	23.0	6.0	0	53%
CARVEL										
ICE CREAM										
'Carvella'	1 serving	164	4.0	16.0	92	na	8.0	na	61	44%
'Thinny-Thin'	1 serving	92	4.0	16.0	80	na	0.0	na	4	0%
ICE CREAM CONE										
plain	1 cone	25	1.0	5.0	25	na	0.0	0.0	na	0%
sugar	1 cone	45	1.0	10.0	30	na	1.0	na	na	20%
YOGURT, FROZEN										
'Lo-Yo'	1 serving	124	4.0	20.0	76	na	4.0	na	16	29%
sugar-free, low-fat	1 serving	104	4.0	20.0	80	na	4.0	na	8	35%
CHICK-FIL-A										
BROWNIE, fudge, w/nuts, 2.8 oz	1 brownie	369	5.0	45.0	213	>.5 c	19.0	na	30	46%
CHEESECAKE										
plain, 3.2 oz	1 slice	299	6.6	24.7	272	>1.0 c	19.1	na	13	57%
w/blueberry topping, 4.3 oz	1 slice	350	6.8	37.3	294	>1.0 c	19.2	na	13	49%
w/strawberry topping, 4.3 oz	1 slice	343	6.9	35.2	309	>1.0 c	19.2	na	13	50%
CHICKEN ENTRÉE, salad plate	11.8 oz	875	29.0	60.0	1839	na	63.0	na	97	65%
CHICKEN NUGGET										
'Chick-Fil-A Nuggets' 8 pack	4 oz	287	28.0	13.0	1326	na	15.0	na	61	47%
'Chick-Fil-A Nuggets' 12 pack	6 oz	430	42.0	19.0	1989	na	23.0	na	92	48%
'Grilled 'n Lites' 2 skewers	1 serving	97	20.0	4.0	280	na	2.0	na	3	19%
CHICKEN SANDWICH										
chargrilled	1 serving	258	30.0	24.0	1121	na	5.0	na	40	17%
chargrilled 'Deluxe' w/lettuce and tomato	1 serving	266	31.0	26.0	1125	na	na	5.0	40	0%
'Chick-Fil-A' w/bun	1 serving	426	42.0	40.0	1174	na	9.0	na	66	19%
'Chick-Fil-A' w/o bun	1 serving	219	36.0	2.0	552	na	7.0	na	42	29%
'Chick-Fil-A Deluxe'	1 serving	368	41.0	30.0	1178	na	9.0	na	66	22%
'Chick-n-Q'	1 serving	409	28.0	41.0	1197	na	15.0	na	10	33%
salad, on wheat bread	5.7 oz	449	10.0	35.0	888	na	26.0	na	50	52%
CHICKEN SOUP										
'Hearty Breast of Chicken' large	17.5 oz	432	52.0	36.0	1746	na	9.0	na	92	19%
'Hearty Breast of Chicken' medium	14 oz	230	27.0	19.0	890	na	5.0	na	80	20%
'Hearty Breast of Chicken' small	1 serving	152	16.0	11.0	530	na	3.0	na	46	18%
COLESLAW	1 cup	175	1.0	11.0	158	na	14.0	na	13	72%
FRENCH FRIES, waffle, small order	3 oz	270	3.0	33.0	45	na	14.0	na	8	47%
ICE CREAM, 'Ice Dream' small cup	4.5 oz	134	4.0	19.0	51	na	5.0	na	24	34%
ICED TEA, unsweetened	9 oz	3	0.0	0.0	0	na	0.0	na	0	0%
LEMON PIE	1 slice	329	8.0	64.0	300	na	5.0	na	7	14%
LEMONADE, regular	10 oz	124	tr	32.0	tr	na	tr	na	tr	0%
ORANGE JUICE	6 oz	82	1.0	20.0	2	na	tr	na	0	0%
SALAD										
carrot-raisin	1 cup	116	1.0	18.0	8	na	5.0	na	6	39%
chargrilled chicken garden, w/o dressing	1 serving	126	20.0	8.0	567	na	2.0	na	28	14%

Food Name	Serving Size	Calories	Prot. gms	Carbs gms	Sod. mgs	Fiber gms	Fat gms	Sat. Fat gms	Chol. mgs	% Fat Cal.
chicken, cup, 4 oz	1 serving	309	12.0	4.0	543	na	28.0	na	21	82%
potato	1 cup	198	3.0	14.0	337	na	15.0	na	6	68%
tossed	1 serving	21	1.0	4.0	19	na	0.0	na	0	0%
tossed, w/blue cheese dressing	6 oz	243	3.0	6.0	475	>2.0 c	24.0	na	38	89%
tossed, w/honey French dressing	6 oz	277	1.0	21.0	396	>2.0 c	21.0	na	0	68%
tossed, w/lite Italian dressing	6 oz	43	1.0	7.0	856	>2.0 c	1.2	na	0	25%
tossed, w/lite ranch dressing	6 oz	114	1.0	13.2	292	>2.0 c	6.3	na	6	50%
tossed, w/ranch dressing	6 oz	298	1.0	6.0	387	>2.0 c	30.0	na	5	91%
tossed, w/Thousand Island dressing	6 oz	250	1.0	12.0	396	>2.0 c	22.0	na	25	79%
SALAD DRESSING, Italian, lite	3 tbsp	43	1.0	7.0	856	na	1.0	na	0	21%

CHURCH'S FRIED CHICKEN

Food Name	Serving Size	Calories	Prot. gms	Carbs gms	Sod. mgs	Fiber gms	Fat gms	Sat. Fat gms	Chol. mgs	% Fat Cal.
APPLE PIE	3.1 oz	280	2.3	40.5	340	1.0	12.3	na	<5	40%
BISCUIT	2.1 oz	250	2.2	25.6	640	1.0	16.4	na	<5	59%
CHICKEN										
breast, boneless, 2.8 oz	1 serving	200	19.0	4.3	510	0	12.4	na	65	56%
breast, fried, 4.3 oz	1 serving	278	21.0	9.0	560	na	17.0	na	na	55%
breast, wing, fried, 4.8 oz	1 serving	303	22.0	9.0	583	na	20.0	na	na	59%
leg, 2.9 oz	1 serving	147	13.0	5.0	286	na	9.0	na	na	55%
leg, boneless, 2 oz	1 serving	140	12.7	2.4	160	0	9.1	na	45	59%
thigh, 4.2 oz	1 serving	306	19.0	9.0	448	na	22.0	na	na	65%
thigh, boneless, 2.8 oz	1 serving	230	16.2	5.3	520	0	16.2	na	80	63%
wing, boneless, 3.1 oz	1 serving	250	18.5	7.7	540	0	16.1	na	60	58%
CHICKEN FILLET										
breast	1 serving	608	27.0	46.0	725	na	34.0	na	na	50%
breast, w/cheese	1 serving	661	30.0	47.0	921	na	38.0	na	na	52%
COLESLAW	3 oz	92	4.2	8.4	230	2.0	5.5	na	0	54%
CORN										
on the cob	5.7 oz	190	7.8	32.4	15	4.0	5.4	na	0	26%
on the cob, w/butter oil	1 ear	237	4.0	33.0	20	na	9.0	na	na	34%
DESSERT, frozen	1 serving	180	4.0	27.0	65	na	6.0	na	na	30%
FISH FILLET										
regular	1 serving	430	20.0	45.0	675	na	18.0	na	na	38%
w/cheese	1 serving	483	23.0	46.0	870	na	22.0	na	na	41%
FRENCH FRIES										
large order	1 serving	320	3.0	40.0	185	na	16.0	na	na	45%
regular order, 2.7 oz	1 serving	210	3.3	28.5	60	2.0	10.5	na	0	45%
HOT DOG										
super	1 serving	520	17.0	44.0	1365	na	27.0	na	na	47%
super, w/cheese	1 serving	580	22.0	45.0	1605	na	34.0	na	na	53%
super, w/chili	1 serving	570	21.0	47.0	1595	na	32.0	na	na	51%
w/cheese	1 serving	330	15.0	21.0	990	na	21.0	na	na	57%
w/chili	1 serving	320	13.0	23.0	985	na	20.0	na	na	56%
HUSHPUPPY	2 pieces	156	3.0	23.0	110	na	6.0	na	na	35%
OKRA	2.8 oz	210	2.7	19.1	520	4.0	16.1	na	0	69%
ONION RINGS	1 serving	280	4.0	31.0	140	na	16.0	na	na	51%
POTATOES, MASHED, w/gravy	3.7 oz	90	1.2	14.0	520	1.0	3.3	na	0	33%
RICE, Cajun	3.1 oz	130	1.3	15.6	260	<1.0	7.0	na	5	48%

COLOMBO
YOGURT, FROZEN

Food Name	Serving Size	Calories	Prot. gms	Carbs gms	Sod. mgs	Fiber gms	Fat gms	Sat. Fat gms	Chol. mgs	% Fat Cal.
lite, nonfat	4 oz	95	4.0	21.0	70	na	0.0	na	0	0%
low-fat	4 oz	99	3.0	18.0	35	na	2.0	na	10	18%

Food Name	Serving Size	Calories	Prot. gms	Carbs gms	Sod. mgs	Fiber gms	Fat gms	Sat. Fat gms	Chol. mgs	% Fat Cal.
DAIRY QUEEN/BRAZIER										
BANANA SPLIT	13 oz	510	9.0	93.0	250	(mq)	11.0	8.0	30	19%
BARBECUE SANDWICH, beef	4.5 oz	225	12.0	34.0	700	(mq)	4.0	1.0	20	16%
BARBECUE SAUCE	1 pkg	41	0.0	9.0	130	na	0.0	na	0	0%
BROWNIE, hot fudge, 'Brownie Delight' 10.8 oz	1 serving	710	11.0	102.0	340	na	29.0	14.0	35	37%
CAKE										
frozen, undecorated	5.8-oz slice	380	6.0	50.0	210	na	18.0	8.0	20	43%
strawberry shortcake	1 serving	540	10.0	100.0	215	na	11.0	na	25	18%
CHEESEBURGER										
double, 8 oz	1 serving	570	37.0	31.0	1070	(mq)	34.0	18.0	120	54%
single, 5.5 oz	1 serving	365	20.0	30.0	800	(mq)	18.0	9.0	60	44%
triple	1 serving	820	58.0	34.0	1010	na	50.0	na	140	55%
CHICKEN NUGGET, all white meat	1 serving	276	16.0	13.0	505	na	18.0	na	39	59%
CHICKEN SANDWICH										
fillet, breaded	6.7 oz	430	24.0	37.0	760	(mq)	20.0	4.0	55	42%
fillet, breaded, w/cheese	7.2 oz	480	27.0	38.0	980	(mq)	25.0	7.0	70	47%
fillet, grilled	6.5 oz	300	25.0	33.0	800	(mq)	8.0	2.0	50	24%
FISH SANDWICH										
fillet	6 oz	370	16.0	39.0	630	(mq)	16.0	3.0	45	39%
fillet, w/cheese	6.5 oz	420	19.0	40.0	850	(mq)	21.0	6.0	60	45%
FRENCH FRIES										
large order	4.5 oz	390	5.0	52.0	200	(mq)	18.0	4.0	0	42%
regular order	3.5 oz	300	4.0	40.0	160	(mq)	14.0	3.0	0	42%
FROZEN DESSERT. See also individual listings.										
'Blizzard' Heath, regular	14.3 oz	820	16.0	114.0	410	na	36.0	17.0	60	40%
'Blizzard' Heath, small	10.3 oz	560	11.0	79.0	280	na	23.0	11.0	40	37%
'Blizzard' strawberry, regular	13.5 oz	740	13.0	92.0	230	na	16.0	11.0	50	19%
'Blizzard' strawberry, small	9.4 oz	500	9.0	64.0	160	na	12.0	8.0	35	22%
'Breeze' Heath, regular	13.4 oz	680	15.0	113.0	360	na	21.0	6.0	15	28%
'Breeze' Heath, small	9.6 oz	450	11.0	78.0	230	na	12.0	3.0	10	24%
'Breeze' strawberry, regular	12.5 oz	590	12.0	90.0	170	na	1.0	<1.0	5	2%
'Breeze' strawberry, small	8.7 oz	400	9.0	63.0	115	na	<1.0	<1.0	5	0%
'Buster Bar'	5.3 oz	450	11.0	40.0	220	na	29.0	9.0	15	58%
'Chipper Sandwich'	1 serving	318	5.0	56.0	170	na	7.0	na	13	20%
'Dilly Bar'	3 oz	210	3.0	21.0	50	na	13.0	6.0	10	56%
'Double Delight'	1 serving	490	9.0	69.0	150	na	20.0	na	25	37%
'DQ Sandwich'	1 serving	140	3.0	24.0	40	na	4.0	na	5	26%
'Float'	1 serving	410	5.0	82.0	85	na	7.0	na	20	15%
'Freeze'	1 serving	500	9.0	89.0	180	na	12.0	na	30	22%
'Fudge Nut Bar'	1 serving	406	8.0	40.0	167	na	25.0	na	10	55%
'Mr. Misty' large	1 serving	340	tr	84.0	10	na	tr	na	0	0%
'Mr. Misty' regular, 11.6 oz	1 serving	250	tr	63.0	10	na	tr	0.0	0	0%
'Mr. Misty Float'	1 serving	390	5.0	74.0	95	na	7.0	na	20	16%
'Mr. Misty Freeze'	1 serving	500	9.0	91.0	140	na	12.0	na	30	22%
'Nutty Double Fudge'	9.7 oz	580	10.0	85.0	170	(mq)	22.0	10.0	35	34%
'Peanut Buster Parfait'	10.8 oz	710	16.0	94.0	410	(mq)	32.0	10.0	30	41%
'QC Big Scoop' chocolate	4.5 oz	310	5.0	40.0	100	na	14.0	10.0	35	41%
'QC Big Scoop' vanilla	4.5 oz	300	5.0	39.0	100	na	14.0	9.0	35	42%
HAMBURGER										
double, 7 oz	1 serving	460	31.0	29.0	630	(mq)	25.0	12.0	95	49%
'Homestyle Ultimate' 9.7 oz	1 serving	700	43.0	30.0	1110	(mq)	47.0	21.0	140	60%
single, 5oz	1 serving	310	17.0	29.0	580	(mq)	13.0	6.0	45	38%
triple	1 serving	710	51.0	33.0	690	na	45.0	na	135	57%

Food Name	Serving Size	Calories	Prot. gms	Carbs gms	Sod. mgs	Fiber gms	Fat gms	Sat. Fat gms	Chol. mgs	% Fat Cal.
HOT DOG										
'DQ Hounder'	1 serving	480	16.0	21.0	1800	na	36.0	na	80	68%
'DQ Hounder' w/cheese	1 serving	533	19.0	22.0	1995	na	40.0	na	89	68%
'DQ Hounder' w/chili	1 serving	575	22.0	25.0	1900	na	41.0	na	89	64%
'1/4 lb Super Dog' 7 oz	1 serving	590	20.0	41.0	1360	(mq)	38.0	16.0	60	58%
regular, 3.5 oz	1 serving	280	9.0	23.0	700	(mq)	16.0	6.0	25	51%
regular, w/cheese, 4 oz	1 serving	330	12.0	24.0	920	(mq)	21.0	9.0	35	57%
regular, w/chili, 4.5 oz	1 serving	320	11.0	26.0	720	(mq)	19.0	7.0	30	53%
super, w/cheese	1 serving	580	22.0	45.0	1605	na	34.0	na	100	53%
super, w/chili	1 serving	570	21.0	47.0	1595	na	32.0	na	100	51%
ICE CREAM CONE										
chocolate, 'Queen's Choice'	1 serving	326	5.0	40.0	84	na	16.0	na	52	44%
chocolate, dipped, large	1 serving	570	9.0	64.0	145	na	24.0	na	30	38%
chocolate, dipped, regular, 5.5 oz	1 serving	330	6.0	40.0	100	(mq)	16.0	8.0	20	44%
chocolate, large, 7.5 oz	1 serving	350	8.0	54.0	170	(mq)	11.0	8.0	30	28%
chocolate, regular, 5 oz	1 serving	230	6.0	36.0	115	(mq)	7.0	5.0	20	27%
vanilla, 'Queen's Choice'	1 serving	322	4.0	40.0	71	na	16.0	na	52	45%
vanilla, large, 7.5 oz	1 serving	340	9.0	53.0	140	(mq)	10.0	7.0	30	26%
vanilla, regular, 5 oz	1 serving	230	6.0	36.0	95	(mq)	7.0	5.0	20	27%
vanilla, small, 3 oz	1 serving	140	4.0	22.0	60	(mq)	4.0	3.0	15	26%
LETTUCE	.5 oz	2	0.0	0.0	1	na	0.0	na	0	0%
MALT										
chocolate, large	1 serving	1060	20.0	187.0	360	na	25.0	na	70	21%
chocolate, regular	1 serving	760	14.0	134.0	260	na	18.0	na	50	21%
chocolate, small	1 serving	520	10.0	91.0	180	na	13.0	na	35	23%
'Queen' large, 21 oz	1 serving	889	16.0	157.0	304	na	21.0	na	60	21%
vanilla, regular, 14.7 oz	1 serving	610	13.0	106.0	230	na	14.0	8.0	45	21%
MILKSHAKE										
chocolate, large	1 serving	990	19.0	168.0	360	na	26.0	na	70	24%
chocolate, regular, 14 oz	1 serving	540	12.0	94.0	290	na	14.0	8.0	45	23%
chocolate, small	1 serving	490	10.0	82.0	180	na	13.0	na	35	24%
'Queen' large, 21 oz	1 serving	831	16.0	140.0	304	na	22.0	na	60	24%
vanilla, large, 16.3 oz	1 serving	600	13.0	101.0	260	na	16.0	10.0	50	24%
vanilla, regular, 14 oz	1 serving	520	12.0	88.0	230	na	14.0	8.0	45	24%
ONION RINGS	3 oz	240	4.0	29.0	135	(mq)	12.0	3.0	0	45%
SALAD										
garden, w/o dressing	10 oz	200	13.0	7.0	240	(mq)	13.0	7.0	185	59%
side order, w/o dressing	4.8 oz	25	1.0	4.0	15	(mq)	0.0	0.0	0	0%
SALAD DRESSING										
French, reduced calorie	2 oz	90	<1.0	11.0	450	0	5.0	1.0	0	50%
Thousand Island	2 oz	225	<1.0	10.0	570	0	21.0	3.0	25	84%
SUNDAE										
chocolate, large	1 serving	440	8.0	78.0	165	na	10.0	na	30	20%
chocolate, regular, 6.2 oz	1 serving	300	6.0	54.0	100	na	7.0	5.0	20	21%
strawberry, waffle cone, 6.1 oz	1 serving	350	8.0	56.0	220	na	12.0	5.0	20	31%
TOMATO	.5 oz	4	0.0	1.0	10	na	0.0	na	0	0%
YOGURT, FROZEN										
cone, large	7.5 oz	260	9.0	56.0	115	0	<1.0	<1.0	5	<4%
cone, regular	5 oz	180	6.0	38.0	80	0	<1.0	<1.0	5	<5%
cup, regular	5 oz	170	6.0	35.0	70	0	<1.0	<1.0	5	<6%
cup, large	7 oz	230	8.0	49.0	100	0	<1.0	<1.0	5	<4%
strawberry sundae, regular	12.5 oz	200	6.0	43.0	80	na	<1.0	<1.0	5	<5%

Food Name	Serving Size	Calories	Prot. gms	Carbs gms	Sod. mgs	Fiber gms	Fat gms	Sat. Fat gms	Chol. mgs	% Fat Cal.
DEL TACO										
BREAKFAST BURRITO	1 burrito	256	9.0	30.0	409	na	11.0	na	90	39%
BURRITO										
beef, 'Del'	1 serving	440	23.0	43.0	878	na	20.0	na	63	41%
'Big Del'	1 serving	453	22.0	49.0	1047	na	20.0	na	59	40%
chicken	1 serving	264	13.0	32.0	771	na	10.0	na	36	34%
chicken fajita, 'Deluxe'	1 serving	435	22.0	41.0	944	na	22.0	na	84	46%
combination	1 serving	413	21.0	46.0	1035	na	17.0	na	49	37%
green	1 serving	229	9.0	32.0	714	na	8.0	na	15	31%
green, large	1 serving	330	14.0	46.0	1149	na	11.0	na	22	30%
red	1 serving	235	10.0	32.0	656	na	8.0	na	17	31%
red, large	1 serving	342	14.0	46.0	1149	na	11.0	na	22	29%
CHEESEBURGER	1 serving	284	14.0	26.0	852	na	13.0	na	42	41%
FRENCH FRIES	1 serving	242	3.0	32.0	136	na	11.0	na	0	41%
GUACAMOLE	2 tbsp	60	1.0	2.0	130	na	6.0	na	0	90%
HAMBURGER	1 serving	231	11.0	26.0	649	na	8.0	na	29	31%
HOT SAUCE	1 tbsp	2	0.0	1.0	38	0	0.0	na	0	0%
MILK, 1% low-fat	1 serving	126	10.0	15.0	152	na	3.0	na	12	21%
ORANGE JUICE	1 serving	83	1.0	20.0	19	na	0.0	na	0	0%
REFRIED BEANS, w/cheese	1 serving	122	7.0	17.0	890	na	7.0	na	9	52%
SALSA	4 tbsp	14	1.0	3.0	308	na	0.0	na	1	0%
TACO										
chicken fajita, 'Deluxe'	1 serving	211	11.0	18.0	492	na	10.0	na	53	43%
soft	1 serving	146	5.0	17.0	223	na	6.0	na	16	37%
soft, regular	1 serving	211	9.0	19.0	320	na	10.0	na	32	43%
DENNY'S										
BAGEL	1 bagel	240	9.0	47.0	450	na	1.0	na	na	4%
BEANS, green	3 oz	13	0.8	2.6	22	na	0.1	na	na	7%
BEEF BARLEY SOUP	1 bowl	79	5.0	11.0	847	na	2.0	na	na	23%
BISCUIT	1 biscuit	217	4.0	35.0	800	na	7.0	na	na	29%
BREAKFAST										
bacon	1 slice	48	3.0	0.5	142	na	4.0	na	na	75%
egg	1 egg	80	6.0	0.0	0	na	6.0	na	na	68%
eggs Benedict	1 serving	658	32.9	20.2	2197	na	35.6	na	na	49%
French toast	2 slices	729	12.0	46.0	275	na	56.0	na	na	69%
ham	1 slice	156	14.0	1.0	1303	na	7.0	na	na	40%
pancake	1 pancake	136	4.0	26.0	656	na	2.0	na	na	13%
sausage	1 link	113	2.5	0.0	250	na	10.0	na	na	80%
waffle	1 waffle	261	6.0	35.0	62	na	10.0	na	na	34%
CARROTS	3 oz	17	0.4	3.8	31	na	0.0	na	na	0%
CHEESE										
American	1 slice	55	3.0	0.5	230	na	1.5	na	na	25%
Jack	1 slice	52	5.5	0.2	195	na	4.3	na	na	74%
D'LITES OF AMERICA										
BROCCOLI SOUP, cream of	1 serving	180	8.0	21.0	na	na	7.0	na	na	35%
CHEESE, lite	1 slice	53	5.0	2.0	na	na	3.0	na	na	51%
CHEESEBURGER										
w/bacon, on multigrain bun	1 serving	370	32.0	20.0	na	na	18.0	na	na	44%
w/bacon, on sesame seed bun	1 serving	370	32.0	20.0	na	na	18.0	na	na	44%
CHICKEN SANDWICH										
fillet, on multigrain bun	1 serving	280	23.0	24.0	na	na	11.0	na	na	35%
fillet, on sesame seed bun	1 serving	280	23.0	24.0	na	na	11.0	na	na	35%

Food Name	Serving Size	Calories	Prot. gms	Carbs gms	Sod. mgs	Fiber gms	Fat gms	Sat. Fat gms	Chol. mgs	% Fat Cal.
D'LITE SOUP	1 serving	130	14.0	10.0	na	na	4.0	na	na	28%
DESSERT, 'Chocolate D'Lite'	1 serving	203	6.0	36.0	na	na	4.0	na	na	18%
FISH SANDWICH										
fillet, on multigrain bun	1 serving	390	22.0	29.0	na	na	21.0	na	na	48%
fillet, on sesame bun	1 serving	390	22.0	29.0	na	na	21.0	na	na	48%
FRENCH FRIES										
large order	1 serving	320	4.0	42.0	na	na	15.0	na	na	42%
regular order	1 serving	260	3.0	34.0	na	na	12.0	na	na	42%
HAM AND CHEESE SANDWICH										
on multigrain bun	1 serving	280	27.0	26.0	na	na	8.0	na	na	26%
on sesame seed bun	1 serving	280	27.0	26.0	na	na	8.0	na	na	26%
HAMBURGER										
'Double D'Lite' on multigrain bun	1 serving	450	44.0	19.0	na	na	22.0	na	na	44%
'Double D'Lite' on sesame seed bun	1 serving	450	44.0	19.0	na	na	22.0	na	na	44%
'Jr. D'Lite' on multigrain bun	1 serving	200	15.0	19.0	na	na	7.0	na	na	32%
'Jr. D'Lite' on sesame seed bun	1 serving	200	15.0	19.0	na	na	7.0	na	na	32%
'1/4 lb D'Lite' on multigrain bun	1 serving	280	25.0	19.0	na	na	12.0	na	na	39%
'1/4 lb D'Lite' on sesame seed bun	1 serving	280	25.0	19.0	na	na	12.0	na	na	39%
POTATO, BAKED										
'Mexican'	1 serving	510	27.0	61.0	na	na	18.0	na	na	32%
regular	1 serving	230	6.0	50.0	na	na	1.0	na	na	4%
w/bacon and cheddar cheese	1 serving	490	25.0	52.0	na	na	20.0	na	na	37%
w/broccoli and cheddar cheese	1 serving	410	15.0	51.0	na	na	16.0	na	na	35%
POTATO SKINS										
'Mexi Skins'	1 piece	99	4.0	6.0	na	na	7.0	na	na	64%
regular	1 piece	90	3.0	6.0	na	na	6.0	na	na	60%
SALAD BAR PLATTER	1 serving	130	10.0	9.0	na	na	6.0	na	na	42%
SALAD DRESSING, mayonnaise, lite	1 tbsp	40	tr	1.0	na	na	4.0	na	na	90%
TARTAR SAUCE, lite	1 tbsp	60	tr	2.0	na	na	6.0	na	na	90%
VEGETARIAN SANDWICH, 'Vegetarian D'Lite'	1 serving	270	16.0	20.0	na	na	14.0	na	na	47%
DUNKIN' DONUTS										
CORN MUFFIN, 3.4 oz	1 muffin	340	7.0	51.0	560	na	12.0	na	40	32%
CROISSANT										
almond, 3.7 oz	1 croissant	420	8.0	38.0	280	3.0	27.0	(mq)	0	58%
chocolate, 3.3 oz	1 croissant	440	7.0	38.0	220	3.0	29.0	(mq)	0	59%
plain, 2.5 oz	1 croissant	310	7.0	27.0	240	2.0	19.0	(mq)	0	55%
DONUT										
apple filled, w/cinnamon sugar, 2.8 oz	1 donut	250	5.0	33.0	280	1.0	11.0	(mq)	0	40%
Bavarian, filled w/chocolate	1 donut	240	5.0	32.0	260	2.0	11.0	(mq)	0	41%
blueberry filled, 2.4 oz	1 donut	210	4.0	29.0	240	2.0	8.0	(mq)	0	34%
'Boston Kreme'	1 donut	240	4.0	30.0	250	na	11.0	2.0	0	41%
buttermilk, glazed, 2.6 oz	1 donut	290	4.0	37.0	370	1.0	14.0	(mq)	10	43%
chocolate, glazed, 2.5 oz	1 donut	324	3.5	34.0	383	1.9	21.0	(mq)	2	58%
cinnamon, apple filled	1 donut	190	4.0	25.0	220	na	9.0	2.0	0	43%
coffee roll, glazed, 2.9 oz	1 donut	280	5.0	37.0	310	2.0	12.0	(mq)	0	39%
cruller, honey dipped	1 donut	260	4.0	36.0	330	na	11.0	2.0	0	38%
French cruller, w/glaze, 1.3 oz	1 donut	140	2.0	16.0	130	0	8.0	(mq)	30	51%
jelly filled, 2.4 oz	1 donut	220	4.0	31.0	230	1.0	9.0	(mq)	0	37%
lemon filled, 2.8 oz	1 donut	260	4.0	33.0	280	1.0	12.0	(mq)	0	42%
plain, cake, 2.2 oz	1 donut	270	4.0	25.0	330	1.0	17.0	(mq)	10	57%
plain, cake, w/handle	1 donut	240	4.0	26.0	370	na	14.0	3.0	0	53%
powdered, cake	1 donut	270	3.0	28.0	340	na	16.0	3.0	0	53%
whole wheat, glazed, 2.9 oz	1 donut	330	4.0	39.0	380	2.0	18.0	(mq)	5	49%

Food Name	Serving Size	Calories	Prot. gms	Carbs gms	Sod. mgs	Fiber gms	Fat gms	Sat. Fat gms	Chol. mgs	% Fat Cal.
yeast, chocolate frosted, 1.9 oz	1 donut	200	4.0	25.0	190	1.0	10.0	(mq)	0	45%
yeast, glazed, 1.9 oz	1 donut	200	4.0	26.0	230	1.0	9.0	(mq)	0	41%
yeast, honey dipped	1 donut	200	4.0	26.0	230	na	9.0	2.0	0	41%
MUFFIN										
apple and spice, 3.5 oz	1 muffin	300	6.0	52.0	360	2.0	8.0	(mq)	25	24%
banana nut, 3.6 oz	1 muffin	310	7.0	49.0	410	3.0	10.0	(mq)	30	29%
blueberry, 3.6 oz	1 muffin	280	6.0	46.0	340	na	8.0	na	30	26%
bran, w/raisins, 3.7 oz	1 muffin	310	6.0	51.0	560	4.0	9.0	(mq)	15	26%
cranberry nut	1 muffin	290	6.0	44.0	360	na	9.0	na	25	28%
oat bran, plain, 3.4 oz	1 muffin	330	7.0	50.0	450	na	11.0	na	0	30%
EL POLLO LOCO										
BEANS, 4 oz	1 serving	100	5.0	16.0	460	8.0	2.5	0.5	0	23%
BURRITO										
bean, rice, cheese	9 oz	530	18.0	86.0	730	na	13.0	5.0	15	22%
chicken	7 oz	310	23.0	30.0	510	4.0	11.0	2.0	65	32%
chicken, 'Classic'	9.5 oz	560	31.0	66.0	1170	na	20.0	8.0	75	32%
chicken, 'Loco Grande'	13.2 oz	680	34.0	70.0	1290	na	30.0	12.0	90	40%
chicken, spicy hot	10 oz	570	31.0	66.0	1180	na	20.0	8.0	75	32%
chicken, whole wheat	10.5 oz	510	25.0	67.0	900	na	16.0	5.0	60	28%
steak	6 oz	450	31.0	31.0	740	4.0	22.0	9.0	70	44%
steak, grilled	11 oz	740	40.0	81.0	1180	na	29.0	13.0	75	35%
vegetarian	6 oz	340	14.0	54.0	360	7.0	7.0	2.0	20	19%
CHEESE, cheddar	1 oz	90	7.0	3.0	180	0	5.0	3.0	27	50%
CHEESECAKE	3.5 oz	310	8.0	30.0	230	0	18.0	9.0	60	52%
CHICKEN										
breast	3 oz	160	26.0	0.0	390	0	6.0	2.0	110	34%
leg	1.75 oz	90	11.0	0.0	150	0	5.0	1.5	75	50%
thigh	2 oz	180	16.0	0.0	230	0	12.0	4.0	130	60%
wing	1.5 oz	110	12.0	0.0	220	0	6.0	2.0	80	49%
COLESLAW	3 oz	90	1.0	7.0	35	1.0	8.0	0.0	0	80%
CORN	3 oz	110	3.0	20.0	110	1.0	2.0	1.0	0	16%
DESSERT										
'Orange Bang'	7 oz	110	0.0	26.0	24	0	0.0	0.0	0	0%
'Pina Colada Bang'	7 oz	110	0.0	26.0	24	0	0.0	0.0	0	0%
FAJITA MEAL										
chicken, w/rice, beans, 3 tortillas, salsa	17.5 oz	780	41.0	120.0	1060	17.0	18.0	3.0	58	21%
steak	17.5 oz	1040	61.0	120.0	1550	17.0	38.0	14.0	100	33%
GUACAMOLE	1 oz	60	1.0	2.0	130	0	6.0	0.0	0	90%
MUSTARD, honey Dijon	1 oz	50	1.0	7.0	440	0	0.5	0.0	0	9%
PASTRY, churro	1.5 oz	140	2.0	4.0	180	0	9.0	1.8	4	58%
RICE	2 oz	110	1.0	19.0	220	0	1.5	0.0	0	12%
SALAD										
chicken, flame-broiled	12 oz	160	22.0	11.0	440	4.0	4.0	1.0	45	23%
potato	4 oz	180	2.0	21.0	340	1.0	10.0	1.5	10	50%
side order	9 oz	50	3.0	10.0	30	4.0	1.0	0.0	0	18%
SALAD DRESSING										
blue cheese	1 oz	80	1.0	4.0	150	0	6.0	1.0	5	68%
French, 'Deluxe'	1 oz	60	<1.0	7.0	160	0	4.0	0.0	0	60%
Italian, reduced calorie	1 oz	25	0.0	2.0	170	0	2.0	0.0	0	72%
ranch	1 oz	75	<1.0	4.0	190	0	6.0	0.0	0	72%
Thousand Island	1 oz	110	<1.0	4.0	240	0	10.0	0.0	5	82%
SALSA	2 oz	10	1.0	3.0	180	1.0	0.0	0.0	0	0%
SOUR CREAM	1 oz	60	1.0	1.0	15	0	6.0	4.0	13	90%

Food Name	Serving Size	Calories	Prot. gms	Carbs gms	Sod. mgs	Fiber gms	Fat gms	Sat. Fat gms	Chol. mgs	% Fat Cal.
TACO										
chicken	5 oz	180	13.0	18.0	300	2.0	7.0	1.0	35	35%
steak	4.5 oz	250	18.0	18.0	410	2.0	12.0	4.0	40	43%
TORTILLA										
corn	1 tortilla	60	1.0	13.0	25	<1.0	0.5	0.0	0	8%
flour	1 tortilla	90	3.0	15.0	150	<1.0	2.5	1.5	0	25%
EVERYTHING YOGURT										
YOGURT, FROZEN										
low-fat	1 serving	95	3.0	18.0	30	na	1.0	na	5	9%
nonfat	1 serving	80	3.0	17.0	40	na	0.0	0.0	0	0%
GODFATHER'S PIZZA										
PIZZA										
Cheese										
golden crust, large	1/10 pie	261	8.0	31.0	314	na	11.0	na	23	38%
golden crust, medium	1/8 pie	229	8.0	28.0	272	na	9.0	na	19	35%
golden crust, small	1/6 pie	213	8.0	27.0	258	na	8.0	na	19	34%
original crust, large	1/10 pie	271	12.0	37.0	329	na	8.0	na	28	27%
original crust, medium	1/8 pie	242	10.0	35.0	285	na	7.0	na	22	26%
original crust, mini	1/4 pie	138	6.0	20.0	159	na	4.0	na	13	26%
original crust, small	1/6 pie	239	10.0	32.0	289	na	7.0	na	25	26%
thin crust, large	1/10 pie	228	11.0	28.0	464	(mq)	7.0	(mq)	16	28%
thin crust, medium	1/8 pie	210	10.0	26.0	410	(mq)	7.0	(mq)	14	30%
thin crust, small	1/6 pie	180	9.0	21.0	370	(mq)	6.0	(mq)	10	30%
Combo										
golden crust, large	1/10 pie	322	14.0	33.0	602	na	15.0	na	34	42%
golden crust, medium	1/8 pie	283	13.0	30.0	526	na	13.0	na	29	41%
golden crust, small	1/6 pie	273	13.0	29.0	542	na	12.0	na	31	40%
original crust, large	1/10 pie	332	16.0	39.0	617	na	12.0	na	39	33%
original crust, medium	1/8 pie	318	16.0	37.0	569	na	12.0	na	38	34%
original crust, mini	1/4 pie	164	8.0	21.0	287	na	5.0	na	17	27%
original crust, small	1/6 pie	299	15.0	34.0	573	na	11.0	na	37	33%
thin crust, large	1/10 pie	336	17.0	31.0	870	(mq)	16.0	(mq)	27	43%
thin crust, medium	1/8 pie	310	15.0	29.0	790	(mq)	14.0	(mq)	25	41%
thin crust, small	1/6 pie	270	13.0	23.0	710	(mq)	13.0	(mq)	25	43%
PIZZA, STUFFED										
cheese, large	1/10 pie	381	16.0	44.0	677	(mq)	16.0	(mq)	32	38%
cheese, medium	1/8 pie	350	14.0	42.0	610	(mq)	13.0	(mq)	25	33%
cheese, small	1/6 pie	310	13.0	38.0	560	(mq)	11.0	(mq)	25	32%
combo, large	1/10 pie	521	23.0	47.0	1204	(mq)	26.0	(mq)	48	45%
combo, medium	1/8 pie	480	21.0	45.0	1105	(mq)	23.0	(mq)	43	43%
combo, small	1/6 pie	430	19.0	41.0	1000	(mq)	20.0	(mq)	40	42%
GOLDEN CORRAL										
BREAD, 'Texas Toast'	1 serving	170	5.0	26.0	230	na	6.0	na	0	32%
CHICKEN, 'Golden Grilled'	1 serving	170	32.0	0.0	520	na	5.0	na	100	26%
CHICKEN FILLET, 'Golden Fried'	1 serving	370	37.0	14.0	570	na	19.0	na	85	46%
POTATO, BAKED	1 serving	220	5.0	46.0	60	na	2.0	na	0	8%
RIBEYE STEAK, regular, 5.11 oz	1 serving	450	34.0	0.0	220	na	35.0	na	120	70%
SHRIMP, 'Golden Fried'	1 serving	250	12.0	24.0	470	na	12.0	na	90	43%
SIRLOIN STEAK	5 oz	230	27.0	0.0	270	na	14.0	na	85	55%
STEAK ENTRÉE										
chopped sirloin, approx 4 oz	1 serving	320	28.0	0.0	160	na	23.0	na	100	65%

Food Name	Serving Size	Calories	Prot. gms	Carbs gms	Sod. mgs	Fiber gms	Fat gms	Sat. Fat gms	Chol. mgs	% Fat Cal.
sirloin tips, w/onions and pepper, approx 8.2 oz	1 serving	290	30.0	8.0	260	na	13.0	na	120	40%
HARDEE'S										
APPLE TURNOVER	3.2 oz	270	3.0	38.0	250	(mq)	12.0	4.0	0	40%
BARBECUE SAUCE										
dipping sauce	.5-oz pkt	14	0.0	4.0	140	0	0.0	0.0	0	0%
dipping sauce	1 oz	30	0.0	8.0	300	0	0.0	0.0	0	0%
BISCUIT										
'Canadian Rise 'N' Shine' 5.8 oz	1 serving	570	24.0	46.0	1860	na	32.0	11.0	175	51%
'Cinnamon 'N' Raisin' 2.8 oz	1 serving	370	3.0	48.0	450	na	18.0	5.0	0	44%
'Rise 'N' Shine'	1 serving	390	6.0	44.0	1000	na	21.0	6.0	0	48%
BREAKFAST										
'Big Country Breakfast' bacon	1 serving	740	25.0	61.0	1800	na	43.0	13.0	305	52%
'Big Country Breakfast' ham, 8.9 oz	1 serving	620	28.0	51.0	1780	(mq)	33.0	7.0	325	48%
'Big Country Breakfast' sausage	1 serving	930	33.0	61.0	2240	na	61.0	19.0	340	59%
'Biscuit 'N' Gravy' 7.8 oz	1 serving	510	10.0	55.0	1500	na	28.0	9.0	15	49%
biscuit, bacon, egg, and cheese	1 serving	530	18.0	45.0	1470	na	31.0	11.0	155	53%
biscuit, bacon, 3.3 oz	1 serving	360	10.0	34.0	950	(mq)	21.0	4.0	10	53%
biscuit, bacon and egg, 4.4 oz	1 serving	490	15.0	44.0	1250	na	27.0	9.0	155	50%
biscuit, chicken	1 serving	510	18.0	52.0	1580	na	25.0	7.0	45	44%
biscuit, country ham	1 serving	430	15.0	45.0	1930	na	22.0	6.0	25	46%
biscuit, country ham and egg, 4.9 oz	1 serving	400	16.0	35.0	1600	(mq)	22.0	4.0	175	50%
biscuit, ham	1 serving	400	9.0	47.0	1340	na	20.0	6.0	15	45%
biscuit, ham, egg, and cheese	1 serving	500	16.0	48.0	1620	na	27.0	10.0	170	49%
biscuit, ham and egg, 4.9 oz	1 serving	370	15.0	35.0	1050	(mq)	19.0	4.0	160	46%
biscuit, sausage, 4.2 oz	1 serving	510	14.0	44.0	1360	na	31.0	10.0	25	55%
biscuit, sausage and egg, 5.3 oz	1 serving	560	18.0	44.0	1400	na	35.0	11.0	170	56%
biscuit, steak	1 serving	580	15.0	50.0	1580	na	32.0	10.0	30	50%
biscuit, steak and egg	1 serving	550	22.0	47.0	1370	na	32.0	8.0	175	52%
pancakes, 3 cakes	1 serving	280	8.0	56.0	890	na	2.0	1.0	15	6%
pancakes, 3 cakes, w/1 sausage patty	1 serving	430	16.0	56.0	1290	na	16.0	6.0	40	33%
pancakes, 3 cakes, w/2 bacon strips	1 serving	350	13.0	56.0	1130	na	9.0	3.0	25	23%
BREAKFAST SANDWICH										
'Frisco Breakfast Sandwich' ham	1 serving	460	20.0	46.0	1320	na	22.0	8.0	175	43%
'Frisco Breakfast Sandwich' w/hash browns	1 serving	230	3.0	24.0	560	na	14.0	3.0	0	55%
CATSUP	.5 oz	14	<1.0	3.0	135	(tr)	<1.0	<1.0	0	0%
CHEESEBURGER										
bacon	1 serving	580	33.0	33.0	980	na	35.0	15.0	50	54%
'Mushroom 'N' Swiss'	1 serving	500	31.0	35.0	1020	na	26.0	13.0	45	47%
quarter pound	1 serving	470	28.0	35.0	890	na	28.0	12.0	35	54%
regular	1 serving	300	13.0	34.0	690	na	13.0	7.0	25	39%
CHICKEN, FRIED										
breast, 5.2 oz	1 serving	370	29.0	29.0	1190	na	15.0	4.0	75	36%
leg, 2.4 oz	1 serving	170	13.0	15.0	570	na	7.0	2.0	45	37%
'Stix'	6 pieces	210	19.0	13.0	680	na	9.0	2.0	35	39%
'Stix'	9 pieces	310	28.0	20.0	1020	(mq)	14.0	3.0	55	41%
thigh, 4.3 oz	1 serving	330	19.0	30.0	1000	na	15.0	4.0	60	41%
wing, 2.3 oz	1 serving	200	10.0	23.0	740	na	8.0	2.0	30	36%
CHICKEN SANDWICH										
breast, grilled, 6.8 oz	1 serving	310	24.0	34.0	890	(mq)	9.0	1.0	60	26%
'Chicken Fillet' 6.1 oz	1 serving	370	19.0	44.0	1060	(mq)	13.0	2.0	55	32%
fillet	1 serving	380	20.0	46.0	1130	na	13.0	3.0	55	31%
grilled, 'Frisco'	1 serving	620	35.0	44.0	1730	na	34.0	10.0	95	49%

Food Name	Serving Size	Calories	Prot. gms	Carbs gms	Sod. mgs	Fiber gms	Fat gms	Sat. Fat gms	Chol. mgs	% Fat Cal.
COLESLAW										
12-oz size	1 serving	710	5.0	38.0	1020	na	60.0	10.0	35	76%
4-oz size	1 serving	240	2.0	13.0	340	na	20.0	3.0	10	75%
COOKIE, 'Big Cookie'	2 oz	280	4.0	41.0	150	na	12.0	4.0	15	39%
FISH SANDWICH, 'Fisherman's Fillet' 7.5 oz	1 serving	480	25.0	49.0	1200	na	22.0	6.0	60	41%
FRENCH FRIES										
big, 5.5 oz	1 serving	500	6.0	66.0	180	(mq)	23.0	5.0	0	41%
'Crispy Curls' 3 oz	1 serving	300	4.0	36.0	840	na	16.0	3.0	0	48%
large order, 6.1 oz	1 serving	430	6.0	59.0	190	na	18.0	5.0	0	38%
medium order, 5 oz	1 serving	350	5.0	49.0	150	na	15.0	4.0	0	39%
small order, 3.3 oz	1 serving	240	4.0	33.0	100	na	10.0	3.0	0	38%
GRAVY										
5-oz serving	1 serving	60	3.0	11.0	850	na	1.0	<1.0	5	15%
1.5-oz serving	1 serving	20	1.0	3.0	260	na	<1.0	<1.0	2	15%
HAM AND CHEESE SANDWICH, 'Hot Ham 'N' Cheese'	1 serving	530	18.0	49.0	1710	na	30.0	9.0	65	51%
HAMBURGER										
'Big Deluxe'	1 serving	510	28.0	35.0	820	na	29.0	12.0	40	51%
'Big Twin' 6.1 oz	1 serving	450	23.0	34.0	580	(mq)	25.0	11.0	55	50%
'Frisco'	1 serving	760	36.0	43.0	1280	na	50.0	18.0	70	59%
regular	1 serving	260	11.0	33.0	460	na	9.0	4.0	20	31%
HONEY SAUCE	.5 oz	45	<1.0	11.0	0	0	<1.0	<1.0	0	<3%
HORSERADISH	.25-oz pkt	25	<1.0	1.0	35	na	2.0	<1.0	5	72%
HOT DOG										
all beef, 4.2 oz	1 serving	300	11.0	25.0	710	(mq)	17.0	8.0	25	51%
6.8 oz	1 serving	450	17.0	52.0	1090	na	20.0	6.0	35	40%
ICE CREAM CONE										
chocolate, 'Cool Twist'	4.2 oz	180	4.0	29.0	85	na	4.0	3.0	15	20%
vanilla, 'Cool Twist'	4.2 oz	180	5.0	29.0	80	na	4.0	3.0	15	20%
vanilla/chocolate, 'Cool Twist'	4.2 oz	170	5.0	29.0	85	na	4.0	3.0	15	21%
MARGARINE-BUTTER BLEND, .2 oz	1 serving	35	0.0	0.0	40	0	4.0	<1.0	5	100%
MAYONNAISE	.5 oz	50	<1.0	1.0	75	0	5.0	1.0	5	90%
MILKSHAKE										
chocolate	11.5 oz	390	15.0	61.0	220	na	10.0	6.0	30	23%
peach	13.3 oz	530	12.0	95.0	220	na	11.0	7.0	45	19%
strawberry	12 oz	390	13.0	65.0	200	na	8.0	5.0	30	18%
vanilla	11.5 oz	370	14.0	59.0	210	na	9.0	6.0	25	22%
MUFFIN										
blueberry	1 muffin	400	7.0	56.0	310	na	17.0	4.0	65	38%
oat bran raisin	1 muffin	410	8.0	59.0	380	na	16.0	3.0	50	35%
MUSTARD	.3-oz pkt	6	<1.0	<1.0	120	(tr)	<1.0	<1.0	0	0%
MUSTARD SAUCE, sweet, dipping sauce	1 oz	50	<1.0	10.0	160	(tr)	<1.0	<1.0	0	<12%
ORANGE JUICE										
11-oz size	1 serving	140	2.0	34.0	5	na	tr	tr	0	0%
6-oz size	1 serving	83	1.0	20.0	5	na	tr	tr	0	0%
POTATOES, HASH BROWN, 'Hash Rounds' 2.8 oz	1 serving	230	3.0	24.0	560	(mq)	14.0	3.0	0	55%
POTATOES, MASHED										
4-oz size	1 serving	70	2.0	14.0	260	na	<1.0	na	0	<9%
12-oz size	1 serving	220	6.0	48.0	760	na	<1.0	0.0	0	<9%
ROAST BEEF SANDWICH										
'Big Roast Beef'	1 serving	350	22.0	33.0	1080	na	15.0	6.0	40	39%
regular	1 serving	270	15.0	28.0	780	na	11.0	5.0	25	37%
SALAD										
chef's, 9.5 oz	1 serving	200	20.0	5.0	910	na	13.0	8.0	45	59%
chicken, grilled, 9.8 oz	1 serving	120	18.0	2.0	520	na	4.0	1.0	60	30%

Food Name	Serving Size	Calories	Prot. gms	Carbs gms	Sod. mgs	Fiber gms	Fat gms	Sat. Fat gms	Chol. mgs	% Fat Cal.
chicken and pasta	14.6 oz	230	27.0	23.0	380	(mq)	3.0	1.0	55	12%
garden, 9.3 oz	1 serving	190	3.0	3.0	280	na	14.0	9.0	40	66%
side order, 5 oz	1 serving	20	1.0	3.0	20	na	tr	tr	0	0%
SALAD DRESSING										
blue cheese	2 oz	210	1.0	10.0	790	0	18.0	3.0	20	77%
French, reduced calorie	2 oz	130	1.0	21.0	480	0	5.0	1.0	0	35%
house	2 oz	290	1.0	6.0	510	na	29.0	4.0	25	90%
Italian, reduced calorie	2 oz	90	<1.0	5.0	310	(tr)	8.0	1.0	0	80%
Thousand Island	2 oz	250	1.0	9.0	540	na	23.0	3.0	35	83%
SAUCE										
'Big Twin'	.5 oz	50	<1.0	4.0	35	na	4.0	<1.0	5	72%
sweet and sour, dipping sauce	1 oz	40	<1.0	10.0	95	0	<1.0	<1.0	0	0%
SUNDAE										
caramel, 'Cool Twist'	6 oz	330	6.0	54.0	290	(tr)	10.0	5.0	20	27%
hot fudge, 'Cool Twist'	6 oz	320	8.0	50.0	260	na	10.0	5.0	25	28%
strawberry, 'Cool Twist'	5.9 oz	260	6.0	48.0	100	na	6.0	3.0	15	21%
SYRUP, pancake	1.5 oz	120	<1.0	31.0	25	0	<1.0	1.0	0	0%
TARTAR SAUCE	.7 oz	90	<1.0	2.0	160	na	9.0	1.0	10	90%
TURKEY SANDWICH, 'Turkey Club' 7.3 oz	1 serving	390	29.0	32.0	1280	(mq)	16.0	4.0	70	37%
HARVEY'S FOODS										
APPLE JUICE	1 serving	80	2.0	20.0	na	na	2.0	na	tr	23%
APPLE TURNOVER	1 serving	179	1.0	28.0	na	na	7.0	na	7	35%
BREAKFAST										
pancakes	1 serving	89	2.0	17.0	na	na	1.0	na	8	10%
sausage	1 serving	167	9.0	3.0	na	na	14.0	na	12	75%
CHEESEBURGER	1 serving	415	22.0	41.0	na	na	18.0	na	30	39%
CHICKEN FINGERS	1 serving	240	15.0	18.0	na	na	12.0	na	57	45%
CHICKEN SANDWICH	1 serving	419	19.0	46.0	na	na	16.0	na	110	34%
FRENCH FRIES	1 serving	478	10.0	56.0	na	na	24.0	na	5	45%
HAMBURGER										
'Double'	1 serving	530	31.0	44.0	na	na	26.0	na	34	44%
regular	1 serving	355	18.0	40.0	na	na	14.0	na	17	35%
'Super'	1 serving	477	37.0	38.0	na	na	19.0	na	112	36%
HOT DOG	1 serving	332	12.0	32.0	na	na	15.0	na	50	41%
MILKSHAKE										
chocolate	1 serving	321	12.0	74.0	na	na	11.0	na	36	31%
strawberry	1 serving	303	11.0	69.0	na	na	10.0	na	36	30%
vanilla	1 serving	305	11.0	69.0	na	na	10.0	na	36	30%
MUFFIN										
blueberry	1 muffin	254	4.0	45.0	na	na	6.0	na	tr	21%
bran	1 muffin	301	5.0	42.0	na	na	13.0	na	tr	39%
ONION RINGS	1 serving	288	4.0	36.0	na	na	14.0	na	5	44%
ORANGE JUICE	1 serving	77	1.0	18.0	na	na	1.0	na	tr	12%
POTATOES, HASH BROWN	1 serving	146	2.0	15.0	tr	na	9.0	na	2	55%
SANDWICH, 'Western'	1 sandwich	347	15.0	58.0	na	na	10.0	na	265	26%
TOAST, plain	1 serving	250	8.0	48.0	na	na	3.0	na	tr	11%
HUNGRY HUNTER										
CHICKEN TERIYAKI, breast, boneless, charbroiled	1 serving	413	71.0	9.0	237	0	8.0	na	193	17%
CRAB										
Alaskan king, w/1 tbsp butter	1 serving	432	73.0	0.0	3436	0	13.0	na	194	27%
Alaskan king, w/o butter	1 serving	332	73.0	0.0	3319	0	2.0	na	163	5%
FILET MIGNON SANDWICH, midwestern, USDA choice	8 oz	539	69.0	0.0	150	0	27.0	na	203	45%

Food Name	Serving Size	Calories	Prot. gms	Carbs gms	Sod. mgs	Fiber gms	Fat gms	Sat. Fat gms	Chol. mgs	% Fat Cal.
LOBSTER										
w/1 tbsp butter	1 serving	241	29.0	2.0	657	0	12.0	na	133	45%
w/o butter	1 serving	139	29.0	2.0	539	0	1.0	na	102	6%
POTATO, BAKED	1 serving	185	4.0	43.0	13	4.0	0.0	0.0	0	0%
RED SNAPPER, fresh, cooked in 1/2 oz butter	1 serving	329	47.0	0.0	262	0	15.0	na	114	41%
RICE PILAF	1 serving	142	4.0	26.0	223	1.0	2.0	na	0	13%
JACK-IN-THE-BOX										
APPLE TURNOVER, 3.9 oz	1 serving	354	3.0	40.0	479	(mq)	19.0	4.4	0	48%
BARBECUE SAUCE	1-oz pkt	44	1.0	11.0	300	0	<1.0	<1.0	0	0%
BEEF SANDWICH, gyro	1 serving	620	27.0	55.0	1310	na	32.0	12.0	65	46%
BEEF TERIYAKI BOWL	1 serving	640	28.0	124.0	930	7.0	3.0	1.0	25	4%
BREADSTICKS, sesame, .5 oz	1 serving	70	2.0	12.0	110	(mq)	2.0	na	<1	26%
BREAKFAST										
pancake platter, 8.1 oz	1 serving	612	15.0	87.0	888	(mq)	22.0	8.6	99	32%
scrambled egg platter, 7.5 oz	1 serving	559	18.0	50.0	1060	(mq)	32.0	8.7	378	52%
BREAKFAST SANDWICH										
'Breakfast Jack' 4.4 oz	1 serving	307	18.0	30.0	871	(mq)	13.0	5.1	203	38%
crescent, Canadian bacon, 4.7 oz	1 serving	452	19.0	25.0	851	(mq)	31.0	9.7	226	62%
crescent, sausage, 5.5 oz	1 serving	584	22.0	28.0	1012	(mq)	43.0	15.5	187	66%
crescent, supreme, 5.1 oz	1 serving	547	20.0	27.0	1053	(mq)	40.0	13.2	178	66%
sausage, 5.5 oz	1 serving	584	22.0	28.0	1012	(mq)	43.0	15.5	187	66%
scrambled egg pocket, 6.5 oz	1 serving	431	29.0	31.0	1060	(mq)	21.0	7.5	354	44%
sourdough bread, egg, ham, and cheese, 5.2 oz	1 serving	381	21.0	31.0	1120	(mq)	20.0	7.1	236	47%
CHEESEBURGER										
'Bacon Bacon Cheeseburger' 8.5 oz	1 serving	705	35.0	41.0	1240	(mq)	45.0	14.9	113	57%
'Jumbo Jack' 8.5 oz	1 serving	677	32.0	46.0	1090	(mq)	40.0	14.0	102	53%
double, 5.3 oz	1 serving	467	21.0	33.0	842	(mq)	27.0	12.3	72	52%
patty melt, 'Old Fashioned' 7.6 oz	1 serving	713	33.0	42.0	1360	(mq)	46.0	14.8	92	58%
regular, 4 oz	1 serving	315	15.0	33.0	746	(mq)	14.0	5.7	41	40%
Swiss cheese and bacon, 6.6 oz	1 serving	678	31.0	34.0	1458	(mq)	47.0	20.0	92	62%
'Ultimate' 9.9 oz	1 serving	942	47.0	33.0	1176	(mq)	69.0	26.4	127	66%
CHEESECAKE, 3.5 oz	1 serving	309	8.0	29.0	208	na	18.0	9.4	63	52%
CHICKEN SANDWICH										
grilled, fillet, 7.4 oz	1 serving	431	29.0	36.0	1070	(mq)	19.0	4.7	65	40%
smoked chicken, cheddar, and bacon	1 serving	540	30.0	37.0	1520	9.0	30.0	11.0	80	50%
spicy crispy chicken	1 serving	560	24.0	55.0	1020	na	27.0	5.0	50	43%
supreme, 8.6 oz	1 serving	641	27.0	47.0	1470	(mq)	39.0	10.0	85	55%
w/mushrooms, 7.8 oz	1 serving	438	28.0	40.0	1340	(mq)	18.0	4.9	61	37%
CHICKEN STRIPS										
4 pieces	4 oz	285	25.0	18.0	695	(mq)	13.0	3.1	52	41%
6 pieces	6.2 oz	451	39.0	28.0	1100	(mq)	20.0	4.9	82	40%
CHICKEN TERIYAKI BOWL	1 serving	580	28.0	115.0	1220	6.0	1.5	na	30	2%
CHICKEN WINGS										
9 pieces	11 oz	1270	51.0	117.0	2560	(mq)	66.0	16.0	272	47%
6 pieces	7.3 oz	846	34.0	78.0	1710	(mq)	44.0	10.7	181	47%
CHIMICHANGA										
mini, 4 pieces	7.3 oz	571	22.0	57.0	633	(mq)	28.0	8.6	64	44%
mini, 6 pieces	11 oz	856	34.0	85.0	949	(mq)	42.0	13.0	95	44%
COCKTAIL SAUCE	1 oz	32	<1.0	6.8	206	na	<1.0	<1.0	0	0%
COFFEE, small	8 oz	2	0.0	0.0	26	0	0.0	0.0	0	0%
DESSERT, double fudge, 3.0 oz	1 serving	288	4.0	49.0	259	(mq)	9.0	2.2	20	28%
EGG ROLL, 5 pieces	10 oz	753	5.0	92.0	1640	(mq)	41.0	11.7	49	49%

Food Name	Serving Size	Calories	Prot. gms	Carbs gms	Sod. mgs	Fiber gms	Fat gms	Sat. Fat gms	Chol. mgs	% Fat Cal.
FAJITA SANDWICH										
beef fajita pita, 6.2 oz	1 serving	333	24.0	27.0	635	(mq)	14.0	5.9	45	38%
chicken fajita pita, 6.7 oz	1 serving	292	24.0	29.0	703	(mq)	8.0	2.9	34	25%
FISH SANDWICH, supreme, 7.7 oz	1 serving	510	24.0	44.0	1040	(mq)	27.0	6.1	55	48%
FRENCH FRIES										
curly, seasoned, 3.8 oz	1 serving	358	5.0	39.0	1030	(mq)	20.0	4.7	0	50%
jumbo order, 4.3 oz	1 serving	396	5.0	51.0	219	(mq)	19.0	4.5	0	43%
regular order, 3.8 oz	1 serving	351	4.0	45.0	194	(mq)	17.0	4.0	0	44%
small order, 2.4 oz	1 serving	219	3.0	28.0	121	(mq)	11.0	2.5	0	45%
GUACAMOLE	1 oz	30	1.0	2.0	128	(mq)	3.0	<1.0	0	90%
HAMBURGER										
'Jumbo Jack' 7.8 oz	1 serving	584	26.0	42.0	733	(mq)	34.0	11.0	73	52%
regular, 3.4 oz	1 serving	267	13.0	28.0	556	(mq)	11.0	4.1	26	37%
HOT SAUCE, .5 oz	1 serving	4	<1.0	1.0	112	0	0.0	0.0	0	0%
ICED TEA, small	16 oz	4	1.0	<1.0	6	0	0.0	0.0	0	0%
ITALIAN SAUCE	1.5 oz	28	<1.0	6.0	176	0	<1.0	<1.0	<1	0%
JELLY, grape	.5 oz	38	0.0	9.0	3	0	0.0	0.0	0	0%
MAYO-MUSTARD SAUCE	.7 oz	124	0.5	2.0	247	0	13.0	na	10	94%
MAYO-ONION SAUCE	.7 oz	143	0.3	1.0	140	0	15.0	na	20	94%
MILK, 2%	8.6 oz	122	8.0	12.0	122	0	5.0	2.9	18	37%
MILKSHAKE										
chocolate	11.4 oz	330	11.0	55.0	270	(tr)	7.0	4.3	25	19%
strawberry	11.6 oz	320	10.0	55.0	240	(tr)	7.0	4.3	25	20%
vanilla	11.2 oz	320	10.0	57.0	230	0	6.0	3.6	25	17%
ONION RINGS, 3.6 oz	1 serving	380	5.0	38.0	451	(mq)	23.0	5.5	0	54%
ORANGE JUICE	6.5 oz	80	1.0	20.0	0	0	0.0	0.0	0	0%
POTATOES, HASH BROWN, 2.0 oz	1 serving	156	1.0	14.0	312	(mq)	11.0	2.6	0	63%
RAVIOLI										
toasted, 7 pieces	5.8 oz	537	15.0	57.0	639	(mq)	28.0	8.0	36	47%
toasted, 10 pieces	8.3 oz	768	22.0	81.0	913	(mq)	40.0	11.4	52	47%
SALAD										
chef's, 11.7 oz	1 serving	325	30.0	10.0	900	(mq)	18.0	8.4	142	50%
Mexican chicken, 14.6 oz	1 serving	442	28.0	30.0	1500	(mq)	23.0	8.6	89	47%
side order, 4 oz	1 serving	51	7.0	<1.0	84	(mq)	3.0	2.0	<1	53%
taco, 14.2 oz	1 serving	503	34.0	28.0	1600	(mq)	31.0	13.4	92	55%
SALAD DRESSING										
blue cheese	2.5-oz pkt	262	<1.0	14.0	918	0	22.0	4.0	18	76%
buttermilk, house	2.5-oz pkt	362	<1.0	8.0	694	0	36.0	5.8	21	90%
French, reduced calorie	2.5-oz pkt	176	<1.0	26.0	600	0	8.0	1.2	0	41%
Italian, low calorie	2.5-oz pkt	25	<1.0	2.0	810	0	2.0	<1.0	0	72%
Thousand Island	2.5-oz pkt	312	<1.0	12.0	700	(tr)	30.0	5.0	23	87%
SALSA	1 oz	8	<1.0	2.0	27	(mq)	<1.0	<1.0	0	0%
SHRIMP										
15 pieces	4.4 oz	404	15.0	34.0	1003	(mq)	24.0	10.8	126	53%
10 pieces	3.0 oz	270	10.0	22.0	669	(mq)	16.0	7.2	84	53%
SOFT DRINK										
Coca-Cola, small	16 oz	192	0.0	48.0	19	0	0.0	0.0	0	0%
Diet Coke, small	16 oz	1	0.0	<1.0	35	0	0.0	0.0	0	0%
Dr. Pepper, small	16 oz	192	0.0	49.0	24	0	0.0	0.0	0	0%
Ramblin' Root Beer, small	16 oz	235	0.0	61.0	27	0	0.0	0.0	0	0%
Sprite, small	16 oz	192	0.0	48.0	61	0	0.0	0.0	0	0%
STEAK SANDWICH										
country-fried, 5.4 oz	1 serving	450	14.0	42.0	891	(mq)	25.0	6.9	36	50%
sirloin, 8.4 oz	1 serving	517	29.0	49.0	1050	(mq)	23.0	5.0	66	40%

Food Name	Serving Size	Calories	Prot. gms	Carbs gms	Sod. mgs	Fiber gms	Fat gms	Sat. Fat gms	Chol. mgs	% Fat Cal.
SWEET AND SOUR SAUCE	1 oz	40	<1.0	11.0	160	0	<1.0	<1.0	<1	0%
SYRUP, pancake	1.5 oz	121	0.0	30.0	6	0	0.0	0.0	0	0%
TACO										
regular, 3 oz	1 serving	187	7.0	15.0	414	(mq)	11.0	3.7	18	53%
super, 4.5 oz	1 serving	281	12.0	22.0	718	(mq)	17.0	5.9	29	54%
TAQUITO										
5 pieces	5 oz	363	16.0	40.0	467	(mq)	16.0	5.6	37	40%
7 pieces	7 oz	508	22.0	56.0	654	(mq)	22.0	7.9	52	39%
TORTILLA CHIPS	1 oz	139	2.0	18.0	134	(mq)	6.0	na	<1	39%
VEGETABLE OIL SPREAD, 'Country Crock'	.2 oz	25	0.0	0.0	40	(mq)	2.8	<1.0	0	100%

KENTUCKY FRIED CHICKEN

Food Name	Serving Size	Calories	Prot. gms	Carbs gms	Sod. mgs	Fiber gms	Fat gms	Sat. Fat gms	Chol. mgs	% Fat Cal.
BARBECUE SAUCE	1 oz	35	0.3	7.1	450	na	0.6	0.1	<1	15%
BEANS										
barbecue baked	3.9 oz	132	5.0	24.0	535	4.0	2.0	1.0	3	14%
green	3.6 oz	36	1.0	5.0	563	2.0	1.0	0.0	3	25%
BISCUIT										
buttermilk, 2.3 oz	1 biscuit	232	4.2	27.1	539	(mq)	11.9	2.8	1	46%
regular, 2.2 oz	1 biscuit	220	5.0	26.0	530	na	12.0	3.0	<5	49%
BREADSTICKS, 1.2 oz	1 breadstick	110	3.0	17.0	15	0	3.0	0.0	0	25%
CHICKEN										
breast, center, 'Extra Tasty Crispy' 4.8 oz	1 serving	342	33.0	11.7	790	(mq)	19.7	4.8	114	52%
breast, center, 'Hot & Spicy' 4.3 oz	1 serving	382	24.3	16.0	905	na	25.0	6.0	84	59%
breast, center, 'Original Recipe' 3.6 oz	1 serving	260	25.0	8.0	609	na	14.0	4.0	na	48%
breast, center, 'Skinfree Crispy'	1 serving	296	24.0	11.0	435	na	16.0	3.1	59	49%
breast, side, 'Extra Tasty Crispy' 3.9 oz	1 serving	343	21.7	14.0	748	(mq)	22.3	5.5	81	59%
breast, side, 'Hot & Spicy' 4.1 oz	1 serving	398	20.5	18.0	922	na	27.0	7.0	83	61%
breast, side, 'Original Recipe'	1 piece	276	20.0	10.0	654	na	17.0	na	na	55%
breast, side, 'Skinfree Crispy'	1 serving	293	22.0	11.0	410	na	17.0	3.5	63	52%
dark meat quarter, w/skin, 'Rotisserie Gold' 5.1 oz	1 serving	333	30.0	1.0	980	na	23.7	6.6	163	64%
dark meat quarter, w/o skin, 'Rotisserie Gold' 4.1 oz	1 serving	217	27.0	0.0	772	na	12.2	3.5	128	51%
drumstick, 'Extra Tasty Crispy' 2.4 oz	1 serving	204	13.6	6.1	324	(mq)	13.9	3.4	71	61%
drumstick, 'Hot & Spicy' 2.5 oz	1 serving	207	10.5	10.0	406	na	14.0	3.0	75	61%
drumstick, 'Original Recipe'	1 piece	147	14.0	4.0	269	na	9.0	na	na	55%
drumstick, 'Skinfree Crispy'	1 serving	166	13.0	8.0	256	na	9.0	1.9	42	49%
'Hot Wings' 6 pieces, 4.8 oz	1 serving	471	27.0	18.0	1230	na	33.0	8.0	150	63%
'Spicy Chicken Bites' small 4.3 oz	1 serving	248	28.7	4.7	344	na	12.4	3.8	143	45%
thigh, 'Extra Tasty Crispy' 4.2 oz	1 serving	406	20.0	14.4	688	(mq)	29.8	7.7	129	66%
thigh, 'Hot & Spicy' 4.2 oz	1 serving	412	19.3	16.0	750	na	30.0	8.0	105	66%
thigh, 'Original Recipe'	1 piece	278	18.0	8.0	517	na	19.0	na	na	62%
thigh, 'Skinfree Crispy'	1 serving	256	17.0	9.0	394	na	17.0	3.6	68	60%
white meat quarter, w/o skin and wing, 'Rotisserie Gold' 4.1 oz	1 serving	199	37.0	0.0	667	na	5.9	1.7	97	27%
white meat quarter, w/skin and wing, 'Rotisserie Gold' 6.2 oz	1 serving	335	40.0	1.0	1104	na	18.7	5.4	157	50%
wing, 'Extra Tasty Crispy' 2.3 oz	1 serving	254	12.4	9.3	422	(mq)	18.6	4.4	67	66%
wing, 'Hot & Spicy' 2.2 oz	1 serving	244	12.1	9.0	459	na	18.0	4.0	65	66%
wing, 'Original Recipe'	1 piece	181	12.0	6.0	387	na	12.0	na	na	60%
CHICKEN NUGGETS										
'Kentucky Nuggets' .6 oz	1 nugget	46	2.8	2.2	140	(mq)	2.9	0.7	12	57%
'Kentucky Nuggets' .6 oz	6 nuggets	284	15.5	15.0	865	na	18.0	4.0	66	57%
CHICKEN SANDWICH										
'Chicken Littles'	1.7 oz	169	5.7	13.8	331	(mq)	10.1	2.0	18	54%
'Colonel's'	5.9 oz	482	20.8	38.6	1060	(mq)	27.3	5.7	47	51%

Food Name	Serving Size	Calories	Prot. gms	Carbs gms	Sod. mgs	Fiber gms	Fat gms	Sat. Fat gms	Chol. mgs	% Fat Cal.
COLESLAW	3.2 oz	114	1.0	13.0	177	na	6.0	1.0	<5	47%
CORN, on the cob	5.3 oz	222	4.0	27.0	76	8.0	12.0	2.0	0	49%
CORNBREAD, 2 oz	1 serving	228	3.0	25.0	194	1.0	13.0	2.0	42	51%
FRENCH FRIES										
'Crispy' 2.5 oz	1 serving	210	3.0	24.0	493	3.0	11.0	3.0	4	47%
'Kentucky Fries'	1 serving	268	5.0	33.0	81	na	13.0	na	na	44%
regular, 2.7 oz	1 serving	244	3.2	31.1	139	(mq)	11.9	2.6	2	44%
GRAVY, chicken	1 serving	59	2.0	4.0	398	na	4.0	na	na	61%
HONEY SAUCE	.5 oz	49	0.0	12.1	15	0	<.1	<.1	<1	<2%
MACARONI AND CHEESE	4 oz	162	7.0	15.0	531	0	8.0	3.0	16	44%
MUSTARD SAUCE	1 oz	36	0.9	6.0	346	na	0.9	0.1	<1	23%
POTATO WEDGES	3.3 oz	192	3.0	25.0	428	3.0	9.0	3.0	3	42%
POTATOES, MASHED										
plain	1 serving	59	2.0	12.0	228	na	tr	na	na	0%
w/gravy	4.2 oz	70	3.0	15.0	370	na	1.0	<1.0	<5	13%
RED BEANS AND RICE	3.9 oz	114	4.0	18.0	315	3.0	3.0	1.0	4	24%
RICE, garden	3.8 oz	75	2.0	15.0	576	1.0	1.0	0.0	0	12%
ROLL, sourdough, 1.7 oz	1 roll	128	4.0	24.0	236	1.0	2.0	0.0	0	14%
SALAD										
garden	3.1 oz	16	1.0	3.0	10	1.0	0.0	0.0	0	0%
macaroni	3.8 oz	248	4.0	20.0	6	1.0	17.0	3.0	12	62%
pasta	3.8 oz	135	2.0	14.0	663	1.0	8.0	1.0	1	53%
potato	4.4 oz	180	3.0	18.0	423	2.0	11.0	2.0	11	55%
vegetable medley	4 oz	126	1.0	21.0	240	3.0	4.0	1.0	0	29%
SALAD DRESSING										
Italian	1 oz	15	0.0	2.0	420	0	1.0	0.0	0	60%
ranch	1 oz	170	0.0	1.0	250	0	18.0	3.0	10	95%
SWEET AND SOUR SAUCE	1 oz	58	0.1	13.0	140	na	0.6	0.1	<1	9%
KRYSTAL										
BISCUIT	3.2 oz	289	5.0	35.0	777	na	14.0	3.0	1	44%
BREAKFAST, gravy biscuit	8.2 oz	445	9.0	43.0	1306	na	26.0	5.0	13	53%
BREAKFAST SANDWICH										
bacon biscuit	3.6 oz	355	9.0	36.0	1055	na	20.0	5.0	14	51%
country ham biscuit	4.5 oz	379	15.0	36.0	1488	na	19.0	5.0	23	45%
egg biscuit	4.8 oz	372	10.0	36.0	813	na	21.0	5.0	133	51%
sausage biscuit	4.3 oz	429	10.0	37.0	987	na	27.0	7.0	29	57%
CHEESEBURGER										
bacon	6.4 oz	583	36.0	34.0	935	na	35.0	14.0	114	54%
'Burger Plus'	7 oz	545	33.0	37.0	962	na	31.0	12.0	105	51%
double	1 serving	214	11.0	22.0	674	na	8.0	2.0	16	34%
regular	1 serving	189	11.0	16.0	456	na	10.0	4.0	30	48%
CHICKEN SANDWICH	6.4 oz	392	21.0	44.0	707	na	16.0	na	33	37%
CHILI										
large, 12 oz	1 serving	322	17.0	33.0	1012	na	11.0	na	25	31%
regular, 8 oz	1 serving	214	11.0	22.0	674	na	8.0	na	16	34%
DONUT										
plain	1.3 oz	100	1.0	17.0	130	na	9.0	2.0	6	81%
w/chocolate icing	1.8 oz	162	1.0	27.0	149	na	11.0	3.0	6	61%
w/vanilla icing	1.8 oz	148	1.0	29.0	130	na	9.0	2.0	6	55%
FRENCH FRIES										
'Krys Kross'	2.6 oz	242	3.0	33.0	589	na	11.0	5.0	10	41%
'Krys Kross' w/cheese	3.6 oz	292	4.0	35.0	789	na	15.0	6.0	11	46%
large order, 5 oz	1 serving	615	5.0	111.0	191	na	17.0	8.0	15	25%

Food Name	Serving Size	Calories	Prot. gms	Carbs gms	Sod. mgs	Fiber gms	Fat gms	Sat. Fat gms	Chol. mgs	% Fat Cal.
medium order, 3.9 oz	1 serving	474	4.0	86.0	147	na	13.0	6.0	12	25%
small order, 2.8 oz	1 serving	338	3.0	61.0	105	na	9.0	na	8	24%
HAMBURGER										
'Big K'	7.3 oz	608	40.0	35.0	1281	na	36.0	14.0	125	53%
'Burger Plus'	6.4 oz	488	30.0	36.0	709	na	27.0	9.0	90	50%
double, 4 oz	1 serving	276	18.0	24.0	532	na	14.0	5.0	43	46%
small, 2.2 oz	1 serving	158	9.0	15.0	339	na	7.0	na	21	40%
HOT DOG										
'Chili Cheese Pup'	2.6 oz	203	8.0	15.0	623	na	13.0	5.0	24	58%
'Chili Pup'	2.5 oz	184	7.0	14.0	593	na	12.0	4.0	19	59%
'Corn Pup'	2.3 oz	214	6.0	17.0	566	na	14.0	6.0	24	59%
plain	1.9 oz	164	6.0	14.0	469	na	10.0	4.0	15	55%
MILKSHAKE, chocolate	12.8 oz	271	8.0	41.0	175	na	10.0	5.0	32	33%
PIE										
apple	4.5 oz	320	3.0	45.0	420	na	14.0	4.0	0	39%
lemon meringue	4 oz	340	7.0	60.0	130	na	9.0	3.0	45	24%
pecan	4 oz	450	5.0	61.0	290	na	24.0	6.0	55	48%
LITTLE CAESARS										
BREAD, 'Crazy Bread'	1 serving	98	4.0	18.0	119	na	1.0	na	2	9%
HAM AND CHEESE SANDWICH	1 serving	520	28.0	55.0	1045	.5	21.0	(mq)	45	36%
PIZZA										
'Baby Pan!Pan!'	1 serving	525	28.0	53.0	1180	na	22.0	na	60	38%
cheese, round 'Pizza!Pizza!' large pie	1 serving	169	11.0	18.0	240	na	6.0	na	15	32%
cheese, round 'Pizza!Pizza!' medium pie	1 serving	154	10.0	16.0	220	na	5.0	na	15	29%
cheese, round 'Pizza!Pizza!' small pie	1 serving	138	9.0	14.0	200	na	5.0	na	15	33%
cheese, single slice, 2.2 oz	1 serving	170	9.0	20.0	285	.2	6.0	(mq)	10	32%
cheese, square 'Pizza!Pizza!' large pie	1 serving	188	10.0	22.0	380	na	6.0	na	20	29%
cheese, square 'Pizza!Pizza!' medium pie	1 serving	185	10.0	22.0	370	na	6.0	na	20	29%
cheese, square 'Pizza!Pizza!' small pie	1 serving	188	10.0	22.0	380	na	6.0	na	20	29%
pepperoni combination, single slice	1 serving	190	10.0	20.0	340	.8	7.0	(mq)	15	33%
PIZZA ENTRÉE										
cheese pizza, w/individual tossed salad	1 serving	600	30.0	73.0	1605	3.0	21.0	(mq)	35	32%
vegetable pizza, w/individual tossed salad	1 serving	640	34.0	76.0	1715	3.6	22.0	(mq)	40	31%
SALAD										
antipasto, w/low-calorie dressing, 12 oz	1 serving	170	10.0	12.0	1145	(mq)	9.0	(mq)	40	48%
Greek, small	1 serving	85	4.0	6.0	400	na	5.0	na	10	53%
Greek, w/low-calorie dressing, 11 oz	1 serving	140	8.0	8.0	1075	(mq)	8.0	(mq)	25	51%
tossed, small	1 serving	37	2.0	7.0	85	na	1.0	na	0	24%
tossed, w/low-calorie dressing, 11 oz	1 serving	80	4.0	11.0	745	(mq)	2.0	(mq)	0	23%
SAUCE, 'Crazy Sauce'	1 serving	63	3.0	11.0	360	na	1.0	na	0	14%
SUBMARINE SANDWICH, Italian	1 serving	590	29.0	55.0	1230	1.7	28.0	(mq)	60	43%
TUNA MELT SANDWICH	1 serving	700	34.0	58.0	825	.6	37.0	(mq)	65	48%
TURKEY SANDWICH	1 serving	450	24.0	49.0	1590	na	17.0	na	45	34%
VEGETARIAN SANDWICH	1 serving	620	30.0	58.0	1000	1.3	30.0	(mq)	55	44%
LONG JOHN SILVER'S										
BEANS, green, 3.5 oz	1 serving	20	1.0	3.0	320	na	<1.0	<.3	0	0%
BREADSTICKS, 1.2 oz	1 serving	110	3.0	18.0	120	na	3.0	na	0	25%
BROWNIE, walnut, 3.4 oz	1 brownie	440	5.0	54.0	150	na	22.0	5.4	20	45%
CATFISH ENTRÉE, fillet, w/fries, 2 hushpuppies, and coleslaw	1 serving	860	28.0	90.0	990	na	42.0	10.0	65	44%
CATFISH FILLET, 2.7 oz	1 serving	203	12.0	13.0	469	na	12.0	na	na	53%
CHEESECAKE, pineapple cream	3.2 oz	310	4.0	34.0	105	na	18.0	9.0	10	52%

Food Name	Serving Size	Calories	Prot. gms	Carbs gms	Sod. mgs	Fiber gms	Fat gms	Sat. Fat gms	Chol. mgs	% Fat Cal.
CHICKEN										
light herb, 3.5 oz	1 serving	120	22.0	<1.0	570	na	4.0	1.2	60	30%
'Plank' 1 piece	2 oz	120	8.0	11.0	400	na	3.0	1.6	15	23%
'Planks' 2 pieces	4 oz	240	16.0	22.0	790	na	12.0	3.2	30	45%
'Planks' 2 pieces, w/fries, hushpuppies, coleslaw	6.9 oz	490	19.0	50.0	1290	na	26.0	5.7	30	48%
CHICKEN ENTRÉE										
'Kids Meal' 2 pieces, w/fries, hushpuppy	7.8 oz	560	21.0	60.0	1310	na	29.0	6.3	30	47%
'Planks' 3 pieces, w/fries, hushpuppies, coleslaw	14.1 oz	890	32.0	101.0	2000	na	44.0	9.5	55	44%
'Planks' 4 pieces, w/fries, coleslaw	1 serving	940	39.0	94.0	1390	na	44.0	10.0	70	42%
w/rice, green beans, coleslaw, roll w/o margarine	15.9 oz	590	32.0	82.0	1620	na	15.0	3.3	75	23%
CHICKEN SANDWICH										
1 piece, batter-dipped, w/o sauce, 4.5 oz	1 serving	280	14.0	39.0	790	na	8.0	2.1	15	26%
CHOWDER										
clam, w/cod	1 serving	140	11.0	10.0	590	na	6.0	2.0	20	39%
seafood, w/cod, 7 oz	1 serving	140	11.0	10.0	590	na	6.0	1.8	20	39%
CLAM ENTRÉE, w/fries, hushpuppies, coleslaw	12.7 oz	990	24.0	114.0	1830	na	52.0	10.9	75	47%
CLAMS, breaded, 4.7 oz	1 serving	526	17.0	48.0	1170	na	31.0	na	na	53%
COLESLAW	1 serving	140	1.0	20.0	260	na	6.0	1.0	15	39%
COMBINATION ENTRÉE										
fish, scallops, w/fries, 2 hushpuppies, coleslaw	1 serving	970	30.0	109.0	1540	na	46.0	10.0	70	43%
'Fish, Shrimp & Chicken' w/fries, hushpuppies, coleslaw	18.1 oz	1160	45.0	113.0	2590	na	65.0	14.2	135	50%
'Fish, Shrimp & Clams' w/fries, hushpuppies, coleslaw	18.1 oz	1240	44.0	123.0	2630	na	70.0	15.2	140	51%
'Fish & Chicken' w/fries, hushpuppies, coleslaw	15.2 oz	950	36.0	102.0	2090	na	49.0	10.6	75	46%
'Fish & Chicken Kids Meal' w/fries, hushpuppies	8.9 oz	620	24.0	61.0	1400	na	34.0	7.4	45	49%
'Fish & Shrimp' w/fries, hushpuppies, coleslaw	17.2 oz	1140	40.0	108.0	2440	na	65.0	14.1	145	51%
1 piece fish, 1 piece chicken, w/fries	8.1 oz	550	23.0	51.0	1380	na	32.0	6.8	45	52%
COOKIE										
chocolate chip	1.0 oz	230	3.0	35.0	170	na	9.0	5.7	10	35%
oatmeal raisin	1.8 oz	160	3.0	15.0	150	na	10.0	2.0	15	56%
CORN, cobbette, 3.3 oz	1 cob	140	3.0	18.0	0	na	8.0	na	0	51%
CRACKER, saltine, 1 pkg	2 crackers	25	<1.0	4.0	75	na	1.0	na	0	36%
FISH. See also individual listings.										
baked, w/sauce, 5.5 oz	1 serving	151	33.0	0.0	361	na	2.0	na	na	12%
batter-dipped, 1 piece	3.1 oz	180	12.0	12.0	490	na	11.0	2.7	30	55%
crispy, 1.8 oz	1 serving	150	8.0	8.0	240	na	8.0	2.2	20	48%
kitchen breaded, 2 oz	1 serving	122	9.0	8.0	374	na	5.0	na	na	37%
lemon crumb, 3 pieces, 5 oz	1 serving	150	29.0	4.0	370	na	1.0	na	110	6%
light paprika, 3 pieces, 4.7 oz	1 serving	120	28.0	<1.0	120	na	<1.0	na	110	<7%
scampi sauce, 3 pieces, 5.2 oz	1 serving	170	28.0	2.0	270	na	5.0	na	110	26%
FISH ENTRÉE. See also individual listings.										
baked, w/sauce, coleslaw, mixed vegetables	1 serving	387	36.0	19.0	1298	na	19.0	na	na	44%
'Crispy Fish' 3 pieces, w/fries, hushpuppies, coleslaw	13.5 oz	980	31.0	92.0	1530	na	50.0	11.3	70	46%
'Fish & Fries Kids Meal' 1 piece, w/fries, hushpuppy, 7 oz	1 serving	500	16.0	50.0	1010	na	28.0	5.8	30	50%
'Fish & Fries' 3 pieces, w/ fries, 2 hushpuppies	1 serving	810	42.0	77.0	1630	na	38.0	9.0	85	42%
'Fish & Fries' 2 pieces, w/ fries, 9.2 oz	1 serving	610	27.0	52.0	1480	na	37.0	7.9	60	55%
'Fish & More' 2 pieces, w/fries, hushpuppies, coleslaw	14.4 oz	890	31.0	92.0	1790	na	48.0	10.1	75	49%
'Homestyle' 6 pieces, w/fries, 2 hushpuppies, coleslaw	1 serving	1260	49.0	124.0	1590	na	64.0	14.0	130	46%
kitchen breaded, 3 pieces, w/fries, hushpuppies, coleslaw	1 serving	940	35.0	84.0	1900	na	52.0	na	na	50%
kitchen breaded, 2 pieces, w/fries, hushpuppies, coleslaw	1 serving	818	26.0	76.0	1526	na	46.0	na	na	51%
lemon crumb, 2 pieces, w/rice, salad, 'Light' 11.8 oz	1 serving	290	24.0	40.0	690	na	5.0	na	75	16%
light paprika, 2 pieces, w/rice and small salad	10 oz	300	24.0	45.0	650	na	2.0	na	70	6%
3 pieces, w/fries, 2 hushpuppies, coleslaw	1 serving	960	43.0	97.0	1890	na	44.0	10.0	100	41%
3 pieces, w/rice, green bean, coleslaw, roll w/o butter	17.4 oz	610	39.0	86.0	1420	na	13.0	2.2	125	19%

Food Name	Serving Size	Calories	Prot. gms	Carbs gms	Sod. mgs	Fiber gms	Fat gms	Sat. Fat gms	Chol. mgs	% Fat Cal
FISH SANDWICH										
'Homestyle'	1 serving	510	22.0	58.0	780	na	22.0	5.0	48	39%
'Homestyle Platter' w/fries, coleslaw	1 serving	870	26.0	108.0	1110	na	38.0	8.0	55	39%
1 piece, batter-dipped, w/o sauce, 5.6 oz	1 serving	340	18.0	40.0	890	na	13.0	3.2	30	34%
FRENCH FRIES, 3 oz	1 serving	220	3.0	30.0	60	na	10.0	3.0	5	41%
HONEY MUSTARD SAUCE	1 oz	56	tr	14.0	315	na	tr	na	na	0%
HUSHPUPPY	1 piece	70	2.0	10.0	25	na	2.0	1.0	5	26%
MALT VINEGAR	1 oz	1	0.0	0.0	15	na	0.0	0.0	na	0%
MIXED VEGETABLES, 4 oz	1 serving	60	2.0	9.0	330	na	2.0	1.0	0	30%
OYSTER ENTRÉE, 6 pieces, w/fries and coleslaw	1 serving	789	17.0	78.0	763	na	45.0	na	na	51%
OYSTERS, 3 pieces, breaded, 2.1 oz	1 serving	180	6.0	18.0	195	na	9.0	na	na	45%
PIE										
apple	4.5 oz	320	3.0	45.0	420	na	13.0	4.5	5	37%
cherry	4.5 oz	360	4.0	55.0	200	na	13.0	4.4	5	33%
lemon	4 oz	340	7.0	60.0	130	na	9.0	3.0	45	24%
pecan	4 oz	446	5.0	59.0	435	na	22.0	na	na	44%
pumpkin	4 oz	251	4.0	34.0	242	na	11.0	na	na	39%
RICE PILAF, 5 oz	1 serving	210	5.0	43.0	570	na	2.0	na	0	9%
ROLL	1.5 oz	110	4.0	23.0	170	na	<1.0	<.3	0	<8%
SALAD										
garden, w/crackers	1 serving	170	9.0	13.0	380	na	9.0	2.0	5	48%
ocean chef, w/crackers	1 serving	250	24.0	19.0	1340	na	9.0	1.0	80	32%
ocean chef, w/o dressing or crackers, 8.3 oz	1 serving	110	12.0	13.0	730	na	1.0	0.4	40	8%
seafood, 1 scoop	1 serving	210	14.0	26.0	570	na	5.0	1.0	90	21%
seafood, w/crackers	1 serving	270	16.0	36.0	670	na	7.0	1.0	90	23%
seafood, w/o dressing or crackers, 9.8 oz	1 serving	380	15.0	12.0	980	na	31.0	5.1	55	73%
shrimp, w/crackers	1 serving	183	27.0	12.0	658	na	3.0	na	na	15%
small, w/o dressing, 1.9 oz	1 serving	8	<1.0	2.0	0	na	0.0	na	0	0%
SALAD DRESSING										
blue cheese	1.5 oz	225	2.0	3.0	na	na	23.0	na	na	92%
Italian, reduced calorie	1.5 oz	20	tr	3.0	882	na	1.0	na	na	45%
sea salad	1.5 oz	220	2.0	5.0	na	na	21.0	na	na	86%
Thousand Island	1.5 oz	225	tr	8.0	422	na	22.0	na	na	88%
SCALLOP ENTRÉE, w/fries and coleslaw	1 serving	747	17.0	66.0	1579	na	45.0	na	na	54%
SCALLOPS, battered, 3 pieces, 2.1 oz	1 serving	159	6.0	12.0	503	na	9.0	na	na	51%
SEAFOOD GUMBO, w/cod	7 oz	120	9.0	4.0	740	na	8.0	2.1	25	60%
SEAFOOD SAUCE	1 oz	34	tr	9.0	357	na	tr	na	na	0%
SHRIMP										
batter-dipped, .4 oz	1 piece	30	1.0	2.0	80	na	2.0	0.5	10	60%
breaded, 4.7 oz	1 serving	388	12.0	33.0	1229	na	23.0	na	na	53%
SHRIMP ENTRÉE										
breaded, 21 pieces, w/fries, hushpuppies, coleslaw	1 serving	1070	25.0	130.0	1790	na	51.0	11.0	125	43%
10 pieces, w/fries, hushpuppies, coleslaw	11.7 oz	840	18.0	88.0	1630	na	47.0	9.7	100	50%
w/scampi sauce	5.2 oz	120	15.0	2.0	610	na	5.0	na	205	38%
SWEET AND SOUR SAUCE	.42 oz	20	<1.0	5.0	45	na	<1.0	<.3	0	0%
TARTAR SAUCE	1 oz	117	tr	5.0	228	na	11.0	na	na	85%
MAZZIO'S PIZZA										
BEEF SANDWICH, barbecue beef and cheddar	1 sandwich	580	39.0	53.0	1260	na	24.0	11.0	95	37%
CHICKEN SANDWICH, chicken and cheddar	1 sandwich	570	33.0	56.0	1350	na	24.0	8.0	70	38%
GARLIC BREAD, w/cheese	2 slices	700	21.0	74.0	1280	na	35.0	7.0	15	45%
HAM AND CHEESE SANDWICH	1 sandwich	790	40.0	71.0	1900	na	39.0	13.0	85	44%
LASAGNA, meat, small	1 serving	460	24.0	26.0	1370	na	25.0	10.0	95	49%
NACHOS, w/meat	4.5 oz	500	21.0	21.0	1200	na	37.0	17.0	75	67%

Food Name	Serving Size	Calories	Prot. gms	Carbs gms	Sod. mgs	Fiber gms	Fat gms	Sat. Fat gms	Chol. mgs	% Fat Cal.
PASTA AND NOODLES										
chicken parmesan	17.5 oz	590	39.0	68.0	1600	na	19.0	3.0	50	29%
fettuccine Alfredo, small	1 serving	440	14.0	34.0	680	na	28.0	16.0	55	57%
spaghetti, small	1 serving	290	11.0	39.0	800	na	10.0	na	5	31%
PIZZA										
cheese, deep pan	1 slice	350	17.0	42.0	620	na	8.0	na	15	21%
cheese, original crust, medium pie	1 slice	260	14.0	33.0	450	na	8.0	na	10	28%
cheese, thin crust	1 slice	220	13.0	22.0	440	na	9.0	na	15	37%
combo, deep pan, medium pie	1 slice	410	19.0	42.0	930	na	18.0	6.0	20	40%
combo, original crust, medium pie	1 slice	320	17.0	34.0	780	na	13.0	6.0	25	37%
'Light' medium pie	1 slice	240	10.0	30.0	460	na	8.0	4.0	20	30%
pepperoni, deep pan, medium pie	1 slice	380	18.0	38.0	740	na	17.0	6.0	25	40%
pepperoni, original crust, medium pie	1 slice	280	16.0	30.0	600	na	11.0	5.0	30	35%
sausage, deep pan, medium pie	1 slice	430	21.0	41.0	1040	na	21.0	8.0	25	44%
sausage, original crust, medium pie	1 slice	350	18.0	34.0	890	na	16.0	7.0	20	41%
SUBMARINE SANDWICH, 'Deluxe'	1 sandwich	810	39.0	68.0	2240	na	43.0	13.0	75	48%
MC DONALD'S										
APPLE JUICE	6 oz	80	0.0	21.0	30	na	0.0	0.0	0	0%
APPLE PIE, 3.0 oz	1 serving	260	2.0	30.0	240	(mq)	15.0	10.0	6	52%
BACON BITS	.1 oz	15	1.0	0.0	95	na	1.0	0.3	1	60%
BARBECUE SAUCE	1 serving	50	0.0	12.0	340	0	0.5	0.2	0	9%
BISCUIT, w/spread, 2.6 oz	1 serving	260	5.0	32.0	730	(mq)	13.0	9.0	1	45%
BREAKFAST										
Cheerios cereal, w/o milk, 3/4 cup	1 serving	80	3.0	14.0	210	na	1.0	0.4	0	11%
eggs, scrambled, 3.5 oz	1 serving	140	12.0	1.0	290	0	10.0	5.0	425	64%
hotcakes, w/margarine and syrup, 6.2 oz	1 serving	440	8.0	74.0	685	(mq)	12.0	5.0	8	25%
sausage, 1.5 oz	1 serving	100	7.0	0.0	310	0	15.0	5.0	43	84%
Wheaties cereal, w/o milk, 3/4 cup	1 serving	90	2.0	19.0	220	na	1.0	0.2	0	10%
BREAKFAST SANDWICH										
biscuit, bacon, egg, and cheese, 5.4 oz	1 serving	440	15.0	33.0	1215	(mq)	26.0	16.0	240	53%
biscuit, sausage and egg, 6.2 oz	1 serving	505	19.0	33.0	1210	(mq)	33.0	20.0	260	59%
biscuit, sausage, 4.2 oz	1 serving	420	12.0	32.0	1040	(mq)	28.0	17.0	44	60%
egg, ham, and cheese, 'Egg McMuffin' 4.8 oz	1 serving	280	18.0	28.0	710	(mq)	11.0	4.0	235	35%
sausage, 'Sausage McMuffin' 4.8 oz	1 serving	345	15.0	27.0	770	(mq)	20.0	11.0	57	52%
sausage, 'Sausage Egg McMuffin' 5.6 oz	1 serving	430	21.0	27.0	920	(mq)	25.0	14.0	270	52%
CHEESEBURGER										
'McLean Deluxe' 7.7 oz	1 serving	370	24.0	35.0	890	(mq)	14.0	8.0	75	34%
'Quarter Pounder' 6.8 oz	1 serving	510	28.0	34.0	1110	(mq)	28.0	16.0	115	49%
regular, 4.1 oz	1 serving	305	15.0	30.0	725	(mq)	13.0	7.0	50	38%
CHICKEN NUGGET, 'Chicken McNuggets' 6 pieces	1 serving	270	20.0	17.0	580	(mq)	15.0	10.0	55	50%
CHICKEN SANDWICH, 'McChicken' 6.6 oz	1 serving	415	19.0	39.0	830	(mq)	19.0	9.0	50	41%
CHOW MEIN NOODLES	1 serving	45	1.0	5.0	60	na	2.0	1.0	2	40%
COOKIE										
'Chocolaty Chip' 2 oz	1 serving	330	4.0	42.0	280	(mq)	15.0	10.0	4	41%
'McDonaldland' 2 oz	1 serving	290	4.0	47.0	300	(mq)	9.0	7.0	0	28%
CROUTONS	.4 oz	50	1.0	7.0	140	(mq)	2.0	1.3	0	36%
DANISH										
apple, 4.1 oz	1 serving	390	6.0	51.0	370	(mq)	17.0	11.0	25	39%
cinnamon raisin, 3.9 oz	1 serving	440	6.0	58.0	430	(mq)	21.0	13.0	34	43%
cheese, iced, 3.9 oz	1 serving	390	7.0	42.0	420	(mq)	21.0	13.0	47	48%
raspberry, 4.1 oz	1 serving	410	6.0	62.0	310	(mq)	16.0	11.0	26	35%
ENGLISH MUFFIN, w/spread, 2.1 oz	1 muffin	170	5.0	26.0	285	(mq)	4.0	2.0	0	21%
FISH SANDWICH, 'Fillet-O-Fish' 5 oz	1 serving	370	14.0	38.0	730	(mq)	18.0	8.0	50	44%

Food Name	Serving Size	Calories	Prot. gms	Carbs gms	Sod. mgs	Fiber gms	Fat gms	Sat. Fat gms	Chol. mgs	% Fat Cal.
FRENCH FRIES										
large order	4.3 oz	400	6.0	46.0	200	(mq)	22.0	15.0	0	50%
large order, unsalted	4.3 oz	400	6.0	46.0	45	(mq)	22.0	15.0	0	50%
medium order	3.4 oz	320	4.0	36.0	150	(mq)	17.0	12.0	0	48%
medium order, unsalted	3.4 oz	320	4.0	36.0	35	(mq)	17.0	12.0	0	48%
small order	2.4 oz	220	3.0	26.0	110	(mq)	12.0	8.0	0	49%
small order, unsalted	2.4 oz	220	3.0	26.0	25	(mq)	12.0	8.0	0	49%
GRAPEFRUIT JUICE	6 oz	80	1.0	19.0	0	na	0.0	0.0	0	0%
HAMBURGER										
'Big Mac' 7.6 oz	1 serving	500	25.0	42.0	890	(mq)	26.0	16.0	100	47%
'McLean Deluxe' 7.3 oz	1 serving	320	22.0	35.0	670	(mq)	10.0	5.0	60	28%
'Quarter Pounder' 5.9 oz	1 serving	410	23.0	34.0	645	(mq)	20.0	11.0	85	44%
regular, 3.6 oz	1 serving	255	12.0	30.0	490	(mq)	9.0	5.0	37	32%
HAMBURGER PATTY, 'McLean Deluxe' 3 oz	1 serving	130	17.0	0.0	110	0	7.0	3.0	60	48%
HONEY SAUCE	1 serving	45	0.0	12.0	0	0	0.0	0.0	0	0%
MILK, 1%	8 oz	110	9.0	12.0	130	na	2.0	0.3	10	16%
MILKSHAKE										
chocolate, low-fat	10.4 oz	320	11.0	66.0	240	(tr)	1.7	0.9	10	5%
strawberry, low-fat	10.4 oz	320	11.0	67.0	170	(tr)	1.3	0.6	10	4%
vanilla, low-fat	10.4 oz	290	11.0	60.0	170	0	1.3	0.6	10	4%
MUFFIN										
apple bran, fat-free, 2.6 oz	1 muffin	180	5.0	40.0	200	(mq)	0.0	0.0	0	0%
blueberry, fat-free, 2.6 oz	1 muffin	170	3.0	40.0	220	na	0.0	0.0	0	0%
MUSTARD SAUCE, hot	1 serving	70	0.0	8.0	250	0	3.6	1.2	5	46%
ORANGE JUICE	6 oz	80	1.0	19.0	0	na	0.0	0.0	0	0%
POTATOES, HASH BROWN 1.9 oz	1 serving	130	1.0	15.0	330	(mq)	7.0	4.0	0	48%
SALAD										
chef's, 9.5 oz	1 serving	170	17.0	8.0	400	(mq)	9.0	4.0	111	48%
chunky chicken, 9.0 oz	1 serving	150	25.0	7.0	230	(mq)	4.0	2.0	78	24%
garden, 6.7 oz	1 serving	50	4.0	6.0	70	(mq)	2.0	1.0	65	36%
side order, 3.7 oz	1 serving	30	2.0	4.0	35	(mq)	1.0	0.5	33	30%
SALAD DRESSING										
blue cheese, 1 tbsp	.5 oz	50	0.0	1.0	150	na	4.0	1.0	7	72%
French, red, reduced calorie, 1 tbsp	.5 oz	40	0.0	5.0	115	na	2.0	0.5	0	45%
Oriental	.5 oz	24	tr	6.0	180	na	tr	0.0	0	0%
ranch, 1 tbsp	.5 oz	55	0.0	1.0	130	na	5.0	0.5	5	82%
Thousand Island, 1 tbsp	.5 oz	78	0.0	2.0	100	na	8.0	2.0	8	92%
vinaigrette, 1 tbsp	.5 oz	12	0.0	2.0	60	na	0.5	0.1	0	38%
SOFT DRINK										
Coca-Cola Classic, extra large, w/ice	32 oz	380	0.0	101.0	40	na	0.0	0.0	0	0%
Coca-Cola Classic, large, w/ice	22 oz	260	0.0	70.0	25	na	0.0	0.0	0	0%
Coca-Cola Classic, medium, w/ice	16 oz	190	0.0	50.0	20	na	0.0	0.0	0	0%
Coca-Cola Classic, small, w/ice	12 oz	140	0.0	38.0	15	na	0.0	0.0	0	0%
Diet Coke, extra large, w/ice	32 oz	3	0.0	0.6	80	na	0.0	0.0	0	0%
Diet Coke, large, w/ice	22 oz	2	0.0	0.5	60	na	0.0	0.0	0	0%
Diet Coke, medium, w/ice	16 oz	1	0.0	0.4	40	na	0.0	0.0	0	0%
Diet Coke, small w/ice	12 oz	1	0.0	0.3	30	na	0.0	0.0	0	0%
orange, extra large, w/ice	32 oz	360	0.0	88.0	25	na	0.0	0.0	0	0%
orange, large, w/ice	22 oz	240	0.0	60.0	20	na	0.0	0.0	0	0%
orange, medium, w/ice	16 oz	180	0.0	44.0	20	na	0.0	0.0	0	0%
orange, small, w/ice	12 oz	130	0.0	33.0	10	na	0.0	0.0	0	0%
Sprite, extra large, w/ice	32 oz	380	0.0	96.0	40	na	0.0	0.0	0	0%
Sprite, large, w/ice	22 oz	260	0.0	66.0	25	na	0.0	0.0	0	0%
Sprite, medium, w/ice	16 oz	190	0.0	48.0	20	na	0.0	0.0	0	0%

Food Name	Serving Size	Calories	Prot. gms	Carbs gms	Sod. mgs	Fiber gms	Fat gms	Sat. Fat gms	Chol. mgs	% Fat Cal.
Sprite, small, w/ice	12 oz	140	0.0	36.0	15	na	0.0	0.0	0	0%
SWEET AND SOUR SAUCE	1 serving	60	0.0	14.0	190	0	0.2	0.1	0	3%
YOGURT, FROZEN										
cone, vanilla, low-fat	3 oz	105	4.0	22.0	80	(mq)	1.0	0.3	3	9%
hot caramel sundae, low-fat	6 oz	270	7.0	59.0	180	(tr)	3.0	1.0	13	10%
hot fudge sundae, low-fat	6 oz	240	7.0	50.0	170	(tr)	3.0	0.5	6	11%
strawberry sundae, low-fat	6 oz	210	6.0	49.0	170	(tr)	1.0	0.5	6	4%
MRS. WINNER'S										
BAKED BEANS	1 serving	149	5.0	31.0	436	na	na	na	1	0%
BISCUIT	1 serving	245	4.0	45.0	503	na	5.0	na	tr	18%
BREAKFAST										
country ham	1 serving	60	4.0	tr	565	na	1.0	na	14	15%
sausage patty	1 serving	200	6.0	tr	400	na	10.0	na	8	45%
CHICKEN										
breast, fried, skin-free	4 oz	280	23.0	14.0	480	na	15.0	na	115	48%
dark meat quarter, 'Rotisserie'	4 oz	216	29.0	2.0	590	na	10.0	na	140	42%
fillet, baked	1 serving	120	10.0	tr	360	na	2.0	na	33	15%
leg, fried, skin-free	1.7 oz	110	10.0	5.0	115	na	6.0	na	50	49%
white meat quarter, 'Rotisserie'	5 oz	242	38.0	2.0	700	na	9.0	na	139	33%
CHICKEN SANDWICH										
breaded	1 serving	203	19.0	12.0	1000	na	10.0	na	37	44%
fillet	1 serving	379	12.0	45.0	541	na	7.0	na	28	17%
salad	1 serving	313	10.0	33.0	599	na	6.0	na	1	17%
COLESLAW	1 serving	188	1.0	9.0	549	na	16.0	na	1	77%
FRENCH FRIES	1 serving	225	6.0	27.0	214	na	9.0	na	1	36%
POTATO WEDGES, oven roasted	1 serving	139	4.0	31.0	132	na	1.0	na	1	6%
POTATOES, MASHED, w/gravy	1 serving	148	3.0	22.0	823	na	3.0	na	2	18%
ROLL, honey yeast	1 roll	200	8.0	35.0	290	na	4.0	na	7	18%
SALAD										
chicken	1 serving	583	9.0	39.0	875	na	8.0	na	3	12%
seafood	1 serving	553	5.0	41.0	756	na	9.0	na	4	15%
tossed	1 serving	6	1.0	1.0	439	na	tr	na	1	0%
STEAK ENTRÉE, country-fried	1 serving	220	12.0	tr	205	na	14.0	na	7	57%
STEAK SANDWICH	1 serving	429	11.0	43.0	644	na	11.0	na	21	23%
ORANGE JULIUS										
JUICE DRINK										
orange, regular	16 oz	265	1.0	66.0	15	na	1.0	na	na	3%
pina colada, regular	16 oz	300	2.0	71.0	15	na	1.0	na	na	3%
raspberry cream supreme, regular	16 oz	510	4.0	76.0	40	na	23.0	na	na	41%
strawberry, regular	16 oz	340	1.0	82.0	15	na	1.0	na	na	3%
tropical cream supreme, regular	16 oz	510	5.0	67.0	40	na	25.0	na	95	44%
PERKINS										
BROCCOLI, raw	4 oz	31	3.4	5.9	31	na	0.4	na	0	12%
CARROTS, raw	4 oz	49	1.2	11.5	39	na	0.2	na	0	4%
CAULIFLOWER, raw	4 oz	27	2.2	5.6	16	na	0.2	na	0	7%
CHICKEN DINNER, lemon pepper, w/rice pilaf, broccoli, salad	1 serving	620	59.4	59.6	1364	na	12.5	na	136	18%
FISH DINNER, orange roughy, w/rice pilaf, broccoli, salad	1 serving	467	33.0	60.0	1387	na	7.0	na	133	13%
FRUIT CUP, cantaloupe, honeydew, blueberries, 4.5 oz	1 serving	48	0.8	11.9	12	na	0.3	na	0	6%
MARGARINE	1 scant tbsp	60	0.0	0.0	60	na	6.5	na	0	98%
MUFFIN										
apple, 6.5 oz pre-baked wt	1 muffin	543	9.0	76.0	728	na	24.0	na	95	40%

Food Name	Serving Size	Calories	Prot. gms	Carbs gms	Sod. mgs	Fiber gms	Fat gms	Sat. Fat gms	Chol. mgs	% Fat Cal.
banana nut, 6.5 oz pre-baked wt	1 muffin	586	9.0	75.0	702	na	29.0	na	92	45%
blueberry, 6.5 oz pre-baked wt	1 muffin	506	7.0	71.0	671	na	23.0	na	88	41%
bran, 6.5 oz pre-baked wt	1 muffin	478	9.0	83.0	572	na	17.0	na	0	32%
carrot, 6.5 oz pre-baked wt	1 muffin	560	7.0	88.0	780	na	23.0	na	81	37%
chocolate chocolate chip, 6.5 oz pre-baked wt	1 muffin	546	10.0	73.0	629	na	26.0	na	83	43%
corn, 6.5 oz pre-baked wt	1 muffin	683	12.0	121.0	1550	na	17.0	na	33	22%
cranberry nut, 6.5 oz pre-baked wt	1 muffin	558	9.0	71.0	671	na	28.0	na	88	45%
oat bran, 6.5 oz pre-baked wt	1 muffin	513	10.0	87.0	588	na	16.0	na	0	28%
plain, 6.5 oz pre-baked wt	1 muffin	586	9.0	81.0	797	na	26.0	na	104	40%
plain, 98% fat-free, 6.5 oz pre-baked wt	1 muffin	495	11.8	111.0	802	na	1.2	na	5	2%
MUSHROOMS, raw	4 oz	29	2.4	5.3	3	na	0.5	na	0	16%
OMELETTE										
country club	1 serving	932	47.2	5.8	1134	<1.0	79.1	na	1154	76%
country club, w/3 oz hash browns	1 serving	1033	48.7	22.5	1162	<1.0	81.7	na	1154	71%
deli ham and cheese	1 serving	962	53.4	8.2	1832	<1.0	79.1	na	864	74%
deli ham and cheese, w/3 oz hash browns	1 serving	1063	54.9	24.9	1860	<1.0	81.7	na	864	69%
'Denver' w/fruit cup	1 serving	235	23.0	22.3	795	na	6.5	na	154	25%
'Everything'	1 serving	697	44.5	8.6	870	na	53.4	na	814	69%
'Everything' w/3 oz hash browns	1 serving	798	46.0	25.3	898	<2.0	56.0	na	814	63%
Granny's country	1 serving	941	42.9	6.9	786	<1.0	81.5	na	810	78%
Granny's country, w/9 oz hash browns	1 serving	1245	47.5	56.9	869	<1.0	89.2	na	810	64%
ham and cheese	1 serving	644	40.9	2.6	832	0	51.3	na	743	72%
ham and cheese, w/3 oz hash browns	1 serving	745	42.4	19.3	860	0	53.9	na	743	65%
mushroom and cheese	1 serving	687	32.0	4.9	925	<1.0	59.9	na	744	78%
mushroom and cheese, w/3 oz hash browns	1 serving	788	33.5	21.6	953	<1.0	62.5	na	744	71%
seafood, w/fruit cup	1 serving	271	28.6	27.5	595	na	5.7	na	197	19%
ONION, raw	4 oz	38	1.3	8.3	3	na	0.3	na	0	7%
PANCAKES										
buttermilk	3 pancakes	442	13.1	69.6	988	na	12.0	na	24	24%
'Harvest Grain' w/1.5 oz low-calorie syrup	5 pancakes	473	11.3	93.0	1640	na	3.4	na	0	6%
'Short Stack Harvest Grain'	3 pancakes	268	6.8	55.7	1020	na	2.0	na	0	7%
PIE										
apple	1 slice	521	3.0	72.0	457	na	26.0	na	0	45%
apple, w/Equal	1 slice	420	3.0	55.0	371	na	24.0	na	0	51%
cherry	1 slice	571	4.0	84.0	702	na	26.0	na	0	41%
cherry, w/Equal	1 slice	425	4.0	55.0	513	na	24.0	na	0	51%
coconut cream	1 slice	437	6.0	56.0	488	na	33.0	na	5	68%
French silk	1 slice	551	4.0	59.0	478	na	37.0	na	53	60%
lemon meringue,	1 slice	395	2.0	63.0	528	na	16.0	na	0	36%
peanut butter brownie	1 slice	455	9.0	44.0	436	na	35.0	na	29	69%
pecan	1 slice	669	7.0	106.0	670	na	26.0	na	17	35%
POTATOES, HASH BROWN	3 oz	101	1.5	16.7	28	na	2.6	na	na	23%
SALAD										
chef's, mini	1 serving	214	22.9	6.8	643	na	11.0	na	55	46%
dinner, 'Lite & Healthy'	1 serving	103	3.4	14.7	496	na	2.1	na	0	18%
SYRUP, low-calorie	1.5 oz	26	0.0	6.6	0	na	0.0	na	na	0%
TOAST, w/.5 oz margarine, .75 oz grape jelly	1 slice	219	2.3	27.7	224	1.0	12.2	na	8	50%
VEGETABLE SANDWICH										
pita, stir-fry	1 serving	308	43.7	41.1	752	na	9.2	na	26	27%
pita, stir-fry, w/coleslaw	1 serving	441	44.7	53.9	877	na	17.8	na	36	36%
pita, stir-fry, w/coleslaw and pasta salad	1 serving	626	49.0	62.9	1395	na	32.5	na	37	47%
pita, stir-fry, w/pasta salad	1 serving	493	48.0	50.1	1270	na	23.9	na	27	44%
mixed vegetables	6 oz	49	2.9	10.3	23	na	0.4	na	0	7%
ZUCCHINI, raw	4 oz	22	1.2	4.7	1	na	0.1	na	0	4%

Food Name	Serving Size	Calories	Prot. gms	Carbs gms	Sod. mgs	Fiber gms	Fat gms	Sat. Fat gms	Chol. mgs	% Fat Cal.
PETER PIPER PIZZA										
PIZZA										
Beef										
express lunch pizza	1 slice	165	9.0	21.0	257	na	5.0	na	13	27%
extra large pie	1 slice	280	15.0	36.0	446	na	8.0	na	20	26%
large pie	1 slice	296	15.0	39.0	482	na	8.0	na	20	24%
medium pie	1 slice	222	12.0	29.0	359	na	6.0	na	15	24%
small pie	1 slice	194	10.0	25.0	319	na	5.0	na	14	23%
Cheese										
express lunch pizza	1 pie	608	32.0	83.0	609	na	16.0	na	47	24%
express lunch pizza	1 slice	152	8.0	21.0	152	na	4.0	na	12	24%
extra large pie	1 pie	3078	160.0	437.0	3113	na	73.0	na	211	21%
extra large pie	1 slice	257	13.0	36.0	260	na	6.1	na	18	21%
large pie	1 pie	2159	111.5	311.4	2176	na	49.4	na	140	21%
large pie	1 slice	270	14.0	39.0	271	na	6.2	na	18	21%
medium pie	1 pie	1622	84.0	235.0	1614	na	37.0	na	105	21%
medium pie	1 slice	203	11.0	29.0	201	na	5.0	na	13	22%
small pie	1 pie	1059	60.0	152.0	1073	na	25.0	na	70	21%
small pie	1 slice	177	9.0	25.0	179	na	4.0	na	12	20%
w/black olives, large pie	1 serving	259	24.0	22.0	407	na	8.0	na	12	28%
w/black olives, medium pie	1 serving	193	18.0	17.0	303	na	6.0	na	9	28%
w/black olives, small pie	1 serving	171	16.0	15.0	276	na	6.0	na	8	32%
w/green pepper, large pie	1 serving	245	24.0	22.0	339	na	7.0	na	12	26%
w/green pepper, medium pie	1 serving	183	18.0	17.0	256	na	5.0	na	9	25%
w/green pepper, small pie	1 serving	163	16.0	15.0	283	na	4.0	na	8	22%
w/ham, large pie	1 serving	258	26.0	22.0	473	na	7.0	na	17	24%
w/ham, medium pie	1 serving	194	19.0	16.0	356	na	6.0	na	13	28%
w/ham, small pie	1 serving	172	17.0	15.0	317	na	5.0	na	11	26%
w/jalapeño, large pie	1 serving	244	24.0	22.0	424	na	7.0	na	12	26%
w/jalapeño, medium pie	1 serving	183	18.0	17.0	319	na	5.0	na	9	25%
w/jalapeño, small pie	1 serving	163	16.0	15.0	283	na	4.0	na	8	22%
w/mushroom, large pie	1 serving	245	24.0	22.0	379	na	7.0	na	12	26%
w/mushroom, medium pie	1 serving	183	18.0	17.0	283	na	5.0	na	9	25%
w/mushroom, small pie	1 serving	162	16.0	15.0	245	na	4.0	na	8	22%
w/onion, large pie	1 serving	243	24.0	22.0	341	na	7.0	na	12	26%
w/onion, medium pie	1 serving	183	18.0	17.0	257	na	5.0	na	9	25%
w/onion, small pie	1 serving	162	16.0	15.0	228	na	4.0	na	8	22%
w/pineapple, large pie	1 serving	246	23.0	23.0	341	na	7.0	na	12	26%
w/pineapple, medium pie	1 serving	185	18.0	17.0	256	na	5.0	na	8	24%
w/pineapple, small pie	1 serving	164	16.0	15.0	228	na	4.0	na	8	22%
Salami										
express lunch pizza	1 slice	164	9.0	21.0	199	na	5.0	na	15	27%
extra large pie	1 slice	273	14.0	37.0	322	na	7.5	na	22	25%
large pie	1 slice	288	15.0	39.0	342	na	8.0	na	23	25%
medium pie	1 slice	216	11.0	29.0	254	na	6.0	na	17	25%
small pie	1 slice	189	8.0	25.0	223	na	5.0	na	15	24%
PIZZA HUT										
PIZZA										
Beef										
hand-tossed	1 slice	261	15.0	28.0	795	2.0	10.0	3.0	25	34%
'Pan Pizza' medium pie	1 slice	288	10.0	27.0	675	3.0	18.0	3.0	25	56%
'Thick 'n Chewy' 10-inch pie	3 slices	620	38.0	73.0	na	na	20.0	na	na	29%
'Thin 'n Crispy' 10-inch pie	3 slices	490	29.0	51.0	na	na	19.0	na	na	35%

Food Name	Serving Size	Calories	Prot. gms	Carbs gms	Sod. mgs	Fiber gms	Fat gms	Sat. Fat gms	Chol. mgs	% Fat Cal.
Cheese										
'Bigfoot'	1 slice	179	9.0	24.0	959	2.0	5.0	3.0	14	25%
hand-tossed, medium pie	1 slice	253	15.0	27.0	593	2.0	9.0	4.0	25	32%
'Pan Pizza' medium pie	1 slice	279	14.0	26.0	473	2.0	13.0	5.0	25	42%
'Thick 'n Chewy' 10-inch pie	3 slices	560	34.0	71.0	na	na	14.0	na	na	23%
'Thin 'n Crispy' medium pie	1 slice	223	13.0	19.0	503	2.0	10.0	5.0	25	40%
'Thin 'n Crispy' 10-inch pie	3 slices	450	25.0	54.0	na	na	15.0	na	na	30%
'Chunky Combo'										
hand-tossed, medium pie	1 slice	280	14.8	28.0	823	2.5	11.6	4.8	29	37%
'Pan Pizza' medium pie	1 slice	306	13.8	26.0	703	2.5	15.5	5.2	29	46%
'Thin 'n Crispy' medium pie	1 slice	250	12.7	20.0	736	2.0	12.7	5.0	29	46%
'Chunky Meat'										
hand-tossed, medium pie	1 slice	325	16.8	28.0	970	2.6	16.0	6.0	40	44%
'Pan Pizza' medium pie	1 slice	352	15.7	27.0	850	2.6	20.0	7.0	40	51%
'Thin 'n Crispy' medium pie	1 slice	295	14.7	20.0	882	2.2	17.0	6.0	40	52%
Italian sausage										
hand-tossed, medium pie	1 slice	313	16.0	27.0	871	2.0	15.0	6.0	38	43%
'Pan Pizza' medium pie	1 slice	399	15.0	26.0	751	2.0	24.0	6.0	38	54%
'Thin 'n Crispy' medium pie	1 slice	282	14.0	20.0	781	2.0	17.0	6.0	38	54%
'Meat Lovers'										
hand-tossed, medium pie	1 slice	321	16.0	28.0	1106	3.0	15.0	4.0	42	42%
'Pan Pizza' medium pie	1 slice	347	15.0	27.0	986	3.0	23.0	5.0	42	60%
'Thin 'n Crispy' medium pie	1 slice	297	14.0	20.0	1068	2.0	16.0	4.0	44	48%
Pepperoni										
'Bigfoot'	1 slice	195	10.0	24.0	1022	2.0	7.0	3.0	17	32%
hand-tossed, medium pie	1 slice	253	20.0	28.0	738	2.0	10.0	3.0	25	36%
'Pan Pizza' medium pie	1 slice	280	8.0	26.0	618	2.0	18.0	3.0	25	58%
'Personal Pan Pizza' 9-oz pie	1 pie	675	37.0	76.0	1335	8.0	29.0	12.5	53	39%
'Thick 'n Chewy' 10-inch pie	3 slices	560	31.0	68.0	na	na	18.0	na	na	29%
'Thin 'n Crispy' medium pie	1 slice	230	12.0	20.0	678	2.0	11.0	3.0	27	43%
'Thin 'n Crispy' 10-inch pie	3 slices	430	23.0	45.0	na	na	17.0	na	na	36%
Pepperoni, mushroom, Italian sausage, 'Bigfoot'	1 slice	213	10.0	25.0	1208	2.0	9.0	4.0	21	38%
'Pepperoni Lovers'										
hand-tossed, medium pie	1 slice	335	19.0	28.0	981	3.0	16.0	4.0	43	43%
'Pan Pizza' medium pie	1 slice	362	14.0	27.0	861	3.0	25.0	5.0	34	62%
'Thin 'n Crispy' medium pie	1 slice	320	18.0	20.0	949	2.0	19.0	4.0	46	53%
Pork										
hand-tossed	1 slice	270	15.0	28.0	803	3.0	11.0	3.0	25	37%
'Pan Pizza'	1 slice	296	10.0	27.0	683	3.0	19.0	3.0	25	58%
'Thick 'n Chewy' 10-inch pie	3 slices	640	36.0	71.0	na	na	23.0	na	na	32%
'Thin 'n Crispy' medium pie	1 slice	240	13.0	20.0	713	2.0	12.0	3.0	25	45%
'Thin 'n Crispy' 10-inch pie	3 slices	520	27.0	51.0	na	na	23.0	na	na	40%
'Super Supreme'										
hand-tossed, medium pie	2 slices	463	29.0	44.0	1336	5.0	21.0	10.3	56	41%
hand-tossed, medium pie	1 slice	276	17.0	28.0	980	3.0	10.0	3.0	32	33%
'Pan Pizza' medium ple	1 slice	302	12.0	27.0	860	3.0	19.0	4.0	32	57%
'Thin 'n Crispy' medium pie	1 slice	253	16.0	20.0	700	2.0	12.0	3.0	35	43%
'Supreme'										
hand-tossed, medium pie	1 slice	289	17.0	28.0	894	3.0	12.0	3.0	29	37%
'Pan Pizza' medium pie	1 slice	315	16.0	27.0	774	3.0	16.0	3.0	29	46%
'Personal Pan Pizza' 9.3-oz pie	1 pie	647	33.0	76.0	1313	9.0	28.0	11.2	49	39%
'Thick 'n Chewy' 10-inch pie	3 slices	640	36.0	74.0	na	na	22.0	na	na	31%
'Thin 'n Crispy' medium pie	1 slice	262	15.0	20.0	819	3.0	14.0	3.0	31	48%
'Thin 'n Crispy' 10-inch pie	3 slices	510	27.0	51.0	na	na	21.0	na	na	37%

Food Name	Serving Size	Calories	Prot. gms	Carbs gms	Sod. mgs	Fiber gms	Fat gms	Sat. Fat gms	Chol. mgs	% Fat Cal.
'Veggie Lovers'										
hand-tossed, medium pie	1 slice	222	13.0	28.0	641	3.0	7.0	3.0	17	28%
'Pan Pizza'	1 slice	249	7.0	27.0	521	3.0	15.0	3.0	17	54%
'Thin 'n Crispy' medium pie	1 slice	192	11.0	20.0	551	3.0	8.0	3.0	17	38%
PONDEROSA										
ALFALFA SPROUTS	1 oz	10	1.0	1.0	0	(mq)	0.0	0.0	0	0%
APPLE										
canned	4 oz	90	0.0	22.0	15	(mq)	0.0	0.0	0	0%
rings, spiced	4 oz	100	0.0	24.0	20	(mq)	0.0	0.0	0	0%
whole, raw	1 med	80	0.0	20.0	1	(mq)	1.0	na	0	11%
APPLESAUCE	4 oz	80	0.0	20.0	20	(mq)	0.0	0.0	0	0%
BANANA										
chips	.2 oz	25	0.2	3.3	tr	(mq)	1.3	na	0	47%
whole, raw	1 med	87	1.1	22.6	1	(mq)	0.2	(tr)	0	2%
BARBECUE SAUCE	1 tbsp	25	0.0	5.0	260	na	0.0	0.0	0	0%
BEAN SPROUTS	1 oz	10	1.1	1.9	1	(mq)	tr	0.0	0	0%
BEANS										
baked	4 oz	170	6.0	21.0	330	(mq)	6.0	(mq)	0	32%
garbanzo	1 oz	102	6.0	17.0	7	na	0.0	na	0	0%
green	3.5 oz	20	1.0	3.0	391	na	0.0	na	0	0%
BEETS, diced	4 oz	55	0.4	12.5	307	(mq)	0.4	na	0	7%
BREADSTICKS										
Italian	1 breadstick	100	4.0	19.0	200	(mq)	1.0	na	0	9%
sesame	2 breadsticks	35	1.0	6.0	60	na	0.0	na	0	0%
BROCCOLI, raw	1 oz	9	1.0	1.7	4	(mq)	0.9	na	0	90%
CABBAGE										
green, raw	1 oz	9	1.0	1.9	7	(mq)	0.0	0.0	0	0%
red, raw	1 oz	1	0.1	0.3	1	(mq)	0.0	0.0	0	0%
CANTALOUPE	1 wedge	13	0.3	3.3	5	(mq)	0.0	0.0	0	0%
CARAMEL TOPPING	1 oz	100	0.4	26.2	72	na	0.7	na	2	6%
CARROTS										
raw	3.5 oz	31	1.0	7.0	33	na	0.0	na	0	0%
raw	1 oz	12	0.3	2.8	13	(mq)	0.1	(tr)	0	8%
CAULIFLOWER										
breaded	4 oz	115	4.0	23.0	446	na	1.0	na	1	8%
raw	1 oz	8	0.8	1.5	4	(mq)	0.1	(tr)	0	11%
CELERY, raw	1 oz	4	0.3	1.1	36	(mq)	0.0	0.0	0	0%
CHEESE, imitation, shredded	1 oz	90	6.0	1.0	420	na	7.0	na	5	70%
CHEESE SAUCE	2 oz	52	1.2	6.4	355	na	2.0	(mq)	4	35%
CHEESE SPREAD	1 oz	98	4.0	4.0	188	na	7.0	na	26	64%
CHEESE TOPPING, herb and garlic	1 tbsp	100	0.0	0.0	120	na	10.0	na	0	90%
CHICKEN										
breast	5.5 oz	98	20.0	1.0	400	na	2.0	na	54	18%
wing	2 pieces	213	11.0	11.0	610	na	9.0	na	75	38%
CHOCOLATE TOPPING	1 oz	89	0.5	24.3	37	na	0.3	na	0	3%
CHOPPED STEAK										
5.3-oz size	1 serving	296	25.0	1.0	296	na	22.0	na	105	67%
4-oz size	1 serving	225	19.0	1.0	150	na	16.0	na	80	64%
CHOW MEIN NOODLES	.2 oz	25	0.6	3.0	42	(mq)	1.2	na	0	43%
COCKTAIL SAUCE	1 oz	34	0.4	6.2	453	na	1.0	na	0	26%
COCONUT, shredded	.2 oz	25	0.2	2.0	14	(mq)	1.9	(mq)	0	68%
COFFEE	6 oz	2	0.0	0.5	26	0	0.0	0.0	0	0%
COOKIE, vanilla wafer	2 wafers	35	0.0	6.0	25	na	1.0	na	5	26%

Food Name	Serving Size	Calories	Prot. gms	Carbs gms	Sod. mgs	Fiber gms	Fat gms	Sat. Fat gms	Chol. mgs	% Fat Cal.
CORN	3.5 oz	90	3.0	21.0	5	(mq)	0.4	na	0	4%
COTTAGE CHEESE	4 oz	120	15.0	5.0	330	na	5.0	na	17	38%
CRACKER										
Melba snacks	2 crackers	18	1.0	4.0	60	(mq)	0.0	0.0	0	0%
'Ritz'	2 crackers	40	0.0	4.0	50	na	2.0	na	0	45%
sesame, 'Meal Mate'	2 crackers	45	1.0	6.0	95	na	2.0	na	0	40%
CROUTONS	1 oz	115	4.0	18.0	351	na	4.0	na	0	31%
CUCUMBER, raw	1 oz	4	0.3	1.0	2	(mq)	0.0	0.0	0	0%
EGG, boiled, diced	2 oz	93	7.0	1.0	74	na	7.0	na	260	68%
FISH. See also individual listings.										
baked, 'Bake 'R Broil'	5.2 oz	230	19.0	10.0	330	na	13.0	na	50	51%
fried	3.2 oz	190	9.0	17.0	170	na	9.0	na	15	43%
nugget	1 nugget	31	1.7	1.9	52	(mq)	1.7	(mq)	8	49%
FRENCH FRIES	3 oz	120	2.0	17.0	39	na	4.0	na	3	30%
FRUIT COCKTAIL	4 oz	97	0.5	25.1	7	(mq)	0.2	(tr)	0	2%
GELATIN DESSERT, plain	4 oz	71	1.0	17.0	73	na	0.0	na	0	0%
GRANOLA	.2 oz	24	0.6	3.1	na	(mq)	1.0	na	0	38%
GRAPES	10 grapes	34	0.3	8.7	2	(mq)	0.2	(tr)	0	5%
GRAVY										
brown	2 oz	25	0.6	3.9	167	na	1.0	na	0	36%
turkey	2 oz	25	0.7	5.1	228	na	0.2	na	0	7%
HALIBUT, broiled	6 oz	170	35.0	0.0	68	0	2.4	(mq)	(mq)	13%
HAM, diced	2 oz	120	9.0	1.0	780	na	10.0	na	76	75%
HONEYDEW MELON	1 wedge	25	0.6	5.8	9	(mq)	0.2	(tr)	0	7%
HOT DOG	1.6 oz	144	5.0	1.0	460	na	13.0	na	27	81%
ICE MILK										
chocolate	3.5 oz	152	4.0	30.0	70	na	3.0	na	22	18%
vanilla	3.5 oz	150	4.0	30.0	58	na	3.0	na	20	18%
ICED TEA	6 oz	2	0.1	0.5	0	0	0.0	0.0	0	0%
LEMON	1 wedge	3	0.1	0.8	0	(mq)	0.1	(tr)	0	30%
LETTUCE	1 oz	5	0.0	2.0	5	na	0.0	na	0	0%
MACARONI AND CHEESE	1 oz	17	0.7	4.4	80	(mq)	0.5	na	1	26%
MARGARINE										
liquid	1 tbsp	100	0.0	0.0	110	0	11.0	(mq)	0	99%
whipped	1 tbsp	34	0.0	0.0	65	0	1.2	(mq)	0	32%
MEATBALLS	2 pieces	115	5.0	2.0	16	na	4.0	na	21	31%
MILK										
chocolate	8 oz	208	7.9	25.9	149	0	8.5	(mq)	33	37%
whole	8 oz	159	8.5	12.0	122	0	8.6	(mq)	34	49%
MOUSSE										
chocolate	4 oz	312	0.0	28.0	72	na	18.0	na	0	52%
chocolate	1 oz	78	0.0	6.9	18	na	4.4	(mq)	0	51%
strawberry	4 oz	297	0.0	25.0	68	na	18.0	na	0	55%
strawberry	1 oz	74	0.0	6.3	17	na	4.6	(mq)	0	56%
MUSHROOMS, raw	1 oz	8	0.8	1.3	4	(mq)	0.1	(tr)	0	11%
OKRA, breaded	4 oz	124	3.0	23.0	483	na	1.0	na	1	7%
OLIVES										
black	1 piece	4	0.0	0.1	24	(mq)	0.4	na	0	90%
green	1 piece	4	0.0	0.0	69	(mq)	0.4	na	0	90%
ONION										
green, raw	1 piece	7	0.2	1.6	1	(mq)	0.1	(tr)	0	13%
red, raw	1 oz	11	0.4	2.5	3	(mq)	0.0	0.0	0	0%
yellow, raw	1 oz	11	0.4	2.5	3	(mq)	0.0	0.0	0	0%
ONION RINGS, breaded	4 oz	213	3.0	30.0	620	na	9.0	na	2	38%

Food Name	Serving Size	Calories	Prot. gms	Carbs gms	Sod. mgs	Fiber gms	Fat gms	Sat. Fat gms	Chol. mgs	% Fat Cal.
ORANGE	1 piece	45	1.2	11.3	1	(mq)	0.1	(tr)	0	2%
ORANGE ROUGHY, broiled	5 oz	139	tr	21.0	88	na	5.0	na	28	32%
PASTA. See also individual listings.										
	2 oz	78	2.4	16.1	1	(mq)	0.3	na	0	3%
PEACH, canned	4 oz	70	0.0	18.0	10	(mq)	0.0	0.0	0	0%
PEANUT TOPPING, granulated	.2 oz	30	1.2	1.1	0	(mq)	2.3	(mq)	0	69%
PEAR, canned	4 oz	98	0.5	25.0	7	(mq)	0.5	na	0	5%
PEAS	3.5 oz	67	5.0	12.0	120	na	0.0	na	0	0%
PEPPER, CHERRY, raw	2 pieces	7	0.2	1.4	415	(mq)	0.2	(tr)	0	26%
PEPPER, GREEN, raw	1 oz	6	0.3	1.4	4	(mq)	0.1	(tr)	0	15%
PICKLE										
dill, spear	.14 oz	1	0.0	0.1	54	(mq)	0.0	0.0	0	0%
sweet, chips	.14 oz	4	0.1	1.0	1	(mq)	0.0	0.0	0	0%
PINEAPPLE										
fresh	1 wedge	11	0.1	2.9	tr	(mq)	0.1	(tr)	0	8%
tidbits	4 oz	95	0.4	24.8	2	(mq)	0.2	na	0	2%
PORTERHOUSE STEAK										
choice	16 oz	640	57.0	3.0	1130	na	31.0	na	82	44%
non-graded	13 oz	440	43.0	1.0	1844	na	30.0	na	67	61%
POTATO, BAKED	7.2 oz	145	4.0	33.0	6	na	0.0	na	0	0%
POTATO WEDGES	3.5 oz	130	3.0	16.0	170	na	6.0	na	na	42%
POTATOES, MASHED	4 oz	62	2.0	13.0	191	na	0.0	na	20	0%
PUDDING										
banana	4 oz	207	1.0	27.0	114	na	10.0	na	0	43%
banana	1 oz	52	0.4	6.4	29	na	2.4	(mq)	0	42%
RADISH, raw	1 oz	4	0.3	0.9	5	(mq)	0.0	0.0	0	0%
RIB EYE STEAK										
choice	6 oz	282	29.0	1.0	570	na	14.0	na	60	45%
non-graded	5 oz	219	25.0	1.0	1130	na	13.0	na	77	53%
RICE PILAF	4 oz	160	4.0	26.0	450	na	4.0	na	22	23%
ROLL										
dinner	1 piece	184	5.0	33.0	311	na	3.0	na	0	15%
sourdough	1 piece	110	4.0	22.0	230	(mq)	1.0	na	0	8%
SALAD										
chicken	3.5 oz	212	11.0	8.0	334	na	15.0	na	42	64%
chicken macaroni	3.5 oz	335	8.0	49.0	431	na	12.0	na	9	32%
macaroni	3.5 oz	335	7.6	49.2	431	(mq)	11.7	(mq)	9	31%
pasta	3.5 oz	268	6.0	34.0	441	na	12.0	na	0	40%
potato	3.5 oz	126	2.0	16.0	300	na	6.0	na	7	43%
turkey-ham	3.5 oz	186	7.5	10.1	655	na	12.8	(mq)	12	62%
SALAD DRESSING										
blue cheese	1 oz	130	1.0	1.0	266	na	14.0	na	27	97%
coleslaw	1 oz	150	tr	6.0	284	na	14.0	na	31	84%
creamy Italian	1 oz	103	0.0	3.0	373	na	10.0	na	0	87%
cucumber, reduced calorie	1 oz	69	tr	3.0	315	na	6.0	na	0	78%
Italian, reduced calorie	1 oz	31	0.0	1.0	371	na	3.0	na	0	87%
Parmesan pepper	1 oz	150	1.0	2.0	281	na	15.0	na	9	90%
ranch	1 oz	147	tr	1.0	297	na	15.0	na	3	92%
salad oil	1 tbsp	120	0.0	0.0	0	0	13.3	(mq)	0	100%
sweet and tangy	1 oz	122	tr	8.0	347	na	10.0	na	1	74%
Thousand Island	1 oz	113	tr	8.0	405	na	10.0	na	9	80%
SALMON, broiled	6 oz	192	37.0	3.0	72	na	3.0	na	60	14%
SCROD, baked	7 oz	120	27.0	0.0	80	na	1.0	na	65	8%

Food Name	Serving Size	Calories	Prot. gms	Carbs gms	Sod. mgs	Fiber gms	Fat gms	Sat. Fat gms	Chol. mgs	% Fat Cal.
SHRIMP										
fried	7 pieces	230	22.0	31.0	612	na	1.0	na	105	4%
mini	6 pieces	47	5.0	6.0	125	na	1.0	na	22	19%
SIRLOIN STEAK, choice	7 oz	241	35.0	1.0	570	na	11.0	na	63	41%
SOUR CREAM	1 tbsp	26	0.4	0.5	6	0	2.5	(mq)	5	87%
SPAGHETTI, w/sauce	6 oz	188	5.0	33.0	520	na	5.0	na	0	24%
SPAGHETTI ENTRÉE	2 oz	78	2.4	16.1	1	(mq)	0.3	na	0	3%
SPAGHETTI SAUCE	4 oz	110	2.0	17.0	520	na	4.0	(mq)	0	33%
SPINACH, raw	1 oz	7	0.9	1.2	20	(mq)	0.1	(tr)	0	13%
STEAK ENTRÉE. See individual listings.										
STEAK KABOBS, meat only	3 oz	153	26.0	2.0	280	na	5.0	na	67	29%
STEAK SANDWICH	4 oz	208	20.0	2.0	850	na	11.0	na	62	48%
STRAWBERRIES	2 oz	14	0.3	3.1	61	(mq)	0.2	(tr)	tr	13%
STRAWBERRY GLAZE	1 oz	37	0.0	9.5	4	na	0.0	0.0	0	0%
STRAWBERRY TOPPING	1 oz	71	0.1	23.6	29	na	0.2	na	0	3%
STUFFING	4 oz	230	6.0	27.0	800	na	11.0	na	22	43%
SWEET AND SOUR SAUCE	1 oz	37	na	8.0	80	na	na	na	0	0%
SWORDFISH, broiled	5.9 oz	271	44.0	0.0	0	na	10.0	na	84	33%
T-BONE STEAK										
choice	10 oz	444	44.0	2.0	850	na	18.0	na	80	36%
non-graded	8 oz	178	24.7	1.6	850	0	8.5	(mq)	71	43%
TARTAR SAUCE	1 oz	85	0.1	11.1	477	na	9.3	(mq)	9	98%
TERIYAKI STEAK	5 oz	174	32.0	5.0	1420	na	3.0	na	64	16%
TOMATO	1 oz	6	0.3	1.3	1	(mq)	0.1	(tr)	0	15%
TORTILLA CHIPS	1 oz	150	3.0	16.0	80	(mq)	8.0	(mq)	0	48%
TROUT, broiled	5 oz	228	30.0	1.0	51	na	4.0	na	110	16%
TURKEY, julienne	1 oz	29	5.0	1.0	192	na	1.0	na	15	31%
WATERMELON	1 wedge	111	2.1	27.3	4	(mq)	0.9	na	0	7%
WHIPPED TOPPING	1 oz	80	0.0	5.0	16	na	7.0	na	0	79%
YOGURT, FROZEN										
fruit	4 oz	115	5.0	23.0	70	na	1.0	na	5	8%
vanilla	4 oz	110	5.0	18.0	75	0	2.0	na	6	16%
ZUCCHINI										
breaded	4 oz	102	3.0	18.0	584	na	1.0	na	1	9%
raw	1 oz	5	0.3	1.0	tr	(mq)	0.0	0.0	0	0%

POPEYES

Food Name	Serving Size	Calories	Prot. gms	Carbs gms	Sod. mgs	Fiber gms	Fat gms	Sat. Fat gms	Chol. mgs	% Fat Cal.
APPLE PIE	3.1 oz	290	2.5	36.6	820	2.0	15.8	na	10	49%
BISCUIT	2.3 oz	250	3.7	26.1	430	1.0	14.9	na	<5	54%
CHICKEN										
breast, mild	3.7 oz	270	23.1	9.2	660	2.0	15.9	na	60	53%
breast, spicy	3.7 oz	270	23.1	9.2	590	2.0	15.9	na	60	53%
leg, mild	1.7 oz	120	10.3	4.4	240	0	7.3	na	40	55%
leg, spicy	1.7 oz	120	10.3	4.4	240	0	7.3	na	40	55%
nugget	4.2 oz	410	17.1	17.9	660	3.0	31.9	na	55	70%
thigh, mild	3.1 oz	300	14.7	9.3	620	<1.0	22.7	na	70	68%
thigh, spicy	3.1 oz	300	14.7	9.3	450	<1.0	22.7	na	70	68%
wing, mild	1.6 oz	160	9.3	6.6	290	0	10.7	na	40	60%
wing, spicy	1.6 oz	160	9.3	6.6	290	0	10.7	na	40	60%
COLESLAW	4 oz	149	0.9	13.6	271	3.0	11.2	na	3	68%
CORN, on the cob	5.2 oz	90	4.0	21.4	20	9.0	2.9	na	0	29%
FRENCH FRIES	3 oz	240	3.5	30.8	610	3.0	12.2	na	10	46%
ONION RINGS	3.1 oz	310	4.9	31.1	210	2.0	19.3	na	25	56%
RED BEANS AND RICE	5.9 oz	270	7.5	29.7	680	7.0	16.9	na	10	56%

Food Name	Serving Size	Calories	Prot. gms	Carbs gms	Sod. mgs	Fiber gms	Fat gms	Sat. Fat gms	Chol. mgs	% Fat Cal.
QUINCY'S										
BEANS, green, 4.3 oz	1 serving	40	2.0	7.0	500	(mq)	1.0	na	0	23%
BROCCOLI, cream of, 9.2 oz	1 serving	193	3.0	13.0	1045	(mq)	14.0	(mq)	na	65%
CATFISH FILLET, 2 pieces, 6.9 oz	1 serving	309	26.0	19.0	101	(mq)	12.0	(mq)	(mq)	35%
CHEESEBURGER, 1/4-lb patty	1 serving	451	28.0	32.0	432	(mq)	23.0	(mq)	(mq)	46%
CHICKEN, breast, grilled, 5 oz	1 serving	145	35.0	0.0	140	0	0.4	(mq)	72	2%
CHICKEN STRIPS, 4 pieces, 4.5 oz	1 serving	318	39.0	4.0	(mq)	(mq)	15.0	(mq)	(mq)	42%
CHILI, w/beans, 9.2 oz	1 serving	346	20.0	32.0	1380	(mq)	16.0	(mq)	(mq)	42%
CHOPPED STEAK										
5.8-oz size	1 serving	466	40.0	0.0	96	0	34.0	(mq)	(mq)	66%
luncheon, 4-oz size	1 serving	350	30.0	0.0	72	0	25.0	(mq)	(mq)	64%
CHOWDER, clam, 9.2 oz	1 serving	198	6.0	15.0	1185	(mq)	14.0	(mq)	(mq)	64%
COLESLAW, 2.1 oz	1 serving	60	<1.0	4.0	75	(mq)	5.0	(mq)	na	75%
CORNBREAD, 1.9 oz	1 serving	178	4.0	28.0	263	(mq)	6.0	(mq)	na	30%
FRENCH FRIES, steak fries, 5.5 oz	1 serving	426	7.0	56.0	90	(mq)	21.0	(mq)	na	44%
HAMBURGER, 1/4-lb patty	1 serving	403	25.0	32.0	284	(mq)	19.0	(mq)	(mq)	42%
MARGARINE, 1 oz	1 serving	204	<1.0	<1.0	268	0	22.0	(mq)	0	97%
MUSHROOM SAUCE, 3 oz	1 serving	27	1.0	5.0	366	na	<1.0	na	na	0%
PEPPERS AND ONIONS, 4 oz	1 serving	80	1.0	8.0	11	(mq)	5.0	(mq)	na	56%
POTATO, BAKED, w/o butter, 8.8 oz	1 serving	181	5.0	41.0	8	(mq)	<1.0	na	0	0%
POTATOES, MASHED, w/gravy, 3.8 oz	1 serving	100	5.0	10.5	460	3.0	6.0	na	<5	54%
RIB EYE STEAK, 7.3 oz	1 serving	665	31.0	0.0	205	0	60.0	(mq)	(mq)	81%
RICE, Cajun, 3.9 oz	1 serving	150	10.0	17.4	1260	3.0	5.4	na	25	32%
SHRIMP										
7 pieces, 3.9 oz	1 serving	248	22.0	11.0	205	(mq)	12.0	(mq)	(mq)	44%
2.8 oz	1 serving	250	15.6	13.2	650	3.0	16.4	na	110	59%
SIRLOIN STEAK										
large, 7.7 oz	1 serving	852	50.0	0.0	241	0	70.0	(mq)	(mq)	74%
petite, 4 oz	1 serving	446	26.0	0.0	118	0	37.0	(mq)	(mq)	75%
regular, 5.9 oz	1 serving	649	38.0	0.0	206	0	54.0	(mq)	(mq)	75%
sirloin club, 4.8 oz	1 serving	283	44.0	0.0	160	0	10.0	(mq)	(mq)	32%
sirloin tips, 4 oz	1 serving	236	37.0	0.0	113	0	9.0	(mq)	(mq)	34%
STEAK. See also individual listings.										
country style, w/mushroom sauce, 6 oz	1 serving	288	18.0	17.0	315	(mq)	19.0	(mq)	(mq)	59%
STEAK FILLET, 5.6 oz	1 serving	331	51.0	0.0	159	0	12.0	(mq)	(mq)	33%
T-BONE STEAK, 7.8 oz	1 serving	1045	43.0	0.0	222	0	95.0	(mq)	(mq)	82%
VEGETABLE BEEF SOUP, 8.6 oz	1 serving	78	5.0	10.0	1045	(mq)	2.0	(mq)	(mq)	23%
RALLY'S										
CHEESEBURGER										
'Bacon Cheeseburger'	1 sandwich	622	33.0	34.5	1629	na	40.3	na	99	58%
'Double Cheeseburger'	1 sandwich	733	42.4	33.9	1473	na	49.1	na	92	60%
'Rallyburger' w/cheese	1 sandwich	486	24.2	33.4	1185	na	29.4	na	79	54%
CHESEBURGER MEAL										
'Large Combo' w/soft drink	1 meal	1018	29.3	129.4	1645	na	45.0	na	89	40%
'Small Combo' w/soft drink	1 meal	764	32.6	84.7	1416	na	37.2	na	84	44%
CHICKEN SANDWICH	1 sandwich	531	18.1	39.5	364	na	30.8	na	18	52%
CHILI	8 oz	340	22.2	21.3	1199	na	19.0	na	67	50%
FRENCH FRIES										
large order	1 serving	317	5.1	39.0	439	na	15.6	na	10	44%
regular order	1 serving	158	2.5	19.5	219	na	7.8	na	5	44%
HAMBURGER, 'Rallyburger'	1 sandwich	436	21.2	32.9	955	na	24.9	na	67	51%
HAMBURGER MEAL										
'Large Combo' w/ soft drink	1 meal	968	26.3	128.9	1415	na	40.5	na	76	38%

Food Name	Serving Size	Calories	Prot. gms	Carbs gms	Sod. mgs	Fiber gms	Fat gms	Sat. Fat gms	Chol. mgs	% Fat Cal.
'Small Combo' w/soft drink	1 meal	714	23.8	84.1	1186	na	32.7	na	71	41%
ICED TEA										
16-oz size	1 serving	3	0.0	0.0	0	0	0.0	0.0	0	0%
32-oz size	1 serving	6	0.0	0.0	0	0	0.0	0.0	0	0%
MILKSHAKE										
chocolate	1 serving	411	9.7	72.5	262	na	11.8	na	38	26%
strawberry banana	1 serving	399	9.4	69.5	223	na	11.3	na	38	25%
vanilla	1 serving	320	9.4	49.0	197	na	11.3	na	38	32%
SAUSAGE										
'Smokin' Sausage'	1 serving	724	28.0	31.0	1998	na	55.0	na	40	68%
'Smokin' Sausage' w/chili	1 serving	830	34.8	35.0	2163	na	62.0	na	67	67%
SOFT DRINK										
Coca-Cola, 32-oz size	1 serving	216	0.0	57.0	21	0	0.0	0.0	0	0%
Coca-Cola, 16-oz size	1 serving	120	0.0	32.0	12	0	0.0	0.0	0	0%
Diet Coke, 32-oz size	1 serving	1	0.0	0.5	39	0	0.0	0.0	0	0%
Diet Coke, 16-oz size	1 serving	1	0.0	0.3	22	0	0.0	0.0	0	0%
Dr. Pepper, 32-oz size	1 serving	216	0.0	57.0	27	0	0.0	0.0	0	0%
Dr. Pepper, 16-oz size	1 serving	120	0.0	32.0	15	0	0.0	0.0	0	0%
Fanta Orange, 32-oz size	1 serving	264	0.0	69.0	21	0	0.0	0.0	0	0%
Fanta Orange, 16-oz size	1 serving	147	0.0	38.4	12	0	0.0	0.0	0	0%
Fanta Root Beer, 32-oz size	1 serving	234	0.0	60.0	30	0	0.0	0.0	0	0%
Fanta Root Beer, 16-oz size	1 serving	130	0.0	33.0	17	0	0.0	0.0	0	0%
Ramblin' Root Beer, 32-oz size	1 serving	264	0.0	69.0	30	0	0.0	0.0	0	0%
Ramblin' Root Beer, 16-oz size	1 serving	147	0.0	38.4	17	0	0.0	0.0	0	0%
Sprite, 32-oz size	1 serving	213	0.0	54.0	69	0	0.0	0.0	0	0%
Sprite, 16-oz size	1 serving	119	0.0	30.0	12	0	0.0	0.0	0	0%
TACO, soft	1 taco	223	12.1	17.0	377	na	9.9	na	36	40%
RAX										
ALFALFA SPROUTS	1 oz	8	<1.0	2.0	<1	(mq)	<1.0	(tr)	0	0%
ALFREDO SAUCE	3.5 oz	80	2.0	12.0	70	(mq)	3.0	(mq)	10	34%
APPLESAUCE	1 cup	100	<1.0	26.0	5	(mq)	<1.0	(tr)	0	0%
BACON BITS	.5 oz	40	5.0	<1.0	427	0	2.0	(mq)	12	45%
BARBECUE MEAT TOPPING	3.25 oz	140	13.0	13.0	898	na	4.0	(mq)	24	26%
BARBECUE SANDWICH, 5.7 oz	1 serving	420	21.0	53.0	1343	(mq)	14.0	(mq)	24	30%
BARBECUE SAUCE	.5 oz	11	0.0	3.0	158	na	0.0	0.0	0	0%
BEANS										
garbanzo	1/2 cup	360	20.0	60.0	26	(mq)	5.0	(mq)	0	13%
kidney	1 cup	220	14.0	40.0	8	(mq)	1.0	(mq)	0	4%
BEEF SANDWICH										
'BBC' beef, bacon, chicken, 8 oz	1 serving	720	30.0	40.0	1873	(mq)	49.0	(mq)	137	61%
Philly beef and cheese, 8.25 oz	1 serving	480	25.0	44.0	1346	(mq)	22.0	(mq)	49	41%
BEETS	1 cup	60	2.0	12.0	73	(mq)	<1.0	(tr)	0	0%
BREADSTICK, sesame	1 oz	150	3.0	13.0	405	(mq)	10.0	(mq)	0	60%
BROCCOLI, raw	1/2 cup	16	2.0	2.0	7	(mq)	<1.0	(tr)	0	0%
BROCCOLI SOUP, cream of	3.5 oz	50	1.0	6.0	219	(mq)	2.0	(mq)	<1	36%
CABBAGE										
green, raw	1 cup	16	<1.0	4.0	18	(mq)	<1.0	(tr)	0	0%
red, raw	1/4 cup	4	<1.0	<1.0	6	(mq)	<1.0	(tr)	0	0%
CANTALOUPE	2 pieces	16	<1.0	4.0	6	(mq)	<1.0	(tr)	0	0%
CARROT, raw	1/4 cup	8	<1.0	2.0	<1	(mq)	<1.0	(tr)	0	0%
CATSUP	1 tbsp	6	<1.0	2.0	50	(mq)	<1.0	(tr)	0	0%
CAULIFLOWER, raw	1/2 cup	16	<.0	2.0	6	(mq)	<1.0	(tr)	0	0%
CELERY, raw	1 tbsp	1	<1.0	<1.0	10	(mq)	<1.0	(tr)	0	0%

Food Name	Serving Size	Calories	Prot. gms	Carbs gms	Sod. mgs	Fiber gms	Fat gms	Sat. Fat gms	Chol. mgs	% Fat Cal.
CHEESE										
cheddar, imitation, shredded	1 oz	90	6.0	2.0	310	na	6.0	(mq)	6	60%
cheddar, tidbits	1 oz	160	3.0	12.0	445	0	11.0	(mq)	<1	62%
Parmesan, substitute	1 oz	80	8.0	2.0	1000	(mq)	4.0	(mq)	<1	45%
CHEESE SAUCE										
nacho	3.5 oz	470	10.0	57.0	190	na	22.0	na	11	42%
regular	3.5 oz	420	10.0	58.0	365	na	17.0	na	11	36%
CHICKEN NOODLE SOUP	3.5 oz	40	2.0	8.0	1040	(mq)	<1.0	(mq)	10	0%
CHILI TOPPING	3 oz	80	8.0	8.0	221	(mq)	2.0	(mq)	18	23%
CHOW MEIN NOODLES	1 oz	140	4.0	17.0	242	(mq)	6.0	(mq)	<1	39%
COCONUT	1 oz	160	<1.0	15.0	<1	(mq)	11.0	(mq)	0	62%
COLESLAW	3.5 oz	70	1.0	8.0	187	(mq)	4.0	(mq)	<1	51%
COOKIE, chocolate chip	1 cookie	130	1.0	17.0	65	(mq)	6.0	(mq)	<1	42%
COTTAGE CHEESE	1 cup	250	33.0	7.0	561	(mq)	10.0	(mq)	47	36%
CRACKER, 'Saltines'	2 crackers	16	<1.0	4.0	70	(mq)	<1.0	(mq)	<1	0%
CROUTONS	.5 oz	40	2.0	8.0	155	(mq)	<1.0	(mq)	<1	0%
CUCUMBER	2 slices	2	<1.0	<1.0	<1	(mq)	<1.0	(tr)	0	0%
EGG, boiled, salad topping	1.5 oz	70	6.0	<1.0	32	0	5.0	(mq)	267	64%
FISH SANDWICH, 7 oz	1 serving	460	14.0	58.0	935	(mq)	17.0	(mq)	<1	33%
FRENCH FRIES										
large order, 4.5 oz	1 serving	390	3.0	50.0	104	(mq)	20.0	(mq)	16	46%
large order, unsalted, 4.5 oz	1 serving	390	3.0	50.0	66	(mq)	20.0	(mq)	16	46%
regular order, 3 oz	1 serving	260	2.0	33.0	69	(mq)	13.0	(mq)	10	45%
regular order, unsalted, 3 oz	1 serving	260	2.0	33.0	44	(mq)	13.0	(mq)	10	45%
GELATIN										
lime	1/2 cup	90	2.0	20.0	90	0	<1.0	(tr)	0	0%
strawberry	1/2 cup	90	2.0	20.0	90	0	<1.0	(tr)	0	0%
GRAPEFRUIT, sections	1 cup	80	2.0	19.0	10	(mq)	<1.0	(tr)	0	0%
GRAPE	1 cup	100	<1.0	25.0	5	(mq)	<1.0	(tr)	0	0%
HAM AND CHEESE SANDWICH, w/Swiss cheese, 7.9 oz	1 serving	430	23.0	42.0	1737	(mq)	23.0	(mq)	37	48%
HONEYDEW MELON	2 pieces	25	<1.0	6.0	5	(mq)	<1.0	(tr)	0	0%
HOT CHOCOLATE	6 oz	110	2.0	<1.0	120	(mq)	11.0	(mq)	<1	90%
KALE	1 oz	16	2.0	2.0	21	(mq)	<1.0	(tr)	0	0%
LETTUCE	1 leaf	2	0.0	0.0	<1	(mq)	0.0	(tr)	0	0%
MARGARINE, liquid	1 tbsp	100	<1.0	<1.0	100	0	11.0	(mq)	0	99%
MILKSHAKE										
chocolate, w/o whipped topping	1 serving	560	13.0	97.0	239	(tr)	13.0	(mq)	63	21%
strawberry, w/o whipped topping	1 serving	560	13.0	97.0	226	(tr)	13.0	(mq)	62	21%
vanilla, w/o whipped topping	1 serving	500	13.0	81.0	286	0	14.0	(mq)	58	25%
MUSHROOM SAUCE	1 oz	16	1.0	1.0	113	na	<1.0	0.0	0	0%
MUSHROOMS, raw	1/4 cup	4	<1.0	<1.0	<1	(mq)	<1.0	(tr)	0	0%
OLIVES	3.5 oz	110	<1.0	6.0	880	(mq)	10.0	(mq)	0	82%
ONION										
diced	.5 oz	10	<1.0	1.0	1	(mq)	<1.0	(tr)	0	0%
green	1/4 cup	10	<1.0	2.0	1	(mq)	<1.0	(tr)	0	0%
raw	1/4 cup	12	<1.0	3.0	3	(mq)	<1.0	(tr)	0	0%
PASTA AND NOODLES. See also individual listings.										
pasta shells	3.5 oz	170	7.0	27.0	2	(mq)	4.0	(mq)	0	21%
pasta/vegetable blend	3.5 oz	100	4.0	12.0	11	(mq)	4.0	(mq)	0	36%
rainbow rotini	3.5 oz	180	6.0	30.0	9	(mq)	4.0	(mq)	2	20%
PEACH	2 slices	16	<1.0	4.0	<1	(mq)	<1.0	(tr)	0	0%
PEAS	1 oz	25	2.0	4.0	35	(mq)	<1.0	(tr)	0	0%
PEPPER, BANANA, rings	1 tbsp	2	<1.0	<1.0	20	(mq)	<1.0	(tr)	0	0%
PEPPER, CHERRY	1 tbsp	6	<1.0	<1.0	180	(mq)	<1.0	(tr)	0	0%

Food Name	Serving Size	Calories	Prot. gms	Carbs gms	Sod. mgs	Fiber gms	Fat gms	Sat. Fat gms	Chol. mgs	% Fat Cal.
PEPPER, GREEN	1/4 cup	8	<1.0	1.0	5	(mq)	<1.0	(tr)	0	0%
PEPPER, JALAPEÑO	1 oz	6	<1.0	1.0	231	(mq)	<1.0	(tr)	0	0%
PICKLE	1 spear	8	<1.0	2.0	928	(mq)	<1.0	(tr)	0	0%
PINEAPPLE										
canned	3.5 oz	100	<1.0	25.0	10	(mq)	<1.0	(tr)	0	0%
fresh	3-oz slice	45	<1.0	12.0	1	(mq)	<1.0	(tr)	0	0%
POTATO, BAKED										
barbecue, w/2 oz cheese	1 serving	730	24.0	104.0	1071	(mq)	24.0	(mq)	18	30%
chili, w/2 oz cheese	1 serving	700	22.0	101.0	599	(mq)	23.0	(mq)	25	30%
plain, 8.8 oz	1 serving	270	8.0	60.0	70	(mq)	<1.0	(mq)	0	0%
plain, w/margarine, 9.3 oz	1 serving	370	8.0	60.0	170	(mq)	11.0	(mq)	0	27%
w/sour cream topping	1 serving	400	11.0	65.0	149	na	11.0	na	tr	25%
w/3 oz cheese and bacon	1 serving	780	22.0	110.0	910	(mq)	28.0	(mq)	23	32%
w/3 oz cheese and broccoli	1 serving	760	19.0	112.0	489	(mq)	26.0	(mq)	11	31%
POTATO SALAD	1 cup	260	7.0	41.0	127	(mq)	17.0	(mq)	7	59%
PUDDING										
butterscotch	3.5 oz	140	2.0	20.0	150	(tr)	6.0	(mq)	2	39%
chocolate	3.5 oz	140	2.0	20.0	120	(tr)	6.0	(mq)	2	39%
vanilla	3.5 oz	140	2.0	20.0	120	(tr)	6.0	(mq)	2	39%
RADISH	.5 oz	2	<1.0	<1.0	<1	(mq)	<1.0	(tr)	0	0%
REFRIED BEANS	3 oz	120	6.0	16.0	375	(mq)	4.0	(mq)	2	30%
RICE, Spanish	3.5 oz	90	3.0	20.0	442	(mq)	<1.0	na	0	0%
ROAST BEEF, 2.8-oz	1 serving	140	14.0	<1.0	524	0	9.0	(mq)	36	58%
ROAST BEEF SANDWICH										
large, 8 oz	1 serving	570	22.0	41.0	1169	(mq)	35.0	(mq)	36	55%
regular, 5.25 oz	1 serving	320	20.0	33.0	969	(mq)	11.0	(mq)	36	31%
small, 'Uncle Al' 3.1 oz	1 serving	260	12.0	21.0	562	(mq)	14.0	(mq)	19	48%
SALAD										
chef's, w/o dressing, 12.5 oz	1 serving	230	22.0	4.0	1048	(mq)	14.0	(mq)	322	55%
garden w/o dressing, 10.5 oz	1 serving	160	12.0	4.0	362	(mq)	11.0	(mq)	273	62%
garden, gourmet 'Lighterside'	1 serving	134	7.0	13.0	350	na	6.0	na	2	40%
macaroni	3.5 oz	160	2.0	21.0	216	(mq)	7.0	(mq)	<1	39%
pasta	3.5 oz	80	2.0	16.0	322	(mq)	1.0	(mq)	<1	11%
potato	1 cup	260	7.0	41.0	tr	(mq)	7.0	(mq)	7	24%
three-bean	1/2 cup	100	3.0	23.0	450	(mq)	<1.0	(mq)	0	0%
SALAD DRESSING										
blue cheese	1 tbsp	50	<1.0	1.0	110	na	5.0	(mq)	8	90%
blue cheese, 'Lite'	1 tbsp	35	<1.0	2.0	240	na	3.0	(mq)	3	77%
French	1 tbsp	60	<1.0	6.0	140	na	4.0	(mq)	0	60%
Italian	1 tbsp	50	<1.0	3.0	159	na	4.0	(mq)	0	72%
Italian, 'Lite'	1 tbsp	30	<1.0	1.0	152	na	3.0	(mq)	0	90%
oil	1 tbsp	130	<1.0	<1.0	<1	0	14.0	(mq)	0	97%
poppy seed	1 tbsp	60	<1.0	5.0	107	na	4.0	(mq)	6	60%
ranch	1 tbsp	45	<1.0	<1.0	103	na	5.0	(mq)	5	100%
Thousand Island	1 tbsp	70	<1.0	6.0	110	na	6.0	(mq)	8	77%
Thousand Island, 'Lite'	1 tbsp	40	<1.0	3.0	143	na	3.0	(mq)	5	68%
vinegar	1 tbsp	2	<1.0	<1.0	5	0	<1.0	(tr)	0	0%
SOUR CREAM, imitation	3.5 oz	130	3.0	5.0	79	na	11.0	(mq)	<1	76%
SOY NUTS	1 oz	120	10.0	5.0	151	(mq)	7.0	(mq)	0	53%
SPAGHETTI	3.5 oz	140	3.0	23.0	1	(mq)	4.0	(mq)	0	26%
SPAGHETTI SAUCE										
regular	3.5 oz	80	1.0	19.0	635	(mq)	<1.0	(mq)	<1	0%
w/meat	3.5 oz	150	7.0	12.0	419	(mq)	8.0	(mq)	<1	48%
SPICY MEAT SAUCE	3.5 oz	80	5.0	6.0	751	na	4.0	(mq)	12	45%

Food Name	Serving Size	Calories	Prot. gms	Carbs gms	Sod. mgs	Fiber gms	Fat gms	Sat. Fat gms	Chol. mgs	% Fat Cal.
STRAWBERRIES	2 oz	18	<1.0	4.0	<1	(mq)	<1.0	(tr)	0	0%
SUNFLOWER SEEDS, w/raisins	1 oz	130	5.0	6.0	5	(mq)	10.0	(mq)	0	69%
TACO SAUCE	3.5 oz	30	1.0	6.0	806	na	<1.0	(tr)	0	0%
TACO SHELL	1 shell	40	<1.0	6.0	53	(mq)	2.0	(mq)	0	45%
TOMATO	1 oz	6	<1.0	2.0	6	(mq)	<1.0	(tr)	0	0%
TORTILLA	1 tortilla	110	3.0	19.0	284	(mq)	2.0	(mq)	0	16%
TORTILLA CHIPS	1 oz	140	2.0	17.0	100	(mq)	7.0	(mq)	0	45%
TURKEY BITS	2 oz	70	10.0	<1.0	686	0	3.0	(mq)	49	39%
TURKEY SANDWICH, turkey bacon club, 9 oz	1 sandwich	670	29.0	41.0	1878	(mq)	43.0	(mq)	87	58%
WATERMELON	2 pieces	18	<1.0	4.0	<1	(mq)	<1.0	(tr)	0	0%
WHIPPED TOPPING	1 dollop	50	<1.0	4.0	6	0	4.0	(mq)	2	72%

RED LOBSTER

Food Name	Serving Size	Calories	Prot. gms	Carbs gms	Sod. mgs	Fiber gms	Fat gms	Sat. Fat gms	Chol. mgs	% Fat Cal.
CALAMARI										
breaded, fried, dinner portion, 10 oz	1 serving	720	26.0	60.0	2300	na	42.0	12.0	280	53%
breaded, fried, 5 oz	1 serving	360	13.0	30.0	1150	na	21.0	6.0	140	53%
CATFISH										
breast, 4 oz	1 serving	120	24.0	0.0	60	na	3.0	1.0	65	23%
dinner portion, 10 oz raw wt	1 serving	340	40.0	0.0	100	na	20.0	6.0	170	53%
lunch portion, 5 oz raw wt	1 serving	170	20.0	0.0	50	na	10.0	3.0	85	53%
CLAM										
cherrystone, dinner portion, 10 oz raw wt	1 serving	260	36.0	22.0	1080	na	4.0	tr	160	14%
cherrystone, lunch portion, 5 oz raw wt	1 serving	130	18.0	11.0	540	na	2.0	tr	80	14%
COD FILLET										
Atlantic, dinner portion, 10 oz raw wt	1 serving	200	46.0	0.0	400	na	2.0	tr	140	9%
Atlantic, lunch portion, 5 oz raw wt	1 serving	100	23.0	0.0	200	na	1.0	tr	70	9%
CRAB LEGS										
'King' 1 lb	1 serving	170	32.0	6.0	000	na	2.0	tr	100	11%
'Onow' 1 lb	1 serving	150	33.0	1.0	1630	na	2.0	1.0	130	12%
FLOUNDER										
dinner portion, 10 oz raw wt	1 serving	200	42.0	2.0	190	na	2.0	tr	140	9%
lunch portion, 5 oz raw wt	1 serving	100	21.0	1.0	95	na	1.0	tr	70	9%
GROUPER										
dinner portion, 10 oz raw wt	1 serving	220	52.0	0.0	140	na	2.0	tr	130	8%
lunch portion, 5 oz raw wt	1 serving	110	26.0	0.0	70	na	1.0	tr	65	8%
HADDOCK										
dinner portion, 10 oz raw wt	1 serving	220	48.0	4.0	360	na	2.0	tr	170	8%
lunch portion, 5 oz raw wt	1 serving	110	24.0	2.0	180	na	1.0	tr	85	8%
HALIBUT										
dinner portion, 10 oz raw wt	1 serving	220	50.0	2.0	210	na	2.0	tr	120	8%
lunch portion, 5 oz raw wt	1 serving	110	25.0	1.0	105	na	1.0	tr	60	8%
HAMBURGER, 1/3 lb	1 serving	320	27.0	0.0	70	na	23.0	11.0	105	65%
LANGOSTINO										
dinner portion, 10 oz raw wt	1 serving	240	52.0	4.0	820	na	2.0	tr	420	8%
lunch portion, 5 oz raw wt	1 serving	120	26.0	2.0	410	na	1.0	tr	210	8%
LOBSTER										
Maine, 1 1/4 lb	1 serving	240	36.0	5.0	550	na	8.0	2.0	310	30%
rock, 1 tail	1 serving	230	49.0	2.0	1090	na	3.0	1.0	200	12%
MACKEREL										
dinner portion, 10 oz raw wt	1 serving	380	2.0	40.0	500	na	24.0	8.0	200	57%
lunch portion, 5 oz raw wt	1 serving	190	1.0	20.0	250	na	12.0	4.0	100	57%
MONKFISH										
dinner portion, 10 oz	1 serving	220	0.0	48.0	190	na	2.0	tr	160	8%
lunch portion, 5 oz	1 serving	110	0.0	24.0	95	na	1.0	tr	80	8%

Food Name	Serving Size	Calories	Prot. gms	Carbs gms	Sod. mgs	Fiber gms	Fat gms	Sat. Fat gms	Chol. mgs	% Fat Cal.
MUSSEL, 3 oz	1 serving	70	9.0	3.0	150	na	2.0	tr	50	26%
OCEAN PERCH										
Atlantic, dinner portion, 10 oz raw wt	1 serving	260	48.0	2.0	380	na	8.0	2.0	150	28%
Atlantic, lunch portion, 5 oz raw wt	1 serving	130	24.0	1.0	190	na	4.0	1.0	75	28%
OYSTER, raw, on half shell, 6 pieces	1 serving	110	8.0	11.0	90	na	4.0	2.0	60	33%
POLLACK										
dinner portion, 10 oz raw wt	1 serving	240	56.0	2.0	180	na	2.0	tr	180	8%
lunch portion, 5 oz raw wt	1 serving	120	28.0	1.0	90	na	1.0	tr	90	8%
RED ROCKFISH										
dinner portion, 10 oz raw wt	1 serving	180	42.0	0.0	190	na	2.0	tr	170	10%
lunch portion, 5 oz raw wt	1 serving	90	21.0	0.0	95	na	1.0	tr	85	10%
RED SNAPPER										
dinner portion, 10 oz raw wt	1 serving	220	50.0	0.0	280	na	2.0	tr	140	8%
lunch portion, 5 oz raw wt	1 serving	110	25.0	0.0	140	na	1.0	tr	70	8%
SALMON										
Norwegian, dinner portion, 10 oz raw wt	1 serving	460	54.0	6.0	120	na	24.0	6.0	160	47%
Norwegian, lunch portion, 5 oz raw wt	1 serving	230	27.0	3.0	60	na	12.0	3.0	80	47%
Sockeye, dinner portion, 10 oz raw wt	1 serving	320	56.0	6.0	120	na	8.0	2.0	100	23%
Sockeye, lunch portion, 5 oz raw wt	1 serving	160	28.0	3.0	60	na	4.0	1.0	50	23%
SCALLOP										
calico, dinner portion, 10 oz raw wt	1 serving	360	64.0	16.0	320	na	4.0	tr	230	10%
calico, lunch portion, 5 oz raw wt	1 serving	180	32.0	8.0	260	na	2.0	tr	115	10%
deep sea, dinner portion, 10 oz raw wt	1 serving	260	52.0	4.0	520	na	4.0	tr	100	14%
deep sea, lunch portion, 5 oz raw wt	1 serving	130	26.0	2.0	260	na	2.0	tr	50	14%
SHARK										
blacktip, dinner portion, 10 oz raw wt	1 serving	300	70.0	0.0	180	na	2.0	tr	120	6%
blacktip, lunch portion, 5 oz raw wt	1 serving	150	35.0	0.0	90	na	1.0	tr	60	6%
mako, dinner portion, 10 oz raw wt	1 serving	280	68.0	0.0	120	na	2.0	tr	200	6%
mako, lunch portion, 5 oz raw wt	1 serving	140	34.0	0.0	60	na	1.0	tr	100	6%
SHRIMP, 8-12 pieces	1 serving	120	25.0	0.0	110	na	2.0	tr	230	15%
SOLE										
lemon, dinner portion, 10 oz raw wt	1 serving	240	54.0	2.0	180	na	2.0	tr	130	8%
lemon, lunch portion, 5 oz raw wt	1 serving	120	27.0	1.0	90	na	1.0	tr	65	8%
STRIP STEAK, 7 oz	1 serving	690	29.0	0.0	70	na	64.0	27.0	140	83%
SWORDFISH										
dinner portion, 10 oz raw weight	1 serving	200	34.0	0.0	280	na	8.0	2.0	200	36%
lunch portion, 5 oz raw weight	1 serving	100	17.0	0.0	140	na	4.0	1.0	100	36%
TILEFISH										
dinner portion, 10 oz raw wt	1 serving	200	40.0	0.0	120	na	4.0	2.0	160	18%
lunch portion, 5 oz raw wt	1 serving	100	20.0	0.0	60	na	2.0	1.0	80	18%
TROUT										
rainbow, dinner portion, 10 oz raw wt	1 serving	340	46.0	0.0	180	na	18.0	6.0	180	48%
rainbow, lunch portion, 5 oz raw wt	1 serving	170	23.0	0.0	90	na	9.0	3.0	90	48%
TUNA										
yellowfin, dinner portion, 10 oz raw wt	1 serving	360	64.0	0.0	140	na	12.0	4.0	140	30%
yellowfin, lunch portion, 5 oz raw wt	1 serving	180	32.0	0.0	70	na	6.0	2.0	70	30%
ROUND TABLE PIZZA										
pizza, cheese, pan, large pie	1 slice	310	13.0	40.0	631	na	11.0	na	30	32%
pizza, cheese, thin crust, large pie	1 slice	166	8.0	18.0	332	na	7.0	na	21	38%
ROY ROGERS										
ALFALFA SPROUTS	2 tbsp	1	tr	tr	<1	(mq)	tr	(tr)	0	0%
BACON BITS	1 tsp	33	3.0	2.0	189	na	1.0	na	0	27%

Food Name	Serving Size	Calories	Prot. gms	Carbs gms	Sod. mgs	Fiber gms	Fat gms	Sat. Fat gms	Chol. mgs	% Fat Cal.
BEAN SPROUTS	2 tbsp	4	tr	1.0	<1	(mq)	tr	(tr)	0	0%
BEETS, sliced	1/4 cup	18	1.0	4.0	162	(mq)	tr	(tr)	0	0%
BISCUIT	1 serving	231	4.0	26.0	575	(mq)	12.0	(mq)	5	47%
BREAKFAST										
egg and biscuit platter	1 serving	557	18.0	44.0	1020	(mq)	34.0	(mq)	417	55%
egg and biscuit platter, w/bacon	1 serving	607	21.0	44.0	1236	(mq)	39.0	(mq)	424	58%
egg and biscuit platter, w/ham	1 serving	605	25.0	44.0	1442	(mq)	36.0	(mq)	437	54%
egg and biscuit platter, w/sausage	1 serving	713	25.0	44.0	1345	(mq)	49.0	(mq)	458	62%
pancake platter, w/syrup and butter	1 serving	386	5.0	63.0	547	(mq)	13.0	(mq)	51	30%
pancake platter, w/syrup and butter, w/bacon	1 serving	436	8.0	63.0	763	(mq)	17.0	(mq)	58	35%
pancake platter, w/syrup and butter, w/ham	1 serving	434	11.0	64.0	969	(mq)	15.0	(mq)	71	31%
pancake platter, w/syrup and butter, w/sausage	1 serving	542	11.0	63.0	872	(mq)	28.0	(mq)	92	46%
BREAKFAST SANDWICH										
crescent	1 serving	408	13.0	28.0	820	(mq)	27.0	(mq)	207	60%
crescent, w/bacon	1 serving	446	15.0	28.0	982	(mq)	30.0	(mq)	212	61%
crescent, w/ham	1 serving	456	20.0	29.0	1243	(mq)	29.0	(mq)	227	57%
crescent, w/sausage	1 serving	564	19.0	28.0	1145	(mq)	42.0	(mq)	248	67%
BROCCOLI, raw	1/4 cup	6	1.0	1.0	6	(mq)	tr	(tr)	0	0%
CABBAGE, raw	1/4 cup	5	tr	1.0	2	(mq)	tr	(tr)	0	0%
CANTALOUPE, cubed	1/4 cup	14	tr	3.0	4	(mq)	tr	(tr)	0	0%
CARROT, raw, shredded	1/4 cup	12	tr	3.0	2	(mq)	tr	(tr)	0	0%
CAULIFLOWER, raw	1/4 cup	6	1.0	1.0	4	(mq)	tr	(tr)	0	0%
CHEESE, cheddar	1/4 cup	100	7.0	tr	275	0	8.0	(mq)	15	72%
CHEESEBURGER										
'Express'	1 serving	613	30.0	42.0	1122	(mq)	37.0	(mq)	82	54%
'Express' w/bacon	1 serving	641	33.0	36.0	1317	(mq)	41.0	(mq)	89	58%
regular	1 serving	525	29.0	37.0	830	(mq)	29.0	(mq)	76	50%
small	1 serving	275	15.0	24.0	558	(mq)	13.0	(mq)	36	43%
w/bacon	1 serving	552	32.0	31.0	1025	(mq)	33.0	(mq)	83	54%
CHICKEN										
breast, fried	1 serving	412	33.0	17.0	609	(mq)	24.0	(mq)	118	52%
breast and wing, fried	1 serving	604	44.0	25.0	894	(mq)	37.0	(mq)	165	55%
breast and wing, w/o skin, 'Roy's Roaster'	1 serving	190	32.0	2.0	na	na	6.0	na	na	28%
leg, fried	1 serving	140	12.0	6.0	190	(mq)	8.0	(mq)	40	51%
leg and thigh, fried	1 serving	436	30.0	17.0	596	(mq)	28.0	(mq)	125	58%
nugget, fried, 6 pieces	1 serving	288	10.0	21.0	548	(mq)	18.0	(mq)	63	56%
thigh, fried	1 serving	296	18.0	12.0	406	(mq)	20.0	(mq)	85	61%
wing, fried	1 serving	192	11.0	9.0	285	(mq)	13.0	(mq)	47	61%
CHICKEN SALAD, grilled	1 serving	120	18.0	2.0	520	na	4.0	na	60	30%
CHINESE NOODLES	1/4 cup	55	2.0	7.0	113	(mq)	3.0	(mq)	1	49%
COLESLAW	1 serving	110	1.0	11.0	261	(mq)	7.0	(mq)	5	57%
COTTAGE CHEESE	2 tbsp	29	4.0	<1.0	114	0	1.0	(mq)	4	31%
CROUTONS	2 tbsp	14	1.0	3.0	50	(mq)	tr	(tr)	0	0%
CUCUMBER, raw	5-6 slices	4	tr	1.0	2	(mq)	0.0	0.0	0	0%
DANISH										
apple swirl	1 serving	328	5.0	62.0	279	(mq)	7.0	(mq)	na	19%
cheese swirl	1 serving	383	8.0	54.0	369	(mq)	15.0	(mq)	na	35%
EGG, boiled, chopped	2 tbsp	55	4.0	1.0	41	0	4.0	(mq)	(mq)	65%
FISH SANDWICH	1 serving	514	18.0	58.0	857	(mq)	24.0	(mq)	62	42%
FRENCH FRIES										
large order, 5.5 oz	1 serving	440	6.0	54.0	225	(mq)	22.0	(mq)	19	45%
regular order, 4 oz	1 serving	320	4.0	39.0	164	(mq)	16.0	(mq)	13	45%
small order, 3 oz	1 serving	238	3.0	29.0	122	(mq)	12.0	(mq)	10	45%
FRUIT COCKTAIL	1/4 cup	46	tr	12.0	1	(mq)	tr	(tr)	0	0%

Food Name	Serving Size	Calories	Prot. gms	Carbs gms	Sod. mgs	Fiber gms	Fat gms	Sat. Fat gms	Chol. mgs	% Fat Cal.
GARBANZO BEANS	1/4 cup	55	3.0	9.0	240	(mq)	1.0	(mq)	0	16%
GELATIN, parfait	1/4 cup	50	1.0	10.0	23	(tr)	2.0	(mq)	0	36%
GRANOLA	1/4 cup	65	2.0	9.0	8	(mq)	3.0	(mq)	0	42%
GRAPES	5 grapes	20	tr	5.0	<1	(mq)	tr	(tr)	0	0%
GREEK PASTA	1/4 cup	159	3.0	19.0	328	(mq)	9.0	(mq)	na	51%
HAMBURGER										
'Express'	1 serving	561	27.0	42.0	899	(mq)	32.0	(mq)	70	51%
regular	1 serving	472	26.0	37.0	607	(mq)	25.0	(mq)	64	48%
'Roy Rogers Bar'	1 serving	573	36.0	38.0	1252	(mq)	31.0	(mq)	96	49%
small	1 serving	222	12.0	23.0	336	(mq)	9.0	(mq)	26	36%
HONEYDEW MELON, cubed	1/4 cup	15	tr	4.0	4	(mq)	tr	(tr)	0	0%
LEMONADE	12 oz	150	tr	39.0	na	na	tr	na	na	0%
LETTUCE										
iceberg	1 cup	7	1.0	1.0	5	(mq)	tr	(tr)	0	0%
romaine	1 cup	9	1.0	1.0	5	(mq)	tr	(tr)	0	0%
MACARONI SALAD	1/4 cup	93	2.0	10.0	301	(mq)	5.0	(mq)	na	48%
MILK, 2%	8 oz	120	8.0	11.0	130	na	5.0	na	18	38%
MILKSHAKE										
chocolate	1 serving	358	8.0	61.0	290	(tr)	10.0	(mq)	37	25%
strawberry	1 serving	315	8.0	49.0	261	(tr)	10.0	(mq)	37	29%
vanilla	1 serving	306	8.0	45.0	282	0	11.0	(mq)	40	32%
ONION, raw, chopped	2 tbsp	7	tr	2.0	tr	(mq)	tr	(tr)	0	0%
ORANGE JUICE	8 oz	120	2.0	32.0	na	na	tr	na	na	0%
PASTA AND NOODLES. See individual listings.										
PASTRY, cinnamon rod	1 serving	376	5.0	55.0	339	(mq)	15.0	(mq)	na	36%
PEACH, sliced	1/4 cup	48	tr	13.0	5	(mq)	tr	(tr)	0	0%
PEAS, green	1/4 cup	28	2.0	5.0	41	(mq)	tr	(tr)	0	0%
PEPPER, GREEN	2 tbsp	3	tr	1.0	tr	(mq)	tr	(tr)	0	0%
PINEAPPLE										
chunks, canned	1/4 cup	48	tr	12.0	5	(mq)	tr	(tr)	0	0%
chunks, fresh	1/4 cup	19	tr	5.0	<1	(mq)	tr	(tr)	0	0%
POTATO, BAKED, plain 'Hot Topped'	1 serving	211	6.0	48.0	65	na	0.0	na	0	0%
POTATO SALAD	1/4 cup	54	1.0	5.0	348	(mq)	3.0	(mq)	na	50%
RADISH, sliced	2 tbsp	2	tr	1.0	4	(mq)	tr	(tr)	0	0%
ROAST BEEF SANDWICH										
large	1 serving	373	35.0	31.0	840	(mq)	12.0	(mq)	82	29%
large, w/cheese	1 serving	427	38.0	31.0	1062	(mq)	17.0	(mq)	94	36%
regular	1 serving	350	26.0	37.0	732	(mq)	11.0	(mq)	68	28%
w/cheese	1 serving	403	29.0	37.0	954	(mq)	15.0	(mq)	70	33%
ROLL, crescent	1 serving	287	5.0	27.0	547	(mq)	18.0	(mq)	5	56%
SALAD DRESSING										
bacon and tomato	2 tbsp	136	tr	6.0	150	na	12.0	(mq)	na	79%
blue cheese	2 tbsp	150	2.0	2.0	153	na	16.0	(mq)	na	96%
Italian, low-calorie	2 tbsp	70	0.0	2.0	100	na	6.0	na	na	77%
ranch	2 tbsp	155	tr	4.0	100	na	14.0	(mq)	na	81%
Thousand Island	2 tbsp	160	tr	4.0	150	na	16.0	(mq)	na	90%
STRAWBERRIES, fresh	1/4 cup	11	tr	3.0	<1	(mq)	tr	(tr)	0	0%
SUNDAE										
caramel	1 serving	293	7.0	52.0	193	(tr)	9.0	(mq)	23	28%
chocolate	1 serving	358	8.0	61.0	290	na	10.0	na	37	25%
hot fudge	1 serving	337	7.0	53.0	186	(tr)	13.0	(mq)	23	35%
strawberry	1 serving	216	6.0	33.0	99	(tr)	7.0	(mq)	23	29%
vanilla	1 serving	306	8.0	45.0	282	na	11.0	na	40	32%
TOMATO	3 slices	20	1.0	5.0	1	(mq)	tr	(tr)	0	0%

Food Name	Serving Size	Calories	Prot. gms	Carbs gms	Sod. mgs	Fiber gms	Fat gms	Sat. Fat gms	Chol. mgs	% Fat Cal.
WATERMELON, diced	1/4 cup	13	tr	3.0	1	(mq)	tr	(tr)	0	0%

SHAKEY'S PIZZA
CHICKEN ENTRÉE

Food Name	Serving Size	Calories	Prot. gms	Carbs gms	Sod. mgs	Fiber gms	Fat gms	Sat. Fat gms	Chol. mgs	% Fat Cal.
5 pieces, fried, w/potatoes	1 serving	1700	97.0	130.0	5327	(mq)	90.0	(mq)	(mq)	48%
3 pieces, fried, w/potatoes	1 serving	947	57.0	51.0	2293	(mq)	56.0	(mq)	(mq)	53%
HAM AND CHEESE SANDWICH, 'Hot Ham & Cheese'	1 sandwich	550	36.0	56.0	2135	na	21.0	na	na	34%
HERO SANDWICH, 'Super Hot Hero'	1 sandwich	810	36.0	67.0	2688	(mq)	44.0	(mq)	(mq)	49%

PIZZA

Food Name	Serving Size	Calories	Prot. gms	Carbs gms	Sod. mgs	Fiber gms	Fat gms	Sat. Fat gms	Chol. mgs	% Fat Cal.
cheese, 'Homestyle Pan Crust' 12-inch pie	1/10 pie	303	14.1	31.0	591	(mq)	13.7	(mq)	21	41%
cheese, thick crust, 12-inch pie	1/10 pie	170	9.0	21.6	421	(mq)	4.8	(mq)	13	25%
cheese, thin crust, 12-inch pie	1/10 pie	133	8.4	13.2	323	(mq)	5.2	(mq)	14	35%
pepperoni, 'Homestyle Pan Crust' 12-inch pie	1/10 pie	343	15.8	31.1	740	(mq)	15.4	(mq)	27	40%
pepperoni, thick crust, 12-inch pie	1/10 pie	185	10.1	21.8	422	(mq)	6.4	(mq)	17	31%
pepperoni, thin crust, 12-inch pie	1/10 pie	148	8.4	13.2	403	(mq)	6.9	(mq)	14	42%
sausage and mushroom, 'Homestyle Pan Crust' 12-inch pie	1/10 pie	343	16.4	31.4	677	(mq)	16.9	(mq)	24	44%
sausage and mushroom, thick crust, 12-inch pie	1/10 pie	179	10.2	21.8	420	(mq)	5.6	(mq)	15	28%
sausage and mushroom, thin crust, 12-inch pie	1/10 pie	141	8.5	13.3	336	(mq)	6.0	(mq)	13	38%
sausage and pepperoni, 'Homestyle Pan Crust' 12-inch pie	1/10 pie	374	17.4	31.2	676	(mq)	19.9	(mq)	24	48%
sausage and pepperoni, thick crust, 12-inch pie	1/10 pie	177	11.1	21.7	424	(mq)	8.0	(mq)	19	41%
sausage and pepperoni, thin crust, 12-inch pie	1/10 pie	166	9.4	13.2	397	(mq)	8.4	(mq)	17	46%
'Shakey's Special' 'Homestyle Pan Crust' 12-inch pie	1/10 pie	384	17.9	31.6	878	(mq)	20.7	(mq)	29	49%
'Shakey's Special' thick crust, 12-inch pie	1/10 pie	208	13.1	22.3	423	(mq)	8.3	(mq)	18	36%
'Shakey's Special' thin crust, 12-inch pie	1/10 pie	171	13.3	13.5	475	(mq)	8.7	(mq)	16	46%
vegetable, 'Homestyle Pan Crust' 12-inch pie	1/10 pie	320	14.7	32.1	652	(mq)	14.7	(mq)	21	41%
vegetable, thick crust, 12-inch pie	1/10 pie	162	9.1	22.2	418	(mq)	4.1	(mq)	13	23%
vegetable, thin crust, 12-inch pie	1/10 pie	125	7.2	13.8	313	(mq)	4.5	(mq)	11	32%
POTATO WEDGES	15 pieces	950	17.0	120.0	0700	(mq)	36.0	(mq)	na	34%
SPAGHETTI ENTRÉE, w/meat sauce and garlic bread	1 serving	940	26.0	134.0	1904	(mq)	33.0	(mq)	(mq)	32%

SHONEY'S

Food Name	Serving Size	Calories	Prot. gms	Carbs gms	Sod. mgs	Fiber gms	Fat gms	Sat. Fat gms	Chol. mgs	% Fat Cal.
BARBECUE SAUCE, soufflé cup	1 serving	41	0.1	8.2	232	0	1.0	na	0	22%
BEAN SOUP	6 oz	63	3.8	9.8	479	1.4	1.1	(mq)	4	16%
BEEF SOUP, w/cabbage	6 oz	86	6.1	9.4	503	2.3	3.0	(mq)	13	31%
BISCUIT	1 serving	170	2.7	21.6	364	0	8.1	(mq)	0	43%
BREAD, Grecian	1 serving	80	2.0	13.2	94	0	2.2	(mq)	0	25%

BREAKFAST

Food Name	Serving Size	Calories	Prot. gms	Carbs gms	Sod. mgs	Fiber gms	Fat gms	Sat. Fat gms	Chol. mgs	% Fat Cal.
bacon	3 strips	109	5.8	0.1	303	0	9.4	(mq)	16	78%
egg, fried	1 egg	159	6.1	0.6	69	0	14.7	(mq)	274	83%
grits	3 oz	57	0.7	6.2	62	0	3.2	(mq)	0	51%
ham	2 slices	59	7.2	0.6	526	0	2.1	(mq)	28	32%
pancake, 6-inch diam	1 pancake	91	1.8	19.9	522	0	0.2	(mq)	0	2%
sausage	1 patty	103	3.7	0.2	161	0	9.6	(mq)	17	84%
BROCCOLI SOUP, cream of	6 oz	75	1.8	10.5	415	.4	4.6	(mq)	1	55%
BROCCOLI-CAULIFLOWER SOUP	6 oz	124	3.8	11.9	560	.5	9.2	(mq)	12	67%
BROWNIE, walnut, à la mode	1 serving	576	9.6	60.6	435	0	33.7	(mq)	35	53%

CAKE

Food Name	Serving Size	Calories	Prot. gms	Carbs gms	Sod. mgs	Fiber gms	Fat gms	Sat. Fat gms	Chol. mgs	% Fat Cal.
carrot	1 serving	500	9.0	56.0	476	0	26.0	(mq)	37	47%
hot fudge	1 serving	522	7.4	81.9	485	0	19.7	(mq)	27	34%

CHEESE SANDWICH

Food Name	Serving Size	Calories	Prot. gms	Carbs gms	Sod. mgs	Fiber gms	Fat gms	Sat. Fat gms	Chol. mgs	% Fat Cal.
grilled	1 sandwich	454	17.0	29.0	1519	na	29.0	na	na	57%
grilled, w/bacon	1 sandwich	440	18.2	27.9	1200	1.3	28.2	(mq)	36	58%
CHEESE SOUP, Florentine, w/ham	6 oz	110	3.7	11.8	890	.6	7.8	(mq)	11	64%

Food Name	Serving Size	Calories	Prot. gms	Carbs gms	Sod. mgs	Fiber gms	Fat gms	Sat. Fat gms	Chol. mgs	% Fat Cal.
CHEESEBURGER										
'Mushroom/Swiss Burger'	1 sandwich	616	31.6	28.8	1135	.7	41.7	(mq)	106	61%
patty melt	1 sandwich	640	38.8	29.5	826	6.7	41.7	(mq)	121	59%
CHICKEN ENTRÉE										
charbroiled, 'LightSide'	1 serving	239	39.0	1.0	592	na	7.0	na	85	26%
tenders, 'America's Favorites'	1 serving	388	34.9	16.6	239	0	20.4	(mq)	64	47%
CHICKEN SANDWICH										
charbroiled	1 sandwich	451	43.2	28.1	1002	.5	17.0	(mq)	90	34%
fillet	1 sandwich	464	29.7	38.9	585	.5	21.2	(mq)	51	41%
CHICKEN GUMBO	6 oz	60	4.0	7.0	1050	na	2.0	(mq)	(mq)	30%
CHICKEN NOODLE SOUP	6 oz	62	3.1	9.2	127	na	1.4	(mq)	14	20%
CHICKEN RICE SOUP	6 oz	72	3.0	13.3	117	.5	0.5	(mq)	6	6%
CHICKEN SOUP, cream of	6 oz	136	4.6	13.5	1164	.3	8.9	(mq)	11	59%
CHICKEN VEGETABLE SOUP, cream of	6 oz	79	3.5	13.4	714	na	1.3	(mq)	(mq)	15%
CHOWDER										
cheddar	6 oz	91	3.0	14.4	948	na	2.3	(mq)	(mq)	23%
clam	6 oz	94	1.7	9.6	66	0	5.4	(mq)	0	52%
corn	6 oz	148	4.0	22.1	510	0	4.7	(mq)	na	29%
COCKTAIL SAUCE, soufflé cup	1 serving	36	0.4	8.7	260	0	0.1	na	0	3%
COMBINATION ENTRÉE										
'Fish N' Shrimp'	1 serving	487	28.1	36.5	644	.3	25.5	(mq)	127	47%
shrimp, charbroiled 'Steak N' Shrimp'	1 serving	361	36.5	1.0	198	0	22.6	(mq)	141	56%
shrimp, fried 'Steak N' Shrimp'	1 serving	507	36.5	15.0	249	.1	32.7	(mq)	150	58%
rib eye steak and chicken, charbroiled	1 serving	605	35.2	0.0	211	0	50.5	(mq)	141	75%
sirloin steak and chicken, charbroiled	1 serving	357	31.9	0.0	160	0	24.5	(mq)	99	62%
steak, charbroiled, and Hawaiian chicken	1 serving	262	39.1	7.4	593	.3	7.4	(mq)	85	25%
steak and chicken, charbroiled	1 serving	239	39.0	1.3	592	0	7.4	(mq)	85	28%
steak and chicken, charbroiled, 8 oz	1 serving	435	31.1	0.0	280	0	34.4	(mq)	123	71%
CROISSANT	1 serving	260	5.0	22.0	260	0	16.0	(mq)	2	55%
FISH										
baked, 'LightSide'	1 serving	170	35.0	2.0	1641	0	1.0	na	83	5%
fried, 'Light'	1 serving	297	19.8	21.5	536	.1	14.4	(mq)	65	44%
FISH AND CHIPS ENTRÉE, w/fries	1 serving	639	32.3	50.4	873	2.9	34.8	na	103	49%
FISH SANDWICH	1 sandwich	323	12.2	41.0	740	.4	12.7	(mq)	21	35%
FRENCH FRIES										
4-oz order	1 serving	252	3.9	38.6	364	3.6	9.9	(mq)	0	35%
3-oz order	1 serving	189	2.9	28.9	273	2.7	7.5	(mq)	0	36%
home fries, 3 oz	1 serving	115	2.0	18.7	53	0	3.7	(mq)	0	29%
GRAVY, country	3 oz	114	1.2	5.7	358	0	9.8	(mq)	2	77%
HAM SANDWICH										
baked	1 sandwich	290	19.2	28.2	1263	1.8	10.3	(mq)	42	32%
club, on whole wheat	1 sandwich	642	37.0	45.2	2105	10.5	35.5	(mq)	78	50%
HAMBURGER										
'All-American'	1 sandwich	501	25.0	26.8	597	.5	32.6	(mq)	86	59%
'Old-Fashioned Burger'	1 sandwich	470	25.1	25.6	681	.6	28.2	(mq)	82	54%
'Shoney Burger'	1 sandwich	498	23.4	22.2	782	.2	35.7	(mq)	79	65%
w/bacon	1 sandwich	591	28.7	28.6	801	.5	40.0	(mq)	86	61%
HAMBURGER PATTY, beef, light	1 serving	289	20.7	0.0	187	0	22.9	(mq)	82	71%
ITALIAN FEAST ENTRÉE	1 serving	500	37.5	43.8	369	1.1	19.6	(mq)	74	35%
LASAGNA ENTRÉE										
'America's Favorites'	1 serving	297	8.3	44.9	870	2.8	9.8	(mq)	26	30%
'LightSide'	1 serving	297	8.0	45.0	870	na	10.0	na	26	30%
LIVER AND ONIONS ENTRÉE, 'America's Favorites'	1 serving	411	34.9	15.4	321	.8	22.9	(mq)	529	50%
MUSHROOMS, sautéed	3 oz	75	1.6	4.3	968	1.3	6.5	(mq)	0	78%

Food Name	Serving Size	Calories	Prot. gms	Carbs gms	Sod. mgs	Fiber gms	Fat gms	Sat. Fat gms	Chol. mgs	% Fat Cal.
ONION, sautéed	2.5 oz	37	0.8	4.3	221	.5	2.1	(mq)	0	51%
ONION RINGS	1 ring	52	0.9	5.0	102	.4	3.1	(mq)	2	54%
ONION SOUP	6 oz	29	1.1	1.5	88	.1	2.0	(mq)	1	62%
PASTA AND NOODLES. See SALAD and individual listings.										
PASTRY, honey bun	1 bun	265	4.0	32.0	33	0	14.0	(mq)	3	48%
PIE										
apple, 'À la mode'	1 serving	492	6.0	67.0	574	na	23.0	(mq)	35	42%
strawberry	1 serving	332	2.1	44.5	247	2.3	16.7	(mq)	0	45%
POTATO, BAKED	10 oz	264	5.6	61.1	16	6.8	0.3	na	0	1%
POTATO SOUP	6 oz	102	1.4	16.8	335	1.6	3.4	(mq)	0	30%
POTATOES, HASH BROWN	3 oz	90	1.6	14.1	50	0	3.1	(mq)	0	31%
REUBEN SANDWICH	1 sandwich	596	32.7	31.5	3873	6.3	34.7	(mq)	138	52%
RICE, 3.5 oz	1 serving	137	2.4	23.1	765	.1	3.7	(mq)	1	24%
SALAD										
ambrosia	1/4 cup	75	0.8	11.5	167	.8	3.3	(mq)	0	40%
apple grape surprise	1/4 cup	19	0.0	4.9	2	.1	0.0	0.0	0	0%
beet onion	1/4 cup	25	0.6	3.0	167	.8	1.3	(mq)	0	47%
broccoli cauliflower	1/4 cup	98	2.3	4.0	478	.9	8.5	(mq)	0	78%
broccoli cauliflower carrot	1/4 cup	53	1.1	2.7	193	.9	4.4	(mq)	1	75%
broccoli cauliflower ranch	1/4 cup	65	0.9	1.6	12	.9	6.4	(mq)	9	89%
carrot apple	1/4 cup	99	0.6	4.2	10	.9	9.1	(mq)	8	83%
coleslaw	1/4 cup	69	1.1	5.1	106	.9	5.1	(mq)	7	67%
cucumber, lite	1/4 cup	12	0.2	2.7	344	.2	0.1	na	0	8%
Don's pasta	1/4 cup	82	1.8	8.6	223	.2	4.6	(mq)	0	50%
fruit delight	1/4 cup	54	0.6	10.1	2	.7	1.6	(mq)	0	27%
Italian vegetable	1/4 cup	11	0.4	2.5	110	.7	0.1	na	0	8%
kidney bean	1/4 cup	55	2.6	6.8	154	1.9	2.1	(mq)	2	34%
macaroni	1/4 cup	207	4.2	17.0	382	.2	10.9	(mq)	14	60%
mixed fruit	1/4 cup	37	0.4	9.3	3	.2	0.1	na	0	2%
mixed squash	1/4 cup	49	1.1	2.3	230	.3	4.1	(mq)	0	75%
Oriental	1/4 cup	79	0.8	13.4	31	.5	2.7	(mq)	1	31%
pea	1/4 cup	73	2.5	3.5	89	2.4	5.5	(mq)	42	68%
rotelli pasta	1/4 cup	78	1.4	8.9	82	.2	4.0	(mq)	0	46%
Seigan	1/4 cup	72	2.3	8.1	122	1.2	3.6	(mq)	5	45%
snow	1/4 cup	72	0.6	9.0	18	.1	4.1	(mq)	0	51%
spaghetti	1/4 cup	81	1.6	8.7	20	.2	4.6	(mq)	0	51%
spring	1/4 cup	38	0.8	2.4	162	.7	2.9	(mq)	0	69%
summer	1/4 cup	114	1.1	2.2	233	.9	11.6	(mq)	0	92%
three bean	1/4 cup	96	1.4	11.9	189	1.3	5.1	(mq)	0	48%
Waldorf	1/4 cup	81	0.9	8.5	68	.8	5.2	(mq)	2	58%
SALAD DRESSING										
Biscayne, low-calorie	2 tbsp	62	6.0	1.0	334	0	1.0	na	0	15%
blue cheese	2 tbsp	113	0.0	0.0	109	0	12.6	(mq)	15	100%
French	2 tbsp	124	2.0	2.0	204	0	12.0	(mq)	12	87%
French, rue	2 tbsp	122	5.0	2.0	364	0	10.0	(mq)	0	74%
honey mustard	2 tbsp	165	2.4	2.4	5	0	17.0	(mq)	18	93%
Italian, creamy	2 tbsp	135	0.0	1.0	454	0	14.5	(mq)	0	97%
Italian, golden	2 tbsp	141	0.0	1.0	302	0	15.0	(mq)	0	96%
Italian, nonfat	2 tbsp	10	0.0	2.4	615	0	0.0	0.0	0	0%
ranch	2 tbsp	95	0.0	0.0	10	0	10.0	(mq)	15	95%
Thousand Island	2 tbsp	130	1.0	2.0	179	0	13.0	(mq)	12	90%
SEAFOOD ENTRÉE, platter	1 serving	566	32.8	45.7	893	.3	28.0	(mq)	127	45%
SHRIMP										
bite-size	1 serving	387	16.4	24.7	1266	0	24.7	(mq)	140	57%

Food Name	Serving Size	Calories	Prot. gms	Carbs gms	Sod. mgs	Fiber gms	Fat gms	Sat. Fat gms	Chol. mgs	% Fat Cal.
charbroiled	1 serving	138	24.7	3.0	170	0	3.0	(mq)	162	20%
SHRIMP ENTRÉE										
boiled	1 serving	93	19.6	0.0	210	0	1.0	(mq)	182	10%
sampler	1 serving	412	25.5	26.1	783	.1	22.7	(mq)	217	50%
'Shrimper's Feast'	1 serving	383	16.5	29.9	216	.3	22.2	(mq)	125	52%
'Shrimper's Feast' large	1 serving	575	24.8	44.9	324	.4	33.3	(mq)	188	52%
SIRLOIN STEAK, charbroiled	6 oz	357	31.9	0.0	160	0	24.5	(mq)	99	62%
SLIM JIM SANDWICH	1 sandwich	484	27.4	40.4	1620	.5	23.9	(mq)	57	44%
SPAGHETTI ENTRÉE										
'America's Favorites'	1 serving	496	24.2	63.4	387	2.2	16.3	(mq)	55	30%
'LightSide'	1 serving	248	12.0	32.0	194	na	8.0	na	28	29%
STEAK ENTRÉE, country-fried, 'America's Favorites'	1 serving	449	19.4	33.9	1177	.9	27.2	(mq)	27	55%
STEAK SANDWICH										
country-fried	1 sandwich	588	24.5	67.0	1501	1.4	25.8	(mq)	29	39%
Philly	1 sandwich	673	31.8	37.2	1242	.1	44.0	(mq)	103	59%
SUNDAE										
hot fudge	1 serving	451	7.0	60.0	226	0	22.0	(mq)	60	44%
strawberry	1 serving	380	6.0	47.7	145	.3	19.0	(mq)	69	45%
SWEET AND SOUR SAUCE, soufflé cup	1 serving	58	0.0	14.7	5	0	0.0	0.0	0	0%
SYRUP, low-calorie	2.2 oz	98	0.0	24.4	0	0	0.0	0.0	0	0%
TARTAR SAUCE, soufflé cup	1 serving	84	0.2	3.6	177	0	7.7	(mq)	11	83%
TOAST, buttered	2 slices	163	4.2	24.6	296	1.2	5.2	(mq)	0	29%
TOMATO SOUP										
Florentine	6 oz	63	2.3	11.0	683	0	1.1	(mq)	0	16%
vegetable	6 oz	46	1.9	9.8	314	.4	0.3	(mq)	0	6%
TURKEY SANDWICH, turkey club, on whole wheat	1 sandwich	635	43.5	44.1	1289	10.2	32.7	(mq)	100	46%
VEGETABLE BEEF SOUP	6 oz	82	3.5	14.1	1254	.3	1.5	(mq)	5	16%
SIZZLER										
ALFALFA SPROUTS	1/4 cup	2	0.0	0.0	0	0	0.0	0.0	0	0%
AVOCADO	1/2 avocado	153	2.0	6.0	11	3.0	15.0	2.0	0	88%
BACON BITS	1 tbsp	27	2.0	2.0	165	1.0	2.0	0.0	0	67%
BEAN SPROUTS	1/4 cup	8	1.0	2.0	2	0	0.0	0.0	0	0%
BEANS										
garbanzo	1/4 cup	63	3.0	11.0	255	3.0	1.0	0.0	0	14%
kidney	1/4 cup	52	3.0	10.0	222	4.0	0.0	0.0	0	0%
BEEF PATTY										
ground, 8-oz size	1 serving	530	42.0	0.0	150	na	38.0	15.4	156	65%
ground, 5.33-oz size	1 serving	353	28.0	0.0	100	na	28.0	10.2	104	71%
BEETS	1/4 cup	13	0.0	3.0	117	1.0	0.0	0.0	0	0%
BREAD, focaccia	2 pieces	108	2.0	9.0	134	0	7.0	1.0	1	58%
BREADSTICKS, garlic, soft	1 oz	75	2.3	15.2	112	na	0.5	na	na	6%
BROCCOLI, raw	1/2 cup	12	1.0	2.0	12	1.0	0.0	0.0	0	0%
BROCCOLI CHEESE SOUP	4 oz	139	3.0	10.0	355	0	9.0	2.0	8	58%
CABBAGE, red, raw	1/4 cup	5	0.0	1.0	2	0	0.0	0.0	0	0%
CANTALOUPE	1/2 cup	28	1.0	7.0	7	1.0	0.0	0.0	0	0%
CARROTS, raw	1/4 cup	12	0.0	3.0	10	1.0	0.0	0.0	0	0%
CAULIFLOWER, battered, unprepared, approx 3.5 oz	1 serving	184	3.1	21.1	49	na	10.3	0.0	1	50%
CHEESE										
cheddar, imitation, shredded	1 oz	85	2.0	4.5	375	na	6.5	1.5	0	69%
Parmesan, grated	1 oz	110	11.0	2.0	550	na	7.0	4.8	4	57%
Swiss, sliced	1 oz	100	8.0	1.0	74	na	8.0	na	25	72%
CHEESE SAUCE, nacho	2 oz	120	5.0	3.0	600	0	10.0	5.0	30	75%
CHEESE TOAST	1 slice	273	6.0	16.0	494	1.0	21.0	5.0	5	69%

Food Name	Serving Size	Calories	Prot. gms	Carbs gms	Sod. mgs	Fiber gms	Fat gms	Sat. Fat gms	Chol. mgs	% Fat Cal.
CHICKEN										
breast, lemon herb	5 oz	151	27.0	27.0	na	na	4.0	na	na	24%
patty, Malibu	1 patty	368	27.0	12.0	na	na	25.0	na	na	61%
wings	1 oz	73	4.0	4.0	136	0	4.0	1.0	20	49%
wings, disjointed, Cajun	3 oz	201	15.9	1.8	435	na	14.4	na	111	64%
wings, disjointed, Southern style	1 oz	73	4.7	3.7	135	na	6.0	1.1	20	74%
wings, whole, Southern style	1 oz	74	3.9	3.7	285	na	4.8	1.7	18	58%
CHICKEN ENTRÉE, w/noodles	6 oz	164	13.0	20.0	524	na	4.0	0.7	40	22%
CHICKEN NOODLE SOUP	4 oz	31	2.0	4.0	495	0	1.0	0.0	7	29%
CHICKEN STRIPS, breaded	1 oz	68	3.6	na	130	na	4.6	0.9	9	61%
CHILI, w/beans, 'Grande'	6 oz	100	5.0	18.0	1190	na	1.0	na	0	9%
CHOCOLATE SYRUP	1 oz	90	0.0	21.0	15	0	0.0	0.0	0	0%
CHOWDER, clam	4 oz	118	3.0	11.0	511	0	6.0	0.0	6	46%
COCKTAIL SAUCE	1.5 oz	40	0.0	8.0	396	0	0.0	0.0	0	0%
CORN NUGGETS	3 oz	117	2.5	22.0	325	na	8.4	na	0	65%
CORNED BEEF, sliced	1 oz	45	7.5	0.2	55	na	1.5	na	na	30%
COTTAGE CHEESE										
low-fat	1/2 cup	100	14.0	4.0	390	na	2.0	1.0	8	18%
regular	2 oz	51	8.0	2.0	230	0	1.0	1.0	5	18%
CRAB										
imitation, shredded, approx 3.5 oz	1 serving	104	12.0	14.0	864	na	<1.0	na	22	0%
snow, legs and claws, scored	3.5 oz	91	20.6	0.0	539	na	1.1	0.1	55	11%
CRACKER, saltine	2 crackers	25	1.0	4.0	74	na	1.0	0.0	2	36%
CREAMER, nondairy	.5 oz	12	0.0	1.0	<5	na	0.8	na	0	60%
CROISSANT, mini	1 croissant	120	2.0	12.0	95	na	8.0	2.5	4	60%
CUCUMBER, raw	2 oz	7	0.0	2.0	1	1.0	0.0	0.0	0	0%
DESSERT, parfait salad, approx 3.5 oz	1 serving	84	1.5	16.5	66	na	1.7	1.7	0	18%
EGG										
cooked, diced	2 oz	85	7.1	0.7	71	na	5.7	na	242	60%
cooked, salad topping	1 oz	44	4.0	0.0	35	0	3.0	1.0	122	61%
FETTUCCINE										
whole egg	2 oz	80	3.0	15.0	5	0	1.0	0.0	5	11%
FILET MIGNON STEAK, 7 oz	3 oz	179	2.0	0.0	54	na	na	na	71	0%
FISH NUGGETS	1 oz	40	4.0	5.0	100	na	0.0	na	10	0%
FRENCH FRIES	4 oz	358	5.0	45.0	245	4.0	12.0	6.0	0	30%
GRAPES	1/2 cup	29	0.0	8.0	1	1.0	0.0	0.0	0	0%
GUACAMOLE										
extra chunky, approx 3.5 oz	1 serving	285	3.0	7.4	na	na	18.4	na	0	58%
regular	1 oz	42	0.0	2.0	425	0	4.0	1.0	0	86%
HALIBUT STEAK										
8-oz size	1 serving	240	48.0	0.0	137	na	3.0	0.7	114	11%
6-oz size	1 serving	180	36.0	0.0	103	na	2.0	0.5	86	10%
HAMBURGER, w/lettuce and tomato	1 serving	626	45.0	36.0	335	1.0	33.0	12.0	142	47%
HONEYDEW MELON	1/2 cup	30	0.0	8.0	9	1.0	0.0	0.0	0	0%
JICAMA	2 oz	13	1.0	3.0	1	0	0.0	0.0	0	0%
KIWIFRUIT	2 oz	35	1.0	8.0	3	2.0	0.0	0.0	0	0%
LASAGNA										
meat	8 oz	327	21.0	23.0	657	na	13.0	6.0	37	36%
vegetable	8 oz	245	15.0	29.0	553	na	8.0	5.0	19	29%
LETTUCE										
iceberg	1 cup	7	1.0	1.0	5	1.0	0.0	0.0	0	0%
romaine	1 cup	9	1.0	1.0	4	1.0	0.0	0.0	0	0%
MACARONI AND CHEESE	6 oz	214	10.0	22.0	590	na	9.0	5.0	26	38%
MARGARINE, whipped	1.5 tbsp	105	0.0	0.0	146	0	11.7	2.0	0	100%

Food Name	Serving Size	Calories	Prot. gms	Carbs gms	Sod. mgs	Fiber gms	Fat gms	Sat. Fat gms	Chol. mgs	% Fat Cal.
MARINARA SAUCE	1 oz	13	0.0	3.0	90	0	0.0	0.0	0	0%
MEATBALLS	4 meatballs	157	9.0	5.0	461	1.0	11.0	5.0	30	63%
MILK, low-fat	1 cup	140	10.0	13.0	150	na	5.0	2.8	10	32%
MINESTRONE SOUP	4 oz	36	1.0	7.0	443	2.0	0.0	0.0	1	0%
MUSHROOMS, raw	1/4 cup	4	0.0	1.0	1	0	0.0	0.0	0	0%
OKRA, breaded, unprepared, approx 3.5 oz	1 serving	105	3.3	24.4	503	na	0.5	0.0	<1	4%
OLIVES	1 oz	47	1.0	1.0	181	1.0	4.0	1.0	0	77%
ONION, red, raw	2 tbsp	8	0.0	2.0	1	0	0.0	0.0	0	0%
ONION RINGS, steak cut, breaded, unprepared, approx 3.5 oz	1 serving	395	4.8	39.0	558	na	24.4	0.0	0	56%
PASTA AND NOODLES. See SALAD and individual listings.										
PEACH	1/4 cup	34	0.0	9.0	3	1.0	0.0	0.0	0	0%
PEAS	1/4 cup	31	2.0	6.0	35	2.0	0.0	0.0	0	0%
PEPPER, BELL	2 oz	8	1.0	2.0	1	1.0	0.0	0.0	0	0%
PINEAPPLE	1/2 cup	38	0.0	10.0	1	1.0	0.0	0.0	0	0%
PIZZA, 'Supreme' round, 5-inch pie	6.5 oz	524	18.0	51.8	1057	na	27.1	na	14	47%
POLLACK, breaded	4 oz	140	14.0	18.0	280	na	1.0	na	35	6%
POTATO, BAKED, pulp only	4 oz	105	2.0	24.0	6	2.0	0.0	0.0	0	0%
POTATO SKINS	2 oz	160	2.0	22.0	463	3.0	8.0	1.0	0	45%
RAVIOLI, CHEESE	4 oz	260	10.0	47.0	270	na	4.0	2.0	20	14%
REFRIED BEANS	3 oz	120	5.0	16.0	320	na	4.0	1.5	2	30%
RICE PILAF	6 oz	256	4.0	47.0	866	1.0	5.0	1.0	0	18%
ROAST BEEF, sliced	2/3 oz	17	3.3	0.3	276	na	0.3	0.1	8	16%
SALAD										
beef, teriyaki, 2 oz	1 serving	49	4.0	5.0	136	1.0	2.0	1.0	7	37%
carrot and raisin, 2 oz	1 serving	130	1.0	10.0	104	1.0	10.0	2.0	10	69%
chicken, Chinese, 2 oz	1 serving	54	4.0	6.0	119	1.0	2.0	0.0	10	33%
four bean, approx 3.5 oz	1 serving	104	2.6	18.8	226	na	2.5	0.4	0	22%
fruit, 'Mediterranean Minted' 2 oz	1 serving	29	1.0	7.0	11	0	0.0	0.0	0	0%
jicama, spicy, 2 oz	1 serving	16	0.0	4.0	28	0	0.0	0.0	0	0%
macaroni and cheddar, approx 3.5 oz	1 serving	185	3.2	15.7	476	na	12.5	3.8	14	61%
'Mexican Fiesta' 2 oz	1 serving	54	2.0	10.0	99	1.0	1.0	0.0	0	17%
pasta, Italian, approx 3.5 oz	1 serving	90	3.9	18.3	352	na	0.6	0.1	0	6%
pasta, Oriental, approx 3.5 oz	1 serving	114	3.7	22.6	781	na	1.6	0.2	<1	13%
pasta, seafood Louis, 2 oz	1 serving	64	3.0	9.0	139	1.0	2.0	0.0	17	28%
pasta, shell, approx 3.5 oz	1 serving	112	3.2	19.4	591	na	2.7	0.5	1	22%
pasta, tuna, 2 oz	1 serving	133	6.0	6.0	188	0	10.0	1.0	10	68%
pasta, tuna, chunky, approx 3.5 oz	1 serving	186	6.0	14.5	365	na	11.0	2.8	17	53%
potato, German, approx 3.5 oz	1 serving	115	2.2	23.1	666	na	2.0	0.5	1	16%
potato, old fashioned, approx 3.5 oz	1 serving	150	1.6	17.0	416	na	8.7	1.3	23	52%
potato, red herb, approx 3.5 oz	1 serving	213	1.5	15.4	437	na	16.2	2.4	15	68%
potato and egg, approx 3.5 oz	1 serving	140	1.6	16.0	340	na	7.8	1.2	28	50%
seafood, 2 oz	1 serving	56	3.0	4.0	255	0	3.0	1.0	7	48%
tuna, approx 3.5 oz	1 serving	353	8.1	7.3	296	na	32.9	5.0	44	84%
SALAD DRESSING										
blue cheese	1 oz	111	1.0	1.0	168	0	12.0	4.0	8	97%
honey mustard	1 oz	160	0.0	4.0	110	0	16.0	2.0	10	90%
hot bacon	1 tbsp	40	0.0	5.8	90	na	2.0	na	na	45%
Italian, lite	1 oz	14	0.0	2.0	350	0	0.0	0.0	0	0%
Japanese rice vinegar, fat-free	1 oz	10	0.0	2.0	172	0	0.0	0.0	0	0%
Malibu	1 tbsp	100	0.0	0.0	125	na	11.0	2.0	10	99%
Parmesan Italian	1 oz	100	0.0	2.0	450	0	10.0	2.0	0	90%
ranch	1 oz	120	0.0	2.0	240	0	12.0	2.0	10	90%
ranch, reduced calorie	1 oz	90	0.0	4.0	270	0	8.0	2.0	10	80%

Food Name	Serving Size	Calories	Prot. gms	Carbs gms	Sod. mgs	Fiber gms	Fat gms	Sat. Fat gms	Chol. mgs	% Fat Cal.
sour	2 tbsp	60	0.0	0.0	30	0	6.0	5.0	0	90%
Thousand Island	1 oz	143	0.0	3.0	125	0	15.0	2.0	11	94%
SALMON										
8-oz portion	1 serving	247	32.0	0.0	232	0	12.0	2.0	41	44%
3.5-oz portion	1 serving	125	20.0	0.0	50	na	5.0	1.0	70	36%
SALSA	1 oz	7	0.0	2.0	156	0	0.0	0.0	0	0%
SAUCE										
buttery dipping	1.5 oz	330	0.0	0.0	0	0	36.7	7.0	0	100%
hibachi	1.5 oz	57	0.0	11.0	707	0	0.0	0.0	0	0%
Malibu	1.5 oz	283	0.0	0.0	354	0	31.0	6.0	28	99%
SCALLOP, breaded, approx 30-40	4 oz	160	14.0	24.0	393	na	1.0	na	18	6%
SHRIMP										
broiled	5 oz	150	23.0	0.0	377	0	6.0	1.0	218	36%
scampi	5 oz	143	27.0	0.0	386	0	3.0	1.0	150	19%
tempura batter, approx 21-25	3 oz	155	10.0	13.0	442	na	8.0	3.0	74	46%
SIRLOIN STEAK										
9.25-oz size	1 serving	655	80.0	0.0	309	0	35.0	18.0	175	48%
6.25-oz size	1 serving	447	55.0	0.0	245	0	34.0	12.0	120	68%
top sirloin	1 oz	55	8.6	na	19	na	2.0	0.7	25	33%
SPAGHETTI	2 oz	80	3.0	16.0	1	1.0	0.0	0.0	0	0%
SPINACH, raw	1/2 cup	6	1.0	1.0	22	1.0	0.0	0.0	0	0%
STRAWBERRIES	1/2 cup	22	0.0	5.0	1	2.0	0.0	0.0	0	0%
STRAWBERRY TOPPING	1 oz	70	0.0	18.0	5	0	0.0	0.0	0	0%
STRIP STEAK, New York, 12 oz	1 serving	600	70.0	5.0	200	na	35.0	na	180	53%
SWORDFISH	8 oz	315	45.0	0.0	331	0	14.0	3.0	89	40%
TACO SHELL	1 shell	50	1.0	7.0	20	1.0	2.0	0.0	0	36%
TARTAR SAUCE	1.5 oz	170	0.0	6.0	453	0	17.0	3.0	14	90%
TOMATO, cherry	1/4 cup	12	0.0	3.0	5	1.0	0.0	0.0	0	0%
TUNA, yellowfin, approx 3.5 oz	1 serving	125	15.0	0.0	50	na	4.0	1.0	65	29%
TURKEY HAM	1 oz	62	4.0	0.0	376	0	5.0	2.0	19	73%
VEGETABLE SIRLION SOUP	4 oz	60	6.0	6.0	364	0	2.0	1.0	10	30%
VEGETABLE SOUP, vegetarian	6 oz	50	2.0	6.0	630	na	1.0	0.2	0	18%
WATERMELON	1/2 cup	26	0.0	6.0	2	0	0.0	0.0	0	0%
WHIPPED TOPPING	1 tbsp	12	0.0	1.0	0	0	1.0	1.0	0	75%
YOGURT, FROZEN										
chocolate, soft-serve	4 oz	136	1.0	24.0	100	0	4.0	4.0	0	26%
vanilla, soft-serve	4 oz	136	1.0	24.0	100	0	4.0	4.0	0	26%
ZUCCHINI										
beer-battered, unprepared, approx 3.5 oz	1 serving	205	2.8	23.1	229	na	11.8	0.0	<1	52%
raw	1/4 cup	5	0.0	1.0	1	1.0	0.0	0.0	0	0%
SKIPPER'S										
BARBECUE SAUCE	1 tbsp	25	0.0	5.0	226	na	1.0	na	0	36%
CHICKEN ENTRÉE										
tenderloin strips, 5 pieces, w/fries	1 serving	793	44.0	69.0	798	(mq)	38.0	(mq)	77	43%
3 pieces, w/small green salad, 'Lite Catch'	1 serving	305	26.0	17.0	673	(mq)	15.0	(mq)	58	44%
CHICKEN SANDWICH, 'Create A Catch'	1 serving	606	31.0	44.0	976	(mq)	32.0	(mq)	82	48%
CHICKEN STRIPS, 'Create A Catch'	1 serving	82	8.0	4.0	150	(mq)	4.0	(mq)	15	44%
CHOWDER										
'Alder Smoked Salmon'	6 oz	166	13.0	14.0	73	na	7.0	na	na	38%
clam, 'Create A Catch' cup	1 serving	100	3.0	14.0	525	(mq)	3.5	(mq)	12	32%
clam, 'Create A Catch' pint	1 serving	200	5.0	19.0	1050	(mq)	7.0	(mq)	24	32%
CLAM ENTRÉE, strips, w/fries 'Basket'	1 serving	1003	22.0	90.0	569	(mq)	70.0	(mq)	14	63%
COCKTAIL SAUCE	1 tbsp	20	0.0	5.0	216	na	0.0	0.0	0	0%

Food Name	Serving Size	Calories	Prot. gms	Carbs gms	Sod. mgs	Fiber gms	Fat gms	Sat. Fat gms	Chol. mgs	% Fat Cal.
COD ENTRÉE										
thick cut, 3 pieces, w/fries	1 serving	665	27.0	68.0	1054	(mq)	32.0	(mq)	38	43%
thick cut, 4 pieces, w/fries	1 serving	759	34.0	74.0	1388	(mq)	36.0	(mq)	50	43%
thick cut, 5 pieces, w/fries	1 serving	853	42.0	80.0	1723	(mq)	41.0	(mq)	62	43%
COLESLAW, 'Create A Catch' 5 oz	1 serving	289	2.0	10.0	329	(mq)	27.0	(mq)	50	84%
COMBINATION ENTRÉE										
chicken strips, 1 piece fish, and fries	1 serving	805	80.0	72.0	858	(mq)	40.0	(mq)	100	45%
chicken strips, shrimp, and fries	1 serving	800	36.0	77.0	1036	(mq)	39.0	(mq)	97	44%
clam strips, 1 piece fish, and fries, 'Combos'	1 serving	868	25.0	81.0	667	(mq)	54.0	(mq)	61	56%
jumbo shrimp, 1 piece fish, and fries, 'Combos'	1 serving	720	24.0	75.0	1268	(mq)	36.0	(mq)	91	45%
1 piece fish, 2 pieces chicken, and small green salad, 'Lite Catch'	1 serving	399	29.0	24.0	880	(mq)	21.0	(mq)	96	47%
shrimp, 1 piece fish, and fries, 'Combos'	1 serving	728	24.0	77.0	943	(mq)	37.0	(mq)	105	46%
oysters, 1 piece fish, and fries, 'Combos'	1 serving	885	25.0	95.0	809	(mq)	44.0	(mq)	80	45%
FISH ENTRÉE. See also individual listings.										
1 fish fillet, w/fries	1 serving	558	17.0	51.0	408	(mq)	28.0	(mq)	55	45%
2 fish fillets, w/fries	1 serving	733	28.0	71.0	765	(mq)	38.0	(mq)	108	47%
2 fish fillets, w/small green salad, 'Lite Catch'	1 serving	409	25.0	27.0	937	(mq)	23.0	(mq)	119	51%
3 fish fillets, w/fries	1 serving	908	39.0	82.0	1122	(mq)	48.0	(mq)	160	48%
FISH FILLET, 'Create A Catch'	1 serving	175	11.0	11.0	357	(mq)	10.0	(mq)	53	51%
FISH SANDWICH										
'Create A Catch'	1 serving	524	19.0	43.0	1191	(mq)	33.0	(mq)	86	57%
double, 'Create A Catch'	1 serving	698	30.0	54.0	1548	(mq)	73.0	(mq)	139	94%
FRENCH FRIES, 'Create A Catch'	1 serving	383	6.0	50.0	51	(mq)	18.0	(mq)	2	42%
GELATIN DESSERT, Jell-O, 'Create A Catch'	1 serving	55	1.0	12.0	35	0	0.0	0.0	0	0%
MILK, low-fat	12 oz	181	15.0	32.0	225	na	10.0	na	0	50%
OYSTER ENTRÉE, w/fries, 'Basket'	1 serving	1038	28.0	118.0	853	(mq)	51.0	(mq)	52	44%
POTATO, BAKED	1 serving	145	4.0	32.0	6	na	0.0	na	0	0%
ROOT BEER FLOAT	1 serving	302	3.0	33.0	66	na	10.0	(mq)	10	30%
SALAD										
green, small, 'Lite Catch'	1 serving	59	3.0	6.0	223	(mq)	3.0	(mq)	13	46%
shrimp and seafood	1 serving	167	23.0	15.0	657	na	3.0	na	80	16%
side order	1 serving	24	0.0	4.0	8	na	0.0	na	0	0%
SALAD DRESSING										
blue cheese, premium	1 pouch	222	1.0	4.0	240	na	23.0	(mq)	8	93%
Italian, gourmet	1 pouch	140	0.0	2.0	200	na	15.0	(mq)	0	96%
Italian, low-calorie	1 pouch	17	0.0	2.0	680	na	1.0	na	0	53%
ranch house	1 pouch	188	1.0	2.0	302	na	20.0	(mq)	0	96%
Thousand Island	1 pouch	160	0.0	8.0	415	na	14.0	(mq)	6	79%
SALMON, baked	4.4 oz	270	39.0	1.0	504	na	11.0	na	70	37%
SEAFOOD ENTRÉE, w/fries, 'Skipper's Platter Basket'	1 serving	1038	32.0	97.0	1202	(mq)	63.0	(mq)	111	55%
SHRIMP ENTRÉE										
jumbo, w/fries, 'Basket'	1 serving	707	20.0	79.0	911	(mq)	35.0	(mq)	73	45%
original, w/fries, 'Basket'	1 serving	723	20.0	82.0	1121	(mq)	36.0	(mq)	102	45%
w/seafood salad, 'Lite Catch'	1 serving	167	23.0	15.0	657	(mq)	3.0	(mq)	80	16%
TARTAR SAUCE	1 tbsp	65	0.0	0.0	102	na	7.0	(mq)	4	97%
SONIC										
BACON, LETTUCE, AND TOMATO SANDWICH 'B-L-T'	1 sandwich	327	8.3	26.5	600	na	19.3	na	9	53%
CHEESE SANDWICH, grilled	1 sandwich	288	11.9	25.3	841	na	17.0	na	36	53%
CHEESEBURGER										
bacon	1 serving	548	27.7	23.0	839	na	38.6	na	87	63%
double meat and cheese, w/mayonnaise, 'Super Sonic'	1 serving	730	43.8	23.9	1023	na	51.5	na	144	63%
double meat and cheese, w/mustard, 'Super Sonic'	1 serving	644	43.8	23.9	1128	na	40.7	na	136	57%

Food Name	Serving Size	Calories	Prot. gms	Carbs gms	Sod. mgs	Fiber gms	Fat gms	Sat. Fat gms	Chol. mgs	% Fat Cal.
jalapeño, double meat, and cheese	1 serving	638	43.6	21.6	1358	na	40.6	na	136	57%
mini	1 serving	281	16.5	20.3	644	na	14.4	na	45	46%
#2 cheeseburger	1 serving	70	4.4	0.3	267	na	5.8	na	18	75%
CHICKEN SANDWICH										
	1 serving	319	21.0	41.0	890	na	9.0	na	47	25%
breaded	1 serving	455	22.7	36.4	755	na	24.7	na	42	49%
grilled	1 serving	265	21.0	23.0	716	na	10.0	na	63	34%
grilled, w/o dressing	1 serving	215	21.0	23.3	716	na	4.3	na	63	18%
CHILI PIE	1 serving	327	11.5	20.1	313	na	22.6	na	28	62%
FISH SANDWICH	1 serving	277	17.0	38.0	655	na	7.0	na	6	23%
FRENCH FRIES										
large order	1 serving	315	4.5	49.5	67	na	11.2	na	11	32%
large order, w/cheese	1 serving	420	10.5	50.5	468	na	20.2	na	38	43%
regular order	1 serving	233	3.0	37.0	50	na	8.0	na	8	31%
HAMBURGER										
hickory	1 serving	314	19.9	23.3	459	na	15.7	na	50	45%
mini	1 serving	246	14.4	20.1	510	na	11.5	na	36	42%
HOT DOG										
corn dog	1 serving	280	7.0	30.0	700	na	15.0	na	35	48%
extra long, 'Cheese Coney'	1 serving	635	24.4	45.4	632	na	39.0	na	65	55%
extra long, w/onions, 'Cheese Coney'	1 serving	640	25.0	47.0	632	na	39.2	na	65	55%
#2 hot dog	1 serving	323	19.9	23.3	549	na	15.7	na	50	44%
regular	1 serving	258	8.2	21.3	241	na	15.3	na	23	53%
regular, 'Cheese Coney'	1 serving	358	14.0	23.1	341	na	23.3	na	40	59%
regular, w/onions, 'Cheese Coney'	1 serving	361	14.0	23.7	341	na	23.3	na	40	58%
ONION RINGS										
large order	1 serving	577	7.6	54.1	532	na	37.8	na	na	59%
regular order	1 serving	404	5.3	37.9	372	na	26.5	na	na	59%
POTATO NUGGETS										
Tater Tots	1 serving	150	2.0	19.0	330	na	7.0	na	10	42%
Tater Tots, w/cheese	1 serving	220	6.0	19.3	569	na	13.0	na	28	53%
STEAK SANDWICH, breaded	1 serving	631	18.6	46.4	1047	na	41.6	na	50	59%
SPAGHETTI WAREHOUSE										
MINESTRONE SOUP	1 serving	56	3.0	8.0	155	2.0	1.0	na	3	16%
SPAGHETTI W/MARINARA SAUCE										
dinner portion	1 serving	403	13.0	75.0	303	5.0	5.0	na	0	11%
lunch portion	1 serving	298	10.0	56.0	210	4.0	4.0	na	0	12%
SPAGHETTI W/TOMATO SAUCE										
dinner portion	1 serving	410	13.0	76.0	454	6.0	5.0	na	0	11%
lunch portion	1 serving	301	10.0	56.0	303	4.0	3.0	na	0	9%
STEAK 'N SHAKE										
APPLE DANISH	1 pastry	391	6.0	35.0	352	na	24.0	na	na	55%
BAKED BEANS	1 serving	173	9.0	27.0	656	na	4.0	na	na	21%
BREAKFAST SANDWICH										
egg	1 serving	275	12.0	33.0	490	na	10.0	na	na	33%
ham, w/egg	1 serving	434	36.0	33.0	1850	na	17.0	na	na	35%
BROWNIE	1 brownie	258	3.0	39.0	165	na	12.0	na	na	42%
CHEESE SANDWICH, toasted	1 serving	250	9.0	24.0	606	na	13.0	na	na	47%
CHEESEBURGER										
steakburger	1 serving	353	23.0	33.0	658	na	13.0	na	na	33%
steakburger, super	1 serving	451	35.0	33.0	680	na	18.0	na	na	36%
steakburger, triple	1 serving	626	52.0	34.0	934	na	30.0	na	na	43%

Food Name	Serving Size	Calories	Prot. gms	Carbs gms	Sod. mgs	Fiber gms	Fat gms	Sat. Fat gms	Chol. mgs	% Fat Cal.
CHEESECAKE										
plain	1 serving	368	7.0	61.0	294	na	11.0	na	na	27%
w/strawberries	1 serving	386	7.0	65.0	294	na	11.0	na	na	26%
CHILI										
'Chili Mac' w/4 saltines	1 serving	310	15.0	34.0	1301	na	12.0	na	na	35%
'Chili 3 Ways' w/4 saltines	1 serving	411	19.0	45.0	1734	na	16.0	na	na	35%
w/oyster crackers	1 serving	337	16.0	37.0	1157	na	14.0	na	na	37%
COTTAGE CHEESE	1/2 cup	93	12.0	3.0	198	na	4.0	na	na	39%
DESSERT										
'Coca-Cola Float'	1 serving	514	16.0	76.0	230	na	17.0	na	na	30%
'Lemon Float'	1 serving	555	18.0	82.0	248	na	19.0	na	na	31%
'Lemon Freeze'	1 serving	548	15.0	69.0	213	na	25.0	na	na	41%
'Orange Float'	1 serving	502	16.0	74.0	224	na	17.0	na	na	30%
'Orange Freeze'	1 serving	516	14.0	63.0	198	na	24.0	na	na	42%
'Root Beer Float'	1 serving	529	17.0	78.0	237	na	17.0	na	na	29%
FRENCH FRIES	1 serving	211	3.0	28.0	297	na	10.0	na	na	43%
HAM SANDWICH, baked	1 serving	451	29.0	37.0	1858	na	22.0	na	na	44%
HAMBURGER										
steakburger	1 serving	277	18.0	33.0	425	na	7.0	na	na	23%
steakburger, super	1 serving	375	30.0	33.0	447	na	12.0	na	na	29%
steakburger, triple	1 serving	474	43.0	33.0	468	na	17.0	na	na	32%
HOT CHOCOLATE	1 serving	686	17.0	129.0	669	na	19.0	na	na	25%
ICE CREAM, vanilla	1 serving	213	1.0	23.0	70	na	12.0	na	na	51%
MILKSHAKE										
chocolate	1 serving	608	13.0	57.0	178	na	38.0	na	na	56%
strawberry	1 serving	648	16.0	62.0	191	na	40.0	na	na	56%
vanilla	1 serving	619	13.0	58.0	181	na	38.0	na	na	55%
PIE										
apple	1 serving	407	4.0	61.0	479	na	18.0	na	na	40%
apple 'À la mode'	1 serving	549	4.0	76.0	525	na	25.0	na	na	41%
cherry	1 serving	334	6.0	48.0	268	na	14.0	na	na	38%
cherry 'À la mode'	1 serving	476	6.0	63.0	314	na	22.0	na	na	42%
SALAD										
chef's	1 serving	313	41.0	6.0	1582	na	18.0	na	na	52%
lettuce and tomato, w/1 oz Thousand Island dressing	1 serving	168	1.0	7.0	223	na	15.0	na	na	80%
STEAK ENTRÉE, platter, low-calorie	1 serving	293	37.0	3.0	242	na	14.0	na	na	43%
SUNDAE										
fudge brownie	1 serving	645	7.0	81.0	262	na	35.0	na	na	49%
hot fudge nut	1 serving	530	5.0	51.0	121	na	34.0	na	na	58%
strawberry	1 serving	330	2.0	29.0	81	na	22.0	na	na	60%
SUBWAY										
SALAD										
chef's, small	1 serving	189	19.0	6.0	479	na	10.0	na	na	48%
garden, large	1 serving	46	2.0	10.0	634	na	0.0	na	0	0%
ham, small	1 serving	170	14.0	6.0	479	na	10.0	na	na	53%
roast beef, small	1 serving	185	18.0	6.0	479	na	10.0	na	na	49%
seafood and crab, small	1 serving	198	12.0	13.0	946	na	11.0	na	na	50%
tuna, small	1 serving	212	20.0	8.0	545	na	12.0	na	na	51%
turkey, small	1 serving	167	15.0	4.0	479	na	9.0	na	na	49%
SALAD DRESSING, Italian, lite	4 tbsp	23	1.0	4.0	952	na	<1.0	na	<1	0%
SUBMARINE SANDWICH										
club, Italian, 12-inch	1 sandwich	693	46.0	83.0	2716	na	22.0	na	84	29%
club, Italian, on honey wheat roll, 12-inch	1 sandwich	722	47.0	89.0	2776	na	23.0	na	84	29%

Food Name	Serving Size	Calories	Prot. gms	Carbs gms	Sod. mgs	Fiber gms	Fat gms	Sat. Fat gms	Chol. mgs	% Fat Cal.
ham, 6-inch	1 sandwich	360	20.0	45.0	839	na	11.0	na	na	28%
ham and cheese, Italian, 12-inch	1 sandwich	643	38.0	81.0	1709	na	18.0	na	73	25%
ham and cheese, on honey wheat roll, 12-inch	1 sandwich	673	39.0	86.0	2508	na	22.0	na	73	29%
Italian cold cut combo, 12-inch	1 sandwich	853	46.0	83.0	2218	na	40.0	na	166	42%
Italian cold cut combo, on honey wheat roll, 12-inch	1 sandwich	882	48.0	88.0	2278	na	41.0	na	166	42%
meatball, 6-inch	1 sandwich	429	26.0	45.0	876	na	16.0	na	na	34%
meatball, Italian, 12-inch	1 sandwich	917	42.0	96.0	2022	na	44.0	na	88	43%
meatball, on honey wheat roll, 12-inch	1 sandwich	947	44.0	101.0	2082	na	45.0	na	88	43%
roast beef, 6-inch	1 sandwich	375	24.0	45.0	839	na	11.0	na	na	26%
roast beef, Italian, 12-inch	1 sandwich	689	42.0	84.0	2287	na	23.0	na	75	30%
roast beef, on honey wheat roll, 12-inch	1 sandwich	717	41.0	89.0	2347	na	24.0	na	75	30%
seafood and crab, 6-inch	1 sandwich	388	18.0	52.0	1306	na	12.0	na	na	28%
steak, 6-inch	1 sandwich	423	28.0	46.0	883	na	14.0	na	na	30%
steak and cheese, Italian, 12-inch	1 sandwich	765	43.0	83.0	1556	na	32.0	na	82	38%
steak and cheese, on honey wheat roll, 12-inch	1 sandwich	711	41.0	89.0	1615	na	33.0	na	82	42%
subway club, 6-inch	1 sandwich	379	25.0	45.0	839	na	11.0	na	na	26%
tuna, 6-inch	1 sandwich	402	26.0	45.0	905	na	13.0	na	na	29%
turkey, 6-inch	1 sandwich	357	21.0	46.0	839	na	10.0	na	na	25%
turkey breast, Italian, 12-inch	1 sandwich	645	40.0	83.0	2459	na	19.0	na	67	27%
turkey breast, on honey wheat roll, 12-inch	1 sandwich	674	42.0	88.0	2520	na	20.0	na	67	27%
veggies and cheese, Italian, 12-inch	1 sandwich	535	20.0	81.0	1076	na	17.0	na	19	29%

SWENSEN'S
ICE CREAM

Food Name	Serving Size	Calories	Prot. gms	Carbs gms	Sod. mgs	Fiber gms	Fat gms	Sat. Fat gms	Chol. mgs	% Fat Cal.
'Almond Praline Delight' low-fat	1/2 cup	130	3.0	25.0	85	0	2.0	1.0	5	14%
'Caramel Apple Crisp' low-fat	1/2 cup	130	3.0	26.0	75	0	1.0	0.5	<5	7%
'Caramel Turtle Fudge' light	1 serving	120	3.0	18.0	50	na	4.0	na	10	30%
'Caramel Turtle Fudge' low-fat	1/2 cup	140	3.0	26.0	70	0	2.5	1.0	5	16%
'Chocolate Chocolate Chip Cheesecake' low-fat	1/2 cup	130	3.0	26.0	80	0	2.5	1.0	<5	17%
'Chocolate Fudge Brownie' low-fat	1/2 cup	120	3.0	24.0	70	0	2.5	1.0	<5	19%
'Cookies 'n' Cream' light	1 serving	130	3.0	20.0	60	na	4.0	na	10	28%
'Cookies 'n' Cream' low-fat	1/2 cup	130	3.0	25.0	80	0	2.5	0.5	<5	17%
'Vanilla' light	1 serving	110	3.0	15.0	50	na	4.0	na	10	33%

YOGURT, FROZEN

Food Name	Serving Size	Calories	Prot. gms	Carbs gms	Sod. mgs	Fiber gms	Fat gms	Sat. Fat gms	Chol. mgs	% Fat Cal.
'Black Forest Cake'	1 serving	95	3.0	21.0	130	na	1.0	na	5	9%
'Black Forest Cake' low-fat	1/2 cup	110	4.0	22.0	55	1.0	1.5	1.0	0	12%
'Blueberry 'n' Cream' gourmet, sugar-free	1 serving	110	3.0	17.0	90	na	4.0	na	10	33%
'Butter Pecan' low-fat	1/2 cup	120	4.0	20.0	55	0	3.0	0.5	<5	23%
'Cherry' nonfat	1/2 cup	90	3.0	20.0	45	0	0.0	0.0	0	0%
'Chocolate Raspberry Truffle' gourmet, sugar-free	1 serving	130	3.0	18.0	80	na	5.0	na	8	35%
'Coconut Pineapple'	1 serving	120	4.0	26.0	65	na	1.0	na	5	8%
'Hazelnut Amaretto' low-fat	1/2 cup	120	4.0	20.0	50	0	3.0	0.0	0	23%
'Mocha Chip' low-fat	1/2 cup	110	4.0	22.0	50	0	1.5	1.0	0	12%
'Strawberry Banana 'n' Cream' nonfat	1/2 cup	90	3.0	20.0	45	0	0.0	0.0	0	0%
'Triple Chocolate' low-fat	1/2 cup	120	4.0	24.0	50	1.0	1.5	1.0	0	11%
'Triple Chocolate' nonfat	1 serving	100	4.0	21.0	65	na	0.0	0.0	0	0%
'Vanilla' nonfat	1/2 cup	90	3.0	20.0	60	0	0.0	0.0	0	0%
'Vanilla Swiss Almond' gourmet, sugar-free	1 serving	140	4.0	15.0	100	na	7.0	na	10	45%

SWISS CHALET
CAKE

Food Name	Serving Size	Calories	Prot. gms	Carbs gms	Sod. mgs	Fiber gms	Fat gms	Sat. Fat gms	Chol. mgs	% Fat Cal.
Black Forest	1 piece	278	3.0	36.0	na	na	14.0	na	na	45%
fudge nut	1 piece	346	4.0	48.0	na	na	16.0	na	na	42%
CHICKEN	1/2 chicken	634	72.0	1.0	na	na	38.0	na	na	54%

Food Name	Serving Size	Calories	Prot. gms	Carbs gms	Sod. mgs	Fiber gms	Fat gms	Sat. Fat gms	Chol. mgs	% Fat Cal.
CHICKEN SALAD	1 serving	500	42.0	23.0	na	na	42.0	na	na	76%
CHICKEN SANDWICH										
cold	1 sandwich	360	33.0	42.0	na	na	5.0	na	na	13%
hot	1 sandwich	310	30.0	30.0	na	na	6.0	na	na	17%
CHICKEN SOUP, 'Chalet'	1 serving	97	9.0	11.0	na	na	2.0	na	na	19%
COLESLAW, 'Chalet'	1 serving	56	2.0	10.0	na	na	1.0	na	na	16%
FRENCH FRIES	1 serving	478	10.0	57.0	na	na	24.0	na	na	45%
GRAVY, sandwich	1 serving	35	1.0	5.0	na	na	1.0	na	na	26%
ICE CREAM, vanilla	1 serving	195	3.0	16.0	na	na	14.0	na	na	65%
PASTRY, chocolate éclair	1 serving	205	2.0	27.0	na	na	10.0	na	na	44%
PIE										
apple	1 serving	394	3.0	45.0	na	na	23.0	na	na	53%
coconut	1 serving	292	2.0	40.0	na	na	14.0	na	na	43%
POTATO, BAKED	1 serving	227	8.0	52.0	na	na	tr	na	na	0%
ROLL	1 roll	116	3.0	24.0	na	na	1.0	na	na	8%
TACO BELL										
BURRITO										
bean	7.3 oz	447	15.0	63.0	1148	(mq)	14.0	4.0	9	28%
beef	7.3 oz	493	25.0	48.0	1311	(mq)	21.0	8.0	57	38%
beef, double, 'Supreme'	1 serving	451	23.0	40.0	928	na	22.0	10.0	59	44%
beef, 'MexiMelt'	3.7 oz	266	13.0	19.0	689	(mq)	15.0	8.0	38	51%
'Cheesarito'	1 serving	312	12.0	37.0	451	na	13.0	7.0	29	38%
chicken	6 oz	334	17.0	38.0	880	(mq)	12.0	4.0	52	32%
chicken, 'MexiMelt'	3.8 oz	257	14.0	19.0	779	(mq)	15.0	7.0	48	53%
combination	7 oz	407	18.0	46.0	1136	(mq)	16.0	5.0	33	35%
'Supreme'	9 oz	503	20.0	55.0	1181	(mq)	22.0	8.0	33	39%
CHEESE SAUCE, nacho	2 oz	103	4.0	5.0	393	0	8.0	3.0	9	70%
FAJITA, chicken	1 serving	226	14.0	20.0	619	na	10.0	4.0	44	40%
FAJITA TACO										
steak	1 serving	235	15.0	20.0	507	na	11.0	5.0	14	42%
steak, w/guacamole	1 serving	269	15.0	23.0	620	na	13.0	5.0	14	43%
steak, w/sour cream	1 serving	281	15.0	21.0	507	na	15.0	7.0	14	48%
GREEN SAUCE	1 oz	4	0.0	1.0	136	na	0.0	0.0	0	0%
GUACAMOLE	.75 oz	34	1.0	3.0	113	(mq)	2.0	0.0	0	53%
NACHOS										
'Nachos Bellgrande'	10.1 oz	649	22.0	61.0	997	(mq)	35.0	12.0	36	49%
'Nachos Supreme'	5.1 oz	367	12.0	41.0	471	(mq)	27.0	5.0	18	66%
regular	3.7 oz	346	7.0	37.0	399	(mq)	18.0	6.0	9	47%
PASTRY, 'Cinnamon Twists'	1.2 oz	171	2.0	24.0	234	(mq)	8.0	3.0	0	42%
PEPPER, JALAPEÑO	3.5 oz	20	1.0	4.0	1370	(mq)	0.0	0.0	0	0%
PINTO BEANS, w/cheese and red sauce	4.5 oz	190	9.0	19.0	642	(mq)	9.0	4.0	16	43%
PIZZA, Mexican	7.9 oz	575	21.0	40.0	1031	(mq)	37.0	11.0	52	58%
RED SAUCE	1 oz	10	0.0	2.0	261	na	0.0	0.0	0	0%
RELISH, 'Pico de Gallo'	.7 oz	6	0.0	1.0	66	na	0.0	0.0	0	0%
SALAD										
seafood, w/ranch dressing	1 serving	884	25.0	49.0	1489	na	66.0	34.0	117	67%
seafood, w/o dressing	1 serving	648	24.0	47.0	917	na	42.0	30.0	82	58%
seafood, w/o dressing, w/o shell	1 serving	217	18.0	12.0	693	na	11.0	6.0	81	46%
taco, 21 oz	1 serving	905	34.0	55.0	910	(mq)	61.0	19.0	80	61%
taco, w/ranch dressing	1 serving	1167	37.0	61.0	1959	na	87.0	45.0	121	67%
taco, w/o beans	1 serving	822	31.0	47.0	1368	na	57.0	38.0	81	62%
taco, w/o salsa	1 serving	931	35.0	60.0	1387	na	62.0	40.0	85	60%
taco, w/o shell, 18.3 oz	1 serving	484	28.0	22.0	680	(mq)	31.0	14.0	80	58%

Food Name	Serving Size	Calories	Prot. gms	Carbs gms	Sod. mgs	Fiber gms	Fat gms	Sat. Fat gms	Chol. mgs	% Fat Cal.
SALAD DRESSING, ranch	2.6 oz	236	2.0	1.0	571	(mq)	25.0	5.0	35	95%
SALSA	.34 oz	18	1.0	4.0	376	na	0.0	0.0	0	0%
SOUR CREAM	.75 oz	46	1.0	1.0	0	0	4.0	2.0	31	78%
TACO										
'Bellgrande'	5.7 oz	335	18.0	18.0	472	(mq)	23.0	11.0	56	62%
chicken	3 oz	171	12.0	11.0	337	(mq)	9.0	3.0	52	47%
chicken, soft	3.8 oz	213	14.0	19.0	615	(mq)	10.0	4.0	52	42%
platter, light	1 serving	1062	38.0	97.0	2068	na	58.0	34.0	82	49%
regular	2.75 oz	183	10.0	11.0	276	(mq)	11.0	5.0	32	54%
regular, soft	3.25 oz	225	12.0	18.0	554	(mq)	12.0	5.0	32	48%
steak, soft	3.5 oz	218	14.0	18.0	456	(mq)	11.0	5.0	30	45%
'Supreme'	3.25 oz	230	11.0	12.0	276	(mq)	15.0	8.0	32	59%
'Supreme,' soft	4.4 oz	272	13.0	19.0	554	(mq)	16.0	8.0	32	53%
TACO SAUCE										
hot	1 pkt	3	0.0	0.0	82	na	0.0	0.0	0	0%
regular	1 pkt	2	0.0	0.0	126	na	0.0	0.0	0	0%
TOSTADA										
beef	1 serving	322	15.0	22.0	764	na	20.0	10.0	40	56%
chicken, w/red sauce	5.8 oz	264	12.0	20.0	454	(mq)	15.0	7.0	37	51%
w/red sauce	5.5 oz	243	9.0	27.0	596	(mq)	11.0	4.0	16	41%
TACO JOHN'S										
BURRITO										
bean	5 oz	249	10.0	36.0	636	(mq)	6.0	(mq)	na	22%
beef	5 oz	355	16.0	25.0	666	(mq)	18.0	(mq)	na	46%
chicken, super, w/o sour cream or cheese	1 serving	366	30.0	40.0	844	na	14.0	na	na	34%
chicken, w/o sour cream or cheese	1 serving	227	27.0	19.0	639	na	10.0	na	na	40%
combo	5 oz	302	11.0	00.0	651	(mq)	12.0	(mq)	na	36%
super	8.3 oz	434	17.0	66.0	1022	(mq)	11.0	(mq)	na	23%
super, w/o sour cream or cheese	1 serving	389	18.0	51.0	856	na	16.0	na	na	37%
w/green chili	12.3 oz	405	18.0	38.0	995	(mq)	24.0	(mq)	na	53%
w/green chili, w/o sour cream or cheese	1 serving	367	20.0	40.0	998	na	18.0	na	na	44%
w/Texas chili	12.3 oz	518	23.0	48.0	746	(mq)	24.0	(mq)	na	42%
CHICKEN SANDWICH, fillet, 'Sierra'	8.5 oz	500	31.0	46.0	1493	23.0	21.0	na	41	38%
CHILI, Texas	9.5 oz	430	23.0	35.0	1580	(mq)	22.0	(mq)	(mq)	46%
CHIMICHANGA, 'Chimi'	12 oz	487	16.0	54.0	1226	(mq)	19.0	(mq)	(mq)	35%
DANISH, 'Apple Grande'	3 oz	257	5.0	44.0	231	(mq)	8.0	(mq)	na	28%
ENCHILADA	7 oz	379	19.0	33.0	431	(mq)	18.0	(mq)	(mq)	43%
NACHOS										
regular	4 oz	407	11.0	42.0	307	(mq)	19.0	(mq)	(mq)	42%
super	11.25 oz	657	23.0	57.0	857	(mq)	34.0	(mq)	(mq)	47%
PASTRY, 'Churro'	1.2 oz	122	1.7	12.0	153	na	7.0	(mq)	na	52%
POTATO, BAKED, 'Potato Ole' large	6 oz	414	6.0	96.0	1595	(mq)	6.0	(mq)	na	13%
REFRIED BEANS	9.5 oz	331	19.0	79.0	1195	(mq)	6.0	(mq)	na	16%
RICE, Mexican	1 serving	340	7.0	59.0	1280	na	8.0	na	na	21%
SALAD										
chicken taco, super, w/o dressing or sour cream	1 serving	377	26.0	56.0	882	na	15.0	na	na	36%
taco, super, 12.3 oz	1 serving	450	16.0	48.0	880	(mq)	18.0	(mq)	na	36%
taco, super, w/o shell, dressing, or sour cream	1 serving	428	21.0	59.0	900	na	20.0	na	na	42%
taco, w/o shell, dressing, sour cream, or cheese	1 serving	228	13.0	30.0	440	na	13.0	na	na	51%
TACO										
chicken, soft shell	1 serving	180	18.0	20.0	490	na	8.0	na	na	40%
regular	4.3 oz	228	11.0	15.0	347	(mq)	13.0	(mq)	(mq)	51%
soft shell	5 oz	276	13.0	23.0	505	(mq)	13.0	(mq)	(mq)	42%

Food Name	Serving Size	Calories	Prot. gms	Carbs gms	Sod. mgs	Fiber gms	Fat gms	Sat. Fat gms	Chol. mgs	% Fat Cal.
'Taco Bravo' super	8 oz	485	18.0	51.0	1006	(mq)	20.0	(mq)	(mq)	37%
'Taco Bravo' w/o sour cream	1 serving	319	16.0	42.0	658	na	14.0	na	na	39%
taco burger	6 oz	332	14.0	31.0	660	(mq)	14.0	(mq)	(mq)	38%
TOSTADA	4.3 oz	228	11.0	15.0	347	(mq)	13.0	(mq)	na	51%

TACO TIME

BURRITO

Food Name	Serving Size	Calories	Prot. gms	Carbs gms	Sod. mgs	Fiber gms	Fat gms	Sat. Fat gms	Chol. mgs	% Fat Cal.
bean, soft	1 serving	547	22.0	68.0	1027	na	21.0	na	20	35%
bean, soft, w/o cheese	1 serving	462	17.0	65.0	895	na	14.0	na	0	27%
'Casita' w/o sour cream or cheese	1 serving	427	23.0	46.0	1243	na	17.0	na	25	36%
combo, soft	1 serving	550	30.0	55.0	1227	na	24.0	na	48	39%
combo, soft, w/o cheese	1 serving	462	17.0	65.0	1095	na	14.0	na	0	27%
meat, soft, w/o cheese	1 serving	467	32.0	40.0	1295	na	19.0	na	53	37%
veggie	1 serving	535	21.0	71.0	890	na	20.0	na	20	34%
veggie, w/o sour cream	1 serving	502	21.0	71.0	883	na	17.0	na	14	30%
veggie, w/o sour cream or cheese	1 serving	477	18.0	69.0	798	na	13.0	na	0	25%
CHEESEBURGER, taco, w/o dressing or cheese	1 serving	397	20.0	49.0	1071	na	13.0	na	17	29%
REFRIED BEANS, 'Refritos' w/o cheese	1 serving	293	11.0	38.0	834	na	11.0	na	0	34%
RICE, brown, Mexican	1 serving	160	2.0	28.0	540	na	2.0	na	0	11%

SALAD

Food Name	Serving Size	Calories	Prot. gms	Carbs gms	Sod. mgs	Fiber gms	Fat gms	Sat. Fat gms	Chol. mgs	% Fat Cal.
chicken taco, w/o dressing	1 serving	436	31.0	35.0	521	na	19.0	na	70	39%
chicken taco, w/o dressing or cheese	1 serving	381	29.0	33.0	436	na	15.0	na	56	35%
side order, w/o dressing or cheese	1 serving	302	12.0	36.0	715	na	13.0	na	0	39%
taco, w/o dressing	1 serving	347	23.0	22.0	720	na	16.0	na	35	41%
veggie, w/o dressing or cheese	1 serving	302	12.0	36.0	715	na	13.0	na	0	39%

SAUCE

Food Name	Serving Size	Calories	Prot. gms	Carbs gms	Sod. mgs	Fiber gms	Fat gms	Sat. Fat gms	Chol. mgs	% Fat Cal.
casa	1 oz	40	0.0	10.0	180	na	0.0	0.0	0	0%
enchilada	1 oz	14	0.0	3.0	115	na	0.0	0.0	0	0%
hot	1 oz	10	0.0	2.0	120	na	0.0	0.0	0	0%
ranchero	2 oz	18	1.0	3.0	115	na	1.0	na	0	50%

TACO

Food Name	Serving Size	Calories	Prot. gms	Carbs gms	Sod. mgs	Fiber gms	Fat gms	Sat. Fat gms	Chol. mgs	% Fat Cal.
chicken, soft	1 serving	390	31.0	34.0	322	na	12.0	na	70	28%
chicken, soft, w/o cheese	1 serving	335	29.0	32.0	237	na	8.0	na	56	21%
flour, soft, w/o cheese	1 serving	331	19.0	34.0	599	na	12.0	na	26	33%
TOSTADA, meat, 'Delight' w/o sour cream or cheese	1 serving	410	22.0	42.0	916	na	17.0	na	25	37%

TCBY

YOGURT, FROZEN, all flavors

Fat-free

Food Name	Serving Size	Calories	Prot. gms	Carbs gms	Sod. mgs	Fiber gms	Fat gms	Sat. Fat gms	Chol. mgs	% Fat Cal.
giant	31.6 oz	869	32.0	182.0	356	na	0.0	0.0	0	0%
super	15.2 oz	418	15.0	87.0	171	na	0.0	0.0	0	0%
large	10.5 oz	289	10.0	60.0	118	na	0.0	0.0	0	0%
regular	8.2 oz	226	8.0	47.0	92	na	0.0	0.0	0	0%
small	5.9 oz	162	6.0	34.0	66	na	0.0	0.0	0	0%
kiddie	3.2 oz	88	3.0	18.0	36	na	0.0	0.0	0	0%

Fat-free, sugar-free

Food Name	Serving Size	Calories	Prot. gms	Carbs gms	Sod. mgs	Fiber gms	Fat gms	Sat. Fat gms	Chol. mgs	% Fat Cal.
giant	31.6 oz	632	32.0	142.0	316	na	0.0	0.0	0	0%
super	15.2 oz	304	15.0	68.0	152	na	0.0	0.0	0	0%
large	10.5 oz	210	10.0	47.0	105	na	0.0	0.0	0	0%
regular	8.2 oz	164	8.0	37.0	82	na	0.0	0.0	0	0%
small	5.9 oz	118	6.0	27.0	59	na	0.0	0.0	0	0%
kiddie	3.2 oz	64	3.0	14.0	32	na	0.0	0.0	0	0%

Regular, 96% fat-free

Food Name	Serving Size	Calories	Prot. gms	Carbs gms	Sod. mgs	Fiber gms	Fat gms	Sat. Fat gms	Chol. mgs	% Fat Cal.
giant	31.6 oz	1027	32.0	182.0	474	na	24.0	16.0	79	21%

Food Name	Serving Size	Calories	Prot. gms	Carbs gms	Sod. mgs	Fiber gms	Fat gms	Sat. Fat gms	Chol. mgs	% Fat Cal.
super	15.2 oz	494	15.0	87.0	228	na	11.0	8.0	38	20%
large	10.5 oz	342	10.0	60.0	156	na	8.0	5.0	26	21%
regular	8.2 oz	267	8.0	47.0	126	na	6.0	4.0	20	20%
small	5.9 oz	192	6.0	34.0	90	na	4.0	3.0	15	19%
kiddie	3.2 oz	104	3.0	18.0	48	na	2.0	2.0	8	17%
WENDY'S										
ALFALFA SPROUTS	1 oz	8	1.0	tr	na	na	tr	na	0	0%
ALFREDO SAUCE	2 oz	35	1.0	5.0	300	na	1.0	0.8	tr	26%
APPLE TOPPING	1 serving	130	tr	32.0	120	na	tr	na	0	0%
BACON BITS, imitation	1/8 oz	10	1.0	tr	100	na	tr	na	tr	0%
BARBECUE SAUCE	1 oz	50	<1.0	11.0	100	na	<1.0	tr	0	0%
BISCUIT, buttermilk	1 serving	320	5.0	37.0	860	na	17.0	na	tr	48%
BLUEBERRIES	1 tbsp	6	1.0	1.0	na	na	tr	na	0	0%
BLUEBERRY TOPPING	1 serving	60	tr	15.0	65	na	tr	na	0	0%
BREADSTICKS										
	1 stick	130	4.0	24.0	250	na	3.0	na	5	21%
salad bar item	2 sticks	35	1.0	6.0	60	na	1.0	na	0	26%
BREAKFAST										
bacon	1 strip	30	2.0	tr	125	na	2.0	na	5	60%
breakfast sandwich	1 serving	370	17.0	33.0	770	na	19.0	na	200	46%
breakfast sandwich, w/bacon	1 serving	430	21.0	33.0	1020	na	23.0	na	na	48%
breakfast sandwich, w/sausage	1 serving	570	25.0	33.0	1175	na	37.0	na	na	58%
eggs, scrambled	2 eggs	190	14.0	7.0	160	na	12.0	na	450	57%
French toast	2 slices	400	11.0	45.0	850	na	19.0	na	115	43%
omelet, ham and cheese	1 serving	290	18.0	7.0	570	na	21.0	na	355	65%
omelet, ham, cheese, and mushroom	1 serving	290	18.0	7.0	570	na	21.0	na	355	65%
omelet, ham, cheese, onion, and green pepper	1 serving	280	10.0	7.0	405	na	19.0	na	525	61%
omelet, mushroom, green pepper, and onion	1 serving	210	14.0	7.0	200	na	15.0	na	460	64%
potatoes	1 serving	360	4.0	37.0	745	na	22.0	na	20	55%
sausage patty	1 patty	200	8.0	tr	405	na	18.0	na	45	81%
BROCCOLI, raw	1/2 cup	12	2.0	2.0	5	na	tr	na	0	0%
BUN										
Kaiser	1 bun	180	7.0	32.0	390	na	2.0	na	5	10%
multigrain	1 bun	140	5.0	25.0	215	na	3.0	na	tr	19%
white	1 bun	140	4.0	26.0	255	na	2.0	na	tr	13%
CABBAGE, red, raw	1/4 cup	4	2.0	tr	5	na	tr	na	0	0%
CANTALOUPE	2 pieces	18	tr	4.0	5	na	tr	na	0	0%
CARROTS, raw	1/4 cup	12	0.0	2.0	10	na	0.0	0.0	0	0%
CATSUP	1 tsp	6	tr	1.0	50	na	tr	na	0	0%
CAULIFLOWER, raw	1/2 cup	12	1.0	2.0	10	na	tr	na	0	0%
CELERY, raw	1 tbsp	0	1.0	tr	5	na	tr	na	0	0%
CHEESE										
American, salad bar item	1 oz	90	6.0	tr	365	na	7.0	na	5	70%
American, sandwich topping	1 slice	60	4.0	tr	295	na	6.0	na	15	90%
cheddar, shredded	1 oz	110	7.0	1.0	175	0	10.0	6.0	30	82%
imitation, shredded	1 oz	90	6.0	1.0	125	na	6.0	4.0	0	60%
mozzarella	1 oz	90	6.0	tr	335	na	7.0	na	tr	70%
Parmesan, grated	1 oz	130	12.0	1.0	510	na	9.0	na	20	62%
Parmesan, imitation	1 oz	80	9.0	4.0	410	na	3.0	3.0	0	34%
provolone	1 oz	90	6.0	tr	335	na	7.0	na	tr	70%
Swiss	1 oz	90	6.0	tr	365	na	7.0	na	5	70%
CHEESE SAUCE	2 oz	39	1.0	5.0	305	0	2.0	1.0	tr	46%

Food Name	Serving Size	Calories	Prot. gms	Carbs gms	Sod. mgs	Fiber gms	Fat gms	Sat. Fat gms	Chol. mgs	% Fat Cal.
CHEESEBURGER										
bacon, 'Jr.' 5.5 oz	1 serving	430	22.0	33.0	840	(mq)	25.0	5.2	50	52%
double	1 serving	620	48.0	26.0	760	na	36.0	na	165	52%
'Jr.' 4.4 oz	1 serving	310	18.0	34.0	770	(mq)	13.0	3.0	35	38%
'Jr. Swiss Deluxe' 5.8 oz	1 serving	360	18.0	35.0	765	(mq)	18.0	3.0	40	45%
'Kids Meal' 4.1 oz	1 serving	300	18.0	33.0	770	(mq)	13.0	3.0	35	39%
CHICKEN NUGGET										
crispy, 6 pieces	1 serving	310	15.0	14.0	660	na	21.0	na	50	61%
crispy, 9 pieces	1 serving	465	23.0	21.0	990	na	32.0	na	75	62%
crispy, 20 pieces	1 serving	1023	50.0	46.0	2178	na	69.0	na	160	61%
CHICKEN SANDWICH										
breast, on white bun	1 serving	340	26.0	30.0	565		12.0	na	60	32%
club, 7.2 oz	1 serving	506	30.0	43.0	930	(mq)	25.0	4.8	70	44%
fried, 6.9 oz	1 serving	440	26.0	43.0	725	(mq)	19.0	2.6	60	39%
grilled, 6.2 oz	1 serving	340	24.0	37.0	815	(mq)	13.0	2.2	60	34%
CHILI										
8-oz size	1 serving	190	19.0	21.0	670	na	6.0	na	40	28%
regular, 9 oz	1 serving	220	21.0	23.0	750	(mq)	7.0	2.6	45	29%
12-oz size	1 serving	290	28.0	31.0	1000	na	9.0	na	60	28%
CHIPS										
cheddar	1 oz	160	3.0	12.0	445	na	11.0	na	na	62%
taco	1.4 oz	260	4.0	40.0	20	(mq)	10.0	0.7	0	35%
CHIVES	1/2 tsp	8	tr	1.0	na	na	tr	na	0	0%
CHOW MEIN NOODLES	.5 oz	70	1.0	8.0	105	na	4.0	na	na	51%
COLESLAW										
'California'	2 tbsp	45	<1.0	5.0	60	na	3.0	<1.0	5	60%
salad bar item	1/4 cup	80	tr	9.0	165	na	5.0	na	40	56%
COOKIE, chocolate chip	2.25 oz	275	3.0	40.0	256	(mq)	13.0	4.2	15	43%
CORN RELISH, 'Old Fashioned'	1/4 cup	35	tr	9.0	215	na	tr	na	na	0%
COTTAGE CHEESE	1/2 cup	110	13.0	3.0	425	na	4.0	na	20	33%
CRACKER, saltines, 2 pieces	1 pkt	25	4.0	1.0	80	na	1.0	na	0	36%
CROUTONS	.5 oz	70	1.0	8.0	105	na	4.0	na	na	51%
CUCUMBER	3 slices	2	1.0	tr	na	na	tr	na	0	0%
DANISH										
apple	1 serving	360	6.0	53.0	380	na	14.0	na	na	35%
cheese	1 serving	430	8.0	52.0	550	na	21.0	na	na	44%
cinnamon raisin	1 serving	430	8.0	52.0	550	na	21.0	na	na	44%
EGG, hard-cooked, salad topping	1 tbsp	30	3.0	tr	25	na	2.0	na	90	60%
FETTUCCINE	2 oz	190	4.0	27.0	3	(mq)	3.0	0.6	10	14%
FISH SANDWICH, fillet, 6 oz	1 serving	460	18.0	42.0	780	(mq)	25.0	4.7	50	49%
FRENCH FRIES										
large order	1 serving	390	6.0	46.0	176	na	20.0	na	7	46%
regular order	1 serving	300	5.0	35.0	135	na	15.0	na	5	45%
small order, 3.2 oz	1 serving	240	3.0	33.0	145	(mq)	12.0	2.5	0	45%
FROZEN DESSERT										
'Frosty Dairy' large	1 serving	680	14.0	100.0	374	na	24.0	na	na	32%
'Frosty Dairy' small	1 serving	400	8.0	59.0	220	na	14.0	na	50	32%
GARLIC TOAST	.6-oz piece	70	2.0	9.0	65	(mq)	3.0	0.6	tr	39%
GRAPEFRUIT	2 oz	10	0.0	2.0	0	na	tr	na	0	0%
GRAPES	1/4 cup	30	tr	7.0	na	na	tr	na	0	0%
HAMBURGER										
'Big Classic' on Kaiser bun	1 serving	470	26.0	36.0	900	na	25.0	na	80	48%
double, 'Big Classic' on Kaiser bun	1 serving	680	46.0	36.0	1005	na	39.0	na	155	52%
double, on white bun	1 serving	560	44.0	26.0	465	na	30.0	na	150	48%

Food Name	Serving Size	Calories	Prot. gms	Carbs gms	Sod. mgs	Fiber gms	Fat gms	Sat. Fat gms	Chol. mgs	% Fat Cal.
'Kid's Meal' 3.7 oz	1 serving	260	15.0	33.0	570	(mq)	9.0	3.0	35	31%
single, 1/4 lb, on white bun	1 serving	350	24.0	26.0	360	na	16.0	na	75	41%
single, plain, 4.4 oz	1 serving	340	24.0	30.0	500	(mq)	15.0	5.5	65	40%
single, w/everything	1 serving	420	25.0	35.0	890	(mq)	21.0	5.5	70	45%
HONEY SAUCE	.5 oz	45	0.0	12.0	tr	0	0.0	0.0	0	0%
HONEYDEW MELON	2 pieces	20	tr	5.0	5	na	tr	na	0	0%
LETTUCE										
iceberg	1 cup	9	tr	1.0	5	na	tr	na	0	0%
romaine	1 cup	9	tr	1.0	5	na	tr	na	0	0%
sandwich topping	1 leaf	2	0.0	0.0	tr	na	0.0	na	0	0%
MARGARINE										
liquid	.5 oz	100	tr	tr	100	na	11.0	na	0	99%
whipped	1 tbsp	70	tr	tr	60	na	8.0	na	0	100%
MAYONNAISE	1 tbsp	90	tr	tr	60	na	10.0	na	10	100%
MILK, 2%	8 oz	110	8.0	11.0	115	na	4.0	na	20	33%
MUSHROOMS, raw	1/4 cup	4	1.0	tr	tr	na	tr	na	0	0%
MUSTARD	1 tsp	4	tr	tr	45	na	tr	na	0	0%
MUSTARD SAUCE, sweet	1 oz	50	<1.0	9.0	140	(mq)	1.0	<1.0	0	18%
ONION										
red, raw	3 rings	2	1.0	tr	tr	na	tr	na	0	0%
sandwich topping	3 rings	2	tr	tr	tr	na	tr	na	0	0%
ORANGE	2 oz	25	tr	7.0	0	na	tr	na	0	0%
ORANGE JUICE	6 oz	80	1.0	19.0	na	na	na	na	0	0%
PASTA AND NOODLES. See also individual listings.										
medley	2 oz	60	2.0	9.0	5	(mq)	2.0	0.3	tr	30%
PEACH	2 pieces	17	tr	4.0	0	na	tr	na	0	0%
PEAS, green	1 oz	25	1.0	4.0	35	na	tr	na	0	0%
PEPPER, rings	1 tbsp	2	tr	tr	200	na	tr	na	0	0%
PEPPER, CHERRY, mild	1 tbsp	6	1.0	tr	180	na	tr	na	0	0%
PEPPER, GREEN	1/4 cup	3	1.0	1.0	5	na	tr	na	0	0%
PEPPER, JALAPEÑO	1 slice	9	tr	2.0	4	na	tr	na	0	0%
PICANTE SAUCE	2 oz	18	<1.0	4.0	5	na	<1.0	<1.0	na	0%
PICKLE, dill	4 slices	2	tr	tr	tr	na	tr	na	0	0%
PINEAPPLE, chunks	1/2 cup	70	tr	18.0	0	na	tr	na	0	0%
POTATO, BAKED										
hot stuffed, w/bacon and cheese	12.8 oz	520	20.0	70.0	1460	(mq)	18.0	5.1	20	31%
hot stuffed, w/broccoli and cheese	12.3 oz	400	8.0	58.0	455	(mq)	16.0	2.9	tr	36%
hot stuffed, w/cheese	11.2 oz	420	8.0	66.0	310	(mq)	15.0	4.0	10	32%
hot stuffed, w/chili and cheese	14.2 oz	500	15.0	71.0	630	(mq)	18.0	4.0	25	32%
hot stuffed, w/sour cream and chives	11.4 oz	500	8.0	67.0	135	(mq)	23.0	9.3	25	41%
plain	8.8 oz	270	6.0	63.0	20	(mq)	<1.0	tr	0	0%
PUDDING										
butterscotch	1/4 cup	90	1.0	11.0	85	na	4.0	na	tr	40%
chocolate	1/4 cup	90	tr	12.0	70	na	4.0	na	tr	40%
RADISH, raw	.5 oz	2	1.0	tr	tr	na	tr	na	0	0%
RAVIOLI, cheese, in sauce	2 oz	45	1.0	8.0	290	(mq)	1.0	0.3	5	20%
REFRIED BEANS	2 oz	70	4.0	10.0	215	(mq)	3.0	0.9	tr	39%
RICE, Spanish	2 oz	70	2.0	13.0	440	(mq)	1.0	0.2	tr	13%
ROTINI	2 oz	90	3.0	15.0	tr	(mq)	2.0	0.3	tr	20%
SALAD										
Caesar, side order	1 serving	160	10.0	18.0	700	na	6.0	na	10	34%
chef's	9.1 oz	130	14.0	8.0	460	(mq)	5.0	1.2	40	35%
chef's, 'Take Out' approx 11.7 oz	1 serving	100	15.0	10.0	140	na	9.0	na	120	45%
chicken, grilled	1 serving	200	25.0	9.0	690	na	8.0	na	55	36%

Food Name	Serving Size	Calories	Prot. gms	Carbs gms	Sod. mgs	Fiber gms	Fat gms	Sat. Fat gms	Chol. mgs	% Fat Cal.
garden	8.1 oz	70	4.0	9.0	60	(mq)	2.0	0.0	0	26%
garden, deluxe	1 serving	110	7.0	9.0	380	na	5.0	na	0	41%
garden, 'Take Out' approx 9.8 oz	1 serving	102	7.0	9.0	110	na	5.0	na	0	44%
pasta	1/4 cup	130	3.0	18.0	190	na	6.0	na	5	42%
pasta, deli	1/4 cup	35	2.0	6.0	120	na	tr	na	na	0%
'Pick-Up-Window'	1 serving	110	8.0	5.0	540	na	6.0	na	0	49%
potato, red bliss	1/4 cup	110	tr	6.0	265	na	9.0	na	na	74%
side order	1 serving	60	4.0	6.0	200	na	3.0	0.0	na	45%
taco	17.3 oz	530	27.0	55.0	825	(mq)	23.0	(mq)	35	39%
three bean, deluxe	1/4 cup	60	1.0	13.0	15	na	tr	na	na	0%
SALAD DRESSING										
bacon and tomato, reduced calorie	1 tbsp	45	<1.0	3.0	190	na	4.0	0.6	<1	80%
blue cheese, 1 ladle = 2 tbsp	1 tbsp	60	tr	1.0	85	na	6.0	na	10	90%
celery seed, 1 ladle = 2 tbsp	1 tbsp	70	tr	3.0	65	na	6.0	na	10	77%
creamy cucumber, reduced calorie, 1 ladle = 2 tbsp	1 tbsp	50	tr	2.0	140	na	5.0	na	5	90%
French, fat-free, 1/2 pkt = 2 tbsp	2 tbsp	35	0.0	8.0	180	na	0.0	na	0	0%
French, sweet red	1 tbsp	70	<1.0	5.0	125	na	6.0	0.8	0	77%
French style, 1 ladle = 2 tbsp	1 tbsp	70	tr	5.0	130	na	5.0	na	0	64%
Italian, golden, 1 ladle = 2 tbsp	1 tbsp	50	tr	3.0	260	na	4.0	na	0	72%
Italian, reduced calorie	1 tbsp	25	<1.0	2.0	185	na	2.0	0.3	0	72%
Italian caesar	1 tbsp	80	<1.0	<1.0	140	na	8.0	1.4	5	90%
oil, 1 ladle = 2 tbsp	1 tbsp	120	tr	tr	0	na	14.0	na	0	100%
ranch, Hidden Valley	1 tbsp	50	<1.0	<1.0	95	na	5.0	1.0	5	90%
Thousand Island, 1 ladle = 2 tbsp	1 tbsp	70	tr	tr	115	na	7.0	na	10	90%
Thousand Island, reduced calorie, 1 ladle = 2 tbsp	1 tbsp	45	tr	2.0	125	na	4.0	na	5	80%
wine vinegar, 1 ladle = 2 tbsp	1 tbsp	2	tr	tr	5	na	tr	na	0	0%
SOUR CREAM										
	1 oz	60	1.0	1.0	15	0	6.0	3.6	10	90%
	2 tsp	20	tr	tr	5	na	2.0	na	5	90%
SOUR CREAM, imitation	1 oz	58	<1.0	2.0	30	0	5.0	5.0	0	78%
SPAGHETTI SAUCE										
regular	1/4 cup	30	1.0	6.0	340	na	<1.0	<1.0	0	0%
w/meat	2 oz	60	4.0	8.0	315	(mq)	2.0	0.7	10	30%
STEAK SANDWICH, country-fried, 5.1 oz	1 serving	440	14.0	45.0	870	(mq)	25.0	5.7	35	51%
STRAWBERRIES	2 oz	18	tr	4.0	tr	na	tr	na	0	0%
SUNFLOWER SEEDS, w/raisins	1 oz	140	5.0	6.0	5	na	10.0	na	0	64%
SWEET AND SOUR SAUCE	1 oz	45	<1.0	11.0	55	na	<1.0	tr	0	0%
SYRUP	1 pkt	140	tr	37.0	5	na	tr	na	0	0%
TACO MEAT	2 oz	110	10.0	4.0	300	na	7.0	1.7	25	57%
TACO SAUCE	1 oz	16	<1.0	3.0	140	na	<1.0	tr	tr	0%
TACO SHELL	.4 oz	45	<1.0	6.0	45	(mq)	3.0	0.7	0	60%
TARTAR SAUCE	1 tbsp	80	tr	tr	75	na	9.0	na	na	100%
TOMATO, 1-oz slice	1 slice	6	1.0	1.0	5	na	tr	na	0	0%
TORTELLINI, cheese, in sauce	2 oz	60	2.0	12.0	280	(mq)	1.0	0.3	5	15%
TORTILLA, flour 1.3 oz	1 tortilla	110	3.0	19.0	220	(mq)	3.0	0.4	na	25%
TURKEY HAM	1/4 cup	50	6.0	tr	na	na	2.0	na	na	36%
WATERMELON	3 pieces	18	tr	4.0	tr	na	tr	na	0	0%
WHATABURGER										
APPLE PIE	1 serving	236	3.0	30.0	265	na	12.0	na	tr	46%
APPLE TURNOVER	1 serving	215	2.4	27.0	241	na	10.8	na	0	45%
BISCUIT, buttermilk	1 serving	280	5.4	36.6	509	na	13.4	na	3	43%
BREAKFAST										
bacon	1 slice	38	2.0	0.0	106	na	3.3	na	6	78%

Food Name	Serving Size	Calories	Prot. gms	Carbs gms	Sod. mgs	Fiber gms	Fat gms	Sat. Fat gms	Chol. mgs	% Fat Cal.
biscuit, w/bacon	1 serving	359	9.6	36.7	730	na	20.2	na	15	51%
biscuit, w/egg and cheese	1 serving	434	13.7	37.5	797	na	26.3	na	202	55%
biscuit, w/egg, cheese, and bacon	1 serving	511	17.8	37.6	1010	na	32.9	na	213	58%
biscuit, w/egg, cheese, and sausage	1 serving	601	20.7	37.9	1081	na	41.6	na	236	62%
biscuit, w/gravy	1 serving	479	8.8	48.3	1253	na	27.4	na	20	51%
biscuit, w/sausage	1 serving	446	12.3	37.0	794	na	28.7	na	37	58%
eggs, scrambled	2 eggs	189	11.3	1.5	842	na	15.0	na	374	71%
pancakes	3 pancakes	259	10.6	39.9	211	na	5.8	na	0	20%
pancakes, w/sausage	3 pancakes	426	17.5	40.3	1127	na	21.1	na	34	45%
pancakes, w/o syrup or butter	1 serving	259	11.0	40.0	842	na	6.0	na	0	21%
platter, w/bacon	1 serving	695	22.1	54.1	1162	na	44.0	na	389	57%
platter, w/sausage	1 serving	785	24.9	54.4	1234	na	52.7	na	412	60%
sausage	1 serving	208	9.0	1.0	355	na	19.0	na	43	82%
BREAKFAST SANDWICH										
'Breakfast on a Bun'	1 serving	520	23.0	29.0	1051	na	34.0	na	234	59%
'Breakfast on a Bun' ranchero	1 serving	530	23.0	32.0	1431	na	35.0	na	236	59%
'Breakfast on a Bun' w/bacon	1 serving	365	17.5	29.4	815	na	19.4	na	210	48%
egg omelette	1 serving	288	13.4	29.4	602	na	12.8	na	198	40%
egg omelette 'Ranchero'	1 serving	322	15.0	31.0	1067	na	16.0	na	191	45%
BUN										
5-inch size	1 bun	290	10.0	56.0	532	na	3.0	na	tr	9%
4-inch size	1 bun	150	5.0	29.0	274	na	2.0	na	tr	12%
BUTTER	1 pkt	36	0.0	0.0	42	na	4.0	na	11	100%
CHEESEBURGER										
double meat	1 serving	895	55.0	59.0	1678	na	49.0	na	180	49%
'Jr. Burger'	1 serving	351	17.0	30.0	921	na	18.0	na	42	46%
'Justaburger'	1 serving	312	15.0	28.0	784	na	16.0	na	37	46%
regular	1 serving	669	36.0	58.0	1474	na	33.0	na	96	44%
CHICKEN SANDWICH										
grilled	1 serving	442	34.3	48.4	1103	na	14.2	na	66	29%
grilled, w/o salad dressing	1 serving	385	34.0	46.0	989	na	9.0	na	66	21%
'Whatachick'n Deluxe'	1 serving	573	34.2	53.0	1338	na	26.9	na	56	42%
COFFEE, small	1 serving	5	0.2	0.9	5	na	0.0	na	0	0%
COOKIE										
chocolate chunk	1 cookie	247	4.0	28.0	75	na	16.0	na	36	58%
macadamia nut	1 cookie	269	3.0	31.0	80	na	16.0	na	34	54%
oatmeal raisin	1 cookie	222	4.0	36.9	70	na	7.0	na	28	28%
peanut butter	1 cookie	262	5.4	30.2	35	na	13.5	na	39	46%
CRACKER, Club	1 pkt	31	0.5	3.9	72	na	1.3	na	0	38%
CREAMER, nondairy	1 pkg	10	0.0	1.0	4	na	1.0	na	0	90%
CROUTONS	1 pkt	29	0.9	4.5	88	na	0.9	na	0	28%
FAJITA TACO										
beef	1 serving	326	21.6	33.6	670	na	11.9	na	28	33%
chicken	1 serving	272	18.2	35.2	691	na	6.7	na	33	22%
FISH SANDWICH										
'Whatacatch'	1 serving	475	14.0	43.0	722	na	27.0	na	34	51%
'Whatacatch' w/cheese	1 serving	522	16.0	43.0	959	na	32.0	na	45	55%
FRENCH FRIES										
junior order	1 serving	221	4.0	25.0	50	na	12.0	na	(tr)	49%
large order	1 serving	442	7.1	49.2	292	na	24.2	na	0	49%
regular order	1 serving	332	5.0	37.0	45	na	18.0	na	(tr)	49%
HAMBURGER										
'Justaburger'	1 serving	265	12.0	28.0	547	na	12.0	na	25	41%
'Whataburger'	1 serving	598	30.2	61.1	1096	na	26.0	na	84	39%

Food Name	Serving Size	Calories	Prot. gms	Carbs gms	Sod. mgs	Fiber gms	Fat gms	Sat. Fat gms	Chol. mgs	% Fat Cal.
'Whataburger' w/double meat	1 serving	823	48.9	61.8	1298	na	42.4	na	168	46%
HAMBURGER PATTY										
ground beef, 1/4 lb	1 patty	226	19.0	1.0	232	na	17.0	na	84	68%
ground beef, 1/10 lb	1 patty	90	8.0	tr	81	na	6.0	na	34	60%
HONEY	1 pkt	27	0.0	7.0	0	na	0.0	na	0	0%
ICED TEA, med	1 serving	3	0.0	1.0	10	na	0.0	na	0	0%
JAM, strawberry	1 pkt	37	0.0	9.0	0	na	0.0	na	0	0%
JELLY, grape	1 pkt	38	0.0	9.0	0	na	0.0	na	0	0%
LEMON JUICE	1 pkt	1	0.0	0.3	1	na	0.0	na	0	0%
MARGARINE	1 pkt	25	0.0	0.0	40	na	3.0	na	0	100%
MILK, 2% butterfat	1 serving	113	8.0	11.0	113	na	4.0	na	18	32%
MILKSHAKE										
chocolate, small	1 serving	333	8.3	56.2	155	na	8.4	na	32	23%
strawberry, small	1 serving	322	7.8	54.9	152	na	8.0	na	31	22%
vanilla, extra large	1 serving	877	25.0	137.0	1168	na	26.0	na	100	27%
vanilla, large	1 serving	657	19.0	102.0	874	na	19.0	na	75	26%
vanilla, medium	1 serving	439	12.0	68.0	230	na	13.0	na	51	27%
vanilla, small	1 serving	322	9.0	50.0	169	na	9.0	na	37	25%
MUFFIN, blueberry	1 muffin	239	6.2	35.6	538	na	7.9	na	0	30%
ONION RINGS										
large order	1 serving	493	8.0	50.7	893	na	28.7	na	0	52%
regular order	1 serving	226	4.0	22.0	410	na	13.0	na	(tr)	52%
ORANGE JUICE	6 oz	77	1.0	18.0	2	na	0.0	na	0	0%
PECAN DANISH	1 serving	270	5.0	28.0	419	na	16.0	na	12	53%
PEPPER, JALAPEÑO	1 pepper	3	0.1	0.6	190	na	0.1	na	0	30%
PICANTE SAUCE	1 pkt	5	0.2	0.9	130	na	0.0	na	0	0%
POTATO, BAKED										
plain	1 serving	310	6.5	71.7	23	na	0.3	na	0	1%
w/broccoli cheese topping	1 serving	453	12.9	79.3	636	na	10.0	na	17	20%
w/cheese topping	1 serving	510	14.6	79.8	863	na	16.3	na	22	29%
w/mushroom topping	1 serving	360	8.0	80.0	778	na	1.6	na	0	4%
POTATOES, HASH BROWN	1 serving	150	1.3	15.9	228	na	9.0	na	0	54%
SALAD										
chicken, grilled	1 serving	150	23.0	14.0	434	na	1.0	na	49	6%
garden	1 serving	56	2.9	11.3	32	na	0.6	na	0	10%
SALAD DRESSING										
French	1 pkt	249	0.0	16.0	729	na	20.0	na	5	72%
ranch	1 pkt	364	0.0	4.0	599	na	37.9	na	5	94%
Thousand Island	1 pkt	280	0.0	9.0	399	na	26.9	na	0	86%
vinaigrette, lite, 2 oz	1 pkt	36	0.0	5.0	878	na	2.0	na	0	50%
SOFT DRINK										
Cherry Coke, medium size	1 serving	151	0.0	39.6	7	na	0.0	na	0	0%
Coca-Cola Classic, medium size	1 serving	141	0.0	37.6	13	na	0.0	na	0	0%
Diet Coke, medium size	1 serving	1	0.0	0.3	17	na	0.0	na	0	0%
Dr. Pepper, medium size	1 serving	138	0.0	34.9	34	na	0.3	na	0	2%
root beer, medium size	1 serving	158	0.0	41.7	17	na	0.0	na	0	0%
Sprite, medium size	1 serving	141	0.0	31.6	30	na	0.0	na	0	0%
SOUR CREAM	2 oz	121	1.8	2.4	30	na	11.9	na	25	89%
STEAK SANDWICH	1 serving	387	35.0	32.0	1164	na	12.0	na	61	28%
SUGAR	1 pkt	15	0.0	4.0	0	na	0.0	na	0	0%
SUGAR SUBSTITUTE, 'Sweet 'n Low'	1 pkt	4	0.0	1.0	0	na	0.0	na	0	0%
SYRUP, pancake	1 pkt	169	0.0	41.8	0	na	0.0	na	0	0%
TAQUITO										
bacon	1 serving	335	14.9	31.7	761	na	16.1	na	286	43%

Food Name	Serving Size	Calories	Prot. gms	Carbs gms	Sod. mgs	Fiber gms	Fat gms	Sat. Fat gms	Chol. mgs	% Fat Cal.
potato	1 serving	446	14.2	47.6	883	na	21.8	na	281	44%
'Ranchero'	1 serving	320	19.0	19.0	1092	na	18.0	na	223	51%
rregular	1 serving	310	19.0	17.0	712	na	19.0	na	223	55%
sausage	1 serving	443	19.8	32.1	790	na	25.9	na	315	53%
w/cheese	1 serving	357	21.0	17.0	949	na	23.0	na	235	58%
w/cheese 'Ranchero'	1 serving	367	21.0	19.0	1329	na	23.0	na	235	56%
TURKEY SANDWICH, grilled	1 serving	439	33.0	49.0	968	na	15.0	na	46	31%

WHITE CASTLE
BREAKFAST SANDWICH

Food Name	Serving Size	Calories	Prot. gms	Carbs gms	Sod. mgs	Fiber gms	Fat gms	Sat. Fat gms	Chol. mgs	% Fat Cal.
sausage, 1.7 oz	1 serving	196	7.0	13.0	488	2.0	12.0	(mq)	(mq)	55%
sausage and egg, 3.4 oz	1 serving	322	13.0	16.0	698	3.0	22.0	(mq)	(mq)	61%
BUN, hamburger, .9 oz	1 bun	74	2.2	13.9	<1	.5	0.9	na	0	11%
CHEESE	.3 oz	31	1.5	2.3	154	.2	1.6	(mq)	na	46%
CHEESEBURGER, 2.3 oz	1 serving	200	8.0	15.0	361	2.7	11.0	(mq)	(mq)	50%
CHICKEN SANDWICH, 2.3 oz	1 serving	186	8.0	21.0	497	1.7	7.0	(mq)	(mq)	34%
CHIPS, 3.3 oz	1 serving	329	4.0	39.0	832	3.5	17.0	(mq)	na	47%
FISH SANDWICH, w/o tartar sauce, 2.1 oz	1 serving	155	6.0	21.0	201	1.4	5.0	(mq)	(mq)	29%
FRENCH FRIES, 3.4 oz	1 serving	301	2.0	38.0	193	4.6	15.0	(mq)	na	45%
HAMBURGER, 2.0 oz	1 serving	161	6.0	15.0	266	2.1	8.0	(mq)	(mq)	45%
ONION RINGS, 2.1 oz	1 serving	245	3.0	27.0	566	2.6	13.0	(mq)	na	48%

ZANTIGO
BURRITO

Food Name	Serving Size	Calories	Prot. gms	Carbs gms	Sod. mgs	Fiber gms	Fat gms	Sat. Fat gms	Chol. mgs	% Fat Cal.
hot cheese, 'Chilito'	1 serving	329	14.0	35.0	466	na	15.0	na	na	41%
mild cheese, 'Chilito'	1 serving	330	14.0	36.0	505	na	15.0	na	na	41%

ENCHILADA

Food Name	Serving Size	Calories	Prot. gms	Carbs gms	Sod. mgs	Fiber gms	Fat gms	Sat. Fat gms	Chol. mgs	% Fat Cal.
beef	1 serving	315	18.0	26.0	904	na	15.0	na	na	43%
cheese	1 serving	390	20.0	26.0	759	na	23.0	na	na	53%

TACO

Food Name	Serving Size	Calories	Prot. gms	Carbs gms	Sod. mgs	Fiber gms	Fat gms	Sat. Fat gms	Chol. mgs	% Fat Cal.
burrito	1 serving	415	21.0	41.0	815	na	19.0	na	na	41%
regular	1 serving	198	10.0	13.0	318	na	12.0	na	na	55%

NUTRiBASE Software for PC's

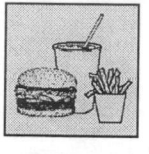 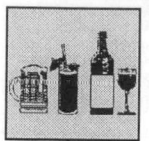 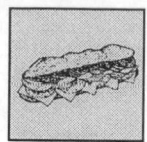 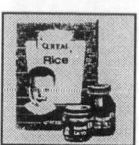 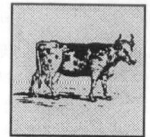 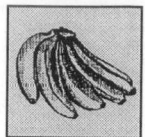 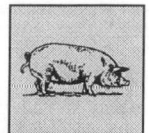

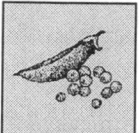 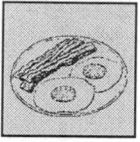 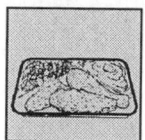 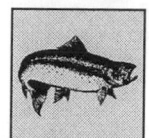 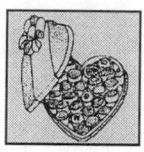 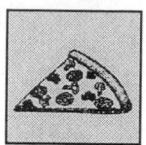 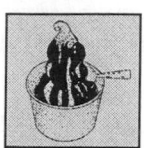

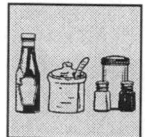 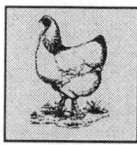 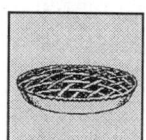 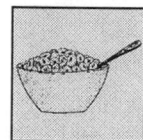 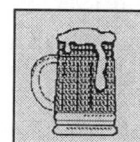 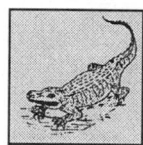 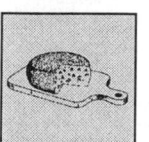

Software Nutrition Managers for Personal and Professional Use

NutriBase software for Windows or DOS provides you with the world's largest database of food items, then helps you set and track your nutritional goals. Goals that help you achieve not only your ideal body weight, but a diet that conforms with national dietary guidelines (or any other guidelines). NutriBase features the nutritional information contained in Dr. Art Ulene's NutriBase Series of books.

NutriBase provides lightning-fast access to nutritional information for 50,000 food items–more than most supermarkets carry. And you can add new food items whenever you wish. Both personal and professional versions feature information for *calories, protein, carbohydrates, total fat, % calories from fat, saturated fat, sodium, cholesterol, fiber,* and *alcohol.* The following capabilities are your keys to a healthier, more nutritious lifestyle:

 Users - NutriBase tracks the progress for up to five users (200 clients in the Professional version). Just answer a few questions (age, sex, body build, etc.) and NutriBase will suggest personal nutrition and body weight goals. After setting these goals, you can track the nutritional information for everything you eat.

 View - Click on this icon to *instantly* display an alphabetized view of food items in a conventional "spreadsheet view" or a convenient "single-screen view." View nutritional information for more than 27,000 brand named foods and 17,000 generic foods, plus well over 3,100 menu items from more than 70 restaurants.

 Rank - *Instantly* rank foods based on their values for any nutrient. For instance, rank the 400 or so ready-to-eat breakfast cereals in NutriBase from high-to-low based on their fiber content. Or rank these foods from low-to-high based on their nutrient value for % calories from fat. Or sodium. Or any other nutrient!

 Query - *Instantly* locate all foods that meet all the criteria you specify. For instance, display all hamburgers and cheeseburgers from Burger King, Hardee's, McDonald's, Wendy's, and Whataburger and sort them from low-to-high based on % calories from fat. Or simply display all the menu items featured at Denny's.

 Footnotes -. NutriBase provides a rich educational experience. This icon displays all footnotes in any current screen. Learn about desirable body weights, food definitions and origins, dieting tips, and much more.

 Jump - Use this icon to instantly "jump" to the first occurrence of any food name or brand name food in NutriBase. This ability makes it even easier to navigate through this tremendous nutritional database.

Tally - One click here provides nutrient information for all the foods you've recorded so far today. This feature displays data for foods you've eaten as a percentage of total calories consumed *and* as a percentage of your target goals.

 New Food Item - Click on this icon to add a new food item. If you find a new food item that isn't already in NutriBase, this is your opportunity to add it yourself. You may add as many new items as you wish.

 Recipes - Simply drag and drop ingredients into this icon to create personal recipes. Click on this icon to edit the ingredients, change serving sizes, specify how many servings the recipe contains, view a tally of the nutritional information, etc. Assign the recipe a name and a comment. Save it for future use.

 Record - Drag and drop ingredients and recipes into this icon to record all the nutritional information for these food items. Click on this icon to edit the items you've dragged in. Recall food items you ate on any day. View and/or edit the information. Copy the food items you recorded for any day to any other day.

 Analyze - Drag and drop any recipe into this icon for an in-depth nutritional analysis. Analyze records from any time period. Generate listings by nutrient intake, % of total calories, % of your target goals, or as an average per-day nutrient intake.

 Graph - Drag and drop ingredients, recipes, and analyses into this icon. Select the graphical analysis you want and NutriBase generates it for you. Pie charts show target goals vs. actual performance to give you an instant snapshot of your progress. Bar charts indicate food intake relative to total calories or to target goals.

 Weight Tracker - Click on this icon to monitor your weight loss (or gain). Graph your progress. Track your actual weight against your target goals. One line shows your desired progress over time–another shows your actual performance.

 Help - Any time you require assistance, click on this icon to access a well-organized and thorough help system. Even if you've never used a PC before, this help system will coach you through any procedure quickly and clearly.

 Alarms - When you select a food item that will cause you to exceed any target goal, you'll trip a warning alarm. You aren't actually going to eat the offending food item, are you? The alarm signals your "moment of truth" and gives you the opportunity to do the right thing.

 Do It! - NutriBase handles virtually everything for you: Goal setting. Record keeping. Graphing. Nutritional analysis. Creating and managing recipes. Adding food items. Weight tracking. Combine all of this capability with the world's largest database of food items and the only thing missing is your willingness to take charge of your nutrition...

Other Exciting Health Titles From Avery